WITHDRAWN

University of Memphis Libraries

Handbook of
Medical
Psychiatry

Medical Psychiatry

Series Editor

William A. Frosch, M.D.

*Weill Medical College of Cornell University
New York, New York*

1. Handbook of Depression and Anxiety: A Biological Approach, *edited by Johan A. den Boer and J. M. Ad Sitsen*
2. Anticonvulsants in Mood Disorders, *edited by Russell T. Joffe and Joseph R. Calabrese*
3. Serotonin in Antipsychotic Treatment: Mechanisms and Clinical Practice, *edited by John M. Kane, H.-J. Möller, and Frans Awouters*
4. Handbook of Functional Gastrointestinal Disorders, *edited by Kevin W. Olden*
5. Clinical Management of Anxiety, *edited by Johan A. den Boer*
6. Obsessive-Compulsive Disorders: Diagnosis • Etiology • Treatment, *edited by Eric Hollander and Dan J. Stein*
7. Bipolar Disorder: Biological Models and Their Clinical Application, *edited by L. Trevor Young and Russell T. Joffe*
8. Dual Diagnosis and Treatment: Substance Abuse and Comorbid Medical and Psychiatric Disorders, *edited by Henry R. Kranzler and Bruce J. Rounsaville*
9. Geriatric Psychopharmacology, *edited by J. Craig Nelson*
10. Panic Disorder and Its Treatment, *edited by Jerrold F. Rosenbaum and Mark H. Pollack*
11. Comorbidity in Affective Disorders, *edited by Mauricio Tohen*
12. Practical Management of the Side Effects of Psychotropic Drugs, *edited by Richard Balon*
13. Psychiatric Treatment of the Medically Ill, *edited by Robert G. Robinson and William R. Yates*
14. Medical Management of the Violent Patient: Clinical Assessment and Therapy, *edited by Kenneth Tardiff*
15. Bipolar Disorders: Basic Mechanisms and Therapeutic Implications, *edited by Jair C. Soares and Samuel Gershon*
16. Schizophrenia: A New Guide for Clinicians, *edited by John G. Csernansky*
17. Polypharmacy in Psychiatry, *edited by S. Nassir Ghaemi*
18. Pharmacotherapy for Child and Adolescent Psychiatric Disorders: Second Edition, Revised and Expanded, *David R. Rosenberg, Pablo A. Davanzo, and Samuel Gershon*
19. Brain Imaging In Affective Disorders, *edited by Jair C. Soares*
20. Handbook of Medical Psychiatry, *edited by Jair C. Soares and Samuel Gershon*

ADDITIONAL VOLUMES IN PREPARATION

Aggression: Psychiatric Assessment and Treatment, *edited by Emil F. Coccaro*

Handbook of Medical Psychiatry

edited by
Jair C. Soares
University of Texas Health Science Center at San Antonio
San Antonio, Texas, U.S.A.

Samuel Gershon
Western Psychiatric Institute and Clinic
University of Pittsburgh School of Medicine
Pittsburgh, Pennsylvania, U.S.A.

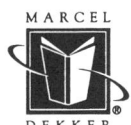

MARCEL DEKKER, INC.   NEW YORK · BASEL

Library of Congress Cataloging-in-Publication Data
A catalog record for this book is available from the Library of Congress.

ISBN: 0-8247-0835-0

This book is printed on acid-free paper.

Headquarters
Marcel Dekker, Inc.
270 Madison Avenue, New York, NY 10016
tel: 212-696-9000; fax: 212-685-4540

Eastern Hemisphere Distribution
Marcel Dekker AG
Hutgasse 4, Postfach 812, CH-4001 Basel, Switzerland
tel: 41-61-260-6300; fax: 41-61-260-6333

World Wide Web
http://www.dekker.com

The publisher offers discounts on this book when ordered in bulk quantities. For more information, write to Special Sales/ Professional Marketing at the headquarters address above.

Copyright © 2003 by Marcel Dekker, Inc. All Rights Reserved.

Neither this book nor any part may be reproduced or transmitted in any form or by any means, electronic or mechanical, including photocopying, microfilming, and recording, or by any information storage and retrieval system, without permission in writing from the publisher.

Current printing (last digit):
10 9 8 7 6 5 4 3 2 1

PRINTED IN THE UNITED STATES OF AMERICA

Series Introduction

In the late 1950s and early 1960s many of the senior professors of psychiatry, including those who were psychoanalysts, also had extensive training in neurology. Some departments, including the one in which I trained, were departments of psychiatry and neurology. To be certified as a psychiatrist, one of the three patients you examined and were questioned about was a patient with primary neurological disease. We were expected to know how to recognize seizure spindles in an EEG, and to be able to point out the anatomy and pathology visible in brain slices. The neurology candidates were similarly examined and questioned in psychiatry. Many practitioners did a bit of both: for example, the senior neurologist in the department in which I trained made his own diagnoses of depression, and administered ECT to the patient in his office.

Outside the "black box" of the skull, our ties to the rest of medicine were not as strong. This was true despite the attempts to promote both concepts of "psychosomatic" medicine and humane care. Unfortunately, neither the concepts nor the data were strong enough to carry the day. More recently, however, the development of new technologies, such as imaging and explication of the genetic code, has resulted in an explosion of knowledge about human biology and pathology. Newer findings have begun to break down the barriers between psychiatry and neurology, and between our understanding of behavioral disorders and the rest of medicine. While I do not believe that we will ever be able to do without a psychology in psychiatry, it is also increasingly clear that psychiatry cannot function without understanding the biology of the brain.

Drs. Soares and Gershon have done an excellent job in bringing together a group of outstanding contributors who bring this new understanding to our field. They have presented the complex material clearly and comprehensively, making it easier to master—a necessary task if we are to continue to help our patients.

William A. Frosch

Foreword

With the publication of the *Handbook of Medical Psychiatry*, Drs. Soares and Gershon have recaptured the traditions of psychiatry over the past century, added the impressive technical capacities of the field in the last decade, and created an important educational resource for this new century. The deceptively simple title of the book belies the scope and depth of the volume. The chapters are organized, in part, by major diagnostic categories (e.g., mood disorders, schizophrenia, and related disorders, etc.), but also by significant crosscutting issues such as research methods and psychopharmacology.

Within this rich composite of important theoretical and practical information the editors have integrated critical themes of modern psychiatry such as:

Classification/nosology. DSM-III and -IV and ICD-10 are clearly interim steps in the development of disease-based classification systems for psychiatry. However, movement from phenomenology to etiolopathogenesis will have many steps along the way. This book examines fundamental issues in diagnosis across the range of psychiatric disorders and will help prepare psychiatrists to better understand strategies to move along that path.

Mechanisms. Ultimately, a disease-based classification will require the elucidation of the basic mechanisms underlying mental disorders. The book presents, in a provocative manner, current leads in neurochemistry, neurocircuitry, molecular biology, and genetics, among other fields.

Tools. Realizing that a more comprehensive understanding of basic mechanisms will evolve over decades, the authors have provided the reader with an understanding of the remarkable tools now available in imaging, molecular biology, and genetics. These new technologies enable researchers to open the "black boxes" of the brain, the cell, and the gene. Understanding how these tools are applied and getting a taste of current findings will enhance the reader's ability to become educated consumers of the barrage of information that is, and will be, emanating from the tremendous growth of research activity in psychiatry.

Evidence. Over the past decades, the values of psychiatry have become more and more closely aligned with the values of science. As such, the ability to interpret and evaluate scientific evidence and augment it with clinical insights is a critical skill. It is a skill that must be not only learned during medical school and residency but also continuously exercised over the course of every psychiatrist's career. The authors have effectively captured the essence of that task in this volume. Readers who engage this important and challenging material will be revitalizing those skills and also preparing themselves for the future. Impressively, Drs. Soares and Gershon have enlisted the talents of many of the world's leading clinicians and scientists in this ambitious work. Even more importantly, they have tapped some of the most promising younger psychiatrists who will be major contributors in expanding our understanding of psychiatric disorders in the future.

Harold Alan Pincus, M.D.
Professor and Executive Vice Chairman
Department of Psychiatry
Western Psychiatric Institute and Clinic
University of Pittsburgh School of Medicine
Pittsburgh, Pennsylvania

Preface

Over the past few decades, increasing emphasis has been given to the study of brain mechanisms that may be dysfunctional in neuropsychiatric illnesses. In recent years, new methodologies from various disciplines in the clinical neurosciences have made available substantially improved and more sophisticated tools for studies of causation of these severe illnesses. For instance, we have seen tremendous progress in knowledge from disciplines such as molecular genetics, neuropsychopharmacology, and brain imaging, which has provided unprecedented tools for studies of the human brain and neuropsychiatric illnesses. These efforts have begun to produce important findings and are beginning to contribute to a better understanding of the basic mechanisms involved in these disorders and the mechanisms of actions of treatments for these conditions, and lead to the development of new therapeutic possibilities.

The *Handbook of Medical Psychiatry* summarizes the main advances in the understanding of the basic mechanisms and therapeutics of the major psychiatric illnesses that have taken place in recent years. The format provides easy access to new information in these areas, making the book of significant interest to academicians, researchers, practitioners, students, residents, and trainees in psychiatry, clinical neuroscience, and the mental health professions. We believe this book will be a helpful, comprehensive, and important resource for individuals in psychiatry and related fields.

Jair C. Soares
Samuel Gershon

Contents

Series Introduction William A. Frosch	*iii*
Foreword Harold Alan Pincus	*v*
Preface	*vii*
Contributors	*xv*

Methodological Issues in Psychiatric Research

1. Animal Models of Neuropsychiatric Disorders: Challenges for the Future   1
   William T. McKinney

2. Methodological Advances in Psychiatric Genetics   13
   Yoav Kohn and Bernard Lerer

3. New Developments in the Regulation of Monoaminergic Neurotransmission   25
   Alan Frazer, David A. Morilak, and Lynette C. Daws

4. Developments in Psychiatric Neuroimaging   43
   Roberto B. Sassi and Jair C. Soares

5. Classification of Childhood and Adolescent Psychiatric Disorders   55
   Norah C. Feeny and Robert L. Findling

6. Classification of Schizophrenia and Related Psychotic Disorders   69
   Tonmoy Sharma and Priya Bajaj

7. Classification of Mood Disorders: Implications for Psychiatric Research   79
   Acioly L. T. Lacerda, Roberto B. Sassi, and Jair C. Soares

8.	Classification of Anxiety Disorders: Implications for Psychiatric Research *Kerrie L. Posey, Susan G. Ball, and Anantha Shekhar*	89
9.	Classification of Dementias and Cognitive Disorders *Frédéric Assal and Jeffrey L. Cummings*	99
10.	Classification of Personality Disorders: Implications for Treatment and Research *Dragan M. Svrakic, Robert Cloninger, Stana Stanic, and Secondo Fassino*	117

Psychiatric Manifestations in Childhood and Adolescence

11.	Mood Disorders in Childhood and Adolescence: Basic Mechanisms and Therapeutic Interventions *Melissa P. DelBello and Robert A. Kowatch*	149
12.	Anxiety Disorders in Childhood and Adolescence: Basic Mechanisms and Therapeutic Interventions *Tiffany Farchione, Shauna N. MacMillan, and David R. Rosenberg*	175
13.	Psychotic Disorders in Childhood and Adolescence: Basic Mechanisms and Therapeutic Interventions *Andrew R. Gilbert and Matcheri S. Keshavan*	197
14.	Neurobiology of Autism and Other Pervasive Developmental Disorders: Basic Mechanisms and Therapeutic Interventions *Antonio Y. Hardan*	205

Schizophrenia and Related Psychotic Disorders

15.	Cognitive Deficits in Schizophrenia *Cameron S. Carter and Stefan Ursu*	223
16.	Neuroimaging Findings in Schizophrenia: From Mental to Neuronal Fragmentation *Lawrence S. Kegeles and Marc Laruelle*	237
17.	The Dopamine Hypothesis of Schizophrenia *Philip Seeman and Mary V. Seeman*	259
18.	Serotonergic Dysfunctions in Schizophrenia: Possible Therapeutic Implications *Johannes Tauscher and Nicolaas Paul Leonard Gerrit Verhoeff*	267
19.	The GABA Cell in Relation to Schizophrenia and Bipolar Disorder *Francine M. Benes and Sabina Berretta*	277
20.	Genetic Findings in Psychotic Disorders *Michael O'Donovan and Michael Owen*	295
21.	Membrane Abnormalities in Psychotic Disorders *Wagner Farid Gattaz and Orestes V. Forlenza*	307
22.	Animal Models of Psychosis *J. David Jentsch, Peter Olausson, and Holly Moore*	317

Contents

Mood Disorders

23. Affective Disorders: Imaging Studies ... 335
    Warren D. Taylor and Ranga R. Krishnan

24. Role of Acetylcholine and Its Interactions with Other Neurotransmitters and Neuromodulators in Affective Disorders ... 347
    David S. Janowsky and David H. Overstreet

25. GABA and Mood Disorders: A Selective Review and Discussion of Future Research ... 363
    Frederick Petty, Prasad Padala, and Surender Punia

26. Signal Transduction Abnormalities in Bipolar Disorder ... 371
    Yarema B. Bezchlibnyk and L. Trevor Young

27. Molecular Genetics and Mood Disorders ... 395
    Daniel Souery and Julian Mendlewicz

28. Biological Distinction Between Unipolar and Bipolar Disorder ... 407
    Xiaohong Wang and Charles B. Nemeroff

Anxiety Disorders

29. Neurobiology of Obsessive-Compulsive Disorder ... 423
    Bavanisha Vythilingum and Dan J. Stein

30. Neurobiology of Panic Disorder ... 433
    Sanjay J. Mathew, Jack M. Gorman, and Jeremy D. Coplan

31. Neurobiology of Posttraumatic Stress Disorder Across the Life Cycle ... 449
    Michael D. De Bellis

32. Genetics of Panic Disorder, Social Phobia, and Agoraphobia ... 467
    Joel Gelernter and Murray B. Stein

Dementia and Cognitive Disorders

33. Imaging Brain Structure and Function in Aging and Alzheimer's Disease ... 477
    Vicente Ibáñez and Stanley I. Rapoport

34. Brain Imaging in Dementia ... 497
    Francesca Mapua Filbey, Robert Cohen, and Trey Sunderland

35. Genetics of Alzheimer's Disease ... 521
    M. Ilyas Kamboh

36. Neurobiology of Alzheimer's Disease ... 537
    Oscar L. Lopez and Steven T. DeKosky

Substance Abuse and Dependence

37. Psychiatric Comorbidity: Implications for Treatment and Clinical Research — 553
    Jack R. Cornelius, Ihsan M. Salloum, Oscar G. Bukstein, and Duncan B. Clark

38. Neurobiology of Alcoholism — 563
    Charles A. Dackis and Charles P. O'Brien

39. Biological Basis of Drug Addiction — 581
    Tony P. George

40. Neuroimaging Abnormalities in Drug Addiction and Alcoholism — 595
    Wynne K. Schiffer, Douglas A. Marsteller, and Stephen L. Dewey

41. Genetics of Addictive Disorders — 615
    Tatiana Foroud and John I. Nurnberger, Jr.

Other Psychiatric Conditions

42. Biological Basis of Eating Disorders — 633
    Walter H. Kaye and Nicole C. Barbarich

43. Biological Basis of Personality Disorders — 643
    Cuneyt Iscan, Charlotte L. Allport, and Kenneth R. Silk

44. Iatrogenic Sexual Dysfunction — 657
    Marlene P. Freeman and Alan J. Gelenberg

45. Neurobiology of Violence and Aggression — 671
    Michael S. McCloskey, Royce J. Lee, and Emil F. Coccaro

46. Pathological Gambling: Clinical Aspects and Neurobiology — 683
    Marc N. Potenza

47. Neurobiology of Suicide — 701
    Leo Sher and J. John Mann

48. Sleep Disorders — 713
    Eric A. Nofzinger

Developments in Pharmacotherapy

49. Perspectives in the Pharmacological Treatment of Schizophrenia — 731
    Larry Ereshefsky

50. Multiple Mechanisms of Lithium Action — 757
    Alona Shaldubina, Robert H. Belmaker, and Galila Agam

51. Mechanisms of Action of Anticonvulsants and New Mood Stabilizers — 767
    Robert M. Post, Elzbieta Chalecka-Franaszek, and Christopher J. Hough

Contents

52. Mechanisms of Action of New Mood-Stabilizing Drugs — 793
    Joseph Levine, Yuly Bersudsky, Carmit Nadri, Yuri Yaroslavsky, Abed Azab, Alex Mishori, Galila Agam, and Robert H. Belmaker

53. Advances in Treatment and Perspectives for New Interventions in Mood and Anxiety Disorders — 807
    Sandeep Patil, Saeeduddin Ahmed, and William Zeigler Potter

54. Perspectives for Pharmacological Interventions in Eating Disorders — 827
    Guido K. Frank

55. Perspectives for New Pharmacological Treatments of Alcoholism and Substance Dependence — 843
    Ihsan M. Salloum, Antoine Douaihy, and Subhajit Chakravorty

56. Perspectives on the Pharmacological Treatment of Dementia — 865
    Bruno P. Imbimbo and Nunzio Pomara

57. Pharmacological Interventions in Psychiatric Disorders Due to Medical Conditions — 899
    E. Sherwood Brown and Dana C. Perantie

58. Perspectives on Treatment Interventions in Paraphilias — 909
    Florence Thibaut

59. Potential of Repetitive Transcranial Magnetic Stimulation in the Treatment of Neuropsychiatric Conditions — 919
    Thomas E. Schlaepfer and Markus Kosel

60. Pharmacokinetic Principles and Drug Interactions — 933
    Ahsan Y. Kahn and Sheldon H. Preskorn

Index — 945

Contributors

Galila Agam, Ph.D.   Psychiatry Research Unit, Ben-Gurion University of the Negev, Beer-Sheva, Israel

Saeeduddin Ahmed, M.D.   Department of U.S. Medical Affairs, Eli Lilly and Company, Indianapolis, Indiana, U.S.A.

Charlotte L. Allport, R.N., B.S.N.   Department of Psychiatry, University of Michigan Health System, Ann Arbor, Michigan, U.S.A.

Frédéric Assal, M.D.   Department of Neurology, David Geffen School of Medicine at UCLA, Los Angeles, California, U.S.A.

Abed Azab, M.Sc.   Department of Clinical Pharmacology, Ben-Gurion University of the Negev, Beer-Sheva, Israel

Priya Bajaj, D.P.M., D.N.B.   Clinical Neuroscience Research Centre, Stonehouse Hospital, Dartford, Kent, England

Susan G. Ball, Ph.D.   Department of Psychiatry, Indiana University School of Medicine, Indianapolis, Indiana, U.S.A.

Nicole C. Barbarich, B.S.   Department of Psychiatry, Western Psychiatric Institute and Clinic, University of Pittsburgh School of Medicine, Pittsburgh, Pennsylvania, U.S.A.

Robert H. Belmaker, M.D.   Department of Psychiatry, Ben-Gurion University of the Negev, Beer-Sheva, Israel

Francine M. Benes, M.D., Ph.D.   Department of Psychiatry, McLean Hospital, Belmont, and Harvard Medical School, Boston, Massachusetts, U.S.A.

Sabina Berretta, M.D.   Department of Psychiatry, McLean Hospital, Belmont, and Harvard Medical School, Boston, Massachusetts, U.S.A.

Yuly Bersudsky, M.D., Ph.D.   Department of Psychiatry, Ben-Gurion University of the Negev, Beer-Sheva, Israel

Yarema B. Bezchlibnyk, B.Sc.   Department of Psychiatry and Behavioral Neurosciences, McMaster University, Hamilton, Ontario, Canada

E. Sherwood Brown, M.D., Ph.D.   Department of Psychiatry, University of Texas Southwestern Medical Center, Dallas, Texas, U.S.A.

Oscar G. Bukstein, M.D., M.P.H.   Department of Psychiatry, Western Psychiatric Institute and Clinic, University of Pittsburgh School of Medicine, Pittsburgh, Pennsylvania, U.S.A.

Cameron S. Carter, M.D.   Department of Psychiatry, Western Psychiatric Institute and Clinic, University of Pittsburgh School of Medicine, Pittsburgh, Pennsylvania, U.S.A.

Subhajit Chakravorty, M.D.   Department of Psychiatry, Western Psychiatric Institute and Clinic, University of Pittsburgh School of Medicine, Pittsburgh, Pennsylvania, U.S.A.

Elzbieta Chalecka-Franaszek, Ph.D.   Department of Psychiatry, Uniformed Services University of the Health Sciences, Bethesda, Maryland, U.S.A.

Duncan B. Clark, M.D., Ph.D.   Department of Psychiatry, Western Psychiatric Institute and Clinic, University of Pittsburgh School of Medicine, Pittsburgh, Pennsylvania, U.S.A.

Robert Cloninger, M.D.   Department of Psychiatry, Washington University School of Medicine in St. Louis, St. Louis, Missouri, U.S.A.

Emil F. Coccaro, M.D.   Department of Psychiatry, University of Chicago, Chicago, Illinois, U.S.A.

Robert Cohen, M.D., Ph.D.   National Institute of Mental Health, Bethesda, Maryland, U.S.A.

Jeremy D. Coplan, M.D.   Department of Psychiatry, SUNY Health Science Center at Brooklyn, and New York State Psychiatric Institute, New York, New York, U.S.A.

Jack R. Cornelius, M.D., M.P.H.   Department of Psychiatry, Western Psychiatric Institute and Clinic, University of Pittsburgh School of Medicine, Pittsburgh, Pennsylvania, U.S.A.

Jeffrey L. Cummings, M.D.   Department of Neurology, David Geffen School of Medicine at UCLA, Los Angeles, California, U.S.A.

Charles A. Dackis, M.D.   Department of Psychiatry, University of Pennsylvania, Philadelphia, Pennsylvania, U.S.A.

Lynette C. Daws, Ph.D.   Department of Psychiatry, University of Texas Health Science Center at San Antonio, San Antonio, Texas, U.S.A.

Michael D. De Bellis, M.D., M.P.H.   Department of Psychiatry and Behavioral Sciences, Duke University Medical Center, Durham, North Carolina, U.S.A.

Steven T. DeKosky, M.D.   Department of Neurology, University of Pittsburgh School of Medicine, Pittsburgh, Pennsylvania, U.S.A.

Contributors

Melissa P. DelBello, M.D. Department of Psychiatry, University of Cincinnati College of Medicine, and Children's Hospital Medical Center, Cincinnati, Ohio, U.S.A.

Stephen L. Dewey, Ph.D. Chemistry Department, Brookhaven National Laboratory, Upton, New York, U.S.A.

Antoine Douaihy, M.D. Department of Psychiatry, Western Psychiatric Institute and Clinic, University of Pittsburgh School of Medicine, Pittsburgh, Pennsylvania, U.S.A.

Larry Ereshefsky, Pharm.D., F.C.C.P. Department of Pharmacotherapy, College of Pharmacy, University of Texas at Austin, Austin, Texas, U.S.A.

Tiffany Farchione, M.D. Department of Psychiatry, Wayne State University, Detroit, Michigan, U.S.A.

Secondo Fassino, M.D. University of Turin, Turin, Italy

Norah C. Feeny, Ph.D. Department of Psychiatry, University Hospitals of Cleveland, and Case Western Reserve University, Cleveland, Ohio, U.S.A.

Francesca Mapua Filbey, Ph.D. National Institute of Mental Health, Bethesda, Maryland, U.S.A.

Robert L. Findling, M.D. Department of Psychiatry, University Hospitals of Cleveland, and Case Western Reserve University, Cleveland, Ohio, U.S.A.

Orestes V. Forlenza, M.D., Ph.D. Department of Psychiatry, Faculty of Medicine, University of São Paulo, São Paulo, Brazil

Tatiana Foroud, Ph.D. Department of Medical and Molecular Genetics, Indiana University School of Medicine, Indianapolis, Indiana, U.S.A.

Guido K. Frank, M.D. Department of Psychiatry, Western Psychiatric Institute and Clinic, University of Pittsburgh School of Medicine, Pittsburgh, Pennsylvania, U.S.A.

Alan Frazer, Ph.D. Department of Pharmacology, University of Texas Health Science Center at San Antonio, San Antonio, and South Texas Veterans Health Care System, San Antonio, Texas, U.S.A.

Marlene P. Freeman, M.D. Department of Psychiatry, University of Arizona College of Medicine, Tucson, Arizona, U.S.A.

Wagner Farid Gattaz, M.D., Ph.D. Department of Psychiatry, Faculty of Medicine, University of São Paulo, São Paulo, Brazil

Alan J. Gelenberg, M.D. Department of Psychiatry, University of Arizona College of Medicine, Tucson, Arizona, U.S.A.

Joel Gelernter, M.D. Department of Psychiatry, Yale University School of Medicine, New Haven, and Veterans Administration Medical Center, West Haven, Connecticut, U.S.A.

Tony P. George, M.D. Department of Psychiatry, Yale University School of Medicine, New Haven, Connecticut, U.S.A.

Andrew R. Gilbert, M.D. Department of Psychiatry, Western Psychiatric Institute and Clinic, University of Pittsburgh School of Medicine, Pittsburgh, Pennsylvania, U.S.A.

Jack M. Gorman, M.D. Department of Psychiatry, Columbia University, and New York State Psychiatric Institute, New York, New York, U.S.A.

Antonio Y. Hardan, M.D. Department of Psychiatry, Western Psychiatric Institute and Clinic, University of Pittsburgh School of Medicine, Pittsburgh, Pennsylvania, U.S.A.

Christopher J. Hough, Ph.D. Department of Psychiatry, Uniformed Services University of the Health Sciences, Bethesda, Maryland, U.S.A.

Vicente Ibáñez, M.D. Division of Neuropsychiatry, University of Geneva, Geneva, Switzerland

Bruno P. Imbimbo, Ph.D. Research and Development, Chiesi Farmaceutici, Parma, Italy

Cuneyt Iscan, M.D. University of Massachusetts Medical School, Worcester, Massachusetts, U.S.A.

David S. Janowsky, M.D. Department of Psychiatry, University of North Carolina at Chapel Hill, Chapel Hill, North Carolina, U.S.A.

J. David Jentsch, Ph.D. Department of Psychology, David Geffen School of Medicine at UCLA, Los Angeles, California, U.S.A.

M. Ilyas Kamboh, Ph.D. Department of Human Genetics, Western Psychiatric Institute and Clinic, University of Pittsburgh School of Medicine, Pittsburgh, Pennsylvania, U.S.A.

Walter H. Kaye, M.D. Department of Psychiatry, Western Psychiatric Institute and Clinic, University of Pittsburgh School of Medicine, Pittsburgh, Pennsylvania, U.S.A.

Lawrence S. Kegeles, M.D., Ph.D. Departments of Psychiatry and Radiology, Columbia University, New York, New York, U.S.A.

Matcheri S. Keshavan, M.D. Department of Psychiatry, Western Psychiatric Institute and Clinic, University of Pittsburgh School of Medicine, Pittsburgh, Pennsylvania, U.S.A.

Ahsan Y. Khan, M.D. Department of Psychiatry, University of Kansas School of Medicine, Wichita, Kansas, U.S.A.

Yoav Kohn, M.D. Department of Psychiatry, Hadassah University Hospital and Hebrew University School of Medicine, Jerusalem, Israel

Markus Kosel, M.D. Department of Psychiatry, University of Bern, Bern, Switzerland

Robert A. Kowatch, M.D. Department of Psychiatry, University of Cincinnati College of Medicine, and Children's Hospital Medical Center, Cincinnati, Ohio, U.S.A.

Ranga R. Krishnan, M.D. Department of Psychiatry and Behavioral Sciences, Duke University Medical Center, Durham, North Carolina, U.S.A.

Acioly L. T. Lacerda, M.D., Ph.D. Department of Psychiatry, Western Psychiatric Institute and Clinic, University of Pittsburgh School of Medicine, Pittsburgh, Pennsylvania, U.S.A.

Marc Laruelle, M.D. Departments of Psychiatry and Radiology, Columbia University, New York, New York, U.S.A.

Contributors

Royce J. Lee, M.D. Department of Psychiatry, University of Chicago, Chicago, Illinois, U.S.A.

Bernard Lerer, M.D. Department of Psychiatry, Hadassah University Hospital and Hebrew University School of Medicine, Jerusalem, Israel

Joseph Levine, M.D. Department of Psychiatry, Ben-Gurion University of the Negev, Beer-Sheva, Israel

Oscar L. Lopez, M.D. Department of Neurology, Western Psychiatric Institute and Clinic, University of Pittsburgh School of Medicine, Pittsburgh, Pennsylvania, U.S.A.

Shauna N. MacMillan, B.S. Department of Psychiatry and Behavioral Neuroscience, Wayne State University, Detroit, Michigan, U.S.A.

J. John Mann, M.D. Department of Psychiatry, Columbia University, New York, New York, U.S.A.

Douglas A. Marsteller, B.A. Chemistry Department, Brookhaven National Laboratory, Upton, New York, U.S.A.

Sanjay J. Mathew, M.D. Department of Psychiatry, Columbia University, and New York State Psychiatric Institute, New York, New York, U.S.A.

Michael S. McCloskey, Ph.D. Department of Psychiatry, University of Chicago, Chicago, Illinois, U.S.A.

William T. McKinney, M.D. The Asher Center for the Study and Treatment of Depressive Disorders, Northwestern University Medical School, Chicago, Illinois, U.S.A.

Julian Mendlewicz, M.D., Ph.D. Department of Psychiatry, Erasme Hospital, Brussels, Belgium

Alex Mishori, M.D. Department of Psychiatry, Ben-Gurion University of the Negev, Beer-Sheva, Israel

Holly Moore, Ph.D. Department of Psychiatry, Columbia University, New York, New York, U.S.A.

David A. Morilak, Ph.D. Department of Pharmacology, University of Texas Health Science Center, San Antonio, Texas, U.S.A.

Carmit Nadri, B.Med.Lab.Sc. Psychiatry Research Unit, Ben-Gurion University of the Negev, Beer-Sheva, Israel

Charles B. Nemeroff, M.D., Ph.D. Department of Psychiatry and Behavioral Sciences, Emory University School of Medicine, Atlanta, Georgia, U.S.A.

Eric A. Nofzinger, M.D. Department of Psychiatry, Western Psychiatric Institute and Clinic, University of Pittsburgh School of Medicine, Pittsburgh, Pennsylvania, U.S.A.

John I. Nurnberger, Jr., M.D., Ph.D. Department of Psychiatry, Indiana University School of Medicine, Indianapolis, Indiana, U.S.A.

Charles P. O'Brien, M.D., Ph.D. Department of Psychiatry, University of Pennsylvania, Philadelphia, Pennsylvania, U.S.A.

Michael O'Donovan, Ph.D., F.R.C.Psych. Department of Psychological Medicine, University of Wales College of Medicine, Cardiff, Wales

Peter Olausson, Ph.D. Department of Psychiatry, Yale University School of Medicine, New Haven, Connecticut, U.S.A.

David H. Overstreet, Ph.D. Department of Psychiatry, University of North Carolina at Chapel Hill, Chapel Hill, North Carolina, U.S.A.

Michael Owen, Ph.D., F.R.C.Psych., F.Med.Sci. Department of Psychological Medicine, University of Wales College of Medicine, Cardiff, Wales

Prasad Padala, M.D. Department of Psychiatry, Creighton University, and Omaha Veterans Administration Medical Center, Omaha, Nebraska, U.S.A.

Sandeep Patil, M.D., Ph.D. Department of Neuroscience, Eli Lilly and Company, Indianapolis, Indiana, U.S.A.

Dana C. Perantie, B.S. Department of Psychiatry, University of Texas Southwestern Medical Center, Dallas, Texas, U.S.A.

Frederick Petty, M.D., Ph.D. Department of Psychiatry, Creighton University, and Omaha Veterans Administration Medical Center, Omaha, Nebraska, U.S.A.

Nunzio Pomara, M.D. Department of Psychiatry, New York University School of Medicine, New York, and Geriatric Psychiatry Program, Nathan S. Kline Institute for Psychiatric Research, Orangeburg, New York, U.S.A.

Kerrie L. Posey, M.D. Department of Psychiatry, Indiana University School of Medicine, Indianapolis, Indiana, U.S.A.

Robert M. Post, M.D. Biological Psychiatry Branch, National Institute of Mental Health, Bethesda, Maryland, U.S.A.

Marc N. Potenza, M.D., Ph.D. Department of Psychiatry, Yale University School of Medicine, New Haven, Connecticut, U.S.A.

William Zeigler Potter, M.D., Ph.D. Neuroscience Therapeutic Area, Eli Lilly and Company, Indianapolis, Indiana, U.S.A.

Sheldon H. Preskorn, M.D. Department of Psychiatry, University of Kansas School of Medicine, Wichita, Kansas, U.S.A.

Surender Punia, M.D. Department of Psychiatry, Creighton University, and Omaha Veterans Administration Medical Center, Omaha, Nebraska, U.S.A.

Stanley I. Rapoport, M.D. National Institute on Aging, National Institutes of Health, Bethesda, Maryland, U.S.A.

David R. Rosenberg, M.D. Department of Psychiatry and Behavioral Neuroscience, Wayne State University, Detroit, Michigan, U.S.A.

Ihsan M. Salloum, M.D., M.P.H. Department of Psychiatry, Western Psychiatric Institute and Clinic, University of Pittsburgh School of Medicine, Pittsburgh, Pennsylvania, U.S.A.

Roberto B. Sassi, M.D. Department of Psychiatry, Western Psychiatric Institute and Clinic, University of Pittsburgh School of Medicine, Pittsburgh, Pennsylvania, U.S.A.

Contributors

Wynne K. Schiffer, Ph.D.   Chemistry Department, Brookhaven National Laboratory, Upton, New York, U.S.A.

Thomas E. Schlaepfer, M.D.   Department of Psychiatry, University of Bern, Bern, Switzerland, and Department of Psychiatry and Behavioral Sciences, Johns Hopkins University School of Medicine, Baltimore, Maryland, U.S.A.

Mary V. Seeman, M.D., D.S.C., F.R.C.P.C.   Department of Psychiatry, University of Toronto, Toronto, Ontario, Canada

Philip Seeman, M.D., Ph.D., D.Sc.   Department of Pharmacology, University of Toronto, Toronto, Ontario, Canada

Alona Shaldubina, M.Sc.   Departments of Psychiatry and Pharmacology, Ben-Gurion University of the Negev, Beer-Sheva, Israel

Tonmoy Sharma, M.B.B.S., M.R.C.Psych.   Clinical Neuroscience Research Centre, Stonehouse Hospital, Dartford, Kent, England

Anantha Shekhar, M.D., Ph.D.   Department of Psychiatry, Indiana University School of Medicine, Indianapolis, Indiana, U.S.A.

Leo Sher, M.D.   Department of Psychiatry, Columbia University, New York, New York, U.S.A.

Kenneth R. Silk, M.D.   Department of Psychiatry, University of Michigan Health System, Ann Arbor, Michigan, U.S.A.

Jair C. Soares, M.D.   Department of Psychiatry, University of Texas Health Science Center at San Antonio, San Antonio, Texas, U.S.A.

Daniel Souery, M.D., Ph.D.   Department of Psychiatry, Erasme Hospital, Brussels, Belgium

Stana Stanic, M.D.   University of Trieste, Trieste, Italy

Dan J. Stein, M.D., Ph.D.   University of Stellenbosch, Cape Town, South Africa, and University of Gainesville, Gainesville, Florida, U.S.A.

Murray B. Stein, M.D.   Department of Psychiatry, University of California, San Diego, La Jolla, and Veterans Affairs San Diego Healthcare System, San Diego, California, U.S.A.

Trey Sunderland, M.D.   National Institute of Mental Health, Bethesda, Maryland, U.S.A.

Dragan M. Svrakic, M.D., Ph.D.   Department of Psychiatry, Washington University School of Medicine in St. Louis, St. Louis, Missouri, U.S.A.

Johannes Tauscher, M.D.   Department of General Psychiatry, University of Vienna, Vienna, Austria

Warren D. Taylor, M.D.   Department of Psychiatry and Behavioral Sciences, Duke University Medical Center, Durham, North Carolina, U.S.A.

Florence Thibaut, M.D., Ph.D.   Department of Psychiatry, Rouen University Hospital, Rouen, France

Stefan Ursu, M.D.   Departments of Neuroscience and Psychiatry, Western Psychiatric Institute and Clinic, University of Pittsburgh School of Medicine, Pittsburgh, Pennsylvania, U.S.A.

Nicolaas Paul Leonard Gerrit Verhoeff, M.D., Ph.D., F.R.C.P.(C) Department of Psychiatry, University of Toronto, and Kunin-Lunenfeld Applied Research Unit, Baycrest Centre for Geriatric Care, Toronto, Ontario, Canada

Bavanisha Vythilingum, M.B., Ch.B. MRC Unit on Anxiety Disorders, University of Stellenbosch, Cape Town, South Africa

Xiaohong Wang, M.D., Ph.D. Department of Psychiatry and Behavioral Sciences, Emory University School of Medicine, Atlanta, Georgia, U.S.A.

Yuri Yaroslavsky, M.D. Department of Psychiatry, Ben-Gurion University of the Negev, Beer-Sheva, Israel

L. Trevor Young, M.D., Ph.D., F.R.C.P.(C) Department of Psychiatry and Behavioral Neurosciences, McMaster University, Hamilton, Ontario, Canada

1

Animal Models of Neuropsychiatric Disorders
Challenges for the Future

WILLIAM T. McKINNEY
Northwestern University Medical School, Chicago, Illinois, U.S.A.

I. INTRODUCTION

The major challenges for future animal modeling research primarily involve conceptual and philosophical issues. Despite the fact that there are a variety of animal models available for many psychiatric disorders [1–3] there are still widespread perceptions that (1) one cannot reasonably study human psychiatric disorders in animals, because psychiatric illnesses are inherently human, and (2) there are no animal models of the various psychiatric disorders available.

In medicine in general, animal models are generally accepted as important for research directed at understanding the mechanisms underlying human disease as well as the development of new treatments. In contrast, modeling of mental disorders in experimental animals has often been regarded as "a highly controversial or outright heretical idea" [4]. There is widespread skepticism regarding animal models in psychiatry, with virtually no organized federal programs/initiatives for encouraging and supporting research in this field. When the active opposition of components of the animal rights movement to research with animals is coupled with the above-mentioned lack of understanding of the role of animal models by leaders in the field (who sometimes have backed off encouraging further developments in this field in the face of the animal rights movement), the stage is set for continuing major problems. This in summary represents the major future challenges for the field of animal modeling research.

The above situation is ironical given the role that research utilizing animal models has played in advancing the understanding of psychiatric disorders. As will be discussed in the historical section, the first data-based integrative theories of psychopathology grew largely out of animal research and/or improving treatment approaches. Since psychiatric disorders need to be understood by using a multivariate approach, animal studies, where variables can be controlled, have the potential for permitting the study of both the main effects of single variables and especially their interaction. Such approaches are highly relevant to what has recently been termed the "biopsychosocial" view of human psychopathology [5].

Research with animals has also been critical in broadening our understanding of human development and in providing empirical support for the importance of early experiences for behavioral and neurobiological development. Work with multiple species has documented the central importance of early social attachment systems and has clarified the behavioral and neurobiological variables mediating the development of these attachment systems [6–10]. Such concepts are by now woven into the fabric of development theory in adult and child psychiatry, and it was experimental animal research that provided the fundamental basis for this knowledge. Furthermore, research with experimental animal systems has documented the devastating and long-term behavioral and neurobiological effects, including effects on brain cytoarchitecture, of never letting such attachment systems develop or of their intermittent disruption at certain developmental stages [11–14].

Studies utilizing animal models have also focused on the interaction between social functioning and neurobiological status and have documented the interactive and reciprocal nature of these relationships in paradigms that would be impossible to implement in human studies [15,16]. In addition, the impact of different types of stress has been extensively explored in animal models and in some instances genetic strains have also been identified or developed which exhibit similarities to clinical syndromes [17,18].

Though there is no perfect animal model with regard to predicting clinical efficacy of pharmacological agents, their use has been critical in the discovery and development of drug treatments [19–22]. There are always false positives and false negatives, but there are experimental paradigms with a high degree of empirical validity. Given a new era of drug discovery and development, there will likely continue to be many challenging issues in this context.

Despite these and many other contributions, acrimonious debates about the validity and/or usefulness of animal models for psychiatric disorders persist. The evaluation of animal models for psychiatric disorders is complex. Unfortunately, there is not yet any single laboratory finding or set of findings for any clinical psychiatric syndrome that one could insist upon as part of the validating criteria. Thus, one largely relies on a combination of behavioral measures and response to known clinically effective agents. Part of the challenge for the future may be to reconsider the validity measures of animal models and to reconceptualize expectations.

There is no "perfect," complete, or comprehensive single animal model for any specific psychiatric disorder. Indeed, there will likely never be an animal model in any field of medicine that is a perfect fit with the human condition; rather the emphasis in the development and study of disease models in animals needs to increasingly focus on specific components of the human illness.

Animal models of diseases in medicine, including psychiatry, need to be understood in a historical and evolutionary perspective and their advantages as well as limitations recognized. Neither overextended cross-species comparisons nor unjustified negativism about animal models seems defensible.

An especially critical challenge in the continuing development and utilization of biobehavioral animal models in psychiatry is their relationship to the molecular neurosciences, including genetics. Given recent advances in the molecular neurosciences relevant to mental disorders, the role of animal models in this context needs to be reconsidered. Failure to do so could lead to an excessively narrow view of animal models or a dismissal of the entire area. Danger signals already exist in this regard. Some contend that, given the new molecular techniques, animal models no longer have a place in psychiatric research. Others have taken the position that since psychiatric illnesses are so difficult to model in animals, we will need to do most of the research on mental disorders in clinical populations [23]. There is also tension between those who think that while one can, with high validity and reliability, measure, for example, receptor functioning in certain brain regions, the measure of behavior in animals lacks comparable scientific precision [24]. Unfortunately, the latter reflects a serious lack of communication between fields because the quantitative assessment of animal behavior is a well-developed science.

With the increasing advances in molecular biology and genetics, functional neuroimaging, and other methods for studying mental disorders, conceptualization of and research on behaviorally based animal models needs to be able to keep pace to maximally enrich psychiatric research. Despite several recent publications about the animal modeling field [25–28], there are many indications that the area remains poorly understood. This paper is an attempt to provide an overview of the past contributions of animal models and to propose some new perspectives that might be helpful in reevaluating the role of animal models in better understanding the major psychiatric illnesses. In an attempt to focus on some fundamental issues and challenges regarding animal models as they relate to neuropsychiatric disorders, a review of available models for each disorder becomes impossible. To attempt such a review would certainly shortchange many important areas, so, rather than attempt this, appropriate references will be provided to articles where such models are discussed.

II. HISTORICAL CONTEXT

Pavlov, often said to have been the originator of research relevant to animal modeling of human psychopathology in general, used clinical terms and experimental techniques that now seem foreign to most clinicians. However, the fact that his work represented one of the first moves away from a strictly correlational method of behavioral analysis to the experimental study of psychopathology is of central importance [29].

Considering Pavlov and other early scientists [30–33], it is difficult to know what conclusions to draw about the early history of the field of experimental psychopathology research. From one standpoint it was not a particularly noteworthy beginning. However, the early pioneers may have been more successful than it appears in developing certain principles that seem to be being rediscovered today, including:

1. Demonstration that psychopathology could be experimentally studied in animals as well as in the strictly correlational studies done previously in humans.
2. Demonstration of the importance of both careful behavioral observations and serendipity. Although most of the early workers did not use the more sophisticated and quantifiable behavioral scoring techniques now available, they were keen observers and literate in their descriptions.
3. The repeated proposal of an interactive model of psychopathology. The role of the temperament of the animals, along with a variety of social and neurobiological variables, was repeatedly stressed in the early literature. The concept of individual variability was part of the early work, and investigation of the sources of such variability continues to be an important area of research.
4. Recognition that there could be a persistent internal response, even after the inducing stimulus was no longer present, a discovery that remains a major contribution to the understanding of a number of forms of psychopathology.
5. Recognition of the importance of unpredictability and uncontrollability of which systematic investigations continue today [5].

III. ETHOLOGICAL CONTEXT

This section touches on some principles of ethology important in evaluating and understanding experimental animal research and a few selected research approaches. Avoidance of misleading clinical labeling based on superficial comparisons across species is critical. However, behavioral profiling in a given species can be done with a degree of precision comparable to other methods in neurobiology. Evolutionary biology principles then need to be understood and applied when it comes to interpretation of these phenomena. Ethology focuses on describing and understanding "animal behavior in the natural habitat and assumes operation of evolutionarily conserved basic plans encoded in the genome. Such basic plans determine behavioral patternings including flexible variants involving learning. Human ethology has emerged as a subdiscipline, including observations of psychiatric patients. The research involved has produced an enormous and varied literature" [34].

Gardner describes this interface as follows:

Sensitive observers have noted that relationship-less psychiatry seems the objective of much current psychiatric practice augmented by the cost-conscious managed care industry. Such a peculiar objective can stand almost unopposed in part because psychiatry has no basic science other than that limited to drug actions on the one hand and venerable, used but unproven and unphysiological theories of psychotherapy on the other hand. Adopting a perspective that shows human relatedness to other animals (near identity of genome) yet human uniqueness (with a massively larger brain) would underline the importance of people for other people that would augment the psychiatric enterprise. Human bonding and human competition shares much in common with other species, yet has its own flavor likely stemming from the human capacity to use stories in many ways. An important step towards psychiatry as a relationship-focused enterprise might come about if there was an explicit label for it. Sociophysiology could furnish that label to emphasize the importance of weighing the following as equally important while interactive: complex behaviors especially communicative ones, ancient reaction patterns, brain functions, cellular actions and genomic mechanisms [35].

Gardner described modeling as depending upon brain-body factors that the animal and humans possess in common. While behavior patterns may be species specific, "core components shared by related animals are typically embroidered through natural selection to produce modified methods of survival and reproduction" [34]. He cites the example of human brains which contrast in size to those of other animals, weighing three times more than brains of surviving large primates or those of human ancestors 3 million years ago. The contrast with other primates especially stems from a massively enlarged neocortex, especially the frontal lobes, with these increases likely stemming from advantages of social functions. Despite differences, the human brain and behavior also show comparability to those of other species through widely shared, conserved features. Gardner contends that this comparability makes continued use of animals important for the study of the pathogenesis, mechanisms, and treatment of mental disease. "Lack of a sufficient database as yet limits other modeling efforts such as computer simulations, mathematical models, and experimentally induced states in hums, and research on animals remains indispensable" [34].

Homology and convergence are important ethological concepts which can serve as frameworks for helping to understand comparative cross species behavior.

> Homology means that a common ancestor once possessed a trait now shared by two species. At points in the past, humans shared common ancestors with monkeys, mice, chickens, fish, insects, and single celled organisms, each such forebear more remote in biological history. In contrast, convergent traits are similar features that stem from environmental shaping through natural selection, although basic plan starting points vary. Wings of insects, bats and birds illustrate this. Ancestors of each animal group had not flown so airborne ability evolved separately and the three kinds of wings illustrate convergent evolution on the level of aerial locomotion. As vertebrate upper extremities, however, wings of bats and birds are homologous to each other but not to the wings of insects. If the starting point of the basic plan generalizes to contractile tissue, however, locomotory body extensions of all three achieve homology [34].

There is great excitement with genome projects of species at different phylogenetic levels and importance. The genome seems to contain at least a partial record of the organism's ancestry, and therefore genomic analysis may help determine evolutionary history (homology) which in turn may foster knowledge of proximal neuronal determinants of behavior. However, this is a very complicated area, and simplistic and overly optimistic expectations will likely fail. As Gardner says, at the behavioral level, redundant, multiply determined brain-behavior adaptations complicate inference, and at the DNA level, genetic transformations such as chromosomal crossovers will reduce certainty about genomic hypotheses [34].

IV. DEFINITIONAL/CONCEPTUAL ISSUES

Animal models are experimental paradigms developed in one species for the purpose of studying specific phenomena occurring in another species. By definition they are not the "real thing." There will always be differences and similarities between models and what is being modeled; otherwise it is not a model. Furthermore, there is no single comprehensive animal model for any mental disorder and probably not for any general medical illness. Thus, animal models should be judged primarily by their relevance to specific questions that they are being used to address rather than their scope. They permit the evaluation of selected aspects of human psychopathology in a systematic and controlled manner and represent simplified and abstracted versions of behavior and physiology, which can be used to develop hypotheses applicable to humans and/or to test hypotheses originating from clinical work [34].

V. TYPES OF ANIMAL MODELS

The following overlapping categories of animal models [29,36–39] have been proposed.

A. Behavioral Similarity Models

These types of models are designed to simulate specific symptoms of a human disorder in animals. The primary intent is to produce a particular set of behaviors that are similar to those shown by humans with a certain illness, rather than to evaluate any specific etiological theory or to study underlying mechanisms or even treatment responsiveness. The validity of these models is judged by how closely the model approximates the human disorder from a phenomenological standpoint [29]. Inducing conditions became secondary.

B. Theory-Driven Models

In these approaches a theory drives the development of specific experimental paradigms. One does not assume the validity of the theory in order to proceed with the research. Rather, the goal is to operationalize the theory one wants to evaluate and study prospectively the efforts of specific manipulations designed to represent putative causative factors.

C. Mechanistic Models

In these kinds of models, animals are used to study mechanisms. With the increasing array of methods for studying pathophysiology, there has been a preoccupation with the molecular and submolecular basis of altered behavior seen in many animal models. Some would consider that the only useful animal models are those which permit these types of studies.

While mechanistic studies can include evaluation of both neurobiological mechanisms as well as social, behavioral, and developmental mechanisms, one cannot necessarily transpose techniques of mechanism studies cross species, i.e., from humans to rodents to primates or vice versa from rodents to monkeys. The study of mechanisms needs to be specific for a particular species. A serious challenge for animal modeling research is the development and utilization of techniques for mechanism studies in socially behaving animals. Some compromises between invasiveness of neurobiological studies and assessment of social behavior may be necessary [29]. Insistence on cross-species mechanistic similarities is premature given that at present we have no mental disorders in humans uniquely linked with a specific mechanism.

D. Empirical Validity Models

Perhaps the best-known and widest use of animal models involves the use of animal preparations to develop and test potential clinically active drugs. In this context, an ideal animal model is one in which there are no false positives and no false negatives; that is, when a drug works in animals it is predictive of its clinical effects in humans, and when it is inactive in animal models it will not have clinical efficacy in humans. Although there are a number of models with high empirical validity, there is never 100% correspondence between the effects of a drug in an animal model and in a clinical condition. The establishment of an animal model as valid on empirical grounds (or on any other grounds) does not necessarily establish its validity on other parameters.

E. Genetic Models

Genetic models involve studying strains that exhibit spontaneous behaviors that mimic a given illness. Through selective breeding, some investigators have developed animal strains that are especially sensitive on certain tests. This topic is discussed more extensively elsewhere in this chapter.

VI. VALIDATION CRITERIA FOR ANIMAL MODELS

In 1969 McKinney and Bunney [36] made explicit the concept of using animal models for studying human depression and proposed for the first time criteria to consider in developing and evaluating animal models in general. Subsequently, modified or expanded sets of criteria were presented [5].

Willner [39] has described three different concepts of validity:

1. *Predictive validity* primarily concerns the correspondence between drug actions in the animal model and in clinical situations. Manipulations which have certain effects in humans should have similar effects in the animal model for that model to be valid from this standpoint. Using this criterion, there will always be false positives and false negatives. Not all agents that work in an animal model will also work in humans, and not all drugs that work in humans will necessarily work in animal models. There is no animal model that has perfect concordance in this regard. In terms of evaluating animal models according to this criteria it is the pharmacological profiling that is critical rather than the response to just one drug.

2. *Face validity* means that there are phenomenological similarities between the model and the illness being studied. In any one model it is never possible to model all the composite patterns of behaviors shown rather than the presence or absence of any one behavior or symptom.

3. *Construct validity* refers to the theoretical rationale for the model, which in turn relates to the theoretical understanding of the clinical condition and its causation. Unfortunately, too many proposed animal models utilize single proposed etiologies rather than a concept involving multiple risk factors. One of the exciting challenges for future animal models is the evaluation of the relative contributions of various risk factors thought to be important in the human syndrome in question.

Geyer [1] makes the point that, before criteria can be considered, it is important to be explicit about the intended purpose of the model which will determine in part the criteria that should be utilized in evaluating its validity. He contends that for a model to be of value in it must satisfy only two criteria: reliability and predictive validity. He does not think that construct validity is essential.

VII. SIGNIFICANCE OF ANIMAL MODELS

As Willner has stated [37,39,40], animal models form an important interface between clinical psychiatry and basic research in behavioral neuroscience. In this context they represent major modalities by which developments at the basic level can be brought into a clinical perspective and clinical theories can be evaluated in a controlled manner. This viewpoint contrasts sharply with the position that animal models have no more use since, for example, we can now discover and design drugs that are very specific and can go directly to testing in humans.

The significance of animal models is also their role in the specification and study of focused components of a clinical syndrome. Experimental paradigms in animals permit evaluation of selected aspects of human psychopathology in a systematic and controlled manner. Their obvious advantage is in the ability to precisely control and alter inducing conditions and to permit the collection of prospective data on both a short- and a long-term basis and permit a broader range of mechanistic studies. For example, in relation to depression, prospective studies examining the effects of developmental events on behavior and on neurobiology can be done much more easily in animals. The timing and exact nature of certain alterations in development can be specified, and the short- and long-term consequences studied. That aspect of modeling research is relevant to the question of developmental vulnerability based on early experiences and the mediating mechanisms of vulnerability.

Animal models make possible the dissection of mechanisms in a more direct way than is possible in human clinical research, and they complement ongoing efforts in human protocols, although such procedures need to be suited to both the species and the overall purpose of the experimental paradigm. The research questions have to be clear and specific.

It is easier in animal studies to isolate and evaluate single variables in terms of their main effects and their interaction with each other. For example, the nature of the interactions among genetic, developmental, social, and biological variables can be studied in various combinations in different species. In human clinical research, multiple variables interact simultaneously, and it has been virtually impossible to sort them out in any quantifiable way.

Of course, animal models are most widely utilized in the preclinical evaluation of drugs. A related aspect is their contribution to a better understanding of the mechanism of the action of drugs in altering specific behavior patterns that goes beyond a mere prediction of whether drugs work or not [29].

Studies utilizing animal models can also help to understand the mechanisms of established treatment techniques, i.e., why do some treatment work in certain paradigms whereas others do not? A type of significance which is often not recognized is that animal modeling research has led to the development of improved behavioral, ethologically based rating methods that are now widely used in clinical research settings.

The following quote is focused on affective disorders but, when considering the significance of animal models for psychopathology in general, contains principles applicable to any psychiatric disorder:

> The traditional difficulties in accepting animal models for psychopathology stem from the argument that there is no evidence for what occurs in the brain of the animal that is equivalent to what occurs in the brain of a human. However, if one models any or some core aspects of affective disorder, this model can become an invaluable tool in the analysis of the multitude of causes, genetic, environmental or pharmacological, that can bring about symptoms homologous to those of patients with affective disorders. Animal models can also allow the study of the mechanisms of specific behaviors, their pathophysiology, and can aid to develop and predict therapeutic response to pharmacological agents.
>
> The use of animal models in the research of affective disorders is multifold. Firstly, these models offer experimental systems that may provide insights into the multitude of causes, genetic, environmental or pharmacological, that can bring about symptoms homologous to those of patients with affective disorders. Models also allow study of the development of specific behaviors and their underlying neuroanatomical substrates and neurochemical mechanisms. Finally, animal models can be utilized to develop and predict therapeutic response to pharmacological agents and investigate their putative mechanisms of action [41].

VIII. CHANGING ROLE OF ANIMAL MODELS

A. Neurosciences

Rapid developments in the basic and clinical neurosciences have presented and will continue to present opportunities yet also serious challenges for animal modeling research. On the positive side has been the general recognition of the importance of having experimental animal models if one is going to better understand the pathophysiology of psychiatric illness and move beyond correlative research. Indeed, some contend that the only useful animal models are those that permit molecular mechanistic studies to be done. However, as important as these types of models are, they are not the only useful types of animal models. There is also a role for more integrative models that will facilitate the study of vulnerability factors in a broader context. Conceptualizing animal models narrowly in a deterministic basic neuroscience context has had some unfortunate consequences in terms of the field's development in that attention to the development and study of new biobehavioral models has been diminished along with critical research on already existing models.

"Mechanisms" should not be viewed as synonymous with "molecular." There is far more involved in understanding mechanism of behavior than molecular genetics and molecular biology. Some animal models will lend themselves to molecular biological studies of mechanisms; others will allow other kinds of contributions. Many major discoveries that have significantly impacted clinical psychiatry have come from either behaviorally oriented studies in animals, e.g., the significant enhancement of our understanding of developmental theories and attachment systems, and/or have been based on empirical observations of animal behaviors in relation to drug treatment, e.g., the initial observations by Cade of lithium's calming effects in guinea pigs [42].

A major challenge/opportunity for the development of animal models in the future relates to alterations of circadian rhythms which remain among the most pervasive and consistent findings in several types of mental disorders, especially the mood disorders. A considerable amount of research needs to be done to understand the mechanisms that underlie this connection. One context to begin to understand these mechanisms is at the interface between development/early experience, social stress, and circadian rhythms. This approach could serve as the nexus of a new approach to animal models which incorporates genetic, developmental, and social stress issues. With the identification and characterization of the first mammalian circadian clock gene [43], some exciting cross-species approaches with high relevance to human disorders are going to become possible.

B. Stress Vulnerability

Early theories of the origins of human psychopathology focused on the importance of a variety of early life relationships and events. With the advent of a new era of neurosciences, interest in such developmental events has waned in many quarters. However, research utilizing animal models over the past 25 years has continued to steadily emphasize that these development stressors are important and can have long-term effects on brain and neurobiological development [44–47]. Obviously such events do not operate in a vacuum. The role of genetic vulnerability and how this interacts with developmental events and their consequences is an extremely important and newly emerging area of research in which experimental animal models can play an increasingly important role. Major theories have been proposed that provide an integrated developmental neurobiological perspective of depressive disorders [48–51] and of schizophrenia [52]. In terms of this approach, animal models have already contributed and have great potential for the future [13,53–59].

C. Clinical Disorders

At present, diagnostic criteria for most human clinical disorders involve both a time dimension and signs and symptoms. Since the defining criteria for animal models of psychiatric disorders rely heavily on observed behaviors, a research challenge is to operationalize in animals what in humans are reported as subjective symptoms. Of course, an animal cannot tell one whether it has a certain symptom or not; however, it is possible to measure in animals such things as motor activity, food and water intake, weight, sleep, a range of social activities, changes in self-rewarding activities, and cognitive behaviors. A collection of changes in such behaviors might be postulated to resemble the symptoms or behavioral changes shown by humans diagnosed as having a certain illness, and by working within proper ethological frameworks cross-species research can aid in the understanding of human illness.

Rather than trying to model an aggregate of symptoms, another approach is to focus on the experimental production of a more limited set of behaviors and to use animal preparations to study these behaviors, e.g., anhedonia, uncontrollability, or changes in social and self-directed behaviors.

What induction techniques to use? There are two broad approaches in utilizing induction procedures. One approach is to use those for which there are data to suggest that they might be important in the etiology of human clinical disorders. An alternative approach is to not worry too much about the cross-species compatibility of inducing conditions, but to use procedures that will produce a set of behaviors in animals that bear some phenomenological similarity to a human illness.

IX. GENETICS

Statements are beginning to appear that the best, or even only, approach to animal models is "genetic," though it is not totally clear what this means. However, with the established importance of genetic vulnerability, experimental paradigms to systematically study genetic variables in animal models are needed as part of an overall approach to the creation and development of animal models. Many techniques are possible. For example, two lines of work, both from the animal models of depression literature, can be summarized as illustrative of this approach. One involves selective breeding and the other study of a specified strain [5].

A. Selective Breeding: Flinders–Sensitive Line (FSL) of Rats

The Flinders line rats [17,60,61] were developed by selective breeding for differences in effects of the anticholinesterase, di-isopropylfluorophosphate (DFP) on temperature, drinking, and body weight. The FSL line rats are more sensitive to DFP as well as cholinergic agonists and have more brain muscarinic receptors in comparison with the Flinders-resistant line (FRL). They were originally proposed as an animal model of depression because of reports that human depressives are also more sensitive to cholinergic agonists. The FSL rats also resemble depressed humans in some other ways: elevated REM sleep, appetite and weight changes, reduced activity and increased anhedonia after exposure to chronic mild stress, and exaggerated immobility in the forced swim test. Imipramine, desipramine, and sertraline have all been shown to reduce immobility in the forced swim test in the Flinders line rats. Lithium, bright lights, and DFP do not. Likewise, amphetamine and scopolamine have no effect in the forced swim paradigm. The calcium channel blockers verapamil and nicardipine were effective in reducing immobility in the forced swim test. Overstreet [62] has also presented data that the FSL rats exhibit altered sensitivity to the locomotor suppressant effects of diazepam; however, anxiolytic effects of diazepam are similar in the FSL. They do not voluntarily drink much alcohol, unlike some depressed individuals. They also do not exhibit any model schizophrenic behavior. They found that swim test immobility cosegregates with serotonergic but not cholinergic sensitivity in cross breeds of Flinders line rats. In conclusion, they present the FSL rat as fulfilling the criteria of face, construct, and predictive validity for an animal model of depression.

B. Specified Strain: Wistar Kyoto (WKY) Rats

Okamoto and Aoki [63] isolated a strain of Wistar rats with spontaneously developed hypertension, the SHR rat. Its normotensive inbred progenitor strain, the WKY rat not only differs from the SHR in respect to resting blood pressure, but also displays smaller stress-induced increases in plasma catecholamines [64], heart rate, and blood pressure [65–67]. In contrast, WKYs show larger endocrine and behavioral responses to stress than SHRs and a heightened susceptibility to stress ulcer. WKY rats [18,68,69] have been proposed as another animal model of depression based on the fact that they (1) exhibit hypoactivity in open field and defensive burying tests (2) readily acquire a learned helplessness task as well as a passive avoidance task; and (3) exhibit more depressive behavior in the Porsolt forced swim test of "behavioral despair" and desipramine reduces the immobility seen in this test. WKY rats also have a heightened susceptibility to stress ulcer and show evidence of heightened emotionality and an exaggerated stress response.

C. Other Genetic Strategies

Another genetic approach would be to utilize targeted mutagenic strategies that rely on transgenic and recombinant DNA-based knockout technologies to create animal models in available biobehavioral tests, thus permitting, within the limitation of these strategies, better understanding of the role of various genes in the control of specific behaviors. A critical research challenge for the future is the question of what specific strategies should be used to develop such models based on current knowledge of the pathophysiology of various mental disorders.

Other genetic approaches could involve genetic manipulation of candidate genes leading to knockout or transgenic mice, chance findings of altered behavioral phenotypes in other, not a priori designed, mouse mutants, or systematic behavioral screening of mutagenized mice to gain novel animal models [41]. A theoretical advantage of the transgenic or knockout approaches is that a specified behavioral alteration can be assigned to a single gene mutation. However, compensatory mechanisms and genetic background are always at work and sometimes obscure the role of a specific gene in a behavior.

A method that will gain influence over the next years is genome-wide or directed mutagenesis followed by screens for relevant phenotypes. The forced swim test has already been used as a pilot behavioral assay in a random mutagenesis screen [70], but the identification of a series of well-defined and well characterized tests with high predictive validity would dramatically increase the efficacy of such an enterprise.

X. NEW THERAPIES

A. New Methods of Discovering and Developing Pharmacological Therapies

Drug discovery is a multidisciplinary effort requiring chemical, structural, and biological approaches. This last includes animal models.

Historically, one of the major uses of animal models has been for the preclinical screening of proposed pharmacological treatment agents. In this context, a variety of experimental animal models have been developed which have reasonable empirical validity. Unfortunately, the presence of false negatives and false positives has led some to sharply criticize animal models and even refuse to use them in drug discovery and development.

A related position is that animal models, in the context of drug discovery and development, are irrelevant given newer molecular techniques for discovering and developing drugs. Newer therapies can be discovered based on hypothesized molecular mechanisms of illness and then moved directly to clinical trials. However, one of the major problems with this approach is that not enough is yet known about the specific pathophysiology of psychiatric illnesses to let that alone drive the therapeutic discovery and development process. Some in vivo testing in animals remains critical to complement drug discovery based on novel mechanisms. Also, since psychiatric disorders are still largely defined by behaviors, it does not intuitively make sense to bypass behavior in the drug discovery and development process [5].

XI. ANIMAL RIGHTS ISSUES

This is one of the foremost challenges with regard to animal modeling research [71,72]. The use of animals for biomedical research in general, and especially for neuropsychiatric disorders, continues under serious threat [73–80]. Detailed discussion of the various groups and strategies is beyond the scope of this chapter; however, the issue is not animal welfare organizations who, in so many invaluable ways, help look after the welfare of needy animals and deserve our enthusiastic support. Likewise, the problem is not the thoughtful groups that share our genuine concern about the welfare of all animals and work to establish reasonable regulations. The problem is with those organizations that are dedicated to stopping animal research at all costs, including violence to researchers and to physical property, and who advocate senseless bureaucracy to discourage researchers from pursuing animal research. We all support the humane treatment of all animals in research and careful and diligent review of all research by independent groups—as is done with human clinical research. However, with the escalating tempo of violence and intimidation in this area that has occurred over the last 10–20 years, some government agencies have hesitated to move ahead with programmatic initiatives in the animal modeling research area, and some universities have been, at best, ambivalent in backing faculty doing animal research. The field has lost productive people as a result, and new, junior people have sometimes hesitated to enter the field. This is a major challenge for the field in the future.

XII. SUMMARY

There are a variety of animal models available for many psychiatric disorders. Just as in any other field of medicine, none are perfect. Indeed, if they were, they would be replicas rather than models. Continuing efforts need to be made to further understand and utilize the models that are available as well as to develop new ones. However, major challenges for the future will also include dealing with the conceptual and philosophical issues that surround animal modeling research in psychiatry. Many of these have been summarized in this chapter.

REFERENCES

1. MA Geyer, A Markou. Animal models of psychiatric disorders. In: FE Bloom, DJ Kupfer, eds. Psychopharmacology: the Fourth Generation of Progress. New York: Raven Press, 1995, pp 787–798.
2. WT McKinney. Models of Mental Disorders: A New Comparative Psychiatry. New York: Plenum, 1988.
3. GF Koob, CL Ehlers, DJ Kupfer, eds. Animal Models of Depression. Boston: Birkaeuser, 1989.
4. BK Lipska, DR Weinberger. To model a psychiatric disorder in animals: schizophrenia as a reality test. Neuropsychopharmacology 23(3):223–239, 2000.
5. WT McKinney. Overview of the past contributions of animal models and their changing place in psychiatry. Semin Clin Neuropsychiatry 6(1):68–78, 2001.
6. J Bowlby. Attachment and Loss: Attachment, Vol. 1. New York: Basic Books, 1969.
7. CL Coe, SP Mendoza, WP Smotherman, S Levine. Mother-infant attachement in the squirrel monkey: adrenal responses to separation. Behav Biol 22:256–263, 1978.
8. GD Jensen and CW Tolman. Mother-infant relationship in the monkey, *Macaca nemestrina*: the effect of brief separation and mother-infant specificity. J Comp Physiol Psychol 55:131–136, 1962.
9. IC Kaufman, LA Rosenblum. The reaction to separation in infant monkeys: anaclitic depression and conservation-withdrawal. Psychosom Med 29:649–675, 1967.
10. WT McKinney Jr, SJ Suomi, HF Harlow. Repetitive peer separations of juvenile-age rhesus monkeys. Arch Gen Psychiatry 27(2):200–203, 1972.
11. RA Hinde, LM Davies. Changes in mother-infant relationship after separation in rhesus monkeys. Nature 239:41–41, 1972.
12. GW Kraemer, MH Ebert, DE Schmidt, WT McKinney. A longitudinal study of the effect of different social rearing conditions on cerebrospinal fluid norepinephrine and biogenic amine metabolites in rhesus monkeys. Neuropsychopharmacology 2(3):175–189, 1989.
13. SJ Siegel, SD Ginsberg, PR Hof, SL Foote, WG Young, GW Kraemer, WT McKinney, JH Morrison. Effects of social deprivation in prepubescent rhesus monkeys: immunohistochemical analysis of the neurofilament protein triplet in the hippocampal formation. Brain Res 619(1–2):299–305, 1993.
14. SJ Suomi, HF Harlow, CJ Domek. Effect of repetitive infant-infant separation of young monkeys. J Abnorm Psychol 76:161–172, 1970.
15. GD Mitchell, DL Clark. Long term effects of social isolation in non-socially adapted rhesus monkeys. J Genetic Psychol 13:117–128, 1968.
16. JM Weiss, HI Glazer, LA Pohorecky, WH Bailey, LH Schneider. Coping behavior and stress-induced behavioral depression: studies of the role of brain catecholamines. In: RA Depue, ed. Psychobiology of Depressive Disorders. New York: Academic Press, 1979, pp 125–160.
17. DH Overstreet. The Flinders sensitive line rats: a genetic animal model of depression. Neurosci Biobehav Rev 17(1):51–68, 1993.
18. WP Pare, E Redei. Depressive behavior and stress ulcer in Wistar Kyoto rats. J Physiol Paris 87(4):229–238, 1993.
19. F Petty, AD Sherman. A pharmacologically pertinent animal model of mania. J Affect Disord 3:381–387, 1981.
20. RD Porsolt. Pharmacological models of depression. In: Dahlem Conference on the Origins of Depression: Current Concepts and Approaches. Berlin: Dahlem University Press, 1982.
21. KA Roth, RJ Katz. Further studies on a novel animal model of depression: therapeutic effects of a tricyclic antidepressant. Neurosci Biobehav Rev 5:253–259, 1981.
22. SJ Suomi, SF Seaman, JK Lewis, RD DeLizio, WT McKinney Jr. Effects of imipramine treatment of separation-induced social disorders in rhesus monkeys. Arch Gen Psychiatry 35(3):321–325, 1978.
23. NIMH. Genetics and Mental Disorders: Report of the National Institute of Mental Health's Genetics Workgroup, 1998.
24. TM Burton. Drug maker's goal: Prozac without the lag. Wall Street Journal, 1998: B1:3.
25. LD Dorn, GP Chrousos. The neurobiology of stress: understanding regulation of affect during female biological transitions. Semin Reprod Endocrinol 15:19–35, 1997.
26. J Flint, R Corley. Do animals models have a place in the genetic analysis of quantitative human behavioral traits? J Mol Med 74(9):515–521, 1996.
27. KP Lesch. Gene transfer to the brain: emerging therapeutic strategy in psychiatry? Biol Psychiatry 45:247–253, 1999.
28. E Sibille, Z Sarnyai, D Benjamin, J Gal, H Baker, M Toth. Antisense inhibition of 5-hydroxytryptamine2a receptor induces an antidepressant-like effect in mice. Mol Pharmacol 52:1056–1063, 1997.
29. WT McKinney. Animal research and its relevance to psychiatry. In: BJ Sadock, VA Sadock, Kaplan and Sadock's Comprehensive Textbook of Psychiatry/VII. eds. Philadelphia: Lippincott Williams and Wilkins, 2000, pp 545–562.

30. DO Hebb. Spontaneous neurosis in chimpanzees: theoretical relations with clinical and experimental phenomena. Psychosom Med 9:3–6, 1947.
31. IP Pavlov. Lectures on Conditioned Reflexes, Vol 1. New York: International Publishers, 1928.
32. IP Pavlov. Lectures on Conditioned Reflexes, Vol 2. New York: International Publishers, 1941.
33. EL Thorndike. Experimental study of rewards. New York: Columbia University Press, 1933.
34. RJ Gardner, WT McKinney. Ethologie und die ansendung von tiermodellen (Ethology and the use of animal models). In: F Henn, ed. Psychiatry der Gegenwart, Heidelberg: Springer-Verlag, 1999, pp. 507–524.
35. RJ Gardner. Evolutionary perspectives on stress and affective disorder. Semin Clin Neuropsychiatry 6(1):32–42, 2001.
36. WT McKinney Jr, WE Bunney Jr. Animal model of depression. I. Review of evidence: implications for research. Arch Gen Psychiatry 21(2):240–248, 1969.
37. P Willner. The validity of animal models of depression. Psychopharmacology 83(1):1–16, 1984.
38. P Willner. Animal models of depression: validity and applications. In: GL Gessa et al., eds. Depression and Mania: From Neurobiology to Treatment. Advances in Biochemical Psychopharmacology. New York: Raven Press, 1995, pp 19–41.
39. P Willner. Animal models of depression: validity and application. Adv Biochem Psychopharmacol 49:19–41, 1995.
40. P Willner. Animal models of depression. In: JA den Boer, A Sitsen, eds. Handbook of Depression and Anxiety: a Biological Approach. New York: Marcel Dekker, 1994, pp 291–316.
41. EE Redei, N Ahmadiyeh, A Baum, D Sasso, J Slone, LC Solberg, C Will, A Volenec. Novel animal models of affective disorders. Semin Clini Neuropsychiatry 6(1):43–67, 2001.
42. JFJ Cade. Lithium salts in treatment of psychotic excitement. Med J Aust 2:349–352, 1949.
43. MH Vitaterna, DP King, AM Chang, JM Kornhauser, PL Lowrey, JD McDonald, WF Dove, LH Pinto, FW Turek, JS Takahashi. Mutagenesis and mapping of a mouse gene, Clock, essential for circadian behavior. Science 264(5159):719–725, 1994.
44. L Arborelius, MJ Owens, PM Plotsky, CB Nemeroff. The role of corticotropin-releasing factor in depression and anxiety disorders. J Endocrinol 160(1):1–12, 1999.
45. AS Clarke, GW Kraemer, DJ Kupfer. Effects of rearing condition on HPA axis response to fluoxetine and desipramine treatment over repeated social separations in young rhesus monkeys. Psychiatry Res 79:91–104, 1998.
46. JD Coplan, LA Rosenblum, JM Gorman. Primate models of anxiety: longitudinal perspectives. Psychiatr Clin North Am 18:727–743, 1995.
47. MA Hofer. On the nature and consequences of early loss. Psychosom Med 58:570–581, 1996.
48. HS Akiskal, WT McKinney Jr. Depressive disorders: toward a unified hypothesis. Science 182(107):20–29, 1973.
49. HS Akiskal, WT McKinney Jr. Overview of recent research in depression. Integration of ten conceptual models into a comprehensive clinical frame. Arch Gen Psychiatry 32(3):285–305, 1975.
50. RM Post. Transduction of psychosocial stress into the neurobiology of recurrent affective disorder. Am J Psychiatry 149(8):999–1010, 1992.
51. PC Whybrow, HS Akiskal, WT McKinney. Mood Disorders: Towards a New Psychobiology. New York: Plenum, 1984, p 228.
52. DR Weinberger. Implications of normal brain development for the pathogenesis of schizophrenia. Arch Gen Psychiatry 44:660–669, 1987.
53. GK Bryan, AH Riesen. Deprived somatosensory-motor experience in stumptailed monkey neocortex: dendritic spine density and dendritic branching of layer IIIB pyramidal cells. J Comp Neurol 286(2):208–217, 1989.
54. MK Floeter, WT Greenough. Cerebellar plasticity: modification of Purkinje cell structure by differential rearing in rhesus monkeys. Science 206:227–228, 1979.
55. SD Ginsberg, PR Hof, WT McKinney, JH Morrison. The noradrenergic innervation density of the monkey paraventricular nucleus is not altered by early social deprivation. Neurosci Lett 158(2):130–134, 1993.
56. SD Ginsberg, PR Hof, WT McKinney, JH Morrison. Quantitative analysis of tuberoinfundibular tyrosine hydroxylase- and corticotropin-releasing factor-immunoreactive neurons in monkeys raised with differential rearing conditions. Exp Neurol 120:95–105, 1993.
57. WT Greenough, JE Black, and CS Wallace. Experience and brain development. Child Dev 58:539–559, 1987.
58. LJ Martin, DM Spicer, MH Lewis, JP Gluck, LC Cork. Social deprivation of infant rhesus monkeys alters the chemoarchitecture of the brain: I. Subcortical regions. J Neurosci 11:3344–3358, 1991.
59. RG Struble, AH Riesen. Changes in cortical dendritic branching subsequent to partial social isolation in stumptail monkeys. Dev Psychobiol 11:479–486, 1978.
60. DH Overstreet. Selective breeding for increased cholinergic function: development of a new animal model of depression. Biol Psychiatry 21(1):49–58, 1986.
61. DH Overstreet, O Pucilowski, V Djuric. Genetic/environment interactions in chronic mild stress. Psychopharmacology 134(4):359–360, 1997.
62. DH Overstreet, O Pucilowski, AH Rezvani, DS Janowsky. Administration of antidepressants, diazepam and psychomotor stimulants further confirms the utility of Flinders sensitive line rats as an animal model of depression. Psychopharmacology 121(1):27–37, 1995.

63. K Okamoto, K Aoki. Development of a strain of spontaneously hypertensive rats. Jpn Circ J 27:282–293, 1963.
64. R McCarty, CC Chiueh, IJ Kopin. Spontaneously hypertensive rats: adrenergic hyperresponsivity to anticipation of electric shock. Behav Biol 23:180–188, 1987.
65. S Knardahl, ED Hendley. Association between cardiovascular reactivity to stress and hypertension or behavior. Am J Physiol 259:H248–257, 1990.
66. JE LeDoux, A Sakaguchi, DJ Reis. Behaviorally selective cardiovascular hyperreactivity in spontaneously hypertensive rats. Hypertension 4:853–863, 1982.
67. R Rettig, MA Geyer, MP Printz. Cardiovascular concomitants of tactile and acoustic startle responses in spontaneously hypertensive and normotensive rats. Physiol Behav 36:1123–1128, 1986.
68. DH Overstreet, DS Janowsky, O Pucilowski, AH Rezvani. Swim test immobility co-segregates with serotonergic but not cholinergic sensitivity in cross-breeds of Flinders line rats. Psychiatric Genet 4(2):101–107, 1994.
69. WP Pare. Open field, learned helplessness, conditioned defensive burying, and forced-swim tests in WKY rats. Physiol Behav 55(3):433–439, 1994.
70. PM Nolan, D Kapfhamer, M Bucan. Random mutagenesis screen for dominant behavioral mutations in mice. Methods 13(4):379–395, 1997.
71. Editorial. In defence of animal research. Nature 407(6805):659, 2000.
72. FK Goodwin, AR Morrison. Science and self-doubt. Reason 32(5):22, 2000.
73. J Kaiser. Animal rights. Activists ransack Minnesota labs [news]. Science 284(5413):410–411, 1999.
74. J Kaiser. Animal rights. Booby-trapped letters sent to 87 researchers. Science 286(5442):1059, 1999.
75. S Nadis. Threats to US primate researchers [news]. Nature 402(6757):7–8, 1999.
76. P Aldhous. Protests force primate farm to close. Nature 404(6775):215, 2000.
77. Editorial. Legal challenges to animal experimentation. Nature Neurosci 3(6):523, 2000.
78. D Malakoff. Animal research. Activists win big on rodent, bird rules [news]. Science 289(5478):377, 2000.
79. N Loder. Britain may boost protection of researchers from intimidation [news]. Nature 407(6800):3, 2000.
80. Q Schiermeier. As German activists wage propaganda war [news]. Nature 407(6800):3, 2000.

2

Methodological Advances in Psychiatric Genetics

YOAV KOHN and BERNARD LERER
Hadassah University Hospital and Hebrew University School of Medicine, Jerusalem, Israel

I. RATIONALE FOR GENETIC RESEARCH IN PSYCHIATRY

Genes play a major role in determining and controlling every phenomenon in life. The inherited potential of the new embryo is encoded in the genes transmitted to him by both his parents. The activation or deactivation of certain genes at certain times governs the differentiation of embryonic stem cells into different tissues and systems. This influence goes on after birth and throughought the life span when the production of enzymes and structural proteins is under genetic control. In this way genes control the activity of cells, tissues, and body systems, produce disorders, and determine programmed cell death. Genes also mediate the influence of the environment. Nutrition, toxins, infectious agents, and psychosocial stresses can all affect the organism by activating or deactivating certain genes. Also, genes may affect the environment that a subject is exposed to. For example, it was found that monkeys with an inborn tendency to have low levels of serotonin metabolite in the CSF were more likely to be subject to violent death in a younger age [1].

When we try to better understand the etiology and pathogenesis of complex phenomena such as behavior, personality traits, and psychiatric disorders, it seems almost impossible to disentangle the numerous factors involved in their development. The situation is very different from research on metabolic disorders, where a biochemical imbalance is obvious and allows rapid characterization of the enzymatic defect and its etiology. In the case of schizophrenia numerous changes probably occur, from the hypothesized maldevelopment of the embryonic central nervous system during the first trimester of pregnancy until the onset of disease at the age of 15–20 years. That psychotic symptoms improve after the administration of dopamine D2 receptor antagonists tells us very little about the beginning of the process two decades before, nor can it help us define the contribution of inherited and environmental factors to the development of the illness.

This complexity of mental phenomena makes genetic research crucial to their understanding. Genes have been implicated in the etiology of almost every psychiatric disorder. The etiological role of environmental and psychosocial factors is also well recognized and, as noted above, may be substantially mediated through genes. Unlike environment, which is constantly changing and always difficult to characterize, genes remain unchanged for the most part from conception until death. Although the level of activation of genes does change throughout life, the DNA sequence remains practically constant. Thus we can find in the adult person with schizophrenia the same inherited predisposing genes that started the process of the disorder in fetal life. Identifying these genes would allow us to understand the unfolding of this process and characterize the relative contribution of environmental factors. Ultimately, this would lead to improvement not only of diagnosis and treatment, but also of prevention. The strategy of starting research on the etiology of disorders by first finding the contributing genes, and then revealing the pathogenesis, is opposite in direction from classical research in medicine and therefore is called "reverse genetics." This methodology will be described in the following sections and is summarized in Table 1.

II. DEFINITION OF PHENOTYPES

Before a search for a disease-causing gene begins, one should correctly define the phenotype—who has the disease and who does not. It is widely acknowledged that psychiatric diagnosis is limited to subjective measures. The identification of genes that cause psychiatric disorders should improve our diagnostic capabilities imensely. The circular problem is that in order to find these genes we should make the correct diagnosis. Broadening the diagnosis to include as many individuals as possible with similar symptoms is doomed to hamper our effort to find the gene. It was shown, for example, that the transmission of schizophrenia is independent of the transmission of bipolar disorder [2]. But even categories such as DSM-IV-defined schizophrenia might be too broad. It is concievable that what we define today as one disorder comprised dozens of different diseases with different etiologies and clinical pictures. Narrowing down the diagnosis is an important step in ensuring that a homogeneous sample with the same genetic etiology is studied. This process should be based not only on theoretical hypotheses but on empirical data. Thus, patients can be subdivided according to clusters of specific symptoms (such as negative or positive ones), neuropsychological tests or imaging studies (e.g., enlarged or nonenlarged ventricles). On the other hand, too much narrowing could lead us to false-negative results and to missing a gene that is expressed differently in different individuals. For example, the genetic liability to develop schizophrenia can also lead to a spectrum of related disorders such as schizotypal and schizoid personality disorders [3].

III. ESTABLISHMENT OF GENETIC ETIOLOGY IN PSYCHIATRIC DISORDERS

A. Family Studies

The first step in genetic research on any disease is to establish its heritability. The most obvious way of doing so is by studying the recurrence rate of the disorder in relatives of affected individuals. This rate should not be measured simply against the rate in the general population. Rather, the comparison should come from the study of relatives of healthy controls, who should be diagnosed using the same instruments. Raters should be blind to the proband's diagnosis. Family studies have revealed increased risk in relatives of probands with schizophrenia [2,4], bipolar disorder [2], major depressive disorder [5], obsessive-compulsive disorder [6], autism [7], attention deficit hyperactivity disorder [8], and anorexia nervosa [9], among others. Increased risk for relatives would suggest that the disorder is familial. This is not equivalent to its being genetic since family members share more than genes. Environmental factors such as nutrition, infections, and psychosocial stressors are also common to family members.

Table 1 Methods of Identifying Genes for Medical Disorders

Establishment of Heritability	Localization of Genes
Family studies	Parametric Linkage Analysis
Adoption studies	Nonparametric methods
Twin studies	Association studies: case control and family based
Segregation analysis	Haplotype relative risk (HRR)
	Transmission disequilibrium test (TDT)
	Allele sharing methods (sibpairs and pedigrees)
	Linkage disequilibrium in genetic isolates
	Quantitative trait loci (QTL)

B. Adoption Studies

Adoption studies are designed to try to disentangle inherited from environmental etiological factors. The rate of the studied disorder is compared between biological and adoptive parents of individuals with a certain disorder. Alternatively, the risk of the disorder can be compared between offspring of affected individuals who were given for adoption and offspring of healthy individuals who were also given for adoption. A third and obviously rare paradigm would be the comparison of offspring of healthy parents who were either adopted by affected individuals or by healthy ones. The last variation is the study of offspring of affected parents who were either reared by them or adopted or reared outside their families (as in foster homes). These methods have mainly been used for the study of schizophrenia [3,10], bipolar disorder, and major depressive disorder [11,12], and have shown the major role of genetics in their etiology.

C. Twin Studies

Twin studies are the gold standard of research on the genetic etiology of disease. The recurrence risk or concordance of a disorder is compared between monozygotic (MZ) and dizygotic (DZ) twins. MZ twins share 100% of their genes while DZ twins share on average 50% of their genes, as do any other pair of siblings. Researchers assume that MZ and DZ twins are similar in the degree to which they share environmental influences. While it is probably true that twins are exposed to the same kind of environment more than nontwin siblings, it is obvious that MZ twins experience a more unique and shared environment than DZ twins.

The only way to overcome this limitation is by comparing concordance rates of MZ twins who were reared together or apart. As this is a rare phenomenon, it is quite impractical for genetic research. Nevertheless, twin studies are considered the best estimate of the heritability of the disorder, which is calculated from the difference in concordance between MZ and DZ twins. Thus, autism is considered to be highly heritable with an MZ concordance rate of 92% compared to 10% for DZ twins [13]. Bipolar disorder has also a high heritabilty rate with MZ concordance of 67% against 20% for DZ twins [14]. In schizophrenia the rates are also suggestive of a strong genetic component in etiology: 48% concordance in MZ twins and 4% in DZ twins [15]. Concordance rates also teach us about the importance of environment in the etiology of disorders. The 48% concordance rate for schizophrenia between MZ twins is a striking example. While a strong genetic influence is suggested, it also means that a person with the genetic predisposition to develop the disorder has >50% chance of avoiding it, perhaps by avoiding a noxious environment or by experiencing some as yet unknown, protective factors. The study of discordant sibs or preferably discordant MZ twins can thus teach us on the role of environment. For example, it was shown that MZ twins with Tourette syndrome (TS), a neuropsychiatric disorder characterized by motor and vocal tics, varied in the severity of symptoms. The twins with a more severe clinical course had a lower birth weight [16].

D. Segregation Analysis

After establishing the role of genetic factors in the etiology of a disorder, the next step is to try to define its mode of inheritance. This is done by studying large pedigrees with multiple affected individuals. The observed inheritance is compared with expected inheritance under various genetic models. The goodness of fit is calculated and certain solutions are rejected. Those that are not rejected are considered consistent with the data, which supports this solution as a possible mode of inheritance (although it does not prove it to be the right one). Using this method, most psychiatric disorders show a complex mode of inheritance. None of them is consistent with simple Mendelian inheritance (i.e., autosomal dominant or recessive, X-linked). Even models of oligogenic or polygenic inheritance (few or many genes with small contribution of each of them) must take into account the role of environment to fit the data. Thus, the model consistent with the inheritance of psychiatric disorders is usually termed multifactorial [17]. The impact of this on the choice of methods for genetic analysis is discussed below.

IV. LOCALIZATION OF GENES THAT PREDISPOSE TO PSYCHIATRIC DISORDERS

A. Parametric Methods

Until a decade ago the most widely used method employed to detect genes for inherited disorders was parametric linkage analysis. In this method large pedigrees with multiple affected members are studied. In each pedigree the inheritance of the studied disorder is compared with the inheritance of DNA markers with a known location on the human genome. The marker can be chosen because of an a priori idea regarding the genetic location of the disease gene. This idea might stem from the study of affected individuals with chromosomal aberrations. This was the case in Douchene muscular dystrophy (DMD). The gene for this X-linked disorder was localized after the study of two females who had the disorder were found to have a deletion and a translocation in a certain region on chromosome X [18]. More frequently there is no idea about the putative location of the disease gene. In this case DNA markers spanning the whole genome are used in what is called a genome scan. These markers are usually DNA sequences with no genetic function known to us, but with slight variations from person to person. These variations, or polymorphisms, serve to mark a specific location on the human genome. Depending on the number of markers (usually in the order of hundreds), some gaps are left unchecked. Nevertheless, as nearby genes and markers are usually transmitted together from parent to offspring, we can compare the inheritance of the marker and of the disease in a certain pedigree. If the studied disease is inherited together with a specific marker, we have a clue about the location of the disease gene.

Take for example the hypothetical pedigree in Figure 1. From looking at the pedigree it seems that the inheritance of the disorder is indeed linked to the inheritance of the studied marker. The affected grandfather (#400) has transmitted the disease coupled with allele 1 of the marker to some of his offspring. The possibility that true linkage exists between the two phenomena is compared with the possibility of observing this by chance. The ratio between these two probabilities is calculated. A ratio of 1000 in favor of linkage is traditionally considered significant. For practical reasons the ratio logarithm is used and called the LOD (logarithm of the odds) score. The LOD scores of different pedigrees can be summed together. Tight linkage (LOD score of >3) implies that the disease gene is located close to the studied marker. LOD score of −2 excludes the region as the possible location for the disease gene. When a genome scan is carried out, multiple testing for hundreds of markers is being done and thus a higher level of significance is needed. A LOD score of 3.3 was shown to correlate to a P value of .05 in this situation and is thus considered significant evidence for linkage in a genome scan [19]. LOD scores of 1.9, the magnitude of most positive findings in psychiatry, are considered only suggestive of linkage.

Recombination, the exchange of DNA between a pair of chromosomes during meiosis, can decrease the evidence for linkage by separating the disease gene from the linked allele. Thus, in our hypothetical pedigree the disease gene can be transmitted by individual #400 to one of his offspring with allele 2 instead of allele 1. This might decrease the evidence for linkage in the pedigree. To overcome the problem, the recombination rate is allowed for in the calculation of the LOD score in relation to the estimated distance between the disease gene and the marker. The recombination rate (or fraction) can vary from 0% if they are in exactly the same location to 50% (or 0.5) if they are on different chromosomes.

As stated above, parametric linkage analysis was the main method of genetic analysis employed until recently. It led to the discovery of genes causing disorders with simple Mendelian inheritance such cystic fibrosis [20] and Huntington's disease [21]. In disorders with a more complex inheritance, such as diabetes, hypertension, and psychiatric disorders, it has not proved to be as useful. The main limitation of this method is that in order to correctly calculate the probability of linkage, certain parameters regarding the inheritance of the disease have to be taken into account. First of all, the mode of inheritance has to be specified. As noted before, in psychiatric disorders, mode of inheritance is probably polygenic with a considerable environmental contribution.

For many years the genes for psychiatric disorders were sought under the incorrect assumption of simple Mendelian inheritance, which yielded mainly negative results or some unreplicable positive results. For exam-

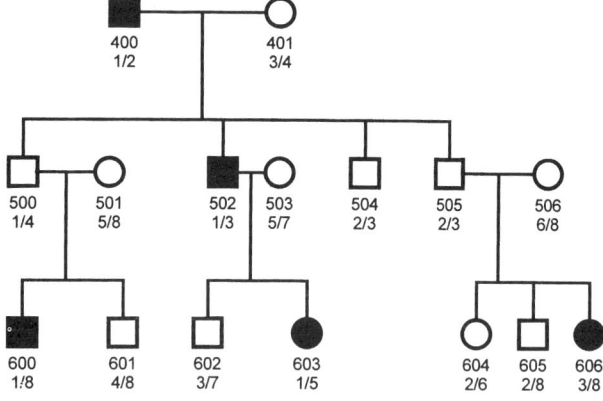

Figure 1 A hypothetical pedigree for linkage analysis. Affected individuals are marked by a dark symbol. Individuals are given identifying numbers from 400 to 606. Genotypes for a certain marker are shown for each individual by the two alleles found in this individual.

ple, researchers who studied Tourette syndrome, were very optimistic at first regarding the chances of finding the gene causing the disorder. It seemed that the inheritance of the disorder was autosomal dominant. It took many years and a great deal of effort with no significant results of parametric linkage analysis to realize that even in TS the inheritance is probably more complex [22,23]. As the exact number of genes that act together to cause psychiatric disorders and the relative role of environment are not known, it is very hard to define the right model for linkage calculations. Unfortunately, the only way to overcome this problem is by finding these genes and isolating their etiological influence from that of environment.

Mode of inheritance is only one of the parameters that linkage analysis is dependent upon. Other parameters are also not known for psychiatric disorders and have to be guessed. Gene frequency, for example, is estimated from disease frequency and the number of implicated genes. The rate of genetic heterogeneity is also estimated. This is the proportion of pedigrees in the studied sample where the disease is caused by different genes. Penetrance has to be taken into account as well. This is the probability that a certain person who carries the disease gene will actually express the disorder. Correct definition of the phenotype is a serious problem that limits the use of parametric linkage in psychiatric genetics, and has been already discussed. But even if we had an accurate diagnostic measure, we would probably still encounter people who carry the gene but for some reason, such as protective factors, do not express the disorder. This might be the case of the person in Figure 1 (#500) who transmitted the disease gene with the linked allele to his affected son from his affected father. Thus, with no correction for penetrance, true linkage can be missed.

Another related parameter that has to be specified in linkage analysis is the rate of phenocopies. These are affected members in the pedigree who acquired their disease because of another, nongenetic factor. This might be the explanation for the occurrence of the disease in individual #606 in the hypothetical pedigree in Figure 1. She has the disease but not the 1 allele. Another possible explanation is that this woman inherited the disease gene or another gene causing the disorder from her mother who is unrelated genetically to the affected grandfather. This phenomenon of disease genes coming from different founders of the pedigree is called bilineality. It is common in pedigrees with psychiatric disorders where assortative mating (between two affected individuals, or between relatives of affected individuals) is common. Bilineality is another parameter that has to be considered to calculate linkage. Usually, researchers attempt to exclude bilineal families from their samples, but absence of bilineality is very difficult to establish with certainty.

Thus, most of the parameters needed for the calculation of linkage are not known for psychiatric disorders and will be known only after the genes for the disorders have been found. When running parametric linkage analyses, many estimates and guesses are made. For each analysis, a specific model composed of the estimated parameters is being used. The many parameters and the numerous different options for each of them make endless numbers of combinations. Examining all of them is impractical and carries the risk of obtaining false-positive results because of multiple testing. Examining only a limited number of models, as is usually done in linkage analysis, is unlikely to include the correct one. This is probably the reason why parametric linkage analysis has been unable as yet to identify a gene for any of the major psychiatric disorders.

Notwithstanding the limitations of parametric linkage analysis in the study of psychiatric disorders, there might be rare instances where its application can be fruitful. Some rare neuropsychiatric disorders such as Rett's disorder, a severe autisticlike X-linked disease, have a more simple Mendelian inheritance. The gene for Rett's disorder was cloned after linkage analysis had been localized to a certain location on chromosome X [24]. The identification of such disease genes, even if rare, could shed light on the pathogenesis of other more common disorders.

B. Nonparametric Methods

Unlike parametric linkage analysis, nonparametric methods are not dependent upon the specification of parameters regarding inheritance. Thus, their use is more suitable for the study of disorders with complex inheritance. Nonparametric methods have been used extensively in the past decade and have shed light on the genetics of disorders such as diabetes, hypertension, Alzheimer's disease, and psychiatric disorders.

1. Association Studies

Case control association studies overcome the problems encountered in genetic analyses of complex disorders by studying a sample of unrelated affected individuals. In this group the frequency of alleles of certain genes is determined and compared to the frequency of the same alleles in a control group of unaffected individuals. Because the affected individuals are not related, increased frequency of a certain allele in them does not usually imply linkage with the disease gene. Rather, it points to a direct role of the studied allele in the etiology of the disorder. Because of that, different alleles or DNA polymorphisms of genes must be studied instead of merely studying DNA markers. This means that the DNA variations that can be used in association studies must occur in the regions of the genome that code for proteins. The variations can occur in an exon, which is the coding region of the gene, meaning that sequence encodes the sequence of amino acids in the product protein. In other cases the polymorphism occurs in a noncoding region of the gene, or intron. As noted above, if a polymorphism occurs in a noncoding region between genes, it is not useful for association studies, as linkage to a nearby gene cannot be studied in a group of unrelated subjects.

Polymorphism can also occur in a regulatory region of the gene, which is a sequence of DNA where certain molecules bind and affect the rate of transcription. A functional DNA polymorphism occurs in a coding region of a gene and affects the function of the product protein. Functional polymorphisms, or those occurring in the regulatory region of the gene, are usually preferred in association studies, as genes with a suspected role in etiology of disorders are investigated in this paradigm.

It was thought until recently that association studies were not suitable for a genome scan because they cannot detect linkage. Now, with the completion of the Human Genome Project, almost the entire DNA sequence of the human genome is known. Thus, theoretically, association can be studied in polymorphism in each and every gene. Practical, technical, and computation limitations make this option not feasible yet.

Many association studies of psychiatric disorders have been performed using candidate genes. These are genes for proteins with a hypothetical function in the pathogenesis of the disorder. In psychiatric genetics these candidate genes are usually genes involved in the production, metabolism, and signal transduction of neurotransmitters. For example, a repeat polymorphism in the gene for the dopamine receptor D4 was found to be associated with ADHD [25] and with the novelty-seeking personality trait [26], and a certain allele of the serotonin transporter gene was associated with anxious personality [27]. These associations were significant but of small magnitude. They explained only a small part of the variance of the studied traits. This means that these genes might have a small contribution to the etiology of the studied phenomena. Combinations of alleles for two different genes were studied and shown to be associated with tardive dyskinesia, for example [28]. Looking at larger numbers of genes simultaneously would yield a greater number of combinations that might be too numerous to study without enormous samples.

The relatively small role of each gene found to be associated with disorders is only one limitation of this study design. As the Human Genome Project has revealed, there are ~30,000 genes (many fewer than once thought, but still an enormous number). A third of these genes are estimated to be expressed in the brain. Most of them are still not known. Moreover, our understanding of the pathogenesis of psychiatric disorders is limited to current processes in the brain of the affected individual. These may be very different from the genetic vulnerability that started the disease many years before. A genomewide association scan might overcome these obstacles but, as stated above, is not feasible yet.

Notwithstanding the above-mentioned difficulties of association studies, their main limitation is the need to find a perfectly matched control group. Controls should resemble affected individuals in every measure that might be related to the studied genes, apart from disease status. The most problematic confounding factor in this regard is ethnicity. Variations of allelic distribution are highly dependent on ethnicity. Significant variations of allelic distribution are found even among ethnic subgroups of a relatively homogeneous population such as Jews [29]. The choice of an ethnically unmatched control group might be the reason for the failure to replicate some of the positive associations reported between psychiatric disorders and certain alleles. Indeed, some of these nonreplications were in studies in which the patient and control group came from a homogeneous population [30]. It is hard to say whether the positive results or the nonreplications were spurious. To overcome this problem researchers are turning more and more to methods that employ unaffected family members as controls. Two widely used family based methods are haplotype relative risk (HRR) and the transmission disequilibrium test (TDT).

2. Haplotype Relative Risk (HRR)

In HRR allele frequencies are studied in a group of affected individuals. The comparison group is made up of hypothetical sibs of these individuals. These made up sibs are presumably healthy and have inher-

Methodological Advances in Psychiatric Genetics

ited from their parents the alleles that were not transmitted to the affected sib (Fig. 2). To be able to make up the control group, both parents of the affected individual must be studied for the same alleles. Thus, HRR requires the ascertainment of "trios" of affected individual and both parents, alive and willing to participate in the study. This makes the research design more complicated. On the other hand, the hypothetical control group in this design is perfectly matched for ethnicity to the patient group.

3. Transmission Disequilibrium Test (TDT)

In TDT, as in HRR, trios are needed for the analysis. In this research design, affected individuals with a parent heterozygous for the allele of interest are studied. In each such case it is determined whether the studied allele was transmitted to the affected offspring or not (Fig. 2). A transmission rate that is significantly higher than the random rate of 50% is considered as evidence for a role of the allele in the etiology of the disorder. The inheritance of multiple genes or haplotypes can be investigated as TDT is studied in families.

Although addressing the issue of ethnicity, both HRR and TDT are limited, as association studies in populations, to the study of candidate genes. Nevertheless, both methods are useful for the attempts to further establish findings from population-based association studies. For example, HRR was used to both replicate and (in other populations) not replicate the association of DRD4 with ADHD [31,32].

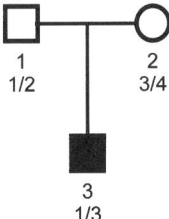

Figure 2 Family based association studies using two different methods. The first method is haplotype relative risk (HRR). Two parents and one offspring (a trio) are studied. The nontransmitted alleles (2 and 4 in this pedigree) comprise the control group of hypothetical healthy sibs made up from many trios. Allele frequencies are compared between groups. The second method is transmission disequilibrium test (TDT). Trios are studied in which one of the parents is heterozygous for a certain allele of the studied marker (1, for example). Transmission of the allele is counted for each trio. The rate of transmission is compared with random rate of transmission, which is 50%.

C. Allele Sharing Methods

1. General Principles

In allele sharing methods of genetic analysis, the degree of sharing of alleles of certain genes or markers is examined in related individuals with the investigated disorder. This can be done either in affected sibs, which is called sibpair analysis, or in affected individuals with a more distant relationship (grandfather and grandson, cousins, etc.). Sharing of alleles can be incidental or can be secondary to inheritance of the same allele from a common ancestor (parent, grandparent, etc.). When the reason for the sharing is not known, it is called "identity by state." When it can be shown that both individuals inherited the same allele from a common source, we use the term "identity by descent." Identity by descent allele sharing is a more powerful tool in genetic analysis. If related individuals with the disorder share the same alleles, identical by descent, more often than expected by chance, an association between the allele and the disease is implied. Alternatively, as the individuals are related, increased sharing can stem from linkage of the marker to the disease gene. Thus a genome scan can be performed with these methods, as well as the study of candidate genes.

When allele sharing is studied, no assumption has to be made about mode of inheritance, genetic heterogeneity, gene frequency, penetrance, rate of phenocopies, and so on. This nonparametric method is model free. This is its great advantage over parametric linkage analysis. On the other hand, parametric linkage under the correct model is much more powerful in the detection of linkage. In order to compare their power to that of parametric linkage, allele sharing methods need to use very large samples of the order of hundreds of sibpairs or dozens of multiplex pedigrees. These are hard to ascertain in one population. Researchers usually combine samples from different populations, which increases the risk of genetic heterogeneity and decreases the chance of finding significant linkage. For this reason allele sharing methods are used in combination with parametric linkage analysis, which means that in the same pedigrees both parametric and nonparametric methods are used. For example, the addition of sibpair analysis to parametric linkage analysis was helpful in supporting suggestive linkage to a locus on chromosome 22q in schizophrenia [33]. Significant linkage between two forms of dyslexia and markers on chromosome 6p and 15p were found using parametric linkage for one form and allele sharing methods for the other [34].

2. Sibpair Analysis

Take for example the sibpair in Figure 3. Affected sibs can either inherit the same two alleles from their parents, one shared allele and one nonshared allele, or two different alleles. If there is no relation between affection status and the studied allele, we expect the probabilities for each of the three cases to be 0.25, 0.5, 0.25, respectively.

The actual allele sharing is studied in many sibpairs, and the observed frequency of sharing of one, two, or zero alleles is compared with the theoretical random frequencies. Any deviance from random distribution is considered evidence for increased allele sharing.

3. Allele Sharing in Pedigrees

In this paradigm allele sharing is compared between affected pedigree members with any degree of relationship apart from parent and offspring (as the allele sharing will always be 0.50 in this case). Observed sharing is compared with expected sharing under no association or linkage. As for parametric linkage analysis, large pedigrees with many affected members are ascertained. But unlike traditional linkage analysis, only allele sharing between affected individuals is studied. Take Figure 1 for example. In allele sharing analysis, only the affected individuals (#400, #502, #600, #603, and #606) will be studied, and allele sharing will be examined in every possible combination of two out of these individuals (apart from parent and child). The other unaffected pedigree members do not contribute to the calculation, apart from verifying that identity between individuals is indeed by descent and not by chance. Thus it is clear that this paradigm is model free, as it is not dependent on the parameters required by parametric linkage. The most widely used software that employs this paradigm is called Genehunter [35], which can also calculate parametric linkage in the same pedigree.

D. Linkage Disequilibrium in Isolated Populations

One of the main limitations of both parametric and nonparametric methods of genetic analysis is the problem of genetic heterogeneity. Researchers use large samples to increase power, and thus run the risk of mixing subpopulations with different genetic etiologies. Studying small populations that are genetically isolated can overcome this obstacle. In such a population, affected individuals are more likely to represent a homogeneous sample, in terms of etiology. It is plausible that most of the affected individuals in a genetic isolate, who have a certain disorder, carry the same disease-causing mutation, which they inherited from a common ancestor. If the mutation process is relatively new, or more possibly if the genetic isolate is relatively young (and the mutation was introduced to it relatively late), we expect that affected individuals share more than the mutation itself. Large regions of DNA on both sides of the mutation should be identical in these individuals, as the short time that elapsed since the isolate was founded did not allow recombination to change them considerably. Thus, these individuals share not merely alleles but large haplotypes identically by descent. The aggregation of certain alleles into haplotypes that are more frequent than what is expected by chance is called "linkage disequilibrium," and is evidence for the presence of a shared mutation in this region.

The main advantage of this paradigm is that only a few affected individuals (as few three or four) need to be examined. These people do not have to be related (apart from being part of the same isolate), and their relatives are not needed for the study. The disadvantages are that these genetic isolates are not easy to find, and are even more difficult to study. Also, genes responsible for psychiatric disorders in these unique populations might be very well specific to them only. Nevertheless, finding one gene for one psychiatric disorder in one population has not yet been achieved by any other method. Linkage disequilibrium in genetic isolates has been used to locate genes for rare medical disorders with simple Mendelian inheritance [36], and

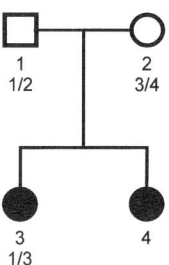

Figure 3 Sibpair analysis: two affected sibs and their parents are studied. In this example one daughter received alleles 1 and 3 from her parents. Her sister can either receive the same two alleles, only one of them (1/4 or 2/3), or the two that were not transmitted to her sister (2/4). The probabilties for each case are equal, and thus for sharing the same two alleles are 0.25, only one allele 0.5, and no sharing 0.25. Actual sharing in many sibpairs is compared to these random probabilities. Significant deviance implies association or linkage.

also for a common disorder with a more complex inheritance such as Hirschprung's disease [37]. Lately, it is being applied to the study of psychiatric disorders as well.

E. Quantitative Trait Loci (QTL)

As implied by its name, QTL is suited for the study of quantitative traits, such as height and weight. It allows the study of many genes, each with a small contribution, to the expression of one continuous variable. QTL is easily applied in laboratory animals, where pure strains can be inbred and the change in the studied trait can be measured under different genetic conditions. Obviously this cannot be done with human beings. Rather, sibs or unrelated subjects with extremely different values of the studied trait are studied and their genotypes compared. It is also debatable whether most psychiatric disorders can be perceived as quantitative traits. Medical psychiatry assumes in most cases a more categorical approach to psychiatric disorders. On the other hand QTL might prove beneficial to the study of personality traits and intelligence [38].

V. ADVANCES IN THE LABORATORY

The significant expansion of DNA marker maps enables the performance of better genome scans. More and more polymorphisms of the human DNA are known. These include single nucleotide polymorphisms (SNP) and certain sequences (from two or three to several dozen nucletodies) that vary in the number in which they are repeated in different individuals. This improved map increases the chances of finding association or linkage with a studied disorder. Data are shared through the Internet and are freely available to any researcher. Technology is improving from day to day. Methods that identify different DNA sequences are much easier to perform and are less time-consuming.

The recent completion of the Human Genome Project opens new and endless horizons for the study of psychiatric genetics. One aspect is the further improvement of marker maps. Moreover, in a short while we should be able (with sufficient computation power) to study association of disorders with each and every of the human genes. Thus we will be able to desert the study of candidate genes that were chosen merely because of our limited knowledge. In this way association studies (both case control and family-based paradigms) will be used for the purpose of hunting genes in genome scans.

When the location of a gene for a psychiatric disorder is eventually found, the new map of the human genome will enable its rapid identification and cloning. The mutations that cause the disorders will be characterized shortly thereafter, and shorten the way to the study of pathogenesis and the application to diagnosis, prevention, and treatment.

VI. SUMMARY AND FUTURE DIRECTIONS

Finding a significant linkage between a psychiatric disorder and a DNA marker, which is replicated consistently, is an objective that has not yet been accomplished. The further objectives of mapping actual disease genes, cloning them, and determining their protein structure and function, are more distant.

The inherent obstacles have been described in this chapter, as well as newer methods of genetic analysis that aim to overcome them. Advances in molecular technology constantly improve our technical tools. Eventually one gene for one psychiatric disorder in (at least) one population will be found. And then? The journey just begins.

The gene for Huntington's disease (HD) was discovered a decade ago [21]. No dramatic change has occurred in the treatment and prognosis of HD patients since then, even though diagnosis is now possible before the onset of the disorder. This has raised painful ethical questions. Is it justified to test young healthy individuals for a dreadful, incurable disease? When we finally find genes for schizophrenia won't we be in the same position? We will have to deal with difficult ethical questions regarding prenatal diagnosis of susceptibility to a disorder with a variable clinical course that has its onset 15–20 years later.

We will also be at the very beginning of the long road which will need to be traversed in order to understand how genes start the process that eventually culminates in psychiatric disorder. Apart from the complexities inherent to the field of psychiatric genetics, there are additional ones. These are related to the fact that interposed between the gene and the protein for which it codes are variations in transcription, translation, and posttranslational modifications that prevent us from being able to assume a simple relationship between gene and disease. Also, epigenetic factors modify expression of genes in ways that can be time specific and tissue specific. Thus, even when a gene for a psychiatric disease is eventually found, a long route will have to be traversed before we undertand how it affects the disease process.

REFERENCES

1. JD Higley, PT Mehlman, SB Higley, B Fernald, J Vickers, SG Lindell, DM Taub, SJ Suomi, M Linnoila. Excessive mortality in young free-ranging male nonhuman primates with low cerebrospinal fluid 5-hydroxyindoleacetic acid concentrations. Arch Gen Psychiatry 53(6):537–543, 1996.
2. W Maier, D Lichtermann, J Minges, J Hallmayer, R Heun, O Benkert, DF Levinson. Continuity and discontinuity of affective disorders and schizophrenia. Results of a controlled family study. Arch Gen Psychiatry 50(11):871–883, 1993.
3. PA Lowing, AF Mirsky, R Pereira. The inheritance of schizophrenia spectrum disorders: a reanalysis of the Danish adoptee study data. Am J Psychiatry 140(9):1167–1171, 1983.
4. KS Kendler, M McGuire, AM Gruenberg, A O'Hare, M Spellman, D Walsh. The Roscommon family study. I. Methods, diagnosis of probands, and risk of schizophrenia in relatives. Arch Gen Psychiatry 50(7):527–540, 1993.
5. W Maier, J Hallmayer, D Lichtermann, M Philipp, T Klingler. The impact of the endogenous subtype on the familial aggregation of unipolar depression. Eur Arch Psychiatry Clin Neurosci 240(6):355–362, 1991.
6. DL Pauls, JP Alsobrook 2nd, W Goodman, S Rasmussen, JF Leckman. A family study of obsessive-compulsive disorder. Am J Psychiatry 152(1):76–84, 1995.
7. P Bolton, H Macdonald, A Pickles, P Rios, S Goode, M Crowson, A Bailey, M Rutter. A case-control family history study of autism. J Child Psychol Psychiatry 35(5):877–900, 1994.
8. J Biederman, SV Faraone, K Keenan, D Knee, MT Tsuang. Family-genetic and psychosocial risk factors in DSM-III attention deficit disorder. J Am Acad Child Adolescent Psychiatry 29(4):526–533, 1990.
9. M Strober, W Morrell, J Burroughs, B Salkin, C Jacobs. A controlled family study of anorexia nervosa. J Psychiatr Res 19(2–3):239–246, 1985.
10. KS Kendler, AM Gruenberg, DK Kinney. Independent diagnoses of adoptees and relatives as defined by DSM-III in the provincial and national samples of the Danish adoption study of schizophrenia. Arch of Gen Psychiatry 51(6):456–468, 1994.
11. J Mendlewicz, JD Rainer. Adoption study supporting genetic transmission in manic-depressive illness. Nature 268(5618):327–329, 1977.
12. PH Wender, SS Kety, D Rosenthal, F Schulsinger, J Ortmann, I Lunde. Psychiatric disorders in the biological and adoptive families of adopted individuals with affective disorders. Arch Gen Psychiatry 43(10):923–929, 1986.
13. A Bailey, A Le Couteur, I Gottesman, P Bolton, E Simonoff, E Yuzda, M Rutter. Autism as a strongly genetic disorder: evidence from a British twin study. Psychol Medi 25(1):63–77, 1995.
14. A Bertelsen, B Harvald, M Hauge. A Danish twin study of manic-depressive disorders. Br J Psychiatry 130:330–351, 1977.
15. S Onstad, I Skre, S Torgersen, E Kringlen. Twin concordance for DSM-III-R schizophrenia. Acta Psychiatr Scand 83(5):395–401, 1991.
16. JF Leckman, RA Price, JT Walkup, S Ort, DL Pauls, DJ Cohen. Nongenetic factors in Gilles de la Tourette's syndrome. Arch Gen Psychiatry 44(1):100, 1987.
17. GP Vogler, II Gottesman, MK McGue, DC Rao. Mixed-model segregation analysis of schizophrenia in the Lindelius Swedish pedigrees. Behav Genet 20(4):461–472, 1990.
18. AH Burghes, C Logan, X Hu, B Belfall, RG Worton, PN Ray. A cDNA clone from the Duchenne/Becker muscular dystrophy gene. Nature 328(6129):434–437, 1987.
19. E Lander, L Kruglyak. Genetic dissection of complex traits: guidelines for interpreting and reporting linkage results. Nat Genet 11(3):241–247, 1995.
20. JM Rommens, MC Iannuzzi, B Kerem, ML Drumm, G Melmer, M Dean, R Rozmahel, JL Cole, D Kennedy, N Hidaka. Identification of the cystic fibrosis gene: chromosome walking and jumping. Science 245(4922):1059–1065, 1989.
21. Huntington's Disease Collaborative Research Group. A novel gene containing a trinucleotide repeat that is expanded and unstable on Huntington's disease chromosomes. Cell 72(6):971–983, 1993.
22. CL Barr, KG Wigg, AJ Pakstis, R Kurlan, D Pauls, KK Kidd, LC Tsui, P Sandor. Genome scan for linkage to Gilles de la Tourette syndrome. Am J Med Genet 88(4):437–445, 1999.
23. JT Walkup, MC LaBuda, HS Singer, J Brown, MA Riddle, O Hurko. Family study and segregation analysis of Tourette syndrome: evidence for a mixed model of inheritance. Am J Hum Genet 59(3):684–693, 1996.
24. RE Amir RE, IB Van den Veyver, M Wan, CQ Tran, U Francke, HY Zoghbi. Rett syndrome is caused by mutations in X-linked MECP2, encoding methyl-CpG-binding protein 2. Nat Genet 23(2):185–188, 1999.
25. GJ LaHoste, JM Swanson, SB Wigal, C Glabe, T Wigal, N King, JL Kennedy. Dopamine D4 receptor gene polymorphism is associated with attention deficit hyperactivity disorder. Mol Psychiatry 1(2):121–124, 1996.
26. J Benjamin, L Li, C Patterson, BD Greenberg, DL Murphy, DH Hamer. Population and familial association between the D4 dopamine receptor gene and measures of novelty seeking. Nat Genet 12(1):81–84, 1996.

27. KP Lesch, D Bengel, A Heils, SZ Sabol, BD Greenberg, S Petri, J Benjamin, CR Muller, DH Hamer, DL Murphy. Association of anxiety-related traits with a polymorphism in the serotonin transporter gene regulatory region. Science 274(5292):1527–1531, 1996.
28. RH Segman, U Heresco-Levy, B Finkel, R Inbar, T Neeman, M Schlafman, A Dorevitch, A Yakir, A Lerner, T Goltser, A Shelevoy, B Lerer. Association between the serotonin 2C receptor gene and tardive dyskinesia in chronic schizophrenia: additive contribution of 5-HT2Cser and DRD3gly alleles to susceptibility. Psychopharmacology (Berl) 152(4):408–413, 2000.
29. Y Kohn, RP Ebstein, U Heresco-Levy, B Shapira, L Nemanov, I Gritsenko, M Avnon, B Lerer. Dopamine D4 receptor gene polymorphisms: relation to ethnicity, no association with schizophrenia and response to clozapine in Israeli subjects. Eur Neuropsychopharmacol 7(1):39–43, 1997.
30. Z Hawi, M McCarron, A Kirley, G Daly, M Fitzgerald, M Gill. No association of the dopamine DRD4 receptor (DRD4) gene polymorphism with attention deficit hyperactivity disorder (ADHD) in the Irish population. Am J Med Genet 96(3):268–272, 2000.
31. M Swanson, GA Sunohara, JL Kennedy, R Regino, E Fineberg, T Wigal, M Lerner, L Williams, GJ La Hoste, S Wigal. Association of the dopamine receptor D4 (DRD4) gene with a refined phenotype of attention deficit hyperactivity disorder (ADHD): a family-based approach. Mol Psychiatry 3(1):38–41, 1998.
32. J Eisenberg, A Zohar, G Mei-Tal, A Steinberg, E Tartakovsky, I Gritsenko, L Nemanov, RP Ebstein. A haplotype relative risk study of the dopamine D4 receptor (DRD4) exon III repeat polymorphism and attention deficit hyperactivity disorder (ADHD). Am J Med Genet 96(3):258–261, 2000.
33. M Gill, H Vallada, D Collier, P Sham, P Holmans, R Murray, P McGuffin, S Nanko, M Owen, S Antonarakis, D Housman, H Kazazian, G Nestadt, AE Pulver, RE Straub, CJ MacLean, D Walsh, KS Kendler, L DeLisi, M Polymeropoulos, H Coon, W Byerley, R Lofthouse, E Gershon, CM Read. A combined analysis of D22S278 marker alleles in affected sib-pairs: support for a susceptibility locus for schizophrenia at chromosome 22q12. Schizophrenia Collaborative Linkage Group (Chromosome 22). Am J Med Genet 67(1):40–45, 1996.
34. EL Grigorenko, FB Wood, MS Meyer, LA Hart, WC Speed, A Shuster, DL Pauls. Susceptibility loci for distinct components of developmental dyslexia on chromosomes 6 and 15. Am J of Hum Genet 60(1):27–39, 1997.
35. L Kruglyak, MJ Daly, MP Reeve-Daly, ES Lander. Parametric and nonparametric linkage analysis: a unified multipoint approach. Am J Hum Genet 58(6):1347–1363, 1996.
36. RHJ Houwen, S Baharloo, K Blankenship, P Raeymaekers, J Juyn, LA Sandkuijl, NB Freimer. Genome screening by searching for shared segments: mapping a gene for benign recurrent intrahepatic cholestasis. Nat Genet 8:380–386, 1994.
37. EG Puffenberger, ER Kauffman, S Bolk, TC Matice, SS Washington, M Angrist, J Weissenbach, KL Garver, M Mascari, R Ladda, SA Slaugenhaupt, A Chakravarti. Identity-by-descent and association mapping of a recessive gene for Hirschprung disease on human chromosome 13q22. Hum Mole Genet 3(8):1217–1225, 1994.
38. PJ Fisher, D Turic, NM Williams, P McGuffin, P Asherson, D Ball, I Craig, T Eley, L Hill, K Chorney, MJ Chorney, CP Benbow, D Lubinski, R Plomin, MJ Owen. DNA pooling identifies QTLs on chromosome 4 for general cognitive ability in children. Hum Mol Genet 8(5):915–922, 1999.

3

New Developments in the Regulation of Monoaminergic Neurotransmission*

ALAN FRAZER
University of Texas Health Science Center at San Antonio, and South Texas Veterans Health Care System, San Antonio, Texas, U.S.A.

DAVID A. MORILAK and LYNETTE C. DAWS
University of Texas Health Science Center at San Antonio, San Antonio, Texas, U.S.A.

I. INTRODUCTION

The process of synaptic transmission is the key target for all psychoactive drugs. Transmission may be influenced by drugs affecting the synthesis, storage, release, inactivation, and postsynaptic effects of transmitter substances. Further, drugs effective in major psychiatric illnesses such as depression and schizophrenia have prominent effects on transmission mediated by biogenic amines such as dopamine (DA), norepinephrine (NE), and 5-hydroxytryptamine (5HT; serotonin). The past decade has seen marked advances in our understanding of key features of the transmission process mediated by these amines. Of particular importance is the emerging concept that transmission mediated by these substances appears, at least in part, to occur through diffusion-mediated signaling, termed extrasynaptic or volume transmission (VT). Also, it is now recognized that the inactivation process of reuptake, mediated by specific transporters located in the plasma membrane, plays the key role in regulating the concentration of these amines in the extracellular fluid (ECF). Furthermore, these protein transporters are not merely constitutive membrane components but undergo a variety of regulatory processes. Finally, in the past decade it has become more accepted, even if still not completely understood, that effects of released amines can be influenced by other peptide transmitters colocalized in the same neurons. Our emerging concepts of the functioning of transporters and the processes of cotransmission and VT have not been well integrated into current views of psychoactive drug action. Yet it is likely that they influence profoundly the effects produced by such drugs. Because of this, it is appropriate to view such processes from the perspective of their potential neuropsychopharmacologic impact.

II. HARD-WIRED VS. PARACRINE OR VOLUME TRANSMISSION

The most widely accepted model for synaptic transmission, including that which occurs in brain, was devel-

---

*Some of the material in this chapter was presented in a review article by Frazer A, Gerhardt GA, and Daws LC: New views of biogenic amine transporter function: implications for neuropsychopharmacology. Int J Neuropsychopharmacol 2:305–320, 1999.

oped from studies involving cholinergic transmission through nicotinic receptors, particularly at the neuromuscular junction. This model was derived in part from the morphological characteristics of such synapses, involving a presynaptic knob with specialized features, a cleft of ~ 40–60 nm, and the postsynaptic membrane containing both receptors and invaginations. Such specialized features within the synapse pose barriers to transmitter diffusion and help to ensure that the transmitter acts only within the strict confines of such conventional synapses. Further contributing to acetylcholine (ACh) having only synaptic effects is the presence of its degradative enzyme acetylcholinesterase within the synapse. This type of transmitter process has been termed "hard-wired."

However, in the mid-1970s, anatomic studies on brain tissue generated data that were interpreted as favoring a different model of synaptic transmission. This model has been referred to as extrasynaptic communication or paracrine transmission (which, historically, relates to a hormone affecting the function of cells at a distance from its site of release) or volume transmission (VT). The essence of such transmission is the passage of chemical messages along multiple, largely unpredictable channels such that transmitters may pervade the extracellular space to act at distant receptors outside the strict confines of conventional synapses. Although there are attractive features of this concept, it has been elusive and difficult to prove. It is outside the scope of this chapter to review this subject in detail. The interested reader is referred to comprehensive reviews of this topic in a recent volume [1]. Since the mid-1970s, anatomic, physiologic, and pharmacologic data have been generated that are consistent with VT, although not proving it. If such transmission does occur in the brain, it could have profound neuropsychopharmacologic implications.

The original observation that there may be nontraditional types of transmission in brain was that of Descarries et al. [2]. These investigators, using ^{3}H-5HT autoradiography in the neocortex of rats, claimed that serotonergic terminals were rarely engaged in morphologically differentiated synapses and speculated about "nonsynaptic" release of 5HT in this brain area. Subsequently, Beaudet and Descarries [3] suggested that 5HT acted on a large number of cortical cells rather than just a restricted number of postsynaptic targets. Their notion was of a predominantly nonjunctional serotonergic innervation of the cortex having paracrine-like properties. Although this work has been criticized [4] and others have found much higher percentages of typical synaptic specializations for 5HT [5,6], there does seem to be a body of data showing a reasonable percentage of nonsynaptic varicosities for biogenic amines in brain [7–9]. The presence of nontraditional synapses may be specific to certain brain regions [10], indicating that these biogenic amines may function both at conventional synapses and nontraditional ones. Further, in different brain regions the extent to which VT is involved in, for example, dopaminergic transmission may vary [11].

Consistent with the view of diffusion of transmitter to act at distant, nonsynaptic receptors is the realization that channels between cells are of sufficient width to allow the passage by diffusion of neuroactive compounds [12]. Although fraught with a variety of assumptions, it has been estimated that DA can diffuse at least 10 μm and 5HT 20 μm from its release site in brain tissue within one half-life [13,14], distances that would permit action at extrasynaptic receptors. Also, in a series of elegant investigations, Wightman and his colleagues [13–15] showed the concentration of either DA or 5HT in ECF to be directly proportional to the number of electrical pulses in an electrical train, a result not consistent with the buffered diffusion that occurs with hard-wired transmission. Further, peak extracellular concentration of either transmitter after a single stimulus was not altered by uptake inhibitors, suggesting that the uptake process is not altering the efflux of these transmitters into the extrasynaptic space. As is discussed in the section on transporters, one explanation for such data is that the uptake sites are extrasynaptic.

If DA or 5HT can "escape" from the synapse and diffuse in ECF some distance from the synapse, is there any evidence that they will encounter appropriate receptors outside the synapse? There appears to be. Although certainly not conclusive, much has been made of, and considerable controversy has been generated by, the many observations showing a "mismatch" in brain between areas receiving very little innervation by a specific type of neuron yet having a high density of receptors for the particular transmitter [16]. For example, in rat cerebral cortex, only the $5HT_2$ receptor has a distribution that appears to match the regional and laminar density of serotonergic innervation [17]. More convincing, though, are studies carried out with electron microscopy which reveal receptor immunoreactivity outside of synapses. This has been found for both D_1 and D_2 dopamine receptors [18,19], $5HT_{1A}$ [20] and $5HT_{2A}$ [21] receptors.

The foregoing lends credence to the view that DA, 5HT, and perhaps NE can spill out from synapses to diffuse to distal sites in concentrations that may be sufficient to activate extrasynaptic receptors [13,14]. This issue and its neuropsychopharmacologic implications are highlighted in the sections dealing with the localization of transporters and their regulation.

III. BIOGENIC AMINE REUPTAKE AND TRANSPORTERS

It has been 40 years since the initial observation that tritiated NE could be taken up from blood into organs containing sympathetic nerves [22], due to an active transport process contained in these nerves. Further research revealed that the primary means of terminating synaptic activity of NE, DA, or 5HT was by these active transport processes. Key neuropsychopharmacological discoveries were that many antidepressants inhibited the uptake of NE and 5HT [23,24], whereas psychostimulants, such as cocaine and methylenedioxymethamphetamine (MDMA; "Ectasy"), blocked the uptake of DA as well as that of 5HT, and, for some of the drugs in this class, uptake of NE was also inhibited [25–27]. The inhibition of uptake was thought to be responsible for the efficacy of antidepressants, whereas the inhibition of DA uptake was linked to the euphoric and reinforcing properties of psychostimulants.

Although the uptake processes for these three amines had similar characteristics, the uptake of each amine is mediated by a specific protein termed a transporter. Furthermore, the transporter proteins were presumed to have a synaptic localization to account for the enhancement of synaptic transmission thought to occur when pharmacological agents inhibited the uptake process. In other words, reuptake (and diffusion) altered the magnitude, duration, and spatial domain of transmitter-induced receptor activation and, in so doing, modified neurotransmission. More recent work [28] has substantiated the idea that these transporters are the *key* cellular elements regulating the concentrations of biogenic amines in ECF. The cloning of biogenic amine transporters in the early 1990s [29–32] and the development of selective radioligands for them at about the same time permitted a range of studies not possible previously. These studies have begun to provide important information about transporter function and regulation that in some cases expands and amplifies our previously held concepts, but in other ways, fundamentally changes them.

A. Structure of Monoamine Transporters

The dopamine transporter (DAT), norepinephrine transporter (NET), and 5-hydroxytryptamine transporter (5HTT) are part of a family of neuronal plasma membrane transporters that include the monoamines and certain amino acids such as gamma-aminobutyric acid (GABA), glycine, and proline [33]. These three transporters share considerable structural homology. They are all Na^+ and Cl^- dependent, have 12 membrane-spanning domains, N- and C-termini located intracellularly and a large extracellular loop with glycosylation sites which may alter trafficking and/or function of the transporters. The extracellular and intracellular portions of the proteins have phosphorylation sites that likely contribute to the functional properties of the transporters. The DAT, NET and 5HTT are each believed to represent a single gene product [33]. Since they represent single gene products, this means that posttranslational or other intracellular regulatory mechanisms must play a role in regulation of the function of these transporters. Data, reviewed below, are starting to appear that support the theory that phosphorylation of transporters through a variety of protein kinases and phosphatases causes changes in their function and plays a role in the trafficking and incorporation of transporters into the plasma membrane.

B. Models of Transporter Function

Current ideas about the function of monoamine transporters have led to proposals that transporters may operate in at least two modes: (1) as an alternating access carrier [34], or (2) in a channel mode [35]. In the more standard alternating access carrier mode (Fig. 1) [36], the protein is first in a conformation such that the cotransported ions, Na^+ and Cl^-, and the substrate (e.g., DA, NE, or 5HT) bind to a cleft in the transporter that is open to the extracellular space. The transporter then converts to a form that is accessible to the intracellular space, allowing the cotransported ions and the substrate access to the cytoplasm. This internal-facing form releases the transported substances into the cytoplasm and then interconverts so as to expose the now empty binding sites to the extracellular environment. This is the transport cycle. In the case of the 5HTT [34], K^+ ion binds to the transporter protein when it is open to the cytoplasm and may facilitate the interconversion of the protein to the form that exposes binding sites to the extracellular space to reinitiate the transport process. According to this model, the rate of influx of extracellular solute determines the rate of efflux of intracellular solute; i.e., influx and efflux rates are modulated equivalently. Data have been obtained recently with the 5HTT and the DAT showing independent modulation of inward and outward transport [38–40]. Thus, some features of transport seem inconsistent with the classical alternating access carrier model.

By contrast, in the channel mode, which is thought to be a low probability event, the transporter protein functions as an ion channel (Fig. 1). Evidence in support of the channel mode of conductance is that the 5HTT and NET have transmitter-activated currents that are not linked stoichiometrically to substrate movement [35, 36, 41–45]. For example, if charge movement were merely linked to coupled transport for the NET, then one would predict one charge/NE molecule. What has been found for the human NET expressed in cultured cells is 200 charges/NE molecule. Such data have been interpreted to mean that these charges are carried by the positively charged NE molecules and cotransported ions [41]. Moreover, when the transporter is in the channel mode, a single transport event carries many more NE molecules than would be predicted by the classic alternating access model [46]. One way this could occur would be if the transporter acted as a channel permitting bulk flow of substrate through the open pore. This behavior of the transporter may be explained by the existence of two gates, one directed intracellularly and one extracellularly. In the case of the alternating access model, the two gates open sequentially during the transport cycle to allow the exchange of ions and substrate between ECF and cytosol by alternating access to the cleft of the transporter [36]. On occasion, the "gates" on both the extracellular and cytoplasmic sides of the transporter open simultaneously, permitting bulk flow of substrate and associated ions through an "ion" channel. It seems possible that transporters are really combined carriers and channels.

One implication of transporters acting as ion channels is that it should be possible to develop drugs that change the probability of the transporter acting in the channel mode, akin to the effect of benzodiazepines at the $GABA_A$ receptor. Such drugs should markedly influence the effect of synaptically released transmitter. If, for example, some psychotic states are linked to excessive dopaminergic transmission, drugs that change the probability of the DAT acting in the channel mode might be effective in these states. Another interesting aspect of the realization of transport-associated currents is that it permits analysis of the effects

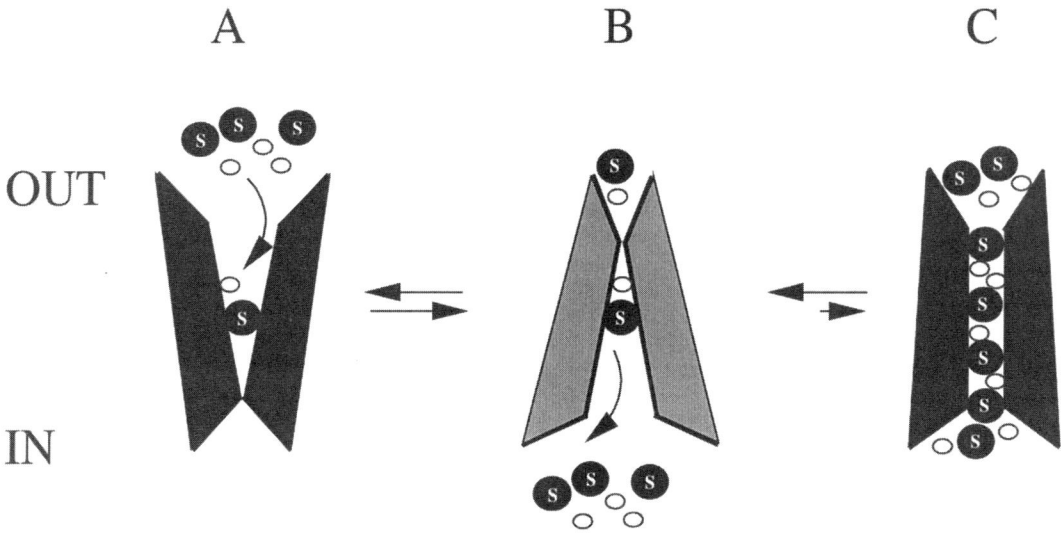

Figure 1 Schematic for biogenic amine transport in the alternating access and channel mode. In the alternating access model, the carrier has an aqueous lumen or cleft that exposes alternatively to the extracellular or intracellular environments. This transition state (A) ⇔ (B) results in transport of the substrate (S) and co-transported ions (empty circles) that is coupled stoichiometrically. The channel mode (C) is a low probability event, in which the ions and substrate move through the channel pore down their electrochemical gradients. The constrictions indicated on the cytoplasmic (A) or extracellular (B) domains of the transporter may be viewed as "gates", both of which are open simultaneously to form a pore (C). (Diagram courtesy of Dr. Aurelio Galli, Department of Pharmacology, University of Texas Health Science Center, San Antonio TX.).

of psychoactive drugs on such currents. These analyses may provide some explanation for differences in the pharmacological properties of "similar" drugs. For example, amphetaminelike compounds (including the neurotoxin 1-methyl-4-phenylpyridinium (MPP$^+$) acted like DA and caused transport-associated currents at DATs whereas cocainelike drugs (including methylphenidate) blocked such currents [47].

C. Electrogenic Processes

The DA, NE, and 5HT transport cycles involve cotransport of ions and therefore the processes are potentially electrogenic. One or two Na$^+$ ions and one Cl$^-$ ion are cotransported, resulting in a net inward flux of positive charge [45,48]. In general, the electrogenic processes involved in transport may contribute substantially to the resting membrane potential of a given nerve terminal and affect not only the relative activity of the transporters but also other processes such as transmitter release. Flux of charges associated with substrate uptake has been demonstrated for all of the monoamine transporters [41,44,46,49]. Consistent with this is the finding that depolarization decreased whereas hyperpolarization enhanced DA uptake in xenopus oocytes [47]. It seems that the DAT is regulated similarly in a voltage-dependent fashion in the mammalian CNS [48,50–53].

The implication of this is that when DA neurons are depolarized, DAT will decrease its transporter activity, allowing for greater diffusion of DA to its receptors [54,55], perhaps distant from a synapse or varicosity (see above). By contrast, hyperpolarization of DA neurons would enhance uptake of DA so as to decrease its receptor-mediated effects. This scheme makes sense physiologically since, for example, situations that would call for depolarization-induced release of DA would "turn off" its inactivation mechanism (i.e., the DAT) in order to facilitate dopaminergic transmission. This regulatory process now appears likely for DA-containing neurons, and may also occur for the NET and 5HTT as well [41,46,56].

D. Anatomical Localization of Transporters

Although transporters were presumed to have a localization within the synapse, results of studies visualizing either the DAT or 5HTT by electron microscopy have revealed the presence of these transporters outside the synapse. For example, Zhou et al. [57] found the majority of 5HTTs to exist in small unmyelinated axons, suggesting 5HT uptake to be mainly extrasynaptic; they found also that 5HTTs on axons outside synapses were engaged in high-affinity uptake of 5HT. They speculated that 5HT can spill out from the synaptic cleft and that the 5HTT located just outside the synapse can take up 5HT near the synapse whereas axonal 5HTT takes up 5HT that has diffused to more distal sites. Evidence for extrasynaptic localization of 5HTTs has also been found in both the shell and core of the nucleus accumbens [21]. Similarly, Nirenberg et al. [58,59] visualized the DAT under electron microscopy in the substantia nigra, the dorsolateral striatum, and the nucleus accumbens, and found evidence in all areas for the DAT being outside of synapses.

The extrasynaptic localization of transporters, coupled with the idea of VT, means, for example, that DA may come into contact with NETs. This is of importance as it has been shown that the NET transports DA even better than NE [60]. By contrast, the DAT does not transport NE, but it has been demonstrated that 5HT can be taken up by the DAT in the striatum [61]. Much earlier work of Shaskan and Snyder [62] showed, using rat brain slices, that noradrenergic nerves could take up 5HT, albeit much less potently than they transported NE; however, their capacity to take up 5HT was much greater than that for NE.

Thus, transporter "promiscuity" coupled with VT could result, for example, in DA reaching NETs in sufficient concentrations so as to be taken up into noradrenergic nerves, or 5HT reaching DATs or NETs so as to be removed by these transporters. There is evidence in support of this concept. For example, in the ventral mesencephalon ^{3}H-DA can be taken up by serotonergic neurons and this effect is partially blocked by fluoxetine [63]. Results with in vivo microdialysis have shown that systemic administration of selective inhibitors of the NET raise DA in the prefrontal cortex [64], and local application into the nucleus accumbens of selective inhibitors of the NET raised extracellular levels of 5HT and DA in addition to NE [65]. Using in vivo voltametry, we also obtained evidence for the uptake of 5HT into noradrenergic nerves [66]. In the dentate gyrus of the hippocampus, where the density of NETs outnumbers 5HTTs by roughly 2:1 (unpublished observations), exogenously administered 5HT was taken up by both serotonergic and noradrenergic nerves. By contrast, in the CA$_3$ region, where 5HTTs outnumber NETs about fourfold (unpublished observations) no evidence of 5HT uptake into noradrenergic nerves was obtained.

Relevant to this issue is an interesting result of Bel and Artigas [67]. These investigators measured the concentration of 5HT in the ECF of the frontal cortex, obtained by microdialysis. Systemic administration of desipramine alone did not raise the concentration of 5HT whereas administration of fluoxetine did. However, when the concentration of 5HT was elevated by a dose of fluoxetine that produced a maximal effect, administration of desipramine was able to raise further the concentration of 5HT. One explanation for this result is that blockade of the 5HTT permitted 5HT to reach noradrenergic nerves where it was taken up by NETs located on them.

All the results cited above have certain limitations which make their extrapolation to the clinical situation problematic. Nevertheless, such results are consistent with data showing that depressed patients treated with selective inhibitors of the 5HTT show decreases not only in the concentration of 5-hydroxyindoleacetic acid (5HIAA) in spinal fluid but in the norepinephrine metabolite 3,4,dehydroxyphenylglycol (MHPG) as well; similarly, treatment of patients with selective noradrenergic uptake inhibitors results in decreases in both MHPG and 5HIAA in spinal fluid [68]. One implication, then, of VT and extrasynaptic localization of transporters is that administration of selective uptake inhibitors could facilitate the uptake of a specific transmitter into other types of nerves producing as yet unknown effects. Another implication is that administration of dual uptake inhibitors (e.g., imipramine, which inhibits the uptake of both NE and 5HT) could result in even greater diffusion of NE or 5HT from their release sites so as to reach receptors on targets that they would not if only one transporter was inhibited. The consequences of this are not clear, but this could be an important area for future research.

Thus, even though uptake inhibitors were developed for clinical use because of the idea that they would prolong "synaptic" transmission (and they may do so by inhibiting perisynaptic transporters), they may produce many other effects as well, both on the membrane potential and intracellular processes of the nerves containing the transporter that they inhibit and on other nerves at a distance from the site of transmitter release.

E. Regulation of Transporter Function

Because transporters for the biogenic amines both are critical in regulating the extracellular concentrations of these amines, and are key targets for a number of psychotherapeutic drugs, understanding how their function is regulated has come under intense scrutiny in recent years. Once the mechanisms for regulation of the biogenic amine transporters are understood, there is great potential for developing new classes of drugs for the treatment of disorders such as depression, mania, anxiety, schizophrenia, and drug abuse. It is becoming clear that transport of biogenic amines is not simply a constitutive property of synaptic membranes but a dynamically regulated component of aminergic signaling.

1. Acute Regulation of Transporter Function

Acute changes in transporter function can occur rapidly (within minutes). Consequently, it is unlikely that such changes are mediated via alterations in gene expression given that at least several hours are required for increases in transporter mRNA to translate into increased transporter expression in the plasma membrane [69]. Commensurate with the finding that transporters for the biogenic amines contain sites for protein phosphorylation by a number of kinases [33], several groups reported rapid changes in transport capacity following activation of cellular kinases. The most common observation was that activation of protein kinase C (PKC) led to a reduction in amine transport capacity [70–72]. There are also considerable data implicating a role for calcium, calmodulin, and other kinase-dependent as well as kinase-independent pathways in the acute regulation of transporter function [73–78]. The decrease in transport capacity ensuing PKC activation is due to a reduction in V_{max} with K_m remaining largely unaltered. The reduction in V_{max} is associated with a decline in the number of transport proteins in the cell membrane [75,79]. This seems to result from sequestration of the transporter for recycling rather than degradation [77,79–81].

New techniques have enabled researchers to track changes in the distribution of transporters within cells. The most extensive studies to date have been carried out in cell lines transfected with the DAT and have consistently demonstrated PKC activation to evoke internalization of this transporter [82–85]. The fate of internalized DATs remains under debate, with evidence for both recycling [85] and degradation [82]. Nevertheless, it is apparent that cell surface redistribution of biogenic amine transporters is a mechanism that contributes to regulation of extracellular levels of transmitter. Such cell surface redistribution has pharmacological significance. For example, Saunders et al. [86] showed that amphetamine, a substrate for the DAT, caused trafficking of the human DAT (*h*DAT) from the plasma membrane to the cytosol of cultured cells. Callaghan and coworkers [87] subsequently showed that cocaine exerted the opposite effect, that is, mobilization of the hDAT from the cytosol to plasma membrane of cultured cells. Determining the pathways through which such psychotropic drugs are able to alter the distribution of transporters on the plasma membrane will have important ramifications for the development of new drug therapies for the treatment of numerous psychiatric disease states and drug abuse.

2. Mechanisms for Trafficking of Biogenic Amine Transporters

One way in which protein kinases can be activated is via presynaptic receptors. Apparsundaram and coworkers [79,81] demonstrated that activation of muscarinic acetylcholine receptors linked to PKC rapidly and selectively decreased the transport capacity (V_{max}) of the NET. In another study, Miller and Hoffman [88] reported that activation of A_3 adenosine receptors in cells increased 5HT uptake. This increase could be blocked by inhibitors of nitric oxide synthase and cGMP-dependent kinases, providing evidence for a nitric oxide–cGMP pathway in the acute regulation of the 5HTT.

In vivo studies have also provided evidence for receptor-mediated pathways in acute transporter regulation. For example, using high-speed chronoamperometry, Daws et al. [89,90] reported that antagonism of the $5HT_{1B}$ autoreceptor prolonged clearance of 5HT in rat hippocampus. Importantly, antagonism of the $5HT_{1B}$ autoreceptor in 5HTT knockout mice failed to alter clearance of 5HT, indicating that the presence of both proteins is required for this effect [91]. These observations are consistent with the idea that activation of $5HT_{1B}$ autoreceptors enhances 5HTT function. Similarly, blockade of the dopamine D2 receptor has been shown to inhibit clearance of DA from extracellular fluid [50,51], an effect that was absent in mice lacking the D2 receptor [52]. Whether autoreceptor regulation of transporter activity leads to transporter trafficking is unknown, as are the signal transduction pathways linking receptor to transporter.

Many signaling proteins, including receptors and ion channels, are modulated via direct protein phosphorylation, and there is evidence that this is also true for biogenic amine transporters [for a recent review, 72]. Blakely and colleagues [92] demonstrated that 5HT reduced phosphorylation of the 5HTT both under basal conditions and following PKC activation. These effects could be blocked by paroxetine, a selective serotonin reuptake inhibitor (SSRI), suggesting that the effects of 5HT were mediated by an action on the transporter and not on 5HT receptors. Ramamoorthy and Blakely [77] later showed that PKC-induced transporter internalization was reduced in the presence of 5HT [77]. The inhibitory effect of 5HT on phosphorylation of the 5HTT is due to its binding to the 5HTT and/or its translocation by it. This indicates that phosphorylation of the 5HTT occurs when it is in the plasma membrane, and further suggests that such phosphorylation serves as a signal for its trafficking and internalization. The ability of 5HT to suppress phosphorylation may be a mechanism to maintain high transporter function when extracellular levels of 5HT are elevated [71]. In contrast to the 5HTT, direct phosphorylation of the DAT does not appear to be involved in PKC-mediated regulation of DAT function [93]. Further, it now appears that phosphatases are also involved in regulating the state of phosphorylation of amine transporters [72,94], providing yet another approach to regulating the function of transporters in vivo.

3. Long-Term Regulation of Transporter Function

Several lines of evidence, including changes in transporter activity and/or expression in response to environmental perturbations (e.g., altered photoperiods) [73], fluctuations in hormone levels (e.g. corticosteroids, estrogen) [95–97], and as a consequence of aging [98,99], suggest that biogenic amine transporters also undergo long-term regulation.

Most relevant to the present review are the changes in transporter activity/expression observed in certain disease states and as a consequence of therapeutic intervention. For example, reductions in both 5HTT and NET binding have been reported in patients with depression [100–102], and significant reductions of 5HTT binding and DAT immunoreactivity have been observed in patients with Parkinson's disease [reviewed in 103]. Depressive disorders are commonly treated with selective inhibitors of 5HT and/or NE uptake. Pharmacologic inhibition of transporters occurs rapidly. However, maximal therapeutic benefit takes weeks to occur, so adaptive changes induced by such drugs on biogenic amine systems have been investigated extensively. Although much of this work focused on receptors and receptor-mediated responses [104], data on transporter function have also been obtained. Numerous studies have assessed the effect of chronic antidepressant treatment on the density of binding sites for the 5HTT and NET. The results have not been consistent [reviewed in 73,105]. Similarly, although several studies have shown no effect of chronic treatment with antidepressants on mRNAs for the 5HTT and NET, others have reported increases and still others, no change [101,105,106]. Obviously, differences in the duration of chronic drug dosage and route of drug delivery, which inevitably exist in such in vivo studies, make firm conclusions regarding alterations in gene expression by chronic drug treatment difficult.

Using high-speed chronoamperometry, we [107] measured the ability of an SSRI, fluvoxamine, applied locally to the hippocampus, to inhibit uptake of exogenously applied 5HT in rats treated for 21 days by osmotic minipump with the SSRI paroxetine. The more constant level of drug in plasma obtained by administration via minipump may better model clinical administration of uptake inhibitors. Acute local administration of fluvoxamine did not inhibit uptake of 5HT in chronically treated rats (as it did in non-treated rats). This lack of an inhibitory effect of fluvoxamine may be due to a robust decrease in 5HTT-binding sites in paroxetine-treated rats [107]. Pineyro et al. [108] also found chronic administration of paroxetine by minipump to cause a decrease in 5HTT function and density. More recently, we [109] showed that the time course for decreased 5HTT function following chronic treatment of rats with an SSRI was gradual. This functional decrease was paralleled by a decrease in 5HTT density but not by mRNA levels for the 5HTT. These data suggest that posttranscriptional events mediate changes in 5HTT function caused by long-term administration of SSRIs. One implication of these data for the clinical setting is that antidepressant-induced decreases in 5HTT density may need to reach a "critical" level before therapeutic benefits are seen. In keeping with this, Alvarez et al. [102] reported that platelet 5HTTs were decreased in patients treated with fluoxetine. Thus, if transporter density can be reduced more rapidly, perhaps clinical improvement can be accomplished in a shorter time frame.

F. Genetic Knockout and Polymorphisms of Biogenic Amine Transporters

Perhaps the most striking demonstration of the importance of transporters in regulating extracellular fluid concentrations of biogenic amines comes from studies using transporter deficient mice. In vivo studies using voltametric recording techniques show that homozygous 5HTT knockout (KO) [91], DAT KO [110], and NET KO [111] mice have a profoundly reduced ability to clear 5HT, DA and NE, respectively, from ECF. However, in most cases, clearance remains more rapid than simple diffusion would predict. This implies that other mechanisms must compensate, at least to some extent, for the loss of transporter. One possibility is that transporters other than the specific transport protein for a given biogenic amine are able to compensate. As has been discussed, transporters for the biogenic amines exhibit some "promiscuity" for transmitters. In addition, the presence of nonneuronal monoamine transporters, such as the extraneuronal monoamine transporter and organic cation transporter 2 (OCT2), in brain [112] may also account for clearance of biogenic amines from ECF in 5HTT-, DAT- and NET-deficient mice. Indeed, OCT2 is reportedly increased in the brains of 5HTT KO mice [113] and may represent an adaptive response to the loss of 5HTT.

The advent of transporter-deficient mice and their altered responses to drugs as well as inherent differences in amine levels, receptors, and behavior [28,111,114], prompted researchers to look for genetic variants in transporter proteins that may predispose to psychiatric disorders. Variants have now been uncovered in the promoter region of the gene encoding the 5HTT that alter mRNA and protein expression both in vitro and in vivo. An association between these variants and a number of disorders, including anxiety, affective disorder, autism, and alcoholism, have been reported. Such associations include a predisposition for the disorder and altered sensitivity to drugs used to treat the disorder [115–118]. Clearly, this is an area for active research which should lend important insights into the underlying etiology of such disorders and improved treatments for them.

G. Implications for Neuropsychopharmacology

Our changing views on modes of neurotransmission (hard-wired vs. VT) and on transporter function (carrier vs. channel mode), together with the marked advances in our understanding of transporter regulation, have paved the way for the development of new drugs. For example, drugs that cause immediate activation of certain protein kinases (or inhibition of certain phosphatases) may speed or enhance the therapeutic efficacy of current antidepressant treatments by either (1) causing a rapid reduction in the number of active transporters at the plasma membrane (e.g., through sequestration) and/or (2) bringing about more rapid changes in transporter gene expression. Likewise, the development of drugs that alter the probability of transporters acting in channel mode, or of drugs that allow greater diffusion of transmitter from their release sites, is also an area for active research because of their therapeutic potential. In addition, understanding the regulation of transporters and the consequences of VT may result in determination of the mechanisms that underlie the reinforcing properties of cocaine, amphetamine, and other drugs of abuse.

Although our understanding of the role of transporters and of diffusion in regulating monoaminergic neurotransmission has increased tremendously in recent years, these remain more "classical" concepts. More recently the idea of peptidergic regulation of monoaminergic neurotransmission has emerged. In particular, there is new evidence that neuropeptide receptors may be novel targets for antidepressant and anxiolytic drugs. Therapeutic efficacy induced by antagonists of certain neuropeptide receptors is thought to be due to changes in noradrenergic and serotonergic activity. Because of this it is timely to review our current understanding of neuropeptide regulation of monoaminergic neurotransmission.

IV. NEUROPEPTIDE MODULATION OF MONOAMINERGIC NEUROTRANSMISSION

In the late 1970s and early 1980s, much fanfare hailed the emergence of a "new" class of brain neurotransmitter, the neuropeptides. Every year, more peptides were isolated, identified, quantified, and mapped anatomically in the brain. There was much excitement and anticipation that this era would generate a new understanding of neurotransmission and regulation of brain function. A noteworthy feature of neuropeptides that emerged from this period of research is that they seem invariably to be colocalized in the same nerve terminals with other neurotransmitters, including the monoamines [119], essentially forcing an obligatory inteaction between the two transmitter classes. Nonetheless, the nature of this interaction and the contexts in which it occurs must be determined by the complement of receptor subtypes expressed by the postsynaptic target neuron, and also by the differential release characteristics of the colocalized peptidergic and monoaminergic neurotransmitters.

A. Neuropeptides Are "Slow" Modulatory Transmitters

The general characteristics of peptide neurotransmission differ in many important respects from those of monoamines [see 120]. Unlike monoamine transmitters, which are derived from a single amino acid by enzymatic synthesis, neuropeptides are small proteins comprising a chain of several amino acids. As such, they are synthesized in the cell body by ribosomal translation of messenger RNA. Like other proteins, they are usually synthesized first in the form of a precursor protein, which is then further cleaved and modified before the peptide is shipped via axonal transport to the nerve terminal. There it is incorporated into large dense-core synaptic vesicles [121]. Thus, unlike the relatively rapid changes that can be induced in the rate of enzymatic synthesis of monoamines directly in the nerve terminal, regulatory induction of neuropeptide synthesis is a slow process, requiring hours or even days for the activation of gene expression, *de novo* protein synthesis, and axonal transport before any change in releasable peptide becomes available to the nerve terminal.

The localization of peptide transmitters in large, dense-core synaptic vesicles, as opposed to the small, clear vesicles in which monoamines are found, also confers unique release characteristics on peptides. These large vesicles are situated father from the so-called active zones [122], than are the small clear vesicles. Thus, they are farther from vesicle docking and release sites, and farther from calcium entry sites, rendering them less sensitive to low levels of electrical activity in the nerve terminal. The practical implication of this is that monoamines show a fairly graded relationship between firing rate in the presynaptic fiber and the amount of neurotransmitter released into the synapse, whereas neuropeptides are preferentially released under conditions of intense activation or burst firing [123]. Thus, whatever regulatory interactions the peptides may have with monoamines, they are likely to occur preferentially under conditions of intense activation of the neuron in which the two transmitters are colocalized.

Unlike the monoamines, for which reuptake by specific transporters is so important to the regulation of synaptic effects, no such reuptake transporters have been identified for neuropeptides in the brain. Rather, termination of the synaptic action of peptides appears to depend upon bulk diffusion and extracellular enzymatic degradation by general peptidases, which can be located at some distance from the synapse [124]. Thus, not only is the synthesis and release of neuropeptides slower than that of monoamines, but the termination of action is slower as well. Moreover, the lack of transporter-mediated reuptake means that peptides are likely to engage in VT, as defined earlier in this chapter. This is supported, perhaps even more strongly than with monoamines, by frequent "mismatches" between the distribution of peptide-containing nerve terminals and appropriate postsynaptic receptors in the brain [reviewed in 125]. These characteristics have all led to the general view that neuropeptides function primarily as neuromodulators, altering effects exerted by other neurotransmitters on the activity of target brain circuits.

The monoamines have themselves been described as serving neuromodulatory functions in the brain [126]. Thus, the corelease of neuropeptides and monoamines during stress, arousal, reward, etc., confers a much higher level of complexity on this modulatory process. With increasing neuronal activity, proportionately more monoaminergic transmitter is released, and its modulatory effect is presumably increased accordingly. However, at some threshold level of activity, the release of a neuropeptide cotransmitter may be progressively recruited. The peptide may itself have modulatory effects on the same target, or it may modify the presynaptic release or the postsynaptic effects of the monoamine with which it has been coreleased.

B. Potential Modes of Interaction Between Neuropeptides and Monoamines in the Brain

There are several ways that neuropeptides and monoamines may interact in the brain. They can be colocalized and coreleased onto common targets, whereby they may exert their respective postsynaptic modulatory effects independently, cooperatively, synergistically, or in opposition, depending on the physiological context and the complement of receptors expressed by the post-synaptic target neuron (see reviews [120,127] for general discussions of colocalized transmitter interactions). Alternatively, they may originate in different afferents that converge onto a common target. In this case, the possibilities for postsynaptic interaction are the same, though independent activation of the different afferent pathways allows for more context specificity in the modulatory interaction. Finally, peptidergic neurons may innervate monoaminergic neurons or terminals, thereby affecting the firing rate or release of the monoamine transmitter in its target region.

The recent development of new tools and techniques, together with the novel application of established approaches, is just now providing both the means and the mindset for making substantive progress in understanding the functional interaction between brain neuropeptides and monoamine transmitters [128]. As this understanding progresses, we are forging a richer understanding of the potential contribution of neuropeptides, and their interaction with monoamine transmitters, in the development or treatment of affective disorders, including depression and anxiety [see reviews 129–133].

C. Substance P Antagonists as Novel Antidepressant/Anxiolytic Drugs

Substance P (SP) and its receptors are present in high concentrations in many forebrain limbic areas that have been implicated in affect and anxiety, including the hypothalamus, septal region, amygdala, and bed nucleus of the stria terminalis, as well as the periaqueductal gray, locus coeruleus, and raphe nuclei [134]. As for its relationship with NE and 5HT, the monoamines most implicated in the etiology and treatment of affective disorders, the substrates exist for many potential modes of interaction between these transmitters. Substance P terminals and receptors overlap those of both NE and 5HT. Likewise, SP fibers innervate serotonergic neurons of the dorsal raphe and noradrenergic neurons of the locus coeruleus. Finally, SP is colocalized with 5HT in ascending projections innervating the limbic forebrain in humans, other primates, and certain other species such as guinea pigs, though apparently not in rats or mice [135].

Surprisingly, whereas SP itself exerts primarily excitatory effects, blockade of SP receptors enhances both noradrenergic and serotonergic activity, most likely through a process of multisynaptic disinhibition [136]. Thus, SP antagonists may have an effect on monoaminergic transmission that is similar, at least acutely, to the effect of classical antidepressants that block monoamine reuptake. In preclinical behavioral assays, systemic or intraventricular administration of a SP antagonist attenuated anxietylike behaviors [137]. In animal models of anxiety- or depressive-like behavior, SP antagonist administration had effects similar to those of established antidepressant and antianxiety compounds [138]. These experiments on the affective response to SP antagonist administration culminated in a clinical study of the antidepressant and antianxiety efficacy of a centrally active SP antagonist in depressed patients [137]. The results of this study showed that the SP antagonist exerted both antidepressant and antianxiety effects, comparable to those of the SSRI paroxetine. This study showed great promise for the establishment of a novel antidepressant agent. Caution is necessary, though, until these clinical results can be replicated. Nonetheless, should SP antagonists ultimately prove useful and efficacious against depression, their targeting a specific neuropeptide that interacts in a novel way with monoamines opens a new possibility for more widely effective, more efficient, or faster treatment of affective disorders.

D. Interaction of Neuropeptide Y and Galanin with Norepinephrine in Modulating Behavioral Reactivity to Stress

Two neuropeptides are prominently colocalized with NE in the locus coeruleus (LC)—neuropeptide Y (NPY) and galanin (GAL). Galanin is expressed in nearly all noradrenergic neurons in the locus coeruleus [139]; thus it likely serves as a cotransmitter in the many limbic forebrain sites innervated by the LC. By contrast, NPY is found in a much smaller proportion of noradrenergic neurons in the LC, but is extensively colocalized with NE in medullary noradrenergic neurons [140].

The central nucleus of the amygdala and the bed nucleus of the stria terminalis, two closely related components of the extended amygdala, are targets of dense noradrenergic innervation, and both have been implicated in fear and anxiety [141]. In a recent series of experiments, we demonstrated that the stress-induced release of NE in these regions facilitates the expression of anxietylike behavioral responses to acute stress [142,143]. This is consistent with the role proposed for NE in modulating affective components of the stress response, including vigilance, arousal, and anxiety [144–146]. By contrast, administration of NPY into the central nucleus exerts distinct anxiolytic effects [147–148], while local administration of NPY antagonist drugs into LC target regions can be anxiogenic [149].

Much like the autoinhibitory effects of NE acting on presynaptic alpha-2 adrenergic autoreceptors, it has been shown that NPY also acts on presynaptic NPY autoreceptors, reducing the release of both NE and NPY [150,151]. In addition, NPY receptors located on noradrenergic cell bodies inhibit the activity of these cells [152,153]. Thus, corelease of NPY with NE invoked when high levels of activity have been stimulated in noradrenergic neurons, may attenuate the anxiogenic effects of NE released in the limbic forebrain, exerting direct anxiolytic effects postsynaptically while at the same time acting presynaptically to inhibit the further release of NE.

Even more than NPY, galanin is extensively coexpressed with NE in the LC [139]. Like NPY, NE neuronal activity is also inhibited by galanin [154,155], and galanin receptors located on NE terminals, which may function either as postsynaptic heteroreceptors or as inhibitory autoreceptors that limit the release of galanin from those terminals, also inhibit the release of NE [151]. In a recent series of studies, we have shown that galanin exerts an anxiety-buffering effect in the central amygdala, attenuating the anxiogenic effects of acute stress that we showed were attributable to NE [156]. In this case, however, the galanin-mediated anxiolytic effect was elicited specifically when stress-induced activation of the noradrenergic system had been accentuated by prior administration of the autoreceptor antagonist yohimbine [158,159].

Along with this context specificity in the CeA related to the level of activation of the noradrenergic system, additional studies revealed that the functional interaction between NE and galanin in other regions of the limbic forebrain during stress were more complicated. In the bed nucleus, acute stress also induced NE release to facilitate anxietylike behavioral responses, but in this region, galanin facilitated these same behavioral responses [156,157], thus acting in the same direction as NE. Moreover, this facilitatory effect of galanin in the BST did not require prior treatment with yohimbine, as did the anxiolytic NE-buffering effects of galanin in the CeA. This is perhaps due to the fact that the major source of noradrenergic innervation in the bed nucleus arises from caudal medullary noradrenergic cell groups rather than the LC. Unlike the LC, these other noradrenergic cell groups do not show a high degree of galanin colocalization [139]. Thus, anxiolytic effects in the CeA may have originated from the corelease of galanin and NE from noradrenergic terminals, while anxiogenic effects in the bed nucleus may have originated from the activation of galanin-synthesizing neurons within the nucleus itself.

These neurons may themselves be targets of noradrenergic innervation [160], which would explain why their activity was elicited specifically in response to stress. Thus, depending on the level of activation of the noradrenergic system, the specific physiological context in which that activation occurred, and the specific brain region involved, galanin could either act in concert with or oppose the stress-induced behavioral effects of NE. Likewise, any drug that mimicked or blocked the effects of galanin in the brain could have anxiogenic, anxiolytic, or mixed effects depending on the context and the circumstance by which the behavioral response had been elicited.

Such complex interactions between transmitters of different classes may be subject to modification by a number of factors, including prior exposure to stress, chronic drug treatment, or genetic predisposition. Given the nature of this interaction, it is clear that drugs that affect monoaminergic neurotransmission could induce regulatory changes in both neuropeptide and monoaminergic functions, disrupting or resetting the delicate balance between these modulatory transmitters, either contributing to or interfering with their clinical effects.

In summary, then, the past decade has witnessed tremendous increases in our understanding of the complexity of the process of monoaminergic transmission and its regulation. This increased understanding has not yet been translated into substantial therapeutic advances but clearly has the potential to do so.

REFERENCES

1. Agnati LF, Fuxe K, Nicholson C, Sykova E. Progress in Brain Research, Vol 125: Volume Transmission Revisited. Amsterdam: Elsevier, 2000.
2. Descarries L, Beaudet A, Watkins KC. Serotonin nerve terminals in adult rat neocortex. Brain Res 1975;100:563–588.
3. Beaudet A, Descarries L. Quantitative data on serotonin nerve terminals in adult rat neocortex. Brain Res 1976;111:301–309.
4. Bloom FE. An integrative view of information handling in the CNS. In: Fuxe K, Agnati LF, eds. Volume Transmission in the Brain: Novel Mechanisms for Neural Transmission. New York: Raven Press, 1991:11–23.
5. Molliver ME, Grzanna R, Lidov HGW, Morrison JH, Olschowka JA. Monoamine systems in the cerebral cortex. In: Chan-Palay V, Palay SL, eds. Cytochemical Methods in Neuroanatomy. New York: Alan R. Liss, 1982:255–277.
6. Papadopoulos GC, Parnavelas JG, Buijs RM. Monoaminergic fibers form conventional synapses in the cerebral cortex. Neurosci Lett 1987;76:275–279.
7. Maley BE, Engle MG, Humphreys S. Monoamine synaptic structure and localization in the central nervous system. J Electron Microsc Technol 1990;15:20–33.
8. Seguela P, Watkins KC, Descarries L. Ultrastructural relationships of serotonin axon terminals in the cerebral cortex of the adult rat. J Comp Neurol 1989;289:129–142.
9. Smiley JF, Goldman-Rakic PS. Serotonergic axons in monkey prefrontal cerebral cortex synapse predominantly on interneurons as demonstrated by serial section electron microscopy. J Comp Neurol 1996;367:431–443.
10. Moukhles H, Bosler O, Bolam JP, Vallee A, Umbriaco D, Geffard M, Doucet G. Quantitative and morphometric data indicate precise cellular interactions between serotonin terminals and postsynaptic targets in rat substantia nigra. Neuroscience 1997;76:1159–1171.
11. Rice ME. Distinct regional differences in dopamine-mediated volume transmission. In: Agnati LF, Fuxe K, Nicholson C, Sykova E, eds. Progress in Brain Research, Vol 125: Volume Transmission Revisited. Amsterdam: Elsevier, 2000:277–290.
12. Nicholson C, Chen KC, Hrabetova S, Tao L. Diffusion of molecules in brain extracellular space: theory and experiment. In: Agnati LF, Fuxe K, Nicholson C, Sykova E, eds. Progress in Brain Research, Vol 125: Volume Transmission Revisited. Amsterdam: Elsevier, 2000:125–154.
13. Bunin MA, Wightman RM. Quantitative evaluation of 5-hydroxytryptamine (serotonin) neuronal release and uptake: an investigation of extrasynaptic transmission. J Neurosci 1998;18:4854–4860.
14. Garris PA, Ciolkowski EL, Pastore P, Wightman RM. Efflux of dopamine from the synaptic cleft in the nucleus accumbens of the rat brain. J Neurosci 1994;14:6084–6093.
15. Bunin MA, Prioleau C, Mailman RB, Wightman RM. Release and uptake rates of 5-hydroxytryptamine in the dorsal raphe and substantia nigra reticulata of the rat brain. J Neurochem 1998;70:1077–1087.
16. Herkenham M. Mismatches between neurotransmitter and receptor localization: implications for endocrine functions in the brain. In: Fuxe K, Agnati LF, eds. Volume Transmission in the Brain: Novel Mechanisms for Neural Transmission. New York: Raven Press, 1991:63–87.
17. Blue ME, Yagaloff KA, Mamounas LA, Hartig PR, Molliver ME. Correspondence between 5-HT$_2$ receptors and serotonergic axons in rat neocortex. Brain Res 1988;453:315–328.
18. Sesack SR, Aoki C, Pickel VM. Ultrastructural localization of D$_2$ receptor-like immunoreactivity in midbrain dopamine neurons and their striatal targets. J Neurosci 1994;14:88–106.
19. Smiley JF, Levey AI, Ciliax BJ, Goldman-Rakic PS. D$_1$ dopamine receptor immunoreactivity in human and monkey cerebral cortex: predominant and extrasynaptic localization in dendritic spines. Proc Natl Acad Sci USA 1994;91:5720–5724.
20. Kia HK, Brisorgueil M-J, Hamon M, Calas A, Verge D. Ultrastructural localization of 5-hydroxytryptamine$_{1A}$ receptors in the rat brain. J Neurosci Res 1996;46:697–708.
21. Pickel VM. Extrasynaptic distribution of monoamine transporters and receptors. In: Agnati LF, Fuxe K,

Nicholson C, Sykova E, eds. Progress in Brain Research, Vol 125: Volume Transmission Revisited. Amsterdam: Elsevier, 2000:267–276.
22. Whitby LG, Axelrod J, Weil-Malherbe H. The fate of 3H-norepinephrine in animals. J Pharmacol Exp Ther 1961;132:193–201.
23. Glowinski J, Axelrod J. Effect of drugs on the disposition of H-3-norepinephrine uptake in the rat brain. Pharmacol Rev 1966;18:775–785.
24. Ross SB, Renyi AL. Inhibition of the uptake of tritiated 5-hydroxytryptamine in brain tissue. Eur J Pharmacol 1969;7:270–277.
25. Amara SG, Sonders MS. Neurotransmitter transporters as molecular targets for addictive drugs. Drug Alcohol Depend 1998;51:87–96.
26. Seiden LS, Sabol KE, Ricaurte GA. Amphetamine: effects on catecholamine systems and behavior. Annu Rev Pharmacol Toxicol 1993;33:639–677.
27. Wall SC, Gu H, Rudnick G. Biogenic amine flux mediated by cloned transporters stably expressed in cultured cell lines: amphetamine specificity for inhibition and efflux. Molecular Pharmacol 1995;47:544–550.
28. Giros B, Jaber M, Jones SR, Wightman RM, Caron MG. Hyperlocomotion and indifference to cocaine and amphetamine in mice lacking the dopamine transporter. Nature 1996;379:606–612.
29. Blakely RD, Berson HE, Fremeau RTJ, Caron MG, Peek MM, Prince HK, Bradley CC. Cloning and expression of a functional serotonin transporter from rat brain. Nature 1991;354:66–70.
30. Giros B, Caron MG. Molecular characterization of the dopamine transporter. Trends Pharmacol Sci 1993;14:43–49.
31. Hoffman BJ, Mezey E, Brownstein MJ. Cloning of a serotonin transporter affected by antidepressants. Science 1991;254:579–580.
32. Pacholczyk T, Blakely RD, Amara SG. Expression and cloning of a cocaine and antidepressant sensitive human noradrenaline transporter. Nature 1991;350:350–354.
33. Borowsky B, Hoffman BJ. Neurotransmitter transporters: molecular biology, function and regulation. Int Rev Neurobiol 1995;38:139–199.
34. Rudnick G, Clark J. From synapse to vesicle: the uptake and storage of biogenic amine neurotransmitters. Biochim Biophys Acta 1993;1144:249–263.
35. DeFelice LJ, Blakely RD. Pore models for transporters? Biophys J 1996;70:579–580.
36. Lester HA, Mager S, Quick MW, Corey JL. Permeation properties of neurotransmitter transporters. Annu Rev Pharmacol Toxicol 1994;34:219–249.
37. Sitte HH, Hiptmair B, Zwach J, Pifl C, Singer EA, Scholze P. Quantitative analysis of inward and outward transport rates in cells stably expressing the cloned human serotonin transporter: inconsistencies with the hypothesis of facilitated exchange diffusion. Molecular Pharmacol 2001;59:1129–1137.
38. Browman KE, Kantor L, Richardson S, Badiana A, Robinson TE, Gnegy ME. Injection of the protein kinase C inhibitor Ro31–8220 into the nucleus accumbens attenuates the acute response to amphetamine: tissue and behavioral studies. Brain Res 1998;814:112–119.
39. Kantor L, Gnegy ME. Protein kinase C inhibitors block amphetamine-mediated dopamine release in rat striatal slices. J Pharmacol Exp Ther 1998;284:592–598.
40. Chen N, Justice JB. Differential effect of structural modifications of human dopamine transporter on the inward and outward transport of dopamine. Brain Res Mol Brain Res 2000;75:208–215.
41. Galli A, Petersen CI, De Blaquiere M, Blakely RD, DeFelice LJ. *Drosophila* serotonin transporters have voltage-dependent uptake coupled to a serotonin-gated ion channel. J Neurosci 1997;17:3401–3411.
42. Lester HA, Cao Y, Mager S. Listening to neurotransmitter transporters. Neuron 1996;17:807–810.
43. Lin F, Lester HA, Mager S. Single channel currents produced by the serotonin transporter and analysis of a mutation affecting ion permeation. Biophys J 1996;71:3126–3135.
44. Mager S, Min C, Henry DJ, Chavkin C, Hoffman BJ, Davidson N, Lester HA. Conducting states of a mammalian serotonin transporter. Neuron 1994;12:845–859.
45. Sonders MS, Amara SG. Channels in transporters. Curr Opin Neurobiol 1996;6:294–302.
46. Galli A, Blakely RD, DeFelice LJ. Patch-clamp and amperometric recordings from norepinephrine transporters: channel activity and voltage-dependent uptake. Proc Natl Acad Sci USA 1998;95:13260–13265.
47. Sonders MS, Zhu SJ, Zahniser NR, Kavanaugh MP, Amara SG. Multiple ionic conductances of the human dopamine transporter: the actions of dopamine and psychostimulants. J Neurosci 1997;17:960–974.
48. Krueger BK. Kinetics and block of dopamine uptake in synaptosomes from rat caudate nucleus. J Neurochem 1990;55:260–267.
49. Rudnick G. Bioenergetics of transmitter transport. J Bioenerg Biomem 1998;30:173–185.
50. Meiergerd SM, Patterson TA, Schenk JO. D2 receptors may modulate the function of the striatal transporter for dopamine: kinetic evidence from studies in vitro and in vivo. J Neurochem 1993;61:764–767.
51. Cass WA, Gerhardt GA. Direct *in vivo* evidence that D2 dopamine receptors can modulate dopamine uptake. Neurosci Lett 1994;176:259–263.
52. Dickinson SD, Sabeti J, Larson GA, Giardina K, Rubinstein M, Kelly MA, Grandy DK, Low MJ, Gerhardt GA, Zahniser NR. Dopamine D2 receptor deficient mice exhibit decreased dopamine transporter function but no changes in dopamine release in the dorsal striatum. J Neurochem 1999;72:148–156.

53. Hoffman AF, Zahniser NR, Lupica CR, Gerhardt GA. Voltage-dependency of the dopamine transporter in the rat substantia nigra. Neurosci Lett 1999;260:105–108.
54. Cass WA, Gerhardt GA. In vivo assessment of dopamine uptake in rat medial prefrontal cortex: comparison with dorsal striatum and nucleus accumbens. J Neurochem 1995;65:201–207.
55. Garris PA, Wightman RM. Different kinetics govern dopaminergic transmission in the amygdala, prefrontal cortex, and striatum: An in vivo voltametric study. J Neurosci 1994;14:442–450.
56. Corey JL, Quick MW, Davidson N, Lester HA, Guastella J. A cocaine-sensitive Drosophila serotonin transporter: cloning, expression, and electrophysiological characterization. Proc Natl Acad Sci USA 1994;91:1188–1192.
57. Zhou FC, Tao-Cheng JH, Segu L, Patel T, Wang Y. Serotonin transporters are located on the axons beyond the synaptic junctions: anatomical and functional evidence. Brain Res 1998;805:241–254.
58. Nirenberg MJ, Vaughan RA, Uhl GR, Kuhar MJ, Pickel VM. The dopamine transporter is localized to dendritic and axonal plasma membranes of nigrostriatal dopaminergic neurons. J Neurosci 1996;16:436–447.
59. Nirenberg MJ, Chan J, Pohorille A, Vaughan RA, Uhl GR, Kuhar MJ, Pickel VM. The dopamine transporter: comparative ultrastructure of dopaminergic axons in limbic and motor compartments of the nucleus accumbens. J Neurosci 1997;17:6899–6907.
60. Povlock SL, Amara SG. The structure and function of norepinephrine, dopamine, and serotonin transporters. In: Reith MEA, ed. Neurotransmitter Transporters. Totowa, NJ: Humana Press, 1997:1–28.
61. Jackson BP, Wightman RM. Dynamics of 5-hydroxytryptamine released from dopamine neurons in the caudate putamen of the rat. Brain Res 1995;674:163–166.
62. Shaskan EG, Snyder SH. Kinetics of serotonin accumulation into slices from rat brain: relationship to catecholamine uptake. J Pharmacol Exp Ther 1970;175:404–418.
63. Chen NH, Reith MEA. Role of axonal and somatodendritic monoamine transporters in action of uptake blockers. In: Reith MEA, ed. Neurotransmitter Transporters: Structure, Function, and Regulation. Totowa, NJ: Humana Press, 1997:345–391.
64. Carboni E, Chiara GD. Serotonin release estimated by transcortical dialysis in freely-moving rats. Neuroscience 1989;32:637–645.
65. Li M-Y, Yan Q-S, Coffey LL, Reith MEA. Extracellular dopamine, norepinephrine, and serotonin in the nucleus accumbens of freely moving rats following local cocaine and other monoamine uptake blockers. J Neurochem 1996;66:559–568.
66. Daws LC, Toney GM, Gerhardt GA, Frazer A. In vivo chronoamperometric measures of extracellular serotonin clearance in rat dorsal hippocampus: contribution of serotonin and norepinephrine transporters. J Pharmacol Exp Ther 1998;286:967–976.
67. Bel N, Artigas F. In vivo effects of the simultaneous blockade of serotonin and norepinephrine transporters on serotonergic function. Microdialysis studies. J Pharmacol Exp Ther 1996;278:1064–1072.
68. Little JT, Ketter TA, Mathe AA, Frye MA, Luckenbaugh D, Post RM. Venlafaxine but not bupropion decreases cerebrospinal fluid 5-hydroxyindoleacetic acid in unipolar depression. Biol Psychiatry 1999;45:285–289.
69. Melikian HE, McDonald JK, Gu H, Rudnick G, Moore KR, Blakely RD. Human norepinephrine transporter: biosynthetic studies using a site-directed polyclonal antibody. J Biol Chem 1994;269:12290–12297.
70. Vaughan RA, Huff RA, Uhl GR, Kuhar MJ. Protein kinase C–mediated phosphorylation and functional regulation of dopamine transporters in striatal synaptosomes. J Biol Chem 1997;272:15541–15546.
71. Blakely RD, Ramamoorthy S, Schroeter S, Qian Y, Apparsundaram S, Galli A, DeFelice LJ. Regulated phosphorylation and trafficking of antidepressant-sensitive serotonin transporter proteins. Biol Psychiatry 1998;44:169–178.
72. Blakely RD, Bauman AL. Biogenic amine transporters: regulation in flux. Curr Opin Neurobiol 2000;10:328–336.
73. Blakely RD, Ramamoorthy S, Qian Y, Schroeter S, Bradley C. Regulation of antidepressant-sensitive serotonin transporters. In: Reith MEA, ed. Neurotransmitter Transporters: Structure, Function and Regulation. Totowa, NJ: Humana Press, 1997:29–72.
74. Reith MEA, Xu C, Chen NH. Pharmacology and regulation of the neuronal dopamine transporter. Eur J Pharmacol 1997;324:1–10.
75. Batchelor M, Schenk JO. Protein kinase A activity may kinetically upregulate the striatal transporter for dopamine. J Neurosci 1998;18:10304–10309.
76. Uchida J, Kiuchi Y, Ohno M, Yura A, Oguchi K. Ca^{++}-dependent enhancement of [^{3}H]noradrenaline uptake in PC12 cells through calmodulin-dependent kinases. Brain Res 1998;809:155–164.
77. Ramamoorthy S, Blakely RD. Phosphorylation and sequestration of serotonin transporters differentially modulated by psychostimulants. Science 1999;285:763–766.
78. Doolen S, Zahniser NR. Protein tyrosine kinase inhibitors alter human dopamine transporter activity in Xenopus Oocytes. J Pharmacol Exp Ther 2001;296:931–938.
79. Apparsundaram S, Galli A, DeFelice LJ, Hartzell HC, Blakely RD. Acute regulation of norepinephrine transport: I. Protein kinase C–linked muscarinic receptors influence transport capacity and transporter density in SK-N-SH cells. J Pharmacol Exp Ther 1998;287:733–743.

80. Qian Y, Galli A, Ramamoorthy S, Risso S, De Felice LJ, Blakely RD. Protein kinase C activation regulates human serotonin transporters in HEK-293 cells via altered cell surface expression. J Neurosci 1997;17:45–57.

81. Apparsundaram S, Schroeter S, Giovanetti E, Blakely RD. Acute regulation of norepinephrine transport. II. PKC-modulated surface expression of human norepinephrine transporter proteins. J Pharmacol Exp Ther 1998;287:744–751.

82. Daniels GM, Amara SG. Regulated trafficking of the human dopamine transporter. Clathrin-mediated internalization and lysosomal degradation in response to phorbol esters. J Biol Chem 1999;274:35794–35801.

83. Zhu SJ, Kavanaugh MP, Sonders MS, Amara SG, Zahniser NR. Activation of protein kinase C inhibits uptake, currents and binding associated with the human dopamine transporter expressed in *Xenopus* oocytes. J Pharmacol Exp Ther 1997;282:1358–1365.

84. Pristupa ZB, McConkey F, Liu F, Man HY, Lee FJS, Wang YT, Niznik HB. Protein kinase-mediated bi-directional trafficking and functional regulation of the human dopamine transporter. Synapse 1998;30:79–87.

85. Melikian HE, Buckley K. Membrane trafficking regulates the activity of the human dopamine transporter. J Neurosci 1999;19:7699–7710.

86. Saunders C, Ferrer JV, Shi L, Chen JX, Merrill G, Lamb ME, Leeb-Lundberg LMF, Carvelli L, Javitch JA, Galli A. Amphetamine-induced loss of human dopamine transporter activity: an internalization-dependent and cocaine-sensitive mechanism. Proc Natl Acad Sci USA 2000;97:6850–6855.

87. Callaghan PD, Daws LC, Kahlig K, Carvelli L, Moron J, Shippenberg S, Javitch JA, Galli A. Cocaine-evoked trafficking of the dopamine transporter causes a time-dependent increase in dopamine uptake. Soc Neurosci Abstr 2001;27:1866.

88. Miller KJ, Hoffman BJ. Adenosine A3 receptors regulate serotonin transport via nitric oxide and cGMP. J Biol Chem 1994;269:27351–27356.

89. Daws LC, Gerhardt GA, Frazer A. 5-HT1B antagonists modulate clearance of extracellular serotonin in rat hippocampus. Neurosci Lett 1999;266:165–168.

90. Daws LC, Gould GG, Teicher SD, Gerhardt GA, Frazer A. Serotonin 5-HT$_{1B}$ receptor-mediated regulation of serotonin clearance in rat hippocampus in vivo. J Neurochem 2000;75:2113–2122.

91. Daws LC, Montanez S, Gould GG, Owens WA, Frazer A, Murphy DL. Influence of genetic knockout (KO) of the serotonin transporter (5-HTT) on kinetics of 5-HT clearance and 5-HT1B receptor regulation of 5-HT clearance in vivo. Soc Neurosci Abstr 2001;27:2155.

92. Ramamoorthy S, Giovanetti E, Blakely RD. 5-HT modulated phosphorylation of the human serotonin transporter. Soc Neurosci Abstr 1997;23:1132.

93. Chang MY, Lee SH, Kim JH, Lee KH, Kim YS, Son H, Lee YS. Protein kinase C–mediated functional regulation of dopamine transport is not achieved by direct phosphorylation of the dopamine transporter protein. J Neurochem 2001;77:754–761.

94. Bauman AL, Apparsundaram S, Ramamoorthy S, Wadzinski VRA, Blakely RD. Cocaine- and antidepressant-sensitive biogenic amine transporters exist in regulated complexes with protein phosphatase 2A. J Neurosci 2000;20:7571–7578.

95. Mendelson SD, McKittrick CR, McEwen BS. Autoradiographic analyses of the effects of estradiol benzoate on [^{3}H]paroxetine binding in the cerebral cortex and dorsal hippocampus of gonadectomized male and female rats. Brain Res 1993;601:299–302.

96. Wakade AR, Wakade TD, Poosch M, Bannon MJ. Noradrenaline transport and transporter mRNA of rat chromaffin cells are controlled by dexamethasone and nerve growth factor. J Physiol (Lond) 1996;494:67–75.

97. Bosse R, Rivest R, Di Paolo T. Ovariectomy and estradiol treatment affect the dopamine transporter and its gene expression in the rat brain. Brain Res Mol Brain Res 1997;46:343–346.

98. Fumagalli F, Jones SR, Caron MG, Seidler FJ, Slotkin TA. Expression of mRNA coding for the serotonin transporter in aged vs. young rat brain: differential effects of glucocorticoids. Brain Res 1996;719:225–228.

99. Herbert MA, Larson GA, Zahniser NR, Gerhardt GA. Age-related reductions in [^{3}H]WIN 35,428 binding to the dopamine transporter in nigrostriatal and mesolimbic brain regions of the Fischer 344 rat. J Pharmacol Exp Ther 1999;288:1334–1339.

100. Klimek V, Stockmeier C, Overholser J, Meltzer HY, Kalka S, Dilley G, Ordway GA. Reduced levels of norepinephrine transporters in the locus coeruleus in major depression. J Neurosci 1997;17:8451–8458.

101. Owens MJ, Nemeroff CB. The serotonin transporter and depression. Depress Anxiety 1998;8(suppl 1):5–12.

102. Alvarez JC, Gluck N, Arnulf I, Quintin P, Leboyer M, Pecquery R, Launay JM, Perez-Diaz F, Spreux-Varoquaux O. Decreased platelet serotonin transporter sites and increased platelet inositol triphosphate levels in patients with unipolar depression: effects of clomipramine and fluoxetine. Clin Pharmacol Ther 1999;66:617–624.

103. Hoffman BJ, Hansson SR, Mezey E, Palkovits M. Localization and dynamic regulation of biogenic amine transporters in the mammalian central nervous system. Front Neuroendocrinol 1998;19:187–231.

104. Mongeau R, Blier P, deMontigny C. The serotonergic and noradrenergic systems of the hippocampus: their interactions and the effects of antidepressant treatment. Brain Res Rev 1997;23:145–195.

105. Zhu M, Blakely RD, Apparsundaram S, Ordway GA. Down-regulation of the human norepinephrine trans-

porter in intact 293-hNET cells exposed to desipramine. J Neurochem 1998;70:1547–1555.

106. Shores MM, Szot P, Veith RC. Desipramine-induced increase in norepinephrine transporter mRNA is not mediated via α2 receptors. Brain Res Mol 1994;27:337–341.

107. Benmansour S, Cecchi M, Morilak DA, Gerhardt GA, Javors MA, Gould GG, Frazer A. Effects of chronic antidepressant treatments on serotonin transporter function, density, and mRNA level. J Neurosci 1999;19:10494–10501.

108. Pineyro G, Blier P, Dennis T, De Montigny C. Desensitization of the neuronal 5-HT carrier following its long-term blockade. J Neurosci 1994;14:3036–3047.

109. Benmansour S, Owens WA, Cecchi M, Morilak DA, Frazer A. Onset of sertraline induced down regulation of the SERT and time course of recovery of the SERT. Soc Neurosci Abstr 2001;27:584.

110. Jones SR, Gainetdinov RR, Wightman RM. Mechanisms of amphetamine action revealed in mice lacking the dopamine transporter. J Neurosci 1998;18:1979–1986.

111. Xu F, Gainetdinov RR, Wetsel WC, Jones SR, Bohn LM, Miller GW, Wang Y-M, Caron MG. Mice lacking the norepinephrine transporter are supersensitive to psychostimulants. Nat Neurosci 2000;3:465–471.

112. Gründermann D, Schmig E. Gene structures of the human non-neuronal monoamine transporters EMT and OCT2. Hum Genet 2000;106:627–635.

113. Li Z, Chen JX, Murphy DL, Pan H, Koepsell H, Gershon MD. Expression and distribution of transporters (SERT, DAT and OCTS 1, 2, and 3) able to mediate 5-HT uptake in the bowel: analysis in single and double knockout mice lacking the SERT and/or DAT. Soc Neurosci Abstr 2000;26:399.

114. Bengel D, Murphy DL, Andrews AM, Wichems CH, Feltner D, Heils A, Mossner R, Westphal H, Lesch K-P. Altered brain serotonin homeostasis and locomotor insensitivity to 3,4-methylenedioxymethamphetamine ("ecstasy") in serotonin transporter-deficient mice. Mol Pharmacol 1998;53:649–655.

115. Lesch K-P, Bengel D, Heils A, Sabol SZ, Greenberg BD, Petri S, Benjamin J, Muller CR, Hamer DH, Murphy DL. Association of anxiety-related traits with a polymorphism in the serotonin transporter gene regulatory region. Science 1996;274:1527–1531.

116. Furlong RA, Ho L, Walsh C, Rubinsztein JS, Jain S, Paykel ES, Easton DF, Rubinsztein DC. Analysis and meta-analysis of two serotonin transporter gene polymorphisms in bipolar and unipolar affective disorders. Am J Med Genet 1998;81:58–63.

117. Smeraldi E, Zanardi R, Benedetti F, Di Bella D, Perez J, Catalano M. Polymorphism within the promoter of the serotonin transporter gene and antidepressant efficacy of fluvoxamine. Mol Psychiatry 1998;3:508–511.

118. Pollock BG, Ferrell RE, Mulstant BH, Mazumdar S, Miller M, Sweet RA, Davis S, Kirshner MA, Houck PR, Stack J, Reynolds CF, Kupfer DJ. Allelic variation of the serotonin transporter promoter affects onset of paroxetine treatment in response to late-life depression. Neuropsychopharmacology 2000;23:587–590.

119. Lundberg JM, Hokfelt T. Coexistence of peptides and classical neurotransmitters. Trends Neurosci 1983;6:325–333.

120. Hokfelt T, Broberger C, Xu Z-QD, Sergeyev V, Ubink R, Diez M. Neuropeptides—An overview. Neuropharmacology 2000;39:1337–1356.

121. Bartfai T, Iverfeldt K, Fisone G, Serfozo P. Regulation of the release of coexisting neurotransmitters. Annu Rev Pharmacol Toxicol 1988;28:285–310.

122. Han W, Ng Y-K, Axelrod D, Levitan ES. Neuropeptide release by efficient recruitment of diffusing cytoplasmic secretory vesicles. Proc Natl Acad Sci USA 1999;96:14577–14582.

123. Lundberg JM, Rudehill A, Sollevi A, Theodorsson-Norheim E, Hamberger B. Frequency- and reserpine-dependent chemical coding of sympathetic transmission: differential release of noradrenaline and neuropeptide Y from pig spleen. Neurosci Lett 1986;63:96–100.

124. Konkoy CS, Davis TP. Ectoenzymes as sites of peptide regulation. Trends Pharmacol Sci 1996;17:288–294.

125. Zoli M, Jansson A, Sykova E, Agnati LF, Fuxe K. Volume transmission in the CNS and its relevance for neuropsychopharmacology. Trends Pharmacol Sci 1999;20:142–150.

126. Bloom FE. The functional significance of neurotransmitter diversity. Am J Physiol 1984;246:C184-C194.

127. Nusbaum MP, Bllitz DM, Swensen AM, Wood D, Marder E. The roles of co-transmission in neural network modulation. Trends Neurosci 2001;24:146–154.

128. Hokfelt TGM, Castel M-N, Morino P, Zhang X, Dagerlind A. General overview of neuropeptides. In: Bloom FE, Kupfer DJ, ed. Psychopharmacology: The Fourth Generation of Progress. New York: Raven Press, 1995:483–492.

129. Arborelius L, Owens MJ, Plotsky PM, Nemeroff CB. The role of corticotropin-releasing factor in depression and anxiety disorders. J Endocrinol 1999;160:1–12.

130. Heilig M, Widerlov E. Neurobiology and clinical aspects of neuropeptide Y. Crit Rev Neurobiol 1995;9:115–136.

131. Rupniak NMJ, Kramer MS. Discovery of the antidepressant and anti-emetic efficacy of substance P receptor (NK$_1$) antagonists. Trends Pharmacol Sci 1999;20:485–490.

132. Stout SC, Owens MJ, Nemeroff CB. Neurokinin1 receptor antagonists as potential antidepressants. Annu Rev Pharmacol Toxicol 2001;41:877–906.

133. Wrenn CC, Crawley JN. Pharmacological evidence supporting a role for galanin in cognition and affect.

134. Mantyh PW, Hunt SP, Maggio JE. Substance P receptors: localization by light microscopic autoradiography in rat brain using [³H]SP as the radioligand. Brain Res 1984;307:147–165.
135. Baker KG, Halliday GM, Hornung JP, Geffen LB, Cotton RG, Tork I. Distribution, morphology and number of monoamine-synthesizing and substance P–containing neurons in the human dorsal raphe nucleus. Neurosci. 1991;42:757–775.
136. Hadjerri N, Blier P. Effect of neurokinin-I receptor antagonists on the function of 5-HT and noradrenaline neurons. Neuroreport 2000;11:1323–1327.
137. Kramer MS, Cutler N, Feighner J, Shrivastava R, Carman J, Sramek JJ, Reines SA, Liu G, Snavely D, Wyatt-Knowles E, Hale JJ, Mills SG, MacCoss M, Swain CJ, Harrison T, Hill RG, Hefti F, Scolnick EM, Cascieri MA, Chicchi GG, Sadowski S, Williams AR, Hewson L, Smith D, Carlson EJ, Hargreaves RJ, Rupniak NMJ. Distinct mechanism for antidepressant activity by blockade of central substance P receptors. Science 1998;281:1640–1645.
138. Rupniak NM, Carlson EC, Harrison T, Oates B, Seward E, Owen S, De Felipe C, Hunt SP, Wheeldon A. Pharmacological blockade or genetic deletion of substance P (NK(1)) receptors attenuates neonatal vocalisation in guinea-pigs and mice. Neuropharmacology 2000;39:1413–1421.
139. Melander T, Hokfelt T, Rokaeus A, Cuello AC, Oertel WH, Verhofstad A, Goldstein M. Coexistence of galanin-like immunoreactivity with catecholamines, 5-hydroxytryptamine, GABA and neuropeptides in the rat CNS. J Neurosci 1986;6:3640–3654.
140. Sawchenko PE, Swanson LW, Grzanna R, Howe PRC, Bloom SR, Polak JM. Colocalization of neuropeptide Y immunoreactivity in brainstem catecholaminergic neurons that project to the paraventricular nucleus of the hypothalamus. J Comp Neurol 1985;241:138–153.
141. Walker DL, Davis M. Double dissociation between the involvement of the bed nucleus of the stria terminalis and the central nucleus of the amygdala in startle increases produced by conditioned versus unconditioned fear. J Neurosci 1997;17:9375–9383.
142. Cecchi M, Khoshbouei H, Helesic G, Morilak DA. Stress-induced norepinephrine release in lateral bed nucleus of the stria terminalis modulates anxiety and ACTH secretion through α_1 adrenergic receptors. Soc. Neurosci. Abstr. 2000;26:29.
143. Cecchi M, Khoshbouei H, Morilak DA. Norepinephrine release in the lateral bed nucleus of the stria terminalis facilitates behavioral and neuroendocrine components of the acute response to stress. Neurosci (in press).
144. Aston-Jones G, Rajkowski J, Kubiak P, Alexinsky T. Locus coeruleus neurons in monkey are selectively activated by attended cues in a vigilance task. J Neurosci 1994;14:4467–4480.
145. Charney DS, Woods SW, Goodman WK, Heninger GR. Neurobiological mechanisms of panic anxiety: biochemical and behavioral correlates of yohimbine-induced panic attacks. Am J Psychiatry 1987;144:1030–1036.
146. Jacobs BL, Abercrombie ED, Fornal CA, Levine ES, Morilak DA, Stafford IL. Single-unit and physiological analyses of brain norepinephrine function in behaving animals. Prog. Brain Res 1991;88:159–165.
147. Heilig M, Koob GF, Ekman R, Britton KB. Corticotropin-releasing factor and neuropeptide Y: role in emotional integration. Trends Neurosci 1994;17:80–85.
148. Sajdyk TJ, Vandergriff MG, Gehlert DR. Amygdalar neuropeptide Y Y_1 receptors mediate the anxiolytic-like effects of neuropeptide Y in the social interaction test. Eur J Pharmacol 1999;368:143–147.
149. Kask A, Rago L, Harro J. Anxiogenic-like effect of the NPY Y_1 receptor antagonist BIBP3226 administered into the dorsal periaqueductal gray matter in rats. Regul Pept 1998;75–76:255–262.
150. Martire M, Pistritto G, Mores N, Agnati LF, Fuxe K. Region-specific inhibition of potassium-evoked [³H]noradrenaline release from rat brain synaptosomes by neuropeptide Y-(13–36). Involvement of NPY receptors of the Y_2 type. Eur J Pharmacol 1993;230:231–234.
151. Tsuda K, Yokoo H, Goldstein M. Neuropeptide Y and galanin in norepinephrine release in hypothalamic slices. Hypertension 1989;14:81–86.
152. Illes P, Finta EP, Nieber K. Neuropeptide Y potentiates via Y2-receptors the inhibitory effect of noradrenaline in rat locus coeruleus neurones. Naunyn Schmied Arch Pharmacol 1993;348:546–548.
153. Kask A, Rago L, Harro J. Anxiolytic-like effects of neuropeptide Y (NPY) and NPY$_{13-36}$ microinjected into vicinity of locus coeruleus in rats. Brain Res 1998;788:345–348.
154. Pieribone VA, Xu ZQ, Zhang X, Grillner S, Bartfai T, Hokfelt T. Galanin induces a hyperpolarization of norepinephrine-containing locus coeruleus neurons in the brainstem slice. Neurosci 1995;64:861–874.
155. Seutin V, Verbanck P, Massotte L, Dresse A. Galanin decreases the activity of locus coeruleus neurons in vitro. Eur J Pharmacol 1989;164:373–376.
156. Khoshbouei H, Cecchi M, Javors M, Morilak DA. Behavioral reactivity to stress: amplification of stress-induced noradrenergic activation elicits a galanin-mediated anxiolytic effect in central amygdala. Pharmacol Biochem Behav 2002;71:407–417.
157. Khoshbouei H, Cecchi M, Morilak DA. Modulatory effects of galanin in the lateral bed nucleus of the stria terminalis on stress-induced behavioral reactivity and ACTH secretion. Soc Neurosci Abstr 2001;27:850.

158. Khoshbouei H, Cecchi M, Morilak DA. Amplifying noradrenergic activation by stress elicits a galanin-mediated anxiolytic response in central amygdala opposing the anxiogenic effects of norepinephrine. Soc Neurosci Abstr 2000;26:1154.
159. Khoshbouei H, Cecchi M, Morilak DA. Modulatory effects of galanin in the lateral bed nucleus of the stria terminalis on behavioral and neuroendocrine responses to acute stress. Neuropsychopharmacology, 2001 (in press).
160. Kozicz T. Synaptic interactions between galanin and axon terminals immunopositive for tyrosine hydroxylase and dopamine β-hydroxylase in the bed nucleus of the stria terminalis in the rat. Soc Neurosci Abstr 1999;25:2220.

4

Developments in Psychiatric Neuroimaging

ROBERTO B. SASSI
Western Psychiatric Institute and Clinic, University of Pittsburgh School of Medicine, Pittsburgh, Pennsylvania, U.S.A.

JAIR C. SOARES
University of Texas Health Science Center at San Antonio, San Antonio, Texas, U.S.A.

I. INTRODUCTION

The scientific inquiry into the human mind seeks to decode how brain structure and activity result in the vast range of cognitive and emotional processes each of us experiences. It also attempts to identify the anatomical and functional correlates of abnormal mental activity, as represented in the neurological and psychiatric disorders. In this perspective, neuroimaging has effected a radical change on the study of the connection between brain and mind.

Early investigations of brain function had to depend on indirect approaches. Lesion experiments on animals and postmortem clinicopathological correlations were the usual methods to investigate cerebral function, with obvious limitations. It was only at the end of the 18th century that the idea that different structures of the nervous system could perform distinct functions began to predominate. During the 19th century, the notion of functionally distinct cortical areas became well established, initially with the controversial works of Gall and the Phrenology school, and later with the discovery of the association of frontal cortex lesion and aphasia by Paul Broca [1]. Afterward, the conceptualization of the neuron, the discovery of specific cytoarchitectonics of different cortical areas, and the electrophysiological experiments on animal and later human cortex have set up the theory of cortical localization of mental functions as the mainstream scientific framework for brain investigation. Event-related potentials and single-neuron recording, 50 years ago, provided further experimental support for cortical localization. But it was only in the early 1970s, with the advent of X-ray computed axial tomography (CT), that it was possible to visualize the brain parenchyma in vivo [2]. Since then, the field of neuroimaging has undergone astonishing developments, and these new methods have rapidly become the most powerful tools to contribute to the understanding of neural organization and mechanisms underlying the mental phenomenon.

The present chapter does not intend to be an exhaustive review of the various neuroimaging techniques currently in use. The specific findings of neuroimaging studies in various psychiatric disorders will be presented in other sections of this book. In this chapter, we have focused on the imaging methods of highest relevance for investigations of the neural basis of behavior, providing an overview of the physiological rationale underlying each method. Each available method assesses a specific feature of the intricate cerebral machinery, with its typical resolution on the spatial and temporal domains, and characteristic methodological limitations. For didactical reasons, we grouped the various techniques into three groups: structural neuroimaging, including the methods designed to explore brain anatomy and structure; chemical neuroimaging, for the methods dedicated to evaluate cell metabolites, neurotransmitters, and receptors in the brain; and functional neuroimaging, encompassing the techniques that evaluate cerebral perfusion, metabolism, and neuronal activation.

II. STRUCTURAL NEUROIMAGING

Before the first CT studies, only highly invasive radiological approaches could be utilized to evaluate brain structural abnormalities in human subjects. Pneumoencephalography, which consisted of an X-ray after air injection into the encephalon through a lumbar puncture, was utilized during the first half of the 20th century to examine the ventricular system. This technique has provided the first in vivo indications of enlarged ventricles and cortical atrophy on schizophrenic patients [3]. The advent of CT yielded a booming interest on structural neuroimaging of psychiatric disorders. Measurements of ventricular dilatation and cortical and cerebellar atrophy could then be performed in several psychiatric disorders [4]. But the evaluation of specific brain structures was still challenging, due to the limited contrast between gray and white matter observed in the CT images. Also, artifacts on the posterior fossa were relatively common owing to dense bone structures surrounding this region, which made brainstem and cerebellum more difficult to evaluate with CT scans. Most of the shortcomings in the earlier structural brain imaging studies were overcome with the advent of magnetic resonance imaging (MRI).

The first commercially available MRI scans appeared in the early 1980s, but the phenomenon of nuclear magnetic resonance has been under study since the 1930s, through the landmark works of the American physicist Isaac Rabi [5], who received the Nobel Prize in physics in 1944. Structural MRI is one of the several brain-imaging technologies that explore the magnetic properties of the atomic nucleus. The MR method is based on the property of some atoms, whose nuclei present an odd number of either protons or neurons, to posses "spin"—i.e., a net magnetic charge, like a small bar magnet. Only the atoms that have this property will be "visible" through nuclear magnetic resonance (NMR). Some biologically relevant examples include ^{1}H, ^{31}P, and ^{23}Na. Also, ^{7}Li and ^{19}F can be detected using NMR. Although present in negligible concentrations in the human brain, these atoms have important pharmacological relevance. On the other hand, atoms such as ^{12}C and ^{16}O are invisible to NMR.

The atoms visible to NMR present a random distribution of the orientation of their nuclear magnetic moment when no external magnetic field is applied. However, when under an external magnetic field (B_0), the nuclei of these atoms tend to align with this field, in the same (lower energy) or the opposite direction (higher energy) (see **Fig. 1**). This is the first step in the acquisition of MR images: to immerse the brain in a strong magnetic field, usually ~ 0.5–3 Tesla. For comparison, 1 Tesla is $\sim 20,000$ times the Earth's magnetic field. Under the action of the magnetic field, the nuclei will spin and generate a movement of precession (see **Fig. 2**), whose frequency is characteristic for each

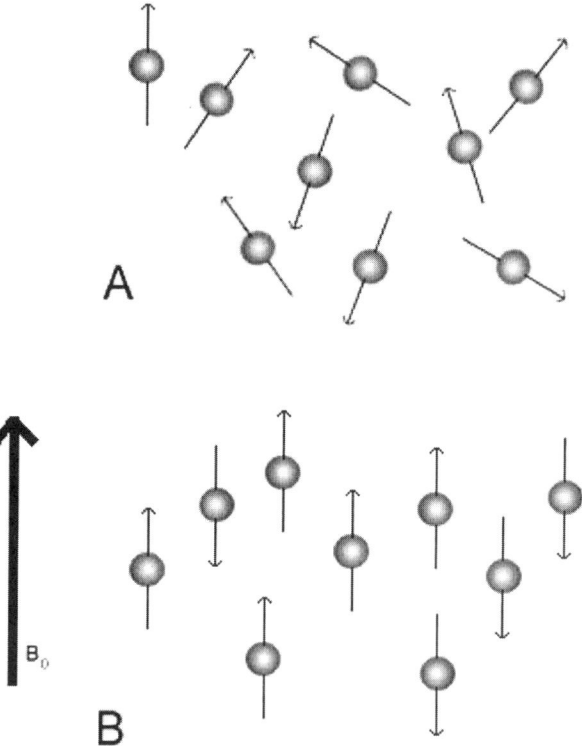

Figure 1 The nuclei of the individual atoms have a random distribution of their magnetic moment (A), with no net direction. When an external magnetic field B_0 is applied (B), all spins align either against or on the same direction of the field.

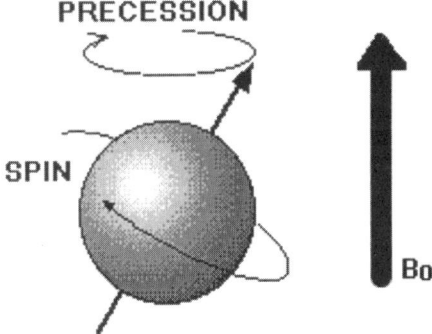

Figure 2 Spinning and precession.

atomic nucleus, and is proportional to B_0 strength. The next step is to expose these nuclei to a short-duration electromagnetic field (B_1, orthogonal to B_0), usually in the radio frequency range. This pulse excites the nuclei, disturbing the previous equilibrium state and inducing a transient phase coherence among the nuclei. This resonance can then be detected as a radio signal through a receiver coil. After turning off B_1, all nuclei return to equilibrium, i.e., from high-energy (excited) to low-energy (equilibrium) state. This process is associated with exponential loss of energy to surrounding nuclei; the time required for the magnetization to return to 63% of its original value is called T1. Since the process is exponential, the spins are usually completely relaxed after 3–5 T1 times. When returning to equilibrium, spins with high and low energy can also exchange energy without loosing it to surrounding nuclei. This phenomenon is termed spin-spin relaxation, and it is related to exponential loss in the transverse magnetization. Similarly, the time required for 63% of transverse magnetization to subside is called T2. For pure water, T1 and T2 are practically the same, around 2–3 secs. However, for most biological materials T2 is far shorter than T1. By varying parameters such as the repetition time or echo time of the radio-frequency signal, it is possible to acquire T1- or T2-weighted images, and consequently obtain distinct information from the biological tissues under analysis. Of course, this is a very simplified explanation of the mechanisms underlying the NMR phenomenon. Nonetheless, it is important to keep in mind that NMR can provide a varied range of information in a noninvasive fashion, from hemodynamics to cell chemistry. In the case of MRI, the resonance of large amounts of ^{1}H in the brain provides high-quality structural image, with spatial resolution of < 1 mm^3, allowing the identification of small brain structures.

Most morphometric studies with MRI utilize an approach known as region of interest (ROI). Basically, the area of a specific brain structure is manually "traced" directly in the image, and the final volume is estimated from the number of slices that intersect the structure under study (see **Fig. 3**). Usually this is done in a blind fashion; i.e., the researcher is not aware of the diagnosis of the subject whose brain MRI is being evaluated. Standardized protocols defining the boundaries of the structure are utilized, which enables reliable reproduction of these methods among different researchers. In some cases, semiautomated procedures can be used to detect the border of particular brain structures, or to derive three-dimensional volumes from the tracings. Also, algorithms are used to segment the brain into gray and white matter and CSF, allowing more specific measurements. ROI-based morphometry has provided extremely important contributions over the past several years, allowing the study of relationship between structural anatomy and psychopathology.

However, this method presents some limitations. Certain arbitrariness is necessary to set the boundaries of structures that do not have well-defined edges. Another limitation of ROI-based analysis is that struc-

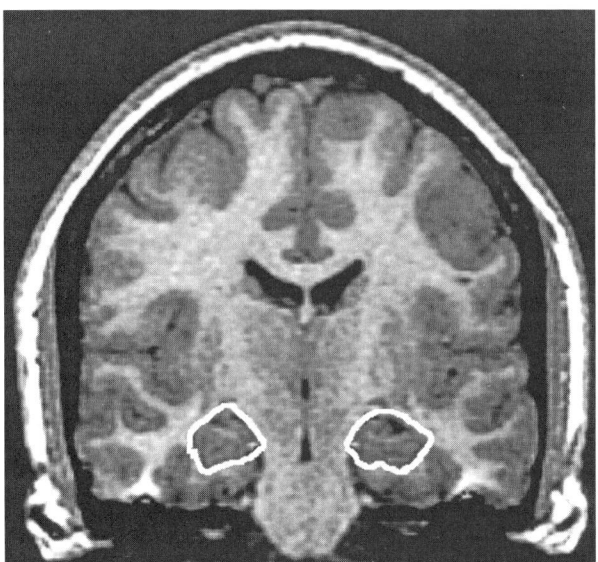

Figure 3 Example of a structural MRI, with the hippocampus traced bilaterally in a coronal slice. In the region-of-interest analysis, an anatomical structure is usually traced in several slices, and the volume is derived from the sum of the areas multiplied by the slice thickness. For the hippocampus, semiautomated procedures are utilized to include in the analysis only the pixels identified as gray matter.

tures with different shapes can have the same volume. Thus, if the shape of an anatomical structure is different between patients and controls, but with similar final volumes, no differences between the groups will be detected. As an attempt to minimize these shortcomings, new experimental designs have been developed. For instance, it is possible to compare the content of gray matter between two groups of subjects in a voxel-by-voxel basis. Voxel is the three-dimensional graphic unit of an MR image, and through a specific mathematical approach, it is possible to examine the whole brain and identify areas that present a lower density of gray matter (voxel-based morphometry), or to compare the relative position (deformation-based morphometry), or local shape (tensor-based morphometry) of certain brain structures among different groups [6]. These statistical parametric methods have been used for functional data, and now are being validated for structural neuroimaging studies.

Nonetheless, a basic shortcoming underlies most of these morphometric methods: the links between the volume of a specific structure and the pathophysiology are still tentative. Data from other neuroimaging methodologies should be considered together to provide a better insight into the relevance of a volumetric finding. The cellular abnormalities underlying an atrophic cortex, for instance, can only be assessed directly through postmortem studies, or indirectly with MR spectroscopy (see below). Also, brain areas that are dysfunctional, but that maintain the same final volume and gray matter density of a healthy structure, will not be identified with morphometric studies, only with functional neuroimaging approaches. Moreover, typical MR images have a limited capacity to discriminate distinct white matter tracts. A very interesting and complementary morphometric approach, diffusion tensor imaging (DTI), has provided new possibilities to examine white-matter fibers. This MR methodology is based on the fact that water molecules inside axons have restricted diffusion; i.e., they diffuse faster in the direction of the axonal fibers than perpendicular to them. This property can be used to map white-matter tracts in vivo, and study the integrity of the connections among different brain areas [7].

The clinical application of MRI in psychiatry is limited, in most cases, to rule out neurologic abnormalities that might be responsible for the psychiatric symptoms, such as stroke or brain tumors. Even with the vast advances in structural neuroimaging observed in recent decades, it is still not possible to individually identify subjects with psychiatric disorders based on brain imaging. Typically, there is a considerable overlap among the structural measurements of patients and healthy controls, even when the patients, as a group, present a statistically significant difference from the control group. Nevertheless, anatomical abnormalities identified with structural neuroimaging studies are helping to develop, in parallel with other neuroimaging approaches, integrated models of pathophysiology of mental disorders.

III. CHEMICAL NEUROIMAGING

Abnormalities in the signaling among neurons have been implied in virtually every neurobiological model for psychiatric disorders. The mechanism of action of drugs with profound effects on behavior, such as antidepressants and antipsychotics, has supported the idea of an imbalance in specific neurotransmitter systems in mental illnesses, e.g., the dopamine hypothesis in schizophrenia, and the monoaminergic theories in depression. However, most of the studies on neurotransmitter functioning were restricted to postmortem brain tissue or peripheral blood cells. This picture has changed drastically with the advent of positron emission tomography (PET) and single-photon emission computed tomography (SPECT). These techniques can provide in vivo anatomically localized information about several parameters of neural transmission, metabolism, and pharmacology.

PET and SPECT are imaging techniques that can quantify and localize biologically relevant molecules, marked with a radionuclide. The brain uptake of the molecule of interest can be ascertained by measuring the amount of the radiotracer in each specific brain region. PET and SPECT are based on different properties of radioactive decay. Basically, in PET the radiotracer decays emitting a positron, which collides with an adjacent electron. This leads to the annihilation of both particles and to the release of two gamma rays (photons) which exact opposite directions [8]. The radiation detector surrounding the brain can detect this coincident emission (see **Fig. 4**). A computer registers that the marked molecule was present at some point along this imaginary line, and later rebuilt a three-dimensional map of the amount of radiotracer for the whole brain. On the other hand, in SPECT, the radiotracer absorbs an electron when decaying, which results in an unstable nucleus that emits a single gamma-photon in this process [8]. The detector, also called *collimator*, rotates 360° around the subject's head, and later translates this information into a picture of the distribution of the radionuclide in the brain

Developments in Psychiatric Neuroimaging

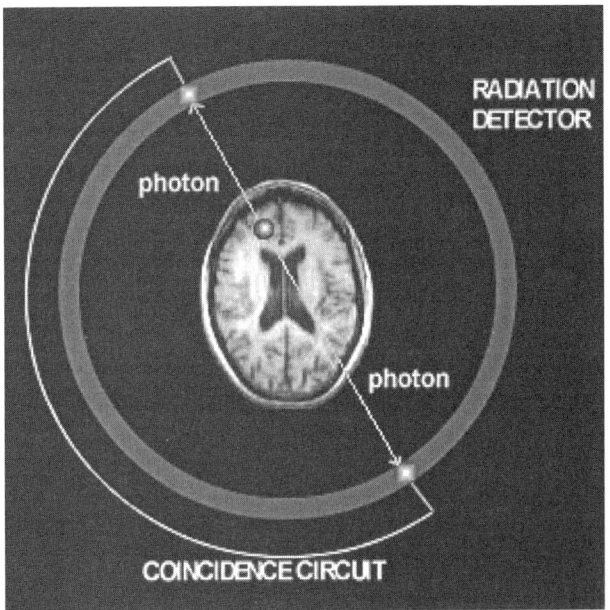

Figure 4 Schematic representation of a PET scanner.

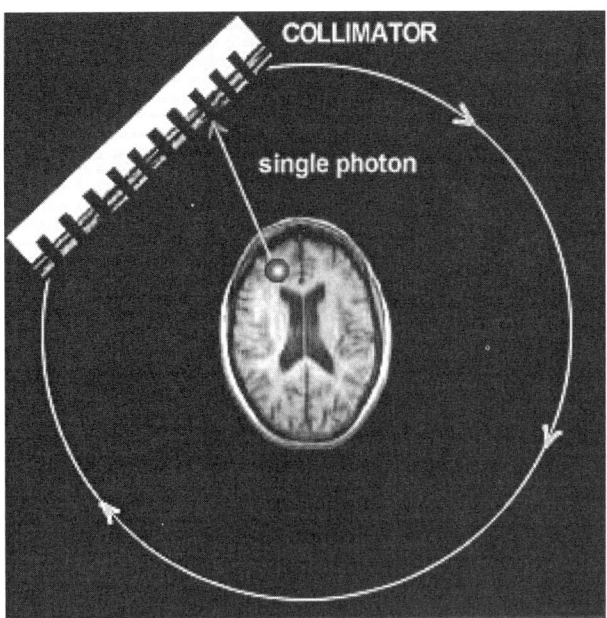

Figure 5 Schematic representation of a SPECT scanner.

(Fig. 5). Owing to these differences in the physical principles, PET and SPECT utilize radiotracers with distinct intrinsic properties, with PET usually providing better spatial resolution than SPECT.

Several aspects of in vivo neurochemical functioning can be assessed with either PET or SPECT. Numerous radiotracers have been developed to identify specific targets in the brain, including neurotransmitter synthesis and release, receptor occupancy and density, monoamine transporters and metabolism [9–11]. Dopaminergic, serotonergic, GABAergic (see **Fig. 6**), opioid, and cholinergic pathways have been studied through PET and SPECT radiotracers in several neuropsychiatric disorders; extensive reviews of available findings can be found elsewhere [12]. Also, PET and SPECT receptor studies have proven informative about the in vivo brain actions of several medications during clinical treatment. For instance, typical and atypical antipsychotics present a distinct pattern of occupancy of dopaminergic and serotonergic receptor subtypes [13,14]. These studies are particularly relevant to the investigation of links between side effects and response to treatment and receptor occupancy, and can aid in the development of new drugs.

Although the amount of radiation in the radiotracers currently utilized for research is minimal, the utilization of radioactivity represents a disadvantage of PET and SPECT techniques, since it limits the number of sessions in which a subject can participate. Better spatial resolution and a greater diversity of available radiotracers make PET a more attractive methodology than SPECT for in vivo brain investigations in neuropsychiatry. However, PET radioligands typically have very short half-lives, so a cyclotron located near the PET scanner is required to the production of these tracers. This makes PET scan a very expensive technology: about US$5 million is necessary to install a PET center, not including the costs related to the extremely specialized and multidisciplinary staff [15]. Since SPECT costs a fraction of PET, and is more widely available, it is expected that improvements in tracer development and technical complexity will result in further advances of SPECT studies in psychiatry.

Measures of brain chemistry can also be obtained through the phenomenon of nuclear magnetic resonance. As stated in the previous section, several different atoms have nuclei with magnetic moment and can therefore be visualized through NMR. For instance, in MRI the images are formed through the resonance of huge amounts of ^1H atoms in water and fat. However, ^1H is also present in several other metabolites, and the resonance frequency of hydrogen is different depending on the molecule it is found. This occurs because nuclear resonance frequency is influenced by the magnetic fields of the nearby electrons and nuclei; i.e., the molecular environment of a certain nucleus produces a resonance frequency for this nucleus that is slightly different than the resonance of the nucleus alone.

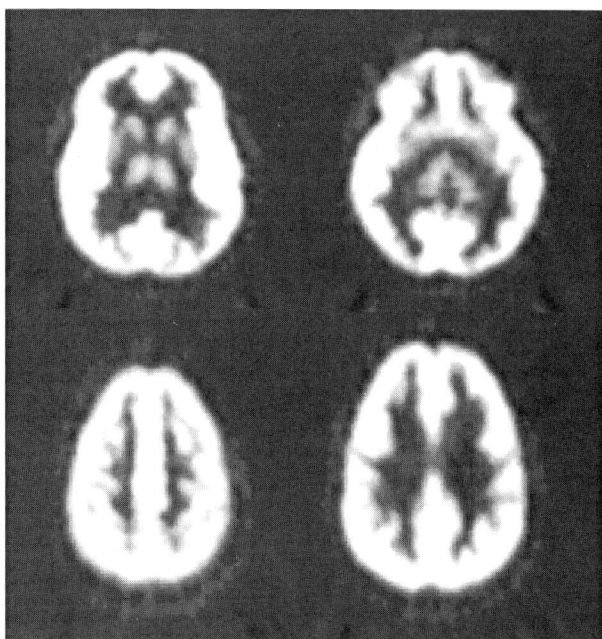

Figure 6 PET scan image showing the brain distribution of GABA A / benzodiazepine receptors using the radiotracer [11C]-Flumazenil. Brighter areas indicate higher concentration of the tracer, and higher receptor densities.

This resonance is characteristic of each molecule, and can be represented in a scale called *chemical shift*, expressed in parts per million (ppm). For instance, the protons in water and fat exhibit two different frequencies, separated by approximately 3.5 ppm [16].

Several different ^{1}H-containing molecules will result in a spectrum of frequencies. This is the principle of magnetic resonance spectroscopy (MRS), a technique that has been used for decades in chemistry and physics to provide information about molecular structure and dynamics [17], and more recently has been employed in the study of in vivo brain chemistry. Given that different nuclei such as ^{1}H, ^{31}P, ^{23}Na, ^{13}C, ^{7}Li, and ^{19}F can be visualized in MRS, this technique allows measurements of molecules containing these nuclei in a noninvasive fashion, and without using radiation.

Since the concentration of most metabolites of interest in the brain is ~10,000 times smaller than the concentration of water, the signal of these metabolites is much weaker. Therefore, MRS studies usually exchange spatial resolution for chemical information. Although MRS procedures are evolving toward improvements on spatial resolution, most studies still utilize a volume-of-interest (VOI) approach; i.e., voxels usually ranging from 1 to 8 mL are placed in relevant anatomical locations, and a spectrum is acquired from each VOI. A spectrum is a plot of intensity versus frequency, with each peak representing a different resonance frequency, i.e., different metabolites, whose concentrations can be estimated from the area under the peaks (see **Fig. 7**).

A varied range of chemical information relevant to research in psychiatry can be acquired from the in vivo brain with MRS [18]:

1. ^{31}P MRS studies enable measurement of pH, inorganic P, adenosine diphosphate (ADP) and triphosphate (ATP), phosphocreatine (PCr), phosphomonoesters, and phosphodiesters. Thus, information on cell membrane integrity and high-energy phosphate metabolism can be obtained.

2. ^{1}H MRS can quantify metabolites involved in neurotransmission (glutamate and choline), energy metabolism (PCr, creatine, lactate, and acetate), second messenger systems (myoinositol), membrane metabolism (phosphocholine and phosphoethanolamine), and neuronal viability (N-acetyl aspartate).

3. Pharmacokinetic and pharmacodynamic data can be obtained through ^{7}Li (brain lithium concentra-

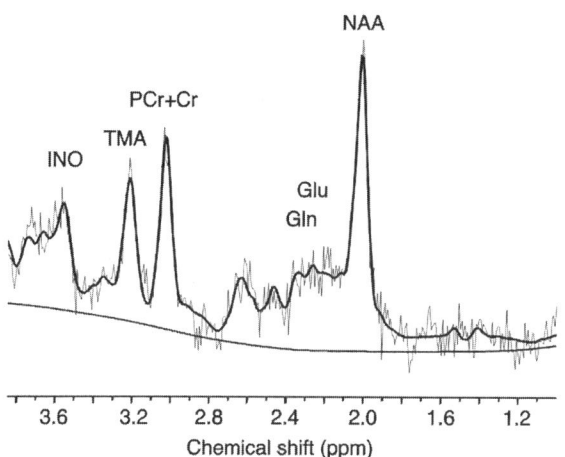

Figure 7 After the processing of the raw MRS data, a mathematical model allows the identification of the peaks corresponding to the ^{1}H resonance frequencies in each distinct molecule. The concentration of each metabolite is then derived from the area under the respective peak. In ^{1}H MRS, the resonance signal of water is suppressed to permit the quantification of other ^{1}H-containing metabolites. The most important metabolites assessed with ^{1}H-MRS are: N-acetyl aspartate (NAA), phosphocreatine + creatine (PCr + Cr), trimethylamines (TMA; commonly referred to as choline containing molecules, which mainly includes phosphorylcholine and glycerophosphocholine), myoinositol (INO), glutamate (Glu), and glutamine (Gln).

tion and distribution, and its correlation with outcome/side effects) and ^{19}F MRS (measurement of the brain concentration of fluorinated compounds, such as fluoxetine and fluphenazine).

4. Glucose metabolism and its relation with the glutamate/GABA cycle can be assessed with ^{13}C MRS [19].

Thus, MRS provides noninvasive measurements of a variety of chemical species *in vivo*, and has the potential to bring important contributions for the investigation of brain chemistry in neuropsychiatric disorders. However, the current MRS methodology still presents significant limitations. MRS signals are weaker than those used by MRI, and the proper acquisition of the spectrum generally requires relatively large voxel sizes (poor spatial resolution) and long acquisition times (poor temporal resolution). Also, several compounds are not MRS visible, even when containing MRS-visible nuclei, owing to intrinsic molecular dynamics. Nonetheless, the ability to provide unique neurochemical information not accessible through other brain-imaging methodologies makes MRS an important tool in psychiatric research, and it is expected that future technical improvements will likely overcome some of the current shortcomings.

Another technique that makes use of the phenomenon of NMR to obtain neurochemical information is the magnetization transfer imaging (MTI). As MRS, this novel MR methodology utilizes the same magnets used to obtain structural MR images. While MRI explores the resonance of ^{1}H in free water to produce brain images, MTI identifies the resonance of protons that are bound to macromolecular structures, such as myelin, and therefore less mobile. The integrity of these macromolecular structures can be assessed through the exchange of magnetization between bounded protons and free water, denominated magnetization transfer ratio (MTR). MTR appears to be a sensitive methodology to identify subtle white-matter abnormalities that do not involve gross loss of volume, or an obvious focal lesion, and therefore are not detected on structural MRI [20]. Reductions in MTR have been reported in neurological conditions that involve white-matter lesions such as multiple sclerosis, and more recently this technique has also been applied to investigations in schizophrenia [21].

IV. FUNCTIONAL NEUROIMAGING

While structural and chemical brain imaging methodologies have remarkably bolstered our knowledge on the pathophysiological process involved in neuropsychiatric disorders, only functional neuroimaging can fully explore the temporal dynamics and regional neural activation underlying specific cognitive functions. Functional neuroimaging is at the forefront of scientific efforts to understand the mental phenomenon. Currently, this is the best method to evaluate the relationship between brain activation and a vast range of mental processes, from problem solving to consciousness. Based on the physiological rationale underlying the methods, we can divide the functional imaging technologies in two groups: those that evaluate an indirect measure of brain activation, such as regional blood flow and energy consumption, and those that directly assess the electrical and magnetical components of neural activity.

The connection between brain functioning and regional increases in blood flow was first proposed in the 19th century, but the scientific attention to this phenomenon had waxed and waned up to the 1950s, when the first measurements of regional blood flow with a diffusible radioactive tracer were made in animals (for a historical perspective of functional brain imaging, see Raichle [22]). Although the relationship of blood flow and neuronal activation is not fully understood, it is postulated that synaptic firing of a group of neurons results in a transient increase in the energetic demands of these cells, and in the local production of some metabolites that, eventually, will lead to local blood vessel response and consequent increased flow [23]. The spatial correlation between neural activation and hemodynamic changes is relatively precise, but the hemodynamic response is somewhat sluggish compared to the actual neuronal firing: blood flow begins to increase ~ 2 seconds after neuronal activation, reaching its peak ~ 5–7 sec [24]. Nonetheless, this robust physiological relationship was successfully explored initially through PET and SPECT methods, and more recently with functional MRI (fMRI).

Regional cerebral blood flow (rCBF) can be accurately and quickly measured with PET. Several radiotracers are available for these measurements, and $H_2^{15}O$ is the most widely used owing to, among other reasons, its short half-life (123 sec), which allows multiple repeat measurements in the same subject [15]. On the other hand, SPECT tracers only allow steady-state assessment of rCBF due to longer half-lives, with a relatively poorer spatial resolution when compared to PET [25]. However, the high costs involved in these procedures (particularly with PET) and the use of radioactive tracers represent relevant limitations to their use. These shortcomings are helping to establish fMRI as the favored technique for rCBF measurements. fMRI is based on the fact that the hemodynamic response to neural activation usually surpasses the local oxygen needs, resulting in higher amounts of oxygenated and lower amounts of deoxygenated hemoglobin when compared with other surrounding areas. Since deoxygenated hemoglobin has more distinct magnetic properties than oxygenated hemoglobin, it may be unambiguously identified through NMR. Thus, neural activation leads to an increased rCBF, which results in a decrease in the content of deoxyhemoglobin in this specific brain region that can be quickly measured by the MRI scanner. This effect is termed BOLD (blood oxygen level dependent), and represents the most common fMRI approach to study brain activation [26]. Like PET, fMRI has the ability to map brain activation in the order of a few seconds, but with the advantages of having better spatial resolution, and being less expensive, noninvasive, and safer (no radiation involved).

fMRI has extended the work initiated with PET, due to its unique qualities, and has now a pivotal role in the functional mapping of the brain. Currently, the most important framework for the design of functional studies and interpretation of data is derived from cognitive neuroscience. In particular, the most widely used strategy consists of dissecting a simple cognitive task to its basic subunits, and to subtract the pattern of brain activation observed during the task of interest from a control task. For instance, one can subtract the map of activation after seeing a happy face from the activation after seeing a neutral face, in order to exclude brain activation related to the visual system, representation of human faces, etc., thus obtaining the activation correlated only with the identification of the emotion of happiness [27]. This methodology permits one to outline, either spatially and/or temporally, neural circuits that are active during specific cognitive processes. Cognitive subtraction is a powerful tool to examine the living brain, but is subject to some criticism, and more integrative and connectionist methodological approaches are now being utilized to address aspects of the mental phenomena that theoretically present less functional segregation [28]. A large number of studies have reported abnormal rCBF at rest or task-related for a variety of psychiatric syndromes and symptoms. An examination of all these findings is beyond the scope of this chapter; reviews of rCBF studies in mental disorders can be found elsewhere [12,29].

Increase in regional blood flow to the brain is not the only indirect physiological measurement of neuronal activation. Increased consumption of glucose is usually bound to increased rCBF in discrete neuronal areas. In fact, the first studies with PET utilized labeled glucose (^{18}F-2-fluoro-2-deoxy-D-glucose, or FDG) to map neural activation. It soon became clear, however, that the long half-life of FDG (110 min) would not allow quick and repeated measurements of discrete cognitive tasks. Nonetheless, interesting task-related regional changes in brain glucose metabolism could be identified with PET studies [30]. The increased blood flow in active brain areas is also correlated with localized tiny increases in temperature. A noninvasive methodology to record thermal information of cortical areas (thermoencephaloscopy; TES) is under investigation, and can potentially be a useful tool for functional neuroimaging [31].

Nonetheless, all methodologies assessing secondary physiological responses to neural activation, such as blood flow or glucose consumption, experience a critical weakness: these methods are not able to unambiguously track the time course of neural events. Neuronal activation occurs within milliseconds, while secondary increases in blood flow and energy consumption happen within a few seconds. Only direct recordings of the electric currents and magnetic fields that accompany the synaptic firing can provide such precise temporal resolution. Neuroelectrical brain measurements are based on the fact that synchronous activation of anatomically localized neurons results in electrical current strong enough to be detected at the surface of the head. Noninvasive recording of this effect is done by placing electrodes on the scalp surface; the more electrodes, the better spatial resolution. In essence, two basic types of neuroelectrical recordings can be performed: electroencephalography (EEG), comprising the examination of brain spontaneous electrical activity, and event-related potentials (ERP), which involves techniques to extract the characteristics of electrical events that are time-related to specific sensory, motor, or cognitive events [32]. ERP studies represent an essential methodology to evaluate functional integrity of sensory systems; moreover, this methodology allowed the identification of electrical potentials that are not directly related to sensory stimuli. These "endogenous" ERPs, such as P300 [33], have played a critical role in the examination of temporal and anatomical sequencing of neural activation related to cognitive processes such as attention, stimuli perception, and memory [34,35].

However, EEG and ERP can not be considered imaging methods in the same way that PET and

MRI. Although exhibiting superb temporal resolution, traditional electrophysiological methods provide poor spatial detail, which limits substantially the anatomical localization of neural activation. The distortion of the electrical signal caused by surrounding brain tissue, skull, and scalp is one of the reasons that account for the lack of detailed anatomical information of EEG/ERPs. On the other hand, the recording of the tiny magnetic fields that result from neuronal electrical activity can potentially provide better spatial resolution, since magnetic fields are not affected by the tissues and fluids they need to cross over.

This technique, named magnetoencephalography (MEG), requires more specialized facilities than EEG, such as a magnetically shielded room, and superconducting technology to record the in vivo brain magnetic fields, but offers similar temporal resolution with improved spatial definition. However, even with MEG, the anatomical resolution of electromagnetical technologies is strikingly inferior to PET or fMRI. Also, electrical or magnetic activities from structures below the surface of the cerebral cortex are difficult to register. Recent methodological strategies have been developed to combine the outstanding anatomical resolution of MRI with the unrivaled temporal definition of EEG/MEG. Brain electrical activity mapping (BEAM), quantitative EEG, and high-density electrical mapping (involving even 256 electrodes) are some of the methodologies utilized to provide a topographical analysis of the EEG/ERP signal. Multichannel MEG and magnetic-evoked field (the magnetic representation of the ERPs) studies have focused in source localization of neural activity by deriving coordinate transformations that permit one to locate magnetic fields in three-dimensional MR images; this technique is called magnetic source imaging (MSI).

These combined functional imaging techniques have been utilized to establish presurgical functional maps for the treatment of pathologies such as brain neoplasms and epilepsy, and more recently have been applied to the characterization of information processing in psychiatric disorders [36,37].

A novel and promising functional technique that may potentially provide insight on both hemodynamic and electrophysiological components of neural response is known as optical imaging. Initially utilized only on exposed living brain cortex [38], optical imaging has evolved into a noninvasive technique capable of mapping brain activity in vivo by way of measuring changes in the properties of light as it crosses different brain tissues. A basic assumption in this approach is that neuronal firing leads to rapid changes in the optical characteristics of the brain region under activation [39]. Malonek and Grinvald have shown that localized changes in light *scattering* have a strong temporal association with cortical activation [40], whereas localized changes in light *absorption* appear to follow a temporal pattern strikingly similar to the slow hemodynamic response of neural activity [41]. Although the physiological mechanisms underlying these phenomena are not completely clear, it is believed that hemoglobin is the major factor responsible for photon absorption [42], while changes in light scattering may be directly related with alterations on the neural membrane potential [43].

Near-infrared spectroscopy (NIRS) is currently the most common form of noninvasive functional optical imaging [44], employing light of long wavelength that characteristically crosses farther through brain tissue than visible light. Investigations combining NIRS with fMRI, PET, and evoked-potential methodologies [39,45] have been validating NIRS and demonstrating its ability to evaluate in vivo changes in rCBF and neuronal activation in humans. Although the spatial resolution of NIRS is still limited [44], it is expected that technical advances will bring further improvements for this promising neuroimaging methodology.

V. DISCUSSION

The elucidation of brain mechanisms involved in formation of the human mind, and how it emerges from the activation of billions of neural cells, is one of the most interesting and challenging scientific endeavors of our day. Currently, in vivo neuroimaging methods have allowed unprecedented studies of the living human brain in health and disease. Available imaging methods can provide a vast range of information, such as detailed anatomical resolution, accurate studies of distribution and function of neurotransmitter systems and intracellular metabolites, and functional activation maps describing the temporal and spatial features of information processing in the brain in virtually real time.

Nonetheless, significant questions still remain to be addressed in the understanding of brain functioning. Conceptual theories on how the brain works are extremely important in the interpretation of neurobiological data. Substantial evidence of functional segregation of several brain functions has been provided from lesion deficit studies, and the identification of "hot spots"— i.e., brain regions unambiguously activated during specific cognitive processes—seems to provide support to theoretical approaches that try to localize mental tasks to discrete anatomical regions. However, the brain is a massively interconnected structure, with reciprocal communications linking practically every anatomical region. A connectionist view of human brain function proposes that several brain regions must be integrated to perform elaborate cognitive functions such as thinking and emotion. Although not excluding modular processing, an integrative framework may be more promising to raise the most critical hypotheses to be examined with neuroimaging studies in psychiatric disorders [28].

Another major challenge in designing neuroimaging studies is the precise definition of the mental processes being tested. Concepts such as emotion, attention, and perception are clearly broad and complex terms, based on psychological models that have been debated over the years. This point is of crucial interest for neuroimaging studies in mental illness, since most psychiatric syndromes present myriad symptoms that may be potentially related to distinct neuropathological processes. Also, the blurred boundaries between some psychiatric diagnoses represent another thorny issue when conceiving an experimental imaging approach. In this sense, brain imaging studies can play a formidable role by helping to dissect the neural processes involved in each component of cognitive processing. This knowledge may eventually allow the development of more precise definitions of mental functions and psychiatric symptoms. Moreover, neuroimaging can potentially provide very important contributions to the development of new models to explain the pathophysiology of mental disorders, and ultimately characterize, for instance, neurobiological markers of illness vulnerability or psychopathology severity. These developments could eventually result in more effective treatments for psychiatric illnesses.

It is essential to understand the weakness and strengths of imaging methodologies, though. Significant efforts are being directed to the improvement of the spatial and temporal resolution of these techniques, and also to be able to examine various neurotransmitter and intracellular signaling systems. Techniques that blend different methodologies, such as MEG + MRI (MSI), seem especially promising. Furthermore, the appreciation of pathological brain functioning will not be complete without a thorough investigation of the healthy brain. In this direction, the development of detailed brain atlases comprising different imaging modalities (anatomical, neurochemical, and functional) is crucial. However, most brain measurements are continuous instead of categorical, and there is an enormous interindividual variability, and consequent overlap of these measurements among psychiatric patients and healthy controls. To consider these issues, population-specific, diagnostic-specific, and developmental probabilistic atlases are in progress [46]. Moreover, the systematic brain mapping of nonhuman primates, and even other species, plays a vital role in setting the findings into an evolutionary perspective, providing a relevant theoretical framework for the identification of specialized neural systems in the human brain [47].

In summary, neuroimaging studies are helping to narrow the gap between clinical psychiatric manifestations and the underlying neuronal pathology. Numerous investigations have confirmed the presence of identifiable brain pathology in mental illness, from gross anatomical abnormalities to dysfunctional task-induced activation of cortical areas. Although no pathognomonic lesions have been identified so far, neuroimaging represents one of the most powerful and versatile methodologies for the study of the living human brain, and has started to provide significant advances in our knowledge of the neurobiology of mental illnesses.

ACKNOWLEDGMENTS

This work was partially supported by grants MH 01736, MH 29618, and MH 30915; the Theodore and Vada Stanley Foundation; the National Alliance for Research in Schizophrenia and Affective Disorders (NARSAD); the American Foundation for Suicide Prevention; and CAPES Foundation (Brazil). Dr. Soares was the 1999–2000 Selo NARSAD Investigator.

REFERENCES

1. Finger S. The era of cortical localization. In: Finger S, ed. Origins of Neuroscience. New York: Oxford University Press, 1994:32.
2. Mazziotta JC, Frackowiak RSJ. The study of human disease with brain mapping methods. In: Mazziotta JC, Toga AW, Frackowiak RSJ, eds. Brain Mapping: The Disorders. New York: Academic Press, 2000:3.
3. Haug JO. Pneumoencephalographic evidence of brain atrophy in acute and chronic schizophrenic patients. Acta Psychiatr Scand 1982; 66(5):374.
4. Ghanem MHM. CT scan in psychiatry. L'Encephale 1986; 12:3.
5. Rabi II, Millman S, Kusch P. A new method of measuring nuclear magnetic moment. The magnetic moments of 3Li6, 3Li7 and 9F19. Physiol Rev 1939; 55:526.

6. Ashburner J, Friston KJ. Voxel-based morphometry—the methods. Neuroimage 2000; 11(6 Pt 1):805.
7. Le Bihan D, Mangin JF, Poupon C, et al. Diffusion tensor imaging: Concepts and applications. J Magn Reson Imaging 2001; 13(4): 534.
8. Malison RT, Laruelle M, Innis RB. Positron and single photon emission tomography: principles and applications in psychopharmacology. In: Bloom FE, Kupfer DJ, eds. Psychopharmacology: The Fourth Generation of Progress. New York: Raven Press, 1995:865.
9. Laakso A, Hietala J. PET studies of brain monoamine transporters. Curr Pharm Des 2000; 6(16):1611.
10. Heinz A, Jones DW, Raedler T, Coppola R, Knable MB, Weinberger DR. Neuropharmacological studies with SPECT in neuropsychiatric disorders. Nuclear Med Biol 2000; 27:677.
11. Kegeles LS, Mann JJ. In vivo imaging of neurotransmitter systems using radiolabeled receptors ligands. Neuropsychopharmacology 1997; 17(5):293.
12. Krishnan KRR, Doraiswamy PM. Brain Imaging in Clinical Psychiatry. New York: Marcel Dekker, 1997.
13. Kapur S. A new framework for investigating antipsychotic action in humans: lessons from PET imaging. Mol Psychiatry 1998; 3(2):135.
14. Kapur S, Zipursky R, Jones C, Remington G, Houle S. Relationship between dopamine D(2) occupancy, clinical response, and side effects: a double-blind PET study of first-episode schizophrenia. Am J Psychiatry 2000; 157(4):514.
15. Hartshorne MF. Positron emission tomography. In: Orrison WW, Lewine JD, Sanders JA, Harshorne MF, eds. Functional Brain Imaging. St Louis: Mosby, 1995:187.
16. Sanders JA. Magnetic resonance spectroscopy. In: Orrison WW, Lewine JD, Sanders JA, Harshorne MF, eds. Functional Brain Imaging. St Louis: Mosby, 1995:419.
17. Macomber RS. A complete introduction to modern NMR spectroscopy. New York: John Wiley & Sons, 1998.
18. Soares JC, Krishnan KR, Keshavan MS. Nuclear magnetic resonance spectroscopy: new insights into the pathophysiology of mood disorders. Depression 1996; 4(1):14.
19. Schulman RG. Functional imaging studies: linking mind and basic neuroscience. Am J Psychiatry 2001; 158:11.
20. Silver NC, Barker GJ, MacManus DG, Tofts PS, Miller DH. Magnetisation transfer ratio of normal brain white matter: a normative database spanning four decades of life. J Neurol Neurosurg Psychiatry 1997; 62(3):223.
21. Foong J, Symms MR, Barker GJ, et al. Neuropathological abnormalities in schizophrenia: evidence from magnetization transfer imaging. Brain 2001; 124(Pt 5):882.
22. Raichle ME. A brief history of human functional brain mapping. In: Toga AW, Mazziotta JC, eds. Brain Mapping: The Systems. San Diego: Academic Press, 2000:33.
23. Jueptner M, Weiller C. Does measurement of regional cerebral blood flow reflect synaptic activity? Implications for PET and fMRI. Neuroimage 1995; 2:148.
24. Rosen BR, Buckner RL, Dale AM. Event-related functional MRI: past, present, and future. Proc Natl Acad Sci USA 1998; 95:773.
25. Reba RC. PET and SPECT: opportunities and challenges for psychiatry. J Clin Psychiatry 1993; 54(Suppl):26.
26. Ogawa S, Lee TM, Kay AR, Tank DW. Brain imaging magnetic resonance imaging with contrast dependet on blood oxygenation. Proc Natl Acad Sci USA 1990; 87:9868.
27. Kesler-West ML, Andersen AH, Smith CD, et al. Neural substrates of facial emotion processing using fMRI. Brain Res Cogn Brain Res 2001; 11(2):213.
28. Dolan RJ, Friston KJ. Functional imaging and neuropsychiatry. Psychol Med 1997; 27(6):1241.
29. Callicott JH, Weinberger DR. Neuropsychiatric dynamics: the study of mental illness using functional magnetic resonance imaging. Eur J Radiol 1999; 30:95.
30. Phelps ME, Mazziotta JC. Positron emission tomography: human brain function and biochemistry. Science 1985; 228(4701):799.
31. Shevelev IA. Functional imaging of the brain by infrared radiation (thermoencephaloscopy). Prog Neurobiol 1998; 56(3):269.
32. Lewine JD, Orrison WW Jr. Clinical electroencephalography and event-related potentials. In: Orrison WW Jr., Lewine JD, Sanders JA, Hartshorne MF, eds. Functional Brain Imaging. St. Louis: Mosby, 1995:327.
33. Polich J. P300 clinical utility and control of variability. J Clin Neurophysiol 1998; 15(1): 14.
34. Coull JT. Neural correlates of attention and arousal: insights from electrophysiology, functional neuroimaging and psychopharmacology. Prog Neurobiol 1998; 55(4): 343.
35. Polich J, Kok A. Cognitive and biological determinants of P300: an integrative review. Biol Psychol 1995; 41(2): 103.
36. Reite M, Teale P, Rojas DC. Magneto-encephalography: applications in psychiatry. Biol Psychiatry 1999; 45:1553.
37. Hughes JR, John ER. Conventional and quantitative electroencephalography in psychiatry. J Neuropsychiatry Clin Neurosci 1999; 11:190.
38. Grinvald A, Lieke E, Frostig RD, Gilbert CD, Wiesel TN. Functional architecture of cortex revealed by optical imaging of intrinsic signals. Nature 1986; 324:361.

39. Gratton G, Fabiani M, Corballis PM, et al. Fast and localized event-related optical signals (EROS) in the human occipital cortex: comparisons with the visual evoked potential and fMRI. Neuroimage 1997; 6(3):168.
40. Malonek D, Grinvald A. Interactions between electrical activity and cortical microcirculation revealed by imaging spectroscopy: implications for functional brain mapping. Science 1996; 272:551.
41. Cannestra AF, Blood AJ, Black KL, Toga AW. The evolution of optical signals in human and rodent cortex. Neuroimage 1996; 3:202.
42. Villringer A, Chance B. Non-invasive optical spectroscopy and imaging of human brain function. Trends Neurosci 1997; 20:435.
43. Stepnoski RA, LaPorta A, Raccuia-Behling F, Blonder GE, Slusher RE, Kleinfeld D. Noninvasive detection of changes in membrane potential in cultured neurons by light scattering. Proc Natl Acad Sci USA 1991; 88:9382.
44. Dale AM, Halgren E. Spatiotemporal mapping of brain activity by integration of multiple imaging modalities. Curr Opin Neurobiol 2001; 11:202.
45. Hock C, Villringer K, Muller-Spahn F, et al. Decrease in parietal cerebral hemoglobin oxygenation during performance of a verbal fluency task in patients with Alzheimer's disease monitored by means of near-infrared spectroscopy (NIRS)—correlation with simultaneous rCBF-PET measurements. Brain Res 1997; 755(2): 293.
46. Toga AW, Thompson PM. An introduction to maps and atlases of the brain. In: Toga AW, Mazziotta JC, eds. Brain Mapping: The Systems. San Diego: Academic Press, 2000:3.
47. Duchaine B, Cosmides L, Tooby J. Evolutionary psychology and the brain. Curr Opin Neurobiol 2001; 11(2):225.

5

Classification of Childhood and Adolescent Psychiatric Disorders

NORAH C. FEENY and ROBERT L. FINDLING
University Hospitals of Cleveland and Case Western Reserve University, Cleveland, Ohio, U.S.A.

I. INTRODUCTION

In the past 20 years, the classification and diagnosis of psychiatric disorders in children and adolescents have undergone substantial change. For example, though long disputed, we now know that depressive disorders can and do occur in youths, as well as in adults [e.g., 1–3]. In general, we use classification systems to reduce complexity, to create order, and, in psychiatry and psychology, to inform treatment. They are heuristic systems that assume general similarities across individuals in particular groups (e.g., depressed vs. not; anxious vs. not) who show similar symptoms. For a psychiatric classification system to be optimally useful, it must reliably differentiate between groups based on established criteria, serve a practical function, predict future behavior, and adequately capture the construct it was intended to. In short, it must be reliable and valid. The Diagnostic and Statistical Manual of Mental Disorders, Fourth Edition (DSM-IV) [4] is the most commonly used diagnostic system in the United States. It utilizes a categorical (as opposed to dimensional) classification system organized by symptom clusters and grounded in empirical findings. In this paper, the DSM-IV disorders will be reviewed as they relate to children and adolescents. First, we will discuss disorders typically diagnosed in infancy and childhood. Second, we will review syndromes that are generally diagnosed in adulthood and how they manifest in children. Specifically, for each diagnostic category, we will review information related to the definition and prevalence of the disorder, comorbidity with other psychiatric disorders, course and developmental considerations relevant to the disorder.

II. DISORDERS TYPICALLY DIAGNOSED IN CHILDHOOD

A. Disruptive Behavior Disorders

In DSM-IIIR [5], attention, conduct, and oppositional behaviors were newly grouped together under the rubric of disruptive behavior disorders. This diagnostic reorganization was partly due to accumulating evidence that the separation of attention and behavior problems was not empirically supported (e.g., 6). DSM-IV maintained this overall organization, but made some major changes to the classification of these disorders: (1) the creation of an overarching category for patients who experience difficulties with restlessness, impulsivity, and inattention: attention deficit hyperactivity disorder (ADHD) with three resultant subtypes; and (2) the creation of two subtypes for conduct disorder based on age of onset.

1. Attention Deficit Hyperactivity Disorder (ADHD)

ADHD is characterized by a persistent and developmentally inappropriate pattern of inattention and/or hyperactivity-impulsivity that is present before age 7 and causes functional impairment in at least two settings (e.g., school and home). Symptoms must be present for at least 6 months. In the DSM-IV, there are three ADHD subtypes: predominantly hyperactive-impulsive, predominantly inattentive, and combined type. Diagnosis of the subtypes should be based on the predominant symptoms for the last 6 months. These subtypes were developed empirically from the DSM-IV field trials, but little is known regarding how valid and valuable they are clinically. In support of their usefulness, in the field trials the subtypes were shown to have differing clinical pictures: inattentive patients were more likely to be female, and were older than the combined types. Combined-type youths were older than the hyperactive impulsive patients and showed greater clinical impairment than the other two types.

The prevalence of ADHD is estimated to be 3–5% in school-age children [4,7]. With the new DSM-IV criteria, preliminary studies suggest that rates have increased owing to the definition of the three subtypes. While much is unknown about the etiology of ADHD, there is now a fair amount of evidence from twin and family-genetic studies that suggest that this disorder runs in families [e.g., 8,9].

Comorbidity is very common among youths with ADHD, most commonly with conduct disorder [10,11,12] and oppositional defiant disorder [13]. Conduct disorder is characterized by serious and pervasive aggressive and antisocial behavior. The overlap between ADHD and conduct disorder has been found consistently in studies of children with both disorders and estimates suggest that 40%–60% of teens with ADHD meet criteria for conduct disorder. The prognosis is worse for those youths who have both ADHD and conduct disorder; these youths are at increased risk for substance abuse, school failure, and future occupational failure.

In regard to the course of the disorder, ADHD is most typically diagnosed in children and adolescents, and symptoms usually decrease in later adolescent and adult years. Although ADHD severity decreases on average with age, symptoms are persistent for many children; in one study, 4 years after initial diagnosis 80% of youths continued to meet criteria for ADHD [14]. Although ADHD is usually diagnosed in childhood, the disorder can be diagnosed in adults as long as symptoms were present before the age of 7. The concept of adult ADHD is not without controversy, however; some claim that adult ADHD is very rare [e.g., 15], while a growing body of evidence suggests that ADHD often persist in adulthood [16]. Some data that support the validity of ADHD in adulthood come from studies that show the children of ADHD adults to have increased prevalence of the disorder [17]. Other support comes from studies showing parents of youths with "persistent" ADHD being much more likely to have ADHD than parents of youths with remitted ADHD [18]. As noted in DSM-IV [4], ADHD's symptom pattern changes with development, often making diagnosis more difficult in adults. For example, disorganization and inattention rather than hyperactivity, are often prominent in adults. Predictors of a good outcome for adulthood include: mild initial severity of ADHD, a supportive family environment, higher intelligence, and a lack of comorbid conduct disorder.

2. Oppositional Defiant Disorder (ODD) and Conduct Disorder (CD)

ODD and CD are childhood disorders characterized by a stable pattern of defiant and/or aggressive behavior that causes functional impairment at home, at school, or in both settings. The diagnosis of CD requires that at least three characteristic behaviors (e.g., stealing, threatening, fighting, cruelty to animals or people) be present in the last 12 months, with at least one symptom present in the last 6 months. Children with this disorder often violate the rights of others, break serious rules, and are destructive and deceitful. DSM-IV criteria specify two subtypes of CD: childhood onset and adolescent onset.

Children with ODD are characteristically negativistic, defiant, and hostile toward authority figures. For a diagnosis of ODD, four defiant behaviors (e.g., temper outbursts, talking back, breaking rules) must be present frequently over a period of 6 months. There are no identified subtypes for ODD.

Prevalence rates for CD appear to be on the rise in the recent decades and may be higher in urban than in rural settings [4]. However, prevalence rates differ dramatically depending on the sample being studied and the assessment method used: for males younger than 18, rates range from 6% to 16%; for females, rates range from 2% to 9%. Similarly, depending on the sample and assessment method, rates of ODD from 2% to 16% have been found [4]. Rates for both behavior disorders are higher in boys than in girls, though after puberty, rates for ODD become roughly equal.

As discussed above, comorbidity between CD and ADHD is quite common. CD and ODD are also commonly comorbid. Indeed, there is significant diagnostic overlap among the disruptive behavior disorders (particularly among very young children) as well as genuine cooccurrence of these conditions [19,20]. It has been suggested by some that hyperactivity is a necessary part of CD [21]. Thus, to appropriately guide treatment, thorough, multimethod, multi-informant evaluations are necessary to attempt to determine which children meet criteria for CD, ODD, and/or ADHD.

In terms of the course of these disorders, there is a good amount of support for the continuity between externalizing problems in preschoolers and CD in children who are school aged and older [e.g., 19,22]. In a review of longitudinal studies examining preschoolers with behavior problems, Campbell [23] showed that at least 50% with moderate to severe behavior problems continued to manifest such problems when they were school aged. Similarly, Richman, et al. [24] showed that almost 70% of preschoolers with disruptive behavior problems continued to have aggression problems when assessed 5 years later.

However, studies of young adults suggest that CD symptoms decline with age; in a longitudinal study of children with ADHD, Manuzza et al. [25] reported that the prevalence of CD dropped from 25% at age 18 to 15% at age 25. In a similar study of youths (6–17 years) with ADHD, Biederman et al. [14] found that CD symptoms persisted in only 42% of those originally diagnosed with subthreshold or full CD. Consistent with these findings are those of CD samples documenting similar decreases in CD symptoms over time [e.g., 26,27]. It may be that significant conduct problems still remain for most, but that previously obvious and overt behaviors become more covert with age and thus are less readily discerned using standard assessment procedures. When looking at the course of ODD, symptoms appear to be stable over time [28]. Importantly, ODD does appear to be validly distinct from CD: the developmental profile, sex distribution, and factor analytically derived behavioral dimensions differ between the two disorders [29–31].

B. Mental Retardation

Many definitions of mental retardation (MR) have been utilized over the years, differing primarily in emphasis, rather than specific content. According to the DSM-IV, MR is defined by intellectual functioning that is significantly below average (IQ of 70 or below) existing prior to age 18, with associated deficits in adaptive functioning. This definition incorporates all of the elements of the widely accepted description of MR developed by the American Association of Mental Retardation (AAMR). In the DSM-IV, MR is further classified according to severity: mild (IQ of 50–55 to 70), moderate (IQ of 35–40 to 50–55) severe (IQ of 20–25 to 35–40), and profound (IQ below 20–25). The AAMR recently abandoned such severity classifications in favor of classification based on the specific needs of individuals with MR. Despite such classification differences, it is widely accepted that the core features of MR are low intelligence and deficits in developmentally appropriate life skills.

Mental retardation occurs in ~ 1% of children and adolescents. However, prevalence estimates vary significantly depending on how mental retardation is defined, the sample selected, and the assessment tools used. Early research suggests that MR is more common with increasing age [32], in males [33], and in minority groups [34], though this last finding may be related to bias in assessment tools. Additionally, research indicates that the prevalence of MR decreases with age as functional impairment due to low cognition reduces with age [4]. Recent reviews of the literature related to the prevalence of MR have suggested that large gaps remain in our knowledge and have called for standardization of MR definitions and research methodologies [e.g., 35].

Comorbidity of psychiatric disorders among individuals with MR is significantly more common than in the general population [4]. For example, a recent study of >6000 children identified 1.5% as having some sort of intellectual deficiency; of these, 32% were also identified as having a comorbid psychiatric disturbance [36]. The rates of comorbidity were significantly higher among those with intellectual deficiencies than among those who were not intellectually disabled [32% vs. 13.5%). Similarly, in an investigation of all children identified with MR in a Norwegian county, 37% were diagnosed with a comorbid psychiatric disorder, most commonly a pervasive developmental disorder [37]. Rates obtained were higher for those with severe MR than with those with mild MR: 42% and 33%, respectively. This pattern is consistent with the adult literature where those with more severe MR have significantly higher rates of comorbidity as well [e.g., 38].

The course of MR varies somewhat depending on the severity of the disorder, associated medical conditions, and environmental opportunities. As mentioned above, a diagnosis of MR necessitates that the disorder be present prior to 18 years of age. More severe retardation tends to be diagnosed at younger ages, especially when associated with a characteristic, syndromal presentation (e.g., trisomy 21) [4]. MR is only diagnosed when clear deficits in adaptive behavior, judged within a developmental context, are present (assessed using standardized tools such as the Vineland Adaptive Behavior Scales). Such deficits can include impaired self-help skills, communication, academics, safety, and work performance. Less severe cases are often not diagnosed until children are old enough to have noticeable difficulties in school. Academic deficits are among the most easily documented and measured, perhaps accounting for the relatively high prevalence of MR during the school years [39]. Indeed, in adulthood, many individuals previously diagnosed with MR may be able to function adaptively enough outside of the academic arena that they are no longer classifiable as MR. That is to say, MR is not necessarily a lifelong disorder; for those adults who can develop good adaptive life skills in various domains (e.g., self-care and work), their level of functioning precludes an MR diagnosis [4].

C. Learning, Communication, and Motor Disorders

This group of disorders is characterized by academic, motor, or communication skills that are below developmental and intellectual expectations. Learning disorders are a fairly heterogeneous group of difficulties distinguished by academic achievement that is substantially below that expected for one's age, intellect, and/or schooling [4]. As a group they include: reading disorder, mathematics disorder, disorder of written expression, and learning disorder not otherwise specified. In the DSM-IV [4], it is specified that achievement deficits be measured by a standardized, individualized test and that they significantly interfere with academic performance or daily life.

Developmental coordination disorder, the only motor skills disorder, is characterized by a significant impairment in motor coordination that causes functional impairment; the specific manifestations of this disorder vary with age and development. The communication disorders include expressive language disorder, mixed expressive-receptive language disorder, phonological disorder, stuttering, and communication disorder not otherwise specified (NOS). Those diagnosed with expressive language disorder have deficient expressive language skills, including small vocabularies, few multiple-word combinations, and idiosyncratic word ordering. Mixed expressive-receptive disorder is characterized by delays in both expressive language and receptive language (i.e., comprehension). Phonological disorder is defined as the failure to develop typical speech sounds (e.g., ch, bu) at the expected age, and stuttering is characterized by speech dysfluency, syllable and sound repetition, and disrupted speech timing.

The prevalence of these disorders is thought to be relatively high, but estimates vary according to sample characteristics and measures used. According to most estimates, 5–15% of school-age children have learning disabilities [40], and these are diagnosed more commonly in boys than in girls [41]. Approximately 6% of young children have developmental coordination disorder [42], and 5–10% of children are estimated to have communication disorders [4,43]. Among the communications disorders, expressive language delays have been found to be the most common. Stuttering, in particular, is much more common in boys than in girls [3:1].

Many children with learning disorders also have associated comorbidities. Conversely, 10–15% of those with conduct disorder, oppositional defiant disorder, ADHD, and depressive disorder also have learning disorders [4]. Although developmental coordination disorder has not been well researched yet, associated difficulties are thought to include other developmental delays, in particular language delays [4]. More research has focused on communication disorders, and at this point, it is fairly well established that young children with communication difficulties are at increased risk for continued language problems, learning disorders, and psychiatric difficulties [e.g., 44–46].

Learning disorders as a group are thought to have a similar course over time. They are most commonly diagnosed in the elementary school years when academic challenges begin to go unmet. The school dropout rate for children with learning disabilities is 40%, significantly higher than the rate for those without such disorders [4]. Higher IQ is associated with better outcome for those with learning disorders. Depending on severity, learning disabilities may persist until adulthood and cause impaired occupational functioning [47].

Among the communication disorders, the course is more variable. Age of identification is predictive of language disorder severity, with later-identified children typically having more severe and persistent delays. Phonological difficulties that are not severe are the most likely to resolve. Among those with expressive language difficulties, ~ 50% will "recover" and the rest will continue to manifest significant language difficulties [e.g., 48–50]. We know very little about the course of developmental coordination disorder; future research should examine the longitudinal course of significant motor skills deficits.

D. Pervasive Developmental Disorders

The pervasive developmental disorders (PDDs) are characterized by severe impairment in several crucial areas of development: communication, social interaction skills, and/or the presence of stereotyped behavior, play, or interests. These disorders are often diagnosed in the first years of life and are typified by behaviors and skills that are grossly developmentally delayed and/or inappropriate. PDDs as defined by the DSM-IV include autistic disorder (autism), Rett's disorder, childhood disintegrative disorder, Asperger's disorder, and pervasive developmental disorder not otherwise specified (PDD NOS) [4].

Autism's essential features include abnormal or impaired social interaction and communication and a severely restricted inventory of interests and activities. Delays or abnormalities must be present before the age of 3 in at least one of the following areas: social interaction, language in social communications, or symbolic/imaginative play. Most children with autism are also mentally retarded [4]. Rett's disorder, which has only been seen in girls, is distinguished by a period of typical functioning followed by the development of multiple specific deficits. For these children, head growth decelerates between 5 and 48 months, previously acquired hands skills are lost between 5 and 30 months, and subsequently, stereotyped hand movements similar to hand-wringing or hand-washing appear. In addition, interest in social interaction diminishes, expressive and receptive language are impaired, psychomotor retardation develops, and poorly coordinated gait or trunk movements appear. Childhood disintegrative disorder (CDD) is similar to Rett's disorder in that severe regression occurs after a period of typical development, but normal development must have lasted at least 2 years. A diagnosis of CDD requires that after the age of 2 (but before 10) there is a clinically significant loss of previously acquired skills in at least two of the following areas: expressive and receptive language, social skills or adaptive behavior, bowel or bladder control, and/or play or motor skills. Children with CDD exhibit social and communication deficits that are similar to those observed in children with autism. Asperger's disorder like autism, is characterized by persistent and severe impairments in social interaction and restricted, repetitive behavior, interests, and activities. However, with Asperger's disorder there are no characteristic language delays or deficits, nor are there cognitive impairments or deficits in age-appropriate adaptive behavior. PDD NOS is a diagnosis for those children who exhibit many, but not all, of the specific features required for a diagnosis of a specific PDD.

In terms of prevalence, PDDs are quite rare. Epidemiological studies suggest a rates of autism to be two to five cases per 10,000 individuals [4]. Data specific to prevalence for the other PDDs are very limited. Rett's disorder has only been discussed in limited case studies and only seen in females. Childhood disintegrative disorder (CDD) is thought to be very rare (much less common than autism) and more common in males than females. Asperger's disorder is also thought to be very rare, and also appears to be more common in males than in females.

PDDs are typically lifelong disorders with characteristic developmental shifts in symptom patterns. However, with early, intensive behavioral treatment some children with autism, Asperger's, or PDD NOS may benefit significantly enough that they lose their PDD diagnosis [51]. Unfortunately, this is not the case for most children; this sort of treatment is not widely available, and is variable in its success depending on factors such as severity of initial symptoms, comorbid mental retardation, and other individual differences that we do not yet well understand. Children with autism typically develop better functioning with age and often show some improvements in language and social interaction. For children with Rett's disorder there are characteristic developmental changes: between 1 and 3 years symptoms are very similar to those of autism, between 2 and 10 years of age, social interest increases somewhat, and after age 10, there are worsening motor problems [52]. For children with CDD, the long-term outcome is typically not very good, with little improvement in specific skills over time. Across the PDDs the prognosis is typically best for those with Asperger's, as they have communicative and cognitive skills that enable them to function well despite substantial social skill deficits. In adulthood, Asperger's (or mild autism) might be confused with schizoid or schizotypal personality disorders because of the overlapping social deficits [4].

III. PSYCHIATRIC DISORDERS USUALLY DIAGNOSED IN ADULTHOOD

A. Mood Disorders

1. Major Depressive Disorder (MDD) and Dysthymia

Although depression was not officially recognized as a disorder of childhood until 1980, at this point it is relatively well established that the clinical presentation of depressive disorders in children is similar to that seen in adults [4,53]. The DSM-IV uses adult criteria to diagnose depressive disorders in children, but places a greater emphasis on the developmental course of the disorder than DSM-III or DSM-III-R. Documented developmental differences in the presentation of MDD include increased suicide attempts and impairment in functioning with age, and decreased somatic complaints, phobias, and behavioral problems, which occur more in childhood than adulthood [e.g., 54].

In the DSM-IV [4], a diagnosis of MDD is made in individuals who demonstrate at least one major depressive episode (MDE) without previous experience of a manic, mixed, or hypomanic episode. Two weeks of a depressed mood or the loss of interest or pleasure in nearly all activities characterizes an MDE. In children, irritability rather than sadness can be the predominant emotion. In addition to a mood disturbance, at least four other symptoms from the following list must be present: changes in sleep, appetite/weight, or psychomotor activity; reduced energy; feelings of worthlessness or guilt; difficulty thinking concentrating or making decisions; and thoughts of death or suicidal ideation, intent, or plan. To be considered symptoms of MDD, these difficulties must represent a clear change from previous functioning.

Dysthymia is a more chronic depressive disorder characterized by similar symptoms of a lessor severity and longer duration (at least 2 years). In the following sections, we will focus primarily on MDD, as the majority of research data pertains to this diagnosis rather than dysthymia.

Depressive disorders in youths are not rare: population studies estimate that between 0.04% and 2.5% of children and 0.04% and 8.3% of adolescents have MDD [54] and $\sim 3\%$ have dysthymia. In a large-scale study of adolescent psychopathology, MDD had the highest lifetime prevalence rate (20%) of all disorders surveyed, and a point prevalence rate of 2.92 [55]. These findings are consistent with other studies of adolescent depression, and with lifetime rates of MDD found among adults [e.g., 56,57]. In childhood, rates of depression are similar for girls and boys; in adolescence, however, the female-to-male ratio jumps to 2:1, which is comparable with ratios found in adult depression [e.g., 3,58).

MDD in youths is often comorbid with other psychiatric disorders. Rates of comorbidity in youths are comparable with, or slightly higher than, rates seen among adults with depression [59]. Epidemiological studies have shown that 40–70% of depressed children and adolescents have a comorbid psychiatric disorder, and that approximately 20–50% have more than one comorbid condition [e.g., 60–62]. Dysthymia cooccurs with depression in $\sim 30\%$ of youths and adults [59]. Diagnoses that are most commonly comorbid with depression in youths include anxiety disorders (30–80%), disruptive behavior disorders (10–80%), and substance abuse (20–30%) [63]. Indeed, anxiety disorders so commonly co-occur with depression that some have argued that they are manifestation of the same, not distinct disorders [64]. Others have cogently argued that although anxiety and depression do share some overlapping symptoms, the absence of positive affect is characteristic of depression, not anxiety [see 65].

Depression in youths is disabling and chronic, though perhaps somewhat less so than among adults. In a large, randomly selected sample of high school students, those who were identified as depressed were likely to have moderate to severe depression (88.6%) and to be judged in need of treatment (93.2%) [55]. The average length of a depressive episode is 9 months in youths [66], while on average 12 months for adults. Relapse rates are disturbingly high for children and adolescents with depression; $\sim 70\%$ will relapse within 5 years [55,59). Moreover, follow-up studies of depressed youths indicate that 20–40% will go on to develop bipolar disorder within 5 years of the onset of their depression [e.g., 67,68).

2. Bipolar Disorders

Though not without controversy, in recent years it has become more recognized that children can manifest symptomatology that is consistent with a diagnosis of mania, or bipolar disorder (BPD). Indeed, several exhaustive reviews of the literature have supported the validity of this diagnosis in youths [69–71]. According to DSM-IV, the occurrence of one or more manic or mixed episodes determines BPD. A manic episode is characterized by a distinct period of an abnormally elevated, irritable, or expansive mood that lasts at least a week. In addition to this mood disturbance, three symptoms from the following list must be present: inflated self-esteem or grandiosity, decreased need for sleep, pressured speech, increased activity or psychomotor agitation, distractibility, flight of ideas or racing thoughts, or involvement in pleasurable activities with a high potential for negative consequences (e.g., buying sprees or indiscriminant sexual encounters). A mixed episode is defined as a period of at least 1 week during which criteria for both a manic and depressed episode are met. Often there is also a history of depressive episodes in these individuals. As classified in DSM-IV, bipolar disorders include: bipolar I, bipolar II, cyclothymic disorder, and bipolar disorder not otherwise specified. These disorders are differentiated based on the duration of symptoms and presence or absence of a full-blown manic or mixed episode.

Empirical work suggests that while bipolar disorder is difficult to diagnose in children, in part because it differs from adult mania in presentation, prevalence rates are higher than previously thought in youths, particularly among inpatients. However, few well-done studies of the prevalence of BPD exist. In one recent study of > 250 consecutively referred preadolescent children, Wozniak and colleagues [72] found that a surprising 16% met diagnostic criteria (DSM-III-R) for mania. In light of such high rates of mania documented by some researchers in specialty mood clinics and low rates seen in epidemiological studies (lifetime prevalence rate of 0.58) [73], the "real" prevalence of BPD in youths and how to best diagnose the disorder is still a hotly debated topic [see, 74–76]. To resolve this debate, more well-designed research needs to be conducted in the area of diagnosis and prevalence of pediatric bipolarity.

Comorbidity with childhood mania is the rule rather than the exception. However, the exact nature of the relationship between childhood mania and other disorders, in particular, attention deficit hyperactivity disorder (ADHD), is still being debated [77]. Indeed, symptom overlap with ADHD (e.g., impulsivity, concentration problems) is one of the most challenging aspects of accurately assessing and diagnosing bipolar disorder in children. Studies have shown rates of ADHD ranging from 60% to up to 90% among children with mania [72,78,79]. Studies involving children with bipolar disorder have also documented a high degree of overlap with conduct disorder [72,80,81]. For example, Kovacs and Pollack [81] reported that among children with BPD, an astonishing 69% also had conduct disorder. A recent epidemiological study also documented high rates of cooccurrence between these disorders [73]. Such complicating comorbidities, as is typical with other disorders, predict a worse course for these youths [e.g., 81].

Age of onset for a first manic episode is typically during late adolescence, but, as alluded to above, some cases start in early adolescence or childhood [4]. The course and presentation of pediatric mania is often atypical when compared to adult mania. Adult and adolescent mania is typically episodic with an acute onset, and is characterized by the presence of euphoric mood. With children, on the other hand, some have asserted that mania during childhood is characterized by a chronic, mixed mood state [72,76] and that the mood disturbance often manifests as irritability rather than euphoria [82,83]. In a recent review of the empirical literature related to pediatric bipolar disorder, it was concluded that, "pre-pubertal BPD is a non-episodic, chronic, rapid cycling, mixed manic state." [70]. This suggests that BPD in youths is indeed atypical when compared to adult BPD, but that it is predictably atypical.

B. Anxiety Disorders

Excessive fear, distress, and/or avoidance of particular situations or objects, thoughts/memories, or physical sensations characterize anxiety disorders. In the DSM-III-R, three anxiety disorders were listed in the child section: overanxious disorder (OAD), separation anxiety disorder, and avoidant anxiety disorder. In DSM-IV, questions regarding the validity of these diagnostic categories led to a reorganization so that only separation anxiety disorder currently remains in the childhood disorders section (in the category "other disorders of childhood"). In addition, the criteria for social phobia and generalized anxiety disorder were modified so that they incorporated the symptoms of children who would have been previously diagnosed with avoidant or overanxious disorder. As such, according to DSM-IV, the general anxiety disorders include: panic disorder with and without agoraphobia, specific phobia, social phobia, obsessive-compulsive disorder (OCD), posttraumatic stress disorder (PTSD), acute stress disorder (ASD), generalized anxiety disorder (GAD), anxiety disorder due to a general medical condition, substance-induced anxiety disorder, and anxiety disorder NOS. After describing each disorder, we will focus on those that are most relevant to children and adolescents and for which the most research exists: social phobia (previously avoidant disorder in children), generalized anxiety disorder (formerly overanxious disorder in children), and separation anxiety disorder. Although, as previously mentioned, separation anxiety disorder is not formally classified with the anxiety disorders, we will discuss it in this section because of the considerable theoretical and clinical overlap it shares with the anxiety disorders as listed in DSM-IV.

In terms of the features that are specific to each disorder, panic disorder with and without agoraphobia is characterized by panic attacks (sudden onset of intense fear and physical symptoms such as racing heart, shortness of breath, feeling dizzy or faint) about which there is persistent concern. Avoidance of or anxiety about places from which escape would be difficult or embarrassing in the event of panic characterizes agoraphobia. Specific phobias are defined by significant anxiety related to a specific object (e.g., insects or needles) or situation (e.g., elevators or flying) which often leads to avoidance. Social phobia is characterized by anxiety and resultant avoidance related to social or performance situations. OCD is defined by the presence of intrusive, upsetting thoughts (obsessions) and compulsions (repetitive or ritualized behaviors or mental acts) designed to reduce anxiety. PTSD is characterized by reexperiencing (e.g., in nightmares or intrusive thoughts) a traumatic event accompanied by avoidance of trauma-related stimuli and increased arousal (e.g., sleep and concentration difficulties). Acute stress disorder is defined by symptoms that are similar to those of PTSD (with an emphasis on dissociative symptoms) that occur very soon after the traumatic event. GAD is typified by persistent worry and anxiety that is difficult to control that lasts at least 6 months. Separation anxiety disorder is characterized by developmentally inappropriate anxiety (lasting at least 4 weeks) regarding separation from the home or people to whom the child is attached.

Anxiety disorders are among the most commonly diagnosed psychiatric disorders in both children and adults [84]. Epidemiological studies show rates of anxiety disorders ranging from 5.7% to 17.7% in children and adolescents [e.g., 57,61,85,86]. Additionally, these studies show a trend for rates of anxiety disorders to increase with age. Looking at specific disorders, epidemiological studies show prevalence rates as follows: social phobia, 0.06%–7.9%; GAD/OAD, 2.9–10.8%; and separation anxiety disorder, 2.0–4.7%. Though there is a good deal of variability in these estimates, GAD appears to be most common in youths, followed by social phobia, which is also very common.

Anxiety disorders in children (specifically social phobia, GAD, and separation anxiety disorder) are often comorbid with other psychiatric disorders. Indeed, for most children with significant anxiety, comorbidity is the rule rather than the exception. As mentioned previously, depression and anxiety in particular very commonly cooccur; anxiety disorders are three to four times as likely to occur in youths with depressive disorders as in youths without such disorders [e.g., 85,86]. Anxiety disorders are also often comorbid with disruptive behavior disorders. Several studies have found them to be two to three times more common among children with ODD and CD [e.g., 85–87].

Data regarding the course of anxiety disorders in youths are scarce. In a recent study, children diagnosed with an anxiety disorder were followed up 3–4 years later [88]. Eighty percent of the children had recovered from the originally diagnosed disorder, and only a small percentage (8%) experienced a relapse of their disorder. However, these children were likely to develop new disorders. These results are consistent with findings from a 5-year follow-up study of children and adolescents initially diagnosed with anxiety disorders; at follow-up, most of the children had either recovered from the initial diagnosis or had developed a different disorder—most typically, a different anxiety disorder [28]. To date, two studies have found that continuity of anxiety disorders is more common among girls than among boys [85,89].

C. Psychotic Disorders

Psychotic disorders are characterized by the presence of hallucinations or delusions, and grossly disorganized behavior or speech. As with affective disorders, the assumption in DSM-IV is that adult criteria for psychotic disorders should be extended downward to apply to children. However, it has been suggested that the lack of specific attention to developmental issues and the focus in DSM-IV on disorganized speech may lead to errors of overdiagnosis in children [90,91]. In DSM-IV, the psychotic disorders include schizophrenia, schizophreniform disorder, schizoaffective disorder, delusional disorder, brief psychotic disorder, shared psychotic disorder, psychotic disorder due to a medical condition, substance-induced psychotic disorder, and psychotic disorder NOS.

The psychotic syndromes are differentiated based on duration and pattern of presenting symptoms. Schizophrenia is characterized by the presence of at least two of the following symptoms present for at least 1 month: hallucinations, delusions, disorganized speech or behavior, and negative symptoms (e.g., anhedonia, avolition). The disturbance must last at least 6 months overall and cause significant clinical impairment. In terms of symptoms, schizophreniform disorder is the same as schizophrenia, but does not last as long (1–6 months) and need not cause functional impairment. Schizoaffective disorder is typified by a mood disturbance that occurs simultaneously with the positive symptoms of schizophrenia, and is preceded by at least 2 weeks of delusions or hallucinations without concomitant mood disturbance. Delusional disorder is characterized by at least 1 month of delusions that are not bizarre in content. Shared psychotic disorder is a disturbance that develops in one person owing to the influence of another person with a similar delusion.

Psychotic disorders in children are considered rare, but few studies have been conducted in this area, and most focus exclusively on schizophrenia. The prevalence of schizophrenia in very young children (12 years old and younger) has been estimated at rates of 1.6–1.9 per 100,000 [92,93]. Among adolescents, rates of schizophrenia are estimated at 0.23% in the general population, 1% among outpatients [94], and 5% among inpatients [95]. Among adults, estimates of schizophrenia prevalence rates range from 0.2% to 2% [4]. Schizophrenia with onset at a very young age is about twice as likely in males as in females [96].

In youths with psychotic disorders it is thought that comorbidity is fairly common, particularly with disorders of behavior, attention, and motor skills. However, little empirical work exists in this area. Histories that are suggestive of premorbid pervasive developmental disorders are common [97,98], as are comorbid behavior and attention problems [99]. Results of one study indicated that among youths diagnosed with schizophrenia, ~13% had a history suggesting preexisting attention or motor skills deficits [100].

Psychotic disorders are typically first diagnosed in the late teens through early 30s, with onset before the teen years being uncommon [4]. Age of onset has been found to be prognostic: children with very early onset schizophrenia tend to have a very poor prognosis [91,101]. In general, studies of adult schizophrenia show a variable course of the disorder, with some individuals remaining chronically ill, and others experiencing periods of remission and exacerbation [4]. There are some common developmental variations in symptoms: in children, visual hallucinations may be more common than in adults, and hallucinations/delusions may be less elaborate. Delusions are only seen in ~50% of cases of childhood schizophrenia [102,103]. Additionally, disorganized speech is common to several disorders typically seen in children (e.g., pervasive developmental disorders, communication disorders), so this symptom is less indicative of a psychotic disorder in this group then when seen in adults. Acute onset of the disorder is more likely the older the age of the child [96].

IV. CONCLUSIONS

This chapter has reviewed many of the major diagnostic classifications as listed in DSM-IV and highlighted diagnostic issues that pertain to children and adolescents. Overall, psychiatric disorders are common in youths and typically increase in prevalence with age. Comorbidity is also quite common in children and adolescents, and is associated with poor outcome. The course of the various psychiatric disorders is variable, but on average, early age of identification predicts a more chronic course, and as such, may serve as a proxy for severity. In terms of developmental sensitivity, in the DSM-IV, there are very few diagnostic criteria differences across the life cycle, but the presentation of symptoms is modified and mediated by developmental influences. As such, we have attempted to outline characteristic developmental symptom patterns for each disorder.

As we noted at the start of this chapter, the classification and diagnosis of psychiatric disorders in children and adolescents have undergone substantial change and progress in the past 20 or so years. We, as a field, have begun to accumulate empirical work that to varying degrees support or make us question our diagnostic categories as they now stand. More research that examines the presentation, course, and outcome of various psychiatric disorders in youth is needed, particularly in the area of bipolar disorders, pervasive developmental disorders, and psychotic disorders.

REFERENCES

1. Kashani JH, Carson GA, Beck NC, et al. Depression, depressive symptoms, and depressed mood among a community sample of adolescents. Am J Psychiatry 144:931–934, 1987.
2. Kovacs M, Beck AT. The wish to die and the wish to live in attempted suicides. J Clin Psychol 33:361–365, 1977.
3. Lewinsohn, PM, Clarke, GN, Seeley, MS, Rohde P. Major depression in community adolescents: age at onset, episode duration, and time to recurrence. J Am Acad Child Adolesc Psychiatry 33(6):809–818, 1994.

4. American Psychiatric Association. Diagnostic and Statistical Manual of Mental Disorders, 4th ed. Washington: Author, 1994.
5. American Psychiatric Association. Diagnostic and Statistical Manual of Mental Disorders, 3rd ed., revised. Washington: Author, 1987.
6. Taylor, EA, Schachar R, Thorley G, Wieselberg, M. Conduct disorder and hyperactivity. I. Separation of hyperactivity and antisocial conduct in British child psychiatric patients. Br J Psychiatry 149:760–767, 1986.
7. Szatmari, P. The epidemiology of attention-deficit hyperactivity disorders. Child Adolesc Psychiatr Clin North Am 1:361–371, 1982.
8. Faraone S, Biederman J. Do attention deficit hyperactivity disorder and major depression share familiar risk factors? J Nerv Mental Dis 185(9):533–540, 1994.
9. Samuel VJ, George P, Thornell A, Curtis S, Taylor A, Brome D, Mick E, Faraone SV, Biederman J. A pilot controlled family study of DSM-IV ADHD in African-American children. J Am Acad Child Adolesc Psychiatry 38(1):34–39, 1999.
10. Biederman J, Munir K, Knee D. Conduct and oppositional disorder in clinically referred children with attention deficit disorder: a controlled family study. J Am Acad Child Adolesc Psychiatry 26:724–727, 1987.
11. Biederman J, Newcorn J, Sprich S. Comorbidity of attention-deficit/hyperactivity disorder with conduct, depressive, anxiety, and other disorders. Am J Psychiatry 148:564–577, 1991.
12. Caron C, Rutter M. Comorbidity in child psychopathology: concepts, issues and research strategies. J Child Psychol Psychiatry 32:1063–1080, 1991.
13. Jensen, PS, Hinshaw, SP, Kraemer, HC, Lenora N, Newcorn JH, Abikoff HB, March JS, Arnold LE, Cantwell DP, Connors CK, Elliott GR, Greenhill LL, Hechtman L, Hoza B, Pelham WE, Severe JB, Swanson JM, Wells KC, Wigal T, Vitiello B. ADHD comorbidity findings from the MTA study: comparing comorbid subgroups. J Am Acad Child Adolesc Psychiatry 40(2):147–158, 2001.
14. Biederman J, Mick E, Faraone S, Burback M. Patterns of remission and symptom decline in conduct disorder: a four-year prospective study of an ADHD sample. J Am Acad Child Adolesc psychiatry 40(3):290–298, 2001.
15. Hill J, Schoener E. Age-dependent decline of attention deficit hyperactivity disorder. Am J Psychiatry 153:1143–1146, 1996.
16. Barkley R. Age-dependent decline in ADHD: true recovery of statistical illusion? ADHD Rep 5:1–5, 1997.
17. Faraone SV, Tsuang Ddd, Tsuang MT. Genetics and Mental Disorders: A Guide for Students, Clinicians, and Researchers. New York: Guilford Press, 1999.
18. Biederman J, Faraone S, Milberger S, Curtis S, et al. Predictors of persistence and remission of ADHD into adolescnece: results from a four-year prospective follow-up study. J Am Acad Child Adolesc Psychiatry 35(3):343–351, 1996.
19. Campbell SB, Pierce EW, March CL, Ewing LJ, Szumowski EK. Hard-to-manage preschool boys: symptomatic behavior across contexts and time. Child Dev 65:836–851, 1994.
20. Campbell SB. Behavior problems in preschool children: a review of recent research. J Child Psychol Psychiatry 36:113–149, 1995.
21. Loeber R, Schmaling KB. Empirical evidence for overt and covert patterns of antisocial conduct problems: a meta-analysis. J Abnorm Child Psychol 13:337–352, 1985.
22. Rutter M. Resilience in the face of adversity: protective factors and resistance to psychiatric disorder. Br J Psychiatry 147:598–611, 1985.
23. Campbell SC. Longitudinal studies of active and aggressive preschoolers: individual differences in early behavior and outcome. In D Cicchetti, SL Toth, eds. Rochester Symposium on Developmental Psychopathology: Internalizing and Externalizing Expressions of Dysfunction. Hillsdale, NJ: Lawrence Erlbaum Associates, 1991, pp 57–90.
24. Richman N, Stevenson J, Graham PJ. Preschool to School: A Behavioral Study. New York: Academic Press, 1982.
25. Mannuzza S, Klein RG, Bessler A, Malloy P, LaPadula M. Adult outcome of hyperactive boys: educational achievement, occupational rank and psychiatric status. Arch Gen Psychiatry 50:565–576, 1993.
26. Lahey B, Loeber R, Hart E, et al. Four-year longitudinal study of conduct disorder in boys: patterns and predictors of persistence. J Abnorm Psychol 13:337–352, 1995.
27. Offord DR, Boyle MH, Racine YA, et al. Outcome, prognosis and risk in a longitudinal follow-up study. J Am Acad Child Adolesc Psychiatry 31:916–923, 1992.
28. Cantwell, DP, Baker L. stability and natural history of DSM-III childhood diagnoses. J Am Acad Child Adolesc Psychiatry 29:691–700, 1989.
29. Lahey BB, Applegate B, Barkley RA, Garfinkel B, McBurnett K, Kerdyk L, Greenhill L, Hynd GW, Frick PJ, Newcorn J, Biederman J, Ollendick T, Hart EL, Perez D, Waldman Shaffer D. DSM-IV field trials for oppositional defiant disorder and conduct disorder in children and adolescents. Am J Psychiatry 151:1163–1171, 1994.
30. Loeber R, Lahey BB, Thomas C. Diagnostic conundrum of oppositional defiant disorder and conduct disorder. J Abnorm Psychol 100:379–390, 1991.
31. Rey JM. Oppositional defiant disorder. Am J Psychiatry 150:1769–1778, 1993.
32. Mercer JR. Labeling the Mentally Retarded. Berkeley: University of California Press, 1973.

33. Mumpower DL. Sex ratios found in various types of referred exceptional children. Except Child 36:621–622, 1970.
34. Mercer JR. Sociological perspectives on mild mental retardation. In: MC Haywood, ed. Sociocultural Aspects of Mental Retardation. New York: Appleton-Century-Croft, 1970.
35. Roeleveld N, Zielhuis GA, Gabreels F. The prevalence of mental retardation: a critical review of recent literature. Dev Med Child Neurol 39(2):125–132, 1997.
36. Linna S, Moilanen I, Ebeling H, Piha J, Kumpulainen K, Tamminen T, Almqvist F. Psychiatric symptoms in children with intellectual disability. Eur Child Adolesc Psychiatry 8(suppl 4):77–82, 1999.
37. Stromme P, Diseth TH. Prevalence of psychiatric diagnoses in children with mental retardation: data from a population-based study. Dev Med Child Neurol 42(4):266–270, 2000.
38. Gostason R. Psychiatric illness among the mentally retarded. A Swedish population study. Acta Psychiatr Scand 71(suppl 318), 1985.
39. Baumeister AA, Baumeister AA. Mental retardation: causes and effects. In: M Hersen, RT Ammerman, eds. Advanced Abnormal Child Psychology, 2nd ed. Mahwah, NJ: Lawrence Erlbaum Associates, 2000.
40. Taylor HG. Learning disabilities. In: EJ Mash, LG Terdal, eds. Behavioral Assessment of Childhood Disorders, 2nd ed. New York: Guilford Press, 1988:402–450.
41. Finucci J, Childs B. Are there really more dyslexic boys than girls? In: A Ansara, N Geschwind, A Galaburda, M Albert, N Gartrell, eds. Sex Differences in Dyslexia. Townson, MD: Orton Dyslexia Society, 1981:1–9.
42. Arnold LE. Learning disorders. In: BD Garfinkle, GA Carlson, EB Weller, eds. Psychiatric Disorders in Children and Adolescents. Philadelphia: Saunders, 1990:237–256.
43. Silva P. The prevalence, stability and significance of developmental language delay in preschool children. Dev Med Child Neurol 22:768–777, 1980.
44. Bishop D, Adams C. A prospective study of the relationship between specific language impairment, phonological disorders, and reading retardation. J Child Psychol Psychiatry 30:1027–1050, 1987.
45. Cantwell D, Baker L. Developmental Speech and Language Disorders. New York: Guilford Press, 1987.
46. Tallal P. Developmental language disorders. In: JF Kavanagh, TJ Truss Jr, eds. Learning Disabilities: Proceedings of the National Conference. Parkton, Md: York Press, 1988: 181–272.
47. Spreen O. Adult outcome of reading disorders. In: RN Malatesha, PG Aaron, eds. Reading Disorders: Varieties and Treatments. New York: Academic Press, 1982: 473–498.
48. Fischel J, Whitehurst G, Caulfield M, DeBaryshe B. Language growth in children with expressive language delay. Pediatrics 82:218–227, 1989.
49. Rescorla L, Schwartz E. Outcome of toddlers with expressive language delay. Appl Psycholing 11:393–407, 1990.
50. Thal D, Tobias S, Morrison D. Language and gesture in late talkers: a 1-year follow-up. J Speech Hearing Res 34:604–612, 1991.
51. Lovaas OI. Behavioral treatment and normal educational and intellectual functioning in young autistic children. J Consult Clin psychol 55:3–9, 1987.
52. Perry A. Rett syndrome: a comprehensive review of the literature. Am J Ment Retard 96:275–290, 1991.
53. Roberts RE, Lewinsohn PM, Seeley Jr. Symptoms of DSM-III-R major depression in adolescence: evidence from an epidemiological study. J Am Acad Child Adolesc Psychiatry 34:1608–1617, 1995.
54. Kashani J, Burback D, Rosenberg T. Perceptions of family conflict resolution and depressive symptomatology in adolescents. J Am Acad Child Adolesc Psychiatry 27:42–48, 1988.
55. Lewinsohn PM, Hops H, Roberts RE, Seeley JR, Andrews JA. Adolescent psychopathology. I. Prevalence and incidence of depression and other DSM-III-R disorders in high school students. J Abnorm Psychol 102:133–144, 1993.
56. Lewinsohn PM, Duncan EM, Stanton AK, Hautziner M. Age at onset for first unipolar depression. J Abnorm Psychol 95:378–383, 1986.
57. Kessler R, McGonagle K, Zhao S, Nelson C, Hughes M, Eshleman S, Wittchen H, Kendler K. Lifetime and 12-month prevalence of DSM-II-R psychiatric disorders in the United States: results from the national comorbidity survey. Arch Gen Psychiatry 51:8–19, 1994.
58. Kessler RC, McGonagle KA, Nelson CB, Hughes M, Swartz M, Blazer DG. Sex and depression in the national comorbidity survey. II. Cohort effects. J Affect Disord 30:15–26, 1994.
59. Kovacs M. Presentation and course of major depressive disorder during childhood and later years of the life span. J Am Acad Child Adolesc Psychiatry 35:705–715, 1996.
60. Anderson JC, McGee R. Comorbidity of depression in children and adolescents. In: WM Reynolds, HF Johnson, eds. Handbook of Depression in Children and Adolescents. New York: Plenum, 1994: 581–601.
61. Kashani JH, Beck NC, Hoeper EW, Fallahi C, Corcoran CM, McAllister JA, Rosenberg TK, Reid JC. Psychiatric disorders in a community sample of adolescents. Am J Psychiatry 144:584–589, 1987.
62. Rohde P, Lewinsohn PM, Seeley JR. Comorbidity of unipolar depression. II. Comorbidity with other mental disorders in adolescents and adults. J Abnorm Psychol 100:214–222, 1991.

63. Birmaher B, Ryan N, Willamson DE, Brent DA, Kaufman J. Childhood and adolescent depression: a review of the past 10 years. Part II. J Am Acad Child Adolesc Psychiatry 35(12):1575–1583, 1996.
64. Kendall PC, Ingram RE. The future of the cognitive assessment of anxiety: let's get specific. In: L Michelson, M Ascher, eds. Anxiety and Stress Disorders: Cognitive-Behavioral Assessment and Treatment. New York: Guilford, 1987: 89–104.
65. Clark LA, Watson D. Tripartite model of anxiety and depression: psychometric evidence and taxonomic implications. J Abnorm Psychol 100(3):316–336, 1991.
66. McCauley E, Myers K, Mitchell J, Calderon R, Schloredt K, Treder R. Depression in young people: Initial presentation and clinical course. J Am Acad Child Adolesc Psychiatry 32:714–722, 1993.
67. Geller B, Fox L, Clark K. Rate and predictors of prepubertal bipolarity during follow-up of 6- to 12-year-old depressed children. J Am Acad Child Adolesc Psychiatry 33:461–468, 1994.
68. Kovacs M, Gatsonis C. Stability and change in childhood-onset depressive disorders. Longitudinal course as a diagnostic validator. In: LN Robins, JE Barrett, eds. The Validity of Psychiatric Diagnosis. New York: Raven Press, 1989: 57–75.
69. Faedda G, Baldessarini R, Suppes T, Tondo L, Becker I, Lipschitz D. Pediatric-onset bipolar disorder: a neglected clinical and public health problem. Harvard Rev Psychiatry 3:171–195, 1995.
70. Geller B, Luby J. Child and adolescent bipolar disorder: a review of the past 10 years. J Am Acad Child Adolesc Psychiatry 36:1168–1176, 1997.
71. Weller E, Weller R, Fristad M. Bipolar disorder children: misdiagnosis, underdiagnosis, and future direction. J Am Acad Child Adolesc Psychiatry 34:709–714, 1995.
72. Wozniak J, Biederman J, Mundy E, Mennin D, Faraone SV. A pilot family study of childhood-onset mania. J Am Acad Child Adolesc Psychiatry 34:1577–1583, 1995.
73. Lewinsohn P, Klein D, Seeley J. Bipolar disorders in a community sample of older adolescents: prevalence, phenomenology, comorbidity, and course. J Am Acad Child Adolesc Psychiatry 34:454–463, 1995.
74. Biederman J. Resolved: mania is mistaken for ADHD in prepubertal children. Affirmative. J Am Acad Child Adolesc Psychiatry 37:1091–1093, 1998.
75. Klein RG, Pine DS, Klein DF. Resolved: mania is mistaken for ADHD in prepubertal children. Negative. J Am Acad Child Adolesc Psychiatry 37:1093–1095, 1998.
76. Faraone SV, Biederman J, Wozniak J, Mundy E, Mennin D, O'Donnell D. Is comorbidity with ADHD a marker for juvenile onset mania? J Am Acad Child Adolesc Psychiatry 36:1046–1055, 1997.
77. Biederman J, Russell R, Soriano J, Wozniak J, Faraone S. Clinical features of children with both ADHD and mania: does ascertainment source make a difference? J Affect Disord 51:101–112, 1998.
78. Borchardt CM, Bernstein GA. Comorbid disorders in hospitalized bipolar adolescents compared with unipolar depressed adolescents. Child Psychiatry Hum Dev 26:11–18, 1995.
79. Geller B, Sun K, Zimmerman B, Luby J, Frazier J, Williams M. Complex and rapid-cycling in bipolar children and adolescents: a preliminary study. J Affect Disord 34:259–268, 1995.
80. Biederman J, Faraone SV, Mick E, Wozniak J, Chen L, Ouellette C, et al. Attention deficit hyperactivity disorder and juvenile mania: an overlooked comorbidity? J Am Acad Child Adolesc Psychiatry 35:997–1008, 1996.
81. Kovacs M, Pollack M. Bipolar disorder and comorbid conduct disorder in childhood and adolescence. J Am Acad Child Adolesc Psychiatry 34:715–723, 1995.
82. Carlson GA. Classification issues of bipolar disorders in childhood. Psychiat Dev 2:273–285, 1984.
83. Davis RE. Manic depressive variant syndrome of childhood: a preliminary report. Am J Psychiatry 136:702–706, 1979.
84. March JS. Anxiety Disorders in Children and Adolescents. New York: Guilford, 1995.
85. Costello EJ, Stouthamer-Loeber, DeRosier M. Continuity and change in psychopathology from childhood to adolescence. Paper presented at the Annual Meeting of the Society for Research in Child and Adolescent Psychopathology, Santa Fe, NM, 1993.
86. Fergusson DM, Horwood LJ, Lynskey MT. Prevalence and comorbidity of DSM-III-R diagnoses in a birth cohort of 15 years olds. J Am Acad Child Adolesc Psychopathol 32:1127–134, 1993.
87. Costello EJ, Costello AJ, Edelbrock C, Burns BJ, et al. Psychiatric disorders in pediatric care: prevalence and risk factors. Arch Gen Psychiatry 45(12):1107–1116, 1988.
88. Last CG, Perrin S, Hersen M, Kazdin AE. A prospective study of childhood anxiety disorders. J Am Acad Child Adolesc Psychiatry 35:1502–1510, 1996.
89. McGee R, Feehan M, Williams S, Anderson J. J Am Acad Child Adolesc Psychiatry 31(1):50–59, 1992.
90. Volkmar FR, Schwab-Stone M. Childhood disorders in DSM-IV. J Child Psychol Psychiatry Allied Disciplines 37(7):779–784, 1996.
91. Werry JS. Childhood schizophrenia. In: F Volkmar, ed. Psychoses and Pervasive Development Disorders in Childhood and Adolescence. Washington: American Psychiatric Press, 1996:1–48.
92. Burd L, Fisher W, Kerbeshian J. A prevalence study of pervasive developmental disorders in North Dakota. J Am Acad Child Adolesc Psychiatry 26:704–710, 1987.
93. Gillberg C, Steffenburg S. Outcome and prognostic factors in infantile autism and similar conditions: a popu-

lation-based study of 46 cases followed through puberty. J Autism Dev Disord 17:273–287, 1987.
94. Evans J, Acton WP. A psychiatric service for the disturbed adolescent. Br J Psychiatry 120:429–432, 1972.
95. Steinberg D, Galhenage DP, Robinson SC. Two years' referrals to a regional adolescent unit: some implications for psychiatric services. Soc Sci Med Part E Med Psychol 15:113–122, 1981.
96. Werry JS. Child and adolescent (early onset) schizophrenia: a review in light of DSM-III-R. J Autism Dev Disord 22:601–624, 1992.
97. Asarnow JR, Ben-Meir S. Chidren with schizophrenia spectrum and depressive disorders: a comparative study of premorbid adjustment, onset pattern and severity of impairment. J Child Psychol Psychiatry Allied Disciplines 29:477–488, 1988.
98. Watkins JM, Asarnow RF, Tanguay PE. Symptom development in childhood onset schizophrenia. J Child Psychol Psychiatry 29:865–878, 1988.
99. Asarnow JR. Annotation: childhood-onset schizophrenia. J Child Psychol Psychiatry 35:1345–1371, 1994.
100. Hellgren L, Gillberg IC, Bagenholm A, Gillberg C. Children with deficits in attention, motor control and perception (DAMP) almost grown up: psychiatric and personality disorders at age 16 years. J Child Psychol Psychiatry 35:1255–1271, 1994.
101. Asarnow RF, Asarnow JR, Strandburg R. Schizophrenia: a developmental perspective. In: D Cicchetti, ed. Rochester Symposium on Developmental Psychology. New York: Cambridge University Press, 1989: 189–220.
102. Green WH, Campbell M, Hardesty AS, Grega DM, Padron-Gaylor M, Shell J, Erlenmeyer-Kimling L. A comparison of schizophrenic and autistic children. J Am Acad Child Adolesc Psychiatry 4:399–409, 1984.
103. Russell AT, Bott L, Sammons C. The phenomenology of schizophrenia occurring in childhood. J Am Acad Child Adolesc Psychiatry 28:399–407, 1989.

6

Classification of Schizophrenia and Related Psychotic Disorders

TONMOY SHARMA and PRIYA BAJAJ
Clinical Neuroscience Research Centre, Stonehouse Hospital, Dartford, Kent, England

I. INTRODUCTION

The need for a classification of mental disorders has been clear throughout the history of medicine, but there has been little agreement on which disorders should be included and the optimal method for their organization. The many nomenclatures that have been developed during the past two millennia have differed in their relative emphasis on phenomenology, etiology, and course as defining features. Some systems have included only a handful of diagnostic categories whereas others have included thousands. Moreover, the various systems for categorizing mental disorders have differed with respect to whether their principal objective was for use in clinical, research, or statistical settings [1].

Attitudes to psychiatric classification have also undergone a revolution in the last generation. In the 1950s and 1960s, psychiatric diagnoses did not occupy center stage in clinical practice. Their reliability was known to be low; it was known that key diagnostic terms like schizophrenia had different meanings in different parts of the world. On the other extreme, there were some who argued that diagnostic categories should be abandoned and they believed that all patients require the same treatment—the "moral regime" of the asylum for Neumann and Prichard in the 19th century, and psychotherapy of Rogers and Menninger in the 20th century [2].

However, a clear definition and accurate classification of a disorder are the first steps in any systematic attempt to understand the pathophysiology and etiology of the disorder. The revolution in biological psychiatry can, in part, be attributed to advances in nosology [3].

II. EVOLUTION OF CLASSIFICATION SYSTEMS

Ethnographic studies have demonstrated that schizophrenia is present in all existing cultures, from the preliterate to the most advanced. Psychotic symptomatology and schizophrenialike syndromes were clearly present in ancient civilizations. However, more accurate and systematized classifications of psychological disturbances began to evolve only in the 1st and 2nd centuries AD. The physician Aretaeus of Cappadocia defined a state of melancholy, which included depression as well as schizophrenialike withdrawal. In the 1700s there was an increasing emphasis on detailed and accurate descriptions of abnormal mental processes and states. Philippe Pinel, a French physician, considered to be one of the founders of modern psychiatry, argued for an objective medicophilosophical approach to psychological disorders. Jean Etienne Esquirol, a student of Pinel, defined hallucinations and identified "monomania", a clinical syndrome similar to modern descriptions of paranoid schizophrenia.

Attempts were also being made to divide the clinical landscape into syndromes sharing both clinical features and course. Benedict Augustin Morel was the first to use the term dementia praecox (*dementia precoce*). Other symptom complexes identified included delusional states (France) and paranoid states, as described by the German physician Vogel in 1764. Johann Christian Augusts Heinroth outlined 48 distinct disease entities and thereby epitomized the general inability to develop straightforward, reliable criteria. These theoretical controversies and confusion led Heinrich Neumann to reject all systems of classifications and suggest that it was necessary to "throw overboard the whole business of classifications" to bring order to the field. He suggested that "there is but one type of mental disturbance, and we call it insanity." Nevertheless, despite the intermittent sense of frustration and confusion, classificatory efforts continued unabated [4].

III. 20TH CENTURY CLASSIFICATORY SCHEMAS OF KRAEPLIN AND BLEULER

It was in the latter part of the 19th century that Emil Kraeplin was able to integrate the diverse clinical phenomena into a coherent and far-reaching classificatory system. His synthetic formulation included the identification of "dementia praecox" to refer to the clinical entity we now call schizophrenia. "Dementia" referred to the progressive deteriorating course of both emotional and cognitive processes; "praecox" indicated the early age of onset in previously healthy individuals. Thus, fundamental to the diagnosis were both cross-sectional and longitudinal components. Importantly, he differentiated the generally deteriorating course of dementia praecox from the more episodic and customarily better outcome seen in manic-depressive disorder. He furthermore divided it into four subtypes: paranoid, hebephrenic, catatonic, and simple.

Eugen Bleuler used Kraeplin's systematic classification of psychoses and a theoretical model of etiological processes to reformulate dementia praecox as "schizophrenia," derived from the Greek words for "split" and "mind" [5]. He asserted that there were four cardinal features almost invariably present in schizophrenia patients, the "four A's": blunted affect, loosening of association, ambivalence, and autism.

He viewed schizophrenia as being composed of several different entities rather than a single disease state as Kraeplin conceptualized. Other symptoms of schizophrenia include delusions, catatonia, negativism, and stupor. These were thought to be "secondary" symptoms and to present in reaction to the individual's intentions, drives, psychotic state, and environmental conditions. Bleuler noted that these secondary symptoms were present in schizophrenia as well as in other disorders. He also asserted that despite the secondary nature of these symptoms, they formed the basis of Kraeplin's classificatory system.

It is noteworthy that two psychotic features emphasised by today's Diagnostic and Statistical Manual (DSM)—hallucinations and delusions—were not crucial for Bleuler's diagnosis of schizophrenia. His emphasis on theory as a means for determining the diagnostic relevance of signs and symptoms contrasted sharply with Kraeplin's reliance on empirical observations. Bleuler's approach was also notable for three other reasons. First, his reformulation of dementia praecox as "the group of schizophrenia" foreshadowed the contemporary view that schizophrenia is a heterogeneous group of disorders with similar clinical presentations. Second, he included defects in affect as a core feature of the disorder. Third, his view of schizophrenia allowed for the possibility of recovery.

Other clinicians also advocated a hierarchical system of symptom classification like Bleuler. In 1959, Kurt Schneider termed the core features "first-rank symptoms". These symptoms included: hearing one's thoughts spoken aloud; auditory hallucinations commenting on one's behavior; thought withdrawal, insertion, and broadcasting; and somatic hallucinations, or the experience of one's thoughts as being controlled or influenced from the outside.

Manifestations of first-rank symptoms in the absence of organic disease, persistent affective disorder, or drug intoxication, were sufficient for a diagnosis of schizophrenia. Second-rank symptoms included other forms of hallucinations, depressive or euphoric mood changes, emotional blunting, perplexity, and sudden delusional ideas. When first-rank symptoms were absent, schizophrenia might still be diagnosed if a sufficient number of second-rank symptoms were present. Although the schneiderian criteria have been criticized as being nonspecific, they have been incorporated into clinical diagnostic tools such as the Research Diagnostic Criteria (RDC) and Diagnostic and Statistical Manual of Mental Disorders (DSM) classificatory systems [4].

IV. CLASSIFICATION ON THE BASIS OF SYMPTOMS

It is widely believed that classification of diseases should, wherever possible, be based on etiology. Unfortunately, the same principle does not apply to psychiatric disorders, since the etiology of most is still unknown or all that is known for certain is that both genetic and environmental factors are involved. For this reason, most contemporary classifications of psychiatric disorders are largely based on clinical symptoms. This state of affairs has a number of important consequences. Decisions about the presence or absence of symptoms are relatively unreliable; and because few psychiatric conditions have pathognomonic symptoms, most conditions have to be defined by the presence of some or most of a group of symptoms rather than the presence of one key symptom. In the jargon of nosology, they are polythetic rather than monothetic. This invites ambiguity and lowers reliability still further, unless operational definitions are adopted. Another important consequence is that most psychiatric diagnoses can never be confirmed or refuted, for there is no external criterion to appeal to.

For these and other reasons it has often been suggested that symptoms should be ignored and a new classification developed on an entirely different basis. Psychoanalysts have frequently advocated a classification based on psychodynamic defense mechanisms and stages of libidinal development. In the 1950s, clinical psychologists extolled the advantages of a classification based on scores on batteries of cognitive and projective tests. More recently, learning theorists have argued that we should classify patients on the basis of a comprehensive analysis of their total behavioral repertoire. In principle, all of these approaches are perfectly legitimate. In practice, however, none of them has ever progressed beyond the stage of advocacy. Two other alternatives proposed are (1) classification on the basis of treatment response, and (2) classification on the basis of the course or outcome of the illness. Unfortunately, neither is feasible since there are few if any specific treatments available in psychiatry, and most disorders can have a wide range of outcomes. It is sometimes assumed that Kraeplin's classification or at least his distinction between dementia praecox and manic-depressive insanity, was based on long term outcome, but this is a misunderstanding. Kraeplin certainly emphasized the difference in the lifetime course of his two great rubrics, and perhaps subdivided the functional psychosis in the way he did to maximize the difference in outcome between them. But he used outcome as a validating criterion (i.e., as evidence that his two rubrics were fundamentally different disorders), not as a defining characteristic. Thus, when patients with dementia praecox recovered completely, he would automatically have changed their diagnosis [2].

As things stand, we have no choice but to use a classification, which is largely based on symptoms, despite its shortcomings and imperfections, because no practical alternative has yet been developed. Kraeplin's and Bleuler's observations evolved into today's psychiatric classification: the International Classification of Diseases (ICD) and the American Psychiatric Association's Diagnostic and Statistical Manual (DSM) [5].

V. DIAGNOSTIC CRITERIA: DIAGNOSTIC AND STATISTICAL MANUAL OF MENTAL DISORDERS (DSM)

In this chapter we shall discuss the evolution of the different classification systems over time using the diagnosis of schizophrenia as an example. We will first address the reliability and validity of DSM and then address how ICD later synchronized with the DSM system.

A. DSM-I

In 1949, the American Psychiatric Association in collaboration with the New York Academy of Medicine began an initiative to standardize the diagnostic system throughout the United States. The result was the Diagnostic and Statistical Manual of Mental Disorders-1 (DSM-I), published in 1952. It was influenced by the theories of Adolf Meyer, and psychiatric disorders were viewed as reactions of the personality to psychological, social, and biological factors [4]. In addition to its use of Kraeplin's and Bleuler's views on the signs and symptoms of schizophrenia, the first DSM defined schizophrenia in a way that at least implied environmental causes. For example, all schizophrenic (and other psychiatric) diagnoses included the term "reaction" (as in "schizophrenic reaction, simple type"). Moreover, definitions were vague and did not discuss differential diagnosis. Such imprecise definitions allowed clinicians much discretion in making a diagnosis. As a result, in the United States, schizophrenia became the diagnosis of choice for psychotic conditions that lacked a clear "organic aetiology" [5].

B. DSM-II

The manual had gone through several major revisions. The DSM-II was published in 1968, but did not differ significantly from its predecessors [4]. It dropped the term "reaction" from its diagnoses and added some discussion of differential diagnoses, but continued the DSM-I tradition of brief, vague descriptions of schizophrenia disorders, without specific operational criteria. Interestingly, both of these early systems viewed psychosis as the key feature of the disorder. DSM-II did not contain a category ("schizophrenia latent type") to describe people with "clear symptoms of schizophrenia but no history of a psychotic schizophrenia episode." This category was intended to encompass individuals with a variety of conditions (e.g., "incipient," "prepsychotic," and "borderline schizophrenia," as well as "schizophrenic reaction, chronic undifferentiated type," from DSM-I). This did not reflect an important attempt to clarify the role of psychosis in schizophrenia illness [5]. Thus, the diagnosis, with schizophrenia as an example, lacked validity and was too vague in its description.

C. DSM-III

DSM-III was radically different from any previous classification. Published in 1980, it brought about a sea change in psychiatric classification, spearheaded by the "neo-Kraeplinian" movement in the 1960s and 1970s and by investigators in psychiatry and clinical psychology who emphasized the importance of empirical, psychometric validation of psychiatric syndromes. Its innovations were a response to the evidence that had accumulated over the previous 20 years that psychiatric diagnoses were generally unreliable, that there were systematic differences in the usage of key terms like "schizophrenia" between the United States and other parts of the world [2]. It contained several innovations, including field tests of diagnostic reliability, specific inclusion and exclusion criteria for diagnoses, multiaxial diagnosis, and a focus on the description of syndromes and course of disorders rather than inferences about their etiology. This last point made psychiatric diagnosis more explicitly consistent with the diagnosis of other medical disorders of unknown etiology.

The traditional distinction between neuroses and psychoses was abandoned to allow all affective disorders to be brought together. Also, in the absence of data to support diagnostic hierarchies, the system encourages comorbidity. DSM-III's use of clearly defined criteria limited the clinician's discretion and narrowed the construct of schizophrenia. This development improved the clinical homogeneity of the disorder, better delimited it from other serious mental illnesses, and raised diagnostic reliability to respectable levels. Nevertheless, DSM-III retained the view that psychosis was fundamental to the definition of schizophrenia. Fewer patients now had the diagnosis of schizophrenia, and more were diagnosed as having unipolar or bipolar affective disorder.

However, many senior American psychiatrists criticized this classification and its principal architect Robert Spitzer for introducing what they regarded as a crude "Chinese menu" approach to diagnoses, with a theoretical bias and phenomenology being favored over mental processes.

D. DSM-III-R

DSM-III was replaced by an extensive revision DSM-III-R (revised) in 1987. In this classification schizoaffective disorders were given an operational definition for the first time; the definition of paranoid disorders was enlarged to include patients with grandiose, somatic, and erotomanic delusions as well as with delusions of persecution and jealousy, and the inappropriate stipulation that schizophrenia must start before the age of 45 years was dropped. Being introduced only 7 years after DSM-III, this classification was criticized for disrupting research and practice because of the evolution of new definitions [2].

E. DSM-IV and DSM-IV-TR

The primacy of psychosis defining schizophrenia also survived DSM-III's revision and its evolution into DSM-IV (published in 1994) and DSM-TR (text revision published in 2000) [6]. DSM-IV was published in 1987 with the following goals [3]:

1. To develop criteria that are more constant with ICD-10, with regard to schizophrenia. Primarily, this had to do with changing the required duration of the psychotic symptoms from 1 week (as in DSM-III-R) to 1 month (as in ICD-9 and ICD-10)
2. To provide a simplified criterion of symptoms by reducing redundancy in the items of criterion A.
3. To include symptoms with proven reliability.
4. To include symptoms only with acceptable prevalence.
5. To provide maximum coverage (sensitivity) for existing cases, thus reducing the reclassification rate.

These goals were met by adopting a "thorough process" by the Psychotic Disorders Work Group, which consisted of comprehensive reviews of literature, reanalyses of previously collected data, input from the field, and issue-focused field trials that included testing of alternative sets of diagnostic criteria. Changes proposed ranged from minor modifications in the DSM-III-R criteria to more weightage for negative symptoms, expansion of the minimum duration of symptoms to 2 weeks or 4 weeks, to the introduction of a concept of "schizophrenia spectrum disorders."

Psychosis was deemphasized in DSM-IV, in that a patient could receive a diagnosis of schizophrenia according to DSM-IV criteria without having delusions or hallucinations. In that case, however, gross disorganization of speech and/or behavior, which are also psychotic symptoms, would still be required because criterion A (i.e., characteristic symptoms) requires at least two of the five symptoms in the category. Thus, four of the five symptoms are still related to psychosis (negative symptoms are the fifth symptom in the category). Moreover, delusions alone can satisfy the criterion if they are bizarre, and hallucinations alone can satisfy the criterion if they involve one or more voices engaging in running commentary or ongoing conversation. Diagnostic changes in DSM-IV thus expanded the nature of the required psychotic symptoms more than they deemphasized psychosis itself [5]. In the DSM-IV "Schizophrenia and other related disorders" include schizophrenia, delusional disorder, and schizoaffective disorder. Schizophrenia is divided into five subtypes including paranoid, disorganized, catatonic, undifferentiated, and residual [4]. The criteria for schizoaffective disorder has been changed to focus on an uninterrupted period of illness rather than on the lifetime pattern of symptoms. In Brief Psychotic Disorder, eliminating the requirement for a sever stressor has broadened the DSM-III-R construct of Brief Reactive Psychosis, and the minimum duration of the psychotic symptoms has been increased from a few hours to 1 day.

The importance of psychotic symptoms in diagnosis extends to other diagnostic systems. Schneider's first-rank symptoms, which form the basis of "nuclear schizophrenia," are types of hallucinations and delusions that have come (more than other, "second-rank" symptoms) to characterize the nature of psychosis in the disorder. More important, they have helped to define the disorder itself, although Schneider himself reviewed them more as diagnostic tools than as theoretical constructs about the etiology of the disorder. First-rank symptoms heavily influenced the development of Research Diagnostic Criteria for schizophrenia, which in turn formed the basis of DSM-III criteria for schizophrenia. These criteria, particularly, continue to influence ICD-10 in the first three symptom groups "that have special importance for the diagnosis" for schizophrenia [5].

VI. DIAGNOSTIC CRITERIA: INTERNATIONAL CLASSIFICATION OF DISEASES (ICD)

The Mental Disorders section of ICD-6 was primarily a classification of "psychoses and mental deficiency." The eighth revision of the International Classification of Diseases, Injuries and Causes of Death (ICD-8) came into use in 1969, owing to strenuous efforts by the World Health Organization. It was replaced by ICD-9 a decade later, in 1979. However, the definitions provided in ICD-8 and ICD-9 were not operational definitions [2].

A. Preparation of ICD-10

The process of drafting ICD-10 started in 1983 but it came into use in United Kingdom and most other countries in 1993. It had a new title, the International Statistical Classification of Diseases and Related Health Problems, and a new alphanumeric format. The main purpose of the latter is to provide more categories and so leave space for future expansion without the whole classification having to be changed. It incorporates many of the radical innovations introduced in DSM-III. Most categories are provided with both diagnostic guidelines for everyday clinical use and separate "diagnostic criteria for research," providing unambiguous rules of application. There is also provision for multiple axes, as in DSM-III and its predecessors.

Field trials of the 1986 draft text were held in 194 different centers in 55 different countries, and the final text benefited greatly from the comments of users in these varied settings and the evidence they provided of the acceptability, coverage, and interrater reliability of the provisional categories and definitions of the draft [2].

B. Differences between ICD-9 and ICD-10

F20–F29, which included schizophrenia, schizotypal states, and delusional disorders have been expanded by the introduction of new categories such as undifferentiated schizophrenia, postschizophrenic depression, and schizotypal disorder. The classification of acute short-lived psychoses, which are commonly seen in most developing countries, is considerably expanded compared with that in the ICD-9 [7].

VII. OTHER PSYCHOTIC DISORDERS: DSM AND ICD DEFINITIONS

A. Schizoaffective Disorder

The study of Schizoaffective Disorder, since it has generally been ill defined, has always presented unique problems due to the lack of producing comparable populations. Several conceptual models of schizoaffective disorder exist, e.g., the episode-based versus the course-based co-occurrence of mood and psychotic symptoms. Both the ICD and the DSM use a common definition of episode-based coexistence of symptoms and are very similar in the other criteria. A rare, small subgroup of patients may, however, be diagnosed as Schizophrenia by the DSM-IV, and Schizoaffective Disorder by the ICD-10. This occurs because the ICD requires that at least 2 weeks of psychosis precede any concurrent psychotic and mood symptoms of schizophrenia, whereas the DSM does not. A patient presenting with concurrent psychotic and mood symptoms from the onset of the episode could be diagnosed Schizophrenia by DSM-IV if satisfying all the other criteria, but might be diagnosed Schizoaffective by ICD-10.

B. Delusional Disorder

For delusional disorder it is likely that some difference in subject selection will persist between the two major symptoms because of differing requirement in duration, i.e., 1 month in DSM versus 3 months in ICD.

C. Acute/Brief Psychotic Disorder

Although termed differently, acute psychotic disorders provide substantially the same coverage in the two systems. In DSM, the terms brief psychotic disorder and schizophreniform disorder are used, while the ICD uses the terms acute and transient disorder with and without schizophrenialike symptoms [3].

VIII. INTERNATIONAL DIFFERENCES IN DIAGNOSTIC CRITERIA

A. Diagnostic Hierarchies

In ICD-10, schizophrenia and affective disorders are at the same level. A diagnosis of schizophrenia cannot be made if the full depressive/manic syndrome is also present "unless it is clear" that schizophrenic symptoms antedated the affective disturbance.

However, in the DSM classification, schizophrenia traditionally follows the "organic psychosis," and the third place in the hierarchy is occupied by the affective disorders. A very similar sequence is involved in the decision pathway of computer programs like Catego [2].

B. Threshold for Diagnosis

Comparative studies carried out by the US/UK diagnostic project in 1960s established that, in comparable series of patients, psychiatrists in New York diagnosed schizophrenia twice as frequently as their counterparts in London. The International Pilot Study of Schizophrenia confirmed that American psychiatrists had an unusually broad concept of schizophrenia, and also showed that the same was true of Russian psychiatrists. The very broad American concept of schizophrenia was psychoanalytic in origin, and the decline of psychoanalytic influence in the 1970s, together with a renewed interest in descriptive psychopathology and classification, led to rapid change. The widespread adoption of the operational definitions of DSM-III and DSM-III-R by research workers in many different parts of the world has also played an important role in reducing the international differences in usage [2].

IX. RELIABILITY AND VALIDITY: THE PREREQUISITES OF A CLINICAL DIAGNOSES

The introduction of structured interviews and operational definitions has improved the reliability and validity of psychiatric diagnosis over the years. But the existing evidence for the validity of most psychiatric diagnoses is rather meager. It is considerably better for the major syndromes like schizophrenia in comparison to sub-categories of major syndromes such as catatonic schizophrenia [2].

A. Reliability and Field Trials

Modern classification schemes such as ICD-10 and DSM-IV have made it possible to assign psychiatric patients reliably to different diagnostic categories [8]. A classificatory system, which has little reliability, has little practical utility [9]. Field trials have been conducted at seven USA sites (each of which contributed 50 subjects) to assess the concordance and symptom reliability within different systems, namely, DSM-III, DSM-III-R, and ICD-10 [1]. Some of the major highlights of the results were:

1. Concordance between diagnostic systems.
2. Symptom reliability.
3. Reliability of diagnostic criteria.
4. Agreement between ICD and DSM-III-R was high (87.6%) for schizophrenia, but 13% of DSM-III-R schizophrenia was classified by ICD as schizoaffective, acute and transient psychotic disorder, schizotypal, or none of the above.
5. Reliability of schneiderian symptoms was similar to that of other symptoms. Likewise, bizarre delusions were as reliably rated as nonbizarre, and even negative symptoms had good reliability in the trial.
6. The length of symptoms is a principal difference in criteria between ICD and DSM. The field trial demonstrated that ~ 5% of DSM-III-R schizophrenia and > 30% of schizophreniform disorder would have to be reclassified to psychosis not otherwise specified (NOS) when the required duration of symptoms is changed to 1 month.

B. Validity of Classification Systems

As yet no clinical or pathological gold standard exists for the diagnosis of schizophrenia. The uncertain validity of the diagnostic categories assigned to the patients is a matter of serious concern because the usefulness of a particular diagnostic construct is greatly reduced if it carries no therapeutic implications.

The validity of diagnostic classification rests to some extent on its ability to predict outcome. In a study by Mason et al. [10], it was found that DSM-III-R and ICD-10 diagnosis of schizophrenia had high predictive validity and were superior to ICD-9. ICD-10, however, had superior sensitivity to DSM-III-R. This study thus suggests that ICD-10 should be preferred for studies needing high sensitivity as well as specificity for the diagnosis of schizophrenia in the acute phase, such as studies of incidence. It also suggests that dropping the 6-month duration criterion should be considered for a future DSM-V [10].

In another study, by Van Os et al. [8], the introduction of a "treatment-relevant" classification of psychiatric disorders such as the functional psychoses was explored. In a sample of 706 patients aged 16–65 years with chronic psychosis, psychopathology was measured using the Comprehensive Psychopathological Rating Scale (CPRS). The principal component factor analysis of the 65 CPRS items on cross-sectional psychopathology yielded four dimensions of positive, negative, depressive, and manic symptoms. The authors concluded that although it was possible to reliably label combinations of psychopathological phenomena, the resulting diagnostic entities reveal very little about the patients. In patients with chronic psychosis, the dimensional approach constitutes a treatment-relevant alternative or complementary strategy. Its use in clinical practice, research, and service evaluation was in need of further investigation [8].

C. International Pilot Study of Schizophrenia: Symptom Frequencies in Cross-Cultural Groups

Computerized statistics have often been used to select diagnostic criteria. Such an approach will seek to select a set of symptoms that are relevant and distinct. The symptoms selected would be required to satisfy the following conditions: They should be common in a representative sample of the population under investigation. Thus, catatonia is not useful, although it's quite a striking symptom, because it is relatively infrequent; they require a high interrater reliability, and this eliminates symptoms that are difficult to identify consistently to serve well as diagnostic criteria the symptoms should be nonredundant; that is, they should be fairly independent of each other but necessary for the diagnosis (this means that they should not have high mutual intercorrelation to avoid tautology); and symptoms to be preferred should have discriminant value for the purpose of differential diagnoses, occurring quite often in concordant cases and rarely, if at all, in discordant cases with an alternative diagnosis. All these conditions define the following statistical criteria for the evaluation of symptoms characteristic of the illness: an adequate rate of occurrence, good interrater reliability, low intercorrelation of symptoms, and a high frequency ratio for concordant versus discordant groups.

Symptom frequencies in concordant and discordant groups from large-scale cross-cultural investigations were published in the International Pilot Study of Schizophrenia (IPSS). Those data can be used to explore the potential for establishing the new diagnostic rules or criteria for schizophrenia.

The IPSS teams found that >40% of patients in concordant and <10% of patients in discordant groups had "experiences of control" (delusions of uncommon mental or physical external influences on the patients). "Auditory hallucinations" met the same conditions. If a less stringent criterion is used (at least 40% of members of concordant groups), flatness (flat affect) appears as a relevant marker. Some other symptoms (e.g., lack of insight, patient-related cooperation difficulties) appeared equally promising on the basis of their high incidence in the concordant group, but were too frequently observed in the discordant group [11].

X. FUTURE RESEARCH AND NEWER CLASSIFICATIONS

A. Reactive Psychosis: A Classical Category Revisited

Reactive psychosis was a category included in ICD-8 and ICD-9 as "reactive depression, reactive excitation, reactive confusion, acute paranoid reaction and unspecified reactive psychosis," and as "brief reactive psychosis" in DSM-III and DSM-III-R. However, in ICD-10 and DSM-IV it no longer occupies a separate category; instead it is subsumed as a subcategory in "acute and transient psychotic disorders" and "brief psychotic disorder," respectively, as "acute and transient psychotic disorder with marked stressor." ICD-10 and DSM-IV only require specifying the presence of a stressor prior to the outbreak of a usually brief, acute psychosis. However, Ungvari et al. [12] have reviewed the diagnostic concept and felt that the classical psychopathological concept of reactive psychosis goes beyond this by stipulating the temporal and contextual continuity between the stressful situation and the ensuing psychosis, taking into account the patient's personality and life history including individual vulnerability to psychological trauma. This diagnostic category featured in the psychiatric literature for several decades mostly on the basis of clinical experience. However, the original form of reactive psychosis had faded away before serious attempts were made to validate this diagnostic category. Currently the concept is not acknowledged or used in clinical practice outside Scandinavia. The wider recognition of reactive psychosis and its delimitation from other acute psychotic disorders would be important for providing clinically more homogenous samples of subjects for psychiatric research [12].

B. Refining "Acute Brief Psychoses"

One of the proposals for ICD-11 and DSM-V has been focused on the diagnostic classification of nonaffective acute remitting psychosis (NARP), also termed acute brief psychosis. The authors have suggested that this category can be delineated from both schizophrenia and the affective psychosis and be considered as a single diagnosis. They have proposed that four criteria be considered central to the diagnosis:

1. Nonaffective
2. Acute onset (over <2 weeks)
3. Recovery within a brief duration (<6 months)
4. Psychosis broadly defined.

The authors felt that both the ICD-10 and the DSM-IV lacked a firm empirical grounding in their classification of acute psychosis. Studies have indicated that the model duration of acute psychoses in the developing country setting is 2–4 months, whereas both ICD-10 and DSM-IV offered diagnoses that excluded psychoses of >1 month's duration. Furthermore, NARP is a highly distinct entity, as evidenced by studies on its demographic distribution, incidence, duration, and long-term course. The clinical characteristics are atypical for schizophrenia and affective psychoses, and it has a stable long-term course. Following recovery from the initial psychotic episodes, the cases rarely evolve into chronic disorders. Even on relapse, the subsequent psychotic episodes tend to be acute in onset and brief in duration. The diagnosis of NARP rests upon criteria, which could be reliably and comparably rated across diverse settings, and offer to bring the nosology of acute psychoses into far closer accord with current empirical data [13].

In summary, diagnostic criteria have evolved over the past five decades from vague concepts based on ideological viewpoints to field trials tested criteria which have high reliability across cultures. We have used schizophrenia as an example to illustrate the evolution of the changes in the DSM and ICD systems, but these evolutionary changes are true to a large extent of other diagnoses as well. Unfortunately, we still have to rely on signs and symptoms assessed clinically to come to a diagnosis. The lack (as yet) of biological markers in assisting clinicians to make a diagnosis can be seen as a drawback in psychiatry today. However, the rapid advances being made in the neurobiology of psychiatric disorders may, one day, lead us to the Holy Grail and establish biological markers as anchors on which psychiatric diagnoses can be made.

REFERENCES

1. American Psychiatric Association. Diagnostic and Statistical Manual of Mental Disorders. 4th ed. Washington; American Psychiatric Association, 1994, pp 13–25.
2. RE Kendell. Diagnosis and classification. In: RE Kendell, AK Zealley, eds. Companion to Psychiatric Studies. 5th ed. New York: Churchill Livingstone, 1993, pp 277–294.
3. AK Pandurangi. Schizophrenia in DSM-IV and implications for biological psychiatry research. In: S Khanna, SM Channabasavanna, MS Keshavan, eds. Methods in Biological Psychiatric Research. New Delhi: Tata McGraw-Hill, 1995, pp 1–9.
4. ML Korn. Historical roots of schizophrenia. Medscape Psychiatry Clinical Management Modules 05:1–19, 2001.
5. MT Tsuang, WS Stone, SV Faraon. Towards reformulating the diagnosis of schizophrenia. Am J Psychiatry 157:1041–1050, 2000.
6. American Psychiatric Association. Diagnostic and Statistical Manual of Mental Disorders, 4th text revision ed. Washington; American Psychiatric Association, 2000, pp 13–25.
7. World Health Organization. The ICD-10 Classification of Mental and Behavioural Disorders, Clinical descriptions and diagnostic guidelines. Geneva: World Health Organization, 1992, pp 9–13.
8. J Van Os, C Gilvarry, R Bale, E Van Horn, T Tattan, I White, R Murray. A comparison of the utility of dimensional and categorical representation of psychosis. Psychol Med 29:595–606, 1999.
9. P Ash. The reliability of psychiatric Diagnoses. J Abnorm Soc Psychol 44:272–277, 1949.
10. P Mason, G Harrison, T Croudace T. DSM-III-R and ICD-10 diagnoses of schizophrenia had higher predictive validity than that of ICD-9 and CATEGO-S+ diagnoses (abstr). Evidence-based Mental Health 1(1):26, 1998.
11. J Landmark, H Merskey, Z Cernovsky, E Helmes. The positive triad of schizophrenic symptoms, its statistical properties and its Relationship to 13 traditional diagnostic systems. Br J Psychiatry 156:388–394, 1990.
12. GS Ungvari, HCM Leung, W Tang. Reactive psychosis: a classical category nearing extinction? Psychiatry Clin Neurosci 54:621–624, 2000.
13. E Susser, MT Finnerty, N Sohler. Acute psychoses: a proposed diagnosis for ICD-11 and DSM-V. Psychiatr Q 67(3):165–176, 1996.

7

Classification of Mood Disorders
Implications for Psychiatric Research

ACIOLY L. T. LACERDA and ROBERTO B. SASSI
Western Psychiatric Institute and Clinic, University of Pittsburgh School of Medicine, Pittsburgh, Pennsylvania, U.S.A.

JAIR C. SOARES
University of Texas Health Science Center, San Antonio, Texas, U.S.A.

1. INTRODUCTION

Several attempts to categorize the various mental disorders have been reported over the years. The first efforts to develop systematic diagnostic classifications were initially put forth by the so-called alienists, during the 19th century [1]. During the first half of the 20th century, psychiatry was strongly influenced by psychoanalysis. While psychoanalytic-oriented thinking initially brought advances to clinical practice by stressing the importance of an individual's personal history and reducing the social stigma of mental illnesses [2], important advances in neuropsychiatry were neglected, and communication among psychiatrists became difficult due to a lack of diagnostic uniformity.

The return of psychiatry to the mainstream of academic medicine, initiated after the early psychopharmacological advances in the 1960s, generated a crucial need for development of a valid and reliable diagnostic classification system that would serve clinical and research purposes [3]. In fact, the relative lack of a medical framework for psychiatry, when compared to other medical specialties, probably had its origins, at least in part, in a delay to have valid and reliable diagnostic classification systems [4]. After several individual attempts to categorize the various mental conditions in the 19th and 20th centuries, the DSM-III classification [5], published in 1980, constituted an important milestone, as it marked a definitive return of psychiatry to the medical model. The DSM-III was a landmark in operational psychiatric classifications, and also had important impact in research financing in the United States, as the absence of operational criteria and the resulting difficulty to accumulate reliable information on the major mental illnesses discouraged potential sponsors of research on this field [6,7]. A lot has changed since that time, with the development and widespread use of well-accepted diagnostic systems, which have substantially contributed to foster psychiatric research and improve clinical practice in this area, as reflected in subsequent revisions of the DSM and ICD classifications.

The phenomenological paradigm utilized for psychiatric diagnosis, which had been initiated in the asylum settings, is still hegemonic in currently available classifications, and therefore is very influential on research and clinical practice. The two most commonly utilized international diagnostic schemes (ICD-10 [8] and DSM-IV [9]) are largely based on Kraepelinian classifications of mental disorders, relying on the observed symptoms, course of illness, and outcome [10]. Although of unquestionable value to psychiatric practice and research, these classifications still have important weaknesses for taking into account only the presence and variation of symptoms over time to define a diagnostic category, without contribution from research findings on biological mechanisms or treatment response. Obviously, because the pathophysiological mechanisms underlying these disorders are largely unknown, those important dimensions are therefore excluded from currently available diagnostic formulations. This lack of mechanistic evidence to support currently available classifications presents a very substantial difficulty for psychiatric research and clinical practice, and is clearly a very important area for future development.

Mood disorders have been included as a diagnostic category in eventually all major psychiatric classifications, as a reflection of their prevalence and significance as major mental illnesses [11]. Nevertheless, the diagnostic criteria utilized for mood disorders has evolved substantially through various diagnostic classifications. This chapter will present a brief historical overview of diagnostic classifications of mood disorders, critically review the available classification systems, and discuss prospects for new diagnostic classifications that would incorporate information on neurobiological mechanisms and treatment response, and possibly be of more assistance to research and clinical efforts.

II. DIAGNOSIS OF MOOD DISORDERS

In 1970, Robins and Guze [12] proposed specific criteria to establish the validity of a psychiatric diagnosis. According to these authors, in order to be valid, a psychiatric diagnosis should: (1) provide an adequate clinical description of the disorder; (2) be consistent with research findings; (3) be well delimited, excluding other disorders; (4) be reasonably related to prognosis; and (5) identify a family pattern, if applicable. Validity refers to the capacity to achieve the correct diagnosis, and reliability refers to the agreement on a specific diagnosis by two or more raters, or by one rater at distinct times [13].

As happened with other psychiatric diagnoses, the reliability of the diagnosis of mood disorders has significantly increased with the availability of operational diagnostic classifications, and with the utilization of structured diagnostic interviews. Since DSM-III was published in 1980, the reported reliability for mood disorders as a diagnostic entity has varied from 0.59 to 0.93. However, when assessing "other affective disorders"—i.e., dysthymia and cyclothymia—lower reliability rates are generally reported [14–16]. When analyzed separately, a classic manic episode presents the highest test-retest reliability among all axis I psychiatric disorders, probably because the behavioral abnormalities and symptoms of this syndrome are unique [17]. On the other hand, major depression presented only moderately high reliability in DSM-IV field trials accross distinct clinical sites. Possibly, the differences in reliability between a full manic episode and depressive disorders are a consequence of the various nonspecific symptoms that are part of the depressive syndrome, and also a reflection of the fact that depression or subthreshold depressive syndromes are largely present as comorbid conditions in many axis I diagnoses. Moreover, in spite of the moderate to high reliability rates achieved for the diagnoses included under "mood disorders," the particular syndromes (mania, depression, dysthymia, cyclothymia, and especially "other mood disorders") included under this large category have significant heterogeneity, with substantial variability on illness course, prognosis, treatment response, and biological abnormalities [18–23]. Furthermore, there are several minor clinical syndromes classified within the "mood disorders" category that are substantially distinct among themselves, even though they do not constitute at this point a separate diagnostic entity. Mixed mania, rapid-cycling bipolar disorder, atypical depression, melancholic depression, late-life depression, seasonal affective disorder, and psychotic depression are examples of subcategories of mood disorders with blurred diagnostic boundaries. Even the classic distinction between unipolar and bipolar depression may not be trivial in clinical settings, since the two syndromes are not easily differentiated if there is no clear history of a manic or hypomanic episode. At the outset of these illnesses, since most bipolar patients present initially with a depressive episode [24,25], a precise clinical distinction between unipolar and bipolar depression may be difficult. However, such a differentiation would be very relevant, from a clinical standpoint, since the administration of antidepressants as monotherapy to bipolar patients may induce a manic episode, or even be related to a rapid-cycling course [26–28].

There is a clear need to develop a diagnostic classification in psychiatry that would provide more homogeneous groups and subcategories that could assist with both clinical and research purposes. Even though there are useful diagnostic research instruments in this field, such as the Schedule of Affective Disorders and Schizophrenia (SADS) [11], Structured Clinical Interview for DSM (SCID) [29], and Composite International Diagnostic Interview (CIDI) [30], all of them have the particular caveat of not including any information from biological research and pathophysiological mechanisms. With recent advances in methods for clinical neuroscience investigations, including developments in genetics, neuroimaging, and neuropsycho- pharmacology, promising new avenues to investigate the pathophysiology of these illnesses have become available and are now leading to studies that attempt to unravel the neurobiological underpinnings of these various conditions. As an example of a recent advance in this field, Steffens and Krishnan [31] proposed the term "vascular depression," based largely on neuroimaging findings, to describe a specific subtype of depression that includes the signs and symptoms of apathy, psychomotor retardation, cognitive impairment, functional disability, and lack of family history as the core clinical manifestations of vascular brain changes. According to the authors, this new proposed diagnostic sub-type is clinically distinguishable from other clinical presentations of depression, besides carrying an etiologic significance. Such advances are very timely and constitute a very welcome new development, and our hope is that, as research in this area continues to evolve, these diagnostic formulations will become increasingly more common.

III. INTEGRATING BASIC RESEARCH AND CLINICAL PROPOSALS

Various biological treatments have been established as effective modalities in the clinical management of mood disorders [32,33]. Furthermore, some preliminary studies have suggested the presence of specific biological markers that could possibly be useful in predicting outcome in a subset of mood disorder patients [34,35]. Nonetheless, despite promising advances in clinical neurosciences research applied to mental illnesses, current psychiatric classifications have had to rely exclusively on psychopathologic features, with no contribution from available findings from clinical neurosciences research or treatment response. This is a reflection of the fact that the pathophysiological mechanisms involved in these various conditions are largely unknown, and that none of the available neurobiological findings as of yet have been proven to have diagnostic or prognostic value. Additionally, another difficulty relates to the fact that basic and clinical research in this area utilize currently available clinical psychopathology definitions and classifications to attempt to address pathophysiological mechanisms. This constitutes a potentially significant problem, as there are reasons to suggest that currently available classifications based only on psychopathological categories may not be fully adequate.

Nonetheless, the current psychiatric diagnostic paradigm brought on with DSM-III represented a real revolution in the field of mental disorders, and resulted on important advances in classification, epidemiology, and treatment, as it established a "common language" absolutely necessary for psychiatry as a medical specialty. However, classifications solely based on psychopathology may have been a limiting factor to further advances in our understanding of pathophysiology of various psychiatric conditions. Even though the main goal of biological psychiatry is to elucidate the pathophysiological mechanisms involved in the major psychiatric illnesses, the establishment of the diagnosis of these illnesses has been an important deterrent to further advances in this field. Although psychiatry can now offer effective pharmacological treatments for several diseases, it has clearly lagged behind other medical specialties concerning the understanding of the etiology and pathophysiology of its most prevalent illnesses, and considerable amount of additional research in this field and related areas is clearly needed.

As proposed by Van Praag [36], it is possible to improve the biological relevance of diagnostic classifications by: (1) using more accurate phenomenological definitions; (2) being cautious in incorporating new diagnoses; (3) establishing landmarks between normal and pathological; (4) not ignoring major domains of psychopathology; and (5) eliminating hierarchical elements from diagnostic process. Still, these measures represent only palliative remedies, since the diagnostic paradigm that focuses exclusively on clinical presentation, and does not include information on pathophysiological mechanisms, has not changed.

IV. A POSSIBLE NEW PARADIGM BASED PRIMARILY ON PATHOPHYSIOLOGY

Othmer et al. [37] proposed that a diagnostic model evolves through four sequential phases. In phase 1, diagnosis is made based on the presence or absence of a key symptom, and its presence confirms, and absence discards, the disease in question. In phase 2 diagnosis is described as a group of associated symptoms constituting a syndrome, which has a known natural history; in phase 3 there is a detectable underlying pathophysiology of the disorder, and in phase 4, beyond a simple understanding about pathophysiology, etiology is also known. Given the complexity of mental disorders, psychiatry still faces tremendous challenges in diagnostic development, despite improvements in knowledge of neurobiological mechanisms involved in some of these disorders in the last decades. Although most psychiatric disorders are still on phase 2 of diagnostic achievement, there is a considerable amount of emerging evidence linking major psychiatric diagnosis, e.g., mood disorders, to identifiable underlying pathophysiological changes. Even though the etiology of these disorders is far from clear, recent neurobiological investigations are beginning to bring the field of psychiatry closer to the possibility of phase 4 diagnoses [37].

In the past three decades, clinical and basic research in the field of mood disorders has allowed important developments in the understanding of pathophysiology and treatment. Not surprisingly, available findings suggest that the pathophysiology of these illnesses is probably multifactorial. In fact, in less than five decades, pharmacological research on antidepressants has advanced from accidental discoveries of nonselective agents to specifically designed drugs that act selectively in target receptors potentially implicated in the pathophysiology of depression [38]. It is relevant to recognize that antidepressant drugs have their mechanisms of action dependent on modulation of specific neurotransmitter systems [38,39]. This fact has led several investigators to hypothesize a central role of neurotransmitter regulation in mood disorders, such as the pioneer works of Kety et al. in the 1950s and Schildkraut in the 1960s [40–42]. The documented therapeutic efficacy of these medications on depression generated a multitude of basic and clinical neurobiological studies attempting to investigate the postulated role of neurotransmitters on mood regulation. Over the past several years, research conducted in this field has indicated that at least three major neurotransmitter systems are likely to be involved in the pathophysiology of mood disorders, and in mechanisms involved in some of the symptomatic dimensions present in these illnesses:

1. Serotonin. There is evidence that serotonin depletion is associated with depression in people predisposed to it, in accordance with the catecholamine theory of depression [42]. Serotonin is a neurotransmitter involved in processes as distinct as cardiovascular and respiratory activities, sleep, sexual and aggressive behaviors, eating, anxiety, mood, motor behavior, hormonal secretion, nociception, and analgesia [43]. The strongest evidence linking depression and serotonergic dysfunction resulted from the introduction of the new antidepressant class, serotonin-selective reuptake inhibitors (SSRIs). SSRIs have demonstrated efficacy in a wide range of psychiatric disorders like depression, obsessive-compulsive disorder, panic disorder, social phobia, eating disorders, and premenstrual dysphoric disorders [38]. Besides this important clinical confirmation, most investigations that addressed the concentration of serotonin, its major metabolites, and different receptors also suggested a serotonergic dysfunction in mood disorders [44–49].

2. Norepinephrine. There is compelling evidence implicating norepinephrine dysfunction in mood disorders, largely originated from depletion studies [41,50–52], and studies of noradrenergic metabolites [53,54] and receptors [55–57]. The strongest evidence linking noradrenergic dysfunction to mood disorders also came from clinical studies with nonspecific antidepressants like the heterocyclic agents [58–60], the partially selective agent venlafaxine (serotonin and norepinephrine reuptake inhibitor) [61,62], bupropion (noradrenergic and dopaminergic effects) [63,64], mirtazapine [65–67], and the most selective norepinephrine reuptake inhibitor, reboxetine [68,69].

3. Dopamine. Although less robust than the findings indicating abnormalities in the serotonin and noradrenergic systems, the possible implication of dopaminergic mechanisms in mood disorders is supported by some evidence. In depression, the theory was initially supported by observation of subcortical brain dopamine reduction in animals exposed to unpredictable stressful situations (animal model of depression). Subsequent studies confirmed this initial finding [70]: clinical effects of dopamine agonists (improving depressive symptoms, e.g., bromocriptine) and antagonists (worsening depressive symptomatology, e.g., classical antipsychotics) in a subgroup of patients [23,71]; measurement of the dopamine metabolite, homovanillic acid (HVA) [72,73]; and the therapeutic effects of bupropion, which possibly has dopamine reuptake blockade as one of its most important mechanisms of action [64]. The evidence for dopaminergic dysfunction in mania originated mainly from clinical studies that demonstrated the efficacy of neuroleptics (potent dopamine antagonists) in the treat-

ment of mania [23,74]. Additional evidence came from measurements of the dopamine metabolite HVA, which appears to be increased in manic states [75].

Despite important limitations, the monoamine theory of mood disorders is still the most accepted theory to attempt to explain pathophysiology of these disorders. It is largely based on the proven clinical efficacy of medications that modulate serotonergic, noradrenergic, or dopaminergic systems, separately or concomitantly, in treating either depression or mania.

Based on available research findings, Petty et al. [76] proposed a "neurotransmitter balance" theory, where psychiatric diagnosis would be determined not only by symptomatology, but also by its relation with neurotransmitter dysfunction. In this way, for instance, thought disorder would be associated with dopaminergic dysfunction, anxiety with noradrenergic dysfunction, and depressive symptoms with both. All systems would be integrated, with the serotonergic system as the most important in the maintenance and reestablishment of "brain homeostasis." In this way, a depressive disorder could therefore be classified as presenting either serotonergic, noradrenergic, or dopaminergic dysfunction, or a combination of them (it would be referred to as a depressive disorder with highlighted serotonergic, noradrenergic, or dopaminergic dysfunction, or a combination of them). Disruption of biological homeostasis could be triggered by environmental factors, which could be secondarily normalized by administration of serotonergic agents. In fact, given the broad efficacy of SSRIs in a wide range of psychiatric disorders—e.g., depression, social phobia, panic disorder, eating disorders, and obsessive-compulsive disorder—serotonin is probably a key neurotransmitter system possibly involved in the pathophysiology of various related mental illnesses. Nonetheless, such propositions still fail to capture the instances where dysfunction in several interrelated neurotransmitter systems and intracellular signal transduction pathways may be involved.

Basic research and clinical studies have provided important new insights about the behavioral manifestations of specific neurotransmitter dysfunction. There have been over the past several years proposals that specific behavioral dimensions would be linked to specific neurotransmitter dysfunction:

1. "Serotonergic syndromes." Although there is a well-described and clinically serious serotonergic syndrome that may be induced by potent serotonin reuptake inhibitors, we here use the term serotonergic syndromes only to refer to possible behavioral representations of a serotonergic dysfunction in the brain. Mood regulation, appetite regulation, anxiety, and sexual functioning are among the specific behavioral dimensions shown to be heavily modulated by serotonergic mechanisms [77–80].

2. "Noradrenergic syndromes." In vitro and in vivo studies have demonstrated an important role of norepinephrine in specific behavioral dimensions such as sleep-wake cycle, attention, learning, memory, and anxiety [81,82].

3. "Dopaminergic syndromes." Dopaminergic dysfunction has been proposed to be associated with some specific core behavioral symptoms, including motor symptoms/signs, motivation, thought abnormalities, and sexual and feeding behavior [83,84].

Obviously, the separation of behavioral manifestations among the distinct neurotransmitter systems discussed above is presented this way for didactical reasons, since it is impossible to isolate the functioning of a single neurotransmitter in human brain, as these various systems are interrelated. It is not possible to act in any neurotransmitter system without a repercussion in virtually all others; thus, a set of symptoms may be more related to a certain neurotransmitter system, but at the same time such abnormalities are generally not specific. Also, research conducted over the past decades has increasingly revealed the complexities of intracellular signaling and signal transduction processes, as well as related transcription mechanisms and gene expression, which are later events in the cascade triggered after a neurotransmitter couples to a receptor system. Therefore, the examination of specific neurotransmitter systems with an aim at improving diagnosis, as research in this area currently stands, may not necessarily result in substantial advances in diagnostics or therapeutics. Additional effects in intracellular processes and downstream mechanisms are being investigated, and their potential clinical relevance should also be examined as specific knowledge in this area continues to accumulate.

Despite all these provisions, it is expected that a dimensional approach to psychiatric diagnoses that takes into account other sources of information like neurochemical disturbances and neuroimaging findings, may become feasible in the next few years. By that time, we would have reached the third phase of evolution of psychiatric diagnoses, as proposed by Othmer et al. [37], and would then be able to treat mood disorders in a more complete manner, perhaps not only treating symptoms but also addressing the real underlying pathophysiology. In this paradigm change, we would have incorporation of new diagnostic criteria that will hopefully be more meaningful and better reflect core aspects of the neurobiology of these illnesses. As a matter of fact, one could have a progressive incorporation of the most relevant research findings as they become available, and this gradual approach would constitute a more rational and productive way to try to integrate new information and foster future developments in this field.

With recent advances in clinical neurosciences, including advances in genetics, neuroimaging, and neuropsychopharmacology, we now have a formidable arsenal of powerful tools that are being applied to investigations in these specific areas, with very encouraging indications that substantial advances are very likely to be forthcoming in the next few years. Because of the probable insufficiency or inadequacy of the current diagnostic constructs for neurobiological investigations in this area, we have seen over recent years proposals to utilize new constructs related to a mood/anxiety disorder continuum of manifestations, or a continuum of psychotic disorders. Such proposals will generate newer and more specific phenotypes that may eventually be elucidative to the understanding of specific neurobiological mechanisms underlying psychiatric symptoms and clinical conditions. These new approaches to neurobiological investigations of symptoms and syndromes in psychiatry constitute a significant departure from prevailing diagnostic thinking, and we will see in future years whether such approaches will result in significant contributions to our field.

V. CONCLUSIONS

The achievement of high diagnostic validity and reliability in psychiatry has allowed significant advances in clinical and research endeavors in this field. In this sense, the DSM-III was a crucial milestone by providing a common language to psychiatric clinical care and research. Moreover, it allowed unquestionable advance by defining relatively homogeneous patient subgroups, a fundamental first step for both research and clinical initiatives. According to the model of "diagnostic evolution" proposed by Othmer et al. [37], the process of establishing a psychiatric diagnosis utilized nowadays is in the "second phase", i.e., the phase where we can identify "syndromic status," with a known natural history but without any specific information on underlying mechanisms or etiology.

Certainly, the progress in psychiatric classifications over the past few decades has allowed extremely relevant achievements, especially important advances in psychopharmacology. However, the currently utilized paradigm in this area is insufficient to assist contemporary clinical and research demands, since it leaves pathophysiology and etiology largely and intentionally neglected in the conceptualization of all currently valid psychiatric diagnoses. Very substantial advances are likely to result when a paradigm change that would incorporate meaningful information about pathophysiology and etiology of these illnesses in current diagnostic classifications becomes feasible. Nonetheless, there are not yet enough available findings that could have diagnostic or prognostic relevance, which hinders possible attempts to develop newer classification models. Because research in this area is advancing at a very fast pace, continued advances that would result in more meaningful psychiatric classifications are clearly expected in the near future. Because of the impossibility of changing immediately to the "next phase" of diagnostic evolution, our field could benefit largely from a "transitional phase," where a gradual incorporation of the most robust research findings into diagnostic classifications would become feasible.

ACKNOWLEDGMENTS

This work was supported by grants MH 01736 and MH 30915 from the National Institute of Mental Health, the Theodore and Vada Stanley Foundation, the American Foundation for Suicide Prevention, and NARSAD. Dr. Soares was the 1999–2001 Selo NARSAD Investigator.

REFERENCES

1. Berrios GE. Classifications in psychiatry: a conceptual history. Aust NZ J Psychiatry 1999; 33:145–60.
2. Braslow JT. Therapeutics and the history of psychiatry. Bull Hist Med 2000; 74:794–802.
3. Tien AY, Gallo JJ. Clinical diagnosis: a marker for disease? J Nerv Ment Dis 1997; 185:739–747.
4. Pfohl B, Andreasen NC. Development of classification systems in psychiatry. Comp Psychiatry 1978; 19:197–207.
5. Diagnostic and Statistical Manual of Mental Disorders, 3rd ed (DSM-III). Washington: American Psychiatric Association, 1980.

6. Wilson M. DSM-III and the transformation of American psychiatry: a history. Am J Psychiatry 1993; 150:399–410.
7. Jablensky A. The nature of psychiatric classification: issues beyond ICD-10 and DSM-IV. Aust N Z J Psychiatry 1999; 33:137–144.
8. The ICD-10 Classification of Mental and Behavioural Disorders. Geneva: WHO, 1992.
9. Diagnostic and Statistical Manual of Mental Disorders, 4th ed (DSM-IV). Washington: American Psychiatric Association, 1994.
10. Compton WM, Guze SB. The neo-Kraepelinian revolution in psychiatric diagnosis. Eur Arch Psychiatry Clin Neurosci 1995; 245:196–201.
11. Endicott J, Spitzer RL. A diagnostic interview: the schedule for affective disorders and schizophrenia. Arch Gen Psychiatry 1978; 35:837–844.
12. Robins E, Guze SB. Establishment of diagnostic validity in psychiatric illness: its application to schizophrenia. Am J Psychiatry 1970; 126:983–987.
13. Holzer CE 3rd, Nguyen HT, Hirschfeld RM. Reliability of diagnosis in mood disorders. Psychiatr Clin North Am 1996; 19:73–84.
14. Spitzer RL, Forman JB, Nee J. DSM-III field trials. I. Initial interrater diagnostic reliability. Am J Psychiatry 1979; 136:815–817.
15. Riskind JH, Beck AT, Berchick RJ, Brown G, Steer RA. Reliability of DSM-III diagnoses for major depression and generalized anxiety disorder using the structured clinical interview for DSM-III. Arch Gen Psychiatry 1987; 44:817–820.
16. Williams JB, Gibbon M, First MB, et al. The Structured Clinical Interview for DSM-III-R (SCID). II. Multisite test-retest reliability. Arch Gen Psychiatry 1992; 49:630–636.
17. Bowden CL. Classification of bipolar and related disorders—implications for biological research in this field. In: Soares JC, Gershon S, eds. Bipolar Disorders—Basic Mechanisms and Therapeutic Implications. New York: Marcel Dekker, 2000:1–12.
18. Merikangas KR, Wicki W, Angst J. Heterogeneity of depression. Classification of depressive subtypes by longitudinal course. Br J Psychiatry 1994; 164:342–348.
19. Soares JC, Mann JJ. The functional neuroanatomy of mood disorders. J Psychiatr Res 1997; 31:393–432.
20. Arias B, Collier DA, Gasto C, et al. Genetic variation in the 5-HT(5A) receptor gene in patients with bipolar disorder and major depression. Neurosci Lett 2001; 303:111–114.
21. Ban TA. Pharmacotherapy of mental illness—a historical analysis. Prog Neuropsychopharmacol Biol Psychiatry 2001; 25:709–727.
22. Arias B, Gutierrez B, Pintor L, Gasto C, Fananas L. Variability in the 5-HT(2A) receptor gene is associated with seasonal pattern in major depression. Mol Psychiatry 2001; 6:239–242.
23. Lacerda ALT, Soares JC, Tohen M. O papel do antipsicoticos atipicos no tratamento do transtorno bipolar (in Portuguese). Rev Bras Psiquiatr 2001; submitted.
24. Lewinsohn PM, Klein DN, Seeley JR. Bipolar disorders in a community sample of older adolescents: prevalence, phenomenology, comorbidity, and course. J Am Acad Child Adolesc Psychiatry 1995; 34:454–463.
25. Parker G, Roy K, Wilhelm K, Mitchell P, Hadzi-Pavlovic D. The nature of bipolar depression: implications for the definition of melancholia. J Affect Disord 2000; 59:217–224.
26. Kruger S, Braunig P, Young LT. Biological treatment of rapid-cycling bipolar disorder. Pharmacopsychiatry 1996; 29:167–175.
27. Walden J, Schaerer L, Schloesser S, Grunze H. An open longitudinal study of patients with bipolar rapid cycling treated with lithium or lamotrigine for mood stabilization. Bipolar Disord 2000; 2:336–339.
28. Henry C, Sorbara F, Lacoste J, Gindre C, Leboyer M. Antidepressant-induced mania in bipolar patients: identification of risk factors. J Clin Psychiatry 2001; 62:249–255.
29. Spitzer RL, Williams JBW, Gibbons M, First MB. Structured Clinical Interview for the DSM-III-R. Washington: American Psychiatric Press, 1990.
30. The Composite International Diagnostic Interview (CIDI). Geneva: WHO, 1990.
31. Steffens DC, Krishnan KR. Structural neuroimaging and mood disorders: recent findings, implications for classification, and future directions. Biol Psychiatry 1998; 43:705–712.
32. Spigset O, Martensson B. Fortnightly review: drug treatment of depression. BMJ 1999; 318:1188–1191.
33. Daly JJ, Prudic J, Devanand DP, et al. ECT in bipolar and unipolar depression: differences in speed of response. Bipolar Disord 2001; 3:95–104.
34. Yatham LN, Srisurapanont M, Zis AP, Kusumakar V. Comparative studies of the biological distinction between unipolar and bipolar depressions. Life Sci 1997; 61:1445–1455.
35. Lestra C, d'Amato T, Ghaemmaghami C, et al. Biological parameters in major depression: effects of paroxetine, viloxazine, moclobemide, and electroconvulsive therapy. Relation to early clinical outcome. Biol Psychiatry 1998; 44:274–280.
36. Van Praag HM. Over the mainstream: diagnostic requirements for biological psychiatric research. Psychiatry Res 1997; 72:201–212.
37. Othmer E, Othmer JP, Othmer SC. Brain functions and psychiatric disorders. A clinical view. Psychiatr Clin North Am 1998; 21:517–566.
38. Feighner JP. Mechanism of action of antidepressant medications. J Clin Psychiatry 1999; 60:4–11; discussion 12–13.

39. Lenox RH, Hahn CG. Overview of the mechanism of action of lithium in the brain: fifty-year update. J Clin Psychiatry 2000; 61:5–15.
40. Schildkraut JJ. The catecholamine hypothesis of affective disorders: a review of supporting evidence. Am J Psychiatry 1965; 122:509–522.
41. Schildkraut JJ, Gordon EK, Durell J. Catecholamine metabolism in affective disorders. I. Normetanephrine and VMA excretion in depressed patients treated with imipramine. J Psychiatr Res 1965; 3:213–228.
42. Lacerda ALT. Transtorno Obsessivo Compulsivo: Um Estudo Psicopatologico, Neuropsicologico e de Fluxo Sanguineo Cerebral Regional (^{99m}Tc-HMPAO). Departamento de Psicologia Medica e Psiquiatria. Campinas: Universidade Estadual de Campinas, 2000:200.
43. Azmitia EC, Whitaker-Azmitia PM. Anatomy, cell biology, and plasticity of the serotonergic system: neuropsychopharmacological implications for the actions of psychotropic drugs. In: Bloom FE, Kupfer DJ, eds. Psychopharmacology—The Fourth Generation of Progress. New York: Raven Press, 1995.
44. Van Praag HM, Korf J, Dols LC, Schut T. A pilot study of the predictive value of the probenecid test in application of 5-hydroxytryptophan as antidepressant. Psychopharmacologia 1972; 25:14–21.
45. Asberg M, Thoren P, Traskman L, Bertilsson L, Ringberger V. Serotonin depression—a biochemical subgroup within the affective disorders? Science 1976; 191:478–480.
46. Salomon RM, Miller HL, Delgado PL, Charney D. The use of tryptophan depletion to evaluate central serotonin function in depression and other neuropsychiatric disorders. Int Clin Psychopharmacol 1993; 8(suppl 2):41–46.
47. Shiah IS, Yatham LN. Serotonin in mania and in the mechanism of action of mood stabilizers: a review of clinical studies. Bipolar Disord 2000; 2:77–92.
48. Serretti A, Lorenzi C, Lilli R, Smeraldi E. Serotonin receptor 2A, 2C, 1A genes and response to lithium prophylaxis in mood disorders. J Psychiatr Res 2000; 34:89–98.
49. Spillmann MK, Van der Does AJ, Rankin MA, et al. Tryptophan depletion in SSRI-recovered depressed outpatients. Psychopharmacology (Berl) 2001; 155:123–7.12
50. Goodwin FK, Bunney WE Jr. Depressions following reserpine: a reevaluation. Semin Psychiatry 1971; 3:435–448.
51. Delgado PL, Miller HL, Salomon RM, et al. Monoamines and the mechanism of antidepressant action: effects of catecholamine depletion on mood of patients treated with antidepressants. Psychopharmacol Bull 1993; 29:389–396.
52. Charney DS. Monoamine dysfunction and the pathophysiology and treatment of depression. J Clin Psychiatry 1998; 59:11–14.
53. Maas JW, Fawcett JA, Dekirmenjian H. Catecholamine metabolism, depressive illness, and drug response. Arch Gen Psychiatry 1972; 26:252–262.
54. Muscettola G, Potter WZ, Pickar D, Goodwin FK. Urinary 3-methoxy-4-hydroxyphenylglycol and major affective disorders. A replication and new findings. Arch Gen Psychiatry 1984; 41:337–342.
55. Charney DS, Heninger GR, Sternberg DE, et al. Presynaptic adrenergic receptor sensitivity in depression. The effect of long-term desipramine treatment. Arch Gen Psychiatry 1981; 38:1334–1340.
56. Charney DS, Menkes DB, Heninger GR. Receptor sensitivity and the mechanism of action of antidepressant treatment. Implications for the etiology and therapy of depression. Arch Gen Psychiatry 1981; 38:1160–1180.
57. Karege F, Bovier P, Widmer J, Gaillard JM, Tissot R. Platelet membrane alpha 2-adrenergic receptors in depression. Psychiatry Res 1992; 43:243–252.
58. Wilson IC, Rabon AM, Merrick HA, Knox AE, Taylor JP, Buffaloe WJ. Imipramine pamoate in the treatment of depression. Psychosomatics 1966; 7:251–253.
59. Roy JY, Pinard G, Hillel J, Gagnon MA, Tetreault L. Comparative study of dibencycladine (Ludiomil) and imipramine in the treatment of psychotic depression. Int J Clin Pharmacol 1973; 7:54–61.
60. Hirschfeld RM, Russell JM, Delgado PL, et al. Predictors of response to acute treatment of chronic and double depression with sertraline or imipramine. J Clin Psychiatry 1998; 59:669–675.
61. Feighner JP. The role of venlafaxine in rational antidepressant therapy. J Clin Psychiatry 1994; 55(suppl A):62–68; discussion 69–70, 98–100.
62. Schweitzer I, Burrows G, Tuckwell V, et al. Sustained response to open-label venlafaxine in drug-resistant major depression. J Clin Psychopharmacol 2001; 21:185–189.
63. Sachs GS, Lafer B, Stoll AL, et al. A double-blind trial of bupropion versus desipramine for bipolar depression. J Clin Psychiatry 1994; 55:391–393.
64. Ascher JA, Cole JO, Colin JN, et al. Bupropion: a review of its mechanism of antidepressant activity. J Clin Psychiatry 1995; 56:395–401.
65. Stahl S, Zivkov M, Reimitz PE, Panagides J, Hoff W. Meta-analysis of randomized, double-blind, placebo-controlled, efficacy and safety studies of mirtazapine versus amitriptyline in major depression. Acta Psychiatr Scand Suppl 1997; 391:22–30.
66. Stimmel GL, Dopheide JA, Stahl SM. Mirtazapine: an antidepressant with noradrenergic and specific serotonergic effects. Pharmacotherapy 1997; 17:10–21.
67. Holm KJ, Jarvis B, Foster RH. Mirtazapine. A pharmacoeconomic review of its use in depression. Pharmacoeconomics 2000; 17:515–534.
68. Schatzberg AF. Clinical efficacy of reboxetine in major depression. J Clin Psychiatry 2000; 61:31–38.

69. Kasper S, el Giamal N, Hilger E. Reboxetine: the first selective noradrenaline re-uptake inhibitor. Expert Opin Pharmacother 2000; 1:771–782.
70. Diehl DJ, Gershon S. The role of dopamine in mood disorders. Compr Psychiatry 1992; 33:115–120.
71. Waehrens J, Gerlach J. Bromocriptine and imipramine in endogenous depression. A double-blind controlled trial in out-patients. J Affect Disord 1981; 3:193–202.
72. Aberg-Wistedt A, Wistedt B, Bertilsson L. Higher CSF levels of HVA and 5-HIAA in delusional compared to nondelusional depression. Arch Gen Psychiatry 1985; 42:925–926.
73. Faustman WO, King RJ, Faull KF, et al. MMPI measures of impulsivity and depression correlate with CSF 5-HIAA and HVA in depression but not schizophrenia. J Affect Disord 1991; 22:235–239.
74. Cookson J, Silverstone T, Wells B. Double-blind comparative clinical trial of pimozide and chlorpromazine in mania. A test of the dopamine hypothesis. Acta Psychiatr Scand 1981; 64:381–397.
75. Chou JC, Czobor P, Tuma I, et al. Pretreatment plasma HVA and haloperidol response in acute mania. J Affect Disord 2000; 59:55–59.
76. Petty F, Davis LL, Kabel D, Kramer GL. Serotonin dysfunction disorders: a behavioral neurochemistry perspective. J Clin Psychiatry 1996; 57:11–16.
77. Peirson AR, Heuchert JW. Correlations for serotonin levels and measures of mood in a nonclinical sample. Psychol Rep 2000; 87:707–716.
78. Halford JC, Blundell JE. Separate systems for serotonin and leptin in appetite control. Ann Med 2000; 32:222–232.
79. Kent JM, Coplan JD, Gorman JM. Clinical utility of the selective serotonin reuptake inhibitors in the spectrum of anxiety. Biol Psychiatry 1998; 44:812–824.
80. Paredes RG, Contreras JL, Agmo A. Serotonin and sexual behavior in the male rabbit. J Neural Transm 2000; 107:767–777.
81. Lapierre YD. Norepinephrine in psychiatry. In: Villeneuve A, ed. Brain Neurotransmitters and Psychiatry. Quebec City: Astra Pharmaceuticals Canada, 1985:42–48.
82. Robbins TW, Everitt BJ. Central norepinephrine neurons and behavior. In: Bloom FE, Kupfer DJ, eds. Psychopharmacology—The Fourth Generation of Progress. New York: Raven Press, 1995:363–372.
83. Moal ML. Mesocorticolimbic dopaminergic neurons—functional and regulatory roles. In: Bloom FE, Kupfer DJ, eds. Psychopharmacology—The Fourth Generation of Progress. New York: Raven Press, 1995:283–294.
84. Becker JB, Rudick CN, Jenkins WJ. The role of dopamine in the nucleus accumbens and striatum during sexual behavior in the female rat. J Neurosci 2001; 21:3236–3241.

8

Classification of Anxiety Disorders
Implications for Psychiatric Research

KERRIE L. POSEY, SUSAN G. BALL, and ANANTHA SHEKHAR
Indiana University School of Medicine, Indianapolis, Indiana U.S.A.

I. INTRODUCTION

From the momentary stage fright to the everyday worry, fear and anxiety are universally shared phenomena. Fear is experienced as the subjective emotion whereas anxiety refers to the construct of physiological symptoms, behaviors, and thoughts that occur in the context of fear. In this chapter, the adaptive and maladaptive features of anxiety will be presented along with a description of the most common anxiety disorders. The research base that has been used to design the current classification will be reviewed as well as the challenges that remain for the DSM diagnostic system. Finally, future directions for conceptualizing anxiety based on a neurobiological framework will be suggested for further consideration in this evolving area of psychiatry.

To understand anxiety as a disorder, one needs to consider the development and purpose of anxiety. The bioevolutionary theory of anxiety proposes that anxiety has developed as an alarm system that occurs in response to danger or threat [1]. The original types of threat that occurred within the natural environment were predominantly physical, e.g., the wild animal, or social challenges, e.g., group and interpersonal dynamics. Confronted with these types of threat, survival depended on the development of effective defensive responses to counter these dangers—defenses such as escape behaviors, avoidance, aggression, and submission [2]. For each type of defensive behavior, there is a corresponding physiological substrate to support the activation and mobilization of resources. The sympathetic activity that is characterized as the "fight-or-flight" mode is neither dangerous nor harmful, but is intended to be aversive, so that a response will be initiated, resulting in a defensive maneuver.

As an alarm system then, three components become necessary for successful functioning: the ability to detect a threat, the ability to identify the threat as a danger, and the ability to respond appropriately to the danger. An optimal alarm system will have a sensitivity that is balanced between the costs of false alarms, e.g., an escape response when there is not a danger, versus the cost of missing a true alarm, failure to respond to an actual danger. Given the relatively low costs of false versus true alarms in the context of danger, a biological alarm system will therefore be biased toward a "better safe than sorry" mechanism for both detection and response components [2]. In addition, the strength of the response should be associated directly with the strength of the perceived threat. The system may maintain a constant level of "hypervigilance" when the environment is generally perceived to be hostile and danger cues are considered to be probable. When the actual danger cues are detected as present, the system then intensifies into a "response" status, whereupon the body is mobilized for a direct action. The "response" is expressed as the panic attack where each symptom either supports the escape behavior (e.g., increases in respiratory rate to support oxygen to muscles) or conserves physical resources (e.g., slowing down salivation and digestion).

Anxiety as an illness or disorder develops when there is a dysregulation in any of the three components of threat detection, threat interpretation, or threat response. A state of persistent hypervigilance will result in overdetection of threats; catastrophic thinking patterns can result in false perceptions of threat; and avoidance and escape behaviors may become over-utilized, resulting in maintenance of fears. The Diagnostic and Statistical Manual for Mental Disorders, 4th edition (DSM-IV) [3], for anxiety disorders classifies seven major areas of illness: generalized anxiety disorder, panic disorder, social phobia, specific phobia, obsessive-compulsive disorder, posttraumatic stress disorder, and acute stress disorder [4]. In the alarm system analogy, these syndromes can be viewed as a predominant disturbance in one or more of the components of threat detection, interpretation, or response. For example, generalized anxiety disorder is a perturbed alarm system, whose threshold for threat detection is set too low. Sharing a low threshold for threat detection, individuals with obsessive-compulsive disorder are also likely to perceive harm with a greater sensitivity than others. Once a stimulus has been detected, threat interpretation becomes problematic in the cases of panic disorder, social phobia, specific phobias, and obsessive-compulsive disorder wherein information is misperceived or processed erroneously (e.g., panic attack symptoms are interpreted as an impending heart attack). Panic disorder, acute stress disorder, and posttraumatic stress disorder develop from the response component of the alarm system, where the response either occurs in the absence of danger (i.e., spontaneous panic attacks) or continues to be triggered despite the cessation of the true danger.

II. CURRENT CLASSIFICATION OF ANXIETY DISORDERS

In the following section, each of the DSM-IV anxiety disorders will be reviewed for their conceptual and defining features. Similar to the other DSM-IV categories, the anxiety disorders diagnostic criteria are empirically descriptive rather than etiologically determined. However, the diagnostic criteria have been strongly influenced by bioevolutionary and cognitive models for anxiety that were developed during the 1980s and 1990s, which have served as the predominant research basis for anxiety disorders.

A. Generalized Anxiety Disorder

Often characterized as the "basic anxiety disorder," generalized anxiety disorder is defined by worry that is pervasive and uncontrollable to the extent that it interferes with daily functioning or causes marked distress. The development of criteria for generalized anxiety disorder was mainly concerned with discriminating pathological worry from the normal adaptive process of worry, which alerts the individual to potential, probable threats. Some of the key findings from research studies were that pathological worry and normal worry could be differentiated on the basis of the difficulty with controlling worry as well as by the accompanying physiological symptoms [5].

Excessive worry was best discriminated from other anxiety disorders by being associated with at least three of the following symptoms: feeling keyed up/on edge, restlessness, easy fatigability, difficulty concentrating, irritability, and difficulty sleeping [6]. Again, consistent with a model of hypervigilance or "heightened threat detection," generalized anxiety disorder criteria require at least 6 months' duration, as "normal worry" typically resolves with the cessation of an episode of stress, but pathological worry persists despite stress resolution. More recent studies, however, such as one conducted by Bienvenu et al. [7], have suggested that the severity of associated symptoms rather than the duration of worry is a better discriminator along the continuum of nonclinical to clinical worry.

B. Panic Disorder

Panic disorder has been a complicated diagnosis that has undergone numerous changes in the DSM classification system. In DSM-III-R, the definition of a panic attack was first defined as the acute onset of at least four cognitive or sympathetic symptoms with a peak onset of 10 min. Although it was useful to have a definition to discriminate the "panic response" from the anxiety pattern of generalized and other anxiety disorders, the exclusive inclusion of the definition of panic attacks within the diagnosis proved problematic. Many of the individuals meeting criteria for other types of anxiety disorders also present with panic attacks, approximately 80% of those with different disorders [8].

Further, panic attacks have different functional significance within different anxiety disorders. Spontaneous attacks (no apparent trigger) may be driven by an underlying false alarm mechanism whereas situationally predisposed (attacks likely in the presence of the trigger) or situationally bound (attack always occurs in the presence of the trigger) are derived from learning or conditioning [9]. In addition, some people experience panic attacks but are not unduly distressed or impaired by them. In recognition of these limitations, the DSM-IV system separated the definition of panic attack from the definition of panic disorder. The panic attack criteria remained the same in requiring that four of 13 symptoms must occur and peak within 10 min to denote the acute intensity and sympathetic activity. The defining symptoms of a panic attacks are heart palpitations/pounding, sweating, trembling/shaking, shortness of breath, feeling of choking, chest pain/discomfort, nausea/abdominal distress, dizziness/unsteadiness, derealization, fear of losing control/going crazy, fear of dying, paresthesias, and chills/hot flushes. With this separate definition, panic attacks were now viewed as simply the "defensive response" that can occur in the context of a perceived imminent, severe threat and thus be diagnosed as occurring within any anxiety disorder [10].

Panic disorder, on the other hand, has been conceptualized to develop as a two-part process [11,12]. Initially, panic disorder may result from the occurrence of "false alarms"; the alarm system becomes triggered in the absence of any objective danger. This false alarm may arise from genetic, biological, and life stress vulnerabilities. For the person who is experiencing the false alarm, however, the phenomenon is inexplicable. The absence of an external source of danger to associate with the alarm results in an internal scanning for the threat. The person then misperceives the occurrence of the alarm as an indication of an internal danger, such as heart attack, loss of control, or fainting. Further focus on the perception that the attacks themselves are dangerous results in a secondary process that maintains the panic attacks. Fear of the attack triggers the alarm system, which then perpetuates further fear, i.e., "the fear of fear." In recognition of the necessity for both initial attacks and the developed fear of the attacks, the DSM-IV criteria for panic disorder requires the occurrence of recurrent panic attacks followed by either worry about the attacks, worry about the implications or consequences of the attacks, or a significant behavioral change due to the attacks.

A common complication of panic disorder is agoraphobia, which is avoidance of situations associated with the fear of having a panic attack and/or being unable to obtain assistance or to escape. Most common types of agoraphobia include situations associated with restriction of movement, e.g., standing in line, being in a barber's chair, or with travel, e.g., driving. One diagnostic controversy has been whether agoraphobia occurs only secondary to panic disorder or whether it can occur without a history of panic. Research that has fueled this controversy has focused on the findings that clinical samples of patients who report agoraphobia typically have an onset of panic disorder prior to the avoidance behavior [13]. However, in the Epidemiological Catchment Study survey, community respondents did meet agoraphobia without having panic disorder [14]. Although this study has been criticized for confounding the diagnoses between agoraphobia and specific phobias [15], the DSM-IV allows the diagnosis of agoraphobia independently of the presence of panic disorder. Clinical studies of patients meeting criteria for agoraphobia without panic disorder typically show that the agoraphobia develops in the context of limited symptom attacks, usually with a predominant gastrointestinal focus [16]. For example, nausea and diarrhea may provoke avoidance of public situations for fear of being unable to leave a place or to get to bathroom facilities adequately. Again, the avoidance strategies become a defensive response for the perception that the symptoms themselves are dangerous and the trigger point for the alarm.

C. Social Phobia

In DSM-IV, social phobia is defined by the cognitive component of an excessive fear of social or performance situations in which the person may be evaluated or the focus of attention [17]. Typical social situations that trigger this anxiety include performance types of situations, such as speaking in front of groups, or interactional types of situations, such as initiating and maintaining conversations. Most individuals (2/3) who have lifetime social phobia report having multiple situations associated with their anxiety [18]. Within these situations, the predominant trigger is a perception that one is going to be evaluated negatively because of one's own failings, which can include the demonstration of anxiety signs, e.g., blushing or sweating. Similarly to panic disorder, the anxiety symptoms themselves may become a focus of the fear. However, while the patient with panic disorder fears the anxiety symptoms for its potential physical (stroke) or psychological (going crazy) consequences, the person with social phobia fears the symptoms for their potential for public embarrassment, as the person often believes that these symptoms are detectable and that others will view them as a sign of weakness or peculiarity.

Social phobia is often viewed by the person as being related to shyness. Although shyness is a common development process that occurs within children and adolescents, it is typically transient and less severe [19]. Similar to generalized anxiety disorder, pathological shyness is differentiated from "normal" shyness by its interference and duration [20]. Situations that trigger the fear must be sufficiently anxiety provoking and/or interfering to warrant the clinical diagnosis. Social phobia is commonly being renamed in the literature as social anxiety disorder to emphasize that it is not the external situation per se that triggers the alarm, as in phobic illness, but rather the internal cognitive processes of perceived negative evaluation [21].

D. Specific Phobias

Most individuals can easily identify specific situations or objects that they associate with danger. The fears that are common to all of us are usually dealt with by simple avoidance. For the person who has an alarm reaction to the stimulus of a dog, the easiest defense is avoidance of dogs. When avoidance strategies fail as a defense, e.g., the person is not able to avoid the situation because of occupational or social factors, the fears then typically meet criteria for a specific phobia. The essential diagnostic defining feature is an alarm response to the object or situation that is excessive or unreasonable, resulting in distress and/or impairment. Often, it is the presence of multiple specific phobias that prompts a person to seek out clinical treatment [22] as the aggregation of several fears begin to impact daily functioning or social relationships.

Interestingly, although the names of various phobias range into the hundreds, most common specific phobias fall into four categories: animal type; natural environment, such as heights; blood/injection/injury type; and situational (claustrophobia). Biological preparedness theory propose that these situations and objects are more easily predisposed to become a conditioned fear object owing to their evolutionary significance to the species, but the empirical support for this theory has been limited [23]. More recently, the development of specific phobias has been associated with a greater underlying fear of anxiety as well as the situation [24].

E. Obsessive-Compulsive Disorder

Although the diagnosis of obsessive-compulsive disorder can be made by meeting the diagnostic criteria for obsessions or compulsions, research supporting the DSM-IV criteria have found that most individuals will meet criteria for both components of the illness [25]. The definition of obsessions recognizes that these may not only be thoughts, but can also be other types of mental phenomenon, including imagery or impulses. For the person who experiences this phenomenon, the thoughts or impulses are perceived as dangerous, thus triggering the alarm system. Unlike an external situation that has been labeled as threatening, when a person is faced with a thought, he or she cannot rely on a simple avoidance. In fact, attempts at thought suppression are likely to increase the frequency of a specific thought. Wegner et al. [26] demonstrated that subjects asked to suppress thoughts about a neutral stimulus, "white bear," actually experienced more intrusions than subjects who were given the directive to think about white bears. Exacerbating the problem of thought suppression, most patients with obsessive-compulsive disorder also have an overly developed perception of responsibility, especially with regard for being able to control one's thoughts [27,28].

Given the inability to suppress the thought and their sense of responsibility for having the thought, the person will then develop a neutralization strategy that will defend against the thought. Compulsions are defined as physical or mental acts that are designed to escape or avoid a thought. Initially, most compulsions have a logical connection with the thought, e.g., washing to neutralize contamination fears, but for some thoughts, the neutralization strategy may simply rely on a magical or superstitious connection, e.g., if I touch something three times, then nothing bad will happen. Mental rituals can also serve this same function. For example, for intrusive unwanted religious thoughts, such as blasphemy, compulsive praying may be viewed as a way to escape the consequence of having these thoughts.

The DSM-IV criteria for OCD highlight these essential features of this illness. The obsessions must be perceived as repetitive/recurrent, anxiety provoking, and ego-dystonic at some point, e.g., an intrusive thought that the person does not want. The person must then also make some effort to neutralize or avoid the thought. To differentiate from psychotic spectrum illness, the person has to recognize that these are his or her own thoughts. Further, the amount of time spent in response to these thoughts, either worrying or compulsing to rid oneself of them, must be sufficiently distressing or interfering. To discriminate between worries that are also anxiety provoking and repetitive, the obsession criterion also includes recognition that the person's thoughts are not simply real-life concerns, but rather are viewed as being inappropriate content, e.g., thoughts of harming someone, or very low probability, e.g., getting contaminated from objects on the floor [29].

F. Acute Stress/Posttraumatic Stress Disorder

Unlike the above DSM anxiety disorders, where the triggers associated with anxiety are typically false signals or misperceptions of threat, acute and posttraumatic stress disorders occur following the experience of a "true alarm", e.g., actual physical threat or danger. Although physically traumatic events, such as assaults or accidents, are commonly considered to be the type of stressor that may result in difficulties with recovery, several studies have also shown that subjective or perceived threat can be as anxiety provoking as objective threat [30].

Most persons who experience a threat of serious physical injury will experience transient emotional and behavioral responses as they adjust to the recognition that they have survived the threat. However, in some cases, a person may experience an alarm reaction that causes significant distress or impairment in functioning, especially with regard to mobilizing resources to respond to the aftermath of the trauma. In recognizing that these types of alarm responses may require direct intervention, acute stress disorder was introduced in DSM-IV [4].

The main diagnostic criteria for acute stress disorder are the experience of a traumatic stressor of both objective or subjective threat; the experience of fear, helplessness, and horror; at least three dissociative symptoms (numbing of emotion, reduction in awareness, derealization, depersonalization, and amnesia), usually some form of reoccurrence of the trauma (images, thoughts, dreams, flashbacks); increased arousal (difficulty sleeping, irritability, exaggerated startles response, motor restlessness, poor concentration); and avoidance of stimuli associated with the trauma.

Posttraumatic stress disorder criteria share several of the same features as acute stress disorder, but there are a couple of key differences. Acute stress disorder requires at least three dissociative symptoms whereas PTSD allows, but does not require, the presence of dissociation. In addition, the PTSD criteria specify that more than one symptom must occur in the areas of reexperiencing, avoidance, and arousal, whereas acute stress disorder does not dictate the number of symptoms but rather focuses on severity as defined by the term "marked." A further difference is the time course, with acute stress disorder occurring between 2 days posttrauma and no longer than 4 weeks, whereas posttraumatic stress is diagnosed 4 weeks following a trauma to denote the chronic alarm response as a disorder.

In developing diagnostic criteria for classifying traumatic responses, several dilemmas have occurred concerning pathologizing normal responses to stressful events as well as whether there is a quantitative or qualitative continuum from the nonclinical to the clinical state. [31]. Although acute stress disorder may be a precursor to posttraumatic stress disorder [32], the emphasis on dissociation within the acute stress criteria makes it a qualitatively different disorder from PTSD [33]. Many individuals who meet criteria for PTSD do not necessarily experience the dissociative symptoms at the time of the trauma, but nonetheless experience impairment from the other symptom clusters [34]. Given these conceptual considerations, further empirical work needs to clarify as to whether the difficulty to integrate a traumatic experience resulting in posttraumatic stress disorder is actually a disorder of magnitude or severity of the alarm response, e.g., a stronger response due to individual vulnerabilities [35], or it is a disorder of the alarm response failing to cease in a normative time course.

III. CHALLENGES TO THE DSM DIAGNOSTIC SYSTEM

One of the primary missions of the DSM-IV task force was to develop a classification system that was supported by an empirical base and that also could be utilized widely to produce reliable diagnoses. Using structured clinical interviews, such as the Anxiety Disorders Interview Schedule for the DSM-IV, researchers have demonstrated good reliability for most of the DSM-IV anxiety disorders [36]. However, another important objective for a classification system is the utility of the diagnoses in predicting clinical profiles, treatment response, or identifying a shared etiology [37] Considering these functions of a diagnostic system, the DSM-IV classification system is challenged by the issues of high degree of comorbidity among the different disorders, a lack of good discrimination by available treatments, and an overlap in neurobiological and genetic diatheses.

A. Comorbidity Among the Different Disorders

In studies utilizing structured clinical interviews, most patients who meet criteria for one anxiety disorder are also likely to meet criteria for a second or third anxiety disorder [38]. Given the DSM-IV emphasis on the diagnosis by the type of threatening stimuli, it is not surprising that comorbidity occurs as a person who overperceives threat in one domain may also be likely to have misperceptions of threat in other domains. For example, a person with panic attacks may fear not only the physical consequences of the panic symptoms, but also the social/evaluative component and therefore meet criteria for panic disorder and social phobia. Similarly, generalized anxiety disorder in which hypervigilance is the primary mode may lead one to worry about physical consequences of symptoms, social performance, and daily responsibilities, resulting in diagnoses of generalized anxiety, panic disorder, and social phobia. Further, across the life span the focus of fear may change from one domain to another resulting in even higher comorbidity when examining lifetime prevalence.

Similarly, the comorbidity of anxiety and depressive illness is also quite high. Several studies have found that the cooccurrence of the diagnostic syndromes of anxiety and depression within clinical samples occurs in the majority of patients, especially when considering lifetime prevalence. Estimates have shown that this cooccurrence is present in both primary anxiety populations as well as primary depressive populations. Thirty percent to 60% of patients with anxiety disorders meet criteria for a current depressive disorder with lifetime estimates ranging to 80% [39,40]. The cooccurrence and risk for comorbidity is not limited solely to clinical populations. In the National Comorbidity Sample, 8000 community respondents were assessed by lay interviewers using the Composite Interview based on DSM-III-R criteria. The odds ratio for having panic attacks with the presence of a depression was 6.2 whereas the odds ratio for having panic disorder with depression, was 6.8. From the patterns found in this study, the presence of a primary panic disorder appeared to be a marker for a secondary depression, whereas primary depression is a risk factor for secondary panic attacks, but not panic disorder [41].

In considering the problem of anxiety and depression comorbidity, the focus of the literature has been on three possibilities: anxiety and depression are viewed as being two distinct illnesses, they are different expressions of a common underlying pathophysiology, or the comorbid condition is its own unique disorder. Further complicating these issues are the diagnostic criteria as defined by the DSM. Many of the symptoms that are included for the anxiety disorder diagnoses are also incorporated into the depressive disorder diagnoses. For example, generalized anxiety disorder and major depressive episode criteria share the symptoms of sleep disturbance, fatigability, and difficulty concentrating. Clinically, irritability has long been associated with depression as has rumination, making the distinction between these disorders more difficult [6].

One of the more influential models in recent years has tried to sort out the symptoms that are shared between the anxiety disorders and depression as well as the unique components. In the tripartite model, anxiety and depression share a common dimension, described as general negative affectivity, representing negative valence emotions and general distress [42]. Symptoms consistent with general negative affectivity include fear, sadness, and tension. Anxiety is proposed to have the unique component of the physiological hyperarousal of the "fight-or-flight" response whereas depressive disorders are suggested to be distinct by the dimension of low positive affectivity, described as the ability to experience pleasure and/or engage in the environment. Patients with anxiety disorders are described as having high levels of general negative affectivity accompanied by physiological hyperarousal; patients with depressive disorders have high general negative affectivity; and low positive affectivity; and those with the comorbid condition would have high general negative affectivity, low positive affectivity, and hyperarousal symptoms.

In the initial presentation of the model, Clark and Watson [42] demonstrated the dimensions of general and positive affectivity through administering multiple questionnaires to 483 outpatients seeking treatment for anxiety or depression, 516 college students, and 453 patients seeking treatment for substance abuse. They argued through the use of structured equation modeling that the responses were consistent with the tripartite model. However, different authors have countered that that the appropriate analyses for this data should be confirmatory factor analyses rather than structured equation modeling [43]. Using the same dataset, Burns and Eidelson [43] found that the responses supported a two-factor model because the nonspecific symptoms of anxiety and depression did not load onto a single general distress factor. Although the tripartite model has provoked an intriguing line of research and discussion, the relationship between anxiety and depression models continues to remain complex and controversial.

B. Lack of Discrimination by Pharmacological Treatment/Biological Challenges

A second challenge to the DSM classification system includes the lack of discrimination in selecting effective treatment modalities based on the diagnoses. Both pharmacotherapy and cognitive-behavioral psychotherapy have been demonstrated to be efficacious for the treatment of anxiety disorders [44]. Within the spectrum of pharmacotherapy, the treatment options can be broadly categorized into two major classes of drugs: antidepressants and the benzodiazepines. The antidepressants can be further subclassified into serotonergic and nonserotonergic groups. As a first line of treatment, the serotonergic reuptake inhibitor (SRI) antidepressants appear to have a broad range of efficacy across the anxiety disorders, including OCD, panic disorder, GAD, social anxiety, and PTSD [45]. Thus, the specific anxiety diagnosis as defined by the current DSM system provides little utility for influencing the decision of SRI treatment. Similarly, benzodiazepines have also demonstrated a ubiquitous positive effect of the pharmacotherapy for anxiety. Initially, benzodiazepines were considered to be differentially more effective in reducing the hypervigilance "threat detection" associated with generalized anxiety than in reducing the "defensive response" of the panic attack. However, the development of high-potency benzodiazepines that were effective in ameliorating panic attacks suggested that this distinction was not as germane [46].

In considering the interaction between the DSM system and lack of treatment differentiation, part of the problem is clearly related to the broad nature of the neurochemical systems that are targeted by these drugs. The serotonin system is a global modulator pathway that affects almost every central nervous system function. Similarly, the benzodiazepines receptors are associated with the gamma-aminobutyric acid (GABA), another pervasive neurotransmitter. Some noradrenergic agents have shown some differential efficacy between panic disorder and obsessive-compulsive disorders, but these agents, too, demonstrate a broad base of efficacy for anxiety [47]. Given the pervasiveness of these neurotransmitter systems, it is not surprising that drugs that work through these neurotransmitters have a broad range of effects across multiple diagnostic categories. Novel treatments based on less global systems, such as peptides, GABA receptor partial agonists and NMDA receptor antagonists may have a better ability to discriminate between diagnostic categories [48].

Not only have pharmacological treatments been nonspecific to different anxiety disorders, but biological challenges that have been used to elicit panic responses in patients have also failed to discriminate among the different disorders. Intravenous sodium lactate and other provocative agents (e.g., carbon dioxide, caffeine, yohimbine) elicit panic attacks in patients with panic disorder but not in normal controls [49]. These agents were thought to be initially be fairly selective for triggering symptoms in panic disorder. However, recent studies suggest that lactate infusions may provoke symptoms in patients with posttraumatic stress disorder [50] as well as premenstrual dysphoric disorder [51]. Therefore, the specificity of these challenges to panic disorder alone has been questioned. While these provocation agents have been of great help in elucidating some of the underlying neurobiology of anxiety symptoms, they have not exhibited adequate selectivity to be of assistance in the classification of the different anxiety disorders.

IV. FUTURE DIRECTIONS

A. Impact of Neuroimaging on Classification

Over the past decade, a number of seminal neuroimaging studies have been conducted in patients with anxiety disorders. Neuroimaging has considerable potential for reorganizing the classifications of psychiatric disorders [52]. Structural and functional imaging studies using psychiatric patients are beginning to identify neuroanatomical systems and neurotransmitters that are disrupted in the anxiety disorders. Studies in normal subjects continue to identify brain regions where activity is modified during presentation of fearful stimuli. For example, results of a recent functional imaging study examining amygdala activation during exposure to neutral or fearful faces revealed greater activation of the amygdala in normal adults during fearful face exposures. In contrast, children demonstrated amygdala activation to both neutral and fearful faces [53]. Furthermore, amygdala activation of male but not female children was decreased with repeated face presentations. These imaging studies clearly indicate that age and sex are both important factors in determining anxious responses in the brain, and these findings are consistent with epidemiological data on anxiety disorders, in which prevalence rates tend to favor women [14]. Eventually, similar neuroimaging approaches may be used to identify individuals at risk for developing disorders.

Some general outlines of the central nervous system pathways involved in the different anxiety states are emerging based on neuroimaging studies of clinical populations, demonstrating specific anxiety symptoms [54,55]. For example, several reports have implicated the orbitofrontal cortex–striatum–thalamic pathway as being a critical component of the pathophysiology in OCD [56,57]. This pathway is quite distinct from areas often implicated in panic disorder, such as the parahippocampal and amygdala regions. However, these areas implicated in panic disorder, especially the amygdala, may also be implicated in phobias, PTSD, and GAD. For example, studies have implicated the amygdala and anterior cingulate cortex in PTSD [58,59]. Some brain regions are consistently activated across several anxiety disorders. For example, symptom provocation paradigms have consistently been shown to activate the amygdala and the right side of the prefrontal cortex across anxiety patient populations [55]. Thus, once again, OCD separates out as a much different pathophysiological entity compared to the other anxiety disorders. With more refined imaging methodologies, it is hoped that greater discriminations can be made within the other anxiety disorders.

B. Impact of Genetic Studies on Classification

Genetic studies are another important approach to elucidating the pathophysiology of psychiatric disorders. Ideally, distinct disorders would be predicted to cluster separately in population genetic studies and eventually be linked to one or more susceptibility genes. There is clear evidence that the major anxiety disorders do exhibit familial patterns with significant genetic components in their etiology [60]. However, the ability to discriminate between the different anxiety disorders based on genetic predisposition has proven to be elusive. For example, there is considerable evidence that generalized anxiety disorder and major depression have common genetic risk factors [61]. Similarly, there are significant overlapping genetic factors between generalized anxiety and panic disorders [62]. Studies have also suggested that perhaps there are several common genetic susceptibility factors for anxiety disorders, some of which are common to anxiety susceptibility in general and others more specific to individual anxiety syndromes [63,62]. Others have suggested that rather than try to find genetic factors for complex syndromes like the anxiety disorders, which are likely to involve a large number of genes, it may be better to define specific markers and endophenotypes (e.g., hypothalamic-pituitary response in posttraumatic stress disorder, respiratory reactivity in panic disorder) as better targets for genetic analysis. [64,65]. Thus, more sophisticated genetic studies are likely to provide other approaches to classification of anxiety syndromes.

C. Impact of Neurobiological Insights

Better elucidation of the underlying neurobiological mechanisms of emotions will undoubtedly have a major impact on our future classification of psychiatric disorders. With regard to the anxiety disorders, determining the neural basis of key components of anxiety disorders, such as threat detection, threat evaluation and defensive responses, will shed new light on classification. For example, the response system to a threatening stimulus involves a series of interconnected pathways extending from the medial amygdala, medial hypothalamus, periaqueductal gray, and the brainstem autonomic centers. Disorders that are clearly related to a disturbed response system such as panic and posttraumatic stress disorders would be expected to show pathological changes in these pathways. Current neuroimaging studies, in fact, suggest that it is indeed the case. Similarly, the functions of threat detection and assessment are likely to involve prefrontal, cingulated, and other cortical areas, the striatum and thalamus, as the key components. Disorders of these functions, such as obsessive-compulsive disorder and generalized anxiety disorder are likely to involve abnormalities in these circuits, which is again supported by current neuroimaging studies. Thus, such informed neurobiological approaches will in the future help to categorizing anxiety disorders at a pathophysiological level rather than at a symptomatic level.

In conclusion, like most psychiatric diagnoses, anxiety disorders are currently classified according to the symptom clusters and the primary focus or source of the anxiety. This empirical system has been extremely helpful in providing uniformity of clinical definition of syndromes, enabling us begin a systematic study of these syndromes. However, such a descriptive system will eventually need to be refined by information gathered from genetic, neurobiological, and treatment outcome studies. Such efforts will perhaps lead in the future to better-defined syndromes that are grouped according to pathophysiological processes rather than purely descriptive similarities.

REFERENCES

1. Nesse R. Emotional disorders in evolutionary perspective. Br J of Med Psychol 1998; 71(4):397–415.
2. Dixon AK. Ethological strategies for defence in animals and humans: their role in some psychiatric disorders. Br J Med Psychol 1998; 71:417–445.
3. American Psychiatric Association. Diagnostic and Statistical Manual for Mental Disorders: DSM-IV, 4th ed. Washington: American Psychiatric Association, 1994.
4. DSM-IV Sourcebook. Washington: American Psychiatric Association, 1994.
5. Abel J, Borkovec TD. Generalizability of DSM-III-R generalized anxiety disorder to proposed DSM-IV criteria and cross-validation of proposed changes. J Anxiety Disord 1995; 9:303–315.
6. Brown T, Marten P, Barlow D. Discriminant validity of the symptoms constituting the DSM-III-R and DSM-IV associated symptom criterion of generalized anxiety disorder. J Anxiety Disord 1995; 1995(9):317–328.
7. Bienvenu OJ, Nestadt G, Eaton WW. Characterizing generalized anxiety: temporal and symptomatic thresholds. J Nerv Ment Dis 1998; 186:51–56.
8. Sanderson WC, DiNardo PA, Rapee RM, Barlow DH. Syndrome comorbidity in patients diagnosed with a DSM-III-R anxiety disorder. J Abnorm Psychol 1990; 99(3):308–312.
9. Rapee RM, Sanderson WC, McCauley PA, DiNardo PA. Differences in reported symptom profile between panic disorder and other DSM-III-R anxiety disordres. Behav Res Ther 1992; 30(1):45–52.
10. Barlow DH, Brown TA, Craske MG. Definitions of panic attacks and panic disorder in the DSM-IV: implications for research. J of Abnorm Psychol 1994; 103(3):553–564.
11. Barlow DH. Unraveling the mysteries of anxiety and its disorders from the perspective of emotion theory. Am Psychol 2000; 55(11):1247–1263.
12. Clark DM. Anxiety disorders: whey they persist and how to treat them. Behav Res Ther 1999; 37:S5–S27.
13. Goisman RM, Warshaw MG, Steketee GS, Fierman EJeal. DSM-IV and the disappearance of agoraphobia without a history of panic disorder: new data on a controversial diagnoses. Am J Psychiatry 1995; 152(10): 1438–1443.
14. Regier DA, Narrow WE, Rae DS. The epidemiology of anxiety disorders: the epidemiologic catchment area (ECA) experience. J Psychiatr Res 1990; 24(suppl 2):3–14.
15. Horwath E, Lish J, Johnson J, Hornig C. Agoraphobia without panic: clinical reappraisal of an epidemiological finding. Am J Psychiatry 1993; 150(10):1496–1501.
16. Pollard AC, Tait RC, Meldrum D et al. Agoraphobia without panic: case illustrations of an overlooked syndrome. J Nerv Ment Dis 1996; 184(1):61–62.
17. Lang AJ, Stein MB. Social phobia: prevalence and diagnostic threshold. J Clin Psychiatry 2001; 62(suppl 1):5–9.
18. Kessler R, Stein M, Berglund P. Social phobia subtypes in the National Comorbidity Survey. Am J Psychiatry 1998; 155(5):613–618.
19. Turner SM, Beidel DC, Borden JW, Stanley MAeal. Social phobia: axis I and axis II correlates. J Abnorm Psychol 1991; 100(1):102–106.
20. Davidson J, Hughes D, George L, et al. The boundary of social phobia: exploring the threshold. Arch Gen Psychiatry 1994; 51:975–983.
21. Stein MB, Gorman JM. Unmasking social anxiety disorder. J Psychiatry Neurosci 2001; 26(3):185–189.
22. Curtis GC, Magee WJ, Eaton WW, et al. Specific fears and phobias: epidemiology and classifcation. Br J Psychiatry 1998; 173:212–217.
23. McNally R. Preparedness and phobias: a review. Psychol Bull 1987; 101(2):283–303.
24. Hofmann SG, Lehman CL, Barlow DH. How specific are specific phobias? Journal of Behav Ther Exp Psychiatry 1997; 28(3):233–240.
25. Foa EB, Kozak MJ. DSM-IV field trial: obsessive-compulsive disorder. Am J Psychiatry 1995; 152(1):90–101.
26. Wegner DM, Schneider DJ, Carter SR, White TL. Paradoxical effects of thought suppression. J Personality Soc Psychol 1987; 53(1):5–13.
27. Salkovskis P, Freeston MH. Obsessions, compulsions, motivation, and responsibility for harm. Aust J Psychol 2001; 53(1):1–6.
28. Foa EB. Inflated perception for harm in obsessive-compulsive disorder. J Anxiety Disord 2001; 15(4): 259–275.
29. Brown TA, Moras K, Zinbarg RE, Barlow DH. Diagnostic and symptom distinguishability of generalized anxiety disorder and obsessive-compulsive disorder. Behav Ther 1993; 24(2):227–240.
30. Tomb DA. The phenomenology of post-traumatic stress disorder. Psychiatr Clin North Am 1994; 17(2): 237–250.
31. Davidson JR, Foa EB. Diagnostic issues in posttraumatic stress: considerations for DSM-IV. J Abnorm Psychol 1991; 100(3):346–355.
32. Classen C, Koopman C, Hales R, Spiegel D. Acute stress disorder as a predictor of post-traumatic stress symptoms. Am J Psychiatry 1998; 155(5):620–624.
33. Bryant RA, Harvey AG. Acute stress disorder: a critical review of diagnostic issues. Clin Psychol Rev 1997; 17(7):757–773.

34. Marshall RD, Spitzer R, Liebowitz MR. Review and critique of the new DSM-IV diagnosis of acute stress disorder. Am J Psychiatry 1999; 156(11):1677–1685.
35. Bowman ML. Individual differences in posttraumatic distress: problems with the DSM-IV model. Can J Psychiatry 1999; 44(1):21–33.
36. Brown TA, Di Nardo PA, Lehman CL, Campbell LA. Reliability of DSM-IV anxiety and mood disorders: Implications for the classification of emotional disorders. J Abnorm Psychol 2001; 110(1):49–58.
37. Nathan PE, Langenbucher JW. Psychopathology: description and classification. Annu Rev Psychol 2000; 50:79–107.
38. Brown TA, Barlow DH. Comorbidity among the anxiety disorders: implications for treatment and DSM-IV. J Consult Clin Psychol 1992; 60(6):835–844.
39. Clark LA. The anxiety and depressive disorders: descriptive psychopathology and differential diagnosis. In: Kendall P, Watson D, eds. Anxiety and Depression: Distinctive and Overlapping Features. New York: Academic Press, 1989.
40. Laberge B, Gauthier J, Cote G, et al. Cognitive-behavioral therapy of panic disorder with secondary major depression: a preliminary investigation. J Anxiety Disord 1993; 6:169–180.
41. Kessler RC, Stang PE, Wittchen HU, et al. Lifetime panic-depression comorbidity in the National Comorbidity Survey. Arch of Gen Psychiatry 1998; 55(9):801–808.
42. Clark LA, Watson D. Tripartite model of anxiety and depression: psychometric evidence and taxonomic implications. J Abnorm Psychol 1991; 100:316–336.
43. Burns DD, Eidelson RJ. Why are depression and anxiety correlated?: A test of the tripartite model. J Consult Clin Psychol 1998; 66(3):461–473.
44. Ballenger JC. Current treatments of the anxiety disorders in adults. Biol Psychiatry 1999; 46(11):1579–1594.
45. Rivas-Vazquez RA. Antidepressants as first-line agents in the current pharmacotherapy of anxiety disorders. Prof Psychol Res Pract 2001; 32(1):101–104.
46. Klerman GL. Treatments for panic disorder. J Clin Psychiatry 1992; 53(suppl 3):14–19.
47. Sullivan GM, Coplan JD, Kent JM, Groman JM. The noradrenergic system in pathological anxiety: a focus on panic with relevance to generalized anxiety. Biol Psychiatry 1999; 46(9):1205–1218.
48. Hood SD, Argyropoulos SV, Nutt DJ. Agents in development for anxiety disorders: current status and future potential. CNS Drugs 2000; 13(6):421–431.
49. Bourin M, Baker GB, Bradwejn J. Neurobiology of panic disorder. J Psychosom Res 1998; 44(1):163–180.
50. Jensen CF, Keller TW, Peskind ER, McFall ME. Behavioral and neuroendocrine responses to sodium lactate infusion in subjects with post-traumatic stress disorder. Am J Psychiatry 1997; 154(2):266–268.
51. Facchinetti F, Tarabusi M, Nappi G. Premenstrual syndrome and anxiety disorder: a psychobiological link. Psychother Psychosom 1998; 67(2):57–60.
52. Malizia AL. What do brain imaging studies tell us about anxiety disorders? J Psychopharmacol 1999; 13(4):372–378.
53. Thomas KM, Drevets WC, Whalen PJ, et al. Amygdala response to facial expressions in children and adults. Biol Psychiatry 2001; 49(4):309–316.
54. Dager SR, Swann AC. Advance in brain metabolism research: towards a moving picture of neural activity. Biol Psychiatry 1996; 39(4):231–233.
55. Davidson RJ, Abercrombie H, Nitschke JB, Putnam K. Regional brain function, emotion, and disorders of emotion. Curr Opin Neurobiol 1999;(9):2–228.
56. Baxter LR, Phelps ME, Mazziotta JC, Guze BH. Local cerebral glucose metabolism rates in obsessive-compulsive disorder: a comparison with rates in unipolar depression and in normal controls. Arch of Gen Psychiatry 1987; 44(3):211–218.
57. Saxena S, Brody AL, Maidment KM, et al. Localized orbitofrontal and subcortical metabolic changes and predictors of response to paroxetine treatment in obsessive-compulsive disorder. Neuropsychopharmacology 1999; 21(6):683–693.
58. Liberzon I, Taylor SF, Amdur R, et al. Brain activation in PTSD in response to trauma-related stimuli. Biol Psychiatry 1999; 45(7):817–826.
59. Rauch SL, Whalen PJ, Shin LM, et al. Exaggerated amygdala response to masked facial stimuli in post-traumatic stress disorder: a functional MRI study. Biol Psychiatry 2000; 47(9):769–776.
60. Smoller JW, Finn C, White C. The genetics of anxiety disorders: An overview. Psychiatric Ann 2000; 30(12):745–753.
61. Kendler KS. Major depression and generalised anxiety disorder: same genes, (partly) different enviornments—revisited. Br J Psychiatry 1996; 168(suppl 30):68–75.
62. Scherrer JF, True WR, Xian H, et al. Evidence for genetic influences common and specific to symptoms of generalized anxiety and panic. J Affect Disord 2001; 57(1):25–35.
63. Weissman MM. Panic and generalized anxiety: are they separate disorders? J Psychiatr Res 1990; 24(suppl 2):157–162.
64. Goldsmith HH, Lemery KS. Linking temperamental fearfulness and anxiety symptoms: a behavior-genetic perspective. Biol Psychiatry 2000; 48(12):1199–1209.
65. Radant A, Tsuang D, Peskind ER, et al. Biological markers and diagnostic accuracy in the genetics of post-traumatic stress disorder. Psychiatry Res 2001; 102(3):203–215.

9

Classification of Dementias and Cognitive Disorders

FRÉDÉRIC ASSAL and JEFFREY L. CUMMINGS
David Geffen School of Medicine at UCLA, Los Angeles, California, U.S.A.

I. INTRODUCTION

There are multiple ways to classify dementias and cognitive disorders. Both may result from a variety of disorders according to their etiology, genetic features, pathophysiology, or clinical signs. Following these different classifications, this chapter will focus on clinically relevant disorders for clinicians or basic scientists who want an overview of current clinical knowledge of this evolving field of clinical neuroscience.

Multidimensional cognitive disorders include delirium and dementia. Single-dimensional cognitive disorder includes focal neuropsychological symptoms like aphasia, apraxia, or agnosia. For didactic reasons, this chapter will focus on dementia and include cognitive disorders related to dementia when they bear as differential diagnosis as augment understanding of dementia.

The term dementia refers to a clinical syndrome of acquired intellectual disturbance meeting criteria defined by the Diagnostic and Statistical Manual of Mental Disorders, 4th edition, Text Revision (DSM-IV-TR) [1] or the International Classification of Disease (ICD)-10 [2]. The essential diagnostic features include impairment in social and occupational functioning and disturbance of memory and one or more other domain (aphasia, apraxia, agnosia, executive functions). Alternative criteria were suggested by Cummings and Benson [3], where they define dementia as an acquired persistent disturbance in neuropsychological function involving at least three of the following spheres of mental activity: language, memory, visuospatial functions, executive functions, personality, and emotion. This definition allows for the possibility that memory disturbance may not be the presenting feature of a dementia. Most definitions identify similar patient groups with shared cognitive features

II. ETIOLOGY

Dementias can be classified into degenerative and nondegenerative etiologies. This classification is relevant in the differential diagnosis and is summarized in Table 1. The nondegenerative dementias encompass almost any neurological disease (vascular, traumatic, demyelinating, neoplastic, infectious, inflammatory, hydrocephalic, systemic and toxic conditions) and are often referred as secondary causes of dementia, some of which may be reversible. Secondary causes are relatively rare. In a cohort of 2915 community inhabitants aged 65 years and over, Alzheimer's disease (AD), vascular dementia (VaD), and mixed dementias encompassed 90.4% of all cases of dementia [4]. Reversible dementia may be even less frequent and account for < 1% of causes in the most recent studies [5]. Nevertheless, these disorders should be recognized and treated. For that reason, the American Academy of Neurology (AAN) has stated that workup of dementia should include structural neuroimaging,

Table 1 Classification of Dementias and Related Cognitive Disorders According to Their Etiology

Degenerative	Nondegenerative
Alzheimer's disease	Vascular dementias
Dementia with Lewy Bodies	Multi-infarct dementia
Frontotemporal dementia	Strategic infarct
Primary progressive aphasia	Lacunar state
Parkinson's disease	Binswanger's disease
Progressive supranuclear palsy	CADASIL
Corticobasal degeneration	Infectious dementias
Multiple system atrophy	AIDS dementia complex
Huntington's disease	Whipple's disease
Wilson's disease	Neurosyphillis
Neuroacanthocytosis	Creutzfeldt-Jakob disease
Idiopathic basal ganglia calcification	Demyelinating dementia
Neurodegeneration with brain iron accumulation type 1	Multiple sclerosis
	Neoplastic conditions
Spinocerebellar ataxias	Brain tumors (primary or secondary)
Leukodystrophies	Meningeal carcinomatosis
Neuronal ceroid lipofuscinosis	Paraneoplastic limbic encephalitis
Amyotrophic lateral sclerosis	Miscellaneous
Cerebral amyloid angiopathy	Nutritional deficiencies (vitamin B_{12}, thiamine, niacin)
	Toxic-metabolic disorders (thyroid, medication, alcohol, polysubstance abuse, heavy metal)
	Normal pressure hydrocephalus

screening for depression, B_{12} deficiency, and hypothyroidism [6].

A. Degenerative Dementia

1. Alzheimer's Disease

Alzheimer's disease is a progressive degenerative disorder that afflicts an estimated 4 million Americans. The sporadic form of AD is the leading cause of dementia among those over age 65. Common diagnostic criteria include those of the National Institute of Neurological and Communication Disorders and Stroke and the Alzheimer's Disease and Related Disorders Association (NINCDS-ADRDA) [7] and the DSM-IV-TR [1]. Both sets of clinical criteria specify that the deficits must be gradually progressive, must not be limited to a period of delirium, and cannot have an alternative explanation. The core clinical syndrome of AD is relatively stereotyped and includes severe impairments in recent memory, mild to moderate language deficits, and visuospatial disturbances including environmental disorientation. Nevertheless, there is substantial variation in the degree of impairment in these domains in individual patients. Cognitive impairment occurs first. Behavioral symptoms including delusions often related to theft or infidelity, misidentification syndromes such as Capgras syndrome, or agitation occur frequently during the middle stages and become more common as the disease progresses. Hallucinations are unusual. Motor problems occur only in the latter stage of the disease; these impair movement, and eventually the inability to swallow leads to aspiration pneumonia, and death.

Besides neuronal loss, senile plaques (SPs) and neurofibrillary tangles (NFTs) constitute the two major neuropathological lesions in AD. Their distribution can be really contrasted. SPs are found in the isocortex, the hippocampus being relatively spared, and their density increases with the severity of the disease. NFTs involve an increasing number of areas in a stereotyped order: entorhinal area, hippocampus-subiculum, isocortex. The occurrence of these two lesions explains why two systems of neuropathological criteria may be used with similar outcomes: the counting of plaques in the isocortex (Consortium to Establish a

Registry for Alzheimer's Disease, or CERAD, criteria) [8] or the mapping of the areas involved by the neurofibrillary pathology (Braak and Braak stages) [9]. These neuropathological lesions explain the progression of the clinical symptoms: entorhinal area and hippocampus causing the episodic memory loss and the associative posterior parietal isocortex, causing the visuospatial and language impairments. They also correlate with the structural and functional neuroimaging findings (medial temporal lobe atrophy, hypoperfusion, or hypometabolism in multimodal association parietal cortex).

2. Dementia with Lewy Bodies

Dementia, parkinsonism, hallucinations, and fluctuations in cognition are part of the Consensus Criteria of Dementia with Lewy Bodies (DLB) [10]. Cognitive deficits of DLB are characterized by prominent deficits in visuospatial skills, and relative sparing of memory. However, neuropsychological tests do not reliably differentiate DLB from either AD or VaD [11], and hallucinations and delusions occur in AD as well. This explains the low sensitivities of the diagnostic criteria when applied against neuropathological findings [12]. Promising tools for the diagnosis of DLB are MRI showing less temporal atrophy than patients with AD [13], functional neuroimaging disclosing more hypoperfusion in the occipital lobes [14,15], and a good response to cholineesterase inhibitors [16].

The neuropathologic hallmarks of DLB are intracytoplasmic inclusions (Lewy bodies; LBs) which are widely distributed throughout paralimbic and neocortical regions as well as the brainstem. Pure LB pathology may occur, but in most cases of DLB they coexist with a plaque-predominant AD (17). High NFT densities sufficient to meet AD pathological criteria are not frequent.

3. Frontotemporal Dementia

Frontotemporal dementia (FTD) is a clinical syndrome with a younger age of onset than AD, and a family history often suggests a dominantly inherited illness [18]. The consensus diagnostic criteria for FTD [19] include both behavioral and cognitive features. Using an earlier version of the consensus criteria [20], behavioral features such as early loss of personal awareness, early loss of social awareness, hyperorality, and stereotyped, perseverative behavior were found to be sensitive (63–73%) and highly specific (97–100%) for differentiating FTD and AD [21], although the study was without autopsy confirmation. Cognitive functions such as speech and language, executive functions, and preserved posterior functions were less useful for differentiating FTD and AD. An autopsy-based class II study (using retrospective clinical diagnosis determined from review of medical records) showed that most patients with FTD fulfilled diagnostic criteria for AD [22]. One study found that the FAS word fluency test was the best neuropsychological test to differentiate the two conditions, and was more altered in FTD [23].

Functional brain imaging, showing decreased frontotemporal perfusion or metabolism, is a promising diagnostic tool which requires rigorous validation. Pathological findings are heterogeneous and complex, and include positive tau and ubiquitin inclusions [24,25]. Grossly, the brain has frontal and/or frontal and anterotemporal atrophy often associated with atrophy of the basal ganglia, substantia nigra, and amygdala. Histologically, neuronal loss, gliosis, and spongiform changes are found primarily in the top three layers of the cortex. Plaques and tangles do not occur beyond what is seen in normal elderly. Pick bodies or argentophilic cytoplasmic inclusions that fill inflated neurons and swollen achromatic cells are found in Pick's disease per se but are not required for the diagnosis of FTD since FTD may occur in the absence of these inclusion types. There are no clinical features that are useful for establishing histologic subtypes.

4. Parkinson's Disease

Parkinson's disease (PD) includes tremor, bradykinesia, rigidity, and postural abnormalities. Evidence of disease progression, parkinsonism, asymmetry of signs and of onset, marked response to levodopa, and absence of clinical feature of alternative diagnosis and of an etiology known to cause similar features have been proposed as research criteria for idiopathic PD [26]. Their validity and reliability remain to be assessed. Besides behavioral symptoms like hallucinations, delusions, mania, anxiety, depression, and obsessive-compulsive features, some of which may be secondary to drug treatment, patients with PD show a prevalence of dementia of ~40% [27]. The risk for developing dementia in patients with PD relative to controls, according to DSM-II-R criteria, after adjusting for age, sex, and education, was 5.9 (95% CI, 3.9–9.1) in a recent prospective study [28].

Several types of dementia have been identified in PD. A frequent pattern of dementia corresponds to a frontosubcortical profile of dysfunctions, characterized by bradyphrenia (mental slowing), executive deficits, memory disturbance with retrieval deficit, and visuospatial deficits [29,30]. Significant disorientation, impairment of memory with an encoding deficit, or naming difficulties that develop in the course of PD are indicative of other degenerative pathology, most commonly of the Alzheimer's type [31].

Characteristic pathologic findings of PD include loss of pigmented neurons and LB in the pars compacta of the substantia nigra, and various other subcortical nuclei. Cortical LB are better correlated with cognitive impairment in patients with PD than AD-type histological findings [32,33]. The contributions of cortical LB, AD-type pathology, and the PD pathology to the dementia of PD are uncertain.

B. Nondegenerative

1. Vascular Dementia

Vascular dementia is a group of disorders resulting from the effects of vascular disease on the brain. The various location, type, and extension of the lesions express heterogeneous clinical symptoms. Recent criteria for VaD are the National Institute of Neurologic Disorders and Stroke and the Association Internationale pour la Recherche et l'Enseignement en Neurosciences (NINDS-AIREN) [34] criteria, and the DSM-IV criteria [1]. Diagnostic criteria typically require the presence of dementia, the demonstration of cerebrovascular disease, and onset of dementias following stroke or with a stepwise pattern of progression. In studies that compared clinical diagnosis and neuropathologic findings, these criteria had low sensitivities and high specificities [35,36].

Most of the autopsy data showed that vascular pathology was rarely sufficient to account for all cognitive symptoms and was frequently accompanied by AD pathology [37,38]. On the other hand, recent studies focus on the additive or even synergistic effect of vascular burden on AD [39].

Lacunar state and Binswanger's disease are both small-vessel diseases. Lacunar state has been defined as the presence of numerous lacunes in the basal ganglia, pons, and white matter of the centrum semiovale. The number of lacunes, the extent of periventricular luency, and the severity of ventricular enlargement were associated with cognitive deficits dependant on frontal executive function [40]. Frontal lobe hypometabolism on functional neuroimaging predicted cognitive decline in patients with lacunar state [41]. Binswanger's disease (BD) is a gradually progressive dementia [42] caused by ischemic injury to the deep periventricular white matter of the cerebral hemispheres. Other usual clinical findings include pseudobulbar palsy, small-stepped gait, and urinary urgency.

Multi-infarct dementia (MID) [42] is the consequence of multiple large cortical infarctions throughout the distributions of the anterior, middle, or posterior artery circulations, usually secondary to atheroscerotic thrombosis or cardiac embolization. Abrupt onset, patchiness of cognitive deficits, associated focal neurological signs, and stepwise progression are the hallmarks of the dementia, and as the disease progresses, most intellectual functions become affected. Modern studies combining these neuropsychological aspects and recent neuroimaging techniques (MRI and functional imaging) are lacking.

Strategic infarcts include small infarctions located so as to disrupt multiple cognitive domains [42]. Angular gyrus syndrome exhibits fluent aphasia, alexia with agraphia, and Gerstmann syndrome (acalculia, right-left disorientation, dysgraphia, finger agnosia). Caudate infarcts produce executive deficits and behavioral symptoms (either disinterest or disinhibition). Executive deficits also occur with pallidum infarctions. When they are bilateral, the infarcts result in profound inertia and loss of psychic self-activation often with obsessive-compulsive features [43].

2. Normal Pressure Hydrocephalus

Normal pressure hydrocephalus (NPH) results from impaired absorption of cerebrospinal fluid at the level of the arachnoid granulations and causes dementia (often with bradyphrenia and executive dysfunctions), gait instability, and urinary incontinence [44]. NPH is a rare cause of dementia, accounting for < 2% of cases [45]. Diagnostic procedures (MRI, radioisotope cisternography, spinal fluid removal, and pressure monitoring) are nonstandardized, and predictive tests for surgical outcomes are still lacking. Recent data showed that AD pathology at biopsy was a frequent finding, contributed to the clinical impairment associated with NPH, and did not seem to strongly influence the clinical response to shunt surgery [46]. These findings require confirmation.

3. Infectious and Prion Diseases

AIDS Dementia Complex (ADC), or HIV dementia, reflects injury induced by HIV-1 viral proteins and the subsequent release of chemokines, cytokines, and toxins, predominantly in the frontal lobe and the basal ganglia [47]. The topography of those lesions explains the clinical features of ADC (slowed mentation, apathy, and absence of aphasia, alexia, or agraphia). ADC occurs most often at moderate and advanced degrees of immunodeficiency. However, with the advent of highly active antiretroviral tharapy, ADC may occur at higher CD4 cell counts than previously [48].

Creutzfeldt-Jakob disease (CJD) is the most common human transmissible subacute spongiform encephalopathy or prion disease (49). Approximately 85% of cases are sporadic. The remaining 15% consist of genetic forms (familial CJD, Gerstmann-Sträussler-Scheinker disease, fatal familial insomnia) and acquired forms (iatrogenic forms transmitted by human growth hormone therapy, surgical procedures, and ingestion of contaminated material—Kuru, and new-variant CJD). New-variant CJD (vCJD) is caused by the same agent as bovine spongiform encephalopathy and was described in 1996 [50].

CJD results in a rapidly progressive dementia with frontal features evolving rapidly into profound aphasia then akinetic mutism. Most patients develop myoclonic jerks, ataxia, visual impairment, and frequent nonspecific symptoms such as anorexia, insomnia, mood changes, and malaise. During the disease course, patients have a characteristic electroencephalogram with periodic or pseudo-periodic complexes. Detection of the 14-3-3 protein in the CSF may be helpful in the diagnosis [51]. Spongiosis, neuronal loss and marked gliosis, and positive PrP immunostaining at autopsy make the diagnosis definite.

4. Neoplastic

Almost any brain tumor can cause simple or multiple cognitive signs such as dementia, but frequently the evolution is acute or subacute and signs of increased intracranial pressure may occur. One study of 119 cases referred for memory loss found that only one patient with significant structrural lesion had no features in the history or examination that would have predicted the lesions [52]. The AAN recommends structural nonconstrast neuroimaging examination at the time of the initial dementia assessment, to identify uncommon causes of dementias such as tumors as well as more common conditions that may cause dementia or coexist with AD such as cerebrovascular disease [6].

Seizures, personality changes, irritability, memory changes, and dementia preceding the diagnosis of the cancer are the most frequent signs of paraneoplastic limbic encephalitis. Although this is a rare condition, the combination of these symptoms, MRI abnormalities in the medial temporal lobes, and paraneoplastic antibodies establish the diagnosis in 78% of patients [53].

5. Metabolic and Toxic

Any kind of systemic illness, nutritional deficiency, and toxin exposure may affect cognitive functions and cause dementia if their effects persist for an extended period of time. Cyanocobalamin or vitamin B_{12} deficiency and hypothyroidism are common in the elderly but are rarely associated with dementia [54,55]. Elevated TSH levels carry an increased risk for dementia [56]. These findings suggest that the presence of these conditions could exaggerate cognitive deficits, rather than cause dementia per se. Treatment may partially reverse the cognitive symptoms [57].

Thiamine deficiency associated with chronic alcoholism or other nutritional deficiency leads to Wernicke-Korsakoff syndrome [58]. After a period of confusional state with ataxia and oculomotor abnormalities, such patients show a profound inability to learn new information (anterograde amnesia) with confabulations. This rare syndrome has been a valuable model for the neuropsychology and the neuropathology of medial diencephalic amnestic syndromes, showing lesions in the mammillary bodies and dorsomedial nucleus of the thalamus.

Marchiafava-Bignami (disconnexion syndrome secondary to corpus callosum pathology) and alcoholic dementia (prominent executive deficits due to frontal involvement) are other alcohol-related cognitive disorders [58].

6. Traumatic Brain Injury

Traumatic brain injury (TBI) is a leading cause of death and cognitive dysfunction among individuals under the age of 50 in the United States [59]. Focal and/or diffuse damage may occur, depending on the mechanisms of the injury. The clinical presentation is therefore heterogeneous, but slowed information processing and impaired concentration and memory, often with impulsivity and disinhibition, are typical [60]. Even in the absence of focal structural lesions of the brain, functional neuroimaging showed decreased metabolism in prefrontal and cingulate cortex [61]. TBI increases the risk for AD in later life [62].

7. Demyelinating disorders

Multiple sclerosis (MS) is the most common demyelinating disorder of the central nervous system. Its etiology is still unknown. The clinical course of MS has three forms: relapsing-remitting, acute progressive, and chronic progressive. Cognitive dysfunction occurs in > 40% of patients with MS, and manifests primarily executive deficits [63,64], correlated with the lesion burden in the frontal lobe [65].

III. GENETICS

Defects in various genes have long been speculated to be the cause of several neurodegenerative diseases, mainly in autosomal-dominant inherited diseases. In the example of Huntington's disease (HD), discovery of the causative mutations helped the clinician in the diagnosis of familial choreiform movements as well as in genetic counseling. In the example of a subset of familial FTD, the discovery of the gene defect was rapidly linked to the protein aggregates that were involved in the disease, and this is helping substantially basic neuroscientists understand the pathophysiology of the disorder. The bulk of neurodegenerative diseases are sporadic and cannot be explained by single gene defects, but causative mutations and risk genes have been discovered for several dementing illnesses.

A. Alzheimer's Disease

Much of the progress in elucidating the genetics and the biology of AD derives from analysis of the two major neuropathological hallmarks of AD (SPs and NFTs). SP contain extracellular deposits of the amyloid-beta protein (A-beta), mainly of A-beta42 peptide, as opposed to A-beta40 peptide. The amyloid precursor protein (APP) is processed into several peptides through select cellular proteases (alpha, beta, and gamma secretases). While some products of this cleavage (A-beta42) form aggregates and eventually give rise to SPs, what other products (A-beta40) do is unclear. The A-beta42 peptide probably initiates a complex cellular response that results in neuronal cell death through calcium-mediated excitotoxicity, free radical–induced oxidative stress, and inflammation [66].

The NFTs are composed of insoluble forms of the microtubule-associated protein tau which are abnormally phosphorylated. This insoluble tau aggregates in the NFTs, and as tau phosphrylation increases, the density and number of NFTs increase.

It has been known for several decades that AD can occur in a familial form that appears to be transmitted as an autosomal-dominant trait. In these families, the symptomatology tends to appear much earlier than sporadic AD (typically in the 40s or 50s, but sometimes earlier). Estimates of the proportion of genetically based AD are < 5%, but may increase with disclosure of additional mutations. There are three well-confirmed genes in which mutations result in AD.

Several missense mutations in the APP gene (chromosome 21) have been described: they account for < 0.1% of all AD cases [67,68] but have been very informative in terms of AD pathogenesis. Most of these mutations are clustered at the beta or gamma secretase site. Inducing cleavage by these secretases leads to increased A-beta42 production.

Many mutations have been identified in presenilin 1 (PS1) on chromosome 14q24.3 [67,68]. PSs are membrane proteins, expressed in all cell types. PS1 mutations alter the processing of APP toward the release of the amyloidogenic A-beta42 peptides, through regulation of the gamma-secretase and other complex mechanisms [69]. PS1 mutations are the most genetic causes of AD and account for more than half of the cases of early-onset familial AD.

A few mutations have been described in the presenilin 2 (PS2) gene on chromosome 1q42.1. In contrast to the frequency of PS1 mutations, screening of large datasets reveal that PS2 mutations are likely to be rare and their phenotype much more variable [70].

Inheritance of one or two epsilon4 alleles of apolipoprotein E (APOE4) on chromosome 19 increases the risk of AD. APOE4 lowers the typical age of onset of sporadic late-life AD to approximately age 65 [71]. APOE4 is considered a risk factor for AD since some subjects who are homozygous for this isoform still show no symptoms in their ninth decade of life. The AAN does not recommend APOE testing as a diagnostic test for AD [6].

Another AD locus was identified in chromosome 12 [72] and 10 [73,74] whose identity at the moment is unclear.

B. Frontotemporal Dementias

In 1994, the first autosomal-dominant inherited FTD, associated with parkinsonism and amyotrophy, was described [75]. A genetic linkage was demonstrated between this pathology and a mutation on chromosome 17q21-22. Several additional families sharing a mutation on 17q21-22 have been reported and been included in a group of pathologies referred to as FTD with parkinsonism linked to chromosome 17 (FTDP-17). Finally, FTDP-17 has been related to mutations in the tau gene [76]. Several mutations have been found in the tau gene among the different families with members diagnosed as FTDP-17 [77]. There are major differences in the phenotype and age of onset within families having the same mutations [78]. Mutations of the tau gene and their involvement in FTDP-17 indicate that abnormal tau protein plays a central role in the etiopathogenesis of neurodegenerative disorders, without the presence of the amyloid cascade.

Tau mutations on chromosome 17 explain only a small proportion of FTD, and alternate genetic loci have also been reported on chromosome 3 [79] and chromosome 9 [80]. These findings suggest that the pathology observed in these tau-negative FTD cases results from mechanisms unrelated to tau or alternative tau functions by different mechanisms [81,82].

Accumulating data suggest that the tau gene on chromosome 17q21-22 is associated with progressive supranuclear palsy (PSP) and corticobasal degeneration (CBD) [83,84]. Different phenotypes have been described within a family with the same tau mutation [85]. In this family one member presented with FTD and another one with CBD.

C. Huntington's Disease

Huntington's disease (HD) is a progressive, autosomal-dominant neurodegenerative disorder with 100% penetrance, caused by an increased number of CAG trinucleotide repeats affecting the IT15 gene at chromosome 4p16.3 [86]. Normal alleles contain 34 or fewer CAG repeats, whereas repeats of 37–150 or more occur in affected individuals. A negative correlation has been observed between the number of repeats and the age of onset of disease. Chorea and cognitive and behavioral changes are the main clinical features [87]. A large survey including 1238 individuals with symptomatic HD revealed that involuntary movements were the earliest reported symptoms, then respectively mental and emotional symptoms. As the disease progressed, behavioral and cognitive symptoms were experienced [88].

D. Wilson's Disease

Wilson's disease (WD), or hepatolenticular degeneration, is an inherited disorder of copper metabolism. Mutations of the gene ATP7B on chromosome 13q14 alter a copper-transporting protein resulting in copper accumulation leading to cellular toxicity [89]. WD is characterized clinically by liver, ocular (Kayser-Fleischer ring), and neurological signs. The latter include extrapyramidal features due to putaminal changes and mainly executive deficits with personality and mood disturbances [90,91].

E. Cerebral Autosomal-Dominant Angiopathy with Subcortical Infarcts and Leucoencephalopathy

Cerebral autosomal-dominant angiopathy with subcortical infarcts and leucoencephalopathy (CADASIL) is an autosomal-dominant disorder due to severe alterations of vascular smooth muscle cells secondary to mutations of the Notch3 gene on chromosome 19q12 [92]. The patients usually present with migraine and recurrent ischemic episodes leading to gait disturbances, urinary urgency, pseudo-bulbar palsy, and psychiatric disturbances without other vascular risk factors [93]. Extensive white matter changes are evident on MRI. The main diseases according to their genetic basis are listed in Table 2.

IV. PATHOPHYSIOLOGY

Most of neurodegenerative diseases that manifest dementia or cognitive disorders are characterized by neuronal loss; intracellular inclusions such as LBs, Pick bodies, or NFTs; or extracellular deposits forming SPs. Intracellular inclusions (in neurons and sometimes in glial cells) and extracellular material are made of different insoluble fibrillar proteins that normally exist in soluble form. These tau, alpha-synuclein, or A-beta protein aggregates differentiate the most common neurodegenerative diseases and subserve this classification. These diseases thus share the deposition of insoluble fibrillar proteins that play an important role in the pathophysiology of neurodegeneration and the expression of the clinical symptoms. The main protein accumulations and their relationships with principal neurodegenerative diseases are summarized in Table 3.

A. Tauopathies

Tauopathies include neuropathological disorders composed of insoluble forms of microtubule-associated protein tau which are abnormally phosphorylated. This insoluble tau aggregates in the filamentous tau lesions, and as tau phosphorylation increases, so do the density and number of tau lesions. In normal brain, tau plays a role in the

Table 2 Classification of Dementias and Related Cognitive Disorders According to Their Genetic Basis

	Chromosome	Gene defect	Comment
Familial AD	14	PS1	Many mutations
	1	PS2	Few mutations
	21	APP	Several mutations
	12	?	
	10	?	
Sporadic AD	19	ApoE	E4 allele as a risk factor
Familial FTD	17	Tau	Several mutations
	3, 9	?	
Huntington's disease	4	IT15	Increase CAG repeats
Parkinson's disease	4	alphaS	Several mutations
	2, 1	?	
Wilson's disease	13	ATP7B	Several mutations
Idiopathic basal ganglia calcification	14	?	
CADASIL	19	Notch 3	Several mutations
Cerebral amyloid angiopathy	21	APP, CST3	Few mutations
Leukodystrophies	X, 22, 10	various	Several mutations
Neuronal ceroid lipofuscinosis type 3	16	CLN3	Several mutations
Mitochondrial encephalomyopathy			Several mutations in mitochondrial DNA
Prion diseases		PRNP	Several mutations

stabilization of neuronal microtubules by interacting with tubulin. Microtubules maintain the cell shape and serve as tracks for axonal transport. Six tau isoforms are produced from a single gene located on chromosome 17q21 by alternative mRNA splicing. The spliced products give rise to three tau isoforms with three repeats (3R) and three other tau isoforms having four repeats (4R). These repeats and their adjacent domains constitute the microtubule-binding domains of tau [94].

Major tauopathies include AD, Pick's disease, FTDP-17, PSP, and CBD, whereas the morphology

Table 3 Protein Aggregations in Major Dementias and Related Cognitive Disorders

Disease	Protein
Alzheimer's disease	A-beta, tau
Frontotemporal dementia, Pick's disease	Tau
Progressive supranuclear palsy	Tau
Corticobasal degeneration	Tau
Parkinson's disease	Alpha-synuclein
Multiple system atrophy	Alpha-synuclein
Huntington's disease	Huntingtin
Prion disease	Prion protein
Spinocerebellar ataxias	Ataxin

and isoform composition of the filamentous tau lesions and their regional brain distribution differ. Most common tauopathies are listed in Table 4.

In Pick's disease, intraneuronal tau aggregates assemble into characteristic spherical Pick bodies in nonpyramidal neurons of layers 2, 3, and 6 of the cerebral cortex and in the dentate granule cells [95]. They consist of paired and straight filaments and are formed of only 3R-tau isoforms [96].

In FTDP-17 (see Sec. III.B), the morphology and isoform composition of tau lesions varies in the different families [97]. In some families, they consist of paired helical filaments or straight filaments, and contain all six major isoforms, similarly to AD. In other families, the lesions resemble twisted ribbons and consist mainly of 4R-tau isoforms.

Although the accumulation of abnormal tau is the hallmark of major tauopathies like Pick's disease and FTDP-17, aggregates of tau are uncommon in sporadic FTD. Loss or reduction of tau has been described recently in sporadic FTD and in a familial form known as hereditary dysphasic dementia 2 [98]. This "tauless" tauopathy is characterized by loss or reduction of all six tau isoforms, but not tau mRNA, suggesting that the level of tau protein is controlled postranscriptionally, at the level of either translation or mRNA stability. The mechanisms by which reduced levels of brain tau cause neurodegeneration remain unknown, but it is

Table 4 Classification of Dementias and Relative Cognitive Disorders According to Their Pathophysiology

Tauopathies	Alpha-synucleinopathies	A-Beta
FTDP-17	Sporadic Parkinson's disease (PD)	Sporadic AD
ALS/parkinsonism-dementia complex	Familial PD	Down syndrome
Pick's disease	Dementia with Lewy bodies	Cerebral amyloid angiopathy (familial and sporadic)
Corticobasal degeneration	Sporadic AD (about 60%)	Prion disease
Alzheimer's disease (AD)	Familial AD	
Dementia pugilistica	Down syndrome	
Down syndrome	Multiple system atrophy	
Multiple system atrophy	Shy-Drager syndrome	
Progressive supranuclear palsy	Striatonigral degeneration	
Gerstmann-Sträussler-Scheinker disease	Olivopontocerebellar atrophy	
Creutzfeldt-Jakob disease	Neurodegeneration with brain iron accumulation, type 1	

likely that loss of functional tau protein leads to death of affected neurons.

In PSP, tau lesions form NFTs and consist of straight and paired helical filaments. They are localized in subcortical regions [99], and in the cortex as well [100]. In contrast to AD, they contain the 4R-tau isoforms [101].

In CBD, neuropathological examination reveals severe glial and neuronal lesions predominantly in the frontoparietal regions and often in basal ganglia and substantia migra [102]. The glial pathology is constituted of astrocytic plaque or conglomerations of tau-positive astrocytes and tau-positive inclusions in oligodendrocytes. Abnormal achromatic ballooned neurons are composed of tau positive filaments. These filaments contain the 4R-tau isoforms [101].

The clinical presentation of CBD is characterized by asymmetric and progressive parkinsonism, alien limb phenomena, ideomotor apraxia, and myoclonus, followed by cognitive impairment (executive deficits and memory disturbance with retrieval deficit) [103,104]. Dementia is not infrequent [104,105]. The clinical diagnosis is often difficult because of overlapping features with PSP, FTD, and cerebrovascular disorder, and clinical findings considered characteristic of CBD are associated with heterogeneous pathologies (AD, PSP, Pick's disease, nonspecific changes, CJD) [106].

In AD, abnormally phosphorylated tau proteins form NFTs, which are composed predominantly of aggregated paired helical filaments and contain all six tau isoforms [96]. Despite these prominent tau accumulations, the tau gene has not been found to be the site of mutations in familial AD. Therefore AD is not considered a primary tauopathy. In this respect, many tauopathies listed in Table 4 may be related to secondary disturbances of tau metabolism rather than primary genetic defects.

B. Alpha-Synucleinopathies

Alpha-synucleinopathies are disorders of one the four currently known members of the synuclein family (alpha, beta, gamma, and synoretin), and are listed in Table 4. These neuronal cytosolic proteins are enriched at presynaptic terminals and may play a role in synaptic plasticity. Alpha-synuclein (alphaS) was mapped on chromosome 4q21.3-22q [107]. The first described autosomal-dominant PD was caused by a missense mutation in the alphaS gene [108]. AlphaS filaments in the cytoplasm of nerve cells form a major component of Lewy bodies (LBs) and Lewy neurites in sporadic PD and DLB. These changes probably result in the loss of neuronal function [109] and are the most specific and sensitive markers for dementia in patients with PD and DLB [33]. AlphaS-positive inclusions (mainly but not exclusively LBs) have been found in > 60% of familial AD with mutations in PS and APP genes [110], and more recently in 48–60% of sporadic AD [111,112].

Unlike PD and DLB, alphaS-positive inclusions in multiple system atrophy (MSA) are found in cytoplasm and nuclei of both nerve cells and glial cells, mainly oligodendrocytes. From the clinical point of view, MSA includes striatonigral degeneration, Shy-Drager syndrome, and olivopontocerebellar atrophy, depending on the predominant symptom (respectively axial parkinsonism and gait disturbances, postural hypotension, cerebellar syndrome) [113]. Dementia is usually absent [113], but patients frequently exhibit executive deficits with no impairment in language or visuospatial skills [114]. These symptoms reflect frontal and cerebellar involvement of alphaS-positive inclusions [115].

C. Amyloid-Beta Protein Pathologies

Both the biochemistry and the genetics of the amyloid-beta protein (A-beta) are described above. Main disorders of A-beta are listed in Table 4.

Cerebral amyloid angiopathy (CAA) may cause lobar cerebral hemorrhages and, less frequently, ischemic brain lesions, especially in nonhypertensive elderly [116]. It thus shares features with VaD. Nevertheless, the pathology (fibrillar amyloid gradually replacing the arteriolar media) and its increasing prevalence with age are characteristics shared with degenerative disorders [117]. Sporadic CAA is common in AD, and several mutations of the APP gene have been described in familial CAA [118–120]. Therefore, it has been suggested that CAA was the microvascular link between parenchymal (AD) and VaD [121].

V. CLINICAL CLASSIFICATION

This classification is based on using clinical phenomena to classify diseases. It derives from more than a century of classic brain lesion studies in humans, and more recently from structural and functional neuroimaging. These data allow clinical neuroscientists to distinguish between two patterns of CNS involvement: cortical and subcortical. Together with the neurological examination, these two major syndromes aid clinicians in making a clinical diagnosis of dementia or other cognitive disorders.

A. Subcortical Dementias

The term subcortical dementia has been replaced by frontosubcortical dementia (FSCD) because of the advances of our understanding in the basic circuitry of basal ganglia and frontal lobes. The striatum, globus pallidus, anterior and medial thalamus, and substantia nigra are interconnected with the prefrontal cortex in multiple parallel circuits with unique functional properties [122–124]. The broad dichotomy between cortical dementia and frontosubcortical dementia has been challenged [125–128], but is a very useful tool for the clinician in terms of diagnosis and understanding some of the basic processing of cognitive functions.

A third category has emerged since the original descriptions of subcortical dementia. FTD, DLB, and CBD have both cortical and frontosubcortical features. Compared to patients with the classic cortical dementia of AD, patients with FSCD show prominent executive deficits, explicit memory impairment with retrieval deficit and no significant aphasia, apraxia, agnosia or encoding memory impairment [29,30,129]. These deficits are presented in Table 5, where differential characterisitics of FSCD and AD are summarized. As an example, one disease is presented here. Other FSCDs are summarized in Table 6.

Progressive supranuclear palsy (PSP) is characterized by supranuclear ophthalmoplegia, axial dystonia, pseudobulbar palsy, bradykinesia, postural instability, and dysarthria [99]. Historically and clinically, PSP is the quintessential example of FSCD [130], but early severe dementia is rare [131]. Recently, a clinicopathologic analysis of nine patients with PSP showed greater frontal lobe atrophy compared to controls, which correlated with increasing NFT densities, and a correlation with clinical dementia [132]. These findings concur

Table 5 Main Symptoms of Frontosubcortical Dementias Compared to Alzheimer's Disease

Feature	FSCD	AD
Attention	Normal (slow)	Normal
Speed of cognitive processing	Slow	Normal
Language	Most often preserved	Impaired
Speech	Dysarthric	Normal
Visuospatial skills	Impaired (poor planning, perseveration errors)	More impaired
Executive functions:		
Set planning and shifting	Severely impaired	Impaired late
Verbal fluency	Severely impaired (especially letter fluency)	Impaired (especially category fluency)
Memory impairment	Retrieval deficit	Encoding deficit

Table 6 Classification of Dementias and Related Cognitive Disorders According to Their Clinical Profile

Frontosubcortical dementia	Cortical dementia	Both
Degenerative		
PSP	Alzheimer's disease	Frontotemporal dementia
Multiple system atrophy		Dementia with Lewy Bodies
Spinocerebellar ataxias		Corticobasal degeneration
Idiopathic basal ganglia calcification		Leukodystrophies
Wilson's disease		
Huntington's disease		
Neuroacanthocytosis		
Vascular		
Binswanger	Multi-infarct dementia	Multi-infarct dementia
Lacunar state		
Strategic infarcts (pallidum and caudate)	Strategic infarct (angular gyrus syndrome)	
Infectious		
AIDS Dementia Complex		Others
Whipple		Normal pressure
Neurosyphilis		Hydrocephalus
Creutzfeldt-Jakob disease		Toxic-metabolic
Demyelinating		Post-traumatic
Multiple sclerosis		Vasculitis

with neuroimaging data showing a reduced frontal perfusion or metabolism in PSP and impaired executive functions [133,134].

B. Cortical Dementias

Cortical dementias, mostly AD, have been discussed above. FTD can present with features of FSCD or with cortical dementia syndrome. Primary progressive aphasia syndrome (PPA) was described relatively recently by Mesulam [135,136] and is a cortical form of FTD. The main core of PPA is a fluent or nonfluent aphasia, starting as an anomia with phonemic paraphasias, unlike AD [137]. There are no significant apathy, disinhibition, memory, visuospatial or visual recognition impairments within the initial 2 years of the disease. Mild acalculia and ideomotor apraxia may be present in the first 2 years. The neuropathology lacks AD-type changes. Neuronal loss, gliosis, mild spongioform changes within superficial layers in the left perisylvian cortex with ubiquitin-positive, tau-negative inclusion bodies or rarely tau-positive neuronal and glial inclusions, and sometimes Pick bodies have been described.

VI. CONCLUSION

These different classifications by etiology, genetics, pathophysiology, and clinical features have had their importance in the history of dementia and behavioral neuroscience, and all of them are still relevant in the 21st century. Increasingly they are converging to provide a molecular pathogenesis relevant to clinical presentations. The clinical classification is crucial in terms of which cognitive systems are involved and gives clues to the anatomical basis of the disease. Together with the associated neurological signs, it allows the clinician to make a diagnosis.

The most recent classifications (genetics and pathophysiology) offer new insights in the dementias and cognitive disorders. Although familial AD comprises only a small proportion of all dementias, it has provided considerable information about the biochemical pathways involved in sporadic forms and how to develop new drugs, such as the antiamyloid vaccine [138], and other mechanism-based strategies.

Selective vulnerability of brain regions and subpopulations of neurons and glial cells is one of major issue of most of dementias and cognitive disorders. The pattern of vulnerability determines the clinical presentation. The pathophysiology of this selective cellular risk has not yet been explained, and will be the critical next step in linking pathophysiology to clinical syndrome.

The issue of phenotypic differences not only between families with different mutations but also within families having the same mutation, remains unsettled. This may suggest that other genetic and/or environmental factors play a role in the pathogenesis of these diseases.

Similarities at the clinical, pathological, and molecular levels among different diseases imply the existence of common pathways in all neurodegenerative disorders. Cell death pathways, for example, appear to involve similar apoptotive cascade across disease entities, and oxidative stress appears to be a common contributive factor to many disorders. Protein aggregation increasingly links many disorders.

More basic and translational research is needed to understand both relationships and differences of major cognitive disorders and dementias. The resolution of issues in basic neuroscience will enhance with our understanding of molecular genetics and our ability to provide effective treatments of affected patients.

ACKNOWLEDGMENTS

This project was supported by an NIA Alzheimer's Disease grant (AG16570), an Alzheimer's Disease Research Center of California grant, the Sidell-Kagen Foundation (J.L.C), and a scholarship from the University Hospital, Geneva, Switzerland (F.A.).

REFERENCES

1. American Psychiatric Association. Diagnostic and Statistical Manual of Mental Disorders, Text Revision: DSM-IV-TR, 4th ed. Washington: American Psychiatric Association, 2000, pp 147–177.
2. World Health Organization. The ICD-10 Classification of Mental and Behavioural Disorders: Clinical Descriptions and Diagnostic Guidelines, 4th ed. Geneva: World Health Organization, 1992, pp 45–46.
3. JL Cummings, DF Benson, SJ LoVerme. Reversible dementia. JAMA 243:2434–2439, 1980.
4. CK Liu, CL Lai, CT Tai, RT Lin, YY Yen, SL Howng. Incidence and subtypes of dementia in southern Taiwan. Impact of socio-demographic factors. Neurology 6:1572–1579, 1998.
5. MD Weytingh, PMM Bossuyt, H van Crevel. Reversible dementia: more than 10% or less than 1%? A quantitative review. J Neurol 242:466–471, 1995.
6. DS Knopman, ST DeKosky, JL Cummings, H Chui, J Cory-Bloom, N Relkin, GW Small, B Miller, JC Stevens. Practice parameter: diagnosis of dementia (an evidence-based review). Report of the Quality Standards Subcommittee of the American Academy of Neurology. Neurology 56:1143–1153, 2001.
7. G McKhann, D Drachman, M Folstein, R Katzman, D Price, EM Stadlan. Clinical diagnosis of Alzheimer's disease: report of the NINCDS-ADRDA work group under the auspices of department of health and human services task force on Alzheimer's disease. Neurology 34:939–944, 1984.
8. SS Mirra, A Heyman, D McKeel, SM Sumi, BJ Crain, LM Brownlee, FS Vogel, JP Hughes, G van Belle, L Berg. The consortium to establish a registry for Alzheimer's disease (CERAD). Part II. Standardization of the neuropathologic assessment of Alzheimer's disease. Neurology 41:479–486, 1991.
9. H Braak, E Braak. Neuropathological staging of Alzheimer-related changes. Acta Neuropathol 82:239–259, 1991.
10. IG McKeith, D Galasko, K Kosaka, EK Perry, DW Dickson, LA Hansen, DP Salmon, J Lowe, SS Mirra, EJ Byrne, G Lennox, NP Quinn, JA Edwardson, PG Ince, C Bergeron, A Burns, BL Miller, S Lovestone, D Collerton, EN Jansen, C Ballard, RA de Vos, GK Wilcock, KA Jellinger, RH Perry. Consensus guidelines for the clinical and pathologic diagnosis of newly proposed clinical criteria for dementia with Lewy bodies (DLB): report of the consortium on DLB international workshop. Neurology 47:1113–1124, 1996.
11. CG Ballard, G Ayre, J O'Brien, A Sahgal, IG McKeith, PG Ince, RH Perry. Simple standardised neuropsychological assessments aid in the differential diagnosis of dementia with Lewy bodies from Alzheimer's disease and vascular dementia. Dement Geriatr Cogn Disord 10:104–108, 1999.
12. OL Lopez, I Litvan, KE Catt, R Stowe, W Klunk, DI Kaufer, JT Becker, ST DeKosky. Accuracy of four clinical diagnostic criteria for the diagnosis of neurodegenerative dementias. Neurology 53:1292–1299, 1999.
13. R Barber, IG McKeith, C Ballard, A Gholkar, JT O'Brien. A comparison of medial temporal lobe atrophy in dementia with Lewy bodies and Alzheimer's disease: magnetic resonance imaging volumetric study. Dement Geriatr Cogn Disord 12:198–205, 2001.
14. K Ishii, S Yamaji, H Kitagaki, T Inamura, N Hirono, E Mori. Regional cerebral blood flow difference between dementia with Lewy bodies and AD. Neurology 53:413–416, 1999.

15. K Lobotesis, JD Fenwick, A Phipps, A Ryman, A Swann, C Ballard, IG McKeith, JT O'Brien. Occipital hypoperfusion on SPECT in dementia with Lewy bodies but not AD. Neurology 56:643–649, 2001.
16. I McKeith, T Del Ser, PF Spano, M Emre, K Wesnes, R Anand, A Cicin-Sain, R Ferrara, R Spiegel. Efficacy of rivastigmine in dementia with Lewy bodies: a randomised, double blind, placebo-controlled international study. Lancet 356:2031–2036, 2000.
17. LA Hansen, E Masliah, D Galasko, RD Terry. Plaque-only Alzheimer disease is usually the Lewy body variant, and vice versa. J Exp Neurol 52:648–654, 1993.
18. M Stevens, CM van Duijn, W Kamphorst, P de Knijff, P Heutink, WA van Gool, P Scheltens, R Ravid, BA Oostra, MF Niermeijer, JC van Swieten. Familial aggregation in frontotemporal dementia. Neurology 50:1541–1545, 1998.
19. D Neary, JS Snowden, L Gustafson, U Passant, D Stuss, S Black, M Freedman, A Kertesz, PH Robert, M Albert, K Boone, BL Miller, J Cummings, DF Benson. Frontotemporal lobar degeneration. A consensus on clinical diagnostic criteria. Neurology 51:1546–1554, 1998.
20. The Lund and Manchester Groups. Clinical and neuropathological criteria for fronto-temporal dementia. J Neurol Neurosurg Psychiatry 57:416–418, 1994.
21. BL Miller, C Ikonte, M Ponton, M Levy, K Boone, A Darby, N Berman, I Mena, JL Cummings. A study of the Lund-Manchester research criteria for frontotemporal dementia: clinical and single-photon emission CT correlations. Neurology 48:937–942, 1997.
22. AR Varma, JS Snowden, JJ Lloyd, PR Talbot, DM Mann, D Neary. Evaluation of the NINCDS-ADRDA criteria in the differentiation of Alzheimer's disease and frontotemporal dementia. J Neurol Neurosurg Psychiatry 66:184–188, 1999.
23. M Lindau, O Almkvist, SE Johansson, LO Wahlund. Cognitive and behavioral differentiation of frontal lobe degeneration of the non-Alzheimer type and Alzheimer's disease. Dement Geriatr Cogn Disord 9:205–213, 1998.
24. M Jackson, J Lowe. The new neuropathology of degenerative frontotemporal dementias. Acta Neuropathol 91:127–134, 1996.
25. DM Mann. Dementia of frontal type and dementias with subcortical gliosis. Brain Pathol 8:325–338, 1998.
26. WC Koller, EB Montgomery. Issues in the early diagnosis of Parkinson's disease. Neurology 49(suppl 1):S10–S25, 1997.
27. JL Cummings, A Darklins, M Mendez, MA Hill, DF Benson. Alzheimer's disease and Parkinson's disease: comparison of speech and language alterations. Neurology 38:680–684, 1988.
28. D Aarlsand, K Andersen, JP Larsen, A Lolk, H Nielsen, P Kragh-Sorensen. Risk of dementia in Parkinson's disease: a community-based, prospective study. Neurology 56:730–736, 2001.
29. SJ Huber, EC Shuttleworth, GW Paulson, MJ Bellchambers, LE Clapp. Cortical vs subcortical dementia. Neuropsychological differences. Arch Neurol 43:392–394, 1986.
30. B Pillon, B Dubois, F Lhermitte, Y Agid. Heterogeneity of cognitive impairment in progressive supranuclear palsy, Parkinson's disease, and Alzheimer's disease. Neurology 36:1179–1185, 1986.
31. F Boller, R Mizutani, U Roessmann, P Gambetti. Parkinson's disease, dementia, and Alzheimer's disease: clinicopathologic correlations. Ann Neurol 7:329–335, 1980.
32. PM Mattila, JO Rinne, H Helenius, DW Dickson, M Roytta. Alpha-synuclein-immunoreactive cortical Lewy bodies are associated with cognitive impairment in Parkinson's disease. Acta Neuropathol 100:285–290, 2000.
33. HI Hurtig, JQ Trojanowski, J Galvin, D Ewbank, ML Schmidt, VM Lee, CM Clark, G Glosser, MB Stern, SM Gollomb, SE Arnold. Alpha-synuclein cortical Lewy bodies correlate with dementia in Parkinson's disease. Neurology 54:1916–1921, 2000.
34. GC Roman, TK Tatemichi, T Erkinjuntti, JL Cummings, JC Masdeu, JH Garcia, L Amaducci, JM Orgogozo, A Brun, A Hofman, DM Moody, MD O'Brien, T Yamaguchi, J Grafman, BP Drayer, DA Bennett, M Fisher, J Ogata, E Kokmen, F Bermejo, PA Wolf, PB Gorelick, KL Bick, AK Pajeau, MA Bell, C DeCarli, A Culebras, AD Korczyn, J Bogousslavsky, A Hartmann, P Scheinberg. Vascular dementia: diagnostic criteria for research studies. Report of the NINDS-AIREN International Workshop. Neurology 43:250–260, 1993.
35. C Holmes, N Cairns, P Lantos, A Mann. Validity of current clinical criteria for Alzheimer's disease, vascular dementia and dementia with Lewy bodies. Br J Psychiatry 174:45–50, 1999.
36. G Gold, P Giannakopoulos, C Montes-Paixao Jr, FR Herrmann, R Mulligan, JP Michel, C Bourras. Sensitivity and specificity of newly proposed clinical criteria for possible vascular dementia. Neurology 49:690–694, 1997.
37. C Hulette, D Nochlin, D McKeel, JC Morris, SS Mirra, SM Sumi, A Heyman. Clinical-neuropathologic findings in multi-infarct dementia: a report of six autopsied cases. Neurology 48:668–672, 1997.
38. KA Nolan, MM Lino, AW Seligmann, JP Blass. Absence of vascular dementia in an autopsy series from a dementia clinic. J Am Geriat Soc 46:597–604, 1998.
39. DA Snowdon, LH Greiner, JA Mortimer, KP Riley, PA Greiner, WR Markesbery. Brain infarction and

40. AJ Corbett, H Bennet, S Kos. Cognitive dysfunction following subcortical infarction. Arch Neurol 51:999–1007, 1994.
41. BR Reed, JL Eberling, D Mungas, M Weiner, WJ Jagust. Frontal lobe hypometabolism predicts cognitive decline in patients with lacunar infarcts. Arch Neurol 58:493–497, 2001.
42. SE McPherson, JL Cummings. Neuropsychological aspects of vascular dementia. Brain Cogn 31:269–282, 1996.
43. D Laplane, M Levasseur, B Pillon, B Dubois, M Baulac, B Mazoyer, S Tran Dinh, G Sette, F Danze, JC Baron. Obsessive-compulsive and other behavioural changes with bilateral basal ganglia lesions. A neurospychological, magnetic resonance imaging and positron tomography study. Brain 112:699–725, 1989.
44. RD Adams, CM Fisher, S Hakim, RG Ojemann. Symptomatic occult hydrocephalus with "normal" cerebrospinal fluid pressure. A treatable syndrome. N Engl J Med 273:126–165, 1965.
45. AM Clarfield. Normal-pressure hydrocephalus: saga or swamp? JAMA 262:2592–2593, 1989.
46. J Golomb, J Wisoff, DC Miller, I Boksay, A Kluger, H Weiner, J Salton, W Graves. Alzheimer's disease comorbidity in normal pressure hydrocephalus: prevalence and shunt response. J Neurol Neurosurg Psychiatry 68:778–781, 2000.
47. BJ Brew. AIDS dementia complex. Neurol Clin 17:861–881, 1999.
48. N Sacktor, RH Lyles, R Skolasky, C Kleeberger, OA Selnes, EN Miller, JT Becker, B Cohen, JC McArthur. HIV-associated neurologic disease incidence changes: multicenter AIDS cohort study, 1990–1998. Neurology 56:257–260, 2001.
49. CC Weihl, RP Roos. Creutzfeldt-Jakob disease, new variant Creutzfeldt-Jakob disease, and bovine spongiform encephalopathy. Neurol Clin 17:835–859, 1999.
50. RG Will, JW Ironside, M Zeidler, SN Cousens, K Estibeiro, A Alperovitch, S Poser, M Pocchiari, A Hofman, PG Smith. A new variant of Creutzfeldt-Jakob disease in the UK. Lancet 347:921–925, 1996.
51. G Hsich, K Kenney, CJ Gibbs, KH Lee, MG Harrington. The 14-3-3 brain protein in cerebrospinal fluid as a marker for transmissible spongiform encephalopathies. N Engl J Med 335:924–930, 1996.
52. H Chui, Q Zhang. Evaluation of dementia: a systematic study of the usefulness of the American Academy of Neurology's practice parameters. Neurology 49:925–935, 1997.
53. S Humayun Gultekin, MR Rosenfeld, R Voltz, J Eichen, JB Posner, J Dalmau. Paraneoplastic limbic encephalitis: neurological symptoms, immunological findings and tumor association in 50 patients. Brain 123:1481–1494, 2000.
54. J Lindenbaum, IH Rosenberg, PW Wilson, SP Stabler, RH Allen. Prevalence of cobalamin deficiency in the Framingham elderly population. Am J Clinical Nutr 60:2–11, 1994.
55. RD Lindemann, DS Schade, A LaRue, LJ Romero, HC Liang, RN Baumgartner, KM Koehler, PJ Garry. Subclinical hypothyroidism in a biethnic, urban community. J Am Geriat Soc 47:703–709, 1999.
56. M Ganguli, LA Burmeister, EC Seaberg, S Belle, ST DeKosky. Association between dementia and elevated TSH: a community-based study. Biol Psychiatry 40:714–725, 1996.
57. N Goebels, M Soyka. Dementia associated with vitamin B_{12} deficiency: presentation of two cases and review of the literature. J Neuropsychiatry Clin Neurosci 12:389–394, 2000.
58. ME Charness, RP Simon, DA Greenberg. Ethanol and the nervous system. N Engl J Med 321:442–454, 1989.
59. JF Kraus. Epidemiologic aspects of brain injury. Neurol Clin 14:435–450, 1996.
60. TW McAllister. Neuropsychiatric sequelae of head injuries. Psychiatr Clin North Am 15:395–413, 1992.
61. A Fontaine, P Azouvi, P Remy, B Bussel, Y Samson. Functional anatomy of neuropsychological deficits after severe traumatic brain injury. Neurology 53:1963–1968, 1999.
62. AB Graves, E White, TD Koepsell, BV Reifler, G van Belle, EB Larson, M Raskind. The association between head trauma and Alzheimer's disease. Am J Epidemiol 131:491–501, 1990.
63. ED Caine, KA Bamford, RB Schiffer, I Shoulson, S Levy. A controlled neuropsychological comparison of Huntington's disease and multiple sclerosis. Arch Neurol 43:249–254, 1986.
64. SM Rao, GJ Leo, L Bernardin, F Unverzagt. Cognitive dysfunction in multiple sclerosis. I. Frequency, patterns, and prediction. Neurology 41:685–691, 1991.
65. M Rovaris, M Filippi. MRI correlates of cognitive dysfunction in multiple sclerosis. J Virol 6 (suppl 2):172–175, 2000.
66. T Harkany, I Abraham, C Konya, C Nyakas, M Zarandi, B Penke, PG Luiten. Mechanisms of beta-amyloid neurotoxicity: perspectives of pharmacotherapy. Rev Neurosci 11:329–382, 2000.
67. DJ Selkoe. The genetics and molecular pathology of Alzheimer's disease. Neurol Clin 18:903–922, 2000.
68. PH St George-Hyslop. Molecular genetics of Alzheimer's disease. Biol Psychiatry 47:183–199, 2000.
69. C Czech, G Tremp, L Pradier. Presenilins and Alzheimer's disease: biological functions and pathogenic mechanisms. Prog Neurobiol 60:363–384, 2000.

70. R Sherrington, S Froelich, S Sorbi, D Campion, H Chi, EA Rogaeva, G Levesque, EI Rogaev, C Lin, Y Liang, M Ikeda, L Mar, A Brice, Y Agid, ME Percy, F Clerget-Darpoux, S Piacentini, G Marcon, B Nacmias, L Amaducci, T Frebourg, L Lannfelt, JM Rommens, PH St George-Hyslop. Alzheimer's disease associated mutations in presenilin 2 is rare and variably penetrant. Hum Mol Genet 5:985–988, 1996.

71. AM Saunders, WJ Strittmatter, D Schmechel, PH George-Hyslop, MA Pericak-Vance, SH Joo, BL Rosi, JF Gusella, DR Crapper-MacLachlan, MJ Alberts, C Hulette, B Crain, D Goldgaber, AD Roses. Association of apolipoprotein E allele epsilon 4 with late-onset familial and sporadic Alzheimer's disease. Neurology 43:1467–1472, 1993.

72. E Rogaeva, S Premkumar, S Song, S Sorbi, N Brindle, A Paterson, R Duara, G Levesque, G Yu, M Nishimura, M Ikeda, C O'Toole, T Kawarai, R Jorge, D Vilarino, AC Bruni, LA Farrer, PH St George-Hyslop. Evidence for an Alzheimer disease susceptibility locus on chromosome 12 and for further locus heterogeneity. JAMA 280:614–618, 1998.

73. L Bertram, D Blacker, K Mullin, D Keeney, J Jones, S Basu, S Yhu, MG McInnis, RC Go, K Vekrellis, DJ Selkoe, RE Tanzi. Evidence for genetic linkage of Alzheimer's disease to chromosome 10q. Science 290:2302–2303, 2000.

74. N Ertekin-Taner, N Graff-Radford, LH Younkin, C Eckman, M Baker, J Adamson, J Ronald, J Blangero, M Hutton, SG Younkin. Linkage of plasma Abeta42 to a quantitative locus on chromosome 10 in late-onset Alzheimer's disease pedigrees. Science 290:2303–2304, 2000.

75. KC Wilhelmsen, T Lynch, E Pavlou, M Higgins, TG Nygaard. Localization of disinhibition-dementia-parkinsonism-amyotrophy complex to 17q21–22. Am J Hum Genet 55:1159–1165, 1994.

76. P Poorkaj, TD Bird, E Wijsman, E Nemens, RM Garruto, L Anderson, A Andreadis, WC Wiederholt, M Raskind, GD Schellenberg. Tau is a candidate gene for chromosome 17 frontotemporal dementia. Ann Neurol 43:815–825, 1998.

77. LA Reed, ZK Wszolek, M Hutton. Phenotypic correlations in FTDP-17. Neurobiol Aging 22:89–107, 2001.

78. TD Bird, D Nochlin, P Poorkaj, M Cherrier, J Kaye, H Payami, E Peskin, TH Lampe, E Nemens, PJ Boyer, GD Schellenberg. A clinical pathological comparison of three families with frontotemporal dementia and identical mutations in the tau gene (P301L). Brain 122:741–756, 1999.

79. J Brown, A Ashworth, S Gydesen, A Sorensen, M Rossor, J Hardy, J Collinge. Familial non-specific dementia maps to chromosome 3. Hum Mol Genet 4:1625–1628, 1995.

80. BA Hosler, T Siddique, PC Sapp, W Sailor, MC Huang, A Hossain, JR Daube, M Nance, C Fan, J Kaplan, WY Hung, D McKenna-Yasek, JL Haines, MA Pericak-Vance, HR Horvitz, RHJ Brown. Linkage of familial amyotrophic lateral sclerosis with frontotemporal dementia to chromosome 9q21-q22. JAMA 284:1664–1669, 2000.

81. H Houlden, M Baker, J Adamson, A Grover, S Waring, D Dickson, T Lynch, B Boeve, RC Petersen, S Pickering-Brown, F Owen, D Neary, D Craufurd, J Snowden, D Mann, M Hutton. Frequency of tau mutations in three series of non-Alzheimer's degenerative dementia. Ann Neurol 46:243–248, 1999.

82. P Poorkaj, M Grossman, E Steinbart, H Payami, A Sadovnick, D Nochlin, T Tabira, JQ Trojanowski, S Borson, D Galasko, S Reich, B Quinn, G Schellenberg, TD Bird. Frequency of tau gene mutations in familial and sporadic cases of non-Alzheimer dementia. Arch Neurol 58:383–387, 2001.

83. M Baker, I Litvan, H Houlden, J Adamson, D Dickson, J Perez-Tur, J Hardy, J Lynch, E Bigio, M Hutton. Association of an extended haplotype in the tau gene with progressive supranuclear palsy. Hum Mol Genet 8:711–715, 1999.

84. H Houlden, M Baker, HR Morris, N MacDonald, S Pickering-Brown, J Adamson, AJ Lees, MN Rossor, NP Quinn, A Kertesz, MN Khan, J Hardy, PL Lantos, P St George-Hyslop, DG Munoz, D Mann, AE Lang, C Bergeron, EH Bigio, I Litvan, KP Bhatia, D Dickson, NW Wood, M Hutton. Corticobasal degeneration and progressive supranuclear palsy share a common tau haplotype. Neurology 56:1702–1705, 2001.

85. O Bugiani, JR Murrell, G Giaccone, M Hasegawa, G Ghigo, M Tabaton, M Morbin, A Primavera, F Carella, C Solaro, M Grisoli, M Savoiardo, MG Spillantini, F Tagliavini, M Goedert, B Ghetti. Frontotemporal dementia and corticobasal degeneration in a family with P301S mutation in tau. J Neuropathol Exp Neurol 58:667–677, 1999.

86. Huntington's Disease Collaborative Research Group. A novel gene containing a trinucleotide repeat that is expanded and unstable on Huntington's disease chromosomes. Cell 72:971–983, 1993.

87. JL Cummings. Behavioral and psychiatric symptoms associated with Huntington's disease. Adv Neurol 65:179–186, 1995.

88. SC Kirkwood, JL Su, PM Conneally, T Foroud. Progression of symptoms in the early and middle stages of Huntington disease. Arch Neurol 58:273–278, 2001.

89. M Frydman. Genetic aspects of Wilson's disease. J Gastroenterol Hepatol 5:483–490, 1990.

90. A Medalia, K Isaacs-Glaberman, IH Scheinberg. Neuropsychological impairment in Wilson's disease. Arch Neurol 45:502–504, 1988.
91. EC Lauterbach, JL Cummings, J Duffy, CE Coffey, D Kaufer, M Lovell, P Malloy, A Reeve, DR Royall, TA Rummans, SP Salloway. Neuropsychiatric correlates and treatment of lenticulostriatal diseases: a review of the literature and overview of research opportunities in Huntington's, Wilson's, and Fahr's disease. J Neuropsychiatry Clin Neurosci 10:249–266, 1998.
92. MG Bousser, E Tournier-Lasserve. Cerebral autosomal dominant arteriopathy with subcortical infarcts and leukoencephalopathy: from stroke to vessel wall physiology. J Neurol Neurosurg Psychiatry 70:285–287, 2001.
93. M Dichgans, M Mayer, I Uttner, R Bruning, J Muller-Hocker, G Rungger, M Ebke, T Klockgether, T Gasser. The phenotypic spectrum of CADASIL: clinical findings in 102 cases. Ann Neurol 44:731–739, 1998.
94. G Lee, RL Neve, KS Kosik. The microtubule binding domain of tau protein. Neuron 2:1615–1624, 1989.
95. J Constantinidis, J Richard, R Tissot. Pick's disease. Histological and clinical correlations. Eur Neurol 11:208–217, 1974.
96. A Delacourte, N Sergeant, A Wattez, D Gauvreau, Y Robitaille. Vulnerable neuronal subsets in Alzheimer's and Pick's disease are distinguished by their tau isoform distribution and phosphorylation. Ann Neurol 43:193–204, 1998.
97. MG Spillantini, TD Bird, B Ghetti. Frontotemporal dementia and parkinsonism linked to chromosome 17: a new group of tauopathies. Brain Pathol 8:387–402, 1998.
98. V Zhukareva, V Vogelsberg-Ragalia, VMD Van Deerlin, J Bruce, T Shuck, M Grossman, CM Clark, SE Arnold, E Masliah, D Galasko, JQ Trojanowski, VM-Y Lee. Loss of brain tau defines novel sporadic and familial tauopathies with frontotemporal dementia. Ann Neurol 49:165–175, 2001.
99. JC Steele, JC Richardson, J Olszewski. Progressive supranuclear palsy. A heterogeneous degeneration involving the brainstem, basal ganglia, and cerebellum with vertical gaze and pseudobulbar palsy, nuchal dystonia, and dementia. Arch Neurol 10:333–358, 1964.
100. JJ Hauw, M Verny, P Delaere, P Cervera, Y He, C Duyckaerts. Constant neurofibrillary changes in the neocortex in progressive supranuclear palsy—basic differences with Alzheimer's disease and aging. Neurosci Lett 119:182–186, 1990.
101. N Sergeant, A Wattez, A Delacourte. Neurofibrillary degeneration in progressive supranuclear palsy and corticobasal degeneration: tau pathology with exclusively "exon 10" isoforms. J Neurochem 72:1243–1249, 1999.
102. M Feany, L Mattiace, D Dickson. Neuropathologic overlap of progressive supranuclear palsy, Pick's disease and corticobasal degeneration. J Neuropathol Exp Neurol 55:53–67, 1996.
103. I Litvan, Y Agid, C Goetz, J Jankovic, GK Wenning, JP Brandel, EC Lai, M Verny, K Ray-Chaudhuri, A McKee, K Jellinger, RKB Pearce, JJ Bartko. Accuracy of the clinical diagnosis of corticobasal degeneration: a clinicopathologic study. Neurology 48:119–125, 1997.
104. B Pillon, B Dubois. Memory and executive processes in corticobasal degeneration. Adv Neurol, 82:91–101, 2000.
105. DA Grimes, AE Lang, CB Bergeron. Dementia as the most common presentation of cortico-basal ganglionic degeneration. Neurology 53:1969–1974, 1999.
106. BF Boeve, DM Maraganore, JE Parisi, JE Ahlskog, N Graff-Radford, RJ Caselli, DW Dickson, E Kokmen, RC Petersen. Pathologic heterogeneity in clinically diagnosed corticobasal degeneration. Neurology 53:795–800, 1999.
107. MG Spillantini, A Divane, M Goedert. Assignment of human alpha-synuclein (SNCA) and beta-synuclein (SNCB) genes to chromosome 4q21 and 5q35. Genomics 27:379–381, 1995.
108. MH Polymeropoulos, C Lavedan, E Leroy, SE Ide, A Dehejia, A Dutra, B Pike, H Root, J Rubenstein, R Boyer, ES Stenroos, S Chandrasekharappa, A Athanassiadou, T Papapetropoulos, WG Johnson, AM Lazzarini, RC Duvoisin, G Di Iorio, LI Golbe, RL Nussbaum. Mutations in the alpha-synuclein gene identified in families with Parkinson's disease. Science 276:2045–2047, 1997.
109. DW Dickson. Tau and synuclein and their role in neuropathology. Brain Res 9:657–661, 1999.
110. CF Lippa, H Fujiwara, DM Mann, B Giasson, M Baba, ML Schmidt, LE Nee, B O'Connell, DA Pollen, P St George-Hyslop, B Ghetti, D Nochlin, TD Bird, NJ Cairns, VM Lee, T Iwatsubo, JQ Trojanowski. Lewy bodies contain altered alpha-synuclein in brains of many familial Alzheimer's disease patients with mutations in presenilin and amyloid precursor protein genes. Am J Pathol 153:1365–1370, 1998.
111. RL Hamilton. Lewy bodies in Alzheimer's disease: a neuropathological review of 145 cases using alpha-synuclein immunochemistry. Brain Pathol 10:378–384, 2000.
112. Y Arai, M Yamazaki, O Mori, H Muramatsu, G Asano, Y Katayama. Alpha-synuclein-positive structures in cases with sporadic Alzheimer's disease: morphology and its relationship to tau aggregation. Brain Research 888:287–296, 2001.
113. GK Wenning, Y Ben-Shlomo, A Hughes, SE Daniel, A Lees, NP Quinn. What clinical features are most useful to distinguish definite multiple system atrophy

114. TW Robbins, M James, KW Lange, AM Owen, NP Quinn, CD Marsden. Cognitive performance in multiple system atrophy. Brain 115:271–291, 1992.
115. MG Spillantini, RA Crowther, R Jakes, NJ Cairns, PL Lantos, M Goedert. Filamentous alpha-synuclein inclusions link multiple system atrophy with Parkinson's disease and dementia with Lewy bodies. Neurosci Lett 251:205–208, 1998.
116. SM Greenberg. Cerebral amyloid angiopathy. Prospects for clinical diagnosis and treatment. Neurology 51:690–694, 1998.
117. SM Greenberg, JP Vonsattel. Diagnosis of cerebral amyloid angiopathy. Sensitivity and specificity of cortical biopsy. Stroke 28:1418–1422, 1997.
118. L Hendriks, CM van Duijn, P Cras, M Cruts, W Van Hul, F van Harskamp, A Warren, MG McInnis, SE Antonorakis, JJ Martin, A Hofman, C Van Broeckoven. Presenile dementia and cerebral haemorrhage linked to a mutation at codon 692 of the beta-amyloid precursor protein gene. Nat Genet 1:218–221, 1992.
119. G Roks, F Van Harskamp, I De Koning, M Cruts, C De Jonghe, S Kumar-Singh, A Tibben, H Tanghe, MF Niermeijer, A Hofman, JC Van Swieten, C Van Broeckhoven, CM Van Duijn. Presentation of amyloidosis in carriers of the codon 692 mutation in the amyloid precursor protein gene (APP692). Brain 123:2130–2140, 2000.
120. TJ Grabowski, HS Cho, JP Vonsattel, GW Rebeck, SM Greenberg. Novel amyloid precursor protein mutation in an Iowa family with dementia and severe cerebral amyloid angiopathy. Ann Neurol 49:697–705, 2001.
121. H Vinters. Cerebral amyloid angiopathy: a microvascular link between parenchymal and vascular dementia. Ann Neurol 49:691–693, 2001.
122. GE Alexander, MR DeLong, PL Strick. Parallel organization of functionally segregated circuits linking basal ganglia and cortex. Ann Rev Neurosci 9:357–381, 1986.
123. GE Alexander, MD Crutcher, MR DeLong. Basal ganglia-thalamocortical circuits: parallel substrates for motor, oculomotor, "prefrontal" and "limbic" functions. Prog Brain Res 85:119–146, 1990.
124. MS Mega, JL Cummings, S Salloway, P Malloy. The limbic system: an anatomic, phylogenetic, and clinical perspective. J Neuropsychiatry Clin Neurosci 6:315–330, 1997.
125. PJ Whitehouse. The concept of subcortical dementia: another look. Ann Neurol 19:1–6, 1986.
126. R Mayeux, Y Stern. Subcortical dementia. Arch Neurol 34:642–646, 1987.
127. TJ Rosen. Cortical vs. subcortical dementia: neuropsychological similarities. Arch Neurol 44:131, 1987.
128. J Parvizi, GW Van Hoesen, A Damasio. The selective vulnerability of brainstem nuclei to Alzheimer's disease. Ann Neurol 49:53–66, 2001.
129. SJ Huber, EC Shuttleworth, DL Freidenberg. Neuropsychological differences between the dementias of Alzheimer's and Parkinson's disease. Arch Neurol 46:1287–1291, 1989.
130. ML Albert, RG Feldman, AL Willis. The "subcortical dementia" of progressive supranuclear palsy. J Neurol Neurosurg Psychiatry 37:121–130, 1974.
131. I Litvan, Y Agid, D Calne, G Campbell, B Dubois, RC Duvoisin, CG Goetz, LI Golbe, J Grafman, JH Growdon, M Hallet, J Jankovic, NP Quinn, E Tolosa, DS Zee. Clinical research criteria for the diagnosis of progressive supranuclear palsy (Steele-Richardson-Olszewski syndrome): report of the NINDS-SPSP International Workshop. Neurology 47:1–9, 1996.
132. NJ Cordato, GM Halliday, AJ Harding, MA Hely, JG Morris. Regional brain atrophy in progressive supranuclear palsy and Lewy body diseases. Ann Neurol 47:718–728, 2000.
133. J Blin, JC Baron, B Dubois, B Pillon, H Cambon, J Cambier, Y Agid. Positron emission tomography study in progressive supranuclear palsy. Brain hypometabolic pattern and clinico-metabolic correlations. Arch Neurol 47:747–752, 1990.
134. KA Johnson, RA Sperling, BL Holman, JS Nagel, JH Growden. Cerebral perfusion in progressive supranuclear palsy. J Nucl Med 33:704–709, 1992.
135. MM Mesulam. Slowly progressive aphasia without generalized dementia. Ann Neurol 11:592–598, 1982.
136. MM Mesulam. Primary progressive aphasia. Ann Neurol 49:425–432, 2001.
137. S Weintraub, NP Rubin, MM Mesulam. Primary progressive aphasia. Longitudinal course, neuropsychological profile, and language features. Arch Neurol 47:1329–1335, 1990.
138. C Janus, J Pearson, J McLaurin, PM Mathews, Y Jiang, SD Schmidt, MA Chishti, P Horne, D Heslin, J French, HT Mount, RA Nixon, M Mercken, C Bergeron, PE Fraser, P St George-Hyslop, D Westaway. A beta petpide immunization reduces behavioural impairment and plaques in a model of Alzheimer's disease. Nature 408:915–916, 2000.

10

Classification of Personality Disorders
Implications for Treatment and Research

DRAGAN M. SVRAKIC and ROBERT CLONINGER
Washington University School of Medicine in St. Louis, St. Louis, Missouri, U.S.A.

STANA STANIC
University of Trieste, Trieste, Italy

SECONDO FASSINO
University of Turin, Turin, Italy

I. INTRODUCTION

Modern psychobiological theory conceptualizes personality as a self-organizing, complex adaptive system involving a bidirectional interaction between heritable neurobiological dispositions to behavior (temperament) and developing concepts about self and external objects (character). As introduced by the seven-factor psychobiological model of personality in 1993 [1,2], the concepts of temperament and character synthesize advances from a wide variety of scientific disciplines—evolutionary biology, genetics, neuroscience, theory of learning, sociology, philosophy—each contributing from its specific angle to the present eclectic understanding of personality development and structure. "Biological" temperament traits and "conceptual" character traits, two distinct but interacting components of personality, are distinguished based on the corresponding neurobiological and psychological mechanisms underlying behavior. These mechanisms provide guidelines for testable hypotheses about etiology and treatment of personality disorder. Clinically, the temperament and character traits are used to classify and diagnose personality disorder and to differentiate its clinical subtypes.

In this paper, we first review the basic aspects of the seven-factor psychobiological model of personality and then outline treatment implications, based on this model, for extreme personality variants classified as personality disorder.

II. TEMPERAMENT AND CHARACTER (NATURE AND NURTURE)

Structurally, the seven-factor model describes four temperament traits (Harm Avoidance, Novelty Seeking, Reward Dependence, and Persistence) and three character traits (Self-Directedness, Cooperativeness, and Self-Transcendence) (Tables 1 and 2).

The temperament traits are largely heritable (up to 60%), relatively stable over lifetime, and universal across cultures and ethnic groups. These traits are

Table 1 Descriptors of Individuals Who Score High and Low on the Four Temperament Dimensions

Temperament dimension	Descriptors of extreme variants	
	High	Low
Harm Avoidance	pessimistic fearful shy fatigable	optimistic daring outgoing energetic
Novelty Seeking	exploratory impulsive extravagant irritable	reserved deliberate thrifty stoical
Reward Dependence	sentimental open warm affectionate	detached aloof cold independent
Persistence	industrious determined enthusiastic perfectionist	lazy spoiled underachiever pragmatist

etiologically associated with basic (or primary) emotions of fear (Harm Avoidance), anger (Novelty Seeking), attachment (Reward Dependence), and perseverance (Persistence). In contrast, character

Table 2 Descriptors of Individuals Who Score High and Low on the Three Character Dimensions

Character dimension	Descriptors of extreme variants	
	High	Low
Self-Directedness	responsible purposeful resourceful self-accepting disciplined	blaming goal-less passive wishful undisciplined
Cooperative	tender-hearted empathic helpful compassionate principled	intolerant insensitive selfish revengeful opportunistic
Self-Transcendent	imaginative intuitive acquiescent spiritual idealistic	conventional logical doubtful materialistic relativistic

traits are weakly heritable, tend to change with age and maturation, and are associated with social (or secondary) emotions, such as honor, integrity, morality, altruism, respect. Roughly, temperament is what we are born with, character is what we make out of ourselves.

The Temperament and Character Inventory (TCI) has been developed to measure the above temperament and character traits (Table 3). As described in the TCI Manual [3], the psychobiological model has been translated into many languages, its psychometric validity confirmed in clinical and nonclinical samples, its

Table 3 Temperament and Character Inventory (TCI)

Harm Avoidance (HA)
  HA1: worry and pessimism vs. uninhibited optimism
  HA2: fear of uncertainty
  HA3: shyness with strangers
  HA4: fatigability and asthenia
Novelty Seeking (NS)
  NS1: exploratory excitability vs. stoic rigidity
  NS2: impulsiveness vs. reflection
  NS3: extravagance vs. reserve
  NS4: disorderliness vs. orderliness
Reward Dependence (RD)
  RD1: sentimentality
  RD2: sociability vs. aloofness
  RD3: attachment vs. detachment
  RD4: dependence vs. independence
Persistence (PS)
  PS1: eagerness of effort vs. laziness
  PS2: work hardened vs. spoiled
  PS3: ambitiousness vs. underachieving
  PS4: perfectionism vs. pragmatism

Self-Directedness (SD)
  SD1: responsibility vs. blaming
  SD2: purposefulness vs. lack of goal direction
  SD3: resourcefulness vs. helplessness
  SD4: self-acceptance vs. self-striving
  SD5: congruent second nature
Cooperativeness (CO)
  C1: social acceptance vs. social intolerance
  C2: empathy vs. social disinterest
  C3: helpfulness vs. unhelpfulness
  C4: compassion vs. revengefulness
  C5: pure hearted vs. self-serving
Self-Transcendence (ST)
  ST1: self-forgetful vs. self-conscious
  ST2: transpersonal identification vs. Self-differentiation
  ST3: spiritual acceptance vs. rational materialism
  ST4: enlightened vs. objective
  ST5: idealistic vs. practical

III. TEMPERAMENT AND CHARACTER: TWO DISTINCT MEMORY AND LEARNING SYSTEMS

Temperament (or the "emotional core" of personality) involves heritable dispositions to early emotions (such as fear, anger, and attachment), and related automatic behavior reactions (such as inhibition, activation, and maintenance of behavior) in response to specific environmental stimuli (danger, novelty, and reward, respectively). Temperament traits are based on presemantic perceptual processing of visuospatial information and affective valence regulated by the corticostriatolimbic system, primarily the sensory cortical areas, amygdala, and the caudate and putamen (the so-called procedural memory). In other words, temperament traits are heritable biases in procedural learning that underlie associative conditioning of automatic behavior responses to danger, novelty, and reward. Temperament traits are genetically homogeneous, independently inherited, relatively stable over lifetime, and cross-culturally universal [4].

Character (or the "conceptual core" of personality) involves higher cognitive functions, such as abstraction and symbolic interpretation, analytical and inductive logic, symbolism, etc., regulated by the hippocampus and neocortex. These functions (also called propositional memory) are critical for cognitive processing of sensory percepts and affects regulated by temperament, leading to the development of abstract conceptual and volitional processes. Character traits reflect one's developing concepts about oneself and the external world [2].

Basic differences between character and temperament are presented in Table 4.

Table 4 Key Differences Between Temperament (associative or procedural learning) and Character (conceptual or propositional learning)

Variable properties	Temperament	Character
Awareness level	automatic	intentional
Memory form	percepts procedures	concepts propositions
Learning principles	associative conditioning	conceptual insight
Role of subject in mental activity	passive reproductive	active constructive
Key brain system	Limbic system Striatum	Temporal cortex Hippocampus
Form of mental representation	stimulus-response sequences varying additively in strength	interactive networks (conceptual schema) varying qualitatively in configuration
Etiological components		
Genetic heritability	40–60%	10–15%
Family environment	0%	30–35%
Random environment	40–60%	40–60%

IV. INTEGRATED VIEW OF PERSONALITY: TEMPERAMENT AND CHARACTER INTERACT TO PRODUCE PERSONALITY

Personality is conceptualized as a self-organizing, complex adaptive system characterized by multiple internal and external, constraining and facilitating factors, interacting nonlinearly to finally funnel into only one (out of several possible) developmental outcome [4]. Personality development is graphically presented as a fitness landscape, where hills and valleys represent high and low adaptive levels, respectively. Periods of stability (i.e., local adaptive optima represented by hills) alternate with relatively rapid transitions (through the valleys) to new adaptive levels [4].

Heritable biological dispositions develop into actual temperament traits, amenable to observation and measurement (i.e., avoidant, exploratory, persistent, or sociable behaviors) as a nonlinear function of the relative strength of the underlying disposition and the characteristics of the interacting environment (e.g., suppression or facilitation of certain behaviors).

With growing perceptual and cognitive capacities, early percepts and affects based on temperament are transformed into more complex concepts about self and the external world. This internalization of new concepts and their associated social emotions (honor, pride, altruism) further neutralizes raw temperament traits, most importantly fear and anger, and provides the stage for personality to crystallize around positive, gratifying experiences associated with attachment. In other words, through this bidirectional interaction of temperament and character, developing concepts about self and the external world modify the significance and the salience of sensory percepts and affects regulated by temperament, and vice versa. Temperament regulates what we notice, and, in turn, character modifies its meaning, so that the salience and significance of all experience depend on both temperament and character.

V. DIFFERENTIATING NORMAL FROM DEVIANT PERSONALITY: WHEN TO TREAT AND WHO NEEDS TREATMENT

The distinction between temperament and character, i.e., between biological and psychological mechanisms underlying behavior, provides guidelines for testable hypotheses about etiology, diagnosis, and treatment of personality disorder. This is not possible for models that confound temperament and character. The TCI has repeatedly proven useful to predict categorical diagnoses of personality disorder in numerous clinical and nonclinical samples, cross-culturally, in patients with and without personality disorder and varying mood and anxiety states [3].

The concepts of temperament and character are essential to decompose the symptoms of personality disorder into *common features* shared by all subtypes (used for diagnosis) and *distinguishing features* unique for each subtype (used for differential diagnosis) [4]. The following major findings are noteworthy:

Low scores on Self-Directedness and Cooperativeness correlate highly with the number of symptoms for personality disorder (Tables 5 and 6) The TCI character traits predict the presence or absence of

Table 5 Correlations Between TCI Scales and Total No. of Symptoms for PDs, Cluster A, Cluster B, and Cluster C Inpatients ($N = 136$)

	Total No. of symptoms	Cluster A symptoms	Cluster B symptoms	Cluster C symptoms
Novelty Seeking	**.22**[c]	.02	**.44**[a]	−.06
Harm Avoidance	**.31**[b]	**.23**[b]	.08	**.43**[a]
Reward Dependence	−.14	−**.37**[a]	−.08	−.04
Persistence	.00	−.07	.04	−.01
Self-Directedness	−**.56**[a]	−**.35**[a]	−**.43**[a]	−**.50**[a]
Cooperativeness	−**.44**[a]	−**.44**[a]	−**.40**[a]	−**.28**[b]
Self-Transcendence	.02	−.08	.03	.04

[a] $< .0001$; [b] $< .001.$; [c] $< .01$.

Table 6 Correlations Between Temperament and Character Dimensions and Symptoms for Individual Personality Disorder

| | TCI temperament and character scale scores |||||||
| | Temperament |||| Character |||
PD symptoms	HA	NS	RD	PS	SD	C	ST
Antisocial	.11	**.51**[a]	−.11	.06	**−.46**[a]	**−.50**[a]	.11
Histrionic	.04	.10	.12	**−.49**[a]	**−.43**[a]	**.28**[c]	**.40**[a]
Borderline	**.45**[a]	**.37**[a]	−.09	.12	**−.67**[a]	**−.43**[a]	**.25**[c]
Narcissistic	.17	**.31**[b]	−.03	.09	**−.49**[a]	**−.44**[a]	**.25**[c]
Avoidant	**.65**[a]	.00	**−.20**[c]	.07	**−.64**[a]	**−.44**[a]	−.07
Obsessive	**.42**[a]	.09	−.13	**.19**[c]	**−.62**[a]	**−.38**[a]	.10
Dependent	**.54**[a]	**.20**[c]	**.18**[c]	.03	**−.61**[a]	**−.22**[c]	.13
Schizoid	**.31**[b]	−.10	**−.46**[a]	−.04	**−.36**[a]	**−.33**[b]	−.16
Schizotypal	**.53**[a]	.09	**−.28**[b]	.00	**−.64**[a]	**−.48**[a]	**.31**[b]
Paranoid	**.33**[b]	**.21**[c]	**−.25**[b]	**.20**[c]	**−.54**[a]	**−.50**[a]	**.28**[c]

[a] < .0001; [b] < .001; [c] < .05.
HA, Harm Avoidance; NS, Novelty Seeking; RD, Reward Dependence; PS, Persistence; SD, Self-Directedness; C, Cooperativeness; ST, Self-Transcendence; PD, Personality Disorder.

any personality disorder (Table 7). In other words, poorly developed character traits, especially low Self-directedness and Cooperativeness, represent the core feature of personality disorder, extending across all clinical subtypes. This accounts for chronic difficulties in accepting responsibility, setting long-term goals, fragile self-esteem, lack of capacity to be alone, unstable self-image, uncertain identity, etc., so typical of personality disorder. Usually, these patients are also uncooperative (revengeful, opportunistic, unhelpful, without stable ethical principles). As shown in Table 6, Self-Transcendence correlates with borderline, narcissistic, and histrionic symptoms (accounting for dissociative tendencies in these cases) and schizotypal and paranoid symptoms (accounting for magical thinking and rich imaginary life in these patients). On the other hand, when coupled with high Self-Directedness and Cooperativeness, Self-Transcendence indicates maturity, spirituality, and creativity rather than psychopathology.

Once the probability for the presence of personality disorder is established based on character, temperament is used for differential diagnosis. In this regard:

1. Each DSM cluster is differentiated based on one of the TCI temperament dimensions (Table 5).
2. The A cluster, which includes schizoid, schizotypal, and paranoid personality (i.e., the "aloof" cluster), is characterized by low Reward Dependence (detached, cold, independent individuals).

Table 7 Temperament and Character Predictors of Personality Disorder Symptoms (controlling for age, depression, and anxiety)

	PD symptoms Partial R²
PD symptoms	
Age/depression/anxiety	**.45***
TCI personality scales	
Novelty Seeking	ns
Harm Avoidance	ns
Reward Dependence	ns
Persistence	ns
Self-Directedness	**.20***
Cooperativeness	**.05***
Self-Transcendence	**.05***
Cumulative R²	**.30***
Model R²	**.75***

*P < .0001.

3. The B cluster, which includes borderline, antisocial, histrionic, and narcissistic personality (i.e., the "impulsive" cluster), is characterized by high Novelty Seeking (exploratory, impulsive, extravagant, irritable individuals).

4. The C cluster, which includes avoidant, dependent, self-defeating and obsessive-compulsive personality (i.e., the "fearful" cluster), is characterized by high Harm Avoidance (fearful, shy, pessimistic individuals).

5. The fourth temperament trait, Persistence, predicts Obsessive-Compulsive traits especially when coupled with high Harm Avoidance.

6. Categorical subtypes of personality disorder are distinguished based on their unique pattern of correlations with temperament traits of Harm Avoidance, Novelty Seeking, Reward Dependence, and Persistence (the temperament traits interact in all possible factorial combinations to produce symptoms for each of the 11 DSM clinical subtypes of personality disorder) (Table 6).

VI. MATURE CHARACTER IS PROTECTIVE AGAINST PERSONALITY DISORDER

Maladaptation is predominantly a function of character, not temperament. Extreme temperament variants alone do not reliably distinguish between normal adaptation and maladapted personality. Some individuals with low Reward Dependence are socially withdrawn, disinterested, and detached, but these features cause no obvious impairment in professional functioning and no signs of personal suffering and distress. Also, neither low nor high temperament scores inherently mean better adaptation, as each extreme has specific adaptive advantages and disadvantages (e.g., high Harm Avoidance is adaptively advantageous when hazard is likely, and not so when hazard is unlikely but still anticipated).

Extreme temperament traits are associated with long-term personal, social, and/or occupational impairments (i.e., maladaptation) only when accompanied by low character traits. In other words, mature character reduces the risk of maladaptation and personality disorder. Individuals high in Novelty Seeking and low in Harm Avoidance may have an impulsive or antisocial personality disorder if they are low in Self-Directedness and Cooperativeness, or may be energetic businessmen or inquisitive scientists without personality disorder if their character is mature, i.e., if they are self-directed and cooperative.

VII. SOME TEMPERAMENT TYPES PROTECT AGAINST PERSONALITY DISORDER

Temperament and character dimensions interact to create composite types or configurations (Figs. 1 and 2). These composite types manifest a number of behaviors directly associated with one of the underlying traits (e.g., impulsivity reflects Novelty Seeking, social attachment reflects Reward Dependence), but also a number of qualitatively new behaviors or emerging properties created by the interactions (e.g., high Harm Avoidance interacts with high Persistence to create obsessive symptoms).

Each of the composite temperament types affects differentially one's risk of immature character and personality disorder (Table 8). Temperament types with high Reward Dependence are protective against personality disorder, presumably because dependency, attachment, sentimentality, and responsivity to social reward facilitate behaviors that conform to local sociocultural norms. In addition, high Reward Dependence facilitates character development, especially Cooperativeness, as indicated by their positive intercorrelation. Accordingly, the "reliable" temperament type (high Reward

Temperament type	Harm Avoidance	Novelty Seeking	Reward Dependence
Cautious	high	low	high
Methodical	high	low	low
Passive-Aggressive	high	high	high
Explosive (Borderline)	high	high	low
Antisocial	low	high	low
Histrionic	low	high	high
Reliable	low	low	high
Schizoid	low	low	low

Figure 1 Temperament traits interact to create composite types (three traits produce eight possible combinations).

Classification of Personality Disorders

Character type	Self-directedness	Cooperativeness	Self Transcendence
Organized	high	high	low
Auticratic	high	low	low
Dependent (irritable)	low	high	low
Downcast (melancholic)	low	low	low
Disorganized (Schizotypal)	low	low	high
Fanatical (paranoid)	high	Low	high
Moody (cyclothymic)	low	high	high
Creative	high	high	high

Figure 2 Character traits interact to create composite types (three traits produce eight possible combinations).

Dependence, low Harm Avoidance, low Novelty Seeking) is at the lowest risk of personality disorder.

In contrast, some temperament types, especially those with high Harm Avoidance and/or high Novelty Seeking, increase the risk for personality disorder, presumably because proneness to anxiety and depression (Harm Avoidance) and impulsivity and anger (Novelty Seeking) interferes with character maturation (especially with the development of Self-Directedness, which is negatively correlated with Harm Avoidance. The explosive (or borderline) type, with high Novelty Seeking, high Harm Avoidance, but low Reward Dependence, has the highest risk of personality disorder. This type is characterized by susceptibility to anxiety and depression, impulsivity, and indifference to sociocultural pressures.

Contrary to the common belief, the "flexible" or "adaptable" personalities, i.e., those with average

Table 8 Relative Risk of Immature Character as a Function of Temperament Type in a General Community Sample ($N = 300$)

Temperament type	Mild i/N	Mild immature %	Pronounced i/N	Pronounced immature %	All immature %	RR
Reliable (nhR)	2/24	8	0/12	0	6	0.2
Histrionic (NhR)	5/32	16	1/18	6	12	0.4
Schizoid (nhr)	5/22	23	0/9	0	16	0.5
Passive-Dependent (nHR)	4/19	21	1/11	9	17	0.5
Flexible (average)			5/15	33	33	1.0
Passive-Aggressive (NHR)	8/20	40	4/10	40	40	1.2
Antisocial (Nhr)	10/19	53	2/6	33	48	1.4
Obsessional (nHr)	22/35	63	4/9	44	59	1.8
Borderline (NHr)	20/29	69	8/10	80	72	2.1

RR = Relative Risk or ratio of observed proportion to that in general population.
i/N = immature characters/number of cases (immature character defined as combined score of Self-Directedness and Cooperativeness > 58 (33rd centile in the sample).
Mild types = at least one temperament trait low or high in terms of percentile scores, i.e., lowest or highest one-third (low = 0–33%, high = 67–100%), other traits low-average (34–50%) or high-average (50–66%).
Pronounced types = all temperament traits low or high.
Lowercase letters (h, n, r) and capital letters (H, N, R) indicate low and high values for temperament traits

scores on all three temperament traits, are not protected against maladaptation. They have an average (not a decreased) risk of personality disorder (Table 8).

VIII. INTEGRATION OF CATEGORICAL AND DIMENSIONAL ASSESSMENT OF PERSONALITY DISORDER

The DSM system conceptualizes personality disorder as categorical, mutually exclusive syndromes of deviant behavior classified as separate diagnostic categories. These categories, however, overlap to the extent that psychometric tests based on the DSM criteria always yield multiple personality diagnoses for one patient. In contrast, the TCI temperament traits differentiate categorical DSM diagnoses without any overlap [5].

The TCI integrates elements of categorical diagnosis into its dimensional assessment of personality disorder. Note that each of the composite temperament types presented in Figure 3 corresponds clinically to one of the traditional DSM categories of personality disorder. Physicians use these "dimensional categories" for time-efficient and vivid clinical portrayal of individual cases. At the same time, the TCI temperament and character dimensions are easily extracted from any particular composite type for independent diagnostic analyses and treatment planning. In summary, the TCI captures more information about severity of impairment and patterns of behavior in terms of quantitative ratings than does the DSM system, and does so without sacrificing the utility of traditional categorical labels.

IX. PERSONALITY DISORDER: SOCIAL OR CLINICAL DIAGNOSIS?

The DSM clinical definition of personality disorder has a significant social connotation, as one of the general criteria is that maladaptive behavior "deviates markedly from the expectations of sociocultural norms." Indeed, clinicians frequently diagnose personality disorder based solely on the extent to which one's behavior is adjusted to the local society.

As noted, temperament profiles with high Reward Dependence have a low incidence of diagnosed personality disorder, whereas those with high Harm Avoidance and/or high Novelty Seeking increase the incidence substantially. Sociocultural pressures are always norm favoring, promoting phenotypes within

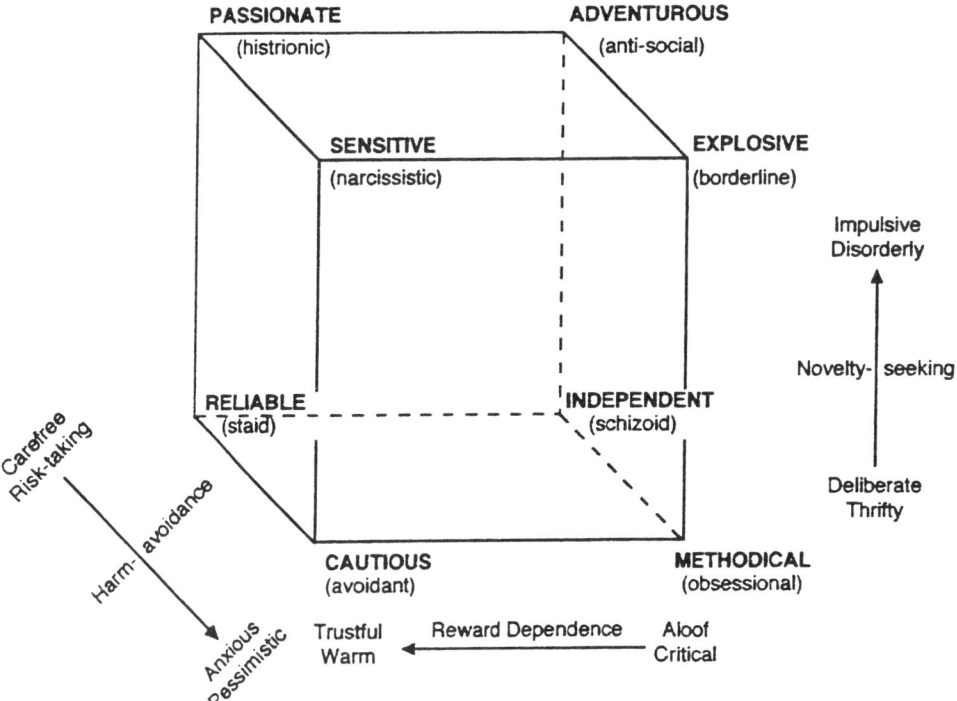

Figure 3 Temperament configuration.

the range of accepted norms. In our society, the normative phenotype is not the one with average personality traits (as one would expect given the adaptive flexibility of such configurations) but the one with high Reward Dependence, presumably due to easy conditioning of socially accepted behaviors compared to other temperament traits. Adults with high Harm Avoidance and/or high Novelty Seeking are more likely to be diagnosed as "personality disorder" and to be treated to change or eliminate behaviors associated with their temperament traits (Table 9).

Similarly, child psychiatry classifies three broad groups of mental disorders in children with high Novelty Seeking (e.g., Attention Deficit Hyperactivity Disorder, Conduct Disorder), or high Harm Avoidance (e.g., Depression, Anxiety Disorders), or low Reward Dependence (e.g., Schizophrenia, Autism). These children are diagnosed as "cases" and treated early in life. In contrast, children with high Reward Dependence (i.e., those sociable, attached, and dependent) are selectively permitted to develop without psychiatric intervention.

At the present level of human civilization, natural selection of biologically dominant and adaptable phenotypes has become almost irrelevant for our survival and reproduction. The latter appear to be now more associated with social dominance and successful behavioral adaptation to the society (achieved primarily by social selection targeting our personality features). Through its selective permissiveness for specific personality traits, modern society appears to be relying (at least partly) on psychiatry to selectively funnel individuals into a relatively narrow spectrum of desired psychological phenotypes.

X. MULTIFINALITY OF OUTCOMES: ONE TEMPERAMENT TYPE HAS MORE THAN ONE CHARACTER OUTCOME

Each of the eight composite character outcomes (Fig. 4) can be predicted from the initial temperament traits, taking into account temperament-character interactions, sociocultural norms, random events

Table 9 Four Dissociable Brain Systems Influencing Stimulus-Response Patterns Underlying Temperament

Brain system (related personality dimension)	Principal neuromodulators	Relevant stimuli	Behavioral response
Behavioral activation (Novelty Seeking)	Dopamine	Novelty CS of reward CS or UCS of relief of monotony or punishment	Exploratory pursuit Appetitive approach Active avoidance Escape
Behavioral inhibition (Harm Avoidance)	GABA serotonin (dorsal raphe)	Aversive conditioning (pairing CS-UCS) Conditioned signals for punishment, novelty, frustrative nonreward	Formation of aversive CS Passive avoidance, extinction
Social attachment (Reward Dependence)	Norepinephrine serotonin (median raphe)	Reward conditioning (pairing CS-UCS)	Formation of appetitive CS
Partial reinforcement (Persistence)	Glutamate serotonin (dorsal raphe)	Intermittent reinforcement	Resistance to extinction

CS, conditioned signals; UCS, unconditioned signals.
Source: Ref. 6.

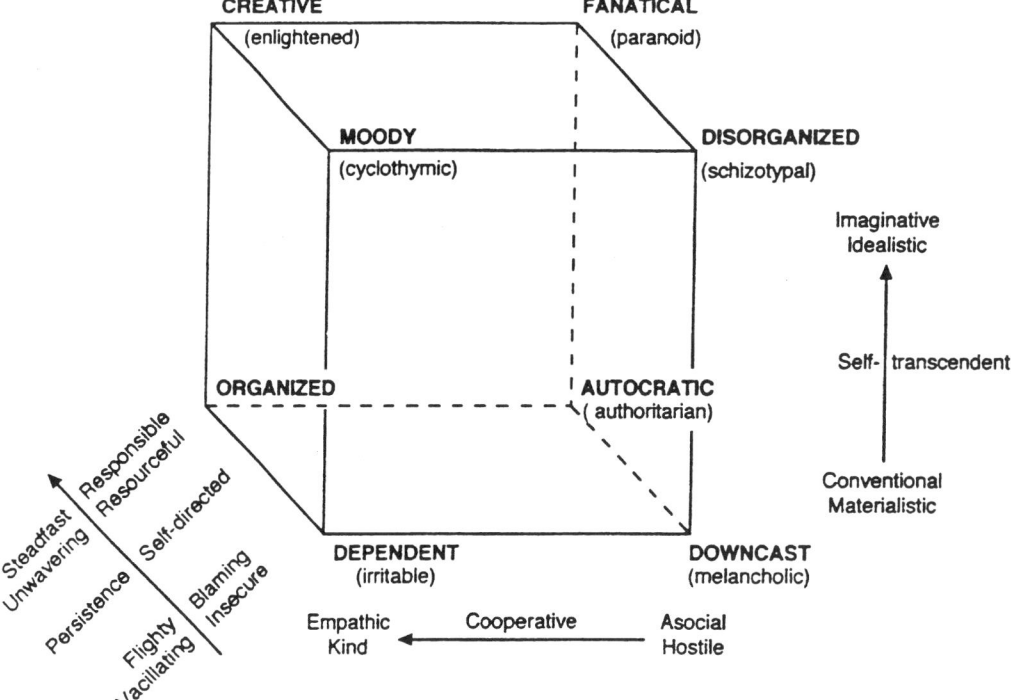

Figure 4 Character configuration.

unique to the individual, and social learning within the family [4]. With all this taken into account, it turns out that a single initial temperament configuration may lead to several different character outcomes. This aspect of development is referred to as *multifinality* [4].

The spectrum of possible character outcomes for each antecedent temperament type ranges from those more mature (achieved under optimal conditions) to those less mature (achieved under suboptimal conditions). For example, computer-simulated character development for the explosive (borderline) temperament type (i.e., high Harm Avoidance, high Novelty Seeking, low Reward Dependence), with all of the above contributing factors taken into account, is restricted to the development of only two character outcomes—both immature, but one relatively more mature (the melancholic character) than the other (the disorganized character). The most likely outcome is the melancholic character, prone to chronic depression and severe personality disorder (all three character traits are poorly developed). A small number of individuals with borderline temperament will develop the disorganized (or schizotypal) character outcome with high Self-Transcendence, but low Self-Directedness and Cooperativeness (this type is characterized by magical thinking, perceptual aberration, and proneness to suicide and psychosis). Chances for other character outcomes for this temperament type are relatively low. Computer-simulated character development for other temperament types have been defined as well.

XI. CHARACTER (IM)MATURITY AND MENTAL (DIS)ORDER

Following the subscale structure of the TCI character traits (a total of 15 subscales for the three traits), full character development involves a sequence of 15 successive developmental steps, corresponding to the 15 subscales. Each new step in development emerges as a result of complex nonlinear facilitating and inhibitory interactions among heritable predispositions, social learning, and individual experiences (Table 10).

These 15 steps in character development are a theoretical ideal, leading to maximal scores on all three character dimensions. As character development depends on many internal and external, antecedent and

Classification of Personality Disorders

Table 10 Fifteen-Step Personality Development

Steps	Self-Directed	Cooperative	Self-Transcendent
TCI Tier 1			
1. co1		tolerant vs. suspicious (trustful vs. mistrustful)	
2. sd1	responsible vs. blaming (confident vs. shameful)		
3. st1			obedient vs. intractable (respectful vs. judgmental)
TCI Tier 2			
4. sd2	purposeful vs. aimless (moderate vs. indulgent)		
5. co2		empathic vs. cruel (prudent vs. scornful)	
6. st2			conscientious vs. unjust (worshipful vs. defiant)
TCI Tier 3			
7. sd3	resourceful vs. inept (hopeful vs. helpless)		
8. co3		generous vs. disagreeable (kind vs. hostile)	
9. st3			spiritual vs. materialistic (contemplative vs. greedy)
TCI Tier 4			
10. sd4	self-accepting vs. vain (humble vs. impatient)		
11. co4		forgiving vs. revengeful (compassionate vs. callous)	
12. st4			enlightened vs. possessive (joyfully free vs. controlling)
TCI Tier 5			
13. sd5	integrity vs. conflict (peaceful vs. undisciplined)		
14. co5		wise vs. unprincipled (loving vs. harsh)	
15. st5			creative vs. dualistic (idealistic vs. practical)

concomitant, facilitating and inhibitory factors, for some individuals full character development of all three traits is simply not possible.

Clinically, the 15 steps are organized into seven hierarchical levels of character disorder (divisions are made at points where developmental failures occur most frequently) (Table 11).

This hierarchical model of underlying character defects is used to classify progressive severity of mental order vs. disorder and provides a theoretical framework for treatment planning (discussed below).

A. Severely Disorganized Behaviors and Psychoses

Problems at the first level, involving basic trust (step 1) and confidence (step 2), are characteristic of individuals with history of sexual or physical abuse, and is associated with *highly disorganized disorders and psychosis*. Following Karasu [7], such patients have severe borderline and narcissistic disorders with "dyadic deficits" if they are arrested at character step 1 (which leads to impairments in the sense of self along with impaired mother-child relations) or

Table 11 A Hierarchical Model of Mental Order and Disorder Based on Level of Personality Development

Character deficits	Associated mental health features
Level I "Walking Together"	(disorganized disorders)
1. co1—mistrust	self-injurious behavior
2. sd1—doubt & shame	sado-masochistic sexuality
Level II "Working Together"	(severe personality disorder)
3. st1—poor impulse control	bipolar affective lability
4. sd2—aimlessness	unemployment, criminality
5. co2—lack of empathy	polysubstance abuse
Level III "Feeling Together"	(mild personality disorder)
6. st2—no conscience	
7. sd3—low self-esteem	social dysfunction
8. co3—selfishness	frequent negative emotions
Level IV "Spiritual Together"	
9. st3—materialism	personal dissatisfaction
10. sd4—arrogance	lack of generativity
11. co4—revengefulness	occasional negative emotions
Level V "Minds Thinking as One"	
12. st4—possessiveness	mature but lack of joy &
13. sd5—integrated	lack of serenity
Level VI "Listening in Silence"	mature but lack of
14. co5—unloving at times	intuitive wisdom
Level VII "Experiencing in Unity"	mature but judgmental
15. st5—dualistic	& not fully harmonious

Subscales are designated by sd (Self-Directedness), co (Cooperativeness), st (Self-Transcendence), and the number of the subscale shown in Table 7 (1–5).

"dyadic conflicts" if they are arrested at character step 2 (which leads to severely impaired object relations, such as difficulty of the child separating from the mother). Such fundamental impairments predispose to vulnerability to psychosis.

B. Severe Personality Disorders

Problems at the second level involve *severe personality disorders* with negativism, disobedience, and lack of purposefulness and empathy. This level, characterized by problematic three-person (i.e., mother-child-father) relationships, includes patients with "triadic deficits" if they are arrested at step 3 (which leads to poor impulse control and reduced capacity for intimacy and social commitment) or "triadic conflicts" (arrested at step 4 or 5, leading to milder Oedipal conflicts, such as inhibited sexuality or impaired internalization of group values [7]. Such individuals have severe problems in working, socialization, and impulse control.

C. Mild Personality Disorder, Alcoholism, Anxiety Disorder, Major Depression

Problems at the third level, with low conscientiousness, low self-confidence, low resourcefulness, and little generosity, are typical of individuals with *mild personality disorder, type 1 alcoholism, anxiety disorder, or major depression*, which are associated with mild problems in self-esteem, and lack of social intimacy or group identification.

D. Higher Levels of Maturity and Well-Being

The fourth and higher levels involve progressive steps in cognitive and spiritual development, predominantly observed with mature individuals seeking fulfillment with better health and happiness. Such overall personality integration can be measured by the sum of scores on all three character dimensions, consistent with Jung's notion of the self-transcendent leader. These higher levels of personality integration may be associated with psychopathology at times of existential crisis.

The above hierarchical model of mental order and disorder is essential to custom-tailor treatment strategies for individual patients (see later).

E. Age and Immaturity

Character immaturity is associated with younger age. This indicates maturation (i.e., remission of maladaptive and most extreme behaviors) with increasing age. In general, three dimensions of personality change substantially with age. Novelty Seeking decreases with age by ~18%, so that older individuals become less impulsive (more reflective), less rule breaking (more orderly), and less quick tempered (more stoical). Cooperativeness increases markedly in most children during school age and then increases by 12% on average after age 18. Self-Directedness increases markedly in most people during adolescence and young adulthood, increasing on average by 9% after age 18.

The decreasing prevalence of personality disorder with age is attributable to the increased development of both Self-Directedness and Cooperativeness with age. The additional tendency for Novelty Seeking to decrease with age explains the finding that, without intervention, patients with impulsive personality disorders (e.g., Antisocial, Histrionic) show more improvement with time than those with anxious or eccentric personality disorders.

Age, therefore, is taken into account in evaluating character development. For example, teenagers and young adults are often still developing in Self-Directedness and Cooperativeness. Here, their low character scores suggestive of a personality disorder may improve owing to continued character development through family, education, and personal effort. Older adults, with fully developed Self-directedness and Cooperativeness, may still not be fully satisfied. They may need to develop a firm basis for transpersonal meaning in their life, which is unaffected by their inevitable morbidity and mortality. Accordingly, they may need to develop higher Self-Transcendence for fuller self-knowledge and serenity. If so, a more appropriate measure of character development for individuals > 35 years of age can be based on the sum of all three character dimensions.

XII. PSYCHOBIOLOGICAL SUMMARY OF CHARACTER TRAITS

As one would intuitively expect, empirical data are more impressive for the "biological" temperament traits than for the "social" character traits. Yet, recent data are beginning to shed more light on the neuropsychological mechanisms underlying character traits as well [2]. Specifically, psychophysiological markers of neocortical processing, such as the P300 event-related potential and Contingent Negative Variation, are correlated with measures of character, but not temperament. For example, Self-Directedness, but not temperament traits, correlates moderately with the evoked potential P300 in parietal leads ($r = .4$, $P > .002$). Likewise, Cooperativeness, but not temperament, correlates with the Contingent Negative Variation (this was particularly obvious for the Empathy subscale, $r = .4$). These are the first empirical findings to associate character, but not temperament, to higher cortical functions in the CNS.

XIII. PSYCHOBIOLOGY OF TEMPERAMENT

Four major temperament traits are now understood as genetically independent dimensions, with distinct learning and neurophysiological features. These are discussed below.

A. Psychobiology of Harm Avoidance

1. Definition

Harm Avoidance involves a heritable bias in the inhibition of behavior in response to signals of punishment and frustrative nonreward.

2. Psychobiological Data for Harm Avoidance

Recent findings suggest that both GABA and serotonergic projections from the dorsal raphe underlie individual differences in behavioral inhibition as measured by the temperament trait of Harm Avoidance. Ascending serotonergic projections from the dorsal raphe nuclei to the substantia nigra inhibit nigrostriatal dopaminergic neurons and are essential for conditioned inhibition of activity by signals of punishment and frustrative nonreward. PET studies show that Harm Avoidance is associated with increased activity in the anterior paralimbic circuit, specifically the right amygdala and insula, the right orbitofrontal cortex, and the left medial prefrontal cortex. This activation pattern corresponds well to the 5HT2 terminal projections of the dorsal raphe. However, 5HT2 receptor numbers have been correlated with Harm Avoidance only in studies of platelets.

Benzodiazepines disinhibit passive avoidance conditioning by GABA-ergic inhibition of serotonergic neurons originating in the dorsal raphe nuclei. Higher plasma GABA levels have also been correlated with low Harm Avoidance. Plasma GABA has also been correlated with other measures of anxiety proneness, and correlates highly with brain GABA levels.

Recent neuropsychological studies confirm that Harm Avoidance is associated with individual differences in classical aversive conditioning and other aspects of behavior inhibition, whereas other dimensions of personality are uncorrelated.

A gene on chromosome 17q12 that regulates the expression of the serotonin transporter has been found to account for 4–9% of the total variance in Harm Avoidance in four of six tests of this relationship.

Psychobiology of Harm Avoidance is summarized in Table 12.

B. Psychobiology of Novelty Seeking

1. Definition

Novelty Seeking reflects a heritable bias in the initiation or activation of appetitive approach in response to novelty, approach to signals of reward, active avoidance of conditioned signals of punishment, and skilled escape from unconditioned punishment.

2. Psychobiological Data for Novelty Seeking

Mesolimbic and mesofrontal dopaminergic projections have been shown to have a crucial role in incentive activation of each aspect of Novelty Seeking in animals. In humans, individuals at risk for Parkinson's disease have low premorbid scores in Novelty Seeking, but not other dimensions of personality, supporting the importance of dopamine in incentive activation of pleasurable behavior.

Table 12 Reported Psychobiological Correlates of Harm Avoidance

Variable	Effect
Neuroanatomy (PET)	
Medial prefrontal (L)	increased activity (behavioral inhibition)
Anterior paralimbic (R)	increased activity (sensitivity to threat)
Neuropsychology	
Aversive conditioning	greater associative pairing with punishment ($r = .4$)
Eyeblink startle reflex	potentiation of response to aversive stimulus (effect size 1.9)
Posner validity effect	greater slowing of responses after invalid cues ($r = +.3$)
Spatial delayed response	better ability to delay responses after ingesting amphetamines ($r = +.5$)
Neurochemistry	
Platelet 5HT2 receptor	fewer receptors ($r = -.6$)
Plasma GABA	lower level ($r = -.5$)
Neurogenetics	
5HT transporter promoter	greater reuptake activity

The association of increased striatal activity with high Novelty Seeking is more specifically associated with higher density of the dopamine transporter, suggesting that Novelty Seeking involves increased reuptake of dopamine at presynaptic terminals, thereby requiring frequent stimulation to maintain optimal levels of postsynaptic dopaminergic stimulation. Novelty Seeking leads to various pleasure-seeking behaviors, including cigarette smoking, which may explain the frequent observation of low platelet MAO B activity because cigarette smoking has the effect of inhibiting MAO B activity in platelets and in brain.

Studies of candidate genes regulating dopamine transmission, such as the dopamine transporter (DAT1) and the type 4 dopamine receptor (DRD4), have provided evidence of association with Novelty Seeking and no other dimension of temperament. The dopamine transporter, which is responsible for presynaptic reuptake of dopamine and a major site of action of drugs including stimulants like methylphenidate and the antidepressant bupropion, is encoded by locus SLC6A3 (alias DAT1) on chromosome 5p. Polymorphisms at this gene locus are associated with Attention Deficit Disorder and other disorders related to variation in Novelty Seeking. Likewise polymorphisms at the DRD4 locus have been associated with Attention Deficit Disorder, opioid dependence, and other traits related to Novelty Seeking.

Psychobiology of Novelty Seeking is summarized in Table 13.

C. Psychobiology of Reward Dependence

1. Definition

Reward Dependence reflects a heritable bias in the maintenance of behavior in response to cues of social reward.

Table 13 Reported Psychobiological Correlates of Novelty Seeking

Variable	Effect
Neuroanatomy (PET)	
Medial Prefrontal(L)	decreased activity (behavioral disinhibition)
Dorsolateral Prefrontal	decreased activity (behavioral disinhibition)
Cingulate	increased activity (behavioral activation)
Caudate (L)	increased activity (behavioral activation)
Neuropsychology	
Reaction time	slower to respond if not reinforced (neutral stimuli, $r = -.4$)
Stimulus intensity (N1/P2 ERP)	augmentation of intensity of cortical responses to novel auditory stimuli ($r = .5$)
Sedation threshold	more easily sedated by diazepam (lower threshold, $r = -.3$)
Rey word list memory	deterioration of verbal memory when excited (after ingesting amphetamine, $r = .6$)
Neurochemistry	
Dopamine transporter	higher density observed in striatum
Platelet MAO B	lower activity (associated with cigarette smoking)
Neurogenetics	
Dopamine receptor D4	association with long alleles of exon III variant
Dopamine transporter	greater reuptake activity

2. Psychobiological Data for Reward Dependence

Reward Dependence is associated with individual differences in formation of conditioned responses to signals of reward. This is also supported by its association with individual differences in paired-associate learning. Noradrenergic projections from the locus ceruleus and serotonergic projections from the median raphe are thought to influence conditioning of responses to signals of reward. In humans, short-term reduction of norepinephrine release by acute infusion of the alpha-2 presynaptic agonist clonidine selectively impairs paired-associate learning, particularly the acquisition of novel associations.

The noradrenergic locus coeruleus is located at the same posterior level of the brain stem as the serotonergic median raphe, and both of these posterior monoamine cells innervate structures important to formation of paired associations, such as the thalamus, neocortex, and hippocampus. High Reward Dependence is associated with serotonergic increased activity in the thalamus, which is consistent with proposals about the importance of serotonergic projections to the thalamus from the median raphe in modulation of social communication.

Noradrenergic mechanisms are also supported by the finding of low levels of urinary MHPG (a norepinephrine metabolite) with high Reward Dependence.

High Reward Dependence is associated with hypercortisolemia in patients with melancholia, but not in nondepressed individuals.

Psychobiology of Reward Dependence is summarized in Table 14.

D. Psychobiology of Persistence

1. Definition

Persistence reflects a heritable bias in the maintenance of behavior despite frustration, fatigue, and intermittent reinforcement.

2. Psychobiological Data for Persistence

Less work is available about Persistence than the other three temperament dimensions, because it has been distinguished as an independently inherited dimension only since 1993. It can be objectively measured by the partial reinforcement extinction effect (PREE) in which persistent individuals are more resistant to the extinction of previously intermittently rewarded

Table 14 Reported Psychobiological Correlates of Reward Dependence

Variable	Effect
Neuroanatomy (PET)	
Thalamus	increased activity (facilitates sensory processing)
Neuropsychology	
Reward conditioning	increased associative pairing with rewards ($r = .3$)
Paired Associates	better learning of novel associations ($r = .5$)
Posner Validity Effect	faster resonses after valid cues ($r = -.4$)
Neurochemistry	
Urinary MHPG	less excretion of norepinephrine metabolite ($r = -.4$)
Plasma cortisol	higher morning cortisol when depressed ($r = .3$)
Urinary Harman	greater excretion of indoleamine product in alcoholics high in reward dependence ($r = .7$)
Neurogenetics	
5HT-2c receptor	allelic association (effect size 2.0)

behavior than other individuals who have been continuously reinforced. Recent work in rodents showed that the integrity of the PREE depends on projections from the hippocampal subiculum to the nucleus accumbens. This glutaminergic projection may be considered as a short circuit from the behavioral inhibition system to the behavioral activation system, thereby converting a conditioned signal of punishment into a conditioned signal of anticipated reward. This connection is probably disrupted in humans by lesions of the orbitomedial cortex that may have a specific antipersistence effect of therapeutic benefit to some severely obsessive-compulsive patients. Bilateral cingulotomy, which reduces Harm Avoidance only, is less effective in reducing persistent compulsive behavior than cingulotomy combined with orbitomedial lesions.

Psychobiology of Persistence is summarized in Table 15.

XIV. TEMPERAMENT AND CHARACTER ARE TREATED SIMULTANEOUSLY

Roughly speaking, "hard-wired" temperament traits are primarily treated by pharmacological intervention. Some psychotherapeutic correction is possible, especially with behavior therapy, because associative conditioning has a pivotal role in the development of temperament traits. In contrast, commonly used psychotropic drugs rarely induce significant changes in the internalized concepts about self and external objects. Character, in other words, is more amenable to psychotherapeutic intervention.

Temperament and character are optimally treated simultaneously with combined psychotherapy and pharmacotherapy, where drug treatment of the biological disposition is combined with psychotherapy of associated psychological mechanisms. In other words, medications are used to temporarily reduce anxiety, anger, impulsivity, or obsessionality related to temperament traits, setting the stage for long-term conceptual changes and character maturation in psychotherapy.

XV. PSYCHOTHERAPY GUIDELINES FOR LOW CHARACTER VARIANTS

In clinical practice, the TCI temperament and character scores are reviewed with the patient to identify their patterns of automatic behavior reactions (i.e., their temperament profile) and their cognitive concepts of themselves and others (their character profile). This is used to guide treatment planning for both pharmacotherapy and psychotherapy.

Psychotherapy guidelines presented here refer to patients with low Self-Directedness and low Cooperativeness, with mild to severe personality disorder (levels II and III in Table 10). Our approach is

Table 15 Reported psychobiological correlates of Persistence

Variable	Effect
Neuroanatomy	
Orbitomedial cortex	disconnection reduces perseveration
Neuropsychology	
Gambling style	perserveration in bet size despite continuing losses
Key word list learning	learning without reinforcement ($r = .5$)
Neurochemistry	
Glutaminergic connection Subiculum to N. accumbens	essential for PREE[a] in rodents
Neurogenetics	
5HT2c receptor	allelic association (effect size 2.0)

[a]Partial reinforcement extinction effect (PREE) is persistence or increased resistance to extinction following intermittent reinforcement.

integrative and eclectic, involving technical synthesis (eclecticism) and theoretical synthesis (integration) of various schools of psychotherapy and a variety of treatment techniques.

As an exception to the above eclecticism, we rarely recommend supportive psychotherapy for immature individuals with personality disorder, because it focuses at strengthening their existing coping mechanisms (which are by definition maladaptive in personality disorder) and thus only reinforces personal and social problems of these patients. Pure supportive-realistic therapy is recommended in most severe cases of personality pathology and psychoses, where safety and survival are of primary concern (these are described in level I in Table 10).

XVI. TREATMENT GOALS AND OUTCOME PLANNING

Patients are asked to identify their expectations and treatment goals in psychotherapy as autonomously as possible. Frequently, this is accomplished by reviewing with them the TCI temperament and character scores, which helps them identify targets for work. There has to be at least one area in which the therapist and patient are in agreement regarding treatment goals.

Not every patient with immature character can be helped to achieve his or her desired level of maturity. In addition to some general indicators of poor prognosis (e.g., low capacity for insights), one of the most important prognostic factors is the compatibility of the desired character outcome with the actual temperament type. As noted before, one initial temperament configuration may lead to several, but not all, of the eight possible character outcomes. Some character outcomes are *incompatible* with some initial temperaments and are therefore not achievable in therapy.

XVII. PREVENTION OF IMMATURITY: ENVIRONMENT IS CRITICAL

The effect of sociocultural factors on personality is less specific than that of genetic factors, influencing success in adaptation rather than its form or personality style. This is consistent with recent findings about the importance of family and local culture in character development. Family environment does not influence temperament, but explains about 35% of variability of character traits. Hence, psychosocial disorganization in the rearing environment of a child has a substantial influence on the risk of personality disorder. This is essential for preventive strategies as even temperament configurations with high risk of personality disorder might be overcome in the early stages in homes and communities that provide security and limits on behavior in a warm, compassionate manner, as well as encouraging self-directed choice and the value of respect for other people.

XVIII. IF EVERYTHING ELSE FAILS, EVERYDAY LIFE EVENTS CAN HELP

As noted, some patients are not likely to benefit from psychotherapy. For those patients, many aspects and events of everyday life, acting randomly, sometimes positive and inspiring (such as illuminating interpersonal contacts, work-related progress), but sometimes negative and destabilizing (such as tragic events, personal downfalls), may initiate character maturation by challenging the present level of adaptation. Often, the emergent changes are sudden and associated with a new perspective on life and new goals and values, which cannot be achieved by logic, medication, or advice alone.

XIX. IDEAL, OPTIMAL, AND COMPROMISE OUTCOMES

Treatment outcomes range from ideal to optimal to compromise. *Ideal* outcomes correspond to the ideally mature personality, with maximal development of all three character traits. These outcomes are not always possible, especially for patients with personality disorder who usually have initial temperament configurations incompatible with high scores on all character dimensions. However, whenever possible, ideal outcomes are pursued as the ultimate standard of maturity.

More frequently, treatment is planned to enable the patient to achieve the best possible adaptation for the present temperament traits and local social circumstances. This is called an *optimal* character outcome.

If, for any reason, the optimal outcome can not be achieved, we chose the *compromise* outcome, i.e., we work with the patient to raise the level of his or her adaptation compared to that at baseline, but do not attempt to reach the maximal adaptation possible for that patient.

XX. "BACK TO THE FUTURE" RECOVERY COURSE

In the fitness landscape of personality development, the hills represent developmental points of more or less successful local adaptation and are thus relatively stable. In contrast, the valleys represent brief transition periods and are thus relatively unstable. The "U-shaped" developmental pattern (see below) explains why extreme temperament types and their associated extreme behaviors, which are clearly not optimal (i.e., are maladaptive relative to the possible maximum for that individual), tend to be stable.

Personality disorder represents a point of developmental stability for many individuals. By definition, it involves maladaptation, i.e., less than optimal adaptation or poor adaptation, but still some adaptation, to the local environment. In other words, personality disorder represents a suboptimal developmental outcome, with established, although maladaptive, personal and social roles, support network, etc. Each new step in development must increase one's adaptation to be more successful in balancing multiple internal and external constraints. Search for higher adaptive hills, however, is discouraged by the necessity of initially regressing to an unstable, transitional developmental level (a valley). This is referred to as the U-shaped developmental pattern, and is commonly observed in complex dynamic systems.

In psychotherapy, patients are expected to give up their current (although maladaptive) personal and social stability in the local environment (i.e., their present hill). They first have to regress (to take a step down) to an unstable, transitional level of development, and then, based on more mature concepts about self and the external world (developed in psychotherapy), to "climb" to a higher adaptive hill with new personal and social roles and better overall adaptation. This "regressive progression" or "back to the future" course derives directly from the U-shaped developmental pattern mentioned earlier, and accounts for both the chronicity and the treatment resistance of individuals with personality disorder.

XXI. STEPWISE CHARACTER DEVELOPMENT: NEVER TOO LATE FOR HEALING

The subscale structure of the TCI was formulated to specify character in terms of 15 component steps of its development, each reflecting one component subscale of three major character traits. As shown in Table 9, stepwise character development follows a spiral pattern, where each revolution around the spiral and each new step of character development introduces a new triad of developmental tasks. For example, during the first revolution around the spiral, a person encounters problems of trust vs. mistrust (Cooperativeness/subscale 1), confidence vs. shame (Self-Directedness/subscale 1), and obedience vs. rebelliousness (Self-Transcendence/subscale 1). As character matures, individuals successively face new developmental tasks associated with other component subscales of Self-Directedness, Cooperativeness, and Self-Transcendence.

This spiral pattern of character development provides the opportunity to correct "developmental errors" that have occurred at any of the previous steps. For example, as character develops to reach a new step in Self-Directedness (e.g., Resourcefulness/subscale 3), one gets "in line" historically with issues of purposefulness and responsibility (subscales 1 and 2 of Self-Directedness), encountered earlier in development. This alignment facilitates retrospective revisions ("retrospective healing") of errors at these earlier developmental steps in psychotherapy. Such retrospective revisions are possible for previous steps within the same trait for all character traits.

XXII. PSYCHOTHERAPY OF CHARACTER: PRACTICAL PEARLS

1. The central message is "Do something with the patient, not something to the patient." This way, the patient feels somewhat in control and this might help keep him or her in treatment.

2. Immature patients usually want psychotherapy "their way," with many conditions and demands. Flexibility in approach, but firmness in basic values, with creativity and readiness to step away from the "rules" is essential to resolve these "no way out" situations.

3. Reflecting their unstable self-image (i.e., low Self-Directedness), patients with personality disorder alternatively feel inferior and omnipotent, assaultive and self-destructive, sensitive to rejection but usually provoking it. These and similar tendencies may cause countertransference problems with a potential loss of professional objectivity; constant supervision and a

support network are therefore necessary. (*Reassuring note for psychotherapists*: These patients are almost never as good as they look when they are doing well, and almost never as bad as they look when they are not doing well.)

4. Psychotherapy of patients with personality disorder takes place constantly (during any and every kind of contact with the patient), not only during the psychotherapy sessions proper. Frequently, what is happening between sessions may be as important for the favorable outcome as the sessions themselves.

5. At least initially, the therapy is supplemented by as much structuring of the patient's life as needed. This may range from simple direction, via day hospital programs, to inpatient hospitalization. Structuring is not expected to generate personality change but to temporarily improve behavior control. Prolonged structuring robs the patient of the opportunity to become more self-reliant and to learn from experience. With very immature patients, psychotherapy means "reparenting"—focusing on some very basic psychological and physical issues, such as general health, diet, social skills, education, help with real life problems, and encouragement.

6. Individuals with personality disorder tend to minimize their own symptoms and problems, even the most serious ones, such as suicide attempts or medical illnesses. These "blind spots" for their own problems reflect mechanisms they have developed since early age to avoid disturbing feelings and thoughts. Hence, they generally feel a much lower level of distress with their own symptoms than people around them. Confrontations (not explanations!) are used to increase their level of discomfort with their own symptoms, which improves their recognition of these symptoms and their motivation to change them. These patients tolerate confrontations very well, provided they trust their therapist. They need an extraordinarily high level of stimulation (sometimes achieved through confrontations) in any relationship, including therapy. This "hunger" for stimuli indicates an early exposure to either lack of stimulation (neglect) or extreme stimulation (abuse) by their caretakers.

7. The greater the character development at baseline, the better the response to psychotherapy is likely to be. High degrees of cognitive dysfunction, as indicated by low character development and/or extensive cognitive distortion in personal authenticity (see the section on the performance scales in the TCI), make improvement in psychotherapy difficult but not impossible.

XXIII. TREATMENT PLANNING

Baseline temperament configurations are carefully reviewed and taken into account for psychotherapy planning as well, not just in pharmacotherapy.

A. High Reward Dependence and High Harm Avoidance (Passive-Aggressive and Cautious Temperaments)

When both Reward Dependence and Harm Avoidance are high, there is a great risk of facilitating dependency in patients if directive techniques are used. Nondirective brief, time-limited therapies should be closely maintained in these cases. Reduction of anxiety, by relaxation or antidepressant therapy, is critical to set the stage for work on character development.

B. Low Harm Avoidance and High Reward Dependence (Passionate and Cyclothymic Type)

In these cases, although the therapist should be nondirective about the patient's basic treatment goals, directive techniques can be safely utilized. Patients who are also high in Cooperativeness are likely to do well with brief directive psychotherapy focused on solving specific interpersonal problems. Such cooperative patients are likely to have good social skills in general or to have the basis for developing them quickly.

C. High Reward Dependence and Low Self-Directedness (Dependent Personalities).

These patients are considered good candidates for dynamic therapy despite their personality dysfunction because of their good capacity for transference associated with high Reward Dependence. However, it is unclear whether the results with psychodynamic techniques are more effective here than other techniques.

High Persistence is usually an asset in achieving character development, provided it is not extreme, as in Obsessive-Compulsive personality, when it interferes with treatment.

Low Reward Dependence may limit development of Cooperativeness unless special attention is devoted to developing empathy and compassion.

Low Novelty Seeking may limit development of Self-Transcendence unless special attention is devoted to insight-based meditation techniques.

XXIV. PSYCHOTHERAPY OF CHARACTER: SPECIFIC TECHNIQUES FOR SPECIFIC TRAITS.

Cognitive-behavioral therapy, psychoanalysis, transactional analysis, and reality therapy focus primarily at developing Self-Directedness.

Some experiential techniques that facilitate acceptance of others or development of cooperative behavior include Rogerian counseling, logotherapy, and interpersonal psychosynthesis..

Attainment of Self-Transcendence is a goal of Jungian analysis, Assaglioli's psychosynthesis, insight meditation as practiced in Buddhism and mystical forms of other religions, and relaxation-based meditation techniques of advanced autogenic training.

XXV. ADVANCED STAGES OF PSYCHOTHERAPY

In the course of successful therapy, as character matures and new concepts and associated secondary or social emotions develop, patients neutralize extreme temperament traits and the related basic emotions of fear and anger. Behaviors change accordingly, from being primarily reactive, i.e., steered by basic emotions and automatic responses regulated by temperament, to being primarily proactive, i.e., steered by secondary emotions and active symbolic constructs regulated by character.

XXVI. PHARMACOTHERAPY GUIDELINES FOR EXTREME TEMPERAMENT VARIANTS

Pharmacological therapy of extreme behaviors can be either *symptomatic*, aimed at correcting target clinical symptoms, or *causal* aimed at correcting neurobiological dispositions underlying deviant traits.

XXVII. SYMPTOMATIC PHARMACOTHERAPY OF EXTREME TEMPERAMENT VARIANTS

Pharmacotherapy cannot be usefully organized around discrete subtypes of personality disorder. These subtypes are described as clinical syndromes (each involving clusters of symptoms, i.e., single acts of deviant behaviors). The efficiency of drug treatments is more accurately observed at a symptom level than at the syndrome level. Also, the target symptoms are not unique to any categorical subtype, but are shared by other subtypes of personality disorder as well. Next, some of the classified personality disorder subtypes are heterogeneous composites that can be further decomposed into one or more subcategories, each potentially requiring specific pharmacotherapy.

Another problem with symptomatic treatments is that they are based on the phenotypic similarity between some Axis I and Axis II syndromes (i.e., treatments established for Axis I symptoms are used to treat "similar" behaviors observed on Axis II). Yet, common pathogenesis for Axis I and Axis II disorders has not been established, leaving open to question the validity of these treatments "by analogy."

However, at the present level of psychiatric theory and practice, symptomatic treatments are considered standard for patients with personality disorder. Most pharmacological trials are focused on acute symptoms (e.g., suicidality, paranoia, depression), but an increasing number of authors advocate long-term pharmacotherapy of chronic pathology as well (e.g., impulsiveness, affective dysregulation) in addition to acute treatments. In that regard, most authors agree that the following four **symptom domains** underlie chronic pathology of personality disorder: (1) aggression and behavioral dyscontrol; (2) affective symptoms and mood dyscontrol; (3) anxiety; and (4) cognitive-perceptual distortions including psychotic symptoms.

Note that these four symptom domains represent behavioral (clinical) correlates of the *underlying* temperament and character dimensions: high Novelty Seeking corresponds to the symptom domain of impulsiveness and aggression, high Harm Avoidance to the symptom domain of anxiety and depression), low Reward Dependence to the symptom domain of affective dysregulation and detachment, and low character traits to the symptom domain of cognitive disturbances. In other words, the identification of these four target symptom domains has narrowed the gap between categorical and dimensional approach to personality disorder and between causal and symptomatic pharmacotherapy of these patients. In the remainder of this chapter, we discuss the causal therapy of personality disorder. Symptomatic pharmacotherapy is described elsewhere in detail [2].

XXVIII. CAUSAL PHARMACOTHERAPY OF EXTREME TEMPERAMENT VARIANTS

Causal pharmacotherapy of extreme temperament traits derives from fundamental neurobiological processes underlying personality and mental disorder. Responses to antidepressants in major depression, e.g., can be predicted by temperament traits to a substantial degree, and not by the number, type, severity, or course of depressive symptoms. Patients who are dysphoric and highly sensitive to social approval (i.e., who are high in Harm Avoidance and Reward Dependence) are most likely to improve on selective serotonin uptake inhibitors (SSRIs). In contrast, those who are highly fearful but not socially dependent are most likely to improve on noradrenergic uptake inhibitors, like desipramine. Likewise, children with Attention Deficit Hyperactivity Disorder are high in Novelty Seeking (i.e., low in central dopaminergic function) and are efficiently treated with drugs that increase dopamine release and inhibit its reuptake, such as methylphenidate. (*Note*: Treatment strategies suggested below are still tentative and need further systematic study.)

XXIX. PHARMACOLOGICAL GUIDELINES FOR CLINICAL SYNDROMES WITH EXTREME UNDERLYING TEMPERAMENT DIMENSIONS

A number of clinical and personality syndromes involve extreme deviation of a single temperament trait. For example, most cases of major depression are characterized by elevated Harm Avoidance (i.e., symptoms of anxiety, pessimism, fatigability), without comorbid deviation of other temperament or character traits. Here, pharmacological manipulation of high Harm Avoidance with SSRIs is indicated (high 5HT2 activity in the prefrontal cortex is postulated to underlie Harm Avoidance, and SSRIs eventually downregulate 5HT2 receptors, leading to symptomatic improvement).

When more than one extreme temperament trait underlies clinical symptoms, treatment planning is more complex. Harm Avoidance is usually the strongest motivator of behaviors and the first temperament trait to develop in the phylogeny of learning in animals, from invertebrates to man, followed by Novelty Seeking, and Reward Dependence. Hence, a person with the so-called approach-avoidance conflict (where both Harm Avoidance and Novelty Seeking are high) will usually tend to inhibit behavior to avoid danger (Harm Avoidance) rather than to activate behavior in pursue of novelty (Novelty Seeking) in response to novel situations. Such motivational hierarchy is used to prioritize pharmacotherapy in clinical syndromes with more than one underlying extreme temperament trait: behaviors associated with high Harm Avoidance (e.g., depression, anxiety) are usually clinically more urgent than disorderliness or impulsivity associated with Novelty Seeking or dependency associated with Reward Dependence, etc. One exception to this is hazardous behaviors associated with high Novelty Seeking which are for safety reasons always treated first.

Most psychotropics are not very specific, adding to the complexity of pharmacological intervention in personality disorder. The selected drug usually affects not only the targeted underlying dimension, but also other dimensions and symptom domains (e.g., SSRIs improve both the symptom domain of anxiety and the symptom domain of aggression). This nonspecificity may reflect the multifinality phenomenon (where different behaviors derive from the same underlying antecedent), or multiple action sites of a single drug affecting several neurophysiological systems at the same time. When carefully manipulated, this nonspecificity may be advantageous in treatment of clinical cases with multiple underlying extreme temperament dimensions (see below).

Psychobiological planning of pharmacotherapy also involves other factors (e.g., social, cultural, family) to customize treatment for individual patients. Even the patient's character structure is taken into account for pharmacological intervention. For example, if Self-Directedness is low (with consequent intolerance, blaming, and revengefulness), mood stabilizers are used to prevent acting out, self-injury, and assaultive behaviors.

XXX. PHARMACOLOGICAL TREATMENT OF PERSONALITY SYNDROMES DOMINATED BY EXTREME HARM AVOIDANCE

The following temperament types and their corresponding traditional personality syndromes are characterized by high Harm Avoidance:

Methodical temperament type (corresponding to the traditional category of Obsessive personality)
Explosive temperament type (corresponding to the traditional category of Borderline personality)
Sensitive temperament type (corresponding to the traditional category of Passive-Aggressive personality)
Cautious temperament type (corresponding to the traditional category of Avoidant personality).

A. Methodical Temperament Type/ Obsessive Personality

High Harm Avoidance, high Persistence, low Novelty Seeking, and low Reward Dependence underlie the *methodical* or *obsessive* temperament type. The majority of methodical individuals, even severe variants, are well adjusted in the society (e.g., as accountants or administrators). Those who also have poor character development are almost invariably maladapted and diagnosed as *obsessive-compulsive* personality disorder (described as inflexible; devoted to work to the exclusion of pleasure; preoccupied with details, rules, and regulations; unable to relax; no sense of humor; etc).

Harm Avoidance is associated with high central 5HT2 activity. Accordingly, OCD patients show increased central serotonergic activity, most prominently in the serotonin pathway from midbrain raphe nuclei to the basal ganglia. Pharmacological treatment of these patients involves "serotonergic" drugs, usually SSRIs (e.g., fluoxetine, fluvoxamine, citalopram, paroxetine, sertraline). The SSRIs increase the amount of active serotonin in all major serotonergic pathways by inhibiting its reuptake into the presynaptic terminal. The increased serotonin affects presynaptic somatodendritic 5HT1A receptors, leading to the disinhibition of serotonergic neurons, increased release of serotonin in the synapse, and downregulation of postsynaptic 5HT2 receptors. Clinically, this is expected to reduce anxiety, depression, and obsessive symptoms.

Drugs that block 5HT2 receptors and also inhibit serotonin and norepinephrine reuptake, such as nefazodone, are useful for obsessive temperaments as well. Similarly, some of the "old-timers," such as chlomipramine, efficiently improve clinical syndromes with high Harm Avoidance, but also syndromes with high Reward Dependence, presumably by affecting both central serotonergic and noradrenergic transmitter systems.

Augmentation strategies, with pindolol (a 5HT1A antagonist) or buspirone (a 5HT1A agonist leading to 5HT1A down regulation and ultimately 5HT2 downregulation) are frequently indicated either to speedup the onset of action of SSRIs or to reestablish the efficacy of SSRIs for patients who have reached a plateau after initially responding.

Benzodiazepines are efficiently used for composite temperament types with dominant Harm Avoidance, including Obsessive personality. These drugs increase GABA-ergic inhibition of serotonergic neurons originating in the dorsal raphe nuclei and facilitate symptomatic improvement. Similarly, gabapentin, a GABA analog, might be helpful for obsessive patients as well.

Severe obsessive temperaments, with low character and extremely high Harm Avoidance, are sometimes treated with antipsychotics, preferably those with significant 5HT2 antagonism (such as risperidone, olanzapine, quetiapine, clozaril, ziprasidone). High activity of these receptors has been demonstrated in OCD symptoms, panic, depression, anxiety, and sexual dysfunction, but also in psychosis and hallucinations.

As a general note for all personality and mood syndromes with high Harm Avoidance, high Harm Avoidance at baseline predicts poorer responses to antidepressants, and vice versa.

Psychotherapy tips: Obsessive temperaments are alexithymic (unable to recognize own emotions), with low capacity for attachment (reflecting their low Reward Dependence), and with a characteristic tendency to dissociate from own symptoms and engage in endless rational analyses of their behavior, a form of flabbergasting to avoid disturbing emotions (this is sometimes called "pseudo-intellectualization"). These features make them more likely to benefit from cognitive behavior techniques (which are more directive, focused on identifiable symptoms, and on the here-and-now). In contrast, mild and moderate obsessive temperaments (high Harm Avoidance, but only mild decrease in Reward Dependence), are candidates for dynamic psychotherapy because of their capacity for attachment and transference, which makes therapy less "academic", more personalized and thus more likely to yield results.

B. Explosive Temperament Type/ Borderline Personality

High Harm Avoidance, high Novelty Seeking, and low Reward Dependence underlie the Explosive (borderline) temperament type. This type has the highest risk of immature character outcome, leading to symptoms diagnosed as Borderline personality disorder. Mild variants are dysphoric, opportunistic, and alienated, whereas moderate and severe variants manifest chronic depression, chronic feelings of emptiness and boredom, low frustration tolerance, distrust of others, impulsivity, unstable relationships, labile mood, frequent acting outs, suicidal gestures, etc.).

Pharmacological treatment of borderline personality is complex. This syndrome is characterized by more than one extreme temperament trait: Harm Avoidance motivates cautious behaviors and passive avoidance of danger; Novelty Seeking motivates active exploratory behaviors, impulsivity, and disorderliness; whereas low Reward Dependence underlies their detachment and insensitivity to social pressures. These conflicting motivations invariably generate a stalemate between activation and inhibition of behavior (the earlier mentioned approach-avoidance conflict).

Recent advances in the psychobiological understanding of the approach-avoidance conflict (high Harm Avoidance coupled with high Novelty Seeking) point to the importance of anterior serotonergic cells in the dorsal raphe nucleus which intermingle with the dopaminergic cells of the ventral tegmental area. Both cell groups innervate the same structures (e.g., basal ganglia, accumbens, amygdala), providing opposing dopaminergic-serotonergic influences in the modulation of approach and avoidance behavior.

High Harm Avoidance generates chronic anxiety, depression, fatigability, dissatisfaction. High Novelty Seeking makes these patients unpredictable, with frequent acting outs, impulsivity, and self-injurious behaviors, drug/ETOH abuse (many of them need detoxification). Finally, because of their usually very low character traits, these individuals are chronically struggling with basic issues of trust, self-esteem, identity, purpose and meaning of life, etc.

Treatments of choice for the explosive temperament type are SSRIs, which are used here to treat not only the underlying high Harm Avoidance, but other symptoms as well. Namely, the SSRIs have been shown to be effective in several symptom domains: depression, anxiety, impulsivity, anger, hostility, mood reactivity, psychoticism, hyperphagia, rejection sensitivity. These symptoms correspond well to the distribution of 5HT2 receptors in the prefrontal cortex (depression) and hypothalamus (impulsivity and bulimia). Treatment with SSRIs downregulates these receptors and decreases Harm Avoidance symptoms. Another explanation for this multifinality of action is that SSRIs activate feedback loops involving multiple neurotransmitter systems and leading to symptomatic improvement in several symptom domains (e.g., the earlier mentioned dopaminergic-serotonergic loop in the modulation of approach and avoidance behaviors). Finally, some of these drugs, originally thought to specifically affect the serotonin system only, affect other transmitter systems as well, accounting for the multifinality of their effects (e.g., paroxetine has been recently postulated to inhibit both serotonin and norepinephrine reuptake). Augmentation strategies, with pindolol or buspirone, are indicated here for patients who plateau after initial good response.

SSRI's' are frequently combined with mood stabilizing GABA analogs (e.g., gabapentin) to treat mood swings and affective reactivity so typical of borderlines. GABA analogs are likely to be efficient because higher plasma GABA levels correlate with low Harm Avoidance. Other mood stabilizers (lithium, valproate, and lamotrigine) have been used nonspecifically here to reduce impulsivity, depression, and self-injury.

Most of the explosive symptoms are caused by the approach-avoidance conflict between high Harm Avoidance and high Novelty Seeking. Hence, SSRIs are frequently combined with dopamine agonists (to reduce symptoms associated with high Novelty Seeking), such as psychostimulants, which increase dopamine release and inhibit its reuptake (e.g., methylphenidate) or with antidepressants with dopaminergic agonism (bupropion). Similarly, pramipexole (a selective D3 agonist) has been postulated to be efficient in treatment of "unstable" and chronic depression.

Depressed patients with volatile or borderline temperaments have average improvement (54%) on antidepressants. Women particularly may respond better to noradrenergic drugs to the extent that they are much higher in Harm Avoidance than in Reward Dependence.

Severely explosive temperaments, especially those with very high Harm Avoidance, are sometimes treated with antipsychotics, preferably 5HT2 receptor antagonists to reduce symptoms associated with 5HT2 hyperactivity (anxiety, depression, sexual dysfunction, bulimia, OCD symptoms, psychotic decompensation).

Psychotherapy tips for explosive individuals: Supportive-realistic therapy ("reparenting") is recommended for severe cases, cognitive-behavior techniques for moderate and mild cases. Psychotherapy focuses on the development of more realistic concepts of the self and the world (while aggression and anxiety are temporarily controlled by medication). These internalized concepts are expected to provide long-term neutralization of aggression and depression.

C. Avoidant Personality/Cautious Temperament Type

High Harm Avoidance, high Reward Dependence, and low Novelty Seeking underlie the Cautious temperament type. Mild variants are high-strung, shy, careful, and cautious. When character development is also low, this type is diagnosed as Avoidant personality disorder (i.e., preoccupation of being criticized or rejected in social situations, feelings of inadequacy, social inhibition, hyperscrupulousness, passive-dependency). However, owing to their high sensitivity to social pressures (associated with high Reward Dependence), Cautious individuals are relatively rarely diagnosed as immature or maladapted (hence, their anxiety and shyness are more accurately diagnosed as Social Phobia).

These patients are primarily treated with SSRIs, because of the dominant Harm Avoidance in the background of their presentation. They respond well to antidepressants in a relatively high proportion of cases (71%). One study has shown superiority of predominantly noradrenergic antidepressants (desipramine) over predominantly serotonergic antidepressants (chlomipramine) in Harm Avoidance and Reward Dependent females with the Cautious temperament type). The exact mechanism of this effect is not clear. One explanation is that desipramine activates alpha-1 noradrenergic mechanisms, resulting in the excitation of serotonergic neurons and down regulation of 5HT2 receptors, with improved Harm Avoidance behaviors. Another possibility is that desipramine activates alpha-2 presynaptic inhibitory receptors, decreasing *temporarily* postsynaptic serotonergic activity, this leading to initial improvement of symptoms (the study lasted only 6 weeks, leaving open the possibility that a more continual noradrenergic inhibition of serotonin release could have caused upregulation of 5HT2 receptors and worsening of the symptoms after initial response). Finally, via its noradrenergic activity, desipramine might have harmonized the Reward Dependence of these women, reducing their problems associated with dependency and leading to symptomatic improvement in their mood and anxiety. Clearly, serotonergic and noradrenergic mechanisms underlying Harm Avoidance and Reward Depend- ence need further systematic study. The above discussion also illustrates that our treatment proposals ought to be interpreted as a theoretical framework only, not as finalized algorithms to treat personality and its disorders.

Psychotherapy tips: Depending on the degree of their character development, cautious individuals are treated with supportive-realistic approach (for those with personality disorder) or dynamic and insight-oriented approach (for mild and moderate variants).

D. Passive-Aggressive Personality/Sensitive Temperament Type

High Harm Avoidance, high Novelty Seeking, and high Reward Dependence constitute the Sensitive temperament type. Mild variants are easily upset (frustrated or distressed), attention-seeking, submissive, and anxious. When character development is also low, this temperament type is diagnosed as Passive-Aggressive personality disorder (with symptoms of procrastination, obstruction, negativism, and other forms of camouflaged aggression and dysphoria).

Passive-aggressive personality is unique because all three temperament traits are elevated, leading to potentially numerous motivational conflicts. Usually, passive-aggressive symptoms reflect underlying conflicts between high Harm Avoidance (fear of punishment) and high Reward Dependence (need for approval and support). High Novelty Seeking contributes to the presentation with symptoms of disorderliness and irritability. Venlafaxine (with serotonergic, noradrenergic, and dopaminergic effects sequentially activated with increased dosing) is usually efficient for individuals with Sensitive temperaments. Venlafaxine is mostly affecting Harm Avoidant behaviors with its serotonergic activity, but is also expected to harmonize Novelty Seeking and

Reward Dependence with its dopaminergic and noradrenergic activity, respectively. Similarly, a trial of bupropion (a noradrenergic-dopaminergic agonist) might be useful in these cases. These "dirty" drugs affect multiple neurotransmitter systems. In temperament profiles, such as the Sensitive type, where more than one temperament trait is generating clinical symptoms, such drug nonspecificity might be advantageous.

Depressed patients with Sensitive type respond well to antidepressants in a relatively high proportion of cases (73%). As noted, Harm Avoidance superordinates hierarchically the other temperament traits and usually dominates the clinical picture, even in cases when other temperament traits are also high (such as Passive-Aggressive personality). Hence, passive-aggressive patients respond to SSRIs by improving fearfulness, dysphoria, anxiety, etc. SSRIs are also useful here to harmonize their anger associated with high Novelty Seeking (see earlier). This "toning down" of Harm Avoidance and Novelty Seeking usually sets the stage for more sociable behaviors, empathy and compassion, associated with high Reward Dependence.

The demonstrated superiority of noradrenergic TCAs (desipramine) over serotonergic TCAs (chlomipramine) in Harm Avoidant females with high Reward Dependence is the basis for trying noradrenergic noradrenergic TCAs (desipramine, nortriptyline), especially in nonresponders to SSRIs. It is noteworthy that some authors found no evidence for differential response to noradrenergic or serotonergic drugs.

Augmentation with lithium carbonate, dopaminergic agonists, or switching to monoamine oxidase inhibitors may be helpful if high Novelty Seeking is considered problematic. These adjunctive medications are indicated to decrease impulsiveness and increase rational planning.

XXXI. PHARMACOLOGICAL TREATMENT OF PERSONALITY SYNDROMES AND TEMPERAMENT TYPES DOMINATED BY HIGH NOVELTY SEEKING

Adventurous temperament type (corresponding to the traditional category of Antisocial Personality)
Passionate temperament type (corresponding to the traditional category of Histrionic Personality)

A. ADVENTUROUS TEMPERAMENT TYPE / ANTISOCIAL PERSONALITY

Low Harm Avoidance, high Novelty Seeking, and low Reward Dependence constitute the Adventurous temperament type. Mild variants tend to be impulsive, careless, disorderly, extravagant, daring, adventurous, unconventional, oppositional, etc. When character traits are also low, severe variants are diagnosed as Antisocial Personality Disorder, where the above symptoms are complicated by active antisocial acts and crime.

Antisocial disorder is an exception to the rule that high Self-Directedness always protects against personality disorder. In fact, many antisocial individuals can be quite resourceful, self-disciplined, and successful in their antisocial activities (i.e., they are self-directed), but their low Cooperativeness (i.e., intolerance, revengefulness, low empathy), together with their social deviation and frequent criminality, makes them maladapted.

The dominant behavior motivator in adventurous temperaments is high Novelty Seeking with symptoms of impulsivity, disorderliness, extravagance, various pleasure-seeking behaviors, alcoholism, food addiction, and use of stimulating drugs. As noted, Novelty Seeking is associated with higher density of the dopamine transporter, suggestive of increased reuptake of dopamine at presynaptic terminals, thereby requiring frequent stimulation to maintain optimal levels of postsynaptic dopaminergic stimulation. Indeed, double-blind trials have shown that psychostimulants, such as methylphenidate, which increase central dopaminergic function, are beneficial in the treatment of inattentive and hyperactive adults who are impulsive and aggressive, especially when the symptoms have begun in childhood.

SSRIs improve impulsivity and "affective aggression" ("hot temper") in antisocial individuals, presumably because increased serotonergic function downregulates 5HT receptors, with subsequent increase in dopamine release in the mesocortical and mesolimbic dopaminergic neurons (behaviorally, this is observed as reduction in symptoms associated with high Novelty Seeking).

Multiple double-blind trials have shown that lithium reduces affective display and aggression in both normal subjects and impulsive-aggressive individuals. Lithium blocks the firing rate of rapidly firing neurons by reducing their ability to restore normal levels of phosphatidylinositol biphosphate (PIP2) after its hydrolization. As noted, dopaminergic mesolimbic neurons in high Novelty Seeking individuals require frequent stimulation ("stimulus hunger") to maintain normal dopaminergic postsynaptic function. Lithium appears to be able to dampen the ability of these neurons to fire rapidly, thus reducing impulsivity and other Novelty Seeking symptoms. Lithium should not be given to antisocial persons without aggression and impulsivity; it does not diminish nonaggressive antisocial behaviors (such as lying or stealing).

Benzodiazepines and alcohol have a disinhibitory effect on avoidance behavior, facilitate violence, and further impair passive avoidance learning in impulsive antisocial persons. This effect is attributed to the reduction of Harm Avoidance (already low in these cases), leaving Novelty Seeking completely unopposed to motivate behavior.

Psychotherapy tips for adventurous individuals: Group therapy is generally considered useful for these patients. This setting is therapeutic for the social deviance, low cooperativeness, lack of empathy, and disregard of others.

B. Passionate Temperament Type/ Histrionic Personality

High Novelty Seeking, high Reward Dependence, and low Harm Avoidance constitute the Passionate temperament type. Mild variants tend to be versatile, attention seeking, pleasure seeking, and impulsive, but trusting and sensitive to cues of social reward. When character development is also low, the Passionate type is diagnosed as Histrionic personality disorder (i.e., these individuals tend to be impulsive, ambitious, self-indulgent, sexually seductive, manipulative, insecurely vain, gullible, and self-centered, with rapidly shifting shallow emotions and frequent episodes of "reactive" dysphoria).

The Passionate temperament type is unique in that their dominant motivation, i.e., hunger for stimulation associated with high Novelty Seeking (manifested as sensation seeking, attention seeking, and pleasure seeking), is *not* conflicting, but is synergistic with their other important motivator, high Reward Dependence (i.e., need for approval, attention, support).

Histrionic individuals are optimally treated with medications targeting not only their high Novelty Seeking, but also their high Reward Dependence, such as bupropion, which inhibits reuptake of both norepinephrine and dopamine. Increased synaptic dopamine optimizes dopaminergic activity in the ventral tegmentum—mesolimbic "pleasure pathway"—and reduces pleasure-seeking behaviors. In addition, through its noradrenergic effect on Reward Dependence, bupropion reduces these patient's need for external gratification.

As with adventurous individuals, SSRIs and psychostimulants are frequently used. SSRIs improve impulsivity and hot temper, presumably by manipulating the underlying high Novelty Seeking (increased 5HT2A function initially inhibits mesocortical and mesolimbic dopaminergic neurons). Psychostimulants, such as methylphenidate, also increase central dopaminergic function and could be beneficial in the treatment of passionate individuals. Mood stabilizers (especially topiramate and gabapentin) are used here nonspecifically, to reduce extreme reactivity of mood and rapid mood swings of Passionate individuals.

Adventurous (antisocial) and passionate (histrionic) symptoms tend to run in the same family and to co-occur in the same person. These two phenotypes share the underlying high Novelty Seeking and low Harm Avoidance. Reward Dependence, however, is low in adventurous and high in passionate individuals. As noted earlier, Reward Dependence facilitates conditioning of behaviors under social pressure. This explains the decrease in the severity of antisocial symptoms from Antisocial Personality (with low Reward Dependence and "major" violent and property criminality) to Histrionic Personality, with high Reward Dependence and "minor" criminality (promiscuity, manipulation). The same factor, high Reward Dependence in passionate individuals, explains their better response to psychotherapy and their greater likelihood to achieve character maturation in psychotherapy than antisocial individuals.

XXXII. PHARMACOLOGICAL TREATMENT OF PERSONALITY SYNDROMES AND TEMPERAMENT TYPES DOMINATED BY HIGH REWARD DEPENDENCE

A. Reliable Temperament Type/ Cyclothymic-Dependent Personality

High Reward Dependence, low Harm Avoidance, and low Novelty Seeking constitute the Reliable temperament type. Mild variants tend to be composed (rarely frustrated or distressed), careful, and trusting, whereas severe variants are described as very susceptible to social pressure, sensitive to rejection, sentimental, attached, trusting. When character development is also low, this temperament type is diagnosed as Dependent (cyclothymic) personality disorder. These patients are hyperthymic ("moody"), scrupulous, gullible, and prone to reactive depression, and to lack initiative and depend on others for reassurance and own decisions.

Noradrenergic projections from the locus ceruleus and serotonergic projections from the median raphe are thought to influence reward conditioning. High Reward Dependence is associated with low levels of urinary MHPG (a norepinephrine metabolite). In addition, high Reward Dependence is associated with increased serotonergic activity in the thalamus, which is consistent with proposals about the importance of serotonergic projections to the thalamus from the median raphe in modulation of social communication.

Most people with even marked variation of the reliable temperament type are well adjusted and well functioning. In fact, this temperament type is associated with the lowest risk of immaturity and maladaptation. Reliable individuals are very responsive to social pressure and are easily conditioned to acquire socially acceptable behaviors. Usually, they seek help when depressed (which is their typical response to frustration and nonreward). In contrast to endogenomorphic depression, their depression is exogenomorphic (also called "characterological"); i.e., biological markers are usually not found (such as decreased REM latency, increased REM frequency, positive Dexamethasone Suppression Test). Their response to antidepressants is poor (<40%), but they respond (improve) to positive events (the so-called good-news depression).

Patients with this temperament type are most likely to respond to SSRIs, and sometimes to MAOIs and TCAs. Bupropion is sometimes effective in reducing their symptoms, presumably by optimizing dopaminergic activity in the mesolimbic "pleasure" pathway and through its noradrenergic inhibitory effect on Reward Dependence (which reduces their dependency on external gratification). Mood stabilizers with some antidepressant properties (e.g., lamotrigine) are sometimes helpful.

Psychotherapy tips: Individuals with reliable temperaments respond exceptionally well to psychotherapy, and equally well to psychodynamic and cognitive behavior approaches.

XXXIII. PHARMACOLOGICAL TREATMENT OF PERSONALITY SYNDROMES AND TEMPERAMENT TYPES WITH LOW REWARD DEPENDENCE:

A. Independent Temperament Type/ Schizoid Personality

Low Harm Avoidance, low Novelty Seeking, and low Reward Dependence constitute the Autonomous temperament type. Mild variants tend to be composed (rarely frustrated or distressed), private, and oppositional. Moderate and severe variants, with very low scores on all temperament traits, are described as isolative, detached, noninvolved, solitary, indifferent to praise or criticism, and emotionally cold and aloof. When character traits are also low, this temperament type maladapted and diagnosed as Schizoid Personality Disorder (characterized by social detachment, restricted range of expressed emotions in interpersonal settings, indifference to praise and criticism, no close friends or confidants other than family members, and preference for solitary activities and fantasy ("loners").

The "negative symptoms" of schizoid individuals (emotional detachment, indifference, aloof emotions) respond well to antidepressants and atypical neuroleptics. In fact, these patients have excellent responses to antidepressant drugs of *any type* in a higher proportion of cases (88%) than any other temperament type. In addition, the so-called atypical neuroleptics, with serotonin-dopamine antagonism (the "SDAs"), like risperidone, olanzapine, or quetiapine, are used in refractory cases. In schizophrenia, the above negative symptoms are believed to reflect dopamine deficiency in the mesocortical pathway. Serotonin-dopamine antagonists increase dopamine in this pathway and reduce the negative symptoms.

Psychotherapy tips: These patients are mostly treated with behavior modification techniques, because of their low capacity for attachment and poor motivation.

XXXIV. PSYCHOBIOLOGICAL INTEGRATION OF TREATMENT

The seven-factor psychobiological model distinguishes components of personality that differ in terms of their etiology, pattern of development, and responses to psychotherapy and pharmacotherapy. This provides a foundation for integrating clinical diagnosis and treatment planning in a manner that is both general (as a theoretical framework) and specific (sensitive to differences among individual patients). Based on the structural, clinical, and neurochemical characteristics of temperament and character, pharmacotherapy and psychotherapy can be systematically matched to the observed temperament structure and actual stage of character development of each individual. This is clearly a unique advantage over other available approaches. The choice of techniques likely to benefit the patient depends on the stage of personality integration. A brief outline of this integrative psychobiological approach is given in Table 16.

Treatment is organized into seven levels corresponding to the seven underlying problem levels described in Table 10. With respect to personality disorder of particular interest are levels 2 and 3 and, somewhat less frequently, levels 1 and 4.

A. First Treatment Level: Walking Together

The first treatment level involves supportive and reality-based techniques, including basic trust building, encouragement, and teaching of basic living skills. The goal here is to assure the safety of patients with severe disorganization and destructive impulses. Trust-building and encouragement within safe limits are basic components of all therapy, and are essential at this level because patients are overwhelmed with negative emotions, such as most patients with explosive (borderline) temperaments and severely immature character (melancholic or schizotypal). However, if the patient is psychotic or prepsychotic, therapy is limited to supportive function. Such supportive intervention may require concomitant somatic therapies like electroconvulsive therapy or antipsychotic medication. The "holding" or reparenting aspects of the psychotherapeutic environment are crucial at this level, including the therapist's being dependable, nonretaliatory, and compassionate despite frequent crises, and able to provide a more optimistic understanding of the patient's needs and opportunities than the patient. This allows the patient to build trust, some optimism, and self-confidence.

B. Second Treatment Level: Working Together

The second treatment level involves direction and cognitive-behavioral techniques that emphasize rational cognitive analysis and repetitive behavioral drills to improve impulse control and discipline. This level involves initial treatment of individuals with moderately severe personality and mood disorders with poor impulse control and emotional lability, such as most antisocial, severe obsessional, or mild borderline patients. Pharmacotherapy for labile affect and impulsivity, such as mood stabilizers, and for hostility, including low-dose neuroleptic, may be beneficial. Discussion of personality structure and emotional needs in such patients is focused on their understanding of their temperament structure and basic emotional needs, along with education about mature ways of satisfying those needs. For example, hatha yoga and martial-arts training are appealing methods for teaching self-control at this level, leading to enhancement of self-esteem and impulse control. Such structured approaches minimize conflict about setting limits, but there must be much patient repetition of practical problem-solving skills and encouragement by discussion of attractive role models. This makes constructive use of such patient's craving for pleasure and power.

C. Third Treatment Level: Feeling Together

The third treatment level involves nondirective dynamic, humanistic, and interpersonal techniques to foster increases in conscientiousness, resourcefulness, and generosity. At this stage direction is counterproductive because the patient needs to internalize group values and to develop confidence in his or her self-willed action. Depression and anxiety are common at this level and may be treated with antidepressants as needed in combination with the non-directive therapy. The standard six exercises of autogenic training are useful at this level, providing relaxation and preparation for meditative exercises at more advanced levels.

D. Fourth Treatment Level: Spiritual Together

The fourth treatment level involves experiential and existential therapy techniques such as meditation and spiritual identification exercises. This involves a conscious expansion of the self-concept to include a transpersonal (i.e., spiritual) component in addition to the mind and body. Antidepressant or antianxiety medication may be useful at times of existential crisis, but are used sparingly and transiently because strong motiva-

Table 16 Integrative Psychobiological Treatment of Personality and Psychopathology

Level	Developmental steps	Methods of treatment
I. Supportive-realistic therapy		
	1. Trust	Acceptance, trust-building Establish supportive environment Antipsychotic medication if needed Detoxification if needed
	2. Stop denial & vain self-sufficiency	Maintain safety and support Teach basic living skills and social interdependence
II. Directive rational-expressive-behavioral therapy		
	3. Obedience, stop defiance	Instruction about temperament Set limits and respect for boundaries

	4. Purposefulness	Explore goals and role models
		  & make a searching personal inventory
		Model problem-solving skills
		  for analysis and imitation

	5. Empathy	Encourage sharing of personal feelings
		Empathy training & teamwork
		+ objectively monitor treatment compliance
		+ pharmacotherapy of impulsivity,
		   violence, craving
		   (e.g. lithium, Tegretol, valproate)
		+ treatment of comorbid depression
		+ conditioning of impulse control
		   by repetitive drills & homework

III. Nondirective dynamic-humanistic-interpersonal therapy		
	6. Conscientiousness	Discursive reflection on goals & values as motivation to adapt Identification with role models

	7. Resourcefulness	Non-directive discussion of options
		  for coping with problems,
		  then self-willed action
		Persistence/resourcefulness training

	8. Generosity	Making amends, helping others Sharing, accepting help from others + monitor treatment compliance by self-report + education about character steps + cognitive analysis of basic emotions, defenses, and virtues + antidepressant medication if needed
IV. Experiential-existential therapy		
	9. Spirituality	Charitable action Mindful meditation with undistracted body scanning & automatic breathing Disidentification with mind-body Identification as mind-body-spirit Spiritual empowerment/communion

Level	Developmental steps	Methods of treatment
	10. Humility, patience	Self-knowledge, disclosure, acceptance—letting go of unimportant expectations
	11. Compassion	Recognize social interdependence Identification in spirit with others Consider work with support groups + cognitive analysis of mature character development
V. Transcendence therapy	12. Detachment, freedom (unconditional joy and trust)	Whole-hearted compassionate activity Contemplation with automatic devout vocalization All-inclusive identification
	13. Integrity, power, peace, courage	Spirit-guided contemplation (Ego-less channeling) Integration of personal goals and values, eliminating distractors Empowerment of Mind (integrating of mind and spirit) Mind-body healing practices + cognitive analysis of conditions for joy & peace
VI. Advanced spiritual guidance	14. Unity of wisdom & love	Social integration for love with enhanced intuitive awareness Superconscious contemplation the intuitive source of transpersonal guidance of (spirit = all-inclusive self) + cognitive analysis of unity and obstacles to integration
VII. Full integration	15. Creativity, bliss	Maintain contemplative awareness in all daily activities Objectless contemplation (nondual consciousness) with creative visualization + integrated creative development

tion is needed to promote the leaps of faith needed to transform consciousness and self-concepts.

E. Advanced Levels (V, VI, and VII) of Development and Maturity

The fifth and higher developmental and treatment levels involve advanced guidance in meditation and other techniques needed to transcend ordinary self-concepts. Such individuals' mature personality developments are seldom impaired by ordinary standards, but seek superior character integration, emotional fulfillment, and healthy longevity.

REFERENCES

1. Cloninger CR, Svrakic DM, Przybeck TR. A Psychobiological Model of Temperament and Character. Arch Gen Psychiatry 1993; 50:975–990

2. Cloninger CR, Svrakic D. Personality disorder. In: Sadock B, Kaplan H, eds. Comprehensive Textbook of Psychiatry, Baltimore: Williams and Wilkins, 7th ed, 1999, pp 1567–1588.
3. Cloninger CR, Przybeck TR, Svrakic DM, Wetzel R. The Temperament and Character Inventory (TCI): A Guide to Its Development and Use, St. Louis, Washington University School of Medicine, Department of Psychiatry, 1944.
4. Svrakic NM, Svrakic DM, Cloninger CR. A general quantitative theory of personality: fundamentals of a self-organizing psychobiological complex. Dev Psychopathology 1996; 8:247–272.
5. Svrakic DM, Whitehead CA, Przybeck TR, Cloninger CR. Differential diagnosis of personality disorders by the seven-factor temperament and character inventory. Arch Gen Psychiatry 1993; 50:991–999.
6. Cloninger CR. A systematic method for clinical description and classification of personality variants. Arch Gen Psychiatry 1987; 44:573–588.
7. Karasu TB. A developmental metatheory of psychopathology. Am J Psychother, 1994; 48(4):581–599.

11

Mood Disorders in Childhood and Adolescence
Basic Mechanisms and Therapeutic Interventions

MELISSA P. DELBELLO and ROBERT A. KOWATCH
University of Cincinnati College of Medicine, and Children's Hospital Medical Center, Cincinnati, Ohio, U.S.A.

I. INTRODUCTION

Child and adolescent mood disorders are complicated in their clinical presentations, and little is known regarding their neurobiology. These disorders commonly manifest with abnormalities in cognition, affective regulation, vegetative behaviors, and perception. Furthermore, children and adolescents who are diagnosed with mood disorders are at high risk for suicide attempts [1,2]. The developmental course and presentation of pediatric mood disorders and the presence of co-occurring disorders may vary with the age and pubertal status of the child [3–5]. Bipolar disorders are particularly complex since their initial presentation is often one of a severe, sometimes psychotic depression that later develops into mania or hypomania. The neurobiology of pediatric mood disorders involves multiple neurotransmitter and neuroendocrine systems and several brain regions. However, compared to adult mood disorders, little is known about the biological basis of pediatric mood disorders. Nonetheless, understanding the neuropathophysiology of pediatric mood disorders is essential so that effective treatment strategies may be developed.

II. EPIDEMIOLOGY AND CLINICAL CHARACTERISTICS

Psychoanalytic theory once taught that children could not experience depression before adolescence [6]. Subsequent research has demonstrated that children develop internal mood states between the ages of 12–18 months [7]. Children who are diagnosed with a mood disorder are commonly referred to clinicians because of "bad behavior" or a decline in school performance. Often children will present with irritability, oppositional and negative behavior, school refusal, and severe outbursts. Sometimes children will present with unexplained physical complaints in excess of a clear medical cause. A child who has a mood disorder might present with hyperactive, impulsive, and severely aggressive behavior, as if driven by a motor, and at the same time deny that anything is wrong. None of these pictures is the layperson's perception of a child who has a mood disorder, and yet the first two presentations are typical for depression and the third is typical for bipolar disorder [8].

A. Epidemiology

Prevalence rates of major depressive disorder (MDD) in children and adolescents range from 0.4% to 8.3% [9–16]. Depressive disorders occur more frequently in adolescents than in children. Prevalence rates of depressive disorders in children and adolescents are only slightly lower than in adults [17], for which 12-month prevalence of major depression is reported to be 10%. MDD in childhood appears to occur at approximately the same rate in girls and boys. However, during adolescence the gender differences observed in adult populations become apparent, with the approximately 2:1 female to male ratio [18]. Prevalence rates for dysthymia are 0.6–1.7% in children and 8% in adolescents [19,20].

Wozniak and colleagues [21] reported that of 262 consecutively referred children to a pediatric psychopharmacology clinic, 16% met DSM-III-R criteria for mania. Bipolar disorders are as prevalent in adolescents as they are in adults, with an estimated prevalence of 1% [2,11,12,22]. Recently, Lewinsohn and colleagues administered diagnostic assessments to a large randomly selected community sample of adolescents (n = 1507) and a subset was again assessed at age 24 years. They found that the lifetime prevalence of bipolar disorder was 1% during adolescence and 2% during young adulthood. Lifetime prevalence of subsyndromal bipolar disorder was 5%. Less than 1% of adolescents who had MDD switched to bipolar disorder by age 24 years [2]. This is in contrast to the results of others who have found "switch" rates of 33% in prepubescent children with MDD [23].

B. Signs and Symptoms

1. Depressive Disorders

Depressive disorders are characterized according to the Diagnostic and Statistical Manual, Fourth Edition (DSM-IV), as major depressive disorder (MDD), depressive disorder not otherwise specified (NOS), or dysthymic disorder [24].

According to DSM-IV, for a diagnosis of MDD, there must be a disturbance of mood (sadness and/or in children, irritability) most of the day, nearly every day, *or* there must be loss of interest or pleasure in all, or almost all, activities most of the day, nearly every day. In addition to a disturbance of mood and/or a loss of interest, five or more of the seven other associated symptoms must be present. The symptom complex must be present for at least 2 weeks. MDD tends to be episodic with either full or partial recovery between episodes (a cyclical disorder). Episodes of MDD cause significant deficits in the child's usual functioning that might be evidenced by a decline in school performance, withdrawal from peers, or conflict with peers and siblings. In depressive disorder NOS, the disorder is episodic, but the episodes will be below the criteria for MDD because of fewer symptoms or shorter duration. Episodes of depressive disorders NOS may be precursors of future MDD episodes or occur independently. Dysthymic disorder refers to a chronically depressed mood, less intense than MDD but with no prolonged well states. The duration of the illness is of at least 1 year in children, and irritability may be present instead of depressed mood. Seventy percent of children who have dysthymic disorder will develop MDD [25].

Although the diagnostic criteria for mood disorders in children and adolescents are generally the same as those for adults, differences in symptomatic expression are substantial, and are outlined below:

1. *Irritability (depressed mood)*. Dysphoria may be characterized by statements and appearance of sadness, loneliness, unhappiness, hopelessness, irritability, hypersensitivity, negative attitude, and being difficult to please. DSM-IV allows children to have irritability instead of a "depressed mood."

2. *Self-deprecation (guilt and worthlessness)*. Self-deprecatory thinking is manifest by thoughts of worthlessness, guilt, persecution, death, and suicidal ideation. In this age group, it is common to project feelings of lowered self-esteem into beliefs of persecution, i.e., "everyone hates me" or "I am not a good kid." Cognitively, it may be difficult for children to express guilt, but feelings of worthlessness and self-blame are evident in their behavior and in their statements.

3. *Agitation (psychomotor changes)*. Agitation is evident by difficulty getting along with others, including fighting, disrespect for authority, and excessive hostility. The increased conflict with others as a result of agitation is what often leads to the referral of a child. The presence of agitation and oppositional behavior can result in misdiagnosis of attention deficit hyperactivity disorder (ADHD) or oppositional defiant disorder. The oppositional or inattentive behavior will typically resolve with treatment of the depression.

4. *Sleep disturbance (insomnia or hypersomnia)*. Sleep problems include initial, middle, and terminal

insomnia, difficulty awakening in the morning, and excessive sleepiness (hypersomnolence). Depressed children will often experience the subjective feeling of initial insomnia, which is not always objectively confirmed. Middle insomnia is not uncommon in small children (getting in bed with parents and siblings). Terminal insomnia is less common in depressed children and adolescents than in depressed adults.

  5. *Change in school performance (poor concentration)*. Teachers may complain about daydreaming, poor concentration and attention, poor motivation, loss of interest in school activities, incomplete schoolwork and homework, and lowered grades. Because of poor concentration, children and adolescents may be misdiagnosed with ADHD. However, their history will often reveal no difficulty with attention prior to the episode of depression

  6. *Decreased socialization (loss of interest or pleasure)*. Children and adolescents with MDD might not seek out friends or participate in social activities.

  7. *Change in attitude regarding school (loss of interest)*. Children and adolescents with MDD may present with school refusal as the primary problem for referral. Although some of these children may have separation anxiety disorder, many have lost interest and pleasure in school.

  8. *Somatic complaints*. Although "somatic complaints" is not a DSM-IV symptom of depression, in children it is a common symptom of MDD. Children with MDD often present to pediatricians with vague complaints of headaches, stomachaches, or other physical symptoms for which the physician can find no cause.

  9. *Fatigue*. The depressed child or adolescent frequently complains of mental and physical fatigue and becomes less active. A child who was active in sports may complain of tiredness, less energy, and even boredom, resulting in diminished participation. Frequently there will be substantial overlap in the vegetative symptoms of loss of energy, sleepiness, and loss of interest.

  10. *Change in appetite and/or weight*. Children will typically become "picky" eaters, crave sweets, or become overeaters. Commonly, depressed children will not demonstrate expected developmental weight gain—rather, actual weight loss.

  11. *Suicidal ideation*. Children and adolescents may demonstrate suicidal plans and intent similar to that of adults. More typically, younger children describe passive suicidal ideation, such as wishing they were dead, but they do not have a plan.

2. Bipolar Disorders

A child or adolescent who has at least one episode of mania is classified as having bipolar I disorder. However, a child or adolescent who has had one or more episodes of major depression, no episodes of mania, and at least one episode of hypomania, is classified according to DSM-IV as having bipolar II disorder [24]. Cyclothymia is a disorder of at least 1-year duration, in which there are periods of hypomanic and depressive symptoms that do not meet criteria for mania or major depression. The child or adolescent is not without symptoms for more than 2 months at a time. Bipolar not otherwise specified (NOS) is a diagnostic category frequently used in children and adolescents since their mood episodes might not meet full DSM-IV criteria for duration of symptoms, or they might have recurrent hypomanic episodes without depression.

Pediatric bipolar disorder often presents differently from in adults. Most commonly, children and adolescents present with irritability, ultrarapid cycling, and mixed manic states. Disruptive behavioral disorder and ADHD are typically comorbid. Prepubertal-onset MDD with a family history of bipolar disorder may also be an early sign of pediatric bipolar disorder [3–5,23].

The following are examples of DSM-IV criteria for mania in children and adolescents.

  1. *Elevated or expansive mood*. The child may be much happier than their situation warrants. Inappropriate "goofiness" and silliness are common. During a manic phase, patients will often have no insight about the inappropriateness of their moods.

  2. *Irritability*. The child may become very belligerent, highly irritable with frequent, intense, and prolonged temper tantrums or "affective storms." An adolescent may appear extremely oppositional, belligerent, short, curt, or hostile, accounting for the common misdiagnosis of oppositional defiant or conduct disorder.

  3. *Inflated self-esteem or grandiosity*. The child or adolescent may think he or she has "superpowers" or "can beat up anyone in the world" or "can teach the class better than any of the teachers," despite failing school.

  4. *Decreased need for sleep*. The child or adolescent may refuse to go to bed before 1 or 2 AM and only sleep 3–4 hours a night without tiring.

  5. *More talkative than usual*. The child or adolescent may repeatedly blurt out answers during class and appear to "know more than the teacher." Their speech

may become very rapid and pressured to the point where it is continuous, and at times unintelligible or difficult to follow.

6. *Fight of ideas or racing thoughts.* The child or adolescent may report that he or she have "too many ideas and can't get them out fast enough." They may describe "thinking faster than others".

7. *Distractibility.* The manic child or adolescent may report that he or she cannot pay attention in class because their thoughts are moving along too fast or there is too much going on around them.

8. *Increase in goal-directed activity.* The child or adolescent will appear very restless and shift from activity to activity rapidly, without necessarily completing any of them.

9. *Excessive involvement in pleasurable activities that have a high potential for painful consequences.* The child may become hypersexual and inappropriately touch dolls, peers, or adults in an attempt to engage them in "sex". Adolescents may display promiscuous sexual behavior, or binges of drinking, drugging, or shopping.

C. Comorbidity

Mood disorders in children and adolescents are often masked by the presence of other co-occurring psychiatric diagnoses. In a recent epidemiological study, 50% of children and adolescents who had a psychiatric disorder had at least one co-occurring disorder [26]. In those with an affective disorder, 24% also had conduct or oppositional disorders, 17% had ADHD, and 17% had an anxiety disorder. Kovacs and colleagues found that the second most common diagnosis in children with affective illness is conduct disorder (23%) [27]. In one study, half of hospitalized adolescents diagnosed with a substance use disorder were found to also have a mood disorder [28].

The most common comorbid diagnoses in children with MDD are anxiety (30–80%), disruptive (10–80%) and substance use (20–30%) disorders [19]. Anxiety disorders commonly co-occur in children with MDD (41%) and typically persist even after the depressive episode remits [29]. Furthermore, the presence of social anxiety disorder in adolescence predicts MDD in young adulthood [30]. Also common in children with MDD is ADHD. Weinberg and Emslie found that 33% of children diagnosed with MDD also met criteria for ADHD [31].

Half of children diagnosed with dysthymic disorder have a co-occurring disorder [25]. Anxiety disorders are commonly comorbid in children and adolescents with dysthymic disorder, especially separation anxiety disorder in children (33%) and generalized anxiety disorder in adolescents (67%) [32]. Conduct disorder (30%), ADHD (24%), and enuresis or encoporesis (15%) are also common in children with dysthymic disorder [19].

The most common comorbid diagnosis among bipolar youth is ADHD. Despite the high co-occurrence of juvenile mania and ADHD, which has been reported in several studies, the relationship between these disorders remains unclear [5,21,33–39]. Explanations for this high comorbidity include juvenile mania with ADHD being a distinct form of early-onset bipolar disorder [34], ADHD being a prodrome of juvenile mania, or simply misclassification due to symptom overlap between the two conditions [35]. Several studies have demonstrated that ADHD is more common in prepubertal-onset bipolar disorder than in adolescent-onset bipolar disorder, suggesting that ADHD may be a marker for a developmentally early form of bipolarity [3,34,40]. Milberger and colleagues investigated whether ADHD with comorbid bipolar or major depressive disorder was two separate disorders or secondary to diagnostic overlap, and found that after overlapping diagnostic criteria were accounted for statistically, 79% maintained their diagnosis of MDD and 56% maintained their diagnosis of bipolar disorder [41]. Other reports support that children and adolescents with bipolar disorder with ADHD have two distinct disorders [42,43]. Faraone and colleagues assessed familial risk in children with ADHD with and without bipolar disorder and healthy volunteer children. They found that both ADHD groups had elevated familial rates of ADHD compared with healthy volunteers. However, a five times elevated risk for bipolar disorder was found among relatives when the proband had bipolar disorder but not when the proband had ADHD alone. Additionally, they reported an elevated risk for severe MDD in relatives of the ADHD+ bipolar probands and that both ADHD and bipolar disorder occurred in the same relatives more often than expected by chance, suggesting that ADHD with comorbid bipolar disorder is a familial distinct form of ADHD related to pediatric bipolar disorder [34,44].

Another disorder that is frequently comorbid in children with bipolar disorder is conduct disorder. Kovacs and Pollock found among 26 bipolar children and adolescents 69% were also diagnosed with conduct disorder. Several studies report that conduct disorder in youth with bipolar disorder predicts a worse clinical course [4,45]. Adolescents with bipolar disorder are five times more likely to develop a substance use disorder than those without bipolar disorder [46]. Recently, Biederman and colleagues [47] used familial risk analysis to disentangle the association between bipolar, substance use, and conduct disorder and reported that bipolar disorder in children and adolescents was a risk factor for substance use disorders, independent of conduct disorder. Furthermore, they found that the effects of bipolar and conduct disorders in probands combined additively to predict the risk for substance use disorders in relatives and therefore, that bipolar and conduct disorder are two distinct illnesses that commonly co-occur. Finally, children and adolescents with pervasive developmental disorders may be at increased risk for developing mania [48,49].

D. Differential Diagnosis

The differential diagnoses for pediatric mood disorders include ADHD, oppositional defiant disorder, conduct disorder, anxiety disorders, including posttraumatic stress disorder (PTSD), and pervasive developmental disorders. However, pediatric mood disorders commonly present with comorbid disruptive behavior, attention deficit, and pervasive developmental and anxiety disorders. Therefore, the assessment of a child or adolescent for a pediatric mood disorder should include identifying age-specific clinical manifestations of mood disorders. Children and adolescents with ADHD without a mood disorder do not have grandiosity, elation, euphoria, extreme irritability, hypersexuality, feelings of guilt or worthlessness, or suicidal ideation. With careful delineation of specific symptoms, these disorders can be separated. Fristad and colleagues used the adult Mania Rating Scale to evaluate a group of prepubertal children with either mania or ADHD [50]. They found this scale to be useful in differentiating manic children from the hyperactive children with the manic children reporting an elevated mood, increased motor activity/energy, decreased need for sleep, increased irritability, pressured speech, flight of ideas, disruptive behavior, thought disorders, and a lack of insight.

Children and adolescents with conduct disorder and without a mood disorder typically do not feel remorseful for their predatory actions. Like children and adolescents with mood disorders, those with PTSD might also present with mood lability and difficulty with sleep and concentration. However, the presence of nightmares, startle and avoidance behaviors, flashbacks, and severe anxiety with a history of trauma suggests PTSD as a primary diagnosis. Although the hypersexuality associated with bipolar disorder might be confused with PTSD, <1% of bipolar children with hypersexual behaviors have been sexually abused [51]. Additionally, although substance use and mood disorders commonly co-occur, it is important to assess for substance-induced mood disorders. The presence of mood symptoms during periods of abstinence, drug screens, and duration and severity of mood symptoms might be helpful in determining the relationship between mood symptoms and substance use.

Medical illnesses can cause mood disturbances and need to be investigated prior to assuming a primary psychiatric etiology. For example, symptoms of thyroid disease, infectious mononucleosis, systemic lupus, temporal lobe epilepsy, or anemia may mimic those of MDD or bipolar disorder.

E. Natural Course

The developmental course of mood disorders suggests that there is a continuum of pathology from childhood to adulthood. Similar to adults with depressive disorder, children and adolescents with MDD often have a chronic course.

Most studies report that the average length of a MDD episode in children and adolescents is 7–9 months [52–55]. In a study of 42 child outpatients with MDD, Kovacs and colleagues found that 59% had recovered (asymptomatic for 2 months) by 1 year and 92% had recovered by 18 months [52]. Similarly, Strober and colleagues found that 81% of 58 adolescent inpatients with MDD had recovered by 1 year and 98% by 2 years from the time of admission, with the average time to recovery of 27.5 weeks from admission [54]. McCauley and colleagues found that 80% of predominantly outpatient children with MDD recovered by 1 year [56].

However, once recovered, children and adolescents with MDD have a high rate of relapse. Recurrence (i.e., a new episode of depression) has been reported in up to 72% of depressed children and adolescents followed for 3–8 years, with similar rates seen in inpatients and outpatients (55–60). For example, Poznanski and colleagues reported that 50% of outpatient adolescents with MDD were depressed when contacted 6.5 years later [61]. Eastgate and Gilmour contacted 19 of 36 child inpatients with depression 7–8 years after their episode and reported that 42% were psychiatrically ill, 21% with MDD [62].

Furthermore, 70% of children and adolescents with early-onset MDD continue having episodes of MDD into adulthood. Kandal and Davies [63] described poor adult outcomes in a large sample of adolescents (n = 1004) identified as having depressive symptoms using a self-report scale. Similarly, in a retrospective, long-term follow-up study of 80 depressed and 80 nondepressed outpatient adolescents, Harrington and colleagues [64] reported that depressed adolescents were more likely than nondepressed adolescents to have MDD in adulthood; however, they noted that most adult depressions are not preceded by adolescent depression. Weissman and colleagues studied 73 patients with adolescent onset MDD into adulthood and found that while 37% survived without an episode of major depression in adulthood, there was substantial increased risk of suicide and adult MDD in those with as compared to those without adolescent MDD [65].

Although there are few investigations of the outcome of childhood-onset dysthymic disorder, children with dysthymic disorder are likely to develop depressive disorders and recurrent affective illnesses [25]. Moreover, the presence of an externalizing disorder predicts a worse outcome in children with dysthymia [25]. Mean episode length is typically 4 years, and children with dysthymia usually develop their first episode of MDD within 2–3 years after the onset of dysthymic disorder [25,52,60].

According to one study, prepubertal-onset depression has been associated with high rates (up to 33%) of bipolar disorder in adolescence and adulthood [23]. However, adolescent depression is only associated with a 1% risk of switching to bipolar disorder [2]. Strober and colleagues followed 58 adolescents who had been admitted to a psychiatric unit for MDD and found that during the 24-month follow-up period, mania occurred in 28% of those patients who had a psychotic depression [54]. Predictors of bipolarity included a depressive syndrome that consisted of rapid onset, psychomotor retardation, mood-congruent psychotic features, a family history of bipolar disorder, the presence of bipolar disorder in three successive generations, and pharmacologically induced mania [66]. In a similar follow-up study of depressed prepubertal children, Geller and colleagues reported that bipolarity was predicted by a family history of major mood disorders or schizoaffective disorder [67].

The outcome of bipolar disorder in children and adolescents has received little study. McGlashen interviewed 62 adult patients who met DSM-III criteria for mania and divided them into two groups—35 with adolescent-onset mania, and 31 with adult-onset mania [68]. He reported that the adolescent-onset group had more hospitalizations, displayed more psychotic symptoms, and were more frequently misdiagnosed with schizoaffective disorder than the adult-onset group. Surprisingly, the adolescent-onset group had a superior outcome to the adult-onset group in terms of social relationships and ability to work.

In contrast, Geller and colleagues reported diagnostic stability in 91 prepubescent and early adolescent subjects. At 6 months, 86% continued to have mania and only 14% recovered. The presence of conduct disorder predicted worse outcome [4]. At 1-year follow-up, 89 of the patients were assessed and rate of recovery was 37%; however, the rate of relapse after recovery was 38% [69]. In these studies recovery was defined as no mania or hypomania for at least 2 weeks, and relapse was defined as having full DSM-IV criteria for mania or hypomania and a Childhood Global Assessment Scale score of ≤60 for at least 2 weeks.

There are very few outcome studies of adolescent mania. Retrospective studies have indicated poor outcomes with high rates of suicide [70]. In the largest and to our knowledge the only, prospective follow-up studies of adolescent mania, Strober and colleagues found 96% of adolescents with bipolar disorder recovered from index affective episode at 5 years and 44% of those had one or more relapses by 5 years. A pure depressive episode at index hospitalization was associated with longer time to recovery. Mixed manic states and cycling index episodes were associated with multiple relapses [71].

In summary, until fairly recently it was commonly believed that pediatric mood disorders did not exist. However, there are now data to support that pediatric mood disorders are highly prevalent and associated with high rates of suicide and comorbid disorders [5,72,73]. Furthermore, children and adolescents with mood disorders will generally exhibit a chronic course and continue to have a mood disorder into adulthood.

III. BIOLOGY

As compared to mood disorders in adults, there have been relatively few investigations of the biology of childhood and adolescent mood disorders. Moreover, these studies are difficult to implement in children and adolescents since they often require several blood draws, subjects remaining still over long periods of time, and the cooperation of the children and adolescents. Owing to the recent data-based characterization of the clinical manifestations of pediatric mood disorder, there has been an increase in biological studies of children and adolescents with bipolar and major depressive disorders.

A. Genetics

Although there have been few molecular genetic studies of children with mood disorders, familial risk studies suggest that early-onset MDD may be a more familial form of the illness than adult-onset MDD. Based on twin studies, childhood and adolescent MDD is significantly heritable (0.50–0.65) in both boys and girls [74]. Children of depressed parents are three times more likely to have a lifetime episode of MDD. Furthermore, early-onset MDD is associated with an increased familial risk of MDD as compared to late-onset MDD [75–77]. However, a family history of MDD is associated with recurrence and continuity of MDD into adulthood in patients with prepubertal-onset MDD and not adolescent-onset MDD [78]. Although the molecular basis of pediatric MDD remains to be determined, there is a familial component to early-onset MDD, particularly in patients who have a more protracted illness course (79).

Overall, family studies have confirmed an increased risk of bipolar disorder, ADHD, and alcoholism in relatives of probands with pediatric bipolar disorder as compared to adult bipolar probands. For example, Biederman and colleagues [33] reported that a family history of affective disorders predicted development of bipolar disorder in children with ADHD at 4-year follow-up. Todd and colleagues found an elevated rate of alcoholism in adult male relatives of bipolar children as compared to relatives of children with MDD and healthy volunteers. Paternal affective disorder and alcoholism predicted offspring affective disorder. The authors suggest that corisk for the two disorders in an individual may interact to lower the observed age at onset of one of the two disorders, potentially through genetic and/or environmental interactions [80].

Children who have a parent with bipolar disorder are also at an increased risk for developing mood disorder. In a review of BP offspring studies that included only investigations that evaluated children and adolescents, rates of mood disorders ranged from 5% to 67% compared to rates in offspring of healthy volunteers of 0–38% [81].

Two molecular genetic studies have been reported in children with bipolar disorder [82,83]. The first study examined the linkage disequilibrium of catechol-O-methyltransferase (l-COMT) in bipolar children since the children described in the sample have high rates of rapid and ultradian cycling (75%), and in adults rapid cycling has been associated with the low-activity allele of l-COMT. Transmission disequilibrium tests were not significant for preferential transmission of l-COMT for the ultradian rapid-cycling subgroup or for the entire sample. The authors suggest several explanations for their finding, including the possibility that ultradian cycling in this pediatric sample may be genetically heterogeneous from the phenomenon in bipolar adults, the ultradian cycling in children may not persist in all of the bipolar children when they reach adulthood, or their sample size may be too small [82]. In the second study, the transmission disequilibrium test for the serotonin transporter-linked promoter region (HTTLPR) short and long alleles was negative in the children with bipolar disorder, suggesting either a lack of involvement of this locus or insufficient power in the study to detect differences [83].

The relationship between velocardiofacial syndrome and pediatric bipolar disorder is of particular interest to understanding the genetic basis of bipolar disorder in children. Velocardiofacial syndrome, a genetic syndrome involving >40 somatic anomalies, as well as learning disabilities and behavioral disorders, is associated with a microdeletion on chromosome 22q11. In a series of patients with velocardiofacial syndrome, 64% met DSM-III-R criteria for a spectrum of bipolar disorder with full syndromal onset in late childhood or early adolescence (mean age at onset 12 years). Given the high prevalence of childhood-onset bipolar disorder in this population, further genetic investigations of chromosome 22 are warranted in the search for a molecular basis of pediatric bipolar disorder [84].

Future familial risk studies, in conjunction with molecular genetic investigations, may help identify the mode of genetic transmission for pediatric mood disorders. Children and adolescents who have a mood disorder and a family history of mood disorders may be the ideal population for performing molecular genetics studies, since this group may have a particularly genetic form of illness.

B. Neurotransmitter Studies

The neurobiological basis of mood disorders involves a range of disturbances in noradrenergic, serotonergic, dopaminergic, cholinergic, GABA-ergic, and other neurotransmitter systems [85]. Evidence from neuroanatomic, neurophysiologic, neurochemical, and behavioral studies in humans and animals supports that mood disorders are modulated by interacting neural networks that are often widely spatially distributed [86–90].

Peripheral studies of neurotransmitters have primarily focused on norepinephrine, serotonin, and acetylcholine [91–94]. Norepinephrine has been the most-studied catacholamine in adults with MDD [95–97]. However, DeVilliers and colleagues [98] found no difference in noradrenergic function between MDD adolescents and healthy controls.

Serotonin (5-hydroxytryptamine) regulation has also been evaluated in adults with MDD [99–102]. Studies measuring baseline CSF 5-hydroxyindole acetic acid (5HIAA) are equivocal. The most comprehensive studies suggest that there is a subgroup (30–40%) of depressed adults with low CSF 5HIAA; this subgroup may show more aggression, anxiety, impulsivity, and suicidality. Ryan and colleagues [103] reported that in response to L-5-hydroxytryptophan (5HT), prepubertal children with MDD (N = 37) secreted less cortisol and more prolactin than normal controls (N = 23), suggesting a dysregulation of central serotonergic systems in childhood MDD. This finding has been confirmed in a more recent study that reported children with a high familial risk for developing MDD secreted similar levels of prolactin in response to a 5HT infusion as MDD children, but significantly more than healthy volunteer children who did not have a family history of mood disorders, suggesting that abnormalities in serotonergic neurons may be a trait marker for childhood MDD [104].

Future studies are necessary to confirm the theoretical framework for the neurotransmitter systems involved in child and adolescent MDD, which was proposed by Rogeness and colleagues [105]. They suggested that dopaminergic function is low (facilitory neurotransmission) and noradrenergic and serotonergic (inhibitory neurotransmission) functions are high.

C. Neuroendocrine Studies

Abnormalities of the hypothalamic-pituitary-adrenal (HPA) axis, the hypothalamic-pituitary-thyroid (HPT) axis, and the hypothalamic-pituitary-growth-hormone (HPGH) axis have been reported in MDD adults. However, abnormal cortisol secretion, as measured by repeated samples over a 24-hour period or by nocturnal sampling, has not been identified in most studies of children and adolescents with MDD [106–109]. In contrast, at the approximate time of sleep onset, MDD adolescents exhibited cortisol elevation [110,111]. In one study, there was a trend toward elevated cortisol levels near sleep onset in adolescents who had recurrent MDD as compared to those who had no further MDD episodes [111]. De Bellis and colleagues [112] reported that prepubertal MDD children had *lower* cortisol levels during the first 4 hours of sleep compared that did healthy controls.

In contrast to studies involving MDD adults, Birmaher and colleagues [113] found no significant difference in baseline or postcorticotropin-releasing hormone (CRH) stimulation values of cortisol or adrenocorticotropin-releasing hormone (ACTH) between prepubertal children with MDD and healthy controls. Post-CRH ACTH may be elevated in MDD children who have been abused as compared to those who have no history of abuse [114], suggesting that increased ACTH may be associated with stressful life events and not MDD. Nonsuppression of cortisol by dexamethasone has been reported in several studies of MDD children and adolescents [115–119].

Kutcher and colleagues [109] reported that nocturnal growth hormone (GH) secretion was significantly elevated in MDD adolescents as compared to controls. However, this finding has not been replicated [112]. In one study, MDD adolescents did not differ from healthy controls in 24-hour GH measures; however, blunting of GH secretion was evident in MDD adolescents with suicidal ideation but not those without suicidal ideation [120]. Blunting of growth hormone-release in response to hypoglycemia, desipramine, clonidine, and growth hormone-releasing hormone (GHRH) in MDD children and adolescents has been reported, even after the depression remits, suggesting that this may be a trait, rather than state, marker for pediatric MDD [121–123]. Furthermore, in a recent study, Birmaher and colleagues [124] demonstrated blunted GH secretion in response to GHRH in children with a high familial risk for developing MDD as compared to healthy controls without a familial risk for MDD, providing additional support that the decreased growth hormone response is a trait marker for pediatric MDD. While these are among the most replicated neuroendocrine findings in pediatric MDD, GH is regulated by many neurotransmitters, limiting the interpretability of these findings. Moreover, the specificity of these findings remains uncertain [19].

There are several studies examining thyroid abnormalities in children and adolescents with mood disorders. Kutcher and colleagues [109] reported that nocturnal thyroid-stimulating hormone (TSH) values were elevated in children with mood disorder as compared to healthy volunteers, but there was no significant difference in total amount of TSH secreted throughout the night. In a study assessing thyroid hormones in MDD children, Dorn and colleagues [125] reported that all subjects were euthyroid. However, boys with MDD exhibited lower thyroxine (T4) and TSH levels than control boys. No differences were found between girls with MDD and control girls. Tri-iodothyronine (T3) uptake was lower in the MDD children compared with healthy controls. West and colleagues [126] found that mean serum thyroxine (T4) concentrations were significantly lower in bipolar adolescents with ADHD than in those without ADHD, suggesting that bipolar disorder with ADHD may be a distinct illness.

In summary, neuroendocrine studies provide preliminary data which suggest that some of the abnormalities involved in adult MDD may also be present in childhood and adolescent MDD. However, further research is necessary to determine state, trait, and developmental factors that may contribute to these findings.

D. Sleep Studies

Sleep studies involving children and adolescents with MDD have not consistently found the same changes that have been reported in adults with MDD. Only one of four studies to evaluate sleep in MDD *children* [127–130] identified decreased rapid eye movement (REM) latency and increased sleep latency in MDD children [127]. Puig-Antich and colleagues [131] found that children who had recovered from an episode of MDD had shorter first REM latencies and a greater number of REM periods compared with themselves when depressed and normal children, suggesting that this may be a marker for a prior MDD episode.

Sleep studies of *adolescents* with major depression have inconsistently reported reduced REM latency and prolonged sleep latency in MDD adolescents as compared to healthy volunteers [132–139].

E. Neuroimaging Studies

Brain-imaging techniques available to study mood disorders may be broadly divided into two groups: those that image the *structure* of the central nervous system, which include computed tomography (CT) and magnetic resonance imaging (MRI), and those that image the *function* of the central nervous system, including positron emission tomography (PET), single-photon emission computed tomography (SPECT), magnetic resonance spectroscopy (MRS), and functional magnetic resonance imaging (fMRI). Despite recent advances in MRI techniques permitting high-resolution thin-slice images for more valid morphometric analyses and the development of noninvasive functional methodologies such as fMRI and MRS, there are few neuroimaging investigations involving children and adolescents with mood disorders.

1. Structural Neuroimaging

There have been few structural neuroimaging studies of children and adolescents with MDD. Hendren and colleagues used MRI to study a mixed group of 37 psychiatric inpatients between the ages of 8 and 12 years, three of whom were hospitalized for treatment of MDD [140]. Two of the three adolescents with MDD had clinical abnormalities on MRI, which included asymmetrical lateral ventricles and a small area of abnormal signal intensity in the "left anterior basal ganglia or medial temporal lobe." In the only published study to examine brain morphometry in pediatric MDD, Steingard and colleagues [141] retrospectively evaluated the MRI scans of children with MDD or dysthymia (N=65) and found that frontal lobe volume was decreased and lateral ventricular volume was increased as compared to hospitalized psychiatric controls (N=18). No group difference was found in total cerebral volume. These results are similar to findings from MRI studies of adults with MDD that suggest prefrontal abnormalities [142,143].

Botteron and colleagues [144] compared bipolar children and adolescents to healthy subjects using MRI and found reduced structural asymmetry of the cerebral hemispheres. Additionally, four of the eight bipolar subjects had ventricular abnormalities or deep white matter hyperintensities as compared to one of five control subjects, although the sample size was too small to provide statistical power. To our knowledge, there are only two additional published brain morphometry studies of adolescents with bipolar disorder, both from the same research group [145,146]. The first study compared cortical regions of adolescents with schizophrenia and bipolar disorder and then combined patient groups and compared them to healthy volunteer adolescents. When patient groups were combined, they had significantly reduced intracranial volumes, elevated frontal and temporal fluid fractions, and decreased brain circumferences and thalamic volumes as compared to healthy volunteers; however, there were no differences between patient groups. Furthermore, the authors examined effect sizes for the differences in structures between bipolar adolescents and healthy controls, and found enlarged frontal and temporal fluid, lateral ventricular volumes, and decreased intracranial volumes (large effect sizes) in bipolar adolescents. Because of multiple comparisons, the authors caution the interpretability of these results. In summary, these studies suggest that, similar to findings from morphometric studies of adults with bipolar disorder, frontal-temporal abnormalities may also be present in bipolar adolescents. Studies of adults with mood disorders have also found abnormalities in the hippocampus, amygdala, thalamus, caudate, putamen, globus pallidus, and cerebellar vermis [147]. Future morphometric studies of these brain regions in children and adolescents with mood disorders are necessary.

2. *Functional Neuroimaging*

PET and SPECT studies in adults with mood disorders have produced variable results, possibly owing to differences in subject selection criteria, diagnostic procedures, severity of illness, medication status, demographic characteristics, imaging techniques, and analytic methods. FMRI is a newer functional imaging technique that does not involve exposure to ionizing radiation and thus is repeatable and noninvasive, making it particularly advantageous for studies involving children and adolescents.

To our knowledge, there have been only three published functional neuroimaging studies in children or adolescents with mood disorders. Kowatch and colleagues [148] used technetium-99m hexamethylpropylene amine oxime (^{99m}Tc-HMPAO) single photon emission tomography (SPECT) to compare relative regional cerebral blood flow (rCBF) between unmedicated MDD adolescents (N=7) and normal controls (N=7). The authors describe relative increases in rCBF in the mesial, right superior-anterior, and left inferolateral temporal lobe and decreases in the left parietal lobe, anterior thalamus, and right caudate in MDD adolescents. These findings suggest that adolescents with MDD exhibit rCBF abnormalities similar to those found in adults with MDD with involvement of the limbic-thalamic-cortical circuit and portions of the basal ganglia [88,89].

In another ^{99m}Tc-HMPAO SPECT study, evaluating untreated MDD adolescents (N=14) and age-matched normal controls (N=11), Tutus and colleagues [149] calculated a relative perfusion index (PI) as the ratio of regional cortical activity to the whole brain activity and reported significant reduced PI in the left anterofrontal and left temporal cortical regions of untreated MDD adolescents. SPECT scans repeated after MDD adolescents were treated and their depression remitted demonstrated a return toward normal.

This study suggests that adolescents with MDD may have state-dependent regional cerebral blood flow deficits in frontal and temporal regions and right-left perfusion asymmetry compared with normal subjects, similar to results in studies of MDD adults [87].

In a more recent study, Dahlstrom and colleagues [150] used SPECT to study serotonin and dopamine transporter levels in drug-naïve children and adolescents with MDD (N=31) and children and adolescents without depression (N=10). They found significantly higher serotonin transporter availability in MDD children in the hypothalamic/midbrain region suggesting that abnormalities in serotonin might play a role in the physiology of pediatric MDD.

Proton magnetic resonance spectroscopy (MRS) is a noninvasive neuroimaging technique that allows in vivo measurement of brain neurochemistry. The major components observed in a proton spectrum of the brain are N-acetylaspartate (NAA), glutamate/glutamine/GABA (Glx), creatine (Cr), choline (Cho), and *myo*-inositol (mI). Steingard and colleagues [151] found elevated Cho/Cr ratios in the medial frontal gray matter of MDD adolescents as compared to healthy volunteers, providing additional evidence for frontal abnormalities in MDD adolescents. Castillo and colleagues [152] found increased prefrontal and temporal Glx concentrations in children with bipolar disorder, suggesting that in addition to structural abnormalities, neurochemical dysfunction may be present in these brain regions.

Although the exact mechanism by which lithium exerts its antimanic and antidepressant effects is unknown, at therapeutic concentrations, lithium is an inhibitor of inositol monophosphatase and polyphosphate-1-phosphatase, which are involved in replenishing *myo*-inositol supplies. Thus, it is postulated that the therapeutic effects of lithium are mediated through depletion of *myo*-inositol [153]. Davanzo and colleagues [154] compared anterior cingulate *myo*-inositol levels in manic children (N=11) before and 1 week after lithium treatment and found that acute lithium treatment was associated with a significant reduction in the *myo*-inositol/Cr ratio, particularly in lithium responders as compared to nonresponders. The authors also reported that at baseline bipolar children had an elevated *myo*-inositol/Cr ratio as compared to demographically matched healthy volunteers. However, many of the bipolar children were taking several concomitant medications during the study. Nonetheless, to our knowledge, this is the first study in bipolar youth to provide support for lithium-induced modification of the phosphoinositide cycle.

Additional structural and functional neuroimaging investigations are necessary to further characterize the neurophysiology of pediatric mood disorders. Furthermore, combining longitudinal imaging and outcome studies will maximize the interpretability of the imaging data and identify neurobiological predictors of illness course and treatment response.

IV. TREATMENT

A. Depressive Disorders

During the past 10 years there have been several treatment studies that have provided important information regarding the treatment of MDD in children and adolescents. In general, tricyclic antidepressants (TCAs), i.e., imipramine, amitriptyline, and nortriptyline, are not more efficacious than placebo for treating MDD in children or adolescents and are not indicated as first-line agents for this disorder. Moreover, selective serotonin reuptake inhibitors (SSRIs), i.e., fluoxetine, paroxetine, and sertraline, have been show to be effective in treating both children and adolescents with MDD. However, there are very few placebo-controlled studies of SSRIs for the treatment of children and adolescents with MDD. Although there are several ongoing studies assessing the long-term efficacy of SSRIs for the treatment of pediatric depression, there are currently no published maintenance treatment studies. Specific psychotherapies such as cognitive behavior therapy and interpersonal psychotherapy may also be helpful in treating children and adolescents with MDD. However, it is unclear how best to integrate psychotherapy and antidepressant treatment.

1. Pharmacotherapy

There have been six double-blind trials of TCAs for the treatment of MDD in children and six double-blind trials in adolescents. The consensus from these 12 trials is that TCAs are no more effective than placebo in child and adolescent MDD and are thus not indicated as first-line treatments for MDD in children or adolescents [155]. However, these studies generally were of small samples of patients with mild to moderate depression. Additionally, some of the studies included patients with secondary depression who are more likely to respond to placebo. In fact, placebo response in most of these studies was 50–70%, greater than that observed in placebo-controlled studies of depressed adults. Moreover, small dosages were administered for possibly too short a period of time to observe large response rates [155]. There have been six reports of sudden cardiac death in children and adolescents treated with the TCA desipramine, which also limits the use of these agents in child and adolescent MDD [156,157]. Current recommendations are to use TCAs as fourth- or fifth-line treatments after adequate trials of other agents [158]. Monoamine oxidase inhibitors (MAOIs) may also be effective for MDD adolescents who are partial responders to TCAs. However, side effects may be severe and include hypertensive crisis if a patient is noncompliant with a low-tyramine diet [159].

The SSRIs are well tolerated in children and adolescents and have many fewer side effects than TCAs [160]. There have two double-blind trials of fluoxetine and several open studies that have shown fluoxetine to be efficacious in the treatment of MDD in children and adolescents. In the first study, Simeon and colleagues treated 40 adolescents with MDD with fluoxetine in a placebo-controlled double-blind study. They reported that approximately two-thirds of the patients showed marked or moderate clinical global improvement with both fluoxetine and placebo, and fluoxetine was superior to placebo on all clinical measures except for sleep disorder [161]. In 1997, Emslie and colleagues [162] reported the results of a second double-blind placebo-controlled study of fluoxetine in children and adolescents (ages 8–18 years) with MDD [162]. There were 96 subjects randomized, and 27/48 (56%) were rated as much or very much improved on fluoxetine compared with 16/48 (33%) on placebo (P = .02). There have been two open-label prospective studies in which sertraline was reported to be effective in treating adolescent MDD [163,164]. Results from the largest double-blind study to date of an SSRI in children and adolescents with MDD (N = 285) found paroxetine was superior to both imipramine and placebo [165]. All of the SSRIs have side effects, including mild gastrointestinal upset, sedation, and behavioral activation.

Less information is available regarding the use of other "atypical" antidepressant agents in MDD children and adolescents. Some promising results have been reported with nefazodone [166], but a small placebo-controlled trial of venlafaxine found no difference from placebo [167].

There are several studies of lithium in children and adolescents with MDD. Geller and colleagues [168] evaluated the efficacy of lithium vs. placebo in the treatment of adolescents with MDD who were refractory to tricyclics and who had a family history of bipolar disorder. The rationale for this study was that prepubescent children with MDD and a family history of bipolar disorder commonly develop bipolar disorder. However, they found no group difference in response, suggesting that lithium may not be effective in the treatment of patients with prepubescent MDD who are at high familial risk for developing bipolar disorder. However, there are two open studies suggesting that lithium may be effective in the augmentation of tricyclics for refractory MDD in children and adolescents [169,170]. Bupropion may be effective for treating depressive disorders with comorbid ADHD, although controlled trials are needed [171].

2. Psychotherapy

There have been no controlled trials of psychoanalytic therapy for the treatment of children and adolescents with MDD. However, recent research has demonstrated that certain types of short-term psychotherapy, particularly cognitive behavior therapy (CBT), are effective for treating MDD in children and adolescents [172]. Brent and colleagues studied 107 adolescent patients with MDD who were randomly assigned to individual CBT, systemic behavior family therapy, or individual nondirective supportive therapy [173]. They found that the adolescents who were treated with CBT had a lower rate of MDD at the end of treatment that those who were treated with supportive therapy. Moreover, adolescents with MDD treated with CBT had higher remission rates that the two other groups. However, when the same subjects were evaluated 2 years after this trial, there were no long-term differences in rates of recovery or recurrence of MDD [174].

Another short-term psychotherapy, interpersonal therapy (IPT), focuses on working through disturbed personal relationships that may contribute to depression. Mufson and colleagues recently performed a controlled, 12-week trial of IPT in which 48 MDD adolescents were randomly assigned to either weekly IPT or clinical monitoring, which was the control condition [175]. In their intent-to-treat sample, 75% who received IPT compared with 46% who received the control condition met recovery criteria at the end of 12 weeks of treatment. They concluded that IPT is efficacious for reducing depressive symptoms and improving social functioning and interpersonal problem-solving skills in MDD adolescents.

3. Treatment Guidelines for Child and Adolescent MDD

A consensus conference was held in 1998 in which a group of national experts in child and adolescent mood disorders developed a consensus algorithm (the Texas Medication Algorithm Project; TMAP) for the treatment of MDD in children and adolescents [176]. The TMAP MDD treatment is illustrated in Figure 1. The first stage in this algorithm is monotherapy with a SSRI. If the child or adolescent does not respond to the first SSRI, then the recommendation is to switch to an alternative SSRI. The seventh and last step of this algorithm is to use ECT. This TMAP algorithm is very useful, as it embodies the current state of knowledge for the treatment of child and adolescent MDD and offers clinicians a rational way to proceed in treating this disorder.

B. Bipolar Disorders

Treatment of pediatric bipolar disorder consists of two phases—treatment of the acute affective episode and maintenance treatment. There have been very few controlled studies of acute treatment for mania in children and adolescents bipolar disorder [177]. Furthermore, there has only been one maintenance treatment study [178]. The American Psychiatric Association issued their "Practice Guideline for the Treatment of Patients with Bipolar Disorder" in which the treatment of bipolar disorder in children and adolescents is also reviewed. These practice guidelines are useful for a further review of several topics that are beyond the scope of this chapter [179].

1. Lithium

Lithium is the most studied treatment for pediatric bipolar disorder and is the only Food and Drug Administration (FDA)-approved medication for the treatment of acute mania and bipolar disorder in adolescents or children (ages 12–18 years). In a survey of the literature, Youngerman and Canino [180] found that in open trials of lithium in children with bipolar disorder, the positive response rate was 66%, similar to that seen in adults treated with lithium. There have been four [181–184] crossover studies of lithium in pediatric bipolar disorder. The average number of subjects in these studies was 18 and response rates ranged from 33% to 80%. In the only placebo-controlled prospective study of a mood stabilizer in pediatric bipolar disorder, Geller and colleagues [177] administered lithium in a double-blind fashion to 25

Mood Disorders in Childhood and Adolescence

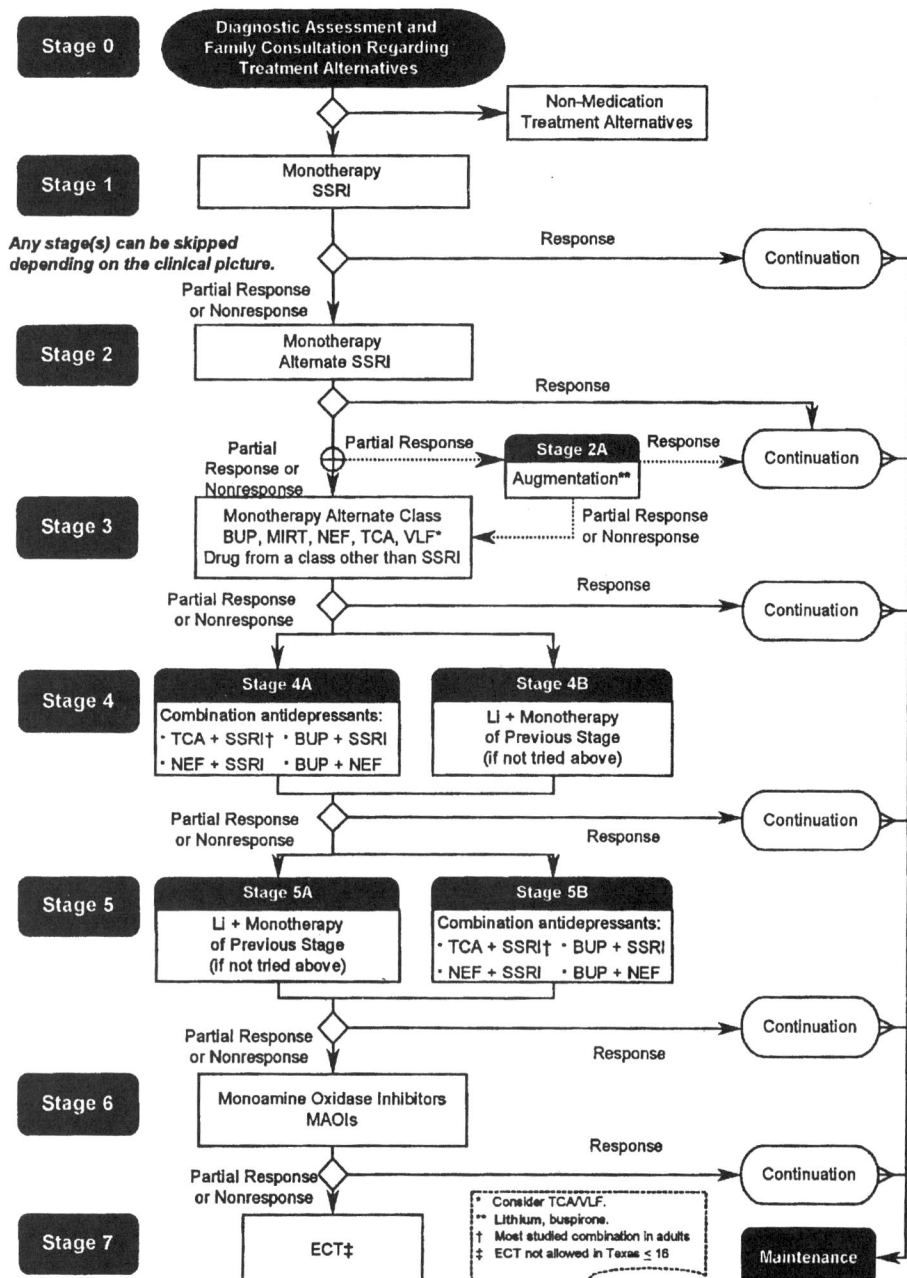

Figure 1 Medication algorithm for treating children and adolescents who meet *DSM-IV* criteria for major depressive disorder. The Children's Medication Algorithm Project algorithms are in the public domain and may be reproduced without permission, but with appropriate citation. The authors bear no responsibility for the use of these guidelines by third parties. SSRI = selective serotonin reuptake inhibitor; BUP = bupropion; MIRT = mirtazapine; NEF = nefazodone; TCA = tricyclic antidepressant; VLF = venlafaxine; ECT = electroconvulsive therapy. Adapted from Crismon et al. (1999).

adolescents with bipolar disorder and substance dependence. After 6 weeks of treatment, subjects treated with lithium showed a significant decrease in substance use and a significant improvement in global assessment of functioning (46% in the lithium-treated group vs. 8% in the placebo group). This report clearly demonstrated the efficacy of lithium carbonate for the treatment of bipolar adolescents. Predictors of poor lithium response in children and adolescents include prepubertal onset [185], presence of co-occurring ADHD [186], personality disorders [187], and mixed mania [188]. In general, for the treatment of an acute mood episode in children and adolescents, lithium should be titrated to a dose of 30 mg/kg/day in three divided doses, which will typically produce a level of 0.8–1.2 mEq/L.

Lithium may also be useful for the maintenance treatment of bipolar disorder in children and adolescents. Since the majority of patients with bipolar disorder experience recurrent episodes of illness, maintenance treatment is generally advised. In the only maintenance treatment study for pediatric bipolar disorder, Strober and colleagues [178] conducted an 18-month naturalistic follow-up study of 37 adolescents whose bipolar disorder had been stabilized with lithium during hospitalization. Despite intensive follow-up, 35% of these patients discontinued lithium, and 92% of those who discontinued subsequently relapsed as compared to 38% of those who were lithium compliant, supporting the possible prophylactic effect of lithium [178].

Common side effects of lithium in children and adolescents include hypothyroidism, nausea, polyuria, polydipsia, tremor, acne, and weight gain. Lithium levels and thyroid function tests should be carefully monitored, and thyroid supplementation should be initiated when indicated [189].

2. Antiepileptics

Response rate to divalproex in open-label studies involving manic adolescents has ranged from 53% to 82% [39,190–193]. The successful use of carbamazepine as monotherapy and adjunctive treatment has also been reported in children and adolescents with bipolar disorder [39,194,195].

In the only study to directly compare mood stabilizers, Kowatch and colleagues [39] compared lithium, divalproex, and carbamazepine for the treatment of 42 acutely manic or hypomanic children and adolescents during a 6-week random-assignment, open prospective investigation. The mean response rates of the intent to treat sample were 40% and 53% for divalproex sodium, 46% and 38% for lithium, and 31% and 38% for carbamazepine as measured by a CGI change score of 1 or 2 and a >50% change from baseline Young Mania Rating Scale, respectively. Divalproex demonstrated the largest effect size (1.63), followed by lithium (1.06) and carbamazepine (1.00). All three drugs were fairly well tolerated, with nausea being the most common side effect for each of the medications. In general, divalproex should be titrated to a dose of 20 mg/kg/day, which will typically produce a serum level of 80–120 µg/ml, and carbamazepine should be titrated to a dose of 15 mg/kg/day to produce a serum level of 7–10 µg/mL [39].

Common side effects of divalproex in children are weight gain, sedation, and tremor [196]. There has been considerable concern regarding the possible association between divalproex and polycystic ovarian syndrome (PCOS). Initially, the reports of PCOS were in women with epilepsy who were taking divalproex [197]. It was unclear whether this association was from divalproex-induced obesity, which might lead to elevated androgen levels, a direct effect of divalproex, or related to epilepsy. Recently, Bauer and colleagues reported that epilepsy, and not the medications may be associated with increased risk for PCOS [198]. Further investigations of the risk of developing PCOS for female bipolar adolescents are necessary. Carbamazepine is less commonly used in children because of the potential for developing aplastic anemia and severe dermatological reactions, such as Stevens-Johnson syndrome. Other frequent side effects include hyponatremia, nausea, and sedation [39].

Since 1990 there have been several new anticonvulsants developed for the treatment of epilepsy. Although data are limited regarding the efficacy and tolerability of these agents for the treatment of bipolar disorder, they are of potential interest because of decreased side effects and drug interactions. There have been two positive reports with a total of 17 bipolar children and adolescents who were treated with lamotrigine as adjunctive therapy [199,200]. Lamotrigine was well tolerated, and none of the children developed a rash. The most common side effects of lamotrigine are dizziness, tremor, somnolence, nausea, asthenia, and headache in 8–20% of patients. Rarely, severe cutaneous reactions such as Stevens-Johnson syndrome and toxic epidermal necrolysis have been described [201]. The risk of serious rashes is approximately three times greater in children and adolescents <16 years old compared with adults and is higher in patients taking concomitant valproate

[202]. Therefore, its use in treating children and adolescents is somewhat limited.

Although preliminary evidence from open studies in adults suggested gabapentin was effective as adjunctive therapy and monotherapy for the treatment of bipolar mania and depression and as an augmenting agent in the maintenance phase of bipolar disorder [203], more recent double-blind controlled studies of gabapentin as adjunctive therapy to lithium or valproate and as monotherapy suggest it is no more effective than placebo for the treatment of mania [204,205]. There has been one case report suggesting that gabapentin may be useful for the treatment of adolescent mania, however, further controlled studies are necessary [206]. Gabapentin is generally well tolerated in children and adolescents [207,208] and may therefore be particularly useful for treating bipolar youth who also have an anxiety disorder [204].

Preliminary data from open studies suggest that topiramate has antimanic properties when used as adjunctive treatment and as monotherapy [209]. There is one case report of a bipolar child who was treated with topiramate and divalproex and experienced significant cognitive dysfunction [210]. Word-finding difficulties have been reported in up to one third of patients treated with topiramate [211]. Encephalopathy has also been reported in patients treated with topiramate, particularly when it is used concomitantly with valproate [212,213]. In contrast to other medications used to treat bipolar disorder, topiramate is associated with anorexia and weight loss [203,209], which is advantageous in some children and adolescents who have gained weight from treatment with other psychotropics.

Preliminary uncontrolled data suggest effectiveness of other new antiepileptics, including tiagabine, oxcabamazepine, and zonisamide in adults with bipolar disorder. Currently, there are no reports of the effectiveness of these medications for the treatment of children and adolescents with bipolar disorder. Other new antiepileptic agents, which have not yet been investigated in the treatment of patients with bipolar disorder, include levetiracetam and vigabatrin.

3. Atypical Antipsychotics

There have been several case series and open-label reports suggesting that atypical antipsychotics such as clozapine [214–216] olanzapine [217–219], risperidone [220], and quetiapine [221,222] are effective for the treatment of pediatric bipolar disorder. In a more recent double-blind placebo-controlled study of 30 manic or mixed adolescents, quetiapine in combination with divalproex was found to reduce symptoms of mania, depression, and psychosis better than divalproex monotherapy, suggesting that quetiapine is effective for the treatment of adolescents with bipolar disorder. In this study, quetiapine was titrated to a dose of 450 mg/day and was well tolerated. Sedation was the most common side effect reported in both treatment groups [223].

4. Other Pharmacological Agents

Although open-label and controlled data are lacking, other psychotropic medications such as nimodipine, a calcium channel blocker [224] melatonin [225], and omega-3 fatty acids may be effective for the treatment of pediatric bipolar disorder.

Stimulant medications may be effective for the treatment of comorbid ADHD in children and adolescents with bipolar disorder; however, adequate mood stabilization with the other pharmacological treatments is necessary prior to initiating stimulant medications [43,226].

5. Treatment of Bipolar Disorders

It is reasonable to maintain a child or adolescent who has had a single manic episode on a mood-stabilizing agent for 12–18 months, and then if he or she is euthymic and asymptomatic to gradually reduce the mood stabilizing agent over 2–3 months [227]. If manic symptoms recur, the mood-stabilizing agent should be reintroduced. If the child is not responding or partially responding to a mood stabilizer, the addition of a second mood stabilizer or an atypical antipsychotic might be required.

Some bipolar children and adolescents maintained on a mood-stabilizing agent may develop a depressive episode after an acute manic episode and while maintained on a mood-stabilizing agent. The role of antidepressants in the treatment of bipolar depression remains unclear. Lithium is considered the first-line therapy for the treatment of acute bipolar depression in adults, since recent evidence supports that typical antidepressants may exacerbate the course of bipolar disorder by precipitating mixed or manic states [228]. However, in children and adolescents the efficacy of lithium in the treatment of bipolar depression is unclear. Recently, in a retrospective chart review and the only report to assess the treatment of bipolar depression in children and adolescents, Biederman and colleagues [229] found that depressive symptoms were 6.7 times more likely to improve when patients received an SSRI than when they did not. In contrast, tricyclics, stimulants, mood stabilizers, and typical antipsychotics were not significantly associated with improvement in depressive symptomatology. SSRIs may have mood-destabilizing effects; however, because too few subjects were being treated with mood stabilizers at the time when manic symptoms reemerged, the authors did not evaluate the protective effects of mood stabilizers in preventing the destabilizing effects.

Other antidepressants, such as bupropion, may be less likely to precipitate manic symptoms [230], although some reports suggest that this may not be the case [231]. Nonetheless, when treating a bipolar child with antidepressants, it is important to monitor the patient's mood and behavior carefully for any signs of mania, since these agents may sometimes precipitate a manic episode.

There have been no treatment studies involving children and adolescents with hypomania (bipolar II disorder), cyclothymia, or bipolar NOS. Mood stabilizers, as well as antidepressants, may be effective in treating these disorders; however, future investigations are necessary [232].

A multimodal treatment approach, combining psychopharmacological and psychotherapeutic therapies for pediatric bipolar disorders, is almost always useful. The psychotherapeutic strategies previously discussed for depressive disorders in children and adolescents may also be indicated for the management of bipolar disorders. However, psychotherapeutic interventions have not been systematically studied in bipolar youth. It is necessary to educate children and adolescents and their families and teachers about bipolar illness, the importance of medication compliance, and the need for regular monitoring of mood stabilizer serum levels and other laboratory measures. Instructing patients and/or their parents to keep a daily record of the level of depressive and manic symptoms ("mood charting") is a tool that may help monitor symptom presence and recurrence [233].

V. FUTURE DIRECTIONS

The recognition and treatment of pediatric mood disorders remains a major challenge for clinicians. Despite recent advances in the field, investigations in the areas of outcome, neurobiology, and treatments are necessary to advance our understanding of depressive and bipolar disorders in children and adolescents.

REFERENCES

1. DA Brent. Depression and suicide in children and adolescents. Pediatr Rev 14:380–388, 1993.
2. PM Lewinsohn, DN Klein, JR Seeley. Bipolar disorder during adolescence and young adulthood in a community sample. Bipolar Disord 2:281–293, 2000.
3. B Geller, B Zimerman, M Williams, K Bolhofner, JL Craney, MP DelBello, CA Soutullo. Diagnostic characteristics of 93 cases of a prepubertal and early adolescent bipolar disorder phenotype by gender, puberty and comorbid attention deficit hyperactivity disorder. J Child Adolesc Psychopharmacol 10:157–164, 2000.
4. B Geller, B Zimerman, M Williams, K Bolhofner, JL Craney, MP DelBello, CA Soutullo. Six-month stability and outcome of a prepubertal and early adolescent bipolar disorder phenotype. J Child Adolesc Psychopharmacol 10:165–173, 2000.
5. B Geller, J Luby. Child and adolescent bipolar disorder: a review of the past 10 years. J Am Acad Child Adolesc Psychiatry 36:1168–1176, 1997.
6. HE Rie. Depression in childhood. A survey of some pertinent contributions. J Am Acad Child Psychiatry 5:653–685, 1966.
7. D Cicchetti, FA Rogosch, SL Toth, M Spagnola. Affect, cognition, and the emergence of self-knowledge in the toddler offspring of depressed mothers. J Exp Child Psychol 67:338–362, 1997.
8. RA Kowatch, GJ Emslie, BD Kemmard. Mood disorders In: DX Parmelee, ed. Child and Adolescent Psychiatry. St. Louis: Mosby–Year Book, 1996, pp 121–140.
9. K Burke, J Burke, D Rae, D Regier. Comparing age at onset of major depression and other psychiatric disorders by birth cohorts in five US community populations. Arch Gen Psychiatry 48:789–795, 1991.
10. J Fleming, D Offord. Epidemiology of childhood depressive disorders: a critical review. J Am Acad Child Adolesc Psychiatry 29:571–580, 1990.
11. JH Kashani, NC Beck, EW Hoeper, C Fallahi, CM Corcoran, JA McAllister, TK Rosenberg, JC Reid. Psychiatric disorders in a community sample of adolescents. Am J Psychiatry 144:584–589, 1987.
12. J Kashani, G Carlson, N Beck, E Hoeper, C Corcoran, J McAllister, C Fallahi, T Rosenberg, J Reid. Depression, depressive symptoms, and depressed mood among a community sample of adolescents. Am J Psychiatry 144:931–934, 1987.
13. P Lewinsohn, E Duncan, A Stanton, M Hantzine. Age at onset for first unipolar depression. J Abnorm Psychol 95:387–393, 1986.
14. P Lewinsohn, H Hops, R Roberts, J Seeley, J Andrews. Adolescent psychopathology. 1. Prevalence and incidence of depression and other DSM-III-R disorders in high school students. J Abnorm Psychol 102:133–144, 1993.

15. P Lewinsohn, G Clarke, J Seeley, P Rhodes. Major depression in community adolescents: age at onset, episode duration, and time to recurrence. J Am Acad Child Adolesc Psychiatry 33:809–818, 1994.
16. D Shaffer, P Fisher, M Dulcan, M Davies, J Piacentini, M Schwab-Stone, B Lahey, K Bourdon, P Jensen, H Bird, G Canino, D Regier. The NIMH diagnostic interview schedule for children version 2.3 (DISC-2.3): description, acceptability, prevalence rates, and performance in the MECA study. Methods for the epidemiology of child and adolescent mental disorders study. J Am Acad Child Adolesc Psychiatry 35:865–877, 1996.
17. R Kessler, K McGonagle, C Nelson, M Hughes, M Swartz, D Blazer. Sex and depression in the national comorbidity survey. II. Cohort effects. J Affect Disord 30:15–26, 1994.
18. G Emslie, W Weinberg, A Rush, R Adams, J Rintelmann. Depressive symptoms by self report in adolescence: phase I of the development of a questionnaire for depression by self-report. J Child Neurol 3:114–121, 1990.
19. B Birmaher, ND Ryan, DE Williamson, DA Brent, J Kaufman, RE Dahl, J Perel, B Nelson. Childhood and adolescent depression: a review of the past 10 years. Part I. J Am Acad Child Adolesc Psychiatry 35:1427–1439, 1996.
20. EB Weller, RA Weller. Depression in adolescents growing pains or true morbidity? J Affect Disord 61(suppl 1):9–13, 2000.
21. J Wozniak, J Biederman, K Kiely, JS Ablon, SV Faraone, E Mundy, D Mennin. Mania-like symptoms suggestive of childhood-onset bipolar disorder in clinically referred children. J Am Acad Child Adolesc Psychiatry 34:867–876, 1995.
22. PM Lewinsohn, DN Klein, JR Seeley. Bipolar disorders in a community sample of older adolescents: prevalence, phenomenology, comorbidity, and course. J Am Acad Child Adolesc Psychiatry 34:454–463, 1995.
23. B Geller, B Zimerman, M Williams, K Bolhofner, JL Craney. Bipolar disorder at prospective follow-up of adults who had prepubertal major depressive disorder. Am J Psychiatry 158:125–127, 2001.
24. American Psychiatric Services. Diagnostic and Statistical Manual of Mental Disorders, 4th ed. Washington; DC: Author, 1994.
25. M Kovacs, HS Akiskal, C Gatsonis, PL Parrone. Childhood-onset dysthymic disorder. Clinical features and prospective naturalistic outcome. Arch Gen Psychiatry 51:365–374, 1994.
26. H Bird, G Canino, M Rubio-Stipec, M Gould, J Ribera, A Sanchez-Lacay, M Moscoso. Estimates of the prevalence of childhood maladjustment in a community survey on Puerto Rico: the use of combined measures. Arch Gen Psychiatry 45:1078–1084, 1988.
27. M Kovacs, S Paulauskas, C Gatsonis, C Richards. Depressive disorders in childhood. III. A longitudinal study of comorbidity with and risk for conduct disorders. J Affect Disord 15:205–217, 1988.
28. O Bukstein, L Glancy, Y Kaminer. Patterns of affective comorbidity in a clinical population of dually diagnosed adolescent substance abusers. J Am Acad Child Adolesc Psychiatry 31:1041–1045, 1992.
29. M Kovacs, C Gatsonis, SL Paulauskas, C Richards. Depressive disorders in childhood. IV. A longitudinal study of comorbidity with and risk for anxiety disorders. Arch Gen Psychiatry 46:776–782, 1989.
30. M Stein, M Fuetsch, N Muller, M Hofler, R Lieb, H Wittchen. Social anxiety disorder and the risk of depression: a prospective community study of adolescents and young adults. Arch Gen Psychiatry 58:251–256, 2001.
31. WA Weinberg, GJ Emslie. Attention deficit hyperactivity disorder: the differential diagnosis. J Child Neurol 6:S23–36, 1991.
32. G Masi, L Favilla, M Mucci, P Poli, R Romano. Depressive symptoms in children and adolescents with dysthymic disorder. Psychopathology 34:29–35, 2001.
33. J Biederman, S Faraone, E Mick, J Wozniak, L Chen, C Ouellette, A Marrs, P Moore, J Garcia, D Mennin, E Lelon. Attention-deficit hyperactivity disorder and juvenile mania: an overlooked comorbidity? J Am Acad Child Adolesc Psychiatry 35:997–1008, 1996.
34. SV Faraone, J Biederman, D Mennin, J Wozniak, T Spencer. Attention-deficit hyperactivity disorder with bipolar disorder: a familial subtype? J Am Acad Child Adolesc Psychiatry 36:1378–1387, 1997.
35. JN Giedd. Bipolar disorder and attention-deficit/hyperactivity disorder in children and adolescents. J Clin Psychiatry 61:31–34, 2000.
36. SM Schneider, DR Atkinson, RS el-Mallakh. CD and ADHD in bipolar disorder. J Am Acad Child Adolesc Psychiatry 35:1422–1423, 1996.
37. SA West, SL McElroy, SM Strakowski, PE Keck Jr, BJ McConville. Attention deficit hyperactivity disorder in adolescent mania. Am J Psychiatry 152:271–273, 1995.
38. MP DelBello, CA Soutullo, W Hendricks, RT Niemeier, SL McElroy, SM Strakowski. Prior stimulant treatment in adolescents with bipolar disorder: association with age at onset. Bipolar Disord 3:53–57, 2001.
39. RA Kowatch, T Suppes, TJ Carmody, JP Bucci, JH Hume, M Kromelis, GJ Emslie, WA Weinberg, AJ Rush. Effect size of lithium, divalproex sodium, and carbamazepine in children and adolescents with bipolar disorder. J Am Acad Child Adolesc Psychiatry 39:713–720, 2000.
40. SV Faraone, J Biederman, J Wozniak, E Mundy, D Mennin, D O'Donnell. Is comorbidity with ADHD a

marker for juvenile-onset mania? J Am Acad Child Adolesc Psychiatry 36:1046–1055, 1997.
41. S Milberger, J Biederman, SV Faraone, J Murphy, MT Tsuang. Attention deficit hyperactivity disorder and comorbid disorders: issues of overlapping symptoms. Am J Psychiatry 152:1793–1799, 1995.
42. B Geller, M Williams, B Zimerman, J Frazier, L Beringer, KL Warner. Prepubertal and early adolescent bipolarity differentiate from ADHD by manic symptoms, grandiose delusions, ultrarapid or ultradian cycling. J Affect Disord 51:81–91, 1998.
43. J Biederman, R Russell, J Soriano, J Wozniak, SV Faraone. Clinical features of children with both ADHD and mania: does ascertainment source make a difference? J Affect Disord 51:101–112, 1998.
44. SV Faraone, J Biederman, MC Monuteaux. Attention deficit hyperactivity disorder with bipolar disorder in girls: further evidence for a familial subtype? J Affect Disord 64:19–26, 2001.
45. M Kovacs, M Pollock. Bipolar disorder and comorbid conduct disorder in childhood and adolescence. J Am Acad Child Adolesc Psychiatry 34:715–723, 1995.
46. TE Wilens, J Biederman, RB Millstein, J Wozniak, AL Hahesy, TJ Spencer. Risk for substance use disorders in youths with child- and adolescent-onset bipolar disorder. J Am Acad Child Adolesc Psychiatry 38:680–685, 1999.
47. J Biederman, SV Faraone, J Wozniak, MC Monuteaux. Parsing the association between bipolar, conduct, and substance use disorders: a familial risk analysis. Biol Psychiatry 48:1037–1044, 2000.
48. J Wozniak, J Biederman. Mania in children with PDD. J Am Acad Child Adolesc Psychiatry 36:1646–1647, 1997.
49. J Wozniak, J Biederman, SV Faraone, J Frazier, J Kim, R Millstein, J Gershon, A Thornell, K Cha, JB Snyder. Mania in children with pervasive developmental disorder revisited. J Am Acad Child Adolesc Psychiatry 36:1552–1559, 1997.
50. MA Fristad, EB Weller, RA Weller. The Mania Rating Scale: can it be used in children? A preliminary report. J Am Acad Child Adolesc Psychiatry 31:252–257, 1992.
51. B Geller, K Bolhofner, JL Craney, M Williams, MP DelBello, K Gundersen. Psychosocial functioning in a prepubertal and early adolescent bipolar disorder phenotype. J Am Acad Child Adolesc Psychiatry 39:1543–1548, 2000.
52. M Kovacs, TL Feinberg, MA Crouse-Novak, SL Paulauskas, R Finkelstein. Depressive disorders in childhood. I. A longitudinal prospective study of characteristics and recovery. Arch Gen Psychiatry 41:229–237, 1984.
53. V Warner, MM Weissman, M Fendrich, P Wickramaratne, D Moreau. The course of major depression in the offspring of depressed parents. Incidence, recurrence, and recovery. Arch Gen Psychiatry 49:795–801, 1992.
54. M Strober, C Lampert, S Schmidt, W Morrell. The course of major depressive disorder in adolescents. I. Recovery and risk of manic switching in a follow-up of psychotic and nonpsychotic subtypes. J Am Acad Child Adolesc Psychiatry 32:34–42, 1993.
55. U Rao, ND Ryan, B Birmaher, RE Dahl, DE Williamson, J Kaufman, R Rao, B Nelson. Unipolar depression in adolescents: clinical outcome in adulthood. J Am Acad Child Adolesc Psychiatry 34:566–578, 1995.
56. E McCauley, K Myers, J Mitchell, R Calderon, K Schloredt, R Treder. Depression in young people: initial presentation and clinical course. J Am Acad Child Adolesc Psychiatry 32:714–722, 1993.
57. J Garber, M Kriss, M Koch, L Lindholm. Recurrent depression in adolescents: a follow-up study. J Am Acad Child Adolesc Psychiatry 27:49–54, 1988.
58. J Asarnow, M Goldstein, G Carlson, S Perdue, S Bates, J Keller. Childhood-onset depressive disorders. A follow-up study of rates of rehospitalization and out-of-home placement among child psychiatry inpatients. J Affect Disord 15:245–253, 1988.
59. G Emslie, A Rush, W Weinberg. Recurrence of major depressive disorder in hospitalized children and adolescents. J Am Acad Child Adolesc Psychiatry 36:785–792, 1997.
60. M Kovacs, T Feinberg, M Crouse-Novak. Depressive disorders in childhood. II. A longitudinal study of the risk for a subsequent major depression. Arch Gen Psychiatry 41:643–649, 1984.
61. EO Poznanski, V Krahenbuhl, JP Zrull. Childhood depression. A longitudinal perspective. J Am Acad Child Psychiatry 15:491–501, 1976.
62. J Eastgate, L Gilmore. Long-term outcome of depressed children: a follow-up study. Dev Med Child Neurol 26:67–72, 1984.
63. D Kandal, M Davies. Adult sequela of adolescent depressive symptoms. Arch Gen Psychiatry 43:255–262, 1986.
64. R Harrington, H Fudge, M Rutter, J Hill. Adult outcomes of childhood and adolescent depression. Arch Gen Psychiatry 47:465–473, 1990.
65. MM Weissman, S Wolk, RB Goldstein, D Moreau, P Adams, S Greenwald, CM Klier, ND Ryan, RE Dahl, P Wickramaratne. Depressed adolescents grown up. JAMA 281:1707–1713, 1999.
66. M Strober, G Carlson. Bipolar illness in adolescents with major depression: clinical, genetic, and psychopharmacologic predictors in a three- to four-year prospective follow-up investigation. Arch Gen Psychiatry 39:549–555, 1982.
67. B Geller, LW Fox, KA Clark. Rate and predictors of prepubertal bipolarity during follow-up of 6- to 12-

year-old depressed children. J Am Acad Child Adolesc Psychiatry 33:461–468, 1994.
68. T McGlashen. Adolescent versus adult onset of mania. Am J Psychiatry 145:221–223, 1988.
69. B Geller, JL Craney, K Bolhofner, MP DelBello, M Williams, B Zimerman. One-year recovery and relapse rates of children with a prepubertal and early adolescent bipolar disorder phenotype. Am J Psychiatry 158:303–305, 2001.
70. M Bashir, J Russell, G Johnson. Bipolar affective disorder in adolescence: a 10-year study. Aust NZ J Psychiatry 21:36–43, 1987.
71. M Strober, S Schmidt-Lackner, R Freeman, S Bower, C Lampert, M DeAntonio. Recovery and relapse in adolescents with bipolar affective illness: a five-year naturalistic, prospective follow-up. J Am Acad Child Adolesc Psychiatry 34:724–731, 1995.
72. D Shaffer, M Goud, P Fisher, P Trautman, D Moreau, M Kleinman, M Flory. Psychiatric diagnosis in child and adolescent suicide. Arch Gen Psychiatry 53:339–348, 1996.
73. GA Carlson, EJ Bromet, S Sievers. Phenomenology and outcome of subjects with early- and adult-onset psychotic mania. Am J Psychiatry 157:213–219, 2000.
74. T Todd, AC Heath, KN Botteron, RJ Neuman, W Reich. Heritability of adolescent onset major depressive disorder: a longitudinal perspective. Mol Psychiatry 4:169, 1999.
75. J Puig-Antich, D Goetz, M Davies, T Kaplan, S Davies, L Ostrow, L Asnis, J Twomey, S Iyengar, ND Ryan. A controlled family history study of prepubertal major depressive disorder. Arch Gen Psychiatry 46:406–418, 1989.
76. MM Weissman, P Wickramaratne, KR Merikangas, JF Leckman, BA Prusoff, KA Caruso, KK Kidd, GD Gammon. Onset of major depression in early adulthood. Increased familial loading and specificity. Arch Gen Psychiatry 41:1136–1143, 1984.
77. MM Weissman, V Warner, P Wickramaratne, BA Prusoff. Early-onset major depression in parents and their children. J Affect Disord 15:269–277, 1988.
78. PJ Wickramaratne, S Greenwald, MM Weissman. Psychiatric disorders in the relatives of probands with prepubertal-onset or adolescent-onset major depression. J Am Acad Child Adolesc Psychiatry 39:1396–1405, 2000.
79. M Kovacs, B Devlin, M Pollock, C Richards, P Mukerji. A controlled family history study of childhood-onset depressive disorder. Arch Gen Psychiatry 54:613–623, 1997.
80. RD Todd, B Geller, R Neuman, LW Fox, J Hickok. Increased prevalence of alcoholism in relatives of depressed and bipolar children. J Am Acad Child Adolesc Psychiatry 35:716–724, 1996.

81. MP DelBello, B Geller. Review of studies of child and adolescent offspring of bipolar parents. Bipolar Disord 3:325–334, 2001.
82. B Geller, EH Cook, Jr. Ultradian rapid cycling in prepubertal and early adolescent bipolarity is not in transmission disequilibrium with val/met COMT alleles. Biol Psychiatry 47:605–609, 2000.
83. B Geller, EH Cook Jr. Serotonin transporter gene (HTTLPR) is not in linkage disequilibrium with prepubertal and early adolescent bipolarity. Biol Psychiatry 45:1230–1233, 1999.
84. C Carlson, D Papolos, RK Pandita, GL Faedda, S Veit, R Goldberg, R Shprintzen, R Kucherlapati, B Morrow. Molecular analysis of velo-cardio-facial syndrome patients with psychiatric disorders. Am J Hum Genet 60:851–859, 1997.
85. AJ Rush, R Stewart, D Garver, D Waller. Neurobiological bases for psychiatric disorders. In: R Rosenberg, D Pleasure, eds. Comprehensive Neurology. New York: John Wiley & Sons, 1998, pp 887–919.
86. M Mesulan. Large-scale neurocognitive networks and distributed processing for attention, language, and memory. Ann Neurol 28:597–613, 1990.
87. HA Sackeim, I Prohovnik, JR Moeller, RP Brown, S Apter, J Prudic, DP Devanand, S Mukherjee. Regional cerebral blood flow in mood disorders. I. Comparison of major depressives and normal controls at rest. Arch Gen Psychiatry 47:60–70, 1990.
88. JC Soares, JJ Mann. The functional neuroanatomy of mood disorders. J Psychiatr Res 31:393–432, 1997.
89. JC Soares, JJ Mann. The anatomy of mood disorders—review of structural neuroimaging studies. Biol Psychiatry 41:86–106, 1997.
90. SM Strakowski, MP DelBello, C Adler, DM Cecil, KW Sax. Neuroimaging in bipolar disorder. Bipolar Disord 2:148–164, 2000.
91. J Coyle. Biochemical development of the brain: neurotransmitters and child psychiatry. In: Psychiatric Pharmacosciences of Children and Adolescents. Washington; American Psychiatric Press, 1987.
92. P Gold, F Goodwin, G Chrousos. Clinical and biochemical manifestations of depression: relation to the neurobiology of stress. N Engl J Med 319:348–353, 413–420, 1988.
93. P Willner. Depression: A Psychobiological Synthesis New York; John Wiley & Sons, 1985.
94. G Zubenko, J Moossy, U Kopp. Neurochemical correlates of major depression in primary dementia. Arch Neurol 47:209–214, 1990.
95. W Bunney, J Davis. Norepinephrine in depressive reactions: a review. Arch Gen Psychiatry 13:483–494, 1965.
96. R Golden, W Potter. Neurochemical and neuroendocrine dysregulation in affective disorders. Psychiatr Clin North Am 9:313–327, 1986.

97. A Schatzberg, P Orsulak, A Rosenbaum, M Salomon, J Lerbinger, P Kizuka, J Cole, J Schildkraut. Toward a biochemical classification of depressive disorders. V. Herterogeneity of unipolar depression. Am J Psychiatry 139:471–475, 1982.

98. A DeVilliers, V Russell, M Carstens, J Searson, AV Zyl, C Lonbard, J Taljaard. Noradrenergic function and hypothalamic-pituitary-adrenal axis activity in adolescents with major depressive disorder. Psychiatry Res 27:101–109, 1989.

99. H Agren. Symptom patterns in unipolar depression correlating with monoamine metabolites in cerebrospinal fluid. I. General patterns. Psychiatry Res 3:211–223, 1980.

100. R Glennon. Central serotonin receptors as targets for drug research. J Med Chem 30:1–12, 1987.

101. A Prange, I Wilson, C Lynn, L Alltop, R Stikeleather. L-tryptophan in mania: contribution to a permissive hypothesis of affective disorders. Arch Gen Psychiatry 30:56–62, 1974.

102. H VanPraag. Depression and Schizophrenia: A Contribution on Their Chemical Pathologies. New York: Spectrum Publications, 1977.

103. ND Ryan, B Birmaher, JM Perel, RE Dahl, V Meyer, M al-Shabbout, S Iyengar, J Puig-Antich. Neuroendocrine response to L-5-hydroxytryptophan challenge in prepubertal major depression. Depressed vs normal children. Arch Gen Psychiatry 49:843–851, 1992.

104. B Birmaher, J Kaufman, DA Brent, RE Dahl, JM Perel, M al-Shabbout, B Nelson, S Stull, U Rao, GS Waterman, DE Williamson, ND Ryan. Neuroendocrine response to 5-hydroxy-L-tryptophan in prepubertal children at high risk of major depressive disorder. Arch Gen Psychiatry 54:1113–1119, 1997.

105. GA Rogeness, MA Javors, SR Pliszka. Neurochemistry and child and adolescent psychiatry. J Am Acad Child Adolesc Psychiatry 31:765–781, 1992.

106. B Birmaher, RE Dahl, ND Ryan, H Rabinovich, P Ambrosini, M al-Shabbout, H Novacenko, B Nelson, J Puig-Antich. The dexamethasone suppression test in adolescent outpatients with major depressive disorder. Am J Psychiatry 149:1040–1045, 1992.

107. B Birmaher, ND Ryan, R Dahl, H Rabinovich, P Ambrosini, DE Williamson, H Novacenko, B Nelson, ES Lo, J Puig-Antich. Dexamethasone suppression test in children with major depressive disorder. J Am Acad Child Adolesc Psychiatry 31:291–297, 1992.

108. J Puig-Antich, R Dahl, N Ryan, H Novacenko, D Goetz, J Twomey, T Klepper. Cortisol secretion in prepubertal children with major depressive disorder. Arch Gen Psychiatry 46:801–809, 1989.

109. S Kutcher, D Malkin, J Silverberg, P Marton, P Williamson, A Malkin, J Szalai, M Katic. Nocturnal cortisol, thyroid stimulating hormone, and growth hormone secretory profiles in depressed adolescents. J Am Acad Child Adolesc Psychiatry 30:407–414, 1991.

110. R Dahl, J Puig-Antich, N Ryan, B Nelson, H Novacenko, J Twomey, D Williamson, R Goetz, PJ Ambrosini. Cortisol secretion in adolescents with major depressive disorder. Acta Psychiatr Scand 80:18–26, 1989.

111. U Rao, RE Dahl, ND Ryan, B Birmaher, DE Williamson, DE Giles, R Rao, J Kaufman, B Nelson. The relationship between longitudinal clinical course and sleep and cortisol changes in adolescent depression. Biol Psychiatry 40:474–484, 1996.

112. M De Bellis, R Dahl, J Perel. Nocturnal ACTH, cortisol, growth hormone, and prolactin secretion in prepubertal depression. J Am Acad Child Adolesc Psychiatry 35:1130–1138, 1996.

113. B Birmaher, RE Dahl, J Perel, DE Williamson, B Nelson, S Stull, J Kaufman, GS Waterman, U Rao, N Nguyen, J Puig-Antich, ND Ryan. Corticotropin-releasing hormone challenge in prepubertal major depression. Biol Psychiatry 39:267–277, 1996.

114. J Kaufman, B Birmaher, J Perel, RE Dahl, P Moreci, B Nelson, W Wells, ND Ryan. The corticotropin-releasing hormone challenge in depressed abused, depressed nonabused, and normal control children. Biol Psychiatry 42:669–679, 1997.

115. E Poznanski, J Carroll, M Banegas, S Cook, J Grossman. The dexamethasone suppression test in prepubertal depressed children. Am J Psychiatry 139:321–324, 1982.

116. I Extein, G Rosenberg, A Pottash, M Gold. The dexamethasone suppression test in depressed adolescents. Am J Psychiatry 139:1617–1619, 1982.

117. D Robbins, N Alessi, G Yanchyshyn, M Colfer. Preliminary report on the dexamethasone suppression test in adolescents. Am J Psychiatry 139:942–943, 1982.

118. M Doherty, D Madansky, J Kraft. Cortisol dynamics and test performance of the dexamethasone suppression test in 97 psychiatrically hospitalized children aged 3–16 years. J Am Acad Child Psychiatry 25:400–408, 1986.

119. G Emslie, W Weinberg, A Rush, J Weissenburger, L Parkin-Feigenbaum. Depression and dexamethasone suppression testing in children and adolescents. J Child Neurol 2:31–37, 1987.

120. RE Dahl, ND Ryan, DE Williamson, PJ Ambrosini, H Rabinovich, H Novacenko, B Nelson, J Puig-Antich. Regulation of sleep and growth hormone in adolescent depression. J Am Acad Child Adolesc Psychiatry 31:615–621, 1992.

121. ND Ryan, RE Dahl, B Birmaher, DE Williamson, S Iyengar, B Nelson, J Puig-Antich, JM Perel. Stimulatory tests of growth hormone secretion in prepubertal major depression: depressed versus normal children. J Am Acad Child Adolesc Psychiatry 33:824–833, 1994.

122. RE Dahl, B Birmaher, DE Williamson, L Dorn, J Perel, J Kaufman, DA Brent, DA Axelson, ND Ryan. Low growth hormone response to growth hormone-releasing hormone in child depression. Biol Psychiatry 48:981–988, 2000.
123. J Puig-Antich, R Goetz, M Davies, M Fein, C Hanlon, WJ Chambers, MA Tabrizi, EJ Sachar, ED Weitzman. Growth hormone secretion in prepubertal children with major depression. II. Sleep-related plasma concentrations during a depressive episode. Arch Gen Psychiatry 41:463–466, 1984.
124. B Birmaher, RE Dahl, DE Williamson, JM Perel, DA Brent, DA Axelson, J Kaufman, LD Dorn, S Stull, U Rao, ND Ryan. Growth hormone secretion in children and adolescents at high risk for major depressive disorder. Arch Gen Psychiatry 57:867–872, 2000.
125. LD Dorn, RE Dahl, B Birmaher, DE Williamson, J Kaufman, L Frisch, JM Perel, ND Ryan. Baseline thyroid hormones in depressed and non-depressed pre- and early-pubertal boys and girls. J Psychiatr Res 31:555–567, 1997.
126. SA West, KW Sax, SP Stanton, PE Keck Jr, SL McElroy, SM Strakowski. Differences in thyroid function studies in acutely manic adolescents with and without attention deficit hyperactivity disorder (ADHD). Psychopharmacol Bull 32:63–66, 1996.
127. GJ Emslie, AJ Rush, WA Weinberg, JW Rintelmann, HP Roffwarg. Children with major depression show reduced rapid eye movement latencies. Arch Gen Psychiatry 47:119–124, 1990.
128. RE Dahl, ND Ryan, B Birmaher, M al-Shabbout, DE Williamson, M Neidig, B Nelson, J Puig-Antich. Electroencephalographic sleep measures in prepubertal depression. Psychiatry Res 38:201–214, 1991.
129. J Puig-Antich, R Goetz, C Hanlon, M Davies, J Thompson, WJ Chambers, MA Tabrizi, ED Weitzman. Sleep architecture and REM sleep measures in prepubertal children with major depression: a controlled study. Arch Gen Psychiatry 39:932–939, 1982.
130. W Young, JB Knowles, AW MacLean, L Boag, BJ McConville. The sleep of childhood depressives: comparison with age-matched controls. Biol Psychiatry 17:1163–1168, 1982.
131. J Puig-Antich, R Goetz, C Hanlon, MA Tabrizi, M Davies, ED Weitzman. Sleep architecture and REM sleep measures in prepubertal major depressives. Studies during recovery from the depressive episode in a drug-free state. Arch Gen Psychiatry 40:187–192, 1983.
132. RR Goetz, J Puig-Antich, N Ryan, H Rabinovich, PJ Ambrosini, B Nelson, V Krawiec. Electroencephalographic sleep of adolescents with major depression and normal controls. Arch Gen Psychiatry 44:61–68, 1987.
133. J Appleboon-Fondu, M Kerkofs, J Mendlewicz. Depression in adolescents and young adults: polysomnographic and neuroendocrine aspects. J Affect Disord 14:35–40, 1988.
134. RE Dahl, J Puig-Antich, ND Ryan, B Nelson, S Dachille, SL Cunningham, L Trubnick, TP Klepper. EEG sleep in adolescents with major depression: the role of suicidality and inpatient status. J Affect Disord 19:63–75, 1990.
135. RE Dahl, ND Ryan, MK Matty, B Birmaher, M al-Shabbout, DE Williamson, DJ Kupfer. Sleep onset abnormalities in depressed adolescents. Biol Psychiatry 39:400–410, 1996.
136. GJ Emslie, AJ Rush, WA Weinberg, JW Rintelmann, HP Roffwarg. Sleep EEG features of adolescents with major depression. Biol Psychiatry 36:573–581, 1994.
137. A Kahn, S Todd. Polysomnographic findings in adolescents with major depression. Psychiatry Res 33:313–320, 1990.
138. S Kutcher, P Williamson, P Marton, J Szalai. REM latency in endogenously depressed adolescents. Br J Psychiatry 161:399–402, 1992.
139. HW Lahmeyer, EO Poznanski, SN Bellur. EEG sleep in depressed adolescents. Am J Psychiatry 140:1150–1153, 1983.
140. RL Hendren, JE Hodde-Vargas, LA Vargas, WW Orrison, L Dell. Magnetic resonance imaging of severely disturbed children—a preliminary study. J Am Acad Child Adolesc Psychiatry 30:466–470, 1991.
141. RJ Steingard, PF Renshaw, D Yurgelun-Todd, KE Appelmans, IK Lyoo, KL Shorrock, JP Bucci, M Cesena, D Abebe, D Zurakowski, TY Poussaint, P Barnes. Structural abnormalities in brain magnetic resonance images of depressed children. J Am Acad Child Adolesc Psychiatry 35:307–311, 1996.
142. WC Drevets, JL Price, JR Simpson Jr, RD Todd, T Reich, M Vannier, ME Raichle. Subgenual prefrontal cortex abnormalities in mood disorders. Nature 386:824–827, 1997.
143. CE Coffey, WE Wilkinson, RD Weiner, IA Parashos, WT Djang, MC Webb, GS Figiel, CE Spritzer. Quantitative cerebral anatomy in depression. A controlled magnetic resonance imaging study. Arch Gen Psychiatry 50:7–16, 1993.
144. KN Botteron, MW Vannier, B Geller, RD Todd, BC Lee. Preliminary study of magnetic resonance imaging characteristics in 8- to 16-year-olds with mania. J Am Acad Child Adolesc Psychiatry 34:742–749, 1995.
145. M Dasari, L Friedman, J Jesberger, TA Stuve, RL Findling, TP Swales, SC Schulz. A magnetic resonance imaging study of thalamic area in adolescent patients with either schizophrenia or bipolar disorder as compared to healthy controls. Psychiatry Res 91:155–162, 1999.
146. L Friedman, RL Findling, JT Kenny, TP Swales, TA Stuve, JA Jesberger, JS Lewin, SC Schulz. An MRI

study of adolescent patients with either schizophrenia or bipolar disorder as compared to healthy control subjects. Biol Psychiatry 46:78–88, 1999.
147. SM Strakowski, CM Adler, MP DelBello. Volumetric MRI studies of mood disorders: do they distinguish unipolar and bipolar disorder? Bipolar Disord 4:80–88, 2002.
148. RA Kowatch, MD Devous Sr, DC Harvey, TL Mayes, MH Trivedi, GJ Emslie, WA Weinberg. A SPECT HMPAO study of regional cerebral blood flow in depressed adolescents and normal controls. Prog Neuropsychopharmacol Biol Psychiatry 23:643–656, 1999.
149. A Tutus, M Kibar, S Sofuoglu, M Basturk, AS Gonul. A technetium-99m hexamethylpropylene amine oxime brain single-photon emission tomography study in adolescent patients with major depressive disorder. Eur J Nucl Med 25:601–606, 1998.
150. M Dahlstrom, A Ahonen, H Ebeling, P Torniainen, J Heikkila, I Moilanen. Elevated hypothalamic/midbrain serotonin (monoamine) transporter availability in depressive drug-naive children and adolescents. Mol Psychiatry 5:514–522, 2000.
151. RJ Steingard, DA Yurgelun-Todd, J Hennen, JC Moore, CM Moore, K Vakili, AD Young, A Katic, WR Beardslee, PF Renshaw. Increased orbitofrontal cortex levels of choline in depressed adolescents as detected by in vivo proton magnetic resonance spectroscopy. Biol Psychiatry 48:1053–1061, 2000.
152. M Castillo, L Kwock, H Courvoisie, SR Hooper. Proton MR spectroscopy in children with bipolar affective disorder: preliminary observations. AJNR 21:832–838, 2000.
153. HK Manji, G Chen, JK Hsiao, ED Risby, MI Masana, WZ Potter. Regulation of signal transduction pathways by mood-stabilizing agents: implications for the delayed onset of therapeutic efficacy. J Clin Psychiatry 57:34–46, 1996.
154. P Davanzo, MA Thomas, K Yue, T Oshiro, T Belin, M Strober, J McCracken. Decreased anterior cingulate myo-inositol/creatine spectroscopy resonance with lithium treatment in children with bipolar disorder. Neuropsychopharmacology 24:359–369, 2001.
155. B Birmaher, ND Ryan, DE Williamson, DA Brent, J Kaufman. Childhood and adolescent depression: a review of the past 10 years. Part II. J Am Acad Child Adolesc Psychiatry 35:1575–1583, 1996.
156. MA Riddle, JC Nelson, CS Kleinman, A Rasmusson, JF Leckman, RA King, DJ Cohen. Sudden death in children receiving Norpramin: a review of three reported cases and commentary. J Am Acad Child Adolesc Psychiatry 30:104–108, 1991.
157. MA Riddle, B Geller, N Ryan. Another sudden death in a child treated with desipramine. J Am Acad Child Adolesc Psychiatry 32:792–797, 1993.

158. B Geller, D Reising, HL Leonard, MA Riddle, BT Walsh. Critical review of tricyclic antidepressant use in children and adolescents. J Am Acad Child Adolesc Psychiatry 38:513–516, 1999.
159. RL Findling, MD Reed, JL Blumer. Pharmacological treatment of depression in children and adolescents. Paediatr Drugs 1:161–182, 1999.
160. GJ Emslie, JT Walkup, SR Pliszka, M Ernst. Nontricyclic antidepressants: current trends in children and adolescents. J Am Acad Child Adolesc Psychiatry 38:517–528, 1999.
161. JG Simeon, VF Dinicola, HB Ferguson, W Copping. Adolescent depression: a placebo-controlled fluoxetine treatment study and follow-up. Prog Neuropsychopharmacol Biol Psychiatry 14:791–795, 1990.
162. GJ Emslie, AJ Rush, WA Weinberg, RA Kowatch, CW Hughes, T Carmody, J Rintelmann. A double-blind, randomized, placebo-controlled trial of fluoxetine in children and adolescents with depression. Arch Gen Psychiatry 54:1031–1037, 1997.
163. PJ Ambrosini, MD Bianchi, H Rabinovich, J Elia. Antidepressant treatments in children and adolescents. I. Affective disorders. J Am Acad Child Adolesc Psychiatry 32:1–6, 1993.
164. BJ McConville, KL Minnery, MT Sorter, SA West, LM Friedman, K Christian. An open study of the effects of sertraline on adolescent major depression. J Child Adolesc Psychopharmacol 6:41–51, 1996.
165. MB Keller, ND Ryan, M Strober, RG Klein, SP Kutcher, B Birmaher, OR Hagino, H Koplewicz, GA Carlson, GN Clarke, GJ Emslie, D Feinberg, B Geller, V Kusumakar, G Papatheodorou, WH Sack, M Sweeney, KD Wagner, E Weller, NC Winters, R Oakes, JP McCafferty. Efficacy of paroxetine in the treatment of adolescent major depression: a randomized, controlled trial. J Am Acad Child Adolesc Psychiatry 40:762–772, 2001.
166. PJ Goodnick, CA Jorge, T Hunter, AM Kumar. Nefazodone treatment of adolescent depression: an open-label study of response and biochemistry. Ann Clin Psychiatry 12:97–100, 2000.
167. MW Mandoki, MR Tapia, MA Tapia, GS Sumner, JL Parker. Venlafaxine in the treatment of children and adolescents with major depression. Psychopharmacol Bull 33:149–154, 1997.
168. B Geller, TB Cooper, B Zimmerman, K Sun, M Williams, J Frazier. Double-blind, placebo controlled study of lithium for depressed children with bipolar family histories. Neuropsychopharmacology 10(S-122):541S, 1994.
169. N Ryan, V Meyer, S Dachille, D Mazzie, J Puig-Antich. Lithium antidepressant augmentation in TCA-refractory depression. J Am Acad Child Adolesc Psychiatry 27:371–376, 1988.
170. M Strober, R Freeman, J Rigali, S Schmidt, R Diamond. The pharmacotherapy of depressive illness

in adolescence. II. Effects of lithium augmentation in nonresponders to imipramine. J Am Acad Child Adolesc Psychiatry 31:16–20, 1992.
171. WB Daviss, P Bentivoglio, R Racusin, KM Brown, JQ Bostic, L Wiley. Bupropion sustained release in adolescents with comorbid attention-deficit/hyperactivity disorder and depression. J Am Acad Child Adolesc Psychiatry 40:307–314, 2001.
172. R Harrington, J Whittaker, P Shoebridge, F Campbell. Systematic review of efficacy of cognitive behaviour therapies in childhood and adolescent depressive disorder. BMJ 316:1559–1563, 1998.
173. DA Brent, D Holder, D Kolko, B Birmaher, M Baugher, C Roth, S Iyengar, BA Johnson. A clinical psychotherapy trial for adolescent depression comparing cognitive, family, and supportive therapy. Arch Gen Psychiatry 54:877–885, 1997.
174. B Birmaher, DA Brent, D Kolko, M Baugher, J Bridge, D Holder, S Iyengar, RE Ulloa. Clinical outcome after short-term psychotherapy for adolescents with major depressive disorder. Arch Gen Psychiatry 57:29–36, 2000.
175. L Mufson, MM Weissman, D Moreau, R Garfinkel. Efficacy of interpersonal psychotherapy for depressed adolescents. Arch Gen Psychiatry 56:573–579, 1999.
176. CW Hughes, GJ Emslie, M Crismon, KD Wagner, B Birmaher, B Geller, SR Pliszka, ND Ryan, M Strober, MH Trivedi, M Toprac, A Sedillo, M Llana, M Lopez, AJ Rush. The Texas Children's Medication Algorithm Project: report of the Texas Consensus Conference Panel on Medication Treatment of Childhood Major Depressive Disorder. J Am Acad Child Adolesc Psychiatry 38:1442–1454, 1999.
177. B Geller, TB Cooper, K Sun, B Zimerman, J Frazier, M Williams, J Heath. Double-blind and placebo-controlled study of lithium for adolescent bipolar disorders with secondary substance dependency. J Am Acad Child Adolesc Psychiatry 37:171–178, 1998.
178. M Strober, W Morrell, C Lampert, J Burroughs. Relapse following discontinuation of lithium maintenance therapy in adolescents with bipolar I illness: a naturalistic study. Am J Psychiatry 147:457–461, 1990.
179. J McClellan, J Werry. Practice parameters for the assessment and treatment of children and adolescents with bipolar disorder. J Am Acad Child Adolesc Psychiatry 36:157S-176S, 1997.
180. J Youngerman, I Canino. Lithium carbonate use in children and adolescents: a survey of the literature. Arch Gen Psychiatry 34:216–224, 1978.
181. L Gram, J Rafaelson. Lithium treatment of psychotic children and adolescents. A controlled clinical trial. Acta Psychiatr Scand 48:253–260, 1972.
182. B Lena, S Surtees, R Maggs. The efficacy of lithium in the treatment of emotional disturbances in children and adolescents. In: Johnson FN, Johnson S, eds. Lithium in Medical Practice. Lancaster, Eng. MTP Press 79–83, 1978.
183. D McKnew, L Cytryn, B MD, J Hammovit, M Lamour, J Rappoport, E Gershon. Lithium in children of lithium responding parents. Psychiatry Res 4:171–180, 1981.
184. G DeLong, G Nieman. Lithium-induced behavior changes in children with symptoms suggesting manic-depressive illness. Psychopharmacol Bull 19:258–265, 1983.
185. M Strober, W Morrell, J Burroughs, C Lampert, H Danforth, R Freeman. A family study of bipolar I disorder in adolescence. Early onset of symptoms linked to increased familial loading and lithium resistance. J Affect Disord 15:255–268, 1988.
186. M Strober, M DeAntonio, S Schmidt-Lackner, R Freeman, C Lampert, J Diamond. Early childhood attention deficit hyperactivity disorder predicts poorer response to acute lithium therapy in adolescent mania. J Affect Disord 51:145–151, 1998.
187. SP Kutcher, P Marton, M Korenblum. Adolescent bipolar illness and personality disorder. J Am Acad Child Adolesc Psychiatry 29:355–358, 1990.
188. JM Himmelhoch, ME Garfinkel. Sources of lithium resistance in mixed mania. Psychopharmacol Bull 22:613–620, 1986.
189. MP DelBello, RA Kowatch. Lithium. In: D Rosenberg, P Davanzo, S Gershon, eds. Textbook of Pharmacotherapy for Child and Adolescent Psychiatric Disorders. Brunner Mazel, (in press).
190. S West, P Keck, S McElroy, S Strakowski, K Minnery, B McConville, M Sorter. Open trial of valproate in the treatment of adolescent mania. J Child Adolesc Psychopharmacol 4:263–267, 1994.
191. G Papatheodorou, SP Kutcher. Divalproex sodium treatment in late adolescent and young adult acute mania. Psychopharmacol Bull 29:213–219, 1993.
192. G Papatheodorou, SP Kutcher, M Katic, JP Szalai. The efficacy and safety of divalproex sodium in the treatment of acute mania in adolescents and young adults: an open clinical trial. J Clin Psychopharmacol 15:110–116, 1995.
193. KD Wagner, E Weller, J Biederman, G Carlson, J Frazier, P Wozniak, C Bowden. Safety and efficacy of divalproex in childhood bipolar disorder in 47th Annual American Academy of Child & Adolescent Psychiatry Scientific Proceedings, New York, 2000, p 116.
194. JL Woolston Case study: carbamazepine treatment of juvenile-onset bipolar disorder. J Am Acad Child Adolesc Psychiatry 38:335–338, 1999.
195. LK Hsu. Lithium-resistant adolescent mania. J Am Acad Child Psychiatry 25:280–283, 1986.
196. CJ McDougle, AE Stern, ME Bangs. Bipolar disorder in children and adolescents. Part II. Valproate and

other newer treatments. Int Drug Ther News 36:1–8, 2001.
197. JI Isojarvi, TJ Laatikainen, AJ Pakarinen, KT Juntunen, VV Myllyla. Polycystic ovaries and hyperandrogenism in women taking valproate for epilepsy. N Engl J Med 329:1383–1388, 1993.
198. J Bauer, A Jarre, D Klingmuller, CE Elger. Polycystic ovary syndrome in patients with focal epilepsy: a study in 93 women. Epilepsy Res 41:163–167, 2000.
199. MW Mandoki. Lamotrigine/valproate in treatment resistant bipolar disorder in children and adolescents. Biol Psychiatry 41(suppl 7):321, 1997.
200. V Kusumakar, LN Yatham. Lamotrigine treatment of rapid cycling bipolar disorder. Am J Psychiatry 154:1171–1172, 1997.
201. A Sabers, L Gram. Newer anticonvulsants: comparative review of drug interactions and adverse effects. Drugs 60:23–33, 2000.
202. JA Messenheimer. Rash in adult and pediatric patients treated with lamotrigine. Can J Neurol Sci 25:S14–S18, 1998.
203. SL McElroy, PE Keck Jr. Pharmacologic agents for the treatment of acute bipolar mania. Biol Psychiatry 48:539–557, 2000.
204. AC Pande, JG Crockatt, CA Janney, JL Werth, G Tsaroucha. Gabapentin in bipolar disorder: a placebo-controlled trial of adjunctive therapy. Bipolar Disord 2:249–255, 2000.
205. MA Frye, TA Ketter, TA Kimbrell, RT Dunn, AM Speer, EA Osuch, DA Luckenbaugh, G Cora-Ocatelli, GS Leverich, RM Post. A placebo-controlled study of lamotrigine and gabapentin monotherapy in refractory mood disorders. J Clin Psychopharmacol 20:607–614, 2000.
206. CA Soutullo, LS Casuto, PE Keck Jr. Gabapentin in the treatment of adolescent mania: a case report. J Child Adolesc Psychopharmacol 8:81–85, 1998.
207. MJ McLean. Gabapentin. Epilepsia 36:S73–86, 1995.
208. DS Khurana, J Riviello, S Helmers, G Holmes, J Anderson, MA Mikati. Efficacy of gabapentin therapy in children with refractory partial seizures. J Pediatr 128:829–833, 1996.
209. SL McElroy, T Suppes, PE Keck, MA Frye, KD Denicoff, LL Altshuler, ES Brown, WA Nolen, RW Kupka, J Rochussen, GS Leverich, RM Post. Open-label adjunctive topiramate in the treatment of bipolar disorders. Biol Psychiatry 47:1025–1033, 2000.
210. P Davanzo, E Cantwell, J Kleiner, C Baltaxe, B Najera, G Crecelius, J McCracken. Cognitive changes during topiramate therapy. J Am Acad Child Adolesc Psychiatry 40:262–263, 2001.
211. P Crawford. An audit of topiramate use in a general neurology clinic. Seizure 7:207–211, 1998.
212. HM Hamer, S Knake, U Schomburg, F Rosenow. Valproate-induced hyperammonemic encephalopathy in the presence of topiramate. Neurology 54:230–232, 2000.
213. GE Solomon. Valproate-induced hyperammonemic encephalopathy in the presence of topiramate. Neurology 55:606, 2000.
214. G Masi, A Milone. Clozapine treatment in an adolescent with bipolar disorder. Panminerva Med 40:254–257, 1998.
215. DC Fuchs. Clozapine treatment of bipolar disorder in a young adolescent. J Am Acad Child Adolesc Psychiatry 33:1299–1302, 1994.
216. RA Kowatch, T Suppes, SK Gilfillan. Clozapine treatment of children and adolescents with bipolar disorder and schizophrenia: a clinical case series. J Child Adolesc Psychopharmacol 5:241–253, 1995.
217. CA Soutullo, MT Sorter, KD Foster, SL McElroy, PE Keck. Olanzapine in the treatment of adolescent acute mania: a report of seven cases. J Affect Disord 53:279–283, 1999.
218. KD Chang, TA Ketter. Mood stabilizer augmentation with olanzapine in acutely manic children. J Child Adolesc Psychopharmacol 10:45–49, 2000.
219. J Frazier, J Biederman, T Jacobs. Olanzapine in the treatment of bipolar disorder in juveniles. Int J Neuropsychopharmacol 3:S330, 2000.
220. JA Frazier, MC Meyer, J Biederman, J Wozniak, TE Wilens, TJ Spencer, GS Kim, S Shapiro. Risperidone treatment for juvenile bipolar disorder: a retrospective chart review. J Am Acad Child Adolesc Psychiatry 38:960–965, 1999.
221. J Schaller, D Behar. Quetiapine for refractory mania in a child. J Am Acad Child Adolesc Psychiatry 38:498–499, 1999.
222. BJ McConville, LA Arvanitis, PT Thyrum, C Yeh, LA Wilkinson, RO Chaney, KD Foster, MT Sorter, LM Friedman, KL Brown, JE Heubi. Pharmacokinetics, tolerability, and clinical effectiveness of quetiapine fumarate: an open-label trial in adolescents with psychotic disorders. J Clin Psychiatry 61:252–260, 2000.
223. MP DelBello, HL Rosenberg, M Schulers, SM Strakowski. Quetiapine as adjunctive treatment for adolescent mania: a double blind placebo-controlled study. J Am Acad Child Adolesc Psychiatry (in press).
224. PA Davanzo, N Krah, J Kleiner, J McCracken. Nimodipine treatment of an adolescent with ultradian cycling bipolar affective illness. J Child Adolesc Psychopharmacol 9:51–61, 1999.
225. JM Robertson, PE Tanguay. Case study: the use of melatonin in a boy with refractory bipolar disorder. J Am Acad Child Adolesc Psychiatry 36:822–825, 1997.
226. J Biederman, E Mick, J Prince, JQ Bostic, TE Wilens, T Spencer, J Wozniak, SV Faraone. Systematic chart review of the pharmacologic treatment of comorbid attention deficit hyperactivity disorder in youth with bipolar disorder. J Child Adolesc Psychopharmacol 9:247–256, 1999.
227. KD Chang, TA Ketter. Special issues in the treatment of paediatric bipolar disorder. Expert Opin Pharmacother 2:613–622, 2001.

228. MT Compton, CB Nemeroff. The treatment of bipolar depression. J Clin Psychiatry 61:57–67, 2000.
229. J Biederman, E Mick, TJ Spencer, TE Wilens, SV Faraone. Therapeutic dilemmas in the pharmacotherapy of bipolar depression in the young. J Child Adolesc Psychopharmacol 10:185–192, 2000.
230. GS Sachs, B Lafer, AL Stoll, M Banov, AB Thibault, M Tohen, JF Rosenbaum. A double-blind trial of bupropion versus desipramine for bipolar depression. J Clin Psychiatry 55:391–393, 1994.
231. J Goldberg, A Rabin, J Whiteside. Prevalence and risks associated with antidepressant-induced mania. Bipolar Disord 3:38, 2001.
232. GM MacQueen, LT Young. Bipolar II disorder: symptoms, course, and response to treatment. Psychiatr Serv 52:358–361, 2001.
233. KD Denicoff, EE Smith-Jackson, ER Disney, RL Suddath, GS Leverich, RM Post. Preliminary evidence of the reliability and validity of the prospective life-chart methodology (LCM-p). J Psychiatr Res 31:593–603, 1997.

12

Anxiety Disorders in Childhood and Adolescence
Basic Mechanisms and Therapeutic Interventions

TIFFANY FARCHIONE, SHAUNA N. MacMILLAN, and DAVID R. ROSENBERG
Wayne State University, Detroit, Michigan, U.S.A.

I. INTRODUCTION

Anxiety can be defined as dread or apprehension [1]. Anxiety in and of itself is not considered a disorder and is seen across the age span and may even be adaptive in certain situations (e.g., anxiety one might feel in a threatening environment such as during an earthquake). In contrast, anxiety disorders are characterized by pathologic anxiety, in which anxiety interferes with achievement of goals or quality of life. Thus, to diagnose a particular anxiety disorder in a person, interference in psychosocial and/or academic/occupational functioning must be present. In the pediatric population, anxiety disorders are relatively common (5–18%) [see 2 for review], with prevalence rates comparable to some physical disorders, such as asthma and diabetes [3].

Nonetheless, recognition of child and adolescent anxiety disorders has been slow in coming. In the first edition of the *Diagnostic and Statistical Manual of Mental Disorders* [4], there were few references to childhood anxiety disorders. "Overanxious reaction of childhood" first appeared in the *DSM-II* [5]. Then, in the *DSM-III* [6], four childhood anxiety disorders were recognized (overanxious disorder, separation anxiety disorder, simple phobia, and social phobia), as well as other childhood disorders with prominent anxiety symptoms. That edition also acknowledged that adult anxiety disorders could begin in childhood. Finally, in the *DSM-IV* [7], the terminology used to describe childhood anxiety disorders was changed, and became more consistent with the adult terminology. For instance, "overanxious disorder" was changed to "generalized anxiety disorder with childhood onset." Although these changing criteria have facilitated the assessment and treatment of childhood anxiety disorders, they have left researchers with a "moving target," making it difficult to apply earlier research to current diagnoses [8].

Neurobiologic and clinical trials in pediatric anxiety disorders have lagged far behind adult studies. For instance, recent reviews of the literature reveal a paucity of neuroimaging data in childhood anxiety disorders [9–11], and most of these studies have been conducted in the past 10 years. However, through the usetremendous strides are now being made toward better characterizing the developmental neurological underpinnings of these debilitating illnesses. Studying these disorders in children near the onset of illness also has tremendous advantages. Specifically, many potentially confounding factors are eliminated including central nervous system (CNS) active medications and long-term illness duration. Recent investigation suggests that pediatric and adult anxiety may have distinct functional brain activation patterns (Fig. 1). It should be noted, however, that several unique challenges are involved in studying children and adolescents with anxiety disorders. For instance, there are inadequate normative data and imprecise definition of groups (note the changing definition of overanxious disorder/generalized anxiety disorder). Also, a lack of well-standardized and reliable methods of neurobiologic measurements has made comparisons from lab to lab problematic. Moreover, without rapid, standardized, automated methods of measuring, analysis of large samples is difficult [9].

Not only has research examining the neurobiologic basis of childhood anxiety lagged behind adult studies, but treatment studies have only recently begun to focus on children. Treatment research is admittedly often more complex in children although the U.S. government is now mandating that medications used in pediatric populations undergo rigorous testing. It is no longer acceptable for pharmaceutical companies to develop a particular compound, test it exclusively in adults, and then extrapolate the data to child populations. This has enormous implications for the psychopharmacologic study of pediatric anxiety disorders and will undoubtedly lead to more effective treatment of these children. Pediatricians have long recognized that children are not simply "little adults." Recent determination that the tricyclic antidepressants, while very effective in treating adults with major depressive disorder (MDD), are no more effective than placebo in treating child and adolescent MDD [12] underscores this point.

There are currently few controlled trials of either psychotherapeutic or psychopharmacologic interventions for children with anxiety disorders. With regard to psychotherapeutic treatments, cognitive behavioral therapy (CBT) is currently regarded by many as the therapy of choice because, among the various psycho-

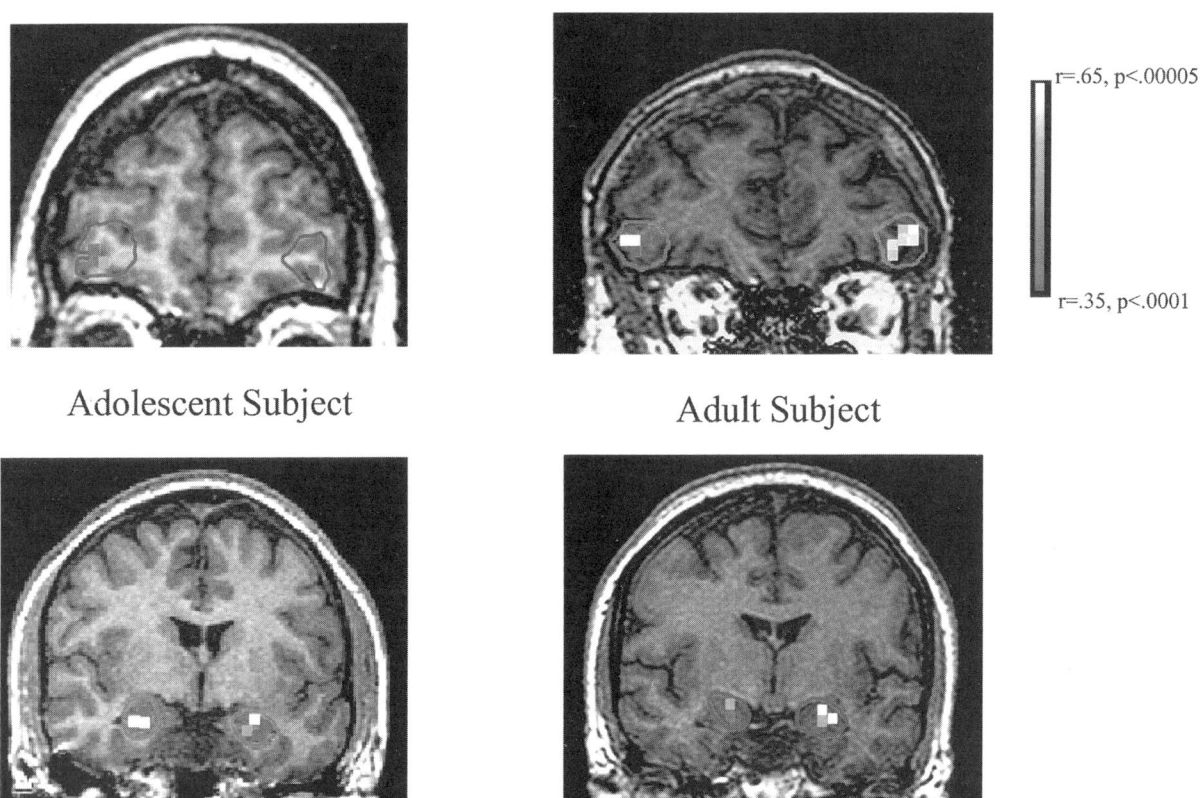

Figure 1. Coronal slices illustrating activation differences between healthy adolescent and adult subjects during the presentation of a facial affect discrimination task. The regions outlined include the dorsolateral prefrontal cortex (above) and the amygdala (below). The gray shades indicate the magnitude of signal intensity change in these regions. The lighter shades of gray are indicative of greater activation than the red color. (Courtesy of Dr. Deborah Yurgelun-Todd, Cognitive Neuroimaging and Neuropsychology Laboratory, McLean Hospital.)

social approaches, it is the only treatment with controlled data supporting its efficacy [13]. CBT has been shown to be effective both immediately posttreatment [14–19] and at 6- or 12-month follow-up [17–19].

II. CHILDHOOD ANXIETY DISORDERS

A. Separation Anxiety Disorder

Separation anxiety disorder (SAD) is characterized by excessive anxiety concerning separation from the home or a major attachment figure [7]. It is one of the most common childhood anxiety disorders, with estimates of prevalence ranging from 3.5% to 5.4% [20]. As many as 33% of children presenting to outpatient anxiety disorder clinics will have SAD as their primary diagnosis [21]. Although separation anxiety is considered developmentally normal beginning $\sim$ 10 months of age, it typically wanes by $\sim$ 18 months [3]. Most children can accept the temporary absence of their primary attachment figure, usually their mother, and be comforted by others by age 3 years [22]. By definition, SAD must have its onset before age 18 years, although some suggest that an adult-onset form of this disorder may exist [23]. SAD is seen most often in prepubertal children [24], with an average age of onset of $\sim$ 7.5 years [25]. Clinical samples suggest an equal prevalence in boys and girls [25], but epidemiologic studies point to a female predominance [26].

Children with SAD may refuse to go to school, be reluctant to sleep alone, have nightmares about separation, or have physical complaints. Different symptoms are more prominent depending on the age of the child. Children under 8 years old typically exhibit school refusal and excessive fear that harm will come to a parent; those 9–12 years of age have excessive distress at the time of separation; those aged 13–16 years have school refusal and physical complaints [3].

As with all anxiety disorders, comorbidity is common in SAD. For instance, in children with comorbid tic disorders and anxiety, Coffey et al. [27] demonstrated that SAD, in particular, may be associated with tic severity. In addition to comorbidity, SAD may be a risk factor for developing other anxiety disorders. In a retrospective survey of adults with anxiety disorders, Lipsitz et al. [28] found a higher prevalence of childhood SAD in adults with two or more anxiety disorders, suggesting that SAD may be a risk factor for multiple anxiety disorders. A number of recent studies have focused on a potential role for SAD as a predictive factor in the development of panic disorder in adolescence and adulthood. Silove et al. [29] found that women with panic disorder reported a higher rate of childhood SAD, and Battaglia et al. [30] suggested that SAD may be a predictor for early onset of panic disorder.

Some studies have suggested that SAD is more common in young children, while other anxiety disorders emerge in adolescence [31,32]. Westenberg et al. [33] have suggested that SAD is more likely to develop in children with lower levels of psychosocial maturity, generalized anxiety disorder (GAD) is more likely in children with higher levels of psychosocial maturity, irrespective of chronological age.

Little is known about the biological processes underlying SAD. Recently, however, studies have begun to implicate abnormal carbon dioxide (CO_2) sensitivity in the pathogenesis of SAD and other anxiety disorders [34–38]. Pine et al. [34] suggested that level of anxiety was related to perceived elevations in CO_2. To test this hypothesis, they compared anxiety symptoms in children with congenital hypoventilation syndrome, children with other chronic illnesses, and healthy controls. Children with congenital hypoventilation syndrome had significantly fewer anxiety symptoms than controls, and controls had fewer than the chronically ill group. For children meeting criteria for an anxiety disorder, the greatest difference in prevalence was between the congenital hypoventilation group (15%) and children with asthma (47%). To examine the underlying physiology of these differences, Pine et al. [35,36] compared ventilatory function in children with anxiety disorders to healthy controls during CO_2 inhalation and while breathing room air. Children with anxiety disorders had larger minute ventilation and higher respiratory rate during CO_2 inhalation, and more variable breathing on room air. These differences correlated with subjective symptom ratings, and findings were consistent with adult studies in patients with panic disorder. Of note, the changes experienced by anxious children during CO_2 inhalation were considered similar to physiologic changes experienced by adults during panic attacks, and these changes were especially pronounced in children with SAD.

Stress-induced increases in catecholamines and glucocorticoids have been implicated in the pathogenesis of many illnesses, including anxiety disorders. In addition to metabolic responses, emotional and cognitive responses to stressors may be mediated by adrenal hormones and central corticotropin-releasing factor (CRF) systems [39]. In an animal model of separation anxiety, Lyons et al. [40] showed that, upon separation from a group, squirrel monkeys had increased plasma cortisol and adrenocorticotropic hormone (ACTH), as well as higher levels of cerebrospinal fluid (CSF) homovanillic acid (HVA). In a review of preclinical data, Heim and Nemeroff [41] found a suggestion in the literature that early-life stress results in persistent central CRF hyperactivity and increased stress reactivity in adulthood. Consistent with these data, women who were sexually abused in childhood have increased pituitary-adrenal and autonomic responses [42].

To date, there are few double-blind, placebo-controlled studies of psychopharmacologic treatment for SAD. However, data suggest that the tricyclic antidepressant (TCA) imipramine may be an effective treatment for SAD [43]. Three children with severe SAD and comorbid panic disorder and agoraphobia improved on a combination of imipramine and alprazolam [44]. In a study conducted by Gittelman-Klein and Klein (45) comparing 6 weeks of treatment with imipramine + a special psychosocial treatment program vs. placebo + psychosocial treatment for 6 weeks in 20 children 7–15 years of age with school refusal, a phenomenon closely associated with SAD [24], school attendance and anxiety were significantly improved in patients treated with imipramine as compared to placebo. They were not able to confirm this finding in subsequent investigation [46]. Berney et al. [47] also reported no superiority of clomipramine vs. placebo in treating children with school phobia. In a 4-week double blind, placebo-controlled study of clonazepam (0.5–2 mg/day) in 15 anxious children suffering primarily from SAD, Graae et al. [48] reported that clonazepam treatment was not superior to treatment with placebo. It should be noted that many clinicians use buspirone for SAD either alone or in combination with other medication and behavioral treatments. While there has been no controlled study of its use for SAD, there are case studies suggesting possible efficacy [49,50].

More recent investigation of imipramine vs. placebo in combination with CBT suggests efficacy and safety of the imipramine + CBT combination over placebo + CBT [51]. This study defined 75% school attendance as representing treatment remission. Over 50% of patients treated with imipramine achieved remission, whereas only 16% treated with placebo achieved remission.

In spite of the aforementioned possible benefit of the TCA imipramine in combination with CBT, in recent years, the selective serotonin reuptake inhibitors (SSRIs) are becoming the first-line treatment for all anxiety disorders including SAD. This reflects their more favorable side-effects profile and recent investigation suggesting efficacy in non–obsessive-compulsive disorder (OCD) anxiety disorders. Open-label fluoxetine was reported to be effective in children with non-OCD anxiety disorders including SAD [52]. More recently, the Research Units of Pediatric Psychopharmacology (RUPRP) Anxiety Group [53] compared fluvoxamine to placebo in a double-blind 8-week comparison of 128 children and adolescents with GAD, SAD, and social phobia. Fluvoxamine was superior to placebo in reducing anxiety in all three conditions, with 79% of patients responding to fluvoxamine as compared to < 30% responding to placebo. Mean doses of fluvoxamine were 100 mg/day with doses started at 25 mg/day and titrated to a maximum of 250 mg/day in 6 to 12-year-old children and 300 mg/day in teenagers 13–17 years of age. It is particularly noteworthy that the improvement in pediatric anxiety disorder patients receiving fluvoxamine was greater than improvement reported in adults treated with benzodiazepines or TCAs. Walkup [54] has recently reported that long-term treatment with fluvoxamine of non-OCD anxiety can be effective with additional benefit being noted after the initial acute trial of the SSRI. It is unlikely that fluvoxamine will be FDA approved on the basis of this study, since the FDA requires that investigations of medication be targeted toward one specific disorder rather than the three anxiety disorders studied by the RUPP Anxiety Group [55]. While many clinicians continue to prescribe benzodiazepines either prior to or during the titration phase of SSRIs (whose effect can be delayed 6–8 weeks), caution is indicated, particularly if there is a history of substance abuse in the child and/or family. Short-term use of benzodiazepines such as alprazolam or clonazepam is recommended. There are no published data on the other SSRIs.

B. Generalized Anxiety Disorder (formerly Overanxious Disorder)

Generalized anxiety disorder (GAD) is characterized by excessive fear or worry about a number of different events or activities for at least 6 months [7]. In previous versions of the DSM, GAD was known as overanxious disorder (OAD), and, while most of the diagnostic criteria are comparable, the OAD criteria for excessive self-consciousness and need for reassurance are not required to diagnose GAD. Prevalance estimates for GAD/OAD range from 2.4% to 6% of children [56,57]. In one of the largest samples, Whitaker et al. [58] reported a lifetime prevalence of GAD in adolescents of 3.7%. There is an approximately equal prevalence of GAD in boys and girls until adolescence, at which time GAD becomes more prevalent in females [59].

GAD can be differentiated from other anxiety disorders based on the diffuse nature of the anxiety symptoms. In GAD, fear and anxiety are experienced in a number of situations. In contrast, the primary fear in SAD is of separation and, in panic disorder, anxiety centers around the fear of having a panic attack [60]. Among the primary worries experienced by children with GAD are concerns about competence and performance in school and athletic activities [7]. Anxiety is often accompanied by somatic symptoms such as restlessness, fatigability, difficulty concentrating, irritability, muscle tension, or sleep disturbance [7]. Finally, children with GAD tend to present at an older age than those with SAD [3].

Given that children with GAD tend to present with a variety of somatic complaints, the differential diagnosis contains multiple medical causes that must be ruled out. In adolescence, excessive use of caffeine or other stimulants is particularly common and easily ruled out by careful history [61]. In the context of a suggestive history or physical exam, one must be wary of hyperthyroidism, hypoglycemia, lupus, and pheochromocytoma [61].

There are few neurobiologic studies in pediatric patients with GAD. In the only neuroimaging study to date of childhood GAD, De Bellis and colleagues [62] reported increased right and total amygdala volumes in 12 children 8–16 years of age suffering from GAD as compared to 24 age- and sex-matched normal controls (two matched controls per GAD patient) (Fig. 2). This finding, however, was not correlated with severity of anxiety.

The amygdala is, in fact, considered a key structure in processing of fear and anxiety information [see 63 for review]. The amygdala receives extensive connections from thalamic and cortical exteroceptive systems, as well as subcortical visceral afferent pathways, making it a central structure in the fear processing pathways (Fig. 3).

A number of studies have investigated potential physiologic markers for GAD. As with SAD, GAD is associated with CO_2 hypersensitivity [35]. Some studies suggest that there is a differential hypersensitivity among the anxiety disorders and that, in fact, patients with GAD are significantly less sensitive to the effects of CO_2 than are patients with panic [64–66]. In a study examining neuroendocrine markers of anxiety in 20 male adolescents (14 of whom had GAD, 6 had GAD

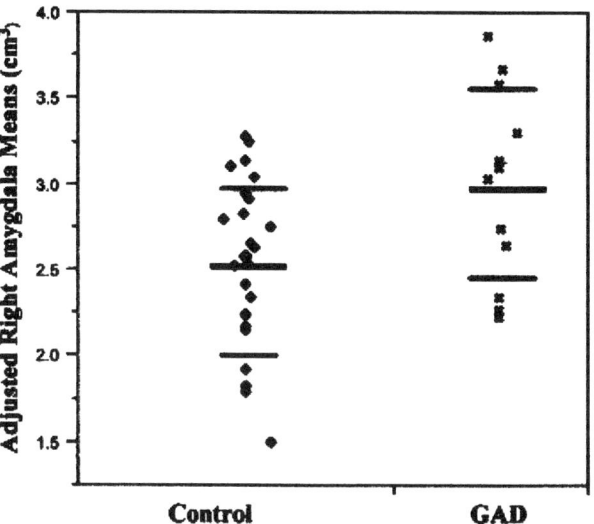

Figure 2 Right [$t(1,33) = 2.44$, $p = .02$] amygdala volume means (cm^3) and standard deviations adjusted for intracranial volume of children and adolescents with generalized anxiety disorder (GAD) and matched comparison subjects. (Reprinted by permission of Elsevier Science. A Pilot Study of Amygdala Volumes in Pediatric Generalized Anxiety Disorder, by DeBellis, Casey, Dahl et al., Biological Psychiatry 48(1):51–57, 2000, by the Society of Biological Psychiatry.)

and SAD), Gerra and colleagues [67] demonstrated that anxious subjects have significantly higher levels of growth hormone (GH), prolactin (PRL), beta-endorphin (beta-ED), and ACTH at baseline. Following a series of psychological stressors, anxious subjects had significantly higher levels of norepinephrine, GH, and testosterone and their nonanxious controls. Beta-EP and PRL decreased significantly in the anxious subjects following the stressor, but remained unaffected in the healthy control subjects. Taken together with adult data [68–70], these studies suggest a role for hypothalamic-pituitary-adrenal axis dysregulation in the pathogenesis of GAD.

With regard to treatment of GAD, data are very limited. There have been no published double-blind, placebo-controlled studies examining the medications commonly prescribed to treat this disorder. However, as mentioned above, one such trial of fluvoxamine for treatment of social phobia, SAD, and GAD was recently completed and found that fluvoxamine is superior to placebo [53]. There is also an ongoing multicenter, double-blind, placebo-controlled industry-sponsored trial of sustained-release venlafaxine (ER) in children and adolescents with GAD. Additionally, there is a large, industry-sponsored trial

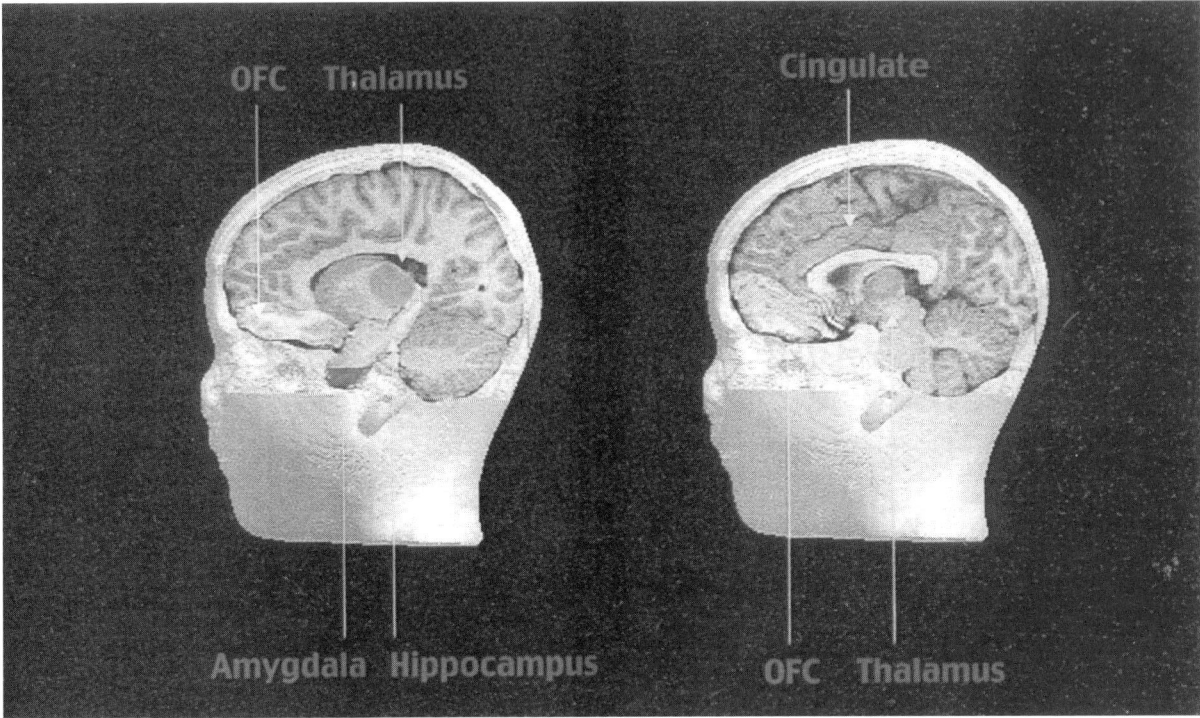

Figure 3 Structures such as the thalamus, cingulate, amygdala, hippocampus and the orbital frontal cortex (OFC) are activated in the emotion fear. (Created by Frank P. MacMaster.) (Reprinted with permission from Cambridge Press. Neuroimaging of Childhhood Onset Anxiety Disorders, Rosenberg, Paulson, MacMaster, Moore. In: Ernest and Rumsey eds. Functional Neuroimaging in Child Psychiatry, 2000, 224–241.)

in progress of the 5HT1A agonist buspirone for GAD in young people aged 5–17 which had recruited 350 subjects within 5 months [13]. The results of this study have not yet been analyzed.

With respect to psychotherapeutic interventions, a number of studies have shown that CBT is superior to no treatment and to nondirective therapy [see 71 for review]. Additionally, Barrett and colleagues [72] demonstrated that, in 52 adolescents (age 14–21) who had undergone cognitive behavioral therapy for anxiety an average of 6 years prior to this study, 85.7% no longer met diagnostic criteria for any anxiety disorder. These patients had been treated with either CBT alone or CBT in combination with family management, both of which were equally effective at long-term follow-up.

C. Social Phobia (Social Anxiety Disorder)

Social phobia (SP) is characterized by a marked fear of social or performance situations in which the child may be observed or evaluated [7]. Patients fear that they will embarrass or humiliate themselves; thus, exposure to the feared situation almost invariably causes anxiety. In severe cases, this anxiety may take the form of a panic attack. SP can be either discrete or generalized. The qualification of generalized is added to the diagnosis if the patient fears most social situations [7]. Among 15 to 54-year-olds, there is a 7–8% 1-year prevalence and 13–14% lifetime prevalence. However, the onset of this disorder is typically prior to or during adolescence [73]. Recent prevalence estimates in children and adolescents range from 0.5% to 4.0% [74]. In community samples, SP is more common in women than men. The opposite has been found in clinical samples [75].

SP is a serious, disabling disorder associated with a decreased quality of life [76]. While most of the reported quality-of-life measures are more specific to adult populations, the fact that 38.1% of SP patients do not graduate high school (compared to 30.1% without SP) is of particular concern in adolescents [76]. Also, a lifetime diagnosis of SP was associated with greater likelihood of having failed at least one grade.

Comorbidity is particularly problematic in SP, as 70–80% of SP patients have at least one comorbid mental disorder [73]. Also, low scores on SP scales in childhood may predict development of conduct disorder in adolescence [77]. Although patients with comorbidity are more likely to seek treatment than those with only SP (51% seek treatment, compared to 20% in SP alone), these patients are also more likely to attempt suicide (15.7% vs. 1%) [78].

With regard to etiology, some studies suggest that *behavioral inhibition* may be a marker for anxiety proneness. Behavioral inhibition is a term first used by Kagan and colleagues [79] to describe a pattern of withdrawal from unfamiliar stimuli. In a 3-year follow-up study of children with behavioral inhibition, Biederman et al. [80] found that inhibited children were at risk for the development of anxiety disorders, with significantly greater risk for multiple diagnoses. A more recent study suggested that inhibited temperament in childhood was associated with generalized social anxiety in adolescence, but not separation anxiety, specific fears, or performance anxiety [81]. Inhibited children can also be distinguished from noninhibited children based on several physiological parameters, including elevated heart rates, urinary catecholamines, and salivary cortisol [82]. Similar physiologic markers are present in several childhood anxiety disorders [67,83]. Additionally, children are more likely to have behavioral inhibition if a parent suffers from MDD or panic [84]. In fact, having a parent who suffered from both MDD and panic conferred a twofold risk for behavioral inhibition in the child.

Unlike some of the other anxiety disorders, neuroendocrine studies have failed to offer insight in the biology of SP. In a study of girls with SP (mean age 15.6 years ± 1.5 years), Martel et al. [85] found no difference in salivary cortisol levels between SP patients and controls either at baseline or during a stressor.

To date, there are no data from double-blind, placebo-controlled studies specific to pediatric SP. As mentioned previously, the RUPP Anxiety Group [53] found fluvoxamine to be superior to placebo in treating children with anxiety disorders including social phobia. Paroxetine was recently FDA approved for treating SP in adults, and Glaxo SmithKline has initiated a multicenter double-blind, placebo-controlled study of paroxetine for SP in children and adolescents. Wyeth-Ayerst has also initiated a multicenter double-blind, placebo-controlled study of sustained-release venlafaxine ER in children and adolescents with SP. The sedative side effects of benzodiazepines typically contraindicate their use for SP. While there are no controlled studies of buspirone for SP, a recent case study suggested possible efficacy in an adolescent with SP [86].

Beta blockers are commonly prescribed to treat SP, especially the subtype with performance anxiety, or "stage fright." In spite of this common clinical practice, there are currently no FDA-approved indications for the use of beta-blockers in psychiatric disorders, and there have been no controlled studies of these medications in children and adolescents. Among the beta blockers, propranolol has been the most studied in neuropsychiatric disorders. Some evidence suggest that may be effective in the treatment of anxiety [87,88]; however, this effect seems to be due more to propranolol's peripheral actions (e.g., decreasing heart rate) than its effect on central noradrenergic beta receptors.

Psychotherapeutic interventions, particularly CBT, have been shown to be effective in the treatment of social phobia [see 89 for review]. In children, it appears that CBT combined with family management may be superior to CBT alone [19], both acutely and at 12-month follow-up. This may be due, in part, to an effect on parental anxiety. In a study examining the role of parental anxiety on treatment outcome in children with anxiety disorder, Cobham and colleagues [90] showed that children of anxious parents did better if parent anxiety management was combined with child CBT.

D. Panic Disorder

Until fairly recently, panic was considered a diagnosis to be made strictly in adults. In fact, some controversy still exists as to whether this diagnosis can be made in children and adolescents [91–93]. However, several cases of adolescent-onset panic have been described, both in current cases [94,95] and in retrospective repots [96,97]. As in adults, panic disorder is characterized by recurrent panic attacks and persistent concerns about having future attacks [7]. While patients with adult-onset and early-onset panic disorder do not seem to differ in symptom severity or social functioning, the early-onset form tends to carry with it higher comorbidity and is possibly a result of greater familial loading for anxiety disorders [98]. For instance, children of parents with panic disorder are significantly more likely to have the disorder themselves [99].

Some studies have indicated that normal and pathologic anxiety may be mediated by different mechanisms. For instance, Sinha et al. [37] showed that, in response to CO_2-induced panic, cortisol levels in panicking patients with panic disorder decreased, while those of healthy comparison subjects and nonpanicking panic disorder patient did not. It is likely that childhood and adult anxiety may have different mechanisms as well. For example, in contrast to adult studies, children with anxiety do not have a blunting of growth hormone (GH) response to clonidine [100]. However, in response to the α_2 agonist yohimbine children with anxiety disorders had increased subjective anxiety, increased adrenergic reactivity, and a decreased GH response, all consistent with literature in adults [101]. Yohimbine is known to increase norepinephrine (NE) release in the hippocampus via increased locus ceruleus firing, leading to behavioral and biologic correlates of anxiety. According to Sallee et al. [10], the combined yohimbine and clonidine data suggest that presynaptic NE sensitivity may be present in early-onset anxiety disorders, but that the overactive noradrenergic system is not necessarily accompanied by the α_2 downregulation seen in adults.

E. Obsessive-Compulsive Disorder

Obsessive-compulsive disorder (OCD) is a chronically disabling condition characterized by repetitive ritualistic behavior and recurrent intrusive thoughts [7]. Frequent obsessions include fears of contamination (35%) and thoughts of harming oneself or loved ones (30%). The most commonly reported compulsions in children and adolescents are washing and cleaning (75%), checking (40%), and straightening (35%) [3]. The lifetime prevalence of OCD is ∼ 2–3% [102], with > 80% of cases having their onset in childhood and adolescence [103]. OCD onset tends to be earlier in boys than girls, with a peak in puberty and in early adulthood [102]. In a study examining comorbidity in 70 children with OCD. Thirty percent of these patients had a comorbid tic disorder. Other common comorbid diagnoses were MDD (26%) and developmental disorders (24%).

As was the case in SP, OCD illustrates again that not all anxiety disorders have known neuroendocrine correlates. Using electrodermal activity and heart rate as markers of autonomic activity, Zahn et al. [105] found no differences between children with OCD and normal controls.

In contrast to other anxiety disorders, more information has been gleaned from neuroimaging studies of children and adolescents with OCD. Neurobiologic studies have implicated a pharmacologically reversible glutamatergic thalamocortico-striatal dysfunction in pediatric OCD [10].

1. Volumetric Studies

An early study using quantitative x-ray computerized tomography (CT) found reduced caudate volumes in young males with OCD [106]. Behar et al. [107] also reported significantly increased ventricular brain ratios suggestive of decreased striatal volume in 16 adolescent OCD patients. Using morphometric magnetic resonance imaging (MRI), Rosenberg and colleagues [108] found that 19 treatment-naïve OCD patients age 7–17 had significantly smaller striatal volumes than did age- and sex-matched healthy comparison subjects (Fig. 4). Reduced striatal volumes were correlated with increased OCD symptom severity but not with increased illness duration. This is consistent with Rauch et al.'s [109] suggestion that striatal dysfunction represents a primary locus of pathology in OCD.

Interestingly, OCD symptoms seen in patients with pediatric autoimmune neuropsychiatric disorders associated with group A beta-hemolytic streptococal (GABHS) infections, called PANDAS, have been found to have increased basal ganglia volumes [110–112]. In these patients, increased antibody titers of antistreptolysin O and antideoxyribonuclease B have been reported to be correlated with increased basal ganglia volumes [112]. Remarkably, immunotherapy (e.g., plasmapheresis) has been reported to be effective in reducing OCD symptoms in some patients with PANDAS [113] and reducing basal ganglia volumes [114].

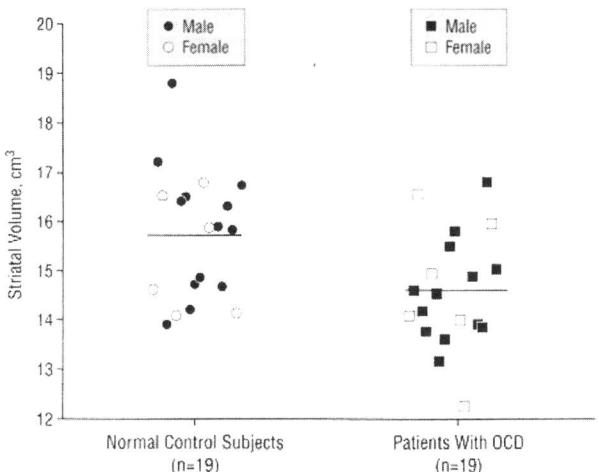

Figure 4 Reduced striatal volume in obsessive compulsive disorder (OCD) patients vs. controls. Lines indicate means. (Reprinted from Rosenberg, Keshavan, O'Hearn et al., 1997. Fronto-Striatal Measurement of Treatment-Naïve Pediatric Obsessive-Compulsive Disorder. Arch Gen Psychiatry 54:824–830.)

These findings underscore the need for precise neurobiological studies to identify possibly distinct subtypes of OCD with different patterns of brain abnormality. Ultimately, such work has the potential to determine differential treatment intervention in pediatric OCD patients based on different patterns of brain abnormality [10]. Moreover, perturbation of specific neural networks in either direction (e.g., increased or decreased) may result in emergence of OCD symptoms.

Abnormalities in the striatum in pediatric OCD patients have prompted investigation in ventral prefrontal cortex and the striatum. The ventral prefrontal cortex sends dense efferent projections to the striatum and thalamus [115–119]. Neuropsychological and neurocognitive studies of tasks purported to probe ventral prefrontal cortical function had suggested abnormalities in pediatric OCD patients compared to controls [120]. Subsequent volumetric MRI investigation demonstrated increased ventral prefrontal cortical volumes in anterior cingulate cortex in pediatric OCD patients compared to controls, particularly younger pediatric OCD patients, with no abnormalities observed in posterior cingulate cortex or in dorsolateral prefrontal cortex [121] (Fig. 5). Specifically, the normal age-related increase in anterior cingulate volume observed in controls was absent in childhood OCD patients. In these OCD patients, increased anterior cingulate volumes were

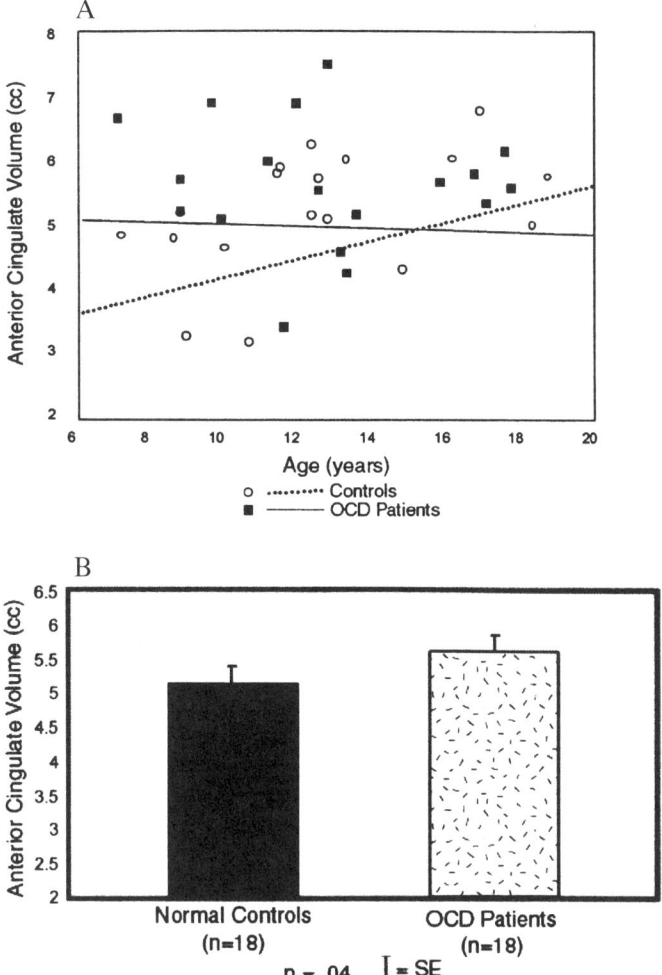

Figure 5 (A) Anterior cingulate volume vs. age in pediatric obsessive compulsive disorder patients and healthy comparison subjects. Note that the age-related increase in anterior cingulate volume observed in healthy children is absent in pediatric patients with obsessive compulsive disorder. (B) Anterior cingulate volume by group. (Reprinted by permission of Elsevier Science. Toward a Neurodevelopmental Model of Obsessive-Compulsive Disorder, by Rosenberg and Keshavan, Biological Psychiatry 43(9):623–640, 1998, by the Society of Biological Psychiatry.)

positively correlated with severity of OCD but not duration of illness.

The thalamus serves as the final subcortical input to frontal cortex [122]. A previous volumetric MRI study [123] found no significant differences in thalamic volume between adult OCD patients and controls. The patients studied in this report, however, had been treated with SSRIs. This led Gilbert et al. [124] to conduct a volumetric MRI study in 21 treatment-naïve pediatric OCD patients and 21 age- and sex-matched controls. Increased thalamic volumes were observed in treatment-naïve pediatric OCD patients compared to controls. A significant decrease in thalamic volume was observed after 12 weeks of monodrug therapy with the SSRI paroxetine (Fig. 6). Decrease in OCD symptom severity was highly correlated with reduction in thalamic volume (Fig. 7). Specifically, increased thalamic volume before treatment with paroxetine predicted better response to the medication. There was no significant reduction in thalamic volume in pediatric OCD patients treated with CBT [125]. Recent investigation by Nolan et al. [2001] found that this decrease in thalamic volume was primarily localized to medial, not lateral, thalamus. Using a newer and more sophisticated technique of brain chemistry, proton magnetic resonance spectroscopy (1-H MRS), functional neurochemical marker abnormalities were localized to medial but not lateral thalamus in pediatric OCD patients compared to controls [126,127]. Amponsah et al. [128] presented data suggesting a trend for increased N-acetyl-aspartate (NAA) concentrations as measured by 1-H MRS in pediatric OCD patients after 12 weeks of treatment with paroxetine. NAA is known to be a reliable indicator of neuronal viability [129].

2. Brain Chemistry/Glutamate

Alterations in glutamatergic-serotonin interactions in ventral prefrontal-striatal-thalamic circuitry in pediatric OCD were suggested by several basic science reports in the literature. Becquet et al. [130] demonstrated that the caudate nucleus, a primary locus of abnormality in OCD [109], receives an especially high glutamate innervation from the prefrontal cortex. Indeed, most of the axon terminals in the caudate nucleus are glutamatergic afferents [116,117]. Glutamate concentrations in the striatum are markedly reduced after ablation of frontal cortex [118,119]. An

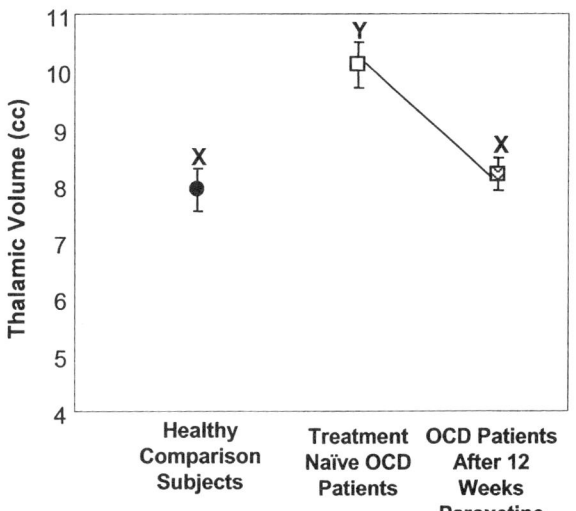

Figure 6 Thalamic volume by diagnostic and treatment condition with groups not sharing the same letter are significantly different at $P < .05$. (Adapted from Gilbert, Moore, Keshavan et al., 2000. Decrease in Thalamic Volumes of Pediatric Obsessive-Compulsive Disorder Patients Taking Paroxetine. Arch Gen Psychiatry 57(5):449–456.)

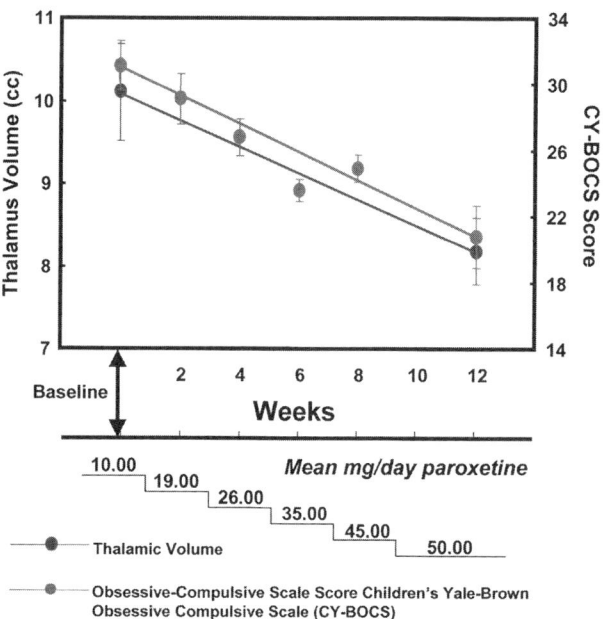

Figure 7 Decrease in thalamic volume associated with reduction in Obsessive-Compulsive Score of the Children's Yale-Brown Obsessive Compulsive Scales. (Reprinted from Gilbert, Moore, Keshavan et al., 2000. Decrease in Thalamic Volumes of Pediatric Obsessive-Compulsive Disorder Patients Taking Paroxetine. Arch Gen Psychiatry 57(5):449–456.)

in vivo glutamate control over presynaptic serotonin release in the caudate nucleus has also been demonstrated [115,131], while serotonergic neurons impact on striatal glutamate concentrations [132].

Using 1-H MRS, Rosenberg et al. [133] found significant elevations in left caudate but not occipital glutamatergic concentrations in OCD patients compared to controls (Figs. 8 and 9). After 12 weeks of monodrug therapy with the SSRI paroxetine, caudate glutamatergic concentrations decreased to levels not significantly different from those in controls. Reduction in glutamergic concentrations in the left caudate nucleus was robustly correlated with reduction in OCD symptom severity (Fig. 10). Pretreatment caudate glutamatergic concentrations tended to predict treatment response with higher pretreatment concentrations predictive of better response to paroxetine. Taken together, these findings suggest that OCD in children and adolescents may be associated with reversible, glutamate-mediated dysfunction of a ventral prefrontal-striatal-thalamic system.

Most of the research guiding current prescribing practices in children and adolescents comes from studies in adults [134]. Pediatric OCD is an exception

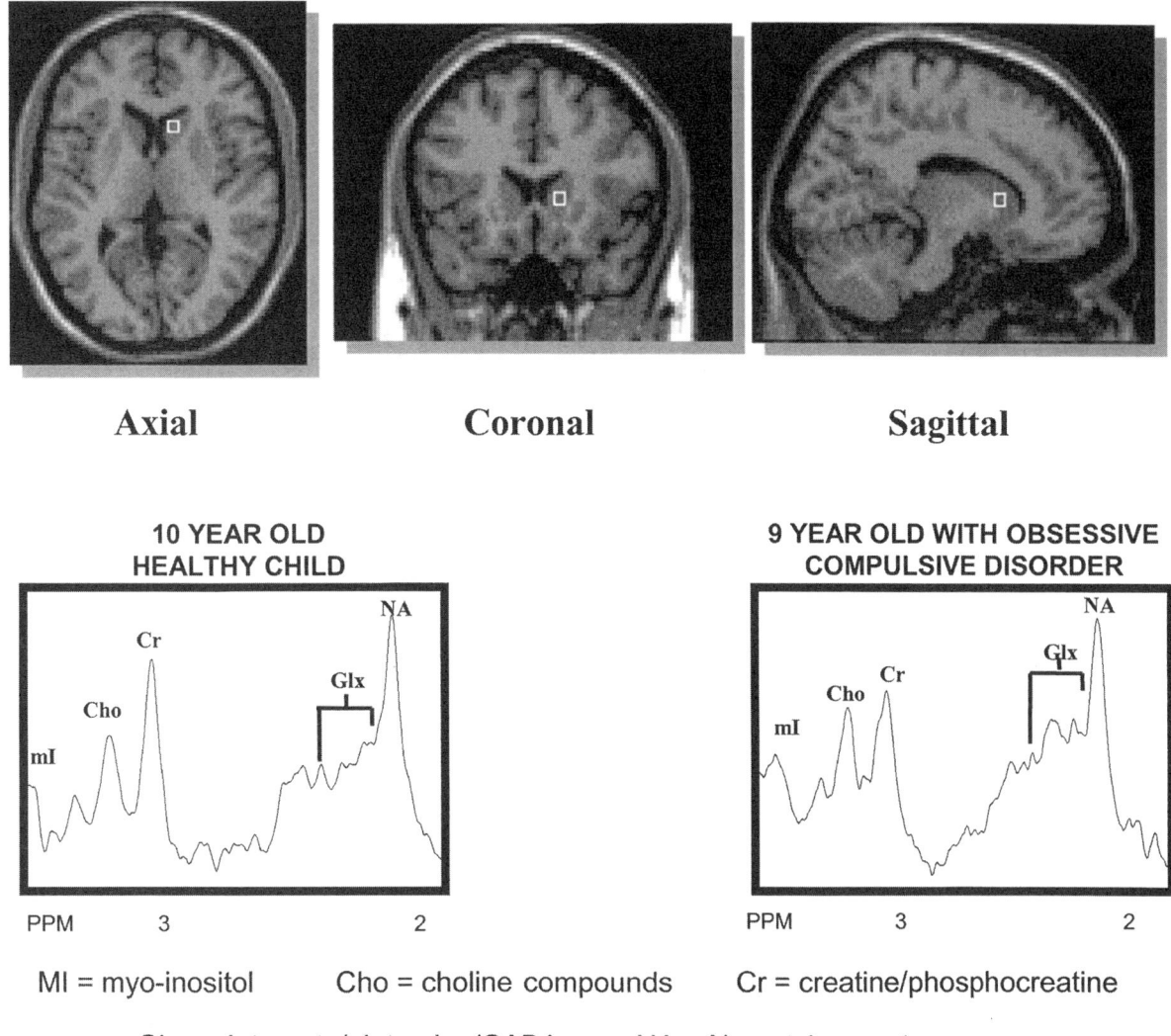

Figure 8 Illustration of voxel placement in left caudate nucleus. 1-H MRS of a 0.7-mL volume of interest centered in the left caudate in a 10-year-old healthy control and a 9-year-old treatment-naïve patient with obsessive-compulsive disorder as shown on the T1-weighted MR images. (Adapted from Rosenberg, MacMillan, Moore, 2001. Brain Anatomy and Chemistry May Predict Treatment Response in Pediatric Obsessive-Compulsive Disorder. Intl J Neuropsychopharmacology 4:179–190.)

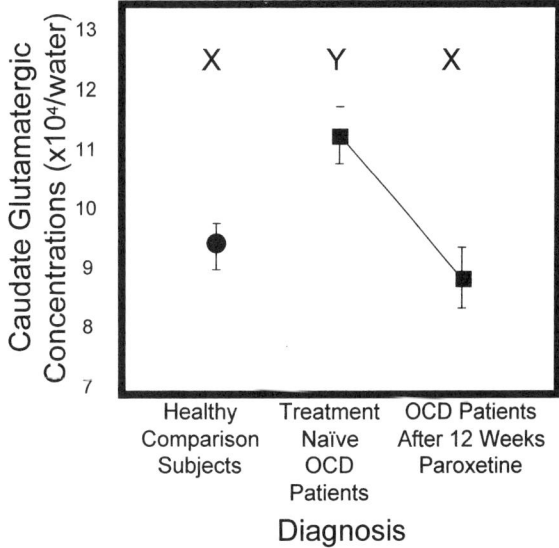

Figure 9 Caudate glutamatergic concentration by diagnostic and treatment condition. Groups not sharing the same letter are significantly different at $P < .05$. (Adapted from Rosenberg, MacMaster, Keshavan et al., 2000. Decrease in Caudate Glutamatergic Concentrations in Pediatric Obsessive-Compulsive Disorder Patients Taking Paroxetine. J Am Acad Child Adolesc Psychiatry 39(9):1096–1103.)

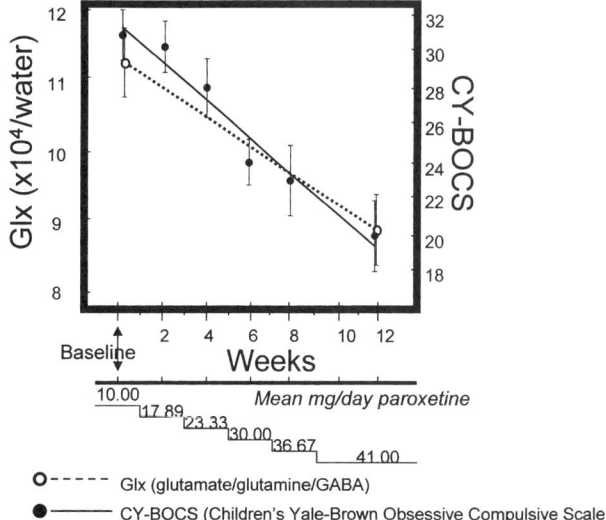

Figure 10 Decrease in left caudate glutamatergic concentrations associated with reduction in Obsessive-Compulsive Score of the Children's Yale-Brown-Obsessive-Compulsive Scales. (Reprinted by permission of Elsevier Science. Genetic and Imaging Strategies in Obsesssive-Compulsive Disorder: Potential Implications for Treatment, by Rosenberg and Hanna, Biological Psychiatry 48(12):1210–1222, 1998, by the Society of Biological Psychiatry.)

to this. There are currently three FDA-approved medications for treatment of child and adolescent OCD—fluvoxamine, sertraline, and clomipramine. A recent 13-week multicenter placebo-controlled investigation of fluoxetine conducted by Eli Lilly in 103 child and adolescent OCD patients 7–17 years old [135] found that fluoxetine was associated with significantly greater reduction in OCD symptom severity than was placebo. SmithKline Beecham also recently conducted a large multicenter study of paroxetine in pediatric OCD [136] and found that paroxetine was safe and effective in treating pediatric OCD patients. While citalopram has not been studied in pediatric OCD, it is likely to be effective in OCD patients. Because of their more favorable side-effects profiles, the SSRIs are typically used as first-line treatment before clomipramine.

In treatment-refractory OCD patients, combination of an SSRI with risperidone has been shown to be superior to placebo in adult patients [139,140]. Double-blind placebo-controlled studies augmenting SSRI therapy with lithium and thyroid hormone [141], trazadone [142], buspirone [143], and clonazepam [144] have not demonstrated benefit of augmentation with active medication over that of placebo augmentation. In adults augmentation of SSRI with haloperidol is superior to augmentation of placebo in treatment-refractory OCD patients with coexistent tics [145,146]. This combination was not effective in OCD patients without coexistent tics. Augmentation of an SSRI regimen with pimozide in refractory OCD patients has also been shown to be superior to placebo in OCD patients with coexistent chronic tic disorders or schizotypical personality disorders [146]. It should be noted that haloperidol and pimozide have potentially irreversible side effects, including tardive dyskinesia. This limits their use in children and adolescents. The atypical neuroleptics are being used more commonly in the clinical setting in refractory OCD patients.

It should be noted that CBT is recognized to be an effective treatment for children and adolescents with OCD [147–150]. A recent National Institute of Mental Health investigation is comparing SSRI (sertraline), CBT, combination therapy, and placebo in children and adolescents with OCD (personal communication, John March, M.D.). The results of this study have not yet been presented. Recent investigation has also found relatively high response rates with relaxation therapy (personal communication, John Piacentini, Ph.D.).

F. Posttraumatic Stress Disorder

Much like panic disorder, the diagnosis of posttraumatic stress disorder (PTSD) has only recently been applied to children. In 1891, Terr's [151] report of the Chowchilla school bus kidnapping was one of the first to describe PTSD in children. PTSD can occur at any age, as it is precipitated by an extreme stressor [152]. Based on the DSM-VI, there are four major criteria that must be met for the diagnosis of PTSD. These include exposure to a stressor, reexperiencing the event, avoidance of stimuli, and persistent increased arousal [7]. The stressor itself must be of a life-threatening or involve the threat of serious injury. PTSD can result from direct, witnessed, or verbal exposure to the stressor [153].

A number of comorbidities and associated symptoms can occur with PTSD. Separation anxiety is fairly common, in part because children may be responding to prior threats to loved ones, but also because most children react to traumatic events with attachment behavior [154]. Among the most common comorbidities are depression spectrum conditions, ranging from demoralization to melancholic MDD [155,156]. This corresponds with recent data from Breslau et al. [157] that suggest a marked increase in risk for MDD in patients with PTSD. Conversely, patients with PTSD following traumatic exposure were at increased risk for depression, while those with exposure who did not develop PTSD were also at risk for depression, suggesting that there may be a common underlying mechanism in PTSD and MDD.

In PTSD, neuroendocrine data in adults and children are fairly consistent. In adults, PTSD is associated with high levels of urinary cortisol; in fact, urinary cortisol following a traumatic event (motor vehicle accident) has been shown to predict the development and severity of PTSD [158]. Urinary catecholamine concentrations reflect plasma and peripheral sympathetic nervous system activity, tonic stimulation of the adrenal medulla, and metabolic breakdown of norepinephrine. De Bellis and colleagues [83] showed that children with PTSD had higher urinary catecholamine excretion than either healthy children or children with GAD/OAD, suggesting that this may be specific to PTSD rather than a marker of anxiety disorders in general. In a study of adult women who had been sexually abused in childhood, Helm et al. [42] showed that perturbations of the hypothalamic-pituitary- adrenal axis and autonomic hyperactivity that result from trauma can persist over time.

Thus far, there have been two neuroimaging studies of PTSD in children and adolescents—one morphometric study, and one spectroscopic. In a study of 44 maltreated children with PTSD, De Bellis et al. [159] found that children with PTSD had an overall reduction in brain volume that correlated with level of environmental stress, smaller medial and posterior corpus callosum, and increased volume of right and left lateral ventricles. In contrast to studies in adults, some with childhood onset of their illness [160–163], children with PTSD did not have reduced hippocampal volume. However, these findings are consistent with models of early-life stress in nonhuman primates [164]. In a sample of 11 children with PTSD, De Bellis et al. [165] found that maltreated children with PTSD had significantly lower NAA levels than healthy controls in the anterior cingulate, suggesting possible neuronal dysfunction in pediatric PTSD. Recent data suggest that 1-H MRS NAA assessment may be more sensitive for detecting neuronal abnormalities than conventional volumetric MRI studies [166].

Until very recently, there were no approved medications for the treatment of PTSD in children or adults. Sertraline has been shown to be effective in double-blind, placebo-controlled studies in adults, particularly with regard to the avoidance/numbing symptom cluster [167]. It was recently approved by the FDA for use in adults. Given the similarities between adult- and childhood-onset PTSD with regard to neuroendocrine factors [83], trials of this drug in children with PTSD are warranted. Future directions for medication development seem to be focused on matching therapy more closely with the pathophysiology of individual disorders. For instance, Friedman [168] suggests that, in PTSD, there are a number of physiologic targets for drug development. He discusses possible roles for CRF antagonists, neuropeptide-Y enhancers, drugs that downregulate glucocorticoid receptors, and more— many of which either are being developed or are in preclinical trials.

As with the other anxiety disorders, the psychotherapeutic intervention for PTSD that has the most empirical support is CBT [see 169 for review]. A study by March and colleagues [170] suggests that CBT is effective both accurately and at 6-month follow-up in children with PTSD.

G. Specific Phobia

Specific phobia is characterized by marked and persistent fear of a particular object or situation. This fear must be excessive and unreasonable and may be cued by the presence or anticipation of the feared stimulus, and the onset of anxiety symptoms occurs immediately [7]. Estimated prevalence rates for specific phobias range from < 1% to 9.2% [171,172]. Although there are a number of different theories suggesting that negative life experiences have an impact on phobia onset, a recent study by Magee [173] found that, of 12 discrete events and 10 chronic stressors, only assault by a relative and verbal aggression between parents influenced the onset of specific phobias. Specific phobias can generally be classified into three categories: (1) environmental/situational; (2) animal; and (3) blood/injection/injury [174]. These classifications also apply to phobias in children and adolescents [175]. While some studies suggest age and gender differences in frequency of particular phobias [174,176], no such studies have been performed in children. The most successful treatments for specific phobia are behavioral desensitization techniques such as systematic desensitization, modeling, and flooding [171]. To date, there is no evidence to support pharmacologic treatment of specific phobias. However, in the case of severe, disabling phobias, SSRIs such as fluvoxamine may be effective [177].

III. FUTURE RESEARCH DIRECTIONS

Although we are learning more about the brain circuits involved in anxiety disorders (Fig. 3), much remains to be done. To date, there has been very little family/genetic research in childhood-onset anxiety disorders. In part, this is because of the lack of psychometrically sound instruments for assessing anxiety, along with prior misconceptions regarding the nature of childhood anxiety [178]. However, two recent observations have spurred an interest in the heritability of anxiety. First, although better characterized in psychotic and mood disorders, there is evidence that there may be heritable forms of adult anxiety disorders that are characterized by onset in childhood [179]. The idea that SAD may be a heritable form of panic is one example [30]. Second, rather than inheriting a disorder, children may inherit a predisposition for that disorder [180]. In this context, neuroendocrine and neuroimaging findings may point toward candidate susceptibility genes. However, it is unlikely that neuroimaging and neuroendocrine data can be used to identify putative markers in the immediate future, primarily owing to the difficulties in replicating findings of susceptibility loci [10].

Pharmacogenetics is another area of genetic research that holds great promise in the study of childhood anxiety disorders. In this discipline, genetic information is used to guide drug design, thus taking individual variation in drug metabolism and response into account [10]. It is likely that this field will eventually intersect with imaging studies [181], especially given recent spectroscopic findings related to treatment response [128,133].

REFERENCES

1. The New Lexicon: Webster's Dictionary of the English Language. New York: Lexicon Publications, 1988.
2. EJ Costello, A Angold. Epidemiology. In: J March, ed. Anxiety Disorders in Children and Adolescents. New York: Guilford Press, 1995:109–124.
3. D Castellanos, T Hunter. Anxiety disorders in children and adolescents. South Med J 92:946–954, 1999.
4. American Psychiatric Association. Diagnostic and Statistical Manual of Mental Disorders. Washington: American Psychiatric Association, 1952.
5. American Psychiatric Association. Diagnostic and Statistical Manual of Mental Disorders, 2nd ed. Washington: American Psychiatric Association, 1968.
6. American Psychiatric Association. Diagnostic and Statistical Manual of Mental Disorders, 3rd ed. Washington: American Psychiatric Association, 1980.
7. American Psychiatric Association. DSM-IV: Diagnostic and Statistical Manual of Mental Disorders, 4th ed. Washington: American Psychiatric Press, 1994.
8. AJ Allen, H Leonard, SE Swedo. Current knowledge of medications for the treatment of childhood anxiety disorders. J Am Acad Child Adolesc Psychiatry 34(8):976–986, 1995.
9. RL Hendren, GJ Pandina. Review of neuroimaging studies of child and adolescent psychiatric disorders from the past 10 years. J Am Acad Child Adolesc Psychiatry 39:815–828, 2000.
10. DR Rosenberg, GL Hanna. Genetic and imaging strategies in obsessive-compulsive disorder: potential implications for treatment development. Biol Psychiatry 48:1210–1222, 2000.
11. R Schultz, DR Rosenberg, K Pugh, DS Pine, B Peterson, J Kaufmann, W Kates, L Jacobsen, J Giedd, X Castellanos, A Anderson. Pediatric neuroimaging. In: M Lewis, ed. Textbook of Child Psychiatry, 2001.

12. ND Ryan, D Varma. Child and adolescent mood disorders-experience with serotonin based therapies. Biol Psychiatry 44:336–340, 1998.
13. MJ Labellarte, GS Ginsburg, JT Walkup, MA Riddle. The treatment of anxiety disorders in children and adolescents. Biol Psychiatry 46:1567–1578, 1999.
14. PC Kendall. Treating anxiety disorders in children: results of a randomized clinical trial. J Consult Clin Psychol 62:100–110, 1994.
15. PC Kendall, E Flannery-Schroeder, SM Panichelli-Mindel, M Southam-Gerow, A Henin, M Warman. Therapy for youths with anxiety disorders: a second randomized clinical trial. J Consult Clin Psychol 65:366–380, 1997.
16. NJ King, BJ Tonge, D Heyne, M Pritchard, S Rollings, D Young, N Myerson, TH Ollendick. Cognitive-behavioral treatment of school-refusing children: a controlled evaluation. J Am Acad Child Adolesc Psychiatry 37:395–403, 1998.
17. MR Dadds, SH Spence, DE Holland, PM Barrett, KR Laurens. Prevention and early intervention for anxiety disorders: a controlled trial. J Consult Clin Psychol 65:627–636, 1997.
18. MR Dadds, DE Holland, KR Laurens, M Mullins, PM Barrett, SH Spence. Early intervention and prevention of anxiety disorders in children: results at 2-year follow-up. J Consult Clin Psychol 67:145–150, 1999.
19. PM Barrett, MR Dadds, RM Rapee. Family treatment of childhood anxiety: a controlled trial. J Consult Clin Psychol 64:333–342, 1996.
20. EJ Costello. Developments in child psychiatric epidemiology. J Am Acad Child Adolesc Psychiatry 28:836–841, 1989.
21. CG Last, CC Strauss, G Francis. Comorbidity among childhood anxiety disorders. J Nerv Ment Dis 175:726–730, 1987.
22. ME Lamb, A Nash, DM Tetli, et al. Infancy. In: Lewis M, ed. Child and Adolescent Psychiatry: Comprehensive Textbook. Baltimore: Williams & Wilkins, 1996:241–270.
23. V Manicavasagar, D Silove, J Curtis, R Wagner. Continuities of separation anxiety from early life into adulthood. J Anxiety Disord 14:1–18, 2000.
24. GA Bernstein, CM Borchardt. Anxiety disorders of childhood and adolescence: a critical review. J Am Acad Child Adolesc Psychiatry 30:519–532, 1991.
25. CG Last, S Perrin, M Hersen, AE Kazdin. DSM-III-R anxiety disorders in children: sociodemographic and clinical characteristics. J Am Acad Child Adolesc Psychiatry 31:1070–1076, 1992.
26. G Francis, CG Last, CC Straus. Expression of separation anxiety disorder: the roles of age and gender. Child Psychiatry Hum Dev 18:82–89, 1987.
27. BJ Coffey, J Biederman, JW Smoller, DA Geller, P Sarin, S Schwartz, GS Kim. Anxiety disorders and tic severity in juveniles with Tourette's disorder. J Am Acad Child Adolesc Psychiatry 39:562–568, 2000.
28. JD Lipsitz, LY Martin, S Mannuzza, TF Chapman, MR Liebowitz, DF Klein, AJ Fyer. Childhood separation anxiety disorder in patients with adult anxiety disorders. Am J Psychiatry 151:927–929, 1994.
29. D Silove, M Harris, A Morgan, P Boyce, V Manicavasagar, D Hadzi-Pavlovic, K Wilhelm. Is early separation anxiety a specific precursor of panic disorder–agoraphobia? A community study. Psychol Med 25:405–411, 1995.
30. M Battaglia, S Bertella, E Politi, L Bernardeschi, G Perna, A Gabriele, L Bellodi. Age at onset of panic disorder: influence of familiar liability to the disease and of childhood separation anxiety disorder. Am J Psychiatry 152:1362–1364, 1995.
31. SN Compton, AH Nelson, JS March. Social phobia and separation anxiety symptoms in community and clinical samples of children and adolescents. J Am Acad Child Adolesc Psychiatry 39:1040–1046, 2000.
32. JH Kashani, H Orvaschel. Anxiety disorders in mid-adolescence: a community sample. Am J Psychiatry 145:960–964, 1988.
33. PM Westenberg, BM Siebelink, NJ Warmenhoven, PD Treffers. Separation anxiety and overanxious disorders: relations to age and level of psychosocial maturity. J Am Acad Child Adolesc Psychiatry 38:1000–1007, 1999.
34. DS Pine, DE Weese-Mayer, JM Silvestri, M Davies, AH Whitaker, DF Klein. Anxiety and congenital central hypoventilation syndrome. Am J Psychiatry 151:864–870, 1994.
35. DS Pine, PG Klein, JD Coplan, LA Papp, CW Hoven, J Martinez, P Kovalenko, DJ Mandell, D Moreau, DF Klein, JM Gorman. Differential carbon dioxide sensitivity in childhood anxiety disorders and nonill comparison group. Arch Gen Psychiatry 57:960–967, 2000.
36. DS Pine, JD Coplan, LA Papp, RG Klein, JM Martinez, P Kovalenko, N Tancer, D Moreau, ES Dummit III, D Shaffer, DF Klein, JM Gorman. Ventilatory physiology of children and adolescents with anxiety disorders. Arch Gen Psychiatry 55:123–129, 1998.
37. SS Sinha, JD Coplan, DS Pine, JA Martinez, DF Klein, JM Gorman. Panic induced by carbon dioxide inhalation and lack of hypothalamic-pituitary-adrenal axis activation. Psychiatry Res 86:93–98, 1999.
38. G Vila, C Nollet-Clemencon, J de Blic, MC Mouren-Simeoni, P Scheinmann. Prevalance of DSM IV anxiety and affective disorders in a pediatric population of asthmatic children and adolescents. J Affect Disord 58:223–231, 2000.
39. C Caldji, J Diorio, MJ Meaney. Variations in maternal care in infancy regulate the development of stress reactivity. Biol Psychiatry 48:1164–1174, 2000.

40. DM Lyons, OJ Wang, SE Lindley, S Levine, NH Kalin, AF Schatzberg. Separation induced changes in squirrel monkey hypothalamic-pituitary-adrenal physiology resemble aspects of hypercortisolism in humans. Psychoneuroendocrinology 24:131–142, 1999.
41. C Heim, CB Nemeroff. The impact of early adverse experiences on brain systems involved in the pathophysiology of anxiety and affective disorders. Biol Psychiatry 46:1509–1522, 1999.
42. C Heim, DJ Newport, S Heit, YP Graham, M Wilcox, R Bonsall, AH Miller, CB Nemeroff. Pituitary-adrenal and autonomic responses to stress in women after sexual and physical abuse in childhood. JAMA 284:592–597, 2000.
43. D Klein, R Gitelman, F Quitkin, et al. Diagnosis and Drug Treatment of Psychiatric Disorders: Adults and Children. Baltimore: Williams & Wilkins, 1980.
44. JC Ballenger, DJ Carek, JJ Steele, D Cornish-McTighe. Three cases of panic disorder with agoraphobia in children [see comments]. Am J Psychiatry 146:922–924, 1989.
45. R Gittelman-Klein, D Klein. Controlled imipramine treatment of school phobia. Arch Gen Psychiatry 47:298–300, 1971.
46. R Klein, H Koplewicz, A Kanner. Imipramine treatment of children with separation anxiety disorder. J Am Acad Child Adolesc Psychiatry 31:21–28, 1992.
47. T Berney, I Kolvin, SR Bhate, RF Garside, J Jeans, B Kay, L Scarth. School phobia: a therapeutic trial with clomipramine and short-term outcome. Br J Psychiatry 138:110–118, 1981.
48. F Graae, J Milner, L Rizzotto, RG Klein. Clonazepam in childhood anxiety disorders. J Am Acad Child Adolesc Psychiatry 33:372–376, 1994.
49. R Balon. Buspirone in the treatment of separation anxiety in an adolescent boy. Can J Psychiatry 39:581–582, 1994.
50. H Kranzler. Use of buspirone on an adolescent with overanxious disorder. J Am Acad Child Adolesc Psychiatry 27:789–790, 1988.
51. GA Bernstein, CM Borchardt, AR Perwien, RD Crosby, MG Kushner, PD Thuras, CG Last. Imipramine plus cognitive-behavioral therapy in the treatment of school refusal. J Am Acad Child Adolesc Psychiatry 39:276–283, 2000.
52. B Birmaher, GS Waterman, N Ryan, M Cully, L Balach, J Ingram, M Brodsky. Fluoxetine for childhood anxiety disorders. J Am Acad Child Adolesc Psychiatry 33:993–999, 1994.
53. Research Units of Pediatric Psychopharmacology (RUPP) Anxiety Group. Fluvoxamine for anxiety in children. N Eng J Med 2001.
54. J Walkup. The RUPP Anxiety Study Group. Long-term treatment of childhood anxiety. Scientific Proceedings of the 47th Annual Meeting of the American Academy of Child and Adolescent Psychiatry 19B, 44, 2000, New York.
55. G Borzo. Fluvoxamine treats anxiety in children, teens. Clin Psychiatry News 28(6):10, 2000.
56. RC Bowen, DR Offord, MH Boyle. The prevalence of overanxious disorder and separation anxiety disorder: results from the Ontario Child Health Study. J Am Acad Child Adolesc Psychiatry 29:753–758, 1990.
57. D Shaffer, P Fisher, MK Dulcan, M Davies, J Piacentini, ME Schwab-Stone, BB Lahey, K Bourdon, PS Jensen, HR Bird, G Canino, DA Regier. The NIMH Diagnostic Interview Schedule for Children Version 2.3 (DISC-2.3): description, acceptability, prevalence rates, and performance in the MECA Study. Methods for the Epidemiology of Child and Adolescent Mental Disorders Study. J Am Acad Child Adolesc Psychiatry 35:865–877, 1996.
58. A Whitaker, J Johnson, D Shaffer, JL Rapoport, K Kalikow, BT Walsh, M Davies, S Braiman, A Dolinsky. Uncommon troubles in young people: prevalence estimates of selected psychiatric disorders in a nonreferred adolescent population. Arch Gen Psychiatry 47(5)487–496, 1990.
59. JS Werry. Overanxious disorder: a review of its taxonomic properties. J Am Acad Child Adolesc Psychiatry 30;533–544, 1991.
60. GA Bernstein, K Shaw. Practice parameters for the assessment and treatment of children and adolescents with anxiety disorders. American Academy of Child and Adolescent Psychiatry: J Am Acad Child Adolesc Psychiatry 36:69S–84S, 1997.
61. R Livingston. Anxiety disorders. In: M Lewis, ed. Child and Adolescent Psychiatry: A Comprehensive Textbook. Baltimore: Williams and Wilkins, 1996:674–683.
62. MD De Bellis, BJ Casey, RE Dahl, B Birmaher, DE Williamson, KM Thomas, DA Axelson, K Frustaci, AM Boring, J Hall, ND Ryan. A pilot study of amygdala volumes in pediatric generalized anxiety disorder. Biol Psychiatry 48:51–57, 2000.
63. DS Charney, A Deutch. A functional neuroanatomy of anxiety and fear: implications for pathophysiology and treatment of anxiety disorders. Crit Rev Neurobiol 10:419–446, 1996.
64. G Perna, R Bussi, L Allevi, L Bellodi. Sensitivity to 35% carbon dioxide in patients with generalized anxiety disorder. J Clin Psychiatry 60:379–384, 1999.
65. K Verburg, E Griez, J Meijer, H Pols. Discrimination between panic disorder and generalized anxiety disorder by 35% carbon dioxide challenge. Am J Psychiatry 152:1081–1083, 1995.
66. R Rapee. Differential response to hyperventilation in panic disorder and generalized anxiety disorder. J Abnorm Psychol 95:24–28, 1986.

67. G Gerra, A Zaimovic, U Zambelli, M Timpano, N Reali, S Bernasconi, F Brambilla. Neuroendocrine respones to psychological stress in adolescents with anxiety disorder. Neuropsychobiology 42:82–92, 2000.
68. O Brawman-Mintzer, RB Lydiard. Biological basis of generalized anxiety disorder. J Clin Psychiatry 58(suppl 3):6–25, 1997.
69. JL Abelson, D Glitz, OG Cameron, MA Lee, M Bronzo, GC Curtis. Blunted growth hormone response to clonidine in patients with generalized anxiety disorder. Arch Gen Psychiatry 48;157–162, 1991.
70. JW Tiller, N Biddle, KP Maguire, BM Davies. The dexamethasone suppression test and plasma dexamethasone in generalized anxiety disorder. Biol Psychiatry 23:261–270, 1988.
71. TD Borkovec, AM Ruscio. Psychotherapy for generalized anxiety disorder. J Clin Psychiatry 62(suppl 11):37–42, 2001.
72. PM Barrett, AL Duffy, MR Dadds, RM Rapee. Cognitive-behavioral treatment of anxiety disorders in children: long-term (6-year) follow-up. J Consult Clin Psychol 69:135–141, 2001.
73. L Sareen, M Stein. A review of the epidemiology and approaches to the treatment of social anxiety disorder. Drugs 59:497–509, 2000.
74. DA Chavira, MB Stein. Recent developments in child and adoelscent social phobia. Curr Psychiatry Rep 2:347–352, 2000.
75. WJ Magee, WW Eaton, HU Wittchen, KA McGonagle, RC Kessler. Agoraphobia, simple phobia, and social phobia in the National Comorbidity Survey. Arch Gen Psychiatry 53:159–168, 1996.
76. MB Stein, YM Kean. Disability and quality of life in social phobia: epidemiologic findings. Am J Psychiatry 157:1606–1613, 2000.
77. DS Pine, E Cohen, P Cohen, JS Brook. Social Phobia and the persistence of conduct problems. J Child Psychol Psychiatry 41:657–665, 2000.
78. FR Schneier, J Johnson, CD Hornig, MR Liebowitz, MM Weissman. Social phobia. Comorbidity and morbidity in an epidemiologic sample. Arch Gen Psychiatry 49:282–288, 1992.
79. J Kagan, JS Reznick, C Clarke, et al. Behavioral inhibition to the unfamiliar. Child Dev 55:2212–2225, 1984.
80. J Biederman, JF Rosenbaum, EA Bolduc-Murphy, SV Faraone, J Chaloff, DR Hirshfeld, J Kagan. A 3-year follow-up of children with and without behavioral inhibition. J Am Acad Child Adolesc Psychiatry 32:814–821, 1993.
81. CE Schwartz, N Snidman, J Kagan. Adolescent social anxiety as an outcome of inhibited temperament in childhood. J Am Acad Child Adolesc Psychiatry 38:1008–1015, 1999.
82. J Kagan, JS Reznick, N Snidman. Biological bases of childhood shyness. Science 240;167–171, 1988.
83. MD De Bellis, AS Baum, B Birmaher, ND Ryan. Urinary catecholamine excretion in childhood overanxious and posttraumatic stress disorders. Ann NY Acad Sci 821:451–455, 1997.
84. JF Rosenbaum, J Biederman, DR Hirshfeld-Becker, J Kagan, N Snidman, D Friedman. A Nineberg, DJ Gallery, SV Faraone. A controlled study of behavioral inhibition in children of parents with panic disorder and depression. Am J Psychiatry 157:2002-2010, 2000.
85. FL Martel, C Hayward, DM Lyons, K Sanborn, S Varady, AF Schatzberg. Salivary cortisol levels in socially phobic adolescent girls. Depress Anxiety 10:25–27, 1999.
86. KJ Zwier, U Rao. Buspirone use in an adoelscent with social phobia and mixed personality disorder (cluster a type). J Am Acad Child Adolesc Psychiatry 33:1007–1011, 1994.
87. RG Kathol, R Noyes, DJ Slymen, RR Crowe, J Clancy, RE Kerber. Propranolol in chronic anxiety disorders. A controlled study. Arch Gen psychiatry 37:1361–1365, 1980.
88. KL Granville-Grossman. Propranolol, anxiety, and the central nervous system. Br J Pharmacol 1:361, 1974.
89. RG Heimberg. Current status of psychotherapeutic interventions for social phobia. J Clin Psychiatry 62(suppl 1):36–42, 2001.
90. VE Cobham, MR Dadds, SH Spence. The role of parental anxiety in the treatment of childhood anxiety. J Consult Clin Psychol 66:893–905, 1998.
91. JL Abelson, NE Alessi. Discussion of "Child panic revisited." J Am Acad Child Adolesc Psychiatry 31:114–116, 1992.
92. DF Klein, S Mannuzza, T Chapman, AJ Fyer. Child panic revisited. J Am Acad Child Adolesc Psychiatry 31(1):112–114, 1992.
93. WB Nelles, DH Barlow. Do children panic? Clin Psychol Rev 8:359–372, 1988.
94. B Black, DR Robbins. Panic disorder in children and adolescents [see comments]. J Am Acad Child Adolesc Psychiatry 29:36–44, 1990.
95. D Moreau, MM Weissman. Panic disorder in children and adolescents: a review. Am J Psychiatry 149:1306–1314, 1992.
96. BA Thyer, RT Parrish, GC Curtis, RM Nesse, OG Cameron. Ages of onset of DSM-III anxiety disorders. Comp psychiatry 26:113-122, 1985.
97. MR Von Korff, WW Eaton, PM Keyl. The epidemiology of panic attacks and panic disorder. Results of three community surveys. Am J Epidemiol 122:970–981, 1985.
98. J Segui, M Marquez, L Garcia, J Canet, L Salvador-Carulla, M Ortiz. Differential clinical features of early-

onset panic disorder. J Affect Disord 54:109–117, 1999.
99. J Biederman, SV Faraone, DR Hirshfeld-Becker, D Friedman, JA Robin, JF Rosenbaum. Patterns of psychopathology and dysfunction in high-risk children of parents with panic disorder and major depression. Am J Psychiatry 158:49–57, 2001.
100. FR Sallee, H Richman, G Sethuraman, D Duogherty, L Sine, S Altman-Hamamdzic. Clonidine challenge in childhood anxiety disorder. J Am Acad Child Adolesc Psychiatry 37:655–662, 1998.
101. FR Sallee, G Sethuraman, L Sine, H Liu. Yohimbine challenge in children with anxiety disorders. Am J Psychiatry 157:1236–1242, 2000.
102. AH Zohar. The epidemiology of obsessive-compulsive disorder in children and adolescents. Child Adolesc Psychiatric Clin North Am 8;445–460, 1999.
103. DL Pauls, JP Alsobrook, M Phil, W Goodman, S Rasmussen, JF Leckman. A family study of obsessive-compulsive disorder. Am J Psychiatry 152:76–84, 1995.
104. SE Swedo, JL Rapoport, H Leonard, M Lenane, D Cheslow. Obsessive-compulsive disorder in children and adolescents. Arch Gen Psychiatry 46:335–341, 1989.
105. TP Zahn, HL Leonard, SE Swedo, JL Rapoport. Autonomic activity in children and adolescents with obsessive-compulsive disorder. Psychiatry Res 60:67–76, 1996.
106. JS Luxenberg, SE Swedo, MF Flament, RP Friedland, J Rapoport, SI Rapoport. Neuroanatomical abnormalities in obsessive-compulsive disorder determined with quantitative x-ray computed tomography. Am J Psychiatry 145[9], 1089–1093, 1988.
107. D Behar, JL Rapoport, CJ Berg, MB Denckla, L Mann, C Cox, P Fedio, T Zahn, MG Wolfman. Computerized tomography and neuropsychological test measures in adolescents with obsessive-compulsive disorder. Am J Psychiatry 141:363–369, 1984.
108. DR Rosenberg, MS Keshavan, KM O'Hearn, EL Dick, WW Bagwell, AB Seymor, DM Montrose, JN Pierri, B Birmaher. Fronto-striatal measurement of treatment-naive pediatric obsessive compulsive disorder. Arch Gen Psychiatry 54:824–830, 1997.
109. SL Rauch, PJ Whalen, DD dougherty, MA Jenike. Neurobiological Models of Obsessive Compulsive Disorders. Obsessive Compulsive Disorders: Practical Management. Boston: Mosby, 1998:222–253.
110. JN Giedd, JL Rapoport, MJP Kruesi, C Parker, MB Schapiro, AJ Allen, HL LEonard, D Kaysen, DP Dickstein, WL Marsh, PL Kozuch, AC Vaituzis, SD Hamburger, SE Swedo. Sydenham's chorea: magnetic-resonance-imaging of the basal ganglia. Neurology 45:2199–2202, 1995.
111. JN Giedd, JL Rapoport, MA Garvey, S Perlmutter, SE Swedo. MRI assessment of children with obsessive-compulsive disorder or tics associated with streptococcal infection. Am J Psychiatry 157(2):281–283, 2000.
112. BS Peterson, JF Leckman, D Tucker, L Scahill, L Staib, H Zhang, R King, DJ Cohen, JC Gore, P Lombroso. Preliminary findings of antistreptococcal antibody titers and basal ganglia volumes in tic, obsessive-compulsive, and attention deficit/hyperactivity disorders. Arch Gen Psychiatry 57:364–372, 2000.
113. AJ Allen, HL Leonard, SE Swedo. case study: a new infection-triggered, autoimmune subtype of pediatric OCD and tourett'e syndrome. J Am Acad Child Adolesc Psychiatry 34:307–311, 1995.
114. JN Giedd, JL Rapoport, HL Leonard, D Richter, SE Swedo. Case study: acute basal ganglia enlargement and obsessive-compulsive symptoms in an adolescent boy. J Am Acad Child Adolesc Psychiatry 35(7):913–915, 1996.
115. D Becquet, M Faudon, F Hery. In vivo evidence for an inhibitory glutamatergic control fo serotonin release in the cat caudate nucleus: involvement of GABA neurons. Brain Res 519:82–88, 1990.
116. A Parent, PY Cote, B Lavoie. Chemical anatomy of primate basal ganglia. Prog Neurobiol 46:131–197, 1995.
117. A Parent, LN Hazrati. Functional anatomy of the basal ganglia. I. The cortico–basal ganglia–thalamo-cortical loop. Brain Res 20:91–127, 1995.
118. JS Kim, R Hassler, P Haug, KS Paik. Effect of frontal cortex ablation on striatal glutamic acid level in rat. Brain Res 132:370–374, 1977.
119. P Calabresi, A Pisani, NB Mercuri, G Bernardi. The corticostriatal projection: from synaptic plasticity to dysfunction of the basal ganglia. Trends Neurosci 19:279–280, 1996.
120. DR Rosenberg, EL Dick, KM O'Hearn, JA Sweeney. Response inhibition defcits in obsessive compulsive disorder: an indicator of dysfunction in fronto-striatal circuits. J Psychiatry Neurosci 22:29–38, 1997.
121. DR Rosenberg, MS Keshavan. Toward a neurodevelopmental model of obsessive compulsive disorder. Biol Psychiatry 43(9):623–640, 1998.
122. LR Baxter, S Saxena, AL Brody, RF Ackermann, M Colgan, JM Schwartz, Z Allen-Martinez, JM Fuster, ME Phelps. Brain mediation of obsessive-compulsive disorder symptoms: evidence from functional brain imaging studies in the human and nonhuman primate. Semin Clin Neuropsychiatry 1:32–47, 1996.
123. MA Jenike, HC Breiter, L Baer, DN Kenendy, CR Savage, MJ Olvares, RL O'Sullivan, DM Shera, SL Rauch, N Keuthen, BR Rosen, VS Caviness, PA Filipek. Cerebral structural abnormalities in obsessive-compulsive disorder: a quantitative morphometric magnetic resonance imaging study. Arch Gen Psychiatry 53:625–632, 1996.

124. AR Gilbert, GJ Moore, MS Keshavan, LD Paulson, V Narula, FP MacMaster, CM Stewart, DR Rosenberg. Decrease in thalamic volumes of pediatric obsessive compulsive disorder patients taking paroxetine. Arch Gen Psychiatry 57(5):449–456, 2000.
125. DR Rosenberg, NR Benazon, AR Gilbert, A Sullivan, GJ Moore. Thalamic volume in pediatric obsessive compulsive disorder patients before and after cognitive behavioral therapy. Biol Psychiatry, 2000.
126. KD Fitzgerald, GJ Moore, LD Paulson, CM Stewart, DR Rosenberg. Proton spectroscopic imaging of the thalamus in treatment-naive pediatric obsessive compulsive disorder. Biol Psychiatry 47:174–182, 2000.
127. DR Rosenberg, A Amponsah, A Sullivan, S MacMillan, GJ Moore. Increased medial thalamic choline in pediatric obsessive compulsive disorder as detected by quantitative in vivo spectrosopic imaging. J Child Neurol 16(9):636–641, 2001.
128. AA Amponsah, GJ Moore, AM Sullivan, DR Rosenberg. Localized changes in medial thalamic neurochemistry in pediatric patients with obsessive compulsive disorder who are taking paroxetine. Biol Psychiatry 49:89, 2001.
129. DL Birken, WH Oldendorf. N-acetyl-L-aspartic acid: a literature review of a compound prominent in 1H-NMR spectroscopic studies of brain (review). Neurosci Biobehav Rev 13:23–31, 1989.
130. D Becquet, F Hery, M Hery, MJ Drian, M Faudon, N Konig. Population-specific modulation of 5-HT expression in cultuers of embryonic rat rhombencephalon. J Neurosci Res 29:42–50, 1991.
131. T Reeisine, P Soubrie, F Artaud, J Glowinski. Application of L-glutamic acid and substance P to the substantia nigra modulates in vivo [3H] serotonin release in the basal ganglia of the cat. Brain Res 236(2):317–327, 1982.
132. E Edwards, E Hampton, CR Ashby, J Zhang, RY Wang. 5-HT3-like receptors in the rat medial prefrontal cortex: further pharmacological characterization. Brain Res 733(1):21–30, 1996.
133. DR Rosenberg, FP MacMaster, M Keshavan, KD Fitzgerald, CM Stewart, GJ Moore. Decrease in caudate glutamatergic concentrations in pediatric obsessive compulsive disorder patients taking paroxetine. J Am Acad Child Adolesc Psychiatry 39(9):1096–1103, 2000.
134. PS Jensen. Links among theory, research, and practice: cornerstones of clinical scientific progress. J Clin Guild psychol 28:553–557, 1999.
135. DA Geller, SL Hoog, JH Heiligenstein, RK Ricardi, R Tamura, S Kluszynski, JG Jacobson. Fluoxetine treatment for obsessive-compulsive disorder in children and adolescents: a placebo-controlled clinical trial. J Am Acad Child Adolesc Psychiatry 40:773–779, 2001.
136. GJ Emslie, KD Wagner, B Birmaher, DA Geller, MA Riddle, SL Kaplan, J Busner, WK Goodman, JT Macken, DJ Carpenter. Safety and efficacy of paroxetine in the treatment of children and adolescent with OCD. Scientific Proceedings of the 47th Annual Meeting of the American Academy of Child and Adolescent Psychiatry 110, 9, 2000, New York.
137. CJ McDougle, CN Epperson, GH Pelton, S Wasylink, LH Price. A double-blind, placebo-controlled study of risperidone addition in serotonin reuptake inhibitor-refractory obsessive-compulsive disorder. Arch Gen Psychiatry 57:794–801, 2000.
138. KD Fitzgerald, CM Stewart, V Tawile, DR Rosenberg. Risperidone augmentation of serotonin reuptake inhibitor treatment of pediatric obsessive compulsive disorder. J Child Adolesc Psychopharmacol 9:115–123, 1999.
139. Y Figueroa, DR Rosenberg, B Birmaher, MS Keshaven. Combination treatment with clomipramine and selective serotonin reuptake inhibitors for obsessive-compulsive disorder in children and adolescents. J Child Adolesc Psychopharmacol 8(1):61–67, 1998.
140. JG Simeon, S Thatte, D Wiggins. Treatment of adolescent obsessive-compulsive disorder with a clomipramine-fluoxetine combination. Psychopharmacol Bull 26:285–290, 1990.
141. TA Pigott, MT Pato, F L'Heureux, JL Hill, GN Grover, SE Bernstein, DL Murphy. A controlled comparison of adjuvant lithiumc arbonate or thyroid hormone in clomipramine-treated patients with obsessive compulsive disorder. J Clin Psychopharmacol 11(4):242–248, 1991.
142. TA Piggott, F L'Heureux, CS Rubenstein, SE Bernstein, JL Hill, DL Murphy. A double-blind, placebo controlled study of trazodone in patients with obsessive-compulsive disorder. J Clin Psychopharmacol 12(3):156–162, 1992.
143. TA Pigott, F L'Heureux, JL Hill, K Bihari, SE Bernstein, DL Murphy. A double-blind study of adjuvant buspirone hydrochloride in clomipramine-treated patients with obsessive compulsive disorder. J Clin Psychopharmacol 12(1):11–18, 1992.
144. TA Pigott, F L'Heureux, CS Rubenstein, JL Hill, DL Murphy. A controlled trial of clonazepam augmentation in OCD patients treated with clomipramine or fluoxetine. New Research Program and Abstracts of the 14th Annual Meeting of the American Psychiatric Association, 82, 1992. Washington: American Psychiatric Association.
145. CJ McDougle, WK Goodman, JF Leckman, NC Lee, GR Heninger, LH Price. Haloperidol addition in fluvoxamine-refractory obsessive compulsive disorder. Arch Gen Psychiatry 51:302–308, 1994.
146. CJ McDougle, WK Goodman, LH Price, PL Delgado, JH Krystal, DS Charney, GR Heninger. Neuroleptic addition in fluvoxamine-refractory obsessive-compulsive disorder. Am J Psychiatry 147(5):652–654, 1990.

147. JS March. Cognitive-behavioral psychotherapy for children and adolescents with OCD: a review and recommendations for treatment. J Am Acad Child Adolesc Psychiatry 34:7–18, 1995.
148. JS March, M Franklin, A Nelson, E Foa. Cognitive-behavioral psychotherapy for pediatric obsessive-compulsive disorder. J Clin Child Psychol 30:8–18, 2001.
149. JS March, K Mulle, B Herbel. Behavioral psychotherapy for children and adolescents with obsessive-compulsive disorder: an open trial of a new protocol-driven treatment package. J Am Acad Child Adolesc Psychiatry 33:333–341, 1994.
150. JS March, K Mulle. OCD in Children and Adolescents: A Cognitive Behavioral Treatment Manual. New York: Guilford Press, 1998.
151. LC Terr. Psychic trauma in children: observations following the Chowchilla school-bus kidnapping. Am J Psychiatry 138:14–19, 1981.
152. JH Kashani, AC Dandoy, H Orvaschel. Current perspectives on anxiety disorders in children and adolescents: an overview. Comp Psychiatry 32:481–495, 1991.
153. PA Saigh. The development of posttraumatic stress disorder following four different types of traumatization. Behav Res Ther 29:213–216, 1991.
154. HL Leonard, J March, KC Rickler, AJ Allen. Pharmacology of the selective serotonin reuptake inhibitors in children and adolescents. J Am Acad Child Adolesc Psychiatry 36:725–736, 1997.
155. W Yule. Post-traumatic stress disorder in child survivors of shipping disasters: the sinking of the 'Jupiter.' Psychother Psychosom 57:200–205, 1992.
156. W Yule, R Canterbury. The treatment of post traumatic stress disorder in children and adolescents. Int Rev Psychiatry 6:141–151, 1994.
157. N Breslau, GC Davis, EL Peterson, LR Schultz. A second look at comorbidity in victims of trauma: the posttraumatic stress disorder–major depression connection. Biol Psychiatry 48:902–909, 2000.
158. DL Delahanty, AJ Raimonde, E Spoonster. Initial posttraumatic urinary cortisol levels predict subsequent PTSD symptoms in motor vehicle accident victims. Biol Psychiatry 48:940–947, 2000.
159. MD De Bellis, A Baum, B Birmaher, M Keshavan, CH Eccard, AM Boring, FJ Jenkins, ND Ryan. Developmental traumatology. Part I. Biological stress systems. A.E. Bennett Research Award paper. Biol Psychiatry 45(10):1271–1284, 1999.
160. JD Bremner, P Randall, TM Scott, RA Bronen, JP Seibyl, SM Southwick, RC Delaney, G McCarthy, DS Charney, RB Innis. MRI-based measurement of hippocampal volume in patients with combat-related posttraumatic stress disorder. Am J Psych 152(7):973–981, 1995.
161. JD Bremner, P Randall, E Vermetten, L Staib, RA Bronen, C Mazure, S Capelli, G McCarthy, RB Innis, DS Charney. Magnetic resonance imaging-based measurement of hippocampal volume in posttraumatic stress disorder related to childhood physical and sexual abuse—a preliminary report. Biol Psychiatry 41(1):23–32, 1997.
162. TV Gurvits, ME Shenton, HH Hokama, H Ohta, NB Lasko, MW Gilbertson, SP Orr, R Kikinis, FA Jolesz, RW McCarley, RK Pitman. Magnetic resonance imaging study of hippocampal volume in chronic combat-related posttraumatic stress disorder. Biol Psychiatry 40(11):1091–1099, 1996.
163. MB Stein, MS Koverola, GL Hanna, MG Torchia, B McClart. Hippocampal volume in women victimized by childhood sexual abuse. Psychol Med 27:1–9, 1997.
164. MM Sanchez, EF Hearn, D Do, JK Rilling, JG Herndon. Differential rearing affects corpus callosum size and cognitive function of rhesus monkeys. Brain Res 812:38–49, 1998.
165. MD De Bellis, MS Keshavan, S Spencer, J Hall. N-Acetylaspartate concentration in the anterior cingulate of maltreated children and adolescents with PTSD. Am J Psychiatry 157:1175–1177, 2000.
166. R Bartha, MB Stein, PC Williamson, DJ Drost, RW Neufield, TJ Carr, G Canaran, M Densmore, G Anderson, AR Siddiqui. A short echo 1H spectroscopy and volumetric MRI study of the corpus striatum in patients with obsessive compulsive disorder and comparison subjects. Am J Psychiatry 155(11):1584–1591, 1998.
167. T Pearlstein. Antidepressant treatment of posttraumatic stress disorder. J Clin Psychiatry 61(suppl 7):40–43, 2000.
168. MJ Friedman. What might the psychobiology of post-tramatic stress disorder teach us about future approaches to pharmacotherapy? J Clin Psychiatry 51:44–51, 2000.
169. EA Hembree, EB Foa. Posttraumatic stress disorder: psychological factors and psychosocial interventions. J Clin Psychiatry 61(suppl 7):33–39, 2000.
170. JS March, L Amaya-Jackson, MC Murray, A Schulte. Cognitive-behavioral psychotherapy for children and adolescents with posttraumatic stress disorder after a single-incident stressor. J Am Acad Child Adolesc Psychiatry 37:585–593, 1998.
171. B Black, HL Leonard, JL Rapoport. Specific phobia, panic disorder, social phobia, and selective mutism. In: JM Weiner, ed. Textbook of Child and Adolescent Psychiatry. Washington: American Psychiatric Press, 1997.
172. CA Essau, J Conradt, F Petermann. Frequency, comorbidity, and psychosocial impairment of specific phobia in adolescents. J Clin Child Psychol 29:221–231, 2000.
173. WJ Magee. Effects of negative life experiences on phobia onset. Soc Psychiatry Psychiatr Epidemiol 34:343–351, 1999.

174. M Fredrikson, P Annas, H Fischer, G Wik. Gender and age differences in the prevalence of specific fears and phobias. Behav Res Ther 34:33–39, 1996.
175. P Muris, H Schmidt, H Merckelbach. The structure of specific phobia symptoms among children and adolescents. Behav Res Ther 37:863–868, 1999.
176. GC Curtis, WJ Magee, WW Eaton, HU Wittchen, RC Kessler. Specific fears and phobias. Epidemiology and classification. Br J Psychiatry 173:212–217, 1998.
177. R Balon. Fluvoxamine for phobia of storms. Acta Psychiatr Scand 100:244–245, 1999.
178. DS Pine. Pathophysiology of childhood anxiety disorders. Biol Psychiatry 46:1555–1566, 1999.
179. RB Goldstein, PJ Wickramaratne, E Horwath, MM Weismann. Familial aggregation and phenomenology of "early"-onset (at or before age 20 years) panic disorder. Arch Gen Psychiatry 54:272–278, 1997.
180. C Grillon, L Dierker, KR Merikangas. Startle modulation in children at risk for anxiety disorders and/or alcoholism. J Am Acad Child Adolesc Psychiatry 36:925–932, 1997.
181. GM Anderson, EH Cook. Pharmacogenetics. Promise and potential in child and adolescent psychiatry. Child Adolesc Psychiatr Clin North Aam 9:23–42, viii, 2000.

13

Psychotic Disorders in Childhood and Adolescence
Basic Mechanisms and Therapeutic Interventions

ANDREW R. GILBERT and MATCHERI S. KESHAVAN
Western Psychiatric Institute and Clinic, University of Pittsburgh School of Medicine, Pittsburgh, Pennsylvania, U.S.A.

I. INTRODUCTION

Once considered a form of autism, childhood-onset psychosis is currently described as a condition continuous with and, perhaps, more severe than adult-onset schizophrenia. Advances in treatment and research have improved our understanding, diagnosis, and management of childhood-onset psychosis. Childhood-onset psychosis was often compared to early infantile autism [1], but later described by Kolvin as a distinct pediatric condition [2]. Several studies since Kolvin's work have examined childhood psychosis, greatly contributing to the classification and elucidation of the disorder [3–5].

Currently, childhood-onset psychosis is defined by the same criteria used for adult schizophrenia. Therefore, there must be positive symptoms—hallucinations, delusions, and/or thought disorder. No single finding is pathognomonic, as any of these overall symptoms can be observed in patients suffering from disorders of affect or organic brain disease. A primary psychosis in childhood and adolescence generally manifests itself in the form of childhood-onset schizophrenia, a rare form of schizophrenia. There are certain characteristics of childhood-onset schizophrenia, however, that are different from the adult-onset illness. First, while a decline from a previous level of functioning is a necessary prerequisite for the diagnosis of schizophrenia beginning in childhood, childhood-onset schizophrenia patients may have never achieved the expected level of functioning. Second, the content of the psychotic symptoms in childhood-onset schizophrenia differs according to the developmental level and age of the patient [6]. Furthermore, others have reported that patients with childhood-onset schizophrenia have considerably less frequent systematic delusions than adult schizophrenics [7]. Another study reported that the ratings of premorbid adjustment for schizophrenic children are poorer than those for adult schizophrenics [8].

In light of the observation that early age of onset is associated with poorer premorbid adjustment, Asarnow and Ben-Meir suggested that childhood-onset schizophrenia may represent an early-onset form of adult schizophrenia [8]. Murray proposed that early-onset schizophrenia might reflect a form of illness with a greater genetic loading, male preponderance, and possibly a greater contribution by neurodevelopmental pathology [9]. Others have pursued investigations of patients with onset of schizophrenia close to the "sensitive" periods of development, such as the peripubertal period, in order to better elucidate the proposed neurodevelopmental pathogenesis of the illness [10].

Since hallucinations and delusions are frequently seen in pediatric populations and may result from a variety of disorders, the diagnosis of childhood-onset psychosis is a difficult one. Often, patients with psychotic symptoms secondary to affective disorders are misdiagnosed with a primary psychosis [11]. Recently, a subgroup from the larger population of children with nonschizophrenic nonaffective psychoses, "multidimensionally impaired" disorder (MDI), has been described and studied [12]. Children with MDI have no thought disorder, but may experience transient hallucinations or delusions and emotional lability, and may demonstrate poor interpersonal skills [11].

As suggested above, it is important to consider the developmental phase of individuals with the illness when making a diagnosis. Furthermore, the developmental stage significantly influences treatment; medications, educational and family interventions, and supportive psychotherapy are often tailored to the developmental capacity of the patient as well as the stage of the illness.

In this chapter, we will review the clinical features, course, outcome, and management of childhood-onset psychosis, with particular emphasis on childhood-onset schizophrenia.

II. HISTORICAL BACKGROUND

Psychotic disorders have been described as far back as 1000 BC [13]. Modern descriptions of schizophrenia, however, began to appear in the literature only in the late 18th and early 19th centuries. Morel first described a condition, dementia praecoce, as an illness beginning in adolescence and leading to a gradual deterioration. Kraepelin later integrated several descriptions of schizophrenialike illnesses into a single entity he labeled dementia praecox [14]. The occurrence of schizophrenia in childhood was also described at the time of Kraepelin. However, childhood-onset psychosis was generally considered a type of autistic or pervasive developmental disorder. Kolvin later demonstrated that autism was a disorder distinct from "later onset" psychoses of childhood [2].

Although few have studied childhood-onset schizophrenia, several studies have recently examined the disorder [3,7,15–19]. An understanding of the neurodevelopmental course of schizophrenia has likely inspired much of this research. Currently, schizophrenia in youth appears to be a more severe form of the same heterogeneous disorder as in adults. The outcomes of current studies, and future studies of children with MDI and atypical psychoses, should better explain the condition and approaches toward treatment.

Schizophrenia is very rare in children below the age of 9. It is about 50 times more prevalent in the general population than in children under 12 years of age. At the beginning of adolescence, there is a sharp increase in the onset of cases, and the number of new cases increases throughout the teenage years. The estimated incidence of schizophrenia in children under 12 years is 3:10,000 [20]. Childhood-onset schizophrenia has a slight male predominance, ~1.5 or 2 males:1 female. There is some evidence that schizophrenic children may be more commonly observed in families of lower socioeconomic status [21].

III. CLINICAL PICTURE

The symptoms of childhood-onset schizophrenia are similar to but often more severe than the symptoms of schizophrenia. Recent studies have suggested that the diagnosis of schizophrenia can be made in children using the same criteria as applied to adults [3,5,22,23]. Both positive and negative symptoms are observed in childhood-onset schizophrenia. Positive symptoms are considered to result from an excessive activity of certain brain processes; in contrast, negative symptoms are suggestive of deficient functioning in specific neuronal systems. Positive symptoms include hallucinations, delusions, "positive" formal thought disorder, and disorganized and bizarre behaviors. Negative symptoms are enduring traits of poverty of speech and thought, affective flattening, inability to experience pleasure, diminution of social contact, inattention, anergia, and lack of persistence in work or social functioning. This distinction has significant implications for diagnosis, prognosis, and treatment [24–26]. DSM-IV suggests that delusions and hallucinations in childhood may be less elaborated than in adulthood, and that visual hallucinations may be more common [27]. Furthermore, disorganized speech and behavior are seen in a variety of more common disorders of childhood, such as Communication Disorders, Pervasive Developmental Disorders, Attention Deficit/Hyperactivity Disorder, and Stereotypic Movement Disorder [27]. The differential diagnosis of childhood-onset psychosis also includes affective disorders, as mood disturbances can often be observed in schizophrenia. It is also important to consider Obsessive-Compulsive Disorder (OCD) when diagnosing childhood-onset psychosis because pediatric patients with OCD may exhibit ideas that are sometimes difficult to distinguish from delusions [21].

In childhood and adolescence, the developmental stage of the patient must be considered when attempting to separate immature fantasy from delusional thinking. Children's tendency to blur the distinction between fantasy and reality, in combination with their inability to fully utilize logical reason, renders it difficult to define delusions in individuals much younger than 5 years old. In general, delusions are found least frequently in children under the age of 10; they tend to be simple, nonsystematized, and centered on disturbances of identity. Hypochondriacal, persecutory, and grandiose delusions appear slightly more often in prepubertal children—and considerably more often in adolescents [2,28–35].

Disturbances in emotions are another hallmark of schizophrenia and become increasingly evident as the illness progresses. Mood disturbance may present as anxiety, perplexity, elevation, or depression. With a loss of ego boundaries and the onset of referential thinking, young schizophrenics often experience marked anxiety early in the illness. They are perplexed by a chaotic inner world that they struggle to understand and articulate. Depression may occur at any time during the illness, but it frequently appears as adolescents gain insight into their growing functional impairments—an awareness that may lead to suicidal behaviors.

The childhood-onset schizophrenia patient often presents with nonspecific somatic complaints, such as constipation, bloating, vague muscle aches, back pain, headaches, disturbed sleep, decreased appetite, fatigue, and listlessness. Objective findings may include avoidance of eye contact, absence or rapidity of eye blinks, staring spells, and a disturbance in eye tracking (i.e., saccades and smooth pursuit eye movements) [36].

Disturbances in neurological maturation, cognition, emotional capacity, and social competency characterize the premorbid condition of schizophrenia [28]. Several studies have suggested that childhood-onset schizophrenia is associated with more severe developmental abnormalities than later-onset schizophrenia [3,4,8,34,37,38]. Adolescents with chronic schizophrenia since childhood or shortly after puberty are likely to have exhibited marked disturbances in neurological growth, with slower motor development, inferior coordination, echolalia, delayed and unclear speech, tactile sensitivity, and nonpurposeful rituals. Such neurodevelopmental findings are nonspecific and do not meet criteria for a pervasive development disorder [2,34,39]. A recent NIMH study of 49 patients with childhood-onset schizophrenia revealed that 55% had language abnormalities, 57% had motor abnormalities, and 55% had social abnormalities years before the onset of psychotic symptoms [3,40]. Cognitive disturbances in early-onset schizophrenia frequently manifest with intellectual impairments, attention deficits, and distractibility [34,41]. Cognitive deficits of this sort commonly give rise to impaired school performance characterized by learning problems, failing grades, truancy, hyperactivity, dropping out of school, and dysfunctional teacher-student relations. The same NIMH study previously mentioned reported that a high percentage (66.3%) of patients had either failed a grade or required special education placement prior to the onset of their illness [3,40]. Other cognitive abnormalities noted include obsessional manifestations, perfectionistic needs, magical thinking, daydreams, and intellectual preoccupations [28,41].

Preschizophrenic individuals have also frequently demonstrated emotional deficits, impaired affective control, angry outbursts, detachment, hypersensitivity, and passivity, as well as depressive features and anxious behaviors [39,42,43]. Other abnormalities observed in the preschizophrenic adolescent include impairment in establishing and maintaining interpersonal relations, poor peer group adjustment, social withdrawal, shyness, introversion, and diffidence. Social isolation and seclusion have been found to result more from the individual being regarded by peers as odd and eccentric than from shyness [43]. Antisocial behaviors are more likely expressed toward family members rather than as a social delinquency [43].

Although premorbid behavioral patterns vary greatly among schizophrenics, clinicians more commonly report these features to be consistent with a schizoid personality type. The schizoid personality of the prepsychotic adolescent is similarly described with traits of passivity, introversion, detachment, and autistic thinking. Preschizophrenic youths are less likely to have intimate friends and social dates, and will choose solitary activities of watching TV, listening to radio, or playing computer games, often to the exclusion of competitive sports and other social activities [44]. Additional personality types described less commonly include avoidant, paranoid, histrionic, and compulsive disorders. Manifestations of a premorbid personality disturbance, which are associated with a poor prognosis, have been observed more often in the earlier-onset schizophrenic syndromes rather than later-onset acute episodes [45].

Schizophrenia has been classified into a variety of subtypes throughout the years. An early study suggested that the majority of children with schizophrenia belong to the undifferentiated subtype [46]. The traditional classification of subtypes outlined below is continued in DSM-IV [27]. A recent study of childhood-onset schizophrenia, however, suggested no significant differences between adults and children when comparing the prevalence of particular subtypes of schizophrenia [16].

Catatonic type is characterized by marked psychomotor disturbance involving stupor, negativism, rigidity, excitement, and posturing. *Disorganized type* is associated with marked loosening of associations, incoherence, grossly disorganized behavior, and flat or grossly inappropriate affect, as well as fragmented delusions and hallucinations lacking a coherent theme. *Paranoid type* is characterized by preoccupation with one or more systematized delusions or presence of frequent hallucinations related to a single theme; symptoms characteristic of disorganized and catatonic types are absent. *Undifferentiated type* is associated with prominent psychotic symptoms that do not meet criteria for other subtypes. *Residual type* is diagnosed by the occurrence of at least one prior episode of schizophrenia with a current clinical picture absent of prominent psychotic symptoms, although signs of the illness persist.

IV. ETIOLOGY AND PATHOPHYSIOLOGY

There is strong evidence that schizophrenia is a neurodevelopmental disorder: the typical onset of the disorder in adolescence, the occurrence of structural and neurofunctional abnormalities at the onset of the illness, and the fact that these abnormalities do not appear to progress with time in most cases [10,47–49]. Several models of the pathophysiology of schizophrenia suggest that causal factors early in development, intra- or perinatally, lead to the brain abnormalities found in the illness. These models further suggest that a "fixed" lesion from early life interacts with normal neurodevelpment occurring later [47,48]. Other models suggest that postnatal developmental abnormalities, like periadolescent synaptic pruning or myelination defects, are responsible for illness pathogenesis [50,51]. These early and late neurodevelopmental models both point to the importance of studying childhood-onset illness; childhood and adolescence may be critical windows of abnormal neurodevelopment in both early- and late-onset schizophrenia.

Understanding the brain mechanisms that regulate neurodevelopment may contribute to our understanding of the pathogenesis of childhood and adult-onset schizophrenia. Excitatory amino acid neurotransmitters such as glutamate are good candidates to be examined in this context. The predominant excitatory neurotransmitter in the mammalian brain, glutamate is responsible for neuronal migration and neuronal survival during early development, neuronal plasticity during adolescence, and neuronal excitability and viability throughout life [52]. Studies of schizophrenia patients have revealed evidence of reduced cerebrospinal fluid glutamate levels, altered glutamate metabolism, and abnormal gene expression of glutamate receptor subunits [53–55]. A glutamatergic hypothesis of schizophrenia has emerged, suggesting that there are the following three critical "windows" of vulnerability: early brain development, adolescence, and early course of illness. The hypothesis suggests that abnormal glutamatergic activity may alter neurodevelopment during these windows [52]. Further study of psychosis in childhood and adolescence may greatly contribute to a better understanding of this hypothesis.

While the etiology of both early- and late-onset schizophrenia remains to be elucidated, biological substrates for the conditions continue to be explored through neuroimaging and genetic studies. As current theory suggests that childhood-onset schizophrenia is continuous with adult-onset schizophrenia, there is great incentive to examine early-onset illness for important etiologic clues [3].

A. Neuroimaging

Recent studies have demonstrated that many of the same morphological differences between adult-onset schizophrenia patients and controls are seen in childhood-onset schizophrenia as well [3,56,57]. A recent NIMH study revealed that patients with childhood-onset schizophrenia had an 8–9% reduction in total cerebral volume as compared to controls [18]. These reduced volumes negatively correlated with total score on the Scale for the Assessment of Negative Symptoms (SANS), leading researchers to consider a more potent neurological basis for childhood-onset schizophrenia [18,58]. In contrast to findings in adult-onset schizophrenia, one study revealed that temporal lobe volumes were larger in childhood-onset schizophrenic patients than in controls. A 2-year follow-up reported significant decreases in hippocampus and superior temporal gyrus (STG) volumes over time during the early course of the illness [18,59,60]. Other studies have reported that hippocampus and amygdala volumes are not reduced in childhood-onset schizophrenia and that limbic structure reductions may be a consequence rather than a cause of schizophrenia [18,61]. Consistent with adult-onset schizophrenia findings, several studies have reported ventricular enlargement in patients with childhood-onset schizophrenia [18]. Rapoport reported that over a 2-year period, childhood-onset cases showed a significantly greater increase in ventricular volume than controls [15]. Rapoport also reported a significant decrease in midsagittal thalamic area over a 2-year period in patients with childhood-onset schizophrenia [15]. Consistent with adult-onset schizophrenia studies, Frazier and colleagues reported increased volumes in the caudate, putamen, and globus pallidus in neuroleptic-treated childhood-onset schizophrenia patients [56].

Functional imaging studies of patients with childhood-onset schizophrenia have revealed similar findings compared to later-onset patients. A positron emission tomography (PET) study revealed hypofrontality in childhood-onset patients [57]. Magnetic resonance spectroscopy (MRS) studies have revealed decreases in n-acetylaspartate (NAA), a putative marker of neuronal integrity in the frontal cortex and hippocampus of childhood-onset schizophrenia patients [62,63].

B. Genetics

Family, twin, and adoption studies have demonstrated that genetic factors play an important role in the etiology of schizophrenia [64,65]. Age of onset may be significantly affected by genetic influences, as one study revealed a higher correlation between concordant monozygotic twins than between affected siblings and concordant dizygotic twins [66]. This study also reported no significant difference in the rates of more disabling psychotic disorders (schizophrenia and schizoaffective disorder) in the relatives of childhood-onset patients than in the relatives of adult-onset patients. However, there was a significant excess of schizotypal and paranoid personality disorders in the relatives of the childhood-onset patients [66]. Recently, a smooth pursuit eye movement study reported that the anticipatory saccades were greater in the relatives of childhood-onset patients than in adult-onset patients [67].

Recent research has revealed an association between a chromosome 22q11 deletion (velocardiofacial syndrome; VCFS) and schizophrenia in adults. The rate of interstitial deletions of chromosome 22q11 has been found to be higher in adult-onset schizophrenia (2.0%) than in the general population [68,69]. A recent study of very early onset schizophrenic patients found that 6.4% of 47 patients studied had 22q11 deletions. The study also found that the patients with deletions had more pronounced premorbid impairments of language, motor, and social development. The authors concluded that the 22q11 deletions may be associated with an earlier age of onset of schizophrenia, possibly as a result of marked neurodevelopmental abnormalities [70].

V. TREATMENT

Current treatment of schizophrenia in adults involves the judicious use of antipsychotic medication to reduce acute symptoms, maintenance medication to sustain the period of recovery, and psychoeducation of both patient and family to ameliorate factors related to relapse. Unfortunately, carefully designed placebo-controlled studies of the efficacy of antipsychotics in childhood and adolescence are few, and studies of psychoeducational approaches are essentially nonexistent. This section briefly reviews current approaches to the pharmacological and psychoeducational treatment of childhood- and adolescent-onset psychoses.

A. Antipsychotic Medication

There are very few drug treatment studies of child and adolescent psychoses. Three controlled trials of first-generation antipsychotics for the treatment of child and adolescent schizophrenia reported the following results: (1) no difference in treatment effect between haloperidol and placebo [71]; (2) ~50% improvement with thiothixene or thioridazine [72]; (3) a significant treatment effect by haloperidol as compared to placebo [73,74]. Two double-blind trials of second-generation antipsychotics in the treatment of child and adolescent schizophrenia revealed the following results: (1) clozapine was superior to haloperidol [75]; (2) olanzapine was superior to risperidone, which was superior to haloperidol (all three were effective) [11]. A recent double-blind haloperidol-clozapine comparison revealed that clozaril significantly reduced negative and positive symptom scores greater than haloperidol following 6 weeks of monotherapy [11].

B. Side Effects

As atypical antipsychotics have replaced typical agents as the first-line treatment approach to childhood-onset psychosis, treatment side effects are more commonly those associated with atypical agents. The most common side effects seen with atypical antipsychotics are weight gain, sedation, and dizziness. Agranulocytosis, seizure disorder, and weight gain are side effects of both first-and second-generation antipsychotic medications that have been reported in children and adolescents [11,76]. Clinical potency differentiates typical neuroleptics' tendency to cause certain side effects. Low-potency agents generally produce more antiadrenergic (e.g., hypotension) and anticholinergic (e.g., dry mouth, sedation, blurred vision) effects, while high-potency antipsychotics tend more frequently to result in extrapyramidal symptoms (EPS) (e.g., acute dystonia, akathisia, and Parkinsonism). EPS, tardive dyskinesia (TD), and neuroleptic malignant syndrome (NMS) can be seen with both typical and atypical antipsychotic use. Recently, several open trials of second-generation antipsychotics have revealed a low incidence of EPS, TD, and NMS in childhood and adolescent psychosis treatment [11].

C. Guidelines for Acute Management

There are no absolute, established guidelines for management of childhood-onset psychoses. Most clinicians apply similar approaches as those used in adult-onset psychoses. A complete biopsychosocial approach to the condition is likely the most salient approach to management. While use of atypical antipsychotics have been found to be effective in a limited number of studies of childhood-onset schizophrenia (as well as anticonvulsants in early-onset bipolar disorder), it is important to recognize that medications are only one part of the treatment plan [11]. Patients and their families need to be educated about the potential severity of the condition and the major life changes that will accompany the illness. Compliance with medications and supportive therapy as well as familial support are critical to the management of psychoses. In general, pharmacological management of childhood-onset psychoses should be approached with the following principles: (1) adding one agent at a time; (2) maximizing the use of one agent before adding another; (3) dosages should be started low; (4) medications should not be stopped abruptly [11].

SUMMARY

Psychosis in childhood and adolescence is very real and disabling, and may be more severe than later-onset forms of the disorder. The concept that childhood-onset schizophrenia is continuous with adult-onset schizophrenia has stimulated child and adolescent research studies examining the neurodevelopmental and genetic etiology of psychosis and schizophrenia. As more patients with childhood psychoses are enrolled in research, structural and functional neuroimaging studies may reveal important differences in brain regions and processes that contribute to the disorder. Furthermore, genetic studies may better elucidate the contribution of other conditions, such as VCFS, which may be risk factors for the development of the disorder. The diagnosis, treatment, and management of pediatric psychosis continue to evolve and develop through prospective research studies and as the condition becomes better recognized and studied by clinical and academic psychiatrists.

ACKNOWLEDGMENT

This paper was supported in part by NIMH grant No. 01180.

REFERENCES

1. Kanner L. Autistic disturbances of affective contact. Nerv Child 1943; 2:217–250.
2. Kolvin I. Studies in the childhood psychoses: I. Diagnostic criteria and classification. Br J Psychiatry 1971; 118:381–384.
3. Rapoport JL et al. Progressive cortical change during adolescence in childhood-onset schizophrenia. A longitudinal magnetic resonance imaging study. Arch Gen Psychiatry, 1999; 56(7):649–654.
4. Alaghband-Rad J et al. Childhood-onset schizophrenia: the severity of premorbid course. J Am Acad Child Adolesc Psychiatry 1995; 34:1273–1283.
5. Russell A. The clinical presentation of childhood-onset schizophrenia. Schizophr Bull 1994; 20:631–646.
6. Gooding DC, WG Iacono. Schizophrenia through the lens of a developmental psychopathology perspective. In: D Cicchetti, DJ Cohen, eds. Developmental Psychopathology: Risk, Disorder, and Adaptation. New York: John Wiley & Sons, 1995:535–580.
7. McClellan J et al. Early-onset psychotic disorders: course and outcome over a 2-year period. J Am Acad Child Adolesc Psychiatry 1999; 38:1380–1388.
8. Asarnow JR. Children at risk for schizophrenia: converging lines of evidence. Schizophr Bull 1988; 14:613–631.
9. Murray RM et al. A neurodevelopmental approach to the classification of schizophrenia. Schizophr Bull 1992; 18:319.

10. Keshavan MS. Neurodevelopment and schizophrenia: quo vadis? In: MS Keshavan, RM Murray, eds. Neurodevelopment and Adult Psychopathology. New York: Cambridge University Press, 1997:267–277.
11. Rapoport, J. Treatment of Pediatric Psychosis. New Orleans: American Psychiatric Association, 2001.
12. Kumra S et al. "Multidimensionally impaired disorder": is it a variant of very early-onset schizophrenia? J Am Acad Child Adolesc Psychiatry 1998; 37:91–99.
13. Jeste DV et al. Did schizophrenia exist before the eighteenth century? Compr Psychiatry 1985; 26:493–503.
14. Kraepelin E. Dementia Praecox and Paraphrenia [1919]. New York: Robert E. Krieger, 1971.
15. Rapoport JL et al. Childhood onset schizophrenia: progressive ventricular change during adolescence. Arch Gen Psychiatry 1997; 54:897–903.
16. Nicolson R, Rapoport JL. Childhood-onset schizohprenia: rare but worth studying. Biol Psychiatry 1999; 46:1418–1428.
17. Nicolson R et al. Children and adolescents with psychotic disorder not otherwise specified: a 2- to 8-year follow-up study. Compr Psychiatry 2001; 42:319–325.
18. Eliez S, AL Reiss. MRI neuroimaging of childhood psychiatric disorders: a selective review. JH Child Psychol Psychiatry 2000; 41(6):679–694.
19. Hollis C. Adult outcomes of child- and adolescent-onset schizophrenia: diagnostic stability and predictive validity. Am J Psychiatry 2000; 157:1652–1659.
20. Sokol M. Schizophrenia in children and adolescents. In: D Parmelee, ed. Child and Adolescent Psychiatry. St. Louis: Mosby, 1996.
21. Volkmar F. Childhood schizophrenia. In: M Lewis, ed. Child and Adolescent Psychiatry. Baltimore: Williams and Wilkins, 1996.
22. Gordon CT et al. Childhood-onset schizophrenia: an NIMH study in progress. Schizophr Bull 1994; 20:697–712.
23. Green WH et al. Schizophrenia with childhood onset: a phenomenological study of 38 cases. J Am Acad Child Adolesc Psychiatry 1992; 31:968–976.
24. Cannon T. Antecedents of predominantly negative- and predominantly positive-symptom schizophrenia in a high risk population. Arch Gen Psychiatry 1990; 47:622–632.
25. Carpenter W, R Buchanan, B Kirkpatrick. The concept of the negative symptoms of schizophrenia. In: TR Greden, ed. Negative schizophrenia symptoms: Pathophysiology and clinical implications., Washington: American Psychiatric Press, 1991.
26. Pogue-Geile M, M Keshavan. Negative symptomatology in schizophrenia: syndrome and subtype status. In: J Greden, R Tandon, eds. Negative Schizophrenia Symptoms: Pathophysiology and Clinical Implications. Washington: American Psychiatric Press, 1991.
27. American Psychiatric Association. Diagnostic and Statistical Manual of Mental Disorders, 4th ed. Washington: American Psychiatric Press, 1994.
28. Beitchman JH. Childhood schizophrenia: a review and comparison with adult-onset schizophrenia. Psychiatr Clin North Am 1985; 8:793–814.
29. Cantor S. Evans, J. Pearce, J. Pezzot-Pearce T. Childhood schizophrenia: present but not accounted for. Am J Psychiatry 1982; 139:758–763.
30. Eggers C. Course and prognosis of childhood schizophrenia. J Autism Child Schizophr 1978. 8:21–36.
31. Garralda ME. Characteristics of the psychoses of late onset in children and adolescents: a comparative study of hallucinating children. J Adolesc 1985; 8:195–207.
32. Jordan K. Prugh DG. Schizophreniform psychosis of childhood. Am J Psychiatry 1971; 128:323–329.
33. Kydd RR. Werry JS. Schizophrenia in children under 16 years. J Autism Dev Disord 1982; 12:343–357.
34. Russell AT, Bott L, Sammons C. The phenomenology of schizophrenia occurring in childhood. J Am Acad Child Adolesc Psychiatry 1989; 28:399–407.
35. Volkmar FR, Cohen DJ, Hoshino Y, Rende RD, Paul R. Phenomenology and classification of the childhood psychoses. Psychol Med 1988; 18:191–201.
36. Holzman PS, DL Levy, LR Proctor. Smooth pursuit eye movements, attention, and schizophrenia. Arch Gen Psychiatry 1976; 33:1415–1420.
37. Hollis C. Child and adolescent (juvenile onset) schizophrenia: a case-control study of premorbid developmental impairments. Br J Psychiatry 1995; 166:489–495.
38. Watkins JM, RF Asarnow, PE Tanguay. Symptom development in childhood-onset schizophrenia. J Child Psychol and Psychiatry 1988; 29:865–878.
39. Holzman P, R Grinker. Schizophrenia in adolescence. J Youth Adolesc 1974; 3:267–270.
40. Nicolson R et al. Premorbid language and motor abnormalities in childhood-onset schizophrenia: association and genetic risk factors. Am Coll Neuropsychopharmacol 1998.
41. Freeman T. Symptomatology, diagnosis and course. In: LL Bellak, ed. The Schizophrenic Syndrome. New York: Grune and Stratton, 1971.
42. Aarkrog T, KV. Mortensen. Schizophrenia in early adolescence. A study illustrated by long-term cases. Acta Psychiatr Scand 1985; 72(5):422–429.
43. Steinberg D. Psychotic and other severe disorders in adolescence. In: M Rutter, L Hersov, eds. Child and Adolescent Psychiatry: Modern Approaches, 1985, Blackwell Scientific: Boston: p. 567–583.
44. Kaplan HI, BJ Saddock, JA Grebb. Synopsis of Psychiatry. Philadelphia: Williams & Wilkins, 1994.
45. Sands D. The psychosis of adolescence. J Ment Sci 1956; 102:308–316.
46. Werry J, J McClellan, L Chard. Childhood and adolescent schizophrenia, bipolar and schizoaffective disor-

ders: a clinical and outcome study. J Am Acad Child Adolesc Psychiatry 1991; 30:457–465.
47. Murray RM, SW Lewis. Is schizophrenia a neurodevelopmental disorder? [editorial]. Br Med J (Clin Res Ed) 1987; 295(6600):681–682.
48. Weinberger DR. Implications of normal brain development for the pathogenesis of schizophrenia. Arch Gen Psychiatry 1987; 44:660–669.
49. Weinberger DR. From neuropathology to neurodevelopment. Lancet 1995; 346:552–557.
50. Feinberg I. Schizophrenia: caused by a fault in programmed synaptic elimination during adolescence? J Psychiatr Res 1982; 17:319–334.
51. Keshavan MS, S Anderson, JW Pettegrew. Is schizophrenia due to excessive synaptic pruning in the prefrontal cortex? J Psychiatr Res 1994; 28:239–265.
52. Keshavan M.S, G.E. Hogarty. Brain maturational processes and delayed onset in schizophrenia. Dev Psychopathol 1999; 11(3):525–543.
53. Kim JS et al. Low cerebrospinal fluid glutamate in schizophrenic patients and a new hypothesis on schizophrenia. Neurosci Lett 1980; 20(3):379–382.
54. Tsai G, JT Coyle. N-acetylaspartate in neuropsychiatric disorders. Prog Neurobiol 1995; 46:531–540.
55. Akbarian S et al. Selective alterations in gene expression for NMDA receptor subunits in prefrontal cortex of schizophrenics. J Neurosci 1996; 16(1):19–30.
56. Frazier JA et al. Brain anatomic magnetic resonance imaging in childhood-onset schizophrenia. Arch Gen Psychiatry 1996; 53(7):617–624.
57. Jacobsen LK et al. Quantitative morphology of the cerebellum and fourth ventricle in childhood-onset schizophrenia. Am J Psychiatry 1997; 154(12):1663–1669.
58. Alaghband-Rad J et al. Childhood-onset schizophrenia: biological markers in relation to clinical characteristics. Am J Psychiatry 1997; 154(1):64–68.
59. Jacobsen LK et al. Temporal lobe morphology in childhood-onset schizophrenia. Am J Psychiatry 1996, 153(3):355–361.
60. Jacobsen LK et al. Progressive reduction of temporal lobe structures in childhood-onset schizophrenia. Am J Psychiatry 1998; 155(5):678–685.
61. Razi K et al. Reduction of the parahippocampal gyrus and the hippocampus in patients with chronic schizophrenia. Br J Psychiatry 1999; 174:512–519.
62. Bertolino A et al. Common pattern of cortical pathology in childhood-onset and adult-onset schizophrenia as identified by proton magnetic resonance spectroscopic imaging. Am J Psychiatry 1998; 155:1376–1383.
63. Thomas MA et al. Preliminary study of frontal lobes 1H MR spectroscopy in childhood-onset schizophrenia. J Magn Reson Imag 1998; 8:841–846.
64. Kendler KS, SR Diehl. The genetics of schizophrenia: a current genetic-epidemiologic perspective. Schizophr Bullet 1993; 19:261–285.
65. McGuffin P, MJ Owen, AE Farmer. Genetic basis of schizophrenia. Lancet 1995; 346(8976):678–82.
66. Kendler KS, MT. Tsuang, P Hays. Age at onset in schizophrenia. A familial perspective. Arch Gen Psychiatry 1987; 44(10):881–90.
67. Ross RG et al. The effects of age on a smooth pursuit tracking task in adults with schizophrenia and normal subjects. Biol Psychiatry 1999; 46(3):383–391.
68. Karayiorgou M et al. Schizophrenia susceptibility associated with interstitial deletions of chromosome 22q11. Proc Natl Acad Sci USA 1995; 92(17):7612–7616.
69. Tezenas Du Montcel S et al. Prevalance of 22q11 microdeletion. J Med Genet 1996; 33:719.
70. Usiskin SI et al. Velocardiofacial syndrome in childhood-onset schizophrenia. J Am Acad Child Adolesc Psychiatry 1999; 38(12):1536–1543.
71. Pool D et al. A controlled evaluation of loxitane in seventy-five adolescent schizophrenic patients. Curr Ther Res Clin Exp 1976; 19(1):99–104.
72. Realmuto GM et al. Clinical comparison of thiothixene and thioridazine in schizophrenic adolescents. Am J Psychiatry 1984; 141:440–442.
73. Spencer EK et al. Haloperidol in schizophrenic children: early findings from a study in progress. Psychopharmacol Bull 1992;28(2):183–186.
74. Spencer EK, M. Campbell. Children with schizophrenia: diagnosis, phenomenology, and pharmacotherapy. Schizophr Bull 1994; 20(4):713–725.
75. Kumra S et al. Childhood-onset schizophrenia. A double-blind clozapine-haloperidol comparison [see comments]. Arch Gen Psychiatry 1996; 53(12):1090–1097.
76. Rancurello, MD, G Vallano, GS Waterman. Psychotropic drug–induced dysfunction in children. In: MS Keshavan, JS Kennedy, eds. Drug Induced Dysfunction in Psychiatry. HPC, 1992; New York: HPC, 1992; 75–92.

14

Neurobiology of Autism and Other Pervasive Developmental Disorders
Basic Mechanisms and Therapeutic Interventions

ANTONIO Y. HARDAN
Western Psychiatric Institute and Clinic, University of Pittsburgh School of Medicine, Pittsburgh, Pennsylvania, U.S.A.

I. INTRODUCTION

Pervasive developmental disorders (PDDs) are described as severe pervasive impairments in several developmental areas such as social interaction, communication, or stereotyped behavior, interests, and activities [1]. Five diagnoses are included under PDD. These are autistic disorder, Asperger's disorder, Rett's disorder (RTT), childhood disintegrative disorder (CDD), and pervasive developmental disorder not otherwise specified (including atypical autism). The validity of autism and RTT disorder as a diagnostic category is well established, but the validity and definition of the other PDDs is more controversial [2]. Autism is the prototypic disorder and will be discussed first.

II. AUTISM

Autism is a neurodevelopmental disorder manifested by 36 months of age and is characterized by abnormalities in social skills and behavior, verbal and nonverbal communications, symbolic and imaginative play, reasoning, and related complex behavior [1]. The prevalence rate is 0.02–0.05% under age 12 [3–4]. However, a more recent survey reported 10-15/10,000 prevalence for PDDs, suggesting that the prevalence may be considerably higher than previously thought [5]. In fact, when using less rigorous criteria prevalence rates ranged from 1/250 to 1/1,000 [6–8]. Further, if severe mental retardation with some autistic features is included, the rate can rise as high as 20/10,000. Autistic disorder is found more frequently in boys than in girls. Three to five times more boys have the disorder, but autistic girls tend to be more seriously affected and more likely to have family histories of cognitive impairment than do boys [9].

Although autistic disorder was first considered to be psychosocial or psychodynamic in origin, evidence has accumulated over the past two decades to support a biological substrate. Autism is currently considered to be a disorder of early brain development involving neuronal organizational events. Studies of brain structure have implicated several aspects of brain development including the elaboration of dendritic and axonal ramifications, the establishments of synaptic connection, and cell death [10]. Even though neuropathologic studies have provided evidence of structural abnormalities in cortical and subcortical structures, theoretical model has focused more on one single structure than on neural systems. In fact, one current debate involves the relative roles played by disturbances of the frontal lobe and the cerebellum in the pathophysiology of autism [11]. The frontal systems models suggest that abnormalities in the prefrontal cortex is expressed functionally as a reduced capacity in shifting attention leading to the cognitive and behavioral symptoms observed in autism. The frontal dysfunction model is supported by functional imaging, neuropsychologic, and neurophysiologic studies [11–13]. In contrast, the cerebellar model proposes that impaired ability to shift attention is originated in the vermis as evidenced by the structural and neurophysiologic abnormalities observed in this structure [14–15]. However, recent structural and functional imaging findings suggest that the anatomic abnormalities are generalized, involving several brain areas and resulting from an abnormal development of connections in yet to be defined functionally disturbed neural networks that include the cerebral cortex, limbic system, and cerebellum [16–18].

A. Pathology

Autopsy studies in autism have failed to show any abnormalities of gross brain structures. There have been, however, several reports of increased brain size and weight [10,19,20]. In a review of 19 autopsy cases with autism, brain weight was found to be increased more in children than in adults [10–19]. Microscopic analysis of cerebral and subcortical regions of a number of autistic individuals revealed increased cell-packing density and decreased cell size in the hippocampus, subiculum, entorhinal cortex, amygdala, mamillary body, and medial septal nucleus bilaterally [10–19]. Outside the forebrain, additional abnormalities have been observed in the cerebellum and include decreased numbers of Purkinje cells, predominantly in the posterior neocerebellar cortex and adjacent archicerebellar cortex, while the vermis is less affected [10,19,20]. These observations suggest abnormalities in neuronal alignment and in the elaboration, pruning, and selective elimination of neuronal processes in the cerebral cortex and cerebellum.

B. Genetic Factors

There is mounting evidence that autism has a strong genetic basis. In several surveys, between 2% and 5% of siblings of those with autism also had autistic disorder, a rate that is 20–60 times greater than in the general population [21,22]. Genetic studies have also reported higher rates of concordance in identical twin pairs, although absolute rates vary from one study to another [23–25]. A recent British twin study showed 60% concordance rate for 25 pairs of monozygotic twins and no concordance for 25 pairs of dizygotic twins [25], with an estimate of heritability of 91–93%. When a broader spectrum of related cognitive and social abnormalities is considered, 92% of monozygotic twins were concordant versus only 10% of dizygotic pairs [25].

Investigators examining the genetics of autism recognize that more than one gene appears to be involved [26], or that several loci are involved with up to 15 loci possible [27]. A broader phenotype of autism has also been suggested which includes milder social and language-based cognitive deficits [25]. In fact, clinical reports and multiple-incidence (multiplex) family studies suggest that the genetic liability for autism may be expressed in some of the non-autistic relatives in a phenotype that is milder but quantitatively similar to the symptoms of autism [28].

C. Biochemical Factors

Studies of the hypothalamic-pituitary and thyroid functioning in autism have not led to consistent results when studied both at baseline and in response to stress or to challenge tests [29]. The noradrenergic functioning appears to be free of marked alterations in most individuals with the possibility of a subgroup of cases exhibiting overresponsiveness to stress [29]. In contrast, abnormalities of the serotoninergic and dopaminergic systems have been reported.

1. Serotonin

The study of peripheral and central levels of serotonin (5-hydroxytryptamine; 5-HT) or its precursors or metabolites has stimulated the most neurochemical research in autism. This interest was originally sparked by an early report of high blood levels of 5-HT in autism [29]. Most subsequent studies have focused on blood levels of 5-HT and have been consistent in reporting elevated plasma 5-HT in at least one-third of patients with autistic disorder [30,31]. However, this finding is not specific to this disorder since people with just mental retardation also display this abnormality. Investigations of the platelet storage of 5-HT has also been conducted but results have not been consistent [31]. A study of hyperserotonemic relatives of children with autism found some suggestive differences in platelets 5-HT uptake and the numbers of platelets 5-HT receptors in subgroups of the relatives [33]. Recent studies have focused on the serotonergic receptor gene. One investigation reported no differences in allele and genotype frequency for the 5-HT$_2$ receptor [34], and another found evidence of linkage and association between the serotonin transporter gene and autism [35]. However, the latter finding could not be replicated [36].

Investigations of the serotoninergic system have also included the examination of tryptophan, a dietary precursor of 5-HT. Tryptophan levels at baseline and after dietary manipulation and challenge tests have been reported with conflicting results [37–40], suggesting that further research is warranted. Levels of 5-hydroxyindoleacetic acid (5-HIAA), the main metabolite of 5-HT has also been examined. Results of studies measuring urinary levels of 5-HIAA have not been concordant with one investigation reporting increased urinary levels of 5-HIAA [41] and others not detecting any differences between autistic subjects and controls [42–43]. Cerebral spinal fluid (CSF) 5-HIAA levels have also been measured with mostly negative findings suggesting that central 5-HT metabolism is minimally if at all affected in autism [44–45].

2. Dopamine

The dopaminergic system has also been investigated in individuals with autism mostly through the measurement of homovanillic acid (HVA) (the major dopamine metabolite) in CSF, plasma, and urine. Studies of CSF HVA levels have not been consistent with some investigators reporting elevated concentration [44–46] and others not [45,47]. In the one study of plasma HVA, no differences were observed between unmedicated autistic subjects and normal controls [43]. In contrast, several studies of urinary levels of HVA have reported that the excretion of this metabolite is elevated in autism, but a more recent and large study was not successful in replicating this finding [29]. Therefore, the peripheral and central levels of dopamine metabolites appear to be unchanged or only slightly altered in autism.

3. Neuropeptides and Neurotrophins

Neuropeptides play an important role in central neurotransmission and neuromodulation which led several investigators to examine the potential function of these substances in the pathophysiology of autism. Initial research has focused on the opioid system in light of early reports of efficacy of opiate antagonist in the treatment of self-injurious behavior in autism [48]. Subsequent treatment studies have failed to replicate these findings and did not support a significant role of this system in autism [50,51]. A recent study examined blood levels of certain neuropeptides and neurotrophins in healthy children and in children with either autism, mental retardation, or cerebral palsy (CP) [52]. Concentrations of substance P and antibodies to myelin basic protein did not differ among the four groups. However, most children with autism (97%) had elevated concentrations of neurotrophin 4, vasoactive intestinal peptide, brain derived neurotrophic factor, and calcitonin-related gene peptide; few (9%) children with CP and none (0%) of the healthy group had elevated levels. Interestingly, most children with mental retardation (92%) also had elevated levels of neuropeptides and neurotrophins, and the pattern of increase of these substances did not distinguish children with autism from those with mental retardation only [52].

D. Electroencephalography and Neurophysiology

The incidence of electroencephalographic (EEG) abnormalities in individuals with autism have ranged from 10% to 83% depending on inclusion criteria, level of mental retardation, and method of interpretation of EEG [53–55]. Common EEG abnormalities include diffuse or focal spikes, slow waves, paroxysmal spike and slow wave activity, and mixed discharges, this last pattern being the most frequently one observed [55]. Epilepsy is also common in autism with a cumulative prevalence by young adulthood of 20–35% [56,57]. The onset of seizures can occur at any age, but its development is more common in early childhood and adolescence [58,59].

Various methods have been used to assess the neurophysiological systems in autism. Studies of evoked potential have essentially been limited to the study of auditory brainstem potential, and results have not been consistent. Early studies have reported a high incidence of abnormalities [60,61]. However, subsequent investigations with more rigorous methodologies that excluded children with underlying neurological conditions and controlled for age and sex did not show differences between autistic children and controls. [62,63]. Studies of attentional abnormalities have demonstrated the integrity of the N_{100} and N_{200} potentials related to basic attentional processes [63–65]. In contrast, studies using contemporary methods have provided evidence of abnormalities in P_{300} in individuals with autism, an event-related potential that is generated by the brain's processing of sensory stimuli [66]. This pattern reflects reliance by the cerebral cortex on less efficient and alternative neural pathways for processing of information [66].

E. Eye Movement

Eye movement studies have originally reported abnormalities in postrotatory nystagmus and nystagmus during REM sleep [67]. These findings were attributed subsequently to poorly designed methodologies [68]. Recent studies have used newly developed paradigms to examine the functional integrity of different systems and structures including the cerebellum, brainstem, basal ganglia, and frontal and parietal cortex. In a study of responses to vestibular stimulation, autistic children exhibited abnormalities suggestive of neurophysiologic dysfunction perhaps involving the brainstem [68]. In a visually guided saccades study to unpredictable targets, normal eye movements, although hypometric horizontally, were reported in mentally retarded individuals with autism in comparison to non-mentally retarded controls [69]. Two well-designed independent studies found no abnormalities of vestibulo-ocular reflexes, or in pursuit of visually-guided saccadic eye movements [70,71]. In a recent eye movement study, visually guided saccades were normal in non-mentally retarded individuals with autism suggesting the absence of functional disturbances in the cerebellar lobules VI and VII, and in automatic shifts of visual attention. However, deficits were observed in two volitional saccade tasks, the oculomotor delayed-response task and the antisaccade task, indicating possible dysfunction in the prefrontal cortex and its connections with the parietal cortex [72].

F. Immunological Factors

Several immunological factors have been identified in individuals with autism, suggesting the pathogenetic role of autoimmunity in this severe developmental disorder. Genetic susceptibility, association with viral infection, and immunologic dysfunction have all been reported [73]. Abnormal cell-mediated immunity and abnormal T-cell subsets have been described in some patients with autism [74,75]. Brain autoantibodies to neural antigens such as myelin basic protein (anti-MBP) and neuron-axon filament protein (anti-NAPF) have been found at higher rates in autistic children than in normal controls [76-79]. Recently, abnormal cytokine profiles with a decrease in TH 1 cytokine-producing cells and an increase in TH 2 cytokine-producing T-cells have been observed [80].

Immune-modulating treatments such as intravenous immunoglobulin have been reported to be beneficial in some but not all children with autism [76,81,82]. Taking into consideration that autoimmune abnormalities have been observed in only a subset of patients with autism, it is unlikely that an immune disorder is the only or primary causal factor. Immunological factors may be contributing to the onset of autism or to some of its clinical features. This observation is supported by the recent report of high correlation between the expression of monoclonal antibody D8/17 and severity of compulsive behaviors in a subgroup of autistic children [83].

G. Neuroimaging

1. Quantitative MRI

Structural imaging studies in autism have found a variety of morphometric alterations involving several brain structures including brain size [84–87], cerebellum [17,18,88], hippocampus and amygdala [89], corpus callosum [90–92], and basal ganglia [93] (Table 1). Initial imaging studies have focused on area measurements of the posterior fossa structures and have led to equivocal and controversial findings. A series of studies reported the existence, in the neocerebellar vermis, of either a generalized hypoplasia [94] or a selective hypo and/or hyperplasia of lobules VI and VII [14,15,95]. However, several replication studies using rigorous methodology failed to detect evidence of either of these findings [17,18,88,96,97]. In contrast to area measurement, volumetric investigations have been more consistent, with most studies reporting increased cerebellar volume [17,18].

Increased cerebellar volume is concordant with recent MRI studies reporting increased brain size in autism [84–87]. These findings are consistent with head circumference studies observing increased head size [98,99] and macrocephaly in autism [100,101]. These findings are the most consistent observations in autism and suggest that brain enlargement may be a biologic marker for this disorder. This increase in brain size appears to be the consequence of enlargement of parietal, temporal, and occipital but not the frontal lobe [84–86], and seems to be more evident in children than in adults [10–87]. Although the pathophysiology of brain enlargement in autism remains unclear, these data suggest that developmental brain processes such as synaptic pruning may be responsible for this abnormal growth.

Table 1 Morphometric Neuroimaging Findings in Autism

Structure	Finding	Replicability
Total brain[a]	Increased	+ +
Cerebellum[a]	Increased	+
Cortical lobes[a]		
Frontal	No differences	0
Temporal	Increased	0
Pareital	Increased	0
Occipital	Increased	0
Amygdala[a]	Decreased	−
Hippocampus[a]	Decreased	−
Basal ganglia[a]		
Caudate	Increased	0
Putamen	No differences	0
Globus pallidus	No differences	0
Total corpus callosum[b]	Decreased	+
Anterior subregions	Decreased	−
Mid body	Decreased	−
Posterior subregions	Decreased	+
Total brainstem[b]		−
Pons	Decreased	−
Midbrain	Decreased	−
Medulla	Decreased	
Total vermis[b]	Decreased	−
Lobules I–V	Decreased	− −
Lobules VI–VII	Decreased	− −
Lobules VIII–X	Decreased	−
Ventricular system[a]		
Lateral ventricles	Increased	+
Third ventricles	Increased	+
Fourth ventricles	Increased	+

[a]Volume.
[b]Area measurement.
Replication key: 0 = no replication; + = one or two replication; + + = several replications; − = one or two articles with different findings; − − = several articles with different findings

2. Magnetic Resonance Spectroscopy

To date, two studies using magnetic resonance spectroscopy (MRS) have been reported in the literature [102,103]. A ^{31}P MRS study of the dorsal prefrontal cortex of 11 non-mentally retarded individuals with autism and 11 age-, IQ-, gender-, race-, and SES-matched healthy controls, found decrease levels of phosphocreatine (PCr) and esterified ends in the autistic group [102]. Interestingly, severity of autism was associated with alterations of MRS metabolites. The second study used ^{1}H MRS to measure N-acetyl aspartate (NAA), creatine + phosphocreatine (Cr + PCr), and choline (Cho) levels in the right medial prefrontal cortex in a group of non–mentally retarded adults with autistic spectrum disorder and matched controls [103]. Higher concentrations of NAA, and Cr + PCr, and Cho were found in the autistic group. NAA concentration was significantly related to the scores on the Yale-Brown Obsessive Compulsive Scale, and Cr + PCr was significantly related to the Autism Diagnostic Interview summary score [103].

3. Positron Emission Tomography and Single-Photon Emission Computed Tomography

Most initial studies with positron emission tomography (PET) or single-photon emission computed tomography (SPECT) in individuals with autism have failed to show focal reductions or elevations in glucose metabolism or oxygen utilization [104–107]. Correlational studies that compared metabolic rates of paired regions in autistic young adult men and controls found unusual metabolic patterns in frontal/parietal regions and the neostriatum and thalamic regions that subserve directed attention [108]. In contrast to the limited findings reported by early studies, recent PET investigations have been able to find localized brain abnormalities in autism. The differences are probably due to the improvement in the spatial resolution of the imaging methods (roughly from 20 mm to 5 mm) and to the application of the whole-brain statistical parametric mapping analysis instead of the region-of-interest method used in the past.

In a PET investigation of the metabolic maturation of the frontal cortex in preschool autistic children, a transient frontal hypoperfusion was found in autistic children (ages 3 and 4), suggesting a delayed frontal maturation consistent with the clinical data and cognitive performance reported in the literature [109]. In a follow-up study of neocortical brain dysfunction, marked bilateral hypoperfusion was found in the temporal lobes, centered in the associative auditory and adjacent multimodal temporal cortex, in a group of autistic children [110]. Thalamic abnormalities have also been reported [111,112]. In a study of subjects performing expressive language tests, alterations of the thalamic blood flow was found in autistic patients relative to that of the healthy control group [112]. Furthermore, autistic subjects differed from controls in the blood flow of the dentatothalamocortical pathway [112], a brain pathway that is important for language production and sensory integration. Finally, in a study of 17 patients with autism, significant metabolic reductions in both the anterior and posterior cingular gyri were observed, but no metabolic abnormalities were observed in the amygdala and the hippocampus [113].

4. Functional MRI

The advent of functional MRI (fMRI) has provided new opportunities to investigate brain functions in pervasive developmental disorders. In a study of social intelligence using fMRI, non–mentally retarded individuals with autism activated the frontotemporal regions but not the amygdala when making mental inferences from the eyes [114], supporting the amygdaloid dysfunction hypothesis [10]. In a subsequent study, the same investigators assessed local processing and visual search abilities in a group of individuals with autism and controls using the Embedded Figures Task [115]. Several cerebral regions were similarly activated in the two groups, but individuals with autism demonstrated greater activation of ventral occipitotemporal regions, while normal controls showed generally more extensive task-related activation including the prefrontal cortical areas [115]. These findings suggest that the cognitive strategies adopted by the two groups are different on a task in which people with autism have been reported to demonstrate superiority over controls [115]. In a study of face discrimination, individuals with autism demonstrated a pattern of brain activity that is consistent with feature based strategies that are more typical of nonface object perception [116]. Results from the face-discrimination task showed that, compared to controls, activation in the fusiform gyrus was decreased in the autistic group, but was increased in the inferior temporal gyri [116]. Recently, a study of eight males with autism and eight matched normal controls reported different patterns of activation between the two groups during visually paced finger movement compared to a control condition that consisted of visual activation in the absence of motor response [117]. Findings from these fMRI studies suggest that individuals with autism when compared to healthy controls depend on different neural systems and sometimes use abnormally large neuronal networks to execute simple and complex cognitive functions.

H. Therapeutic Interventions

Since pharmacotherapy is of limited benefit in targeting the core symptoms of autism, psychosocial interventions are essential in the management of social, communication, and behavioral impairment. Treatment is aimed at increasing prosocial behaviors, decreasing aberrant behaviors, and assisting in the development of verbal and nonverbal communication. Educational and behavioral methods are currently considered the treatments of choice. Behavior modification techniques have proven to be effective in decreasing aberrant behaviors and reinforcing socially acceptable interaction and encouraging self-care skills. Structured classroom training in combination with behavioral approaches and language remediation are effective treatment strategies for a large number of autistic children. These strategies should be complemented and, even better, preceded by the introduction of in-home early intervention. The implementation of such modalities or training programs may yield to gains in the areas of language and cognition and decreases in maladaptive behaviors. These training programs are rigorous, require much of parents' time, and require as much structure as possible and daily program for as many hours as possible. Therefore, careful training of parents and in-home workers is essential to achieve considerable improvement in the target symptoms.

While no drug has been found to treat all the symptoms of autism, psychotropic agents are a valuable adjunct in comprehensive treatment programs to target a wide range of associated symptoms, including aggression, impulsivity, low level of tolerance for frustration, self injurious behaviors, hyperactivity, and obsessive-compulsive symptomatology. Drug therapy is also beneficial in treating comorbid disorders such as depressive and anxiety disorders.

Several studies of the effects of various typical antipsychotics in autistic children have been conducted. The use of typical antipsychotic is hampered by the potential for side effects and specifically tardive dyskinesia in light of the increased incidence of this movement disorder in this population [118]. Haloperidol remains the best-studied agent with several published controlled studies indicating the effectiveness of the agent in targeting hyperactivity, stereotypies, social withdrawal, irritability, and mood lability [119,120]. Pimozide has also been shown to be effective in children with autism in one well-designed study [121]. Recently, risperidone, a high-potency atypical antipsychotic with combined dopamine type 2 and 5-HT$_2$ receptor antagonism has been shown to be effective in several open-label studies and one placebo-controlled study in decreasing the rates of aggressivity, hyperactivity, and self-injurious behavior in children, adolescents, and adults with autism [122,123]. Other novel antipsychotics, such as clozaril and olanzapine, have reportedly been effective in the treatment of individuals with autism, but no controlled trials have been published so far [124–125].

The serotonin reuptake inhibitors (SRIs) have been used to target obsessive-compulsive and stereotyped behaviors. Clomipramine, a tricyclic antidepressant (TCA) with potent inhibition of 5-HT, has been shown in a well-designed study to be more effective than placebo in improving the core symptoms of autism, anger/uncooperativeness, hyperactivity, and obsessive-compulsive symptoms [126]. However, subsequent studies have failed to replicate these findings and have reported a high incidence of side effects including QT_c prolongation [127,128]. Owing to the adverse effects associated with clomipramine, selective SRIs (SSRIs) have been considered to be a safer alternatives with their better tolerability and lack of significant cardiac side effects. To date, only one double-blind placebo-controlled study of fluvoxamine, an SSRI, have been reported to be effective in adults with autism [129]. Fluvoxamine was effective in reducing repetitive thoughts and behaviors, maladaptive behavior, and aggression [129]. In contrast, a well-designed and controlled study using fluvoxamine in children and adolescents with autism failed to show positive results [130]. Other SSRIs, including fluoxetine, paroxetine, and sertraline, have also been shown to be effective in the treatment of individuals with autism, but no controlled trials have yet been conducted [130].

Several others medications have also been used to treat individuals with autism. Two well-designed studies of methylphenidate were found to be effective in decreasing hyperactivity [131,132]. However, adverse effects were observed at high rates, including social withdrawal, dullness, sadness, and irritability. Two alpha 2-adrenergic agonists, clonidine and guanfacine, were found in several trials to be effective in the treatment of related symptoms of autism including hyperactivity and anxiety [130,133,134]. Despite early reports of potential benefit, naltrexone, an opioid receptor antagonist, has failed to demonstrate efficacy in improving the core and related symptoms of autism [51–135]. Finally, data are also available, though limited in some instances, on numerous agents that appear to be either promising such as lamotrigine [136], divalproex sodium [137], mirtazapine [130], buspirone [138], propanolol [139], donepezil [130], and vancomycin [140] or not encouraging in the example of amantadine [141], secretin [142,143], fenfluramine [144], and intravenous immunoglobulin [82].

III. OTHER PERVASIVE DEVELOPMENTAL DISORDERS

A. Asperger's Disorder

Individuals with Asperger's disorder show severe, sustained impairment in social interaction and restricted repetitive pattern of behavior, interests, and activities [1]. Unlike autistic disorder, in Asperger's disorder there are no significant delays in language, cognitive development, or age appropriate self-help skills. Hans Asperger, an Austrian physician, first described a syndrome applied to people with normal intelligence who exhibit qualitative impairment in reciprocal social interaction and behavioral oddities without delays in language development [145]. This syndrome was originally named *autistic psychopathy*, but was later changed to Asperger's disorder or syndrome to avoid misinterpretation with sociopathy [147]. Estimates for the prevalence of the disorder have ranged from 3.6/1000 to 1/10,000 [145,146]. This disorder is more commonly found in boys than in girls, and the male/female ratio is higher than in autism.

The validity of Asperger's disorder as an entity distinct from high-functioning autism or autism has been debated [147], but important differences have been reported [148]. Asperger's disorder is characterized by a later age of onset, a better prognosis, more prominent clumsiness, and less severe social/communicative deficits when compared with individuals with high-functioning autism. Furthermore, evidence from the DSM-IV field trials supports the distinction of Asperger's disorder from both autism and PDD, NOS [149]. Recent studies comparing children with Asperger's disorder and children with autistic disorder reported that children with Asperger's disorder were more likely to look for social interaction and seek vigorously to make friends [149]. The overlap between Asperger's disorder and other diagnostic concepts such as nonverbal learning disabilities (NLD) provide further evidence to support the differences between the Asperger's disorder and high-functioning autism since the former was frequently associated with NLD profile while the latter was not [150].

The cause of Asperger's disorder is unknown, but genetic studies, even though limited, suggest the presence of genetic factors and possible relation to autistic disorder. Originally, Asperger observed that the disorder is more commonly found in fathers of the boys who had the disorder [145]. Several pairs of identical twins have been reported who have Asperger's disorder

[151], and some of the clinical characteristics of this disorder appear to be more common in fathers of affected individuals [152]. Data on birth complications suggest an increased rate of prenatal and perinatal complications [145–151] but not as much as non–mentally retarded individuals with autism [152]. Neurochemical and neurophysiological studies have been limited. A sleep study of eight patients with Asperger's disorder showed decreased sleep time in the first two-thirds of the night, REM sleep disruption, and increased number of shifts into REM sleep from a waking epoch, suggesting a defective sleep control systems in this disorder [153].

Several neuroimaging studies have been reported examining individuals with Asperger's disorder. Structural brain studies have reported focal areas of cortical polymicrogyria and cortical defects [154], left occipital lobe damage [155], thinning of the posterior corpus callosum [154], and enlargement of the right lateral ventricles [156]. Recently, qualitative area measurements of specific brain structures were measured in 8 individuals with Asperger's disorder [157]. In comparison to controls, no abnormalities were found in the midsagittal areas of vermal lobules I–V, and VI and VII, total area of the midsagittal corpus callosum, and the hippocampal body [157]. SPECT studies have reported left occipital hypoperfusion without global or regional differences in blood flow or oxygen metabolism [158], and abnormalities in right hemisphere functioning [156]. A recent PET study examining individuals with Asperger's disorder reported significant reductions in both the anterior and posterior cingulate gyri while performing a serial verbal learning test [113]. No differences were found in the metabolism of the amygdala or the hippocampus between the affected group and controls [113]. Finally, fMRI studies have reported a wide range of findings in Asperger's disorder, including difficulties with face perception [159], no activation in the amygdala while decoding emotional expression [114], and abnormalities in the pattern of brain activation during face discrimination involving increased activity in the inferior temporal gyri and decreased activation in the fusiform gyrus [116].

No controlled trials are available examining the effectiveness of psychosocial or pharmacologic interventions in Asperger's disorder. Treatment strategies have been developed based solely on clinical experience. Specialized educational placements, social and communications skills training, and real-life skills are often necessary [160].

B. Rett's Disorder (RTT)

In 1966, Andreas Rett, an Australian physician, identified a syndrome in 22 girls who appeared to have had a normal development for a period of at least 6 months, followed by severe developmental deterioration [161]. The onset of this disorder is characterized by progressive symptoms in which children developed some behaviors suggestive of autism associated with deceleration of brain growth and aberrant behaviors and symptoms not typical of autism [1]. The symptomatology of RTT include characteristic hand movements (hand washing and hand wringing), severe mental retardation, ataxia, and breath-holding spells [1]. The diagnostic criteria include apparently normal prenatal and perinatal development with normal head circumference at birth followed by decelerated head growth, loss of purposeful hand movements, lack of social engagement, and marked communicative and cognitive delay [1]. The onset of the condition is between 5 and 48 months, and has been essentially observed only in girls, with two exceptions [1]. The estimated prevalence of RTT is 1/10,000 to 1/23,000 live female births [162].

The biologic and genetic foundations of RTT were not clear until recently, when it was reported that mutations in the X-linked MECP$_2$ gene were detected in ~50% of RTT patients [164]. Methyl-CpG-binding protein 2 (MeCP2) is an abundant chromosomal protein that binds specifically to methylated CpG dinucleotides in the genome and mediates the transcription repression through interaction with histon deacetylase and the corepressor SIN3A. Because MECP2 mutations have not been shown in all affected subjects, other genetic factors may be involved in the pathogenesis of RTT including the X chromosome and autosomal loci [165]. Genetic contributions to RTT have previously been suspected because of the existence of a small number of familial cases where higher degrees of concordance in monozygotic than dizygotic twins were reported [166].

Associated features of RTT include seizures in up to 84% of affected children and disorganized EEGs with some epileptiform discharges is observed in almost all young children with RTT, even in the absence of clinical seizures [167]. Nonspecific patterns on EEGs have been reported including rhytmical slowing (most common), diffuse and scattered or bilateral-synchronous spikes or sharp waves, slow spike-wave complexes, and intermittent spike or slow-wave activity followed by suppression of background activity [167,168]. The most common types of seizures are generalized tonic-clonic and partial complex seizures, with overall lower frequency and decrease severity after the teenage years except for partial seizures [169]. An additional associated feature is irregular respiration, with episodes of hyperventilation, apnea, and breath-holding. Interestingly, the disorganized breathing occurs in most patients while they are awake; during sleep, breathing usually normalizes [170]. This pattern suggests normal brainstem control of ventilation and that disordered breathing seen during wakefulness is due to abnormality of cortical influence on ventilation [170].

Several neurobiologic abnormalities have been reported in RTT. Autopsy studies have described decreased brain weight in RTT ranging from 14% to 80% with diffuse cortical atrophy but without degenerative evidence [171]. Further neuropathologic findings include deficient pigmentation of the substantia nigra [172] and locus coeruleus [173], abnormalities of dendritic architecture of pyramidal neurons [174], gernerlized cerebellar atrophy with associated cell loss, gliosis in the granular, Purkinje, and molecular layers [175], and mitochondrial inclusions [174]. Several metabolic abnormalities have been suggested including decreased cortical and subcortical levels of choline acetyltransferase [176], elevated CSF beta-endorphins immunoreactivity, glutamate, and lactate levels [177,178], and decreased CSF brain gangliosides [179]. However, replication studies are either lacking or have failed to support these findings [180,181].

Structural and functional neuroimaging studies have been reported in RTT. Qualitative CT and MRI studies have not been consistent in reporting structural abnormalities in the frontal cortical area, brainstem, and thalamus [182,183]. Recent quantitative morphometric MRI measurements of girls with RTT revealed reduced cerebellar and cerebral volumes which is consistent with the neuropathologic studies [184,185]. Evidence of greater loss of gray matter in comparison with white was also found especially in the caudate, prefrontal, posterior-frontal, and temporal regions [184,185]. Functional imaging studies have been limited. Few reports of magnetic resonance spectroscopy (MRS) have been published, and results are not concordant [186–188]. Most of these studies involved relatively small numbers of subjects and studied one region of the brain (single-voxel); only one study used spectroscopic imaging performed in one slice. Recently, a multislice high-resolution ^{1}H MRS imaging study was conducted in 17 girls with RTT and found metabolic impairments involving both gray and white matter in the cortical lobes and the insular cortex [189]. Average Cho concentrations were higher possibly from gliosis, and average NAA concentrations were lower in the affected subjects, suggesting reduced neuronal and dendritic tree size. Finally, in a SPECT study involving a small number of subjects, decreased cerebral blood flow was observed predominantly in the frontal lobes, indicating the loss of hyperfrontality in RTT [168].

Psychosocial and pharmacologic therapy is aimed at symptomatic intervention. Behavioral therapy is useful to control self-injurious behavior and may help in regulating the breathing disorganization. Many patients become wheelchair-bound with muscle wasting and rigidity. Physiotherapy has been beneficial for the muscular dysfunction. Medications are often necessary for the treatment of seizures and behavioral dyscontrol. Several investigators have demonstrated the efficacy of ketogenic diet and carbamazepine, especially when there is a predominance of partial-complex seizures [190]. Psychiatric symptoms can be treated pharmacologically, but no controlled data are available.

C. Childhood Disintegrative Disorder

CDD is characterized by marked regression in several areas of functioning after at least 2 years of apparently normal development [1]. This condition was originally referred to as *dementia infantilis* and later on was called *disintegrative psychosis*. It was first described by Theodor Heller in 1908 as a deterioration of several months occurring in 3- and 4-year-olds who had normal early development [191]. This deterioration is characterized by a loss of social skills and speech together with a severe disorder of emotions, behavior, and relationships, leading to symptomatology that closely resembles children with autism [1]. Limited epidemiological data are available. CDD is estimated to be at least one-tenth as common as autistic disorder, with an estimated prevalence to be about one case in 100,000 boys [192,193]. The ratio of boys to girls seems to be between four and eight boys to one girl. To date there have been 106 reported cases [192,193].

The pathogenis of CDD is unclear, but neurobiological factors are certainly involved. The unusual and distinctive onset typically prompts a search for general medical conditions. A number of CNS disorders, including the neurolipidoses, adrenoleukodystrophy, and metachromatic leukodystrophy, have been associated with this disorder. Limited family and genetic data are available with no significant family history found in one small study of 10 children with CDD [194]. To date, no investigations have examined neurochemical abnormalities in CDD, and no chromosomal abnormalities have been reported [192,193]. Two autopsy studies of patients who possibly had CDD revealed evidence of cerebral degeneration suggestive of lipidosis [195,196]. The frequent association of EEG abnormalities and seizure disorders has also suggested an unidentified neuropathological process. [192,193]. Several studies have shown high rates of EEG abnormalities and seizure disorders similar to those reported for autism [193]. Finally, a CT scan study of 10 patients with CDD reported that five scans were normal and the reminder showed nonspecific abnormalities [193].

No specific pharmacologic or psychosocial interventions have been identified or developed to treat CDD. The treatment approach is the same as that for autism, taking in consideration the clinical similarity between the two disorders.

D. Pervasive Developmental Disorder, Not Otherwise Specified

PDD NOS is characterized by severe impairment in social interaction or communication skills or the presence of stereotyped behavior, interests, and activities [1]. It represents a subthreshold or residual subclass within the PDD class. It is more common than autism, affecting one in 200 children, and has overall a better prognosis [197]. Limited neurobiological research is available, given the heterogeneity of this group and difficulties with the diagnostic concept. Treatment is very similar to that for other PDDs, combining psychosocial and psychopharmacologic interventions targeting aberrant and disruptive behaviors.

IV. SUMMARY

PDDs are very complex, and our understanding of the pathophysiology of these disorders has increased greatly over the past 15 years, although basic questions have yet to be answered. With the exception of autism and RTT, studies in the phenomenology, epidemiology, natural course, and treatment of these conditions are needed. Genetic and molecular biological studies are promising and have led to significant progress, especially for RTT. Many genes appear to influence the phenotypic manifestations of autism and Asperger's disorder, and the next decade is critical for the identification of specific genes involved in these developmental disorders. Neuroimaging studies using PET, SPECT, fMRI, and MRS will provide the tools to examine in vivo brain functioning and help identify the different neural networks involved in the debilitating symptoms of PDD. Finally, investigations of the plasma concentrations of neuropetides and neurotrophins are potentially useful for understanding the developmental neurobiology of these disorders and monitoring and assessing the efficacy of psychosocial and psychopharmacologic interventions.

REFERENCES

1. American Psychiatric Association. Diagnostic and Statistical Manual of Mental Disorders, 4th ed. Washington: American Psychiatric Press, 1994.
2. FR Volkmar, A Klin, DJ Cohen. Diagnosis and classification of autism and related disorders: consensus and issues. In: D Cohen, F Volkmar, eds. Handbook of Autism and Pervasive Developmental Disorders, 2nd ed. New York: John Wiley, 1997, pp 44–60.
3. V Lotter. Epidemiology of autistic conditions in young children. I. Prevalence. Soc Psychiatry 1:124–137, 1966.
4. L Wing, SR Yeates, LM Brierley, J Gould J. The prevalence of early childhood autism. Comparison of administrative and epidemiological studies. Psychol Med 6:89–100, 1976.
5. National Institute of Neurobiologic Disorders and Strokes. Office of Scientific and Health Reports, U.S. Department of Health and Human Services on the Frequency of Neurologic Disorders, 1983.
6. SE Bryson, BS Clark, IM Smith. First report of a Canadian epidemiological study of autistic syndromes. J Child Psychol Psychiatry 29:433–445, 1988.
7. T Sugiyama, T Abe. The prevalence of autism in Nagoya, Japan: a total population study. J Autism Dev Disord 19:87–96, 1989.
8. S Ehlers, C Gillberg. The epidemiology of Asperger syndrome: a total population study. J Child Psychol Psychiatry 34:1327–1350, 1993.
9. FR Volkmar, A Klin, B Siegel, P Szatmari, C Lord, M Campbell, BJ Freeman, DV Cicchetti, M Rutter, W Kline. Field trial for autistic disorder in DSM-IV. Am J Psychiatry 151:1361–1367, 1994.
10. TL Kemper, ML Bauman. Neuropathology of infantile autism. J Neuropathol Exp Neurol 57:645–652, 1998.
11. NJ Minshew, G Goldstein, DJ Siegel. Neuropsychologic functioning in autism: profile of a complex information processing disorder. J Int Neuropsychol Soc 3:303–316, 1997.
12. S Ozonoff, BF Pennington, SJ Rogers. Executive function deficits in high-functioning autistic individuals: relationship to theory of mind. J Child Psychol Psychiatry 32:1081–1105, 1991.

13. JM Rumsey, SD Hanburger. Neuropsychological divergence of high-level autism and severe dyslexia. J Autism Dev Disord 20:155–169, 1990.
14. E. Courchesne, R Yeung-Courchesne, GA Press, JR Hesselink, TL Jernigan. Hypoplasia of cerebellar vermal lobules VI and VII in autism. N Engl J Med 318:1349–1354, 1988.
15. E Courchesne, J Townsend, O Saitoh. The brain in infantile autism: posterior fossa structures are abnormal. Neurology 44:214–223, 1994.
16. NJ Minshew. Brain mechanisms in autism: functional and structural abnormalities. J Autism Dev Disord 26:205–209, 1996.
17. J Piven, K Saliba, J Bailey, S Arndt. An MRI study of autism: the cerebellum revisited. Neurology 31:491–504, 1997.
18. AY Hardan, NJ Minshew, K Harenski, MS Keshavan. Postrior fossa MRI in autism. J Am Acad Child Adolesc Psychiatry 40:666–672, 2001.
19. ML Bauman, TL Kemper. Neuroanatomic observations of the brain in autism. In: Bauman ML, Kemper TL, eds. The Neurobiology of Autism. Baltimore, Johns Hopkins University Press, 1994, pp 119–145.
20. A Bailey, P Luthert, A Dean, B Harding, I Janota I, M Montgomery, M Rutter, P Lantos. A clinicopathological study of autism. Brain 121:889–905, 1998.
21. S Smalley, R Asarnow, M Spence. Autism and genetics: a decade of research. Arch Gen Psychiatry 45:953–961, 1988.
22. S Folstein, M Rutter. Genetic influences and infantile autism. Nature 265:726–728, 1977.
23. S Folstein, M Rutter. Infantile autism: genetic study of 21 twin pairs. J Child Psychol Psychiatry 18:297–321, 1977.
24. S Steffenburg, C Gillberg, L Hellgren, L Anderson, IC Gillberg, G Jacobsson, M Bohman. A twin study of autism in Denmark, Finland, Ireland, Norway and Sweden. Child Psychol Psychiatry 3:405–416, 1989.
25. A Bailey, A LeCouteur, I Gottesman, O Bolton, E Simonoff, E Yuzda E, M Rutter. Autism as a strongly genetic disorder: evidence from twin study. Psychol Med 25:63–78, 1995.
26. E Maestrini, AJ Marlow, DE Weeks, AP Monaco. Molecular genetic investigations of autism. J Autism Dev Disord 28:427–437, 1998.
27. N Risch, D Spiker, L Lotspeich, N Nouri, H Hinds, J Hallmayer, L Kalaydjieva, P McCague, S Dimiceli, T Pitts, L Nguyen, Y Yang, C Harper, D Thorpe, S Vermeer, H Young, J Hebert, A Lin, J Ferguson, C Chiotti, S Wiese-Slater, T Rogers, B Salmon, P Nicholas, RM Myers RM. A genomic screen of autism: evidence for a multilocus etiology. Am J Hum Genet 65:493–507, 1999.
28. A. Le Couteur, A Bailey, S Goode, A Pickles, S Robertson, I Gottesman, M Rutter. A broader phenotype of autism: the clinical spectrum in twins. J Child Psychol Psychiatry Allied Disc 37:785–801, 1996.
29. GM Anderson, Y Hoshino. Neurochemical studies in autism. In: D Cohen, F Volkmar, eds. Handbook of Autism and Pervasive Developmental Disorders, 2nd ed. New York: John Wiley, 1997, pp 325–343.
30. RER Ritvo, A Yuwiler, E Geller, EM Ornitz, K Saeger, S Plotkin. Increased blood serotonin and platelets in early infantile autism. Arch Gen Psychiatry 23(6):566–572, 1970.
31. GM Anderson, RB Minderaa, PP van Benthem, FR Volkmar, DJ Cohen. Platelet imipramine binding in autistic subjects. Psychiatry Res 11:133–141, 1984.
32. DJ Boullin, HN Bhagavan, M Coleman M, RA O'Brien, MB Youdim. Platelet monoamine oxidase in children with infantile autism. Med Biol 53:210–213, 1975.
33. EH Cook, RC Arora, GM Anderson, EM Berry-Kravis, SY Yan, HC Yeoh, PJ Sklena, DA Charak, BL Leventhal. Platelet serotonin studies in hyperserotonemic relatives of children with autistic disorder. Life Sci 52:2005–2015, 1993.
34. J Heraulrt, E Petit, J Martineau, C Cherpi, A Perrot, C Barthelemy, G Lelord, JP Muh. Serotonin and autism: biochemical and molecular biology features. Psychiatry Res 65:33–43, 1996.
35. EH Cook Jr, R Courchesne, C Lord, NJ Cox, S Yan, A Lincoln, R Haas, E Courchesne, BL Leventhal. Evidence of linkage between the serotonin transporter and autistic disorder. Mol Psychiatry 2:247–250, 1997.
36. SM Klauck, F Poustka, A Benner, KP Lesch, A Poustka. Serotonin transporter (5-HTT) gene variants associated with autism? Hum Mol Genet 6:2233–2238, 1997.
37. Y Hoshino, T Yamamoto, M Kaneko, R Tachibana, M Watanabe, Y Ono, H Kumashiro. Blood serotonin and free tryptophan concentration in autistic children. Neuropsychobiology 11:22–27, 1984.
38. GM Anderson, DX Freedman, DJ Cohen, FR Volkmar, EL Hoder, P McPhedran, RB Minderaa, CR Hansen, JG Young. Whole blood serotonin in autistic and normal subjects. J Child Psychology Psychiatry Allied Disc 28:885–900, 1987.
39. HE Sutton, JH Read, A Arbor. Abnormal amino acid metabolism in a case suggesting autism. Am J Dis Child 96:23–28, 1958.
40. RB Minderaa, GM Anderson, FR Volkmar, D Harcherick, GW Akkerhuis, DJ Cohen. Whole blood serotonin and tryptophan in autism: temporal stability and the effects of medication. J Autism Dev Disord 19:129–136, 1989.
41. HG Hanley, SM Stahl, DX Freedman. Hyperserotonemia and amine metabolites in autistic and retarded children. Arch Gen Psychiatry 34:521–531, 1977.

42. MW Partington, JB Tu, CY Wong. Blood serotonin levels in severe mental retardation. Dev Med Child Neurol 15:616–627, 1973.
43. RB Minderaa, GM Anderson, FR Volkmar, GW Akkerhuis, DJ Cohen DJ. Urinary 5-hydroxyindoleacetic acid and whole blood serotonin and tryptophan in autistic and normal subjects. Biol Psychiatry 22:933–940, 1987.
44. C Gillberg, L Svennerholm. CSF monoamines in autistic syndromes and other pervasive developmental disorders of early childhood. Br J Psychiatry 151:89–94, 1987.
45. M Narayan, S Srinath, GM Anderson, DB Meundi. Cerebrospinal fluid levels of homovanillic acid and 5-hydroxyindoleacetic acid in autism. Biol Psychiatry 33:630–635, 1993.
46. C Gillberg, L Svennerholm, C Hamilton-Hellberg. Childhood psychosis and monoamine metabolites in spinal fluid. J Autism Dev Disord 13: 38–96, 1983.
47. DJ Cohen, JG Young. Neurochemistry and child psychiatry. J Am Acad Child Psychiatry 16:353–411, 1977.
48. PR Barrett, C Feinstein, WT Hole. Effects of naloxone and naltrexone on self-injury: a double-blind placebo-controlled analysis. Am J Ment Retard 93:644–651, 1989.
49. M Leboycr, MP Bouvard, JM Launay, F Tabuteau, D Waller, M Dugas, B Kerdelhue, P Lensing, J Panksepp. A double-blind study of naltrexone in infantile autism. J Autism Dev Disord 22:309–319, 1992.
50. M Campbell, LT Anderson, AM Small, JJ Locascio, NS Lynch, MC Choroco. Naltrexone in autistic children: a double-blind and placebo-controlled study. Psychopharmacol Bull 26:130–135, 1990.
51. BK Kolman, HM Feldman, BK Handen, JE Janosky. Naltrexone in young autistic children: a double-blind, placebo-controlled crossover study. J Am Acad Child Adolesc Psychiatry 34:223–231, 1995.
52. KB Nelson, JK Grther, LA Croen, JM Dambrosia, BF Dickens, RL Hansen TM Philips. Neuropeptides and neurotrophins in neonatal blood of children with autism, mental retardation, or cerebral palsy. Neurology 54:A247, 2000 (Abstract).
53. PT White, W DeMeyer, M DeMeyer. EEG abnormalities in early childhood schizophrenia. Am J Psychiatry 120:950–958, 1964.
54. I Olsson, S Seffenburg, V Gillberg. Epilepsy on autism and autistic-like conditions. Arch General Psychiatry 42:1018–1025, 1988.
55. LY Tsai, MC Tsai, GJ August. Brief report: implications of EEG diagnoses in the subclassification of infantile autism. J Autism Dev Disord 15:339–344, 1985.
56. L Lockyer, M Rutter. A five to fifteen year follow-up study of infantile psychosis: patterns of cognitive ability. Br J Soc Clin Psychol 9:152–163, 1970.
57. C Gillberg, S Steffenburg. Outcome and prognostic factors in infantile autism and similar conditions. A population-based study of 46 cases followed through puberty. J Autism Dev Disord 17:273–287, 1987.
58. FR Volkmar, DS Nelson. Seizure disorders in autism. J Am Acad Child Adolesc Psychiatry 1:127–128, 1990.
59. EY Deykin, G MacMahon. The incidence of seizure, among children with autistic symptoms. Am J Psychiatry 136:1310–1312, 1979.
60. E Courchesne, RY Courchesne, G Hicks, AJ Lincoln. Functioning of the brainstem auditory pathway in non-retarded autistic individuals. Electroencephalogr Clin Neuropysiol 61:491–501, 1985.
61. JM Rumsey. Conceptual problem-solving in highly verbal, nonretarded autistic men. J Autism Dev Disord 1:23,1985.
62. JM Rumsey, AM Grimes, AM Pikus, R Duara, DR Ismond. Auditory brainstem responses in pervasive developmental disorders. Biol Psychiatry 19:1403–1418, 1984.
63. C Grillon, E Courchesne, N Akshoomoff. Brainstem and middle latency auditory evoked potentials in autism and developmental language disorder. J Autism Dev Disord 19:255–269, 1989.
64. E Courchesne, AJ Lincoln BA Kilman, R Galambos. Event-related brain potential correlates of the processing of novel visual and auditory information in autism. J Autism Dev Disord 15:1–17, 1985.
65. E Courchesne, BA Kilman, R Galambos, AJ Lincoln. Autism: processing of novel auditory information assessed by event-related brain potentials. Electroencephalogr Clin Neurophysiol 59:238–248, 1984.
66. B Novick, HG Vaughan Jr, D Kurtzberg, R Simson. An electrophysiologic indication of auditory processing defects in autism. Psychiatr Res 3:107–114, 1980.
67. EM Ornitz, MB Brown, A Mason, NH Putnam. Effect of visual input on vestibular nystagmus in autistic children. Arch Gen Psychiatry 31:369–375, 1974.
68. EM Ornitz, CW Atwell, AR Kaplan, JR Westlake. Brain-stem dysfunction in autism. Results of vestibular stimulation. Arch Gen Psychiatry 42:1018–1025, 1985.
69. U Rosenhall, E Johansson, C Gillberg. Oculomotor findings in autistic children. J Laryngol Otol 102:435–439, 1988.
70. NJ Minshew, JM Furman, G Goldstein, JB Payton. The cerebellum in autism: a central role or epiphenomenon. Neurology 40:173, 1990.
71. NJ Minshew, G Goldstein, DJ Seigel. Neuropsychologic functioning in autism: profile of a complex information processing disorder. J Int Neuropsychol 3:303–316, 1997.
72. NJ Minshew, B Luna, JA Sweeny. Oculomotor evidence for neocortical systems but not cerebellar dysfunction in autism. Neurology 52:917–922, 1999.

73. G DelGiuidce-Asch, E Hollander. Altered immune function in autism. CNS spectrums. Int J Neuropsychiat Medi 2:61–68, 1997.
74. RP Warren, P Cole, JD Odell, CB Pingree, WL Warren, E White, VK Singh. Detection of maternal antibodies in infantile autism. J Am Acad Child Adolesc Psychiatry 29:873–877, 1990.
75. EG Stubbs, ML Crawford, DR Burger, AA Vanderbark. Depressed lymphocyte responsiveness in autistic children. J Autism Child Schizophr 7:49–55, 1977.
76. VK Singh, HH Fudenberg, D Emerson, M Coleman. Immunodiagnosis and immunotherapy in autistic children. Ann NY Acad Sci 540:602–604, 1988.
77. VK Singh, SX Lin, VC Yang. Serological association of measles virus and human herpes virus-6 with brain autoantibodies in autism. Clin Immunol Immunopathol 89:105–108, 1998.
78. RD Todd, JM Hickok, GM Anderson, DJ Cohen. Antibrain antibodies in infantile autism. Biol Psychol 23:644–647, 1988.
79. AM Connolly, MG Chez, G Michael, A Pestronk, ST Arnold, S Mehta, RK Deuel. Serum antibodies to brain in Landau-Kleffner variant, autism, and other neurologic disorders. Pediatrics 134:607–613, 1999.
80. S Gupta, S Aggarwal, B Rashanravan, T Lee. Th1- and Th2-like cytokines in CD4(+) and CD8(+) T cells in autism. J Neuroimmunol 85:106–109, 1998.
81. S Gupta, B Rimland, PD Shilling. Pentoxifylline: brief review and rationale for its possible use in the treatment of autism. J Child Neurol 11:501–4, 1996.
82. G Delgiudice-Asch, L Simon, J Schmeidler, C Cunningham-Rundles, E Hollander. Brief report: a pilot open clinical trial of intravenous immunoglobulin in childhood autism. J Autism Dev Disord 29:157–160, 1999.
83. E Hollander, G DelGiudice-Asch, L Simon, J Schmeidler, C Cartwright, CM DeCaria J Kwon, C Cunningham-Rundles, F Chapman, JB Zabriskie. B lymphocyte antigen D8/17 and repetitive behaviors in autism. Am J Psychiatry 156:317–320, 1999.
84. PA Filipek, C Richelme, DN Kennedy, J Rademacher, DA Pitcher, SY Zidel, VS Caviness. Morphometric analysis of the brain in developmental language disorders and autism. Ann Neurol 32:475, 1992.
85. J Piven, S Arndt, J Bailey, S Havercamp, N Andreason, P Palmer. An MRI study of brain size in autism. Am J Psychiatry 152:1145–1149, 1995.
86. J Piven, S Arndt, J Bailey, N Andreasen. Regional brain enlargement in autism: a magnetic resonance imaging study. J Am Acad Child Adolesc Psychiatry 35:530–536, 1996.
87. AY Hardan, NJ Minshew, M Mallikarjuhn, M Keshavan. Brain volume in autism. J Child Neurol 16:421–424, 2001.
88. J Piven, E Nehme, J Simon, P Barta, G Pearlson, S Folstein. Magnetic resonance imaging in autism: measurement of the cerebellum, pons, and fourth ventricle. Biol Psychiatry 31:491–505, 1992.
89. EH Aylward, NJ Minshew, G Goldstein, NA Honeycutt, AM Augustine, KO Yates, PE Barta, GD Pearlson. MRI volumes of amygdala and hippocampus in non–mentally retarded autistic adolescents and adults. Neurology 53:2145–2150, 1999.
90. B Egaas, E Courchesne, O Saitoh. Reduced size of corpus callosum in autism. Arch Neurol 52:794–801,1995.
91. J Piven, J Bailey, BJ Ranson, S Arndt. An MRI study of corpus callosum in autism. Am J Psychiatry 154:1051–1056, 1997.
92. AY Hardan, NJ Minshew, M Keshavan. Corpus callosum size in autism. Neurology 55:1033–1036, 2000.
93. LL Sears, V Cortney, S Mohamed, J Bailey, BJ Rabson, J Piven. An MRI study of the basal ganglia in autism. Prog Neuro-Psychoparmacol Biol Psychiatry 23:613–624, 1999.
94. T Hashimoto, M Tayama, K Murakawa, T Yoshimoto, M Miyazaki, M Harada, Y Kuroda. Development of the brainstem and cerebellum in autistic children. J Autism Dev Disord 25:1–18, 1995.
95. GB Schaefer, JN Thompson, JB Bodensteiner, JM McConnell, WJ Kimberling, CT Gay, WD Dutton, DC Hutchings, SB Gray. Hypoplasia of the cerebellar vermis in neurogenic syndromes. Ann Neurol 48:1178–1187, 1996.
96. JR Holttum, NJ Minshew, RS Sanders, NE Philips. Magnetic resonance imaging of the posterior fossa in autism. Biol Psychiatry 32:1091–1101, 1992.
97. MD Kleiman, S Neff, NP Rosman. The brain in infantile autism: is the cerebellum really abnormal? Neurology 2:645–652, 1992.
98. P Bolton, H Macdonald, A Pickles, P Rios, S Goode, M Crowson. A case-control family history study of autism. J Child Psychol Psychiatry 35:877–900, 1994.
99. HA Walker. Incidence of minor anomaly in autism. J Autism Child Schizophr 7:165–176, 1977.
100. A Bailey, P Luthert, P Bolton, A LeCouteur, M Rutter. Autism and megalencephaly. Lancet 341:1225–1226, 1993.
101. JE Lainhart, J Piven, M Wzorek, R Landa, SL Santangelo, H Coon, SE Folstein. Macrocephaly in children and adults with autism. J Am Acad Child Adolesc Psychiatry 36:282–290, 1997.
102. NJ Minshew, G Goldstein, SM Dombrowski, K Panchalingam, JW Pettegrew. A preliminary ^{31}P MRS study of autism: evidence for undersynthesis and increased degradation of brain membranes. Biol Psychiatry 33:762–773, 1993.
103. DGM Murphy, D Robertson, TV Amelsvoort, E Daly, P Howlin, S Williams, H Critchley. Asperger syndrome: an fMRI/^{1}H MRS study of brain function

and myelination (abstr). Biol Psychiatry 45(suppl 8S):111, 1999.
104. JM Rumsey, R Duara, C Grady, LJ Rapoport, RA Margolin, ST Rapoport, NR Cutler. Brain metabolism in autism: resting cerebral glucose utilization rates as measured with positron emission tomography. Arch Gen Psychiatry 42:448–455, 1985.
105. A De Volder, A Bol, C Michel, M Congneau, A Goffinet. Brain glucose metabolism in children with the autistic syndrome: positron tomography analysis. Brain Dev 9:581–587, 1987
106. S Herold, RSJ Frackowiak, A Le Couteur, M Rutter, P Howlin. Cerebral blood flow and metabolism of oxygen and glucose in young autistic adults. Psychol Med 18:823–831, 1988.
107. M Zilbovicius, B Garreau, N Tzourio, B Mazoyer, B Bruck, J-L Martinot, C Raynaud, Y Samson, A Syrota, G Lelord. Regional cerebral blood flow in childhood autism: a SPECT study. Am J Psychiatry 149:924–930, 1992.
108. B Horwitz, JM Rumsey, CL Grady, SI Rapoport. The cerebral metabolic landscape in autism: intercorrelations of regional glucose utilization. Arch Neurol 45:749–755, 1988.
109. M Zilbovicius, B Garreau, Y Samson, R Remy Philipe R, C Barthelemy, A Syrota, G Lelord. Delayed maturation of the frontal cortex in childhood. Am J Psychiatry 152:248–252, 1993.
110. M Zilbovicius, N Boddaert, P Belin, JB Poline, P Remy, JF Mangin, L Thivard, C Barthelemy, Y Samson. Temporal lobe dysfunction in childhood autism: a PET study. Am J Psychiatry 157:1988–1993, 2000.
111. DC Chugani, O Muzik, R Rothermel, M Behen, P Chakraborty, T Mangner. Altered serotonin synthesis in the dentatothalamocortical pathway in autistic boys. Ann Neurol 42:666–669, 1997.
112. RA Muller, DC Chugani, ME Behen, RD Rothermel, O Muzik, PK Chakraborty, PK Chugani. Impairment of the dentato-thalamocortical pathway in autistic men: language activation data from the positron emission tomography. Neurosci Lett 245:1–4, 1998.
113. MM Haznedar, MS Buchsbaum, TC Wei, PR Hof, C Cartwright, CA Bienstock, E Hollander. Limbic circuitry in patients with autism spectrum disorders studied with positron emission tomography and magnetic resonance imaging. Am J Psychiatry 154:682–684, 1997.
114. S Baron-Cohen, HA Ring, S Wheelwright, ET Bullmore, MJ Brammer, A Simmons, SC Williams. Social intelligence in the normal and autistic brain: an fMRI study. Eur J Neurosci 11:1891–1898, 1999.
115. HA Ring, S Baron-Cohen, S Wheelwright, SC Williams, M Brammer, C Andrew, ET Bullmore. Cerebral correlates of preserved cognitive skills in autism: a functional MRI study of embedded figures task performance. Brain 122:1305–1315, 1999.
116. RT Schultz, I Gauthier, A Klin, RK Fulbright, AW Anderson, F Volkmar, P Skudlarski, C Lacadie, DJ Cohen, JC Gore. Abnormal ventral temporal cortical activity during face discrimination among individuals with autism and Asperger syndrome. Arch Gen Psychiatry 57:331–340, 2000.
117. RA Muller, K Pierce, JB Ambrose, G Allen, E Courchesne. Atypical patterns of cerebral motor activation in autism: a functional magnetic resonance study. Biol Psychiatry 49:665–76, 2001.
118. M Campbell, JL Armenteros, RP Malone, PB Adams, ZW Eisenberg, JE Overall JE. Neuroleptic-related dyskinesias in autistic children: a prospective, longitudinal study. J Am Acad Child Adolesc Psychiatry 36:835–43, 1997.
119. M Campbell, LT Anderson, M Meier, IL Cohen, AM Small, C Samit, EJ Sachar. A comparison of haloperidol and behavior therapy and their interaction in autistic children. J Am Acad Child Psychiatry 17:640–655, 1978.
120. LT Anderson, M Campbell, P Adams, AM Small, R Perry, J Shell. The effects of haloperidol on discrimination learning and behavioral symptoms in autistic children. J Autism Dev Disord 19:227–239, 1989.
121. H Naruse, M Nagahata, Y Nakane, K Shirahashi, M Takesada, K Yamazaki. A multi-center double-blind trial of pimozide (Orap), haloperidol and placebo in children with behavioral disorders, using crossover design. Acta Paedopsychiatr 48:173–84, 1982.
122. AY Hardan, K Johnson, C Johnson, B Hrecznyj B. Case study: risperidone treatment of children and adolescents with developmental disorders. J Am Acad Child Adolesc Psychiatry 35:1551–6, 1996.
123. CJ McDougle, JP Holmes, DC Carlson, GH Pelton, DJ Cohen, LH Price. A double-blind, placebo-controlled study of risperidone in adults with autistic disorder and other pervasive developmental disorders. Arch Gen Psychiatry 55:633–641, 1998.
124. A Zuddas, MG Ledda, A Fratta, P Muglia, C Cianchetti. Clinical effects of clozapine on autistic disorder. Am J Psychiatry 153:738, 1996.
125. MN Potenza, JP Holmes, SJ Kanes SJ, CJ McDougle. Olanzapine treatment of children, adolescents, and adults with pervasive developmental disorders: an open-label pilot study. J Clin Psychopharmacol 19:37–44, 1999.
126. CT Gordon, RC State, JE Nelson, SD Hamburger, JL Rapoport. A double-blind comparison of clomipramine, desipramine, and placebo in the treatment of autistic disorder. Arch Gen Psychiatry 50:441–447, 1993.
127. ES Brodkin, CJ McDougle, ST Naylor, DJ Cohen, LH Price. Clomipramine in adults with pervasive developmental disorders: a prospective open-label investiga-

128. LE Sanchez, M Campbell, AM Small, JE Cueva, JL Armenteros, PB Adams. A pilot study of clomipramine in young autistic children. J Am Acad Child Adolesc Psychiatry 35:537–544, 1996.
129. CJ McDougle, ST Naylor, DJ Cohen, FR Volkmar, GR Heninger, LH Price. A double-blind, placebo-controlled study of fluvoxamine in adults with autistic disorder. Arch Gen Psychiatry 53:1001–1008, 1996.
130. DJ Posey, CJ McDougle. Pharmacotherapeutic management of autism. Exp Opin Pharmacother 2:587–600, 2001.
131. B Birmaher, H Quintana, LL Greenhill. Methylphenidate treatment of hyperactive autistic children. J Am Acad Child Adolesc Psychiatry 27:248–251, 1988.
132. BL Handen, CR Johnson, M Lubetsky. Efficacy of methylphenidate among children with autism and symptoms of attention-deficit hyperactivity disorder. J Autism Dev Disord 30:245–255, 2000.
133. CA Jaselskis, EH Cook Jr., KE Fletcher, BL Leventhal. Clonidine treatment of hyperactive and impulsive children with autistic disorder. J Clin Psychopharmacol 12:322–327, 1992.
134. MP Fankhauser, VC Karumanchi, ML German, A Yates, SD Karumanchi. A double-blind, placebo-controlled study of the efficacy of transdermal clonidine in autism. J Clin Psychiatry. 53(3):77–82, 1992.
135. M Campbell, LT Anderson, AM Small, P Adams, NM Gonzalez, M Ernst. Naltrexone in autistic children: behavioral symptoms and attentional learning. J Am Acad Child Adolesc Psychiatry 32:1283–1291, 1993.
136. P Uvebrant, R Bauziene. Intractable epilepsy in children. The efficacy of lamotrigine treatment, including non-seizure-related benefits. Neuropediatrics 25:284–289, 1994.
137. E Hollander, R Dolgoff-Kaspar, C Cartwright, R Rawitt, S Novotny. Divalproex sodium in autism spectrum disorders: a pilot trial (NCDEU Abstract). J Child Adolesc Psychopharmacol 10:251–252, 2000
138. JK Buitelaar, RJ van der Gaag, J van der Hoeven. Buspirone in the management of anxiety and irritability in children with pervasive developmental disorders: results of an open-label study. J Clin Psychiatry 59:56–59, 1998.
139. JJ Ratey, E Mikkelsen, P Sorgi, HS Zuckerman, S Polakoff, J Bemporad, P Bick, W Kadish. Autism: the treatment of aggressive behaviors. J Clin Psychopharmacol. 7:35–41, 1987.
140. RH Sandler, SM Finegold, ER Bolte, CP Buchanan, AP Maxwell, ML Vaisanen, MN Nelson, HM Wexler. Short-term benefit from oral vancomycin treatment of regressive-onset autism. J Child Neurol 15:429–435, 2000.
141. BH King, EH Cook, L Sikich, et al. A controlled trial of amantadine in the treatment of autistic children. Scientific Proceedings of the 46th Annual Meeting of the American Academy of Child and Adolescent Psychiatry, Chicago, 2000, p 129.
142. AD Sandler, KA Sutton, J DeWeese, MA Girardi, V Sheppard, JW Bodfish. Lack of benefit of a single dose of synthetic human secretin in the treatment of autism and pervasive developmental disorder. N Engl J Med 341:1801–1806, 1999.
143. MG Chez, CP Buchanan, BT Bagan, MS Hammer, KS McCarthy, I Ovrutskaya, CV Nowinski, ZS Cohen. Secretin and autism: a two-part clinical investigation. J Autism Dev Disord 30:87–94, 2000.
144. M Campbell, M Campbell, P Adams, AM Small, EL Curren, JE Overall, LT Anderson, N Lynch, R Perry. Efficacy and safety of fenfluramine in autistic children. J Am Acad Child Adolesc Psychiatry 27:434–439, 1988.
145. L Wing. Asperger's syndrome: a clinical account. Psychol Med. 11:115–129, 1981.
146. S Ehlers, C Gillberg. The epidemiology of Asperger syndrome. A total population study. J Child Psychol Psychiatry Allied Disc 34:1327–1350, 1993.
147. L Wing. The relationship between Asperger's syndrome and Kanner's autism. In: U Firth, ed. Autism and Asperger's Syndrome. Cambridge: Cambridge University Press, 1991, pp 93–121.
148. A Klin, FR Volkmar. Asperger's syndrome. In : DJ Cohen, FR Volkmar, eds. Handbook of Autism and Pervasive Developmental Disorders, 2nd ed. New York: Wiley, 1997, pp 94–122.
149. FR Volkmar, A Klin, B Siegel, P Szatmari, C Lord, M Campbell, BJ Freeman, DV Cicchetti, M Rutter, W Kline. Field trial for autistic disorder in DSM-IV. Am J Psychiatry, 151:1361–1367, 1994.
150. A Klin, FR Volkmar, SS Sparrow, DV Cicchetti, BP Rourke. Validity and neuropsychological characterization of Asperger syndrome: convergence with nonverbal learning disabilities syndrome. J Child Psychol Psychiatry Allied Dis 36:1127–1140, 1995.
151. P Szatmari, R Bremner, J Nagy. Asperger's syndrome: a review of clinical features. Can J Psychiatry 34:554–560, 1989.
152. C Gillberg. Asperger syndrome in 23 Swedish children. Dev Med Child Neurol 31:520–531, 1989.
153. R Godbout, C Bergeron, E Limoges, E Stip, L Mottron. A laboratory study of sleep in Asperger's syndrome. Neuroreport 11:127–130, 2000.
154. ML Berthier, A Bayes, ES Tolosa. Magnetic resonance imaging in patients with concurrent Tourette's disorder and Asperger's syndrome. J Am Acad Child Adolesc Psychiatry 32:633–639, 1993.
155. PB Jones, RW Kerwin. Left temporal lobe damage in Asperger's syndrome. Br J Psychiatry 156:570–572, 1990.

156. JR McKelvey, R Lambert, L Mottron, MI Shevell. Right-hemisphere dysfunction on Asperger's syndrome. J Child Neurol 10:310–314, 1995.
157. A Lincoln, E Courchesne, M Allen, E Hanson. Neurobiology of Asperger syndrome. In: E Schopler, GB Mesibov, LJ Kunce, eds. Asperger Syndrome or High Functioning Autism. New York: Plenum, 1998, pp 145–163.
158. KR Ozbayrak, O Kapucu, E Erdem, T Aras. Left occipital hypoperfusion in a case with the Asperger syndrome. Brain Dev, 13:454–456, 1991.
159. S Davies, D Bishop, AS Manstead, D Tantam. Face perception in children with autism and Asperger's syndrome. J Child Psychol Psychiatry Allied Disc 35:1033–1057, 1994.
160. A Klin, FR Volkmar. Treatment and intervention guidelines for individuals with Asperger syndrome. In: A Klin, FR Volkmar, Eds. Asperger Syndrome. New York: Guilford Press, 2000, pp 340–366.
161. Rett A. Über ein eigenartiges hirnatrophisches Syndrom bei Hyperammonaemie im Kindesalter. Wien Med Wochenschr 116:723–726, 1966.
162. B Hagberg. Rett syndrome: Swedish approach to analysis of prevalence and cause. Brain Dev 7:276–280, 1985.
163. CA Kozinetz, ML Skender, N MacNaughton, MJ Almes, RJ Schultz RJ, AK Percy, DG Glaze. Epidemiology of Rett syndrome: a population-based registry. Pediatrics 91:445–450, 1993.
164. RE Amir, IB Van den Veyver, M Wan, CQ Tran, U Francke, HY Zoghbi. Rett syndrome is caused by mutations in X-linked MECP2, encoding methy-CpG-binding protein 1. Nat Genet 23:185–188, 1999.
165. EM Bühler, NJ Malik, M Alkan. Another model for the inheritance of Rett syndrome. Am J Med Genet 36:126–131, 1990.
166. AK Percy. The Rett syndrome: the recent advances in genetic studies in the USA. Brain Dev 14(suppl):S104–S105, 1992.
167. E Niedermeyer, A Ret, H Renner, M Murphy, S Naidu. Rett syndrome and the electroencephalogram. Am J Med Genet 1(suppl 1):195–199, 1986.
168. R Lappalainen, K Liewendahl, K. Sainio, P Nikkinen, RS Riikonen. Brain perfusion SPECT and EEG findings in Rett syndrome. Acta Neurol Scand 95:44–50, 1997.
169. U Steffenburg, G Hagberg, B Hagberg. Epilepsy in a representative series of Rett syndrome. Acta Paediatr 90:34–39, 2001.
170. M Segawa, Y Nomura. Polysomnography in the Rett syndrome. Brain Dev 14(suppl):S46–S54, 1992.
171. AK Percy. Meeting report: second International Rett Syndrome Workshop and Symposium. J Child Neurol 8:97–100, 1993.
172. A Lekman, I Witt-Engerstrom, J Gottfries, BA Hagberg, AK Percy, L Svennerholm. Rett syndrome: biogenic amines and metabolites in postmortem brain. Pediatr Neurol 5:357–362, 1989.
173. T Brucke, E Sofic, W Killian, A Rett, P Riederer. Reduced concentration and increased metabolism of biogenic amines in a single case of Rett's syndrome: a postmortem brain study. J Neural Transm 68:315–324, 1988.
174. ME Cornford, M Philippart, B Jacobs, AB Scheibel, HV Vinters. Neuropathology of Rett syndrome: case report with neuronal and mitochondrial abnormalities in the brain. J Child Neurol. 9:424–431, 1994.
175. ML Bauman, TL Kemper, DM Arin. Microscopic observations of the brain in Rett syndrome. Neuropediatrics 26:105–108, 1995.
176. GL Wenk, M O'Leary, CB Nemeroff, G Bissette, H Moser, S Naidu. Neurochemical alterations in Rett syndrome. Dev Brain Res 74:67–72, 1993.
177. SS Budden, EC Myer, IJ Butler. Cerebrospinal fluid studies in the Rett syndrome: biogenic amines and beta-endorphins. Brain Dev 12:81–84, 1990.
178. R Lappalainen, RS Riikonen. Elevated CSF lactate in the Rett syndrome: cause or consequence? Brain Dev 16:399–401, 1994.
179. AY Lekman, BA Hagberg, LT Svennerholm. Cerebrospinal fluid gangliosides in patients with Rett syndrome and infantile neuronal ceroid lipofuscinosis. Eur J Paediat Neurol 3:119–123, 1999.
180. AR Genazzani, M Zappella, A Nalin, Y Hayek, F Facchinetti. Reduced cerebrospinal fluid B-endorphin levels in Rett syndrome. Child Nerv Syst 5:111–113, 1989.
181. C Gillberg, L Terenius, B Hagberg, I Witt-Engerstrom, I Eriksson. CSF beta-endorphins in childhood neuropsychiatric disorders. Brain Dev 12:88–92, 1990.
182. I Krageloh-Mann, G Schroth, G Niemann, R Michaelis. The Rett syndrome: magnetic resonance imaging and clinical findings in four girls. Brain Dev 11:175–178, 1989.
183. Y Nomura, M Segawa, M Hasegawa. Rett syndrome—clinical studies and pathophysiological consideration. Brain Dev 6:475–486, 1984.
184. B Subramaniam, S Naidu, AL Reiss. Neuroanatomy in Rett syndrome: cerebral cortex and posterior fossa. Neurology 48:399–407, 1997.
185. AL Reiss, F Faruque, S Naidu, M Abrams, T Beaty, RN Bryan, H Moser. Neuroanatomy of Rett syndrome: a volumetric imaging study. Ann Neurol 34:227–234, 1993.
186. F Hanefeld, HJ Christen, U Holzbach, B Kruse, J Frahm, W Hanicke. Cerebral proton magnetic resonance spectroscopy in Rett syndrome. Neuropediatrics 26:126–127, 1995.
187. JW Pan, JB Lane, H Hetherington. Rett syndrome: ^{1}H spectroscopic imaging at 4.1 Tesla. J Child Neurol 4:524–528, 1999.

188. T Hashimoto, N Kawano, K Fukuda, S Endo, K Mori, Y Yoneda, T Yamaue, M Harada, K Miyoshi. Proton magnetic resonance spectroscopy of the brain in three cases of Rett syndrome: comparison with autism and normal controls. Acta Neurol Scand 98:8–14, 1998.
189. A Horska, S Naidu, EH Herskovits, PY Wang, WE Kaufmann, PB Barker. Quantitative ^{1}H MR spectroscopic imaging in early Rett syndrome. Neurology 54:715–722, 2000.
190. E Trevathan, S Naidu. The clinical recognition and differential diagnosis of Rett syndrome. J Child Neurol 3(suppl):6–16, 1988.
191. T Heller. Demantia infantilis. Z Erforsch Behandlung Jugenlichen Schwachsinns 2:141–165, 1908.
192. FR Volkmar, A Klin, DJ Cohen, W Marrens. Childhood desintegrative disorder. In: DJ Cohen, FR Volkmar, eds. Handbook of Autism and Pervasive Developmental Disorders, 2nd ed. New York: John Wiley, 1997, pp 47–59.
193. FR Volkmar, DJ Cohen. Disintegrative disorder or "late onset" autism. J Child Psychol Psychiatry Allied Disc 30:717–724, 1989.
194. LG Evans-Jones, L Rosenbloom. Disintegrative psychosis in childhood. Dev Med Child Neurol 20:462–470, 1978.
195. N Malamud. Heller's disease and childhood schizophrenia. Am J Psychiatry 116:215–218, 1959.
196. EM Creak. Childhood psychosis: a review of 100 cases. Br J Psychiatry 109:84–89, 1963.
197. K Towbin. Pervasive developmental disorder not otherwise specified. In: D Cohen, F Volkmar, eds. Handbook of Autism and Pervasive Developmental Disorders, 2nd ed. New York: John Wiley, 1997, pp 123–147.

15

Cognitive Deficits in Schizophrenia

CAMERON S. CARTER and STEFAN URSU
Western Psychiatric Institute and Clinic, University of Pittsburgh School of Medicine, Pittsburgh, Pennsylvania, U.S.A.

I. INTRODUCTION

Since the earliest description of schizophrenia, cognitive deficits have been noted to be a prominent and enduring aspect of the illness [1]. During the past decade, however, there has been a dramatic increase in interest in this aspect of the psychopathology of schizophrenia. There appear to be at least two reasons for this phenomenon. The first reflects an increased awareness of the functional significance of impaired cognition in schizophrenia, and the treatment refractoriness of cognitive deficits [2]. The second factor reflects the emergence of cognitive neuroscience as a major, new, integrative neuroscientific discipline, the tools and constructs of which are being increasingly applied to investigations of the neural basis of cognitive deficits in brain disorders [3,4].

Cognitive dysfunction is a highly clinically relevant aspect of schizophrenia. A number of studies during the past decade [5–8] have strongly suggested that cognitive deficits are highly correlated with poor outcome and functional disability in this illness. Impaired cognition more strongly predicts poor social and occupational functioning than the positive symptoms, such as hallucinations and delusions, which have traditionally been the targets of therapy. Yet it is clear that the typical neuroleptics have no positive impact on this domain of functioning. The existing data for atypical agents are mixed and suggest only limited benefit, at best [2,9–12], with the majority of patients treated with our best atypical agents continuing to be markedly cognitively impaired. The question whether the modest cognitive improvements translate into improved social or occupational functioning of patients has not adequately been addressed, and the evidence for such associations is still unclear [9,13,14]. As a result of this new knowledge regarding the clinical significance of cognitive deficits in schizophrenia, there has been a renewed interest in understanding and treating cognitive deficits in schizophrenia, in an effort to move the treatment of this illness beyond symptom control and relapse prevention and toward rehabilitation and disability reduction.

Accompanying this growing awareness of the functional importance of cognitive impairments has been a dramatic advance in the tractability of the problem, owing to the development of cognitive neuroscience and its application in clinical neuroscience research. In this new field of neuroscience, methods from experimental cognitive psychology are integrated with physiological methods such as human functional neuroimaging or single cell recording in behaving nonhuman primates. As one of the most active areas in neuroscience it has provided a wealth of new knowledge regarding the neural basis of cognition. It has also provided psychiatric investigators with a powerful new methodology for investigating the neural basis of impaired cognition in schizophrenia. A prerequisite for applying these tools, however, is knowledge of the kinds of cognitive deficits which are common in schizophrenia, of their reliable measurement, and of their application in functional imaging and electrophysiological studies in clinical populations.

In this chapter we will discuss the range of cognitive deficits observed in patients with schizophrenia, beginning with a discussion of the involvement of the major cognitive systems of attention, memory, and language processing, as well as deficits in sensory processing. We will then discuss an overarching cognitive theory to account for the range of cognitive deficits present in schizophrenia, namely, the disruption of what has been referred to as cognitive control or executive functions. Finally, we will selectively review the literature relating cognitive dysfunction to specific neural systems in schizophrenia with an emphasis on how this literature might provide clues for future directions in the treatment of cognitive dysfunction in this illness.

II. THE SCOPE OF IMPAIRED COGNITION IN SCHIZOPHRENIA

A range of approaches may be used to study cognitive dysfunction in schizophrenia. Many studies have used batteries of neuropsychological tasks to characterize cognitive deficits in schizophrenia. This approach has a number of strengths, including standardization of test administration and extensive normative data against which to compare the performance of a specific patient. Such assessments remain very valuable tools in clinical assessment.

However, this approach has three major limitations in the investigation of cognitive deficits in schizophrenia. First, the tasks used in neuropsychological batteries are complex and cannot isolate distinct cognitive functions. Second, even when factor analyses are used to identify profiles of deficits, the specificity of such profiles is confounded by differential discriminating power across for domains [15,16]. In the simplest sense this can be understood as the problem that if a patient has poor motivation or is otherwise not engaged with the task, they will show their worst performance on the most difficult tasks. Since factors of clusters of tasks in a neuropsychological battery are not matched for their sensitivity to such a generalized deficit, differential patterns of performance may create a false impression of a specific profile of deficits. It is important to note that many experimental cognitive studies of cognition in schizophrenia are also subject to this confound. However, because of the flexibility of task, design solutions are available within this experimental framework that make it possible to control for this confound and identify deficits in specific cognitive processes in schizophrenia [17,18]. The third limitation of the clinical neuropsychological approach relates again to the complexity of the tasks, which renders them unsuitable for use in neuroscientific studies such as functional brain imaging, which has become a critical tool for the investigation of the neural basis of impaired cognition in schizophrenia.

Because of the above limitations, this review will emphasize those studies which are amenable to analysis and interpretation using the tools and constructs of experimental cognitive psychology. This approach has dominated the empirical study of human cognition for four decades. It promotes the use of a common taxonomy of cognition and provides a theoretical clarity which is grounded in a vast empirical literature. It also permits a mechanistic approach to the investigation of cognitive dysfunction in schizophrenia in which task design is theoretically driven and implemented in a systematic, hypothesis driven manner. Most importantly, this approach can be integrated with human and nonhuman neuroscientific studies. For completeness, we will begin with a brief review of disturbances of perceptual processes in schizophrenia, which have been extensively studied and have potentially important implications for our understanding of the neurobiology of this illness. We will then focus the remainder of the paper on the deficits in higher cognitive functions such as attention and memory, and the executive functions that govern these cognitive systems that appear to be so relevant for functional outcome in this illness.

III. PERCEPTUAL DISTURBANCES IN SCHIZOPHRENIA

Disturbances have been observed at a number of levels of information processing in schizophrenia, including mechanisms which are traditionally considered perceptual or preattentive [19–21]. In addition to psychophysical performance data (e.g., reaction times, accuracy), many of these studies have used cortical evoked potentials (ERP) to index the altered information processing seen in this illness.

Processing of early sensory information in schizophrenia has been studied extensively using paradigms in which two subsequent auditory stimuli are presented at relatively short time intervals (ranging from tens to hundreds of milliseconds). In normal subjects, early sensory gating is manifested as decreased response to the second stimulus, commonly referred to as prepulse inhibition (PPI). Numerous studies have shown decreased prepulse inhibition in schizophrenia patients, measuring behaviors such as the startle response [22,23], or the P50 component of the auditory event-related potential. Several studies have described correlations of these indices with symptoms and/or treatment effects [24–26], but the functional significance of the former is still debated [27–29]. Psychotic manic patients display a similar reduction of P50 suppression, but while antipsychotic treatment normalizes the suppression in these patients, it does not do so in schizophrenia [30], suggesting that the P50 inhibition is a trait deficit in this illness. The mismatch negativity, the earliest attention-independent response to deviant stimuli [31,32], and the amplitude [27,33,34] and PPI [24,35] of the N100 component of the ERP (the earliest attention-dependent index of stimulus selection) are all reduced in schizophrenia.

The impaired sensory gating of auditory stimuli has been proposed as a possible mechanism underlying other cognitive deficits present in schizophrenia, in which the unmodulated processing of sensory information disrupts higher level cognitive functions. However, the corollary to this formulation is that evidence for top-down modulation of early sensory processing [36,37] may offer an alternative explanation for disturbed sensory gating in schizophrenia. According to this hypothesis, disrupted sensory gating may be secondary to impaired attentional modulation of the sensory cortex. Further research is necessary to discriminate between early information-processing disturbances and attentional impairments as underlying the subtle disturbances in perceptual processes observed in this illness.

IV. ATTENTION DEFICITS IN SCHIZOPHRENIA

The construct of attention refers to an array of mental processes which ultimately determine to what degree information is processed and responded to and to what degree it is ignored. Taxonomies of attention have generally sorted these processes into a few broad classes of functions [38,39]. Our conception of attention has become increasingly constrained by our knowledge of brain function, and has emphasized mechanisms by which both perceptual and response

related processes may be modulated by attention [39], as well as the interactive nature and parallel organization of the neural circuitry [40]. Within these widely accepted theoretical frameworks, a common distinction that is made is between executive processes, which are involved in the control of attention in a task appropriate manner, and local changes in the activity of information processing pathways through which attentional modulation of stimulus processing and response selection occur [38,41].

In their taxonomies of attention, cognitive psychologists have generally distinguished among vigilance, or maintaining an attentive state over time, preparation (getting ready for a stimulus to appear), and selective attention [38]. These three elements of attention have been extensively studied in schizophrenia, and a specific pattern of deficits, in which some aspects of attention are impaired while others are preserved, is evident.

The continuous-performance task (CPT) [42] is a cognitive paradigm which has been used repeatedly to investigate attention in schizophrenia over the years. Patients attend to a sequence of stimuli appearing on a monitor and respond when a prespecified target stimulus appears. Schizophrenia patients are impaired on this task, especially when the difficulty of the task is increased by degrading the stimulus to make it harder to discriminate targets from nontargets [43], or by adding a memory load by instructing subjects to respond to targets that are repeats of previous stimuli. Interestingly, impairment on the CPT is evenly distributed across the duration of the testing session; it does not get worse the longer the subjects are performing [2]. Hence, *vigilance* in schizophrenia, defined as the ability to maintain an attentive state over time, is intact.

Preparatory attention refers to the ability to take advantage of a cue warning the subject to prepare for an upcoming stimulus [38]. For example, in a spatial cuing task [44] subjects watch for the occurrence of a simple stimulus, and at a variable interval prior to its appearance a cue (either an arrow pointing to where it will occur, or a brightening of a box marking one of the locations) informs the subject where the stimulus is likely to occur. Normal subjects are faster to respond when the cue correctly predicts the location of the probe. Studies using variants of this task have been conducted in schizophrenia [45–50], and the results are actually very mixed from study to study. One consistent finding with this task is patients *are* able to improve their performance with a cue just like normals. They use the cue to prepare effectively for the target, taking advantage of the prior knowledge to detect the target more quickly. We found a similar result using a task known as the Global/Local task [19] in which subjects are shown a complex visual stimulus consisting of a large letter made up of many copies of a smaller letter. They are asked to decide which of two target letters, one of which is always present, has occurred. The target may be at either the small letter (local) level, or at the large letter (global) level. When patients were instructed that on a given block of trials 80% of the targets would appear at a particular level, they were able to significantly improve their performance for targets at that level, to the same degree as normal subjects. In other words, they were able to use prior knowledge about at which level the target was likely to occur and improve their response time. Hence, one can conclude that as is the case for vigilance, the preparatory aspect of attention is intact in schizophrenia.

The third class of attentional processes that we will consider is *selective* attention. This refers to the processing of information which is relevant for appropriate task performance, but not information that is irrelevant for performance. A selective attention deficit will result in distractibility. The classical experimental paradigm used to investigate selective attention is the Stroop task, one the most widely applied procedures in cognitive science [51,52]. In the Stroop task, subjects are required to name the colors of colored words, which may themselves be the names of colors. Because word reading is automatic, when the word is a color name it affects subjects responses, despite the fact that they are instructed to ignore it. For example, if the word and the color are incongruent (e.g. the word RED printed in blue), then subjects are slower or make errors (they say the word instead of the color), an effect referred to as *interference*. When the word and the color are congruent (e.g., the word RED printed in red), they respond more quickly, an effect referred to as *facilitation*.

The original version of the Stroop task used cards, and many studies using this approach were performed in schizophrenia over the years. The interpretation of most of these studies was unfortunately confounded by a failure to take into account general impairments such as slower overall response times of patients with schizophrenia [53]. More recent studies have used computerized presentation of single stimuli and on line monitoring of response times and accuracy. Compared to controls, patients make more errors in response to incongruent stimuli, and show increased facilitation with congruent stimuli, suggesting that patients with schizophrenia show more of an effect of task irrelevant information, i.e., a selective attention deficit [46,53–55]. Increased distractibility in schizophrenia has also been shown using the antisaccade task, where subjects must overcome the prepotent response to make a saccadic eye movement to the location of onset of visual stimulus, and instead make a saccade to a location in the opposite visual field [56].

The systematic study of attention in schizophrenia suggests that certain aspects of this cognitive domain, such as vigilance and preparation, are intact. However, selective attention, the ability to respond to task-relevant information in the face of distracting, task irrelevant information, is reliably impaired in this illness.

V. MEMORY

As with the construct of attention, the term memory refers to a broad class of cognitive functions. Most models of memory make the broad distinction between short- and long-term memory. The concept of short term memory has best been extensively elaborated by Baddeley [57], who has described a system called *working* memory, which functions on a time scale of just a few seconds. Baddeley's model of the working memory system consists of a set of buffers for the short-term storage of information, and a central executive, which is responsible for manipulating the contents of the system. Information held in working memory may or may not be encoded into long-term memory (for example, a phone number retrieved from a directory may be retained just long enough to dial but not recalled later if the line was busy), depending on the context involved.

Models of long-term memory are based largely on studies of amnestic individuals who have damage to their medial temporal lobes and show a remarkable inability to acquire new memories for events. A common broad distinction which is made is between declarative and nondeclarative memory systems [e.g., 58,59]. Declarative or explicit memory involves the conscious recollection of facts and occurrences. Nondeclarative, or implicit, memory refers to a range of knowledge and abilities including motor and cognitive skills which do not require conscious recollection of the occurrences through which they were learned. Extensive research using memory tasks in schizophrenia has established that, like attention, certain aspects of memory are reliably impaired, while others are preserved.

Working memory has been extensively studied in schizophrenia and shown to be impaired in this illness.

Working memory for spatial information has been shown to be impaired in a number of studies of schizophrenia [60–63]. Working memory for verbal information has also been shown to be impaired [54,64]. Verbal working memory appears to be most evident when patients are challenged with a high information load [65], when distraction is present [61], and when executive functions are engaged by the requirement that patients manipulate, rather than just rehearse, information in working memory [66]. It is unclear whether working memory disturbances in schizophrenia reflect deficits in maintenance processes [62], executive processes [67], or both [60]. Patients are often impaired on tasks that place demands on executive functions (such as the Stroop task) but have minimal working memory demands. Selective attention deficits have been also shown to strongly correlate with working memory impairments in schizophrenia [67]. Our interpretation of these results is that the evidence more strongly supports impairments in executive processes rather than in impairments solely in the buffer systems in working memory. This view is supported by the fact that schizophrenia patients generally perform well on simple span tasks [66,68], which measure the integrity of the buffers. Clarifying the precise mechanisms underlying working memory impairments in schizophrenia is an active area of investigation in the cognitive neuroscience of schizophrenia. Since there is some evidence that different neural systems underlie storage and executive functions of working memory in the human brain, the results of these studies may have important implications for our understanding of the neurobiology of cognitive disability in schizophrenia.

In contrast to the well-established working memory deficits in schizophrenia, whether or not declarative memory is impaired in this illness is controversial. This reflects in part the methodological difficulties of evaluating declarative memory in the presence of deficits in attention and working memory. Patients are undoubtedly impaired on declarative learning and memory tests such as word list learning [10,68–71]. However, impaired executive processes and selective attention could account for these deficits. A classical finding is that patients with schizophrenia show impaired recall but intact recognition performance on list-learning tasks. It has also been shown that schizophrenia patients can actually improve their recall performance into the normal range when they are provided cues for use during the task to facilitate learning [70]. In addition, studies have found that recall is improved in schizophrenia when strategies to improve encoding such as semantic chunking are provided [72].

These studies suggest that schizophrenia patients have difficulties not so much with declarative learning per se, but with executive processes associated with the encoding and retrieval of items from declarative memory. The pattern of performance of patients with schizophrenia is much more like that seen in patients with frontal lobe lesions than with lesions of the medial temporal lobe, an observation that lends weight to the emphasis placed on the frontal lobes in investigations of the neural substrates impaired cognition in schizophrenia.

In contrast to studies of declarative memory in schizophrenia, the results of studies of nondeclarative memory are relatively unambiguous. Compared to normal controls, schizophrenia patients acquire procedural knowledge as well as normal subjects [e.g., 10,68,70]. For example, patients acquire simple motor skills at the same rate and to the same level of precision as do normal subjects.

However, the literature related to one aspect of memory thought to reflect a nondeclarative form of memory, semantic priming, is far from clear. Semantic priming tasks examine the behavioral effects of the strength of associations between related concepts in semantic memory, i.e., knowledge acquired implicitly during development. In one version of a semantic priming task, a lexical decision task, a subject is asked to respond to a letter string by deciding whether it is a word or not, or in other paradigms subjects are asked to by pronounce the word out loud. In these priming tasks the stimulus to which the subject is required to respond (the target) is immediately preceded by another stimulus to which the subject does not respond (the prime). Response times to targets which are words are faster if the prime is a word, rather than a nonword, and faster again if the prime is semantically related to the target than if it is semantically unrelated. Faster reaction times for related, compared to unrelated, prime-target pairs are referred to as the semantic priming effect. An early study using this paradigm [73] suggested that schizophrenia patients showed increased semantic priming. Relative to controls, it was reported that patients showed faster response times to making a lexical decision when it was preceded by a related word (e.g., DOCTOR followed by NURSE). This finding proposed to reflect increased spread of activation in the networks representing semantic knowledge in schizophrenia.

Subsequent studies using this approach have been frustratingly mixed. There have been some replications [74–76] but also a number of nonreplications [77–79].

This has led to the suggestion that increased semantic priming is not a reliable finding in schizophrenia, or may be confounded by clinical state, cohort, or medication effects. It is noteworthy that those studies which have reported this finding all involved medicated patients. Based on the results of many studies of different forms of nondeclarative memory in schizophrenia it appears likely that a number of aspects of nondeclarative memory (procedural learning and priming effects) are preserved in this illness.

VI. UNDERSTANDING IMPAIRED COGNITION IN SCHIZOPHRENIA

A. The Concept of Impaired Executive Functions

The notion that impaired executive functions underlie impaired higher cognition in schizophrenia has formed the basis of many general theories of impaired cognition in schizophrenia [4,67,80–82]. We also believe that this is an informative and parsimonious way of understanding the range of cognitive deficits seen in this illness. However, the term executive functions needs clarification, since it has been used in relationship to a number of domains of cognition in cognitive psychology as well as in relation to a wide range of tasks in clinical neuropsychology. Executive functions encompasses a broad range of mental processes involved in initiating and maintaining controlled information processing and coordinated actions [83]. These processes include goal or context representation and maintenance, strategic processes such as attention allocation and stimulus-response mapping, and performance monitoring [40,65,84]. Deficits in executive functions have been frequently reported in schizophrenia using a range of methodologies from neuropsychology and experimental cognitive psychology. A disturbance in the ability to initiated and maintain controlled information processing can clearly account for the pattern of deficits of selective attention, working memory, and declarative memory performance seen in patients with this illness. We believe that it is important to emphasize the diversity of executive functions and to point out that the *specific* abnormality or abnormalities within the executive system in schizophrenia have yet to be identified. To date, well-articulated theories emphasizing impaired context representation and maintenance [82,85], attention allocation [80], and performance monitoring [86–89] have all been hypothesized, with some data supporting each of these alternatives having been presented. No single theory of impaired executive functions has garnered overwhelming empirical support over other theories to this point. Further research is needed to clarify whether a disruption of one specific aspect of executive functions in schizophrenia is sufficient to account for the range of higher cognitive deficits observed or whether multiple different executive deficits exist, each of which may contribute to different aspects of cognitive disability.

For future investigations directed toward understanding the precise nature of impaired executive functions in schizophrenia, the tools and constructs of cognitive neuroscience are likely to play a critical role. The discrete, elemental processes of executive functions described above have begun to be linked to discrete elements of a distributed neural network serving executive functions in the brain. This new knowledge is allowing us to begin, for the first time, to develop the beginnings of a functional-anatomic understanding of cognitive deficits in schizophrenia.

B. The Neural Basis of Cognitive Deficits in Schizophrenia

It seems fair to say that in recent years more investigation has been undertaken into the neural substrates of cognitive functions in schizophrenia than perhaps any other aspect of the illness. We believe that this reflects in part the fact that, in addition to its increasingly obvious clinical importance, investigation of the neural basis of cognitive deficits is more tractable than is the case for other aspects of the illness. Cognition in schizophrenia can be reliably and objectively measured using methods from experimental cognitive psychology, while assessment of symptoms such as hallucinations and delusions relies on patient self-report and clinical inference. Also, cognitive activation has become a standard method of examining brain behavior relationships in cognitive neuroscience. The methodology is mature and there is a rapidly increasing base of knowledge regarding the neural basis of normal cognition which provides the necessary framework for designing and interpreting results from clinical studies involving patients.

Results to date suggest that patients with schizophrenia do have reliable disturbances in activity in the neural network involved in executive processes, which includes the dorsolateral prefrontal cortex (DLPFC) and the anterior cingulate cortex (ACC) [65,90–95]. This is not to imply that these are the only regions that have been reported to be abnormal in functional imaging studies of schizophrenia. Disturbances have also been reported in temporolimbic regions including the hippocampus [96,97], the superior temporal gyrus [98–101], and the striatum and cerebellum [90,102]. The significance of altered activity in temporolimbic regions of the brain in schizophrenia for cognition remains unclear. It is possible that activity in these regions is related to other aspects of the illness, such a delusions and hallucinations [103]. In this chapter we are focusing on cognition in schizophrenia, and our emphasis on the role of the frontal cortex in this chapter reflects the central role impaired executive functions play in these deficits, the well-established relationship between the function of the frontal lobes and executive control, and the growing literature linking impaired executive functions in schizophrenia to disturbances in the functions of the frontal cortex.

The first functional imaging study in schizophrenia, conducted by Ingvar and Franzden [104], reported that schizophrenia patients showed a loss of the normal hyperfrontal pattern of blood flow while performing a neuropsychological task. Since that time many, but certainly not all, studies of schizophrenia have reported reduced blood flow or metabolism in the DLPFC in schizophrenia [90,102]. This finding is not as reliable when patients are studied at rest [105], and we and others have argued that it is most reliably present when patients are performing tasks which engage cognitive systems known to reflect neural activity in this region of the brain, such as working memory tasks [65,94,106,107].

Much of the focus on hypofrontality in schizophrenia has centered on the DLPFC; however, the ACC, another critical element in the neural network subserving executive functions in the normal brain, has also frequently been found to be functioning abnormally in functional imaging studies of this illness. Tamminga and colleagues [97] found decreased resting ACC (and hippocampal) metabolism in an unmedicated group of schizophrenia patients. Buchsbaum and colleagues [108,109] have also reported cingulate hypometabolism in unmedicated subjects. In a fascinating correlational study between symptoms and resting cerebral blood flow measures using positron emission tomography (PET) [103], blood flow in the ACC correlated specifically with schizophrenia patients' level of behavioral disorganization.

With regard to its function during cognition, a number of studies have examined ACC activity in schizophrenia during cognitive activation. During a single photon emission computer tomography (SPECT) study in which unmedicated subjects performed the Tower of London, a test of executive function, decreased ACC activity was observed [90]. Decreased ACC activation responses in schizophrenia have also been reported during two other classical measures of executive functions—an auditory-verbal supraspan memory task [100], and verbal fluency [98]. Our own group reported that schizophrenia patients showed reduced ACC activation during the Stroop task, a challenging selective attention task which elicits response conflict which must be overcome by the participant [92]. Based on recent work [65,110] using event-related functional magnetic resonance imaging (fMRI) in normal subjects it has been hypothesized that the ACC serves a very specific, evaluative function associated with the executive control of cognition. It appears that the ACC detects, online, cognitive states that may be associated with poor task performance, such as the occurrence of conflicts between simultaneously activated but incompatible response tendencies. Increased activity in this region may then provide a signal to other components of the executive system, indicating the need for increased attentional engagement and more effective controlled processing (e.g., through improved attention allocation). In a recent event-related fMRI study [93] we reported that error-related activity in the ACC is reduced in schizophrenia. We also found in this study that patients failed to show the usual posterror adjustments in performance seen in control subjects. The functional significance of the physiological disturbances in the ACC revealed by the neuroimaging studies described above may be that an impairment in the performance monitoring function of this brain region contributes to impaired executive functions in schizophrenia.

C. The Clinical Significance of Cognitive Deficits in Schizophrenia

As noted in the introduction of this chapter, there is a growing awareness of the clinical significance of impaired cognition in schizophrenia. The association between cognitive deficits in schizophrenia and the relative treatment refractoriness of this aspect of the illness has drawn attention to the need for further understanding of its neurobiological substrates. There has also been a tendency to see cognitive deficits as reflecting an independent dimension of schizophrenia, unrelated to the positive and negative symptoms that have traditionally defined the illness. However, we believe that it is unlikely that impaired cognition is completely independent, either at the behavioral level or at the neural systems level, from the other mental perturbations of schizophrenia, and that an understanding of impaired cognition and its potential relationship to other signs and symptoms will result in a richer clinical understanding of the illness than we have had in the past.

Given the association between executive functions and frontal lobe function, for example, it might be expected that symptoms which would be likely to be associated with frontal deficits, particularly negative symptoms and behavioral disorganization, would be associated with cognitive disability. There is some support for the association between negative symptoms and spatial working memory [60,61]; however, reviews of the literature [2,111,112] show many negative studies, and our own group has not consistently found relationships between impaired executive functions and negative symptoms [54,67]. One factor in the unreliability of associations between negative symptoms and cognitive deficits might reflect the practical difficulty of distinguishing drug-induced parkinsonism from true-negative symptoms in medicated patients.

A second, perhaps even more important, factor underlying the above variability in findings may be the assumptions made in many studies regarding the structure of symptoms in schizophrenia. Many older studies used a two-factor model, classifying symptoms into positive and negative factors. More recently, however, a number of studies have suggested that the factor structure of schizophrenia is more complex, and includes a disorganization factor which is separate from the positive and negative factors and is composed of items previously considered belong to each of the other two dimensions [113–115]. In our own more recent work we have taken this three-factor approach. In both medicated and unmedicated groups of patients we have occasionally found relationships among negative symptoms and deficits in selective attention and verbal working memory. In contrast, we have consistently found robust relationships between these measures of cognitive disability and the syndrome of disorganization [67,116]. This is consistent with previous theories regarding the relationship of disorganization and attentional disturbances [117]. This idea was in fact articulated by Bleuler nearly a century ago [118], when he argued that disturbances in the control of attention were responsible for the associational disturbances that distinguished the schizophrenias from the other major psychoses. Based on these results we suggest that there is in fact some overlap between cognitive symptoms of schizophrenia and other aspects of the clinical syndrome, particularly with behavioral disorganization. This view of a Bleulerian cognition/disorganization dimension to the illness might give clinicians a fresh perspective on the source of some patients functional difficulties and also define a target syndrome for new treatment development.

VII. TREATMENT STRATEGIES TARGETING COGNITIVE DISABILITY IN SCHIZOPHRENIA

The current data on the effects of the currently available antipsychotic treatments suggest at best limited benefits on cognitive dysfunction in schizophrenia [10,11]. There is evidence from a number of clinical trials that atypical antipsychotic agents offer some advantages of typical agents [119]; however, these benefits are limited. Minimizing the use of adjunctive therapies such as anticholinergics, benzodiazpines, beta blockers, and other agents that can worsen cognitive functioning, is also an important aspect of the pharmacotherapy of cognition in schizophrenia. How then do we proceed to address this shortcoming of our current therapy?

The first step toward developing effective treatments for cognitive disability in schizophrenia will be to continue the paradigm shift which is already under way in the field. The emphasis, to date, on positive and more recently negative symptoms as outcome measures for therapies for schizophrenia needs to be expanded to include measures of cognitive function, specifically, measures of attention and memory.

Unlike our treatments for positive symptoms, which were developed serendipitously, the development of treatments for impaired cognition in schizophrenia may proceed based on our developing knowledge of the likely pathophysiological mechanisms underlying this aspect of the illness. Functional neuroimaging studies suggest that disturbances in DLPFC and ACC circuitry related to executive functions may account for many of these deficits. Disturbances in elements of the local circuitry of these regions that have been reported in postmortem brains of schizophrenia patients may provide clues to potential pharmacological strategies for remediating the function of these circuits. Reductions in markers of inhibitory interneuron function, reductions in markers of glutamatergic function, and reductions in afferent dopaminergic modulatory input have been reported in both of these regions [120–123]. New agents which remediate one or more of these disturbances might provide a whole new avenue for disability reduction in schizophrenia. Preliminary work administering glycine cycloserine and D-serine [124–126] to enhance glutamatergic function supports the feasibility of this approach. New agents which enhance glutamatergic effects though more specific mechanisms are under development. Similarly, transient benefits on cognitive function have been observed after stimulant challenge [92,127], which in our study extended beyond effects on working memory to include improvement in measures of the organization of language production. Agents that enhance phasic dopamine in the cortex may also have promise in treating cognitive dysfunction in schizophrenia.

It is possible and even likely that cognitive rehabilitation strategies targeting the potential neuroplasticity of the frontal cortical-based circuits mediating executive functions will also be of benefit in treating cognitive deficits in schizophrenia. Preliminary data using methods adapted from cognitive rehabilitation treatments for closed head injury combined with optimizing pharmacotherapy and other psychosocial interventions support the possible efficacy of this approach [128].

VIII. CONCLUSIONS

Over the past decade there has been a growing awareness of the clinical importance of cognitive disability in schizophrenia. Deficits observed cut across a number of domains of cognitive functioning including selective attention and working memory. These deficits can be understood as a disturbance in executive functions—a complex set of operations required for the efficient execution of each of these cognitive systems. Functional brain-imaging studies also suggest that these higher cognitive deficits are related to physiological dysfunction in circuits underlying executive functions in the brain, including the DLPFC and the ACC. At the local circuit level, disturbances in glutamatergic and GABA-ergic neurotransmission, and the modulation of these by dopamine are likely to be present. The development of therapies targeting these disturbances at the local circuit level in medial and dorsolateral prefrontal cortex promises to begin a new phase in the therapeutics of schizophrenia in which the focus will be on disability reduction in this illness.

ACKNOWLEDGMENTS

We would like to gratefully acknowledge Lynn Rago for her assistance in preparing this manuscript. The first author is supported by federal grants MH59883 and MH64190 and a Burroughs Wellcome Fund Clinical Scientist Award in Translational Research.

REFERENCES

1. Kraepelin E. Dementia Praecox and Paraphrenia. Edinburgh: Livingston (original work published 1919), 1971.
2. Green MF. Schizophrenia from a neurocognitive perspective: probing the impenetrable darkness. Boston: Allyn and Bacon, 1998.
3. Green MF, Neuchterlein KH. Cortical oscillations and schizophrenia: timing is of the essence. Arch Gen Psychiatry 1999; 56:1007–1008.
4. Posner MI, Abdullaev YG. eds. What to Image? Anatomy, Circuitry and Plasticity of Human Brain Function. Brain Mapping: The Methods. New York: Academic Press, 1996.
5. Connor RO, Herman H. Assessment of contributions to disability in people with schizophrenia during rehabilitation. Aust NZ J Psychiatry 1993; 27:595–600.
6. Davidson L, McGlashan TH. The varied outcomes of schizophrenia. Can J Psychiatry 1997; 42:34–43.
7. Green MF. What are the functional consequences of neurocognitive deficits in schizophrenia? Am J Psychiatry 1996; 153:321–330.
8. Klapow JC, Evans J, Patterson TL, Heaton RK, Koch WL, Jeste DV. Direct assessment of functional status in older patients with schizophrenia. Am J Psychiatry, 1997; 154:1022–1024.
9. Cuesta MJ, Peralta V, Zarzuela A. Effects of olanzapine and other antipsychotics on cognitive function in chronic schizophrenia: a longitudinal study. Schizophr Res, 2001; 48(1):17–28.
10. Goldberg TE, Saint-Cyr J, Weinberger DR. Assessment of procedural learning and problem solving in schizophrenia patients using Tower of Hanoi type tasks. J Neuropsychiatry Clin Neurosci 1990; 2:165–173.
11. Green MF, Marshall BD Jr, Wirshing WC, Ames D, Marder SR, McGurk S, Kern RS, Mintz J. Does risperidone improve verbal working memory in treatment-resistant schizophrenia? Am J Psychiatry 1997; 154(6):799–804.
12. Purdon SE, Jones BD, Stip E, Labelle A, Addington D, David SR, Breier A, Tollefson GD. Neuropsychological change in early phase schizophrenia during 12 months of treatment with olanzapine, risperidone, or haloperidol. Arch Gen Psychiatry 2000; 57(3):249–258.
13. Buchanan RW, Holstein C, Breier A. The comparative efficacy and long-term effect of clozapine treatment on neuropsychological test performance. Biol Psychiatry 1994; 36(11):717–725.

14. Galletly CA, Clark CR, McFarlane AC, Weber DL. Relationships between changes in symptom ratings, neurophysiological test performance and quality of life in schizophrenic patients treated with clozapine. Psychiatry Res 1997; 72(3):161-16-6.
15. Chapman LJ, Chapman JP. Problems in the measurement of cognitive deficit. Psychol Bull 1973; 79:380–385.
16. Chapman LJ, Chapman JP. The measurement of differential deficit. Journal of Psychiatric Res 1978; 14:303–311.
17. Knight RA, Silverstein SM. A process-oriented approach for averting confounds resulting from general performance deficiencies in schizophrenia. Journal of Abnormal Psychol 2001; 110:15–30.
18. MacDonald AW, Carter CS. Cognitive experimental approaches to investigating impaired cognition in schizophrenia: a paradigm shift. J Clin Exp Neuropsychol (in press).
19. Carter CS, Robertson LC, Nordahl TE, Chaderjian M, Oshora-Celaya L. Attentional and perceptual asymmetries in schizophrenia: further evidence for a left hemisphere deficit. Psychiatry Res 1996; 62:111–119.
20. Green MF, Neuchterlein KH, Mintz J. Backward masking in schizophrenia and mania: specifying a mechanism. Arch Gen Psychiatry 1994; 51:939–944.
21. Saccusso DP, Braff DL. Early information processing deficits in schizophrenia. Arch Gen Psychiatry 1981; 38:175–179.
22. Braff DL, Grillon C, Geyer MA. Gating and habituation of the startle reflex in schizophrenic patients. Arch Gen Psychiatry 1992; 49(3):206–215.
23. Perry W, Braff DL. Information-processing deficits and thought disorder in schizophrenia. Am J Psychiatry 1994; 151(3):363–367.
24. Bender S, Schall U, Wolstein J, Grzella I, Zerbin D, Oades RD. A topographic event-related potential follow-up study on 'prepulse inhibition' in first and second episode patients with schizophrenia. Psychiatry Res 1999; 90(1):41–53.
25. Kumari V, Soni W, Sharma T. Normalization of information processing deficits in schizophrenia with clozapine. Am J Psychiatry 1999; 156(7):1046–51.
26. Light GA, Geyer MA, Clementz BA, Cadenhead KS, Braff DL. Normal P50 suppression in schizophrenia patients treated with atypical antipsychotic medications. Am J Psychiatry 2000; 157(5):767–771.
27. Adler LE, Waldo MC, Tatcher A, Cawthra E, Baker N, Freedman R. Lack of relationship of auditory gating defects to negative symptoms in schizophrenia. Schizophr Res 1990; 3(2):131–138.
28. Jin Y, Bunney WE Jr, Sandman CA, Patterson JV, Fleming K, Moenter JR, Kalali AH, Hetrick WP, Potkin SG. Is P50 suppression a measure of sensory gating in schizophrenia? Biol Psychiatry 1998; 43(12):873–878.
29. Light GA, Braff DL. Do self-reports of perceptual anomalies reflect gating deficits in schizophrenia patients? Biol Psychiatry 2000; 47(5):463–467.
30. Franks RD, Adler LE, Waldo MC, Alpert J, Freedman R. Neurophysiological studies of sensory gating in mania: comparison with schizophrenia. Biol Psychiatry 1983; 18(9):989–1005.
31. Hirayasu Y, Potts GF, O'Donnell BF, Kwon JS, Arakaki H, Akdag SJ, Levitt JJ, Shenton ME, McCarley RW. Auditory mismatch negativity in schizophrenia: topographic evaluation with a high-density recording montage. Am J Psychiatry 1998; 155(9):1281–1284.
32. Javitt DC, Doneshka P, Grochowski S, Ritter W. Impaired mismatch negativity generation reflects widespread dysfunction of working memory in schizophrenia. Arch Gen Psychiatry, 1995; 52(7):550–558.
33. Ogura C, Nageishi Y, Matsubayashi M, Omura F, Kishimoto A, Shimokochi M. Abnormalities in event-related potentials, N100, P200, P300 and slow wave in schizophrenia. Jpn J Psychiatry Neurol 1991; 45(1):57–65.
34. Waldo MC, Adler LE, Freedman R. Defects in auditory sensory gating and their apparent compensation in relatives of schizophrenics. Schizophr Res 1988; 1(1):19–24.
35. Boutros NN, Belger A, Campbell D, D'Souza C, Krystal J. Comparison of four components of sensory gating in schizophrenia and normal subjects: a preliminary report. Psychiatry Res 1999; 88(2):119–130.
36. Kastner S, Ungerleider LG. Mechanisms of visual attention in the human cortex. Annu Rev Neurosci 2000; 23:315–341.
37. Shulman GL, Corbetta M, Buckner RL, Raichle ME, Fiez JA, Miezin FM, Petersen SE. Top-down modulation of early sensory cortex. Cerebral Cortex 1997; 7(3):193–206.
38. LaBerge D. Attentional Processing. Cambridge, MA: Harvard University Press, 1995.
39. Posner MI, Petersen SE. The attention system of the human brain. Annu Rev Neurosci 1990; 13:25–42.
40. Cohen JD, Dunbar K, McClellend JL. On the control of automatic processes: a parallel distributed processing account of the Stroop effect. Psychol Rev 1990; 97:332–361.
41. Desimone R, Duncan J. Neural mechanisms of selective visual attention. Annu Rev Neurosci 1995; 18:193–222.
42. Rosvold KE, Mirsky AF, Sarason I, Bransome ED, Beck LH. A continuous performance test of brain damage. J Consult Psychol, 1956; 20:343–350.
43. Nuechterlein KH, Dawson ME. Information processing and attentional functioning in the developmental course of schizophrenia disorders. Schizophr Bull, 1984; 10:160–203.

44. Posner MI, Cohen Y. Components of visual orienting, In: Toga AW, Mazziota JC, eds. Brain Mapping: The Methods. Hillsdale, NJ: Erlbaum, 1984:531–556.
45. Bustillo JR, Thaker G, Buchanan RW, Moran M, Kirkpatrick B, Carpenter WT Jr. Visual information-processing impairments in deficit and nondeficit schizophrenia. Am J Psychiatry 1997; 154(5):647–654.
46. Carter CS, Robertson LC, Nordahl TE. Abnormal processing of irrelevant information in schizophrenia: selective enhancement of Stroop facilitation. Psychiatry Res, 1992; 41:137–146.
47. Nestor PG, Faux SF, McCarley RW, Penhune V, Shenton ME, Pollak S. Attentional cues in chronic schizophrenia: abnormal disengagement of attention. J Abnorm Psychol, 1992; 101:682–689.
48. Posner MI, Early TS, Reiman E, Pardo PJ, Dhawan M. Asymmetries of attentional control in schizophrenia. Arch Gen Psychiatry 1988; 45:814–821.
49. Strauss ME, Novakovic T, Tien AY, Bylsma FW, Pearlson GD. Disengagement of attention in schizophrenia. Psychiatry Res, 1991; 37:139–146.
50. Strauss ME, Alphs LD, Boekamp J. Disengagement of attention in chronic schizophrenia. Psychiatry Res, 1992; 43:87–92.
51. Macleod CM. Half a century of research on the Stroop effect: an integrative review. Psychol Bull, 1990; 109:163–203.
52. Stroop JR. Studies of interference in serial verbal reactions. J Exp Psychol (Gen) 1935; 18:643–662.
53. Perlstein WM, Carter CS, Barch DM, Baird JW. The Stroop task and attention deficits in schizophrenia: a critical evaluation of card and single-trial Stroop methodologies. Neuropsychology 1998; 12(3):414–425.
54. Cohen JD, Barch DM, Carter CS, Servan-Schreiber D. Schizophrenic deficits in the processing of context: converging evidence from three theoretically motivated cognitive tasks. J Abnorm Psychol 1999; 108:120–133.
55. Taylor S, Kornblum S, Tandon R. Facilitation and interference of selective attention in schizophrenia. J Psychiat Res 1996; 30:251–259.
56. Crawford TJ, Haeger B, Kennard C, Reveley MA, Henderson L. Psychol Med, 1995; 25(3):461–471.
57. Baddeley AD. Working Memory, New York: Oxford University Press, 1986.
58. Squire L. Declarative and non-declarative memory. Multiple brain systems supporting learning and memory. J Cogn Neurosci, 1992; 4:232–243.
59. Squire L, Zola-Morgan S. Declarative and non-declarative memory: multiple brain systems support learning and memory. Trends Neurosci, 1988; 11:170–175.
60. Carter CS, Robertson LC, Nordahl TE, Kraft L, Chaderjian M, Oshora-Celaya L. Spatial working memory deficits and their relationship to negative symptoms in unmedicated schizophrenia patients. Biol Psychiatry 1996; 40:930–932.
61. Keefe RSE, Roitman SEL, Harvey PD, Blum CS, DuPre RL, Prieto DM, Davidson M, Davis KL. A pen-and-paper human analogue of a monkey prefrontal cortex activation task: spatial working memory in patients with schizophrenia. Schizophr Res, 1995; 17:25–33.
62. Park S, Holtzman PS. Schizophrenics show spatial working memory deficits. Arch Gen Psychiatry 1992; 49:975–982.
63. Stone M, Gabrieli JD, Stebbins GT, Sullivan EV. Working and strategic memory deficits in schizophrenia. Neuropsychologia 1998; 12(2):278–288.
64. Servan-Schreiber D, Cohen J, Steingard S. Schizophrenic deficits in the processing of context: a test of a theoretical model. Arch Gen Psychiatry 1996; 53:1105–1112.
65. Carter CS, Braver TS, Barch DM, Botvinick M, Noll D, Cohen JD. Anterior cingulate cortex, error detection, and the on line monitoring of performance. Science 1998; 280(5364):747–749.
66. Gold JM, Carpenter C, Randolph C, Goldberg TE, Weinberger DR. Auditory working memory and Wisconsin card sorting test performance in patients with schizophrenia. Arch Gen Psychiatry 1997; 54(2):159–165.
67. Barch DM, Carter CS. Selective attention in schizophrenia: relationship to verbal working memory. Schizophr Res, 1998; 33:53–61.
68. Clare L, McKenna PJ, Mortimer AM, Baddeley AD. Memory in schizophrenia, what is impaired and what is preserved. Neuropsychologia 1993; 31:1225–1241.
69. Schmand B, Beand N, Kuipers T. Procedural learning of cognitive and motor skills in psychotic patients. Schizophr Res, 1992; 8:157–170.
70. Schwartz BL, Rosse RB, Deutsch SI. Towards a neuropsychology of memory in schizophrenia. Psychopharmacol Bull, 1992; 28:341–351.
71. Tamlyn D, McKenna PJ, Mortimer AM, Lund CE, Hammond S, Baddeley AD. Memory impairment in schizophrenia: its extent, affiliations and neuropsychological character. Psychol Med, 1992; 22:101–115.
72. Koh SD. Remembering of verbal materials by schizophrenic young adults. In: Schwartz S, ed. Language and Cognition in schizophrenia. Hillsdale, NJ: Lawrence Erlbaum, 1978:55–59.
73. Manschreck TC, Maher BA, Milavetz JJ, Ames D, Weisstein CC, Schneyer ML. Semantic priming in thought disordered schizophrenic patients. Schizophr Res, 1988; 1:61–66.
74. Henik A, Nissimov E, Priel B, Umansky R. Effects of cognitive load on semantic priming in patients with schizoprenia. Abnorm Psychol, 1995; 104:576–584.
75. Kwapil TR, Hegley DC, Chapman LJ, Chapman JP. Facilitation of word recognition by semantic priming in schizophrenia. J Abnorm Psychol, 1990; 3:215–221.

76. Spitzer M. The psychopathology, neuropsychology and neurobiology of associative and working memory in schizophrenia. Eur Arch Psychiatry Clin Neurosci 1993; 243:57–70.
77. Barch DM, Cohen JD, Servan-Schreiber D, Steingard S, Steinhauer S, Van Kammen DP. Semantic priming in schizophrenia: an examination of spreading activation using word pronunciation and multiple SOA's. J Abnorm Psychol, 1996; 105(4):592–601.
78. Henik A, Priel B, Umansky R. Attention and automaticity in semantic processing of schizophrenic patients. Neuropsychiatry Neuropsychol Behav Neurol, 1992; 5:161–169.
79. Vinogradov S, Ober BA, Shenaut GK. Semantic priming of word pronunciation and lexical decision in schizophrenia. Schizophr Res, 1992; 8:171–181.
80. Braff D. Information processing and attention dysfunction in schizophrenia. Schizophr Bull, 1993; 19:233–259.
81. Calloway E, Naghdi S. An information processing model for schizophrenia. Arch Gen Psychiatry 1982; 39:339–347.
82. Cohen JD, Servan-Schreiber D. Context, cortex and dopamine: a connectionist approach to behavior and biology in schizophrenia. Psychol Rev, 1992; 99(1):45–77.
83. Carter CS, Botvinick MM, Cohen JD. The contribution of the anterior cingulate cortex to executive processes in cognition. Rev Neurosci, 1999; 10(1):49–57.
84. Shallice T. From Neuropsychology to Mental Structure. Cambridge: Cambridge University Press, 1988.
85. Shakow D. Segmental set: a theory of the formal psychological deficit in schizophrenia. Arch Gen Psychiatry 1962; 6:1–17.
86. Feinberg I. Efference copy and corollary discharge: implications for thinking and its disorders. Schizophr Bull 1978; 4:636–640.
87. Frith CD, Done DJ. Experiences of alien control in schizophrenia reflect a disorder in the central monitoring of action. Psychol Med, 1989; 19:359–363.
88. Gray J, Feldon J, Rawlins J, Hemsley D, Smith A. The neuropsychology of schizophrenia. Behav Brain Sci, 1990; 14:1–84.
89. Malenka RC, Angel RW, Hampton B, Berger PA. Impaired central error-correcting behavior in schizophrenia. Arch Gen Psychiatry 1982; 39:101–107.
90. Andreasen NC, Rezai K, Alliger R, Swayze V, Flaum M, Kirchner P, Cohen G, O'Leary DS. Hypofrontality in neuroleptic naive patients and in patients with chronic schizophrenia: assessment with xenon 133 single photon emission computed tomography and the Tower of London. Arch Gen Psychiatry 1992; 49:943–958.
91. Barch DM, Carter CS, Braver TS, Sabb FW, MacDonald AW, Noll DC, Cohen JD. Selective deficits in prefrontal cortex function in medication naive patients and schizophrenia. Arch Gen Psychiatry 2001; 58:280–288.
92. Carter CS, Mintun M, Nichols T, Cohen JD. Anterior cingulate gyrus dysfunction and selective attention deficits in schizophrenia: an [^{15}O]H$_2$O PET study during single trial Stroop task performance. Am J Psychiatry 1997; 154(12):1670–1675.
93. Carter CS, MacDonald AW, Ross LL, Stenger AS. Anterior cingulate cortex and impaired self-monitoring of performance in patients with schizophrenia: an event-related fMRI study. Am J Psychiatry 2001; 1423–1428.
94. Perlstein WM, Carter CS, Noll DC, Cohen JD. fMRI evidence of prefrontal cortex dysfunction in schizophrenia during parametric manipulation of working memory load. Am J Psychiatry (in press).
95. Weinberger DR, Berman K, Illowsky B. Physiological dysfunction of the dorsolateral prefrontal cortex. III. A new cohort and evidence for a monoaminergic mechanism. Arch Gen Psychiatry 1988; 45:609–615.
96. Nordahl TE, Kusubov N, Carter CS, Salama S, Cummings AM, O'Shora-Celaya L, Eberling J, Robertson LC, Huesman R, Jagust W, Budinger TF. Temporal lobe glucose metabolic differences in medication free out-patients with schizophrenia via the PET 600. Neuropsychopharmacology 1996; 15:541–554.
97. Tamminga CA, Thaker GK, Buchanan R, Kirkpatrick B, Alphs LD, Chase TN, Carpenter WT. Limbic system abnormalities identified in schizophrenia with fluorodeoxyglucose and neocortical alterations with the deficit syndrome. Arch Gen Psychiatry 1992; 49:522–530.
98. Dolan RJ, Fletcher P, Frith CD, Friston KJ, Frackowiak RS, Grasby PM. Dopaminergic modulation of impaired cognitive activation in the anterior cingulate cortex in schizophrenia. Nature 1995; 378(6553):180–183.
99. Frith CD, Friston KJ, Herold S, Silbersweig D, Fletcher P, Cahill C, Dolan RJ, Frackowiak RJS, Liddle PF. Regional brain activity in chronic schizophrenia patients during the performance of a verbal fluency task. Br J Psychiatry 1995; 167:343–349.
100. Ganguli R, Carter CS, Mintun M, Brar JS, Becker JT, Sarma TN, Bennington E. Abnormal cortical physiology in schizophrenia: a PET blood flow study during rest and supraspan memory performance. Biol Psychiatry 1997.
101. O'Leary DS, Andreasen NC, Hurtig RT, Kesler MI, Rogers M, Arndt S, Cizadlo T, Watkins L, Boles Potno LL, Kirchner PT, Hichwa RD. Auditory attentional deficits in schizophrenia: A positron emission tomography study. Arch Gen Psychiatry 1996; 53:633–641.

102. Buchsbaum M. The frontal lobes, basal ganglia and temporal lobes as sites for schizophrenia. Schizophr Bull, 1990; 16:379–389.
103. Liddle PF, Friston KJ, Frith CD, Hirsch SR, Jones T, Frackowiak RSJ. Patterns of cerebral blood flow in schizophrenia. Br J Psychiatry 1992; 160:179–186.
104. Ingvar DH, Franzen G. Distribution of cerebral activity in chronic schizophrenia. Lancet, 1974; 1484–1486.
105. Gur RC, Gur RE. Hypofrontality in schizophrenia: RIP. Lancet 1995; 345:1383–1340.
106. Goldman-Rakic PS. Circuitry of primate prefrontal cortex and regulation of behavior by representational memory. In: Handbook of Physiology: The Nervous System, Vol 5. Bethesda, MD: American Physiological Society, 1987.
107. Goldman-Rakic PS. Prefrontal cortical dysfunction in schizophrenia: the relevance of working memory. In: Psychopathology and the Brain. New York: Raven Press, 1991:1–23.
108. Hadnezar MM, Buchsbaum MS, Luu C, Hazlett EA, Siegel BV Jr, Lohr J, Wu J, Haier RJ, Bunney WE Jr. Decreased anterior cingulate gyrus metabolic rate in schizophrenia. Am J Psychiatry 1997; 1564(5):682–684.
109. Seigel BV, Buchsbaum MS, Bunney WE Jr, Gottschalk LA, Haier RJ, Lottenberg S, Najafi A, Lohr J, Neuchterlein KH, Potkin SG, Wu J. Cortico-striatal-thalamic circuits and brain glucose metabolism in 70 unmedicated schizophrenic patients. Am J Psychiatry 1993; 150:1325–1336.
110. MacDonald AW 3rd, Cohen JD, Stenger VA, Carter CS. Dissociating the role of the dorsolateral prefrontal and anterior cingulate cortex in cognitive control. Science 2000; 288(5472):1835–1838.
111. Strauss ME. Relations of symptoms to cognitive deficits in schizophrenia. Schizophr Bull, 1993; 19:215–231.
112. Walker E, Lewine RJ. Negative symptom distinction in schizophrenia: validity and etiological relevance. Schizophr Res, 1988; 1:315–328.
113. Andreasen NC, Arndt S, Alliger R, Miller DD, Flaum M. A longitudinal study of symptom dimensions in schizophrenia: prediction and patterns of change. Arch Gen Psychiatry, 1995; 52:341–352.
114. Arndt S, Andreasen NC, Miller DD, Nopoulos P. Symptoms of schizophrenia: methods, meanings, and mechanisms. Arch Gen Psychiatry 1995; 52:352–360.
115. Liddle PF, Barnes TRE. Syndromes of chronic schizophrenia. Br J Psychiatry 1990; 157:558–561.
116. Cohen JD, Barch DM, Carter CS, Servan-Schreiber D. Context-processing deficits in schizophrenia: converging evidence from three theoretically motivated cognitive tasks. J Abnorm Psychol, 1999; 108(1):120–133.
117. Liddle PF, Morris DL. Schizophrenic syndromes and frontal lobe performance. Br J Psychiatry 1991; 158:340–345.
118. Bleuler E. Dementia Praecox or the Group of Schizophrenias. New York: International Universities Press (original work published 1911), 1950.
119. Javitt DC. Treatment of negative and cognitive symptoms. Curr Psychiatry Rep 1999; 1(1):25–30.
120. Akbarian S, Sucher NJ, Bradley D, Tafazzoli A, Trinh D, Hetrick WP, Potkin SG, Sandman CA, Bunney WE Jr, Jones EG. Selective alterations in gene expression for NMDA receptor subunits in prefrontal cortex of schizophrenics. J Neurosci, 1996; 16(1):19–30.
121. Benes FM. Is there a neuroanatomic basis for schizophrenia? Neuroscientist 1995; 1:112–120.
122. Meador-Woodruff JH, Haroutunian V, Pochik P, Davidson M, Davis KL, Watson SJ. Dopamine receptor transcript expression in striatum and prefrontal and occipital cortex: focal abnormalities in orbitofrontal cortex in schizophrenia. Arch Gen Psychiatry 1997; 54(12):1089–1095.
123. Woo T-U, Whitehead RB, Melchitzky DS, Lewis DA. A subclass of prefrontal gamma-aminobutyric acid axon terminals are selectively altered in schizophrenia, Proc Nat Acad Sci USA 1998: 5341–5346.
124. Goff DC, Tsai G, Manoach DS, Flood J, Darby DG, Coyle JT. D-cycloserine added to clozapine for patients with schizophrenia. Am J Psychiatry 1996; 153(12):1628–1630.
125. Heresco-Levy U, Silipo G, Javitt DC. Glycinergic augmentation of NMDA receptor-mediated neurotransmission in the treatment of schizophrenia. Psychopharmacol Bull, 1996; 32(4):731–740.
126. Leiderman E, Zylberman I, Zukin SR, Cooper TB, Javitt DC. Preliminary investigation of high-dose oral glycine on serum levels and negative symptoms in schizophrenia: an open-label trial. Biol Psychiatry 1996; 39(3):213–215.
127. Goldberg TE, Bigelow LB, Weinberger DR, Daniel DG, Kleinman JE. Cognitive and behavioral effects of the coadministration of dextroamphetamine and haloperidol in schizophrenia. Am J Psychiatry 1991; 148:78–84.
128. Hogarty GE, Flesher S. Practice principles of cognitive enhancement therapy for schizophrenia. Schizophr Bull (in press).

16

Neuroimaging Findings in Schizophrenia
From Mental to Neuronal Fragmentation

LAWRENCE S. KEGELES and MARC LARUELLE
Columbia University, New York, New York, U.S.A.

I. INTRODUCTION

Over the last 20 years, the ability to image the living human brain underwent enormous developments, opening direct windows into brain function and cellular processes associated with health and disease. Brain imaging techniques are classically divided into structural, functional, and chemical imaging, although the distinctions among these domains are somewhat arbitrary. These techniques are based either on the injection of radioactive moieties whose distribution is recorded with positron emission tomography (PET) or single photon emission computerized tomography (SPECT), or on the direct detection of molecules based on their intrinsic magnetic properties with magnetic resonance imaging (MRI and fMRI) or spectroscopy (MRS).

This chapter will summarize important results obtained using brain imaging techniques in schizophrenia research, and the various insights on the pathophysiology and treatment of schizophrenia gained by these results. A more detailed technical discussion of these various imaging modalities is found in Chapter 7 of this volume.

II. STRUCTURAL IMAGING

Tomographic imaging, beginning with CT scanning and shortly thereafter MRI, has enabled rapid progress in studying brain structure in vivo. Following the initial CT report of enlarged ventricles in schizophrenia [1], a large number of CT studies replicated this observation [reviewed in 2–4]. This finding is the most replicated and well-established brain imaging finding in schizophrenia, and was historically important in establishing that schizophrenia is a brain disease. It should be noted, however, that the distribution of ventricular-brain ratios in patients with schizophrenia overlaps with the distribution in control subjects, and that this phenomenon is also found, although to a lesser extent, in other psychiatric conditions such as bipolar disorder [5]. As enlarged ventricular-brain ratio appears to be present at onset of illness, this finding was also critical in supporting the hypothesis that schizophrenia might be associated with an abnormal neurodevelopmental process.

These CT findings of enlarged ventricles and cortical sulci in schizophrenia were soon replicated with MRI, a technique which offers spatial and gray-white matter resolution superior to CT and has the additional advantage of requiring no ionizing radiation. For these reasons, it has largely supplanted CT scanning for structural brain research.

A. Findings in Schizophrenia

Notable in the MRI volumetric literature is variability of findings for a given brain region. Sources of this variability in findings for given brain structures include actual subject variability across different study samples, as well as variation in technical aspects of MRI. For example, studies have used a range of MRI pulse sequences, slice thicknesses, and spatial resolution, as well as criteria for defining regional anatomic boundaries [6].

Regarding whole-brain volume, a review of 31 studies found that a minority (19%) reported volume differences, and of these, four reported decreases and one reported a volume increase [6]. Consistent with a small effect, a meta-analysis of 31 studies (946 patients and 921 control subjects) found whole-brain volumes were 98% of control volumes.

The largest and most replicated structural brain finding is increased size of the lateral and third ventricles, but not the fourth ventricle [6]. A meta-analysis of 58 studies [7] drew similar conclusions, showing a larger effect for the left lateral ventricle than the right, marked effects in temporal horns, and again a significant effect in third but not fourth ventricles. Lateral and third ventricular volumes were enlarged as much as 25–30% above healthy controls.

Whole temporal lobe volumes were found in the meta-analysis [7] to be $\sim$ 98% of control volumes—i.e., in line with whole brain reductions—but substructures showed greater volume deficits. Hippocampus and hippocampus-amygdala were found to have $\sim$ 5–6% volume deficits bilaterally. Another meta-analysis found bilateral hippocampal volume reductions of 4% [8]. Superior temporal gyri were reduced several percent except for the right posterior superior temporal gyrus, which was increased $\sim$ 3% in volume. Temporal lobe deficits, the most robust of MRI volumetric findings in schizophrenia, have been found in several studies to correlate with symptoms. Medial temporal lobe reductions have shown correlations with positive symptoms [9,10] and with logical memory impairment [10]. Associations between superior temporal gyrus deficits and hallucinations were reported by Barta et al. [11] and Flaum et al. [12]. Measures of thought disorder and superior temporal gyrus volumes have been shown to be correlated [13].

Frontal lobe volumes were 95% of control values, or 98% adjusted for total brain volume reduction [7]. A review of 33 studies showed that 55% of the studies found volume abnormalities but that 45% did not [6]. These small effects could be consistent with the small (8%) reduction in cortical thickness found in postmortem work [14] that corresponded to significant abnormalities in densities of certain cell types. Frontal lobe deficits, themselves smaller and less replicated than the temporal lobe findings, have shown fewer clinical correlates, but left prefrontal cortical white matter volume deficits were found to be associated with the Scale for Assessment of Negative Symptoms (SANS) [15].

Relative volumes of basal ganglia structures were higher in patients by 2–4% in caudate but by > 20% in globus pallidus [7]. This may be a medication effect, since studies of patients receiving atypical antipsychotic medications show smaller increases than patients taking typical neuroleptics, and patients taking minimal or no antipsychotic medications have no change or even a decrease in basal ganglia volumes [16,17].

Thalami were found to be reduced in relative volume by 3–4% on meta-analysis, consistent with a review that found abnormalities in four of six studies of this region.

B. Summary and Significance

In conclusion, the major findings to date are [1] very minor deficits of whole brain or intracranial volume; [2] consistently replicated enlargement of the lateral and third ventricles; [3] parenchymal deficits in the temporal lobes, including medial temporal lobe structures such as hippocampus and superior temporal gyrus, frequently reported to be more pronounced on the left compared to the right side. While frontal lobes have been implicated functionally in schizophrenia, volumetric deficits have been less reliably found, possibly because any such deficits are near threshold of detectability with MRI methods. Subcortical structures including thalamus and basal ganglia have been reported to show volume changes, with increases in basal ganglia generally thought to be medication related.

These volume deficits have been found to be associated with clinical manifestations of the illness, including positive symptoms, memory impairment, thought disorder, and negative symptoms. Frontal lobe [18] and temporal lobe [19] volume deficits have been found to progress in longitudinal studies, although an earlier study reported absence of cortical or ventricular volume progression [20]. Because of its absence of ionizing radiation, MRI is a modality particularly suited to longitudinal studies, including the prodrome, and this is an area of active research. Such studies will help address the issue of timing of anatomic disturbances relative to symptom onset, and the relative roles of neurodevelopment and neurodegeneration in the illness.

III. FUNCTIONAL IMAGING

Over the last 40 years, measurement of neuronal activity underwent major technical advances, each bringing new insights about alterations in brain regional function in schizophrenia. The main imaging modalities included SPECT studies with the xenon inhalation technique, PET studies measuring rate of glucose utilization with [^{18}F]fluorodeoxyglucose ([^{18}F]FDG) or measuring regional blood flow with $H_2^{15}O$, and more recently fMRI, using blood-oxygen-level-dependent (BOLD) contrast. Each of these techniques provided improvements in terms of spatial and temporal resolution, as discussed in Chapter 7.

A. Resting-State Studies

In 1974, Ingvar and Franzen [21] published a landmark report describing lower flow in anterior compared to posterior regions of the brain, a finding termed hypofrontality. A large number of studies have attempted to replicate this finding [for review see 22,23–29]. Hypofrontality has not been consistently replicated, and the opposite observation (hyperfrontality) has been reported, especially in acutely ill patients. The lack of consistent pattern emerging from these studies has been interpreted as reflecting the heterogeneity of the illness and of the "baseline" or "resting" conditions. Regarding the heterogeneity of the condition, an influential study was the report of Liddle et al. [30], who described several patterns of flow alterations in psychomotor poverty (hypofrontality), disorganization (anterior cingulate overactivity), and reality distortion (underactivity of left temporal lobe). Many of these findings have been replicated; for example, several studies suggested that low prefrontal flow or metabolism at baseline might be associated with severity of negative symptoms. Abnormalities in temporal region have frequently been reported and have been linked with positive symptoms and noted more frequently on the left side. Temporal activation has also be recorded during the experience of hallucinations by several investigators, although the details of anatomical activation patterns differed. Regarding the impact of antipsychotic medications, an increase in basal ganglia activity has been the most reliable finding.

B. Task-Related Activation Studies

Hypofrontality has been more consistently observed during performance of executive and working memory tasks engaging the frontal cortex. For example, lower activation of the frontal cortex has been reported during the Wisconsin card sort task [31], the Tower of London task [32], word generation task [33,34], or n-back task [35]. A general problem with these observations is that the level of performance in the patient group is generally found to be diminished compared to controls, raising questions regarding the interpretation of these data as reflecting a primary abnormality of prefrontal cortex and its connectivity, a lower engagement of the patients during the tasks, or some combination of both factors [see discussion in 36]. Another very interesting approach is to examine patterns of covariance between regions during task performance [37].

The introduction of fMRI, allowing multiple determinations of dorsolateral prefrontal cortex (DLPFC) activation at various WM loads has provided new insights into the relationship between working memory tasks and DLPFC activation in schizophrenia. Increasing working memory load while keeping other aspects of the task constant is easily achieved with parametric tasks such as the n-back test, and, in healthy subjects, a significant relationship is observed between working memory load and DLPFC activation [38,39]. Using this new approach, a more subtle pattern of alterations in DLPFC activation (decreased efficiency and lower disengagement threshold) is emerging from studies in patients with schizophrenia. The concept of efficiency refers to the magnitude of DLPFC activation required to perform a task at a given level. Manoach et al. [40,41] demonstrated that, on a working memory task designed specifically to engage schizophrenic patients, patients showed greater DLPFC activation for a given level of performance than controls. Callicott et al. [42] examined the effect of parametric increases in the n-back test and found that patients with schizophrenia had greater DLPFC activation than controls on the 1-back and 2-back condition (low to moderate working memory load). These data suggest that schizophrenia might be associated with reduced DLPFC efficiency, i.e., with larger metabolic activation to reach a given level of performance in a relatively easy task. Several studies [40–42] also documented that, at high working memory load, patients with schizophrenia show decreased performance and decreased activation compared to controls. This observation also suggests that most earlier brain imaging studies were performed in a range where the complexity or load of the task reached the disengagement threshold for patients, resulting in apparent hypofrontality.

In conclusion, functional imaging studies during resting state as well as during task-related activation documented that schizophrenia is associated with a disrupted pattern of activation in cortico-limbic networks, and that the prefrontal cortex is a critical deficient node in this network.

IV. NEUROCHEMICAL AND NEUROPHARMACOLOGICAL IMAGING

A. PET and SPECT Neurochemical Imaging

The principles of PET and SPECT neurochemical imaging are reviewed elsewhere in this volume. Numerous PET and SPECT radiotracers are currently available to study key proteins in the living brain, such as receptors, transporters, and enzymes. Regarding schizophrenia, the majority of clinical investigations studied various aspects of dopaminergic transmission. Dopamine (DA) D_2 receptors were the first neuroreceptors visualized in the living human brain [43]. Since then, several DA related radiotracers have been developed, allowing the study of many aspects of dopaminergic transmission (DA synthesis, DA release, D_1 and D_2 receptors, DA transporters). Given the availability of these tools and the important role that DA transmission is believed to play in schizophrenia, it is not surprising that most of the research effort focused on this system. Despite marked limitations, these studies provide a relatively consistent picture suggesting that schizophrenia, at least during periods of clinical exacerbation, is associated with dysregulation of DA transmission.

1. Imaging DA Transmission

The classical DA hypothesis of schizophrenia, formulated over 30 years ago, proposed that a hyperactivity of the dopaminergic transmission is associated with this illness [44,45]. This hypothesis was essentially based on the observation that all antipsychotic drugs provided at least some degree of D2 receptor blockade, a proposition that is still true today [46,47]. As D2 receptor blockade is most effective against positive symptoms, the DA hyperactivity model appeared to be most relevant to the pathophysiology of positive symptoms. That sustained exposure to DA agonists such as amphetamine can induce a psychotic state characterized by some salient features of positive symptoms of schizophrenia (emergence of paranoid delusions and hallucinations in the context of a clear sensorium) also contributed to the idea that positive symptoms might be due to sustained excess dopaminergic activity [48,49]. These pharmacological effects indeed suggest, but do not establish, a dysregulation of DA systems in schizophrenia.

On the other hand, negative and cognitive symptoms are generally resistant to treatment by antipsychotic drugs. Functional brain imaging studies suggested that these symptoms are associated with prefrontal cortex (PFC) dysfunction [36]. Studies in nonhuman primates demonstrated that deficits in DA transmission in PFC induce cognitive impairments reminiscent of those observed in patients with schizophrenia [50], suggesting that a deficit in DA transmission in the PFC might be implicated in the cognitive impairments presented by these patients [51,52]. In addition, a recent postmortem study described abnormalities of DA terminals in the PFC associated with schizophrenia [53]. Thus, a current view on DA and schizophrenia is that subcortical mesolimbic DA projections might be hyperactive (resulting in positive symptoms) and that the mesocortical DA projections to the PFC are hypoactive (resulting in negative symptoms and cognitive impairment). Furthermore, these two abnormalities might be related, as the cortical DA system generally exerts an inhibitory action on subcortical DA systems [54,55].

The advent in the early 1980s of techniques based on PET and SPECT for measuring indices of DA activity in the living human brain held considerable promise for investigating these questions.

Striatal DA Transmission

D_2 RECEPTORS. Striatal D_2 receptor density in schizophrenia has been extensively studied with PET and SPECT imaging (Table 1). In a recent meta-analysis [56], we identified 17 imaging studies comparing D_2 receptor parameters in patients with schizophrenia (total of 245 patients, 112 neuroleptic naive, and 133 neuroleptic free), and controls (n = 231), matched for age and sex [57–73]. These studies are summarized in Table 1. Radiotracers included butyrophenones ([^{11}C]N-methyl-spiperone, [^{11}C]NMSP,

Table 1 Imaging Studies of Striatal D_2 Receptor Parameters in Drug Naive and Drug-Free Patients with Schizophrenia

Class radiotracer	Radiotracer	Study	n Controls	n Patients (DN/DF)[a]	Method	Outcome	Controls (mean ± SD)[b]	Patients (mean ± SD)[b]	P	Effect size[c]	Ratio SD
Butyrophenones	[^{11}C]NMSP	[57]	11	15 (10/5)	Kinetic	B_{max}	100 ± 50	253 ± 105	<.05	3.06	2.10
	[^{76}Br]SPI	[58]	8	16 (12/4)	Ratio	S/C	100 ± 14	111 ± 12	<.05	0.79	0.86
	[^{76}Br]SPI	[59]	8	8 (0/8)	Ratio	S/C	100 ± 14	104 ± 14	ns	0.28	1.00
	[^{76}Br]SPI	[60]	12	12 (0/12)	Ratio	S/C	100 ± 11	101 ± 15	ns	0.14	1.41
	[^{11}C]NMSP	[61]	17	10 (8/2)	Kinetic	B_{max}	100 ± 80	173 ± 143	.08	0.91	1.79
	[^{11}C]NMSP	(62)	7	7 (7/0)	Kinetic	B_{max}	100 ± 25	133 ± 63	ns	1.33	2.50
	[^{11}C]NMSP	(63)	18	17(10/7)	Kinetic	k3	100 ± 21	104 ± 16	ns	0.19	0.74
Benzamides	[^{11}C]Raclopride	[64]	20	18 (18/0)	Equilib	B_{max}	100 ± 29	107 ± 18	ns	0.23	0.63
	[^{11}C]Raclopride	[65]	10	13 (0/13)	Equilib	B_{max}	100 ± 22	112 ± 43	ns	0.55	1.99
	[^{123}I]IBZM	[66]	20	20 (17/3)	Ratio	S/FC	100 ± 8	99 ± 7	ns	−0.07	0.82
	[^{123}I]IBZM	[67]	15	15 (1/14)	Equilib	BP	100 ± 26	115 ± 33	ns	0.56	1.25
	[^{123}I]IBZM	[68]	16	21 (1/20)	Equilib	BP	100 ± 29	97 ± 38	ns	−0.12	1.31
	[^{11}C]Raclopride	[69]	12	11 (6/5)	Equilib	BP	100 ± 18	100 ± 30	ns	0.02	1.69
	[^{123}I]IBZM	[70]	15	15 (2/13)	Equilib	BP	100 ± 20	102 ± 49	ns	0.09	2.50
	[^{123}I]IBZM	(71)	18	18 (8/10)	Equilib	BP	100 ± 13	104 ± 14	ns	0.33	1.11
Ergot Alk	[^{76}Br]Lisuride	[72]	14	19 (10/9)	Ratio	S/C	100 ± 10	104 ± 12	ns	0.45	1.21
	[^{76}Br]Lisuride	[73]	10	10 (2/8)	Ratio	S/C	100 ± 10	100 ± 13	ns	0.00	1.29

[a] DN = drug naive; DF = drug free
[b] Mean normalized to mean of control subjects
[c] Effect size calculated as (mean patients − mean controls)/SD controls

n = 4, and [^{76}Br]bromospiperone, n = 3), benzamides ([^{11}C]raclopride, n = 3, and [^{123}I]IBZM, n = 5), or the ergot derivative [^{76}Br]lisuride, n = 2). Only two out of 17 studies detected a significant elevation of D_2 receptor density parameters. However, meta-analysis revealed a small (12%) but significant elevation of striatal D_2 receptors in patients with schizophrenia. No clinical correlates of increased D_2 receptor binding parameters have been reliably identified. The aggregate D_2 receptor increase reported in vivo is much lower than the increase reported in postmortem studies, supporting the idea that postmortem results were affected by antemortem medications. Studies performed with butyrophenones (n = 7) show an effect size of 0.96 ± 1.05, significantly larger than the effect size observed with other ligands (benzamides and lisuride, n = 10, 0.20 ± 0.26, $P = 0.04$). This difference might be due to differences in vulnerability of the binding of these tracers to endogenous DA, and elevation of endogenous DA in schizophrenia [74,75]. Other potential explanations for this difference, such as contributions of D4 receptors or states of receptor oligomerization, have also been proposed but remain largely unsubstantiated.

DOPA DECARBOXYLASE ACTIVITY. Five studies reported rates of DOPA decarboxylase in patients with schizophrenia, using [^{18}F]DOPA (76–79) or [^{11}C]DOPA [80] (Table 2). Four out of five studies reported increased accumulation of DOPA in the striatum of patients with schizophrenia, and the combined analysis yielded an effect size of 0.92 ± 0.45, which is significantly different from zero (p = 0.01). The variability of the DOPA accumulation was larger in the schizophrenic group than in the control group. Several of these studies reported the observation of high DOPA accumulation in psychotic paranoid patients, and low accumulation in patients with negative or depressive symptoms, and catatonia. While the relationship between DOPA decarboxylase and DA synthesis rate is unclear (DOPA decarboxylase is not the rate-limiting step of DA synthesis), these observations are compatible with higher DA synthesis activity of DA neurons in schizophrenia, at least in subjects experiencing psychotic symptoms.

AMPHETAMINE-INDUCED DA RELEASE. As discussed above, endogenous DA competition is a source of errors for *in vivo* measurement of D_2 receptors. On the other hand, the recognition of this phenomenon implies that D_2 receptor imaging, combined with pharmacological manipulation of DA release, enables functional evaluation of DA presynaptic activity. Indeed, over the last decade, numerous groups demonstrated that acute increase in synaptic DA concentration is associated with decreased in vivo binding of [^{11}C]raclopride and [^{123}I]IBZM. These interactions have been demonstrated in rodents, nonhuman primates, and humans, using a variety of methods to increase synaptic DA [for review of this abundant literature, see 81]. It has also been consistently observed that the in vivo binding of spiperone and other butyrophenones are not as affected as the binding of benzamides by acute fluctuations in endogenous DA levels [81].

The decrease in [^{11}C]raclopride and [^{123}I]IBZM in vivo binding following acute amphetamine challenge has been well validated as a measure of the change in D_2 receptor stimulation by DA due to amphetamine-induced DA release. Manipulations that are known to inhibit amphetamine-induced DA release, such as pretreatment with the DA synthesis inhibitor alpha-methyl-para-tyrosine (αMPT) or with the DAT blocker GR12909, also inhibit the amphetamine-induced decrease in [^{123}I]IBZM or [^{11}C]raclopride binding [82,83]. Combined microdialysis and imaging experiments in primates demonstrated that the magnitude of the decrease in ligand binding was correlated with the magnitude of the increase in extracellular DA induced by the challenge [69,83], suggesting that this noninvasive technique provides an appropriate measure of the changes in synaptic DA levels.

Three out of three studies demonstrated that amphetamine-induced decrease in [^{11}C]raclopride or [^{123}I]IBZM binding was elevated in untreated patients with schizophrenia compared to well-matched controls [67,69,70]. A significant relationship was observed between the magnitude of DA release and transient induction or worsening of positive symptoms. The increased amphetamine-induced DA release was observed in both first-episode/drug-naive patients and patients previously treated by antipsychotic drugs [84]. Combined analysis of the results of two studies revealed that patients who were experiencing an episode of illness exacerbation (or a first episode of illness) at the time of the scan showed elevated amphetamine-induced DA release, while patients in remission showed DA release values not different from those of controls [84]. These findings were generally interpreted as reflecting a larger DA release following amphetamine in the schizophrenic group. Another interpretation of these observations would be that schizophrenia is associated with increased affinity of D_2 receptors for

Table 2 Imaging Studies of Striatal Presynaptic DA Parameters in Drug-Naive and Drug-Free Patients with Schizophrenia

Parameter	Study	n Controls	n Patients (DN/DF)[a]	Radiotracer (/challenge)	Method	Outcome	Controls (mean ± SD)[b]	Patients (mean ± SD)[b]	P	Effect size[c]	Ratio SD
DOPA decarboxylase activity	[76]	13	5 (4/1)	[^{18}F]DOPA	Kinetic	k_3	100 ± 23	120 ± 15	<.05	0.91	0.68
	[77]	7	7 (7/0)	[^{18}F]DOPA	Graphical	K_i	100 ± 11	117 ± 20	<.05	1.54	1.82
	[78]	7	6 (2/4)	[^{18}F]DOPA	Graphical	K_i	100 ± 11	103 ± 40	ns	0.30	3.80
	[80]	10	12 (10/2)	[^{11}C]DOPA	Graphical	K_i	100 ± 17	113 ± 12	<.05	0.77	0.70
	[79]	13	10 (10/0)	[^{18}F]DOPA	Graphical	K_i	100 ± 14	115 ± 28	<.05	1.09	1.97
Amphetamine-induced DA release	[67]	15	15 (2/13)	[^{123}I]IBZM/amphetamine	Equilibrium	Delta BP	100 ± 113	271 ± 221	<.05	1.51	1.97
	[69]	18	18 (8/10)	[^{11}C]raclopride/amphetamine	Equilibrium	Delta BP	100 ± 43	175 ± 82	<005	1.73	1.90
	[70]	16	21 (1/20)	[^{123}I]IBZM/amphetamine	Equilibrium	Delta BP	100 ± 88	194 ± 145	<.05	1.07	1.64
Baseline DA concentration	[71]	18	18 (8/10)	[^{123}I]IBZM/αMPT	Equilibrium	Delta BP	100 ± 78	211 ± 122	<.05	1.43	1.57
DAT density	[202]	9	9 (9/0)	[^{18}F]CFT	Ratio	S/C	100 ± 12	101 ± 13	<.05	0.11	1.06
	[93]	22	22 (2/20)	[^{123}I]CIT	Equilibrium	BP	100 ± 17	93 ± 20	<.05	−0.43	1.21

[a] DN = drug naive; DF = drug free
[b] Mean normalized to mean of control subjects
[c] Effect size calculated as (mean patients − mean controls)/SD controls

DA. Development of D_2 receptor imaging with radiolabeled agonists is needed to settle this issue [85].

Direct evidence has been provided that disinhibition of subcortical DA activity might be associated with prefrontal pathology in schizophrenia. In patients with schizophrenia, low NAA concentration in the dorsolateral prefrontal cortex (DLPFC), a marker of DLPFC pathology, is associated with increased amphetamine-induced DA release [86]. Pretreatment with ketamine, an N-methyl-d-aspartate (NMDA) antagonist, is associated with large increase in amphetamine-induced decrease in [^{123}I]IBZM binding [87]. This observation demonstrated that blockade of glutamatergic-mediated regulation of DA release results in increased amphetamine-induced DA release, and provides a link between the classical dopamine hypothesis and the NMDA deficiency hypothesis [88-90] of schizophrenia.

BASELINE DA RELEASE. A limitation of the amphetamine challenge imaging studies is that they measure changes in synaptic DA transmission following a nonphysiological challenge (i.e., amphetamine) and do not provide any information about synaptic DA levels at baseline, i.e., in the unchallenged state. Several laboratories reported that, in rodents, acute depletion of synaptic DA is associated with an acute increase in the in vivo binding of [^{11}C]raclopride or [^{123}I]IBZM to D_2 receptors [for review, see 81]. The increased binding was observed in vivo but not in vitro, indicating that it was not due to receptor upregulation [91], but to removal of endogenous DA and unmasking of D_2 receptors previously occupied by DA. The acute DA depletion technique was developed in humans using αMPT, to assess the degree of occupancy of D_2 receptors by DA [91,92]. Using this technique, higher occupancy of D_2 receptors by DA was recently reported in patients with schizophrenia experiencing an episode of illness exacerbation, compared to healthy controls [71]. Again assuming normal affinity of D2 receptors for DA, the data are consistent with higher baseline DA synaptic levels in patients with schizophrenia. This observation was present in both first-episode/drug-naive and previously treated patients.

DA TRANSPORTERS. The data reviewed above are consistent with higher DA output in the striatum of patients with schizophrenia, which could be explained by increased density of DA terminals. Since striatal DA transporters (DAT) are exclusively localized on DA terminals, this question was investigated by measuring binding of [^{123}I]β-CIT [93] or [^{18}F]CFT [48] in patients with schizophrenia. Both studies reported no differences in DAT binding between patients and controls. In addition, Laruelle et al. [93] reported no association between amphetamine-induced DA release and DAT density. Thus, the increased presynaptic output suggested by the studies reviewed above does not appear to be due to higher terminal density, an observation consistent with postmortem studies that failed to identify alteration in striatal DAT binding in schizophrenia [94-99].

Prefrontal DA Transmission

The majority of DA receptors in the PFC are of the D_1 subtype [100,101]. In postmortem studies, no evidence was found for an alteration in D_1 receptors in the DLPFC of patients with schizophrenia [102,103], and D_1 receptor gene expression is unaltered [104]. A PET study with [^{11}C]SCH 23390 reported decreased density of D_1 receptors in younger patients with schizophrenia [63]. In addition, low PFC D_1 density was associated with the severity of negative symptoms and poor performance on the Wisconsin Card Sort Test (WCST). In contrast, a more recent study using the superior radiotracer [^{11}C]NNC 112 reported increased D_1 receptor availability in the DLPFC of patients with schizophrenia [105]. Furthermore, increased [^{11}C]NNC 112 binding was associated with poor performance at the n-back, a test involving working memory [105]. The reasons for the discrepant results obtained with [^{11}C]SCH 23390 and [^{11}C]NNC 112 remain to be elucidated, but it is interesting to note that the binding of the two radiotracers is differentially affected by endogenous DA competition and receptor trafficking [81].

2. Studies of Nondopaminergic Receptors in Schizophrenia

Receptors related to the GABA and 5HT systems have been studied in vivo in schizophrenia. Postmortem studies reported abnormalities of both systems in schizophrenia. A robust body of findings suggests deficiency of GABA-ergic function in the PFC in schizophrenia [for reviews, see 106,107]. In vivo evaluation of GABA-ergic systems in schizophrenia has so far been limited to evaluation of benzodiazepine receptor densities with SPECT and [^{123}I]iomazenil, and three out of three studies comparing patients with schizophrenia and controls reported no significant regional differences [108-110]. While some significant correlations with symptoms clusters and regional benzodiazepine densities have been observed [108,109,111,112], these relationships have not been replicated by other studies. Thus, together, these studies are consistent with an absence of marked abnormalities of benzodiazepine receptor concentration in the cortex of patients with schizophrenia. Alterations of GABA-ergic systems in schizophrenia might not involve benzodiazepine receptors [113], or be restricted to certain cortical layers or classes of GABA-ergic cells that are beyond the resolution of current radionuclide-based imaging techniques. Recent developments in GABA imaging with MRS described below are a promising new avenue to study in vivo GABA-ergic function in schizophrenia.

Abnormalities of 5HT transporters (SERT), $5HT_{2A}$ receptors, and, more consistently, $5HT_{1A}$ receptors have been described in postmortem studies in schizophrenia [see references in 114]. Given the relatively recent development of radiotracers to study 5HT receptors, only a limited number of imaging studies have been published. The concentration of SERT in the midbrain measured by $[^{123}I]\beta$-CIT is unaltered in patients with schizophrenia [93]. Studies with more specific SERT ligands are warranted to assess the distribution of SERT in other brain areas, such as the PFC, where their density has been reported to be reduced in three out of four postmortem studies [114]. Decrease in $5HT_{2A}$ receptors has been reported in the PFC in 4 out of 8 postmortem studies [114,115]. Three PET studies in drug naive or drug free patients with schizophrenia reported normal cortical $5HT_{2A}$ receptor binding [115–117], while one study reported a significant decrease in PFC $5HT_{2A}$ binding in a small group (n = 6) of drug-naive schizophrenic patients [118]. The most consistent abnormality of 5HT parameters reported in postmortem studies in schizophrenia is an increase in the density of $5HT_{1A}$ receptors in the PFC, reported in seven out of eight studies [114]. Several groups are currently evaluating the binding of this receptor in vivo with PET and $[^{11}C]WAY100907$.

3. Receptor Occupancy by Antipsychotic Drugs

Maybe the most widespread use of neuroreceptor imaging in schizophrenia over the last decade has been the assessment of neuroreceptor occupancy achieved by typical and atypical antipsychotic drugs, a topic that has been the subject of recent reviews [119,120]. Neuroreceptors studied included mainly D2 receptors, but also $5HT_{2A}$ and D1 receptors. The main conclusions from this line of research are as follows:

1. Studies repeatedly confirmed the existence of a threshold of occupancy of striatal D2 receptors (∼ 80%) above which extrapyramidal side effects are likely to occur [121].
2. In general, studies failed to observe a relationship between degree of D2 receptor occupancy and clinical response [122,123]. Yet, most studies were performed at doses achieving > 50% occupancy, and the minimal level of occupancy required for therapeutic response remains undefined. Two studies performed with low doses of relatively selective D_2 receptor antagonists (haloperidol and raclopride) suggested that 50–60% occupancy was required to observe a rapid clinical response [124,125].
3. Clozapine, at clinically therapeutic doses, achieved only 40–60% D_2 receptor occupancy [121,123,126], which, in conjunction with its anticholinergic properties, accounts for its low liability for extrapyramidal symptoms (EPS).
4. Occupancy of $5HT_{2A}$ receptors by "$5HT_{2A}/D_2$ balanced antagonists" such as risperidone does not confer protection against EPS, since the threshold of D_2 receptor occupancy associated with EPS is not markedly different between these drugs and drugs devoid of $5HT_{2A}$ antagonism [127–130].
5. Studies with quetiapine suggested that, at least with this agent, transient high occupancy of D_2 receptors might be sufficient to elicit clinical response [131,132].

An interesting question relates to putative differences in degree of occupancy achieved by atypical antipsychotic drugs in striatal and extrastriatal areas. Pilowsky et al. [133] reported lower occupancy of striatal D_2 receptors compared to temporal cortex D_2 receptors in seven patients treated with clozapine, using the high-affinity SPECT ligand $[^{123}I]$epidipride. In contrast, typical antipsychotics were reported to achieve similar occupancy in striatal and extrastriatal areas, as measured with $[^{11}C]FLB$ 457 [134] or $[^{123}I]$epidipride [135]. It should be noted, however, that these very high affinity ligands do not allow accurate determination of D_2 receptor availability in the striatum. In contrast, $[^{18}F]$fallypride enables accurate determination of D_2 receptor availability in both striatal and extrastriatal areas [136], and preliminary PET experiments in primates with $[^{18}F]$fallypride indicate that clozapine and risperidone achieve similar D_2 receptor occupancy in striatal and extrastriatal regions [137]. Finally, it is important to point out that the most robust evidence regarding the site of therapeutic effect of antipsychotic drugs in rodents points toward the nucleus accumbens [138,139], while the imaging studies reviewed above contrasted striatal versus mesotemporal D_2 receptor binding. Improved resolution of PET cameras currently allows distinguishing signals from ventral and dorsal striatum [140,141], and it is now feasible to specifically study the clinical correlates of D_2 receptor occupancy in ventral striatum in humans.

Another unresolved question is the discrepant values of D_2 receptor occupancy obtained with [^{11}C]raclopride versus [^{11}C]NMSP. The haloperidol plasma concentration associated with 50% inhibition of [^{11}C]NMSP binding (3–5 ng/mL) [142] is 10 times higher than that associated with 50% inhibition of [^{11}C]raclopride binding (0.32 ng/mL) [143]. Quetiapine, at a dose of 750 mg, decreased [^{11}C]raclopride specific binding by 51%, but failed to affect [^{11}C]NMSP specific binding [144]. These observations contribute to the debate regarding differences between benzamide and butyrophenone binding to D_2 receptors.

B. Magnetic Resonance Spectroscopy

Magnetic resonance spectroscopy (MRS) is a noninvasive imaging modality capable of evaluating the chemistry of living tissue. Like magnetic resonance imaging (MRI) and functional MRI (fMRI), it is an application of the basic method of nuclear magnetic resonance (NMR), and as such involves no radioactivity (ionizing radiation) and generally involves the same scanning equipment and environment as MRI. The neurochemical abnormalities of schizophrenia remain an area of active investigation. New information on the neurochemistry of schizophrenia has mainly been derived from phosphorus and proton MRS.

1. Phosphorus Spectroscopy

Phosphorus MRS (^{31}P MRS) can provide an assessment of brain membrane phospholipid and high-energy phosphate metabolism. However, ^{31}P MRS is only ~ 5% as sensitive as proton MRS, primarily because of the lower gyromagnetic ratio of ^{31}P [145], requiring correspondingly greater volumes of interest (often chosen to be 15–36 cm^3). Metabolites detectable in the ^{31}P spectrum include α, β, and γ nucleoside triphosphates (NTP), phosphomonoesters (PME), phosphodiesters (PDE), phosphocreatine (PCr), and inorganic phosphate (Pi). In addition, intracellular magnesium (Mg^{2+}) and intracellular pH can be computed from spectral separation of certain resonant peaks in the ^{31}P spectrum [146,147].

PME and PDE resonances arise from the precursors and breakdown products, respectively, of membrane phospholipids, as well as phospholipid bilayer itself. The observed PME spectrum is composed mainly of the metabolites phosphocholine, phosphoethanolamine, and L-phosphoserine. PDE spectra are primarily comprised of glycerol-3-phosphocholine (GPC), glycerol-3-phosphoethanolamine (GPE), and phospholipid bilayer [148].

PCr, NTP, and Pi resonances are indicators of the state of energy metabolism in the region of interest. In the schizophrenia ^{31}P MRS literature, it has generally been assumed that the predominant contribution to the NTP resonances is adenosine triphosphate (ATP). Calculation of such metabolite concentration ratios as PCr to Pi, NTP to Pi, and PCr to NTP can also offer useful information about the regional energy state.

In an early study, Pettegrew et al. [149] studied membrane phospholipid and high-energy phosphate metabolism in the dorsal prefrontal cortex of first-episode, neuroleptic-naive patients with schizophrenia and matched healthy controls. The study found reductions in PME and Pi, and increases in PDE and βATP, but no significant differences in PCr or intracellular pH in patients relative to controls. The authors proposed that their phospholipid findings may be related to an exaggeration of normal synaptic pruning during adolescence, when PME levels normally decrease [149,150]], and interpreted these findings as reflecting decreased synthesis and increased breakdown of membrane phospholipids in the patients. They interpreted the high-energy phosphate findings as consistent with hypofrontality in schizophrenia as previously found by PET and other methods [21,31,151,152] in that increased ATP and decreased Pi levels suggested decreased ATP utilization.

PME decreases have been replicated in other in vivo ^{31}P MRS studies in treatment-naive, first-episode [153] and chronic medicated patients [154–156], as well as in patients with prominent negative symptoms [157], but were not found by Volz et al. [158] or by Deicken et al. [159] in chronic patients. PDE increases have been replicated in first-episode, treatment-naive patients [153]. However, in chronic medicated patients, PDE changes have been quite variable: increases were found by Deicken et al. [159]; no changes were seen by Williamson et al. [154], Fujimoto et al. [160] or Shioiri et al. [157]; and decreases were found by Volz et al. [158]. Differing MRS methodologies (including voxel size, pulse sequences, localization method, quantification of signal ratios) may account for some or all of these discrepant findings [161,162].

Taken together, the phospholipid findings of Pettegrew et al. [149], Williamson et al. [154], and Stanley et al. [153] have been interpreted as suggesting that as schizophrenia progresses to chronicity, levels of breakdown products may normalize from their early elevated levels, while the precursors of membrane phospholipids remain in deficit as in the earlier stages of illness. However, the study by Potwarka et al. [156] using ^{1}H decoupled ^{31}P MRS methods capable of distinguishing the components of the PDE resonance has suggested an alternative interpretation of the increases in that peak. Their finding in a study of chronic, medicated patients showed an increase only in the mobile or membrane phospholipid component of the PDE peak, but not in the phospholipid breakdown products GPE and GPC, suggesting abnormal membrane structure but not increased phospholipid breakdown.

High-energy phosphate metabolism findings have been inconsistent across studies, perhaps due to variability in the MRS or clinical methodology [161,162]. While Pettegrew et al. [149] and Shioiri et al. [157] observed increased ATP, suggesting hypofrontality, other investigators, including Stanley et al. [153] and Volz et al. [158] found no alterations in these measures. Phosphocreatine (PCr) levels have also been variable, with both increases [155] and decreases [159] being reported.

Temporal lobe findings using ^{31}P MRS have shown considerable variation for high-energy phosphate and membrane phospholipid metabolism [161,162]. In a study of chronic patients, O'Callaghan et al. [163] found no differences in any metabolite levels in the left temporoparietal region, while the studies of Fujimoto et al. [160] and Fukuzako et al. [164] found increases in PDE, and a more recent study [165] found both decreased PME and increased PDE.

Calabrese et al. [166] investigated asymmetry of ^{31}P MRS measures in a group of chronic, mainly medicated patients, and found higher PCr/βATP and PCr/Pi ratios in the right temporal lobe, and elevation in βATP itself on the left. With improved technology, this group [167] later replicated these findings; however, they contrast in laterality to the ATP findings of Fujimoto et al. [160] and Fukuzako et al. [164], and a more recent study [165] found no changes.

2. Proton Spectroscopy

The signals of interest in proton or ^{1}H MRS are derived from protons in compounds other than water, in contrast to MRI, where the proton signal that yields the structural image is derived mainly from water. Indeed, the protons in tissue water and lipids emit extremely intense signals that tend to obscure the ^{1}H spectra of interest. The compounds of interest typically occur in concentrations on the order of mM, or 10^4- to 10^5-fold less than water. The dominant water and lipid signals must therefore be suppressed [168] for the fine spectral structure to emerge, historically a technically demanding requirement but now a routine part of ^{1}H MRS.

The compounds of interest detected by proton MRS include N-acetylaspartate (NAA), an amino acid derivative described as a putative cell marker, found in all structural components of neurons, and found mainly but not exclusively in neurons [169]. The role of NAA in neuronal function is not fully understood; its signal strength is generally regarded as proportional to neuronal density, neuronal function, or neuronal viability, and may undergo reversible changes [170–172]. Proton MRS can also detect choline containing compounds (Cho), creatine/phosphocreatine (Cr), myo-inositol, and lactate. Glutamate (Glu), the major excitatory neurotransmitter in the central nervous system, can also be measured, particularly at shorter echo times, although it is not routinely resolvable from glutamine (Gln) and gamma-aminobutyric acid (GABA) at the clinical magnetic field strength of 1.5 tesla. Other discernible but less reliably quantified peaks are alanine, aspartate, and glucose [173]. In addition to these metabolite peaks, resonances from macromolecules have been shown to contribute to the spectrum in the range 0.9–2.05 parts per million (ppm). These overlap with metabolites in short echo time spectroscopy, complicating the process of spectral assignment and quantification [174,175]. Separation of these resonances by exploiting their differing T1 relaxation times from those of metabolites has been demonstrated [174], allowing both improved identification of metabolites at short echo times and direct investigation of macromolecule resonances in pathological conditions.

The three strongest and most easily quantifiable metabolite peaks are produced by NAA, Cr, and Cho, and these have therefore been the most studied compounds in ^{1}H MRS. Proton (^{1}H) MRS has two distinct advantages over other nuclei: hydrogen atoms are present in almost every compound in living tissue, and hydrogen has the most sensitive of the nuclei studied by MRS, allowing relatively small volumes of interest (fractions of a cm^3 to several cm^3). One difficulty arises from the narrow (10 ppm) range of chemical shifts of ^{1}H spectra [161], making resolution of individual resonances more difficult. For example, glutamine, glutamate, and GABA are difficult to distinguish as noted at conventional 1.5 tesla magnetic field strength because of partially overlapping peaks. Resolution of these peaks is possible with more sophisticated spectroscopic editing acquisition techniques [176,177] and with higher field strengths [178]. These developments are of great interest in psychiatric research, in view of the potential significance of these compounds for the pathophysiology of psychiatric disorders.

Findings in Schizophrenia

Studies of NAA in frontal lobes in schizophrenia have produced mixed results. Stanley et al. reported an absence of NAA change in first-episode patients [179], which was replicated in a later study [180]. However, other groups have found decreased NAA in first-episode patients [181,182]. In chronic schizophrenia, results have been similarly mixed: reduced frontal lobe NAA/Cr ratio was found in some studies [183–185] while others reported no changes [186,187]. A study notable for its large size (47 patients and 66 controls) [188] included subjects of mixed chronicity and found no NAA reduction. These authors provided an effect size estimate for an even larger sample of subjects from their laboratory (103 patients and 71 controls) of ~ 0.2.

These studies have also investigated the amino acid signal (glutamate, GABA, glutamine) in frontal lobes, with mixed results. The ratio of GABA plus glutamate to creatine was found to be elevated by Choe et al. [182,189]. Stanley et al. [179] and Bartha et al. [180] reported no change in glutamate, but an increase in glutamine signal. Stanley et al. [179] interpreted their findings of unaltered glutamate with an increase in the glutamine signal as reflecting altered glutamatergic neurotransmission and suggested that glutamine may be a more sensitive marker of alteration in glutamatergic neurotransmission.

NAA reductions in temporal lobes have been found fairly reliably in schizophrenia. Reduced NAA (or NAA/Cr ratios) were reported by Deicken et al. [190], Fukuzako et al. [187], Lim et al. [191], Bertolino et al. [183,184], Maier et al. [192], Nasrallah et al. [193], and Yurgelun-Todd et al. [194] in medial temporal structures in chronic schizophrenia, but not by Buckley et al. [186] or Heimberg et al. [195]. First-episode psychosis was studied by Renshaw et al. [196], who found a reduction in the NAA/Cr ratio bilaterally.

Clinical and Imaging Correlates

Evidence for an absence of neuroleptic medication effect on NAA has been provided by the studies of Bertolino et al. [184], Choe et al. [182], and Stanley et al. [179].

No consistent correlations have been found between frontal or temporal lobe NAA and cognitive or symptom measures [186] or duration of illness [190]. Frontal lobe NAA reductions have been found in adolescent [197] and older relatives at risk for schizophrenia [188], raising the question whether NAA reductions may characterize individuals at risk for schizophrenia.

Frontal lobe NAA has been compared with other brain imaging and clinical measures in recent studies. NAA exhibited interesting correlations with amphetamine-induced DA release [86] and with a PET measure of cerebral blood flow during cognitive challenge tasks [198], suggesting a relation between frontal lobe neuronal deficits and impaired cognitive function as well as subcortical dopamine dysregulation.

The quite reproducible NAA deficits in temporal lobe and the more variable frontal lobe NAA deficits are consistent with impaired neuronal function across a distributed network already implicated in schizophrenia. The variable reports for frontal lobe, consistent with the effect size indicated by the report of Callicott et al. [188], suggest a quite small yet detectable effect in frontal lobes. The frontal NAA reduction may be substantially larger in chronic patients, as indicated by the positive findings in small samples of chronic patients reported by Bertolino et al. [183,184]. This may place limitations on the generalizability of the frontal NAA reduction and may place constraints on its interpretation, in that this regional deficit may evolve with chronicity, or may be detectable mainly in patients with illness severity sufficient to necessitate long-term hospital care.

3. *Summary*

Considerable progress has been made in utilizing the capabilities of in vivo MRS to study the neurochemistry of schizophrenia. The first generation of MRS studies in schizophrenia has been characterized by a marked diversity of techniques, study populations, and anatomic regions investigated. A corresponding range of results has been obtained; nevertheless, areas have emerged of reproducible findings of alterations in membrane phospholipid metabolism using ^{31}P MRS, and reduction in temporal lobe (and more variably, frontal lobe) NAA using ^{1}H MRS. These findings have both contributed to our understanding of the neurochemistry of schizophrenia and have stimulated continued investigation.

Research into the roles in brain physiology of the metabolites detectable by MRS has been stimulated by the application of this modality; further understanding, including normal values in various regions and brain matter types, is needed to assist in interpreting MRS findings. A methodological advance that would improve data analysis and interpretation would be the establishment of a reliable method for absolute metabolite quantification [199,200], particularly in the ^{1}H case. Interpretability of MRS data would also be improved by the reporting of segmentation analyses of the MRS voxels into distinct brain matter types, since illness may modify not only the neurochemistry but also the relative amounts of brain matter types in the regions under study.

Future investigations of MRS in schizophrenia can be expected to benefit from availability of higher field strengths for human studies, permitting improvements both in spectral and in spatial resolution; application of tracer methods such as ^{13}C label to probe biosynthetic pathways [201]; and spectroscopic editing techniques which allow enhanced peak identification at a given field strength [176,177]. The potential of ^{1}H MRS to examine glutamate, glutamine, and GABA with increasing resolution suggests a future generation of direct studies of these specific neurochemicals.

V. CONCLUSION

Development of sophisticated brain imaging techniques has enabled the study of alterations in brain structure, function, and neurochemistry associated with schizophrenia. Regarding structure, studies showed that subtle morphological abnormalities are consistently observed, involving increased ventricular-brain ratios, and moderate general tissue reduction, the latter being more pronounced in the limbic regions of the mesial temporal lobe. Findings with proton spectroscopy demonstrating reductions in NAA content are generally consistent with the structural abnormalities, and indicate that these volume reductions might be associated with reduction in neuronal density or function. Functional studies are consistent with aberrations of regional connectivity in corticolimbic networks, and implicate the prefrontal cortex as a critically deficient node in these interactions. Imaging of the dopaminergic system is also consistent with the idea of dysconnectivity, as regulation of this system appears to be deficient. Combined with complementary neuropathological findings, these studies have put into images the dysconnectivity of mental processes characterizing this illness. Maybe the most fundamental contribution of brain imaging so far has been to document that neuronal fragmentation underlies the mental fragmentation experienced by the patients. The hope for the future is that refinements in imaging techniques will provide endophenotypes contributing to the elucidation of the genetic and epigenetic etiology of the illness and offer insights for new therapeutic approaches.

ACKNOWLEDGMENTS

Supported by the National Institute of Mental Health (L.K., K08 MH01594-01; M.L., K02 MH01603-01).

REFERENCES

1. Johnstone EC, Crow TJ, Frith CD, Husband J, Kreel L. Cerebral ventricular size and cognitive impairment in chronic schizophrenia. Lancet 1976; 2(7992):924–926.
2. Andreasen NC, Swayze VW, 2nd, Flaum M, Yates WR, Arndt S, McChesney C. Ventricular enlargement in schizophrenia evaluated with computed tomographic scanning. Effects of gender, age, and stage of illness. Arch Gen Psychiatry 1990; 47(11):1008–1015.
3. Raz S, Raz N. Structural brain abnormalities in the major psychoses: a quantitative review of the evidence from computerized imaging. Psychol Bull 1990; 108(1):93–108.
4. Van Horn JD, McManus IC. Ventricular enlargement in schizophrenia. A meta-analysis of studies of the ventricle:brain ratio (VBR). Br J Psychiatry 1992; 160:687–697.
5. Strakowski SM, DelBello MP, Adler C, Cecil DM, Sax KW. Neuroimaging in bipolar disorder. Bipolar Disord 2000; 2(3 Pt 1):148–164.
6. McCarley RW, Wible CG, Frumin M, Hirayasu Y, Levitt JJ, Fischer IA, Shenton ME. MRI anatomy of schizophrenia. Biol Psychiatry 1999; 45(9):1099–1119
7. Wright IC, Rabe-Hesketh S, Woodruff PW, David AS, Murray RM, Bullmore ET. Meta-analysis of regional brain volumes in schizophrenia. Am J Psychiatry 2000; 157(1):16–25.
8. Nelson MD, Saykin AJ, Flashman LA, Riordan HJ. Hippocampal volume reduction in schizophrenia as assessed by magnetic resonance imaging: a meta-analytic study. Arch Gen Psychiatry 1998; 55(5):433–440.
9. Bogerts B, Lieberman JA, Ashtari M, Bilder RM, Degreef G, Lerner G, Johns C, Masiar S. Hippocampus-amygdala volumes and psychopathol-

ogy in chronic schizophrenia. Biol Psychiatry 1993; 33(4):236–246.
10. Goldberg TE, Torrey EF, Berman KF, Weinberger DR. Relations between neuropsychological performance and brain morphological and physiological measures in monozygotic twins discordant for schizophrenia. Psychiatry Res 1994; 55(1):51–61.
11. Barta PE, Pearlson GD, Powers RE, Richards SS, Tune LE. Auditory hallucinations and smaller superior temporal gyral volume in schizophrenia. Am. J. Psychiatry 1990; 147(11):1457–1462.
12. Flaum M, O'Leary DS, Swayze VW, 2nd, Miller DD, Arndt S, Andreasen NC. Symptom dimensions and brain morphology in schizophrenia and related psychotic disorders. J Psychiatr Res 1995; 29(4):261–276.
13. Shenton ME, Kikinis R, Jolesz FA, Pollak SD, LeMay M, Wible CG, Hokama H, Martin J, Metcalf D, Coleman M. Abnormalities of the left temporal lobe and thought disorder in schizophrenia. A quantitative magnetic resonance imaging study. N Engl Med 1992; 327(9):604–612.
14. Selemon LD, Rajkowska G, Goldman-Rakic PS. Elevated neuronal density in prefrontal area 46 in brains from schizophrenic patients: application of a three-dimensional, stereologic counting method. J Comp Neurol 1998; 392(3):402–412.
15. Wible CG, Shenton ME, Hokama H, Kikinis R, Jolesz FA, Metcalf D, McCarley RW. Prefrontal cortex and schizophrenia. A quantitative magnetic resonance imaging study. Arch Gen Psychiatry 1995; 52(4):279–288.
16. Chakos MH, Lieberman JA, Bilder RM, Borenstein M, Lerner G, Bogerts B, Wu HW, Kinon B, Ashtari M. Increase in caudate nuclei volumes of first-episode schizophrenic patients taking antipsychotic drugs. Am J Psychiatry 1994; 151(10):1430–1436.
17. Ohnuma T, Kimura M, Takahashi T, Iwamoto N, Arai H. A magnetic resonance imaging study in first-episode disorganized-type patients with schizophrenia. Psychiatry Clin Neurosci 1997; 51(1):9–15.
18. Gur RE, Cowell P, Turetsky BI, Gallacher F, Cannon T, Bilker W, Gur RC. A follow-up magnetic resonance imaging study of schizophrenia. Relationship of neuroanatomical changes to clinical and neurobehavioral measures. Arch Gen Psychiatry 1998; 55(2):145–152.
19. DeLisi LE, Sakuma M, Tew W, Kushner M, Hoff AL, Grimson R. Schizophrenia as a chronic active brain process: a study of progressive brain structural change subsequent to the onset of schizophrenia. Psychiatry Res 1997; 74(3):129–140.
20. Degreef G, Ashtari M, Wu HW, Borenstein M, Geisler S, Lieberman J. Follow up MRI study in first episode schizophrenia. Schizophr Res 1991; 5(3):204–206.
21. Ingvar DH, Franzen G. Abnormalities of cerebral blood flow dstribution in patients with chronic schizophrenia. Acta Psychiatr Scand 1974; 50:425–462.
22. Cohen RM, Semple WE, Gross M, Nordahl TE. From syndrome to illness: delineating the pathophysiology of schizophrenia with PET. Schizophr Bull 1988; 14(2):169–176.
23. Williamson P. Hypofrontality in schizophrenia: a review of the evidence. Can J Psychiatry 1987; 32(5):399–404.
24. Gur RE, Pearlson GD. Neuroimaging in schizophrenia research. Schizophr Bull 1993; 19(2):337–353.
25. Kotrla KJ, Weinberger DR. Brain imaging in schizophrenia. Ann Rev Med 1995; 46:113 122.
26. Chua SE, McKenna PJ. Schizophrenia—a brain disease: a critical review of structural and functional cerebral abnormality in the disorder. Br J Psychiatry 1995; 166(5):563–582.
27. Liddle PF. Functional imaging—schizophrenia. Br Med Bull 1996; 52(3):486–494.
28. Andreasen NC, O'Leary DS, Flaum M, Nopoulos P, Watkins GL, Boles Ponto LL, Hichwa RD. Hypofrontality in schizophrenia: distributed dysfunctional circuits in neuroleptic-naive patients. Lancet 1997; 349(9067):1730–1734.
29. Buchsbaum MS, Hazlett EA. Positron emission tomography studies of abnormal glucose metabolism in schizophrenia. Schizophr Bull 1998; 24(3):343–364.
30. Liddle PF, Friston KJ, Frith CD, Hirsch SR, Jones T, Frackowiak RS. Patterns of cerebral blood flow in schizophrenia. Br J Psychiatry 1992; 160:179–186.
31. Weinberger DR, Berman KF, Zec RF. Physiological dysfunction of dorsolateral prefrontal cortex in schizophrenia. I. Regional cerebral blood flow evidence. Arch Gen Psychiatry 1986; 43:114–124.
32. Andreasen NC, Rezai K, Alliger R, Swayze VW 2nd, Flaum M, Kirchner P, Cohen G, O'Leary DS. Hypofrontality in neuroleptic-naive patients and in patients with chronic schizophrenia. Assessment with xenon 133 single-photon emission computed tomography and the Tower of London. Arch Gen Psychiatry 1992; 49(12):943–958.
33. Frith CD, Friston KJ, Herold S, Silbersweig D, Fletcher P, Cahill C, Dolan RJ, Frackowiak RS, Liddle PF. Regional brain activity in chronic schizophrenic patients during the performance of a verbal fluency task. Br J Psychiatry 1995; 167(3):343–349.
34. Curtis VA, Bullmore ET, Brammer MJ, Wright IC, Williams SC, Morris RG, Sharma TS, Murray RM, McGuire PK. Attenuated frontal activation during a verbal fluency task in patients with schizophrenia. Am J Psychiatry 1998; 155(8):1056–1063.
35. Carter CS, Perlstein W, Ganguli R, Brar J, Mintun M, Cohen JD. Functional hypofrontality and working memory dysfunction in schizophrenia. Am J Psychiatry 1998; 155(9):1285–1287.

36. Weinberger DR, Berman KF. Prefrontal function in schizophrenia: confounds and controversies. Phil Trans R Soc Lond Ser B. Biol Sci 1996; 351(1346):1495–1503.
37. Friston KJ, Frith CD, Liddle PF, Frackowiak RS. Functional connectivity: the principal-component analysis of large (PET) data sets. J. Cereb. Blood Flow Metab 1993; 13(1):5–14.
38. Braver TS, Cohen JD, Nystrom LE, Jonides J, Smith EE, Noll DC. A parametric study of prefrontal cortex involvement in human working memory. Neuroimage 1997; 5(1):49–62.
39. Barch DM, Braver TS, Nystrom LE, Forman SD, Noll DC, Cohen JD. Dissociating working memory from task difficulty in human prefrontal cortex. Neuropsychologia 1997; 35(10):1373–1380.
40. Manoach DS, Press DZ, Thangaraj V, Searl MM, Goff DC, Halpern E, Saper CB, Warach S. Schizophrenic subjects activate dorsolateral prefrontal cortex during a working memory task, as measured by fMRI. Biol Psychiatry 1999; 45(9):1128–1137.
41. Manoach DS, Gollub RL, Benson ES, Searl MM, Goff DC, Halpern E, Saper CB, Rauch SL. Schizophrenic subjects show aberrant fMRI activation of dorsolateral prefrontal cortex and basal ganglia during working memory performance [in process citation]. Biol Psychiatry 2000; 48(2):99–109.
42. Callicott JH, Bertolino A, Mattay VS, Langheim FJ, Duyn J, Coppola R, Goldberg TE, Weinberger DR. Physiological dysfunction of the dorsolateral prefrontal cortex in schizophrenia revisited. Cereb Cortex 2000; 10(11):1078–1092.
43. Wagner H Jr, Burns HD, Dannals RF, Wong DF, Langstrom B, Duelfer T, Frost JJ, Ravert HT, Links JM, Rosenbloom SB, Lukas SE, Kramer AV, Kuhar MJ. Imaging dopamine receptors in the human brain by positron tomography. Science 1983; 221(4617):1264–1266.
44. Rossum V. The significance of dopamine receptor blockade for the mechanism of action of neuroleptic drugs. Arch Int Pharmacodyn Ther 1966; 160:492–494.
45. Carlsson A, Lindqvist M. Effect of chlorpromazine or haloperidol on formation of 3-methoxytyramine and normetanephrine in mouse brain. Acta Pharmacol Toxicol 1963; 20:140–144.
46. Seeman P, Lee T. Antipsychotic drugs: direct correlation between clinical potency and presynaptic action on dopamine neurons. Science 1975; 188:1217–1219.
47. Creese I, Burt DR, Snyder SH. Dopamine receptor binding predicts clinical and pharmacological potencies of antischizophrenic drugs. Science 1976; 19:481–483.
48. Connell PH. Amphetamine Psychosis. London; Chapman and Hall, 1958.
49. Angrist BM, Gershon S. The phenomenology of experimentally induced amphetamine psychosis—preliminary observation. Biol Psychiatry 1970; 2:95–107.
50. Goldman-Rakic PS, Selemon LD. Functional and anatomical aspects of prefrontal pathology in schizophrenia. Schizophr Bull 1997; 23:437–458.
51. Weinberger DR. Implications of the normal brain development for the pathogenesis of schizophrenia. Arch Gen Psychiatry 1987; 44:660–669.
52. Knable MB, Weinberger DR. Dopamine, the prefrontal cortex and schizophrenia. J Psychopharmacol 1997; 11(2):123–131.
53. Akil M, Pierri JN, Whitehead RE, Edgar CL, Mohila C, Sampson AR, Lewis DA. Lamina-specific alterations in the dopamine innervation of the prefrontal cortex in schizophrenic subjects. Am J Psychiatry 1999; 156(10):1580–1589.
54. Deutch AY. Prefrontal cortical dopamine systems and the elaboration of functional corticostriatal circuits: implications for schizophrenia and Parkinson's disease. J Neural Transm Gen Sect 1993; 91(2–3):197–221.
55. Wilkinson LS. The nature of interactions involving prefrontal and striatal dopamine systems. J Psychopharmacol 1997; 11(2):143–150.
56. Weinberger DR, Laruelle M. Neurochemical and neuropharmacological imaging in schizophrenia. In Neuropsychopharmacology—the fifth generation of progress. Davis KL, Charney DS, Coyle JT, Nemeroff C, eds. Lippincott, New York; Williams and Wilkins, 2001.
57. Wong DF, Wagner HN, Tune LE, Dannals RF, Pearlson GD, Links JM, Tamminga CA, Broussolle EP, Ravert HT, Wilson AA, Toung JK, Malat J, Williams JA, O'Tuama LA, Snyder SH, Kuhar MJ, Gjedde A. Positron emission tomography reveals elevated D_2 dopamine receptors in drug-naive schizophrenics. Science 1986; 234:1558–1563.
58. Crawley JC, Owens DG, Crow TJ, Poulter M, Johnstone EC, Smith T, Oldland SR, Veall N, Owen F, Zanelli GD. Dopamine D_2 receptors in schizophrenia studied in vivo. Lancet 1986; 2(8500):224–225.
59. Blin J, Baron JC, Cambon H, Bonnet AM, Dubois B, Loc'h C, Maziere B, Agid Y. Striatal dopamine D_2 receptors in tardive dyskinesia. PET study. J Neurol Neurosurg Psychiatry 1989; 52(11):1248–1252.
60. Martinot J-L, Peron-Magnan P, Huret J-D, Mazoyer B, Baron J-C, Boulenger J-P, Caillard V, Syrota A. Striatal D2 dopaminergic receptors assessed with positron emission tomography and 76-Br-bromospiperone in untreated patients. Am J Psychiatry 1990; 147:346–350.
61. Tune LE, Wong DF, Pearlson G, Strauss M, Young T, Shaya EK, Dannals RF, Wilson AA, Ravert HT, Sapp J. Dopamine D_2 receptor density estimates in schizophrenia: a positron emission tomography study with ^{11}C-N-methylspiperone. Psychiatry Res 1993; 49(3):219–237.
62. Nordstrom AL, Farde L, Eriksson L, Halldin C. No elevated D_2 dopamine receptors in neuroleptic-naive

schizophrenic patients revealed by positron emission tomography and [^{11}C]N-methylspiperone [see comments]. Psychiatry Res 1995; 61(2):67–83.

63. Okubo Y, Suhara T, Suzuki K, Kobayashi K, Inoue O, Terasaki O, Someya Y, Sassa T, Sudo Y, Matsushima E, Iyo M. Tateno Y, Toru M. Decreased prefrontal dopamine D_1 receptors in schizophrenia revealed by PET. Nature 1997; 385(6617):634–636.

64. Farde L, Wiesel F, Stone-Elander S, Halldin C, Nordsröm AL, Hall H, Sedvall G. D_2 dopamine receptors in neuroleptic-naive schizophrenic patients. A positron emission tomography study with [^{11}C]raclopride. Arch Gen Psychiatry 1990; 47:213–219.

65. Hietala J, Syvälahti E, Vuorio K, Nagren K, Lehikoinen P, Ruotsalainen U,. Räkköläinen V, Lehtinen V, Wegelius U. Striatal D_2 receptor characteristics in neuroleptic-naive schizophrenic patients studied with positron emission tomography. Arch Gen Psychiatry 1994; 51:116–123.

66. Pilowsky LS, Costa DC, Ell PJ, Verhoeff NPLG, Murray RM, Kerwin RW. D_2 dopamine receptor binding in the basal ganglia of antipsychotic-free schizophrenic patients. An I-123-IBZM single photon emission computerized tomography study. Br J Psychiatry 1994; 164:16–26.

67. Laruelle M, Abi-Dargham A, Van Dyck CH, Gil R, De Souza CD, Erdos J, McCance E, Rosenblatt W, Fingado C, Zoghbi SS, Baldwin RM, Seibyl JP, Krystal JH, Charney DS, Innis RB. Single photon emission computerized tomography imaging of amphetamine-induced dopamine release in drug free schizophrenic subjects. Proc Natl Acad Sci USA 1996; 93:9235–9240.

68. Knable MB, Egan MF, Heinz A, Gorey J, Lee KS, Coppola R, Weinberger DR. Altered dopaminergic function and negative symptoms in drug-free patients with schizophrenia. [^{123}I]-iodobenzamide SPECT study. Br J Psychiatry 1997; 171:574–577.

69. Breier A, Su TP, Saunders R, Carson RE, Kolachana BS, deBartolomeis A, Weinberger DR, Weisenfeld N, Malhotra AK, Eckelman WC, Pickar D. Schizophrenia is associated with elevated amphetamine-induced synaptic dopamine concentrations: evidence from a novel positron emission tomography method. Proc Natl Acad Sci USA 1997; 94(6):2569–2574.

70. Abi-Dargham A, Gil R, Krystal J, Baldwin R, Seibyl J, Bowers M, Van Dyck C, Charney D, Innis R, Laruelle M. Increased striatal dopamine transmission in schizophrenia: confirmation in a second cohort. Am J Psychiatry 1998; 155:761–767.

71. Abi-Dargham A, Rodenhiser J, Printz D, Zea-Ponce Y, Gil R, Kegeles L, Weiss R, Cooper T, Mann JJ, Van Heertum R, Gorman J, Laruelle M. Increased baseline occupancy of D_2 receptors by dopamine in schizophrenia. Proc Natl Acad Sci USA 2000; 97(14):8104–8109.

72. Martinot Jl, Paillère-Martinot ML, Loc'h C, Hardy P, Poirier MF, Mazoyer B, Beaufils B, Mazière B, Alliaire JF, Syrota A. The estimated density of D_2 striatal receptors in schizophrenia. A study with positron emission tomography and ^{76}Br-bromolisuride. Br J Psychiatry 1991; 158:346–350.

73. Martinot JL, Paillère-Martinot ML, Loch'H C, Lecrubier Y, Dao-Castellana MH, Aubin F, Allilaire JF, Mazoyer B, Mazière B, Syrota A. Central D_2 receptors and negative symptoms of schizophrenia. Br J Pharmacol. 1994; 164:27–34.

74. Seeman P, Guan H-C, Niznik HB. Endogenous dopamine lowers the dopamine D_2 receptor density as measured by [^{3}H]raclopride: implications for positron emission tomography of the human brain. Synapse 1989; 3:96–97.

75. Seeman P. Brain dopamine receptors in schizophrenia. PET problems. Arch Gen Psychiatry 1988; 45:598–560.

76. Reith J, Benkelfat C, Sherwin A, Yasuhara Y, Kuwabara H, Andermann F, Bachneff S, Cumming P, Diksic M, Dyve SE, Etienne P, Evans AC, Lal S, Shevell M, Savard G, Wong DF, Chouinard G, Gjedde A. Elevated dopa decarboxylase activity in living brain of patients with psychosis. Proc Natl Acad Sci USA 1994; 91:11651–11654.

77. Hietala J, Syvalahti E, Vuorio K, Rakkolainen V, Bergman J, Haaparanta M, Solin O, Kuoppamaki M, Kirvela O, Ruotsalainen U. Presynaptic dopamine function in striatum of neuroleptic-naive schizophrenic patients. Lancet 1995; 346(8983):1130–1131.

78. Dao-Castellana MH, Paillere-Martinot ML, Hantraye P, Attar-Levy D, Remy P, Crouzel C, Artiges E, Feline A, Syrota A, Martinot JL. Presynaptic dopaminergic function in the striatum of schizophrenic patients. Schizophr Res 1997; 23(2):167–174.

79. Hietala J, Syvalahti E, Vilkman H, Vuorio K, Rakkolainen V, Bergman J, Haaparanta M, Solin O, Kuoppamaki M, Eronen E, Ruotsalainen U, Salokangas RK. Depressive symptoms and presynaptic dopamine function in neuroleptic-naive schizophrenia. Schizophr Res 1999; 35(1):41–50.

80. Lindstrom LH, Gefvert O, Hagberg G, Lundberg T, Bergstrom M, Hartvig P, Langstrom B. Increased dopamine synthesis rate in medial prefrontal cortex and striatum in schizophrenia indicated by L-(beta-^{11}C) DOPA and PET. Biol Psychiatry 1999; 46(5):681–688.

81. Laruelle M. Imaging synaptic neurotransmission with in vivo binding competition techniques: a critical review. J Cereb Blood Flow Metab 2000; 20(3):423–451.

82. Villemagne VL, Wong DF, Yokoi F, Stephane M, Rice KC, Matecka D, Clough DJ, Dannals RF, Rothman RB. GBR12909 attenuates amphetamine-induced striatal dopamine release as measured by [(11)C]raclopride continuous infusion PET scans. Synapse 1999; 33(4):268–273.
83. Laruelle M, Iyer RN, Al-Tikriti MS, Zea-Ponce Y, Malison R, Zoghbi SS, Baldwin RM, Kung HF, Charney DS, Hoffer PB, Innis RB, Bradberry CW. Microdialysis and SPECT measurements of amphetamine-induced dopamine release in nonhuman primates. Synapse 1997; 25:1–14.
84. Laruelle M, Abi-Dargham A, Gil R, Kegeles L, Innis R. Increased dopamine transmission in schizophrenia: relationship to illness phases. Biol Psychiatry 1999; 46(1):56–72.
85. Hwang D, Kegeles LS, Laruelle M. (-)-N-[(11)C]propyl-norapomorphine: a positron-labeled dopamine agonist for PET imaging of D(2) receptors. Nucl Med Biol 2000; 27(6):533–539.
86. Bertolino A, Breier A, Callicott JH, Adler C, Mattay VS, Shapiro M, Frank JA, Pickar D, Weinberger DR. The relationship between dorsolateral prefrontal neuronal N-acetylaspartate and evoked release of striatal dopamine in schizophrenia. Neuropsychopharmacology 2000; 22(2):125–132.
87. Kegeles LS, Abi-Dargham A, Zea-Ponce Y, Rodenhiser-Hill J, Mann JJ, Van Heertum RL, Cooper TB, Carlsson A, Laruelle M. Modulation of amphetamine-induced striatal dopamine release by ketamine in humans: implications for schizophrenia. Biol Psychiatry 2000; 48(7):627–640.
88. Javitt DC, Zukin SR. Recent advances in the phencyclidine model of schizophrenia. Am J Psychiatry 1991; 148(10):1301–1308.
89. Olney JW, Farber NB. Glutamate receptor dysfunction and schizophrenia. Arch Gen Psychiatry 1995; 52(12):998–1007.
90. Moghaddam B. Recent basic findings in support of excitatory amino acid hypotheses of schizophrenia. Prog Neuro-Psychopharmacol Biol Psychiatry 1994; 18(5):859–870.
91. Laruelle M, D'Souza CD, Baldwin RM, Abi-Dargham A, Kanes SJ, Fingado CL, Seibyl JP, Zoghbi SS, Bowers MB, Jatlow P, Charney DS, Innis RB. Imaging D-2 receptor occupancy by endogenous dopamine in humans. Neuropsychopharmacology 1997; 17(3):162–174.
92. Fujita M, Verhoeff NP, Varrone A, Zoghbi SS, Baldwin RM, Jatlow PA, Anderson GM, Seibyl JP, Innis RB. Imaging extrastriatal dopamine D(2) receptor occupancy by endogenous dopamine in healthy humans. Eur J Pharmacol 2000; 387(2):179–188.
93. Laruelle M, Abi-Dargham A, Van Dyck C, Gil R, D'Souza CD, Krystal J, Seibyl J, Baldwin R, Innis R. Dopamine and serotonin transporters in patients with schizophrenia: an imaging study with [(123)I]beta-CIT. Biol Psychiatry 2000; 47(5):371–379.
94. Hirai M, Kitamura N, Hashimoto T, Nakai T, Mita T, Shirakawa O, Yamadori T, Amano T, Noguchi-Kuno SA, Tanaka C. [^{3}H]GBR-12935 binding sites in human striatal membranes: binding characteristics and changes in parkinsonians and schizophrenics. Jpn J Pharmacol 1988; 47(3):237–243.
95. Czudek C, Reynolds GP. [^{3}H]GBR 12935 binding to the dopamine uptake site in post-mortem brain tissue in schizophrenia. J Neural Transm 1989; 77(2–3):227–230.
96. Pearce RK, Seeman P, Jellinger K, Tourtellotte WW. Dopamine uptake sites and dopamine receptors in Parkinson's disease and schizophrenia. Eur Neurol 1990; 30(suppl 1):9–14.
97. Joyce JN, Lexow N, Bird E, Winokur A. Organization of dopamine D1 and D2 receptors in human striatum: receptor autoradiographic studies in Huntington's disease and schizophrenia. Synapse 1988; 2(5):546–557.
98. Chinaglia G, Alvarez FJ, Probst A, Palacios JM. Mesostriatal and mesolimbic dopamine uptake binding sites are reduced in Parkinson's disease and progressive supranuclear palsy: a quantitative autoradiographic study using [^{3}H]mazindol. Neuroscience 1992; 49(2):317–327.
99. Knable MB, Hyde TM, Herman MM, Carter JM, Bigelow L, Kleinman JE. Quantitative autoradiography of dopamine-D_1 receptors, D_2 receptors, and dopamine uptake sites in postmortem striatal specimens from schizophrenic patients. Biol Psychiatry 1994; 36(12):827–835.
100. De Keyser J, Ebinger G, Vauquelin G. Evidence for a widespread dopaminergic innervation of the human cerebral neocortex. Neurosci Lett 1989; 104:281–285.
101. Hall H, Sedvall G, Magnusson O, Kopp J, Halldin C, Farde L. Distribution of D_1- and D_2-dopamine receptors, and dopamine and its metabolites in the human brain. Neuropsychopharmacology 1994; 11:245–256.
102. Laruelle M, Casanova M, Weinberger D, Kleinman J. Postmortem study of the dopaminergic D_1 receptors in the dorsolateral prefrontal cortex of schizophrenics and controls. Schizophrenia Res 1990; 3:30–31.
103. Knable MB, Hyde TM, Murray AM, Herman MM, Kleinman JE. A postmortem study of frontal cortical dopamine D_1 receptors in schizophrenics, psychiatric controls, and normal controls. Biol Psychiatry 1996; 40(12):1191–1199.
104. Meador-Woodruff JH, Haroutunian V, Powchik P, Davidson M, Davis KL, Watson SJ. Dopamine receptor transcript expression in striatum and prefrontal and occipital cortex. Focal abnormalities in orbitofrontal cortex in schizophrenia. Arch Gen Psychiatry 1997; 54(12):1089–1095.

105. Abi-Dargham A, Gil R, Mawlawi O, Hwang DR, Kochan L, Lombardo I, Rodenhiser J, Kegeles L, Martinez D, Keilp J, Van Heertum R, Gorman J, Laruelle M. Selective alteration in D1 receptors in schizophrenia: a PET in vivo study. J Nucl Med 2001; 42:17P.
106. Lewis DA. GABAergic local circuit neurons and prefrontal cortical dysfunction in schizophrenia. Brain Res Rev 2000; 31(2–3):270–276.
107. Benes FM. Emerging principles of altered neural circuitry in schizophrenia. Brain Res Rev 2000; 31(2–3):251–269.
108. Busatto GF, Pilowsky LS, Costa DC, Ell PJ, David AS, Lucey JV, Kerwin RW. Correlation between reduced in vivo benzodiazepine receptor binding and severity of psychotic symptoms in schizophrenia. Am J Psychiatry 1997; 154(1):56–63.
109. Verhoeff NP, Soares JC, D'Souza CD, Gil R, Degen K, Abi-Dargham A, Zoghbi SS, Fujita M, Rajeevan N, Seibyl JP, Krystal JH, Van Dyck CH, Charney DS, Innis RB. [^{123}I]Iomazenil SPECT benzodiazepine receptor imaging in schizophrenia. Psychiatry Res 1999; 91(3):163–173.
110. Abi-Dargham A, Laruelle M, Krystal J, D'Souza C, Zoghbi S, Baldwin RM, Seibyl J, Mawlawi O, de Erasquin G, Charney D, Innis RB. No evidence of altered in vivo benzodiazepine receptor binding in schizophrenia. Neuropsychopharmacology 1999; 20(6):650–661.
111. Schröder J, Bubeck B, Demisch S, Sauer H. Benzodiazepine receptor distribution and diazepam binding in schizophrenia: an exploratory study. Psychiat. Res. Neuroimaging 1997; 68(2–3):125–131.
112. Ball S, Busatto GF, David AS, Jones SH, Hemsley DR, Pilowsky LS, Costa DC, Ell PJ, Kerwin RW. Cognitive functioning and GABAA/benzodiazepine receptor binding in schizophrenia: a ^{123}I-iomazenil SPET study. Biol Psychiatry 1998; 43(2):107–117.
113. Benes FM, Wickramasinghe R, Vincent SL, Khan Y, Todtenkopf M. Uncoupling of GABA(A) and benzodiazepine receptor binding activity in the hippocampal formation of schizophrenic brain. Brain Res 1997; 755(1):121–129.
114. Abi-Dargham A, Krystal J. Serotonin receptors as target of antipsychotic medications. In: Neurotransmitter Receptors in Actions of Antipsychotic Medications. Lidow MS, ed. Boca Raton, FL; CRC Press LLC, 2000, pp 79–107.
115. Lewis R, Kapur S, Jones C, DaSilva J, Brown GM, Wilson AA, Houle S, Zipursky RB. Serotonin 5-HT2 receptors in schizophrenia: a PET study using [^{18}F]setoperone in neuroleptic-naive patients and normal subjects. Am J Psychiatry 1999; 156(1):72–78.
116. Trichard C, Paillere-Martinot ML, Attar-Levy D, Blin J, Feline A, Martinot JL. No serotonin 5-HT2A receptor density abnormality in the cortex of schizophrenic patients studied with PET. Schizophr Res 1998; 31(1):13–17.
117. Okubo Y, Suhara T, Suzuki K, Kobayashi K, Inoue O, Terasaki O, Someya Y, Sassa T, Sudo Y, Matsushima E, Iyo M, Tateno Y, Toru M. Serotonin 5-HT2 receptors in schizophrenic patients studied by positron emission tomography. Life Sci 2000; 66(25):2455–2464.
118. Ngan ET, Yatham LN, Ruth TJ, Liddle PF. Decreased serotonin 2A receptor densities in neuroleptic-naive patients with schizophrenia. A PET study using [(18)F]setoperone. Am J Psychiatry 2000; 157(6):1016–1018.
119. Kapur S, Zipursky RB, Remington G. Clinical and theoretical implications of 5-HT2 and D$_2$ receptor occupancy of clozapine, risperidone, and olanzapine in schizophrenia. Am J Psychiatry 1999; 156(2):286–293.
120. Nyberg S, Nilsson U, Okubo Y, Halldin C, Farde L. Implications of brain imaging for the management of schizophrenia. Int Clin Psychopharmacol 1998; 13(suppl 3):S15–S20.
121. Farde L, Nordström AL, Wiesel FA, Pauli S, Halldin C, Sedvall G. Positron emission tomography analysis of central D$_1$ and D$_2$ dopamine receptor occupancy in patients treated with classical neuroleptics and clozapine. Arch Gen Psychiatry 1992; 49:538–544.
122. Wolkin A, Barouche F, Wolf AP, Rotrosen J, Fowler JS, Shiue CY, Cooper TB, Brodie JD. Dopamine blockade and clinical response: evidence for two biological subgroups of schizophrenia. Am J Psychiatry 1989; 146(7):905–908.
123. Pilowsky LS, Costa DC, Ell PJ, Murray RM, Verhoeff NPLG, Kerwin RW. Clozapine, single photon emission tomography, and the D$_2$ dopamine receptor blockade hypothesis of schizophrenia. Lancet 1992; 340:199–202.
124. Nordstrom AL, Farde L, Wiesel FA, Forslund K, Pauli S, Halldin C, Uppfeldt G. Central D$_2$-dopamine receptor occupancy in relation to antipsychotic drug effects: a double-blind PET study of schizophrenic patients. Biol Psychiatry 1993; 33(4):227–235.
125. Kapur S, Zipursky R, Jones C, Remington G, Houle S. Relationship between dopamine D(2) occupancy, clinical response, and side effects: a double-blind PET study of first-episode schizophrenia. Am J Psychiatry 2000; 157(4):514–520.
126. Nordstrom AL, Farde L, Nyberg S, Karlsson P, Halldin C, Sedvall G. D$_1$, D$_2$, and 5-HT2 receptor occupancy in relation to clozapine serum concentration: a PET study of schizophrenic patients [see comments]. Am J Psychiatry 1995; 152(10):1444–1449.
127. Nyberg S, Farde L, Eriksson L, Halldin C, Eriksson B. 5-HT2 and D$_2$ dopamine receptor occupancy in the

living human brain. A PET study with risperidone. Psychopharmacology 1993; 110:265–272.
128. Kapur S, Remington G, Zipursky RB, Wilson AA, Houle S. The D_2 dopamine receptor occupancy of risperidone and its relationship to extrapyramidal symptoms: a PET study. Life Sci 1995; 57(10):L103–L107.
129. Knable MB, Heinz A, Raedler T, Weinberger DR. Extrapyramidal side effects with risperidone and haloperidol at comparable D_2 receptor occupancy levels. Psychiatr Res Neuroimag 1997; 75(2):91–101.
130. Kapur S, Zipursky RB, Remington G, Jones C, DaSilva J, Wilson AA, Houle S. 5-HT2 and D_2 receptor occupancy of olanzapine in schizophrenia: a PET investigation. Am J Psychiatry 1998; 155(7):921–928.
131. Gefvert O, Bergstrom M, Langstrom B, Lundberg T, Lindstrom L, Yates R. Time course of central nervous dopamine-D_2 and 5-HT2 receptor blockade and plasma drug concentrations after discontinuation of quetiapine (Seroquel) in patients with schizophrenia. Psychopharmacology (Berl) 1998; 135(2):119–126.
132. Kapur S, Zipursky R, Jones C, Shammi CS, Remington G, Seeman P. A positron emission tomography study of quetiapine in schizophrenia: a preliminary finding of an antipsychotic effect with only transiently high dopamine D_2 receptor occupancy. Arch Gen Psychiatry 2000; 57(6):553–559.
133. Pilowsky LS, Mulligan RS, Acton PD, Ell PJ, Costa DC, Kerwin RW. Limbic selectivity of clozapine. Lancet 1997; 350(9076):490–491.
134. Farde L, Suhara T, Nyberg S, Karlsson P, Nakashima Y, Hietala J, Halldin C. A PET study of [C-11]FLB 457 binding to extrastriatal D-2-dopamine receptors in healthy subjects and antipsychotic drug-treated patients. Psychopharmacology 1997; 133(4):396–404.
135. Bigliani V, Mulligan RS, Acton PD, Visvikis D, Ell PJ, Stephenson C, Kerwin RW, Pilowsky LS. In vivo occupancy of striatal and temporal cortical D_2/D_3 dopamine receptors by typical antipsychotic drugs. [123I]epidepride single photon emission tomography (SPET) study. Br J Psychiatry 1999; 175:231–238.
136. Abi-Dargham A, Hwang DR, Huang Y, Zea-Ponce Y, Martinez D, Lombardo I, Broft A, Hashimoto T, Slifstein M, Mawlawi O, Van Heertum R, Laruelle M. Reliable quantification of both striatal and extrastriatal D_2 receptors in humans with [^{18}F]fallypride. J Nucl Med 2000; 41:139P.
137. Mukherjee J, Christian BT, Narayanan TK, Shi B, Mantil J. Measurement of striatal and extrastriatal D-2 receptor occupancy by clozapine and risperidone using [^{18}F]fallypride and PET. Neuroimage 2000; 11:S53.
138. Robertson GS, Matsumura H, Fibiger HC. Induction patterns of Fos-like immunoreactivity in the forebrain as predictors of atypical antipsychotic activity. J Pharmacol Exp Ther 1994; 271(2):1058–1066.

139. Deutch AY, Lee MC, Iadarola MJ. Regionally specific effects of atypical antipsychotic drugs on striatal fos expression: the nucleus accumbens shell as a locus of antipsychotic action. Mol Cell Neurosci 1992; 3:332–341.
140. Martinez D, Hwang DR, Broft A, Mawlawi O, Simpson N, Ngo K, Pidcock J, Van Heertum R, Laruelle M. PET imaging of amphetamine-induced endogenous dopamine release in mesolimbic and nigro-striatal dopamine systems in humans. J Nucl Med 2000; 41:105P.
141. Drevets WC, Price JC, Kupfer DJ, Kinahan PE, Lopresti B, Holt D, Mathis C. PET measures of amphetamine-induced dopamine release in ventral versus dorsal striatum. Neuropsychopharmacology 1999; 21(6):694–709.
142. Wolkin A, Brodie JD, Barouche F, Rotrosen J, Wolf AP, Smith M, Fowler J, Cooper TB. Dopamine receptor occupancy and plasma haloperidol levels. Arch Gen Psychiatry 1989; 46(5):482–484.
143. Fitzgerald PB, Kapur S, Remington G, Roy P, Zipursky RB. Predicting haloperidol occupancy of central dopamine D_2 receptors from plasma levels. Psychopharmacology (Berl) 2000; 149(1):1–5.
144. Hagberg G, Gefvert O, Bergstrom M, Wieselgren IM, Lindstrom L, Wiesel FA, Langstrom B. N-[^{11}C]methylspiperone PET, in contrast to [^{11}C]raclopride, fails to detect D_2 receptor occupancy by an atypical neuroleptic. Psychiatry Res 1998; 82(3):147–160.
145. Nasrallah HA, Skinner TE, Schmalbrock P, Robitaille PM. In vivo ^{1}H-NMR-spectroscopy of the limbic temporal lobe in patients with schizophrenia. In: NMR Spectroscopy in Psychiatric Brain Disorders. Nasrallah HA, Pettegrew JW, eds. Washington, D C, American Psychiatric Press, 1995, pp 1–20.
146. Gupta RK, Gupta P, Moore RD. NMR studies of intracellular metal ions in intact cells and tissues. Annu Rev Biophys Bioeng 1984; 13:221–246.
147. Pettegrew JW, Withers G, Panchalingam K, Post JF. Considerations for brain pH assessment by ^{31}P NMR. Magn Reson Imag 1988; 6(2):135–142.
148. Murphy EJ, Rajagopalan B, Brindle KM, Radda GK. Phospholipid bilayer contribution to ^{31}P NMR spectra in vivo. Magn Reson Med 1989; 12(2):282–289.
149. Pettegrew JW, Keshavan MS, Panchalingam K, Strychor S, Kaplan DB, Tretta MG, Allen M. Alterations in brain high-energy phosphate and membrane phospholipid metabolism in first-episode, drug-naive schizophrenics. A pilot study of the dorsal prefrontal cortex by in vivo phosphorus-31 nuclear magnetic resonance spectroscopy [see comments]. Arch Gen Psychiatry 1991; 48(6):563–568.
150. Feinberg I. Schizophrenia: caused by a fault in programmed synaptic elimination during adolescence? J Psychiatr Res 1982; 17(4):319–334.

151. Buchsbaum MS, Ingvar DH, Kessler R, Waters RN, Cappelletti J, Van Kammen DP, King AC, Johnson JL, Manning RG, Flynn RW, Mann LS, Bunney WE Jr, Sokoloff L. Cerebral glucography with positron tomography. Use in normal subjects and in patients with schizophrenia. Arch Gen Psychiatry 1982; 39(3):251–259.

152. Andreasen NC, Rezai K, Alliger R, Swayze VW 2nd, Flaum M, Kirchner P, Cohen G, O'Leary DS. Hypofrontality in neuroleptic-naive patients and in patients with chronic schizophrenia. Assessment with xenon-133 single-photon emission computed tomography and the Tower of London. Arch Gen Psychiatry 1992; 49(12):943–958.

153. Stanley JA, Williamson PC, Drost DJ, Carr TJ, Rylett RJ, Malla A, Thompson RT. An in vivo study of the prefrontal cortex of schizophrenic patients at different stages of illness via phosphorus magnetic resonance spectroscopy. Arch Gen Psychiatry 1995; 52(5):399–406.

154. Williamson P, Drost D, Stanley J, Carr T, Morrison S, Merskey H. Localized phosphorus-31 magnetic resonance spectroscopy in chronic schizophrenic patients and normal controls. Arch Gen Psychiatry 1991; 48(6):578.

155. Kato T, Shioiri T, Murashita J, Hamakawa H, Inubushi T, Takahashi S. Lateralized abnormality of high-energy phosphate and bilateral reduction of phosphomonoester measured by phosphorus-31 magnetic resonance spectroscopy of the frontal lobes in schizophrenia. Psychiatry Res 1995; 61(3):151–160.

156. Potwarka JJ, Drost DJ, Williamson PC, Carr T, Canaran G, Rylett WJ, Neufeld RW. A ^{1}H-decoupled ^{31}P chemical shift imaging study of medicated schizophrenic patients and healthy controls. Biol Psychiatry 1999; 45(6):687–693.

157. Shioiri T, Kato T, Inubushi T, Murashita J, Takahashi S. Correlations of phosphomonoesters measured by phosphorus-31 magnetic resonance spectroscopy in the frontal lobes and negative symptoms in schizophrenia. Psychiatry Res 1994; 55(4):223–235.

158. Volz HP, Rzanny R, Rossger G, Hubner G, Kreitschmann-Andermahr I, Kaiser WA, Sauer H. Decreased energy demanding processes in the frontal lobes of schizophrenics due to neuroleptics? A ^{31}P-magneto-resonance spectroscopic study. Psychiatry Res 1997; 76(2–3):123–129.

159. Deicken RF, Calabrese G, Merrin EL, Meyerhoff DJ, Dillon WP, Weiner MW, Fein G. ^{31}Phosphorus magnetic resonance spectroscopy of the frontal and parietal lobes in chronic schizophrenia. Biol Psychiatry 1994; 36(8):503–510.

160. Fujimoto T, Nakano T, Takano T, Hokazono Y, Asakura T, Tsuji T. Study of chronic schizophrenics using ^{31}P magnetic resonance chemical shift imaging. Acta Psychiatr Scand 1992; 86(6):455–462.

161. Kegeles LS, Humaran TJ, Mann JJ. In vivo neurochemistry of the brain in schizophrenia as revealed by magnetic resonance spectroscopy. Biol Psychiatry 1998; 44:382–398.

162. Keshavan MS, Stanley JA, Pettegrew JW. Magnetic resonance spectroscopy in schizophrenia: methodological issues and findings—part II. Biol Psychiatry 2000; 48(5):369–380.

163. O'Callaghan E, Redmond O, Ennis R, Stack J, Kinsella A, Ennis JT, Larkin C, Waddington JL. Initial investigation of the left temporoparietal region in schizophrenia by ^{31}P magnetic resonance spectroscopy. Biol Psychiatry 1991; 29(11):1149–1152.

164. Fukuzako H, Takeuchi K, Ueyama K, Fukuzako T, Hokazono Y, Hirakawa K, Yamada K, Hashiguchi T, Takigawa M, Fujimoto T. ^{31}P magnetic resonance spectroscopy of the medial temporal lobe of schizophrenic patients with neuroleptic-resistant marked positive symptoms. Eur Arch Psychiatry Clin Neurosci 1994; 244(5):236–240.

165. Fukuzako H, Fukuzako T, Hashiguchi T, Kodama S, Takigawa M, Fujimoto T. Changes in levels of phosphorus metabolites in temporal lobes of drug-naive schizophrenic patients. Am J Psychiatry 1999; 156(8):1205–1208.

166. Calabrese G, Deicken RF, Fein G, Merrin EL, Schoenfeld F, Weiner MW. ^{31}Phosphorus magnetic resonance spectroscopy of the temporal lobes in schizophrenia. Biol Psychiatry 1992; 32(1):26–32.

167. Deicken RF, Calabrese G, Merrin EL, Vinogradov S, Fein G, Weiner MW. Asymmetry of temporal lobe phosphorous metabolism in schizophrenia: a ^{31}phosphorous magnetic resonance spectroscopic imaging study. Biol Psychiatry 1995; 38(5):279–286.

168. Frahm J, Merboldt KD, Hanicke W. Localized proton spectroscopy using stimulated echoes. J Magn Reson Imaging 1987; 72:502–508.

169. Urenjak J, Williams SR, Gadian DG, Noble M. Proton nuclear magnetic resonance spectroscopy unambiguously identifies different neural cell types. J Neurosci 1993; 13:981–989.

170. Simmons ML, Frondoza CG, Coyle JT. Immunocytochemical localization of N-acetyl-aspartate with monoclonal antibodies. Neuroscience 1991; 45:37–45.

171. DeStefano N, Francis G, Antel JP, Arnold DL. Reversible decreases of N-acetylaspartate in the brain of patients with relapsing remitting multiple sclerosis. Proc Soc Magn Res Med 1993; 1:280.

172. Tsai G, Coyle JT. N-Acetylaspartate in neuropsychiatric disorders. Prog Neurobiol 1995; 46:531–540.

173. Maier M. In vivo magnetic resonance spectroscopy. Applications in psychiatry. Br J Psychiatry 1995; 167(3):299–306.

174. Behar KL, Rothman DL, Spencer DD, Petroff OA. Analysis of macromolecule resonances in ¹H NMR spectra of human brain. Magn Reson Med 1994; 32(3):294–302.
175. Hwang JH, Graham GD, Behar KL, Alger JR, Prichard JW, Rothman DL. Short echo time proton magnetic resonance spectroscopic imaging of macromolecule and metabolite signal intensities in the human brain. Magn Reson Med 1996; 35(5):633–639.
176. Rothman DL, Petroff OA, Behar KL, Mattson RH. Localized ¹H NMR measurements of gamma-aminobutyric acid in human brain in vivo. Proc Natl Acad Sci USA 1993; 90(12):5662–5666.
177. Keltner JR, Wald LL, Christensen JD, Maas LC, Moore CM, Cohen BM, Renshaw PF. A technique for detecting GABA in the human brain with PRESS localization and optimized refocusing spectral editing radiofrequency pulses. Magn Reson Med 1996; 36:458–461.
178. Mason GF, Pan JW, Ponder SL, Twieg DB, Pohost GM, Hetherington HP. Detection of brain glutamate and glutamine in spectroscopic images at 4.1 T. Magn Reson Med 1994; 32(1):142–145.
179. Stanley JA, Williamson PC, Drost DJ, Rylett RJ, Carr TJ, Malla A, Thompson RT. An in vivo proton magnetic resonance spectroscopy study of schizophrenia patients. Schizophr Bull 1996; 22(4):597–609.
180. Bartha R, al-Semaan YM, Williamson PC, Drost DJ, Malla AK, Carr TJ, Densmore M, Canaran G, Neufeld RW. A short echo proton magnetic resonance spectroscopy study of the left mesial-temporal lobe in first-onset schizophrenic patients. Biol Psychiatry 1999; 45(11):1403–1411.
181. Cecil KM, Lenkinski RE, Gur RE, Gur RC. Proton magnetic resonance spectroscopy in the frontal and temporal lobes of neuroleptic naive patients with schizophrenia. Neuropsychopharmacology 1999; 20(2):131–140.
182. Choe BY, Suh TS, Shinn KS, Lee CW, Lee C, Paik IH. Observation of metabolic changes in chronic schizophrenia after neuroleptic treatment by in vivo hydrogen magnetic resonance spectroscopy. Invest Radiol 1996; 31(6):345–352.
183. Bertolino A, Nawroz S, Mattay VS, Barnett AS, Duyn JH, Moonen CTW, Frank JA, Tedeschi G, Weinberger DR. Regionally specific pattern of neurochemical pathology in schizophrenia as assessed by multislice proton magnetic resonance spectroscopic imaging. Am J Psychiatry 1996; 153:1554–1563.
184. Bertolino A, Callicott JH, Elman I, Mattay VS, Tedeschi G, Frank JA, Breier A, Weinberger DR. Regionally specific neuronal pathology in untreated patients with schizophrenia: a proton magnetic resonance spectroscopic imaging study. Biol Psychiatry 1998; 43(9):641–648.
185. Deicken RF, Zhou L, Corwin F, Vinogradov S, Weiner MW. Decreased left frontal lobe N-acetylaspartate in schizophrenia. Am J Psychiatry 1997; 154(5):688–690.
186. Buckley PF, Moore C, Long H, Larkin C, Thompson P, Mulvany F, Redmond O, Stack JP, Ennis JT, Waddington JL. ¹H-Magnetic resonance spectroscopy of the left temporal and frontal lobes in schizophrenia: clinical, neurodevelopmental, and cognitive correlates. Biol Psychiatry 1994; 36(12):792–800.
187. Fukuzako H, Takeuchi K, Hokazono Y, Fukuzako T, Yamada K, Hashiguchi T, Obo Y, Ueyama K, Takigawa M, Fujimoto T. Proton magnetic resonance spectroscopy of the left medial temporal and frontal lobes in chronic schizophrenia: preliminary report. Psychiatry Res 1995; 61(4):193–200.
188. Callicott JH, Egan MF, Bertolino A, Mattay VS, Langheim FJ, Frank JA, Weinberger DR. Hippocampal N-acetyl aspartate in unaffected siblings of patients with schizophrenia: a possible intermediate neurobiological phenotype. Biol Psychiatry 1998; 44(10):941–950.
189. Choe BY, Kim KT, Suh TS, Lee C, Paik IH, Bahk YW, Shinn KS, Lenkinski RE. ¹H Magnetic resonance spectroscopy characterization of neuronal dysfunction in drug-naive, chronic schizophrenia. Acad Radiol 1994; 1:211–216.
190. Deicken RF, Zhou L, Schuff N, Fein G, Weiner MW. Hippocampal neuronal dysfunction in schizophrenia as measured by proton magnetic resonance spectroscopy. Biol Psychiatry 1998; 43(7):483–488.
191. Lim KO, Adalsteinsson E, Spielman D, Sullivan EV, Rosenbloom MJ, Pfefferbaum A. Proton magnetic resonance spectroscopic imaging of cortical gray and white matter in schizophrenia. Arch Gen Psychiatry 1998; 55(4):346–352.
192. Maier M, Ron MA, Barker GJ, Tofts PS. Proton magnetic resonance spectroscopy: an in vivo method of estimating hippocampal neuronal depletion in schizophrenia. Psychol Med 1995; 25(6):1201–1209.
193. Nasrallah HA, Skinner TE, Schmalbrock P, Robitaille PM. Proton magnetic resonance spectroscopy (¹H MRS) of the hippocampal formation in schizophrenia: a pilot study. Br J Psychiatry 1994; 165(4):481–485.
194. Yurgelun-Todd DA, Renshaw PF, Gruber SA, Waternaux C, Cohen BM. Proton magnetic resonance spectroscopy of the temporal lobes in schizophrenics and normal controls. Schizophr Res 1996; 19:55–59.
195. Heimberg C, Komoroski RA, Lawson WB, Cardwell D, Karson CN. Regional proton magnetic resonance spectroscopy in schizophrenia and exploration of drug effect. Psychiatry Res 1998; 83(2):105–115.
196. Renshaw PF, Yurgelun-Todd DA, Tohen M, Gruber S, Cohen BM. Temporal lobe proton magnetic reso-

197. Keshavan MS, Montrose DM, Pierri JN, Dick EL, Rosenberg D, Talagala L, Sweeney JA. Magnetic resonance imaging and spectroscopy in offspring at risk for schizophrenia: preliminary studies. Prog Neuropsychopharmacol Biol Psychiatry 1997; 21(8):1285–1295.
198. Bertolino A, Esposito G, Callicott JH, Mattay VS, Van Horn JD, Frank JA, Berman KF, Weinberger DR. Specific relationship between prefrontal neuronal N-acetylaspartate and activation of the working memory cortical network in schizophrenia. Am J Psychiatry 2000; 157(1):26–33.
199. Tofts PS, Wray S. A critical assessment of methods of measuring metabolite concentrations by NMR spectroscopy. NMR Biomed 1988; 1:1–10.

nance spectroscopy of patients with first-episode psychosis. Am J Psychiatry 1995; 152(3):444–446.

200. Shungu DC, Bhujwalla ZM, Li SJ, Rose LM, Wehrle JP, Glickson JD. Determination of absolute phosphate metabolite concentration in RIF-1 tumors in vivo by ^{31}P-^{1}H-^{2}H NMR spectroscopy using water as an internal intensity reference. Magn Reson Med 1992; 28:105–121.
201. Rothman DL, Novotny EJ, Shulman GI, Howseman AM, Petroff OA, Mason G, Nixon T, Hanstock CC, Prichard JW, Shulman RG. ^{1}H-[^{13}C] NMR measurements of [4-^{13}C]glutamate turnover in human brain. Proc Natl Acad Sci USA 1992; 89(20):9603–9606.
202. Laakso A, Vilkman H, Alakare B, Haaparanta M, Bergman J, Solin O, Peurasaari J, Rakkolainen V, Syvalahti E, Hietala J. Striatal dopamine transporter binding in neuroleptic-naive patients with schizophrenia studied with positron emission tomography. Am J Psychiatry 2000; 157(2):269–271.

17

The Dopamine Hypothesis of Schizophrenia

PHILIP SEEMAN and MARY V. SEEMAN
University of Toronto, Toronto, Ontario, Canada

I. INTRODUCTION

The speculation that impairments in dopamine circuitry lie at the heart of the susceptibility to schizophrenia has long been debated but, recently, new evidence has arisen to support it. Dopamine mimetics such as L-dopa, amphetamine, and disulfiram are well known to produce psychotic symptoms de novo or to worsen pre-existing ones. Recent evidence shows that amphetamine causes a twofold higher release of dopamine in individuals with schizophrenia than it does in control subjects [1,2].

At the same time, dopamine-blocking drugs have long been known to reduce psychotic symptoms. It had been thought that the newer or "atypical" drugs exert their action through a different mechanism but, in fact, all antipsychotic agents block D2 receptors. Their clinical potency against positive symptoms of schizophrenia correlates with their ability to block this receptor [3–6].

The therapeutic concentrations of antipsychotic drugs used to derive the receptor occupancies have been summarized elsewhere [6–10]. The prediction that clinical efficacy requires a threshhold of 60–70% receptor occupancy is supported by PET (positron emission tomography) and SPET (single photon emission tomography) studies [11–17]. This range of D2 receptor occupancy correlates with efficacy for all clinically effective compounds.

II. IS CLOZAPINE AN EXCEPTION?

Using PET with a variety of radioligands, clozapine has been reported to occupy only between 0% and 50% of D2 receptors at clinically effective doses [11,12,15,18–25]. This is also true for studies using SPET methods [26–30]. Taken at face value, these results have been interpreted as evidence against the dopamine hypothesis since clozapine is considered one of the most (if not *the* most) effective antipsychotic agents in the treatment of schizophrenia.

The majority of these imaging studies, however, have examined schizophrenia patients at a time point that corresponds with a period of 6–12 h following the last oral dose of the drug. Importantly, recent data by Kapur and colleagues have shown that both clozapine and quetiapine occupy the requisite 60–70% of dopamine receptors as long as the patient is scanned within 2–4 h after the last administered dose [31–33].

The reason time is important is that compounds such as clozapine and quetiapine are loosely bound to the dopamine receptor. This stands in contrast to compounds such as haloperidol, chlorpromazine, remoxipride, olanzapine, raclopride, and sertindole, which are all tightly bound [34].

The loosely bound drugs are easily displaced by endogenous dopamine. A pulse of an endogenous concentration of 100 nM dopamine [35] displaces

D2-bound [³H]clozapine or [³H]quetiapine at least one hundred times faster than it does D2-bound [³H]haloperidol or [³H]chlorpromazine [34]. Thus, the rapidity with which endogenous dopamine supplants clozapine and quetiapine at dopamine D2 receptors contributes to low apparent D2 receptor occupancy.

III. EVIDENCE OF ISOMERS

The three-dimensional molecular configuration of antipsychotic agents is similar to that of dopamine itself, which explains their ability to fit snugly into the receptor and obstruct dopamine transmission. Drugs with very similar structures that do not fit into and block the receptor are not antipsychotics. As an example, the isomer of flupenthixol that blocks dopamine receptors is an effective antipsychotic whereas the isomer that does not is ineffective. Loosely bound drugs (clozapine and quetiapine) fit the receptor, but not snugly, and they are therefore easily displaced and their blockade is brief.

IV. EVIDENCE OF DOPAMINE DEPLETION

Also supporting the dopamine hypothesis are data that show that dopamine depletion by reserpine produces an antipsychotic effect and that blocking dopamine synthesis by alpha-methyl-p-tyrosine (AMPT), for instance, reduces the antipsychotic dose needed to produce an antipsychotic effect.

V. EVIDENCE OF PROLACTIN ELEVATION

All antipsychotics, including clozapine, can be shown to elevate prolactin levels by a direct block of D2 receptors in the anterior pituitary. Prolactin elevations with the loosely bound agents are, however, transient [36], mirroring striatal effects.

VI. EFFECT LAG

One time-honored objection to the dopamine hypothesis of antipsychotic action is the therapeutic time lag. Antipsychotics alter dopamine activity from the first day of treatment whereas clinical improvement does not set in until later, although some clinical effects (calming of agitation, fear reduction, disappearance of catatonic features, attenuation of suspicion/hostility) begin almost immediately, reducing scores on the Brief Psychiatric Rating Scale (BPRS). In the face of postsynaptic blockade, the reaction of a dopamine neuron is to compensate by increasing presynaptic release. This is evidenced by initial increases of dopamine metabolites—i.e., increases in levels of homovanillic acid (HVA). With time, the HVA levels in the cerebrospinal fluid decrease, as the dopamine system accommodates. In patients who respond to antipsychotics, full clinical response occurs at a time that corresponds with the plateau in HVA levels ($\sim$ 3 weeks after initiation of treatment).

VII. WHAT CAN BE LEARNED BY THE NOVEL "ATYPICAL" ANTIPSYCHOTICS?

The block of D2 receptors by antipsychotic drugs elicits parkinsonism and other extrapyramidal signs. Clozapine and quetiapine, however, cause few or no extrapyramidal effects. Few extrapyramidal signs are induced by other novel antipsychotics as well, as long as the dose is kept low.

Does this mean that the D2 blockade of these agents is small relative to other receptor block, and does this undermine the hypothesis that dopamine D2 binding is the primary source of antipsychotic action? For instance, it has been suggested that the blockade of serotonin-2A receptors alleviates the parkinsonism caused by D2 block. But most data do not support this hypothesis. For example, selective serotonin-2A receptor blockade actually enhances the catalepsy of submaximal doses of raclopride in rats (Wadenberg M-LG, Hicks PB, Young KA, 1997, personal communication). Rat catalepsy is the analog of parkinsonism in humans.

Furthermore, the serotonin-2A blocker, ritanserin, (2 mg/kg SC) had no effect on raclopride-induced catalepsy in rats, whether maximal (4 mg/kg SC) or submaximal (0.2 mg/kg SC) doses of raclopride are used [37]. Additionally, in humans, a high degree of serotonin-2A receptor occupancy (95%) by risperidone (6 mg/day) does not prevent extrapyramidal signs in six out of seven patients with schizophrenia [38].

Finally, when it comes to clozapine, this drug is 20 to 50-fold more potent in blocking muscarinic acetylcholine receptors than in blocking dopamine D2 receptors. Clozapine and olanzapine are extremely potent anticholinergic drugs. Clozapine blocks muscarinic receptors between 1.5 nM and 36 nM, and this may contribute to the absence of parkinsonism by clozapine.

More importantly and more generally, antipsychotic drugs which tend to elicit little or no extrapyramidal signs are those that have dissociation constants (K_d values) > 1.5 nM, which is the K_d for dopamine at the high-affinity state of D2. This means that dopamine binds more tightly to D2 than the drugs do, so that the high endogenous dopamine in the human striatum quickly replaces loosely bound antipsychotics at the D2 receptor.

If that is the case, how can loosely bound drugs exert their effect against psychosis? Part of the explanation is that endogenous dopamine in limbic brain regions (e.g., frontal cortex, cingulate gyrus) is one-tenth that of the striatum. These low concentrations of endogenous dopamine in the synapses of limbic brain regions cannot compete against the drug. Thus, the D2 occupancy of these drugs in the limbic regions of the human brain may be high for longer periods than in the striatum. In other words, the higher output of endogenous dopamine in the striatum displaces D2-bound clozapine more quickly than does the low output of dopamine in the cerebral cortex. In corroboration of this theoretical model, Pilowsky et al. [39] have indeed found that clozapine occupies more D2 receptors in the cerebral cortex of patients than in the striatum.

It may also be possible that relatively transient D2 receptor occupancy is all that is needed in order to achieve clinical efficacy and that constant blockage of the receptor is unnecessary.

VIII. CONSEQUENCES OF LOOSE/TIGHT CATEGORIES

It appears that the rapid displacement of clozapine by dopamine is an important part of the explanation for the lack of extrapyramidal effects induced by novel antipsychotic agents. While dopamine can also displace other antipsychotic drugs such as raclopride [40] or [3H]chlorpromazine) [1,41]. such action is not sufficiently rapid to prevent parkinsonism. This is because these drugs are more tightly bound to D2 than is clozapine.

The separation of antipsychotic drugs into "loose" and "tight" D2 binding, relative to that for dopamine, is consistent with the findings by Kalkman et al. [42]. In animal models, these investigators were able to reverse catalepsy that was induced by olanzapine and loxapine (both more loosely bound than dopamine), but were not able to reverse the catalepsy produced by haloperidol (Kalkman HO, Tricklebank MD, 1997, personal communication).

Another consequence is that patients taking clozapine are at risk for quick relapse upon stopping their medication [43,44]. Because clozapine is loosely bound to the dopamine D2 receptor ($K_d = 44$ nM), it is readily displaced by any sudden pulse of endogenous dopamine arising from emotional or physical activity. In fact, both R. Conley [in 43] and Pickar et al. [45] observed that the D2 occupancy by clozapine rapidly decreased upon clozapine withdrawal. This was in contrast to the 2 weeks or more of residual occupancy of D2 by traditional neuroleptics [46]. Any sudden surge of impulse-triggered release of endogenous dopamine will quickly displace residual clozapine and may lead to a precipitate clinical relapse.

IX. FURTHER EVIDENCE FOR THE IMPORTANCE OF ENDOGENOUS DOPAMINE

Low dose clozapine [47–51] or remoxipride [52] effectively treats L-dopa psychosis in Parkinson's disease. The average dose for clozapine for this condition is 55 mg/day, while that for remoxipride is 150 mg/day, much lower doses than those used to treat schizophrenia.

The reason for the effectiveness of these very low doses is the fact that >95% of the brain dopamine has been depleted in Parkinson's disease. Thus, there is virtually no endogenous dopamine to compete against the clozapine or remoxipride. The low dose of clozapine corresponds to a low spinal fluid concentration of clozapine and norclozapine, estimated to be of the order of 60 nM (given that the unbound clozapine is 20% of the total plasma clozapine) [53]. Under these conditions, the fraction of D2 receptors occupied would be ~ 60%*.

X. IS D2 BLOCK A NECESSARY MINIMUM FOR ANTIPSYCHOTIC ACTION?

If serotonin block is not the major reason for the relative absence of extrapyramidal side effects by the novel antipsychotic agents, is it perhaps the reason for the extra efficacy attributed to these drugs, especially to

---

*Where C/(C + K) is 60 nM/(60 nM + 44 nM) = 60% of D2.

clozapine? It seems not. Full blockade of serotonin-2A receptors occurs at doses of risperidone, olanzapine, and clozapine, which are markedly subtherapeutic, indicating that serotonin-2A block contributes little or nothing to antipsychotic action [17].

The consistent finding that all antipsychotic drugs, including clozapine, occupy 60–70% of D2 receptors when clinically effective, suggests that the blockade of D2 is an essential minimal requirement for clinical antipsychotic action in those patients who respond to neuroleptics. It is also true, however, that many schizophrenia patients may not clinically improve despite high drug occupancy (>75%) of their D2 receptors.

The argument has been made that, since 30% of patients who have not responded to traditional D2 blockers such as haloperidol do respond to clozapine, then the drug must work through a different mechanism [54]. Such "treatment-resistant" patients, however, also respond (often dramatically) to remoxipride [55–57], which is extremely selective for D2. In fact, just like clozapine, remoxipride clinically improves at least 30% of treatment-resistant schizophrenia patients [55–57]. The experience with remoxipride indicates that treatment-resistant patients may still improve via D2 block when using a low potency drug such as clozapine ($K_d = 44$ nM at D2) or remoxipride ($K_d = 30$ nM at D2).

XI. DO DOPAMINE RECEPTORS HAVE ANYTHING TO DO WITH SCHIZOPHRENIA?

Although it is important to recognize that the drugs we currently use to control schizophrenia symptoms all act principally through dopamine receptors, does this have anything to tell us about the etiology of schizophrenia? Does the dopamine hypothesis refer only to drug action, or to the pathophysiology of the disease itself? By using D2-blocking isotopes in a PET scanner, it is possible to image striatal dopamine receptors in psychotic patients who are drug free. Some drug-free patients manifest an increase in D2 receptors [58], suggesting a possible early indication of increased sensitivity to dopamine. Other investigators have not been able to replicate this finding [59], but these studies have used different ligands, and different assumptions and the sample sizes have been small, so no definite conclusions are currently possible. The group that finds elevations uses the ligand [11C]methylspiperone [22]; the group that does not, uses [11C]raclopride [60].

The two ligands may bind differently to the D2 receptor. Since D2 receptors exist either in the monomer or the dimer form both in rat and human tissue [61], one ligand may bind only to the monomer and the other may bind to both. There are reasons to believe that raclopride, like nemonapride, binds to both forms of the receptor [62–64] and, thus, the raclopride method may obscure a D2 monomer elevation that, at least speculatively, lies at the heart of schizophrenia susceptibility.

Why would D2 monomers be elevated in schizophrenia? In postmortem tissue, their elevation might be explained as a response to the virtual absence of dopamine in the synaptic cleft [65]. But in vivo studies throw further light on the situation. In the presence of a resting level of neuron firing, the synaptic level of dopamine in subjects with schizophrenia is at least twice that of control subjects [1,2,41]. Presumably, in living subjects, there is a faster turnover, more dopamine being synthesized in response to increased need. In other words, the more monomer-type receptors on the postsynaptic membrane, the more dopamine depletion in the synapse, the more feedback to autoreceptors on the presynaptic cell, and the more dopamine synthesis.

XII. EFFECT OF THE D1 RECEPTOR

There is the further influence of the D1 receptor, which plays a role as yet not well defined. What we do know is that D1 influences D2, possibly in the direction of reducing its high affinity states. The D1-D2 link appears to be reduced or even absent in post mortem tissues in psychosis [66]. Without the moderating influence of D1, more D2 receptors in schizophrenia may exist in their high-affinity (or physiologically active) [67] state, thus further increasing psychosis vulnerability.

XIII. THE DOPAMINE HYPOTHESIS AND MOLECULAR GENETICS

Genetic linkage with dopamine receptor subtypes has, in general, excluded dopamine receptor genes as loci of major effect in schizophrenia [68]. Association studies suggest that variation in the D3 gene may confer a small relative risk to schizophrenia [69]. Incidentally, the same review [69] underscores the important links which exist between impaired cognition in schizophrenia and dopamine pathways, too extensive a literature to include in this chapter. It is important to understand that genetic linkage to the disease may not directly involve dopamine receptor genes but may implicate genetic defects of other proteins responsible for the regulation or modulation of these genes. The increase of D2 monomers found in schizophrenia, and the presence of relatively more D2 high-affinity states, may be a response to as yet unknown genetic variations in other systems. For instance, Kegeles et al. [70] found that ketamine, which blocks N-methyl-D-aspartate (NMDA) receptors, enhances the amphetamine-induced release of endogenous dopamine in healthy volunteers, strongly suggesting an interaction between glutamate and dopamine systems. A confounding factor, however, is that ketamine has equal affinity for NMDA receptors and the high-affinity state of dopamine D2 receptors [71]. This shows the complexity and the interaction potential of neurotransmission systems, which increases the difficulty of candidate gene searches.

REFERENCES

1. M Laruelle, A Abi-Dargham, CH van Dyck, R Gil, CD De Souza, J Erdos, E McCance, W Rosenblatt, C Fingado, SS Zoghbi, RM Baldwin, JP Seibyl, JH Krystal, DS Charney, RB Innis. Single photon emission computerized tomography imaging of amphetamine-induced dopamine release in drug free schizophrenic subjects. Proc Natl Acad Sci USA 93:9235–9240, 1996.
2. A Abi-Dargham, R Gil, J Krystal, RM Baldwin, JP Seibyl, M Bowers, CH van Dyck, DS Charney, RB Innis, M Laruelle. Increased striatal dopamine transmission in schizophrenia: Confirmation in a second cohort. Am J Psychiatry 155:761–767, 1998.
3. P Seeman, M Chau-Wong, J Tedesco, K Wong. Brain receptors for antipsychotic drugs and dopamine: direct binding assays. Proc Natl Acad Sci USA 72:4376–4380, 1975.
4. P Seeman, T Lee, M Chau-Wong, K Wong. Antipsychotic drug doses and neuroleptic/dopamine receptors. Nature 261:717–719, 1976.
5. DR Burt, I Creese, SH Snyder. Properties of [^{3}H]haloperidol and [^{3}H]dopamine binding associated with dopamine receptors in calf brain membranes. Mol Pharmacol 12:800–812, 1976.
6. P Seeman, T Tallerico. Antipsychotic drugs which elicit little or no parkinsonism bind more loosely than dopamine to brain D2 receptors, yet occupy high levels of these receptors. Mol Psychiatry 3: 123–134, 1998.
7. P Seeman. Therapeutic receptor-blocking concentrations of neuroleptics. Int Clin Psychopharmacol 10(suppl 3):5–13, 1995.
8. P Seeman, R Corbett, DNam, HHM Van Tol. Dopamine and serotonin receptors: amino acid sequences, and clinical role in neuroleptic parkinsonism. Jpn J Pharmacol 71:187–204, 1996.
9. P Seeman, R Corbett, HHM Van Tol. Atypical neuroleptics have low affinity for dopamine D2 receptors or are selective for D4. Neuropsychopharmacology 16: 91–110, 1996.
10. P Seeman, HHM Van Tol. Deriving the therapeutic concentrations for clozapine and haloperidol: the apparent dissociation constant of a neuroleptic at the dopamine D2 or D4 receptor varies with the affinity of the competing radioligand. Eur J Pharmacol Mol Pharmacol Section 291:59–66, 1995.
11. L Farde, A-LNordström, F-A Wiesel, S Pauli, C Halldin, G Sedvall. Positron emission tomographic analysis of central D1 and D2 dopamine receptor occupancy in patients treated with classical neuroleptics and clozapine. Arch Gen Psychiatry 49: 538–544, 1992.
12. A-L Nordström, L Farde, S Nyberg, P Karlsson, C Halldin, G Sedvall. D1, D2, and 5-HT2 receptor occupancy in relation to clozapine serum concentration: a PET study of schizophrenic patients. Am J Psychiatry 152: 1444–1449, 1995.
13. S Nyberg, A-L Nordström, C Halldin, L Farde. Positron emission tomography studies on D2 dopamine receptor occupancy and plasma antipsychotic drug levels in man. Int Clin Psychopharmacol 10(suppl 3):81–85, 1995.
14. S Kapur, G Remington, RB Zipursky, AA Wilson, S Houle. The D2 dopamine receptor occupancy of risperidone and its relationship to extrapyramidal symptoms: a PET study. Life Sci 57: PL103–PL107, 1995.
15. S Kapur, G Remington, C Jones, AA Wilson, J DaSilva, S Houle, RB Zipursky. High levels of dopamine D2 receptor occupancy with low-dose haloperidol treatment: a PET study. Am J Psychiatry 153:948–950, 1996.
16. MB Knable, A Heinz, R Coppola, J Gorey, DR Weinberger. IBZM SPECT measurement of D2 receptor occupancy by haloperidol and risperidone (abstr). Biol Psychiatry 39:515, 1996.
17. S Kapur, RB Zipursky, G Remington, C Jones, J DaSilva, AA Wilson, S Houle. 5-HT2 and D2 receptor occupancy of olanzapine in schizophrenia: a PET investigation. Am J Psychiatry 155:921–928, 1998.
18. H Karbe, K Wienhard, K., Hamacher, M Huber, K Herholz, HH Coenen, G Stöcklin, A Lövenich, WD Heiss. Positron emission tomography with (^{18}F)methylspiperone demonstrates D2 dopamine receptor binding differences of clozapine and haloperidol. J Neural Transm 86:163–173, 1991.
19. JW Louwerens, JA Buddingh, S Zijlstra, J Pruim, J., Korf, AMJ Paans, W Vaalburg, CJ Slooff. Dopamine (D2)-receptor occupancy in clozapine-treated patients as measured by positron emission tomography using

18FESP. In: N Brunello, J Mendlewicz, G Racagni, eds. New Generation of Antipsychotic Drugs: Novel Mechanisms of Action, Vol 4. Basel: Karger, 1993, pp 130–135.

20. JW Louwerens, CJ Slooff, J Korf, HJ Coppens, AMJ Paans. Dopamine$_2$- and serotonin$_2$-receptor-antagonism by antipsychotics in man (abstr). Schizophr Res 18:141, 1996.

21. R Conley, D Medoff, D Wong, C Tamminga. ^{11}C NMSP receptor occupancy by clozapine and haloperidol in schizophrenic subjects (abstr). Schizophr Res 1995; 15:80.

22. A L Nordström, L Farde, L Friksson, C Halldin. No elevated D$_2$ dopamine receptors in neuroleptic-naive schizophrenic patients revealed by positron tomography and [^{11}C]N-methylspiperone. Psychiatry Res Neuroimag 61:67–83, 1995.

23. R Conley, M Zhao, D Wong, C Tamminga. ^{11}C NMSP receptor occupancy by clozapine and haloperidol in schizophrenic subjects (abstr). Biol Psychiatry 39:513, 1996.

24. S Kapur, RB Zipursky, C Jones, GJ Remington, AA Wilson, J DaSilva, S Houle. The D2 receptor occupancy profile of loxapine determined using PET. Neuropsychopharmacology 15:562–566, 1996.

25. S Kapur, RB Zipursky, G Remington, C Jones, G McKay, S Houle. PET evidence that loxapine is an equipotent blocker of 5-HT2 and D2 receptors: implications for the therapeutics of schizophrenia. Am J Psychiatry 154:1525–1529, 1997.

26. GF Busatto, LS Pilowsky, DC Costa, PJ Ell, NPLG Verhoeff, R Kerwin. Dopamine D2 receptor blockade in vivo with the novel antipsychotics risperidone and remoxipride—an ^{123}I-IBZM single photon emission tomography (SPET) study. Psychopharmacology 117:55–61, 1995.

27. E Klemm, F Grünwald, S Kasper, C Menzel, K Broich, P Danos, K Reichmann, C Krappel, O Rieker, B Briele, AL Hotze, H-J Möller, H-J Biersack. [^{123}I]IBZM SPECT for imaging of striatal D2 dopamine receptors in 56 schizophrenic patients taking various neuroleptics. Am J Psychiatry 153:183–190, 1996.

28. D Pickar, T-P Su, DR Weinberger, R Coppola, AK Malhotra, MB Knable, KS Lee, J Gorey, J J Bartko, A Breier, J Hsiao. Individual variation in D2 dopamine receptor occupancy in clozapine-treated patients. Am J Psychiatry 153:1571–1578, 1996.

29. LS Pilowsky, GF Busatto, M Taylor, DC, Costa, T Sharma, T Sigmundsson, PJ Ell, V Nohria, RW Kerwin. Dopamine D2 receptor occupancy in vivo by the novel atypical antipsychotic olanzapine—a ^{123}I IBZM single photon emission tomography (SPET) study. Psychopharmacology 124:148–153, 1996.

30. T-P Su, A Breier, R Coppola, K Hadd, L Elman, C Adler, AK Malhotra, E Watsky, J Gorey, DR Weinberger, D Pickar. D2 receptor occupancy in risperidone and clozapine-treated schizophrenics. Biol Psychiatry 39: 512–513, 1996.

31. P Seeman, S Kapur S. Clozapine occupies high levels of dopamine D2 receptors. Life Sci 60:207–216, 1997.

32. S Kapur, RB Zipursky, C Jones, CS Shammi, G Remington, P Seeman. A positron emission tomography study of quetiapine in schizophrenia—a preliminary finding of an antipsychotic effect with only transiently high dopamine D2 receptor occupancy. Arch Gen Psychiatry 57:553–559, 2000.

33. S Kapur, P Seeman. Does fast dissociation from the dopamine D2 receptor explain the action of atypical antipsychotics? A new hypothesis. Am J Psychiatry 158:360–369, 2001.

34. P Seeman, T Tallerico. Clozapine and quetiapine: rapid release from D2 explains low receptor occupancy and early clinical relapse upon drug withdrawal. Am J Psychiatry (submitted).

35. KT Kawagoe, PA Garris, DJ Wiedemann, RM Wightman. Regulation of transient dopamine concentration gradients in the microenvironment surrounding nerve terminals in the rat striatum. Neuroscience 51:55–64, 1992.

36. P Turrone, S Kapur, MV Seeman, A Flint. Elevation of prolactin levels by atypical antipsychotics. Am J Psychiatry 159:133–135, 2002.

37. M-L Wadenberg, P Salmi, P Jimenez, T Svensson, S Ahlenius. Enhancement of antipsychotic-like properties of the dopamine D$_2$ receptor antagonist, raclopride, by the additional treatment with the 5-HT2 receptor blocking agent, ritanserin, in the rat. Eur Neuropsychopharmacol 6:305–310, 1996.

38. S Nyberg, Y Nakashima, A-L Nordström, C Halldin, L Farde. Positron emission tomography of in-vivo binding characteristics of atypical antipsychotic drugs. Review of D2 and 5-HT2 receptor occupancy studies and clinical response. Bri J Psychiatry 168:40–44, 1996.

39. LS Pilowsky, RS Mulligan, PD Acton, PJ Ell, DC Costa, RW Kerwin. Limbic selectivity of clozapine. Lancet 350:490–491, 1997.

40. P Seeman, H-C Guan, HB Niznik. Endogenous dopamine lowers the dopamine D2 receptor density as measured by [^{3}H]raclopride: implications for positron emission tomography of the human brain. Synapse 3:96–97, 1989.

41. M Laruelle, CD D'Souza, RM Baldwin, A Abi-Dargham, SJ Kanes, CL Fingado, JP Seibyl, SS Zoghbi, MB Bowers, P Jatlow, DS Charney, RB Innis. Imaging D$_2$ receptor occupancy by endogenous dopamine in humans. Neuropsychopharmacology 17:162–174, 1997.

42. HO Kalkman, V Neumann, MD Tricklebank. Clozapine inhibits catalepsy induced by olanzapine and loxapine, but prolongs catalepsy induced by SCH

23390 in rats. Naunyn-Schmiedeberg's Arch Pharmacol 355:361–364, 1997.
43. D Shore, S Matthews, J Cott, JA Lieberman. Clinical implications of clozapine discontinuation: report of an NIMH workshop. Schizophr Bull 21:333–338, 1995.
44. HY Meltzer, MA Lee, R Ranjan, EA Mason, PA Cola. Relapse following clozapine withdrawal: effect of neuroleptic drugs and cyproheptadine. Psychopharmacology 124:176–187, 1996.
45. D Pickar, T-P Su, R Coppola, CS Lee, JK Hsiao, A Breier, DR Weinberger. D2 occupancy and dopamine release determined by ^{123}I-IBZM SPECT following clozapine dose reduction (abstr). Schizophr Res 15:96, 1995.
46. JC Baron, JL Martinot, H Cambon, JP Boulenger, MF Poirier, V Caillard, J Blin, JD Huret, C Loc'h, B Maziere. Striatal dopamine receptor occupancy during and following withdrawal from neuroleptic treatment: correlative evaluation by positron emission tomography and plasma prolactin levels. Psychopharmacology 99:463–472, 1989.
47. JH Friedman, MC Lannon. Clozapine in the treatment of psychosis in Parkinson's disease. Neurology 39:1219–1221, 1989.
48. RF Pfeiffer, J Kang, B Graber, R Hofman, J Wilson. Clozapine for psychosis in Parkinson's disease. Mov Disord 5:239–242, 1990.
49. N Kahn, A Freeman, JL Juncos, D Manning, RL Watts. Clozapine is beneficial for psychosis in Parkinson's disease. Neurology 41:1699–1700, 1991.
50. SA Factor, D Brown. Clozapine prevents recurrence of psychosis in Parkinson's disease. Mov Disord 7:125–131, 1992.
51. JM Rabey, TA Treves, MY Neufeld, E Orlov, AD Korczyn. Low-dose clozapine in the treatment of levodopa-induced mental disturbances in Parkinson's disease. Neurology 45:432–434, 1995.
52. P Sandor, AE Lang, S Singal, C Angus. Remoxipride in the treatment of levodopa-induced psychosis. J Clin Psychopharmacol 16:395–399, 1996.
53. C Nordin, B Alm, U Bondesson. CSF and serum concentrations of clozapine and its demethyl metabolite: a pilot study. Psychopharmacology 122:104–107, 1995.
54. J Kane, G Honigfeld, J Singer, HY Meltzer. Clozaril Collaborative Study Group. Clozapine for the treatment-resistant schizophrenic: a double-blind comparison with chlorpromazine. Arch Gen Psychiatry 45:789–796, 1988.
55. HJ Scurlock, PH Robinson. Case report 2: remoxipride in resistant schizophrenia. J Drug Dev 6:71–72, 1993.
56. HJ Scurlock, AN Singh, J Catalan. Atypical antipsychotic drugs in the treatment of manic syndromes in patients with HIV-1 infection. J Psychopharmacol 9:151–154, 1995.
57. H Vartianen, E Leinonen, A Putkonen, S Lang, U Hagert, U Tolvanen. A long-term study of remoxipride in chronic schizophrenic patients. Acta Psychiatr Scand 87:114–117, 1993.
58. DF Wong, HN Wagner Jr, LE Tune, RF Dannals, GD Pearlson, JM Links, CA Tamminga, EP Broussolle, HT Ravert, AA Wilson, JKT Toung, J Malat, JA Williams, LA O'Tuama, SH Snyder, MJ Kuhar, A Gjedde. Positron emission tomography reveals elevated D_2 dopamine receptors in drug-naive schizophrenics. Science 234:1558–1563, 1986.
59. G Sedvall, L Farde, A Persson, F-A Wiesel. Imaging of neurotransmitter receptors in the living human brain. Arch Gen Psychiatry 43:995–1005, 1986.
60. L Farde, F-A Wiesel, S Stone-Elander, C Halldin, A-L Nordström, H Hall, G Sedvall. D_2 dopamine receptors in neuroleptic-naive schizophrenic patients. Arch Gen Psychiatry 47:213–219, 1990.
61. P Zawarynski, T Tallerico, P Seeman, SP Lee, BF O'Dowd, SR George. Dopamine D2 receptor dimers in human and rat brain. FEBS Lett 441:383–386, 1998.
62. GYK Ng, BF O'Dowd, M Caron, M Dennis, MR Brann, SR George. Phosphorylation and palmitoylation of the human D2L dopamine receptor in Sf9 cells. J Neurochem 63:1589–1595, 1994.
63. GYK Ng, BF O'Dowd, SP Lee, HT Chung, MR Brann, P Seeman, SR George. Dopamine D2 receptor dimers and receptor-blocking peptides. Biochem Biophys Res Commun 227:200–204, 1996.
64. GYK Ng, G Varghese, HT Chung, J Trogadis, P Seeman, BF O'Dowd, SR George. Resistance of the dopamine D_{2L} receptor to desensitization accompanies the up-regulation of receptors on to the surface of Sf9 cells. Endocrinology 138:4199–4206, 1997.
65. P Seeman, H-C Guan, HHM Van Tol. Dopamine D4 receptors elevated in schizophrenia. Nature 365:441–445, 1993.
66. P Seeman, HB Niznik, H-C Guan, G Booth, C Ulpian. Link between D1 and D2 dopamine receptors is reduced in schizophrenia and Huntington diseased brain. Proc Natl Acad Sci USA 86:10156–10160, 1989.
67. SR George, M Watanabe, T Di Paolo, P Falardeau, F Labrie, P Seeman. The functional state of the dopamine receptor in the anterior pituitary is in the high-affinity form. Endocrinology 117:690–697, 1985.
68. HW Moises, J Gelernter, LA Giuffra, V Zarcone, L Wetterberg, O Civelli, KK Kidd, LL Cavalli-Sforza, DK Grandy, JL Kennedy. No linkage netween D2 dopamine receptor gene region and schizophrenia. Arch Gen Psychiatry 48:643–647, 1991.
69. G Emilien, J-M Maloteaux, M Geurts, MJ Owen. Dopamine receptors and schizophrenia: contribution of molecular genetics and clinical neuropsychology. Int J Neuropsychopharmacol 2:197–227, 1999.

70. LS Kegeles, A Abi-Dargham, Y Zea-Ponce, J Rodenhiser-Hill, JJ Mann, RL Van Heertum. Modulation of amphetamine-induced striatal dopamine release by ketamine in humans: Implications for schizophrenia. Biol Psychiatry 48:627–640, 2000.

71. S Kapur, P Seeman. Ketamine has equal affinity for NMDA receptors and the high-affinity state of the dopamine D2 receptor. Biol Psychiatry 49:954–957, 2001.

18

Serotonergic Dysfunctions in Schizophrenia
Possible Therapeutic Implications

JOHANNES TAUSCHER
University of Vienna, Vienna, Austria

NICOLAAS PAUL LEONARD GERRIT VERHOEFF
University of Toronto, and Baycrest Centre for Geriatric Care, Toronto, Ontario, Canada

I. INTRODUCTION

There is considerable evidence for a role of the neurotransmitter serotonin (5-hydroxytryptamine; 5HT) in schizophrenia. Numerous studies indicate that the cortical serotonergic signal transduction system is likely to be deficient in that disorder [1–5]. Furthermore, the psychotomimetic actions of 5HT agonists like lysergic acid diathylamide (LSD) and mescaline are well documented and mimic, at least partially, psychotic symptoms seen in schizophrenia [1].

Recent interest in 5HT with regard to antipsychotic drug action has been fueled by the fact that novel antipsychotic drugs such as clozapine, olanzapine, quetiapine, risperidone, sertindole, and ziprasidone are potent $5HT_{2A}$ receptor antagonists and relatively weaker dopamine D_2 antagonists [6]. In addition, $5HT_{1A}$ and $5HT_{2C}$ receptors seem to contribute to clinical effects of some novel antipsychotics [7].

This chapter will provide a selective review of the literature with regard to evidence for serotonergic dysfunctions in schizophrenia. First, we will briefly review the evidence from genetic studies and from challenge experiments with serotonin agonists. Then we will continue with a more detailed description of the possible molecular role of several families of serotonin receptors in schizophrenia, and conclude with an overview about the relevance of serotonin for atypical antipsychotics.

II. GENETICS

While the causes for schizophrenia remain unknown, evidence from family, twin, and adoption studies clearly demonstrates that it aggregates in families. This clustering is largely attributable to genetic rather than cultural or environmental factors. Identifying the genes involved has proved to be a difficult task because schizophrenia is a complex disorder characterized by the existence of phenocopies, low disease penetrance, and an imprecise phenotype. The current working hypothesis for schizophrenia causation is that multiple genes of small to moderate effect confer compounding risk through interactions with each other and with nongenetic risk factors. These same genes may be commonly involved in conferring risk across populations, or they may vary in number and strength among different populations. To search for evidence of such genetic loci, both candidate gene and genome wide linkage studies have been used in clinical cohorts collected from a variety of populations. Collectively, these works provide some evidence for the involvement of a number of specific genes (e.g., the 5HT$_{2A}$ receptor gene [8] and the dopamine D$_3$ receptor gene) and as yet unidentified factors localized to specific chromosomal regions, including 6p, 6q, 8p, 13q, and 22q. These data provide suggestive, but no conclusive, evidence for causative genes. More detailed reviews of the molecular genetics [9] and epigenetics [10] of schizophrenia can be found elsewhere.

III. CHALLENGE STUDIES

Pharmacological challenge with the partial 5HT agonist m-chlorophenylpiperazine (MCPP) significantly increased positive psychotic symptoms in schizophrenic patients but not in healthy controls [11]. This effect appears to be specific for schizophrenia as MCPP has been reported to be anxiogenic but not psychotomimetic in patients with panic disorder, posttraumatic stress disorder, major depressive disorder, obsessive-compulsive disorder, alcohol dependence, or Alzheimer's disease.

IV. SEROTONIN 5HT$_{1A}$ RECEPTORS

Serotonin 5HT$_{1A}$ receptors are located pre- and postsynaptically. The presynaptic 5HT$_{1A}$ receptor is an autoreceptor located on cell bodies of raphe neurons, and its stimulation inhibits firing of 5HT neurons. Stimulation of postsynaptic 5HT$_{1A}$ receptors leads to hyperpolarization of neurons. Human autoradiography revealed the highest density of 5HT$_{1A}$ receptors in temporolimbic cortex, followed by brainstem raphe nuclei, frontal cortex, and other neocortical regions, with very low or undetectable levels in the cerebellum [12]. The brainstem receptors are somatodendritic autoreceptors, while cortical receptors are mainly postsynaptic. The cortical 5HT$_{1A}$ receptors are localized on axon hillocks of pyramidal cells, especially in the layers II, III and V of the cerebral cortex [12]. These receptors are involved in the inhibitory modulation of corticocortical association and corticostriatal efferent fibers [13]. Cortical 5HT$_{1A}$ receptors exert inhibitory control over striatal glutamate release, and 5HT$_{1A}$ antagonists increase glutamate release in the striatum via corticostriatal efferents [14]. In addition, 5HT$_{1A}$ agonists increase the outflow of dopamine in the prefrontal cortex, without a similar change in striatal dopamine release [15]. Stimulation of 5HT$_{1A}$ receptors appears to produce many of the same effects as antagonism of 5HT$_{2A}$ receptors [7].

Earlier efforts to quantitatively analyze 5HT$_{1A}$ receptors were limited by a lack of appropriate ligands. Results obtained with the widely used agonist ligand 8-OH-DPAT were hampered by the fact that it labels 5HT$_{1A}$ receptors only in their high-affinity state. This problem has recently been overcome by the discovery of WAY-100635, a selective high affinity ($K_d < 1$ nM) 5HT$_{1A}$ antagonist, which labels both low- and high-affinity receptors [16].

Postmortem studies showed an elevation in cortical serotonin 5HT$_{1A}$ receptor density in schizophrenia using [^{3}H]8-OH-DPAT as a ligand [17,18]. This finding was subsequently replicated by other groups using 8-OH-DPAT [19–23] and WAY-100635[12] for postmortem quantification of 5HT$_{1A}$ receptors (Table 1).

To adapt WAY-100635 for human studies, it has been labeled at the [*carbonyl*-^{11}C] position [24] and can be used for the quantitative analysis of binding to 5HT$_{1A}$ receptors in humans [25]. Using [*carbonyl*-^{11}C]WAY-100635 and positron emission tomography (PET), cortical 5HT$_{1A}$ binding can be quantitatively analyzed using the cerebellum as input function of a simplified reference tissue model (SRTM) [26].

PET and ^{11}C]WAY-100635 were used to show decreased 5HT$_{1A}$ receptor binding potential (BP) [27] in patients with major depression, [28, 29] as compared to healthy controls. Using PET and ^{11}C]WAY-100635, our group demonstrated an age-dependent decline of cortical 5HT$_{1A}$ receptor BP in healthy volunteers, [30], consistent with postmortem studies which showed a decline in 5HT$_{1A}$ receptor numbers with age [31–33].

Our group recently completed a PET study in 14 neuroleptic-naïve patients with a DSM-IV diagnosis of schizophrenia suffering from a first psychotic episode. On the basis of human postmortem studies, we hypothesized that the in vivo 5HT$_{1A}$ receptor BP as measured with [*carbonyl*-^{11}C]WAY-100635 and PET will be higher in frontal and temporal cortex of schizophrenic patients, as compared to an age-matched control group of healthy volunteers. The 5HT$_{1A}$ BP of 14 antipsychotic naïve patients were compared to 14 age-matched healthy controls [34]. PET data were analyzed using nine cortical regions of interests (ROI), which were delineated on a coregistered MRI scan and transferred to the PET image, with the cerebellum as reference region for a SRTM. Additionally, we

Table 1 Postmortem Studies of Serotonin $5HT_{1A}$ Receptors in Schizophrenia

Study	Pts. vs controls	$5HT_{1A}$ Receptors in prefrontal cortex
Hashimoto et al. [17,18]	10 vs. 11	40% increase in B_{max}[a] in Scz[b] ($P < .05$). No difference in K_d[c]
Joyce et al. [19]	10 vs. 8	20–40% increase in B_{max} in Scz ($P < .01$).
Simpson et al. [20]	12 vs. 18	20–40% increase in B_{max} in male Scz ($P < .05$). No difference in K_d
Burnet et al. [12,21]	9 vs. 8	23% increase in B_{max} in Scz ($P < .01$)
Sumiyoshi et al. [22]	10 vs. 11	79% increase in B_{max} in Scz ($P < .001$). No difference in K_d.
Gurevich et al. [23]	10 vs. 13	20–75% increase in B_{max} in Scz ($P < .05$)

[a] B_{max} = number of $5HT_{1A}$ receptors
[b] Scz = schizophrenic patients
[c] K_d = equilibrium dissociation constant (a measure for affinity)

performed a voxel-wise comparison using Statistical Parametric Mapping (SPM) [35]. The ROI-based analysis revealed a significant mean cortical $5HT_{1A}$ receptor BP increase of 7.1% ((6.4 SD) in schizophrenic patients ($F = 2.975$; $P = .025$); local differences were +20% in left mediotemporal cortex (MTC; $F = 9.339$; $P = .005$) and +13% in right MTC ($F = 4.453$; $P = .045$) [34]. There were no significant differences in regional R_1 values or cerebellar [^{11}C]WAY-100635 uptake. The voxel-based analysis with SPM99 also confirmed a group difference in a small region of the left MTC. In summary, this in vivo PET study revealed a medio-temporal increase of cortical $5HT_{1A}$ receptor BP in patients suffering from a first episode of schizophrenia [34].

All patients in the postmortem studies had received several years of antipsychotic treatment, and all except five in the Hashimoto et al. study [17] were receiving antipsychotics at the time of death. In contrast, all patients in the PET study were antipsychotic naïve. Hence the noted increase in postmortem $5HT_{1A}$ receptors could be an effect of chronic drug treatment. However, there was no correlation between antipsychotic dose at death and the degree of $5HT_{1A}$ elevation, [20–22], and repeated administration of antipsychotics in animals did not alter $5HT_{1A}$ receptor number [17,18].

Another noteworthy confound of the postmortem studies is that patients had an average illness duration of ~ 20 years. In the PET study, the sample consisted of first-episode patients with an average duration of untreated psychosis of 21 months (± 18 SD), ranging from 7 months to 5 years. There is some evidence for an abnormal persistence of $5HT_{1A}$ receptors in schizophrenia, suggesting a failure to regress rather than an abnormal upregulation during the course of the disease [36]. In line with that theory, the PET study was not able to demonstrate any significant correlation between $5HT_{1A}$ receptor BP and duration of the illness.

Most postmortem studies selected limited and often arbitrary brain regions to study. Only two groups studied samples from all cortical regions [17,18,23]. All others investigated only the prefrontal cortex, [12,20–22] or the prefrontal and temporal cortex [19]. While all the postmortem studies report "prefrontal" increases, the data came from Brodmann Areas (BA) 9 [19], 10 [17], 11 and 12 [20], 24, 9a, and 44 [23], or 46 [12,21]. To avoid an unjustified restriction to frontal brain areas in the PET study, $5HT_{1A}$ receptor BP was analyzed in cortical ROI drawn in several cortical regions. Although all ROIs were delineated on the coregistered MRI and were consecutively transferred onto the PET summation image, the process of co-registering introduces another source of error. This also contributes to anatomical inaccuracy of the ROI approach. Moreover, if any given pathology afflicts only parts of an ROI, a possible BP increase or decrease will be diluted. As a result, the chance to miss a group difference is high. With this in mind, the results of the ROI analysis were validated by applying additional voxel-wise analyses with SPM. This approach revealed an elevated $5HT_{1A}$ receptor BP in left MTC of patients, confirming the strongest result of the ROI based approach. Although the left temporal cortex is an anatomical region known to be afflicted in schizophrenia [37], the significance and functional relevance of locally elevated [^{11}C]WAY-100635 uptake in schizophrenic patients is unclear.

V. SEROTONIN 5HT₂ RECEPTORS

The published studies of 5HT$_{2A}$ receptors in schizophrenic patients to date have mainly involved postmortem brain samples, and produced conflicting results. The radioligands [^{3}H]ketanserin, [^{3}H]spiperone, [^{3}H]LSD, and [^{125}I]LSD, which bind to 5HT$_{2A}$ and 5HT$_{2C}$ receptors, were used in 10 studies, and these studies have produced discrepant results: – six studies [18,21,23,38–40] found a reduction in 5HT$_2$ receptor density in the frontal cortex of schizophrenic patients, and the other four did not find significant differences compared to controls [19,41–43]. Limitations of postmortem studies in terms of inaccurate diagnosis, prior medication history, effects of concurrent illnesses and medications at the time of death, different causes of death such as suicide, differences in brain subregions investigated, as well as different radioligands used, further restrict inferences regarding the role of a possible 5HT$_{2A}$ receptor abnormality in schizophrenia. Most of these confounds can be better addressed with in vivo imaging studies.

Among numerous PET tracers developed for 5HT$_{2A}$ receptors, only [^{18}F]altanserin [44–46], ^{18}F]setoperone [47–50], and [^{11}C]MDL 100,907 [51] have demonstrated appropriate in vivo properties for a successful imaging agent in humans. In two recent [^{18}F]setoperone PET studies using ROI analysis no decreases in 5HT$_{2A}$ receptors were observed in neuroleptic-free or neuroleptic-naïve schizophrenic patients [52,53]. However, localized differences may have been diluted in these ROIs if either some areas were considerably smaller than the ROIs or some areas were not or only partially included in the ROIs. Therefore, additional 5HT$_{2A}$ PET studies have been performed using voxel-by-voxel analysis by the application of SPM [35]. One study reanalyzed data from 13 schizophrenic patients obtained in a previous study [53] but compared them with a larger group of 35 age-matched controls [54]. No substantial 5HT$_{2A}$ receptor changes were observed in the schizophrenic patients. Another [^{18}F]setoperone PET study indicated significant 5HT$_{2A}$ receptor decreases in the left and right prefrontal cortex in six schizophrenic patients versus seven age-matched controls [55].

The lack of substantial 5HT$_{2A}$ receptor BP changes observed in vivo is in contrast with the majority of postmortem studies that reported regionally localized 5HT$_{2A}$ decreases in the frontal cortices from schizophrenic patients [18,21,23,38–40]. It is conceivable that the 5HT$_{2A}$ receptor decrease observed in earlier postmortem studies in schizophrenic patients either on antipsychotic medication, or withdrawn from antipsychotics at time of death, was confounded by medication effects. Studies performed in rats suggest that 5HT$_{2A}$ receptor downregulation may be a component of antipsychotic activity not only of atypical antipsychotics (such as clozapine) but of some typical antipsychotics (such as chlorpromazine, thioridazine, and loxapine) as well.[56–59]. Receptor downregulation is less likely to have confounded the results from the in vivo studies as these were performed in neuroleptic-free or neuroleptic-naïve schizophrenic patients with an interval off antipsychotics of at least 1 month, [52], or 7 weeks [53], prior to PET imaging.

However, in one postmortem study that carefully controlled for the use of antipsychotics at time of death, nonsuicidal schizophrenic patients who had been medication free for at least 1 month showed significant 5HT$_2$ receptor decreases in the anterior cingulate and medial and superior parts of the premotor cortex, corresponding to BAs 24 and 6, more pronounced in cortical layer III than in layer VI [23]. Cortical 5HT$_{2A}$ receptors are localized on apical dendrites of pyramidal neurons [60–62] and on certain subclasses of GABAergic interneurons that provide inhibitory input to pyramidal cells [63–66]. Post mortem studies have shown that in the prefrontal cortex of schizophrenic patients selective subclasses of GABAergic interneurons are decreased [67], unchanged [68], or increased [69]. The assessment of 5HT$_{2A}$ receptor BP in vivo is not sufficiently specific or sensitive to detect selective 5HT$_{2A}$ decreases in cortical layers or selective decreases and increases in subclasses of GABA-ergic interneurons expressing 5HT$_{2A}$ receptors.

In addition, the sensitivity of the in vivo studies to detect group differences has been limited. Given the relatively small sample sizes of the schizophrenic patient groups in these studies, reductions in 5HT$_{2A}$ receptor density may not have been detected if these had been minimal, in areas of high 5HT$_{2A}$ receptor density variability, or with an variable location, leading to type 2 errors [70]. Nevertheless, a recent PET study using SPM analysis which showed significant 5HT$_{2A}$ receptor BP decreases in the left and right prefrontal cortex in six schizophrenic patients versus seven controls indicates that such a detection is feasible in vivo [55]. The discrepant findings between the in vivo studies could, similar to the discrepancies among the postmortem studies, be due to heterogeneity in the populations of schizophrenic patients studied.

VI. SEROTONIN 5HT₃ RECEPTORS

In one postmortem study, ^{3}H]LY278584 was used to analyze binding to serotonin 5HT$_3$ receptors in samples of amygdala from schizophrenic and matched control subjects [71]. All of the schizophrenic patients but none of the controls had been treated with neuroleptics. In a first step, the effects of short- and long-term haloperidol administration on limbic 5HT$_3$ receptors were investigated in rodents, and no effect was found. Furthermore, no differences in the maximum number of 5HT$_3$ binding sites or equilibrium dissociation constant between schizophrenics and controls were found in the amygdala. This study did not support the presence of an alteration of 5HT$_3$ receptors in the amygdala in schizophrenic patients [71].

VII. SEROTONIN TRANSPORTERS

Serotonin transporters (SERT) have been implied to play a role in various psychiatric disorders. Single-photon emission computed tomography (SPECT) and the ligand [¹²³I](-CIT revealed a decreased SERT density in depression, [72] and in seasonal affective [73] and eating disorders [74]. However, an in vivo SPECT study investigating potential alterations of striatal dopamine transporters (DAT) and brainstem SERT density in schizophrenia did not find alterations of DAT in the striatum or SERT in the brainstem [75], although one postmortem study in schizophrenic patients had shown decreased SERT in the prefrontal cortex [43].

VIII. SEROTONIN AND ATYPICAL ANTIPSYCHOTICS

Serotonin receptors implicated in the action atypical antipsychotic agents, such as clozapine, or other recently introduced novel antipsychotics include 5HT$_{1A}$, 5HT$_{2A}$, 5HT$_{2C}$, 5HT$_3$, 5HT$_6$, and 5HT$_7$ receptors [76]. These are also of potential value for developing more effective or better-tolerated antipsychotic agents. It was initially thought that a relatively higher 5HT$_{2A}$ receptor affinity as compared to that for the D$_2$ receptor is the basis for the difference between "atypical" and "typical" antipsychotic agents, with "atypical antipsychotic" defined as an agent causing low EPS at doses with demonstrated or putative antipsychotic activity. This hypothesis contributed to the development of newer antipsychotic agents, all of which are consistent with the hypothesis of high affinity for 5HT$_{2A}$ and low affinity for D$_2$ receptors [6]. While some of the atypical antipsychotic drugs also have affinities for 5HT$_{2C}$, 5HT$_6$, or 5HT$_7$ receptors that are in the same range as those for the 5HT$_{2A}$ receptor, it has been found that this is not a common characteristic of these agents and, thus, it is not likely that affinities for 5HT$_{2C}$, 5HT$_6$ or 5HT$_7$ receptors are primary factors contributing to the low EPS profile of the entire class of agents [6,77,78]. However, the low EPS effects of specific drugs, or other actions, could still be dependent on their affinity for one or more of these 5HT receptors, including the 5HT$_{2C}$ and 5HT$_7$ receptors. Among other factors, 5HT$_{1A}$ receptor agonism has also been suggested to be able to contribute to an atypical antipsychotic drug profile [7,79]. Furthermore, there is extensive evidence for interactions among 5HT$_{2A}$, 5HT$_{2C}$, and 5HT$_{1A}$ receptors [80].

Serotonin 5HT$_{2A}$ receptors have been implicated in the genesis and treatment of psychosis, negative symptoms, mood disturbance, and EPS. The antipsychotic effect of clozapine has been attributed, in part, to its ability to block excessive 5HT$_{2A}$ receptor stimulation [81]. This is supported by the high occupancy of 5HT$_{2A}$ receptors produced by clozapine at clinically effective doses and its low occupancy of D$_2$ receptors [80].

Clinical trials of ritanserin, a potent 5HT$_{2A}$ and 5HT$_{2C}$ antagonist, were conducted to test the contribution of 5HT$_{2A}$ receptor antagonism to antipsychotic drug action. The limited data available suggest little or no beneficial effect, and 5HT$_{2C}$ receptor antagonism might even oppose the beneficial effects of 5HT$_{2A}$ receptor blockade. The bell-shaped dose response curve of risperidone, with higher doses being less effective than lower doses, [82], suggests that excessive D$_2$ receptor antagonism may diminish some of the beneficial effects of 5HT$_{2A}$ receptor blockade [78]. The potent D$_4$/5HT$_{2A}$ receptor antagonist fananserin was ineffective in acutely psychotic patients with schizophrenia [83]. Additional evidence supporting the role of 5HT$_{2A}$ receptor blockade in the action of clozapine and possibly other drugs with potent 5HT$_{2A}$ affinities is available from the several reports that the *His452Tyr* allele of the 5HT$_{2A}$ receptor, which is present in 10–12% of the population, is associated with a higher frequency of poor response to clozapine [84]. In summary, the evidence from clinical trial data suggests that 5HT$_{2A}$ receptor blockade may contribute to antipsychotic drug action.

Serotonin 5HT$_{1A}$ receptors may be of interest for the development of novel medications as there is some preclinical evidence to support a role for 5HT$_{1A}$ agonism in the antipsychotic action and extrapyramidal side effects of drugs [7,79,85]. Results of behavioral studies in animals using the $5HT_{1A}$ agonist 8-OH-DPAT first suggested in the late 1980s that stimulation of $5HT_{1A}$ receptors might produce antipsychoticlike effects [86]. Subsequent studies demonstrated that 8-OH-DPAT enhanced the antipsychotic-like effect of the D_2/D_3 antagonist raclopride [87] and haloperidol [88], and antagonized the catalepsy induced by the D_1 agonist SCH23390 in rats [89]. It was recently demonstrated that 8-OH-DPAT inhibited the ability of clozapine and low-dose risperidone, but not haloperidol, to increase extracellular DA levels in the nucleus accumbens and the striatum of conscious rats [85]. Several atypical antipsychotic drugs are partial agonists at the $5HT_{1A}$ receptor, including clozapine, ziprasidone, quetiapine and tiospirone. The affinities of these drugs for $5HT_{1A}$ receptors were similar to their affinities at the human D_2 dopamine receptor [90]. These findings suggest that the combination of D_2 antagonism and $5HT_{1A}$ agonism may produce an atypical antipsychotic agent. S16924 is an example of such a compound. It has atypical properties very similar to those of clozapine in a variety of animal models [91]. Compounds such as ziprasidone and clozapine combine $5HT_{1A}$ agonism and $5HT_{2A}$ antagonism. Clinical studies of adding $5HT_{1A}$ partial agonists such as buspirone, ipsapirone, and tandospirone may help to clarify the possible importance of $5HT_{1A}$ agonism in the treatment of schizophrenia.

REFERENCES

1. Breier A. Serotonin, schizophrenia and antipsychotic drug action. Schizophr Res 1995;14(3):187–202.
2. Huttunen M. The evolution of the serotonin-dopamine antagonist concept. J Clin Psychopharmacol 1995;15 (1 suppl 1):4S–10S.
3. Iqbal N, Van Praag HM. The role of serotonin in schizophrenia. Eur Neuropsychopharmacol 1995; 5(suppl):11–23.
4. Abi-Dargham A, Laruelle M, Aghajanian GK, Charney D, Krystal J. The role of serotonin in the pathophysiology and treatment of schizophrenia. J Neuropsychiatry Clin Neurosci 1997;9(1):1–17.
5. Kroeze WK, Roth BL. The molecular biology of serotonin receptors: therapeutic implications for the interface of mood and psychosis. Biol Psychiatry 1998;44(11):1128–1142.
6. Schotte A, Janssen PF, Gommeren W, Luyten WH, Van Gompel P, Lesage AS, et al. Risperidone compared with new and reference antipsychotic drugs: in vitro and in vivo receptor binding. Psychopharmacology (Berl) 1996;124(1–2):57–73.
7. Meltzer HY. The role of serotonin in antipsychotic drug action. Neuropsychopharmacology 1999;21(2 suppl):106S-15S.
8. Williams J, Spurlock G, McGuffin P, Mallet J, Nothen MM, Gill M, et al. Association between schizophrenia and T102C polymorphism of the 5- hydroxytryptamine type 2a-receptor gene. European Multicentre Association Study of Schizophrenia (EMASS) Group. Lancet 1996;347(9011):1294–1296.
9. Mowry BJ, Nancarrow DJ. Molecular genetics of schizophrenia. Clin Exp Pharmacol Physiol 2001;28(1–2):66–69.
10. Petronis A. The genes for major psychosis: aberrant sequence or regulation? Neuropsychopharmacology 2000;23(1):1–12.
11. Krystal JH, Seibyl JP, Price LH, Woods SW, Heninger GR, Aghajanian GK, et al. m-Chlorophenylpiperazine effects in neuroleptic-free schizophrenic patients. Evidence implicating serotonergic systems in the positive symptoms of schizophrenia. Arch Gen Psychiatry 1993;50(8):624–635.
12. Burnet PW, Eastwood SL, Harrison PJ. [^{3}H]WAY-100635 for 5HT1A receptor autoradiography in human brain: a comparison with [^{3}H]8-OH-DPAT and demonstration of increased binding in the frontal cortex in schizophrenia. Neurochem Int 1997;30(6):565–574.
13. Bowen DM, Francis PT, Pangalos MN, Chessell IP. Neurotransmitter receptors of rat cortical pyramidal neurones: implications for in vivo imaging and therapy. J Reprod Fertil suppl 1993;46:131–143.
14. Dijk SN, Francis PT, Stratmann GC, Bowen DM. NMDA-induced glutamate and aspartate release from rat cortical pyramidal neurones: evidence for modulation by a 5HT1A antagonist. Br J Pharmacol 1995;115(7):1169–1174.
15. Wedzony K, Mackowiak M, Fijal K, Golembiowska K. Ipsapirone enhances the dopamine outflow via 5HT1A receptors in the rat prefrontal cortex. Eur J Pharmacol 1996;305(1–3):73–78.
16. Fletcher A, Cliffe IA, Dourish CT. Silent 5HT1A receptor antagonists: utility as research tools and therapeutic agents. Trends Pharmacol Sci 1993;14(12): 41–48.
17. Hashimoto T, Nishino N, Nakai H, Tanaka C. Increase in serotonin 5HT1A receptors in prefrontal and temporal cortices of brains from patients with chronic schizophrenia. Life Sci 1991;48(4):355–363.
18. Hashimoto T, Kitamura N, Kajimoto Y, Shirai Y, Shirakawa O, Mita T, et al. Differential changes in serotonin 5HT1A and 5HT2 receptor binding in patients with chronic schizophrenia. Psychopharmacology (Berl) 1993;112(1):S35–S39.
19. Joyce JN, Shane A, Lexow N, Winokur A, Casanova MF, Kleinman JE. Serotonin uptake sites and serotonin receptors are altered in the limbic system of schizophrenics. Neuropsychopharmacology 1993;8(4):315–336.

20. Simpson MD, Lubman DI, Slater P, Deakin JF. Autoradiography with [³H]8-OH-DPAT reveals increases in 5HT(1A) receptors in ventral prefrontal cortex in schizophrenia. Biol Psychiatry 1996;39(11): 919–928.
21. Burnet PW, Eastwood SL, Harrison PJ. 5HT1A and 5HT2A receptor mRNAs and binding site densities are differentially altered in schizophrenia. Neuropsychopharmacology 1996;15(5):442–455.
22. Sumiyoshi T, Stockmeier CA, Overholser JC, Dilley GE, Meltzer HY. Serotonin1A receptors are increased in postmortem prefrontal cortex in schizophrenia. Brain Res 1996;708(1–2):209–214.
23. Gurevich EV, Joyce JN. Alterations in the cortical serotonergic system in schizophrenia: a postmortem study. Biol Psychiatry 1997;42(7):529–545.
24. Farde L, Ginovart N, Ito H, Lundkvist C, Pike VW, McCarron JA, et al. PET-characterization of [carbonyl-¹¹C]WAY-100635 binding to 5HT1A receptors in the primate brain. Psychopharmacology (Berl) 1997;133(2):196–202.
25. Farde L, Ito H, Swahn CG, Pike VW, Halldin C. Quantitative analyses of carbonyl-carbon-11-WAY-100635 binding to central 5-hydroxytryptamine-1A receptors in man. J Nucl Med 1998;39(11):1965–1971.
26. Lammertsma AA, Hume SP. Simplified reference tissue model for PET receptor studies. Neuroimage 1996;4 (3 Pt 1):153–158.
27. Mintun MA, Raichle ME, Kilbourn MR, Wooten GF, Welch MJ. A quantitative model for the in vivo assessment of drug binding sites with positron emission tomography. Ann Neurol 1984;15(3):217–227.
28. Drevets WC, Frank E, Price JC, Kupfer DJ, Holt D, Greer PJ, et al. PET imaging of serotonin 1A receptor binding in depression. Biol Psychiatry 1999;46(10): 1375–1387.
29. Sargent PA, Kjaer KH, Bench CJ, Rabiner EA, Messa C, Meyer J, et al. Brain serotonin1A receptor binding measured by positron emission tomography with [¹¹C]WAY-100635: effects of depression and antidepressant treatment. Arch Gen Psychiatry 2000;57(2):174–180.
30. Tauscher J, Verhoeff NPLG, Christensen BK, Hussey D, Meyer JH, Kecojevic A, et al. Serotonin 5HT1A receptor binding potential declines with age as measured by [¹¹C]WAY-100635 and PET. Neuropsychopharmacology 2001;24(5):522–530.
31. Dillon KA, Gross-Isseroff R, Israeli M, Biegon A. Autoradiographic analysis of serotonin 5HT1A receptor binding in the human brain postmortem: effects of age and alcohol. Brain Res 1991;554(1–2): 56–64.
32. Lowther S, De Paermentier F, Cheetham SC, Crompton MR, Katona CL, Horton RW. 5HT1A receptor binding sites in postmortem brain samples from depressed suicides and controls. J Affect Disord 1997;42(2–3):199–207.
33. Matsubara S, Arora RC, Meltzer HY. Serotonergic measures in suicide brain: 5HT1A binding sites in frontal cortex of suicide victims. J Neural Transm Gen Sect 1991;85(3):181–194.
34. Tauscher J, Kapur S, Verhoeff NPLG, Hussey DF, Daskalakis ZJ, Tauscher-Wisniewski S, Wilson AA, Houle S, Kasper S, Zipursky RB. Brain serotonin 5-HT₁A receptor binding in schizophrenia measured by positron emission tomography and [¹¹C]WAY-100635. Arch Gen Psychiatry 2002;6:514–520.
35. Friston KJ, Holmes AP, Worsley KJ, Poline JP, Frith CD, Frackowiack RSJ. Statistical parametric maps in functional imaging: a general linear approach. Hum Brain Mapping 1995;2:189–210.
36. Slater P, Doyle CA, Deakin JF. Abnormal persistence of cerebellar serotonin-1A receptors in schizophrenia suggests failure to regress in neonates. J Neural Transm 1998;105(2–3):305–315.
37. Hirayasu Y, McCarley RW, Salisbury DF, Tanaka S, Kwon JS, Frumin M, et al. Planum temporale and Heschl gyrus volume reduction in schizophrenia: a magnetic resonance imaging study of first-episode patients. Arch Gen Psychiatry 2000;57(7):692–699.
38. Bennett JP Jr, Enna SJ, Bylund DB, Gillin JC, Wyatt RJ, Snyder SH. Neurotransmitter receptors in frontal cortex of schizophrenics. Arch Gen Psychiatry 1979;36(9):927–934.
39. Mita T, Hanada S, Nishino N, Kuno T, Nakai H, Yamadori T, et al. Decreased serotonin S2 and increased dopamine D2 receptors in chronic schizophrenics. Biol Psychiatry 1986;21(14):1407–1414.
40. Arora RC, Meltzer HY. Serotonin2 (5HT2) receptor binding in the frontal cortex of schizophrenic patients. J Neural Transm Gen Sect 1991;85(1):19–29.
41. Whitaker PM, Crow TJ, Ferrier IN. Tritiated LSD binding in frontal cortex in schizophrenia. Arch Gen Psychiatry 1981;38(3):278–280.
42. Reynolds GP, Rossor MN, Iversen LL. Preliminary studies of human cortical 5HT2 receptors and their involvement in schizophrenia and neuroleptic drug action. J Neural Transm suppl 1983;18:273–277.
43. Laruelle M, Abi-Dargham A, Casanova MF, Toti R, Weinberger DR, Kleinman JE. Selective abnormalities of prefrontal serotonergic receptors in schizophrenia. A postmortem study. Arch Gen Psychiatry 1993;50(10):810–818.
44. Biver F, Goldman S, Luxen A, Monclus M, Forestini M, Mendlewicz J, et al. Multicompartmental study of fluorine-18 altanserin binding to brain 5HT2 receptors in humans using positron emission tomography. Eur J Nucl Med 1994;21(9):937–946.
45. Sadzot B, Lemaire C, Maquet P, Salmon E, Plenevaux A, Degueldre C, et al. Serotonin 5HT2 receptor imaging in the human brain using positron emission tomography and a new radioligand, [¹⁸F]altanserin: results in young normal controls. J Cereb Blood Flow Metab 1995;15(5):787–797.

46. Rosier A, Dupont P, Peuskens J, Bormans G, Vandenberghe R, Maes M, et al. Visualisation of loss of 5HT2A receptors with age in healthy volunteers using [^{18}F]altanserin and positron emission tomographic imaging. Psychiatry Res 1996;68(1):11–22.

47. Blin J, Sette G, Fiorelli M, Bletry O, Elghozi JL, Crouzel C, et al. A method for the in vivo investigation of the serotonergic 5HT2 receptors in the human cerebral cortex using positron emission tomography and ^{18}F-labeled setoperone. J Neurochem 1990;54(5):1744–1754.

48. Petit-Taboue MC, Landeau B, Osmont A, Barre L, Luet D, Tillet I, et al. Estimation of cortical 5HT2 receptor (5HT2R) binding parameters from single dose ^{18}F-setoperone data in baboons: comparison of different methods [abstract]. J Cereb Blood Flow Metab 1993;13(suppl 1):S795.

49. Petit-Taboue MC, Landeau B, Osmont A, Tillet I, Barre L, Baron JC. Estimation of neocortical serotonin-2 receptor binding potential by single-dose fluorine-18-setoperone kinetic PET data analysis. J Nucl Med 1996;37(1):95–104.

50. Petit-Taboue MC, Landeau B, Barre L, Onfroy MC, Noel MH, Baron JC. Parametric PET imaging of 5HT2A receptor distribution with ^{18}F-setoperone in the normal human neocortex. J Nucl Med 1999;40(1):25–32.

51. Ito H, Nyberg S, Halldin C, Lundkvist C, Farde L. PET imaging of central 5HT2A receptors with carbon-11-MDL 100,907. J Nucl Med 1998;39(1):208–214.

52. Trichard C, Paillere-Martinot ML, Attar-Levy D, Blin J, Feline A, Martinot JL. No serotonin 5HT2A receptor density abnormality in the cortex of schizophrenic patients studied with PET. Schizophr Res 1998;31(1):13–7.

53. Lewis R, Kapur S, Jones C, DaSilva J, Brown GM, Wilson AA, et al. Serotonin 5HT2 receptors in schizophrenia: a PET study using [^{18}F]setoperone in neuroleptic-naive patients and normal subjects. Am J Psychiatry 1999;156(1):72–78.

54. Verhoeff NP, Meyer JH, Kecojevic A, Hussey D, Lewis R, Tauscher J, et al. A voxel-by-voxel analysis of [^{18}F]setoperone PET data shows no substantial serotonin 5HT(2A) receptor changes in schizophrenia. Psychiatry Res 2000;99(3):123–135.

55. Ngan ET, Yatham LN, Ruth TJ, Liddle PF. Decreased serotonin 2A receptor densities in neuroleptic-naive patients with schizophrenia: a PET study using [(^{18})F]setoperone. Am J Psychiatry 2000;157(6):1016–1018.

56. Lee T, Tang SW. Loxapine and clozapine decrease serotonin (S2) but do not elevate dopamine (D2) receptor numbers in the rat brain. Psychiatry Res 1984;12(4):277–285.

57. Andree TH, Mikuni M, Tong CY, Koenig JI, Meltzer HY. Differential effect of subchronic treatment with various neuroleptic agents on serotonin2 receptors in rat cerebral cortex. J Neurochem 1986;46(1):191–197.

58. Matsubara S, Meltzer HY. Effect of typical and atypical antipsychotic drugs on 5HT2 receptor density in rat cerebral cortex. Life Sci 1989;45(15):1397–1406.

59. Kuoppamaki M, Palvimaki EP, Hietala J, Syvalahti E. Differential regulation of rat 5HT2A and 5HT2C receptors after chronic treatment with clozapine, chlorpromazine and three putative atypical antipsychotic drugs. Neuropsychopharmacology 1995;13(2):139–150.

60. Araneda R, Andrade R. 5-Hydroxytryptamine2 and 5-hydroxytryptamine 1A receptors mediate opposing responses on membrane excitability in rat association cortex. Neuroscience 1991;40(2):399–412.

61. Tanaka E, North RA. Actions of 5-hydroxytryptamine on neurons of the rat cingulate cortex. J Neurophysiol 1993;69(5):1749–1757.

62. Jakab RL, Goldman-Rakic PS. 5-Hydroxytryptamine2A serotonin receptors in the primate cerebral cortex: possible site of action of hallucinogenic and antipsychotic drugs in pyramidal cell apical dendrites. Proc Natl Acad Sci USA 1998;95(2):735–740.

63. Sheldon PW, Aghajanian GK. Excitatory responses to serotonin (5HT) in neurons of the rat piriform cortex: evidence for mediation by 5HT1C receptors in pyramidal cells and 5HT2 receptors in interneurons. Synapse 1991;9(3):208–218.

64. Gellman RL, Aghajanian GK. Pyramidal cells in piriform cortex receive a convergence of inputs from monoamine activated GABAergic interneurons. Brain Res 1993;600(1):63–73.

65. Marek GJ, Aghajanian GK. Excitation of interneurons in piriform cortex by 5-hydroxytryptamine: blockade by MDL 100,907, a highly selective 5HT2A receptor antagonist. Eur J Pharmacol 1994;259(2):137–141.

66. Morilak DA, Somogyi P, Lujan-Miras R, Ciaranello RD. Neurons expressing 5HT2 receptors in the rat brain: neurochemical identification of cell types by immunocytochemistry. Neuropsychopharmacology 1994;11(3):157–166.

67. Woo TU, Whitehead RE, Melchitzky DS, Lewis DA. A subclass of prefrontal gamma-aminobutyric acid axon terminals are selectively altered in schizophrenia. Proc Natl Acad Sci USA 1998;95(9):5341–5346.

68. Woo TU, Miller JL, Lewis DA. Schizophrenia and the parvalbumin-containing class of cortical local circuit neurons. Am J Psychiatry 1997;154(7):1013–1015.

69. Beasley CL, Reynolds GP. Parvalbumin-immunoreactive neurons are reduced in the prefrontal cortex of schizophrenics. Schizophr Res 1997;24(3):349–355.

70. Wright IC, Ellison ZR, Sharma T, Friston KJ, Murray RM, McGuire PK. Mapping of grey matter changes in schizophrenia. Schizophr Res 1999;35(1):1–14.

71. Abi-Dargham A, Laruelle M, Lipska B, Jaskiw GE, Wong DT, Robertson DW, et al. Serotonin 5HT3

receptors in schizophrenia: a postmortem study of the amygdala. Brain Res 1993;616(1–2):53–57.
72. Malison RT, Price LH, Berman R, Van Dyck CH, Pelton GH, Carpenter L, et al. Reduced brain serotonin transporter availability in major depression as measured by [^{123}I]-2 beta-carbomethoxy-3 beta-(4-iodophenyl)tropane and single photon emission computed tomography. Biol Psychiatry 1998;44(11):1090–1098.
73. Willeit M, Praschak-Rieder N, Neumeister A, Pirker W, Asenbaum S, Vitouch O, et al. [^{123}I]-beta-CIT SPECT imaging shows reduced brain serotonin transporter availability in drug-free depressed patients with seasonal affective disorder. Biol Psychiatry 2000;47(6):482–489.
74. Tauscher J, Pirker W, Willeit M, de Zwaan M, Bailer U, Neumeister A, et al. [^{123}I] beta-CIT and single photon emission computed tomography reveal reduced brain serotonin transporter availability in bulimia nervosa. Biol Psychiatry 2001;49(4):326–332.
75. Laruelle M, Abi-Dargham A, Van Dyck C, Gil R, D'Souza DC, Krystal J, et al. Dopamine and serotonin transporters in patients with schizophrenia: an imaging study with [(^{123})I]beta-CIT. Biol Psychiatry 2000;47(5):371–379.
76. Meltzer HY, Nash JF. Effects of antipsychotic drugs on serotonin receptors. Pharmacol Rev 1991;43(4):587–604.
77. Roth BL, Craigo SC, Choudhary MS, Uluer A, Monsma FJ Jr, Shen Y, et al. Binding of typical and atypical antipsychotic agents to 5-hydroxytryptamine-6 and 5-hydroxytryptamine-7 receptors. J Pharmacol Exp Ther 1994;268(3):1403–1410.
78. Meltzer HY, Fatemi SH. The role of serotonin in schizophrenia and the mechanism of action on anti-psychotic drugs. In: Kane JM, Moller HJ, Awouters F, eds. Serotonergic Mechanisms in Antipsychotic Treatment. New York: Marcel Decker; 1996. pp 77–107.
79. Protais P, Chagraoui A, Arbaoui J, Mocaer E. Dopamine receptor antagonist properties of S 14506, 8-OH-DPAT, raclopride and clozapine in rodents. Eur J Pharmacol 1994;271(1):167–177.
80. Kapur S, Remington G. Serotonin-dopamine interaction and its relevance to schizophrenia. Am J Psychiatry 1996;153(4):466–476.
81. Meltzer HY, Matsubara S, Lee JC. Classification of typical and atypical antipsychotic drugs on the basis of dopamine D-1, D-2 and serotonin2 pK$_i$ values. J Pharmacol Exp Ther 1989;251(1):238–246.

82. Marder SR, Meibach RC. Risperidone in the treatment of schizophrenia. Am J Psychiatry 1994;151(6):825–835.
83. Truffinet P, Tamminga CA, Fabre LF, Meltzer HY, Riviere ME, Papillon-Downey C. Placebo-controlled study of the D4/5HT2A antagonist fananserin in the treatment of schizophrenia. Am J Psychiatry 1999;156(3):419–425.
84. Masellis M, Basile V, Meltzer HY, Lieberman JA, Sevy S, Macciardi FM, et al. Serotonin subtype 2 receptor genes and clinical response to clozapine in schizophrenia patients. Neuropsychopharmacology 1998;19(2):123–132.
85. Ichikawa J, Meltzer HY. The effect of serotonin(1A) receptor agonism on antipsychotic drug- induced dopamine release in rat striatum and nucleus accumbens. Brain Res 2000;858(2):252–263.
86. Ahlenius S. Antipsychotic-like properties of the 5HT1A agonist 8-OH-DPAT in the rat. Pharmacol Toxicol 1989;64(1):3–5.
87. Wadenberg ML, Ahlenius S. Antipsychotic-like profile of combined treatment with raclopride and 8-OH-DPAT in the rat: enhancement of antipsychotic-like effects without catalepsy. J Neural Transm Gen Sect 1991;83(1–2):43–53.
88. Prinssen EP, Kleven MS, Koek W. Effects of dopamine antagonists in a two-way active avoidance procedure in rats: interactions with 8-OH-DPAT, ritanserin, and prazosin. Psychopharmacology (Berl) 1996;128(2):191–197.
89. Wadenberg ML. Antagonism by 8-OH-DPAT, but not ritanserin, of catalepsy induced by SCH 23390 in the rat. J Neural Transm Gen Sect 1992;89(1–2):49–59.
90. Newman-Tancredi A, Gavaudan S, Conte C, Chaput C, Touzard M, Verriele L, et al. Agonist and antagonist actions of antipsychotic agents at 5HT1A receptors: a [^{35}S]GTPgammaS binding study. Eur J Pharmacol 1998;355(2–3):245–256.
91. Millan MJ, Schreiber R, Dekeyne A, Rivet JM, Bervoets K, Mavridis M, et al. S 16924 ((R)-2-[1-[2-(2,3-dihydro-benzo[1,4] dioxin-5-yloxy)-ethyl]- pyrrolidin-3yl]-1-(4-fluoro-phenyl)-ethanone), a novel, potential antipsychotic with marked serotonin (5HT)1A agonist properties. II. Functional profile in comparison to clozapine and haloperidol. J Pharmacol Exp Ther 1998;286(3):1356–1373.

19

The GABA Cell in Relation to Schizophrenia and Bipolar Disorder

FRANCINE M. BENES and SABINA BERRETTA
McLean Hospital, Belmont, and Harvard Medical School, Boston, Massachusetts, U.S.A.

I. INTRODUCTION

Neurons that express the compound γ-aminobutyric acid (GABA) are broadly present throughout the central nervous system, although the cerebral cortex shows the most abundant quantities of this neurotransmitter [1]. Over the past several decades, several subtypes of GABA cell have been identified using a combination of anatomical and physiological approaches (Fig. 1). In the discussion that follows, the functional integration of various types of GABA-ergic interneuron [for a review, see 2] in the cortex and hippocampus will be related to recent postmortem studies implicating this transmitter system in the pathophysiology of schizophrenia and its treatment with neuroleptic drugs [for more comprehensive reviews on cortical and hippocampal neurons, see 3–5].

II. FUNCTIONS OF GABA-ERGIC INTERNEURONS IN THE CORTEX AND IN THE HIPPOCAMPUS

A. Feedback and Feedforward Activity

Basic electrophysiological studies have demonstrated that the action of GABA is typically an inhibitory one [6]. It seems obvious from the above discussion, however, that different interneuronal subpopulations play different and highly specialized roles in rather complex circuits. At the most basic level, most inhibitory interneurons in the cortex and hippocampus are involved in either *feedback* or *feedforward* inhibitory mechanisms which are thought to help stabilize the activity of pyramidal neurons. In *feedback inhibition,* an excitatory input activates the pyramidal neuron, which in turn excites inhibitory interneurons through recurrent collateral fibers [7]. The inhibitory interneurons thereby activated inhibit principal projection neurons, including those that directly excited them. Intracellular recordings from cortical pyramidal cells typically show a depolarization of brief duration that is followed by a longer lasting hyperpolarization [8]; it is the latter component of this complex that reflects the action of GABA on the $GABA_A$-chloride ionophore complex expressed by most postsynaptic neurons [for a comprehensive review, see 9]. Such an arrangement provides a "fail safe" mechanism that ensures pyramidal neuron do not fire excessively.

In a *feedforward* system, on the other hand, pyramidal neurons (e.g., in CA3) project downstream to other pyramidal cells in CA1 (Fig. 2, upper panel). In addition, however, these excitatory neurons also project to interneurons of CA1, and this ultimately curtails the excitability of pyramidal neurons in this latter sector [10].

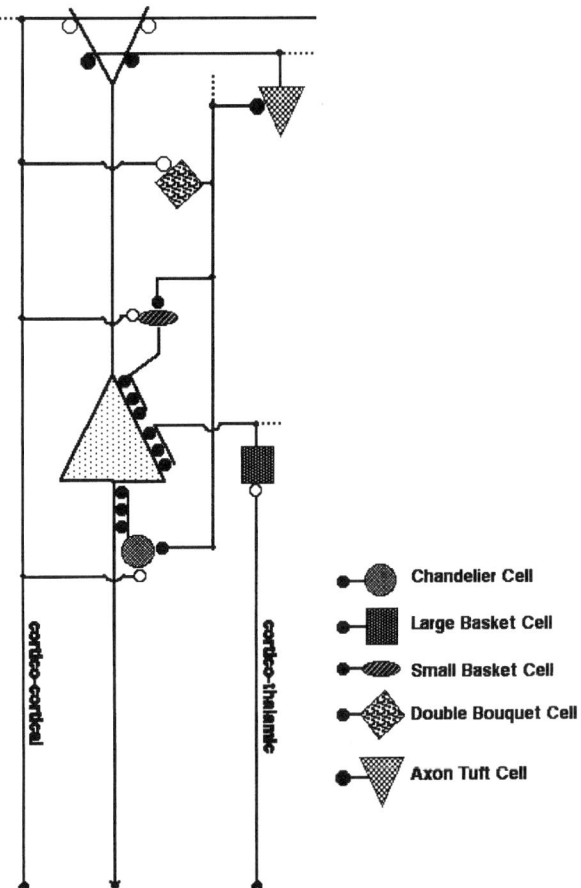

Figure 1 Schematic diagram showing the relationship between various types of GABA-ergic interneurons and a pyramidal cell (black, open circles). Small and large *basket cells*, respectively, form axosomatic contacts with the cell body of the pyramidal neuron. A *chandelier cell* forms axo-axonic synapses with the proximal portion of the pyramidal cell dendrite. A *double bouquet* cell is shown forming GABA-to-GABA synapses with a small basket cell and a large basket cell and a axon tuft cell. A fourth type of interneuron, called a Martinotti cell (MC), is also found predominantly in layer VI and may be excitatory in nature. Not shown are the Cajal-Retzius neurons that are primarily found in layer I and to a lesser extent layer II of the cortex. Interneurons are depicted as receiving excitatory inputs from extrinsic afferents from other regions. (From Ref. 179).

B. Network Oscillations

In both the cortex and the hippocampus, complex interconnections between GABA-ergic interneurons and pyramidal cells have been found to establish and maintain large scale network oscillations, such as those in the theta, gamma (40–100 Hz) and ultra-fast (200 Hz) frequency ranges [3,11–23]. Studies of theta oscillations have demonstrated that both interneurons and pyramidal cells fire during the negative phase of the waveform; however, the interneurons discharge earlier than pyramidal cells. In the cortex, networks of inhibitory interneurons have been found to entrain pyramidal cell discharges. This results in coherent oscillations that have been proposed to "group" or "bind" features detected in different cortical areas into unified perceived objects [19]. In the hippocampus, these oscillations have been proposed to provide the "context" for the "content" coded by excitatory projection neurons [for review see [21,22]. According to this hypothesis, GABA-ergic "supernetworks" may control pyramidal neurons and provide the temporal structure needed to coordinate and maintain the function of neuronal ensembles in the hippocampus. The available evidence suggests that networks of hippocampal interneurons are capable of generating gamma frequency oscillations [24]. For the theta rhythm, basket cells have been found to have regular membrane oscillations, and the occurrence of rhythmic inhibitory postsynaptic potentials are believed to involve GABA-ergic inputs from the septal nuclei [25]. Thus, GABA-to-GABA interactions, albeit ones involving extrinsic afferents, may play a key role in the generation of some rhythmic activity generated by the hippocampus.

C. Discriminative Processing

Growing evidence supports the hypothesis that cortical interneurons can influence the discriminative properties of pyramidal neurons. For example, in the visual system, GABA-ergic interneurons play a key role in modulating geniculate inputs to the primary visual cortex and in defining the orientation selectivity of its neurons [8,26]. Support for a role of interneurons in the shaping of receptive fields has been extended to other cortical areas such as the somatosensory cortex [27–30]. For example, recordings from layer IV neurons of the somatosensory cortex in the presence of GABA receptor antagonists have shown that inhibitory receptive field properties of barrel neurons can be explained by intrabarrel inhibition and that the expansion of receptive field size during GABA blockade is due to an enhanced effectiveness of convergent, multiwhisker thalamocortical inputs [31]. Interestingly, in monkey prefrontal cortex, interneurons have similar receptive fields to those found for pyramidal neurons. This suggests that interneurons carry a specific informational signal that helps in shaping receptive fields [32]. Furthermore, it has been shown that, in the motor cortex, intrinsic inhibitory circuits maintain and adapt motor representations [33]. Inhibitory interneurons appear to be able to unmask latent connections, so that rather than being "hard-wired" somatotopic maps, they show a marked degree of plasticity and can continually reorganize [33]. It can readily be appreciated that similar neurons located in associative cortical regions may play a similar role in defining the nature and integrity of higher cognitive functions, such as motivation, attention, learning, and object recognition. For example, recent findings suggest a role for cortical interneurons in working memory [30,34,35]. In the dorsal prefrontal cortex "fast-spiking" interneurons have been shown to play an important role in shaping "spatial memory fields" in much the same way as they have been found to shape "sensory receptor fields" [34,35]. In addition, blockade of GABA-ergic inhibition in the inferotemporal area has been associated with a disruption of the normal response of neurons selective for particular object features [36].

D. Long-Term Potentiation (LTP) and Depression (LDP)

Intrinsic inhibitory interneurons in the hippocampus have been suggested to control long-term modifications of synaptic strength induced by synaptic transmission [37–42]. Both LTP and LDP play a central role in memory and learning.

E. Phenotypical Differentiation

Of particular interest for the field of schizophrenia research is the fact that interneurons have been shown to regulate the differentiation of hippocampal neurons during development [43]. That many of these functions might involve functional (and presumably structural) neuroplasticity is strongly suggested by the observation that GABA, GAD, and the $GABA_A$ receptors are all regulated in an activity-dependent manner [44,45]. This raises the question whether phenotypic changes in the GABA system seen in schizophrenia might be related to increases or decreases in the flow of afferent activity into the cortex and hippocampus from other regions with which they are connected (see below).

III. THE GABA SYSTEM IN SCHIZOPHRENIA AND BIPOLAR DISORDER

GABA dysfunction is believed to play a role in various neuropsychiatric disorders. For example, as early as 1972, Eugene Roberts postulated that this compound might play a central role in the pathophysiology of schizophrenia [46]. Schizophrenia typically involves disturbances of cognitive functioning that include impaired attentional reponses [47], disruptions of normal information processing [48,49], and a selective impairment in declarative memory [50]. Overall, the thought pattern of schizophrenics has been described as being "overinclusive"; i.e., there is an inability to filter out extraneous information [51–53]. This has lead to the speculation that an impaired central filtering mechanism may be present in this disorder [54], as schizophrenic individuals are unable to distinguish relevant objects in the perceptual field [55]. Using physiological recordings from schizophrenics, a decreased auditory-evoked P50 response to repeated stimuli has been noted [56]. These authors concluded that such a defect may be related not only to sensory gating difficulties, but also to problems with learning efficiency and accuracy. The most consistent electrophysiological abnormalities observed in schizophrenia, however, are a reduced amplitude and increased latency of the P300 evoked potential [57]. These changes are related to a diminished ability to habituate selective attentional responses to a stimulus, and could reflect defective GABA-ergic inhibitory modulation. Consistent with this idea, a recent PET study has demonstrated an increase of basal metabolism in the hippocampal formation of schizophrenic subjects [50], and, as shown in Figure 2 (lower panel), this finding is consistent with a recent model for how the GABA system in this region may be dysfunctional in schizophrenia [58,59]. On a highly speculative level, it could be hypothesized that decreased GABA-ergic transmission in specific cortical areas could result in rearrangement, and possibly enlargement, of sensory, memory, and cognitive fields and thereby lead to overinclusive, disorganized thought processes.

To better understand the functional implications of a dysfunction of the GABA system in schizophrenia, it is necessary to have direct empiric evidence demonstrating alterations of specific markers for this neurotransmitter system. To date, such information has come largely from postmortem investigations as discussed below.

Normal Control

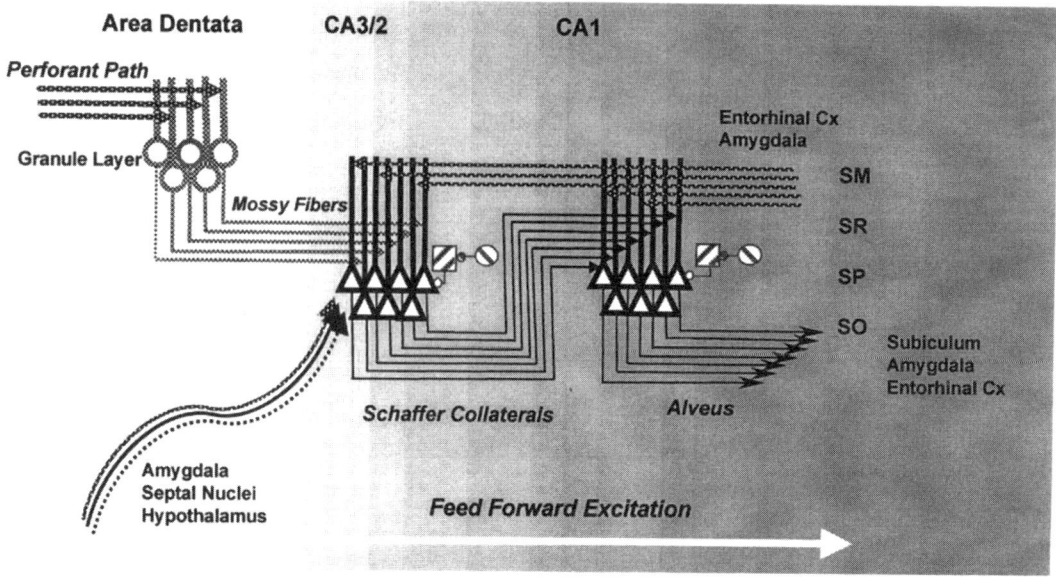

Schizophrenic

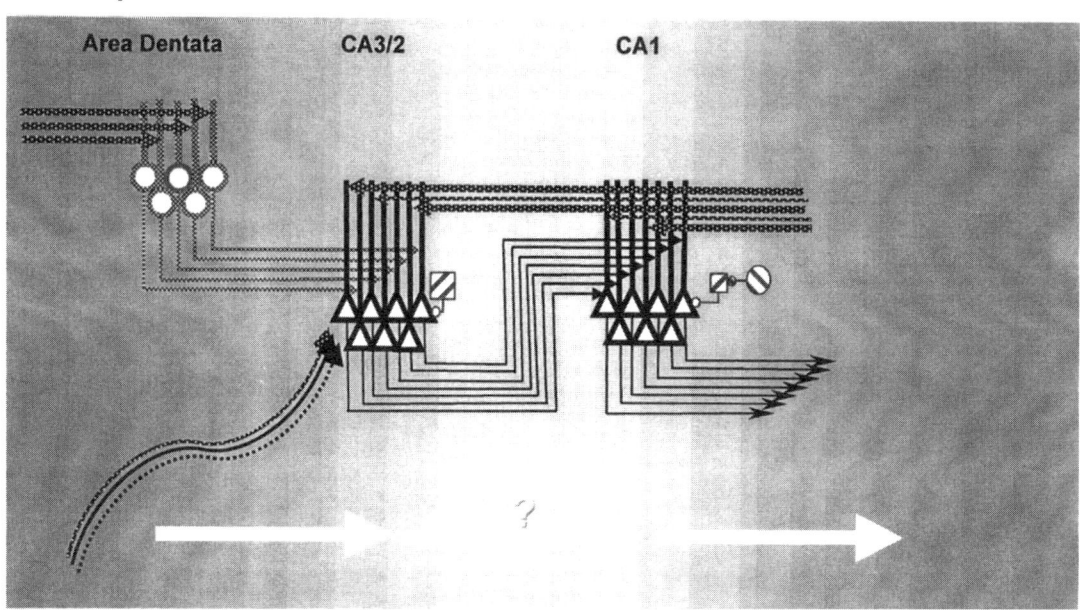

The GABA Cell

A. Postmortem Evidence for a GABA Defect in Schizophrenia

1. Numerical Density of Interneurons

Cell-Counting Studies

CEREBRAL CORTEX. In 1991, a postmortem study in which pyramidal and nonpyramidal neurons were differentially counted in cresyl violet–stained sections revealed a decreased density of nonpyramidal cells in layers II–VI of the anterior cingulate area and layer II only of the prefrontal cortex of schizophrenic and schizoaffective subjects [60]. In the anterior cingulate cortex, however, these changes were primarily significant in the schizoaffective group, suggesting the possibility that they might show a stronger covariation with affective disorder than with schizophrenia. This finding is controversial, however, since several other groups have not demonstrated a similar change in the prefrontal cortex of schizophrenics [61–64] and the anterior cingulate cortex of bipolar subjects [65]. There are significant methodologic factors that may have contributed to these failures to replicate the reduced density of nonpyramidal cells. Not least among these are the difficulties in comparing data obtained with two-dimensional-cell counting methods with those obtained with three-dimensional techniques. Both have their strengths and weaknesses. In evaluating conflicting results, it is important to consider the type of cell counting method employed in studies of schizophrenia [for detailed review, see [66,67].

In a subsequent replication study, a 2D method was employed to study a cohort in which schizophrenics and manic-depressives were included as comparison groups. The results of this study showed a pattern similar to that previously reported [68]. The manic-depressive showed approximately a 30% decrease, while the schizophrenics showed a 16% decrease. It is noteworthy that another study in which tyrosine hydroxylase–immunoreactive fibers were analyzed [69] was found in a post hoc analysis to also show an 18% reduction in the density of nonpyramidal neurons in layer II of ACCx [70]. More recently, the findings from these three studies have been combined and the data indicate that the reduction in the density of nonpyramidal neurons in layer II of ACCx was 16% in the schizophrenics (N = 25), 25% in schizoaffectives (n = 18) and 30% in manic-depressives [71]. Taken together, these data suggest that a loss of interneurons does occur in affective disorder as well as schizophrenia.

HIPPOCAMPUS. In a recent study of the hippocampal formation, a preferential decrease in the number of nonpyramidal neurons was observed in sector CA2 (refer to Fig. 2, lower panel); however, in this region, the change occurred to an equivalent degree in both schizophrenics and bipolars [72]. Based on these

Figure 2 (continued) CA1 (see text for details). There are inhibitory interneurons (square cells with hatched filling) providing GABA-ergic input to pyramidal cells in CA3 and CA1 and to the stratum oriens. Some GABA cells are disinhibitory interneurons (circular cells with hatched filling) that decrease the ability of the GABAergic cell to fire. **Schizophrenics:** A schematic diagram similar to that shown for normal controls, except that there is increased excitatory activity (thickened arrows) entering the trisynaptic pathway from three routes: (1) basolateral nucleus of the amygdala; (2) entorhinal projections to the stratum moleculare of the dentate gyrus; and (3) entorhinal projections to CA1 and CA3 from layers III and II, respectively, that travel along the stratum moleculare of the these subfields (see text for details). In addition, there is a defect of GABA-ergic modulation at various points along the trisynaptic pathway. First, inhibitory GABA-ergic activity appears to be decreased in sectors CA4, CA3, and CA2, but not CA1. There is also a subtle decrease of disinhibitory modulation in the stratum pyramidale of CA3 that would result in an increased inhibition of pyramidal cell firing in this sector. Although it is difficult to understand how a dual defect in inhibitory *and* disinhibitory modulation in CA3 might impact on the flow of activity along the trisynaptic pathway, it seems likely that there would be an overall increase of excitatory activity along most of the trisynaptic pathway. This is indicated as an intensification of the dark shading occurring uniformly from the area dentata through sector CA1. In the area dentata, the feedforward excitatory drive progressively increases as the conduction of impulses passes toward CA1. Since the changes in GABA-ergic integraion in CA3 are complex and the increase of disinhibitory activity may have the ability to offset some of this excitation, the arrow is missing in this sector and is replaced by a question mark (?). In CA1, the excitatory drive would attain its highest level of activity, particularly since a decrease of inhibitory modulation appears to be minimally present in this sector in schizophenics. Taken together, these hypothesized changes would be capable of generating an overall increase of basal metabolism in this region, but an impaired ability to selectively retrieve information when challenged with a specific task. (From Ref. 50.)

results, it has been postulated that a loss of GABA-ergic neurons might be related to a factor (such as stress) that the two disorders would share to an equivalent degree. It is not straightforward to explain why there is a greater decrease in the density of nonpyramidal neurons in ACCx of manic-depressives than in schizophrenics. Nor is it obvious why this parameter shows an equivalent change in the hippocampal formation of both disorders; however, it is conceivable that each disorder may involve region-specific alterations of neural circuitry that impact on GABA-ergic neurons to differing degrees, depending on the specific diagnostic category.

Calcium-Binding Peptides

CEREBRAL CORTEX. A variety of peptides have been found to be associated with various subtypes of nonpyramidal neurons and are being used to identify specific phenotypes of GABA-ergic inteneurons [73]. An ICC localization of the calcium binding protein parvalbumin (PVB) has demonstrated a *decrease* of cells showing this immunoreactivity in the prefrontal cortex of schizophrenics [74]. In another study, however, prefrontal areas 9 and 46 showed no differences in the distribution of neurons expressing detectable levels of immunoreactivity (-IR) for PVB [75]. In the anterior cingulate cortex, on the other hand, an increase of cells immunoreactive for this peptide has been reported in schizophrenics [76]. In attempting to interpret such disparate results, it is important to consider whether differences in the regions studied, tissue handling, and perhaps even subject populations may account for the discrepancies. All of these factors may potentially influence whether the amount of PVB-IR is either above or below the level of detection.

For calbinding (CB) 28k, an increase in the numerical density of neurons showing immunoreactivity for this peptide in the dorsolateral prefrontal cortex was observed, while there was no change in those containing calretinin (CR-IR) [77]. Unfortunately, there has not as yet been another study reporting on this peptide in the prefrontal cortex of schizophrenics.

HIPPOCAMPUS. CB expression has been shown to be increased [77] and CB-IR neurons have been reported to show a marked degree of disarray in sector CA2 [78]. Although an overt decrease in the numerical density of these cells was not detected, it is noteworthy that another study revealed a selective loss of nonpyramidal neurons in sector CA2 of subjects with schizophrenia and bipolar disorder [72].

Taking together the results of cell-counting studies using cresyl violet–stained sections with those processed immunocytochemically with antibodies against various calcium-binding proteins, there does not appear to be a definitive answer as to whether a decrease of interneurons is present in the cortex or the hippocampus of schizophrenic subjects. On the one hand, studies of cresyl violet–Stained sections suffer from significant issues regarding cell-counting methodology. On the other hand, studies that have localized PVB, CB, and CR are impeded by the factors that influence the retention of immunoreactivity in the tissue and the fact that increases or decreases of detectable levels of peptide may occur without any overt change in the actual number of neurons. Thus, the apparent changes in numerical density of such cells can be quite misleading.

2. *Markers for GABA-ergic Terminals*

In the 1970s, perhaps prompted by the speculations of Eugene Roberts [46], a series of neurochemical investigations focused on various markers for the GABA system in schizophrenia. The first study to appear examined the concentrations of GABA in the nucleus accumbens and thalamus of patients with schizophrenia and a group of subjects with Huntington's chorea, and found a reduction of this transmitter in the two disorders [79]. Around the same time, another study reported that the activity of glutamate decarboxylase (GAD) was significantly reduced in schizophrenics [80]. Although it began to appear that a pattern of decreased GABA-ergic activity was emerging, subsequent studies failed to show changes in either GABA levels or GAD activity [81], although one study did show a nonsignificant decrease of GAD in the prefrontal cortex [82]. Because subjects who died suddenly were less apt to show such changes, it was believed by some that decreases in the specific activity of GAD were related to the agonal state [83].

More consistent findings have come from studies of the GABA uptake site where reductions of this marker have been consistently observed in the prefrontal cortex [84], amygdala [85], and hippocampus [86] of the schizophrenic brain. A recent attempt to replicate this finding in prefrontal and temporal cortex, however, did not show any differences in schizophrenics [87].

More recently, the 65-kDa isoform of GAD, a marker for GABA-ergic terminals [88], has been localized immunocytochemically in the anterior cingulate cortex, where schizophrenic patients showed no differences (not shown). In bipolar subjects, on the other hand, a marked decrease was detected on pyramidal neurons in layers II and III (Fig. 3). In the hippocampal formation no overall differences between normal controls and schizophrenics were detected in the density of GAD_{65}-IR terminals on either pyramidal or nonpyramidal cells in any of the subregions or sublaminae [89]. However, a small number of subjects who were neuroleptic free for at least a year prior to death showed a significant reduction on both neuronal subtypes in sectors CA4, CA3, and CA2, but not in sector CA1. The subjects treated with neuroleptics showed a dose-related increase in terminal density in these sectors, particularly in the stratum oriens of CA3 and CA2. These data suggest that there may be an intrinsic reduction of GABA-ergic terminals in the hippocampus of schizophrenics, and the therapeutic efficacy of neuroleptic drugs may involve, at least in part, a trophic sprouting of these terminals. This conclusion is consistent with a controlled study in rat medial prefrontal cortex (anterior cingulate region) in which chronic haloperidol administration was associated with a marked increase of GABA-IR terminals [90]. Whether such changes require blockade of dopamine receptors on GABA cells is not clear; however, the increase in this latter study was most striking in layer II, where the dopaminergic projections to this region are most sparse [91]. Nevertheless, antipsychotic drugs may be capable of inducing changes in GABA cells that are mediated either alone or in combination with other receptors, such as the $5HT_{2A}$ receptor [92], or possibly even by direct trophic changes in synapses [93–95].

Other cytochemical studies have employed in situ hybridization (ISH) to examine the distribution of mRNA for GAD, particularly that for the 67 kDa isoform (GAD_{67}) [88]. In the prefrontal cortex of schizophrenics, a reduction in the number of cells expressing GAD_{67} mRNA has been reported by two different groups [64,96]. More recently, a decreased expression in GAD_{67} mRNA, but not GAD_{65}, its closely related isoform, has again been noted [97]. A variety of studies have suggested that GAD_{67} is regulated through transcriptional mechanisms. For example, increased expression of mRNA for this protein has been found in relation to lesioning of the substantia nigra [98,99], climbing fibers of the cerebellum [100], and in the hippocampus in response to systemic treatment with kainic acid [101]. In contrast, expression of mRNA for GAD_{65} [102] and its translation into protein also appears to be relatively stable [103],

although its regulation may be controlled primarily through posttranslational mechanisms [104]. The postmortem findings obtained using either immunocytochemistry or ISH show decreased expression of GAD_{67}, but not GAD_{65}, as well as stable levels of immunoreactivity for GAD_{65} in terminals of the hippocampal formation [89]. Since mRNA for the two isoforms of GAD are expressed by 95% of the neurons in rat hippocampus [105], it seems likely that complex cellular mechanisms may be influencing the nature of the results observed in these postmortem studies. That changes in GAD_{67} mRNA in prefrontal cortex were observed not only in schizophrenics, but also in subjects with bipolar disorder [97] suggests that these changes may be related to a nonspecific factor associated with both disorders. Interestingly, differential expression of mRNAs associated with the two isoforms of GAD have been reported in relation to both acute and chronic stress [106], although that for GAD_{67} was increased rather than decreased. A recent study in rats has attempted to model for the effects of pre- and/or postnatal stress by injecting rats with corticosterone [107]. Within 24 hr of the last injection, a decreases of mRNA for GAD_{67}, but not GAD_{65}, was observed in the dentate gyrus, CA4, CA2, and CA1 of rats exposed both pre- and postnatally. Five days after the last injection, however, the levels of mRNA for GAD_{67} returned to normal, while those for GAD_{65} were markedly increased. These findings suggest that stress during the prodrome and/or early stages of schizophrenia or bipolar disorder could theoretically influence the regulation of both isoforms, whether or not exposure to stress has occurred early in life. Such an effect should be considered when interpreting changes in GAD mRNA expression.

Another finding supporting the presence of disruption of GABA-ergic networks in schizophrenia is the decrease of "cartridge-like" terminals that are immunopositive for the GABA membrane transporter (GAT-1) in prefrontal cortex [108]. These "cartridges" represent axo-axonic terminations of chandelier neurons (see Fig. 1) and are strategically positioned within cortical circuitry to modulate cortical output. Thus, their decrease is likely to reflect crucial changes in information processing in the cortex. Other terminals with a more conventional punctate appearance did not show differences. This population of GABA terminals accounts for only 1% of the total. It is not known, however, whether GAT-1-containing terminations express GAD_{65}, GAD_{67} or both.

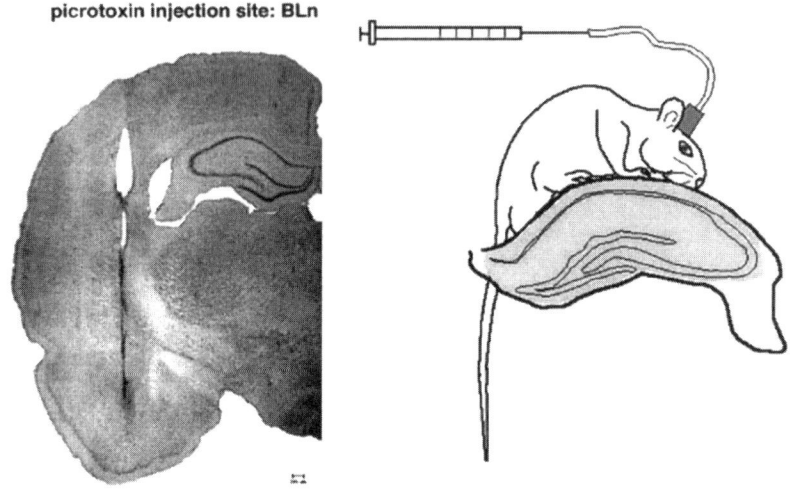

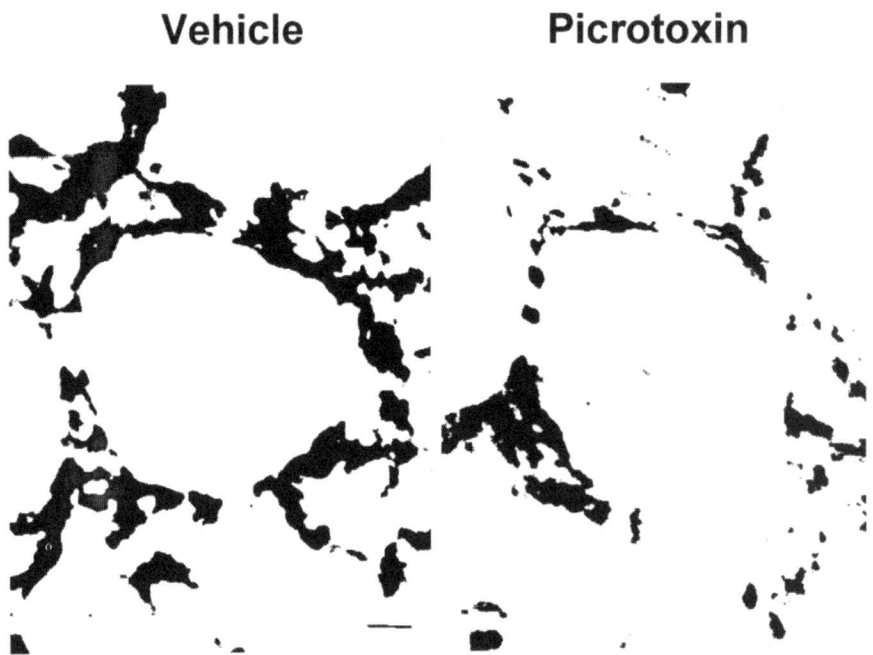

Figure 3 Stereotaxical local infusion of the GABA$_A$ receptor antagonist picrotoxin in the amygdala (needle track shown in upper left panel) of awake freely moving rats (schematic in upper right) induced significant changes in densities of GAD$_{65}$-positive terminals in hippocampus of picrotoxin-treated rats (lower right) when compared to vehicle-treated (lower left). These decreases, detectable around cell bodies of pyramidal neurons, were selectively observed in sectors CA3 and CA2, but not CA1 and therefore showed a subregional distribution of GABA changes remarkably similar to that seen in schizophrenia and bipolar disorder

3. GABA Receptor-Binding Activity

Binding of the selective radiolabeled agonist [^{3}H]muscimol was evaluated in the prefrontal cortex of controls and schizophrenics matched for age, but with an average postmortem interval of 8 and 13 h, respectively [82]. The data indicated that the schizophrenics showed a 48% increase (not significant) in the B$_{max}$, but no difference in affinity for [^{3}H]muscimol binding. Addition of the benzodiazepine diazepam resulted in a greater increase in binding in the schizophrenics. One limitation of this study was the fact that GABA was used as a competitive inhibitor, rather than bicuculline, a specific antagonist of the GABA$_A$ receptor [9]. Thus, it is unclear whether the results reflect changes in this latter receptor, the GABA$_B$ receptor, GAT-1 or perhaps even other GABA transporters.

Subsequent investigations have specifically examined high affinity binding to the GABA$_A$ receptor complex. Using bicuculline as a selective antagonist, [^{3}H]muscimol binding was found to be increased in the hippocampal formation (Fig. 7) [109], anterior cingulate cortex [110], and prefrontal region [111,112] of schizophrenic subjects. It is noteworthy, however, that benzodiazepine receptor activity did not show differences in the hippocampal formation, suggesting that there might be an uncoupling in the regulation of these two sites on the GABA$_A$ chloride ionophore complex [113]. One other study had reported a decrease of benzodiazepine receptor binding in the cortex [114], but it is not clear if the subjects in this study were treated with benzodiazepine agents prior to death. It is also important to note that this pattern does not preclude the presence of an allosteric uncoupling in the regulation of the receptor.

SPECT imaging investigations have also been used to study the GABA$_A$ receptor in schizophrenia using specific ligands, such [^{123}I]iomazenil for the benzodiazepine receptor. While two such studies have found no differences in schizophrenics [115,116], two others have found a reduction in this binding activity [117,118]. In two of these studies, changes in the benzodiazepine receptor correlated with both cognitive impairment [118] and severity of illness [115]. It is important to emphasize that these studies were probably examining only the benzodiazepine site on the GABA$_A$ chloride ionophore complex so that, in the setting of an allosteric uncoupling in its regulation, the status of the GABA$_A$ site cannot be inferred from such imaging data.

A high-resolution microscopic technique has provided specific information regarding the distribution of this receptor binding activity on pyramidal neurons versus nonpyramidal cells (interneurons). In the prefrontal [119] and anterior cingulate [110] cortices, increased GABA$_A$ receptor binding activity has been preferentially found on pyramidal, but not nonpyramidal neurons, particularly in layers II and III. This pattern was thought to be consistent with the hypothesis that a compensatory upregulation of this receptor was occurring in response to a decrease of GABA-ergic neurons and/or activity. When this form of analysis was applied to the hippocampal formation, a similar "classic" pattern was observed on pyramidal neurons in sector CA1 [109]. In sector CA3, however, the increase of GABA$_A$ receptor-binding activity was paradoxically found on nonpyramidal neurons, but not pyramidal cells, suggesting that a decrease of GABA-to-GABA interactions might be occurring in this sector of schizophrenics.

Taken together, these results consistently indicate that a disruption of inhibitory GABA-ergic neurons occurs in selective regions of the cerebral cortex. In the hippocampus, however, there may be more complex alterations that involve both inhibitory and disinhibitory GABA cells along the trisynaptic pathway of schizophrenics [58,120], and these changes would likely result in disruptions of the normal feedforward activity of this region (see Fig. 2).

4. Altered Inputs to GABA Cells

The dopamine system has long been suspected of playing a role in the pathophysiology of schizophrenia [121], even though convincing empiric evidence for a primary defect in this system has been lacking [122]. Seymour Kety was the first to suggest that subtle changes in connectivity could occur in the absence of any discernible biochemical alterations [123]. To determine whether such a defect is present in schizophrenia, it is now possible to visualize dopamine fibers using antibodies against tyrosine hydroxylase (TH) [124–128]. A recent study of the distribution of TH-IR varicosities in the anterior cingulate and prefrontal cortices of schizophrenic brain has suggested that there may be a decrease of these fibers on pyramidal neurons, but an increase on interneurons in layer II of the anterior cingulate; this change was not observed in the prefrontal cortex [69]. In layers V and VI of the cingulate region, there was also a significant reduction in the density of TH-IR varicosities, and this compares favorably with an analysis of fiber length in the prefrontal cortex of schizophrenics where a significant reduction was also found in layer VI [129]. In the anterior cingulate cortex, however, this change was only found in patients treated on neuroleptics, whereas the apparent shift of TH-IR varicosities from pyramidal to nonpyramidal cells of layer II was found in all schizophrenic subjects, whether they were treated with antipsychotic medication or not [69].

A subsequent post hoc analysis in which several different working models were considered suggested that these data might best be explained by a trophic shift of TH-IR fibers from pyramidal to nonpyramidal neurons [70]. A loss of GABA-ergic interneurons was not required for this pattern to occur, although it could coexist with such a shift. If these findings were correct, they would suggest that dopaminergic afferents might be providing a nonadaptive hyperinnervation to a subpopulation of GABA-ergic interneurons. Since dopamine appears to exert an inhibitory effect on cortical GABA cells [130], these findings would predict that an excessive release of dopamine would occur under conditions of stress [131,132]. This could lead to a secondary effect on GABA-ergic function and ultimately to a decompensation of the intrinsic circuitry in layer II of anterior cingulate cortex [133].

B. The Neurodevelopmental Hypothesis

1. Cell Migration

The findings of a variety of changes in layer II of the anterior cingulate and prefrontal cortices suggested the possibility that there might be a disturbance in the migration of neurons in the developing cortex of subjects with schizophrenia [134]. To investigate this possibility further, the distribution of nicotinamide adenine dinucleotide diaphorase (NADPH diaphorase) was examined in the prefrontal cortex of normal controls and schizophrenics [135]. The results demonstrated a significantly higher density of cells positive for this marker in the subcortical white matter when compared to the cortical mantle [136]. Of significance to the current discussion is the fact that NADPH diaphorase has been colocalized to interneurons that are GABA-ergic in nature [137–145].

2. Reelin and Cortical Lamination

Another line of investigation that has pointed to a possible neurodevelopmental mechanism playing a role in the pathophysiology of schizophrenia has come from studies of Reelin, a protein derived from the Reeler mouse mutant. Reelin is believed to be secreted by a subclass of GABA-ergic interneuron called a Cajal-Retzius cell [146,147] that are the first to appear during ontogenesis and are localized in layer I [148]. During fetal development, they interact with Martinotti cells in deeper laminae and are thought to play a role in the formation of laminar patterns [148]. In both schizophrenia and bipolar disorder, both Reelin and GAD_{67} mRNA have been found to be decreased in layer I and, to a lesser extent, layer II [149]. These latter findings are consistent with two other studies, one in which nonpyramidal neurons were counted [150] and another using high resolution analyses of $GABA_A$ receptor binding activity [119], showing preferential changes in layer II of the prefrontal cortex. These authors propose that a downregulation of Reelin expression in this region of schizophrenic and bipolar brain may be due to either a genetic or an epigenetic factor. Since this protein is reduced in both schizophrenia and bipolar disorder, it seems more likely that the changes noted might be related to an environmental factor common to both. In this regard, it is noteworthy that obstetrical complications have been found to occur in both schizophrenia [151] and bipolar disorder [152,153], making it plausible that an insult early in life could influence the subsequent expression of this protein during adulthood.

3. Postnatal Ingrowth of Extrinsic Afferents

Important questions regarding the role of a neurodevelopmental disturbance in the induction of altered phenotypes of GABA cells are when and how such changes become manifest during the life cycle in individuals who carry the susceptibility genes for schizophrenia and bipolar disorder. One possibility is that the GABA cells are abnormal from birth; however, the clinical observation that most subjects with schizophrenia are relatively normal during childhood and early adolescence argues against this possibility. It is important to emphasize, however, that studies in rat suggest that the cortical GABA system continues to develop until the equivalent of early adolescence [90,154–157]. Taking together these various observations, a second possibility is that the GABA cells are relatively normal during childhood when they are also relatively immature [158], but become abnormal as their maturation process is completed. The activation of a putative gene or genes associated with schizophrenia and/or bipolar disorder may "trigger" the appearance of a phenotypic abnormality in GABA-ergic interneurons. In this case, it would be assumed that both disorders might share common genes and that these would be capable of altering the normal functioning of GABA cells. A third possibility is that the GABA cells are either relatively normal or abnormal during childhood, but their activity is quiescent as they await the ingrowth of a fiber system from another region. The dopaminergic afferents to the cortex are a good candidate for playing such a role, as there have been at least three studies demonstrating an increase in medial prefrontal cortex during the equivalent of adolescence [159,160]. These fibers continue forming increased numbers of appositions with GABA-ergic interneurons until the early adult period [161].

4. Influence of Pre- and Postnatal Stress

The potential role that stress might play in the induction of changes in the cortical GABA system is an interesting issue to explore. For example, glucocorticoid hormones have the ability to bind to the $GABA_A$ receptor [162] and have been found to directly increase its activity [163,164]. It is noteworthy that the binding of [^{3}H]corticosterone is greatest in sector CA2 [165,166] where schizophrenics and bipolars both show a marked decrease of nonpyramidal neurons and the largest increase of $GABA_A$ receptor binding (see above). It is important to point out, however, that stress is believed to increase rather than decrease the activity of the GABA system [167–170], although it is possible that chronic stress, particularly when preceded by stress in utero, might result in an eventual decrease in the activity of this transmitter system. This possibility is particularly intriguing when the marked sensitivity of GABA-ergic neurons to excitotoxic injury [171] is considered. It is believed that cell death in this setting probably requires both an increase of excitatory activity and an increase of circulating levels of glucocorticoid hormone [172].

Another important component to the stress response is the increased release of dopamine that occurs in the medial prefrontal cortex (see above). By exposing rats both pre- and postnatally to stress-related doses of corticosterone, an increase of dopamine varicosities forming appositions with GABA-ergic interneurons has been induced [133]. Thus, it is possible that the postnatal maturation of GABA cells in the cortex may be normally influenced by the ingrowth of dopamine fibers, but abnormally affected when this occurs in individuals for whom pre- and postnatal stress are comorbid factors. In this latter case, it would have to be assumed that gene(s) involving the dopamine system and perhaps also cortical GABA cells would be affected by prenatal exposure to stress and would be permanently sensitized in such individuals.

IV. MODELING ACTIVITY-DRIVEN CHANGES IN HIPPOCAMPAL GABA CELLS

A conundrum that has presented itself from postmortem studies of the GABA system in schizophrenia and bipolar disorder is the following: Why are abnormalities preferentially detected in layer II of the prefrontal and anterior cingulate cortices and sectors CA3 and CA2 of the hippocampus? A potentially important clue that will help answer this question comes from studies of the connectivity of these regions. Layer II of the anterior cingulate cortex is known to receive a "massive" projection from the basolateral nucleus of the amygdala [173], while sectors CA3 and CA2 also receive a substantial input from this same complex [174]. Taken together with other evidence [59,175], it seems plausible that the changes in the GABA system described above may potentially be related to an increased inflow of activity from this key limbic region. To explore the possibility that changes in the cortical and hippocampal GABA system in schizophrenia could be related to an increased inflow of activity originating in the amygdala, a "partial" animal model has been developed [120]. When the $GABA_A$ antagonist picrotoxin is infused locally into the basolateral nuclear complex of awake, freely moving rats, within 2 hr, a marked decrease in the density of both the 65- and 67-kDa isoform of GAD-IR terminals can be detected on neuron somata in sectors CA3 and CA2, but not CA1. In anterograde tracer studies, amygdalo-hippocampal projection fibers show a similar distribution. Overall, these results suggest that activation of afferents from the basolateral nucleus is associated with the induction of significant changes in the GABA system in the hippocampus with a subregional distribution that is remarkably similar to that found in schizophrenia. Under pathological conditions, an excessive discharge of excitatory activity emanating from the amygdala could be capable of altering inhibitory modulation along the trisynaptic pathway and may contribute to disturbances of GABA-ergic function in schizophrenia. Such "partial" modeling in rodents will provide an important strategy for deciphering the effect of altered corticolimbic circuits in schizophrenia.

V. CONCLUSIONS

The cortical and hippocampal GABA systems consists of many different subclasses of interneurons, each having unique phenotypes defined by their morphology, neuropeptide content, electrophysiological properties, and synaptic connectivity (Benes and Berretta, 2001). In reviewing the postmortem investigations of schizophrenic brain, it is clear that there have been some inconsistencies, particularly with regard to cell-counting findings. There are many different confounding factors that can be invoked to explain failures to replicate and these vary according to the types of methodology that have been employed. Nevertheless, when this literature is viewed as a totality, not only cell-counting studies, but also those in which immunocytochemistry, receptor-binding autoradiography, and in situ hybridization have indicated that some form of dysfunction in the GABA-ergic system appears in the cortex of schizophrenics. That similar findings are also being reported in bipolar disorder further suggests that such a defect may be related to a common environmental factor, perhaps one that is related to obstetrical complications. Indeed, the neurodevelopmental hypothesis of schizophrenia (and by extrapolation, bipolar disorder) has received its most convincing evidence from studies of the GABA system.

An important question raised by these findings is whether the GABA-ergic interneuron might be a common site for the action of drugs that are used in the treatment of both schizophrenia and bipolar disorder. Indeed, GABA-mimetic drugs, such as mood-stabilizing anticonvulsants, show efficacy in the treatment of both schizophrenia [176] and bipolar disorder [177], although patients with affective disorder show a more striking beneficial effect. Recent studies demonstrating direct interactions between the dopamine and serotonin systems with GABA-ergic neurons in the cortex, as well as the expression of their respective receptor systems in these interneurons [for review, see 178], are also consistent with this idea.

In the years to come, continued investigations of the GABA system in rodent, nonhuman primate, and human brain will undoubtedly provide important new insights into how the integration of macro- and microcircuitry in the corticolimbic system is altered in schizophrenia and bipolar disorder. Most importantly, the use of increasingly sophisticated probes will eventually lead to a precise understanding of how neuroleptic drugs can influence the structural and functional integrity of the GABA system and other neuromodulator systems with which it interacts. Information of this type will ultimately point the way toward novel approaches to the treatment of schizophrenia and bipolar disorder.

ACKNOWLEDGMENTS

This work has been supported by grants from the National Institutes of Health (MH00423, MH42261, MH31862, MH31154) and the Stanley Foundation.

REFERENCES

1. Jones, E.G, GABA-peptide neurons in primate cerebral cortex. J. Mind Behav, 1987, 8: p. 519–536.
2. Benes, F.M., Berretta, S. GABA-ergic interneurons: implications for understanding schizophrenia and bipolar disorder. Neuropsychopharmacology 2001 (in press).
3. Freund, T.F., Buzsaki, G. Interneurons of the hippocampus. Hippocampus 1996, 6(4):347–470.
4. Hof, P.R., et al., Calcium-binding proteins define subpopulations of interneurons in cingulate cortex. In Neurobiology of Cingulate Cortex and Limbic Thalamus: A Comprehensive Handbook. B.A. Vogt, M. Gabriel, eds. Birkhauser, Boston: 1993.
5. Somogyi, P., et al. Salient features of synaptic organisation in the cerebral cortex. Brain Res Brain Res Rev 1998, 26(2–3):113–135.
6. Krnjevic, K. GABAergic inhibition in the neocortex. J Mind Behav, 1987, 8(4):537–548.
7. Andersen, P., J.C. Eccles, and Y. Loyning. Location of synaptic inhibitory synapses on hippocampal pyramids. J Neurophysiol 1964, 27:592–607.
8. Sillito, A.M. The contribution of inhibitory mechanisms to the receptive field properties of neurons in the striate cortex. J Physiol (Lond) 1975, 250:305–329.
9. Rabow, R., Farb, D.H. From ion currents to genomic analysis: recent advances in $GABA_A$ receptor research. Synapse, 1995, 21:189–274.
10. Buzsaki, G. Feed-forward inhibition in the hippocampal formation. Prog Neurobiol 1984, 22(2):131–153.
11. Buzsaki, G., E. Eidelberg. Phase relations of hippocampal projection cells and interneurons to theta activity in the anesthetized rat. Brain Res. 1983. 266(2):334–339.
12. Buzsaki, G., et al. High-frequency network oscillation in the hippocampus. Science 1992,. 256(5059):1025–1027.
13. Fraser, D.D., and B.A. MacVicar. Low-threshold transient calcium current in rat hippocampal lacunosum-moleculare interneurons: kinetics and

modulation by neurotransmitters. J Neurosci 1991, 11(9):2812–2820.
14. Soltesz, I., and M. Deschenes. Low- and high-frequency membrane potential oscillations during theta activity in CA1 and CA3 pyramidal neurons of the rat hippocampus under ketamine-xylazine anesthesia. J Neurophysiol 1993, 70(1):97–116.
15. Bragin, A., et al. Gamma (40–100 Hz) oscillation in the hippocampus of the behaving rat. J Neurosci 1995, 15(1 Pt 1):47–60.
16. Ylinen, A., et al. Sharp wave-associated high-frequency oscillation (200 Hz) in the intact hippocampus: network and intracellular mechanisms. J Neurosci 1995, 15(1 Pt 1):30–46.
17. Ylinen, A., et al. Intracellular correlates of hippocampal theta rhythm in identified pyramidal cells, granule cells, and basket cells. Hippocampus 1995, 5(1):78–90.
18. Jefferys, J.G., R.D. Traub, M.A. Whittington. Neuronal networks for induced '40 Hz' rhythms. Trends Neurosci 1996. 19(5):202–208.
19. Whittington, M.A., R.D. Traub, J.G. Jefferys. Synchronized oscillations in interneuron networks driven by metabotropic glutamate receptor activation. Nature 1995, 373(6515):612–615.
20. Amzica, F., M. Steriade. Disconnection of intracortical synaptic linkages disrupts synchronization of a slow oscillation. J Neurosci 1995, 15(6):4658–4677.
21. Buzsaki, G. Functions for interneuronal nets in the hippocampus. Can J Physiol Pharmacol 1997, 75(5):508–515.
22. Buzsaki, G, J.J. Chrobak. Temporal structure in spatially organized neuronal ensembles: a role for interneuronal networks. Curr Opin Neurobiol 1995, 5(4):504–510.
23. Buzsaki, G., et al. High-frequency network oscillation in the hippocampus. Science 1992, 256(5059):1025–1027.
24. Traub, R.D., Jefferys, J.G., Whittington, M.A. Simulation of gamma rhythms in networks of interneurons and pyramidal cells. J Comput Neurosci, 1997, 4:141–150.
25. Ylinen, A., et al. Intracellular correlates of hippocampal theta rhythm in identified pyramidal cells, granule cells, and basket cells. Hippocampus 1995,5:78–90.
26. Tsumoto, T., Eckart, W., Creutzfeldt, O.D. Modifications of orientation sensitivity of cat visual cortex neurons by removal of GABA-mediated inhibition. Exp Brain Res 1979, 34:351–363.
27. Alloway, K.D., H. Burton. Differential effects of GABA and bicuculline on rapidly- and slowly-adapting neurons in primary somatosensory cortex of primates. Exp Brain Res 1991, 85(3):598–610.
28. Alloway, K.D., P. Rosenthal, H. Burton, Quantitative measurements of receptive field changes during antagonism of GABAergic transmission in primary somatosensory cortex of cats. Exp Brain Res 1989, 78(3):514–532.
29. Kyriazi, H.T., et al. Quantitative effects of GABA and bicuculline methiodide on receptive field properties of neurons in real and simulated whisker barrels. J Neurophysiol 1996, 75(2):547–560.
30. Wilson, F.A., S.P. O'Scalaidhe, P.S. Goldman-Rakic. Functional synergism between putative gamma-aminobutyrate-containing neurons and pyramidal neurons in prefrontal cortex. Proc Natl Acad Sci USA, 1994, 91(9):4009–4013.
31. Kyriazi, H.T., et al. Effects of baclofen and phaclofen on receptive field properties of rat whisker barrel neurons. Brain Res 1996, 712:325–328.
32. Wilson, F., S. O'Scalaidhe, P. Goldman-Rakic. Functional synergism between putative gamma-aminobutyrate-containing neurons and pyramidal neurons in prefrontal cortex. Proc Natl Acad Sci USA, 1994, 91(9):4009–4013.
33. Jacobs, K.M., J.P. Donoghue. Reshaping the cortical motor map by unmasking latent intracortical connections. Science 1991, 251:944–947.
34. Rao, S.G., G.V. Williams, P.S. Goldman-Rakic. Isodirectional tuning of adjacent interneurons and pyramidal cells during working memory: evidence for microcolumnar organization in PFC. J Neurophysiol 1999, 81(4):1903–1916.
35. Rao, S.G., G.V. Williams, P.S. Goldman-Rakic. Destruction and creation of spatial tuning by disinhibition: GABA(A) blockade of prefrontal cortical neurons engaged by working memory. J Neurosci 2000, 20(1):485–494.
36. Wang, Y., I. Fujita, Y. Murayama, Y. Neuronal mechanisms of selectivity for object features revealed by blocking inhibition of inferotemporal cortex. Nat Neurosci, 2000, 3:807–813.
37. Buzsaki, G., et al. Pattern and inhibition-dependent invasion of pyramidal cell dendrites by fast spikes in the hippocampus in vivo. Proc Natl Acad Sci USA, 1996, 93(18):9921–9925.
38. Maccaferri, G., C.J. McBain. Long-term potentiation in distinct subtypes of hippocampal nonpyramidal neurons. J Neurosci 1996, 16(17):5334–5343.
39. Miles, R., et al. Differences between somatic and dendritic inhibition in the hippocampus. Neuron 1996, 16(4):815–823.
40. Tsubokawa, H., W.N. Ross. IPSPs modulate spike backpropagation and associated $[Ca^{2+}]i$ changes in the dendrites of hippocampal CA1 pyramidal neurons. J Neurophysiol 1996, 76(5):2896–2906.

41. McMahon, L.L., J.A. Kauer. Hippocampal interneurons express a novel form of synaptic plasticity. Neuron 1997, 18(2):295–305.
42. Laezza, F., J.J. Doherty, R. Dingledine. Long-term depression in hippocampal interneurons: joint requirement for pre- and postsynaptic events. Science 1999, 285(5432):1411–1414.
43. Marty, S., et al. GABAergic stimulation regulates the phenotype of hippocampal interneurons through the regulation of brain-derived neurotrophic factor. Neuron 1996, 16:565–570.
44. Jones, E.G. GABAergic neurons and their role in cortical plasticity in primates. Cereb Cortex 1993, 3:361–372.
45. Jones, E.G. The role of afferent activity in the maintenance of primate neocorticalfunction. J Exp Biol 1990, 153:155–176.
46. Roberts, E. An hypothesis suggesting that there is a defect in the GABA system in schizophrenia. Neurosci Res Prog Bull, 1972, 10(4):468–482.
47. McGhie, A., J. Chapman. Disorders of attention and perception in early schizophrenia. Br J Med Psychol 1961, 34:103–116.
48. Braff, D.L., et al., The generalized pattern of neuropsychological deficits in outpatients with chronic schizophrenia with heterogeneous Wisconsin Card Sorting Test results. Arch. Gen. Psychiatry, 1991. 48:891–898.
49. Saccuzzo, D.P. and D.L. Braff, Information-processing abnormalities: trait- and state-dependent component. Schizophr Bull., 1986. 12:447–456.
50. Heckers, S., S.L. Rausch, D. Goff, C.R. Savage, D.L. Schacter, A.J. Fischman, N.M. Alpert. Impaired recruitment of the hippocampus during conscious recollection in schizophrenia. Nat Neurosci, 1998, 1:318–323.
51. Cameron, N. Reasoning, regression and communication in schizophrenics. Psychol Rev Monogr, 1938, 50:1–33.
52. Payne, R.W., P. Matussek, and E.I. George. Experimental study of schizophrenic thought disorder. Br J Psychiatry 1961, 108:362–367.
53. Payne, R.W., D. Friedlander. Short battery of simple tests for measuring over-inclusive thinking. J Ment Sci 1962, 108:362–367.
54. Detre, T.P, H.G. Jarecki. Schizophrenic disorders. In: Modern Psychiatric Treatment. J.B. Lippincott, Philadelphia: 1971, pp 108–116.
55. Matussek, P. Untersuchunger uber die wahnwahrenmung. I Mitteilung: Verangerunger der Wahrenhmungswelt bei beginnenden, primaren Wahn. Arch Psychiatr Nervenkl 1951, 189:279–319.
56. Adler, L.A., E. Pachtman, F.D. Franks, M. Pecevich, M.D. Waldo, R. Freedman. Neurophysiological evidence for a defect in neuronal mechanisms involved in sensory gating in schizophrenia. Biol Psychiatry 1982, 17:639–654.
57. Blackwood, D.H.R., et al. Magnetic resonance imaging in schizophrenia: altered brain morphol- ogy associated with P300 abnormalities and eye tracking dysfunction. Biol Psychiatry 1991, 30:753–769.
58. Benes, F.M. Evidence for altered trisynaptic circuitry in schizophrenic hippocampus. Biol Psychiatry 1999, 46(5):589–599.
59. Benes, F.M. Emerging principles of altered neural circuitry in schizophrenia. Brain Res Brain Res Rev 2000, 31(2–3):251 269.
60. Benes, F.M., et al., Deficits in small interneurons in prefrontal and anterior cingulate cortex of schizophrenic and schizoaffective patients. Arch Gen Psychiatry 1991, 48:996–1001.
61. Selemon, L.D., G. Rajkowska, P.S. Goldman-Rakic. Abnormally high neuronal density in the schizophrenic cortex. A morphometric analysis of prefrontal area 9 and occipital area 17. Arch Gen Psychiatry 1995, 52(10):805–818; discussion 819–820.
62. Selemon, L.D., G. Rajkowska, P.S. Goldman-Rakic. Elevated neuronal density in prefrontal area 46 in brains from schizophrenic patients: application of a three-dimensional, stereologic counting method. J Comp Neurol 1998, 392(3):402–412.
63. Arnold, S.E., et al Smaller neuron size in schizophrenia in hippocampal subfields that mediate cortical-hippocampal interactions. Am J Psychiatry 1995, 152(5):738–748.
64. Akbarian, S., et al. Gene expression for glutamic acid decarboxylase is reduced without loss of neurons in prefrontal cortex of schizophrenics. Arch Gen Psychiatry 1995, 52:258–278.
65. Ongur, D., W.C. Drevets, J.L. Price. Glial reduction in the subgenual prefrontal cortex in mood disorders. Proc Natl Acad Sci USA 1998, 95(22):13290–13295.
66. Benes, F.M., N. Lange. Two dimensional versus three dimensional cell counting: a practical perspective. Trends Neurosci 2000 (In press).
67. Benes, F.M. Is there evidence for neuronal loss in schizophrenia? Int Rev Psychiatry 1997, 9:429–436.
68. Vincent, S.L., F.M. Benes. Density of pyramidal and nonpyramidal neurons in anterior cingulate region of control, schizophrenic and manic depressive subjects. Soc Neurosci Abstr 1996, (in press).
69. Benes, F.M., M.S. Todtenkopf, J.B. Taylor. Differential distribution of tyrosine hydroxylase fibers on small and large neurons in layer II of anterior cingulate cortex of schizophrenic brain. Synapse 1997, 25(1):80–92.
70. Benes, F.M. Model generation and testing to probe neural circuitry in the cingulate cortex of postmortem schizophrenic brain. Schizophr Bull 1998, 24(2):219–230.

71. Benes, F.M., M.S. Todtenkopf. Meta-analysis of nonpyramidal neuron (NP) loss in layer II in anterior cingulate cortex (ACCx-II) from three studies of postortem schizophrenic brain. Soc Neurosci Abstr, 1998, 24(2):1275.
72. Benes, F.M., et al. A reduction of nonpyramidal cells in sector CA2 of schizophrenics and manic depressives [see comments]. Biol Psychiatry 1998, 44(2):88–97.
73. Conde, F., et al. Local circuit neurons immunoreactive for calretinin, calbindin D-28k or parvalbumin in monkey prefrontal cortex: distribution and morphology. J Comp Neurol 1994, 341(1):95–116.
74. Beasley, C.L., G.P. Reynolds. Parvalbumin-immunoreactive neurons are reduced in the prefrontal cortex of schizophrenics. Schizophr Res 1997, 24(3):349–355.
75. Woo, T.U., J.L. Miller, D.A. Lewis,. Schizophrenia and the parvalbumin-containing class of cortical local circuit neurons. Am J Psychiatry 1997, 154(7):1013–1015.
76. Kalus, P., D. Senitz, H. Beckmann. Altered distribution of parvalbumin-immunoreactive local circuit neurons in the anterior cingulate cortex of schizophrenic patients. Psychiatry Res 1997, 75(1):49–59.
77. Daviss, S.R., D.A. Lewis. Local circuit neurons of the prefrontal cortex in schizophrenia: selective increase in the density of calbindin-immunoreactive neurons. Psychiatry Res 1995, 59(1–2):81–96.
78. Iritani, S., et al. Calbindin immunoreactivity in the hippocampal formation and neocortex of schizophrenics. Prog Neuropsychopharmacol Biol Psychiatry, 1999. 23(3):409–421.
79. Perry, T.L., et al. Gamma-aminobutyric acid deficiency in brains of schizophrenic patients. Lancet, 1979, 1:237–239.
80. Bird, E.D., et al. Increased brain dopamine and reduced glutamic acid decarboxylase and choline acetyl transferase activity in schizophrenia and related psychoses. Lancet, 1977, Dec 3:1157–1159.
81. Cross, A.J., T.J. Crow, F. Owen. Gamma-aminobutyric acid in the brain in schizophrenia [letter]. Lancet 1979, 1(8115):560–561.
82. Hanada, S., et al., ^{3}H-Muscimol binding sites increased in autopsied brains of chronic schizophrenics. Life Sci 1987, 40:259–266.
83. Bird, E.D., E.G. Spokes, L.L. Iversen. Increased dopamine concentration in limbic areas of brain from patients dying with schizophrenia. Brain 1979, 102(2):347–360.
84. Simpson, M.D., et al. Reduced GABA uptake sites in the temporal lobe in schizophrenia. Neurosci Lett 1989, 107(1–3):211–215.
85. Reynolds, G.P. Increased concentrations and lateral asymmetry of amygdala dopamine in schizophrenia. Nature 1983, 305:527–529.
86. Reynolds, G.P., C. Czudek, H. Andrews. Deficit and hemispheric asymmetry of GABA uptake sites in the hippocampus in schizophrenia. Biol Psychiatry 1990, 27:1038–1044.
87. Simpson, M.D., P. Slater, J.F. Deakin. Comparison of glutamate and gamma-aminobutyric acid uptake binding sites in frontal and temporal lobes in schizophrenia. Biol Psychiatry 1998, 44(6):423–427.
88. Kaufman, D.L., C.R. Houser, A.J. Tobin. Two forms of the γ-aminobutyric acid synthetic enzyme glutamate decarboxylase have distinct intraneuronal distributions and cofactor interactions. J Neurochem 1991, 56(2):720–723.
89. Todtenkopf, M.S., and F.M. Benes. Distribution of glutamate decarboxylase65 immunoreactive puncta on pyramidal and nonpyramidal neurons in hippocampus of schizophrenic brain. Synapse 1998. 29(4):323–332.
90. Vincent, S.L., et al. The effects of chronic haloperidol administration on GABA- immunoreactive axon terminals in rat medial prefrontal cortex. Synapse, 1994, 17(1):26–35.
91. Lindvall, O., A. Bjorklund. General organization of cortical monoamine systems. In: Monoamine Innervation of Cerebral Cortex. T.R. Reader, H.H. Jasper, eds. Alan R. Liss, New York: 1984, pp 9–40.
92. Benes, F.M. Is there a neuroanatomic basis for schizophrenia? Neuroscientist, 1995, 1(2):104–115.
93. Benes, F.M., P.A. Paskevich, V.B. Domesick. Haloperidol-induced plasticity of axon terminals in rat substantia nigra. Science 1983, 221(4614):969–971.
94. Benes, F.M., et al. Synaptic rearrangements in medial prefrontal cortex of haloperidol- treated rats. Brain Res 1985. 348(1):15–20.
95. Kerns, J.M., et al. Synaptic plasticity in the rat striatum following chronic haloperidol treatment. Clin Neuropharmacol 1992, 15(6):488–500.
96. Volk, D.W., et al. Decreased glutamic acid decarboxylase67 messenger RNA expression in a subset of prefrontal cortical gamma-aminobutyric acid neurons in subjects with schizophrenia. Arch Gen Psychiatry 2000, 57(3):237–245.
97. Guidotti, A., J. Auta, J.M. Davis, Y. Dwivedi, D.R. Grayson, F.. Impagnatiello, G. Pandeyh, C. Pesold, R. Sharma, D. Uzunov, E. Costa. Decrease in Reelin and glutamate acid decarboxylase67 (GAD67) expression in schizophrenia and bipolar disorder. Arch Gen Psychiatry 2000 (in press).
98. Vernier, P., et al. Similar time course changes in striatal levels of glutamic acid decarboxylase and proen-

98. kephalin mRNA following dopaminergic deafferentation in the rat. J. Neurochem 1988, 51:1375–1380.
99. O'Connor, L., S. Brene, M. Herrera-Marschitz, H. Persson, U. Ungerstedt. Short-term dopaminergic regulation of GABA release in dopamine deafferentated caudate-putamen is not directly associated with glutamic acid decarboxylase gene expression. Neurosci Lett, 1991. 128:66–70.
100. Litwak, J., M. Mercugliano, M.F. Chesselet, G.A. Oltmans. Increased glutamic acid decarboxylase (GAD) mRNA and GAD activity in cerebellar Purkinje cells following lesion-induced increases in cell firing. Neurosci Lett, 1990, 116:179–183.
101. Feldblum, R.F. Ackerman, A.J. Tobin. Long-term increase of glutamate decarboxylase mRNA in a rat model of temporal lobe epilepsy. Neuron 1990, 5:361–371.
102. Feldblum, S., M. Anoal, S. Lasher, A. Cumoulin, A. Privat. Partial deafferentation of the developing rat spinal cord delays the spontaneous repression of GAD_{67} mRNAs in spinal cells. Perspect Dev Neurobiol, 1998, 5:131–143.
103. Martin, D.L., S.B. Martin, S.J. Wu, N. Expina. Regulatory properties of brain glutamate decarboxylase (GAD): the apoenzyme of GAD is present principally as the smaller of the two molecular forms of GAD in the brain. J Neurosci, 1993, 11:2725–2731.
104. Miller, L.P., J.R. Walters, D.L. Martin. Post-mortem changes implicate adenine nucleotides and puridoxal-5'-phosphate in regulation of brain glutamate decarboxylase. Nature 1991. 266:847–848.
105. Stone, D.J., J. Walsh, F.M. Benes. Localization of cells preferentially expressing GAD(67) with negligible GAD(65) transcripts in the rat hippocampus. A double in situ hybridization study. Brain Res Mol Brain Res 1999, 71(2):201–209.
106. Bowers, G., W.E. Cullinan, J.P. Herman. Region-specific regulation of glutamic acid decarboxylase (GAD) mRNA expression in central stress circuits. J Neurosci 1998, 18(15):5938–5947.
107. Stone, D.J., J.P. Walsh, F.M. Benes. Effects of pre- and postnatal stress on the rat GABA system. Hippocampus 2001 (in press).
108. Pierri, J.N., et al. Alterations in chandelier neuron axon terminals in the prefrontal cortex of schizophrenic subjects. Am J Psychiatry 1999, 156(11):1709–1719.
109. Benes, F.M., et al. Differences in the subregional and cellular distribution of $GABA_A$ receptor binding in the hippocampal formation of schizophrenic brain. Synapse 1996, 22(4):338–349.
110. Benes, F.M., et al. Increased $GABA_A$ receptor binding in superficial layers of cingulate cortex in schizophrenics. J Neurosci 1992, 12(3):924–929.
111. Benes, F.M., et al. Up-regulation of GABAA receptor binding on neurons of the prefrontal cortex in schizophrenic subjects. Neurosci, 1996, 75(4):1021–1031.
112. Dean, B., et al. Changes in serotonin2A and GABA(A) receptors in schizophrenia: studies on the human dorsolateral prefrontal cortex. J Neurochem 1999, 72(4):1593–1599.
113. Benes, F.M., et al. Uncoupling of GABA(A) and benzodiazepine receptor binding activity in the hippocampal formation of schizophrenic brain. Brain Res 1997, 755(1):121–129.
114. Squires, R.F., et al. Reduced [^{3}-H]-Flunitrazepam bindings in cingulate cortex and hippocampus of postmortem schizophrenic brains. Neurochem Res 1993, 18:219–223.
115. Busatto, G.F., et al. Correlation between reduced in vivo benzodiazepine receptor binding and severity of psychotic symptoms in schizophrenia [published erratum appears in Am J Psychiatry 1997 May; 154(5):722] [see comments]. Am J Psychiatry 1997, 154(1):56–63.
116. Abi-Dargham, A., et al. No evidence of altered in vivo benzodiazepine receptor binding in schizophrenia. Neuropsychopharmacology 1999, 20(6):650–661.
117. Verhoeff, N.P., et al., [^{123}I]Lomazenil SPECT benzodiazepine receptor imaging in schizophrenia. Psychiatry Res 1999, 91(3):163–173.
118. Ball, S., et al. Cognitive functioning and $GABA_A$/benzodiazepine receptor binding in schizophrenia: a ^{123}I-iomazenil SPET study. Biol Psychiatry 1998, 43(2):107–117.
119. Benes, F.M., et al. Upregulation of GABA-A receptor binding on pyramidal neurons of prefrontal cortex in schizophrenic subjects. Neuroscience 1996, 75:1021–1031.
120. Berretta, S., D.W. Munno, F.M. Benes. Amygdalar activation alters the hippocampal GABA system: 'partial' modelling for postmortem changes in schizophrenia. J Comp Neurol, 2000 (in press).
121. Kety, S, S. Matthysse. Prospects for research on schizophrenia. An overview. Neurosci Res Bull 1972, 10:456–467.
122. Carlsson, A. Does dopamine have a role in schizophrenia? Biol. Psychiatry 1978, 13:3–21.
123. Kety, S. Biochemical theories of schizophrenia. Part I of a two-part critical review of current theories and of the evidence used to support them. Science 1959, 129:1528–1596.
124. Gaspar, P., et al. Catecholamine innervation of the human cerebral cortex as revealed by comparative immunohistochemistry of tyrosine hydroxylase and dopamine beta-hydroxylase. J Comp Neurol 1989, 279:249–271.

125. Lewis, D.A., et al. The distribution of tyrosine hydroxylase immunoreactive fibers in primate neocortex is widespread but regionally specific. J Neurosci 1987, 7:279–290.
126. Noack, H.J., D.A. Lewis. Antibodies directed against tyrosine hydroxylase differentially recognize noradrenergic axons in monkey neocortex. Brain Res 1989, 500:313–324.
127. Samson, Y., et al. Catecholaminergic innervation of the hippocampus in the cynomolgus monkey. J Comp Neurol 1990., 298:250–263.
128. Williams, S.M., P.S. Goldman-Rakic. Characterization of the dopaminergic innervation of the primate frontal cortex using a dopamine-specific antibody. Cereb Cortex 1993, 3:199–222.
129. Akil, M., et al. Lamina-specific alterations in the dopamine innervation of the prefrontal cortex in schizophrenic subjects. Am J Psychiatry 1999, 156(10):1580–1589.
130. Retaux, S., M.J. Besson, J. Penit-Soria. Synergism between D1 and D2 dopamine receptors in the inhibition of the evoked release of [^{3}H]GABA in the rat prefrontal cortex. Neuroscience 1991, 43(2/3):323–329.
131. Thierry, A.M., et al. Selective activation of the mesocortical DA system by stress. Nature 1976, 263:242–244.
132. Roth, R.H., et al. Stress and the mesocorticolimbic dopamine systems. Ann NY Acad Sci 1988, 537:138–147.
133. Benes, F.M. The role of stress and dopamine-GABA interactions in the vulnerability for schizophrenia. J Psychiatr Res 1997, 31(2):257–275.
134. Benes, F.M. Neurobiological investigations in cingulate cortex of schizophrenic brain. Schizophr Bull 1993, 19(3):537–549.
135. Akbarian, S., et al. Altered distribution of nicotinamide-adenine dinucleotide phosphate-diaphorase cells in frontal lobe of schizophrenics implies disturbances of cortical development. Arch Gen Psychiatry 1993, 50:227–230.
136. Andersen, S.A., D.W. Volk, D.A. Lewis. Increased density of microtubule associated protein 2-immunoreactive neurons in the prefrontal white matter of schizophrenic subjects. Schizophr Res, 1996, 19:111–119.
137. Chesselet, M.F., E. Robbins. Characterization of striatal neurons expressing high levels of glutamic acid decarboxylase messenger RNA. Brain Res 1989, 492(1–2):237–244.
138. Valtschanoff, J.G., et al. Neurons in rat hippocampus that synthesize nitric oxide. J Comp Neurol 1993, 331(1):111–121.
139. Valtschanoff, J.G., et al. Neurons in rat cerebral cortex that synthesize nitric oxide: NADPH diaphorase histochemistry, NOS immunocytochemistry, and colocalization with GABA. Neurosci Lett 1993, 157(2):157–161.
140. Spike, R.C., A.J. Todd, H.M. Johnston. Coexistence of NADPH diaphorase with GABA, glycine, and acetylcholine in rat spinal cord. J Comp Neurol 1993, 335(3):320–333.
141. Davila, J.C., et al. NADPH diaphorase-positive neurons in the lizard hippocampus: a distinct subpopulation of GABAergic interneurons. Hippocampus 1995, 5(1):60–70.
142. Gabbott, P.L., S.J. Bacon. Co-localisation of NADPH diaphorase activity and GABA immunoreactivity in local circuit neurones in the medial prefrontal cortex (mPFC) of the rat. Brain Res 1995, 699(2):321–328.
143. Gabbott, P.L., S.J. Bacon. Local circuit neurons in the medial prefrontal cortex (areas 24a,b,c, 25 and 32) in the monkey. I. Cell morphology and morphometrics. J Comp Neurol 1996, 364(4):567–608.
144. Gabbott, P.L., S.J. Bacon, Local circuit neurons in the medial prefrontal cortex (areas 24a,b,c, 25 and 32) in the monkey. II. Quantitative areal and laminar distributions. J Comp Neurol 1996, 364(4):609–636.
145. Gabbott, P.L., et al. Local-circuit neurones in the medial prefrontal cortex (areas 25, 32 and 24b) in the rat: morphology and quantitative distribution. J Comp Neurol 1997, 377(4):465–499.
146. Pesold, C., F. Impagnatiello, M.G. Pisu, D.P. Uzunov, E. Costa, A. Guidotti. Reelin is preferentially expressed in neurons synthesizing γ-aminobutyric acid in cortex and hippocampus in adult rats. Proc Natl Acad Sci USA 1998, 95:3221–3226.
147. Pesold, C., W.S. Liu, A. Guidotti, E. Costa, H.J. Caruncho. Cortical bitufted, horizontal and martinotti cells preferentially express and secrete reelin into perineuronal nets, nonsynaptically modulating gene expression. Proc Natl Acad Sci USA, 1999, 96:3217–3222.
148. Marin-Padilla, M. Neurons of layer I. A developmental analysis. In: Cerebral Cortex. A. Peter, E.G. Jones, eds. New York: Plenum Press, 1984, pp 447–478.
149. Impagnatiello, F., et al. A decrease of reelin expression as a putative vulnerability factor in schizophrenia. Proc Natl Acad Sci USA 1998, 95(26):15718–15723.
150. Benes, F.M., et al. Deficits in small interneurons in prefrontal and cingulate cortices of schizophrenic and schizoaffective patients. Arch Gen Psychiatry 1991, 48(11):996–1001.

151. Jacobsen, B., D.K. Kinney, Perinatal complications in adopted and non-adopted schizophrenics and their controls: Preliminary results. Acta Psychiatr Scand 1980. 238:103–123.
152. Kinney, D.K., et al. Obstetrical complications in patients with bipolar disorder and their siblings. Psychiatry Res, 1993, 48:47–56.
153. Kinney, D.K., et al. Pre- and perinatal complications and risk for bipolar disorder: a retrospective study. J Affect Disord, 1998. (in press).
154. Johnston, M.V., J.T. Coyle, Ontogeny of neurochemical markers for noradrenergic, GABA-ergic and cholinergic neurons in neocortex lesioned with methylazoxymethanol acetate. J Neurochem 1980, 34:1429–1441.
155. Johnston, M.V. Biochemistry of neurotransmitters in cortical development. In: Cerebral Cortex. A. Peter, E.G. Jones, eds. New York: Plenum Press, 1988, pp 211–236.
156. Coyle, J.T., H.I. Yamamura. Neurochemical aspects of the ontogenesis of GABAergic neurons in the rat brain. Brain Res. 1976, 118:429–440.
157. Candy, J.M., I.L. Martin. The postnatal development of the benzodiazepine receptor in the cerebral cortex and cerebellum of the rat. J Neurochem 1979, 32:655–658.
158. Vincent, S.L., F.M. Benes. Postnatal maturation of GABA-immunoreactive neurons of rat medial prefrontal cortex. J Comp Neurol 1995, 355:81–92.
159. Verney, C., et al. Development of the dopaminergic innervation of the rat cerebral cortex. A light microscopic immunocytochemical study using anti-tyrosine hydroxylase antibodies. Brain Res 1982, 281(1):41–52.
160. Kalsbeek, A., et al. Development of the dopaminergic innervation in the prefrontal cortex of the rat. J Comp Neurol 1988, 269(1):58–72.
161. Benes, F.M., et al. Increased interaction of dopamine-immunoreactive varicosities with GABA neurons of rat medial prefrontal cortex occurs during the postweanling period. Synapse 1996, 23(4):237–245.
162. Sutanto, W., et al. Multifaceted interaction of corticosteroids with the intracellular receptors and with membrane $GABA_A$ receptor complex in the rat brain. J Neuroendocrinol 1989, 1:243–247.
163. Lambert, J.J., J.A. Peters, G.A. Cottrell. Actions of synthetic and endogenous steroids on the GABAA receptor. Trends Pharmacol Sci 1987, 8:224–227.
164. Majewska, M.D., J.-C. Bisserbe, L.R. Eskay. Glucocorticoids are modulators of $GABA_A$ receptors in brain. Brain Res 1985, 339:178–182.
165. Stumpf, W.E., C. Heiss, M. Sar, G.E. Duncan, C. Draver. Dexamethasone and corticosterone receptor sites. Histochemistry 1989, 92:201–210.
166. McEwen, B. Glucocorticoids and hippocampus: receptors in search of a function. In: Adrenal Actions on Brain. D. Ganten, E. Pfaff, eds. Springer-Verlag, Berlin: 1982, 1–22.
167. Woodbury, D.M. Effects of adrenal steroids: separability of anticonvulsant from hormonal effects. J Pharmacol Exp Ther, 1952, 153:337–343.
168. Pfaff, D.W., M.T.A. Silva, J.M. Weiss. Telemeterred recording of hormone effects on hippocampal neurons. Science 1971, 172:394–395.
169. Feldman, W., S. Robinson. Electrical activity of the brain in adrenalectomized rats with implanted electrodes. J Neurol Sci, 1968, 6:1–8.
170. Miller, A.L., C. Chaptal, B.S. Mcewen, J.R.E. Beck. Modulation of high affinity GABA uptake into hippocampal synaptosomes by glucocorticoids. Psychoneuroendocrinology 1978, 3:155–164.
171. Schwarcz, R., J.T. Coyle. Neurochemical sequelae of kainate injections in corpus striatum and substantia nigra of the rat. Life Sci 1977, 20:431–436.
172. Sapolsky, R.M. Stress, the Aging Brain, and the Mechanisms of Neuron Death. Cambridge, MA: MIT Press, 1992.
173. Van Hoesen, G.W., R.J. Morecraft, B.A. Vogt. Connections of the monkey cingulate cortex. In: Neurobiology of Cingulate Cortex and Limbic Thalamus. B.A. Vogt, M. Gabriel, eds. Birkhauser, Boston: 1993, pp 249–284.
174. Pikkarainen, M.S., S Ronkko, V. Savander, R. Insausti, A. Pitkanen. Projections from the lateral, basal and accessory basal nuclei of the amygdalal to the hippocampal formation. J Comp Neurol, 1999. 403:229–260.
175. Longson, D., J.F. Deakin, and F.M. Benes. Increased density of entorhinal glutamate-immunoreactive vertical fibers in schizophrenia. J Neural Transm 1996, 103(4):503–507.
176. Wassef, A.A., et al. Critical review of GABA-ergic drugs in the treatment of schizophrenia. J Clin Psychopharmacol 1999, 19(3):222–232.
177. Bowden, C.L. New concepts in mood stabilization: evidence for the effectiveness of valproate and lamotrigine. Neuropsychopharmacology 1998, 19(3):194–199.
178. Benes, F.M., J.B. Taylor, M.C. Cunningham. Convergence and plasticity of monoaminergic systems in the medial prefrontal cortex during the postnatal period: implications for the development of psychopathology. Cereb Cortex 2000, 10(10):1014–1027.
179. Eccles, J.C. The cerebral neocortex. A theory of its operation. In: Cerbral Cortex. Functional Properties of Cortical Cells. E.G. Jones, A. Peter, eds. New York: Plenum Press, 1984, pp 1–48.

20

Genetic Findings in Psychotic Disorders

MICHAEL O'DONOVAN and MICHAEL OWEN
University of Wales College of Medicine, Cardiff, Wales

I. INTRODUCTION

Hypotheses concerning the etiology and pathophysiology of schizophrenia are legion, but the origins of this disorder remain unknown. Furthermore, as there are no objective, laboratory-based diagnostic tests for schizophrenia; diagnosis is based on patterns of symptoms, signs, and other historical variables. Given these problems, the disorder we know as schizophrenia should be thought of as a syndrome, covering a range of conditions that are heterogeneous in terms of symptoms, course, outcome, response to treatment, and probably etiology. Nevertheless, with the use of structured and semistructured interviews and explicit operational diagnostic criteria, it is possible to diagnose the disorder with a high degree of reliability, and, as we shall show below, the syndrome so defined has a high heritability thus allowing the possibility of dissection of schizophrenia by genetic investigation. However, as in all areas of schizophrenia research, the likely etiological heterogeneity of the disorder poses a formidable obstacle to progress, and disappointments abound in schizophrenia genetic research, particularly in the field of molecular genetics. Nevertheless, progress has been made and we remain optimistic that schizophrenia will succumb to the ever increasingly powerful tools available to geneticists. In this chapter, we review the current state of the field from the perspective of psychiatric geneticists, consider some of the difficulties that lie ahead, and offer our opinion on the likely solutions and the trajectory that future research is likely to follow.

II. GENETIC EPIDEMIOLOGY

A. Familiality and Genetic Risk

The extensive literature in genetic epidemiology contains some of the most robust findings in psychiatric research. In particular, the observation that schizophrenia tends to run in families is no longer open to serious debate. For example, Gottesman and Shields [1], based on data from ~40 family studies spanning much of the 20th century, were able to conclusively show that the risk of schizophrenia is increased in relatives of probands with the disorder. The lifetime risk for schizophrenia in the general population worldwide is generally reported to be around 1%. This contrasts with the risk to siblings (10%) and offspring of affected probands (13%), and although the risk to parents of an affected proband is somewhat lower (6%), this reflects the reproductive disadvantage conferred by schizophrenia. Many of the studies in this analysis predate up-to-date methods, but in a review of seven methodologically modern studies, the finding of an approximately 10-fold increase in risk of schizophrenia in first-degree relatives of schizophrenic probands remains [2].

However, it is well known that in addition to genetic inheritance, infective, cultural, and socioeconomic transmission may explain familial clustering. Fortunately, there is also an unambiguous twin and adoption literature on schizophrenia that permits genetic factors to be differentiated from other causes of familiality. The evidence here is clearcut; shared genes rather than shared environments underlie the increased risk of illness in relatives of those with the disorder [3]. Undoubtedly, unknown environmental factors play an important role in determining liability to schizophrenia, but the major determinant of individual variation in susceptibility is genetic. It is difficult to put an exact figure on the contribution made by genes, but based on the five most recent twin studies (conducted since 1995), the probandwise concordance rate for schizophrenia in monozygotic (MZ) twin pairs is 41–65% compared with 0–28% for dizygotic (DZ) twin pairs. This corresponds to heritability estimates of $\sim$ 80–85% [4].

B. Complex Genetics

Genetic epidemiology provides clear evidence that genes are the major risk factors for schizophrenia, and therefore, if we are to understand the etiology of schizophrenia, we must understand its genetics. Ideally, before seeking a disease-related gene or genes for a given disorder using molecular genetics techniques, it is helpful to define the mode of inheritance of that disorder. Under the simplest genetic models, there is a very strong correlation between phenotype (i.e., affected status) and genotype. For example, if a disease is genetically homogeneous, under a model of simple autosomal-dominant transmission, if a person is affected, then he can be assumed to carry a mutation at the disease locus, and vice versa. Under recessive inheritance, if a person is affected, then he can be assumed to carry a disease mutation in both copies of the gene involved in disease, and vice versa. However, given the fairly high rates of discordance for schizophrenia in MZ twin pairs, it is clear that such strict correlations between genotype and phenotype are not the rule.

The risk of a disease in a defined class of relative compared to that in the general population is often called λ. The λ for siblings is called λs, and in schizophrenia this is $\sim$ 10. The contribution of an individual allelic variant to the familiality of a disorder can be also expressed in these terms. Thus, for a given risk allele, λs is the relative risk to siblings resulting from possession of that disease allele [5]. This measure can be used to test the simplest hypothesis that risk for disease in any given family can be attributed to alleles of a single gene of large effect. By comparing expected with observed recurrence rates for a range of classes of relative, Risch [5] has calculated that the maximum λs for any schizophrenia susceptibility gene is $\sim$ 3 and, unless extreme epistasis exists, multiple loci of $\lambda s \leq 2$ are more plausible. These calculations are based on the assumption that the population of schizophrenics is etiologically homogeneous. Under a model of heterogeneity, it is possible that genes of larger effect are operating in some subpopulations of patients. Nevertheless, these and other analyses [e.g., 6] strongly suggest that schizophrenia is neither a single-gene disorder nor a collection of single-gene disorders. Rather, the mode of transmission is complex; how complex, is unknown.

Complex inheritance implies that susceptibility in any given individual may be conferred by coinheritance of alleles in more than one gene. This may be a small number of alleles of moderate effect (oligogenic inheritance), a large number of alleles of small effect (polygenic inheritance), or a mixture of the two. However, the number of susceptibility loci, the disease risk conferred by each locus, and the degree of interaction between loci all remain unknown. It is also important to note that complex inheritance implies that not all affected individuals will carry a given susceptibility variant, and conversely, many (possibly most) unaffected individuals carry at least one susceptibility variant. This complexity is the second major obstacle faced by those whose goal is identifying genes for schizophrenia.

C. Complex Phenotype

Many of the difficulties in classifying and defining the schizophrenia phenotype have been discussed elsewhere in this book, and we will therefore mention them only briefly. While it is clear that genotype confers liability to schizophrenia, we have no clear idea what form this "liability" actually takes. That is to say, we do not understand the nature of the inherited intermediate phenotypes that predispose to schizophrenia. It follows, then, that unless it is manifest as disorder, we do not know who has inherited high liability or, more accurately, how liability should be measured and quantified.

The situation is made even more complex by the fact that we are unable to demarcate the clinical syndrome to which liability may lead. Family, twin, and adoption studies have shown that the phenotype extends beyond the core diagnosis of schizophrenia to include a spectrum of disorders including, mainly, schizophrenic schizoaffective disorder and schizotypal personality disorder [7]. However, the limits of this spectrum of disorders and its relationship with other psychoses, affective and nonaffective, and nonpsychotic affective disorders remain uncertain [8–10]. Uncertainty, then, about the nature of liability and the limits of the phenotype is the third major obstacle to genetic analysis of schizophrenia.

These difficulties are not unique to schizophrenia or psychiatric genetics, and although it is of little consolation, they are faced to varying degrees by genetic investigators of other common diseases, be it diabetes, cancer, asthma, or heart disease. In spite of the problems and uncertainties we have described and the difficulties that ensue, schizophrenia seems a compelling candidate for molecular genetic approaches. This is because genes make such a strong contribution to its etiology, and, notwithstanding improvements in neuroimaging, the brain is still difficult to study directly, and the interpretation of cause and effect is problematic.

III. MOLECULAR GENETICS

There are two main approaches for identifying disease genes in human populations: linkage, and association. In linkage studies the objective is to identify regions of the genome that are cotransmitted with the disease in families containing two or more affected individuals. Where linkage is appropriate, it can detect the presence of genes within large chromosomal regions. This means that *relatively* few evenly spaced genetic markers (∼ 200–300) are required to screen the whole genome for the presence of disease genes. Therefore, linkage has the potential to locate disease genes by chromosomal position alone without regard to any prior knowledge of disease etiology.

Linkage is ideally suited to detecting genes for simple genetic disorders, but its power to detect genes of moderate to small effect is limited. In association studies, the aim is to detect alleles that are more (or less) common in a series of unrelated cases than in controls. Under most circumstances, association is more powerful for detecting genes of small effect than linkage. However, in outbred populations, many tens, or even hundreds, of thousands of markers are required to screen the whole genome by association. This is currently impractical, and although the hope is that genomewide association screening may be possible with improved technology, the role of association to date is restricted to testing discrete hypotheses except in unusual isolated populations.

A. Linkage

The first wave of systematic molecular genetic studies of schizophrenia in the late 1980s/early 1990s focused on linkage analysis of large pedigrees containing multiple affecteds. This approach had been highly effective for identifying genes of large effect in single-gene disorders. The proponents of this method were aware it was unlikely that such genes accounted for most of the genetic risk for schizophrenia. Instead, the hope was that under a mixed genetic model, the multiplex families, or at least a sufficient proportion of them, were the result of segregation of rare genes of large effect.

This optimistic view proved to be well founded in a number of complex disorders—for example, Alzheimer's disease (AD), where mutations in three genes, APP, PS1, and PS2, are now known to cause rare forms of the disorder. In such cases, the disease is of unusually early onset and is transmitted through multiplex pedigrees as an autosomal-dominant [11–13]. Early studies of large schizophrenia pedigrees also initially produced a strongly positive finding [14]. Unfortunately, this could not be replicated. However, modest evidence for several linked loci has been reported, some of which has received supportive evidence from international collaborative studies. These include chromosome 22q11-12, 6p24-22, 8p22-21, and 6q [15–17]. There are also a number of other promising areas of putative linkage, which have been supported by other individual groups although not from larger, international consortia. These include 13q14.1-q32 [18–20], 5q21-q31 [21,22], and 10p15-p11 [21,23,24]. One other region that is notable for the strength of evidence (maximum heterogeneity LOD score of 6.5) from a single study, rather than the more important convergence of evidence from different sources is 1q21-q22 [25]. The finding on 1q21-q22 more than meets standard criteria for claiming "significant" linkage. Early experience in psychiatric genetics has, however, impressed the need for replication firmly upon the minds of most researchers, and although there have been other reports of linkage to markers on chromosome 1 [26,27], these are distal to 1q21-q22, and it is not yet clear that these findings are consistent with the existence of a single susceptibility locus on 1q. Not surprisingly, this region is now under intense investigation by an international linkage consortium.

While the linkage data based on multiplex families are not definitive, it seems likely that one or more of the above loci are true positives. However, it should be noted that in every case there are negative as well as positive findings, and in only two cases, 13q14.1-q32 and 1q21-q22, did any single study achieve genomewide significance at $P < .05$, that is, a linkage value that is expected less than once by chance in 20 complete genome scans.

As more linkage data from genome scans of schizophrenia and bipolar disorder have emerged, putative linkages to both disorders have been reported in the same regions of the genome, for example 13q22 and 22q11-13 [28]. The observation of common linked loci may indicate at least a partial degree of overlap in the etiologies of these two disorders. However, while we are inclined to be sympathetic to this view, there are several reasons for caution:

1. None of the linkages are as yet definitive, and therefore the strength of the evidence for joint areas of linkage is not conclusive.
2. Similarity is more noticeable than dissimilarity. Until the apparent "clustering" has been subjected to rigorous statistical analysis, the pattern may be coincidence.
3. Even if correct, the regions of linkage contain hundreds or even thousands of genes. It follows that the presence of common linked loci does not prove common genes.
4. It is possible that the joint linkages are to loci that modify the phenotype of both disorders rather than susceptibility genes common to both. An obvious example that might lead to increased ascertainment in linkage studies of both disorders is chronicity.

As an alternative to linkage based on multiplex families, some groups have advocated the use of smaller families with two or more affecteds in a single sibship. This is in the belief that such families may be more suited for the analysis of complex traits, and being much more common, may also be more representative of disease in the general population. This approach has been successful in detecting linkage to several complex diseases. Of most relevance to this readership, these include late-onset AD [29]. We have recently reported the largest systematic search for linkage yet published using a sample of 196 affected sibling pairs (ASPs) [30]. This study was designed to have power > 0.95 to detect a susceptibility locus of $\lambda s = 3$ (the maximum effect size estimated by Risch [5]) with genomewide significance of 0.05. However, no regions of the genome gave linkage results approaching genomewide significance, but we did find modest evidence (at the level expected by chance once per genome scan) for loci on chromosomes 4p, 18p, and the centromeric region of X.

Since, arguably, no definitive linkages have emerged to date from linkage analysis of schizophrenia, the results must be viewed as disappointing. However, as some of the more promising findings described above have only recently emerged, we believe that persistence with the linkage approach is justified. We must also continue to explore different models of disease definition, but also tailor our sample sizes appropriately. For example our own genome scan [30] based on sib pairs was powered predicated on a locus of $\lambda s = 3$, but only had power of 0.7 to detect significant linkage to loci of $\lambda s = 2$. Such loci are still within the detection limits of linkage, using sample sizes of 600–800 sibling pairs [31,32], and in collaboration with colleagues in Sweden, we are currently engaged in such a study. Those engaged in linkage analysis should now give priority to collecting such samples (or equivalently powered samples of multiplex families). Furthermore, clinical methodology must be, as far as is possible, comparable across all interested research groups if "failure to replicate" is to have much meaning. However, if liability to schizophrenia is entirely due to the operation of many genes of small effect, then even these large-scale studies will be unsuccessful. To detect genetic risk factors of this magnitude, we must turn to the second main gene identification strategy based on association designs.

B. Association Studies

As mentioned above, association studies offer a powerful means of identifying genes of small effect. However, because it is impractical at present to screen the whole genome by association, researchers must select specific genes or loci to be tested. This may be on the grounds that a gene is a functional candidate (i.e., it is involved in a biological process that is postulated as relevant to the disorder), because it is a positional candidate gene (i.e., it is located, or maps, to a locus that has been implicated by linkage), or a combination of the two. Because of doubts concerning the robustness of linkage findings in schizophrenia, most studies to date have focused on functional candidate genes. Before considering the most widely debated findings, it is necessary to consider some of the potential problems with association studies.

First, for disorders of unknown etiology such as schizophrenia, the potential choice of candidate genes is limited largely by the number of genes in the human genome ($\sim$ 40,000). This places a heavy burden of proof on positive results because each gene has an extremely low prior probability that it is involved in the disorder [33]. Second, many researchers believe that these studies have a significant potential to generate false positives due to unknown differences in the genetic structure of cases and well-matched control groups. This problem can be addressed by family-based association methods [34], but large enough samples with all relevant family members willing to participate are difficult to collect [35]. The next two problems relate to the interpretation of "failures to replicate" positive findings. This is often interpreted as evidence that the first study is a false positive. However, it is also possible that subsequent studies are false negatives, as to date all association studies of schizophrenia have had insufficient power to reliably detect small genetic effects. Even with larger samples, potential differences in the genetic structure of samples collected by different groups means fresh studies cannot be considered true replication experiments. For these reasons, it is difficult to draw definitive conclusions from conflicting findings [35].

The most obvious candidate genes derive from the neuro-pharmacological literature (see Chapters 0, 0, 0, 0 and 0 in this section). Thus, genes involved in dopaminergic and serotonergic neurotransmission have received a great deal of attention. With recent developments in genome analysis technology and the recent publication of the (almost) complete sequence of the human genome, these data are being rapidly extended to other systems including the glutamatergic, GABA-ergic, and genes involved in neuromodulation and neurodevelopment. It is impossible for us to present the results of the hundreds, possibly thousands, of candidate gene analyses that have been published or reported at meetings. Fortunately for the reader, this can be avoided by noting that for the reasons just outlined, the overwhelmingly negative reports cannot be considered as definitive exclusions of small genetic effects. Moreover, with perhaps the two exceptions we discuss below, no positive finding has received sufficient support from more than one group to suggest a true association with even a modest degree of probability.

C. Serotonin 5HT2a receptor

The serotonergic system is a therapeutic target for several antipsychotic drugs. The first genetic evidence for its involvement in schizophrenia was a report of association with a T > C polymorphism at nucleotide 102 in the HTR2A gene which encodes the 5HT2a receptor [36]. This association was based on a small sample of Japanese subjects. Firmer evidence for association subsequently emerged from a large, multicenter European consortium [37] and a meta-analysis of all the data available in 1997 based on > 3000 subjects [38].

Since the meta-analysis was undertaken, a few further negative reports have followed, none with the sample sizes required. If we assume homogeneity and that the association is correct, the odds ratio (OR) for the C allele is $\sim$ 1.2. Sample sizes of 1000 subjects are required for 80% power to detect an effect of this size even at $P = .05$. However, while the negative studies do not refute the putative association, the evidence presented even in the meta-analysis ($P = .0009$) is well short of genome wide significance (estimated at around $P = 5 \times 10^{-8}$ by Risch and Merikangas [39]). Admittedly, demanding genomewide significance is inappropriate for such a strong candidate gene because the prior probability that it is involved in schizophrenia is greater than a gene selected at random. However, as there is no way of quantifying how much greater the prior probability is, we have no compelling alternative to genomewide significance. Consequently, we believe that the evidence tends to indicate association between HTR2A and schizophrenia, but that the burden of proof has not yet been met. Another reason to be skeptical about the putative association is that there are no variants yet detected in the gene that clearly alter receptor function or expression. However, there is some indirect evidence for the existence of sequence variation elsewhere that alters HTR2A expression in some regions of the brain [40].

D. Dopamine D3 Receptor Gene

The dominant neurochemical hypothesis of schizophrenia involves dysregulation of the dopaminergic system, with disordered transmission at the dopamine D2 receptor widely favored. However, association analyses of DRD2 to date have essentially been negative, although recently, three groups, two Japanese [41,42] and one Swedish [43], have implicated a polymorphism in the promoter which alters DRD2 expression in vitro. Unfortunately, the biggest single study to date found no evidence for association [44]. Furthermore, when the U.K. data from this study were combined with a large dataset from Scotland, the allele that was associated with schizophrenia in the other three studies was actually significantly less common in the patient group [45]. This finding has been interpreted as suggestive that the polymorphism tested in these studies is simply a marker for the true susceptibility variant (i.e., association due to linkage disequilibrium [LD]). While it is reasonable to attribute reversal of allelic association to LD differences between samples of different ethnic origins, the explanation would be more convincing if the same allele were associated in both the U.K. and the Swedish samples. Furthermore, if LD is the explanation, then the fact that this particular polymorphism is functional is no longer relevant. Data from more groups are required before a sensible discussion of the role of this variant can be undertaken.

The dopamine hypothesis has received somewhat stronger, although not robust, support from studies of DRD3 which encodes the dopamine D3 receptor. Association has been reported between schizophrenia and homozygosity for a Ser9Gly polymorphism in exon 1 of this gene [46]. As expected, positive and negative data have emerged, but unlike DRD2, sufficient data are available for meta-analysis. Based on all available data from > 5000 individuals, Williams and colleagues [47] concluded in favor of association although the effect size was extremely small (OR = 1.23) but nominally significant ($P = .0002$). As for HTR2A, for the reasons outlined above, the level of statistical evidence, while supportive, is not conclusive.

IV. ANTICIPATION AND TRINUCLEOTIDE REPEATS

Anticipation is the phenomenon whereby a disease becomes more severe or has an earlier age at onset in successive generations. Numerous studies have now suggested that the pattern of illness in multiplex pedigrees segregating schizophrenia and other psychotic illnesses is at least consistent with anticipation, although ascertainment biases offer an alternative explanation [48].

True genetic anticipation is a hallmark of a particular class of mutation called expanded trinucleotide repeats. The observations in families have therefore been taken as suggestive that such mutations might be involved in the etiology of psychosis [49]. This hypothesis has received support from a number of studies reporting that large but unidentified CAG/CTG trinucleotide repeats are more common in patients with schizophrenia and other psychoses than in unaffected controls [e.g., 50,51]. Unfortunately, these early findings have been followed by numerous failures of replication. Also, the specific loci responsible for ~ 50% of the anonymous CAG/CTG repeats detected in the previous studies have now been identified, but neither is associated with psychosis [e.g., 52,53]. These data have tempered much of the enthusiasm for the CAG/CTG hypothesis, but it is still premature to discard it. Indeed, two independent groups have recently detected the presence of proteins in a small number of schizophrenics that react with an antibody against moderate to large polyglutamine sequences [see 54]. This is of relevance here because polyglutamine sequences are often encoded in DNA by CAG repeats. It remains to be seen whether these proteins are involved in the disease rather than simply chance findings.

V. CYTOGENETIC ABNORMALITIES

A third approach by which investigators have sought to locate susceptibility genes for schizophrenia has been to identify chromosomal abnormalities in affected individuals. Cytogenetic anomalies, such as translocations and deletions, may be pathogenic through several mechanisms; direct disruption of a gene or genes; indirect disruption of the function of neighbouring genes by a so-called position effect; or an alteration of gene dosage in the case of deletions, duplications, and unbalanced translocations. It is also possible for an abnormality merely to be linked with a susceptibility variant in a particular family. Owing to the high prevalence of schizophrenia, a single incidence of a cytogenetic abnormality is insufficient to suggest causality. To warrant further investigation, a cytogenetic abnormality should either be shown to exist in greater frequencies in affected individuals, to disrupt a region already implicated by genetic analyses, or to show co-segregation with the condition in affected families.

There have been numerous reports of associations between schizophrenia and chromosomal abnormalities [55,56], but, with two exceptions, none has yet provided convincing evidence to support the location a gene conferring risk to schizophrenia. The first strongly suggestive finding is a t(1;11) balanced reciprocal translocation found to cosegregate with schizophrenia in a large Scottish family [57], and which has recently been reported to directly disrupt three genes, of unknown function, on chromosome 1 [58]. Interestingly, the breakpoint appears to be located close to the markers implicated in the two Finnish studies mentioned previously [26,27]. However, until mutations have been identified in other families or convincing biological evidence implicating this locus has been obtained, the mechanism by which the translocation confers risk to mental illness remains obscure. The second finding of interest is the association between velocardiofacial syndrome and schizophrenia.

Velocardiofacial syndrome (VCFS), also known as DiGeorge or Shprintzen syndrome, is associated with small interstitial deletions of chromosome 22q11. The phenotype of VCFS is variable, but in addition to characteristic core features of dysmorphology and congenital heart disease, there is strong evidence that individuals with VCFS have a dramatic increase in the risk of psychosis [59–61]. There is still some dispute about the nature of the psychotic phenotype associated VCFS. Thus, the first two of these studies [59,60] suggested the association to be with schizophrenia and schizoaffective disorders, while the third [61] demonstrated a high prevalence of bipolar spectrum disorders. At least some of the differences can be attributed to differing methods of proband ascertainment, the proband age group, and the diagnostic methodology used.

To characterize the psychosis phenotype in VCFS further, we recently evaluated 50 VCFS cases with a structured clinical interview to establish DSM-IV diagnosis [62]. Fifteen individuals with VCFS (30%) had a psychotic disorder, 12 of whom met DSM-IV criteria for schizophrenia. These data strongly suggest that it is schizophrenia and allied disorders that explain the high rates of psychosis in VCFS, but studies based on sounder epidemiological principles are now required to demonstrate this beyond all doubt.

Clearly, with an estimated prevalence of 1 in 4000 live births, one can estimate that VCFS cannot be responsible for more than a small fraction (~1%) of cases, and this estimate is in keeping with empirical data (63). From the practical perspective, clinicians should be vigilant for VCFS especially when psychosis occurs in the presence of other features suggestive of the syndrome such as dysmorphology, mild learning disability, or a history of cleft palate or congenital heart disease [64,65]. However, from the perspective of the genetic researcher, the most pressing question is whether the high rate of psychosis in VCFS provides a short cut to a gene within the deleted region which is involved in susceptibility to schizophrenia in cases without a deletion. To answer this, we are currently screening all the genes that map to the deleted region. However, there are reasons to be optimistic that this will be a route to a general susceptibility gene rather than a blind alley. As we have already seen, some linkage studies suggest the presence of a general schizophrenia susceptibility locus on 22q. While most suggest that this maps outside the VCFS region, linkage mapping in complex diseases is imprecise, and modest evidence for linkage within the VCFS region has also been reported [19,66,67].

VI. RESOLVING THE IMPASSE

The linkage studies to date have shown that genes of major effect are not common causes of schizophrenia and allied psychoses. They have also provided information concerning the *possible* location of some genes of moderate effect. Association studies have provided further mapping information, with VCFS providing fairly strong evidence for a susceptibility locus in 22q11. To a lesser degree, with the proviso that the associations in HTR2A and DRD3 are at best weak and provisional, they also suggest that the dominant neurochemical hypotheses are at least partially correct. It is clear, however, that the findings from molecular genetics are as fragile as those from genetic epidemiology are robust. How are we to make progress?

As in other common diseases, it is hoped that advances in the genetics of schizophrenia will come through the application of detailed information on the anatomy and sequence of the human genome combined with new methods of genotyping and statistical analysis. To take advantage of these developments, collection of large, well-characterized samples is a priority [68]. Samples for genetic studies of schizophrenia are generally ascertained in differing and unsystematic ways, which may be one of the explanations of failures to replicate between studies. For example, if a positive association is detected in one patient group that, by virtue of the method of ascertainment, has been inadvertently selected for chronicity, the putative "risk allele" might actually be an allele that modifies treatment response rather than predisposing to the disorder itself. Unless this is recognized, replication will be difficult except in samples with a bias toward chronicity.

Another possible route forward will be the development of suitable animal models and the possibility of identifying the disease genes in animals by genetic mapping. This may be simpler in animals because, unlike humans, they can be bred under conditions that allow optimal power for gene detection. New technical developments also now permit us to compare the expression of thousands of different mRNAs and proteins between model and control animals, with the goal of identifying clues to novel biological pathways that can be tested in human subjects. Disorders that predominantly involve higher cognitive function such as schizophrenia are likely to prove difficult to model in animals, but there have been some developments that will be discussed in Section B, Chapter 9.

Finally, it is worth reminding ourselves that the effectiveness of molecular genetic studies depends on the genetic validity of the phenotypes studied. We therefore need to focus research on the development and refinement of phenotypic measures and biological markers, which might simplify the task of finding genes. It is possible that genetic validity may be improved by focusing on quantitative aspects of clinical variation such as symptom profiles [e.g., 69] or by identifying biological markers that predict degree of genetic risk or define more homogeneous subgroups. However, it seems unlikely that these phenotypes will provide a rapid solution to the problem. First, we will need measures that can be practically applied to a sufficient number of families or unrelated patients; second, we will need to ensure that the traits identified are highly heritable, which will itself require a return to classic genetic epidemiology and model fitting.

REFERENCES

1. II Gottesman, J Shields. Schizophrenia: The Epigenetic Puzzle. Cambridge: Cambridge University Press, 1982.
2. KS Kendler, SR Diehl. The genetics of schizophrenia: a current, genetic-epidemiologic perspective. Schizophr Bull 19:261–285, 1993.
3. P McGuffin, MJ Owen, MC O'Donovan, A Thapar, II Gottesman. Seminars in Psychiatric Genetics. London; Gaskell Press, 1994.
4. AG Cardno, II Gottesman. Twin studies of schizophrenia: from bow-and-arrow concordances to star wars Mx and functional genomics. Am J Med Genet 97(1):12–17, 2000.
5. N Risch. Linkage strategies for genetically complex traits. 2. The power of affected relative pairs. Am J Hum Genet 46:229–241, 1990.
6. M McGue, II Gottesman. A single dominant gene still cannot account for the transmission of schizophrenia. Arch Gen Psychiatry 46:478–479, 1989.
7. KS Kendler, AM Gruenberg, DK Kinney. Independent diagnoses of adoptees and relatives as defined by DSM-III in the provincial and national samples of the Danish adoption study of schizophrenia. Arch Gen Psychiatry 51(6):456–468, 1994.
8. KS Kendler, MC Neale, D Walsh. Evaluating the spectrum concept of schizophrenia in the Roscommon family study. Am J Psychiatry 152(5):749–754, 1995.
9. KS Kendler, LM Karkowski, D Walsh, TJ Crow. The structure of psychosis: latent class analysis of probands from the Roscommon family study. Arch Gen Psychiatry 55(6):492–509, 1998.
10. AG Cardno, VR Frühling, PC Sham, RM Murray, P McGuffin. A twin study of genetic relationships between psychotic symptoms. (Submitted.)
11. A Goate, MC Chartierharlin, M Mullan, J Brown, F Crawford, L Fidani, L Giuffra, A Haynes, N Irving, L James, R Mant, P Newton, K Rooke, P Roques, C Talbot, M Pericakvance, A Roses, R Williamson, M Rossor, M Owen, J Hardy. Segregation of a missense mutation in the amyloid precursor protein gene with familial Alzheimers disease. Nature 349:704–706, 1991.
12. R Sherrington, EI Rogaev, Y Liang, EA Rogaeva, G Levesque, M Ikeda, H Chi, C Lin, G Li, K Holman, T Tsuda, L Mar, JF Foncin, AC Bruni, MP Montesi, S Sorbi, I Rainero, L Pinessi, L Nee, I Chumakov, D Pollen, A Brookes, P Sanseau, RJ Polinsky, W Wasco, Har Dasilva, JL Haines, MA Pericakvance, RE Tanzi, AD Roses, PE Fraser, JM Rommens, PH Stgeorgehyslop. Cloning of a gene bearing missense mutations in early-onset familial Alzheimers disease. Nature 375:754–760, 1995.
13. E Levy-Lahad, W Wasco, P Poorkaj, DM Romano, J Oshima, WH Pettingell, CE Yu, PD Jondro, SD Schmidt, K Wang, AC Crowley, YH Fu, SY Guenette, D Galas, E Nemens, E Wijsman, TD Bird, GD Schellenberg, RE Tanzi. Candidate gene for the chromosome-1 familial Alzheimers disease locus. Science 269:973–977, 1995.
14. R Sherrington, J Brynjolfsson, H Petursson, M Potter, K Dudleston, B Barraclough, J Wasmuth, M Dobbs, H Gurling. Localization of a susceptibility locus for schizophrenia on chromosome-5. Nature 336:164–167, 1988.
15. M Gill, H Vallada, D Collier, P Sham, P Holmans, R Murray, P McGuffin, S Nanko, M Owen, S Antonarakis, D Housman, H Kazazian, G Nestadt, AE Pulver, RE Straub, CJ Maclean, D Walsh, KS Kendler, L Delisi, M Polymeropoulos, H Coon, W Byerley, R Lofthouse, E Gershon, L Golden, T Crow, R Freedman, C Laurent, S Bodeaupean, T Damato, M Jay, D Campion, J Mallet, DB Wildenauer, B Lerer, M Albus, M Ackenheil, RP Ebstein, J Hallmayer, W Maier, H Gurling, D Curtis, G Kalsi, J Brynjolfsson, T Sigmundson, H Petursson,

D Blackwood, W Muir, D Stclair, L He, S Maguire, HW Moises, HG Hwu, L Yang, C Wiese, L Tao, XH Liu, H Kristbjarnason, DF Levinson, BJ Mowry, H Doniskeller, NK Hayward, RR Crowe, JM Silverman, DJ Nancarrow, CM Read. A combined analysis of D22s278 marker alleles in affected sibpairs — support for a susceptibility locus for schizophrenia at chromosome 22Q12. Am J Med Genet 67:40–45, 1996.

16. Schizophrenia Linkage Collaborative Group for Chromosomes 3, 6, and 8. Additional support for schizophrenia linkage on chromosomes 6 and 8: a multicenter study. Am J Med Genet 67:580–594, 1996.

17. DF Levinson, P Holmans, RE Straub, MJ Owen, DB Wildenauer, PV Gejman, AE Pulver, C Laurent, KS Kendler, D Walsh, N Norton, NM Williams, SG Schwab, B Lerer, BJ Mowry, AR Sanders, SE Antonarakis, J-L Blouin, J-F DeLeuze, J Mallet. Multicenter linkage study of schizophrenia candidate regions on chromosomes 5q, 6q, 10p, and 13q: Schizophrenia Linkage Collaborative Group III. Am J Hum Genet 67:652–663, 2000.

18. MW Lin, D Curtis, N Williams, M Arranz, S Nanko, D Collier, P McGuffin, R Murray, M Owen, M Gill, J Powell. Suggestive evidence for linkage of schizophrenia to markers on chromosome 13q14.1-q32. Psychiatr Genet 5:117–126, 1995.

19. JL Blouin, BA Dombroski, SK Nath, VK Lasseter, PS Wolyniec, G Nestadt, M Thornquist, G Ullrich, J McGrath, L Kascg, M Lamacz, MG Thomas, C Gehrig, U Radhakrishna, SE Snyder, KG Balk, K Neufield, KL Swartz, N Demarchi, GN Papadimitriou, DG Dikeos, CN Stefanis, A Chakravarti, B Childs, DE Housman, HH Kazazian, SE Antonarakis, AE Pulver. Schizo- phrenia susceptibility loci on chromosomes 13q32 and 8p21. Nat Genet 20:70–73, 1998.

20. LM Brzustowicz, WG Honer, EWC Chow, D Little, J Hogan, K Hodgkinson, AS Bassett. Linkage of familial schizophrenia to chromosome 13q32. Am J Hum Genet 65:1096–1103, 1999.

21. SG Schwab, J Hallmayer, M Albus, B Lerer, GN Eckstein, M Borrmann, RH Segman, C Hanses, J Freymann, A Yakir, M Trixler, P Falkai, M Rietschel, W Maier, DB Wildenauer. A genome-wide autosomal screen for schizophrenia susceptibility loci in 71 families with affected siblings: support for loci on chromosome 10p and 6. Mol Psychiatry 5(6):638–649, 2000.

22. RE Straub, CJ Maclean, FA Oneill, D Walsh, KS Kendler. Support for a possible schizophrenia vulnerability locus in region 5q22-31 in Irish families. Mol Psychiatry 2:148–155, 1997.

23. SV Faraone, T Matise, D Svrakic, J Pepple, D Malaspina, B Suarez, C Hampe, CT Zambuto, K Schmitt, J Meyer, P Markel, H Lee, J Harkavy-Friedman, C Kaufmann, CR Cloninger, MT Tsuang. Genome scan of European-American schizophrenia pedigrees: results of the NIMH genetics initiative and millennium consortium. Am J Med Genet 81:290–295, 1998.

24. RE Straub, CJ Maclean, RB Martin, YL Ma, MV Myakishev, C HarrisKerr, BT Webb, FA Oneill, D Walsh, KS Kendler. A schizophrenia locus may be located in region 10p15-p11. Am J Med Genet 81:296–301, 1998.

25. LM Brzustowicz, KA Hodgkinson, EWC Chow, WG Honer, AS Bassett. Location of a major susceptibility locus for familial schizophrenia on chromosome 1q21-22. Science 288:678–682, 2000.

26. I Hovatta, T Varilo, J Suvisaari, JD Terwilliger, V Ollikainen, R Arajärvi, H Juvonen, M-J Kokko-Sahin, L Väisänen, H Mannila, J Lönnqvist, L Peltonen. A genomewide screen for schizophrenia genes in an isolated finnish subpopulation, suggesting multiple susceptibility loci. Am J Hum Genet 65:1114–1125, 2000.

27. J Ekelund, D Lichtermann, I Hovatta, P Ellonen, J Suvisaari, JD Terwilliger, H Juvonen, T Varilo, R Arajärvi, M-L Kokko-Sahin, J Lönnqvist, L Peltonen. Genomewide scan for schizophrenia in the Finnish population: evidence for a locus on chromosome 7q22. Hum Mol Genet 9(7):1049–1057, 2000.

28. WH Berrettini. Susceptibility loci for bipolar disorder: overlap with inherited vulnerability to schizophrenia. Biol Psychiatry 47:245–251, 2000.

29. A Myers, P Holmans, H Marshall, J Kwon, D Meyer, D Ramic, S Shears, J Booth, F Wavrant DeVrieze, R Crook, M Hamshere, R Abraham, N Tunstall, F Rice, S Carty, S Lillystone, P Kehoe, V Rudrasingham, L Jones, S Lovestone, J Perez-Tur, J Williams, MJ Owen, J Hardy, AM Goate. Susceptibility locus for Alzheimer's disease on chromosome 10. Science 290(5500):2304–2305, 2000.

30. NM Williams, MI Rees, P Holmans, N Norton, AG Cardno, LA Jones, KC Murphy, RD Sanders, G McCarthy, MY Gray, I Fenton, P McGuffin, MJ Owen. A two-stage genome scan for schizophrenia susceptibility genes in 196 affected sibling pairs. Hum Mol Genet 8:1729–1739, 1999.

31. ER Hauser, M Boehnke, SW Guo, NJ Risch. Affected sib pair interval mapping and exclusion for complex traits: sampling considerations. Genet Epidemiol 13:117–137, 1996.

32. W Scott, M Pericakvance, J Haines. Genetic analysis of complex diseases. Science 275:1327, 1997.

33. MJ Owen, P Holmans, P McGuffin. Association studies in psychiatric genetics. Mol Psychiatry 2:270–273, 1997.

34. DJ Schaid, SS Sommer. Comparison of statistics for candidate gene association studies using cases and parents. Am J Hum Genet 55:402–409, 1994.

35. MC O'Donovan, MJ Owen. Candidate gene association studies of schizophrenia. Am J Hum Genet 65:587–592, 1999.
36. Y Inayama, H Yoneda, T Sakai, Y Ishida, Y Nonomura, R Kono, J Takahata, J Koh, J Sakai, A Takai, Y Inada, H Asaba. Positive association between a DNA sequence variant in the serotonin 2A receptor gene and schizophrenia. Am J Med Genet 67:103–105, 1996.
37. J Williams, G Spurlock, P McGuffin, J Mallet, MM Nothen, M Gill, H Aschauer, P Nylander, F Macciardi, MJ Owen. Association between schizophrenia and T102C polymorphism of the 5-hydroxytryptamine type 2A-receptor gene. Lancet 347:1294–1296, 1996.
38. J Williams, P McGuffin, M Nothen, MJ Owen, the EMASS Collaborative Group. Meta-analysis of association between the 5-HT2a receptor T102C polymorphism and schizophrenia. Lancet 349:1221, 1997.
39. N Risch, K Merikangas. The future of genetic studies of complex human diseases. Science 273:1516–1517, 1996.
40. R Bunzel, I Blumcke, S Cichon, S Normann, J Schramm, P Propping, MM Nothen. Polymorphic imprinting of the serotonin-2A (5-HT2A) receptor gene in human adult brain. Mol Brain Res 59:90–92, 1998.
41. T Arinami, M Gao, H Hamaguchi, M Toru. A functional polymorphism in the promoter region of the dopamine D2 receptor gene is associated with schizophrenia. Hum Mol Genet 6(4):577–582, 1997.
42. K Ohara, M Nagai, K Tani, Y Nakamura, A Ino, K Ohara. Functional polymorphism of -141C Ins/Del in the dopamine D2 receptor gene promoter and schizophrenia. Psychiatry Res 81(2):117–123, 1998.
43. EG Jonsson, MM Nothen, H Neidt, K Forslund, G Rylander, M Mattila-Evenden, M Asberg, P Propping, GC Sedvall. Association between a promoter polymorphism in the dopamine D2 receptor gene and schizophrenia. Schizophr Res 40(1):31–36, 1999.
44. T Li, X Hu, KG Chandy, E Fantino, K Kalman, G Gutman, JJ Gargus, B Freeman, RM Murray, E Dawson, XH Liu, AT Bruinvels, PC Sham, DA Collier. Transmission disequilibrium analysis of a triplet repeat within the hKCa3 gene using family trios with schizophrenia. Biochem Biophys Res Communs 251:662–665, 1998.
45. G Breen, J Brown, S Maude, H Fox, D Collier, T Li, M Arranz, D Shaw, D St Clair. -141 C Del/Ins polymorphism of the dopamine receptor 2 gene is associated with schizophrenia in a British population. Am J Med Genet Neuropsychiatr Genet 88(4):407–410, 1999.
46. MA Crocq, R Mant, P Asherson, J Williams, Y Hode, A Mayerova, D Collier, L Lannfelt, P Sokoloff, JC Schwartz, M Gill, JP Macher, P McGuffin, MJ Owen. Association between schizophrenia and homozygosity at the dopamine-d3 receptor gene. J Med Genet 29:858–860, 1992.
47. J Williams, G Spurlock, P Holmans, R Mant, K Murphy, L Jones, A Cardno, P Asherson, D Blackwood, W Muir, K Meszaros, H Aschauer, J Mallet, C Laurent, P Pekkarinen, J Seppala, CN Stefanis, GN Papadimitriou, F Macciardi, M Verga, C Pato, H Azevedo, MA Crocq, G Gurling, G Kalsi, D Curtis, P McGuffin, MJ Owen. A meta-analysis and transmission disequilibrium study of association between the dopamine D3 receptor gene and schizophrenia. Mol Psychiatry 3:141–149, 1998.
48. MC O'Donovan, MJ Owen. Dynamic mutations and psychiatric genetics. Psychol Med 28:1–6, 1996.
49. A Petronis, JL Kennedy. Unstable genes — unstable mind? Am J Hum Genet 152:164–172, 1996.
50. MC O'Donovan, C Guy, N Craddock, KC Murphy, AG Cardno, L Jones, MJ Owen, P McGuffin. Expanded CAG repeats in schizophrenia and bipolar disorder. Nat Genet 10:380–381, 1995.
51. AG Morris, E Gaitonde, PJ Mckenna, JD Mollon, DM Hunt. CAG repeat expansions and schizophrenia: association with disease in females and with early age at onset. Hum Mol Genet 4:1957–1961, 1995.
52. JB Vincent, A Petronis, E Strong, SV Parikh, HY Meltzer, J Lieberman, JL Kennedy. Analysis of genome-wide CAG/CTG repeats, and at SEF2-1B and ERDA1 in schizophrenia and bipolar affective disorder. Mol Psychiatry 4:229–234, 1999.
53. T Bowen, CA Guy, AG Cardno, JB Vincent, JL Kennedy, LA Jones, M Gray, RD Sanders, G McCarthy, KC Murphy, MJ Owen, MC O'Donovan. Repeat sizes at CAG/CTG loci CTG18.1, ERDA1 and TGC13-7a in schizophrenia. Psychiatr Genet 10(1): 33–37, 2000.
54. CA Ross. Schizophrenia genetics: expansion of knowledge? Mol Psychiatry 4:4–5, 1999.
55. Bassett AS. Chromosomal aberrations and schizophrenia: autosomes. Br J Psychiatry 161:323–334, 1992.
56. Baron M. Genetics of schizophrenia and the new millennium: progress and pitfalls. Am J Hum Genet 68:299–312, 2001.
57. D St Clair, D Blackwood, W Muir, A Carothers, M Walker, G Spowart, C Gosden, HJ Evans. Association within a family of a balanced autosomal translocation with major mental illness. Lancet 336:13–16, 1990.
58. JK Millar, JC Wilson-Annan, S Anderson, S Christie, MS Taylor, CA Semple, RS Devon, DM Clair, WJ Muir, DH Blackwood, DJ Porteous. Disruption of two novel genes by a translocation co-segregating with schizophrenia. Hum Mol Genet 9:1415–1423, 2000.

59. RJ Shprintzen, RB Goldberg, KJ Golding-Kushner. Late-onset psychosis in the velocardiofacial syndrome. Am J Med Genet 42:141–142, 1992.
60. AE Pulver, G Nestadt, R Goldberg, RJ Shprintzen, M Lamacz, PS Wolyniec, B Morrow, M Karayiorgou, SE Antonarakis, D Housman, R Kucherlapati. Psychotic illness in patients diagnosed with velo-cardio-facial syndrome and their relatives. J Nerv Ment Dis 182:476–478, 1994.
61. DF Papolos, GI Faedda, S Veit, RB Goldberg, B Morrow, R Kucherlapati, R Shprintzen. Bipolar spectrum disorders in patients diagnosed with velo-cardio-facial syndrome: does a hemizygous deletion of chromosome 22q11 result in bipolar affective disorder? Am J Psychiatry 153:1541–1547, 1996.
62. KC Murphy, LA Jones, MJ Owen. High rates of schizophrenia in adults with velo-cardio-facial syndrome. Arch Gen Psychiatry 56:940–945, 1999.
63. M Karayiorgou, MA Morris, B Morrow, RJ Shprintzen, R Goldberg, J Borrow, A Gos, G Nestadt, PS Wolyniec, VK Lasseter, AE Pulver. Schizophrenia susceptibility associated with interstitial deletions of chromosome 22q11. Proc Natl Acad Sci USA 92:7612–7616, 1995.
64. D Gothelf, A Frisch, H Munitz, R Rockah, T Aviram AMozes, M Birger, A Weizman, M Frydman. Velocardiofacial manifestations and microdeletions in schizophrenic patients. Am J Med Genet 72:455–461, 1997.
65. A Bassett, K Hodgkinson, EWC Chow, S Correia, LE Scutt, R Welsberg. 22q11 Deletion syndrome in adults with schizophrenia. Am J Med Genet 81:328–337, 1998.
66. VK Lasseter, AE Pulver, PS Wolyniec, G Nestadt, D Meyers, M Karayiorgou, D Housman, S Antonarakis, H Kazazian, L Kasch, R Babb, M Kimberland, B Childs. Follow-up report of potential linkage for schizophrenia on chromosome 22q3. Am J Med Genet 60:172–173, 1995.
67. SH Shaw, M Kelly, AB Smith, G Shields, PJ Hopkins, J Loftus, SJ Laval, A Vita, M DeHert, LR Cardon, TJ Crow, R Sherrington, LE Delisi. A genome wide search for schizophrenia susceptibility genes. Am J Med Genet 81:364–376, 1998.
68. MJ Owen, AG Cardno, MC O'Donovan. Psychiatric genetics: back to the future. Mol Psychiatry 5:22–31, 2000.
69. AG Cardno, LA Jones, KC Murphy, P Asherson, LC Scott, J Williams, MJ Owen, P McGuffin. Factor analysis of schizophrenic symptoms using the OPCRIT checklist. Schizophr Res 22:233–239, 1996.

21

Membrane Abnormalities in Psychotic Disorders

WAGNER FARID GATTAZ and ORESTES V. FORLENZA
University of São Paulo, São Paulo, Brazil

I. INTRODUCTION

Research into biochemical processes affecting membrane composition and fluidity have generated models that fit relatively well in both the neurodevelopmental hypotheses of schizophrenia and the neurodegenerative mechanisms of dementia. Data from the late 1980s suggesting increased phospholipase A_2 (PLA_2) activity in schizophrenia [1,2], and decreased in Alzheimer's disease [3,4], have been replicated by several groups [5,6]. Abnormalities of PLA_2 metabolism have also been described in other neuropsychiatric diseases such as multiple sclerosis [7] and temporal-lobe epilepsy [8,9].

PLA_2 enzymes participate in a wide variety of physiological processes, including phospholipid digestion, remodeling of cell membranes, and host defense. They also take part in pathophysiological processes by producing precursors of various types of biologically active lipid mediators, such as prostaglandins, leukotrienes, thromboxanes, and platelet-activating factor [10]. Over the past two decades, with advances in molecular biology, numerous PLA_2 subtypes have been identified and characterized [11–16]. According to biochemical features such as their primary structure, cellular localization, requirement of Ca^{2+}, and substrate specificity, these PLA_2s are classified into several families, including low-molecular-weight secretory PLA_2 ($sPLA_2$), Ca^{2+}-sensitive arachidonoyl-specific 85-kDa cytosolic PLA_2, Ca^{2+}-independent PLA_2, and platelet-activating factor-acetylhydrolase [13].

Accordingly to the "phospholipid hypothesis," membrane changes play a primary role in the etiology of schizophrenia. Abnormal regulation of highly unsaturated fatty acid metabolism, mainly at the *sn*-2 position of phospholipid molecules, results in modifications of the neuronal membrane structure, affecting intracellular signalling from neurotransmitter- and ion channel-related functions [17].

A. Short Review on the Biology of Membranes

Biomembranes are major constituents of neural tissue. Membrane integrity is essential for neuronal metabolism, at both the cellular and subcellular levels. The 7-nm-thick outer membrane provides an impermeable barrier for extracellular agents and substances, as well as the ability for the cell to become electrically and chemically excitable. The biophysical and biochemical properties of the membrane are the basis for all message transmission and signal transduction in the mammalian brain. In addition, the distinct roles that organelles undertake through neuronal metabolism are notably dependent on membrane function. One should include nuclear and mitocondrial membranes, the primarily membranous organelles such as smooth and rough endoplasmic reticula, the Golgi complex, and the container membranes required for disposal of catabolic products (lysosomes) and for enclosing intracellular stores of calcium and neurotransmitters (synaptic vesicles).

Membrane remodeling is fundamental for the long-term maintenance of neuronal function, since mammalian neurons are postmitotic from embryonic life and therefore no longer undertake cell division. All neuronal membranes are made up of lipids in which phospholipids, cholesterol, and cholesteryl esters play major roles in structure and function. In neurons, as compared to other nonneuronal cells, the importance of phospholipid metabolism is even greater, bearing in mind the profusion of axons and dendrites—which are mostly membrane-coated cytoskeleton—and the phenomenon of synaptic plasticity.

Biochemical signaling is likewise dependent on membrane function. Neuronal proteins and receptors are mostly embedded in, or attached to, phospholipid-rich membranes. Downstream on signal transduction, the release of second messengers is also highly dependent on the activity of phospholipases. Fatty acids, diacylglycerols, and inositol phosphates, which are central components of intracellular signaling systems, are released from membrane phospholipids during neuronal activation and under the catabolic action of phospholipases A, B, C, and D.

B. Molecular Structure of Phospholipids

Membrane phospholipids are large molecules assembled on a three-carbon backbone of glycerol. The four most important membrane phosphoglycerides—phosphatidylcholine (lecithin), phosphatidylethanolamine (cephalin), phosphatidylserine, and phosphatidylinositol—have two long fatty acid chains starting from carbon atoms at positions sn-1 and sn-2, and a phosphate-bound hydrophilic "characterizing group" (choline, ethanolamine, serine, and inositol) at sn-3 (Fig. 1).

The existence of a hydrophylic head group at one end of the molecule, and two hydrophobic fatty acid tails at the other, yields the amphipathic nature of phosphoglycerides. Such biophysical properties determine the ability of phospholipids to organize themselves as lipid bilayers in the interface of two aqueous solutions, that is, between the intracellular (cytosol) and extracellular environments.

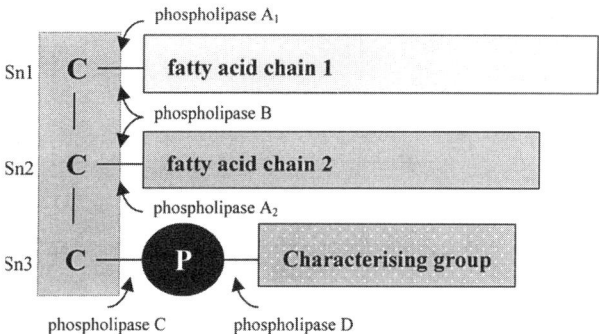

Figure 1 Schematic structure of membrane phospholipids, showing the three-carbon (C) backbone of glycerol (positions sn-1, 2, and 3) bearing two varying fatty acid tails and the phosphate- (P) bound characterizing group (phosphatidylcholine, phosphatidylethanolamine, phosphatidylserine, or phosphatidylinositol). The sites of action of phospholipases A_1, A_2, B, C and D are indicated by arrows. The catalytic activity of phospholipases originates free fatty acids and lysophospholipids (phosphodiesters) from phosphomonoester substrates.

Phospholipids differ from each other not only according to their "characterizing" heads, but also to the varying length of fatty acid chains (ranging from 12 to 20 carbons) and the nature of the bonds between every two carbon atoms within the fatty acid sequence. In other words, carbons may be linked by saturated (single) or unsaturated (double) covalent bonds. Both these features have an effect on the nature of the membrane. The shorter and more unsaturated the fatty acid tail, the greater the fluidity of the membrane, since such properties make the tails more difficult to pack compactly within the membrane's core. The interior of the membrane is thus an organic fluid in which the individual phospholipid molecules continuously exchange places with each other and seldom migrate (or "flip-flop") from one side of the membrane to another. Modifications of membrane fluidity are expected to occur during neuronal metabolism and, indeed, as a consequence of brain maturation and ageing. Indeed, recent data from our laboratory provide indications of altered membrane fluidity in postmortem brains of schizophrenic and Alzheimer's disease patients (in preparation).

C. Role of Phospholipase A_2 in Membrane Phospholipid Metabolism

Phospholipids are substrates for the production of intra- and extracellular signaling molecules, and PLA_2

is one of the major phospholipid-cleaving enzymes. The PLA$_2$ superfamily is a heterogeneous group of enzymes, most of which display high selectivity for sn-2-arachidonoyl-containing phospholipids. Biochemically, PLA$_2$ enzymes are classified based on their molecular size, substrate specificity, aminoacid sequence, and disulfide bond pattern [18]. According to its site of release and action, human PLA$_2$ can be further classified in cytosolic (type IV or cPLA$_2$) and secretory (sPLA$_2$) phospholipase A$_2$, the latter group being additionally subdivided into pancreatic (type I) or nonpancreatic (type II) forms. Recently, several additional members of the PLA$_2$ superfamily have been identified, leading to the inclusion of class V (secretory), VI (80 kDa inducible), VII and VIII (both of which are calcium independent and specific for platelet activating factor), and IX (secretory) [19,20].

Type II sPLA$_2$ are small (13–19 kDa) secretory enzymes characterized by the presence of several disulfide bridges, being thus inhibited by sulfhydryl reducing agents. Secretory PLA$_2$ becomes active following extracellular release and requires micromolar calcium concentrations as a catalytic cofactor. In addition, sPLA$_2$ has no preference for arachidonic acid over other acyl groups at the sn-2 position—rather, it has a broad affinity for phospholipids with different polar head groups and fatty acyl chains [18,21,22]. At present, mammalian sPLA$_2$s are classified into five different groups (groups IB, IIA, IIC, V, and X), depending on the number and positions of cysteine residues and the localization of intramolecular disulfide bridges [14]. Among them, group IIA PLA$_2$ has been thought to be one of the key enzymes in the pathogenesis of inflammatory diseases, owing to its augmented expression under various inflammatory conditions including sepsis, Crohn's disease, and acute pancreatitis. Likewise, the expression of sPLA$_2$-IIA has been shown to correlate well with disease severity in rheumatoid arthritis [23].

Type IV cPLA$_2$ are very distinct enzymes in that they display no detectable sequence homology to sPLA$_2$. The mammalian 85-kDa calcium-dependent cytosolic PLA$_2$ (cPLA$_2$-α) is a well studied example of this class of enzyme [11,24]. It is a monomeric polypeptide of 749 amino acids containing an aminoterminal calcium-dependent regulatory domain responsible for the translocation of the enzyme to membranes of the nuclear envelope upon activation [25–27]. Thus, cPLA$_2$ are larger intracellular molecules, with a clear preference (as compared to sPLA$_2$) for the cleavage of arachidonic acid at the sn-2 position of phospholipids. Whereas some type IV (cPLA$_2$) are calcium-dependent, other forms are not. More recently, three distinct subtypes of cPLA$_2$ have been described—α-, β-, and γ-PLA$_2$. Despite significant homology in both the calcium-dependent lipid-binding domain as well as in the catalytic domain, βPLA$_2$ is markedly less selective for cleavage at position sn-2 of phospholipids [28].

Phospholipases A$_2$ that reside in the cytosol are of particular interest because of their ability to interact directly with signal transduction elements such as G-proteins and kinases. Thus, cPLA$_2$ plays an essential role in neuronal membranes, not only by influencing the physicochemical properties of synaptic membranes, but also in signal transduction [29,30]. Lysophospholipids have several biological properties including membrane lysis, chemotaxy, mithogenesis, smooth muscle fiber contraction [31], and platelet activation factor (PAF) synthesis [32]. In addition, cPLA$_2$ activation leads to the downstream release of arachidonic acid and choline, respective substrates for the synthesis of major inflammatory mediators (eicosanoids) and acetylcholine [33,34] (Figure 2).

Both nonpancreatic sPLA$_2$ and cPLA$_2$ are ubiquitous enzymes and have been found in every cell line so far investigated, including neurons [35,36]. Tissue distribution is likewise wide, including platelets, neutrophils, monocytes, macrophages, skin fibroblasts, and

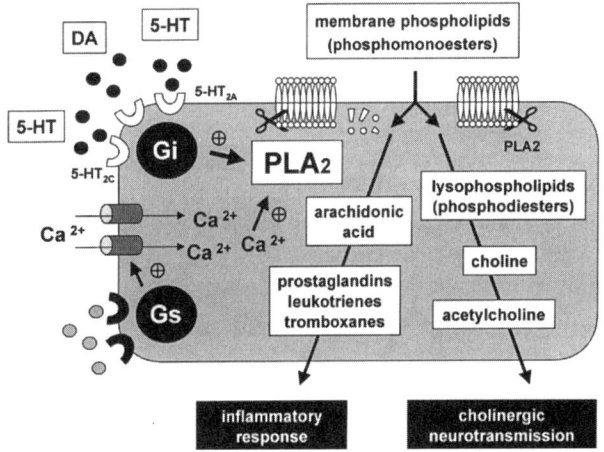

Figure 2 The 85-kDa intracellular enzyme cPLA$_2$ catalyzes the hydrolysis of the acyl group from the position sn-2 membrane glycerophospholipids. Both products of the reaction, fatty acids and lysophospholipids, may act as second messengers in intracellular signaling. Arachidonic acid has a central importance in generating bioactive and proinflammatory lipid components such as eicosanoids (e.g., prostaglandins, leukotrienes, and tromboxanes). The subsequent hydrolysis of lysophosphatidylcholine generates choline for acetylcholine synthesis.

cells of the brain, lung, liver, kidney, and spleen [18]. Although the importance of these enzymes in eicosanoid metabolism and signal transduction is not questioned, much of PLA$_2$ function and regulation remains to be learned. Cellular mechanisms for activation are yet unclear although 85 kDa undergoes translocation to membrane fractions in the presence of physiologically relevant changes in free calcium; an aminoterminal 140 aminoacid fragment of cPLA$_2$ shares this activity, suggesting the existence of a calcium-dependent phospholipid-binding motif [11]. PLA$_2$ activity is modulated by proteins of the PLIP (phospholipase-inhibiting protein) family, of which annexin-I, a calcium-dependent phospholipid-binding protein, has been shown to inhibit both low- and high-molecular-weight PLA$_2$ in a substrate-specific fashion [37].

Cytosolic PLA$_2$ is also a substrate for enzymes of the mitogen-activated protein (MAP) kinase cascade, and the phosphorylation at serine 505 by MAP-kinase increases the enzymatic activity of cPLA$_2$ [38]. In response to growth factors and neurotransmittters, ^{p42}MAP-kinase and protein-kinase C (PKC) activation lead to the phosphorylation of cPLA$_2$ in distinct sites, bearing the involvement of tyrosine kinase and G-protein-linked receptors in the regulation PLA$_2$ metabolism [38,39]. In fact, mechanisms of cross-talk between phospholipase A$_2$ and C have been suggested in studies with bone marrow [40] and thyroid cells [41,42].

Cytosolic PLA$_2$ expression can be influenced by tumor necrosis factor, interleukin-1, transforming growth factor beta, macrophage colony-stimulating factor, and glucocorticoids [18]. In animals, levels of calcium-independent cPLA$_2$ can be elevated by oxidative stress [43]. In the rat brain, it has been shown that PLA$_2$ expression is also developmentally regulated, being highest at embryonic day 12, gradually decreasing toward birth and retaining a constant level into adulthood [44]. This suggests that the enzyme plays an important role in the early development of the nervous system, which adds—at least theoretically—speculative interest in the neurodevelopmental models of schizophrenia.

II. PHOSPHOLIPIDS AND SCHIZOPHRENIA

A. Evidence of Relationship Extrapolated from Basic Research

In tissue culture models, it has been shown that arachidonic acid participates in pathways underlying neurite outgrowth and diferentiation of neuroblastoma cells [45]. Thus, one can speculate that genetically determined abnormalities of PLA$_2$ metabolism, affecting arachidonic acid availability in early stages of embryonic life, are likely to result in abnormal neuronal sprouting and differentiation, leading to cytoarchitectural changes within the brain. In vitro studies show that PLA$_2$ modulates dopamine (DA) synthesis and release [46,47]. The addition of exogenous PLA$_2$ and arachidonate to primary cultures of rat tuberoinfundibular neurones has been shown to stimulate DA release; likewise, the activation of calcium channels by ionophore agents leads to increased arachidonate levels (suggesting PLA$_2$ activation), and results in enhanced DA release [47]. On the other hand, dopamine receptor sensitivity is under negative modulation of PLA$_2$, as shown by the inhibition of the activation of DA-sensitive adenylate cyclase in striatal tissue by the pretreatment with PLA$_2$ [48] and by the PLA$_2$- and lysophosphatidylcholine-induced reduction of [^{3}H]spiperone binding to DA receptors in microsomal membranes isolated from sheep caudate nucleus [49].

Animal models have granted interesting insights on the inhibition of dopaminergic function by PLA$_2$. The in vivo effects of intracerebral injections of the PLA$_2$ were investigated in the model of DA-mediated locomotion behaviour in rats under apomorphine challenge. It is well known that subcutaneous injection of apomorphine increases locomotion in rats by a direct agonism of postsynaptic DA receptors. According to the rotational model presented by Ungerstedt and Arbuthnottin 1970 [50], the direction of circling movements is ipsilateral to the hemisphere with the lowest nigrostriatal dopaminergic activity [51,52]. Both intranigral [53,54] and intracerebroventricular injection of PLA$_2$ [55] resulted in reduced locomotion after apomorphine challenge, as compared to saline-injected controls. The inhibiton of apomorphine-induced locomotion by PLA$_2$ was reversible within 4 weeks after stereotaxic surgery, suggesting a functional inhibition of dopaminergic postsynaptic receptors by PLA$_2$. Unilateral stereotaxic injection of PLA$_2$ into the nigrostriatal area caused an ipsilateral apomorphineinduced rotational asymmetry, whereas intracerebroventricular PLA$_2$ application reduced apomorphine-induced locomotion [56]. Taken together, these data suggest that intracerebral injection of PLA$_2$ inhibits dopaminergic neurotransmission in vivo.

B. From Animal Models to Schizophrenic Patients

How could this inhibitory effect of PLA$_2$ on dopaminergic neurotransmission be involved in the pathophysiology of schizophrenia? Because of the central role of phospholipids in neurons, one could argue that the very large number of neurotransmitter-related abnormalities in schizophrenia may be a secondary consequence of phospholipid changes [57].

In 1971 John Stevens published what is perhaps the first report describing membrane lipid pathology in schizophrenia, after studying the lipid composition of erythrocyte membranes from 101 schizophrenics as compared to 20 normal controls [58]. Of the four major phospholipids studied, he found a marked (50%) increase in the phosphatidylserine content among schizophrenics, and an associated smaller decrease in phosphatidylcholine and phosphatidylethanolamine. Stevens was foresighted in his brief discussion, in which he pointed out that "if these membrane abnormalities extended to the brain, they could change the electrostatic charge at the synapse and thus have an infience on the threshold and transmission of impulses" [58,59].

Evidence of disturbed PLA_2 metabolism in schizophrenia was drawn from our studies at the University of Heidelberg in the late 1980s, bearing indications of increased PLA_2 activity in schizophrenic patients. The activity of PLA_2 was determined in the plasma of 20 drug-free schizophrenic patients, six nonschizophrenic psychiatric control patients, and 21 healthy controls. Schizophrenics showed significantly higher plasma PLA_2 activity than both controls (70% of the schizophrenics had enzyme activity higher than the highest value from the control group), which was reduced to the level of the controls after 3 weeks of neuroleptic treatment [1]. Such findings were subsequently corroborated by postmortem studies of schizophrenic brains, in which Horrobin and collaborators demonstrated significant differences from normal in the fatty acid composition of phosphatidylethanolamine in the frontal cortex [60].

Controversy was raised after negative measurements in the serum of drug-naïve schizophrenics [61], and the specificity of the finding was further questioned by the observation of increased plasmatic PLA_2 both in schizophrenic and nonschizophrenic psychiatric patients. Noponen and collaborators in 1993 found higher than normal PLA_2 activity not only in schizophrenics, but also in a psychiatric control group, including patients with major depression, bipolar disorder, posttraumatic stress disorder, and substance abuse [5]. Although PLA_2 activity values in the nonschizophrenic patients were not as high as among schizophrenics, the authors claimed that such increases should be viewed as nonspecific, in the same fashion as the findings of increased circulating PLA_2 in infectious and inflammatory conditions.

Such controversies were explained by the heterogeneity of plasmatic PLA_2 and the use of methodologies that may have measured the activity of diferent molecular forms of the enzyme [3]. In view of that, Ross and collaborators in 1997 [6] compared the PLA_2 activity simultaneously by means of the distinct protocols that had been used by earlier authors [1,5,61]. Activity of PLA_2 in serum samples obtained from 24 individuals with schizophrenia was compared with serum obtained from 33 age- and sex-matched control subjects, using both fluorometric and radiometric assays with different substrates. They were able to confirm by fluorometric analysis that PLA_2 activity was significantly elevated in schizophrenic patients compared to controls, validating the previous indications of abnormal phospholipid metabolism in schizophrenia. In contrast, radiometric assay of the same serum samples resulted in PLA_2 activity not significantly different between patients and control subjects. Further investigations demonstrated that, whereas the radiometric assay measured activity of a calcium-dependent enzyme, the fluorometric assay detected a calcium-insensitive enzyme possessing an acid-neutral pH optimum [6].

Indeed, calcium-independent $cPLA_2$ activity in schizophrenic patients has been consistently reported to be increased in plasma [1,6], serum [2,5], and platelet membranes [2,62]. In platelets of schizophrenics, phosphatidylcholine concentration (a substrate of PLA_2) was found to be decreased, and lysophosphatidylcholine (a breakdown product of PLA_2 hydrolysis) elevated [63]. These data are suggestive of an accelerated systemic breakdown of membrane phospholipids. However, in a subgroup of schizophrenic patients, the concentration of arachidonic acid was found to be decreased in red blood cell membranes [64].

Further studies from our group, conducted with the University of Turku, Finland [65], compared the concentrations of types I and II PLA_2 in the serum of 43 schizophrenic patients, 32 nonschizophrenic psychiatric patients, and 41 heathy controls. No differences were found among the three groups with respect to pancreatic (type I) PLA_2, whereas nonpancreatic (type II) PLA_2 was significantly elevated in schizophrenics as compared to nonpsychiatric ($P < .05$) and psychiatric controls ($P < .05$). In addition, positive correlations were found between higher PLA_2 levels and scores on negative symptoms.

In a prospective case control study, 31 drug-free schizophrenic patients (half of whom were first-episode and drug-naïve schizophrenics) were compared with sex- and gender-matched nonschizophrenic psychiatric patients and healthy controls [3]. Baseline and weekly determinations of platelet PLA$_2$ activity were respectively obtained prior to and during a 3-week 10-mg/day haloperidol course. PLA$_2$ activity was significantly increased both in the group schizophrenic patients as a whole and in the first-onset subgroup, when compared to nonschizophrenic patients ($P < .03$) and healthy controls ($P < .01$). No differences were found between the two control groups. In addition, haloperidol treatment resulted in decreased PLA$_2$ activity, abolishing the previous difference between schizophrenic cases and controls. Likewise, schizophrenic patients had decreased concentrations of the PLA$_2$ substrate phosphatidylcholine ($P < .006$), and increased concentrations of the metabolite lysophosphatidylcholine ($P < .005$), which reverted to control levels after neuroleptic treatment.

Membrane fluidity studies recently performed in our laboratory reinforce the assumption that enhanced PLA$_2$ activity is related with abnormal fatty acid metabolism in schizophrenia (data in preparation). Synaptosomal-mitochondrial membranes isolated from the frontal cortex and hippocampus of schizophrenic brains (n = 7) were compared to the respective controls (n = 8). Membrane fluidity was examined using four different fluorescent techniques, showing that frontal cortex membranes obtained from schizophrenics had a significantly higher flexibility of fatty acids in the membrane hydrocarbon core and in the hydrophilic region of phospholipid head groups than controls. Conversely, fluidity parameters in hippocampal membranes were unchanged. Taken together, these data indicate alterations of biological properties of membranes that may be specific to frontal areas of schizophrenic brains.

C. Spectroscopy Studies

In addition to biochemical studies, the examination of brain phospholipid metabolism in living patients was made possible with the aid of ^{31}P magnetic resonance spectroscopy (NMR). Several studies suggested that schizophrenic patients have lower prefrontal levels of phosphomonoesters (PME) and higher levels of phosphodiesters (PDE) compared to matched controls [66–73]. Thus, an increased concentration of membrane phospholipid breakdown products (PDE) associated with a decrease in the respective precursors (PME) is suggestive of accelerated phospholipid breakdown—in other words, increased PLA$_2$ cleaving activity—particularly in frontal areas. However, patients with psychotic depression also seem to show lower levels of phosphomonoesters than controls, and furher studies are needed to define whether these findings are specific to schizophrenia or part of a generalized membrane phospholipid abnormality in psychotic disorders [74].

Attempts to correlate psychopathological subtypes and *in vivo* phospholipid metabolism abnormalities suggested that negative symptoms may be associated with higher levels of saturated fatty acids and lower levels of long-chain unsaturates in red blood cell membranes, while the positive symptom patients showed the opposite picture [75]. Maras et al., [65] also described association between higher serum PLA$_2$ levels and negative schizophrenic symptoms. More recently, NMR spectroscopy studies demonstrated that disordered phospholipid metabolism in the prefrontal cortex of schizophrenic patients is correlated with neuropsychological dysfunction [72]. Comparing 16 chronic schizophrenic patients and 13 normal controls, Deicken et al. [72] observed that lower left frontal phosphomonoester levels in the schizophrenics were associated with fewer categories achieved, lower percent conceptual level, and greater total errors in the Wisconsin Card Sort Test. No significant correlations between frontal phospholipid measures and performance on the test were noted in the controls. The results suggest a relationship between altered left frontal phospholipid metabolism and a specific measure of frontal lobe neuropsychological functioning. Since a reduced dopaminergic activity in the prefrontal cortex has been postulated in the hypofrontality hypothesis of schizophrenia [76], increased PLA$_2$ activity may be hypothesized as one of the causes of hypodopaminergic function in the prefrontal system in schizophrenia.

D. Genetic Studies

Few studies have addressed the genetic basis for disordered phospholipid metabolism in schizophrenia. The 85 kDa cPLA$_2$ gene has been sequenced and mapped to the chromosome 1q25 in humans [11,77]. Two simple sequence repeats, i.e., the poly(A) or (dA)n mononucleotide repeat and the (CA)n dinucleotide repeat, were reported at the human PLA$_2$ locus. The poly(A) simple sequence repeat is located at the 5' end of an inverted Alu repeat near the promotor region, and its predicted DNA fragment should contain the (dA)43 repeat sequence. The analysis of length polymorphism within this marker, using a polymerase chain reaction (PCR) method, showed 10 individual alleles with ∼ 76% of heterozygosity due to the poly(A) repeat among unrelated individuals [77]. Hudson and collaborators examined the association of the poly(A) simple sequence repeat in the human PLA_2 gene with the schizophrenic phenotype, and described a genetic variant near the $cPLA_2$ locus in 65 schizophrenics, as compared with a matched normal control population [78]. Out of 10 alleles (A1–A10), the frequency of A1–A6 was significantly lower in patients with schizophrenia than in control subjects. A follow-up haplotype relative-risk study of 44 triads (mother, father, affected offspring), confirmed the results seen in the association study. Such findings suggest that a genetic variant near the promotor region of the gene for $cPLA_2$ may be associated with schizophrenia. However, a similar study was conducted in 58 patients with schizophrenia and 56 control subjects, but the authors failed to demonstrate the allelic association of the poly(A) repeat polymorphism with schizophrenia [79].

More recently, Peet and collaborators [80] identified a dimorphic site on the first intron of the cPLA2 gene, by using a long PCR combined with restriction length fragment polymorphism analysis. Schizophrenic subjects were found to have a significant excess of the A2/A2 homozygote relative to healthy control subjects.

In addition, PLIP genes are located in chromosome 6, not far from major histocompatibility complex (HLA) genes. Evidence of linkage between HLA antigens and schizophrenia [81–83] leads to the speculation that PLIP genes might be involved in the pathogenesis of the disease. Genetic alteration in the $cPLA_2$ gene may be manifested as a membrane abnormality throughout the body. Since a major proportion of neuronal membrane is made up of unsaturated fatty acids, this abnormality will be most pronounced in the brain.

III. CONCLUSIONS

Cytosolic PLA_2 catalyzes the hydrolysis of membrane phospholipids to release cytotoxic products, such as lysophosphatidylcholine. In schizophrenia, increased PLA_2 activity and an accelerated breakdown of membrane phospholipids have been reported. In neuronal membranes, PLA_2 modulates DA release and receptor sensitivity, and has been shown to reduce dopaminergic neurotransmission. Spectroscopy data suggest disorderd phospholipid metabolism in the prefrontal cortex of schizophrenics, which correlates with the occurrence of negative symptoms, consistent with the hypofrontality hypothesis of schizophrenia.

REFERENCES

1. WF Gattaz, M Köllisch, T Thuren, JA Virtanen, PKJ Kinnunen. Increased plasma phospholipase-A_2 activity in schizophrenic patients: reduction after neuroleptic therapy. Biol Psychiatry 22:421-426, 1987.
2. WF Gattaz, CK Hübner, TJ Nevalainen, T Thuren, PKJ Kinnunen. Increased serum phospholipase A_2 activity in schizophrenia: a replication study. Biol Psychiatry 28:495, 1990.
3. WF Gattaz, A Steudle, A Maras. Increased platelet phospholipase A_2 in schizophrenia. Schizophr Res 16:1–6, 1995.
4. WF Gattaz, NJ Cairns, R Levy, H Forstl, DF Braus, A Maras. Decreased phospholipase A2 activity in the brain and in platelets of patients with Alzheimer's disease. Eur Arch Psychiatry Clin Neurosci 246(3):129–131, 1996.
5. M Noponen, M Sanfilipo, K Samanich, H Ryer, G Ko, B Angrist, A Wolkin, J Rotrosen. Elevated PLA_2 activity in schizophrenics and other psychiatric patients. Biol Psychiatry 34:641–649, 1993.
6. BM Ross, C Hudson, J Erlich, JJ Wars, SJ Kish. Increased phospholipid breakdown in schizophrenia. Arch Gen Psychiatry 54:487–494, 1997.
7. M Simonato. A pathogenetic hypothesis of temporal lobe epilepsy. Pharmacol Res 27:217–225, 1993.
8. H Woelk, K Peiler-Ichikawa. Zur Aktivität der Phospholipase A_2 gegenüber verschiedenen 1-Alk-1′-enyl-2-acyl- und 1-Alkyl-2-acyl-Verbindungen während der multiplen Sklerose. J Neurol 207:319–326, 1974.
9. F Visioli, EB Rodriguez-de-Turco, NR Kreisman, NG Bazan. Membrane lipid degradation is related to interictal cortical activity in a series of seizures. Metab Brain Dis 9:161–170, 1994.
10. EA Dennis. Diversity of group types, regulation, and function of phospholipase A_2. J Biol Chem 269:13057–13060, 1994
11. JD Clark, LL Lin, RW Kriz, CS Ramesha, LA Sultzman, AY Lin, N Milona, JL Knopf. A novel arachidonic acid–selective cytosolic PLA2 contains a Ca(2+)-dependent translocation domain with homology to PKC and GAP. Cell 65(6):1043–1051, 1991.
12. J Chen, SJ Engle, JJ Seilhamer, JA Tischfield. Cloning and recombinant expression of a novel human low molecular weight Ca(2+)-dependent phospholipase A2. J Biol Chem 269:2365–2368, 1994.
13. K Hattori, H Adachi, A Matsuzawa, K Yamamoto, M Tsujimoto, J Aoki, M Hattori, H Arai, K Inoue. cDNA Cloning and expression of intracellular platelet-activating factor (PAF) acetylhydrolase II. J Biol Chem 271:33032–33038, 1996.
14. L Cupillard, K Koumanov, MG Mattei, M Lazdunski, G Lambeau. Cloning, chromosomal mapping, and expression of a novel human secretory phospholipase A_2. J Biol Chem 272:15745–15752, 1997.

15. J Tang, RW Kriz, N Wolfman, M Shaffer, J Seehra, SS Jones. A novel cytosolic calcium-independent phospholipase A2 contains eight ankyrin motifs. J Biol Chem 272:8567–8575, 1997.
16. KW Underwood, C Song, RE Kriz, XJ Chang, JL Knopf, LL Lin. A novel calcium-independent phospholipase A2, cPLA2-γ, that is prenylated and contains homology to cPLA2. J Biol Chem 273:21926–21932, 1998.
17. DF Horrobin. The membrane phospholipid hypothesis as a biochemical basis for the neurodevelopmental concept of schizophrenia. Schizophr Res 30(3):193–208, 1998.
18. S Watson, S Arkinstall. The G-Linked Protein Receptor—Facts book. London: Academic Press, 1994, pp 388–390.
19. SK Han, ET Yoon, W Cho. Bacterial expression and characterization of human secretory class V phospholipase A2. Biochem J 331(Pt 2):353–357, 1998.
20. HC Yang, M Mosior, CA Johnson, Y Chen, EA Dennis. Group-specific assays that distinguish between the four major types of mammalian phospholipase A2. Anal Biochem 269(2):278–288, 1999.
21. RJ Mayer, LA Marshall. New insights on mammalian phospholipase A2(s); comparison of arachidonoyl-selective and -nonselective enzymes. FASEB J 7:339–348, 1993.
22. JA Tischfield. A reassessment of the low molecular weight phospholipase A2 gene family in mammals. J Biol Chem 272 (28):17247–17250, 1997.
23. W Pruzanski, EC Keystone, B Sternby, C Bombardier, KM Snow, P Vadas. Serum phospholipase A2 correlates with disease activity in rheumatoid arthritis. J Rheumatol 15(9):1351–1355, 1988.
24. JD Sharp, DL White, XG Chiou, T Goodson, GC Gamboa, D McClure, S Burgett, J Hoskins, PL Skatrud, JR Sportsman, GW Becker, LH Kang, EF Roberts, RM Kramer. Molecular cloning and expression of human Ca(2+)-sensitive cytosolic phospholipase A2. J Biol Chem 266:14850–14853, 1991.
25. EA Nalefski, LA Sultzman, DM Martin, RW Kriz, PS Towler, JL Knopf, JD Clark. Delineation of two functionally distinct domains of cytosolic phospholipase A2, a regulatory Ca(2+)-dependent lipid-binding domain and a Ca(2+)-independent catalytic domain. J Biol Chem 269:18239–18249, 1994.
26. A Schievella, M Regier, W Smith, L Lin. Calcium-mediated translocation of cytosolic phospholipase A2 to the nuclear envelope and endoplasmic reticulum. J Biol Chem 270:30749–30754, 1995.
27. S Glover, T Bayburt, M Jonas, E Chi, MH Gelb. Translocation of the 85-kDa phospholipase A2 from cytosol to the nuclear envelope in rat basophilic leukemia cells stimulated with calcium ionophore or IgE/antigen. J Biol Chem 270:15359–15367, 1995.
28. C Song, XJ Chang, KM Bean, MS Proia, JL Knopf, RW Kriz. Molecular characterization of cytosolic phospholipase A2-beta. J Biol Chem 274(24):17063–17067, 1999.
29. D Piomelli. Arachidonic acid in cell signaling. Curr Opin Cell Biol 5:274–280, 1993.
30. NG Bazan, CF Zorumski, GD Clark. The activation of phospholipase A2 and release of arachidonic acid and other lipid mediators at the synapse: the role of platelet activating factor. J Lipid Mediators 6:421–427, 1993.
31. Y Nishizuka. Intracellular signaling by hydrolysis of phospholipids and activation of protein kinase C. Science 258(5082):607–614, 1992.
32. DJ Hanahan. Platelet activating factor: a biologically active phosphoglyceride. Annu Rev Biochem 55:483–509, 1986.
33. AA Farooqui, Y Hirashima, LA Horrocks. Brain phospholipases and their role in signal transduction. In: NG Bazan, MG Murphy, G Tofano, eds. Neurobiology of Essential Fatty Acids. New York: Plenum Press, 1992, pp 11–26.
34. AA Farooqui, LA Horrocks. Involvement of glutamate receptors, lipases, and phospholipases in long-term potentiation and neurodegeneration. J Neurosci Res 38:6–11, 1994.
35. TJ Nevalainen, TJ Haapanen. Distribution of pancreatic (group I) and synovial-type (group II) phospholipases A2 in human tissues. Inflammation 17(4):453–464, 1993.
36. DT Stephenson, JV Manetta, DL White, XG Chiou, L Cox, B Gitter, PC May, JD Sharp, RM Kramer, JA Clemens. Calcium-sensitive cytosolic phospholipase A2 (cPLA2) is expressed in human brain astrocytes. Brain Res 637:97–105, 1994.
37. KM Kim, DK Kim, YM Park, CK Kim, DS Na. Annexin I inhibits phospholipase A2 by specific interaction, not by substrate depletion. FEBS Lett 343(3):251–255, 1994.
38. LL Lin, MWartmann, AY Lin, JL Knopf, A Seth, RJ Davis. cPLA2 is phosphorylated and activated by MAP kinase. Cell 72:269–278, 1993.
39. RA Nemenoff, S Winitz, NX Qian, V Van Putten, GL Johnson, LE Heasley. Phosphorylation and activation of a high molecular weight form of phospholipase A2 by p42 microtubule-associated protein 2 kinase and protein kinase C. J Biol Chem 268:1960–1964, 1993.
40. D Visnjic, D Batinic, M Marusic, H Banfic. Short-term and long-term effects of phorbol 12-myristate 13-acetate and different inhibitors on the ability of bone marrow cells to form colonies in vitro. Eur J Clin Chem Clin Biochem 33(10):679–686, 1995.
41. S Shimegi, F Okajima, Y Kondo. Permissive stimulation of Ca(2+)-induced phospholipase A2 by an adenosine receptor agonist in a pertussis toxin-sensitive manner in FRTL-5 thyroid cells: a new 'cross-talk' mechanism in Ca^{2+} signalling. Biochem J 299:845–851, 1994.
42. FJ Thomson, MS Johnson, R Mitchell, B Wolbers. Evidence for a role of phospholipase A2 in the mechan-

43. CF Kuo, S Cheng, JR Burgess. Deficiency of vitamin E and selenium enhances calcium-independent phospholipase A_2 activity in rat lung and liver. J Nutr 125:1419–1429, 1995.
44. Y Yoshihara, M Yamaji, M Kawasaki, Y Watanabe. Ontogeny of cytosolic phospholipase A2 activity in rat brain. Biochem Biophys Res Commun 185:350–355, 1992.
45. EJ Williams, FS Walsh, P Doherty. The production of arachidonic acid can account for calcium channel activation in the second messenger pathway underlying neurite outgrowth stimulated by NCAM, N-cadherin, and L1. J Neurochem 62(3):1231–1234, 1994.
46. PG Bradford, GV Marinetti, LG Abood. Stimulation of phospholiopase A_2 and and secretion of catecholamines from brain synaptosomes by potassium and A23187. J Neurochem 41:1684–1693, 1983.
47. M Ohmichi, K Hirota, K Koike, K Kadowaki, A Miyake, H Kiyama, M Tohyama, O Tanizawa. Involvement of extracellular calcium and arachidonate in [^{3}H] dopamine release from rat tuberoinfundibular neurons. Neuroendocrinology 50(4):481–487, 1989.
48. MB Anand-Srivastava, RA Johnson. Role of phospholipids in coupling of adenosine and dopamine receptors to striatal adenylate cyclase. J Neurochem 36:819–1828, 1981.
49. CR Oliveira, EP Duarte, AP Carvalho. Effect of phospholipase digestion and lysophosphatidylcholine on dopamine receptor binding. J Neurochem 43: 455–465, 1984.
50. U Ungerstedt, GW Arbuthnott. Quantitative recording of rotational behavior in rats after 6-hydroxy-dopamine lesions of the nigrostriatal dopamine system. Brain Res 24(3):485–493, 1970.
51. T Zetterstrom, M Herrera-Marschitz, U Ungerstedt. Simultaneous measurement of dopamine release and rotational behaviour in 6-hydroxydopamine denervated rats using intracerebral dialysis. Brain Res 376(1):1–7, 1986.
52. LS Carman, FH Gage, CW Shults. Partial lesion of the substantia nigra: relation between extent of lesion and rotational behavior. Brain Res 553(2):275–283, 1991.
53. JL Cadet, M Hu, V Jackson-Lewis. Behavioral and biochemical effects of intranigral injection of phospholipase-A2. Biol Psychiatry 26(1):106–110, 1989.
54. J Brunner, WF Gattaz. Intracerebral injection of phospholipase A2 inhibits dopamine-mediated behavior in rats: possible implications for schizophrenia. Eur Arch Psychiatry Clin Neurosci 246:13–16, 1995.
55. J Brunner, WF Gattaz. Intracerebroventricular injection of phospholipase A_2 inhibits apomorphine-induced locomotion in rats. Psychiatry Res 58:165–169, 1995.
56. WF Gattaz, J Brunner. Phospholipase A_2 and the hypofrontality hypothesis of schizophrenia. In: M Peet, I Glen, DF Horrobin, eds. Phospholipid Spectrum Disorder in Psychiatry. Carnforth: Marius Press, 1999, pp 39–44.
57. DF Horrobin, CN Bennett. The membrane phospholipid concept of schizophrenia. In: WF Gattaz, H Häfner, eds. Search for the Causes of Schizophrenia. Vol IV, Balance of the Century. Darmstadt: Steinkopff Verlag, 1999, pp 261–277.
58. JD Stevens. Settling characteristics of red cells in mental patients. Dis Nerv Syst 32(8):554–558, 1971.
59. J Rotrosen, A Wolkin. Phospholipid and prostaglandin hypotheses of schizophrenia. In: HY Meltzer, ed. Psychopharmacology: The Third Generation of Progress. New York: Raven Press, 1987, pp 759–764.
60. DF Horrobin, MS Manku, H Hilman, A Iain, M Glen. Fatty acid levels in the brains of schizophrenics and normal controls. Biol Psychiatry 30:795–805, 1991.
61. M Albers, H Meurer, F Märki, J Klotz. Phospholipase A2 activity in serum of neuroleptic-naive psychiatric inpatients. Pharmacopsychiatry 26:4–98, 1993.
62. WF Gattaz, A Schmitt, A Maras. Increased platelet phospholipase A_2 activity in schizophrenia. Schizophr Res 16:1–6, 1995.
63. AM Pangerl, A Steudle, HW Jaroni, R Rüfer, WF Gattaz. Increased platelet membrane lysophosphatidylcholine in schizophrenia. Biol Psychiatry 30:837–840, 1991.
64. M Peet, JDE Laugharne, DF Horrobin, GP Reynolds. Arachidonic acid: a common link in the biology of schizophrenia? Arch Gen Psychiatry 51:665–666, 1994.
65. A Maras, TJ Nevalainen, WF Gattaz. Erhöhte phospholipase A2 - subtyp II korreliert mit negativsymptomatik schizophrener Patienten. Fortsch Neurol-Psychiatrie 62(2):117, 1994.
66. P Williamson, D Drost, J Stanley, T Carr, S Morrison, H Merskey. Localized phosphorous 31 magnetic resonance spectroscopy in chronic schizophrenic patients and normal controls. Arch Gen Psychiatry 48:578, 1991.
67. T Fujimoto, T Nakano, T Takano, Y Hokazono, T Asakura, T Tsuji. Study of chronic schizophrenics using ^{31}P magnetic resonance chemical shift imaging. Acta Psychiatr Scand 86:455–462, 1992.
68. MS Keshavan, RD Sanders, JW Pettegrew, SM Dombrowsky, KS Panchalingam. Frontal lobe metabolism and cerebral morphology in schizophrenia: ^{31}P MRS and MRI studies. Schizophr Res 10:241–246, 1993.
69. JW Pettegrew, MS Keshavan, NJ Minshew. ^{31}P nuclear magnetic resonance spectroscopy: neurodevelopment and schizophrenia. Schizophr Bull 19:35–53, 1993.
70. RF Deicken, G Calabrese, EL Merrin, DJ Meyerhoff, W Dillon, MW Weiner, G Fein. ^{31}Phosphorous magnetic mesonance spectroscopy of the frontal and parietal lobes in chronic schizophrenia. Biol Psychiatry 36:503–551, 1993.

71. H Fukuzako, K Takeuchi, K Ueyama, T Fukuzako, Y Hokazono, K Hirakawa, K Yamada, T Hashiguchi, M Takigawa, T Fujimoto. ^{31}P magnetic resonance spectroscopy of the medial temporal lobe of schizophrenic patients with neuroleptic-resistant marked positive symptoms. Eur Arch Psychiatry Clin Neurosci 244:236–24037, 1994.
72. RF Deicken, EL Merrin, EL, TC Floyd, MW Weiner. Correlation between left frontal phospholipids and Wisconsin Card Sort Test performance in schizophrenia. Schizophr Res 14:177–181, 1995.
73. AD Hinsberger, PC Williamson, TJ Carr, JA Stanley, DJ Drost, M Densmore, GC MacFabe, DG Montemurro. Magnetic resonance imaging volumetric and phosphorus-31 magnetic resonance spectroscopy measurements in schizophrenia. J Psychiatry Neurosci 22 (2):111–117, 1997.
74. PC Williamson, M Brauer, S Leonard, T Thompson, D Drost. ^{31}P magnetic resonance spectroscopy studies in schizophrenia. Prostaglandins Leukot Essent Fatty Acids 55(1–2):115–118, 1996.
75. AI Glen, EM Glen, DF Horrobin, KS Vaddadi, M Spellman, N Morse-Fisher, K Ellis, FS Skinner. A red cell membrane abnormality in a subgroup of schizophrenic patients: evidence for two diseases. Schizophr Res 12(1):53–61, 1994.
76. DR Weinberger. Implications of normal brain development for the pathogenesis of schizophrenia. Arch Gen Psychiatry 44:660–669, 1987.
77. A Tay, JS Simon, J Squire, K Hamel, HJ Jacob, K Skorecki. Cytosolic phospholipase A2 gene in human and rat: chromosomal localization and polymorphic markers. Genomics 26(1):138–141, 1995.
78. JC Hudson, JL Kennedy, A Gotowiec, N King, K Gotjan, F Macciardi, K Skorecki, HY Meltzer, JJ Warsh, DF Horrobin. Genetic variant near cytosolic phospholipase A_2 associated with schizophrenia. Schizophr Res 21:111–116, 1996.
79. SA Price, H Fox, D St Clair, DJ Shaw. Lack of association between schizophrenia and a polymorphism close to the cytosolic phospholipase A_2 gene. Psychiatr Genet 7:111–114, 1997.
80. M Peet, CN Ramchand, J Lee, SD Telang, GK Vankar, S Shah, J Wei. Association of the Ban I dimorphic site at the human cytosolic phospholipase A2 gene with schizophrenia. Psychiatr Genet 8(3):191–192, 1998.
81. WF Gattaz, RW Ewald, H Beckmann. The HLA system and schizophrenia. A study in a German population. Arch Psychiatr Nervenkr 228:205–211, 1980.
82. WF Gattaz, H Beckmann, J Mendlewicz. HLA antigens and schizophrenia: a pool of two studies. Psychiatry Res 5:123–128, 1981.
83. HW Moises, L Yang, H Kristbjarnarson, C Wiese, W Byerley, F Macciardi, V Arolt, D Blacwood, X Liu, B Sjogren. An international two-stage genome-wide search for schizophrenia susceptibility genes. Nat Genet, 11:321–324, 1995.

22

Animal Models of Psychosis

J. DAVID JENTSCH
David Geffen School of Medicine at UCLA, Los Angeles, California, U.S.A.

PETER OLAUSSON
Yale University School of Medicine, New Haven, Connecticut, U.S.A.

HOLLY MOORE
Columbia University, New York, New York, U.S.A.

I. INTRODUCTION

Animal models of human disorders can be invaluable tools for investigating the etiology and underlying pathophysiology of clinical syndromes, including psychiatric disorders. For example, as epidemiological, genetic, or biochemical studies identify a particular factor (e.g., gene, protein, developmental insult, change in the social milieu) that may be causal or contributory for the incidence of a disease such as schizophrenia, animal models can be employed to evaluate the possibility that manipulation of the factor may plausibly result in the occurrence of relevant psychopathology. The contribution of particular biological substrates to symptomatic components of the human disorder can be evaluated in animals with perturbations of discrete physiological functions.

Psychotic disorders have been particularly difficult to model in nonhuman species because the array of affected functions includes processes that are difficult to evaluate in animals, if they are present at all. For example, the objective measurement of animal behaviors thought to model formal thought disorder or hallucinations is abstruse, and other symptoms, such as verbal dysfunction, exist within domains that likely are not reproducible in any nonhuman species. In addition, schizophrenia and related disorders are characterized by spectra of impairments that implicate complex, multivariate dysfunctions. This pathophysiology may be difficult to model using selective, experimental manipulations.

Despite these limitations, important information regarding the pathophysiology of schizophrenia has been developed in animals via two parallel courses of investigation. First, researchers have examined the neurobiological consequences of perturbations that are thought to *evoke* psychotic reactions in otherwise normal humans or to provoke symptoms in schizophrenia patients. As will be discussed below, a variety of approaches have been employed in an attempt to induce schizophrenialike behavior in animals, and despite the disparateness of some of these approaches, it is hoped that understanding what common, vulnerable brain systems are affected by all these psychosis-producing conditions will result in greater insights regarding the pathophysiology of the idiopathic disorder.

Second, analyses of the mechanisms of action of therapeutically antipsychotic drugs in animals have contributed to conceptual hypotheses regarding the neurochemical and structural bases of schizophrenia. The hypothesis here is that the brain substrates targeted by antipsychotic drugs are the systems that are primarily dysfunctional in the diseased condition. Ultimately, these two approaches (studies of pro- and antipsychotic manipulations) may be successfully combined to more fully examine mechanisms underlying effective treatment of the dysfunctional brain [1].

In this chapter we will focus on animal models designed to evoke schizophrenia-like phenotypes. For descriptions of models designed primarily to predict the effects of antipsychotic drugs, the reader is referred to other reviews [2,3]. The use of psychotomimetic drugs (agents that provoke psychotic reactions), neurodevelopmental insults, and genetic manipulations will be reviewed. Ultimately, we will try to go beyond simple description of multiple models and provide some insight into the brain systems that are affected by each of these manipulations. In the end, we expect that understanding the areas of overlap among otherwise etiologically diverse animal models will contribute to understanding the pathophysiology of idiopathic psychotic disorders.

II. WHAT PSYCHOPATHOLOGY SHOULD AN ANIMAL MODEL OF PSYCHOSIS REFLECT?

Schizophrenia is a psychiatric disease that probably involves pathological function in many brain areas and systems (Table 1) [4–8], and the complexity of the syndromatic spectrum reflects that pervasiveness. Nevertheless, for simplicity, the symptoms of schizophrenia have been subdivided into three functional categories: positive, negative, and cognitive symptoms (Fig. 1) [9]. These categories are not arbitrary but are meant to classify symptoms into relational groups. Positive symptoms include motor stereotypy, formal thought disorder, delusions, and hallucinations (psychopathology that otherwise does not appear in normal individuals). Negative symptoms include normative functions that are lost in the disorder, e.g., avolition and flattened affect. In addition, neurocognitive dysfunction is likely to be at the core of the schizophrenic disease process [10,11], and cognitive symptoms include dysfunction of working memory and alterations of attention and executive function. Other symptoms are more difficult to definitively categorize; impaired latent and prepulse inhibition may reflect deficits of attention, stimulus filtering, and motivation, while impairments of social function may reflect subtle cognitive loss as well as decreased desire to engage the social network. The particular symptoms and features of psychotic disorders exhibited in Figure 1 have been provided as examples because they are ones that have been investigated in animal models most fully, and this is discussed in some detail below. Again, these diverse impairments probably point to dysfunction of multiple brain structures and circuits, including (but not limited to) the frontal and temporal cortices and the basal ganglia (Fig. 1, Table 1).

III. DRUG-INDUCED MODELS OF PSYCHOSIS

Certain classes of drugs, including stimulants such as d-amphetamine, serotonin receptor agonists, and noncompetitive N-methyl-D-aspartate (NMDA)/glutamate receptor antagonists, provoke psychoticlike reactions in otherwise normal humans or schizophrenia patients. Though a variety of pharmacological classes of compounds are able to elicit psychotomimetic reactions, the effects of different agents have been interpreted to provide evidence for alterations of different neurotransmitter systems in schizophrenia. d-Amphetamine, which strongly increases the release of dopamine and other monoamines in brain, can induce transient psychotic states in normal humans that strongly resemble the positive symptoms of schizophrenia [12], and these results were interpreted to suggest that a hyperdopaminergic state may underlie some components of the schizophrenic disease process. In addition, most serotonin type-2 (5HT$_2$) receptor agonists, including lysergic acid diethylamide (LSD) and mescaline, produce hallucinations in human beings [13], providing support for a serotonergic component to schizophrenia. Finally, noncompetitive NMDA/glutamate receptor antagonists, such as phencyclidine and ketamine, can evoke the positive, negative, and cognitive components of schizophrenia in normal humans, evidence for hypoglutamatergic function in psychosis [14–16]. For each of these agents, their psychotomimetic effects were first observed in humans; however, animal studies quickly followed. The animal studies were supported by two primary expectations: (1) that the agents would induce repre-

Animal Models of Psychosis

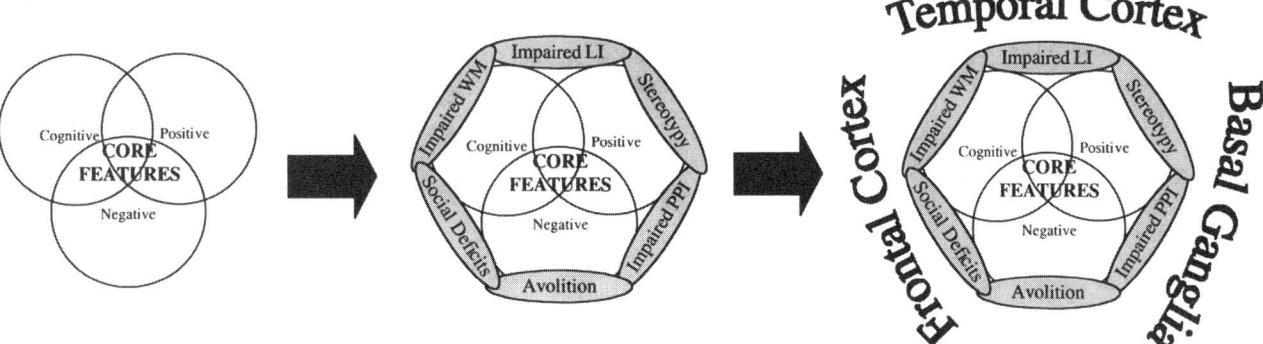

Figure 1 The psychopathology of schizophrenia can be categorized roughly into positive, negative, and cognitive subsyndromes. These groupings are not exclusive, and many symptoms can be considered to fall within more than one grouping. Nevertheless, a variety of behaviors including stereotypy, impaired prepulse inhibition (PPI), avolition, deficits of social function, impaired working memory, and latent inhibition are key to the disorder and can be modeled with some success in animals. These impairments map onto dysfunction of corticostriatal circuits originating in the frontal and temporal cortices and having outputs via the basal ganglia.

Table 1 Variables Currently or Potentially Useful for Assessng Isomorphism of Animal Models with Schizophrenia

Type of evidence	Specific dependent variables	Change in schizophrenia	Refs
Neuropsychological	Working memory tasks	Deficits	69
	Reversal learning	Retarded	70
	Perseverative responding	Increased	70
	Latent inhibition	Impaired	30
	Attention tasks	Impaired	10
Sensorimotor gating:	Prepulse inhibition	Decreased	24
Neurological:	Spontaneous oral dyskinesias	Increased in patients with frontal lobe pathology	90, 111
Brain Morphometric:	Brain volume	Normal or decreased	86
	Cerebral cortical size	Normal or decreased	
	Hippocampal/parahippocampal size	More markedly and reliably decreased	
	Medial frontal cortical size	Slightly decreased	
Cellular:	Cerebral cortical neuronal density/neurophil	Increased/decreased in multiple regions	129
	Cerebral cortical neuronal: size	Decreased	130
	shape	Altered	
	distribution	Altered	
	Number of neurons in thalamus	Decreased anterior, limbic-related thalamus	131
	Expression of genes related to synaptic transmission and plasticity	Decreased in prefrontal and parahippocampal cortices, but also in other cortical regions	132,133

sentative psychopathology that would model key characteristics of the idiopathic disease. and (2) that subsequent, systematic neurobiological studies would reveal the causes for these behavioral abnormalities, and thus indirectly, for the human illness.

A. *d*-Amphetamine

A variety of psychomotor stimulant drugs, including *d*-amphetamine and cocaine, can induce psychotomimetic responses in humans, particularly after high dose or repeated administrations [17]. Progressive augmentations in the behavioral and neurochemical effects of stimulant drugs (termed "sensitization") have been argued to serve as a basis for the induction of psychopathology [17–19], though repeated treatments are not necessary for amphetamine-induced psychosis [12].

Amphetamine produces a number of behavioral abnormalities in animals that are thought to be relevant to schizophrenia. These include motor stereotypies, disruption of latent and prepulse inhibition and abnormalities of social interactions. As described above (Sect. II), these are principal components of the schizophrenia syndrome, and the validity of an animal model of psychosis is dependent upon reflecting some or all of these symptoms.

Motor stereotypy is the perseverative repetition of motor behaviors, particularly those that are very short and/or that require no external feedback [20]. One of the most classically studied effects of amphetamine is the induction of multiple forms of stereotypy [20–25], and the attenuation of amphetamine-induced stereotypy is a common effect of antipsychotic drugs [e.g., 25,26], many of which act as dopamine receptor antagonists [27].

Other behavioral effects of amphetamine may represent more complex forms of psychopathology. Latent inhibition describes a process wherein repeated, noncontingent exposures to a neutral stimulus retard the ability of subjects to subsequently learn a Pavlovian relationship between that stimulus and a contingently paired reinforcer. Schizophrenia patients have been reported to exhibit abnormal latent inhibition in that noncontingent preexposure to the neutral stimulus does not affect subsequent conditioning in psychotic individuals [28, but see 29]. This possible impairment is thought to implicate deficits of selective attention during the noncontingent preexposure period. Amphetamine administration to animals produces impairments of latent inhibition, and these effects are blocked by coadministration of either typical or atypical antipsychotic drugs [reviewed in 30].

Another paradigm that involves attentive processes, as well as subattentional components, is prepulse inhibition [24,31–33]. This measure of sensorimotor gating in humans and animals is assessed in a paradigm in which the delivery of a stimulus that normally causes startle in animals or humans (an air puff or very loud sound) is preceded by a neutral stimulus. In normal subjects, the delivery of the neutral stimulus gates or attenuates the subsequent startle reflex. In contrast, schizophrenia patients exhibit a reduced attenuation of the startle response with the presentation of the neutral "warning" stimulus. The face validity of the prepulse inhibition paradigm for modeling schizophrenic sensorimotor-gating deficits has been well established [24]. Amphetamine administration dose-dependently reduces prepulse inhibition of the startle reflex in rats [34], and both atypical and typical antipsychotic drugs block the amphetamine-induced impairment of prepulse inhibition [32].

Amphetamine produces behavioral abnormalities in socially living nonhuman primates and rodents [35–37]. These drug-induced behavioral alterations are characterized by stereotypy/hyperreactivity together with social withdrawal and anxious responses to social interactions, a behavioral profile similar to that observed in many patients suffering from schizophrenia. The amphetamine-induced changes in social behavior have thus been argued to model some processes relevant to schizophrenia, and to constitute an animal model with face validity for schizophrenia that encompasses both positive (e.g., stereotypy) and negative (e.g., social withdrawal) symptoms. In addition, pharmacological experiments using known antipsychotics have suggested that this model also have some degree of predictive validity [37]. However, it is not clear that social functions in rats and humans bear any relationship to one another (in terms of either the form of the behavior or the motivation to engage in such interactions). Moreover, there is strong evidence that social impairments in schizophrenia may be secondary, for instance, to cognitive dysfunction. Thus, the "face validity" of amphetamine-induced disruptions of social behavior may be misleading.

Above, the evidence that amphetamine administration can produce a spectrum of behavioral abnormalities in animals that are thought to model components of schizophrenia symptomatology was reviewed. The face validity of some of these behavioral effects is supplemented by the modulation of these responses by antipsychotic drugs (predictive validity). However, there are also several key limitations to this model. Perhaps most importantly, amphetamine has variable effects on cognitive functions. At low to moderate doses, amphetamine improves cognition in schizophrenia [38] while exacerbating psychotic symptoms [39]. Therefore, the amphetamine model of psychosis may not provide good insights into the neurocognitive component of schizophrenia.

Morever, the equivalent effects of typical and atypical antipsychotic drugs on amphetamine-induced behaviors have led many to assume that the amphetamine model may not be particularly useful in terms of predicting the unique qualities that are essential in next-generation antipsychotic drugs. Other pharmacological models, including those discussed below, may be more useful in that regard.

B. Serotonin 5HT$_2$ Agonists

Certain 5HT$_2$ receptor agonists (e.g., LSD and mescaline) produce hallucinogenic effects in human subjects [13]; these drug-induced consequences have inspired researchers to use these substances to examine neural mechanisms relevant to psychosis and schizophrenia. These experiments are supported by observations demonstrating 5HT neurotransmission abnormalities in schizophrenic patients [40], as well as evidence indicating that actions at brain 5HT$_2$ receptors contribute to the clinical efficacy of atypical antipsychotic drugs [41]. Although the psychoactive effects produced by 5HT$_2$ agonists in humans in some respects are similar to the symptoms of schizophrenia, there are also important differences. For example, the 5HT$_2$ receptor agonists primarily produce visual hallucinations whereas auditory hallucinations dominate in schizophrenic individuals. Although such differences may limit the usefulness of this animal model for studying schizophrenia, it has been stressed that the use of 5HT$_2$ agonists could yield important information about specific components of the schizophrenia syndrome [24].

One such line of investigation is in the study of prepulse inhibition. As discussed above, schizophrenia patients exhibit disruptions of sensorimotor gating [33], and treatment of experimental animals with hallucinogenic drugs can reproduce this impairment [42]. New research utilizing transgenic murine models has begun to implicate particular serotonin receptor subtypes that contribute to normative prepulse inhibition [43]. Future investigations utilizing these techniques may yield insights into either pathophysiology of schizophrenia or the receptors critical to antipsychotic efficacy.

C. N-Methyl-D-Aspartate/Glutamate Receptor Antagonists

Nearly forty years ago, it was first reported that acute administration of the noncompetitive NMDA-sensitive glutamate receptor antagonist phencyclidine to normal humans induced a psychopathology with "impressive similarity (to) ... certain primary symptoms of the schizophrenic process" [44]. In addition, acute phencyclidine treatment exacerbates the primary symptoms of chronic schizophrenia patients [45]. The pharmacological specificity of these effects is supported by the observations that ketamine, which, like phencyclidine noncompetitively blocks NMDA receptors, also simulates schizophrenic psychopathology in normal humans [46] and exacerbates symptoms in schizophrenic patients [47].

Phencyclidine is distinguishable from both *d*-amphetamine-like stimulant drugs and serotonin receptor agonists in that it can produce both positive and "negative" or deficit state symptoms of schizophrenia, such as emotional lability and social withdrawal [14,15]. In addition, phencyclidine/ketamine administration can lead to substantial cognitive dysfunction [14,15,44], including impaired performance of the Wisconsin Card Sort Test and continuous performance vigilance tasks and deficits in delayed recall, free recall, recognition memory, and verbal fluency [46].

Many attempts have been made to draw parallels between the behaviors exhibited by phencyclidine-treated animals and schizophrenia symptomatology [see 24,15]. The quantified behaviors examined occur within several different domains, including locomotor behavior, sensorimotor gating, latent inhibition, social interactions, and cognitive functions. As mentioned previously, each of these behavioral domains has proved useful to investigating the neural circuitry underlying both psychotomimetic and antipsychotic drug responses.

The ability of phencyclidine, or its congeners, to stimulate locomotor behavior and induce motor stereotypy in animals has been evaluated as a model of some components of schizophrenia psychopathology [48–50]. It is not clear that locomotor behavior in rats bears any relationship to schizophrenic symptomatology; however, dysfunction within corticostriatal circuitry, which may be manifest as locomotor abnormalities in rodents, has been postulated to be a critical pathophysiological substrate of the disease [4,8,51]. Moreover, the modification of phencyclidine-induced locomotion and motor stereotypy by drugs is one classical assay for putative antipsychotic efficacy because these effects are differentially sensitive to atypical versus typical antipsychotic drugs (e.g., clozapine is more potent than haloperidol in terms of preventing phencyclidine-induced hyperlocomotion in rodents) [48,52].

Similarly to amphetamine or serotonin receptor agonists, phencyclidine administration disrupts prepulse inhibition in rats [31]. The face validity of the phencyclidine-induced impairment of sensorimotor gating is strengthened by the manifestation of similar deficits by patients suffering from idiopathic schizophrenia [32,33]. Though stimulant drugs and serotonin receptor agonists likewise disrupt prepulse inhibition of the startle reflex (see above), it is argued that unlike amphetamine-induced alterations of prepulse inhibition, the effects of phencyclidine on startle gating are differentially affected by typical, atypical, and putative antipsychotic drugs [53]. For this reason, phencyclidine-induced disruption of prepulse inhibition may represent an important measure of the therapeutic efficacy of new-generation antipsychotic drugs.

Phencyclidine administration reduces social interactions in rats, and as discussed above, this impairment is thought to model the alterations of social interactions exhibited by schizophrenia patients [49]. In addition to the "face validity" of these effects, the social deficits produced by phencyclidine are amenable to treatment with atypical antipsychotic drugs [54]. However, as discussed above, construct validity for this sort of model is far from assured.

Attempts to study cognitive functions in phencyclidine-treated animals may yield the more informative results for several reasons. The performance of cognitive tasks by animals and patients may depend on similar neural and psychological constructs, and the validity of the particular tasks employed cross-species may be directly assessed. In addition, schizophrenia has been described by some as a fundamentally neurocognitive disorder [10,11], and therefore, the examination of cognitive processes in animals may tap more directly into the core features of the disorder.

Administration of phencyclidine, ketamine, or MK-801 (another noncompetitive NMDA receptor antagonist) to rats produces performance impairments on a variety of tests of learning and memory, including passive avoidance, acquisition of the Morris water maze task or a conditional discrimination, tests of spatial working memory and performance of a spatial continuous-recognition memory task [reviewed in 15,55]. However, administration of noncompetitive NMDA receptor antagonists impairs even simple behavioral measures, evidence for impairments of simple sensory processes and associative learning [15,55]. For this reason, the specificity of "cognitive" deficits in animals acutely treated with phencyclidine/ketamine/MK-801 is questionable.

The effects of chronic, rather than single-dose, exposure to phencyclidine may better represent some facets of schizophrenia. Though both regimens can induce psychosis, thought disorder, delusions, flattened affect, and withdrawal, with the effects of chronic exposure being generally more persistent [44,56,57], there are qualitative differences between the effects of these two dosing regimens. Acute ketamine administration to humans produces delusions and hallucinations, typically within the visual domain [46], similar to LSD intoxication [13] but not schizophrenia [24]. More consistent with symptoms observed in schizophrenia patients, phencyclidine-abusing humans present with religious and paranoid delusions and auditory hallucinations [56,57]. These findings provide support for the argument that long-term phencyclidine abuse is associated with a psychopathology that is remarkably similar to schizophrenia and which may be more isomorphic to the chronic symptoms of schizophrenia (e.g., cognitive and negative symptoms) than those induced by acute phencyclidine exposure.

Long-term phencyclidine treatment may also closely model the cerebral metabolic dysfunction of schizophrenia. Chronic phencyclidine intake by humans has been associated with reduced frontal lobe blood flow and glucose utilization [58,59], a finding consistent with the observation that some components of the cognitive dysfunction of schizophrenia is associated with reduced frontal blood flow, so-called hypofrontality [60]. By contrast, acute ketamine administration markedly increases frontal blood flow [61]. Therefore, there are biological indices that suggest chronic, rather than acute, phencyclidine administration may be a superior model of schizophrenia.

Though less explored, there are a number of behavioral impairments that appear to be as a persistent/long-lasting consequence of single or repeated doses of phencyclidine. These behavioral effects are likely not to be complicated by the "acute" effects of phencyclidine intoxication, and may therefore be more selective and hence relevant to schizophrenia. Augmentations of the locomotor response to stress or d-amphetamine is a persistent consequence of single-dose or chronic phencyclidine administration [62,63], and subchronic ketamine administration leads to greater apomorphine-induced stereotypy [64]. Impaired social interactions have also been reported in rats after cessation of repeated phencyclidine administrations [54,65].

Finally, impaired latent inhibition, but not prepulse inhibition, has been reported to be a long-term consequence of phencyclidine exposure [66,67]. These long-term behavioral effects of phencyclidine exposure may be indicative of corticostriatal dysfunction relevant to schizophrenia.

The cognitive effects of long-term phencyclidine treatment in rats and monkeys have also been investigated. Long-term phencyclidine administration delay-dependently impairs performance of a variable-delay spatial T-maze alternation task (a test of spatial working memory) [68], and these impairments are similar to those observed in schizophrenia patients using analogous tasks [69]. Pronounced deficits of reversal learning (a measure of cognitive control over reward-related behavior) have also been reported in schizophrenia [70] and in rats after repeated phencyclidine treatments [71]. Finally, prolonged administration of phencyclidine to monkeys produces cognitive dysfunction [72], effects that are associated with altered corticostriatal dopaminergic function [73]. Though this is a developing line of investigation, the results suggest that prolonged treatment with phencyclidine produces a pattern of neuroadaptive changes that may ultimately produce behavioral impairments with superior similarity to the primary psychopathology of schizophrenia.

An additional issue pertains the predictive validity of any of these effects. As noted above, many of the "acute" behavioral effects resulting from phencyclidine administration are differentially sensitive to atypical versus typical antipsychotic drugs, and for this reason, the phencyclidine model is hoped to be a mechanism for predicting the efficacy of next-generation antipsychotic drugs with superior therapeutic effects. Recent studies of the cognitive consequences of long-term phencyclidine administration also bear out these differences. For example, the enduring deficits of cognitive control over motor behavior produced by phencyclidine administration to monkeys is attenuated by systemic administration of the atypical antipsychotic clozapine but not the classical neuroleptic haloperidol [72,74]. Similar effects have been observed in rats [75].

The degree to which phencyclidine administration to animals may model the primary symptoms of schizophrenia undoubtedly requires further exploration, and it is likely that both acute intoxication with and chronic administration of phencyclidine will provide important insights into the pathophysiology of psychotic disorders. Much new research has begun to focus on the neural mechanisms that are enduringly affected by phencyclidine exposure [15,76,77], and insights from these studies may ultimately be integrated with observations of clinical pathophysiology in the idiopathic disease.

D. Common Mechanisms Among Pharmacological Models?

What can pharmacological models tell us about the pathophysiology underlying schizophrenia if otherwise pharmacologically diverse compounds produce similar behavioral effects? Do these drug effects indicate that NMDA/glutamatergic, dopaminergic, and serotonergic systems are all dysfunctional in schizophrenia? Or do they indicate that the subtle (and difficult to measure) interactions between these systems, at the neurochemical and physiological levels, are impaired? These questions are made even more challenging when one considers that several other classes of drugs also exhibit psychotomimetic effects, including cannabinoid receptor agonists [78], antidepressant drugs [79], and antiparkinsonian agents [80].

Otherwise different pharmacological classes of psychotomimetic drugs may share among themselves common downstream alterations of corticostriatal circuitry. In the most simplistic sense, almost all psychotomimetic drugs either directly or indirectly affect frontal and temporal cortical and/or striatal metabolic activity [81,82], as well as the impulse-dependent or -independent release of neuromodulatory transmitters within these structures [15,83]. However, the neural mechanisms that are targeted by psychotomimetic drugs are undoubtedly very complex. For example, O'Donnell and Grace [84] have provided evidence that phencyclidine acts, in part, to attenuate the drive of limbic striatal neuron activity by excitatory corticostriatal afferent inputs, and amphetamine is known to likewise reduce the excitatory influence of cortical inputs on striatal neurons [85]. Therefore, further exploration of the common actions of psychotomimetic drugs on corticostriatal functioning, determined both behaviorally and physiologically, seems warranted.

IV. DEVELOPMENTAL MANIPULATIONS AS MODELS OF SCHIZOPHRENIA

Developmental models share the strategy of using manipulations early in brain development in order to produce an adult phenotype that is isomorphic with schizophrenia in critical aspects. These models are based on growing epidemiological, behavioral, and neuroanatomical evidence for abnormal brain,

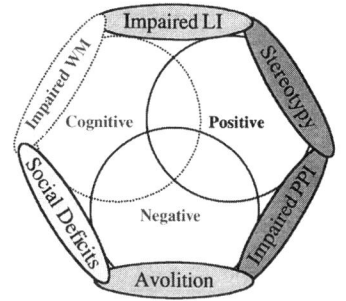
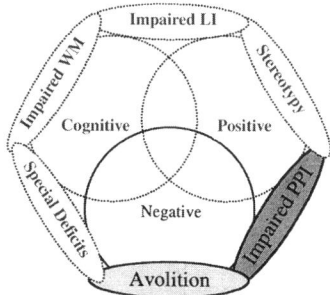

Amphetamine Model   5-HT$_2$ Agonist Model

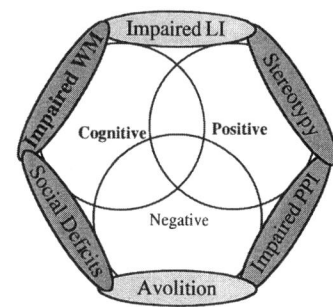

Phencyclidine Model

Figure 2 Schematic representation of the spectra of psychopathology reflected by three principal pharmacological models of schizophrenia. Each model mimics components of psychotic disorders, yet the phencyclidine model is considerably more comprehensive in terms of mimicking the negative, positive, and cognitive components of idiopathic schizophrenia. Dark gray ovals represent symptoms that are successfully modeled by the drug, with white ovals indicating areas in which the models do not accurately represent schizophrenia. Intermediate shades indicate no data or insufficient studies.

especially cerebral cortical, development in a large number of schizophrenia patients. This evidence includes ventricular enlargement and reduced cerebral, especially parahippocampal, volume occurring in the absence of gliosis. The cytoarchitectural abnormalities in cerebral cortex are also consistent with abnormal neuronal differentiation and migration and/or genesis or maintenance of synapses [86,87]. There is also evidence for subtle neurological, neuropsychological, or craniofacial abnormalities in children who later develop schizophrenia, and a significant association of obstetric complications or perinatal stress with severity or age of onset of schizophrenia [88–90]. Importantly, of the hundreds of research findings in schizophrenia, many are difficult to replicate or appear to have a elatively weak association with the risk for the disease. However, hypotheses proposing an early disruption of brain development that initiates a process that retards the development of limbic and prefrontal cortices and/or renders them significantly more vulnerable to environmental stressors most successfully accounts for the plethora of findings and the variance among them.

Thus, whereas as pharmacological models in adult animals model key aspects of the fully manifested behavioral (and, where information is available, neurochemical) phenotypes within schizophrenia, developmental models emphasize other aims, roughly falling into three categories. The first is to make a developmental manipulation, usually directed at limbic forebrain regions, that will model the age of onset of the behaviors and neurochemical changes believed to be closely related to the "positive" symptoms. Another aim is to model a developmental process that leads to the neuroanatomical abnormalities evidenced in the brains of schizophrenia patients. The third, perhaps ultimate, aim is to also model a pathodevelopmental process that, while leading to marked dysfunction prefrontal cortex, limbic-related cortex, and subcortical and cortical dopamine systems in the adult, also leads to the anatomical and neurochemical phenomena that are isomorphic with schizophrenia. To assess the usefulness of these models in understanding schizophrenia, an array of dependent variables have been measured. These variables, shown in Table 1, are considered to be isomorphic with brain and behavioral indices that are altered in schizophrenia. In this section, we describe a number of different experimental methods used to disrupt brain development and evaluate how they address the general aims described above. Genetic manipulations designed to specifically affect cortical development will be included here, while those based on the role of the gene in the mature brain will be covered in the *Genetic Models* section, below.

A. Early Limbic Lesion Models

The use of neonatal lesions of limbic structures to model schizophrenia was pioneered by Lipska and Weinberger [87,91]. The effects of excitotoxic lesions of the ventral hippocampus (VH) on postnatal day 7 in the rat have been most carefully characterized and extensively reviewed. Lesioned rats are tested before puberty (PD 32) and in adulthood (after PD 56). Around PD 32, lesioned rats show few small behavioral differences from controls when psychostimulant or stress-evoked locomotion or prepulse inhibition is assessed. However on or after PD 56, neonatal VH-lesioned rats show increased psychomotor activity evoked by indirect and direct dopamine agonists and psychotomimetic NMDA receptor antagonists, as well as exaggerated effects of these drugs on PPI (relative to control littermates). The hippocampus is largely absent in adult rats having received neonatal lesions; however, lesions of the hippocampus in adulthood do not reproduce the same effects. This has led to the hypothesis that neonatal VH lesions produce consequent dysregulated development of other forebrain structures, most probably the prefrontal cortex [91].

This hypothesis is supported by various findings [91]. Firstly, neonatal VH lesions result in altered N-acetylasparate levels (a measure of neuronal integrity) in prefrontal cortex (similar effects are found in schizophrenia patients). Moreover, subtle alterations of dendritic morphology of prefrontal cortical neurons results from VH lesions; these effects are very similar to that found in schizophrenia. The hypothesis that the alteration of prefrontal cortex is tangibly manifest in the abnormal behaviors exhibited by these rats is supported by the observation that destruction of the prefrontal cortex in adulthood reverses many of the abnormal behaviors produced by neonatal VH lesions. Thus, although a near-complete lesion of the hippocampus is clearly not present in schizophrenia patients, nearly all of the known effects of neonatal hippocampal lesions in rats and primates appear to be highly relevant for the psychopathology of schizophrenia and may be mediated by abnormal prefrontal cortical development and function.

Other early limbic lesions have also been shown to lead to abnormalities in prefrontal structure and function and DA system activity. For example, electrolytic or excitotoxic lesions of the amygdala 2–7 days after birth also increase locomotor sensitivity to DA agonists and produce morphometric changes in the temporal and frontal lobes that are to some extent consistent with morphometric abnormalities in schizophrenia patients [92,93]. Another technique, infusion of a low dose of kainic acid into the ventricles of rats on PD 7, produces a delayed, relatively subtle cell loss in the dorsal hippocampus [94]. However, loss of cortical neurons is not a consistent finding in schizophrenia. It remains to be determined whether intraventricular infusions of kainic acid or amygdala lesion models will show the range of effects observed in neonatal VH lesion model. Though intriguing, it remains to be tested if these other limbic lesion models can model as many aspects of schizophrenia as the Lipska-Weinberger model.

The effects of early developmental limbic lesions have also been characterized in primate by Bachevalier and colleagues [95]. Monkeys with early hippocampal and/or amygdalar lesions display a progression of abnormality in social behaviors that have face validity with the social withdrawal that precedes and progresses through the onset of psychosis in schizophrenia [95]. Neonatal limbic-lesioned monkeys also show decreases in NAA in the prefrontal cortex and altered prefrontal cortical regulation of mesostriatal dopamine [96], findings that are isomorphorphic with the neurochemical phenotype of schizophrenia (Table 1) [97]. However, these monkeys also display cognitive deficits that are not prominent in schizophrenia, resembling hippocampally rather than prefrontally mediated neuropsychological deficits [98]. Taken together, however, all of these models support the notion that early developmental lesions of limbic cortex or amygdala lead to abnormalities in behaviors normally regulated by the prefrontal cortex, limbic cortex, or mesolimbic dopamine in the adult. Moreover, some of these deficits appear to be isomorphic or consistent with behavioral phenotypes in schizophrenia.

B. Perinatal Distress Models

Given the small but significant association with early-life "psychological" stressors and later expression of schizotypal symptoms [88], a number of studies have examined the effect of perinatal or neonatal stress in rats on brain systems implicated in schizophrenia. Repeated stress and nutritional deprivation [99,100] of the dam during gestation have each been shown to lead to delayed and persistent changes in hippocampal neuron morphology and catecholamine systems in the offspring. Similarly, 24-hr isolation of pups at PD 3, 6, or 9 leads to deficits in PPI and enhanced apomorphine-induced motor stereotypy in the adult rat, indicating delayed changes in hippocampal and mesolimbic dopamine circuits [37,101]. Moreover, although the effects of maternal separation on the behavioral response to psychostimulants appear to be inconsistent, these rats show increased amphetamine-evoked striatal DA efflux as adults [102]. Whereas neonatal maternal separation imposes substantial *physiological* stress on rats, social isolation of weanlings is arguably a more *psychological* stressor. This stressor also leads to persistent deficits in prepulse inhibition and amphetamine-evoked striatal dopamine efflux, but has no effect on latent inhibition [103]. Taken together, studies of gestational or early postnatal stressors indicate that striatal dopamine systems are exquisitely sensitive to early-life stressors.

C. Developmental Viral Infections or Evoked Immune Responses

As with early-life stressors, there is a small but significant association between viral infection during gestation and the risk for schizophrenia [88]. Thus, researchers have investigated the effects of perinatal infection or maternal immune responses on brain development and behavior of the offspring. These models are not as widely used as other perinatal manipulations, perhaps because of the indirect relationship between schizophrenia risk and viral infection. Moreover, because of differences in rodent and human gestational periods, viruses would be expected to affect more stages of brain development in rodents than in humans. Accordingly, influenza or Borna infections in rodents cause gross morphological abnormalities in the brains of the offspring that are unlike the relatively subtle morphologic and histologic abnormalities found in brains of schizophrenia patients. Nevertheless, the available studies indicate that gestational exposure to viral infection can result in cytochemical abnormalities in the cerebral cortex [104], as well as deficits in frontal lobe–mediated behaviors [105] and enhanced responsiveness to psychostimulants [106] in the adult offspring. Moreover, it has recently been shown that offspring of dams treated with polyribocytidilic acid, a compound that induces release of cytokines, show a delayed onset of latent inhibition [107]. It has been hypothesized that the cytokines released during the response to viral infection may significantly affect brain development and plasticity and, thus, may be more directly relevant to schizophrenia [108].

D. Genetic Factors

Given the evidence for developmental abnormalities, especially in limbic-related and frontal cortical regions in schizophrenia patients, genes known to regulate cortical development are considered candidates in creating animal models of schizophrenia. The possible roles of some of these genes in schizophrenia have been proposed [109,110]. One fact that may become important in focusing on particular genes in developmental models is that schizophrenia is considered to involve maldevelopment of the cerebral cortex and/or abnormal plasticity within cortical circuits in the adult. Therefore, genes known to play a role in both of these processes may be of the most relevance. Moreover, given that a subset of these genes is preferentially expressed in the cortical regions most affected in schizophrenia, the search could be narrowed further. Alternatively, given the overwhelming evidence that schizophrenia is a "polygenic" disorder, it has been proposed that genes that regulate processes such as methylation which, in turn, regulate multiple chromosomal sites and, thus, multiple genes, may be highly relevant [111]. This argument would be especially important if manipulation of such genes is shown to have a relatively greater impact on development and plasticity of limbic-related and frontal cortices. An example of a genetic model that achieves a subset of the aims described above is genetic manipulation of *reelin*, a protein involved in neuronal migration that is localized in the dendritic spines of mature. *Reelin* is decreased in schizophrenia [112]. Furthermore, mutations of the genes regulating *reelin* expression or function result in decreases in size of the hippocampus and cytoarchitectural changes, mainly neuronal disorganization. However, mutation of *reelin*-related genes also results in marked deformation of the hippocampus, cerebellum, thalamus, and brainstem [113], unlike the subtle structural changes in schizophrenia. More generally, in fact, knockouts of many of the "candidate" genes described above, when not fatal, result in severe brain deformation and/or mental retardation [e.g., 114]. Thus, genetic strategies that are more temporally and anatomically selective than knockouts are likely to be necessary to achieve valid models of schizophrenic phenotypes.

E. Epigenetic Manipulations That Alter the DNA of Developing Neurons

A key issue in animal models of schizophrenia is to be able to understand how a unitary etiological process can produce diffuse histopathological and variable morphological changes in the cerebral cortex coexisting with relatively localized and severe dysfunction of limbic and paralimbic cortical circuits. A recent model employing the neuronal DNA-methylating agent methylazoxymethanol acetate (MAM) addresses this issue [111]. In this model, MAM is administered to pregnant Fischer 344 rats on gestation day (GD) 17, a period during which neuronal proliferation is continuing in limbic-related cortical regions, slowing in other cortical regions, and paused or completed in most other brain regions. Similar to other developmental models the offspring of dams treated with MAM on GD17 show a delayed onset of an enhanced locomotor response to amphetamine [111], indicative of increased amphetamine-evoked DA release in striatum. MAM GD17 offspring also show abnormal spontaneous and drug-induced orofacial behaviors, and deficits in reversal learning and PPI, indicating dysfunction of medial prefrontal cortical, hippocampal/parahippocampal and related dopaminergic circuits (see Table 1).

Single-cell recording in the PFC, ventral striatum, and ventral tegmental area have revealed marked alterations in neurophysiological activity regulated by the limbic or paralimbic afferents to these neurons. Importantly, however, these relatively prominent functional abnormalities occur in the presence of small to moderate reductions in cross-sectional thickness and increases in neuronal density in the cerebral cortex, especially limbic-related regions. Moreover, while medial limbic thalamic regions were also reduced in size, the sizes of nonlimbic thalamus and anterior cerebellum are not affected. Thus, the pattern of anatomical, neurophysiological, and behavioral abnormalities resulting from the disruption of neuronal DNA methylation on GD 17 in the rat is isomorphic with schizophrenia in several critical aspects and may model the pathophysiology subserving a core set of behavioral abnormalities in this disorder.

The effects of MAM administration at earlier time points also appear to be relevant to schizophrenia. Administration of MAM at GD 12–15 affects the fetal brain during the neurogenesis of the majority of neurons destined for the forebrain, including basal ganglia and thalamus, thus producing less selective and more severe hypoplasia than MAM exposure at GD 17 [111]. However, there are some characteristics shared by offspring of dams treated with MAM at GD 12, 15, or 17 that are highly relevant to schizophrenia, including a greater reduction in the size of hippocampal or parahippocampal regions, relative to other cortical regions [115] and behavioral abnormalities such as increased responsiveness to amphetamine [111] and PPI deficits [116]. Thus, the effects of exposure to MAM at one of several points of rat gestation indicate that disruption of DNA methylation can disrupt cortical development, but that limbic cortex is the most affected morphologically. Other methods of disrupting DNA structure, such as radiation exposure, can have similar effects when timed appropriately [115]. Moreover, irradiation can be used in primates to affect DNA structure during specific stages of brain development, in order to produce primate models of thalamic or cortical maldevelopment [117].

In summary, as with nearly all other developmental models, this disruption of DNA methylation or structure results in prefrontal cortical and limbic cortical dysfunction, as well as abnormal cortical regulation of forebrain DA systems in the adult. Importantly, the MAM GD 17 model shows that a pathodevelopmental process can produce these functional abnormalities while causing relatively subtle anatomical abnormalities similar to those observed in the brains of schizophrenia patients.

F. Implications

There is considerable evidence to support the hypothesis that the etiology of schizophrenia begins early in brain development. Developmental models have revealed common etiologic pathways for some of the key neuroanatomical, neurochemical, and behavioral abnormalities observed in schizophrenia. Moreover, there is converging evidence from these models that normal development of limbic cortex is critical to the normal development of the prefrontal cortex and cortical regulation of dopamine transmission. Other commonalities among the models support the notion that the limbic-related cortical neurons are significantly more vulnerable to developmental disruptions than neurons in other cortical regions. This may relate to unique patterns of gene expression in limbic-related regions, or may relate more generally to the stability of expressed regions of the chromosome in these neurons. The findings generated from developmental models do not disprove a degenerative component to the etiology of schizophrenia or negate the possibility that chronic drug administration can induce changes in cortical circuits similar to those resulting from abnormal development. Moreover, the effects of epigenetic manipulations used in these models are not inconsistent with the evidence that the majority of the risk for schizophrenia is inherited.

V. GENETIC MODELS OF SCHIZOPHRENIA

As discussed in the previous section, considerable evidence suggests that schizophrenia depends on a relatively large heritable component [118–121]. Despite this, very little progress has been made in determining candidate polymorphisms or mutations that have a significant load factor associated with them; therefore, it seems likely that schizophrenia is a polygenic disorder that significantly interacts with nongenomic factors [120].

With the advent of transgenic technologies, it is increasingly possible to induce specific genomic effects in animals and to subsequently evaluate the validity of the line as a putative model of psychosis, or other psychiatric disorders [122]. Genetic models have been chiefly targeted toward neurotransmitter systems widely theorized to subserve the behavioral phenotypes within schizophrenia (e.g., alpha 7 nicotinic acetylcholine receptor and sensory gating; catechol-O-methyl transferase [COMT] and working memory) or be involved with neural systems thought to be abnormal in schizophrenia (e.g., dopamine system manipulations, NMDA receptors). Moreover, some experimental genetic manipulations have additional construct validity, given the fact that the targeted gene is located in chromosomal regions that are significantly linked with increased risk for schizophrenia. For example, the alpha 7 nicotinic receptor and COMT protein are located on chromosomes 15 and 22q, respectively, at loci known to be linked with increased risk for schizophrenia [119–121].

The gene for the alpha 7 subunit of the nicotinic cholinergic receptor has been the subject of intense study, since it has been revealed that the expression of this subunit is strongly associated with suppression of the P50 component of a sensory-evoked EEG potential. The decrease in P50 is a phenotype reliably observed schizophrenia patients and their relatives [123]. Freedman and coworkers have selectively bred mice with sensory gating deficits and have found this phenotype to be significantly associated with abnormal nicotinic receptor binding in the hippocampus [124]. Moreover, in the same mouse strains, the deficits can be rescued by selective alpha 7 nicotinic receptor agonists [125].

Based on the observation that there may be hypoglutamatergic function in schizophrenia [14,16,126], Mohn et al. [127] explored the behavioral consequences of knockdown of NR1, an obligatory subunit of the N-methyl-D-asparate/glutamate receptor, in mice. Mice expressing only 5% of normal levels of NR1 display behavioral abnormalities, including increased motor activity and stereotypy and deficits in social and sexual interactions. The responsiveness of the phenotype to administration of the antipsychotic drug clozapine further evidences the usefulness of transgenic models of this type.

In fact, schizophrenia and other disorders characterized by psychosis and pervasive attentional and executive dysfunction may be characterized by at least two sets of "genetic" abnormalities. The first set would involve genes that regulate the maturation of synaptic transmission and plasticity in cortical, especially limbic cortical, circuits. In the mature system, however, a second set of abnormally regulated genes could be associated with schizophrenia: those involved in the real-time pathophysiology underlying the psychopathology of schizophrenia. Dysregulation of the second set of genes could result from developmental pathology mediated by the first set of genes, but could also be secondary to alterations modeled, for example, by the effects of phencyclidine. Whereas prevention of schizophrenia will depend on revelation of the first set of genes and finding ways to normalize the relevant developmental processes, treatment will depend on therapeutic regulation the second set of genes.

VI. FUTURE DIRECTIONS FOR ANIMAL MODELS OF SCHIZOPHRENIA

One advantage of having validated animal models of schizophrenia, particularly etiologically distinct models, is the ability to then test directly whether particular biological mechanisms may be realistically implicated in psychopathology. For example, quantitative trait loci are being developed for schizophrenia, and candidate genes are on the horizon [120]. Having a validated model in hand, we can again utilize behavioral pharmacological approaches, or even transgenic techniques, to question whether the candidate(s) may be *plausibly* related to impaired function. In turn, we can use the same techniques to question whether direct manipulation of these same factors may yield antipsychotic effects.

For example, a substitution mutation in the COMT gene, which putatively results in reduced cortical catecholaminergic function because of *increased* catabolic activity, has been implicated in the neurocognitive component of schizophrenia [128]. Animals with pharmacological or transgenic manipulations of cortical COMT activity can be utilized to [1] evaluate the plausibility that alterations of enzyme activity could produce neurocognitive dysfunction, and [2] to determine the potential antipsychotic effects of directly manipulating COMT activity. This two-pronged approach depends critically on the use of validated and well-understood animal models. It is also strongly supported by the utilization of behavioral procedures in animals with strong construct validity for the symptomatology of schizophrenia.

Undoubtedly, future research will focus on the generation of new animal models and the refinement of behavioral techniques for modeling symptoms of schizophrenia. In addition, the integration of multiple models (to reflect etiological heterogeneity of idiopathic schizophrenia) may assist in the production of more comprehensive reproductions of primary symptomatology. And ultimately, as with any debilitating disease, it is hoped that animal models will generate useful information that will improve the functional outcome of patients with schizophrenia.

REFERENCES

1. JD Jentsch, Roth RH. Effects of antipsychotic drugs on dopamine release and metabolism in the central nervous system. In: M Lidow, ed. Neurotransmitter Receptors in Actions of Antipsychotic Drugs. Boca Raton: CRC Press, 2000, pp 31–41.
2. J Arnt, T Skarsfeldt, J Hyttel. Differentiation of classical and novel antipsychotics using animal models. Int Clin Psychopharmacol 12:S9–S17, 1997.
3. AA Grace, BS Bunney, H Moore, CL Todd. Dopamine-cell depolarization block as a model for the therapeutic actions of antipsychotic drugs. Trends Neurosci 20:31–37, 1997.
4. TW Robbins. The case of frontostriatal dysfunction in schizophrenia. Schizophr Bull 16:391–402, 1990.
5. RE Gur, RC Gur, AJ Saykin. Neurobehavioral studies in schizophrenia: implications for regional brain dysfunction. Schizophr Bull 16:445–451, 1990.
6. HM Moore, AR West, AA Grace. The regulation of forebrain dopamine transmission: relevance to the pathophysiology and psychopathology of schizophrenia. Biol Psychiatry 46:40–55, 1999.
7. NC Andreasen, P Nopoulos, DS O'Leary, DD Miller, T Wassink, M Flaum. Defining the phenotype of schizophrenia: cognitive dysmetria and its neural mechanisms. Biol Psychiatry 46:908–920, 1999.
8. AA Grace. Gating of information flow within the limbic system and the pathophysiology of schizophrenia. Brain Res Brain Res Rev 31:330–341, 2000.
9. GK Thaker, WT Carpenter. Advances in schizophrenia. Nat Med 6:667–671, 2001.
10. MF Green, KH Nuechterlein. Should schizophrenia be treated as a neurocognitive disorder? Schizophr Bull 25:309–319, 1999.
11. B Elvevag, TE Goldberg. Cognitive impairment in schizophrenia is the core of the disorder. Crit Rev Neurobiol 14:1–21, 2000.
12. BM Angrist, S Gershon. The phenomenology of experimentally-induced psychosis—preliminary observations. Biol Psychiatry 2:95–107, 1970.
13. GK Aghajanian, GJ Marek. Serotonin and hallucinogens. Neuropsychopharmacology 21:16S–23S, 1999.
14. DC Javitt, SR Zukin. Recent advances in the phencyclidine model of schizophrenia. Am J Psychiatry 148:1301–1308, 1991.
15. JD Jentsch, Roth RH. The neuropsychopharmacology of phencyclidine: from NMDA receptor hypofunction to the dopamine hypothesis of schizophrenia. Neuropsychopharmacology 20:201–225, 1999.
16. CA Tamminga. Schizophrenia and glutamatergic transmission. Crit Rev Neurobiol 12:21–36, 1998.
17. JA Lieberman, BB Sheitman, BJ Kinon. Neurochemical sensitization in the pathophysiology of schizophrenia: deficits and dysfunction in neuronal regulation and plasticity. Neuropsychopharmacology 17:205–229, 1997.
18. SA Castner, PS Goldman-Rakic. Long-lasting psychotomimetic consequences of repeated low-dose amphetamine exposure in rhesus monkeys. Neuropsychopharmacology 20:10–28, 1999.
19. TE Robinson, JB Becker. Enduring changes in brain and behavior produced by chronic amphetamine administration: a review and evaluation of animal models of amphetamine psychosis. Brain Res 396:157–198, 1986.
20. M Lyon, TW Robbins. The action of central nervous system stimulant drugs: a general theory concerning amphetamine effects. In: WB Essman, L Valzelli, eds. Current Developments in Psychopharmacology, Vol 2. New York: Spectrum, 1975, pp 79–163.

21. I Creese, SD Iversen. The role of forebrain dopamine systems in amphetamine induced stereotyped behavior in the rat. Psychopharmacologia 39:345–357, 1974.
22. TW Robbins. Relationship between reward-enhancing and stereotypical effects of psychomotor stimulant drugs. Nature 264:57–59, 1976.
23. DS Segal, MA Geyer, MA Schuckit. Stimulant-induced psychosis: an evaluation of animal methods. Essays Neurochem Neuropharmacol 5:95–129, 1981.
24. MA Geyer, A Markou. Animal models of psychiatric disorders. In: Psychopharmacology: The Fourth Generation of Progress. New York: Raven Press, 1991, pp 787–798.
25. R Kuczenski, DS Segal. Sensitization of amphetamine-induced stereotyped behaviors during the acute response. J Pharmacol Exp Ther 288:699–709, 1999.
26. JT Tschanz, GV Rebec. Atypical antipsychotic drugs block selective components of amphetamine-induced stereotypy. Pharmacol Biochem Behav 31:519–522, 1988.
27. I Creese, DR Burt, SH Snyder. Dopamine receptor binding predicts clinical and pharmacological potencies of antischizophrenic drugs. Science 192:481–483, 1976.
28. I Baruch, DR Hemsley, JA Gray. Differential performance of acute and chronic schizophrenics in a latent inhibition task. J Nerv Ment Dis 176:598–606, 1988.
29. JH Williams, NA Wellman, DP Geaney, PJ Cowen, J Feldon, JN Rawlins. Reduced latent inhibition in people with schizophrenia: an effect of psychosis or of its treatment? Br J Psychiatry 172:243–249, 1998.
30. PC Moser, JM Hitchcock, S Lister, PM Moran. The pharmacology of latent inhibition as an animal model of schizophrenia. Brain Res Brain Res Rev 33:275–307, 2000.
31. MA Geyer, DS Segal, BD Greenberg. Increased startle responding in rats treated with phencyclidine. Neurobehav Toxicol Teratol 6:1–4, 1984.
32. MA Geyer, DL Braff. Startle habituation and sensorimotor gating in schizophrenia and related animal models. Schizophr Bull 13:643–668, 1987.
33. DL Braff, C Grillon, MA Geyer. Gating and habituation of the startle reflex in schizophrenic patients. Arch Gen Psychiatry 49:206–215, 1992.
34. RS Mansbach, MA Geyer, DL Braff. Dopaminergic stimulation disrupts sensorimotor gating in the rat. Psychopharmacology (Berl) 94:507–514, 1988.
35. DL Garver, RF Schlemmer, JW Maas, JM Davis. A schizophreniform behavioral psychosis mediated by dopamine. Am J Psychiatry 132:33–38, 1975.
36. JD Gambill, C Kornetsky. Effects of chronic amphetamine on social behavior of the rat: implications for an animal model of paranoid schizophrenia. Psychopharmacology 50: 215–223, 1976.
37. BA Ellenbroek, AR Cools. Animal models for the negative symptoms of schizophrenia. Behav Pharmacol 11:223–233, 2000.
38. DG Daniel, DR Weinberger, DW Jones, JR Zigun, R Coppola, S Handel, LB Bigelow, TE Goldberg, KF Berman, JE Kleinman. The effect of amphetamine on regional cerebral blood flow during cognitive activation in schizophrenia. J Neurosci 11:1907–1917, 1991.
39. BM Angrist, J Rotrosen, S Gershon. Differential effects of amphetamine and neuroleptics on negative vs. positive symptoms in schizophrenia. Psychopharmacology (Berl) 72:17–19, 1980.
40. JN Joyce, A Shane, N Lexow, A Winocur, MF Casanova, JE Kleinman. Serotonin uptake sites and serotonin receptors are altered in the limbic system of schizophrenics. Neuropsychopharmacology 8:315–336, 1993.
41. HY Meltzer, S Matsubara, JC Lee. Classification of typical and atypical antipsychotic drugs on the basis of dopamine D-1, D-2 and serotonin2 pKi values. J Pharmacol Exp Ther 251:238–246, 1989.
42. MA Geyer. Behavioral studies of hallucinogenic drugs in animals: implications for schizophrenia research. Pharmacopsychiatry Suppl 31:73–79, 1998.
43. SC Dulawa, C Gross, KL Stark, R Hen, MA Geyer. Knockout mice reveal opposite roles for serotonin 1A and 1B receptors in prepulse inhibition. Neuropsychopharmacology 22:650–659, 2000.
44. ED Luby, BD Cohen, G Rosenbaum, JS Gottlieb, R Kelly. Study of a new schizophrenic-like drug: Sernyl. Arch Neurol Psychiatry 81:363–369, 1959.
45. T Itil, A Keskiner, N Kiremitci, JMC Holden. Effect of phencyclidine in chronic schizophrenics. Can J Psychiatry 12:209–212, 1967.
46. JH Krystal, LP Karper, JP Seibyl, et al. Subanesthetic effects of the noncompetitive NMDA receptor antagonist, ketamine, in humans: psychotomimetic, perceptual, cognitive and neuroendrocrine responses. Arch Gen Psychiatry 51:199–214, 1994.
47. AC Lahti, B Koffel, D Laporte, CA Tamminga. Subanesthetic doses of ketamine stimulate psychosis in schizophrenia. Neuropsychopharmacology 13:9–19, 1994.
48. WJ Freed, DR Weinberger, LA Bing, RJ Wyatt. Neuropharmacological studies of phencyclidine (PCP)-induced behavioral stimulation in mice. Psychopharmacology 71:291–297, 1980.
49. F Sams-Dodd. Phencyclidine-induced stereotyped behaviour and social isolation in rats: a possible animal model of schizophrenia. Behav Pharmacol 7:3–23, 1996.
50. B Moghaddam, BW Adams. Reversal of phencyclidine effects by a group II metabotropic glutamate receptor agonist in rats. Science 281:1349–1352, 1998.
51. JD Jentsch, RH Roth, JR Taylor. Role for dopamine in the behavioral functions of the prefronto-corticos-

triatal system: implications for mental disorders and psychotropic drug action. Prog Brain Res 126:433–453, 2000.
52. S Maurel-Remy, K Bervoets, MJ Millan. Blockade of phencyclidine-induced hyperlocomotion by clozapine and MDL 100,907 in rats reflects antagonism of 5-HT2a receptors. Eur J Pharmacol 280:9–11, 1995.
53. VP Bakshi, NR Swerdlow, MA Geyer. Clozapine antagonizes phencyclidine-induced deficits in sensorimotor gating of the startle response. J Pharmacol Exp Ther 27:787–794, 1994.
54. RE Steinpreis, JD Sokolowski, A Papanikolaou, JD Salamone. The effects of haloperidol and clozapine on phencyclidine- and amphetamine-induced suppression of social behavior in the rat. Pharmacol Biochem Behav 47:579–585, 1994.
55. JD Jentsch, JR Taylor, RH Roth. Phencyclidine model of frontal cortical dysfunction. Neuroscientist 6:263–270, 2000.
56. JM Rainey Jr, MK Crowder MK. Prolonged psychosis attributed to phencyclidine: report of three cases. Am J Psychiatry 132:1076–1078, 1975.
57. RM Allen, SJ Young. Phencyclidine-induced psychosis. Am J Psychiatry 135:1081–1084, 1978.
58. M Hertzman, RC Reba, EV Kotlyarove. Single photon emission computerized tomography in phencyclidine and related drug abuse. Am J Psychiatry 147:255–256, 1990.
59. JC Wu, MS Buchsbaum, W Bunney. Positron emission tomography study of phencyclidine users as a possible drug model of schizophrenia. Jpn J Psychopharmacol 11:47–48, 1991.
60. DR Weinberger, KF Berman. Prefrontal function in schizophrenia: confounds and controversies. Phil Trans R Soc Lond B 351:1495–1503, 1996.
61. A Breier, AK Malhotra, DA Pinals, NI Weisenfeld, D Pickar. Association of ketamine-induced psychosis with focal activation of the prefrontal cortex in healthy volunteers. Am J Psychiatry 154:805–811, 1997.
62. JD Jentsch, JR Taylor, RH Roth. Subchronic phencyclidine administration increases mesolimbic dopaminergic system responsivity and augments stress- and psychostimulant-induced hyperlocomotion. Neuropsychopharmacology 19:105–113, 1998.
63. SM Turgeon, JK Roche. The delayed effects of phencyclidine enhance amphetamine-induced behavior and striatal c-Fos expression in the rat. Neuroscience 91:1265–1275, 1999.
64. B Lannes, G Micheletti, JM Warter, E Kempf, G Di Scala. Behavioural, pharmacological and biochemical effects of acute and chronic administration of ketamine in the rat. Neurosci Lett 128:177–181, 1991.
65. H Qiao, Y Noda, H Kamei, T Nagai, H Furukawa, H Miura, Y Kayukawa, T Ohta, T Nabeshima. Clozapine, but not haloperidol, reverses social behavior deficit in mice during withdrawal from chronic phencyclidine treatment. Neuroreport 12:11–15, 2001.
66. SM Turgeon, EA Auerbach, MA Heller. The delayed effects of phencyclidine (PCP) disrupt latent inhibition in a conditioned taste aversion paradigm. Pharmacol Biochem Behav 60:553–558, 1998.
67. ZA Martinez, GD Ellison, MA Geyer, NR Swerdlow. Effects of sustained phencyclidine exposure on sensorimotor gating of startle in rats. Neuropsychopharmacology 21:28–39, 1999.
68. JD Jentsch, A Tran, D Le, KD Youngren, RH Roth. Subchronic phencyclidine administration reduces mesoprefrontal dopamine utilization and impairs prefrontal cortical–dependent cognition in the rat. Neuropsychopharmacology 17:92–99, 1997.
69. S Park, PS Holzman. Schizophrenics show spatial working memory deficits. Arch Gen Psychiatry 49:975–982, 1992.
70. R Elliott, PJ McKenna, TW Robbins, BJ Sahakian. Neuropsychological evidence for frontostriatal dysfunction in schizophrenia. Psychol Med 25:619–630, 1995.
71. JD Jentsch, JR Taylor. Impaired inhibition of conditioned responses produced by subchronic administration of phencyclidine to rats. Neuropsychopharmacology 24:66–74, 2001.
72. JD Jentsch, DE Redmond Jr, JD Elsworth, JR Taylor, KD Youngren, RH Roth. Enduring cognitive deficits and cortical dopamine dysfunction in monkeys after long-term administration of phencyclidine. Science 277:953–955, 1997.
73. JD Jentsch, JR Taylor, JD Elsworth, DE Redmond Jr, RH Roth. Altered frontal cortical dopaminergic transmission in monkeys after subchronic phencyclidine exposure: involvement in frontostriatal cognitive deficits. Neuroscience 90:823–832, 1999.
74. JD Jentsch, JR Taylor, DE Redmond Jr, JD Elsworth, KD Youngren, RH Roth. Dopamine D4 receptor antagonist reversal of subchronic phencyclidine-induced object retrieval/detour deficits in monkeys. Psychopharmacology (Berl) 142:78–84, 1999.
75. U Schroeder, H Schroeder, H Schwegler, BA Sabel. Neuroleptics ameliorate phencyclidine-induced impairments of short-term memory. Br J Pharmacol 130:33–40, 2000.
76. VL Arvanov, RY Wang. Clozapine, but not haloperidol, prevents the functional hyperactivity of N-methyl-D-aspartate receptors in rat cortical neurons induced by subchronic administration of phencyclidine. J Pharmacol Exp Ther 289:1000–1006, 1999.
77. Y Noda, H Kamei, T Mamiya, H Furukawa, T Nabeshima. Repeated phencyclidine treatment induces negative symptom-like behavior in forced-swimming test in mice: imbalance of prefrontal serotonergic and dopaminergic functions. Neuropsychopharmacology 23:375–387, 2000.

78. MB Bowers Jr, R Imirowicz, B Druss, CM Mazure. Autonomous psychosis following psychotogenic substance abuse. Biol Psychiatry 37:136–137, 1995.
79. A Preda, RW MacLean, CM Mazure, MB Bowers Jr. Antidepressant-associated mania and psychosis resulting in psychiatric admissions. J Clin Psychiatry 62:30–33, 2001.
80. BK Young, R Camicioli, L Ganzini. Neuropsychiatric adverse effects of antiparkinsonian drugs. Characteristics, evaluation and treatment. Drugs Aging 10:367–383, 1997.
81. ED London, G Wilkerson, C Ori, AS Kimes. Central action of psychomotor stimulants on glucose utilization in extrapyramidal motor areas of the rat brain. Brain Res 512:155–158, 1990.
82. S Miyamoto, JN Leipzig, JA Lieberman, GE Duncan. Effects of ketamine, MK-801 and amphetamine on regional brain 2-deoxyglucose uptake in freely moving mice. Neuropsychopharmacology 22:400–412, 2000.
83. AA Grace. Gating of information flow within the limbic system and the pathophysiology of schizophrenia. Brain Res Brain Res Rev 31:330–341, 2001.
84. P O'Donnell, AA Grace. Phencyclidine interferes with the hippocampal gating of nucleus accumbens neuronal activity in vivo. Neuroscience 87:823–830, 1998.
85. CY Yim, GJ Mogenson. Response of nucleus accumbens neurons to amygdala stimulation and its modification by dopamine. Brain Res 239:401–415, 1982.
86. PJ Harrison. The neuropathology of schizophrenia: a critical review of the data and their interpretation. Brain 122:593–624, 1999.
87. DR Weinberger, BK Lipska. Cortical maldevelopment, anti-psychotic drugs, and schizophrenia: a search for common ground. Schizophr Res 16:87–110, 1995.
88. A Jablensky. The 100-year epidemiology of schiozophrenia. Schizophr Res 28:111–125, 1997.
89. C McDonald, RM Murray. Early and late environmental risk factors for schizophrenia. Brain Res Rev 31:130–137, 2000.
90. JL Waddington, E O'Callaghan, P Buckley, et al. Tardive dyskinesia in schizophrenia: relationship to minor physical anomalies, frontal lobe dysfunction and cerebral structure on magnetic resonance imaging. Br J Psychiatry 167: 41–44, 1995.
91. BK Lipska, DR Weinberger. To model a psychiatric disorder in animals: schizophrenia as a reality test. Neuropsychopharmacology 24:66–74, 2000.
92. FM Hanlon, RJ Sutherland. Changes in adult brain and behavior caused by neonatal limbic damage: implications for the etiology of schizophrenia. Behav Brain Res 107:71–83, 2000.
93. G Wolterink, LEWPM Daenen, S Dubbeldam, et al. Early amygdala damage in the rat as a model for neurodevelopmental psychopathological disorders. Eur Neuropsychopharmacol 11:51–59, 2001.
94. EM Montgomery, ME Bardgett, B Lall, CA Csernansky, JG Csernansky. Delayed neuronal loss after administration of intracerebroventricular kainic acid to preweanling rats. Dev Brain Res 112:107–116, 1999.
95. J Bachevalier, MC Alvarado, L Malkova. Memory and socioemotional behavior in monkeys after hippocampal damage incurred in infancy or in adulthood. Biol Psychiatry 46:329–339, 1999.
96. RC Saunders, BS Kolachana, J Bachevalier, DR Weinberger. Neonatal lesions of the medial temporal lobe disrupt prefrontal cortical regulation of striatal dopamine. Nature 393:169–171,1998.
97. A Bertolino, MB Knable, RC Saunders, et al. The relationship between dorsolateral prefrontal N-acetylaspartate measures and striatal dopamine activity in schizophrenia. Biol Psychiatry 45:660–667, 1999.
98. O Pascalis, J Bachevalier. Neonatal aspiration lesions of the hippocampal formation impair visual recognition memory when assessed by paired-comparison task but not by delayed nonmatching-to-sample task. Hippocampus 9:609–616, 1999.
99. WA Debassio, TL Kemper, JR Galler, J Tonkiss. Prenatal malnutrition effect on pyramidal and granule cell generation in the hippocampal formation. Brain Res Bull 35:57–61, 1994.
100. ES Marichich, VA Molina, OA Orsingher. Persistent changes in central catecholaminergic system after recovery of perinatally undernourished rats. J Nutr 109:1045–1050, 1979.
101. BA Ellenbroek, AR Cools. The long-term effects of maternal deprivation depend on the genetic background. Neuropsychopharmacology 23:99–106, 2000.
102. FS Hall, LS Wilkinson, T Humby, TW Robbins. Maternal deprivation of neonatal rats produces enduring changes in dopamine function. *Synapse* 32:37–43, 1999.
103. LS Wilkinson, SS Killcross, T Humby, FS Hall, MA Geyer, TW Robbins. Social isolation in the rat produces developmentally specific deficits in prepulse inhibition of the acoustic startle response without disrupting latent inhibition. Neuropsychopharmacology 10:61–72, 1994.
104. SH Fatemi, ES Emamian, D Kist, et al. Defective corticogenesis and reduction in Reelin immunoreactivity in cortex and hippocampus of prenatally infected neonatal mice. Mol Psychiatry 4:145–154, 1999.
105. MV Solbrig, GF Koob, JH Fallon, S Reid, WI Lipkin. Prefrontal cortex dysfunction in Borna disease virus (BDV)-infected rats. Biol Psychiatry 40:629–636, 1996.
106. DM Rothschild, M O'Grady, L Wecker. Neonatal cytomegalovirus exposure decreases prepulse inhibition in adult rats: implications for schizophrenia. J Neurosci Res 57:429–434, 1999.
107. L Zuckerman, I Winer. Personal communication.

108. H Nawa, M Takahashi, PH Patterson. Cytokine and growth factor involvement in schizophrenia—support for the developmental model. Mol Psychiatry 5:594–603, 2000.
109. BG Bunney, SG Potkin, WE Bunney. Neuropathological studies of brain tissue in schizophrenia. J Psychiatr Res 31:159–173, 1997.
110. CS Weickert, DR Weinberger. A candidate molecule approach to defining developmental pathology in schizophrenia. Schizophr Bull 24:303–316, 1998.
111. HM Moore, ME Ghajarnia, JD Jentsch, MA Geyer, AA Grace. Late gestational disruption of cerebral cortical neurogenesis in the rat leads to structural and functional abnormalities in limbic-related cortical circuits: relevance to schizophrenia. Submitted, 2001.
112. F Impagnatiello,, AR Guidotti, C Pesold, et al. A decrease of reelin expression as a putative vulnerability factor in schizophrenia. Proc Natl Acad Sci USA 95:15718–15723, 1998.
113. DS Rice, T Curran. Mutant mice with scrambled brains: understanding the signaling pathways that control cell positioning in the CNS. Genes Dev 13:2758–2773, 1999.
114. WE Kaufmann, SM MacDonald, CR Altamura. Dendritic cytoskeletal protein expression in mental retardation: an immunohistochemical study of the neocortex in Retts syndrome. Cereb Cortex 10:992–1004, 2000.
115. F Cattabeni, M Di Luca. Developmental models of brain dysfunctions induced by targeted cellular ablations with methylazoxymethanol. Physiol Rev 77:199–215, 1997.
116. LM Talamini, B Ellenbroek, T Koch, J Korf. Impaired sensory gating and attention in rats with developmental abnormalities of the mesocortex. Implications for schizophrenia. Ann NY Acad Sci 911:486–494, 2000.
117. MK Schindler, L Selemon, L Wang, JG Csernansky. Structural variance of thalamus and other cortical structures in normal adult macaques and inter-uterine irratiated macaques. Schizophr Res 49(suppl):49, 2001.
118. TD Cannon, J Kaprio, J Lonnqvist, M Huttunen, M Koskenvuo. The genetic epidemiology of schizophrenia in a Finnish twin cohort. A population-based modeling study. Arch Gen Psychiatry 55:67–74, 1998.
119. MT Tsuang, WS Stone, SV Faraone. Schizophrenia: a review of genetic studies. Harvard Rev Psychiatry 7:185–207, 1999.
120. TD Cannon, TL Gasperoni, TG van Erp, IM Rosso. Quantitative neural indicators of liability to schizophrenia: implications for molecular genetic studies. Am J Med Genet 105:16–19, 2001.
121. R Freedman, SS Leonard. Chromosome 15q linkage for schizophrenia in the NIMH genetics initiative families. Schizophr Res 49:70, 2001.
122. RR Gainetdinov, AR Mohn, MG Caron. Genetic animal models: focus on schizophrenia. Trends Neurosci 24:527–533, 2001.
123. LE Alder, R Freedman, RG Ross, A Olincy, MC Waldo. Elementary phenotypes in the neurbiological and genetic study of schizophrenia. Biol Psychiatry 46:8–18, 1999.
124. KE Stevens, R Freedman, AC Collins, et al. Genetic correlation of hippocampal auditory response and alpha-bungarotoxin binding in inbred mouse strains. Neuropsychopharmacology 15:152–162, 1996.
125. KE Stevens, WR Kem, VM Mahnir, R Freedman. Selective alpha 7-nicotinic agonists normalize inhibition of auditory response in DBA mice. Psychopharmacology 136:320–327, 1998.
126. JW Olney, NB Farber. Glutamate receptor dysfunction and schizophrenia. Arch Gen Psychiatry 52:998–1007, 1995.
127. AR Mohn, RR Gainetdinov, MG Caron, BH Koller. Mice with reduced NMDA receptor expression display behaviors related to schizophrenia. Cell 98:427–436, 1999.
128. MF Egan, TE Goldberg, BS Kolachana, JH Callicott, CM Mazzanti, RE Straub, D Goldman, DR Weinberger. Effect of COMT Val108/158 Met genotype on frontal lobe function and risk for schizophrenia. Proc Natl Acad Sci USA 98:6917–6922, 2001.
129. LD Selemon, G Rajkowska, PS Goldman-Rakic. Abnormally high neuronal density in the schizophrenic cortex. A morphometric analysis of prefrontal area 9 and occipital area 17. Arch Gen Psychiatry 52:805–818, 1995.
130. G Rajkowska, LD Selemon, PS Goldman-Rakic. Neuronal and glial somal size in the prefrontal cortex: a postmortem morphometric study of schizophrenia and Huntington disease. Arch Gen Psychiatry 55:215–224, 1998.
131. GJ Popken, WE Bunney Jr, SG Potkin, EG Jones. Subnucleus-specific loss of neurons in medial thalamus of schizophrenics. Proc Natl Acad Sci USA 97:9276–9280, 2000.
132. SA Anderson, DW Volk, DA Lewis. Increased density of microtubule associated protein 2–immunoreactive neurons in the prefrontal white matter of schizophrenic subjects. Schizophr Res 19:111–119, 1996.
133. K Mirnics, FA Middleton, A Marquez, DA Lewis, P Levitt. Molecular characterization of schizophrenia viewed by microarray analysis of gene expression in prefrontal cortex. Neuron 28:53–67, 2000.

23

Affective Disorders
Imaging Studies

WARREN D. TAYLOR and RANGA R. KRISHNAN
Duke University Medical Center, Durham, North Carolina, U.S.A.

I. INTRODUCTION

The development of new imaging technology, able to more fully visualize the structure and function of specific brain regions, has enabled us to better understand the biological basis of psychiatric disorders. Specific brain regions, including the frontal lobe, the basal ganglia, and the limbic system, are all involved in the regulation of emotions, and injury to these areas can increase the risk of developing a mood disorder. Functional imaging studies demonstrate that mood disorders are associated with impairment in their normal function.

Computed tomography (CT) scans were used for earlier research, but magnetic resonance imaging (MRI) provides several advantages over CT. These higher-resolution images allow for more accurate measurement of structure volumes, which is facilitated by the MRI's ability to distinguish gray and white matter. Additionally, the MRI can discern smaller abnormalities not visible on CT. Further, this work in structural imaging is complementary to research utilizing functional imaging, which can measure regional blood flow or glucose utilization. This chapter will review this research and highlight specific brain regions implicated in mood disorders. When possible, we will attempt to correlate these findings with clinical outcomes.

II. IMAGING STUDIES IN DEPRESSION

Structural imaging research in depression has typically focused on two types of studies: research on structural volumes, and research on the presence, severity or volume of high-intensity lesions (hyperintensities) reflecting pathology. Unlike neuroimaging research in many other psychiatric disorders, imaging research in depression has typically focused on the elderly. This may limit the generalizability of this research, as geriatric depression is often clinically different than depression in younger individuals, but it also allows us to correlate psychiatric findings with injury to specific regions.

Functional imaging studies have mostly examined younger cohorts with smaller numbers of subjects. Many research findings using these techniques appear contradictory, which emphasizes the heterogeneity of disorders that may result in a clinical diagnosis of depression. Regardless, this body of work is highly important as it documents alteration in function of specific regions.

A. Structural Imaging Studies in Depression

1. Global Brain Abnormalities and Normal Aging

Clinically, these studies also have limited utility, as there are no well-established age- and sex-specific normal values [1]. In general, whole-brain volume data are less informative than data on specific regions that distinguish between gray and white matter.

Research clearly demonstrates that the brain's volume decreases with normal aging [2–4], but atrophy may not occur at the same rate in various regions [5]. Both cortical and subcortical regions, such as the caudate, putamen, and thalamus, are affected [6,7]. There are also gender differences, as men exhibit more atrophy with normal aging than women [2,3,5]. These data emphasize the need for age- and sex-matching when performing controlled neuroimaging studies, particularly in the elderly.

The majority of studies comparing whole-brain volumes between elderly depressed subjects and controls showed no significant difference between the two groups. There was no difference between elderly subjects with late-onset depression and controls, [8–12] nor was there a difference between late- and early-onset depressed subjects [8], but these results are not universal [13]. Studies exclusively of depression in women have also demonstrated no total brain volume difference from age-matched controls [14,15]. Also, neither depression severity [9] nor age of depressive symptom onset, after controlling for the subjects' current age [4], exhibited a significant association with total brain volume.

Another persistent finding in depressed elders is increased ventricle size. Subjects with late-onset depression have increased whole-brain CSF fluid volumes, larger ventricle-to-brain ratios, [10,13,16] and larger lateral and third ventricles than controls [10,13,16,17]. These findings have been interpreted as "atrophy" in depressed subjects, but this conclusion conflicts with studies of total brain volume. As CSF is typically easier to measure, this may be a more precise estimate but is also affected by overall head size; longitudinal studies are needed.

2. Regional Brain Measurements

Frontal Lobe

The frontal lobe has long been implicated in the regulation of both emotion and executive functioning. Multiple studies have demonstrated a reduced frontal lobe volume in depressed elders compared with controls [7,18,19], and smaller frontal lobes have also been observed in familial depressed subjects [20]. Only one study found no significant difference in frontal lobe volume between late-onset depression and controls, [13] but these researchers defined late-onset as after age 50, while other studies used an older age. The cause of this reduced volume may be decreased asymmetry in the frontal lobes of depressed subjects. Kumar et al. [21] demonstrated a significant right greater than left volume asymmetry in the frontal lobe of controls and subjects with minor depression. This asymmetry decreased (by diminishing right-sided volume) with increasing depression severity. The group with major depressive disorder did not exhibit a significant difference in volumes of the two lobes.

As the frontal lobe comprises almost a third of the brain, efforts have been made to examine specific regions, particularly the prefrontal cortex (PFC). Late-onset depressed subjects have a smaller PFC volume than controls [9], with an inverse correlation between depression severity and odds ratio for acquiring major depressive disorder, and PFC volume [9,10,21]. The absolute volume of the PFC may also be smaller in subjects with psychotic depression compared with nonpsychotic depression [22]. Specific regions of the PFC have also been studied, noting a decreased volume of gray matter in the subgenual PFC in familial depressed subjects; this finding correlated with decreased blood flow by PET [23]. Depressed subjects also exhibit a decreased orbitofrontal cortex volume compared with controls in imaging studies [24], correlating with atrophy of this region found in postmortem studies [25].

Temporal Lobe

The temporal lobe exhibits no statistically significant reduction in volume when late-onset depressed subjects are compared with controls [10,13]. There are reports of small, statistically insignificant differences in temporal lobe volumes of elders when both major and minor depression are compared with controls [9,26], however, when the small effect size is coupled with the negative studies, the relevance of this observation must be questioned. Although the temporal lobe's total volume may not be associated with late-onset depression, there may be contributory regional atrophy; a comparison of elderly late-onset depressed subjects to early-onset depressed subjects showed the late-onset group had more left medial temporal atrophy [27]. Another study demonstrated greater left sylvian fissure size and greater bilateral temporal sulcal enlargement when compared with controls [28].

Hippocampus and Amygdala

In depression research, the hippocampus has been primarily studied in two populations-women and the elderly. The studies in women intentionally excluded men to eliminate brain differences related to gender [15], and demonstrated smaller hippocampi bilaterally in women with recurrent major depressive disorder [14, 15] and smaller amygdala core nuclei volumes bilaterally [14]. These changes were not associated with age or age of depression onset, but were associated with lifetime duration of depression [14,15]. Other studies of mixed-gender cohorts found a significant 19% decrease in left hippocampal volume in depressed subjects, and a similar insignificant trend on the right hippocampus; there was no correlation with hippocampal volume and duration of depression [29].

Several investigators have hypothesized that the association between hippocampal volume loss and depression duration may be explained by episodes of hypercortisolemia during depressive episodes [15,30]. Animal studies that found the hippocampus to be sensitive to the neurotoxic effect of elevated cortisol levels [31]. One study correlated reduced hippocampal volumes with specific changes in cortisol concentration [32].

Studies in the elderly have been less conclusive. Several research groups failed to demonstrate a significant difference in the amygdala/hippocampal complex volume between late-onset depressed subjects and controls [13,18,32,33], or between late-onset compared with early-onset depressed subjects [33]. One study did find that depressed elders had significantly smaller right hippocampal volumes than controls, with a trend toward smaller left volumes [34]—a finding similar to Bremner et al.'s study in a younger population [29]. These apparently contradictory data are difficult to interpret owing to the amygdala/hippocampal complex's small size and the different techniques used to measure it; many studies measured the amygdala and hippocampus together, which could be a partial explanation of this discrepancy.

If reduced hippocampal volume is confirmed in other depressed, elderly populations, does this mean glucocorticoid toxicity is also responsible? Possibly, but that is not the only conceivable etiology, as neurodegenerative processes may also be involved. Late-onset depression can precede the onset of Alzheimer's dementia, which is itself associated with hippocampal degeneration [35]. Further research is needed to clarify this issue.

Subcortical Gray Matter Structures

Studies examining the basal ganglia's role in depression were initially driven by early observations about the increased frequency of depression seen in diseases that affect the basal ganglia, like Parkinson's disease. Smaller caudate nuclei are consistently found in late-onset depression when compared with controls [6–8] or early-onset subjects [8], although this finding may be specific to the left caudate [27]. The putamen is also smaller in late-onset depressed subjects than controls, and younger age at the first depressive episode correlated with smaller putaminal volumes [6,7]. Thalamic volumes are not different between controls and depressed subjects [6,8]. These findings are not consistent across all ages, as younger individuals may not exhibit volume abnormalities [36].

3. Cerebral Hyperintensities in Depression

General Associations

Hyperintensities, or high-intensity lesions, are bright areas in the brain parenchyma on T2-weighted magnetic resonance images that have strongly been associated with late-onset depression. They are traditionally classified into three major groups based on their location: periventricular hyperintensities (PVH), deep white matter hyperintensities (DWMH), and subcortical gray matter hyperintensities (SCH) (Fig. 1). Large, irregular hyperintense lesions > 5 mm are considered to represent actual infarcts.

Hyperintensities are associated with increased age [4,37] and are seen in normal aging [38]. They are also associated with medical comorbidity, appearing in neurologic diseases such as Alzheimer's dementia [16] and multiple sclerosis. Increased hyperintensity severity also correlates with cerebrovascular risk factors [37,38], including hypertension, diabetes, history of smoking, low cerebral blood flow velocity, carotid artery disease, and prior episodes of cerebral ischemia. However, hyperintensities can occur in many subjects without obvious risk factors. A recent study using diffusion tensor imaging, a MRI variant sensitive to ischemic disease, concluded that hyperintensities had diffusion characteristics similar to ischemic lesions, supporting a cerebrovascular etiology [39].

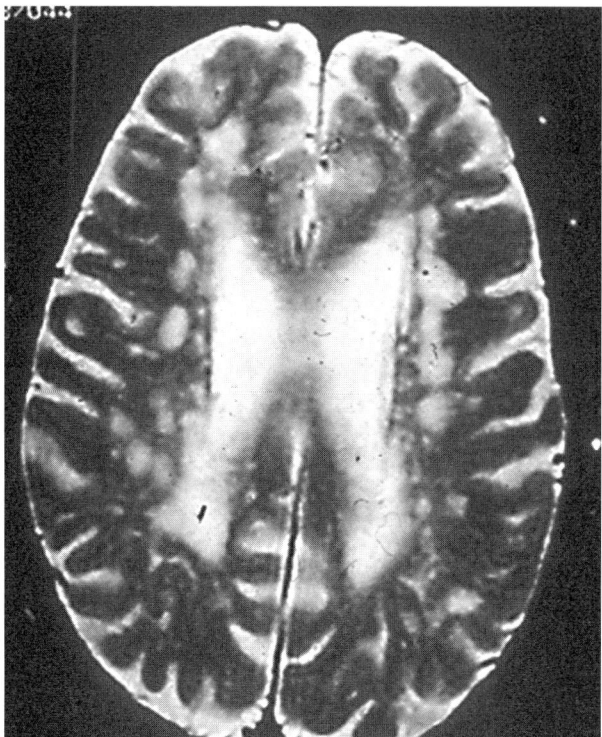 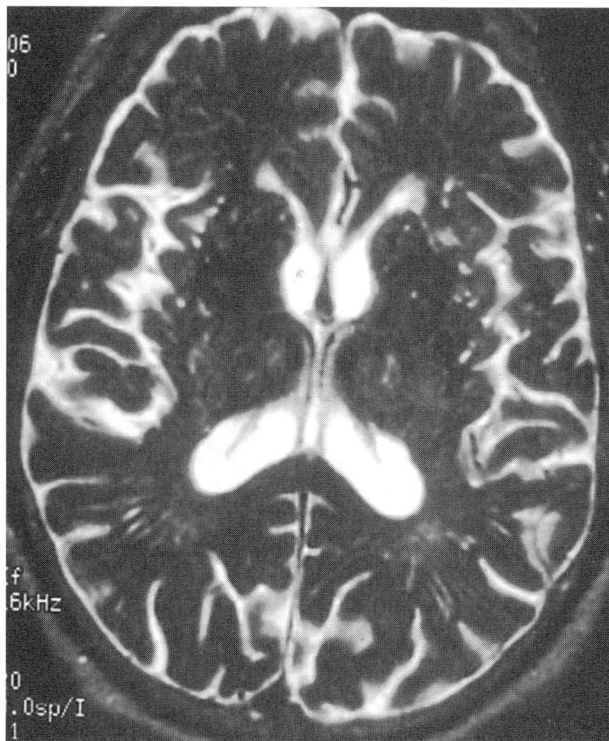

Figure 1 Axial slices exhibiting severe confluent deep white matter (DWMH) and periventricular hyperintensities (PVH) in the left image. PVH tend to hug the ventricle border, while DWMH are further from the ventricles in the white matter. The right image demonstrates smaller, punctate subcortical hyperintensities (SCH) in the basal ganglia and thalamus. (From the Neuropsychiatric Research Imaging Laboratory, Duke University Medical Center, Durham, NC)

Hyperintensity Location

Hyperintensities are more common and more severe in late-onset depressed subjects than in age-matched controls [16,17,40–42]. This is not true for younger depressed individuals.

Does hyperintensity location matter in the development of depression? Evidence is strongest for a contributory effect of SCH, particularly basal ganglia hyperintensities, which are more common in late-onset depressed subjects than controls [17,41,43–45], although this finding is not universal [46]. Results for PVH are more mixed. Although more common in depressed elders [18, 47], there may not be a correlation between PVH and depression [17,43]. The relationship between DWMH and depression is more promising. Late-onset depressed subjects exhibit more significant DWMH disease than do controls [17,26] or early-onset subjects [8,47–49]. Increased DWMH severity is associated with increased depression risk [26], but this finding is not universal [43].

Frontal lobe hyperintensities may be particularly important, as one study found that left frontal hyperintensities predicted assignment into the depressed group [44]. Another study found that increased lesion density in the medial orbital PFC and a region of the left internal capsule correlated with depression severity [45].

4. Clinical Significance of Neuroimaging Findings

Volumetric studies are difficult to translate into clinical relevance, as there are no well-defined "normal volumes" for specific structures. Clinical correlates of hyperintensity presence have been bettered studied. Increased SCH and DWMH severity are associated with poor treatment response to both pharmacotherapy and ECT [50–52]. One author, having previously coined the term "silent cerebral infarction" (SCI) in referring to hyperintensities [53], retrospectively found that individuals with more severe SCI had significantly longer hospitalizations for depression [54]. Lesion severity in younger depressed subjects is not so significantly correlated with outcome as it is in elderly depressed subjects [55].

More severe SCI is also associated with a higher occurrence of adverse central nervous system reactions to antidepressants [54], a finding replicated elsewhere that demonstrates an association with a higher risk of delirium from both antidepressant drug therapy [56] and electroconvulsive therapy [57]. Specifically, caudate hyperintensities are associated with increased risk of antipsychotic-induced parkinsonism [58].

Increased hyperintensity severity, particularly PVH and DWMH, is also associated with neuropsychological deficits [37], including impaired psychomotor speed, executive dysfunction [47,50,51], and impairment in verbal and nonverbal memory [47]. Caudate lesions are specifically associated with impairment on tasks requiring planning and sequencing. Increased severity of gray matter hyperintensities is also associated with the subsequent development of frank dementia [59].

5. Vascular Depression

Because of these findings, various authors have proposed that vascular disease is more than a cause of depression—rather a distinct subtype. Initially coined "arteriosclerotic depression" [60] this described a syndrome of vascular changes associated with depressive symptoms, including apathy, psychomotor retardation, cognitive impairment, functional disability, and lack of a family history of mood disorders [50,60,61]. Later, to be more consistent with the concept of vascular dementia, the term was changed to "vascular depression" [61,62]. Authors have used varying definitions of this syndrome: Krishnan et al. [61] defined it by MRI findings, while Alexopoulos et al. [63] used a broader definition which included depressed patients with any vascular disease. Diagnostic criteria for this subtype, utilizing both MRI findings and clinical symptoms, have been proposed [1].

6. Conclusion

Both volumetric studies and hyperintensity measurements correlate with depression. The frontal lobe, particularly the PFC, and the basal ganglia are most associated not only with depression, but also with neuropsychological deficits and functional impairment. It is very likely that hyperintensities and atrophy in these regions represent two separate pathways to a common clinical syndrome.

B. Functional Imaging Studies in Depression

Functional imaging studies, many examining younger cohorts than do structural studies in depression, demonstrate that the metabolic rate of frontal, striatal, and limbic regions is altered in depression. When results are compared across studies there are occasionally conflictual data, with some studies reporting hypometabolism and others hypermetabolism for the same structure in similar depressed states. It is likely these findings represent the heterogeneous pathogenesis of depression, which is associated with multiple pathophysiological states and subsequent assortment of distinct functional imaging abnormalities [64]. Although specific regional metabolic changes are not yet associated with distinct clinical syndromes, the fact that these regions exhibit an altered metabolism in depression supports their involvement in the pathogenesis of mood disorders. The most implicated regions include the prefrontal cortex (PFC), the cingulate and hippocampus, and the basal ganglia.

1. Resting Studies

Specific PFC regions consistently exhibit metabolic changes in depressed individuals. Most studies examining the dorsolateral PFC found a left-sided decrease in metabolism and blood flow in depressed subjects compared with control subjects [65–67]; a few studies reported bilateral hypometabolism [68,69]. Other studies have found relative dorsolateral PFC hypermetabolism [70]. The ventrolateral PFC, adjacent to the dorsolateral PFC, may also be involved, exhibiting a hypermetabolic rate in depression [66,70,71].

The medial OFC demonstrate hypermetabolism—increased blood flow and glucose metabolism—in depression [64–66, 72]. Studies in older depressed subjects found an opposite result; older subjects had decreased cerebral blood flow in the orbital frontal cortex, in the context of globally reduced cerebral blood flow and glucose metabolism [73,74].

The cingulate gyrus, a limbic structure, also has regional metabolic changes in depression. The anterior cingulate gyrus ventral to the genu of the corpus callosum exhibits decreased blood flow and metabolic rate [23,67,75,76]. This is also seen in older subjects [74], although recent data in a group of young male subjects found a higher metabolic rate in the right pregenual anterior cingulate in depressed subjects than control subjects [77]. Experimentally induced sadness may result in increased blood flow to the subgenual cingulate [78]. Basal ganglia structures also involved, particularly the caudate, which consistently exhibits metabolic changes, either a lower [71,72,74,75,77,79] or higher metabolic rate [65,70].

2. Studies of Antidepressant Response

These studies examined metabolic changes in depressed individuals compared with controls. What about comparing regional metabolic rates before and after treatment? Most research demonstrates that successful antidepressant therapy results in metabolic rate normalization in the dorsolateral PFC [68,70,77,78], but these findings are not universal [76,80]. This is also noted in the ventrolateral PFC [70,76] and medial orbital frontal cortex [76]; decreases in ventrolateral metabolism correlate with decreased depression severity [76].

Changes in the cingulate or basal ganglia are not so clear. Some data demonstrate that specific regions of the cingulate's metabolism may decrease with treatment response [78,81,82], but other research suggests that it may not normalize with treatment [23,76]. The dorsal anterior cingulate may experience an increased metabolic rate with successful antidepressant therapy [77]. The caudate's metabolic rate may normalize, but some studies have found this specific to the right side [70,83]. Other research shows that caudate metabolism may decrease with successful treatment, while putaminal metabolism initially increases, then decreases after several weeks of treatment [81].

Unfortunately, many of these studies provide limited information on neural circuitry that may mediate or predict antidepressant response. There is some evidence that baseline metabolism may predict response to antidepressant therapy; a study of the rostral anterior cingulate found that subjects with hypermetabolism in this region responded better to therapy than did hypometabolic subjects [69]. A recent EEG study utilizing brain electrical tomography analysis replicated this finding [84]. Lower baseline metabolism of the ventral anterior cingulate may also be associated with better response [76]. Clearly more research into how neuroimaging findings may influence treatment response and ultimately guide clinical treatment is needed.

3. Conclusions

Although the heterogeneity of findings in functional imaging makes these results difficult to interpret, this research supports the role of specific regions in the pathogenesis of depression. Although different depressive syndromes and different antidepressant therapies may result in different metabolic changes, the dorsolateral and ventrolateral PFC, the anterior cingulate, the medial orbital frontal cortex, and the basal ganglia continue to be specifically implicated. Functional imaging also has the potential to identify prognostic features supportive of treatment response, but more work is clearly needed.

III. IMAGING STUDIES IN BIPOLAR DISORDER

Historically there has been less structural neuroimaging research of bipolar disorder than depression. Also, in contrast to the research in depression, most neuroimaging studies in bipolar disorder have focused on younger populations, with several recruiting first-episode manic subjects.

There are several confounders when examining this research. Substance abuse is more common in this group than the general population, and bipolar patients more frequently have smoking histories, which qualifies as a cerebrovascular risk factor; both may affect neuroimaging results. Beyond this, there is also the potential confounder of treatment, as chronic lithium use has been associated with an increased volume of certain cortical regions, including the hippocampus [85].

A. Structural Imaging Studies in Bipolar Disorder

1. Volumetric Studies in Bipolar Disorder

There is no evidence of whole brain or cortical atrophy in subjects with bipolar disorder [86–92], but studies examining ventricular enlargement are more mixed, with some studies finding increased ventricle-to-brain ratios [48,89,93,94], and others not [95,96]. Specific cerebellar regions may also be atrophic in bipolar patients with multiple past affective episodes [92].

Bipolar subjects generally exhibit no frontal or parietal lobe volume abnormalities, even when specific regions such as the PFC are measured [1,97], although one study did find a significantly smaller PFC in bipolar subjects than controls [86]. Most research has also shown no difference in temporal lobe volumes [94,98], although this finding is not universal [1]. Late onset bipolar subjects may be different from early-onset or control subjects, as they exhibit increased volume of the left sylvian fissure and bilateral temporal sulcal enlargement [28].

As in depression, the hippocampus is smaller than in controls [97,98], particularly the right hippocampus

[98]. There is a suggestion of increased amygdala volumes in bipolar subjects [90,97], but there was no correlation between amygdala volume and duration or severity of illness [97]. Others have not found significant differences in amygdala volumes [98], or found smaller left amygdala volumes [91].

Data regarding subcortical structure volumes are also mixed. Some studies have reported enlarged thalami and basal ganglia [97]. One report demonstrated larger caudate volumes exclusively in male bipolar patients compared with controls [87]. Other studies have not found increased volumes of the caudate [98], putamen [87,98], or globus pallidus [87].

2. Hyperintensities in Bipolar Disorder

There are significantly fewer studies examining the presence and severity of hyperintensities in bipolar disorder than in depression. Most research shows that hyperintensities are increased in bipolar patients compared with controls, are more common in bipolar patients of all ages [99], and that hyperintensities are stable over time [48,87,96,100–102]. These trends are also true in treatment-naïve subjects [93], but other studies did not find increased hyperintensity frequency in bipolar subjects but did find that the risk of bipolar disorder was significantly greater in those with focal signal hyperintensities [96].

In the studies that reported increased hyperintensity severity in bipolar patients, the most commonly reported region was the deep white matter of the frontal and parietal lobes [48,87,100,102]. Younger bipolar subjects may have an increased frequency of PVH [96,101,102]. Unlike hyperintensities seen in older patients, these hyperintensities are not located in watershed zones, but rather in the deep white matter of the frontal and frontoparietal regions of both hemispheres [88]. Hyperintensities in young bipolar patients are not related to any vascular risk factors, but may be familial [88]. One study examining a family with a strong history of bipolar disorder reported that the majority of family members had MRI hyperintensity findings, including all those individuals with bipolar disorder [103]. Elderly bipolar patients also have increased SCH and DWMH when compared with controls [102].

3. Clinical Significance of Structural Findings in Bipolar Disorder

The clinical correlations of neuroimaging abnormalities have not been as extensively studied as in depression. The presence of hyperintensities is related to the presence of psychosis, the likelihood of rehospitalization in 2 years [102], and the total number of psychiatric hospitalizations [100]. One study classified bipolar subjects as poor outcome or good outcome, and found that poor outcome subjects had a greater number and more severe subcortical hyperintensities than did good outcome or control subjects [104].

As in depression, hyperintensities in bipolar subjects may also correlate with neuropsychological impairment: in this case, deficits on tests of fluency or recall [100], although some research has been unable to correlate white matter lesions in bipolar subjects with cognitive deficits [105]. This area of research desperately needs further study: several studies demonstrate that neurocognitive deficits observed in young bipolar subjects do not fully reverse with remission of mood symptoms [17], and that elderly bipolar patients with cognitive deficits may experience progression of their cognitive impairment [106]. These findings have not been correlated with neuroimaging, nor have they been correlated with treatment options.

4. Conclusion

Given the limited research, it is more difficult to reach firm conclusions about neuroanatomical substrates of bipolar disorder. As in depression, hyperintensities are more common, but unlike depression, are more common at earlier ages. There may be a familial component to hyperintensities in bipolar subjects, and they also appear related to worse treatment outcomes, although data for this conclusion are sparse. Volumetric studies are mixed, and the findings complicated by recent discoveries of the potential neurotrophic effects of mood stabilizers.

B. Functional Imaging in Bipolar Disorder

There have been limited number of studies utilizing functional imaging to study bipolar disorder, however even these preliminary studies may provide insight into involved brain structures. One complication of research utilizing these methods is the current mood state of the subjects; regional brain activity may differ in depression and mania.

Specific regions exhibit changes in glucose metabolism in bipolar disorder. Frontal metabolism is decreased in depressed bipolar subjects compared with controls [23,71,79], and one study has demonstrated reduced metabolism and regional blood flow specifically in the subgenual prefrontal cortex [23]. Manic subjects may exhibit increased glucose metabolism in this region [23]; however, other investigators have not replicated this finding [68,79]. One study examining temporal cortical regions also demonstrated decreased metabolism during depression and increased metabolism during mania [107], but these results have not been replicated. There are also reports of decreased caudate and thalamic metabolism in depressed subjects [79], and decreased metabolism of the left amygdala in manic subjects [108].

Although far from conclusive, this research further supports the involvement of frontal, striatal, and limbic structures in the pathogenesis of both bipolar depression and mania. Further research is needed to examine how the functioning of these regions may change with treatment or with repeated mood episodes and treatment resistance.

IV. CONCLUSIONS

This body of literature clearly demonstrates, in both studies of regional injury (atrophy and hyperintense lesions) and regional metabolism and functioning, that frontal, limbic, and striatal regions are involved in both depression and mania. Further, depression research demonstrates that injury to specific regions is associated with poor or delayed treatment response and increase frequency of adverse events to antidepressant therapies.

This research has started to be applied to therapeutic interventions, but more work is needed. Using neuroimaging techniques to identify individuals who will exhibit a poorer treatment response is the first step, but future use of this research may guide the development of new, more effective interventions. This critical research, along with future work, can help improve treatment outcomes and thus the quality of life for our patients.

REFERENCES

1. Steffens DC, Krishnan KRR. Structural neuroimaging and mood disorders: recent findings, implications for classification, and future directions. Biol Psychiatry 1998; 43:705–712.
2. Coffey CE, Lucke JF, Saxton JA, DPhil GR, Unitas LJ, Billig B, Bryan RN. Sex differences in brain imaging. Arch Neurol 1998; 55:169–179.
3. Passe TJ, Rajagopalan P, Tupler LA, Byrum CE, MacFall JR, Krishnan KRR. Age and sex effects on brain morphology. Prog Neuropsychopharmacol Biol Psychiatry 1997; 21:1231–1237.
4. Kumar A, Bilker W, Jin Z, Udupa J, Gottlieb G. Age of onset of depression and quantitative neuroanatomic measures: absence of specific correlates. Psychiatry Res 1999; 91:101–110.
5. Cowell PE, Turetsky BI, Gur RC, Grossman RI, Shtasel DL, Gur RE. Sex differences in aging of the human frontal and temporal lobes. J Neurosci 1994; 14:4748–4755.
6. Lisanby SH, McDonald WM, Massey EW, Doraiswamy PM, Rozear M, Boyko OB, Krishnan KR, Nemeroff C. Diminished subcortical nuclei volumes in Parkinson's disease by MR imaging. J Neural Trasm Suppl 1993; 40:13–21.
7. Parashos IA, Tupler LA, Blitchington T, Krishnan KRR. Magnetic-resonance morphometry in patients with major depression. Psychiatry Res 1998; 84:7–15.
8. Krishnan KRR, McDonald WM, Doraiswamy PM, Tupler LA, Husain M, Boyko OB, Figiel GS, Ellinwood EHJ. Neuroanatomical substrates of depression in the elderly. Eur Arch Psychiatry Clin Neurosci 1993; 243:41–46.
9. Kumar A, Jin Z, Bilker W, Udupa J, Gottlieb G. Late-onset minor and major depression: early evidence for common neuroanatomical substrates detected by using MRI. Proc Natl Acad Sci USA 1998; 95:7654–7658.
10. Kumar A, Schweizer E, Jin Z, Miller D, Bilker W, Swan LL, Gottlieb G. Neuroanatomical substrates of late-life minor depression. A quantitative magnetic resonance imaging study. Arch Neurol 1997; 54(5):613–617.
11. Palsson S, Aevarsson O, Skoog I. Depression, cerebral atrophy, cognitive performance, and incidence of dementia. Population study of 85-year-olds. Br J Psychiatry 1999; 174:249–253.
12. Palsson S, Larsson L, Tengelin E, Waern M, Samuelsson S, Hallstrom T, Skoog I. The prevalence of depression in relation to cerebral atrophy and cognitive performance in 70- and 74-year-old women in Gothenburg. The Women's Health Study. Psychol Med 2001; 31:39–49.
13. Pantel J, Schroder J, Essig M, Popp D, Dech H, Knopp MV, Schad LR, Eysenbach K, Backenstrab M, Friedlinger M. Quantitative magnetic resonance imaging in geriatric depression and primary degenerative dementia. J Affect Disord 1997; 42:69–83.
14. Sheline YI, Sanghavi M, Mintun MA, Gado MH. Depression duration but not age predicts hippocampal volume loss in medically healthy women with recurrent major depression. J Neurosci 1999; 19:5034–5043.
15. Sheline YI, Wang PW, Gado MH, Csernansky JG, Vannier MW. Hippocampal atrophy in recurrent major depression. Proc Natl Acad Sci USA 1996; 93:3908–3913.

16. Kumar A, Miller D, Ewbank D, Yousem D, Newberg A, Samuels S, Cowell P, Gottlieb G. Quantiative anatomic measures and comorbid medical illness in late-life major depression. Am J Geriatr Psychiatry 1997; 5:15–25.
17. Rabins PV, Pearlson GD, Aylward E, Kumar AJ, Dowell K. Cortical magnetic resonance imaging changes in elderly inpatients with major depression. Am J Psychiatry 1991; 148:617–620.
18. Coffey CE, Wilkinson WE, Weiner RD, Parashos IA, Djang WT, Webb MC, Figiel GS, Spritzer CE. Quantitative cerebral anatomy in depression: a controlled magnetic resonance imaging study. Arch Gen Psychiatry 1993; 50(1):7–16.
19. Krishnan KRR, McDonald WM, Escalona PR, Doraiswamy PM, Na C, Husain MM, Figiel GS, Boyko OB, Ellinwood EH, Nemeroff CB. Magnetic resonance imaging of the caudate nucleus in depression. Preliminary observations. Arch Gen Psychiatry 1992; 49:553–557.
20. Simpson S, Baldwin RC, Jackson A, Burns A. The differentiation of DSM-III-R psychotic depression in later life from nonpsychotic depression: comparisons of brain changes measured by multispectral analysis of magnetic resonance brain images, neuropsychological findings, and clinical features. Biol Psychiatry 1999; 45:193–204.
21. Kumar A, Bilker W, Lavretsky H, Gottlieb G. Volumetric asymmetries in late-onset mood disorders: an attenuation of frontal asymmetry with depression severity. Psychiatry Res 2000; 100:41–47.
22. Kim DK, Kim BL, Sohn SE, Lim SW, Na DG, Paik CH, Krishnan KRR, Carroll BJ. Candidate neuroanatomic substrates of psychosis in old-aged depression. Prog Neuropsychopharmacol Biol Psychiatry 1999; 23:793–807.
23. Drevets WC, Simpson JRJ, Todd RD, Reich T, Vannier M, Raichle ME. Subgenual prefrontal cortex abnormalities in mood disorders. Nature 1997; 386:824–827.
24. Lai TJ, Payne ME, Byrum CE, Steffens DE, Krishnan KRR. Reduction of orbital frontal cortex volume in geriatric depression. Biol Psychiatry 2000; 48(10):971–975.
25. Rajkowska G, Miguel-Hidalgo JJ, Wei J, Dilley G, Pittman SD, Meltzer HY, Overholser JC, Roth BL, Stockmeier CA. Morphometric evidence for neuronal and glial prefrontal cell pathology in major depression. Biol Psychiatry 1999; 45(9):1085–1098.
26. Kumar A, Bilker W, Zhisong J, Jayaram U. Atrophy and high intensity lesions: complementary neurobiological mechanisms in late-life depression. Neuropsychopharmacology 2000; 22:264–274.
27. Greenwald BS, Kramer-Ginsberg E, Bogerts B, Ashtari M, Aupperle P, Wu H, Zeman D, Patel M. Qualitative magnetic resonance imaging findings in geriatric depression. Possible link between later-onset depression and Alzheimer's disease? Psychol Med 1997; 27:421–431.
28. Rabins PV, Aylward E, Holroyd S, Pearlson G. MRI findings differentiate between late-onset schizophrenia and late-life mood disorder. Int J Geriatr Psychiatry 2000; 15:954–960.
29. Bremner JD, Narayan M, Anderson ER, Staib LH, Miller HL, Charney DS. Hippocampal volume reduction in major depression. Am J Psychiatry 2000; 157:115–117.
30. Sapolsky RM. Potential behavioral modification of glucocorticoid damage to the hippocampus. Behav Brain Res 1993; 57:175–182.
31. Sapolsky RM, Uno H, Rebert CS, Finch CE. Hippocampal damage associated with prolonged glucocorticoid exposure in primates. J Neurosci 1990; 10:2897–2902.
32. Axelson(ab) DA, Doraiswamy PM, McDonald WM, Boyko OB, Tupler LA, Patterson LJ, Nemeroff CB, Ellinwood EHJ, Krishnan KRR. Hypercortisolemia and hippocampal changes in depression. Psychiatry Res 1993; 47:163–173.
33. Ashtari M, Greenwald BS, Kramer-Ginsberg E, Hu J, Wu H, Patel M, Aupperle P, Pollack S. Hippocampal/amygdala volumes in geriatric depression. Psychol Med 1999; 29:629–638.
34. Steffens DC, Byrum CE, McQuoid DR, Greenberg DL, Payne ME, Blitchington TF, MacFall JR, Krishnan KRR. Hippocampal volume loss in geriatric depression. Biol Psychiatry 2000; 48:301–309.
35. Laakso MP, Soininen H, Partanen K, Lehtovirta M, Hallikainen M, Hanninen T, Helkala EL, Vainio P, Riekkinen PJS. MRI of the hippocampus in Alzheimer's disease: sensitivity, specificity, and analysis of the incorrectly classified subjects. Neurobiol Aging 1998; 19:23–31.
36. Lenze EJ, Sheline YI. Absence of striatal volume differences between depressed subjects with no comorbid medical illness and matched comparison subjects. Am J Psychiatry 1999; 156:1989–1991.
37. Longstreth WTJ, Manolio TA, Arnold A, Burke GL, Bryan N, Jungreis CA, Enright PL, O'Leary D, Fried L. Clinical correlates of white matter findings on cranial magnetic resonance imaging of 3301 elderly people: the cardiovascular health study. Stroke 1996; 27:1274–1282.
38. Fazekas F, Niederkor K, Schmidt R, Offenbacher H, Honner S, Bertha G, Lechner H. White matter signal abnormalities in normal individuals: correlation with carotid ultrasonography, cerebral blood flow measurements, and cerebrovascular risk factors. Stroke 1988; 19:1285–1288.
39. Taylor WD, Payne ME, Krishnan KRR, Wagner HR, Provenzale JM, Steffens DC, MacFall JR. Evidence of white matter tract disruption in

MRI hyperintensities. Biol Psychiatry 2001; 50:179–183.
40. Coffey CE, Figiel GS, Djang WT, Weiner RD. Subcortical hyperintensity on magnetic resonance imaging: a comparison of normal and depressed elderly subjects. Am J Psychiatry 1990; 147(2):187–189.
41. Greenwald BS, Kramer-Ginsberg E, Krishnan KRR, Ashtari M, Aupperle PM, Patel M. MRI signal hyperintensities in geriatric depression. Am J Psychiatry 1996; 153:1212–1215.
42. Lenze E, DeWitte C, McKeel D, Neuman RJ, Sheline YI. White matter hyperintensities and gray matter lesions in physically healthy depressed subjects. Am J Psychiatry 1999; 156:1602–1607.
43. Steffens DC, Helms MJ, Krishnan KRR, Burke GL. Cerebrovascular disease and depression symptoms in the cardiovascular health study. Stroke 1999; 30(10):2159–2166.
44. Greenwald BS, Kramer-Ginsberg E, Krishnan KRR, Ashtari M, Auerbach C, Patel M. Neuroanatomic localization of magnetic resonance imaging signal hyperintensities in geriatric depression. Stroke 1998; 29(3):613–617.
45. MacFall JR, Payne ME, Provenzale JE, Krishnan KRR. Medial orbital frontal lesions in late-onset depression. Biol Psychiatry 2001; 49:803–806.
46. Sato R, Bryan RN, Fried LP. Neuroanatomic and functional correlates of depressed mood: the cardiovascular health study. Am J Epidemiol 1999; 150:919–929.
47. Salloway S, Malloy P, Kohn R, Gillard E, Duffy J, Rogg J, Tung G, Richardson E, Thomas C, Westlake R. MRI and neuropsychological differences in early- and late-life-onset geriatric depression. Neurology 1996; 46(6):1567–1574.
48. Figiel GS, Krishnan KRR, Rao VP, Doraiswamy M, Ellinwood EH, Nemeroff CB, Evans D, Boyko O. Subcortical hyperintensities on brain magnetic resonance imaging: a comparison of normal and bipolar subjects. J Neuropsychiatry Clin Neurosci 1991; 3:18–22.
49. Lesser IM, Boone KB, Mehringer CM, Wohl MA, Miller BL, Berman NG. Cognition and white matter hyperintensities in older depressed patients. Am J Psychiatry 1996; 153:1280–1287.
50. Hickie I, Scott E, Mitchell P, Wilhelm K, Austin MP, Bennett B. Subcortical hyperintensities on magnetic resonance imaging: clinical correlates and prognostic significance in patients with severe depression. Biol Psychiatry 1995; 37(3):151–160.
51. Simpson S, Baldwin RC, Jackson A, Burns AS. Is subcortical disease associated with a poor response to antidepressants? Neurological, neuropsychological and neuroradiological findings in late-life depression. Psychol Med 1998; 28:1015–1026.
52. Steffens DC, Conway CR, Dombeck CB, Wagner HR, Tupler LA, Weiner RD. Severity of subcortical gray matter hyperintensity predicts ECT response in geriatric depression. J ECT 2001; 17:45–49.
53. Fujikawa T, Yamawaki S, Touhouda Y. Incidence of silent cerebral infarction in patients with major depression. Stroke 1993; 24:1631–1634.
54. Fujikawa T, Yokota N, Muraoka M, Yamawaki S. Response of patients with major depression and silent cerebral infarction to antidepressant drug therapy, with emphasis on central nervous system adverse reactions. Stroke 1996; 27:2040–2042.
55. Krishnan KR, Hays JC, George LK, Blazer DG Six-month outcomes for MRI-related vascular depression. Depress Anxiety 1998; 8(4):142–6.
56. Figiel GS, Krishnan KRR, Breitner JC, Nemeroff CB. Radiologic correlates of antidepressant-induced delirium: the possible significance of basal-ganglia lesions. J Neuropsychiatry Clin Neurosci 1989; 1:188–190.
57. Figiel GS, Coffey CE, Djang WT, Hoffman GJ, Doraiswamy PM. Brain magnetic resonance imaging findings in ECT-induced delirium. J Neuropsychiatry Clin Neurosci 1990; 2:53–58.
58. Figiel GS, Krishnan KRR, Doraiswamy PM, Nemeroff CB. Caudate hyperintensities in elderly depressed patients with neuroleptic-induced parkinsonism. J Geriatr Psychiatry Neurol 1991; 4:86–89.
59. Steffens DC, MacFall JR, Payne ME, Welsh-Bohmer KA, Krishnan KRR. Grey-matter lesions and dementia. Lancet 2000; 356:1686–1687.
60. Krishnan KRR, McDonald WM. Arteriosclerotic depression. Med Hypotheses 1995; 44:111–115.
61. Krishnan KRR, Hays JC, Blazer DG. MRI-defined vascular depression. Am J Psychiatry 1997; 154(4):497–501.
62. Alexopoulos GS, Meyers BS, Young RC, Campbell S, Silbersweig D, Charlson M. 'Vascular depression' hypothesis. Arch Gen Psychiatry 1997; 54(10):915–922.
63. Alexopoulos GS, Meyers BS, Young RC, Kakuma T, Silbersweig D, Charlson M. Clinically defined vascular depression. Am J Psychiatry 1997; 154(4):562–565.
64. Drevets WC. Functional neuroimaging studies of depression: the anatomy of melancholia. Annu Rev Med 1998; 49:341–361.
65. Cohen RM, Gross M, Nordahl TE, Semple WE, Oren DA, Rosenthal N. Preliminary data on the metabolic brain pattern of patients with winter seasonal affective disorder. Arch Gen Psychiatry 1992; 49:545–552.
66. Biver F, Goldman S, Delvenne V, Luxen A, De Maertelaer V, Hubain P, Mendlewicz J, Lotstra F. Frontal and parietal metabolic disturbances in unpolar depression. Biol Psychiatry 1994; 36:381–388.
67. Bench CJ, Friston KJ, Brown RG, Scott LC, Frackowiak RSJ, Dolan RJ. The anatomy of mel-

ancholia—focal abnormalities of cerebral blood flow in major depression. Psychol Med 1992; 22:607–615.
68. Baxter LRJ, Schwartz JM, Phelps ME, Mazziotta JC, Guze BH, Selin CE, Gerner RH, Sumida RM. Reduction of prefrontal cortex glucose metabolism common to three types of depression. Arch Gen Psychiatry 1989; 46:243–250.
69. Mayberg HS, Brannan SK, Mahurin RK, Jerabek PA, Brickman JS, Tekell JL, Silva JA, McGinnis S, Glass TG, Martin CC, Fox PT. Cingulate function in depression: a potential predictor of treatment response. Neuroreport 1997; 8:1057–1061.
70. Brody AL, Saxena S, Stoessel P, Gillies LA, Fairbanks LA, Alborzian S, Phelps ME, Hunag S-C, Wu H-M, Ho ML, Ho MK, Au SC, Maidment K, Baxter LR Jr. Regional brain metabolic changes in patients with major depression treated with either paroxetine or interpersonal therapy. Arch Gen Psychiatry 2001; 59:631–640.
71. Buchsbaum MS, Wu J, DeLisi LE, Holcomb H, Kessler R, Johnson J, King AC, Hazlett E, Langston K, Post RM. Frontal cortex and basal ganglia metabolic rates assessed by positron emission tomography with [^{18}F]2-deoxyglucose in affective illness. J Affect Disord 1986; 10:137–152.
72. Drevets WC, Videen TO, Price JL, Preskorn SH, Carmichael T, Raichle ME. A functional anatomical study of unipolar depression. J Neurosci 1992; 12:3628–3641.
73. Lesser IM, Mena I, Boone KB, Miller BL, Mehringer MC, Wohl M. Reduction of cerebral blood flow in older depressed patients. Arch Gen Psychiatry 1994; 51:677–686.
74. Kumar A, Newberg A, Alavi A, Berlin J, Smith R, Reivich M. Regional cerebral glucose metabolism in late-life depression and Alzheimer disease: a preliminary positron emission tomography study. Proc Natl Acad Sci USA 1993; 90:7019–7023.
75. Mayberg HS, Lewis PJ, Regenold W, Wagner HN Jr. Paralimbic hypoperfusion in unipolar depression. J Nucl Med 1994; 35:929–934.
76. Brody AL, Saxena S, Silverman DHS, Alborzian S, Fairbanks LA, Phelps ME, Huang S-C, Wu H-M, Maidment K, Baxter LR Jr. Brain metabolic changes in major depressive disorder from pre- to post-treatment with paroxetine. Psychiatry Res 1999; 91:127–139.
77. Kennedy SH, Evans KR, Kruger S, Mayberg HS, Meyer JH, McCann S, Arifuzzman AI, Houle S, Vaccarino FJ. Changes in regional brain glucose metabolism measured with positron emission tomography after paroxetine treatment of major depresssion. Am J Psychiatry 2001; 158:899–905.
78. Mayberg HS, Liotti M, Brannan SK, McGinnis S, Malhurin RK, Jerabek PA, Silva JA, Tekell JL, Martin CC, Lancaster JL, Fox PT. Reciprocal limbic-cortical function and negative mood: converging PET findings in depression and normal sadness. Am J Psychiatry 1999; 156:675–682.
79. Baxter LR, Phelps ME, Mazziotta JC, Schwartz JM, Gerner RH, Selin CE, Sumida RM. Cerebral metabolic rates for glucose in mood disorders. Studies with positron emission tomography and fluorodeoxyglucose F 18. Arch Gen Psychiatry 1985; 42:441–447.
80. Nobler MS, Sackeim HA, Prohovnik IM, J.R., Mukherjee S, Schnur DB, Prudic J, Devanand DP. Regional cerebral blood flow in mood disorders. III. Treatment and clinical response. Arch Gen Psychiatry 1994; 51:884–897.
81. Mayberg HS, Brannan SK, Tekell JL, Silva A, Mahurin RK, McGinis S, Jerabek PA. Regional metabolic effects of fluoxetine in major depression: serial changes and relationship to clincal response. Biol Psychiatry 2000; 48:830–843.
82. Smith GS, Reynolds CF, Pollock B, Derbyshire S, Nofzinger E, Dew MA, Houck PR, Milko D, Meltzer CC, Kupfer DJ. Cerebral glucose metabolic response to combined total sleep deprivation and antidepressant treatment in geriatric depression. Am J Psychiatry 1999; 156:683–689.
83. Martin SD, Martin E, Santoch SR, Richardson MA, Royall R, Eng C. Brain blood flow changes in depressed patients treated with interpersonal psychotherapy or venlafaxine hydrochloride. Arch Gen Psychiatry 2001; 58:641–648.
84. Pizzagalli D, Pascual-Marqui RD, Nitschke JB, Oakes TR, Larson CL, Abercrombie H, Schaefer SM, Koger JV, Benca RM, Davidson RJ. Anterior cingulate activity as a predictor of degree of treatment response in major depression: evidence from brain electrical tomography analysis. Am J Psychiatry 2001; 158:405–415.
85. Manji HK, Moore GJ, Chen G. Clinical and preclinical evidence for the neurotrophic effects of mood stabilizers: implications for the pathophysiology and treatment of manic-depressive illness. Biol Psychiatry 2000; 48:740–754.
86. Sax KW, Strakowski SM, Zimmerman ME, DelBello MP, Keck PEJ, Hawkins JM. Frontosubcortical neuroanatomy and the continuous performance test in mania. Am J Psychiatry 1999; 156:139–141.
87. Aylward EH, Roberts-Twille JV, Barta PE, Kumar AJ, Harris GJ, Geer M, Peyser CE, Pearlson GD. Basal ganglia volumes and white matter hyperintensities in patients with bipolar disorder. Stroke 1994; 17:1084–1089.
88. Dupont RM, Jernigan TL, Heindel W, Butters N, Shafer K, Wilson T, Hesselink J, Gillin JC. Magnetic resonance imaging and mood disorders. Localization of white matter and other subcortical abnormalities. Arch Gen Psychiatry 1995; 52:747–755.

89. Zipursky RB, Seeman MV, Bury A, Langevin R, Wortzman G, Katz R. Deficits in gray matter volume are present in schizophrenia but not bipolar disorder. Schizophr Res 1997; 26:85–92.
90. Altshuler LL, Bartzokis G, Grieder T, Curran J, Mintz J. Amygdala enlargement in bipolar disorder and hippocampal reduction in schizophrenia: an MRI study demonstrating neuroanatomic specificity. Arch Gen Psychiatry 1998; 55:663–664.
91. Pearlson GD, Barta PE, Powers RE, Menon RR, Richards SS, Aylward EH, Federman EB. Medial and superior temporal gyral volumes and cerebral asymmetry in schizophrenia versus bipolar disorder. Biol Psychiatry 1997; 41:1–14.
92. DelBello MP, Strakowski SM, Zimmerman ME, Hawkins JM, Sax KW. MRI analysis of the cerebellum in bipolar disorder: a pilot study. Neuropsychopharmacology 1999; 21:63–68.
93. Stradowski SM, Woods BT, Tohen M, Wilson DR, Douglas AW, Stoll AL. MRI subcortical signal hyperintensities in mania at first hospitalization. Biol Psychiatry 1993; 33:204–206.
94. Hauser P, Matochik J, Altshuler LL, Denicoff KD, Conrad A, Li X, Post RM. MRI-based measurements of temporal lobe and ventricular structures in patients with bipolar I and bipolar II disorders. J Affect Disord 2000; 60:25–32.
95. Dupont RM, Jernigan TL, Gllin JC, Butters N, Delis DC, Hesselink JR. Subcortical signal hyperintensities in bipolar patients detected by MRI. Psychiatry Res 1987; 21:357–358.
96. Swayze VW, Andreasen NC, Alliger RJ, Ehrhardt JC, Yuh WT. Subcortical brain abnormalities in bipolar affective disorder. Ventricular enlargement and focal signal hyperintensities. Arch Gen Psychiatry 1990; 47:1054–1059.
97. Strakowski SM, DelBello MP, Sax KW, Zimmerman ME, Shear PK, Hawins JM, Larson ER. Brain magnetic resonance imaging of structural abnormalities in bipolar disorder. Arch Gen Psychiatry 1999; 56:254–260.
98. Swayze VW, Andreasen NC, Alliger RJ, Yuh WT, Ehrhardt JC. Subcortical and temporal structures in affective disorder and schizophrenia: a magnetic resonance imaging study. Biol Psychiatry 1992; 31:221–240.
99. Woods BT, Yurgelun-Todd D, Mikulis D, Pillay SS. Age related MRI abnormalities in bipolar illness: a clinical study. Biol Psychiatry 1995; 38:846–847.
100. Dupont RM, Jernigan TL, Butters N, Delis D, Hesselink JR, Heindel W, Gillin JC. Subcortical abnormalities detected in bipolar affective disorder using magnetic resonance imaging. Clinical and neuropsychological significance. Arch Gen Psychiatry 1990; 47:55–59.
101. Altshuler LL, Curran JG, Hauser P, Mintz J, Denicoff K, Post R. T2 hyperintensities in bipolar disorder: magnetic resonance imaging comparison and literature meta-analysis. Am J Psychiatry 1995; 152:1139–1144.
102. McDonald WM, Tupler LA, Marsteller FA, Figiel GS, DiSouza S, Nemeroff CB, Krishnan KRR. Hyperintense lesions on magnetic resonance images in bipolar disorder. Biol Psychiatry 1999; 45:965–971.
103. Ahearn EP, Steffens DC, Cassidy F, Van Meter SA, Provenzale JM, Seldin MF, Weisler RH, Krishnan KRR. Familial leukoencephalopathy in bipolar disorder. Am J Psychiatry 1998; 155:1605–1607.
104. Moore PB, Shepherd DJ, Eccleston D, MacMillan IC, Goswami U, McAllister VL, Ferrier IN. Cerebral white matter lesions in bipolar affective disorder: relationship to outcome. Br J Psychiatry 2001; 178:172–176.
105. Krabbendam L, Honig A, Wiersma J, Vuurman EF, Hofman PA, Derix MM, Nolen WA, Jolles J. Cognitive dysfunctions and white matter lesions in patients with bipolar disorder in remission. Acta Psychiatr Scand 2000; 101:274–280.
106. Stone K. Mania in the elderly. Br J Psychiatry 1989; 155:220–224.
107. Cohen RM, Semple WE, Gross M, Nordahl TE, King AC, Pickar D, Post RM. Evidence for common alterations in cerebral glucose metabolism in major affective disorders and schizophrenia. Neuropsychopharmacology 1989; 2:241–254.
108. Al-Mousawi AH, Evans N, Ebmeier KP, Roeda D, Chaloner F, Ashcroft GW. Limbic dysfunction in schizophrenia and mania: a study using ^{18}F-labeled fluorodeoxyglucose and positron emission tomography. Br J Psychiatry 1996; 169:509–516.

24

Role of Acetylcholine and Its Interactions with Other Neurotransmitters and Neuromodulators in Affective Disorders

DAVID S. JANOWSKY and DAVID H. OVERSTREET
University of North Carolina at Chapel Hill, Chapel Hill, North Carolina, U.S.A.

I. INTRODUCTION

Most mood disorder hypotheses are limited to focus on a single neurotransmitter, neuromodulator, or postsynaptic messenger. There are viable hypotheses proposing that norepinephrine (NE), dopamine (DA), gamma amino butyric acid (GABA), serotonin, (5HT) acetylcholine (ACh), and/or their respective receptors, as well as postsynaptic mechanisms including G proteins, cyclic AMP, and the inositol system predispose to or regulate mania and depression. Why single-factor hypotheses have dominated the literature is probably due in part to their conceptual simplicity, the relative ease by which they can be pursued, and the rewards an investigator derives from focusing on a specific neurochemical. However, there is considerable evidence that the various neurotransmitters/neuromodulators and related neurochemicals actively interact with each other. Virtually all perturb other systems, leading to the strong possibility that a cascade of neurochemical events, rather than a single neuroactive compound, is related to the mood disorders.

Although neurotransmitter interactions have been found for Parkinson's disease and for a variety of autonomic phenomena such as heart rate, pupillary size, and bowel motility, prior to 30 years ago no widely accepted balance or interactive hypothesis existed for an emotional disorder. In 1972, Janowsky and colleagues proposed the adrenergic-cholinergic balance hypothesis of affective disorders [1]. With an interactive perspective in mind, in this paper we will utilize ACh and its muscarinic receptor effects as a prototype to illustrate how it and its interactions and perturbations may lead to affective phenomena. We will describe the proposed relationship of ACh as such to mood disorders (i.e., a unitary hypothesis). We will also demonstrate how a more complete and complex picture can be obtained by considering how other candidate neurochemicals (i.e., 5HT, DA, GABA, G proteins, cyclic AMP, etc.) can be affected by ACh and/or influence ACh and hence mood.

II. CHOLINERGIC-BEHAVIORAL EFFECTS IN ANIMAL MODELS

Several preclinical animal models of depression have been developed, including the self stimulation model, the hypoactivity model, the learned helplessness model, the chronic stress model, and the behavioral despair or forced swim model [2,3]. Such models are useful in investigating neurochemical hypotheses of affective disorders. When central cholinergic activity is increased with centrally acting cholinomimetic drugs, such as the direct cholinergic agonists arecoline and oxotremorine, and with cholinestrase inhibitors which inhibit the breakdown of ACh, such as physostigmine, the animal behavioral concomitants of depression occur. Thus, centrally acting cholinergic drugs consistently cause lethargy, hypoactivity, decreases in self-stimulation, increases in behavioral despair and decreases in preference for the reinforcing effects of sugar as swell as activation of the hypothalamic pituitary axis [3–6].

A very productive strategy for studying depression has been the development of genetically derived animal models which show enhanced or diminished responses to a given neurochemical perturbation. Such genetically derived animal stains can represent animal analogs of depression. For example, the Roman Low Avoidance rats (RLA) have been bred to ineffectively learn avoidance responses. Interestingly, these animals are relatively more sensitive to cholinergic agonists [7], and are considered to be an animal model for anxiety and depression [8]. Similarly, the Flinders Sensitive Line (FSL) of rats, developed by co-author David Overstreet, were selectively bred to have increased muscarinic responses to the anticholinesterase agent diisopropylfluorophosphate (DFP), an agent which blocks the central and peripheral breakdown of ACh [9].

FSL rats were bred to show increased behavioral toxicity and an exaggerated decrease in temperature after exposure to DFP, and in later generations to the cholinergic agonist oxotremorine. They were developed in parallel with the Flinders Resistant Line (FRL) rat, which does not show such sensitivity to cholinergic drugs. Overstreet and colleagues have proposed that the FSL rat is an animal model of depression, and an increasing and impressive body of evidence supports this contention. Among the many similarities between FSL rats and depressed humans, FSL rats have lower body weight, decreased activity, and decreased locomotion. Very significantly, they have increased REM sleep and reduced REM sleep latency, and given cholinergic stimulation, they have an exaggerated release of cortisterone [9]. FSL rats also demonstrate less interest in drinking saccharin than do controls when exposed to chronic mild stress [3]. This suggests that the FSL rats may have stress-induced anhedonia, another parallel to the symptoms of depression. Very importantly, FSL rats have exaggerated immobility in the forced swim test, a test is considered to be an excellent animal model for depression and for detecting antidepressant drug effects [10]. This phenomenon parallels the increased immobility induced by centrally acting cholinergic agonists, as recently confirmed by Hasey and Hanin [11].

III. MOOD-DEPRESSING EFFECTS OF CHOLINOMIMETICS IN MAN

One of the most dramatic effects of centrally acting ACh-enhancing drugs is their ability to rapidly induce depressed moods. In the early 1950s, Rowntree et al. [12] observed depression in a number of affective disorder patients and in several normals that he treated with DFP. Furthermore, Gershon and Shaw [13] and Bowers et al. [14] and others have reported induction of anxiety and depression by nerve gases and related cholinomimetic insecticides. Building on the above information, Janowsky and colleagues, in 1972, found induction and intensification of depressive symptoms in bipolar manic patients given physostigmine [1]. They also found that depression increased significantly when unipolar depressed patients and schizoaffective depressed patients were given physostigmine. The noncentrally acting cholinesterase inhibitor neostigmine did not cause any such behavioral effects, nor did the noncentrally acting anticholinergic and antimuscarinic agent, methscopolamine. Significantly, the centrally acting anticholinergic and antimuscarinic agent, atropine, did reverse the mood depressing effects of physostigmine [15–17]

This work has been replicated by a number of authors including Davis et al. [18] and Modestin et al. [19,20], who found an increase in depression in manic patients given physostigmine. Risch et al. [21] and Nurnberger et al. [22,23] gave depressed patients the direct-acting cholinergic agonist arecoline and noted that their patients developed increased depression, as well as anxiety and hostility. Oppenheimer et al. [24] also noted that depression was also caused by physostigmine in a majority of euthymic bipolar patients who were receiving lithium. Furthermore, Risch et al. [21,25,26] found a significant increase in negative affect on the Profile of Mood States (POMS) mood rating scale in normals receiving physostigmine or arecoline. Mohs et al. [27] also noted induction of severe depression in an Alzheimer's patient receiving oxotremorine. El-Yousef, Janowsky, and colleagues [28] reported that physostigmine induced extreme depression in individuals who had recently smoked marijuana. This apparently was a central effect, since it was reversible with atropine.

In addition to eliciting depressed mood, physostigmine and other cholinomimetic agents induced a psychomotor depression which was very similar to that occurring in endogenous depression. This observation was consistent with the anergic and behavioral inhibitory effects noted by Rowntree et al. [12], Gershon and Shaw [13], Modestin et al. [19,20], and Janowsky et al. [29]. Indeed, these anergic behavioral-inhibitory effects crossed diagnostic lines, and were not selective for affective disorder patients.

Choline is a precursor of ACh and it or its precursors' administration increases ACh levels. Tamminga et al. [30] and Davis et al. [31] observed an increase in depressive symptoms in a subgroup of schizophrenic patients receiving choline, a phenomenon that was atropine reversible. Similarly, a subgroup of Alzheimer's disease cases developed depressed mood as a side effect of choline and lecithin (a choline precursor) treatments [30]. Furthermore, the choline precursor deanol caused a depressed mood [32].

A growing body of information suggests not only that can muscarinic cholinomimetic drugs induce depression, but that patients with mood disorders are more vulnerable to the depressing effects of these agents than are normals or individuals with other psychiatric diagnoses. Thus, Janowsky et al. [15,16,33] observed that patients with an affective component to their illness (i.e., patients with depression, mania, or schizoaffective disorders), when compared to schizophrenics without a mood component, were vulnerable to becoming depressed or more depressed after receiving physostigmine. Similarly, Oppenheimer et al. [24], giving physostigmine to lithium-treated euthymic bipolar patients, observed a significant percentage who became depressed, while noting that normal controls receiving physostigmine showed anergia, but not depression.

Janowsky et al. [33,34] replicated the above findings using self-rated and observer-rated scales. They showed that greater increases in the anxiety, depression, and hostility and decreases in the elation subscale of the POMS occurred in mood-disordered patients compared to other psychiatric patients or normals following physostigmine infusion. Using the acetylcholine precursor deanol, Casey [32] also found selectively increased depressive symptoms in affective-disorder patients compared to non-affective-disorder patients who had tardive dyskinesia.

In related studies, Steinberg et al. [35] found that patients who had affectively unstable personalities (often Borderline Personality Disorder patients) were more vulnerable to increases in negative affect caused by physostigmine than were individuals who were affectively stable or who had predominantly impulsive personality disorders. Significantly, such individuals with affectively unstable personalities did not show negative affect following noradrenergic, serotonergic, or placebo challenges. Also, Fritze et al. [36,37] noted that behavioral and cardiovascular sensitivity to physostigmine correlated with baseline irritability and emotional lability, and with the degree to which an individual showed habitual passive stress coping strategies. Thus, stress sensitivity and coping profiles, rather than specific affective diagnostic disorders as such, may determine sensitivity to a cholinomimetic agent.

IV. CHOLINOMIMETIC EFFECTS ON SLEEP PARAMETERS

Major depression is associated with such sleep changes as decreased rapid eye movement (REM) sleep latency and increased REM sleep density. Significantly, muscarinic cholinergic agonists such as arecoline, physostigmine, RS86, and pilocarpine shorten REM latency and increase REM density [38–40]. Sitaram et al. [41,42] and Gillin et al. [43] demonstrated that individuals receiving arecoline who had a history of an affective disorder or a family history of affective disorder showed exaggerated shortening of REM latency following arecoline infusion.

Further replication of the phenomena of exaggerated REM latency shortening in affective disorder patients was noted by Berger et al. [44]. These authors found that supershortening of REM latency occurred in patients with endogenous depression following administration of the oral muscarinic agonist RS86. The control group, which showed less shortening, were normals and eating-disorder patients. Significantly, Berger et al. [39] also found that physostigmine-induced arousal and awakening from sleep predominated in affective-disorder patients.

In an extension of the above studies, Gann et al. [45] administered placebo and RS86 to patients with major depression, anxiety disorder patients, and healthy control subjects. RS86 selectively increased the number of REM episodes, the shortening of REM latency, and the increasing of REM density and duration. Riemann et al. [46,47] found that to a lesser extent, schizophrenics showed parallel findings to the affective disorder patients. However, patients with anxiety disorders did not show the degree of cholinomimetic-induced REM or behavioral abnormalities noted in the affective-disorder patients [48,49].

There is evidence, as was noted in the FSL rats [9], that hypersensitivity to cholinomimetics of REM sleep parameters is genetically determined. This relationship has been confirmed in monozygotic/dizygotic twin studies, in which twin pairs received arecoline [50], and in which monozygotic twins showed increased concordance of effects on REM parameters after administration of the cholinomimetic drug compared to dizygotic twins.

Similarly, Schreiber et al. [51] evaluated first-degree relatives of patients with a DSM-III diagnosis of major depression and found enhanced shortening of REM latency and increased sleep-onset REM periods following RS86 administration. Furthermore, early results by Holsboer (personal communication, 1998) suggest that nondepressed relatives of depressives who initially showed prominent decreases in REM latency following RS86 are more likely to become depressed at a later point in time.

V. GROWTH HORMONE SUPERSENSITIVITY IN MOOD DISORDER PATIENTS

There is considerable evidence that centrally acting ACh activation increases growth hormone levels [33,52]. With respect to affective disorders, O'Keane et al. [52] evaluated growth hormone release following administration of the peripherally acting cholinesterase inhibitor pyridostigmine in depressed patients and normals. Their depressed patients, especially males, showed relatively higher serum levels of growth hormone following pyridostigmine infusion. This finding was also observed in manic patients [53], in obsessive-compulsive patients [54], and in schizophrenics [55,56]. However, Cooney et al. [56] observed that schizophrenics with panic disorder and low depression scores did not differ from a control group in their pyridostigmine induced levels of growth hormone.

VI. INCREASED CENTRAL CHOLINE IN IMAGING STUDIES

Clinical in vivo proton magnetic resonance spectroscopy and other techniques including PET scanning offer a relatively direct way of observing cholinergic function in the living individual. These technologies can be used to measure choline-containing substances in the brain, and the amount of measured central choline may reflect central ACh activity, since choline is an ACh precursor. Charles et al. [57] observed an increase in choline in the brains of patients with major depression compared to controls. Significantly, choline levels were state dependent and decreased to those of normal controls after successful drug treatment of the depression. In another study, Renshaw et al. [58] studied the basal ganglia of depressed and control subjects. These authors noted alterations in cytosolic choline in the basal ganglia in depressives, particularly of those who responded to fluoxetine. Similarly, Hankura et al. [59] found higher subcortical choline containing compounds in depressed bipolar disorder patients than in normals. More recently, Moore et al. [60] found that in the left cingulate cortex, bipolar subjects' depression ratings correlated positively with MRSI measures of choline Cr-PCr. In the right cingulate cortex, the choline Cr-PCr ratio was significantly higher in subjects with bipolar disorder than in control subjects. In addition, bipolar subjects not taking antidepressants had a significantly higher right cingulate cortex choline Cr-PCr ratio than patients taking antidepressants or controls. No clinical or drug-related changes were observed for the inositol Cr-PCr ratio. The results of the study suggest that bipolar disorder is associated with alterations in the metabolism of cytosolic, choline-containing compounds in the anterior cingulate cortex.

All of the above imaging studies offer indirect evidence in support of a role for ACh in the phenomenology and/or etiology of mood disorders. However, it must be mentioned that choline has many other functions along with serving as a precursor to ACh. Therefore, proof of a direct relationship between the choline findings and affective disorders awaits further research.

Furthermore, in contrast to the above results, a preliminary study by Soares et al. [61] found no difference in choline/Cr-PCr ratio in the anterior cingulate of depressed patients, compared to controls. Also, they found that depressed subjects had lower rather than higher initial choline levels than normal controls. Therefore, as Moore et al. [60] note, increases and decreases in choline/Cr-PCR have been associated with depressed state or response to therapy. Significantly, however, where inconsistencies occur, they often were in studies of unipolar rather than bipolar subjects.

VII. CENTRALLY ACTING ANTICHOLINERGIC AGENTS AS ANTIDEPRESSANTS

Several studies have pointed out that antiparkinsonian drugs with centrally acting antimuscarinic properties may cause euphoria, feelings of increased well-being, sociability, and a reversal of depressed mood in schizophrenic patients. These compounds are generally quite complex in their effects, and probably affect DA and other neurotransmitters, as well as obviously affecting ACh receptors. Kasper et al. [61] observed that the centrally acting antimuscarinic drug biperiden had antidepressant effects, especially in patients with endogenous depression. However, several studies have shown a lack of antidepressant efficacy for anticholinergic drugs. Thus, Fritze et al. [37] could not demonstrate an advantage to the addition of biperiden over noncentrally acting anticholinergic drugs, where study drugs were added to ongoing antidepressant medications. Similarly, Gillin et al. [62] could find no antidepressant effects for biperiden in depressives. Also, there is little or no evidence that the centrally acting antimuscarinic agent scopolamine is useful in the treatment of depression.

VIII. SUPERSENSITIVE PUPILLARY RESPONSES TO PILOCARPINE

Sokolski and DeMet [63] studied the pupillary miotic response to the muscarinic cholinergic agonist pilocarpine. They found that this response was exaggerated in patients with major depression. This exaggeration represents a shifting in balance to a cholinergic predominance, since the pupil is controlled by reciprocal noradrenergic and cholinergic mechanisms. Sokolski and DeMet [63] suggest that the supersensitive pupillary response may be mediated by M3 muscarinic receptors, working through the G protein-phosphatidyl inositol system. These data support the notion of both peripheral and central muscarinic supersensitivity and noradrenergic hyposensitivity in depressives. In a related study, Fountoulakis and colleagues [64], comparing depressed patients and normal controls, found that depressed patients with melancholic features manifested shorter ACh-induced latency to constriction than did control subjects. These authors suggest that there is NE hypoactivity in melancholic depression and that therefore relatively smaller changes in ACh are needed to balance the NE. Conversely, Sokolski and DeMet [65] found that patients with more severe mania required relatively higher concentrations of pilocarpine in order to effect a 50% decrease in pupillary size. Presumably, the resistance to pilocarpine-induced pupillary constriction represents an overbalancing of cholinergic activity by adrenergic activity, since the mania ratings were linearly related to the effective dose of pilocarpine needed to cause pupillary constriction. Furthermore, DeMet and Sokolski [66] observed that improvements in mania after treatment with valproic acid were closely correlated with a decrease in the amount of pilocarpine needed to cause a 50% reduction in pupillary size, and this relationship was indistinguishable from one previously observed after lithium treatment.

IX. CHOLINERGIC MECHANISMS AND THE HYPOTHALMIC-PITUITARY-ADRENAL AND ADRENOMEDULLARY AXES

In humans, a major characteristic of depression is activation of the hypothalamic-pituitary-adrenal (HPA) axis. Indeed, depression has been considered to be a form of stress. Several studies have shown that increased cortisol, ACTH, and β-endorphin levels exist in depressed patients, and that endogenously depressed patients often fail to suppress cortisol after administration of dexamethasone. A variety of studies have suggested that cholinomimetic drugs and ACh as such can release corticotrophin-releasing factor (CRF), and subsequently a cascade follows in which elevation, activation, and release of ACTH, cortisol, and β-endorphin occurs [33]. In separate studies, physostigmine has been shown to reverse dexamethasone-induced suppression of cortisol in normals and in depressives [67]. Therefore, an HPA axis analog of depression is created by cholinomimetic agents such as physostigmine, and this can be reversed by centrally acting antimuscarinic agents [16].

In addition to effects on the HPA axis, patients with major depressive disorder have been reported to have increased epinephrine excretion and some increases in NE excretion. As with the HPA axis, physostigmine has been found to cause epinephrine release, and to a much lesser extent to cause norepinephrine release. This effect is centrally mediated, being effectively blocked by centrally acting scopolamine but not by noncentrally acting methscopolamine [16]. This represents central muscarinic stimulation leading to the adrenal release of epinephrine. Furthermore, both physostigmine and arecoline have been shown to increase pulse rate and blood pressure in subjects treated with peripherally acting antimuscarinic drugs, probably secondary to epinephrine and norepinephrine release. These physiological effects, almost certainly mediated by sympathetic outflow, can be antagonized by the centrally acting antimuscarinic drug scopolamine but not by the noncentrally acting drug methscopolamine [16].

It is likely that ACh is an important moderator of the body's stress responses, and conversely, that stress activates ACh. Stress is multidimensional and includes gastrointestinal, cardiovascular, behavioral, analgesic, immunological, endrocrinological, psychological-behavioral, and psychopathological changes [33]. Information from animal studies suggests that stress is likely to be mediated by complex alterations of a variety of central neurotransmitters, mostly almost all depression relevant, such as ACh, NE, 5HT, GABA, and DA. A dramatic demonstration of a stress-ACh linkage is the work of Gilad et al. [68] showing increased ACh release and downregulation of muscarinic receptors after exposure to stress, a phenomenon much exaggerated in stress-sensitive rats. Furthermore, Mizuno and Kimura [69] found hippocampal ACh release and cortisol release were increased following stress in young rats, and Mark et al. [70], using microdialysis, showed that inescapable stress caused selective ACh release in rat hippocampus and prefrontal cortex, a phenomenon which was further exaggerated when the stress was lifted. Likewise, Day et al. [71] showed that prenatally stressed rats, as adults, showed greater hippocampal ACh activity when exposed to a mild stress or when given corticotrophin-releasing factor.

X. NICOTINIC AND MUSCARINIC INTERACTIONS AND DEPRESSION

Although the major focus of this chapter has been on muscarinic mechanisms, a number of studies have suggested that there is a relationship between depression and nicotine consumption. Glassman et al. [72] reviewed this information in depth and suggested that tobacco smoking was associated with current major depression and current depressive symptoms. Furthermore, a lifetime history of major depression increases the chances of a person trying nicotine and becoming addicted to it, even if the individual is not depressed at the time of exposure. Furthermore, there is evidence in people with a history of major depression that attempts to stop smoking may precipitate severe depression. Also, Kendler et al. [73], using monozygotic and dyzgotic twin pair data, found that smoking and depression appear to be linked genetically.

Nicotine's stimulating effects on dopaminergic reward systems have been offered as a popular explanation as to why people smoke, and why depressives might be more likely to smoke and/or have trouble stopping smoking. However, it is possible that a relationship or interaction between muscarinic and nicotinic mechanisms may underlie nicotine addiction, since ACh naturalistically stimulates both muscarinic and nicotinic receptors. It is conceivable that stress and/or depression, causing ACh release and activating muscarinic mechanisms, leads to an overall muscarinic predominance. This could be overcome by nicotinic activation via smoking, possibly via the release of dopamine. However, if nicotinic activation ceased owing to acute abstinence, there could be a rapid decrease in dopaminergic activity, leading to a muscarinic predominance and to dysphoria and depression. Furthermore, there is some evidence that activation of nicotinic receptors such as occurs with cigarette smoking leads to muscarinic outflow [74]. Therefore, it is possible that if nicotinic stimulation leads to muscarinic activation, this muscarinic activation remains a predominant effect when nicotine is stopped, leading to depression, anxiety, and other symptoms of nicotine withdrawal.

Paralleling the above possibilities, it should also be pointed out that nicotine has also been reported to have antidepressantlike effects in animal models [75–77]. Importantly, the control strain of rat that was treated chronically with nicotine exhibited a withdrawal depression when observed 2 days after cessation of treatment [75]. Thus, evidence in animal models supports the hypothesized muscarinic basis for humans taking nicotine for its antidepressant effects.

XI. NEUROTRANSMITTER/NEUROMODULATOR/ACETYLCHOLINE INTERACTIONS

Although much information suggests a strong role for ACh in the phenomenology and/or etiology of the affective disorders, there is information that is not supportive of acetylcholine directly effecting depression. As described above, one would expect centrally active antimuscarinic agents such as scopolamine and atropine to be effective antidepressants, but the evidence for this is equivocal at best. Furthermore, many effective antidepressant medications, such as the selective serotonin reuptake inhibitors, lack muscarinic receptor blocking properties.

Thus, there is strong evidence both for cholinergic supersensitivity and for the induction of depression in human depressives by cholinomimetic agents, yet there is also the inability of muscarinic antagonists to ameliorate depression and the lack of effect of several antidepressants on muscarinic receptors. One scenario that might explain the above paradox is as follows: The basic abnormalities underlying depression could be located in serotonergic, dopaminergic, GABA-ergic, or other systems, initially effected by ACh, but later assuming a life of their own. Thus, administration of cholinergic agonists and other cholinomimetic agents might perturb or induce these other systems, resulting in depression, but once perturbed, these systems would be unlinked from muscarinic receptors. Anticholinergic agents would then be unable to counteract depressive symptoms, yet stimulation by ACh would cause an increase in effects.

A second possibility is that the basic abnormalities underlying depression are located in a second-messenger cascade that is downstream from the muscarinic receptor itself. An abnormality in the cascade that amplifies the cholinergic signal could promote supersensitive responses to cholinergic agonists. However, because this abnormality would be beyond the receptor, muscarinic antagonists would not affect its actions and therefore, could not alleviate symptoms of depression. The plausibility of this model is enhanced by recent studies suggesting abnormalities in second-messenger systems in human depressives [78,79].

As a prelude to discussing the clinical and biochemical interactions that occur between ACh and other neurotransmitters, neuromodulators, and second messengers, especially in the mood disorders, it is illustrative to discuss the nature of altered neurochemicals in the brains of the cholinergically derived FSL rats. As mentioned earlier, these rats were developed to be supersensitive to muscarinic cholinergic drugs. They show supersensitivity with respect to vulnerability to the behavioral and hypothermic effects of cholinergic agents. The FSL rats also show decreased persistence in the forced swim test, an animal analog of depression used to screen for antidepressant drugs [9].

In recent years, Overstreet and collaborators have begun to look at secondary neurotransmitters and neuromodulator effects of this primarily hypermuscarinic rat line. They have found that differences in central catecholamines exist between FSL rats and control FRL rats. In a study by Zangen and colleagues [80], NE levels were two- to threefold higher in nucleus accumbens, hippocampus, and median raphe, and DA levels were six times higher in the nucleus accumbens and two times higher in the striatum, hippocampus, and hypothalamus of FSL rats. After administration of antidepressants, catecholamine levels were normalized. Furthermore, Serova et al. [81] observed that catecholamine biosynthetic MRNAs for tyrosine hydroxylase and dopamine beta-hydroxylase were markedly elevated in the FSL rats. Interestingly, Yadid et al. [82] reported that when FSL and control rats were stressed in a forced swim test, DA levels decreased initially in FSL and control rats, but subsequently increased only in control rats. Also, Zangen et al. [83] found that extracellular dopamine levels in the nucleus accumbens of FSL rats were 40% lower than in control rats, and that FSL rats did not respond with an expected release in DA following 5HT administration, a lack of reactivity reversed by antidepressant drug treatment. Thus, FSL rats appear to have more stored catecholamines but to have less that is available.

Like the catecholamine system, 5HT sensitivity is altered in FSL rats. Overstreet et al. [84] found that the FSL rat is hypersensitive not only to cholinergic agents, but to 5HT1A receptor stimulating agents. Supersensitive responses to the 5HT1A agonist 8-OH-DPAT were observed in the FSL rats, and these were not blocked by anticholinergic agents. Conversely, Zangen et al. [85] observed that levels of 5HT and its metabolite 5-hydroxyindolacetic acid (5HIAA) were two- to eightfold higher in the nucleus accumbens, prefrontal cortex, hippocampus, and hypothalamus of FSL rats, an effect which normalized with antidepressant drug treatment. Also, the 5HIAA/5HT ratio was lower in FSL rats, meaning that less metabolism was occurring and more 5HT was stored. The lower ratio was increased after chronic desipramine treatment, while the high tissue levels decreased. Therefore, with respect to DA and 5HT, the observations suggest that there is more intracellular and less extracellular monoamine neurotransmitter in the FSL rats, suggesting a relative cholinergic predominance.

XII. CATECHOLAMINE/ACETYLCHOLINE INTERACTIONS

As suggested in the original 1972 article proposing the adrenergic-cholinergic balance hypothesis of mood disorders [1], considerable information suggests a role for monoaminergic-cholinergic balance in the pathogenesis of mood disorders. In the original hypothesis, the coauthor of this paper, Janowsky, and colleagues [1] proposed that depression was a manifestation of central cholinergic predominance, whereas mania, conversely, was due to a relative monoaminergic (i.e., catecholaminergic) predominance. The original conceptualization of this hypothesis was based on the observation that centrally active cholinergic agonists and cholinesterase inhibitors possess antimanic properties. At the time that the hypothesis was developed, mania was considered, as conceptualized in the catecholamine hypothesis, to be a disease of excessive NE and/or DA. Therefore, turning off mania with a cholinomimetic drug would suggest a shifting of catecholaminergic-cholinergic balance, such as occurs with heart rate, pupillary constriction, and bowel motility [86]. To this end, Rowntree et al. [12] gave the centrally acting cholinesterase inhibitor DFP to several patients who were manic or hypomanic. The manics studied improved with DFP, and one who became less manic relapsed upon DFP withdrawal. Subsequently, Janowsky et al. [1,29,87] in the early 1970s conducted a controlled experiment in which the centrally acting cholinesterase inhibitor physostigmine was compared with placebo, as well as the noncentrally acting cholinesterase inhibitor neostigmine. Neither placebo nor neostigmine produced any behavioral changes, but physostigmine administration caused the manics to become less talkative, active, active, happy, friendly, grandiose, or euphoric, and to effect a decrease in their flight of ideas. These results were replicated by Modestin et al. [19,20], who reported a diminution of manic systems following physostigmine, but not neostigmine infusion. Likewise, Davis et al. [18] reported that physostigmine caused antimanic effects, and these results were replicated by Carroll et al. [88] and Shopsin et al. [89], as well as Berger et al. [44], who used RS86, a relatively specific muscarinic (M_1) receptor agonist.

Several studies have demonstrated antimanic effects using ACh precursors including the choline precursor lecithin [30,90]. The antimanic efficacy of phosphatidyl choline was also demonstrated by Leiva [91]. Most recently, Burt et al. [92] found that the cholinesterase inhibitor and anti-Alzheimer's drug, donepezil (Aricept) was useful in treating 6 of 11 treatment-resistant manic patients who had been maintained on antimanic therapy.

The converse of the above studies is found in the mood effects of antiadrenergic agents. Sympatholytic-antihypertensive medications, including α-methyldopa propranolol, clonidine, and reserpine, can cause depression. These drugs appear to have ACh-releasing/activating properties as well as antiadrenergic properties. They can cause mood depression as well as vivid nightmares, lethargy, and sleeplessness, symptoms very similar to those caused by physostigmine or other cholinomimetic agents, and to those occurring in naturalistic depression and in Parkinson's disease [1,93]. Furthermore, antipsychotic agents, which block central DA receptors, also increase ACh turnover and are quite capable of causing depression [94]; and depression is a frequent concomitant of Parkinson's disease, in which decreased DA and increased ACh activity coexist [95].

There is also evidence that when the central ACh system is activated using cholinesterase inhibitors, ultimately a compensatory antagonistic activation of the noradrenergic/dopaminergic system occurs. To this end, Fibiger et al. [96] demonstrated that the increase in acetylcholine activity caused by the administration of physostigmine initially caused a decrease in locomotion in rats, and eventually led to exaggerated locomotion. This activating effect occurred as physostigmine's effects were wearing off, and was exaggerated when the centrally acting anticholinergic agent scopolamine was given at the onset of the hyperactivity phase. Thus, it would appear that cholinomimetic agents can simultaneously both antagonize and activate central catecholaminergic mechanisms.

The work of Fibiger et al. [96], described above, is paralleled by results in humans. "Rebounding" into a mania after DFP was given was reported by Rowntree et al. [12]. Similarly, Shopsin et al. [89] demonstrated rebounding into hypermania following physostigmine infusion in two of three manic patients, and more recently, donepezil has been observed to cause manic episodes [92]. Thus, Jacobsen and Comas-Diaz [97] observed that donepezil (Aricept), given to nongeriatric affective-disorder patients to treat psychotropic drug-induced anticholinergic symptoms, caused antagonism of these symptoms. In addition, the donezepil caused nausea, vomiting, diarrhea, and mania within hours of starting it in two bipolar patients. Similarly, Benazzi reported donepezil induced mania [98].

A behavioral pharmacological model for naturally occurring adrenergic-cholinergic balance in the regulation of mood may be found in the interaction of psychostimulants and cholinomimetics. Methylphenidate-induced psychostimulation, including increased locomotor activity, stereotyped movement behavior, and stereotyped self-injurious gnawing behavior in rats is antagonized by physostigmine [99]. Furthermore, there is strong evidence that dopaminergic agents stimulate the reward processes [100,101] and that cholinergic agonists inhibit it [102,103]. These findings may have particular relevance to mood disorders, because a cardinal symptom of depression is anhedonia. Thus, it is possible that anhedonia could arise by either an underactive dopamine system or an overactive cholinergic system. Alternatively, the anhedonia associated with an overactive cholinergic system might be overcome by activating the dopaminergic system.

In human studies paralleling the above animal studies, methylphenidate-induced hypertalkativeness, euphoria, and increased thinking is rapidly antagonized by physostigmine but not by noncentrally acting neostigmine [104]. Conversely, physostigmine's inhibitory and mood depressant effects in man are rapidly reversed by methylphenidate administration. This type of reversal is also reflected in the observation that physostigmine can cause a dramatic decrease in 3-methyoxy-4-hydroxphenylglycol (MHPG), a NE metabolite [105]. This decrease was associated with a tearful, depressed state, and a decrease in manic symptoms.

With respect to sleep, we have previously described the central cholinomimetic-muscarinic effects on REM density, frequency, and latency. However, REM parameters appear to reflect a balance between monoaminergic and cholinergic factors. Dopamine and norepinephrine (and serotonin) all increase REM latency and decrease REM density, in marked contrast to the effects of acetylcholine. Related to the above, Schittecatte et al. [106] noted that human depressives are subsensitive to the REM-suppressing effect of the noradrenergic agent clonidine. This would suggest that β-adrenergic (i.e., noradrenergic) subsensitivity might exist in depressives along with cholinergic hypersensitivity.

A reciprocal relationship appears to exist between a subject's response to a psychostimulant and his or her separate response to a cholinomimetic agent. A negative correlation was noted between amphetamine-induced behavioral excitation and the ability of arecoline, given on another occasion, to decrease REM latency [107]. Similarly, Siever et al. [108] showed that in a mixed group of affective-disorder and normal subjects, those with the most dramatic physostigmine- or arecoline-induced anergy and negative affect showed a blunted growth hormone response to the noradrenergic agonist clonidine. This was presumably a reflection of decreased noradrenergic responsiveness. Unfortunately, Siever et al. [108] did not measure growth hormone responses to cholinergic challenges, so a direct comparison of the adrenergic and cholinergic systems in regulating growth hormone could not be made.

Several more direct biochemical studies also suggest that the dopaminergic and cholinergic systems oppose each other. Ikarashi et al. [109] found that DA D2 receptor stimulation in the striatum led to an inhibition in ACh release. In contrast, Downs et al. [110] demonstrated that depletion of brain DA caused a supersensitive ACTH response following physostigmine administration, a finding paralleling the exaggerated ACTH response to physostigmine found in affective-disorder patients [111,112]. There is also evidence that chronic treatment with antipsychotic drugs, which produce dopamine supersensivity, also produces a cholinergic subsensitivity [113]. Thus, several studies suggest opposite changes in dopaminergic and cholinergic systems following specific manipulations. These findings raise the possibility that the cholinergic supersensitivity observed in depressed patients could be due to an indirect consequence of dopamine deficiency, as well as to an innately supersensitive cholinergic system.

Consideration of the second-messenger cascades of the two primary DA and ACh receptors may help understand the mechanisms involved in depressive disorders. The m_1 and m_2 ACh receptors are positively and negatively coupled to the phosphatidyl inositol and adenyl cyclase cascades. A similar arrangement appears to exist for the D_1 and D_2 DA receptors [114]. This information seems paradoxical, because the D_2 and m_2 receptors would be expected to operate in parallel if they operate through the same second-messenger cascade. However, one must also consider neuroanatomy. For example, DA terminals innervate cholinergic interneurons in the striatum and inhibit these neurons via D_2 receptors. The cholinergic neurons in turn disinhibit GABA inhibitory neurons, which then inhibit the dopamine neurons in the substantia nigra. Also, a recent study has also indicated the involvement of GABA-ergic neurons in the effects of cholinergic modulation of locus coeruleus noradrenergic neurons. The direct stimulation of cholinergic neurons projecting to the locus coeruleus inhibits the REM-off neurons, an effect that can be blocked by GABA antagonists [115].

XIII. ACETYLCHOLINE-SEROTONIN INTERACTIONS

At this time, the most widely accepted etiological hypothesis of depression is the 5HT hypothesis, as described elsewhere in this volume. Convincing evidence of the importance of 5HT comes from the fact that selective 5HT reuptake inhibitors have little effect on muscarinic receptors. However, there is considerable information suggesting that there are important interactions between the serotonergic and cholinergic systems, which do not involve their respective receptors as such.

Interactions between the cholinergic and serotonergic systems have been described for a variety of situations, including global interactions at the clinical level, more discrete interactions for specific physiological and behavioral functions, and synaptic and/or molecular interactions that have been observed in vitro as well as in vivo. The current section will present evidence for cholinergic/serotonergic interactions in these three broad categories.

Clinically, there are two major areas where an interaction between the two systems have been demonstrated. These are sleep regulation and hormonal regulation, both of which are abnormal in depressive disorders. With regard to sleep, there is a long history of cholinergic stimulation leading to REM sleep and serotonergic stimulation being associated with slow-wave sleep [38,43,44,46,47,116]. It appears, however, that serotonergic stimulation, via 5HT1A receptors, can also suppress REM sleep [116], suggesting that the cholinergic and serotonergic systems are opposing systems in the regulation of REM sleep. One implication of this balance model is that the apparent cholinergic supersensitivity of REM sleep in depressed individuals [43,116] could be the consequence of a subsensitivity of the serotonergic balancing system. However, no evidence for a reduced inhibitory effect of the 5HT1A receptor agonist ipsapirone on REM sleep in depressed individuals could be found [117].

It has been well established that levels of specific hormones, such as cortisol, prolactin, and growth hormone, can be modified by cholinergic and serotonergic agents [53,54,118,119]. In general, the levels of these hormones are raised by the appropriate agonists. As far as we can tell, there is no information about how these two systems interact in the control of these hormones. No study has given probes from both systems to the same group of subjects.

The literature cited above indicates that the serotonergic and cholinergic systems are opposing systems in the regulation of sleep. However, there is evidence from other sources for parallel systems being involved in other functions. It has been shown that memory can be impaired by the disruption of either system, but the impairments are more severe if both systems are damaged [120]. Similarly, both muscarinic and 5HT1A receptor agonists induce hypothermia in rats [84,121,122].

Although the selective serotonin reuptake inhibitors do not appear to block muscarinic receptors as such, Saito et al. [123] have shown that ACh release appears to be regulated by inhibitory 5HT1B heteroreceptors located on cholinergic nerve terminals. Similarly, Crespi et al. [124] found that 5HT3 receptor agonists decrease ACh release by affecting 5HT3 hetero-receptors located on cortical cholinergic nerve endings.

Consistent with the above, the 5HT1A agonist 8-OH-DPAT turned off cholinergic REM-on neurons which activate REM sleep [125]. Conversely, 8-OH-DPAT enhanced ACh release from rat hippocampus and cerebral cortex [126], and MKC-242, another 5HT1A agonist, likewise increased extracellular ACh [127]. Thus, it is at least possible that the selective 5HT reuptake inhibitors, such as fluoxetine, may in part exert their effects by decreasing ACh availability in some brain regions while increasing it in others.

The studies described above indicate that 5HT could interact positively or negatively with ACh through release mechanisms. However, another mechanism by which the two systems could interact is via postreceptor cascades. The fact that there are at least five muscarinic receptors and at least 20 5HT receptors makes defining such a task daunting. We propose, therefore, to consider the postreceptor cascades for the 5HT1A and 5HT2A and the m_1 and m_2 ACh receptors only in this discussion.

Current evidence suggests that the 5HT1A receptor is negatively coupled to an adenyl cyclase cascade, while the 5HT2A receptor is positively coupled to the phosphatidyl inositol cascade [128]. Likewise, the m_2 and m_1 ACh receptors are negatively and positively coupled to adenyl cyclase and phosphatidyl inositol cascades, respectively [114,128]. Therefore, stimulation of the 5HT1A and m_2 ACh receptors could have a similar effect in those brain regions where these receptors are located postsynaptically on the same neurons. It must be remembered, however, that both 5HT1A and m2 receptors are located on axon terminals as well as on postsynaptic neurons and that their function in those locations is normally to inhibit release of the transmitter. It is also possible that responses mediated by 5HT2A and m_1 receptors could have additive effects. Unfortunately, there are hardly any data to support these ideas at present. However, one study has suggested that 5HT1A and m_2 receptor stimulation may have their effects via different G proteins [119]. This study suggests that it might be possible to develop pharmacological agents that selectively stimulate the serotonergic cascade.

XIV. SECOND-MESSENGER/ ACETYLCHOLINE INTERACTIONS

In the past decade, a number of studies have suggested that second-messenger alterations are linked to the affective disorders and possibly are causative of them. These include alterations in the phosphatidyl inositol system (with evidence that administration of inositol leads to antidepressant and antiobsessional effects), alterations in the cyclic AMP system, and alterations in G proteins. However, what is often not stressed in these papers is that the very neurotransmitters which have been implicated as moderating depression are those which moderate the activities of second messengers, including 5HT, DA, NE and ACh. Thus, ACh activates the phosphatidyl inositol system, turns on cyclic GMP (which antagonizes cyclic AMP), and has effects on G proteins. It is thus quite possible that an interaction between ACh and other neurotransmitters, impacting on appropriate receptors, and leading to second-messenger activation may be significant in inducing a cascade leading to depression. Conceivably, this might explain why activation of such receptors appears important, but blockade of them leaves them in a quiescent phase, and therefore they are not relevant to the treatment or phenomenology of depression. More specifically, Manji and Chen [128] have suggested that guanine nucleotide binding protein coupled signal pathways are regulatory in mood states. Avissar and Schreiber [129] have found that lithium inhibited the coupling of both muscarinic and β-adrenergic receptors, suggesting alterations of G proteins. These results suggest that antidepressant and mood stabilizing treatments attenuate β-adrenergic receptor coupled G protein function [129]. In these studies, m_1 receptors appear especially sensitive to carbamylcholine effects and to the effects of guanine triphosphate (GTP) binding. Similarly, the phosphatidylinositol system, a second-messenger system used by noradrenergic, serotonergic, and cholinergic receptors, has been implicated in unipolar depression and bipolar disorder [78,130], and it would appear that for lithium to exert its effects on the phosphatidyl inositol system, acetylcholine is essential [131].

XV. SUMMARY

As reviewed above, considerable evidence suggests that the cholinergic nervous system, alone or acting in concert with other neurotransmitters, may have an important role in the regulation of affect. Nevertheless, as with all currently proposed biological hypotheses of the etiology of affective disorders, there exist alternative explanations, as well as some data that are inconsistent with the cholinergic hypothesis.

One question concerns the specificity of the cholinergic alterations: Are they confined to patients with affective disorder only or are they also present in other disorders such as schizophrenia, chronic fatigue, or multiple chemical sensitivity? A number of studies have failed to detect any evidence for cholinergic supersensitivity among patients with anxiety disorders [49]. In contrast, several studies suggested an involvement of cholinergic mechanisms in schizophrenia. Early investigators used cholinesterase inhibitors to treat schizophrenia. Others proposed a dopaminergic/cholinergic balance and/or interactive model for schizophrenia [31], and it has been suggested that cholinergic over activity may underlie the negative symptoms of schizophrenia, such as affective flattening, anhedonia, asociality, and apathy [132]. Reduced REM sleep latency has also been observed in schizophrenics [133]. Thus, symptoms of schizophrenia that bear some similarity to key symptoms of depression may also be mediated by cholinergic overactivity.

As described above, it is possible that pharmacologically induced changes in acetylcholine may cause perturbations in depression-relevant systems other than the cholinergic nervous system. Pharmacologically induced acetylcholine alterations could cause a "model depression" by perturbing other potential governing neurotransmitters (e.g., GABA, serotonin, dopamine, or norepinephrine) or second messengers in affect-disordered patients. Furthermore, obviously, the fundamental biochemical changes in depression could be due to a relatively low level of central norepinephrine or serotonin activity, a situation that could explain all of the above observations under the scope of a balance hypothesis. It is also conceivable that the cholinergic supersensitivity observed in many depressives may be a reflection of altered second messengers, including G proteins [93,129,134].

However, even if cholinomimetics can only cause a "model depression" (with such components as low mood, psychomotor depression, elevated ACTH, cortisol, β-endorphin, and epinephrine levels, as well as sleep architecture changes and increased pulse rates and blood pressure), understanding how this pharmacological phenomenon occurs may ultimately offer a window into understanding the pathophysiology of affective disorders and may have useful treatment implications. Thus, at the least, understanding the implications of the mood-depressant and other depressionlike effects of cholinomimetics may give clues as to the actual neurobiology of affective disorders. Alternatively, it is not beyond possibility that acetylcholine actually is directly involved in the etiology and the expression of the affective disorders, alone or acting through other relevant neurotransmitters and/or second messengers.

REFERENCES

1. DS Janowsky, MK El-Yousef, JM Davis, HJ Sekerke. A cholinergic-adrenergic hypothesis of mania and depression. Lancet 2:632–635, 1972.
2. WT. McKinney. Animal models of depression: an overview. Psychiatr Dev 2:77–96, 1984.
3. O Pucilowski, DH Overstreet, AH Rezvani, DS Janowsky. Chronic mild stress-induced anhedonia: greater effect in a genetic rat model of depression. Physiol Behav 54:1215–1220, 1993.
4. P Willner. The validity of animal models of depression. Psychopharmacology 83:1-16, 1984
5. P. Willner. Animal models of depression: an overview. Pharmacol Ther 45:425–455, 1990.
6. DS Janowsky, SC Risch. Role of acetylcholine mechanisms in the affective disorders. In: HY Meltzer, ed. Psychopharmacology. The Third Generation of Progress. New York: Raven Press; 1987,527–534.
7. JR Martin, P Driscoll, C Gentsch. Differential response to cholinergic stimulation in psychogenetically selected rat lines. Psychopharmacology 83:262–267, 1984.
8. CD Walker, ML Aubert, MJ Meaney, P Driscoll. Individual differences in the activity of the hypothalamus-pituitary-adrenocortical system after stress: use of psychogenetically selected rat lines. In: Driscoll P, ed. Genetically Defined Animal Models of Neurobehavioral Dysfunctions. Boston: Birkhauser, 1992: pp. 276–296.
9. DH Overstreet. The Flinders sensitive line rats: a genetic animal model of depression. Neurosci Biobehav Rev 17:51–68, 1993.
10. F Borsini, A Meli. Is the forced swimming test a suitable model for revealing antidepressant activity? Psychopharmacology 94:147–160, 1984.
11. G Hasey, I Hanin. The cholinergic-adrenergic hypothesis of depression reexamined using clonidine, metoprolol, and physostigmine in an animal model. Biol Psychiatry 29:127–138, 1991.
12. DW Rowntree, S Neven, A Wilson. The effect of diisopropylfluorophosphonate in schizophrenia and manic depressive psychosis. J Neurol Neurosurg Psychiatry 13:47–62, 1950.
13. S Gershon, FH Shaw. Psychiatric sequelae of chronic exposure to organophosphorous insecticides. Lancet 1:1371–1374, 1961.
14. MB Bowers, E Goodman, VM Sim. Some behavioral changes in man following anticholinesterase administration. J Nerv Ment Dis 138:383–389, 1964.
15. DS Janowsky, SC Risch, D Parker, LY Huey, LL Judd. Increased vulnerability to cholinergic stimulation in affect disorder patients. Psychopharmacol Bull 16:29–31., 1980.
16. DS Janowsky, SC Risch, B Kennedy, M Ziegler, LY Huey. Central muscarinic effects of physostigmine on mood, cardiovascular function, pituitary, and adrenal neuroendocrine release. Psychopharmacology 89:150–154, 1986.
17. DS Janowsky, SC Risch, LL Judd, LY Huey, DC Parker. Cholinergic supersensitivity in affect disorder patients: behavioral and neuroendocrine observations. Psychopharmacol Bull 17:129–132, 1981.
18. KL Davis, PA Berger, LE Hollister, E DeFraites. Physostigmine in man. Arch Gen Psychiatry 35:119–122, 1979.
19. JJ Modestin, J Hunger, RB Schwartz. Uber die depressogene wirkung von physostigmine. Arch Psychiatrie Nervenkr 218:67–77, 1973.
20. JJ Modestin, RB Schwartz, J Hunger. Zur frage der beeinflussung schizophrener symptom physostigmine. Pharmacopsychiatria 3:300–304, 1973.
21. SC Risch, LJ Siever, JC Gillin JC. Differential mood effects of arecoline in depressed patients and normal volunteers. Psychopharmacol Bull 19:696–698, 1983.
22. JL Nurnberger, DC Jimerson, S Simmons-Alling. Behavioral, physiological and neuroendocrine response to arecoline in normal twins and well state bipolar patients. Psychiatry Res 9:191–200, 1983.
23. JL Nurnberger, W Berrettini, WB Mendelson, B Sack, ES Gershon. Measuring cholinergic sensitivity. I. Arecoline effects in bipolar patients. Biol Psychiatry 25:610–617, 1989.
24. G Oppenheimer, R Ebstein, R Belmaker. Effects of lithium on the physostigmine-induced behavioral syndrome and plasma cyclic GMP. J Psychiatry Res 14:133–139, 1979.
25. SC Risch, PM Cohen, DS Janowsky, NH Kalin, TR Insel, DL Murphy. Physostigmine induction of depressive symptomatology in normal human subjects. Psychiatry Res 4:89–94, 1981.
26. SC Risch, NH Kalin, DS Janowsky. Cholinergic challenge in affective illness: behavioral and neuroendocrine correlates. J Clin Psychopharmacol 1:186–192, 1981.
27. R Mohs, E Hollander, V Haroutunian, M Davidson, T Horvath, KL Davis. Cholinomimetics in Alzheimer's disease. Int J Neurosci 32:775–776, 1987.
28. M El-Yousef, DS Janowsky, JM Davis, JE Rosenblatt. Induction of severe depression in marijuana intoxicated individuals. Br J Addict 68:321–325, 1973.
29. DS Janowsky, MK El-Yousef, JM Davis. Acetylcholine and depression. Psychosom Med 36:248–257, 1974.
30. C Tamminga, RC Smith, S Change, JS Haraszti, KL Davis. Depression associated with oral choline. Lancet 2:905, 1976.

31. KL Davis, LE Hollister, PA Berger. Choline chloride in schizophrenia. Am J Psychiatry 136:1581–1584, 1979.
32. DE Casey. Mood alterations during deanol therapy. Psychopharmacology (Berl) 62:187–191, 1979.
33. DS Janowsky, SC Risch. Cholinomimetic and anticholinergic drugs used to investigate an acetylcholine hypothesis of affective disorder and stress. Drug Dev Res 4:125–142, 1984.
34. DS Janowsky, SC Risch, LL Judd, LY Huey, DC Parker. Brain cholinergic systems and the pathogenesis of affective disorders. In: MM Singh, DM Warburton, H Lal, eds. Central Cholinergic Mechanisms and Adaptive Dysfunction. New York: Plenum; 309–353, 1985.
35. BJ Steinberg, R Trestman, V Mitropoulou, M Serby, J Silverman, E Coccaro, S Weston, M de Vegvar, LJ Siever. Depressive response to physostigmine challenge in borderline personality disorder patients. Neuropsychopharmacology 17(4):264–273, 1997.
36. J Fritze, M Lanczik, E Sofic, M Struc, P Riederer. Cholinergic neurotransmission seems not to be involved in depression but possibly in personality. J Psychiatry Neurosci 20(1):39–48, 1995.
37. J Fritze. The adrenergic-cholinergic imbalance hypothesis of depression: a review and a perspective. Rev Neurosci 4(1):63–93, 1993.
38. A Berkowitz, L Sutton, DS Janowsky, JC Gillin. Pilocarpine, an orally active muscarinic cholinergic agonist, induces REM sleep and reduces delta sleep in normal volunteers. Psychiatry Res 33:113–119, 1990.
39. M Berger, R Lund, T Bronisch, D von Zeerssen. REM latency in neurotic and endogenous depression and the cholinergic REM induction test. Psychiatry Res 10:113–123, 1983.
40. RE Dahl, ND Ryan, J Perel, B Birmaher, M alShabbout, B Nelson, J Puig-Antich. Cholinergic REM induction test with arecoline in depressed children. Psychiatry Res 51(3):269–282, 1994.
41. N Sitaram, D Jones, S Dube, J Bell, P Rivard. Supersensitive ACh REM-induction as a genetic vulnerability marker. Int J Neurosci 32:777–778, 1985.
42. N Sitaram, J Nurnberger, ES Gershon, JC Gillin. Cholinergic regulation of mood and REM sleep. A potential model and marker for vulnerability to depression. Am J Psychiatry 139:571–576, 1982.
43. JC Gillin, L Sutton, C Ruiz, J Kelsoe, RM Dupont, D Darko, SC Risch, S Golshan, D Janowsky. The cholinergic rapid eye movement induction test with arecoline in depression. Arch Gen Psychiatry 48:264–270, 1991.
44. M Berger, D Riemann, D Hochli, R Spiegel. The cholinergic rapid eye movement sleep induction test with RS-86. Arch Gen Psychiatry 46:421–428, 1989.

45. H Gann, D Riemann, F Hohagen, H Dressing, WE Muller, M Berger. The sleep structure of patients with anxiety disorders in comparison to that of healthy controls and depressive patients under baseline conditions and after cholinergic stimulation. J Affect Dis 26:179–190, 1992.
46. D Riemann, F Hohagen, M Bahro, S Lis, G Stadmuller, H Gann, M Berger. Cholinergic neurotransmission, REM sleep and depression. J Psychosom Res 38(1):15–25, 1994.
47. D Riemann, F Hohagen, S Krieger, H Gann, WE Muller, R Olbrich, HJ Wark, M Bohus, H Low, M Berger. Cholinergic REM induction test: muscarinic supersensitivity underlies polysomnographic findings in both depression and schizophrenia. J Psychiatr Res 28(3):195–210, 1994.
48. MH Rapaport, SC Risch, JC Gillin, S Golshan, D Janowsky. The effects of physostigmine infusion on patients with panic disorder. Biol Psychiatry 29:658–664, 1991.
49. S Dube, N Kumar, A Ettedgui, R Pohl, D Jones, N Sitaram. Cholinergic REM induction response: separation of anxiety and depression. Biol Psychiatry 20:408–418, 1985.
50. JI Nurnberger Jr, N Sitaram, ES Gershon, JC Gillin. A twin study of cholinergic REM induction. Biol Psychiatry 18:1161–1173, 1983.
51. W Schreiber, CJ Lauer, K Krumrey, F Holsboer, JC Krieg. Cholinergic REM sleep induction test in subjects at high risk for psychiatric disorders. Biol Psychiatry 32:79–90, 1992.
52. V O'Keane, K O'Flynn, J Lucey, TG Dinan. Pyridostigmine-induced growth hormone responses in healthy and depressed subjects: evidence for cholinergic supersensitivity in depression. Psychol Med 22(1):55–60, 1992.
53. TG Dinan, V O'Keane, J Thakore. Pyridostigmine induced growth hormone release in mania: focus on the cholinergic/somatostatin system. Clin Endocrinol 40(1):93–96, 1994.
54. JV Lucey, G Butcher, AW Clare, TG Dinan. Elevated growth hormone responses to pyridostigmine in obsessive-compulsive disorder: evidence of cholinergic supersensitivity. Am J Psychiatry 150:961–962, 1993.
55. TG Dinan TG. Psychoneuroendocrinology of depression. Growth hormone. Psychiatr Clin North Am 21(2):325–339, 1998.
56. JM Cooney, JV Lucey, V O'Keane, TG Dinan. Specificity of the pyridostigmine/growth hormone challenge in the diagnosis of depression. Biol Psychiatry 42(9):827–833, 1997.
57. HC Charles, F Lazeyras, KRR Krishnan, OB Boyko, M Payne, D Moore. Brain choline in depression: in vivo detection of potential pharmacodynamic effects of antidepressant therapy using hydrogen localized

spectroscopy. Prog Neuro-Psychopharmacol Biol Psychiatry 18:1121–1127, 1993.
58. RF Renshaw, B Lafer, SM Babb, M Fava, AL Stoll, JD Christensen, CM Moore, DA Yurgelun-Todd, CM Bonello, SS Pillay, AJ Rothschild, AA Nierenberg, JF Rosenbaum, BM Cohen. Basal ganglia choline levels in depression and response to fluoxetine treatment: an in vivo proton magnetic resonance spectroscopy study. Biol Psychiatry 41(8):837–843, 1997.
59. H Hankura, T Kato, J Murashita, N Kato. Quantitative proton magnetic resonance spectroscopy of the basal ganglion in patients with affective disorder. Eur Arch Psychiatry Clin Neurosci 248(1):53–58, 1998.
60. CM Moore, JL Breeze, SA Gruber, SM Babb, BF Blaise, RA Villafuerte, AL Stoll, J Hennen, DA Yurgelun-Todd, BM Cohen, PF Renshaw. Choline, myo-inositol and mood in bipolar disorder: a proton magnetic resonance spectroscopic imaging study of the anterior cingulate cortex. Bipolar Disord 2:207–216, 2000.
61. J Soares, F Boada, S Spencer, K Wells, A Mallinger, E Frank, S Gershon, D Kupfer, M Keshaven. NAA and choline measures in the anterior cingulate of bipolar disorder patients. Biol Psychiatry 45s(suppl):119, 1999.
62. JC Gillin, J Lauriello, JR Kelsoe, M Rapaport, S Golshan, WM Kenny, L Sutton. No antidepressant effect of biperiden compared with placebo in depression: a double-blind 6-week clinical trial. Psychiatry Res 58(2):99–105, 1995.
63. KA Sokolski, EM DeMet. Increased pupillary sensivity to pilocarpine in depression. Prog Neuropsychopharmacol Biol Psychiatry 20:253–262, 1996.
64. 64.K Fountoulakis, F Fotiou, A Iacovides, J Tsiptsios, A Goulas, M Tsolaki, C Ierodiakonou. Changes in pupil reaction to light in melancholic patients. Int J Psychophysiol 31(2):121–128, 1999.
65. KN Sokolski, EM DeMet. Cholinergic sensitivity predicts severity of mania. Psychiatry Res 95(3):195–200, 2000.
66. EM DeMet, KN Sokolski. Sodium valproate increases pupillary responsiveness to a cholinergic agonist in responders with mania. Biol Psychiatry 46:432–436, 1999.
67. P Doerr, M Berger. Physostigmine-induced escape from dexamethasone suppression in normal adults. Biol Psychiatry 18:261–268, 1983.
68. GM Gilad. The stress-induced response of the septo-hippocampal cholinergic system. A vectorial outcome of psychoneuroendocrinological interactions. Psychoneuroendocrinology 12(3):167–184, 1987.
69. T Mizuno, F Kimura. Attenuated stress response of hippocampal acetylcholine release and adrenocortical secretion in aged rats. Neurosci Lett 222(1):49–52, 1997.
70. GP Mark, PV Rada, TJ Shorts. Inescapable stress enhances extracellular acetylcholine in the rat hippocampus and prefrontal cortex but not the nucleus accumbens or amygdala. Neuroscience 74(3):767–774, 1996.
71. JC Day, M Koehl, V Deroche, M Le Moal, S Maccari. Prenatal stress enhances stress- and corticotropin-releasing factor–induced stimulation of hippocampal acetylcoline release in adult rats. J Neurosci 18(5):1886–1892, 1998.
72. AH Glassman. Cigarette smoking: implications for psychiatric illness. Am J Psychiatry 150:546–553, 1993.
73. K Kendler, MC Nenale, CL MacLean, AC Heath, LJ Eaves, RC Kessler. Smoking and major depression: a causal analysis. Arch Gen Psychiatry 50:36–43, 1993.
74. ET Iwamoto. Antinociception after nicotine administration into the mesopontine tegmentum of rats: evidence for muscarinic actions. J Pharmacol Exp Ther 251:412–421, 1989.
75. Tizabi, DH Overstreet, AH Rezvani, VA Louis, E Clark Jr, DS Janowsky, MA Kling. Antidepressant effects of nicotine in an animal model of depression. Psychopharmacology 142:193–199, 1999.
76. Y Tizabi, AH Rezvani, LT Russell, KY Tyler, DH Overstreet. Depressive characteristics of FSL rats: involvement of central nicotinic receptors. Pharmacol Biochem Behav 66:63–77, 2000.
77. VJ Djuric, E Dunn, DH Overstreet, A Dragomir, M Steiner. Antidepressant effect of ingested nicotine in female rats of Flinders resistant and sensitive lines. Physiol Behav 67:533–537, 1999.
78. H Ozawa, W Gsell, L Frolich, R Zochlig, P Pantucek, H Beckmann, P Riederer. Imbalance of the Go and Gi/o function in postmortem human brain of depressed patients. J Neural Transm 94:63–69, 1993.
79. KP Lesch, HK Manji. Signal-transducing G proteins and antidepressant drugs: evidence for modulation of alpha subunit gene expression in rat brain. Biol Psychiatry 32:549–579, 1992.
80. A Zangen, DH Overstreet, G Yadid. Increased catecholamine levels in specific brain regions of a rat model of depression: normalization by chronic antidepressant treatment. Brain Res 824:243–250, 1999.
81. L Serova, EL Sabban, A Zangen, DH Overstreet, G Yadid. Altered gene expression for catecholamine biosynthetic enzymes and stress response in rat genetic model of depression. Mol Brain Res 63:133–138, 1998.
82. G Yadid, DH Overstreet, A Zangen. Limbic dopaminergic adaptation to a stressful stimulus in a rat model of depression. Brain Res 896:43–47, 2001.
83. A Zangen, R Nakash, DH Overstreet, G Yadid. Association between depressive behavior and absence of serotonin-dopamine interaction in the nucleus accumbens. Psychopharmacology 155: 434–439, 2001.

84. DH Overstreet, LC Daws, GD Schiller, J Orbach, DS Janowsky. Cholinergic/serotonergic interactions in hypothermia: implications for rat models of depression: Pharmacol Biochem Behav 59:777–785, 1998.
85. A Zangen, DH Overstreet, G Yadid. High serotonin and 5-hydroxyindoleacetic acid levels in limbic regions of a rat model of depression: normalizaton by chronic antidepressant treatment. J Neurochem 69:2477–2483, 1997.
86. Overstreet DH, Pucilowski O, Rezvani AH, Janowsky DS. Administration of antidepressants, diazepam and psychomotor stimulants further confirms the utility of Flinders Sensitive Line rats as an animal model of depression. Psychopharmacology 121:27–37, 1995.
87. DS Janowsky, MK El-Yousef, JM Davis, HJ Sekerke. Parasympathetic suppression of manic symptoms by physostigmine. Arch Gen Psychiatry 28:542–547, 1973.
88. BJ Carroll, A Frazer, A Schless, J Mendels. Cholinergic reversal of manic symptoms. Lancet 427–428, 1973.
89. B Shopsin, DS Janowsky, JM Davis, S Gershon. Rebound phenomena in manic patients following physostigmine. Neuropsychobiology 1:180–187, 1975.
90. BM Cohen, JF Lipinski, RI Altesman. Lecithin in the treatment of mania: double-blind, placebo controlled trials. Am J Psychiatry 139(9):1162–1164, 1982.
91. DB Leiva. The neurochemistry of mania: a hypothesis of etiology and rationale for treatment. Prog Neuropsychopharmacol Biol Psychiatry 14(3):423–429, 1990.
92. T Burt, GS Sachs, C Demopulos. Donepezil in treatment-resistant bipolar disorder. Biol Psychiatry 45:959–964, 1998.
93. BH Guze, JC Barrio. The etiology of depression in Parkinson's disease patients. Psychosomatics 32(4):390–395, 1991.
94. W Powe, Luginger E. Depression in Parkinson's disease: impediments to recognition and treatment. Neurology 52(7 suppl 3):S2–S6, 1999 Review.
95. MP De Parada, MA Parada, P Rada, L Hernandez, BG Hoebel. Dopamine-acetylcholine interaction in the rat lateral hypothalamus in the control of locomotion. Pharmacol Biochem Behav 66(2):227–234, 2000.
96. HC Fibiger, GS Lynch, HP Cooper. A biphasic action of central cholinergic stimulation behavioral arousal in the rat. Psychopharmacologia 20:336–382, 1971.
97. FM Jacobsen, L Domas-Diaz. Donepezil for psychotropic-induced memory loss. J Clin Psychiatry 60(10):698–704, 1999.
98. F Benazzi. Mania associated with donepezil. J Psychiatry Neurosci 24(5):468–469, 1999.
99. DS Janowsky, AA Abrams, GP Groom, LL Judd, P Cloptin. Lithium administration antagonizes cholinergic behavioral effects in rodents. Psychopharmacology 63(2):147–150, 1979.
100. DC German, DM Bowden. Catecholamine systems as the neural substrate for intracranial self-stimulation: A hypothesis. Brain Res 73:381–419, 1974.
101. RA Wise RA. Catecholamine theories of reward. A critical review. Brain Res 152:233–247, 1979.
102. EF Domino, ME Olds. Cholinergic inhibition of self-stimulation behavior. J Pharmacol Exp Ther 164:202–211, 1968.
103. LM Newman. Effects of cholinergic agonists and antagonists on self-stimulation behavior. J Comp Physiol Psychol 79:394–413, 1972.
104. DS Janowsky, MK El-Yousef, JM Davis. Antagonistic effects of physostigmine and methylphenidate in man. Am J Psychiatry 130:13701376, 1973.
105. D Ostrow, A Halaris, M Dysken, E DeMet, M Harrow, J Davis. State dependence of noradrenergic activity in a rapidly cycling bipolar patient. J Clin Psychiatry 45:306–309, 1984.
106. M Schittecatte, G Charles, R Machowsky, J Garcia, J Medelwicz, J Wilmotte. Reduced clonidine rapid eye movement suppression in patients with primary major affective illness. Arch Gen Psychiatry 49:637–642, 1992.
107. JI Nurnberger Jr, ES Gershon, N Sitaram, JC Gillin, G Brown, M Ebert, P Gold, D Jimerson, L Kessler. Dextroamphetamine and arecoline as pharmacogenetic probes in normals and remitted bipolar patients. Psychopharmacol Bul 17:80–82, 1981.
108. LJ Siever, SC Risch, DL Murphy. Central cholinergic-adrenergic balance in the regulation of affective state. Psychiatry Res 5:108–109, 1981.
109. Y Ikarashi, A Takahashi, H Ishimaru, T Arai, Y Maruyama. Suppression of cholinergic activity via the dopamine D2 receptor in the rat striatum. Neurochem Int 30(2):191–197, 1997.
110. NS Downs, KT Britton, DM Gibbs, GF Koob, NR Swerdlow. Supersensitive endocrine response to physostigmine in dopamine-depleted rats: a model of depression? Biol Psychiatry 21(8–9):775–786, 1986.
111. SC Risch, DS Janowsky, NH Kaslin, RM Cohen, JA Aloi, DL Murphy. Cholinergic beta endorphin hypersensitivity associated with depression. In: I Hanin, E Usdin, eds. Biological Markers in Psychiatry and Neurology. Oxford: Pergamon Press, 1982:269–278.
112. SC Risch, DS Janowsky, SJC Gillin. Muscarinic supersensitivity of anterior pituitary ACTH and beta endorphin release in major depressive illness. Peptides 9:789–792, 1981.
113. P Muller, P Seeman. Brain neurotransmitter receptors after long-term haloperidol: dopamine, acetylcholine, serotonin, alpha-noradrenergic and naloxone receptors. Life Sci 21:1751–1759, 1977.
114. ER Kandel, JH Schwartz, TM Jessell. Principles of Neural Science, 4th ed. New York: McGraw-Hill, 2000.

115. Mallick BN. Kaur S. Saxena RN. Interactions between cholinergic and GABAergic neurotransmitters in and around the locus coeruleus for the induction and maintenance of rapid eye movement sleep in rats. Neuroscience 104(2):467–485, 2001.
116. JC Gillin, TW Sohn, SM Stahl, M Lardon, J Kelsoe, M Rapaport. Ipsapirone, a 5HT1A agonist, suppresses REM sleep equally in unmedicated depressed patients and normal controls. Neuropsychopharmacology 15:109–115, 1996.
117. E Seifritz, JC Gillin, MH Rapaport, JR Kelsoe, T Bhatti, SM Stahl. Sleep EEG response to muscarinic and serotonin 1A receptor probes in patients with major depression and in normal controls. Biol Psychiatry 44:21–33, 1998.
118. LD van de Kar. Neuroendocrine aspects of the serotonergic hypothesis of depression. Neurosci Biobehav Rev 13:237–246, 1989.
119. KP Lesch, J Disselkamp-Tietze, A Schmidtke. 5HT1A receptor function in depression: effects of chronic amitriptyline treatment. J Neural Transm 80:157–161, 1990.
120. P Riekkinen Jr. 5HT1A and muscarinic acetylcholine receptors jointly regulate passive avoidance behavior. Eur J Pharmacol 262:77–90, 1994.
121. DH Overstreet, DS Janowsky, O Pucilowski, AH Rezvani. Swim test immobility cosegregates with serotonergic but not cholinergic sensitivity in cross breeds of Flinders Line rats. Psychiatr Genet 4:101–107, 1994.
122. DH Overstreet, AH Rezvani, O Pucilowski, L Gause, DS Janowsky. Rapid selection for serotonin-1A sensitivity in rats. Psychiatr Genet 4:57–62, 1994.
123. H Saito, M Matsumoto, H Togashi, M Yoshioka. Functional interactions between serotonin and other neuronal systems: focus on in vivo microdialysis studies. Jpn J Pharmacol 70(3):203–205, 1996.
124. D Crespi, M Gobbi, T Mennini. 5HT3 serotonin hertero-receptors inhibit ^{3}H acetylcholine release in rat corticol synaptosomes. Phamacol Res 35(4):351–354, 1997.
125. P Sombonnthum, T Matsuda, S Asano, M Sakaue, A Baba. MKC-242, a novel 5HT1A receptor agonist, facilitates cortical acetylcholine release by a mechanism different from that of 8-OH-DPAT in awake rats. Neuropharmacology 36(11–12):1733–1739, 1997.
126. MM Thakkar, RE Strecker, RW McCarley. Behavioral state control through differential serotonergic inhibition in the mesopontine cholinergic nuclei: a simultaneous unit recording and microdialysis study. J Neurosci 18(4):5490–5497, 1998.
127. T Fujii, M Yoshizawa, K Nakai, K Fujimoto, T Suzuki, K Kawashima. Demonstration of the facilitatory role of 8-OH-DPAT on cholinergic transmission in the rat hippocampus using in vivo microdialysis. Brain Res 761(2):244–249, 1997.
128. HK Manji, G Chen. Post-receptor signaling pathways in the pathophysiology and treatment of mood disorders. Curr Psychiatry Rep 2:479–489, 2000.
129. S Avissar, G Schreiber. Muscarinic receptor subclassification and G-proteins: significance for lithium action in affective disorders and for the treatment of extrapyramidal side effects of neuroleptics. Biol Psychiatry 26:113–130, 1989.
130. E Sanders-Bush, H Canton. Serotonin receptors: signal transduction pathways. In: FE Bloom, DJ Kupfer eds. Psychopharmaoclogy. The Fourth Generation of Progress. New York: Raven Press, 1995:431–442.
131. CH Lee, JF Dixon, M Reichman, C Moummi, G Los, LE Hokin. Li$^+$ increases accumulation of inositol 1,4,5-trisphosphate and inositol 1,3,4,5-tetrakisphosphae in cholinergically stimulated cortex slices in guinea pig, mouse and rat. The increases require inositol supplementation in mouse and rat but not in guinea pig. Biochem J 1:377–385, 1992.
132. R Tandon, JF Greden. Cholinergic hyperactivity and negative schizophrenic symptoms: A model of dopaminergic/cholinergic interactions in schizophrenia. Arch Gen Psychiatry 46:745–753, 1989.
133. D Riemann, H Gann, R Fleckenstein, F Hohagen, R Olbrich, M Berger. Effect of RS86 on REM latency in schizophrenia. Psychiatry Res 38:84–92, 1991.
134. Y Odagaki, K Fuxe. 5HT1A, GABA and pirenzepine-insensitive muscarinic receptors are functionally coupled to distinct pools of the same kind of G proteins in rat hippocampus. Brain Res 689:129–135, 1995.

25

GABA and Mood Disorders
A Selective Review and Discussion of Future Research

FREDERICK PETTY, PRASAD PADALA, and SURENDER PUNIA
Creighton University and Omaha Veterans Administration Medical Center, Omaha, Nebraska, U.S.A.

I. INTRODUCTION

Gamma-amino butyric acid (GABA) is a neurotransmitter which is ubiquitous in mammalian brain. About 30–50 % of neurons in the central nervous system use GABA as a neurotransmitter. Thus, a role for GABA in the molecular and neuronal etiopathology of mental illnesses and behavioral disorders is expected. In fact, GABA is thought to be involved in a variety of psychiatric disorders, including personality disorders, anxiety disorder, schizophrenia, addictive disorders, and mood disorders. This review will focus on mood disorders.

II. BACKGROUND

GABA is considered to be an "inhibitory" neurotransmitter. Sometimes this causes confusion regarding its relationship with mental illnesses and behavioral disorders. First, the word inhibitory relates to physiology, not to behavior, in the context of neurotransmitter function. Most GABA neurons are small interneurons which synapse upon other GABA interneurons. Thus, physiological disinhibition is often the net or end result of activation of GABA. From a behavioral perspective, drugs that act to increase GABA activity or function, such as alcohol or benzodiazepines, tend to have a disinhibitory effect, particularly at low doses. Of course, higher doses lead to physiological and behavioral inhibition, such as sedation. Thus, while at a particular receptor, the action of GABA molecules may be inhibitory, at the systems level the effects are much more complex. Additionally, it is worth noting that at some biogenic amine nerve terminals GABA actually facilitates release of norepinephrine and dopamine, adding another level of complexity [1].

The general topic of GABA and mood disorders has been recently, well, and thoroughly reviewed [1–4]. Thus, we will not provide an exhaustive or comprehensive review of the data, rather, we will attempt to highlight and synthesize the most important and provocative features of this work. Also, we will analyze some interesting inconsistencies in the data, and suggest plausible explanations and hypotheses for further exploring the field. Finally, we will attempt to provide an overall theoretical framework and suggest potentially fruitful areas for future further exploration.

Initial interest in GABA in the etiopatholoqy of mood disorders derived from clinical observations made in the 1970s that valproic acid (valproate) was useful in treatment of *both* depression and mania in bipolar patients. In fact, the first published announcement of a "GABA Theory of Affective Illness" was provided by Emrich [5], based on a case series of observations in manic-depressive patients.

Valproate exerts its primary neurochemical effects by increasing GABA in the brain. Hence, the original idea was that low GABA caused, or was related to, bipolar disorder, since the therapeutic effects of valproate were assumed to occur by rectifying this deficit. Subsequently, other agents that increase GABA levels or function were found useful in the treatment of bipolar patients. Interestingly, these medications are effective across a remarkably wide range of symptomatology, including anxiety, depression, irritability, aggression, and mania. In other words, these medications do not just provide symptomatic relief for a particular clinical state, such as mania, but appear to have beneficial action across the broad spectrum of psychopathological manifestations we observe in persons with symptomatic bipolar disorder [6].

III. DEPRESSION

In addition to its role in manic depressive disease, a role for GABA in depressive disorders was also first suggested in the early 1980s by findings from several studies of cerebrospinal fluid (CSF). Most of these studies reported that patients with depression had low GABA, compared to controls. While not all the studies were statistically significant, a meta-analysis revealed an overall high level of statistical significance [2]. Only one study included patients with mania [7]. Manic patients had CSF GABA lower than controls, though this did not achieve statistical significance. Generally, neurotransmitters measured in CSF are thought to originate from brain, though the contributions from spinal cord should not be ignored. Studies with GABA in spinal fluid are complicated by the rostrocaudal gradient of GABA concentration in CSF, and by the fact that GABA levels in CSF are artifactually elevated if samples are not collected on dry ice, because of breakdown of conjugated GABA.

GABA can also be measured in plasma, where its levels are comparable to those in CSF. Our group has studied plasma GABA in mood disorders for two decades. Naturally, the measurement of neurotransmitters in plasma is very controversial, since a presumption is that peripheral sources contribute to most of what is measured in peripheral tissues, such as blood. This, of course, is true for the biogenic amine neurotransmitters, since brain levels of these compounds are relatively low and peripheral sources are prominent in total body metabolism. Serotonin, for example, is the neurotransmitter for only a few hundred thousand neurons, but has high concentrations in platelets. Similarly, norepinephrine is the neurotransmitter for relatively few neurons, but is synthesized by the adrenal. In the case of GABA, however, the largest concentrations are in brain, which accounts for perhaps 98% of total body GABA. It has been thought that GABA does not cross the blood brain barrier. However, like most neutral amino acids, GABA indeed does cross the blood brain barrier if ingested or given intravenously in large doses. Also, it certainly crosses the brain CSF barrier, and the CSF blood barrier, and most GABA measured in plasma is likely to have an origin in brain, judging from experiments performed in laboratory animals [8]. Nevertheless, even a peripheral marker of mental illness can be useful [9].

IV. PLASMA GABA

A consistent and well replicated finding of this research is that GABA levels are low in plasma in patients with primary, unipolar, major depressive disorder [10]. Further, low GABA in depression does not normalize with treatment or with clinical recovery [11]. Nor does low GABA in depressed patients correlate with severity of illness [12]. Taken together, these features suggest low GABA in depression may be a trait marker for the illness. We do not know whether low GABA in depression is an antecedent of illness, or a consequence or "scar." However, we do know that low GABA characterizes only adult depression, since levels of GABA in children and adolescents with mood disorders are not different from controls [1]. Further research should clarify the important question of whether low GABA in adults precedes the onset of depression and represents a vulnerability marker, or is a long-term consequence of depression. Possibly, the neurobiology of the disease process in adolescents and children is different from that in adults.

Low GABA in depression characterizes a subset of patients, about 40%. We have not done a detailed examination of what behavioral, symptomatic, or psychological features differentiate patients with low, versus normal, GABA levels. A post hoc analysis suggested that low-GABA patients had higher levels of endogenicity, based on items from the Hamilton Rating Scale for Depression [10]. Also, a post hoc analysis of data obtained from a family study suggested that GABA levels were inversely correlated with hostility in first-degree relatives of persons with primary unipolar depression who were not themselves depressed [13]. Further research is needed to elucidate whether low GABA in depression has any value in characterizing the illness according to behavioral subtypes, or in selecting treatments.

It is worth emphasizing that plasma GABA will never serve as a diagnostic test for depression, simply because low GABA is not specific for depression and within depression characterizes only a subset of patients. Thus, as a diagnostic test, plasma GABA lacks both sensitivity and specificity. We do not consider this to be a problem. Depression is a heterogeneous illness, with multiple causes, multiple features, multiple treatments, and multiple responses to treatment. The diagnosis of depression is a clinical diagnosis, with an arbitrary cluster of symptoms and no truly pathognomonic features. Hence, we should not expect, and in fact should be skeptical of, any marker which purports to identify all, or even most, depressed patients, and to differentiate them from other mental illnesses. Nevertheless, as a marker for depression, low plasma GABA has some selectivity. Plasma levels of GABA appear normal in patients with anxiety disorders and in patients with eating disorders [14–16]. Both these conditions are associated with high rates of comorbid depression. Mean plasma GABA levels in patients with schizophrenia are similar to control, though with a larger standard deviation [16]. There has not been a detailed study with a large cohort of plasma GABA levels in schizophrenia.

V. SPECIFICITY

Plasma GABA levels are low in patients with alcohol dependence [17]. In patients with alcohol dependence, GABA levels remain low for several months after cessation of drinking and maintenance of sobriety. GABA levels after withdrawal and detoxification predict outcome, in that patients with lower levels are more likely to maintain sobriety at 6-month follow-up. This seems counterintuitive, if a GABA "deficit" corresponds to a feature of illness that alcoholics are "self-medicating" with alcohol, which has its primary action via the GABA-A receptor, by facilitating GABA transmission. On the other hand, one might speculate that higher GABA levels, which are associated with conduct disorder in children and adolescents, may be associated with disinhibition. Thus, persons with higher GABA may be more predisposed to impulsive actions, and a greater likelihood of return to drinking.

Brain GABA levels are inversely correlated with symptom severity, in biopsies from patients undergoing psychosurgery [18]. Brain GABA levels are low in patients with major depressive disorder, as measured by magnetic resonance spectroscopy (MRS) [4,19]. Unlike plasma GABA, brain GABA as measured by MRS levels do seem to increase and return toward normal with treatment and clinical improvement (Sanacora, personal communication, 2001). An interesting facet of the brain GABA research with MRS is that, for technical reasons, levels are measured in the occipital cortex. Generally, our conceptualization of the anatomy of mood disorders involves the limbic system, specifically the frontal cortex, hippocampus, amygdala, hypothalamus, cingulate cortex, and so forth. Thus, finding low GABA in occipital cortex in depression suggests that the GABA deficit in depression is global. Plasma GABA, if we accept that this originates from brain, must reflect some global, probably cortical GABA level. This suggests that the "lesion" involved in low GABA states is not anatomically specific, but occurring throughout much, if not most, of brain, and perhaps in the periphery as well. Thus, the low GABA observed in depression and in bipolar disorder may be due to low activity of an enzyme which regulates GABA levels, rather than a specific receptor.

A small number of neuroendocrine challenge studies with GABA agonists have been reported, mostly with the GABA-B receptor agonist baclofen. These studies are mixed in their results, but the largest and best study reported a positive finding [20]. To our knowledge, no challenge studies with GABA-A agonists, or with valproate, or GABA itself, have been reported.

VI. PHARMACOLOGY

Further support for a "GABA deficit" in depression was provided by the provocative findings that the GABA agonists progabide and fengabine were efficacious in the treatment of major depressive disorder [21]. These medications never achieved widespread clinical use, owing to problems associated with hepatotoxicity. However, the benzodiazepine alprazolam did achieve wide spread clinical use, with an indication for anxiety disorders. About 20 clinical trials of alprazolam for major depressive disorder were conducted, with consistently positive results [22]. Though alprazolam remains the best-studied benzodiazepine in the treatment of major depression, some preliminary studies suggest that the high-potency benzodiazepines lorazepam and clonazepam may also have antidepressant efficacy [23,24]. Since the primary mechanism of action of these compounds involves facilitating the GABA-A receptor, these findings are compatible with a GABA deficit in patients with depression.

We have further tested the GABA deficit hypothesis in depression by treating depressed patients with valproate. In an open-label trial with patients with primary, unipolar depression, valproate led to significant improvement over 8 weeks of treatment [25]. In a recently completed double-blind, placebo-controlled trial, valproate was no different from placebo in symptom reduction in patients with unipolar depression. In patients with bipolar depression, valproate treatment was better than placebo at the trend (P < .1) level [26].

Further research with GABA agonists in the treatment of depression is certainly needed, and the newer anticonvulsants, vigabatrin and tiagabine, should be tested as antidepressant (and antimanic) agents.

VII. ANIMAL MODELS

Recently, techniques of molecular biology have been applied to research in GABA and mood disorders. Table 1 summarizes findings to date. Needless to say, the results of these studies are preliminary, and in need of extension and replication. It is worth noting that no

Table 1 Molecular Genetics of GABA System and Mood Disorders

Author	Year	Study	Finding
De bruyn[a]	1996	Linkage study between bipolar and genes involved in dopaminergic and GABA-ergic neurotransmission	Excluded linkage for DAT1, DRD2, DRD3, DRD5, DBH, GABRA 1 and GABARB1 genes
Duffy[b]	2000	Linkage sudy of candidate genes in GABA-ergic transmission in lithium-responsive bipolar disorder	Significant association between Lithium response and GABA RA3,RA5 and RB3
Oruc[a]	1997	Association between GABRA5 and unipolar recurrent major depression	Positive association of GABRA5 gene in unipolar recurrent major depression
Papadimitriou[d]	2001	Association between GABA-A receptor beta-3 and alpha-5 subunit gene cluster in chromosome 15q11-q13 and bipolar	No difference between bipolar and controls
Papadimitriou[e]	1998	Association GABA-A receptor alpha-5 gene locus and bipolar	Presence or absence of 282-bp allele does not influence the age of onset or severity; More in manic episodes than depression
Puertollano[f]	1997	Association between MDD and a highly polymorphic marker from the GABR-beta-1 gene	No association; significant difference between patients and controls in women subpopulation
Serretti[g]	1999	D2 and D4 genes,GABA A alpha-1 subunit genes, and response to lithium prophylaxis in mood disorders	No association

[a] A De bruyn, D Souery, K Mendelbaum, J Mendlewicz, A Van Broeckhov. A linkage study between bipolar disorder and genes involved in dopaminergic and GABAergic neurotransmission. Psychiatr Genet 6:67–73, 1996.

[b] A Duffy, G Turecki, P Grof, P Cavazzoni, E Grof, R Joober, B Ahrens, A Berghofer, B Muller-Oerlinghausen, M Dvorakoya, E Libigerova, M Voitechovsky, P Zvolsky, A Nilsson, RW Licht, NA Rasmussen, M Schou, P Vestergaard, A Holzinger, C Shumann, K Thau, C Robertson, GA Rouleau, M Alda. Association and linkage studies of candidate genes involved in GABAergic neurotransmission in lithium-responsive bipolar disorder. J Psychiatry Neurosci. 25:353–358, 2000.

[c] L Oruc, GR Verheyen, I Furac, S Ivezic, M Jakovljevic, P Raeymaekers, C Broeckhoven. Positive association between the GABRA5 gene and unipolar recurrent major depression. Neuropsychobiology 36:62–64, 1997.

[d] GN Papadimitriou, DG Dikeos, G Karadima, D Avramopoulos, EG Daksalopoulou, D Vassilopoulos, CN Stefanis. Association between the GABA(A) receptor alpha5 subunit gene locus (GABRA%) and bipolar affective disorder. Am J Med Genet 81:73–80, 1998.

[e] GN Papadimitriou, DG Dikeos, G Karadima, D Avaramopolous, EG Daskalopoulou, CN Stefanis. GABA-A receptor beta3 and alpha5 subunit gene cluster on chromosome 15q11-q13 and bipolar disorder: a genetic association study. Am J Med Genet 105:317–320, 2001.

[f] R Puertollano, G Visedo, C Zapata, J Fernandez-Piqueras. A study of genetic association between manic-depressive illness a: a highly polymorphic marker from the GABRbeta-1 gene. Am J Med Genet 74:342–344, 1997.

[g] A Serreti, R Lilli, Lorenzi C, Franchini, D Di Bella, M Catalano, E Smeraldi. Dopamine receptor D2 and D4 genes (GABA)A alpha-1 subuni genes and response to lithium prophylaxis in mood disorders. Psychiatry Res 87:7–19, 1999.

study to date has attempted to study both the phenotype of low plasma, or CSF, or brain GABA, and genotypes in the same patient cohort.

Research with animal models of depression tends to support a role for GABA in depression. Curiously, to our knowledge, no studies have been done with plasma or brain GABA levels in animal models of depression. Thus, an exact extrapolation or comparison with the clinical data is difficult. An interesting finding of early research with the learned helplessness model and olfactory bulbectomy models was that GABA-B receptors were downregulated in the "depressed" rats, and that chronic treatment with a variety of antidepressants upregulated the GABA-B receptor. "Depressed" rats that received chronic antidepressant treatment had normal density of GABA-B receptors [27]. These findings are provocative, but have proved difficult to replicate. Whether GABA-B agonists have antidepressant properties is not clear. GABA agonists are active in the learned helplessness model, reversing "depressed" behavior [28].

Our research with GABA in the learned-helplessness model has shown decreased GABA release from synaptosomes from hippocampus of helpless rats. This decrease was normalized by repeated treatment with tricyclic antidepressant in a time course which paralleled normalization of helpless behavior [29]. Interestingly, helpless behavior could be prevented by intracerebral microinjection of GABA into frontal cortex and hippocampus, and normalized by injection of GABA into hippocampus of helpless rats [27]. Bicuculine, a GABA-A receptor antagonist, caused helpless behavior in naïve, nonstressed rats when injected into hippocampus [27]. We have recently completed an extensive study of GABA-A and GABA-B receptors in learned helplessness using quantitative receptor autoradiography. Results were surprising, since we found no changes in either GABA-A or GABA-B receptors in frontal cortex, hippocampus, hypothalamus, or amygdala. In lateral septum, GABA-A receptors were upregulated in both helpless rats and rats that received inescapable stress but did not become helpless, but more so in the helpless rats. Also in lateral septum, GABA-B receptors were downregulated in the stressed, nonhelpless rats, but similar to control in helpless rats [30]. Parenthetically, in another study, lateral septum was also the only brain region where expression of the immediate early gene c-fos was decreased in helpless rats exposed to brief stress [31]. This brain region deserves additional study, since it serves as a relay between hippocampus and hypothalamus, two regions of the limbic system clearly implicated both in learned helplessness and in human depressive disorders. Thus, research with animal models supports an important role for GABA in regulating "depressive" behavior, but not a clear "deficit" hypothesis.

However, we should be cautious regarding acceptance of simplistic "neurochemical deficit" theories of mental illnesses. Just because something is found to be low in some patients with depression doesn't mean that this is etiologically related to the cause of illness, or that rectifying the deficit will correct the illness. Also, GABA has known interactions with all other neurotransmitters. The low GABA may not, therefore, be the "primary" lesion. For example, a primary disturbance in, say, glutamate function might lead to a secondary decrease in GABA.

VIII. BIPOLAR DISORDER

Low plasma GABA is found in patients with bipolar disorder, in both the manic and depressed phases of the illness. This means that low GABA is not a "state" marker for illness, since if it were, levels in persons with bipolar disorder would be different in mania from these in depression. "Bipolar disorder" is now widely recognized as a spectrum of related conditions. This spectrum includes psychiatric illnesses, personality disorders, and temperamental variants, ranging from classic Bipolar I (manic-depressive disease), through Bipolar II, Cyclothymia, Recurrent Brief Depression, Borderline Personality Disorder, and Hyperthymic Temperament. These conditions can be manifest by inappropriate, fluctuating mood, disturbed biorhythms, compromised social function, and impulsive aggressive behavior. Notably, when persons with a bipolar spectrum condition are not "symptomatic," they appear normal to most observers; indeed, a hallmark of bipolar disorder is its episodic nature, with good prognosis and interepisode recovery. While the vulnerability for bipolar disorder is clearly genetic, and known to involve several genes, the precise onset, severity, expression, and pattern of illness are influenced by developmental, environmental, toxic, and other factors. Hence, the concept that the phenotype of bipolar disorders will naturally range across a spectrum of clinical syndromes and behavioral manifestations, is coherent and rational.

With this developing knowledge of bipolar disorders has similarly evolved an increasing appreciation for neurotransmitter regulation of the dimensions of temperament and behavior, initially prompted by the clinical utility of selective serotonin reuptake inhibitors across a wide variety of clinical syndromes. Similarly, valproate appears to have beneficial effects for persons with impulsivity and aggression across diagnoses. At the molecular level, alterations in genes regulating biogenic amine transporters and receptors correlate more with dimensions of behavior, such as harm avoidance, novelty seeking, or high anxiety, than with arbitrarily defined syndromes or psychiatric diagnoses. Similarly, further research with GABA may well show low levels in patients across the bipolar spectrum. Thus, concurrent with the conceptualization of bipolar disorders as a spectrum, evolves an understanding that neurotransmitter alterations may influence a variety of temperaments or behaviors across psychiatric diagnoses.

IX. GABA AND MOOD DISORDERS

Hence, the theory that alterations in the neurotransmitter GABA are reflected in several "mental illnesses," as well as in related behaviors that are not clearly pathological, seems intuitive and plausible. The primacy of GABA as a neurotransmitter, regulating most if not all brain synapses, supports an important role for GABA regulation of behavior.

A logical hypothesis derived from these clinical observations is that low GABA represents the phenotype, or expression, of a genetic trait marker of bipolar disorder. Indeed, our laboratory has reported that low GABA is a trait marker for bipolar disorder in a subset of patients. Low GABA is not unique to bipolar disorder, since, as mentioned, a subset of patients with primary unipolar disorder also have low GABA. Since bipolar disorder and unipolar disorder share both symptomatic features and a genetic diathesis, finding a commonality in neurochemical abnormalities in these two conditions is, in fact, to be expected. Not surprisingly, low plasma GABA also occurs in about one-third of males with primary alcoholism. Again, a strong relationship has repeatedly been demonstrated between alcohol dependence and mood disorders, in both clinical and family studies. In addition to the extensive comorbidity between these diagnostic categories, it is of particular importance to the GABA theory of bipolar spectrum that episodes of alcohol abuse frequently precede the onset of first mania in persons with bipolar disorder, particularly males.

An interesting and seemingly counterintuitive observation we have made, in several studies, is that treatments which improve clinical state, in other words, treatments which improve depression and mania, tend to decrease, rather than increase, plasma levels of GABA [32]. In fact, in bipolar patients in the manic phase of the illness, we found an inverse correlation between plasma GABA levels and clinical response to valproate [33]. Again, this seems counterintuitive, since if valproate is rectifying a GABA deficit, one would predict that the patients with low GABA levels should be preferential valproate responders. Superficially, this seems to contradict to the hypothesis that low GABA correlates with psychopathology. However, if low GABA is represent a trait, rather than a state, biomarker of illness, indeed, treatments that improve overall clinical function might well be expected to revert GABA levels toward their premorbid and psychopathologically neutral state, which in a subset of persons with mood disorders is low. Hence, finding that antimanic and antidepressant treatments lead to a decrease in GABA in some symptomatic individuals, in synchrony with clinical improvement, provides an independent confirmation that low GABA is a trait, not a state, biomarker of illness.

X. A GABA THEORY OF MOOD DISORDERS

From these and other observations, we have developed a "GABA theory of mood disorders." This theory postulates that low GABA is a genetically determined trait which creates a vulnerability to development of symptoms of either depression or mania. Then, other factors, such as stress or heavy alcohol use, increase GABA over its baseline, creating an instability in the neuronal circuits of the limbic system. Though elevated above baseline, the levels are still lower than population norms. This instability in the limbic GABA system is accompanied by symptoms and behavioral features characteristic of the state of illness, and described clinically as depression or mania. Then, with mood-stabilizing treatment, cessation of heavy drinking, relief of stress, or with the passage of time, the GABA levels decrease back to the lower, premorbid baseline, in synchrony with clinical recovery and return to euthymia.

This theory is testable. Recently, we found that plasma GABA levels are under genetic control, with an autosomal-recessive, single-gene model [34]. Levels of GABA in brain are regulated by a relatively small number of enzymes, and by the GABA transporter. Thus, the number of candidate genes responsible for low GABA in mood disorders is small. Research in progress will attempt to identify the specific identify mutations that underlie the genetic basis of bipolar disorder.

Finally, we will comment regarding an interesting and probably important discrepancy in the data. Our earliest (1980–84) research studies on plasma GABA in psychiatric patients used a gas chromatography (GC) assay, which measured total GABA levels. In plasma, and in CSF, and, presumably in brain, most (~ 80%) of GABA is conjugated with other amino acids, and exists as di- and tripeptides. Thus, the GC assay measures both free and conjugated GABA in plasma. In these studies, we found that bipolar disorder in the manic phase had elevated levels of GABA, and patients with bipolar depression had levels similar to controls. Patients with primary, unipolar depression, and with alcoholism, had low levels, compared to control. Since 1984, our laboratory has used a high-performance liquid chromatography (HPLC) assay which is specific to measuring free, unconjugated GABA. Of course, the absolute levels reported are about one-fifth those found with the GC assay. Also, with the HPLC assay, we find low GABA in bipolar patients in both the manic and depressed phase of the illness, and in primary unipolar depression. Interestingly, with MRS measuring brain GABA levels, low levels are found in primary unipolar depression and in alcohol dependence, but not in bipolar depression. This suggests that the brain MRS measurements correspond to total GABA, with findings similar to those obtained with the GC assay. Future research should investigate the role of conjugated GABA in mood disorders.

XI. SUGGESTIONS FOR FUTURE RESEARCH

1. Clinical trials of new GABA agonists, and GABA-mimetic compounds, such as gabapentin and pregabalin, in depression and bipolar disorder.
2. Brain imaging with specific ligands for the GABA-A and GABA-B receptors.
3. Molecular genetic analyses of glutamate decarboxylase isoforms in mood disorders, coupled with measures of plasma and/or brain GABA.
4. Animal research measuring plasma or whole brain GABA in learned-helplessness and/or olfactory bulbectomy animal models of depression.
5. Development of a valid animal model for bipolar disorder.
6. Plasma and/or brain GABA measurement in bipolar spectrum conditions, such as borderline personality disorder.

ACKNOWLEDGMENT

Supported in part by the VA Medical Research Service and Creighton University.

REFERENCES

1. J Prosser, CW Hughes, S Sheikha, RA Kowatch, GL Kramer, N Rosenbarger, J Trent, F Petty. Plasma GABA in children and adolescents with mood behavior and comorbid mood and behavior disorders: a preliminary study. J Child Adoles Psychopharmacol 7:181–199, 1997.
2. F Petty. GABA and mood disorders: a brief review and hypothesis. J Affect Disord 34:275–281, 1995.
3. IS Shiah, LN Yatham. GABA function in mood disorders: an update and critical review. Life Sci. 63(15):1289–2303, 1998.
4. G Sanacora, GF Mason, DL Rothman, KL Behar, F Hyder, OA Petroff, RM Berman, DS Charney, JH Krystal. Reduced cortical gamma-aminobutyric acid levels in depressed patients determined by proton magnetic resonance spectroscopy. Arch Gen Psychiatry 56(11):1043–1047, 1999.
5. HM Emrich, D von Zerssen, W Kissling, HJ Moller, A Windorfer. Effect of sodium valproate on mania. The GABA-hypothesis of affective disorders. Arch Psychiatr Nervenkr 229(1):1–16, 1980.
6. LL Davis, W Ryan, B Adinoff, F Petty. Comprehensive review of the psychiatric uses of valproate. J Clin Psychopharmacol 20 (suppl 1)1S–17S, 2000.
7. RH Gerner, L Fairbanks, GM Anderson, JG Young, M Scheinin, M Linnoila, TA Hare, BA Shaywitz, DJ Cohen. CSF neurochemistry in depressed, manic, and schizophrenic patients compared with that of normal controls. Am J Psychiatry 141(12):1533–1540, 1984.
8. F Petty, GL Kramer, M Fulton, FG Moeller, AJ Rush. Low plasma GABA is a trait-like marker for bipolar illness. Neuropsychopharmacology 9:125–132, 1993.
9. F Petty, G Kramer, M Feldman. Is plasma GABA of peripheral origin? Biol Psychiatry 22:725–735, 1987.
10. F Petty, GL Kramer, CM Gullion, AJ Rush. Low plasma GABA in male patients with depression. Biol Psychiatry 32:354–363, 1992.
11. F Petty, GL Kramer, M Fulton, L Davis, AJ Rush. Stability of plasma GABA at four-year follow-up in patients with primary unipolar depression. Biol Psychiatry 37:806–810, 1995.

12. F Petty. Plasma GABA and mood disorders: a blood test for manic depressive disease? Clin Chem 40:296–302, 1994.
13. JM Bjork, FG Moeller, GL Kramer, M Kram, A Suris, AJ Rush, F Petty. Plasma GABA levels correlate with aggressiveness in relatives of patients with unipolar depressive disorder. Psychiatry Res 101:131–136, 2001.
14. PP Roy-Byrne, DS Cowley, D Hommer, DJ Greenblatt, GL Kramer, F Petty. Effect of acute and chronic benzodiazepines on plasma GABA in anxious patients and controls. Psychopharmacology 109:153–156, 1992.
15. AW Goddard, M Narayan, SW Woods, M Germine, GL Kramer, LL Davis, F Petty. Plasma levels of gamma-aminobutyric acid and panic disorder. Psychiatry Res 63:223–225, 1996.
16. F Petty, AD Sherman. Plasma GABA levels in psychiatric illness. J Affect Disord 6:131–138, 1984.
17. JA Coffman, F Petty. Plasma GABA levels in chronic alcoholics. Am J Psychiatry 142 (10)1204–1205, 1985.
18. A Honig, JR Bartlett, N Bouras, PK Bridges. Amino acid levels in depression: a preliminary investigation. J Psychiatr Res 22(3):159–164, 1988.
19. G Sanacora, GF Mason, JH Krystal. Impairment of GABAergic transmission in depression: new insights from neuroimaging studies. Crit Rev Neurobiol 14(1):23–45, 2000.
20. LL Davis, M Trivedi, A Choate, GL Kramer, F Petty. Growth hormone response to the $GABA_B$ agonist baclofen in major depressive disorder. Psychoneuroendocrinology 22:129–140, 1997.
21. KG Lloyd, B Zivkovic, D Sanger, H Depoortere, G Bartholini. Fengabine, a novel antidepressant GABAergic agent. I. Activity in models for antidepressant drugs and psychopharmacological profile. J Pharmacol Exp Ther 241(1):245–250, 1987.
22. F Petty, MH Trivedi, M Fulton, AJ Rush. Benzodiazepines as antidepressants: does GABA play a role in depression? Biol Psychiatry 38:578–591, 1995.
23. G Laakman, M Faltermaier-Temizel, S Bossert-Zaudig, T Baghai, G Lorkowski. Treatment of depressive outpatients with lorazepam, alprazolam, amytriptyline and placebo. Psychopharmacology (Berl).120(1):109–115, 1995.
24. A Kishimoto, K Kamata, T Sughihara, S Ishiguro, H Hazama, R Mizukawa, N Kunimoto. Treatment of depression with clonazepam. Acta Psychiatr Scand 77(1):81–86, 1988.
25. LL Davis, D Kabel, D Patel, AD Choate, C Foslien-Nash, GNM Gurguis, GL Kramer, F Petty. Valproate as an antidepressant in major depressive disorder. Psychopharmacol Bull 32:647–652, 1996.
26. F Petty, LL Davis. Unpublished data.
27. AD Sherman, F Petty. Neurochemical basis of the action of antidepressants on learned helplessness. Behav Neural Biol 30:119–134, 1980.
28. KG Lloyd, PL Morselli, H Depoortere, V Fournier, B Zivkovic, B Scatton, C Broekkamp, P Worms, G Bartholini. The potential use of GABA agonists in
29. M Kram, GL Kramer, M Steciuk, PJ Ronan, F Petty. Effects of learned helplessness on brain GABA receptors. Neuroscience Res 38:193–198, 2000.
30. AD Sherman, JL Sacquitne, F Petty. Specificity of the learned helplessness model of depression. Pharmacol, Biochem Behav 16:449–454, 1982.
31. M Kram, GL Kramer, M Steciuk, PJ Ronan, F Petty. Effects of learned helplessness on brain GABA receptors. Neurosci Res 38:193–198, 2000.
32. M Steciuk, M Kram, GL Kramer, F Petty. Decrease in stress-induced c-Fos-like immunoreactivity in the lateral septal nucleus of learned helpless rats. Brain Res. 822:256–259, 1999.
33. DP Devanand, B Shapira, F Petty, G Kramer, L Fitzsimons, B Lerer, HA Sackeim. Effects of electroconvulsive therapy on plasma GABA. Convuls Ther 11:3–13, 1995.
34. F Petty, AJ Rush, JM Davis, JR Calabrese, SE Kimmel, GL Kramer, JG Small, MJ Miller, AE Swann, PJ Orsulak, ME Blake, CL Bowden. Plasma GABA predicts acute response to divalproex in mania. Biol Psychiatry 39:278–284, 1996.
35. F Petty, M Fulton, GL Kramer, M Kram, LL Davis, AJ Rush. Evidence for the segregation of a major gene for human plasma GABA levels. Mol Psychiatry 4:587–589, 1999.

26

Signal Transduction Abnormalities in Bipolar Disorder

YAREMA B. BEZCHLIBNYK and L. TREVOR YOUNG
McMaster University, Hamilton, Ontario, Canada

I. INTRODUCTION

There is compelling evidence of neurobiological impairment in patients with bipolar disorder (BD). Although the exact biochemical abnormalities underlying this disorder have not been conclusively identified, the multiple neurotransmitter systems involved in regulating mood have directed many researchers to consider the functional balance among these complex, interacting systems. The temporal discrepancy between the pharmacological and clinical effects of mood stabilizers has implicated cellular and molecular processes that occur over time in the mechanism of mood stabilizer action. In the CNS, intracellular signal transduction pathways are uniquely able to mediate the downstream activities of these multiple neurotransmitter systems. They affect both the levels and function of these systems, and link them together to coordinate complex neurobiological events [1,2]. Indeed, higher-order brain functions implicated in BD, such as behavior, mood, and cognition, are critically dependent on signal transduction processes for their proper functioning. Furthermore, post-receptor signaling systems connect immediate synaptic stimuli with long-term changes in gene expression. Consequently, it has been suggested that the dysregulation of one or more intracellular signal transduction processes leads to episode specific alterations in gene expression, and a periodic loss of homeostasis via the activation of existing physiologic feedback mechanisms which may be crucial to the clinical manifestation of BD [3]. Therefore, signal transduction molecules have presented researchers with a wide range of compelling targets for investigating the biological basis of BD and its treatment. In the following sections, we present a brief overview of these intracellular signal transduction pathways, and review some of the major clinical findings implicating these processes in BD.

II. SIGNAL TRANSDUCTION SYSTEMS

Extracellular "first" messengers, which include neurotransmitters, modulators, hormones, growth factors, and ions, activate various neuronal receptors. In turn, these receptors are coupled to diverse intracellular second-messenger systems via different mechanisms, including the activation of receptor-linked guanine-nucleotide binding proteins (G-proteins) [4]; the direct activation of ligand-gated receptor/ion channel complexes [5]; and the stimulation of tyrosine receptor- and nonreceptor-kinase activity [6]. The result is the integration, amplification, and transmission of the extracellular signals to specific intracellular effector enzymes or ion channels, which catalyze the production of an extensive array of cascading "second" messengers that act on various protein kinases [1]. These protein kinases are ultimately responsible for modulating and regulating a diverse set of biologically essential intracellular responses, including gene expression.

A. G-Proteins

Guanine-nucleotide binding proteins (G-proteins) are an integral part of the intracellular signaling pathway, with ~ 80% of all known first messengers eliciting cellular responses through receptors coupled to these molecules. G-proteins are heterotrimers, consisting of an α subunit, which binds and hydrolyzes guanosine triphosphate (GTP), and a tightly but noncovalently linked dimer composed of the regulatory β and γ subunits [7]. The functional diversity of G-proteins is primarily conferred by the α subunits, which form an extensive family consisting of four main classes that selectively regulate different effector enzymes: $G\alpha_s$, $G\alpha_i$, $G\alpha_q$, and $G\alpha_{1/2}$ [8,9]. This functional heterogeneity allows for the coupling of a wide variety of receptors to the same or different signal transduction systems, leading to near-infinite combinations. Recent evidence has also suggested important roles for the $\beta\gamma$ subunits in intracellular signal transduction. Aside from modulating GDP/GTP exchange and serving to anchor the α subunit to the plasma membrane [4], the $\beta\gamma$ subunit has been shown to activate K^+ channels, negatively regulate calcium ion channels, and possibly activate the mitogen activated protein kinase (MAPK) pathways through Ras [10–12]. Furthermore, it has been shown that these molecules variously affect certain members of the adenylyl cyclase (AC) family [13], and directly activate phospholipase C (PLC) [10,14]. Thus, even modest changes in the levels and/or function of the G-proteins have the potential to markedly alter the signal generated by various receptor ligands.

B. Cyclic AMP–Generating Pathway

Following receptor activation, G-proteins interact with a number of effector enzymes. In particular, coupling of either the stimulatory or inhibitory G-protein subunits (α_s or $\alpha_{i1/2}$, respectively) to AC has been extensively characterized (Fig. 1) [7]. There are multiple isoforms of AC which catalyze the production of cyclic adenosine monophosphate (cAMP), a ubiquitous second messenger, from ATP. These can be broadly grouped into three subfamilies depending on whether they are stimulated, inhibited, or unaffected by Ca^{2+}/calmodulin (CaM) binding [15]. Furthermore, these enzymes are differentially susceptible to regulation by the $\beta\gamma$ G-protein subunits [13], as well as phosphorylation by both PKC and PKA [16–18]. The production of cAMP by this enzyme is balanced through rapid degradation by cyclic nucleotide phosphodiesterases, which also exist as multiple subtypes [19]. Cyclic AMP second messengers in turn regulate many cellular functions, such as metabolism and gene transcription by acting through several intracellular targets. Chief among these is AMP-dependent protein kinase, also known as protein kinase A (PKA) [20,21].

The inactive PKA tetramer consists of two catalytic subunits, coupled to a dimer of regulatory subunits. When cAMP levels rise within the cell, the binding of this factor to each of the regulatory subunits induces the dissociation of the holoenzyme, thereby releasing the monomeric catalytic subunits. Once released, these subunits are free to regulate the activity of a number of substrate proteins (including receptors, ion channels, cytoskeletal proteins, phosphatase inhibitors, and transcription factors) by phosphorylating them at specific serine and threonine residues [22,23]. This action continues until the level of cAMP in the cell diminishes, causing the regulatory subunits to regain their high affinity for the catalytic monomers.

C. Phosphoinositide Pathway

The G-protein isoforms G_q/G_{11} couple many neurotransmitter receptors to yet another signaling pathway, via the phosphatidylinositol-specific phospholipase (PLC) enzyme (Fig. 2) [24]. The activation of these receptors stimulates PLC, which in turn induces the hydrolysis of the inositol-containing phospholipid phosphatidylinositol 4,5-bisphosphate (PIP_2) to two second messengers—1,2-diacylglycerol (DAG), and inositol 1,4,5-triphosphate (IP_3) [25]. IP_3 stimulates the release of intracellular stored calcium from the smooth endoplasmic reticulum (ER) into the cytosol, by binding to an IP_3-specific receptor on the ER surface [26]. Metabolism of IP_3 then proceeds either by dephosphorylation to $Ins(1,4)P_2$, or phosphorylation to 1,3,4,5-inositol terakisphosphate (IP_4) by PI3-kinase. This latter isoform may mediate slower and more prolonged responses by enhancing the entry of calcium into the cell from external sources [27]. DAG, on the other hand, typically in conjunction with calcium, activates protein kinase C (PKC), which comprises another family of kinases [25]. Furthermore, because inositol crosses the blood brain barrier poorly, cells must maintain a sufficient supply of myo-inositol for the resynthesis of PIP_2, and the maintenance and

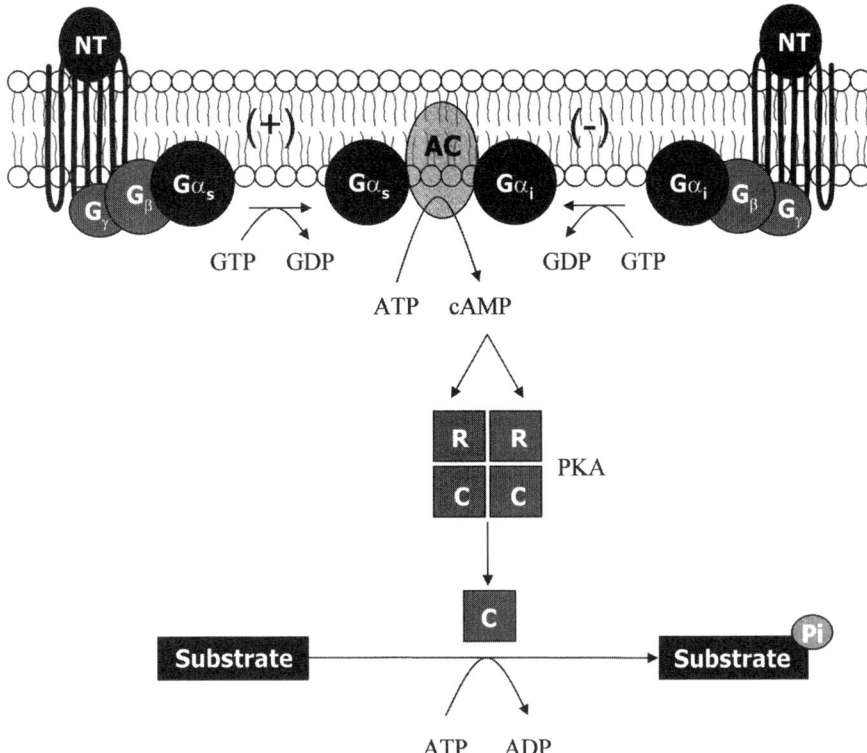

Figure 1 G-protein-coupled cyclic AMP system. Neurotransmitters (NT) bind to G-protein-coupled transmembrane receptors, which interact with G-proteins composed of α, β, and γ subunits. Receptor activation induces a conformational change in receptor associated G-protein, resulting in the exchange of GDP for GTP on the a subunit. The Gα subunit then stimulates (Gα_s) of inhibits (Gα_i) adenylyl cyclase (AC). Activation of AC converts ATP to cAMP. As a second messenger, cAMP activates cAMP-dependent protein kinase A by binding to the regulatory (R) domains and inducing the dissociation of the catalytic (C) domains. The free C moiety in turn phosphorylates various substrates.

efficiency PI-mediated signal transduction. This supply of myo-inositol thus depends on the dephosphorylation of inositol phosphates. The enzyme which catalyzes this reaction, inositol monophosphatase (IMPase), thus plays a crucial role in the PI signaling pathway [28].

PKC is a ubiquitous enzyme that is involved in a diverse array of cellular responses [29]. Together with other kinases, it appears to play a major role in the regulation of synaptic plasticity, learning, and memory [30]. Molecular cloning of this enzyme indicates that it exists as a family of closely related subspecies heterogeneously distributed in the brain, organized into subfamilies based on domain homology and biochemical properties: conventional PKC isozymes that require calcium for activation and are sensitive to phorbol esters; those that are sensitive to phorbol esters but not to calcium; and PKC, which is not responsive to either [29]. Activation involves the binding of DAG (or certain hydrophobic esters) to a specific regulatory site on the enzyme, and the translocation of the enzyme from the cytosol to the particulate fraction of both neuronal tissue and platelets [25,31]. Interestingly, several isoforms of PKC may be co-expressed in a single cell, which together with their differential tissue distribution suggests that each isozyme may exert specific and distinct cellular functions [32]. In addition, PKC negatively regulates the activity of various phospholipases, which along with the degradation of IP$_3$ by activation of IP$_3$ phosphatase, serves to control signaling through the PI and calcium cascades [33].

D. Intracellular Calcium Signaling

Although the importance of the calcium ion in synaptic transmission and neurotransmitter release is well established, it has become increasingly apparent that calcium has a critical role in mediating diverse intracellular events. These include synaptic plasticity, cell survival, and excitotoxic cell death. Increased intracel-

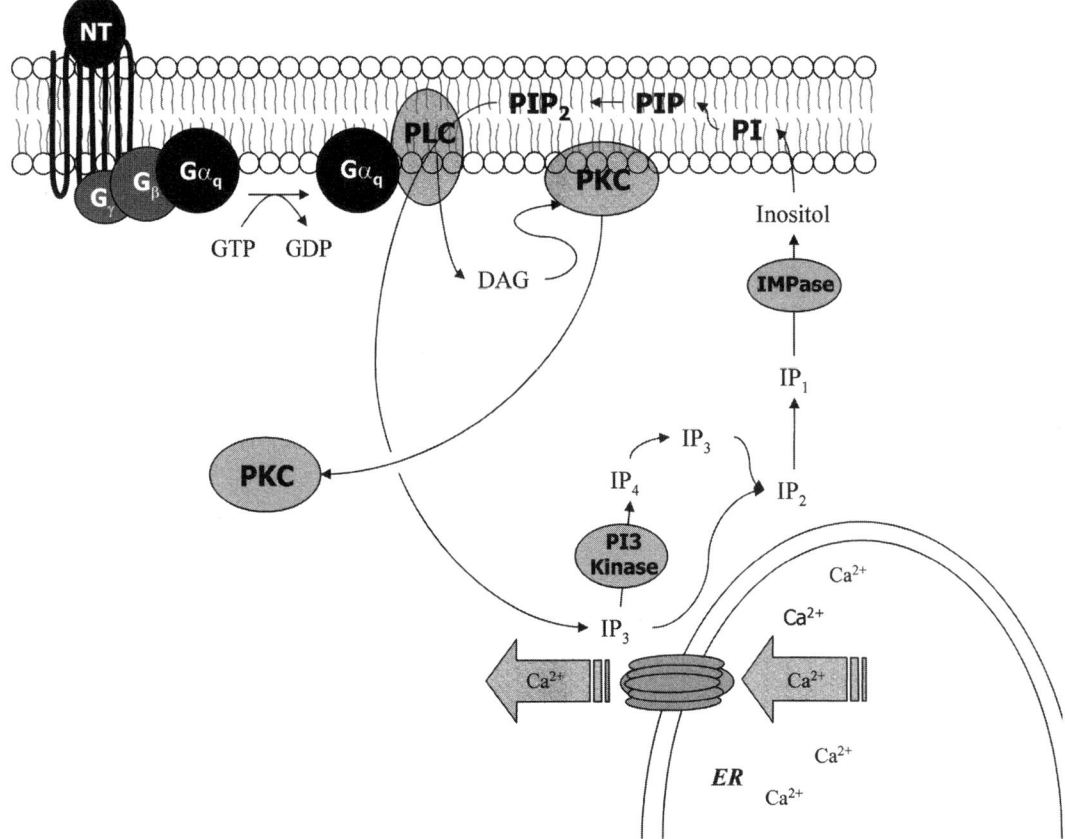

Figure 2 Phosphoinositide-generated second-messenger system. The binding of a ligand activates receptors coupled to a G-protein (G_q) composed of α, β, and γ subunits. The $G\alpha_q$ subunit dissociates and activates PLC, which catalyzes the hydrolysis of phosphatidylinositol 4,5-biphosphate (PIP_2) and generates two second messengers—diacylglycerol (DAG), and 1,4,5-inositol triphosphate (IP_3). IP_3 releases calcium from the endoplasmic reticulum (ER), which increases levels of intracellular calcium. IP_3 is metabolized by either phosphorylation to IP_4 or dephosphorylation to IP_2. Subsequently, PI3-kinase dephosphorylates IP_4. Finally, IMPase dephosphorylates these substrates, producing inositol, which replenishes the phospholipid content of the membrane. DAG, on the other hand, activates PKC (synergistically with Ca^{2+} in most cases), which is then free to phosphorylate various substrate molecules.

lular Ca^{2+} has also been shown to affect protein phosphorylation [34], neuronal periodicity [35], neurotransmitter synthesis and release [36], and the formation of new functional associations [37]. Consequently, the mechanisms by which changes in intracellular calcium levels can lead to diverse, long-lasting biochemical alterations have been a target of directed investigation.

Cells have two major sources of calcium—the extracellular milieu, and the endoplasmic reticulum. Calcium influx from either of these stores into the cytosol is controlled by ion channels, which are regulated in turn by voltage changes or by the binding of various ligands such as NMDA (Fig. 3) [38]. With respect to the stores in the ER, we have already discussed Ca^{2+} release via IP_3 binding to specific ion channel–coupled receptors in the ER. Experiments have also shown that certain calcium ion channels may be regulated by the $\beta\gamma$ G-protein subunit [39,40], and that calcium can autoregulate its own release through the process of Ca^{2+}-induced Ca^{2+} release (CICR) [41]. This process, which occurs upon neuronal excitation, generally involves regional increases in Ca^{2+} concentration providing a triggering pulse of Ca^{2+} that diffuses throughout the cell in a regenerative manner to recruit neighboring Ca^{2+}-sensitive channels, such as the IP_3 receptor in the ER membrane [41]. In any case, with cellular stimulation the concentration of calcium in the cytosol rises rapidly, from approximately 100 nM to values in the mM range [42]. At high intracellular con-

Signal Transduction Abnormalities in Bipolar Disorder

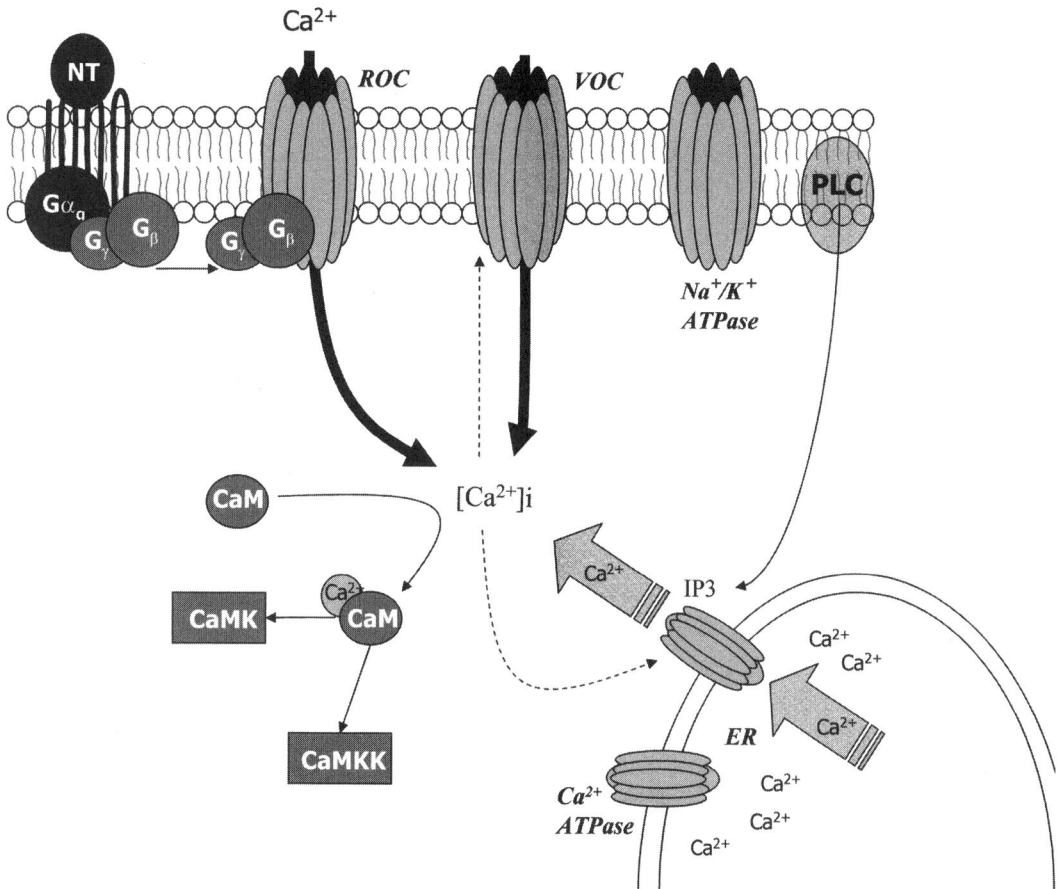

Figure 3 Intracellular calcium signaling. Calcium influx into the cytosol is stimulated by the binding of a ligand to a G-protein-coupled receptor, or by the direct activation of a transmembrane ion channel. In the first case, activation of the receptor frees α and $\beta\gamma$ G-protein subunits, which are variously able to stimulate Ca^{2+} signaling in different tissues and conditions. Both mechanisms open Ca^{2+} ion channels, allowing Ca^{2+} to enter along its gradient, and rapidly increase intracellular Ca^{2+} levels. At low concentrations, Ca^{2+} triggers the activation of ER and transmembrane ion channels. However, when Ca^{2+} concentrations become too high, Ca^{2+} negatively regulates these same channels. Intracellular calcium is bound to calmodulin, which transduces the ionic currents to enzymatic actions on specific substrates. In particular, Ca^{2+}/calmodulin is able to potentiate PKC, PKA, PLC, and various CaM kinases. The calcium concentration gradient is reestablished by Ca^{2+}- and Na^+/K^+-ATPases.

centrations however, Ca^{2+} downregulates its signaling by inhibiting IP_3 receptor sensitivity [26], and stimulating the hydolysis of IP_3 [43]. Return of intracellular free calcium to resting levels terminates many of its cellular effects. This gradient is reestablished and maintained by the action of membrane-associated Ca^{2+} ATPases (Ca^{2+} pumps), which drive Ca^{2+} against a steep concentration gradient either out of the cell or into intracellular stores [42], or through energy-dependent Na^+/Ca^{2+} exchange, which pumps Ca^{2+} out of and Na^+ into the cytosol of the cell [44,45].

After entering the cytosol, Ca^{2+} interacts with a number of regulatory proteins. One of these is calmodulin, a small Ca^{2+}-binding protein which acts as an intracellular Ca^{2+} sensor and is critical in the regulation of diverse cellular events [46]. Following Ca^{2+} binding, the Ca^{2+}/calmodulin (CaM) complex regulates a number of other enzymes. These include the CaM-dependent protein kinases (CaMKs), other Ca^{2+}-sensitive kinase isozymes, certain protein phosphatases, and some members of the adenylate cyclase and PLC families [46]. In addition, CaMK I, IV, and certain CaMK II isoforms may be specifically involved in mediating transcriptional activation of gene expression in response to changes in Ca^{2+} fluctuations in the cytosol [47,48].

E. ERK/MAP Kinase Signaling Pathway

The MAPK cascade is an evolutionarily conserved signaling pathway that plays a crucial role in cell growth and survival in diverse organisms. In vertebrates, at least six MAPK cascades have been identified, each of which transduces signals to a specific serine-threonine kinase subfamily. These subfamilies include ERKs 1 and 2, c-Jun-N-terminal kinases (JNKs), p38 MAPKs, ERK5, ERK7, and MOK [49–51]. The activation of these diverse kinases proceeds from a wide range of extracellular stimuli, of which the growth factors are the most extensively characterized. Growth factors such as nerve growth factor (NGF) exert their cellular effects by binding to a family of receptors known as receptor tyrosine kinases (trks) [52]. Analogous to the G-protein coupled pathways, stimulation of receptor trks by growth factor binding recruits and activates members of the ras family of low-molecular-weight GTP-binding proteins. The ras-signaling pathway subsequently involves the recruitment of a serine-threonine kinase (or MAPK kinase kinase) such as Raf-1 or B-raf, which then phosphorylates MAPK kinase (MEK). In turn, MEK activation results in the phosphorylation and activation of its target, the ERK1/2 members of the MAPK family of serine-threonine kinases [53]. Interestingly, one substrate for these ERKs is the ribosomal protein SG kinase family (RSK1–3), the activation and nuclear translocation of which play an essential role in the inducible expression of many genes [53,54]. However, alternative pathways leading to activation of MAPKs have been uncovered, and each MAPK pathway has its own unique set of related enzymes responsible for transducing signals from the receptors to the effector molecules.

F. Integration of Intracellular Responses

It is increasingly apparent that the various second messenger systems can be markedly influenced by the activity of other transduction pathways. Intracellular signaling is refined at multiple levels by an extensive cross-regulatory network, whereby second messengers linked to one receptor modulate the effector responses at another. For example, the $\beta\gamma$ subunit released upon activation of $G\alpha_i$-coupled receptors may augment the production of cAMP [55]. Furthermore, intracellular calcium balances the production and degradation of cAMP by stimulating or inhibiting AC activity [15], and potentiating Ca^{2+}/CaM-dependent phosphodiesterases (PDEs) [56]. Other studies suggest that Ca^{2+} may affect PKA activity [57] and stimulate the PI-signaling pathway by potentiating PLC and PKC activation. In turn, cAMP regulates intracellular Ca^{2+} by decreasing the sensitivity of IP_3 receptors [58], stimulating the phosphorylation of voltage-dependent ion channels [59], opening receptor-activated Ca^{2+} channels [60], increasing Ca^{2+} removal by stimulating Ca^{2+}-ATPase [61], and inhibiting the activity of $PLC\beta_2$ [62]. Additionally, cAMP inhibits agonist-stimulated hydrolysis of membrane phophoinositides, thus reducing the production of the PI-generated second messengers. In turn, PKC has been shown to stimulate cAMP accumulation by acting on certain ACs [16], and possibly by inhibiting $G\alpha_s$ and $G\alpha_{i2}$ mRNA transription [63].

A fairly extensive body of research also recognizes the intricate cross-communication between these signal transduction pathways and the MAPK system. In particular, the ras-mediated activation of both Raf-1 and B-raf is inhibited by PKA [64,65], whereas this same enzyme serves to activate B-raf through the GTPase Rap1 [66]. Evidence also suggests interaction with the calcium and PI signal transduction cascades. Upon GTP binding, Rap1b recruits PLC-γ to the cell membrane, where it can act on inositol phosphates [67]. Therefore, phosphorylation of Rap1b by PKA or CaMK results in the inhibition of PLC-γ, reducing PI-generated signaling [67,68]. In turn, both second messengers generated by PLC activation, calcium and DAG, are able to induce Rap1 activation [69,70]. PKC is also able to stimulate the ERK/MAPK pathway, by activating MEK1 and ERK1 via raf [71]. Alternatively, Ca^{2+} is able to activate the MAPK pathway through ras, ostensibly via CaMK stimulation of GTP binding and activation of various tyrosine kinases [72,73].

G. Regulation of Gene Expression

The propagation of extracellular stimuli to the nucleus of the cell may result in long-term changes at the genomic level. These changes occur through differential expression of a broad assortment of genes. One way to regulate the expression of these genes is to control the rate of mRNA transcription initiated by RNA polymerases. This action is mediated by *trans*-acting proteins known as transcription factors, which bind to specific *cis*-acting regulatory elements on specific target genes. These transcription factors are a major target for intracellular second messengers and their related protein kinases, which can alter their activity through changes in phosphorylation state, or concentration within the cell [74]. In particular, researchers have focused intensively on two such factors—CREB and activating protein 1 (AP-1) (see Fig. 4).

Cyclic AMP–responsive element–binding (CREB) protein is intimately involved in the regulation of numerous genes, including other transcription factors and key members of the signal transduction pathways [75,76]. The CREB family of transcription factors includes CREB itself, the CRE modulator (CREM), the activating transcription factors (ATF), and the inducible cAMP early repressor (ICER). CREB is expressed constitutively in an inactive form, with activation requiring phosphorylation at Ser-133 by a variety of protein kinases [76,77]. These include PKA, MAPKs (such as RSK1-3), and Ca^{2+}/calmodulin-dependent kinases (CaMKs), which are regulated by the major signal transduction pathways described above. Active phosphorylated CREB (pCREB) proteins then free to regulate gene transcription by binding to a regulatory consensus region in the promoter of certain target genes, known as the cyclic AMP-response element (CRE) [78].

AP-1 is of a collection of homodimeric and heterodimeric complexes composed of the transcription factors Fos and Jun. Each of these is the product of a separate family, and is induced rapidly and transiently by a wide variety of extracellular stimuli—the induction of c-fos is rapid and transient, reaching its maximal levels within 30 min and lasting for 1–2 h [79], while the induction of c-jun, which positively regulates its own transcription, is longer lasting and varies from a few hours to several days in a cell type – and stimulus-dependent manner [79]. Both Fos and Jun are translocated to the nucleus, where they form the dimeric AP-1 complex. AP-1 proteins then bind to a common nucleotide sequence, known as the AP-1 site or the TPA response element (TRE), which is found in

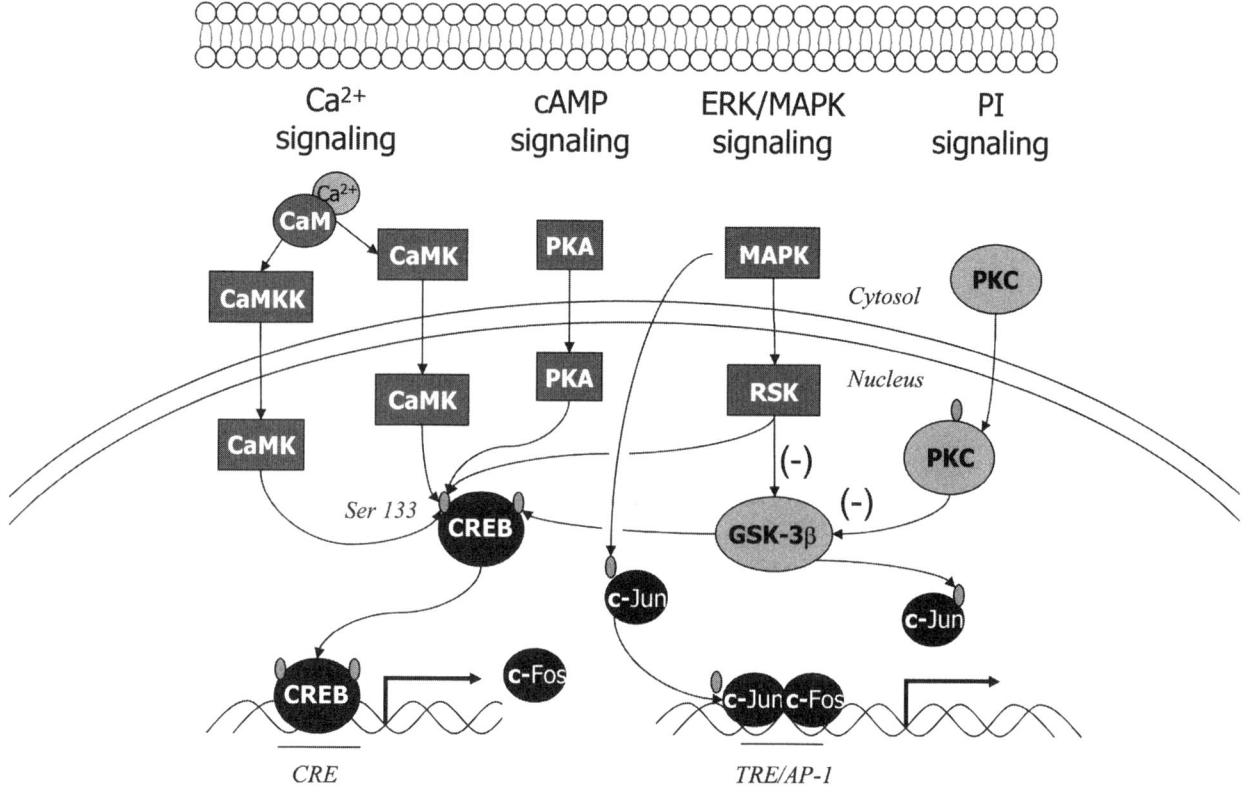

Figure 4 Regulation of gene expression. Signal transduction systems transmit extracellular events to intracellular responses by modulating the activation state of key protein kinases. These protein kinases, which include Ca^{2+}-calmodulin-dependent protein kinases (CaMK), cAMP-dependent protein kinase (PKA), PKC, and elements of the MAPK cascade, in turn modulate the activity of transcription factors such as CREB and AP-1. For example, when CREB is phosphorylated at serine-133, it may bind to a cAMP-response element (CRE) in various target genes. This in turn regulates the transcription of c-fos, which combines with c-jun to form the AP-1 class of transcription factors. AP-1 may then bind to its own consensus sequence, the TRE site. Concomitantly, c-jun and CREB are both regulated by GSK3β.

the regulatory domain of many important genes [79]. These include various neuropeptides, neurotrophins, receptors, transcription factors, enzymes involved in neurotransmitter biosynthesis, and a number of cytoskeletal-binding proteins [79]. Activation and binding of the AP-1 complex can negatively or positively regulate transcription at this site [80,81].

Recently, experiments have revealed another modulator of both pCREB and AP-1 DNA binding activity glycogen synthase kinase 3β (GSK3β). GSK3β is a highly conserved serine-threonine protein kinase which is regulated by at least three signal transduction cascades including the PI3-K cascade [82], the Wnt cascade [83], and the MAP kinase cascade [84], and plays a critical role in regulating long-term nuclear events. It phosphorylates c-jun at three sites adjacent to the DNA-binding motif, thereby reducing AP-1 binding activity [85]. As for CREB, phosphorylation at Ser-133 may make it a substrate for GSK-3β mediated phosphorylation at Ser-129, which could contribute to CREB activation under certain conditions [77]. In addition, it may regulate diverse brain proteins, such as microtubules [86], neurofilaments [87], myelin-basic protein [88], nerve growth factor [89], and tau [90]. As such, GSK3β further refines the complex patterns of gene expression in the CNS.

III. SIGNAL TRANSDUCTION ABNORMALITIES IN BIPOLAR DISORDER

Among the first studies to implicate disturbances in postreceptor signaling in the pathophysiology of BD revealed attenuated β-adrenergic receptor-activated AC activity in peripheral cells (platelets and lymphocytes) from patients with unipolar and bipolar depression [91–94]. Studies confirmed that such changes were not accompanied by changes in βAR density or affinity [95,96], which led these investigators to suggest reduced responsiveness or desensitization rather than diminished number of β adrenergic receptors, perhaps as a result of a defect distal to the receptor complex [95,97]. As a result, a wide variety of techniques and methodologies have been utilized to ascertain the locus of these postreceptor changes. Additionally, research has identified a number of signal transduction molecules as targets of medications that are most effective in the treatment of mood disorders (for review see [30]). In order to determine whether or not these treatments correct an underlying signal transduction abnormality, a number of studies have examined the state of various intracellular transduction molecules in patient samples. These include studies in blood cells (such as platelets and leukocytes) and postmortem brain samples. As will be seen, these studies have generally complemented those drawn on the effects of mood-stabilizing medication, and supported theories of signal transduction abnormalities in the pathobiology of BD.

A. G-Proteins

Numerous independent laboratories have examined G-proteins in patients with BD, in light of their critical role in transducing signals from extracellular events to effectors with the cell (Table 1). Interest in these proteins was stimulated by studies in molecular pharmacology, which suggested that the mood stabilizer lithium attenuates the function of stimulatory G proteins [33,98,99]. In two postmortem brain studies, Young et al. [100,101] described increased immunoreactivity of the G-protein a subunit $G\alpha_s$ (but not $G\alpha_i$, $G\alpha_o$, or $G\beta$) in frontal, temporal, and occipital cortex of subjects with BD. Furthermore, they described increased forskolin-stimulated AC activity in BD temporal and occipital cortices, which was significantly correlated with the elevated $G\alpha_s$ measures. These findings were supported by a more recent postmortem study [102], which also reported elevated immunoreactivity specific to $G\alpha_s$, as well as increased agonist-activated [^{35}S]GTPγS binding to $G\alpha$ subunits in the frontal cortex of BD subjects. These investigators also suggest that the proportion of G-proteins in the trimeric state is significantly increased in bipolar brain, as observed through increases in both pertusis toxin (PTX)- catalyzed ADP ribosylation (a measure dependent on the heterotrimeric state of the substrate G-protein), and coprecipitation of $G\beta$ with $G\alpha$ [102]. Both of these measures were significantly reduced relative to controls upon receptor activation, indicative of enhanced receptor–G-protein coupling. Interestingly, there is also evidence of increased PTX-catalyzed ADP-ribosylation in platelet membranes of lithium-treated BD subjects [103].

Complementary observations in peripheral blood cells have largely confirmed the above findings, and explored the relationship between G-protein signaling and mood state. Indeed, Schreiber and associates [104] first reported enhanced agonist-stimulated binding of a tritiated nonhydrolyzable analog of GTP ([^{3}H]Gpp(NH)p) in mononuclear leukocytes (MNLs) of manic BD patients, implicating increased G-protein levels and/or enhanced receptor-mediated

Table 1 G-Protein Abnormalities

Tissue	Patient group	Physiological change	Ref.
Postmortem cerebral cortex	BD	↑ Gα_s; ↔ Gα_i, Gα_o, and Gβ levels	100, 101
	BD	↔ Gα_s mRNA levels	119
	BD	↑ coupling of 5-HT receptors to membrane G-proteins; ↑ Gα_s levels; ↔ Gα_i, Gα_o, Gα_z, G$\alpha_{q/11}$, Gβ; ↑ ADP-ribosylation of Gα_i and Gα_o; ↑ Gβ coprecipitation with Gα	102
	BD	↓ Gα_s levels in Li-treated subjects;	110
MNLs	BD (depressed)	↑ Gα_s and Gα_i levels	96
	BD (depressed)	↓ agonist-induced Gpp(NH)p binding; ↓ Gα_s levels	109
	BD (manic and depressed)	mania – ↑ agonist-induced Gpp(NH)p binding; depression – ↓; mania – ↑ Gα_s and Gα_i levels; depression – ↓; ↔ Gβ	105
	BD (euthymic)	↓ Gα_s levels in Li-treated patients; ↔ in Haloperidol-treated subjects	112
	BD (Type I Li-treated euthymic)	↔ Gα_s levels	111
Platelets and MNLs	BD (mostly manic, Li-treated euthymic)	↑ Gα_s levels in leukocytes; ↓ G$\alpha_{q/11}$ and ↑ ADP ribosylation in platelets from Li-treated patients	103
	BD I and II (euthymic on medication)	↑ Gα_s levels in platelets of BD types I and II, irrespective of treatment; ↑ in MNLs	106
Granulocytes	BD (depressed and Li-treated euthymic)	↑ Gα_s levels	108

activation of G-proteins in patients with BD. A large body of data strongly suggests an increase in both level and function of G-protein a stimulatory and inhibitory subunits in the manic and euthymic states [103–106], using immunoreactivity and/or [^{3}H]Gpp(NH)p binding assays.

Somewhat conflicting results have been observed in the depressed state, however. Young and associates [107] initially observed elevated Gα_s and Gα_i levels in MNLs from unmedicated depressed bipolar patients, a finding which was recently confirmed in granulocytes by another group [108]. In contrast, a number of studies conducted by Avissar et al. [105,109] show significantly decreased Gα_s and Gα_i levels and function in MNLs from bipolar as compared to manic patients or controls, and a concomitant negative correlation between Gα_s protein function and severity of depression. These observations strongly suggest that changes in G-protein α subunits are a state-related abnormality.

Although the literature has been quite consistent with respect to elevated Gα subunit levels and/or function in patients with BD, recent studies in both postmortem brain [110] and transformed lymphoblasts [111] have not been able to confirm these findings. By way of explanation, it has been suggested that differences in the level and function of this G-protein may be influenced by differences in mood state [105,111]. As a number of studies indicate that lithium treatment [99,103,108,112], antidepressants [113], and ECT [114] may modulate G-protein-a subunit activity, treatment history may also be informative to the G-protein response [110,111,115]. It should also be noted that it has proved more difficult to identify the mechanisms responsible for the observed G-protein abnormalities. Linkage studies of BD with the gene coding for Gα_s have yielded negative results [116–118], and Gα_s mRNA levels do not appear to be altered in postmortem brain from subjects with BD [119]. In any case, the transcriptional and posttranscriptional regulation of G-protein subunits is likely to be complex, and it has yet to be determined whether G-protein abnormalities are directly involved in BD or if they represent a secondary manifestation of dysfunction in some as yet uninvestigated mechanism. On the whole, studies in G-proteins suggest that altered Gα levels and function, perhaps through increased receptor-G-protein coupling, play important roles in the pathophysiology of bipolar disorder, by way of their pivotal roles as an amplifiers, integrators, and transducers of extracellular signals to diverse effector pathways in the CNS.

B. Cyclic AMP Signaling Pathway

As has been described, a substantial body of literature suggests that increased basal and receptor-activated AC activity in BD brain and peripheral cells is linked to disturbances in the G-protein a subunits [91–93,100,101,104,105,109,120]. Furthermore, these changes correlate significantly with treatment or mood state, with a number of studies demonstrating decreased AC activity in depressed [105,109] or lithium-treated euthymic BD patients [120]. As disturbances in activated AC, which catalyzes the formation of cAMP from ATP, may lead to further disturbances in the cAMP second messenger system, several groups have undertaken to determine whether these observations are attended by abnormalities downstream in the cAMP signaling cascade (Table 2).

The cellular effects of cAMP are mediated through cAMP-dependent protein kinase A (PKA). As such, investigations have examined this enzyme extensively. A postmortem study of [^{3}H]cAMP binding to the PKA regulatory (R) subunits [121] was the first to suggest that the proportion of these subunits is reduced in brains of bipolar patients, possibly as a result of altered synthesis or protein degradation stemming from increased cAMP signaling [reviewed by 122]. As the activation state of PKA depends on the dissociation of R subunits following cAMP binding from the catalytic (C) moiety, a more recent postmortem brain study demonstrating increased basal and stimulated cAMP-dependent PKA activity in temporal cortex of patients with BD, as well as increased PKA sensitivity to cAMP, suggests a relative reduction in R subunit levels in BD [123]. Subsequent examination of the

Table 2 Cyclic AMP Signaling Pathway Abnormalities

Tissue	Patient group	Physiological change	Ref.
Postmortem cerebral cortex	BD	↑ forskolin-stimulated cAMP production;	100, 101
	BD	↔ AC levels	202
	BD	↓ [^{3}H]-cAMP binding	121
	BD	↑ maximal and basal cAMP dependent PKA activity; ↓ PKA EC50 for cAMP	123
	BD	↓ forskolin-stimulated AC; ↓ CREB levels in anticonvulsant-treated subjects	110
MNLs	Depressed (including BD)	↓ Isoproterenol-stimulated cAMP production	95, 97
	BD (manic)	↑ agonist-induced Gpp(NH)p binding	104
	BD type I	↑ basal and NaF stimulated ↓ isoproterenol induced cAMP formation in subjects with high Ca^{2+} levels	156
Platelets	Depressed (including BD)	↓ PGE1-stimulated cAMP; ↓ NE inhibition of PGE1-stimulated cAMP production	203
	BD (unmedicated to Li-treated)	↓ forskolin-stimulated AC activity subsequent to Li-treatment in vitro	93
	BD (Li-treated euthymic)	↓ basal and stimulated AC activity	94
	BD (euthymic)	↑ cAMP dependent protein phosphorylation	125, 126
	BD (euthymic untreated—pre and post Li-treatment)	↑ basal and cAMP-stimulated protein phosphorylation following 15 days of Li-treatment in BD; ↔ in controls	127
	BD (unmedicated)	↑ PKA catalytic subunit levels vs. untreated euthymic BD and controls; ↔ PKA regulatory subunit (type I and II) levels; ↑ Rap1 levels	124

PKA subunits, while failing to uncover changes in R subunit levels, revealed significantly elevated PKA C immunolabelling in both manic and depressed BD patients, suggesting that elevated PKA activity in BD is a state-related abnormality resulting from an imbalance in the PKA subunits [124]. In assessing the functional measures of PKA activation, this group showed significantly increased cAMP-dependent phosphorylation of the MAPK-linked GTPase Rap1b in platelets of both lithium-treated and untreated euthymic BD subjects [125,126,127]. However, subsequent analyses of Rap1 immunoreactivity showed that the levels of this protein were significantly higher in platelets from BD patients irrespective of mood state [124,126], suggesting that changes in Rap1 phosphorylation may be due to preexisting changes in Rap1 levels. This highlights the importance of further studies to clarify the relationship between PKA levels and cAMP-dependent phosphorylation.

C. Phosphoinositide Pathway

Studies in peripheral cells and postmortem brain have generally supported the notion of PI abnormalities in bipolar disorder (Table 3). However, initial investigations of free inositol levels failed to uncover significant changes in unmedicated BD patients [128,129], although one study observed reduced incorporation

Table 3 Phosphoinositide Signaling Pathway Abnormalities

Tissue	Patient group	Physiological change	Ref.
Postmortem occipital cortex	BD	↑ $G\alpha_{q/11}$ and PLC-β immunoreactivity; ↔ $G\beta$	142
	BD	↓ GTPγS and NaF-stimulated [^{3}H]PI hydrolysis in BD vs. Li treated and controls; ↔ Ca^{2+} stimulated PLC activity	143
	BD	↓ inositol levels in frontal cortex; ↔ IMPase activity	130
Postmortem frontal cortex	BD	↑ PKC activation; ↑ PMA and phorbol-ester induced PKC translocation; ↑ cytosolic α and membrane associated γ- and ε-PKC isozyme levels; ↓ cytosolic ε-PKC levels	148
	BD (depressed)	↔ IMPase activity	28
Platelets	BD (Li treated euthymic)	↓ PLC activity	94
	BD (manic—pre and post Li treatment)	↑ membrane-bound vs cytosolic PKC activity; ↑ 5-HT elicited PKC translocation; ↓ basal and 5-HT elicited PKC activity following 2 weeks of Li treatment	144
	BD (manic)	↑ PIP_2 levels	133
	BD (single case study)	↑ PIP_2 levels manic vs. untreated euthymia; ↓ Li treated vs. manic; ↔ between Li treated vs. untreated euthymic	135
	BD (Li-treated euthymic)	↓ PIP_2; ↔ in other phospholipids	136
	BD (manic and depressed)	↑ basal PKC activity in manic BD; ↓ PKC responsiveness to PMA/thrombin in depressed BD; ↑ PKC responsiveness to 5-HT; ↔ in PMA induced translocation	145
	BD (type I unmedicated and Li-treated)	↔ PKC-α levels	204
	BD (euthymic untreated—pre and post Li treatment)	↓ PIP_2; following Li treatment; ↔ in other phospholipids	137
	BD (Li-treated euthymic)	↓ PIP_2; ↓ cytosolic PKC-α levels; no correlation between PLC and PIP_2 measures	138
	BD (depressed)	↑ membrane PIP_2 levels; ↔ in other phospholipids	134
Erythrocytes	BD (unmedicated and Li-treated)	↓ inositol 1-phosphatase activity in Li treated BD	131

of tritiated inositol to PI intracellular pools [128]. Subsequent studies in postmortem brain did observe a significant decrease in free inositol levels in the frontal cortex of BD patients, but found no change in IMPase activity [130]. This finding supports an earlier study which found no significant difference in IMPase activity from erythrocytes of unmedicated BD as compared to controls [131]. However, this same study did confirm an inhibitory effect of lithium, consistent with preclinical observations. In addition, recent findings from MRI studies indicate a temporal dislocation between lithium-induced myoinositol depletion and clinical improvement [132]. As the mechanism of lithium therapy does not appear to involve inositol depletion in vivo, this effect may be seen as at best an initiating event. To further evaluate these findings, researchers examined the relative content of membrane phosphoinositides, with a particular emphasis on the major PLC substrate PIP_2, under various mood and treatment states. Brown et al. [133] were the first to show increased levels of PIP_2 in the manic state of BD, a finding that was recently observed in platelets of patients with bipolar depression as well [134]. Since PIP_2 is the precursor of IP_3 and DAG, the authors suggested increased PI signaling as a possible outcome of their findings [133,134]. A subsequent study by the same group reported on a patient whose PIP_2 membrane levels increased in the course of cycling from unmedicated euthymia to mania, and normalized with a return to euthymia subsequent to lithium treatment [135]. This finding was explored further in a number of subsequent studies, which together show significant and specific reduction in platelet PIP_2 levels in lithium treated euthymic BD patients as compared to controls [136–138]. While mood normalization cannot be discounted as a contributing factor, these studies suggest that lithium may blunt PI signaling, at least in part by diminishing the relative abundance of PIP_2 [136].

Regulation of PLC, which hydrolyzes membrane inositol phospholipids (chiefly PIP_2) to yield IP_3 and DAG, is mediated primarily by the G-protein G_q and G_{11} isoforms [24,139,140], although one or more G_i or G_o isoforms may also play a role [4,141]. However, there are few direct analyses of the primary PI-coupled G-proteins in clinical samples. Indeed, while one postmortem study reported increased abundance of both $G\alpha_{q/11}$ and $PLC\beta$ specific to the occipital region of subjects with BD [142], a second study observed decreased PI-coupled G-protein activation in the same region, as determined by GTPγS-stimulated [^{3}H]PI hydrolysis [143]. In an attempt to explain these findings, the authors suggest an adaptive increase in $G\alpha_{q/11}$ expression as a result of deficient PI signaling activity in BD, although long-term lithium treatment could also have confounded the results [143]. Of relevance, an earlier study in peripheral blood cells found no significant differences in $G\alpha_{q/11}$ levels in unmedicated BD subjects, although the levels of these proteins in lithium-treated samples were decreased relative to controls [103]. Together with the observed changes in AC-coupled G-proteins, the data from PLC-coupled $G\alpha_q$ and $G\alpha_{11}$ may be indicative of a functional imbalance between abnormally decreased PI-signaling and elevated cAMP-signaling systems [143].

PKC, the effector molecule in the PI-signaling pathway, is an important intracellular enzyme that has stimulated much interest in recent years. A number of studies published by Friedman and coworkers [144,145] demonstrated increased membrane-bound platelet PKC activity in the manic state of subjects with BD. These findings were seen as further confirmation of impaired PI signaling, as PKC is activated directly in response to intracellular DAG levels. In addition, the earlier study, which assessed platelets obtained from BD patients before and during lithium treatment, showed increased serotonin-stimulated PKC translocation (a measure of stimulated PKC activity) from the cytosolic to the particulate fraction in the manic state [144]. This measure, along with basal PKC activity, was reduced following lithium treatment for 2 weeks [144], and in platelets from euthymic lithium treated BD patients [137,138], similar to preclinical findings [31,146,147]. More recently, investigators from the same laboratory examined the PKC enzyme in postmortem brain from subjects with bipolar disorder [148]. They observed increased PKC activity and translocation to membrane fractions, as well as increased levels of cytosolic α- and membrane-associated γ- and ζ-PKC isozyme levels in frontal cortex from BD subjects relative to tissue from controls. Additional studies by this same laboratory and others suggest that these findings may be specific to BD [144,145,149,150] and may be related to changes in the enzyme protein per se, or to increased expression of membrane RACK (receptor for activated C-kinase) protein, which anchors the enzyme to the membrane [151,152].

Given the relatively consistent findings of elevated PKC activity in bipolar disorder, and related studies showing attenuating effects of lithium treatment on PKC activity, Manji and coworkers have recently suggested that PKC inhibitors may be efficacious in the clinical treatment of this disorder [30]. As such, they have initiated pilot studies with tamoxifen, a synthetic nonsteroidal antiestrogen widely used in the treatment of breast cancer, which was recently found to be a selective PKC inhibitor as well. Interestingly, preliminary findings from a small sample are so far promising, and provide evidence of some antimanic qualities for this medication [153]. However, these results must be interpreted with caution, and conclusions must await results of large-scale, randomized double-blind placebo-controlled studies.

D. Intracellular Calcium Signaling

The calcium signaling system has increasingly been the focus of investigation in mood disorders research. Evidence supports the notion that Ca^{2+} channels may be coupled to $G\alpha_s$ in some tissues [154,155], suggesting that the relatively robust findings of increased $G\alpha_s$ levels associated with BD may result in increased cytosolic Ca^{2+} concentrations. A recent study by Emamghoreishi et al. [156] indicates that trait-dependent disturbances with respect to βAR sensitivity and G-protein-coupled AC activity may occur in conjunction with high concentrations of Ca^{2+}. Specifically, they described decreased isoproterenol-stimulated, and increased basal and NaF-stimulated cAMP formation in β lymphocytes from BD type I patients who had high intracellular Ca^{2+} levels, compared to BD patients with normal Ca^{2+} concentration and controls. As βAR sensitivity is subject to regulation by a number of factors, including PKC and PKA activity (which are in turn sensitive to either direct or indirect modulation by Ca^{2+}), dysfunction at the level of one pathway may disrupt the intricate crosstalk between various signal transduction systems [156].

Furthermore, calcium communicates directly with the primary effector molecules of the PI-signaling pathway, and increased PI signaling might be expected to be accompanied by increased levels of intracellular calcium. As such, although investigators have maintained a long-standing interest in calcium signaling irrespective of these other second-messenger systems, the findings in these two postreceptor signaling systems may be relevant for future and current study. Initial studies in calcium signaling by Carman et al. [157] uncovered a significant relationship between transient increases in serum Ca^{2+} levels and the switch into mania. Direct measurement of intracellular free calcium has largely supported and extended these observations, with Dubovsky and colleagues [158] describing increased baseline Ca^{2+} concentration in platelets and leukocytes from unmedicated bipolar patients in both manic and depressed states (Table 4). Indeed, given that Ca^{2+} is necessary for PKC activation, many of the previously described findings with respect to elevated PKC activity and translocation in patients with BD may be at least partly a consequence of increased affinity of certain PKC isozymes to Ca^{2+} [145]. However, while the aforementioned Ca^{2+} studies are intriguing in that they complement previously described studies in the PI-signaling pathway, other investigators have not been able to confirm these findings [159–163].

On the other hand, treatment of blood cells with various agents has generated more robust observations. Stimulation of platelets from unmedicated depressed and manic BD patients with platelet-activating factor and thrombin significantly increased calcium response relative to euthymic BD, MDD, and controls [164–166]. Likewise, agonist-induced stimulation of serotonin $5HT_{2A}$ receptors produced consistent elevations in Ca^{2+} response in both depressed bipolar and unipolar subjects, as reported in a number of studies by diverse laboratories [159,163,167–169]. These findings were also confirmed in a very recent study including a wide range of psychiatric disorders, although in this case they were found to be specific to platelets from BD patients from a sample [162]. By way of explanation, the authors suggest that some patients classified as MDD in previous studies from their group [163,166,169] have recently been reclassified on follow-up diagnoses, with significantly increased 5HT-induced mobilization over the other "unipolar" patients that may have inadvertently skewed the results in favor of significance [162]. Another study of both unmedicated manic and euthymic bipolar patients further confirms an increase in 5HT-stimulated Ca^{2+} responses in the manic state [170]. While some of these studies suggest that elevated Ca^{2+} concentration and/or response may be a state-dependent variable that normalizes with remission of mood [158], others indicate that the persistence of these findings in euthymia suggests it to be a trait-dependent variable [161,167,169,171,172), and at least one study could not discern a correlation between severity of depressive symptoms and Ca^{2+} response [169]. Finally, while the involvement of the calcium/calmodulin activated kinases in regulating other signal transduction pathways and gene transcription has been well documented in preclinical samples, only one clinical study has been published on this family of enzymes to date. This study, conducted in postmortem cerebral cortex, was unable to associate changes in CaMK immunoreactivity with BD [173].

Table 4 Calcium Signaling Pathway Abnormalities

Tissue	Patient group	Physiological change	Ref.
MNLs	BD types I and II	↑ basal Ca^{2+} concentration; ↓ percent change in phytohemagglutinin stimulated vs. basal Ca^{2+} levels in BD type I	172
	BD type I	↑ basal and NaF stimulated and ↓ isoproterenol stimulated cAMP formation in BD subjects with high basal Ca^{2+} levels;	156
Platelets and MNLs	BD (manic and depressed)	↑ basal and stimulated Ca^{2+} levels in manic and depressed states	158, 205, 206
	BD types I and II, unmedicated and Li-treated	↑ basal and stimulated Ca^{2+} concentration; ↔ between types or med state in BD; no correlation between Ca^{2+} and severity	207
Platelets	BD (unmedicated)	↑ basal and stimulated Ca^{2+} levels in manic and depressed states vs. euthymic and control	165, 164
	BD (manic and depressed)	↑ 5-HT stimulated Ca^{2+} response	159
	BD (Li-treated)	↑ basal Ca^{2+} levels; ↑ thrombin-stimulated Ca^{2+} response; ↑ thrombin-stimulated Ca^{2+} response with Li treatment in vitro	171
	BD (depressed)	↑ 5-HT-stimulated Ca^{2+} response	163
	BD (manic and depressed, Li-treated euthymic)	↑ PAF and thrombin stimulated Ca^{2+} response in unmedicated states	166
	BD (depressed)	↑ 5-HT stimulated Ca^{2+} responses	167, 168
	BD	↔ basal or stimulated Ca^{2+}; ↑ serum and 5-HT stimulated intracellular Ca^{2+} levels in Li treated group	160
	BD (depressed)	↑ 5-HT-stimulated Ca^{2+} response	169
	BD (depressed)	↔ basal or 5-HT/thrombin induced Ca^{2+} response with either in vitro or chronic Li treatment	208
	BD (eythymic)	↔ basal Ca^{2+}	161
	BD (manic)	↑ 5-HT stimulated Ca^{2+} responses	170
	BD (manic and depressed)	↔ Ca^{2+} uptake; ↓ Ca^{2+} uptake following in vitro Li treatment in all samples	209
	BD (depressed to Li treatment—longitudinal study)	↑ 5-HT-stimulated Ca^{2+} response correlated with response to treatement with mood stabilizers	210
	BD	↔ basal or 5-HT induced Ca^{2+}	162
Platelets and Erythrocytes	BD	↔ Ca^{2+} response; ↑ Ca^{2+}-ATPase levels in manic and depressed BD	175
Erythrocytes	BD (depressed)	↓ Na^+/K^+-ATPase activity	177, 178, 211
	BD (manic and depressed)	↑ Ca^{2+}-ATPase activity	174
Neutrophils	BD (depressed and euthymic; Li-treated euthymic)	↑ fLMP-stimulated Ca^{2+} responses in BD vs. controls; ↓ fLMP-stimulated Ca^{2+} responses in Li treated BD	212
	BD (Li-treated euthymic)	↓ fLMP-stimulated Ca^{2+} responses	213

In accounting for the mechanisms behind disrupted calcium signaling, further confirmation of calcium-signaling abnormalities in BD was provided by reports of elevated Ca^{2+} extrusion ATPase activity in red blood cells from manic and depressed [174,175], as well as lithium-treated [176] BD patients in comparison to matched controls. These findings suggest either a compensatory change in Ca^{2+}-ATPase activity as a result of—or a primary change leading to—increased levels of intracellular free Ca^{2+}. As well, some groups have described significantly lower Na^+-K^+-ATPase activity, which regulates Na^+/Ca^{2+} exchange, in red blood cells of depressed patients with BD [177–180].

E. Regulation of Gene Expression

Gene expression is critical to the maintenance of cellular viability and function, and has also been strongly implicated in the neuronal changes thought to underlie the pathobiology as well as pharmacotherapy in subjects with BD. Recently, studies have attempted to associate diagnosis or treatment with changes in gene expression, using a variety of techniques with the ability to simultaneously analyze expression of thousands of genes. These powerful new tools thus hold out the exciting prospect of screening large numbers of genes for differential regulation of factors which may be relevant to the underlying disease process or pharmacotherapy. Differential display, serial analysis of gene expression (SAGE), and cDNA expression arrays are three such techniques which have produced promising results in both clinical and preclinical samples [181–185], including a possible decrease in the inhibitory cytokine transforming growth factor beta in the frontal cortex of subjects with BD [181].

The protein kinases regulated by postreceptor signal transduction pathways have among their targets several transcription factors which are essential to maintaining responsive and accurate gene expression. The observation of signal transduction abnormalities thus suggests that downstream consequences at the level of these transcription factors may play a role in the neuronal changes thought to underlie BD. To this end, many studies have examined the effects of pharmacotherapy on transcription factor activity in cell lines and animal models. It has repeatedly been observed that therapeutic concentrations of both lithium and valproate regulate AP-1 binding activity in these systems [182,186–188]. Likewise, Nibuya et al. [189] demonstrated that chronic AD treatment increased rat hippocampal CREB protein and mRNA levels as well as its binding to the CRE, a finding which was confirmed in postmortem brain samples from subjects with MDD [190]. However, the status of these enzymes in subjects with BD has not been extensively explored. The sole clinical study to this end, by Dowlatshahi et al. [110], measured the levels of CREB in temporal and occipital cortices of subjects with BD, MDD, SCZ, and controls. While they were unable to observe any significant association of CREB levels with BD, decreased levels were observed in subjects who died as a result of suicide, and those treated with anticonvulsants at the time of death. This later finding, which is opposite of that observed with AD treatment, supports studies in both rat brain and cultured cells [187,191,192]. Furthermore, it is consistent with the effects of lithium treatment on the signal transduction pathways (see above) and the clinical effects of ADs and ACs in different states, such as mania and depression.

IV. DISCUSSION

The above data provide convincing evidence of signal transduction abnormalities associated with BD. In summary, the findings supporting cAMP-signaling abnormalities in BD are extensive and suggest increased levels of $G\alpha_s$, at least in the manic state. These reports are supported by observed abnormalities further downstream, in elevated AC-mediated cAMP production and PKA activation. In the PI pathway, a set of findings including increased PIP_2 levels and PKC activity has generally implicated increased signaling along this pathway as well. Indeed, experiments currently in progress are attempting to ascertain the efficacy of PKC inhibitors as antimanic agents. However, the few studies on G-protein-coupled PLC activity have been less conclusive. Finally, increased Ca^{2+} responses have been observed by a number of independent laboratories in both peripheral blood cells and postmortem brain tissue of subjects with BD, broadly supporting the findings in PI signaling. However, in spite of attempts to control for the use of medications, the possibility that treatment with antidepressants and/or mood stabilizers may be at least partly responsible for some of the observed changes cannot be discounted [110]. Furthermore, extensive crosstalk between the AMP and the phosphoinositide- and calcium-signaling pathways confounds the elucidation of clear loci of major effect in this pathway.

Given the complexity of intracellular communication, more recent studies have implicated the involvement of other signal transduction pathways in BD, including the ERK/MAPK cascade. The last few years have witnessed the growth of considerable interest in this pathway, in light of the extensive crosstalk between this and the other signal transduction systems, and the recent focus on neurodevelopmental and kindling models as etiologically relevant in mood disorders research [3,193–196]. Studies by Perez et al. have revealed that the levels of Rap1b are increased in subjects with BD, with a concomitant increase in its active phosphorylated state [124–127]. However, the exact mechanism of Rap1 regulation, and its place in the intracellular milieu in reference to these other signaling pathways, remains highly speculative. In addition, studies of gene expression have directed research to consider novel targets, such as GSK-3β. In 1973, a team of researchers first demonstrated that therapeutic concentrations of lithium inhibit the phosphorylation of glycogen synthase by acting on an enzyme subsequently identified as GSK-3β [197,198]. More recently, VPA has been shown to have a similar effect on GSK-3β activity, further suggesting that this enzyme may play a role in the pathophysiology of BD [199]. Lesort and associates [200] examined the immunoreactivity of GSK-3β and two proteins shown to be modified by this enzyme—tau and β-catenin—in prefrontal cortex from subjects with BD and matched controls. Although no change in any of these measures reached statistical significance, the tau profile was modified in subjects with BD. Similarly, a recent study could find no change in GSK-3β protein levels in frontal cortical samples from subjects with BD [201]. Therefore, these studies suggest that mood stabilizer–mediated GSK-3β regulation may correct pathobiological dysfunction at other loci. However, further study is needed to establish the role of GSK-3β in pharmacotherapy.

V. CONCLUSION

Aggregate findings from a diverse array of clinical samples strongly implicate dysregulation of second-messenger systems in the pathophysiology of BD. In particular, altered levels and function of Gα subunits and effector molecules such as PKA and PKC have consistently been associated with BD in both peripheral cells and postmortem brain, suggesting that these systems may be involved in the complex neurobiological changes believed to underlie this disorder. On the other hand, the continuing inability to establish direct links between clinical abnormalities and specific biochemical insults has recently been attributed to the complex interactions between many, if not all, of these signal transduction systems. Intracellular signaling is refined at multiple levels by an extensive cross-regulatory network, whereby second messengers linked to one receptor modulate the effector responses at another. The integration and modulation of these responses ensure the fidelity of signal transduction, and finely attune signaling to conditions both within and without the cell. This process also ensures that the initiation, timing, and termination of cellular responses are coordinated so as to maintain the functional integrity of the system. Likewise, BD exhibits a marked variability in the symptoms and course of the illness across patients, who also respond differently to pharmacotherapy. As it is unlikely that a single defect could account for these observations, BD may be due to the interaction of many interacting abnormalities. Thus, more recent studies have implicated novel second-messenger systems, such as the ERK/MAPK cascade, in the progression of mood disorders. With the fortuitous advances in molecular techniques such as DD, SAGE, and cDNA array hybridization, it is now possible to visualize the end result of these diverse abnormalities within the nucleus. While the published findings from these studies have for the most part been limited to cell culture and animal models, we have recently published a cDNA array study in postmortem brain samples of subjects with BD [181]. These results, in combination with work in progress at many different research centers, promise to further our understanding of signal transduction abnormalities in the context of a complex, multifactorial disease such as BD.

REFERENCES

1. EM Ross. Signal sorting and amplification through G protein–coupled receptors. Neuron 3:141–152, 1989.
2. CJ Hudson, LT Young, PP Li, JJ Warsh. CNS signal transduction in the pathophysiology and pharmacotherapy of affective disorders and schizophrenia. Synapse 13:278–293, 1993.
3. RM Post. Transduction of psychosocial stress into the neurobiology of recurrent affective disorder. Am J Psychiatry 149:999–1010, 1992.
4. L Birnbaumer, J Abramowitz, AM Brown. Receptor-effector coupling by G proteins. Biochim Biophys Acta 1031:163–224, 1990.
5. J Giraudat, M Dennis, T Heidmann, PY Haumont, F Lederer, and JP Changeux. Structure of the high-affinity binding site for noncompetitive blockers of the

acetylcholine receptor: [³H]chlorpromazine labels homologous residues in the beta and delta chains. Biochemistry 26:2410–2418, 1987.
6. A Ullrich, J Schlessinger. Signal transduction by receptors with tyrosine kinase activity. Cell 61:203–212, 1990.
7. L Birnbaumer. Receptor-to-effector signaling through G proteins: roles for beta gamma dimers as well as alpha subunits. Cell 71:1069–1072, 1992.
8. CW Taylor. The role of G proteins in transmembrane signalling. Biochem J 272:1–13, 1990.
9. JR Hepler, AG Gilman. G proteins. Trends Biochem Sci 17:383–387, 1992.
10. DE Clapham, EJ Neer. New roles for G-protein beta gamma-dimers in transmembrane signalling. Nature 365:403–406, 1993.
11. E Reuveny, PA Slesinger, J Inglese, JM Morales, JA Iniguez-Lluhi, RJ Lefkowitz, HR Bourne, YN Jan, LY Jan. Activation of the cloned muscarinic potassium channel by G protein beta gamma subunits. Nature 370:143–146, 1994.
12. P Crespo, N Xu, WF Simonds, JS Gutkind. Ras-dependent activation of MAP kinase pathway mediated by G-protein beta gamma subunits. Nature 369:418–420, 1994.
13. WJ Tang, AG Gilman. Type-specific regulation of adenylyl cyclase by G protein beta gamma subunits. Science 254:1500–1503, 1991.
14. MR Wing, D Houston, GG Kelley, CJ Der, DP Siderovski, TK Harden. Activation of phospholipase C-epsilon by heterotrimeric G protein beta-gamma-subunits. J Biol Chem 276:48257–48261, 2001.
15. RK Sunahara, CW Dessauer, AG Gilman. Complexity and diversity of mammalian adenylyl cyclases. Annu Rev Pharmacol Toxicol 36:461–480, 1996.
16. O Jacobowitz, J Chen, RT Premont, R Iyengar. Stimulation of specific types of Gs-stimulated adenylyl cyclases by phorbol ester treatment. J Biol Chem 268:3829–3832, 1993.
17. J Kawabe, G Iwami, T Ebina, S Ohno, T Katada, Y Ueda, CJ Homcy, Y Ishikawa. Differential activation of adenylyl cyclase by protein kinase C isoenzymes. J Biol Chem 269:16554–16558, 1994.
18. G Iwami, J Kawabe, T Ebina, PJ Cannon, CJ Homcy, Y Ishikawa. Regulation of adenylyl cyclase by protein kinase A. J Biol Chem 270:12481–12484, 1995.
19. JA Beavo. Cyclic nucleotide phosphodiesterases: functional implications of multiple isoforms. Physiol Rev 75:725–748, 1995.
20. JA Beavo, PJ Bechtel, EG Krebs. Activation of protein kinase by physiological concentrations of cyclic AMP. Proc Natl Acad Sci USA 71:3580–3583, 1974.
21. JD Scott. Cyclic nucleotide–dependent protein kinases. Pharmacol Ther 50:123–145, 1991.
22. EG Krebs, JA Beavo. Phosphorylation-dephosphorylation of enzymes. Annu Rev Biochem 48:923–959, 1979.
23. SI Walaas, P Greengard. Protein phosphorylation and neuronal function. Pharmacol Rev 43:299–349, 1991.
24. AV Smrcka, JR Hepler, KO Brown, PC Sternweis. Regulation of polyphosphoinositide-specific phospholipase C activity by purified Gq. Science 251:804–807, 1991.
25. MJ Berridge. 5-Hydroxytryptamine stimulation of phosphatidylinositol hydrolysis and calcium signalling in the blowfly salivary gland. Cell Calcium 3:385–397, 1982.
26. SH Snyder, S Supattapone. Isolation and functional characterization of an inositol trisphosphate receptor from brain. Cell Calcium 10:337–342, 1989.
27. RF Irvine. Inositol phosphates and Ca^{2+} entry: toward a proliferation or a simplification? FASEB J 6:3085–3091, 1992.
28. JR Atack, HB Broughton, SJ Pollack. Structure and mechanism of inositol monophosphatase. FEBS Lett 361:1–7, 1995.
29. AC Newton. Protein kinase C: structure, function, regulation. J Biol Chem 270:28495–28498, 1995.
30. HK Manji, RH Lenox. Ziskind-Somerfeld Research Award. Protein kinase C signaling in the brain: molecular transduction of mood stabilization in the treatment of manic-depressive illness. Biol Psychiatry 46:1328–1351, 1999.
31. S Weiss, J Ellis, DD Hendley, RH Lenox. Translocation and activation of protein kinase C in striatal neurons in primary culture: relationship to phorbol dibutyrate actions on the inositol phosphate generating system and neurotransmitter release. J Neurochem 52:530–536, 1989.
32. S Stabel, PJ Parker. Protein kinase C. Pharmacol Ther 51:71–95, 1991.
33. S Avissar, G Schreiber, A Danon, RH Belmaker. Lithium inhibits adrenergic and cholinergic increases in GTP binding in rat cortex. Nature 331:440–442, 1988.
34. EG Lapetina, SP Watson, P Cuatrecasas. myo-Inositol 1,4,5-trisphosphate stimulates protein phosphorylation in saponin-permeabilized human platelets. Proc Natl Acad Sci USA 81:7431–7435, 1984.
35. EK Matthews. Calcium and membrane permeability. Br Med Bull 42:391–397, 1986.
36. H Rasmussen. The calcium messenger system (1). N Engl J Med 314:1094–1101, 1986.
37. DL Alkon, M Kubota, JT Neary, S Naito, D Coulter, H Rasmussen. C-kinase activation prolongs Ca^{2+}-dependent inactivation of K^+ currents. Biochem Biophys Res Commun 134:1245–1253, 1986.
38. RW Tsien, D Lipscombe, DV Madison, KR Bley, AP Fox. Multiple types of neuronal calcium channels and

39. HM Colecraft, DL Brody, DT Yue. G-protein inhibition. J Neurosci 21:1137–1147, 2001.
40. M De Waard, H Liu, D Walker, VE Scott, CA Gurnett, KP Campbell. Direct binding of G-protein betagamma complex to voltage-dependent calcium channels. Nature 385:446–450, 1997.
41. V Henzi and AB MacDermott. Characteristics and function of Ca^{2+}- and inositol 1,4,5-trisphosphate-releasable stores of Ca^{2+} in neurons. Neuroscience 46:251–273, 1992.
42. DE Clapham. Intracellular calcium. Replenishing the stores. Nature 375:634–635, 1995.
43. M Eberhard, P Erne. Regulation of inositol 1,4,5-trisphosphate-induced calcium release by inositol 1,4,5-trisphosphate and calcium in human platelets. J Recept Signal Transduct Res 15:297–309, 1995.
44. E Carafoli. Intracellular calcium homeostasis. Annu Rev Biochem 56:395–433, 1987.
45. MP Blaustein. Sodium/calcium exchange and the control of contractility in cardiac muscle and vascular smooth muscle. J Cardiovasc Pharmacol 12(suppl 5):S56-S68, 1988.
46. H Schulman. The multifunctional Ca^{2+}/calmodulin-dependent protein kinases. Curr Opin Cell Biol 5:247–253, 1993.
47. A Ghosh, ME Greenberg. Calcium signaling in neurons: molecular mechanisms and cellular consequences. Science 268:239–247, 1995.
48. RP Matthews, CR Guthrie, LM Wailes, X Zhao, AR Means, GS McKnight. Calcium/calmodulin-dependent protein kinase types II and IV differentially regulate CREB-dependent gene expression. Mol Cell Biol 14:6107–6116, 1994.
49. MK Abe, WL Kuo, MB Hershenson, MR Rosner. Extracellular signal-regulated kinase 7 (ERK7), a novel ERK with a C-terminal domain that regulates its activity, its cellular localization, cell growth. Mol Cell Biol 19:1301–1312, 1999.
50. Y Miyata, E Nishida. Distantly related cousins of MAP kinase: biochemical properties and possible physiological functions. Biochem Biophys Res Commun 266:291–295, 1999.
51. TP Garrington, GL Johnson. Organization and regulation of mitogen-activated protein kinase signaling pathways. Curr Opin Cell Biol 11:211–218, 1999.
52. Y Muragaki, N Timothy, S Leight, BL Hempstead, MV Chao, JQ Trojanowski, VM Lee. Expression of trk receptors in the developing and adult human central and peripheral nervous system. J Comp Neurol 356:387–397, 1995.
53. J Blenis. Signal transduction via the MAP kinases: proceed at your own RSK. Proc Natl Acad Sci USA 90:5889–5892, 1993.
54. J Xing, JM Kornhauser, Z Xia, EA Thiele, ME Greenberg. Nerve growth factor activates extracellular signal-regulated kinase and p38 mitogen-activated protein kinase pathways to stimulate CREB serine 133 phosphorylation. Mol Cell Biol 18:1946–1955, 1998.
55. KD Lustig, BR Conklin, P Herzmark, R Taussig, HR Bourne. Type II adenylylcyclase integrates coincident signals from Gs, Gi, Gq. J Biol Chem 268:13900–13905, 1993.
56. RK Sharma. Signal transduction: regulation of cAMP concentration in cardiac muscle by calmodulin-dependent cyclic nucleotide phosphodiesterase. Mol Cell Biochem 149–150:241–247, 1995.
57. U Dobbeling, MW Berchtold. Down-regulation of the protein kinase A pathway by activators of protein kinase C and intracellular Ca^{2+} in fibroblast cells. FEBS Lett 391:131–133, 1996.
58. S Supattapone, SK Danoff, A Theibert, SK Joseph, J Steiner, SH Snyder. Cyclic AMP–dependent phosphorylation of a brain inositol trisphosphate receptor decreases its release of calcium. Proc Natl Acad Sci USA 85:8747–8750, 1988.
59. J Chad, D Kalman, D Armstrong. The role of cyclic AMP-dependent phosphorylation in the maintenance and modulation of voltage-activated calcium channels. Soc Gen Physiol Ser 42:167–186, 1987.
60. GJ Barritt. Receptor-activated Ca^{2+} inflow in animal cells: a variety of pathways tailored to meet different intracellular Ca^{2+} signalling requirements. Biochem J 337(Pt 2):153–169, 1999.
61. J Helman, BL Kuyatt, T Takuma, B Seligmann, BJ Baum. ATP-dependent calcium transport in rat parotid basolateral membrane vesicles. Modulation by agents which elevate cyclic AMP. J Biol Chem 261:8919–8923, 1986.
62. M Liu, MI Simon. Regulation by cAMP-dependent protein kinease of a G-protein-mediated phospholipase C. Nature 382:83–87, 1996.
63. EA Thiele, BA Eipper. Effect of secretagogues on components of the secretory system in AtT-20 cells. Endocrinology 126:809–817, 1990.
64. J Wu, P Dent, T Jelinek, A Wolfman, MJ Weber, TW Sturgill. Inhibition of the EGF-activated MAP kinase signaling pathway by adenosine 3′,5′-monophosphate. Science 262:1065–1069, 1993.
65. RR Vaillancourt, AM Gardner, GL Johnson. B-Raf-dependent regulation of the MEK-1/mitogen-activated protein kinase pathway in PC12 cells and regulation by cyclic AMP. Mol Cell Biol 14:6522–6530, 1994.
66. MR Vossler, H Yao, RD York, MG Pan, CS Rim, PJ Stork. cAMP activates MAP kinase and Elk-1 through a B-Raf- and Rap1-dependent pathway. Cell 89:73–82, 1997.

67. M Torti, EG Lapetina. Role of rap1B and p21ras GTPase-activating protein in the regulation of phospholipase C-gamma 1 in human platelets. Proc Natl Acad Sci USA 89:7796–7800, 1992.
68. DL Altschuler, SN Peterson, MC Ostrowski, EG Lapetina. Cyclic AMP–dependent activation of Rap1b. J Biol Chem 270:10373–10376, 1995.
69. SJ McLeod, RJ Ingham, JL Bos, T Kurosaki, MR Gold. Activation of the Rap1 GTPase by the B cell antigen receptor. J Biol Chem 273:29218–29223, 1998.
70. B Franke, JW Akkerman, JL Bos. Rapid Ca^{2+}-mediated activation of Rap1 in human platelets. EMBO J 16:252–259, 1997.
71. Y Ueda, S Hirai, S Osada, A Suzuki, K Mizuno, S Ohno. Protein kinase C activates the MEK-ERK pathway in a manner independent of Ras and dependent on Raf. J Biol Chem 271:23512–23519, 1996.
72. CL Farnsworth, NW Freshney, LB Rosen, A Ghosh, ME Greenberg, LA Feig. Calcium activation of Ras mediated by neuronal exchange factor Ras-GRF. Nature 376:524–527, 1995.
73. LB Rosen, DD Ginty, MJ Weber, ME Greenberg. Membrane depolarization and calcium influx stimulate MEK and MAP kinase via activation of Ras. Neuron 12:1207–1221, 1994.
74. PJ Mitchell, and R Tjian. Transcriptional regulation in mammalian cells by sequence-specific DNA binding proteins. Science 245:371–378, 1989.
75. M Sheng, and ME Greenberg. The regulation and function of c-fos and other immediate early genes in the nervous system. Neuron 4:477–485, 1990.
76. TE Meyer, JF Habener. Cyclic adenosine 3′,5′-monophosphate response element binding protein (CREB) and related transcription-activating deoxyribonucleic acid-binding proteins. Endocr Rev 14:269–290, 1993.
77. AJ Shaywitz, ME Greenberg. CREB: a stimulus-induced transcription factor activated by a diverse array of extracellular signals. Annu Rev Biochem 68:821–861, 1999.
78. MR Montminy, KA Sevarino, JA Wagner, G Mandel, RH Goodman. Identification of a cyclic-AMP-responsive element within the rat somatostatin gene. Proc Natl Acad Sci USA 83:6682–6686, 1986.
79. P Hughes, M Dragunow. Induction of immediate-early genes and the control of neurotransmitter-regulated gene expression within the nervous system. Pharmacol Rev 47:133–178, 1995.
80. P Angel, M Imagawa, R Chiu, B Stein, RJ Imbra, HJ Rahmsdorf, C Jonat, P Herrlich, M Karin. Phorbol ester–inducible genes contain a common *cis* element recognized by a TPA-modulated *trans*-acting factor. Cell 49:729–739, 1987.
81. T Curran, JI Morgan. Fos: an immediate-early transcription factor in neurons. J Neurobiol 26:403–412, 1995.
82. M Shaw, P Cohen, DR Alessi. The activation of protein kinase B by H_2O_2 or heat shock is mediated by phosphoinositide 3-kinase and not by mitogen-activated protein kinase-activated protein kinase-2. Biochem J 336(Pt 1):241–246, 1998.
83. J Papkoff, M Aikawa. WNT-1 and HGF regulate GSK3 beta activity and beta-catenin signaling in mammary epithelial cells. Biochem Biophys Res Commun 247:851–858, 1998.
84. SL Pelech, DL Charest. MAP kinase–dependent pathways in cell cycle control. Prog Cell Cycle Res 1:33–52, 1995.
85. WJ Boyle, T Smeal, LH Defize, P Angel, JR Woodgett, M Karin, T Hunter. Activation of protein kinase C decreases phosphorylation of c-Jun at sites that negatively regulate its DNA-binding activity. Cell 64:573–584, 1991.
86. TJ Singh, I Grundke-Iqbal, K Iqbal. Differential phosphorylation of human tau isoforms containing three repeats by several protein kinases. Arch Biochem Biophys 328:43–50, 1996.
87. RJ Guan, BS Khatra, JA Cohlberg. Phosphorylation of bovine neurofilament proteins by protein kinase FA (glycogen synthase kinase 3). J Biol Chem 266:8262–8267, 1991.
88. SD Yang. Identification of the ATP.Mg-dependent protein phosphatase activator (FA) as a myelin basic protein kinase in the brain. J Biol Chem 261:11786–11791, 1986.
89. M Taniuchi, EM Johnson Jr, PJ Roach, JC Lawrence Jr. Phosphorylation of nerve growth factor receptor proteins in sympathetic neurons and PC12 cells. In vitro phosphorylation by the cAMP-independent protein kinase FA/GSK-3. J Biol Chem 261:13342–13349, 1986.
90. CA Grimes, RS Jope. The multifaceted roles of glycogen synthase kinase 3beta in cellular signaling. Prog Neurobiol 65:391–426, 2001.
91. GN Pandey, MW Dysken, DL Garver, JM Davis. Beta-adrenergic receptor function in affective illness. Am J Psychiatry 136:675–678, 1979.
92. I Extein, J Tallman, CC Smith, FK Goodwin. Changes in lymphocyte beta-adrenergic receptors in depression and mania. Psychiatry Res 1:191–197, 1979.
93. RP Ebstein, D Moscovich, S Zeevi, Z Amiri, B Lerer. Effect of lithium in vitro and after chronic treatment on human platelet adenylate cyclase activity: postreceptor modification of second messenger signal amplification. Psychiatry Res 21:221–228, 1987.
94. RP Ebstein, B Lerer, B Shapira, Z Shemesh, DG Moscovich, S Kindler. Cyclic AMP second-messenger signal amplification in depression. Br J Psychiatry 152:665–669, 1988.

95. JJ Mann, RP Brown, JP Halper, JA Sweeney, JH Kocsis, PE Stokes, JP Bilezikian. Reduced sensitivity of lymphocyte beta-adrenergic receptors in patients with endogenous depression and psychomotor agitation. N Engl J Med 313:715–720, 1985.
96. LT Young, PP Li, SJ Kish, JJ Warsh. Cerebral cortex beta-adrenoceptor binding in bipolar affective disorder. J Affect Disord 30:89–92, 1994.
97. JP Halper, RP Brown, JA Sweeney, JH Kocsis, A Peters, JJ Mann. Blunted beta-adrenergic responsivity of peripheral blood mononuclear cells in endogenous depression. Isoproterenol dose-response studies. Arch Gen Psychiatry 45:241–244, 1988.
98. A Mork, A Geisler, P Hollund. Effects of lithium on second messenger systems in the brain. Pharmacol Toxicol 71(suppl 1):4–17, 1992.
99. ED Risby, JK Hsiao, HK Manji, J Bitran, F Moses, DF Zhou, WZ Potter. The mechanisms of action of lithium. II. Effects on adenylate cyclase activity and beta-adrenergic receptor binding in normal subjects. Arch Gen Psychiatry 48:513–524, 1991.
100. LT Young, PP Li, SJ Kish, KP Siu, JJ Warsh. Postmortem cerebral cortex Gs alpha-subunit levels are elevated in bipolar affective disorder. Brain Res 553:323–326, 1991.
101. LT Young, PP Li, SJ Kish, KP Siu, A Kamble, O Hornykiewicz, JJ Warsh. Cerebral cortex Gs alpha protein levels and forskolin-stimulated cyclic AMP formation are increased in bipolar affective disorder. J Neurochem 61:890–898, 1993.
102. E Friedman, HY Wang. Receptor-mediated activation of G proteins is increased in postmortem brains of bipolar affective disorder subjects. J Neurochem 67:1145–1152, 1996.
103. HK Manji, G Chen, H Shimon, JK Hsiao, WZ Potter, RH Belmaker. Guanine nucleotide-binding proteins in bipolar affective disorder. Effects of long-term lithium treatment. Arch Gen Psychiatry 52:135–144, 1995.
104. G Schreiber, S Avissar, A Danon, RH Belmaker. Hyperfunctional G proteins in mononuclear leukocytes of patients with mania. Biol Psychiatry 29:273–280, 1991.
105. S Avissar, Y Nechamkin, L Barki-Harrington, G Roitman, G Schreiber. Differential G protein measures in mononuclear leukocytes of patients with bipolar mood disorder are state dependent. J Affect Disord 43:85–93, 1997.
106. PB Mitchell, HK Manji, G Chen, L Jolkovsky, E Smith-Jackson, K Denicoff, M Schmidt, WZ Potter. High levels of Gs alpha in platelets of euthymic patients with bipolar affective disorder. Am J Psychiatry 154:218–223, 1997.
107. LT Young, PP Li, A Kamble, KP Siu, JJ Warsh. Mononuclear leukocyte levels of G proteins in depressed patients with bipolar disorder or major depressive disorder. Am J Psychiatry 151:594–596, 1994.
108. O Spleiss, D van Calker, L Scharer, K Adamovic, M Berger, PJ Gebicke-Haerter. Abnormal G protein alpha(s)—and alpha(i2)-subunit mRNA expression in bipolar affective disorder. Mol Psychiatry 3:512–520, 1998.
109. S Avissar, L Barki-Harrington, Y Nechamkin, G Roitman, G Schreiber. Reduced beta-adrenergic receptor-coupled Gs protein function and Gs alpha immunoreactivity in mononuclear leukocytes of patients with depression. Biol Psychiatry 39:755–760, 1996.
110. D Dowlatshahi, GM MacQueen, JF Wang, JS Reiach, LT Young. G protein–coupled cyclic AMP signaling in postmortem brain of subjects with mood disorders: effects of diagnosis, suicide, treatment at the time of death. J Neurochem 73:1121–1126, 1999.
111. M Alda, D Keller, E Grof, G Turecki, P Cavazzoni, A Duffy, GA Rouleau, P Grof, LT Young. Is lithium response related to G(s)alpha levels in transformed lymphoblasts from subjects with bipolar disorder? J Affect Disord 65:117–122, 2001.
112. F Karege, J Golaz, M Schwald, A Malafosse. Lithium and haloperidol treatments differently affect the mononuclear leukocyte Galphas protein levels in bipolar affective disorder. Neuropsychobiology 39:181–186, 1999.
113. JA Garcia-Sevilla, C Walzer, X Busquets, PV Escriba, L Balant, J Guimon. Density of guanine nucleotide-binding proteins in platelets of patients with major depression: increased abundance of the G alpha i2 subunit and down-regulation by antidepressant drug treatment. Biol Psychiatry 42:704–712, 1997.
114. S Avissar, Y Nechamkin, G Roitman, G Schreiber. Dynamics of ECT normalization of low G protein function and immunoreactivity in mononuclear leukocytes of patients with major depression. Am J Psychiatry 155:666–671, 1998.
115. F Karege, P Bovier, R Stepanian, A Malafosse. The effect of clinical outcome on platelet G proteins of major depressed patients. Eur Neuropsychopharmacol 8:89–94, 1998.
116. PV Gejman, M Martinez, Q Cao, E Friedman, WH Berrettini, LR Goldin, P Koroulakis, C Ames, MA Lerman, ES Gershon. Linkage analysis of fifty-seven microsatellite loci to bipolar disorder. Neuropsychopharmacology 9:31–40, 1993.
117. F Le, P Mitchell, C Vivero, B Waters, J Donald, LA Selbie, J Shine, P Schofield. Exclusion of close linkage of bipolar disorder to the Gs-alpha subunit gene in nine Australian pedigrees. J Affect Disord 32:187–195, 1994.
118. A Ram, F Guedj, A Cravchik, L Weinstein, Q Cao, JA Badner, LR Goldin, N Grisaru, HK Manji, RH Belmaker, ES Gershon, PV Gejman. No abnormality

in the gene for the G protein stimulatory alpha subunit in patients with bipolar disorder. Arch Gen Psychiatry 54:44–48, 1997.
119. LT Young, V Asghari, PP Li, SJ Kish, M Fahnestock, JJ Warsh. Stimulatory G-protein alpha-subunit mRNA levels are not increased in autopsied cerebral cortex from patients with bipolar disorder. Brain Res Mol Brain Res 42:45–50, 1996.
120. RP Ebstein, B Lerer, ER Bennett, B Shapira, S Kindler, Z Shemesh, N Gerstenhaber. Lithium modulation of second messenger signal amplification in man: inhibition of phosphatidylinositol-specific phospholipase C and adenylate cyclase activity. Psychiatry Res 24:45–52, 1988.
121. S Rahman, PP Li, LT Young, O Kofman, SJ Kish, JJ Warsh. Reduced [3H]cyclic AMP binding in postmortem brain from subjects with bipolar affective disorder. J Neurochem 68:297–304, 1997.
122. SW Spaulding. The ways in which hormones change cyclic adenosine 3′,5′-monophosphate-dependent protein kinase subunits, how such changes affect cell behavior. Endocr Rev 14:632–650, 1993.
123. A Fields, PP Li, SJ Kish, JJ Warsh. Increased cyclic AMP-dependent protein kinase activity in postmortem brain from patients with bipolar affective disorder. J Neurochem 73:1704–1710, 1999.
124. J Perez, D Tardito, S Mori, G Racagni, E Smeraldi, R Zanardi. Abnormalities of cyclic adenosine monophosphate signaling in platelets from untreated patients with bipolar disorder. Arch Gen Psychiatry 56:248–253, 1999.
125. J Perez, R Zanardi, S Mori, M Gasperini, E Smeraldi, G Racagni. Abnormalities of cAMP-dependent endogenous phosphorylation in platelets from patients with bipolar disorder. Am J Psychiatry 152:1204–1206, 1995.
126. J Perez, D Tardito, S Mori, G Racagni, E Smeraldi, R Zanardi. Altered Rap1 endogenous phosphorylation and levels in platelets from patients with bipolar disorder. J Psychiatr Res 34:99–104, 2000.
127. R Zanardi, G Racagni, E Smeraldi, J Perez. Differential effects of lithium on platelet protein phosphorylation in bipolar patients and healthy subjects. Psychopharmacology (Berl) 129:44–47, 1997.
128. RE Banks, JF Aiton, G Cramb, GJ Naylor. Incorporation of inositol into the phosphoinositides of lymphoblastoid cell lines established from bipolar manic-depressive patients. J Affect Disord 19:1–8, 1990.
129. H Mori, T Koyama, I Yamashita. Platelet alpha-2 adrenergic receptor-mediated phosphoinositide responses in endogenous depression. Life Sci 48:741–748, 1991.
130. H Shimon, G Agam, RH Belmaker, TM Hyde, JE Kleinman. Reduced frontal cortex inositol levels in postmortem brain of suicide victims and patients with bipolar disorder. Am J Psychiatry 154:1148–1150, 1997.
131. DG Moscovich, RH Belmaker, G Agam, A Livne. Inositol-1-phosphatase in red blood cells of manic-depressive patients before and during treatment with lithium. Biol Psychiatry 27:552–555, 1990.
132. GJ Moore, JM Bebchuk, JK Parrish, MW Faulk, CL Arfken, J Strahl-Bevacqua, HK Manji. Temporal dissociation between lithium-induced changes in frontal lobe myo-inositol and clinical response in manic-depressive illness. Am J Psychiatry 156:1902–1908, 1999.
133. AS Brown, AG Mallinger, LC Renbaum. Elevated platelet membrane phosphatidylinositol-4,5-bisphosphate in bipolar mania. Am J Psychiatry 150:1252–1254, 1993.
134. JC Soares, CS Dippold, KF Wells, E Frank, DJ Kupfer, AG Mallinger. Increased platelet membrane phosphatidylinositol-4,5-bisphosphate in drug-free depressed bipolar patients. Neurosci Lett 299:150–152, 2001.
135. JC Soares, CS Dippold, AG Mallinger. Platelet membrane phosphatidylinositol-4,5-bisphosphate alterations in bipolar disorder—evidence from a single case study. Psychiatry Res 69:197–202, 1997.
136. JC Soares, AG Mallinger, CS Dippold, E Frank, DJ Kupfer. Platelet membrane phospholipids in euthymic bipolar disorder patients: are they affected by lithium treatment? Biol Psychiatry 45:453–457, 1999.
137. JC Soares, G Chen, CS Dippold, KF Wells, E Frank, DJ Kupfer, HK Manji, AG Mallinger. Concurrent measures of protein kinase C and phosphoinositides in lithium-treated bipolar patients and healthy individuals: a preliminary study. Psychiatry Res 95:109–118, 2000.
138. JC Soares, AG Mallinger, CS Dippold, WK Forster, E Frank, DJ Kupfer. Effects of lithium on platelet membrane phosphoinositides in bipolar disorder patients: a pilot study. Psychopharmacology (Berl) 149:12–16, 2000.
139. M Strathmann, MI Simon. G protein diversity: a distinct class of alpha subunits is present in vertebrates and invertebrates. Proc Natl Acad Sci USA 87:9113–9117, 1990.
140. SJ Taylor, JH Exton. Two alpha subunits of the Gq class of G proteins stimulate phosphoinositide phospholipase C-beta 1 activity. FEBS Lett 286:214–216, 1991.
141. 141. A Kikuchi, O Kozawa, K Kaibuchi, T Katada, M Ui, Y Takai. Direct evidence for involvement of a guanine nucleotide-binding protein in chemotactic peptide-stimulated formation of inositol bisphosphate and trisphosphate in differentiated human leukemic (HL-60) cells. Reconstitution with Gi or Go of the plasma membranes ADP-ribosyl-

142. R Mathews, PP Li, LT Young, SJ Kish, JJ Warsh. Increased G alpha q/11 immunoreactivity in postmortem occipital cortex from patients with bipolar affective disorder. Biol Psychiatry 41:649–656, 1997.
143. RS Jope, L Song, PP Li, LT Young, SJ Kish, MA Pacheco, JJ Warsh. The phosphoinositide signal transduction system is impaired in bipolar affective disorder brain. J Neurochem 66:2402–2409, 1996.
144. E Friedman, YW Hoau, D Levinson, TA Connell, H Singh. Altered platelet protein kinase C activity in bipolar affective disorder, manic episode. Biol Psychiatry 33:520–525, 1993.
145. HY Wang, P Markowitz, D Levinson, AS Undie, E Friedman. Increased membrane-associated protein kinase C activity and translocation in blood platelets from bipolar affective disorder patients. J Psychiatr Res 33:171–179, 1999.
146. HY Wang, E Friedman. Lithium inhibition of protein kinase C activation-induced serotonin release. Psychopharmacology (Berl) 99:213–218, 1989.
147. HY Wang, E Friedman. Protein kinase C translocation in human blood platelets. Life Sci 47:1419–1425, 1990.
148. HY Wang, E Friedman. Enhanced protein kinase C activity and translocation in bipolar affective disorder brains. Biol Psychiatry 40:568–575, 1996.
149. GN Pandey, Y Dwivedi, R Kumari, PG Janicak. Protein kinase C in platelets of depressed patients. Biol Psychiatry 44:909–911, 1998.
150. GN Pandey, Y Dwivedi, SC Pandey, RR Conley, RC Roberts, CA Tamminga. Protein kinase C in the postmortem brain of teenage suicide victims. Neurosci Lett 228:111–114, 1997.
151. D Mochly-Rosen, H Khaner, J Lopez. Identification of intracellular receptor proteins for activated protein kinase C. Proc Natl Acad Sci USA 88:3997–4000, 1991.
152. D Ron, CH Chen, J Caldwell, L Jamieson, E Orr, D Mochly-Rosen. Cloning of an intracellular receptor for protein kinase C: a homolog of the beta subunit of G proteins. Proc Natl Acad Sci USA 91:839–843, 1994.
153. JM Bebchuk, CL Arfken, S Dolan-Manji, J Murphy, K Hasanat, HK Manji. A preliminary investigation of a protein kinase C inhibitor in the treatment of acute mania. Arch Gen Psychiatry 57:95–97, 2000.
154. A Yatani, Y Imoto, J Codina, SL Hamilton, AM Brown, L Birnbaumer. The stimulatory G protein of adenylyl cyclase, Gs, also stimulates dihydropyridine-sensitive Ca^{2+} channels. Evidence for direct regulation independent of phosphorylation by cAMP-dependent protein kinase or stimulation by a dihydropyridine agonist. J Biol Chem 263:9887–9895, 1988.
155. A Yatani, J Codina, Y Imoto, JP Reeves, L Birnbaumer, AM Brown. A G protein directly regulates mammalian cardiac calcium channels. Science 238:1288–1292, 1987.
156. M Emamghoreishi, PP Li, L Schlichter, SV Parikh, R Cooke, JJ Warsh. Associated disturbances in calcium homeostasis and G protein–mediated cAMP signaling in bipolar I disorder. Biol Psychiatry 48:665–673, 2000.
157. JS Carman, RM Post, DC Runkle, WE Bunney Jr, RJ Wyatt. Increased serum calcium and phosphorus with the 'switch' into manic or excited psychotic state. Br J Psychiatry 135:55–61, 1979.
158. SL Dubovsky, J Murphy, M Thomas, J Rademacher. Abnormal intracellular calcium ion concentration in platelets and lymphocytes of bipolar patients. Am J Psychiatry 149:118–120, 1992.
159. S Yamawaki, A Kagaya, Y Okamoto, M Shimizu, A Nishida, Y Uchitomi. Enhanced calcium response to serotonin in platelets from patients with affective disorders. J Psychiatry Neurosci 21:321–324, 1996.
160. RA Bothwell, D Eccleston, E Marshall. Platelet intracellular calcium in patients with recurrent affective disorders. Psychopharmacology (Berl) 114:375–381, 1994.
161. M Berk, W Bodemer, T van Oudenhove, N Butkow. Dopamine increases platelet intracellular calcium in bipolar affective disorder and controls. Int Clin Psychopharmacol 9:291–293, 1994.
162. K Suzuki, I Kusumi, Y Sasaki, T Koyama. Serotonin-induced platelet intracellular calcium mobilization in various psychiatric disorders: is it specific to bipolar disorder? J Affect Disord 64:291–296, 2001.
163. I Kusumi, T Koyama, I Yamashita. Serotonin-stimulated Ca^{2+} response is increased in the blood platelets of depressed patients. Biol Psychiatry 30:310–312, 1991.
164. SL Dubovsky, C Lee, J Christiano, J Murphy. Elevated platelet intracellular calcium concentration in bipolar depression. Biol Psychiatry 29:441–450, 1991.
165. SL Dubovsky, J Christiano, LC Daniell, RD Franks, J Murphy, L Adler, N Baker, RA Harris. Increased platelet intracellular calcium concentration in patients with bipolar affective disorders. Arch Gen Psychiatry 46:632–638, 1989.
166. I Kusumi, T Koyama, I Yamashita. Thrombin-induced platelet calcium mobilization is enhanced in bipolar disorders. Biol Psychiatry 32:731–734, 1992.
167. A Eckert, H Gann, D Riemann, J Aldenhoff, WE Muller. Elevated intracellular calcium levels after 5-HT2 receptor stimulation in platelets of depressed patients. Biol Psychiatry 34:565–568, 1993.
168. A Eckert, H Gann, D Riemann, J Aldenhoff, WE Muller. Platelet and lymphocyte free intracellular cal-

cium in affective disorders. Eur Arch Psychiatry Clin Neurosci 243:235–239, 1994.
169. I Kusumi, T Koyama, I Yamashita. Serotonin-induced platelet intracellular calcium mobilization in depressed patients. Psychopharmacology (Berl) 113:322–327, 1994.
170. Y Okamoto, A Kagaya, H Shinno, N Motohashi, S Yamawaki. Serotonin-induced platelet calcium mobilization is enhanced in mania. Life Sci 56:327–332, 1995.
171. CH Tan, MA Javors, E Seleshi, PA Lowrimore, CL Bowden. Effects of lithium on platelet ionic intracellular calcium concentration in patients with bipolar (manic-depressive) disorder and healthy controls. Life Sci 46:1175–1180, 1990.
172. M Emamghoreishi, L Schlichter, PP Li, S Parikh, J Sen, A Kamble, JJ Warsh. High intracellular calcium concentrations in transformed lymphoblasts from subjects with bipolar I disorder. Am J Psychiatry 154:976–982, 1997.
173. RJ Stewart, B Chen, D Dowlatshahi, GM MacQueen, LT Young. Abnormalities in the cAMP signaling pathway in postmortem brain tissue from the Stanley Neuropathology Consortium. Brain Res Bull 55:625–629, 2001.
174. M Linnoila, E MacDonald, M Reinila, A Leroy, DR Rubinow, FK Goodwin. RBC membrane adenosine triphosphatase activities in patients with major affective disorders. Arch Gen Psychiatry 40:1021–1026, 1983.
175. CL Bowden, LG Huang, MA Javors, JM Johnson, E Seleshi, K McIntyre, S Contreras, JW Maas. Calcium function in affective disorders and healthy controls. Biol Psychiatry 23:367–376, 1988.
176. HL Meltzer, S Kassir, PJ Goodnick, RR Fieve, L Chrisomalis, M Feliciano, D Szypula. Calmodulin-activated calcium ATPase in bipolar illness. Neuropsychobiology 20:169–173, 1988.
177. M Hokin-Neaverson, DA Spiegel, WC Lewis. Deficiency of erythrocyte sodium pump activity in bipolar manic-depressive psychosis. Life Sci 15:1739–1748, 1974.
178. BB Johnston, GJ Naylor, EG Dick, SE Hopwood, DA Dick. Prediction of clinical course of bipolar manic depressive illness treated with lithium. Psychol Med 10:329–334, 1980.
179. GJ Naylor. Reversal of vanadate-induced inhibition of Na-K ATPase. A possible explanation of the therapeutic effect of carbamazepine in affective illness. J Affect Disord 8:91–93, 1985.
180. L Cherry, AC Swann. Cation transport mediated by $Na^+,K(^+)$-adenosine triphosphatase in lymphoblastoma cells from patients with bipolar I disorder, their relatives, unrelated control subjects. Psychiatry Res 53:111–118, 1994.

181. Y B Bezchlibnyk, JF Wang, G MacQueen, LT Young. Gene expression differences in bipolar disorder revealed by cDNA array analysis of postmortem frontal cortex. J Neurochem 79:826–834, 2001.
182. G Chen, WZ Zeng, PX Yuan, LD Huang, YM Jiang, ZH Zhao, HK Manji. The mood-stabilizing agents lithium and valproate robustly increase the levels of the neuroprotective protein bcl-2 in the CNS. J Neurochem 72:879–882, 1999.
183. JF Wang, LT Young. Differential display PCR reveals increased expression of 2′,3′-cyclic nucleotide 3′-phosphodiesterase by lithium. FEBS Lett 386:225–229, 1996.
184. JF Wang, B Chen, LT Young. Identification of a novel lithium regulated gene in rat brain. Brain Res Mol Brain Res 70:66–73, 1999.
185. JF Wang, CD Bown, B Chen, LT Young. Identification of mood stabilizer-regulated genes by differential-display PCR. Int J Neuropsychopharmacol 4:65–74, 2001.
186. RS Jope. A bimodal model of the mechanism of action of lithium. Mol Psychiatry 4:21–25, 1999.
187. N Ozaki, DM Chuang. Lithium increases transcription factor binding to AP-1 and cyclic AMP–responsive element in cultured neurons and rat brain. J Neurochem 69:2336–2344, 1997.
188. PX Yuan, G Chen, LD Huang, HK Manji. Lithium stimulates gene expression through the AP-1 transcription factor pathway. Brain Res Mol Brain Res 58:225–230, 1998.
189. M Nibuya, EJ Nestler, RS Duman. Chronic antidepressant administration increases the expression of cAMP response element binding protein (CREB) in rat hippocampus. J Neurosci 16:2365–2372, 1996.
190. D Dowlatshahi, GM MacQueen, JF Wang, LT Young. Increased temporal cortex CREB concentrations and antidepressant treatment in major depression. Lancet 352:1754–1755, 1998.
191. G Chen, PX Yuan, YM Jiang, LD Huang, HK Manji. Valproate robustly enhances AP-1 mediated gene expression. Brain Res Mol Brain Res 64:52–58, 1999.
192. JF Wang, V Asghari, C Rockel, LT Young. Cyclic AMP responsive element binding protein phosphorylation and DNA binding is decreased by chronic lithium but not valproate treatment of SH-SY5Y neuroblastoma cells. Neuroscience 91:771–776, 1999.
193. RS Duman, J Malberg, S Nakagawa, C D'Sa. Neuronal plasticity and survival in mood disorders. Biol Psychiatry 48:732–739, 2000.
194. RS Duman, GR Heninger, EJ Nestler. A molecular and cellular theory of depression. Arch Gen Psychiatry 54:597–606, 1997.
195. RM Post, SR Weiss. Sensitization, kindling, anticonvulsants in mania. J Clin Psychiatry 50(suppl):23–30, 1989.

196. RM Post, SR Weiss. A speculative model of affective illness cyclicity based on patterns of drug tolerance observed in amygdala-kindled seizures. Mol Neurobiol 13:33–60, 1996.
197. RS Horn, O Walaas, E Walaas. The influence of sodium, potassium and lithium on the response of glycogen synthetase I to insulin and epinephrine in the isolated rat diaphragm. Biochim Biophys Acta 313:296–309, 1973.
198. PS Klein, DA Melton. A molecular mechanism for the effect of lithium on development. Proc Natl Acad Sci USA 93:8455–8459, 1996.
199. G Chen, LD Huang, YM Jiang, HK Manji. The mood-stabilizing agent valproate inhibits the activity of glycogen synthase kinase-3. J Neurochem 72:1327–1330, 1999.
200. M Lesort, A Greendorfer, C Stockmeier, GV Johnson, RS Jope. Glycogen synthase kinase-3beta, beta-catenin, tau in postmortem bipolar brain. J Neural Transm 106:1217–1222, 1999.
201. N Kozlovsky, RH Belmaker, G Agam. Low GSK-3beta immunoreactivity in postmortem frontal cortex of schizophrenic patients. Am J Psychiatry 157:831–833, 2000.
202. JS Reiach, PP Li, JJ Warsh, SJ Kish, LT Young. Reduced adenylyl cyclase immunolabeling and activity in postmortem temporal cortex of depressed suicide victims. J Affect Disord 56:141–151, 1999.
203. LJ Siever, MS Kafka, S Targum, CR Lake. Platelet alpha–adrenergic binding and biochemical responsiveness in depressed patients and controls. Psychiatry Res 11:287–302, 1984.
204. LT Young, JF Wang, CM Woods, JC Robb. Platelet protein kinase C alpha levels in drug-free and lithium–treated subjects with bipolar disorder. Neuropsychobiology 40:63–66, 1999.
205. SL Dubovsky, J Murphy, J Christiano, C Lee. The calcium second messenger system in bipolar disorders: data supporting new research directions. J Neuropsychiatry Clin Neurosci 4:3–14, 1992.
206. SL Dubovsky, M Thomas, A Hijazi, J Murphy. Intracellular calcium signalling in peripheral cells of patients with bipolar affective disorder. Eur Arch Psychiatry Clin Neurosci 243:229–234, 1994.
207. C Hough, SJ Lu, CL Davis, DM Chuang, RM Post. Elevated basal and thapsigargin–stimulated intracellular calcium of platelets and lymphocytes from bipolar affective disorder patients measured by a fluorometric microassay. Biol Psychiatry 46:247–255, 1999.
208. I Kusumi, T Koyama, I Yamashita. Effect of mood stabilizing agents on agonist–induced calcium mobilization in human platelets. J Psychiatry Neurosci 19:222–225, 1994.
209. M Berk, NH Kirchmann, N Butkow. Lithium blocks $45Ca^{2+}$ uptake into platelets in biopolar affective disorder and controls. Clin Neuropharmacol 19:48–51, 1996.
210. I Kusumi, K Suzuki, Y Sasaki, K Kameda, T Koyama. Treatment response in depressed patients with enhanced Ca mobilization stimulated by serotonin. Neuropsychopharmacology 23:690–696, 2000.
211. GJ Naylor, AH Smith, EG Dick, DA Dick, AM McHarg, Chambers CA. Erythrocyte membrane cation carrier in manic–depressive psychosis. Psychol Med 10:521–525, 1980.
212. D van Calker, U Forstner, M Bohus, P Gebicke-Harter, H Hecht, HJ Wark, M Berger. Increased sensitivity to agonist stimulation of the $Ca2+$ response in neutrophils of manic–depressive patients: effect of lithium therapy. Neuropsychobiology 27:180–183, 1993.
213. U Forstner, M Bohus, PJ Gebicke-Harter, B Baumer, M Berger, D van Calker. Decreased agonist–stimulated $Ca2+$ response in neutrophils from patients under chronic lithium therapy. Eur Arch Psychiatry Clin Neurosci 243:240–243, 1994.

27

Molecular Genetics and Mood Disorders

DANIEL SOUERY and JULIAN MENDLEWICZ
Erasme Hospital, Brussels, Belgium

I. INTRODUCTION

Advances toward the understanding of the etiological mechanisms involved in mood disorders provide interesting yet diverse hypotheses and promising models. In this context, molecular genetics has now been widely incorporated into genetic epidemiological research in psychiatry. Affective disorders and, in particular, bipolar affective disorder (BPAD) have been examined in many molecular-genetics studies which have covered a large part of the genome, specific hypotheses such as mutations have also been studied. Decades of research into the genetic etiology of mood disorders provide evidence in favor of complex mode of inheritance unlikely to be determined by single-gene dysfunction, and appear to have non-Mendelian patterns of inheritance. Most recent studies indicate that several chromosomal regions may be involved in the etiology of BPAD. These include genes on chromosomes 18, 21, 4, 5, 12, 11, and X. Genetic heterogeneity and polygenic inheritance may explain the large number of potential genes involved.

This chapter will review the current methodologies and study tools used to search for molecular genetic factors in mood disorders and the chromosomal regions of interest already investigated for bipolar (BPAD) and unipolar (UPAD) mood disorders.

II. GENETIC EPIDEMIOLOGY

The various strategies available to investigate genetic risk factors in psychiatric disorders belong to the wider discipline of genetic epidemiology. This combines both epidemiological and genetic investigations and has the primary objective of identifying the genetic and nongenetic (environmental) causes of a disease. Genetic epidemiological data in affective disorders has come mostly from family, twin, adoption and segregation (within-family) studies. Family, twin, and adoption studies are the mainstay in establishing the genetic basis of affective disorders. These methods first demonstrated that genetic factors are involved in the etiology of these disorders. Twin and adoption data may also be used to investigate the relative contributions of genetic and environmental factors to the etiology of a disease [Vieland et al., 1995]. The exact contribution of these factors is not yet firmly understood for affective disorders, but some recent studies provide contributing findings. The study of adoptees separated from their biological parents has consistently favored the gene-environment hypothesis in the etiology of diverse psychiatric disorders. One study [Cadoret et al., 1996] shows that major depression in females is predicted by an alcoholic diathesis only when combined with an environmental factor that is characterized by a psychiatrically ill adoptive parent. Other possible environmental factors were identified, such as fetal alcohol exposure, age at the time of adoption, and a family with an adopted sibling who had a psychiatric problem. These findings confirm the importance of the gene-environment interactions in the understanding of etiological mechanism in mood disorders. The adoption study design is also used to validate clinical entities throughout the understanding of the gene-environment interactions as etiologic factor. The concept of depression spectrum disease has originally been developed from family studies [Winokur et al., 1971] and further validated in adoption studies. In this model, depressions were divided into pure depressive disease (only depression in the family) and depression spectrum disease (characterized by a family history of alcoholism or antisocial personality). Different adoption studies confirmed this hypothesis, showing that daughters of alcoholics who where not adopted away showed significantly greater depression than control subjects and their female siblings who had been adopted away [Goodwin et al., 1977]. An excess of biological mothers with substance abuse was found among adoptees with depression [Van Knorring et al., 1983], and more alcoholism was observed in the biological relatives of depressed adoptees than in the biological relatives of nondepressed adoptees [Wender et al., 1986]. These results confirm the significant role of gene-environment interactions in depression spectrum disease and further validate the concept.

The diagnostic validation and the structure of the genetic and environmental risk factors in mood disorders are also approached in twin studies. Using a prospective, epidemiologic, and genetically informative sample of adult female twins, Kendler et al., [1996] were able to identify and validate a typology of depressive syndromes characterized by mild typical depression, atypical depression (increased eating, hypersomnia, frequent, relatively short episodes, and a proclivity to obesity), and severe typical depression (comorbid anxiety and panic, long episodes, impairment, and help seeking). The members of twin pairs concordant for depression had the same depressive syndrome more often than expected by chance, and this resemblance was greater in monozygotic than in dizygotic pairs. To clarify the interactions between genetic factors and stressful life events in the etiology of depression, a population-based sample of female-female twin pairs including 2,164 individuals were analyzed in regard to stressful life events and onset of major depressive episodes in the past year [Kendler et al., 1995]. For severe stressful events, the best-fitting model for the joint effect of stressful events and genetic liability on onset of major depression suggested genetic control of sensitivity to the depression-inducing effects of stressful life events. The authors concluded that genetic factors influence the risk of onset of major depression in part by altering the sensitivity of individuals to the depression-inducing effect of stressful life events. In a more complex analysis of comorbidity among different psychiatric disorders, a large epidemiological survey of 1030 female-female twin pairs [Kendler et al., 1995] investigated the influence of major genetic and environmental risk factors (separated into different domains: genes, family environment, and individual-specific environment) on comorbidity between different psychiatric disorders (phobia, generalized anxiety disorder, panic disorder, bulimia, major depression and alcoholism). Each major risk factor domain influenced comorbidity, but in a distinct manner according to the disorders investigated and most of the genetic factors that influence vulnerability to alcoholism in women do not alter the risk for development of other common psychiatric disorders.

Segregation analysis is used to determine the mode of genetic transmission of a disorder by describing the distribution of phenotypes in affected families. The two principal hypotheses that have emerged from these complex analyses in affective disorders are the Single Major Locus (SML) model and the Polygenic Model (PM) involving possible interaction between two or more loci. The exact mode of inheritance is not yet clear [Smeraldi et al., 1995]. The situation is further complicated by the possible presence of anticipation in families with mood disorder [McInnis et al., 1993; Nylander et al., 1995; Engström et al., 1995]. This mode of transmission, which involves dynamic mutations, fits better with the twin and family epidemiological data available in affective disorders and may explain their non-Mendelian pattern of inheritance.

III. LINKAGE METHOD

The initial molecular genetic studies of BPAD, considered the core phenotype of affective disorders, involved the parametric linkage studies of large families. Linkage examines the cosegregation of a genetic marker and disease in affected individuals within families—that is, the nonrandom sharing of marker alleles between affected members of each family

[Smeraldi and Macciardi, 1995]. Two genetic loci are linked if they are located closely together on a chromosome. In linkage analysis, the distance between a marker locus and the gene under investigation is used for gene mapping. This method was originally designed to explore a major single genetic transmission and to evaluate the extent of cosegregation between genetic markers and the phenotype investigated in pedigrees. After initial localization, additional markers in that chromosomal region are typed, and the location of the disease gene may be determined more precisely by further linkage analysis. Linkage studies use Lod score analysis which require the specification of genetic parameters such as gene frequencies, mode of transmission and penetrance [Ott, 1991]. A limitation of this approach is that for affective disorders, the mode of inheritance in unknown, so that a variety of genetic models must be tested. Thus, multiple testing is required which may increase the risk of type I errors. Since the true mode of inheritance is not known, an appropriate model may not be tested at all, so there is a risk of type II errors as well. Furthermore, the linkage approach fails to detect minor gene effects that contribute to genetic susceptibility to the disorder [Propping et al., 1993]. Another limitation in linkage studies is that broad-spectrum phenotypes are often employed, which may be less stable over time and less likely to have the a homogeneous genetic etiology.

Large pedigrees with high density of affected status are often used in linkage studies. Genetic heterogeneity may be present is such large densely affected pedigrees. These supposedly homogeneous groups of individuals are not necessarily sufficient to overcome the possibility that different genes may lead to the disease for different people. Moreover, large pedigrees are rare and thus difficult to collect. Furthermore, since these pedigrees are rare, it is questionable that they actually represent the etiology of the disease in the population at large.

The sib-pair method provides advantages over classical linkage analysis in that specific parameters need not be specified. The sample size, on the other hand, must be relatively large owing to decreased power.

High Lod scores have been observed in single pedigrees but are generally not replicated in others, which may be due to genetic heterogeneity. Even if genetic heterogeneity is present, one should find consistently positive, if not significant, linkage results in other families. Linkage may be present in some families and not in others, and these families may in fact be rare.

IV. ASSOCIATION METHOD

Given the difficulties inherent in detecting genes of small to modest effect using linkage approach, the candidate gene association method offers an alternative strategy of studying genetic factors involved in complex diseases in which the mode of transmission is not known. Association between diseases and marker may be found if the gene itself, or a locus in linkage disequilibrium with the marker, is involved in the pathophysiology of the disease [Hodge, 1994]. Thus, an association may imply a direct effect of the gene tested, or the effect of another gene close to the marker examined. Linkage disequilibrium between the disease locus and the marker tested occurs when the level of concordance between the two loci is higher than that would be expected by chance, the reason for this being their proximity on a chromosome. The major advantage of association studies is that they can detect genes with minor effects. The association method is therefore appropriate for examination of a disorder that may be caused by genes that augment susceptibility but are neither necessary nor sufficient for the development of the disease [Greenberg, 1993; Plomin et al., 1994]. The major limitation is that spurious associations between a genetic marker and a disorder may result from variations in allele frequency between cases and controls if the two populations are ethnically different (population stratification). It is important in this case to test populations that are comparable in ethnic background.

The Haplotype Relative Risk (HRR) strategy uses parental data for the control sample and reduces this type of bias. The HRR method selects nontransmitted alleles from parents of the probands for the control population [Terwilliger and Ott, 1992]. Another limitation encountered in association studies is that small sample sizes do not provide enough statistical power to detect minor gene effects. Caution must be used in the interpretation of the association observed. The result may be interpreted as linkage disequilibrium between the disease locus and the associated marker allele(s), the associated marker may be a susceptibility factor which is directly involved in the disease, or the association may be due to chance. The association method alone cannot determine which interpretation is correct [Hodge, 1994]. Once a positive association is observed, exploration of the allele occurring more frequently with the disease must be carried out to ascertain if it represents a change in gene functioning that might be implicated in the pathophysiology of the disorder. If the observed disease allele leads to reduced function or transcription of an enzyme or receptor involved in neurotransmission, the result would truly enhance our understanding of the etiology of the disease.

The candidate gene approach is a useful method to investigate association between markers and disease. A candidate gene refers to a region of the chromosome which is potentially implicated in the etiology of the disorder concerned. The possibility of false-positive results must be taken into account, as a very large number of candidate genes now exist. The probability that each of these genes is involved in the etiology of the disorder is relatively low.

The candidate gene approach can be extended to phenotypes not directly linked to the diagnoses of mood disorders. The therapeutic effect of psychotropic drugs may be considered to investigate genetic polymorphisms (psychopharmacogenetics). In recent years, research in psychopharmacogenetics has focused on evaluating functional polymorphisms both in genes coding for drug-metabolizing znzymes and in genes coding for other enzymes or receptors involved in the mechanism of action of psychoactive drugs. In this context, the use of new technologies is rapidly evolving. Gene expression patterns in response to drug treatments can be investigated by new techniques such as DNA microarrays. Microarrays are powerful tools for investigating the mechanism of drug action by measuring changes in mRNA levels in brain tissues before and after exposure to treatment [Debouck and Goodfellow, 1999].

V. CANDIDATE CHROMOSOMAL REGIONS AND CANDIDATE GENES

A. Chromosome X

A systematic review of the literature on linkage studies in BPAD (Turecki et al., 1996) indicated that the proportion of positive DNA findings is higher for X markers compared to other chromosomal regions. Mendlewicz et al. (1987) first reported possible genetic linkage between BPAD and coagulation Factor IX (F9) located at Xq27 in 11 pedigrees. The same genetic marker was also tested in a French pedigree where linkage was confirmed [Lucotte et al., 1992]. Linkage with DNA markers on the X chromosome has been excluded, however, in other pedigrees [Berrettini et al., 1990, Gejman et al., 1990, Bredbacka et al., 1993]. A study published in 1987 by Baron et al. [1987] demonstrated positive linkage for glucose-6-phosphate deshydrogenase (G6PD), but later results from the same author did not support this finding [Baron et al., 1993], though G6PD was slightly positive for linkage in one family. In a more recent study [De Bruyn et al., 1994] several DNA markers in the Xq27-28 region were tested in nine bipolar families. Results suggestive of linkage were found in four bipolar I families with the markers F9, F8, and DXS52. Pekkarinen et al. [1995] evaluated 27 polymorphic markers on the X chromosome (Xq25-28 region) in one large Finnish family, and found the highest Lod scores when using a narrower phenotype definition (BPI and BPII only). Linkage was found between a marker located on Xq26 (AFM205wd2) and BPAD. This marker is located ~ 7 cm centromeric to the F9 locus. The initial genome screen for BPAD in the NIMH genetics initiative of 97 pedigrees also revealed positive though small Lod-scores on the X chromosome (Xp22 and Xq26-28) [Stine et al., 1997]. All these results are extremely suggestive of X linkage; in particular, the Xq26-28 should be considered a strong candidate region for genetic studies in BPAD.

The association between BPAD and polymorphic DNA markers in the pseudoautosomal region of the X chromosome have also been investigated. Yoneda et al. [1992] reported an association between the A4 allele of the marker DXYS20 in this chromosomal region in Japanese BPAD patients. This has not been replicated in European populations, however [Nothen et al., 1993; Parsian et al., 1994].

The MAOA and MAOB genes which code for the enzymes that degrade biogenic amines, including neurotransmitters implicated in the pathophysiology of affective disorders such as norepinephrine, dopamine and serotonin, are both located on the X chromosome and tightly linked to each other (Xp11.12–Xp11.4). Lim et al. [1994a, 1995] reported a weak but significant association for 3 different polymorphisms of MAOA, but not for MAOB, in a sample of 57 BPAD patients compared to population controls not assessed for psychiatric status. A weak association was found for MAOA and bipolar disorder by Kawada et al. [1995], but different alleles were more frequent in the patient population compared to the previous report. A series of negative reports followed, leaving the question open as to the usefulness of the MAO genes in psychiatric genetics research [Craddock et al., 1995a, Nothen et al., 1995; Muramatsu et al., 1997).

B. Chromosome 18

Berrettini et al., [1994] first reported linkage of BPAD to chromosome 18 DNA markers in a systematic genome survey of 22 families including 156 subjects with bipolar disorder. Though the overall Lod score for the pedigree series was negative, results of two-point linkage analysis in individual families indicated possible linkage with some marker loci in the 18p11 region. Nonparametric analysis (affected pedigree member and affected sib-pair analysis) of this sample confirmed the observation of linkage [Gershon, 1996]. These results suggested the existence of a susceptibility gene in the pericentromic region that can not be fully evaluated by classic linkage analysis. These results may be of interest because genes coding for the alpha unit of a GTP binding protein involved in neurotransmission, a corticotrophin receptor gene, and RED-1-containing triplet repeats have been mapped to this region. Stine et al. [1996] studied 28 nuclear families for markers on chromosome 18 and also found evidence for linkage and allele sharing between sib-pairs at 18p11.22–p11.21. This study replicated the findings of Berrettini, yet also demonstrated evidence for linkage and parent-of-origin effect in a region located on the long arm of chromosome 18, a sex-averaged distance 30 cm away. An excess of paternally but not maternally transmitted alleles from the D18S41 was observed.

In a study of five rigorously defined, high-density German families, no robust evidence for linkage for the pericentromeric region could be found, though one family showed slightly elevated lod scores under a recessive mode of inheritance for D18S40 [Maier et al., 1995]. Linkage to the pericentromeric region of chromosome 18 was excluded in three large Old Order Amish families [Pauls et al., 1995], and in two large Belgian pedigrees [De Bruyn et al., 1996]. In the Belgian pedigrees, while negative Lod scores were found for a marker located in the pericentromeric region, linkage and segregation analysis in one family suggested that the 18q region of the chromosome (18q21.33–q23) might contain a susceptibility locus for BPAD [De Bruyn et al., 1996]. Freimer et al. [1996], using both linkage and association strategies, reported evidence of linkage with markers in this region (18q22) in a Costa Rican pedigree with a common founder. A subsequent study further supported the interest of the 18q23 region showing linkage among six pedigrees [Coon et al., 1996]. An additional study of 173 affected subjects using the multilocus affected-pedigree member method, demonstrated a susceptiblity gene in the pericentromeric region, and multilocus analysis by affected sib-pair method also showed evidence for linkage [Berrettini et al., 1997]. Yet despite slight allele sharing with two markers on chromosome 18 (D18S40 on 18p and D18S70 on 18q) in the NIMH genetics initiative BPAD pedigrees, linkage to chromosome 18 was not confirmed in this large genome scan [Detera-Wadleigh et al., 1997]. Furthermore, Knowles et al. [1998] found no evidence for significant linkage between bipolar disorder and chromosome 18 pericentromeric markers in another large sample (1013 genotyped individuals) using 10 highly polymorphic markers.

C. Chromosome 5

Preliminary linkage data including three DNA markers on this chromosome (D5S39, D5S43, and D5S62) suggested linkage with BPAD [Coon et al., 1993]. Two of these markers, D5S62 and D5S43, are located on the distal region of the long arm of chromosome 5 (5q35-qter). This region contains candidate genes for affective disorders such as the alpha-1 protein subunit of the GABA A receptor (GABRA1) and the 5HT1A receptor (5HTR1A). These two markers, however, had exclusion Lod scores in a previous study of 14 families [Detera-Wadleigh et al., 1992]. Similarly, strongly negative Lod scores were found in a linkage study covering the 5HTR1A locus in five pedigrees [Curtis et al., 1993]. The dopamine transporter gene (DAT1) is located in a different region of chromosome 5 (5p15.3). This marker has been investigated in association studies with BPAD, yet no association has been found [Souery et al., 1996a; Gomez-Casero et al., 1996; Manki et al., 1996]. Kelsoe et al. [1996] reported possible linkage, however, between a locus near the dopamine transporter (DAT) and BPAD, under a dominant transmission model giving a modest Lod score of 2.38. Replication of this finding was subsequently shown in another linkage analysis [Waldman et al., 1997].

D. Chromosome 11

Chromosome 11 has been thoroughly investigated in affective disorders because of the presence of candidate genes involved in catecholamine neurotransmission such as tyrosine hydroxylase (TH, 11p15), tyrosinase (11q14-21), dopamine receptor D2 (DRD2, 11q22-23), Dopamine receptor D4 (DRD4, 11p15.5), and tryptophan hydroxylase (TPH, 11p15). Overall, results of linkage studies indicate that the TH gene does not contribute a major gene effect to BPAD [Souery et al., 1996b]. A possible role for the TH gene was also examined in BPAD association studies, all on moderate to small sample sizes. Meta-analysis of the results [Furlong et al., 1999] do not support the TH gene having a major role in the etiology of BPAD, while data suggest that this candidate gene should be examined in larger samples of UPAD for which this marker may confer susceptibility to the disease.

Linkage to the dopamine 2 receptor (DRD2) has been excluded in a number of studies [Ewald et al., 1994; Nanko et al., 1994; Kelsoe et al., 1993; Holmes et al., 1991, Byerley et al., 1990]. Most association studies have similarly showed no association between the gene for this receptor and BP [Craddock et al., 1995b; Souery et al., 1996a; Manki et al., 1996].

Linkage to the DRD4 receptor gene has not been definitively excluded [Nanko et al., 1994; Sidenberg et al., 1994], and a few association studies have found positive results. For unipolar patients alone, an excess of short exon III repeats (two to four repeats) has been found to be significantly more frequent than controls [Manki et al., 1996]. The No. 7 repeat allele was associated to bipolar disorder, and an excess of allele 3 among controls in another study, yet negative results were then found in a larger sample by the same group [Lim et al., 1994b]. Serretti et al., [1998] recently reported an excess of allele 7 among affective disorder patients with delusional features, suggesting its importance in psychoses, not necessarily affective disorders.

VI. SEROTONIN MARKERS AND AFFECTIVE DISORDERS

Dysfunction of the serotoninergic system has long been suspected in major depression and related disorders. Depression can be successfully treated with selective drugs which target serotonin receptors. The serotonin transporter may also be involved in susceptibility to affective disorders and in the response to treatment with these drugs. Allelic association has been suggested between the serotonin transporter gene (located on chromosome 17q11.1-12) and UPAD [Ogilvie et al., 1996]. The presence of one allele of this gene was significantly associated with a risk of UPAD. This study also included a group of BPAD patients although no associations were found with this marker in this patient group compared to normal controls. This preliminary finding may add to our understanding of the possibility of polygenic inheritance in affective disorders. These findings were replicated in two different samples, again showing an association between this marker and UPAD (major depression with melancholia) [Gutierrez et al., 1998a] and no association with a group of BPAD patients [Gutierrez et al., 1998b]. A higher frequency of the 12-repeat allele of the Variable Number Tandem Repeat (VNTR) polymorphism has been associated to affective disorders in a number of studies [Collier, 1996; Rees, 1997; Battersby, 1996], with results being the most significant for bipolar subjects. On the other hand, the No. 9 repeat allele has been shown to be significantly associated with unipolar depression, (Battersby, 1996, Olgilvie, 1996].

A linkage study with the functional variant of the serotonin transporter gene in families with BPAD could not exclude linkage [Ewald et al., 1998a]. More interestingly, a polymorphism within the promoter region of the serotonin transporter gene has been associated to treatment response to fluvoxamine, a typical selective serotonin rehuptake inhibitor (SSRI) in major depression with psychotic features [Smeraldi et al., 1999]. This promising preliminary finding remains to be confirmed. The tryptophan hydroxylase (TPH) gene, which codes for the rate-limiting enzyme of serotonin metabolism, is also an important candidate gene for affective disorders and suicidal behavior. Bellivier et al., [1998] reported a significant association between genotypes at this marker and BPAD, but no association was found with suicidal behavior. In a previous study in depressed patients suicidal behavior was associated with one variant of this gene [Mann et al., 1997].

A. Chromosome 4

Possible candidate genes on chromosome 4 include the dopamine receptor D5 (DRD5) and the alpha-adrenergic 2C receptor (ADRA2C) genes. Using both linkage and sib-pair methods to evaluate six families, postive results have been found for the loci for DRD5 and ADRA2C [Byerley et al., 1994], though this was not fully replicated in a later study with a larger sample size [Blackwood et al., 1996]. Linkage was found between a locus on chromosome 4p (D4S394, 4p16) and BPAD in the latter study, yielding a robust two-point Lod score of 4.1 under a model that allowed for heterogeneity. Though the region of 4p16 contains the genes for both DRD5 and ADRA2C, specific markers for these genes were not significant for linkage in this study. Though linkage was not found in the NIMH initiative for any region on chromosome 4, modest elevation of allele frequencies was found for markers on both arms of the chromosome, D4S2397 and D4S391, on 4p and DS1647 4q [Detera-Waldeigh et al., 1997].

Other possible candidate genes mapped to chromosome 4 include those coding for protein subunits of the heteromeric GABA A receptor: the alpha-2 protein subunit (GABRA2) and the beta-1 subunit (GABRB1), located at 4p13-12. This region was exluded for linkage in a large family in Blackwood's [1996] study, but perhaps could be examined more fully.

B. Chromosome 21

Straub et al. [1994] detected linkage with the locus for liver-type phosphofructokinase enzyme (PFLK) on chromosome 21 (21q22.3) in one large, multigenerational bipolar family. Initial results from 47 families assessed in this genome survey did not support linkage with this marker, however. Follow-up linkage analysis of an extended sample of 57 families on the 373 most informative individuals, using markers < 2 cm apart, found evidence of linkage (Lod score 3.35) at marker D21S1260, which is 5 cm proximal to PFKL [Aita et al., 1998]. Linkage between bipolar disorder and the PFLK region has also been confirmed in other studies [Ewald et al., 1996; Smyth et al., 1997], though negative results have also been reported [Byerley et al., 1995, Vallada et al. 1996]. Further confirmation of linkage to this region with a large sample size, and a later report of excess allele sharing of a cluster of markers within a 9 cm interval on 21q (D21S1254, D21S65, D21S1440 and D21S1254), were found in the NIMH Genetics Initiative bipolar pedigrees [Detera-Waldeigh et al., 1996, 1997]. Linkage to a larger region proximal to the gene for PFKL, 21q21-22, has also been reported by a number of groups [Kwok et al., 1999; LaBuda et al, 1996]. Taken together, these results indicate that the region of interest on 21q remains large, though no discrete locus or obvious candidate gene has been identified as of yet.

C. Chromosome 12

Darier's disease (keratosis follicularis), a rare autosomal-dominant skin disorder associated with increased prevalence of epilepsy and mental retardation, whose gene has been mapped to chromosome 12q23-24.1, was found to cosegregate with bipolar disorder in one pedigree [Caddock, 1994). The Darier's disease region has been investigated in several family studies in BPAD, suggesting a possible linkage [Craddock et al., 1994; Dawson et al., 1995; Barden et al., 1996; Ewald et al., 1998]. Two of these studies have been able to report significant Lod scores > 3 [Barden et al., 1996; Ewald et al., 1998b]. To further test the hypothesis that genes containing expanded trinucleotide repeats may contribute to the genetic etiology of BPAD, loci within this region containing CAG/CTG repeat expansions have also been investigated, but no association was found with BPAD [Franks et al., 1999].

VII. ANTICIPATION AND EXPANDED TRINUCLEOTIDE REPEAT SEQUENCES

Anticipation implies that a disease occurs at a progressively earlier age of onset and with increased severity in successive generations. This may explain deviations from Mendelian inheritance observed in some inherited diseases. This phenomenon has been observed in several neurological diseases including myotonic dystrophy, fragile X syndrome, Huntington's disease, and spinobulbar muscle atrophy [Trottier et al., 1995; Paulson and Fischbeck, 1996]. Anticipation has been found to correlate with a new class of mutations, expanded trinucleotide repeat sequences. An expanded repeat sequence is unstable and may increase in size across generations, leading to an increased disease severity of the disorder. CAG repeats are detected by the Repeat Expansion Detection (RED) method. Such unstable mutations could also be an alternative explanation in addition to environmental factors for discordance between monozygotic twins for affective disorders, where the repeat amplification might be different during mitosis in each of the two twins. A shortcoming of anticipation studies involves ascertainment bias. Earlier age of onset and/or increased severity in successive generations may be related to increased sensitivity to diagnosis in offspring of affected parents. It may appear that parents have a later age of onset than children, but perhaps parents with an earlier age of onset were not able to reproduce at all. That social and environmental factors in the younger generation may favor earlier detection and expression of the disease, is not necessarily related to observed repeats. Cohort effects can be controlled for in statistical analyses, however, such as examining age at onset in an entire generation compared to the difference observed between probands and parents.

Most unstable nucleotide repeat diseases showing anticipation also demonstrate imprinting, or parent-of-origin effect. Affective disorders have not yet unequivocally shown such an effect, though this does not necessarily exclude the possibility that anticipation occurs.

Evidence for anticipation has been observed in BPAD [McInnis et al., 1993; Nylander et al., 1995;

Lipp et al., 1995] and in UPAD [Engström et al., 1995]. Correlation between anticipation observed at the phenotypic level with the number of dynamic mutations may be the only way to confirm the implication of this phenomenon in affective disorders. One study highlighted an association between the number of CAG trinucleotide repeats and severity of BPAD illness in Swedish and Belgian patients [Lindblad et al., 1994]. This study, replicated subsequently in a different sample [O'Donovan et al., 1995; Oruc et al., 1997], showed for the first time in a major psychiatric disorder that the length of CAG repeats were significantly higher in BPAD than in normal controls. These molecular genetic findings may indicate a genetic basis for anticipation in BPAD. This hypothesis has recently been tested in a sample of two-generation pairs with BPAD. Globally, no significant differences were found in the mean number of CAG repeats between parent and offspring generations. A significant increase in CAG repeats between parents and offspring was observed, however, when the phenotype increased in severity, i.e., changed from major depression, single-episode or unipolar recurrent depression to BPAD [Mendlewicz et al., 1997]. A significant increase in CAG repeats length between generations was also found in female offspring with maternal inheritance, but not in male offspring. This is the first evidence of genetic anticipation in BPAD families and should be followed by the identification of loci within the genome containing triplet repeats. CTG 18.1 on chromosome 18q21.1 and ERDA 1 on chromosome 17q21.3 are two repeat loci recently identified [Lindblad et al., 1998] which can be investigated in such study.

VIII. ETHICAL POINT OF VIEW

Ethical questions arise from genetic research on complex diseases, such as AD, as well as clinical management of a complex disorder, involving both genetic and environmental components. The approaches and rules on genetic studies vary between countries; informed consent must be obtained (Shore, 1993). That was not the case a few years ago when the Department of Health and Human Services Office for Protection from Research Risks (OPRR) released an evaluation on human subject issues in a study at the University of California at Los Angeles involving outpatients with schizophrenia. Several problems were found with the informed consent documents. In particular, some investigators estimated that people who have mental disorders should be considered incapable of providing valid informed consent. This opinion is not currently accepted in many countries. In a NIMH consensus, it has been established that consent documents, and the process by which informed consent is obtained, are state of the art (Shore, 1996). Parker (2002) recently summarized the difficulties in the enrollment of patients with BPAD. The study of bipolar disorders presents particular challenges due to the uncertainty and stigma that surrounds the disorders and because some of the relevant subjects may have diminished capacity to consent to participation. During a severe manic or depressive episode, the subject will not be able to correctly judge the cost and benefits of the study. Therefore, investigators must wait to approach the patient when his symptoms are controlled by medication. Furthermore, genetic studies do not offer direct benefit to the patient. This point must be taken into account and explained to the patient. The disclosure of familial genetic information has been widely discussed. The clinician has often to decide when or whether an ethical duty to inform at-risk family members about an increased genetic risk overrides the duty to maintain patient confidentiality (Lehmann et al., 2000). Recently, the American Society of Human Genetics argued that confidentiality can be breached in situations in which "serious and foreseeable harm" is highly likely to occur to the at-risk relative, assuming that the relative is identifiable and the disease is preventable, treatable, or can be detected in its early stages (American Society of Human Genetics, 1998). In BPAD, some individuals who have never considered themselves as affected may be found to fit the diagnostic criteria. From our experience, it appears that the clinician must be aware that the disclosure of such information has psychosocial implications for the patient and their family. More generally, the clinicians must take time to explain the nature of the genetic risk, the virtual risk within the family and the consequences in terms of the possibility of pregnancy to avoid miscomprehension and suicide ideation or attempt, present by virtue in BPAD.

IX. CONCLUSIONS

The physical mapping of the human genome provides an immense factory providing thousands of genes which will accelerate the identification of genes responsible for mood disorders and will contribute to significant advances in the awareness of diagnosis (diagnostic process and early recognition), pathophysiology, epidemiology, and treatment issues. During the past two decades, the search for genes for mood disorders has mainly contributed to better understanding and confirmation of the genetic complexities inherent in these disorders. The large amount of results available and the difficulty to digest them corroborate this observation. The major contribution of these findings should be integrated in the context of the worldwide efforts to identify the thousands of genes of the human genome. The majority of these genes will be identified within the next few years. Several consistent hypotheses are currently being tested and will, hopefully, speed up the process of narrowing the important regions when the complete genome map will be available. The most promising chromosomal regions have been localized on chromosomes 4, 5, 11, 12, 18, 21 and X. A number of candidate genes have also been investigated, some of which are directly linked to neurobiological hypotheses of the etiology of affective disorders. In parallel, specific hypotheses have been implicated, such as anticipation and dynamic mutations. Further research should concentrate on these hypotheses and confirm positive findings through interdisciplinary and multicenter projects.

REFERENCES

Aita VM, Liu J, Terwilllinger JD, et al. (1998) A follow-up linkage analysis of chromosome 21 continues to provide evidence for aputative bipolar affective disorder locus. Am J Med Genet (Neuropsychiatr Genet) 81(6):476.

American Society of Human Genetics (1998). Professional disclosure of familial genetic information. Am J Hum Genetics 62:474–483.

Barden N, Plante M, Rochette D, Gagne B, et al. (1996) Genome wide microsatellite marker linkage study of bipolar affective disorders in a very large pedigree derived from a homogeneous population in Quebec points to susceptibility locus on chromosome 12. Psychiatr Genet 6:145–146.

Baron M, Risch N, Hamberge R, et al. (1987) Genetic linkage between X-Chromosome markers and bipolar affective illness. Nature 326:289–292.

Baron, M, Freimer, NF, Risch, N, et al. (1993) Diminished support for linkage between manic depressive illness and X-chromosome markers in three Israeli pedigrees. Nat Genet 3:49–55.

Battersby S, Ogilvie AD, Smyth CA, et al. (1996). Structure of a variable number tandem repeat of the serotonin transporter gene and association with affective disorder. Psychiatr. Genet. 6:177–181.

Bellivier F, Henry C, Szuke A, Schurhoff F, et al. (1998). Serotonin transporter gene polymorphisms in patients with unipolar or bipolar depression. Neurosci Lett Oct 23;255(3):143–146.

Bellivier F, Leboyer M, Courtet P, Buresi C, et al. 1998. Association between the tryptophan hydroxylase gene and manic-depressive illness. Archives of General Psychiatry. 55:33–37

Berrettini WH, Goldin LR, Gelernter J, et al. (1990) X chromosome markers and manic-depressive illness: rejection of linkage to Xq28 in nine bipolar pedigrees. Arch Gen Psychiatry 47:366–373.

Berrettini WH, Ferraro TN, Goldin LR, et al. (1994). Chromosome 18 DNA markers and manic-depressive illness: eidence for a susceptibility gene. Proc Nat Acad Sci USA 91:5918–5922.

Blackwood D, He L, Morris S, et al. (1996). A locus for bipolar affective disorder on chromosome 4p. Nat Genet 12:427–430.

Bredbacka PE, Pekkarinen P, Peltonen L, et al. (1993). Bipolar disorder in an extended pedigree with a segregation pattern compatible with X-linked transmission: exclusion of the previously reported linkage to F9. Psychiatr Genet 3:79–87.

Byerley W, Holik J, Hoff M, et al. (1995). Search for a gene predisposing to manic-depression on chromosome 21. Am J Med Genet 60(3):231–233.

Byerley W, Hoff M, Holik J, et al. (1994). A linkage study with D_5 dopamine and α_{2C}-adrenergic receptor genes in six multiplex bipolar pedigrees. Psychiatr Genet 4:121–124.

Byerley W, Leppert M, O'Connell P, et al., (1990). D_2 dopamine receptor gene not linked to manic-depression in three families. Psychiatr Genet 1:55–62.

Cadoret RJ, Winokur G, Lengbehn D, Troughton E, et al. (1996) Depression spectrum disease. I. The role of gene-environment interaction. Am J Psychiatry 153:892–899.

Collier DA, Stober G, Li T, et al. (1996). A novel functional polymorphism within the promoter of the serotonin transporter gene: possible role in susceptibility to affective disorders. Mol Psychiatry 1:453–460.

Coon H, Hoff M, Holik J, Hadley D, et al. (1996). Analysis of chromosome 18 DNA markers in multiplex pedigrees with manic depression. Biol Psychiatr 39:689–696.

Craddock N, McGuffin P, Owen M. (1994). Darier's disease cosegregating with affective disorder. Br J Psychiatry ;165(2):272.

Craddock N, Daniels J, Roberts E, Rees M, et al. (1995a. No evidence for allelic association between bipolar disorder and monoamine oxidase A gene polymorphisms. Am J Med Genet 60:322–324.

Craddock N, Roberts Q, Williams N, McGuffin P, et al. (1995b). Association study of bipolar disorder using a functional polymorphism (Ser311→Cys) in the dopamine D2 receptor gene. Psychiatr Genet. 5(2):63–65.

Curtis D, Brynjolfsson J, Petursson H, et al. (1993). Segregation and linkage analysis in five manic depression pedigrees excludes the 5HT1a receptor gene (HTR1A). Ann Hum Genet 57:27–39.

Dawson E, Parfitt E, Roberts Q, et al. (1995). Linkage studies of bipolar disorder in the region of Darier's disease gene on chromosome 12q23–24.1 Am J Med Genet (Neuropsychiatr Genet) 60(2):94–102.

Debouck C, Goodfellow PN. (1999) DNA microarrays in drug discovery and development. Nat Genet 21(1 suppl):48–50.

De Bruyn A, Raeymaekers P, Mendelbaum K, et al. (1994). Linkage analysis of bipolar illness with X-chromosome DNA markers: a susceptibility gene in Xq27–28 cannot be excluded. Am J Med Genet 54:411–419.

De Bruyn A, Souery D, Mendelbaum K, et al. 1996. Linkage analysis of 2 families with bipolar illness and chromosome 18 markers. Biol Psychiatry 39:679–688.

Detera-Waldeigh SD, Badner JA, Goldin LR, et al. (1996). Affected sib-pair analyses reveal support of prior evidence for a susceptibility locus for bipolar disorder, on 21q. Am J Hum Genet 58:1279–1285.

Detera-Wadleigh SD, Badner JA, Yoshikawa T, et al. (1997). Initial genome screen for bipolar disorder in the NIMH genetics initiative pedigrees: chromosomes 4, 7, 9, 18. (19, 20 and 21q. Am J Med Genet (Neuropsychiatr Genet) 74:254–262.

Detera-Wadleigh SD, Berrettini WH, Goldin LR, et al. 1992. A systematic search for a bipolar predisposing locus on chromosome 5. Neuropsychopharmacology 6:219–229.

Engstrom C, Thornlund AS, Johansson EL, et al. (1995). Anticipation in unipolar affective disorder. J Affect Disord. 35(1–2):31–40.

Ewald H, Eiberg H, Mors O, et al. (1996). Linkage study between manic-depressive illness and chromosome 21. Am J Med Genet. 67(2):218–224.

Ewald H, Mors O, Friedrich U, et al. (1994). Exclusion of linkage between manic depressive illness and tyrosine hydroxylase and Dopamine D_2 receptor genes. Psychiatr Genet 4: 13–22.

Ewald H, Flint T, Degn B, Mors O, Kruse TA (1998a). A functional variant of the serotonin transporter gene in families with bipolar affective disorder. J Affect Disord 48:135–144.

Ewald H, Degn B, Mors O, Kruse TA. (1998b). Significant linkage between bipolar affective disorder and chromosome 12q24. Psychiatr Genet. 8:131–140.

Franks E, Guy C, Jacobsen N, Bowen T, Owen MJ, et al. (1999). Eleven trinucleotide repeat loci that map to chromosome 12 excluded from involvement in the pathogenesis of bipolar disorder. Am J Med Genet 5:67–70.

Freimer N, Reus V, Escamilla M., et al. (1996). Genetic mapping using haplotype, association and linkage methods suggests a locus for severe bipolar disorder (BPI) at 18q22-q23. Nat Genet 12:436–444.

Furlong RA, Rubinsztein JS, Ho L, Walsh C, Coleman TA, et al. (1999). Analysis and metaanalysis of two polymorphisms within the tyrosine hydroxylase gene in bipolar and unipolar affective disorders. Am J Med Genet 5:88–94.

Gejman PV, Detera-Wadleigh S, Martinez MM, et al. (1990). Manic depressive illness not linked to factor IX in a independent series of pedigrees. Genomics 8:648–655.

Gershon ES, Badner JA, Detera-Waldeigh SD, et al. (1996). Maternal inheritance and chromosome 18 allele sharing in unilineal bipolar illness pedigrees. Am J Med Genet (Neuropsychiatr Genet) 67:202–207.

Gomez-Casero E, Perez de Castro I, Saiz-Ruiz J, et al. (1996). No association between particular DRD3 and DAT gene polymorphisms and manic-depressive illness in a Spanish sample. Psychiatr Genet 6(4):209–212.

Goodwin D, Schulsinger F, Knop J, Mednik S, et al. (1977) Alcoholism and depression in adopted-out daughters of alcoholics. Arch Gen Psychiatry 34; 751–755.

Greenberg DA. (1993). Linkage analysis of "necessary" disease loci versus "susceptibility" loci. Am J Hum Genet 52(1):135–143.

Gutierrez B, Pintor L, Gasto C, Rosa A, et al. (1998a). Variability in the serotonin transporter gene and increased risk for major depression with melancholia. Hum Genet. 103:319–322.

Gutierrez B, Arranz MJ, Collier DA, Valles V, et al. (1998b). Serotonin transporter gene and risk for bipolar affective disorder: an association study in Spanish population. Biol Psychiatry 43:843–847.

Hodge SE. (1994). What association analysis can and cannot tell us about the genetics of complex disease. Am J Med Genet 54:318–323.

Holmes D, Brynjolfsson J, Brett P, et al. (1991). No evidence for a susceptibility locus predisposing to manic depression in the region of the dopamine (D_2) receptor gene. Br J Psychiatry 158:635–641.

Kawada Y, Hattori M, Dai XY, Nanko S, et al. (1995). Possible association between monoamine oxidase A gene and bipolar affective disorder. Am J Hum Genet 56:335–336.

Kelsoe JR, Kristbjanarson H, Bergesch P, et al. (1993). A genetic linkage study of bipolar disorder and 13 markers on chromosome 11 including the D2 dopamine receptor. Neuropsychopharmacology 9(4):293–301.

Kelsoe JR, Sadovnick AD, Kristbjarnarson H, et al. (1996) Possible locus of bipolar disorder near the dopamine transporter on chromosome. Am J Med Genet 67(6):533–540.

Kendler KS, Eaves LJ, Walters EE, et al. (1996) The identification and validation of distinct depressive syndromes in a population-based sample of female twins. Arch Gen Psychiatry 53:391–399.

Kendler KS, Kessler RC, Walters EE, MacLean C, et al. (1995) Stressful life events, genetic liability, and onset of an episode of major depression in women. Am J Psychiatry;152:833–842.

Kendler KS, Walters EE, Neale MC, et al. (1995) The structure of the genetic and environmental risk factors for six major psychiatric disorders in women. Phobia, generalized anxiety disorder, panic disorder, bulimia, major depression, and alcoholism. Arch Gen Psychiatry 52:374–383.

Knowles JA, Rao PA, Cox-Lmatise T, et al. (1998). No evidence for significant linkage between bipolar affective disorder and chromosome 18 pericentromeric markers in a large series of mulitplex pedigrees. Am J Hum Genet 62:916–924.

Kwok JB, Adams LJ, Salmon JA, et al. (1999). Nonparametric simulation-based statistical analyses for bipolar affective disorder locus on chromosome 21q22.3. Am J Med Genet. 88(1):99–102.

LaBuda MC, Maldonado M, Marshall D, Otten K, Gerhard DS. (1996). A follow-up report of a genome search for affective disorder predisposition loci in the Old Order Amish. Am J Hum Genet 59:1343–1362.

Lehmann LS, Weeks JC, Klar N et al. (2000). Disclosure of familial genetic information: perceptions of the duty to inform. Am J Med, 109:705-711.

Lim LCC, Powell JF, Murray R (1994a). Monoamine oxidase A gene and bipolar affective disorder. Am J Hum Genet 54:1122–1124.

Lim LCC, Nöthen MM, Körner J, et al. (1994b). No evidence of association between dopamine D_4 receptor variants and bipolar affective disorder. Am J Med Genet 54:259–263.

Lim LCC, Powell, Sham P, Castle D, Hunt N, Murray R, Gill M. (1995). Evidence for a genetic association between alleles of monoamine oxidase A gene and bipolar disorder. Am J Med Genet 60:325–331.

Lindblad K, Nylander PO, De bruyn A, et al. (1995). Expansion of trinucleotide CAG repeats detected in bipolar affective disorder by the RED (rapid expansion detection) method. Neurobiol Dis 2:55–62.

Lindblad K, Nylander PO, Zander C, et al. (1998). Two commonly expanded CAG/CTG repeat loci: involvement in affective disorders? Mol Psychiatry 3(5):405–410.

Lucotte G, Landoulsi A, Berriche S et al. (1992). Manic depressive illness is linked to factor IX in a french pedigree. Ann Génét 35:93–95.

Maier W, Hallmayer J, Zill P, et al. (1995). Linkage analysis between pericentromeric markers on chromosome 18 and bipolar disorder: a replication test. Psychiatry Res 59:7–15.

Manki H, Shigenobu K, Muramatsu T, et al. (1996). Dopamine D2, D3 and D4 receptor and transporter gene polymorphims and mood disorders. J Affect Disord 40:7–13.

Mann JJ, Malone KM, Nielsen DA, Goldman D, Edos J, Gelernter J. (1997). Possible association of a polymorphism of the tryptophan hydroxylase gene with suicidal behavior in depressed patients. Am J Psychiatry 154:(10):1451–1453.

McInnis MG, McMahon FJ, Chase GA et al. (1993). Anticipation in bipolar affective disorder. Am J Hum Genet 53: 385–390.

Mendlewicz J, Lipp O, Souery D, et al. (1997). Expanded trinucleotide CAG repeats in families with bipolar affective disorder. Biol Psychiatry 42(12):1115–1122.

Mendlewicz J, Simon P, Sevy S, et al. (1987). Polymorphic DNA marker on chromosome and manic-depression. Lancet 1:1230–1232.

Muramatsu T, Matsushita S, Kanba S, et al. (1997). Monoamine oxidase genes polymorphisms and mood disorder. Am J Med Genet 74:494–496.

Nanko S, Fukuda R, Hattori M, et al. (1994). Linkage studies between affective disorder and dopamine D2, D3, and D4 receptor gene loci in four Japanese pedigrees. Psychiatry Res 52(2):149–157.

Nothen MM, Eggermann K, Albus M et al. (1995). Association analysis of the monoamine oxidase A gene in bipolar affective disorder by using family-based internal controls. Am J Hum Genet 57:975–977.

Nöthen MM, Cichon S, Erdmann J, et al. (1993). Pseudoautosomal marker DXYS20 and manic depression. Am J Hum Genet 52:841–842.

Nylander PO, Engström C, Chotai J, et al. (1994). Anticipation in Swedish families with bipolar affective disorder. J Med Genet 9: 686–689.

O'Donovan M.C, Guy C, Craddock N, et al. (1995). Expanded CAG repeats in schizophrenie and bipolar disorder. Nature Genet 1995:10:380–381.

Ogilvie AD, Battersby S, Bubb VJ, et al. (1996). Polymorphism in serotonin transporter gene associated with susceptibility to major depression. Lancet 347:731–733.

Oruc L, Lindblad K, Verheyen G, et al. (1997). CAG expansions in bipolar and unipolar disorders. Am J Hum Genet 60:730–732.

Ott J. (1991). Analysis of Human Genetic Linkage, 2nd ed. Baltimore: Johns Hopkins University Press.

Parker LS (2002). Ethical issues in bipolar disorders pedigree research: privacy concerns, informed consent and grounds for waiver. Bipolar Disord 4:1–16.

Parsian A, Todd RD (1994). Bipolar disorder and the pseudoautosomal region: an association study. Am J Med Genet 54: 5–7.

Pauls DL, Ott J, Paul SM, et al. (1995). Linkage analyses of chromosome 18 markers do not identify a major susceptibility locus for bipolar affective disorder in the Old Order Amish. Am. J. Med. Genet. 57: 636–643.

Paulson HL, Fischbeck KH. (1996). Trinucleotide repeats in neurogenetic disorders.

Annu Rev Neurosci. 19:79–107.

Plomin R, Owen MJ, McGuffin P. (1994). The genetic basis of complex human behaviors. Science 264(5166):1733–1739.

Pekkarinen P, Terwilliger J, Bredbacka P-E, et al. (1995). Evidence of a predisposing locus to bipolar disorder on Xq24-q27.1 in an extended Finnish pedigree. Genome Res 5:105–115.

Propping P, Nothen MM, Fimmers R, et al. (1993). Linkage versus association studies in complex diseases. Pychiatr Genet 3:136.

Rees M, Norton N, Jones I, et al. (1997). Association study of bipolar disorder at the human serotonin transporter gene (hSERT; 5HTT). Mol Psychiatry 2:398–402.

Serretti A, Macciardi F, Cusin C, et al. (1998). Dopamine receptor D4 gene is associated with delusional symptomatology in mood disorders. Psychiatry Res 80(2):129–136.

Shore D. (1993). Legal and ethical issues in psychiatric genetic research. Am J Med Genet 48:17–21.

Shore D. (1996). Ethical principles and informed consent: an NIMH perspective. Psychopharmacol Bull 32:7–10.

Sidenberg DG, King N, Kennedy JL (1994). Analysis of new D_1 Dopamine receptor (DRD4) coding region variants and TH microsatellite in the Old Amish family (00A110). Psychiatr Genet 4:95–99.

Smeraldi E, Macciardi F. (1995). Association and linkage studies in mental illness. In: Papadimitriou GN, Mendlewicz J, eds. Genetics of Mental Disorders Part I: Theoretical Aspects. Bailliere's Clinical Psychiatry, International Practice and Research. London: Bailliere Tindall, 1(1):97–110.

Smeraldi E, Zanardi R, Benedetti F, Di Bella D, et al. (1998). Polymorphism within the promoter of the serotonin transporter gene and antidepressant efficacy of fluvoxamine. Mol Psychiatry 3:508–511.

Smyth C, Kalsi G, Curtis D, et al. (1997). Two-locus admixture linkage analysis of bipolar and unipolar affective disorder supports the presence of susceptiblity loci on chromosomes 11p15 and 21q22. Genomics 39:271–298.

Souery D, Lipp O, Mahieu B, at al. (1996a). Association study of bipolar disorder with candidate genes involved in catecholamine neurotransmission: DRD2, DRD3, DAT1 and TH genes. Am J Med Genet (Neuropsychiatr Genet) 67(6):551–555.

Souery D, Papadimitriou GN, Mendlewicz J. (1996b). New genetic approaches in affective disorders. In: Papadimitriou GN, Mendlewicz J, eds. Genetics of Mental Disorders Part II: Clinical Issues. Baillière's Clinical Psychiatry, International Practice and Research. London: Bailliere Tindall, 2(1).

Stine C, Xu J, Koskela R, et al. (1996). Evidence for linkage of bipolar disorder to chromosome 18 with parent-of-origin effect. Am J Hum Genetic 57:1384–1394.

Stine OC, McMahon FJ, Chen L, et al. (1997). Initial genome screen for bipolar disorder in the NIMH genetics initiative pedigrees: Chromosomes 2, 11, 13, 14 and X. Am J Med Genet 74:263–269.

Straub RE, Lehner Th, Luo Y, et al. (1994). A possible vulnerability locus for bipolar affective disorder on chromosome 21q22.3. Nat Genet 8:291–296.

Terwilliger JD and Ott J (1992). A haplotype-based haplotype relative risk statistic. Hum Heredity 42:337–346.

Trottier Y, Lutz Y, Stevanin G, et al. (1995). Polyglutamine expansion as a pathological epitope in Huntington's disease and four dominant cerebellar ataxias. Nature. 378(6555):403–406.

Turecki G, Rouleau GA, Mari JJ, et al. (1996). A systematic evaluation of linkage studies in bipolar disorder. Acta Scand Psychiatr 93:317–326.

Vallada H, Craddock N, Vasques L, et al. (1996). Linkage studies in bipolar affective disorder with markers on chromosome 21. J Affect Disord 41(3):217–221.

Van Knorring AL, Cloninger C, Bohman M, et al. (1983) An adoption study of depressive disorders and substance abuse. Arch Gen Psychiatry 40:943 950.

Vieland VJ, Susser E, Weissman MM. (1995) Genetic epidemiology in psychiatric research. In: Papadimitriou GN, Mendlewicz J, eds. Genetics of Mental Disorders Part I: Theoretical Aspects. Baillière's Clinical Psychiatry, International Practice and Research. London: Bailliere Tindall, 1(1):19–46.

Waldman ID, Robinson BF, Feigon SA, et al. (1997). Linkage disequilibrium between the dopamine transporter gene (DAT1) and bipolar disorder: extending the transmission disequilibrium test to examine genetic heterogeneity. Genet Epidemiol 14:699–704.

Wender P, Kttzs S, Rosenthal D. (1986) Psychiatr disorders in the biological and adoptive families of adopted individuals with affective disorders. Arch Gen Psychiatry 43:923–950.

Winokur G, Cadoret R, Dorzab J, Baker M. (1971) Depressive disease: a genetic study. Arch Gen Psychiatry 24:135–144.

Yoneda H, Sakai T, Ishida T, et al. (1992). An association between manic-depressive illness and a pseudoautosomal DNA marker. Am J Hum Genet 51:1172–1173.

28

Biological Distinction Between Unipolar and Bipolar Disorder

XIAOHONG WANG and CHARLES B. NEMEROFF
Emory University School of Medicine, Atlanta, Georgia, U.S.A.

I. INTRODUCTION

The DSM-IV and the International Classification of Diseases, 10th revision (ICD-10), provide clear diagnostic criteria for distinguishing bipolar disorder from unipolar disorder. The clinical signs and symptoms of unipolar disorder include loss of interest or pleasure, reduced energy, poor sleep, decreased appetite and weight loss, hopelessness or worthless feeling, and suicidal thoughts. Whereas bipolar disorder includes all of the clinical symptoms of major depression during a depressive episode, it also obviously is characterized by a number of symptoms during the manic phase including an elevated, expansive, or irritable mood as well as grandiosity, decreased sleep and appetite, pressured speech, racing thoughts, and excessive involvement in pleasurable but potentially dangerous activities. Moreover, manic and depressive symptoms often occur together in the so-called mixed state. Although clinicians and investigators concur that these two syndromes are surely distinct entities, in terms of both clinical course and response to treatment, it is not clear what the definitive neurobiological distinctions are between these two disorders. During the last decade, extraordinary advances in both neuroscience and psychopharmacology have provided the field with the tools to further understand the differences between these mood disorders.

II. NEUROENDOCRINE HYPOTHESIS

It has been recognized for many years that certain endocrine disorders are associated with a higher than expected frequency of a wide spectrum of psychiatric symptoms and syndromes, e.g., glucocorticoid-induced depression, mania and psychotic symptoms; hypothyroidism-induced depression, etc. The excessive secretion of cortisol in Cushing's syndrome is also well known to be associated with both anxiety and depressive symptoms. Specific neuroendocrine alterations in response to stressors or pharmacological challenge tests have been shown to be highly associated with certain neuropsychiatric disorders. The majority of studies have scrutinized the hypothalamic-pituitary-adrenal (HPA) and -thyroid (HPT) axes as well as growth hormone and gonadal hormone secretions.

A. Hypothalamic-Pituitary-Adrenal Axis

There are extensive data available on the activity of the HPA axis in patients with mood disorders. A sizable subgroup of patients with unipolar depression exhibits hyperactivity of the HPA axis, characterized by hypercortisolemia, increased urinary free cortisol concentrations, and nonsuppression of cortisol after administration of the synthetic glucocorticoid dexamethasone. Patients with mixed mania exhibit similar HPA axis hyperactivity including elevation of CSF cortisol concentrations [16]. In contrast, patients with euphoric mania have normal HPA function.

Many studies have supported the hypothesis that CRF hyperactivity may contribute to the pathogenesis of depression. CRF is released from neurons in the paraventricular nucleus (PVN) of the hypothalamus and is transported to the anterior pituitary through the hypothalamo-hypophyseal-portal circulation. ACTH is released from the anterior pituitary gland by CRF, and is carried in the peripheral circulation to the adrenal cortex where it releases cortisol.

In drug-free unipolar depressed patients, CSF CRF concentrations are increased. This increase is likely due to the increased activity of CRF-secreting neurons in the hypothalamus, as well as extra-hypothalamic brain regions [1,2]. Interestingly, electroconvulsive therapy (ECT) or treatment with antidepressants such as fluoxetine, desipramine, and venlafaxine reduce CRF concentrations in CSF in depressed patients [3,4]. Normal controls and nonhuman primates with euphoric mania do not exhibit elevation in CSF CRF concentrations.

Assessment of the activity of the HPA axis in depressed patients has been intensively scrutinized. Two tests are widely used, either alone or in combination. The dexamethasone suppression test (DST), though much maligned, has documented HPA axis hyperactivity in patients with unipolar depression and in those with mixed or dysphoric mania [5,6]. The CRF stimulation test is a more sensitive test of HPA axis function. In this test, CRF is administered intravenously (usually in a 1 μg/kg or 100 μg dose), and blood samples are obtained for ACTH and cortisol assay at 30-min intervals over a 2- to 3-hr period. When compared to normal subjects, the ACTH response to exogenous CRF is blunted in drug-free depressed patients, but not in patients with euphoric mania [7–12]. Mixed mania has not yet been studied. The pathophysiology of the blunted ACTH response may be due to chronic hypersecretion of CRF with resultant CRF receptor downregulation and/or the feedback of hypersecreted cortisol on ACTH secretion.

The combination of the dexamethasone (DEX) suppression test and the CRF stimulation test (DEX/CRF test) has the promise of being an even more sensitive measure of HPA axis activity. In the DEX/CRF test, a single dose (1.5 mg) DEX is given to patients at 23:00 hr, and 100 mg CRF is given intravenously at 15:00 hr the following day. In depressed patients, the release of ACTH and cortisol was significantly higher than in nondepressed controls—evidence of the HPA axis hyperactivity. Rybakowski and Twardowska [13] reported that in bipolar depressed patients, DEX/CRF induced much higher elevations of cortisol than in unipolar depressed patients and normal controls. A separate report indicated that bipolar patients in remission had higher baseline and peak ACTH concentration after a single dose of CRF (100 μg) [14]. Acutely manic patients have higher basal cortisol levels as opposed to controls, and DEX challenge showed that these patients had lower DEX-induced growth hormone responses than did controls [15]. Finally, Swann and colleagues [16] have reported elevated CSF cortisol concentrations in patients with mixed, but not euphoric, mania.

B. Hypothalamic-Pituitary-Thyroid Axis

Alterations in the HPT axis have long been associated with higher than expected prevalence rates of all forms of mood disorders. Hypothyroidism has repeatedly been demonstrated in patients with depression, including symptomless autoimmune thyroiditis [17,18]. In clinical studies, T_3 augments the effects of antidepressants in treating depression [19]. Many studies have focused on the potential role of thyrotropin-releasing hormone (TRH), discovered in 1970. Similar to CRF, TRH is released from the hypothalamus and acts on the anterior pituitary via the portal system. TRH binds to the pituitary TRH receptor and induces the release of thyroid-stimulating hormone (TSH). TSH then enters the systemic circulation and binds to TSH receptors on the thyroid gland which causes the release of the two major thyroid hormones (T_3 and T_4). The activity of the HPT axis is controlled through the negative feedback of thyroid hormones on both TSH and TRH secretion.

In addition to its role in the HPT axis, TRH also acts as a CNS neurotransmitter in both hypothalamic and extra-hypothalamic brain areas. Thyroid hormone is well known to be essential for normal neuronal development in the CNS. Primary hypothyroidism is associated with many behavioral symptoms also observed in primary depression including depressed mood, fatigue, decreased sexual drive, psychomotor retardation, increased sleep, and weight gain. In contrast, hyperthyroidism is associated with increased autonomic function, anxiety, psychomotor agitation, and emotional lability. There are two reports of elevated TRH concentrations in CSF in depressed patients, both bipolar and unipolar [20,21]. This elevation may be due to the hypersecretion of TRH in response to relative hypothyroidism. This explanation is supported by the report of low CSF concentrations of the thyroid transport globulin transthyretin in treatment-refractory depressive patients [22,23] and the increased size of the pituitary gland in depressed patients [24], which might be partly due to TRH hypersecretion. Symptoms of depression in patients with primary hypothyroidism do not respond to antidepressant treatment unless thyroid function is normalized. Several studies have found that the addition of T_3 (25–50 μg/day) is effective in converting antidepressant nonresponders to responders [19,25–27].

One of the most sensitive measures of HPT axis is the TRH stimulation test, in which TSH is measured at baseline and at 30-min intervals after IV injection of TRH (200–500 μg). In primary hypothyroidism an exaggerated TSH response is observed, and in primary hyperthyroidism the TSH response is attenuated. Multiple reports have demonstrated that both unipolar and bipolar depressed patients exhibit a blunted TSH response to TRH [18,28–33]. The pathophysiology of this blunted TSH response may well be due to chronic hypersecretion of TRH and the resultant downregulation of the TRH receptor in pituitary thyrotrophs. Other sensitive methods of measuring HPT axis function include the measurement of maximal circadian secretion of TSH between 23:00 hr and 01:00 hr [34,35], and performance of a standard TRH stimulation test at both 08:00 hr and 23:00 hr that was developed by Duval [36]. The differential response at 08:00 hr and 23:00 hr were compared, designated the $\Delta\Delta$TSH. The depressed patients, both unipolar and bipolar, had a significantly lower $\Delta\Delta$TSH than normal controls. Recently, two reports revealed higher TRH-stimulated TSH levels in lithium-naive bipolar II [37] and in bipolar mixed patients [38].

In contrast to the evidence for TRH hypersecretion in depression is the hypothesis that TRH acts as endogenous antidepressant. A recent report, for example, reported that TRH exhibited acute antidepressant effects when injected directly into CSF [39]. In addition, pharmacological doses of T_4 are reportedly effective in treating both the depression and mania in rapid-cycling bipolar disorder [40]. In a recent report of a 3-year treatment study of bipolar disorder with lithium or carbamazepine, a lower mean serum level of free T_4 was associated with more affective episodes and greater severity of depression. This suggests that the lower level of free T_4 may be a causal factor in mood instability, and T_4 replacement may warrant further study [41].

C. Hypothalamic-Growth Hormone Axis

Alterations in the HGH axis have also been reported in patients with mood disorders. Growth hormone is secreted from the basophilic cells of the anterior pituitary. Its secretion is regulated by two hypothalamic peptide hormones, growth—hormone–releasing hormone (GHRH) and somatostatin. GHRH induces GH release whereas somatostatin inhibits GH release. The main function of GH is to promote body growth via the release of insulinlike growth factor 1 (IGF-1) and somatomedins from the liver. GH also directly counteracts insulin's effects. The secretion of GH has a unique circadian pattern, with a peak during stage 4 sleep. GH secretion is also responsive to other factors including stress, exercise, hypoglycemia, and other neurotransmitters, e.g., dopamine, norepinephrine, and acetylcholine.

In depressed patients, nocturnal GH secretion is decreased [42], whereas daytime GH secretion is increased in both unipolar and bipolar patients [43]. GHRH-induced GH release has been reported to be diminished in depressed patients [44–47]. It would be fair to say, however, that the standardized GHRH stimulation test to evaluate HGH axis function in patients with mood disorders has not yet been developed and results obtained thus far are not consistent [48].

To further assess the integrity of HGH axis, several studies using standardized provocative pharmacological challenge tests either with clonidine (an α_2 adrenergic receptor agonist) or apomorphine (a dopamine D_2 receptor agonist) have been utilized. A blunted GH response has repeatedly been obtained in depressed patients [49–52]. In addition, a blunted GH response to other challenges such as insulin-induced hypoglycemia and L-dopa have also been noted in depressed patients [53]. Because depressed patients have repeatedly shown to have decreased CSF somatostatin concentrations [54], which would likely increase GH secretion, alternative mechanisms to explain the blunted response must be involved.

In bipolar patients, blunted GH responses to both noradrenergic stimuli and dexamethasone stimulation has been reported [15,55]. The GH response to baclofen, a GABA-B receptor agonist, was reported to be enhanced in bipolar patients, suggesting upregulation of GABA-B receptors [56]. A blunted GH response in depressed but not bipolar patients to sumatriptan, a $5HT_{1D}$ receptor agonist that stimulates GH secretion, has also been observed [57].

D. Hypothalamic-Pituitary-Gonadal Axis

A significant role for HPG axis alterations in mood disorders has been postulated to explain the inordinately high rate of depression in women, and also its higher incidence during pregnancy and in the puerperium. Similar to the HPA and HPT axes, the HPG axis is also regulated hierarchically, in this case by a releasing hormone secreted from hypothalamus, gonadotropin-releasing hormone (GnRH). This decapeptide, released from hypothalamus, acts on the anterior pituitary to release both luteinizing hormone (LH) and follicle-stimulating hormone (FSH). Both of these gonadotropins are important for sexual development and maintenance of normal sexual function in males and females. Together they are responsible for estrogen and progesterone secretion in women and testosterone in men. GnRH secretion is positively regulated by noradrenergic agonists and negatively regulated by endogenous opioids. Postpartum depression and premenstrual dysphoric disorder (PMDD) may be in part due to disturbances of gonadal steroid regulation and secretion. One recent report revealed that androstenedione, testosterone, and dihydrotestosterone levels are increased in hypercortisolemic women with severe major depression. This study suggested that HPG axis alterations may be associated with hyperactivity of the HPA system [58,59]. In contrast, another study reported that daytime, nighttime, and 24-h mean testosterone levels are significantly lower in depressed men than in normal controls [60]. Leuprolide is a GnRH agonist and is widely used in the treatment of endometriosis and prostate cancer by inducing a "chemical gonadectomy." It is effective in the treatment of PMDD. However, leuprolide has been reported to induce depression, and concomitant sertraline treatment improved these depressive symptoms [61–63]. Plasma levels of LH and GnRH-induced LH secretion have been reported to be increased in mania, but unchanged in depression [64–66].

III. THE IMMUNE SYSTEM AND MOOD DISORDER

Numerous studies have documented that the immune system and the CNS interact and regulate each other. Dysfunction of one system may cause dysfunction in the other. Evidence has accrued that patients with a variety of psychiatric disorders, particularly those that are stress related, cause a wide range of immune alterations including decreased NK cell counts and reduced mitogen-stimulated lymphocyte proliferation. Moreover, agents that alter immune function such as the exogenous use of cytokines or immunosuppressive agents (glucocorticoids) cause significant mood alterations.

A. Interaction Between the CNS and the Immune System

Interactions between the immune and CNS systems have been extensively studied. Immune cells express receptors for a wide spectrum of neurotransmitters, hormones, and neuropeptides. These include monoamines, prolactin, GH, CRF, ACTH, and opioids [67–69]. The immune system is also regulated by the autonomic nervous system, especially the sympathetic division [70]. Limbic and cortical regions may also be involved in the modulation of immune activity. In the rat, CRF, administered intracerebroventricularly, causes activation of the central sympathetic pathway and significantly decreased NK cell number in the spleen [71]. To understand this complex, multidirectional communication, Ader proposed a term, psychoneuroimmunology, to study brain-immune interaction [67]. The advances in neuroscience and related areas suggest that this term, psychoneuroendoimmunology, may more accurately describe the interaction among the CNS, endocrine, and immune systems. Stress and medical or psychiatric illness are associated with neurobiological alterations in certain brain areas. These changes may, as noted above, trigger HPA axis alterations or changes in other hypothalamus–pituitary–end organ axes and/or descending autonomic pathways. The endocrine and sympathetic signals are sent to target immune organs such as the spleen or thymus and further trigger immune responses in vulnerable individuals. Because the interaction is multidirectional, alterations in immune or endocrine system may also induce responses in the CNS and precipitate psychiatric or medical illness.

B. Stress and the Immune Response

In 1977, Bartrop and coworkers reported that stressful life events such as bereavement have exhibited a reduction in mitogen-stimulated lymphocyte proliferation [72]. This finding was replicated in a prospective study by Schleifer et al. [73], who collected lymphocytes from individuals before and after bereavement. Mitogen-stimulated lymphocyte proliferation (MSLP) assays were performed using phytohemagglutinin (PHA), concanavalin A, and pokeweed mitogen.

MSLP was significantly lower during postbereavement when compared with the prebereavement samples. Another immune parameter, NK cell activity, has also been used to study the impact of stress on immune response. Glaser and colleagues have conducted a series of studies in this area [74]. Examination stress in medical students was found to be associated with a decreased in T-cell number, decreased MSLP, and decreased interferon production. NK cell activity was decreased during the final examination period when compared to preexamination [75]. Life stresses also caused alterations in lymphocyte subpopulation, an impaired antibody response to influenza vaccine, and prolonged latency of wound healing [76–78].

C. Mood Disorder and the Immune Response

Similar to the impact of stress on the immune system, depression has also been reported to be associated with decreased MSLP in several studies [79,80] and decreased NK cell activity as well [81]. Subsequent studies have reported discordant results. A variety of factors likely contribute to these discrepancies. One such significant variable is that circulating lymphocyte subpopulations exhibit different circadian rhythms [82]. In one report, NK cell number and activity in depressed patients and normal controls were studied at both diurnal peak (8 AM) and nadir (4 PM) [83]. In depressed patients, a significantly lower diurnal variation in NK cell number and NK activity was noted. Antidepressant treatment reportedly augments NK cell activity both in vivo and in vitro [84]. Depressed patients treated with fluoxetine (20 mg/day) for 4 weeks as outpatients exhibited increased NK cell activity in patients who had low pretreatment NK cell activity, but produced no effects on patients who had normal or high NK cell activity at baseline. Interestingly, treatment of mononuclear cells with fluoxetine and paroxetine in vitro also enhanced NK cell activity. In a separate study [85] 10 depressed cancer patients were treated with fluvoxamine, an SSRI antidepressant, for 28 days; one-half of the patients responded to the treatment with significantly improved HAM-D scores, and the mean NK cell number increased 53%. There was a significant correlation between the change in HAM-D score of the responders and the change in NK cell counts. The specificity of the action of SSRIs on NK cell activity and number was highlighted by Mizruchin and coworkers who confirmed the effects of SSRIs in reversing low NK cell activity in depressed patients associated with concomitant clinical improvement; D_2 receptor antagonists or agonists were without effects [86].

There are a limited number of studies evaluating immune responses in patients with bipolar disorders. Several reports revealed hyperactivity of the immune system. In a recent study of 23 bipolar patients and 23 matched normal controls, the MSLP and serum soluble IL-2 receptor (sIL-2R) levels were significantly higher during acute mania than in remission. There was no difference in the immune measures between normal controls and remitted bipolar patients [87]. In a separate study, lithium treatment normalized the elevation of sIL-2R and sIL-6R in rapid-cycling bipolar patients [88]. Euthymic bipolar patients or those medicated with lithium have normal sIL-2R levels, antithyroid antibody levels, mitogen stimulation responses, and circulating lymphocyte phenotype profiles [89].

D. Mechanism of the Effects of Stress and Mood Disorders on the Immune System

As discussed above, the HPA axis and the autonomic nervous system, two major stress-responsive elements, exert immunoregulatory effects. Corticosteroids, the final product of the HPA axis, produce major effects on immune systems. Immune cells and tissues possess corticosteroid receptors and represent the substrate by which the immune system is regulated by glucocorticoids. Obviously corticosteroids are widely used clinically as immunosuppressive and antiinflammatory agents. Such actions may be mediated through the inhibition of the synthesis of cytokines and other mediators of inflammation [90]. Corticosteroids also produce a shift of immune reaction from primarily a cell-mediated to an antibody-mediated response by the action of certain cytokines [91,92]. In addition to a role for the HPA axis and sympathetic nervous system in regulating immune responses, CRF itself is immunomodulatory. CRF regulates the immune system response not only via the HPA axis but directly as well. CRF-overproducing mice exhibit immune defects with a profound decrease in the number of B-cells and severely impaired primary and memory antibody response [93] though this may be explained by HPA axis hyperactivity. CRF can also increase release of cytokines, specifically IL-1α and IL-2 [94,95]. Taken together, the impact of the HPA axis, sympathetic nervous system, and CRF on immune system responses is indeed very complex.

IV. CYTOKINES AND MOOD DISORDERS

The cytokines, considered as hormones of the immune system, are a group of large peptides/small proteins of low molecular weight that communicate between immune cells and mediate inflammatory or immune response to stress, injury, and infection. A growing body of literature supports the fact that cytokines act not only as immunomodulators but also as neuromodulators. Cytokines are classified into three large groups based on function: proinflammatory (IL-1, IL-6 and TNF), anti-inflammatory (IL-4, IL-10, IL-13), and hematopoietic (IL-3, IL-5, colony-stimulating factor) cytokines. Cytokines not only exist in the immune system, but also within the CNS, where they are secreted from astrocytes and microglia, and perhaps neurons. IL-1 has been found in several brain regions and its function in brain has been studied extensively [96]. Moreover IL-1 is able to stimulate the production of itself, IL-6, TNF-α, and colony-stimulating factor from astroglial cells [97,98]. Intraperitoneal injection of IL-1β into mice increases MHPG (the major norepinephrine metabolite) and 5HIAA (the major serotonin metabolite) in the hypothalamus [99,100]. Injection of IL-1β and TNF-α intracerebroventricularly (icv) causes an elevation of 5-HIAA in the nucleus raphe dorsalis [101]. IL-1 treatment was also associated with increases in CRF, ACTH, and corticosteroids [102,103]. IL-6, TNF, and interferon were reported to produce similar effects on the HPA axis [104].

CRF, administered intravenously in humans, causes a marked increase of plasma IL-1α and IL-2 concentrations [95]. Plasma concentrations of proinflammatory cytokines, IL-1, and IL-6 have been reported to be increased in depressed patients [105–107]. A recent study with a small sample replicated the increased IL-1 concentrations in CSF in depressed patients, but IL-6 concentrations were reduced and TNF-α concentrations unchanged [108]. Plasma soluble IL-6 receptor and soluble IL-2 receptor were reportedly higher in manic patients than in normal controls [109] and a recent report confirmed the latter finding in mania [87]. Interferon-α (IFN-α), an important cytokine in the early immune response to viral infection has both antiproliferative and antiviral properties [110]. IFN-α has been successfully used in the treatment of melanoma and hepatitis C. The treatment with IFN-α has been associated with a high rate of CNS side effects similar to depression (anhedonia, fatigue, anorexia, poor concentration, and sleep disturbance) [111,112]. A recently published study from our group demonstrated that antidepressant treatment with an SSRI prevents IFN-α-induced depression [113]. In a double-blind, placebo-controlled study of 40 patients with malignant melanoma, paroxetine treatment (2 weeks prior to the initiation of IFN-α) significantly decreased the severity of depressive symptoms and the percentage of patients who fulfilled criteria for major depression induced by IFN-α treatment. Paroxetine treatment also significantly reduced the incidence of major depression during IFN-α treatment. Interestingly, several case reports demonstrated that treatment with IFN-α may also cause mania [114–118]. The mechanism of cytokine-induced mood instability may either be a direct effect on the CNS or via stimulatory effects on the HPA axis via CRF as described in Section III.D.

V. ROLE OF NEUROTRANSMITTERS AND NEUROPEPTIDES

Considerable advances in understanding of neurotransmitters and their receptors have occurred over the last decade. Many in psychoneuroendocrinoimmunology research have suggested that neurotransmitter systems function in various CNS sites and in the periphery in a concerted harmonious manner. For example, CRF responds to psychological or physical stresses and stimulates the HPA axis ultimately increasing glucocorticoid secretion and also exerts target immune organs as well. CRF also acts on extra pituitary sites to cause a wide range of biological and behavioral effects. Molecular biology, human genetics, and other research technologies have provided novel information on receptor subfamilies and their differential functions, alternate splicing of pre-prohormones in various physiological states, intracellular signal transduction and related gene transcription, genetic polymorphism of certain neurotransmitter transporters and receptors, and *in vivo* studies by remarkable new functional imaging technologies. The roles of several neurotransmitters in the pathophysiology of depression and bipolar disorder are described below.

A. Norepinephrine

The catecholamine hypothesis of affective disorders originally conceptualized by Schildkraut [42] suggested a relative deficiency of one or more catecholamines within the CNS in depression, and a relative excess in mania. The sympathoadrenal system consists of the adrenal medulla and the sympathetic nervous system (SNS). As early as the 1960s, 3-methoxy-4-hydroxy-phenylglycol (MHPG), a major norepinephrine metabolite, was reported to be elevated in the CSF of a subgroup of patients with mood disorder [42]. Significant elevation of plasma and urinary norepinephrine and its metabolites was also reported in a subgroup of depressed patients by many research groups [119–121]. Results in patients with bipolar disorder were equivocal, probably due to their disease state, i.e., manic, depressed, or euthymic. The excretion of norepinephrine and epinephrine in urine of bipolar depressed patients was consistently lower when compared with unipolar depressed patients [122–124]. Plasma MPHG concentrations were also reported to be lower in bipolar depressed patients than in unipolar depressed patients [125]. Elevated plasma and urinary norepinephrine and epinephrine concentrations were reported in bipolar manic patients [126]. The major difference between bipolar depressed and unipolar depressed patients was the greater urinary MPHG levels in unipolar depressed patients. No significant differences in CSF norepinephrine and its metabolites were noted between bipolar and unipolar patients. Treatment with fluoxetine normalized CSF norepinephrine in depressed patients [4]. A recent study indicated that pretreatment levels of urinary MPHG correlated with improvement of mania [127]. In a recent report, Johnston et al. [128] used plasma norepinephrine levels to predict the outcome of major depressive disorder (MDD). Forty patients with MDD were followed for 8 years. The results revealed that the higher the plasma norepinephrine concentrations, the better the outcome for MDD, and the longer the time to first recurrence.

Reboxetine, the first selective norepinephrine reuptake inhibitor, has provided additional opportunities to evaluate the role of the noradrenergic system in mood disorders. Although controlled data are scant, there is a general consensus among clinicians that antidepressants that block norepinephrine, but not serotonin, reuptake are more likely to cause a switch into mania in depressed bipolar patients.

B. Serotonin

The serotonin hypothesis of depression proposed that a relative deficiency of serotonin in the CNS renders individuals vulnerable to affective illness. Reduced concentrations of CSF 5-hydroxyindoleacetic acid (5HIAA), the major metabolite of serotonin (5-hydroxytryptamine, 5HT), has repeatedly been reported in depressed patients [129–131] as well as in patients with suicidality, increased aggression, and poor impulse control [132]. The significant efficacy of the selective serotonin reuptake inhibitors (SSRIs; e.g., fluoxetine, sertraline, paroxetine, citalopram, and fluvoxamine) in the treatment of depression strongly supports a serotonergic deficiency in CNS, though some SSRIs affect norepinephrine and dopamine uptake as well. A recent study [133] using the tryptophan depletion paradigm in 55 drug-free depressed patients treated with either fluoxetine or desipramine revealed that 53% relapsed in the fluoxetine group vs. only 6% in the desipramine group. The results indicate that antidepressant response to fluoxetine (and probably other SSRIs) appears to be dependent on serotonin availability.

Other serotonergic alterations have been reported in both bipolar and unipolar depression. Platelet 5HT$_2$ receptor number is increased in depressed patients and significantly decreased after antidepressant treatment [134]. Increased platelet serotonin concentrations have been reported in bipolar depressed patients [135]. Unaffected bipolar relatives were found to have lower platelet serotonin transporter function and reduced serotonin transporter-binding sites, and diminished platelet serotonin levels [136]. Levels of urinary 5HIAA were not different in bipolar and unipolar depressed patients [122]. Brain imaging studies, largely using SPECT, have confirmed the reduction in raphe serotonin transporter binding in drug-free depressed patients [137].

C. Dopamine

There are relatively few reports concerning the role of dopamine (DA) in the pathophysiology of mood disorders. Elevation of CNS DA activity may play an important role in the etiology of psychotic depression. However, the effects of some medications with primary actions on DA circuits suggest that DA may still play a pivotal role in the etiology of mood disorders. Although concentrations of urinary and CSF homovanillic acid (HVA), a metabolite of DA, were found to be no different in bipolar and unipolar depressed patients [122] others have noted that CSF HVA levels are decreased in depressed patients [138–141] and increased in agitated or manic patients [142–144]. The purported efficacy of methylphenidate, a psychostimulant which releases DA from presynaptic terminals, in the treatment of depression particularly in depressed patients with medical illness, also supports a role for DA system in mood disorder. For example, treatment of depressed post-stroke patients with methylphenidate caused significant improvement (70–

80%) and a relatively rapid response when compared to nortriptyline [145–147]. Moreover, nomifensine, a selective DA reuptake inhibitor, was shown to be an effective antidepressant, but was withdrawn from the market because of untoward effects on the hematopoietic systems.

Postsynaptic DA agonists also possess antidepressant properties, e.g., pramipexole [148]. A recent report suggests that a deficit of brain DA and norepinephrine occurs in refractory depressed patients [149]. This study, using a catheter placed in the patients' internal jugular vein to estimate the release of brain norepinephrine and DA, showed a significant decrease of the brain venoarterial norepinephrine and DA gradient in the depressed patients compared with normal controls.

Increased dopaminergic activity has been implicated in the pathophysiology of bipolar disorder. An amphetamine challenge to euthymic bipolar patients produced a significant behavioral response as assessed by the Brief Psychiatric Rating Scale, but functional brain imaging (SPECT) failed to demonstrate increased striatal DA release after amphetamine challenge in these bipolar patients [150]. The investigators suggested that their data were consistent with enhanced postsynaptic DA responsiveness in bipolar patients.

D. γ-Aminobutyric Acid (GABA)

GABA plays an important role in the CNS as a major inhibitory neurotransmitter. It interacts with biogenic amine neurotransmitters, including norepinephrine and serotonin. Dysfunction of the GABA system has been postulated to play an important role in mood disorders. Both preclinical and clinical studies suggest that a GABA deficit may occur in depression, whereas elevated GABA activity may occur in mania [151]. Several reports of decreased CSF and plasma GABA concentrations in depressed patients [152–154] have appeared; higher GABA levels were found in bipolar manic and euthymic patients compared with unipolar depressed patients [154]. Using magnetic resonance spectroscopy, medication-free depressed patients exhibited a 52% reduction in occipital cortex GABA concentrations compared with normal controls [155].

Manic patients have been reported to exhibit enhanced growth hormone responses to baclofen, a GABA-B receptor agonist, suggesting elevated hypothalamic GABA-B receptor function in bipolar disorder [56]. In addition, pretreatment plasma GABA levels were related to severity of manic symptoms, especially in women [127]. However, several anti-manic agents (valproic acid, carbamazepine, and lithium) have been reported to exert complex effects on GABA-ergic activity. Thus, valproic acid, carbamazepine, and lithium decrease GABA turnover in the frontal cortex [156] and increase GABA-B receptors in hippocampus after chronic administration [157,158]. Post noted that the GABA-B agonist baclofen exacerbated depression and its discontinuation was associated with mood improvement [159].

E. Glutamate

Glutamate is the major excitatory neurotransmitter in pyramidal neurons. Its postsynaptic signals are mediated through several receptor subtypes (i.e., N-methyl-D-aspartate, quisqualate, and kainate). The well-documented excitatory and neurotoxic effects of glutamate can occur by actions on both NMDA or non-NMDA receptors. A growing body of preclinical research suggests that brain glutamate systems may be involved both in the pathophysiology of mood disorders and the mechanism of action of antidepressants. In one placebo-controlled, double-blind study, a single dose of an NMDA receptor antagonist, ketamine, caused significant improvement in depressed patients after 72 hours [160]. Two recent reports used *in vivo* proton magnetic resonance spectroscopy to study the role of glutamate in both depression and bipolar [161,162]. In severely depressed patients, levels of glutamate and glutamine (Glu/Gln) were decreased in the anterior cingulate, whereas Glu/Gln levels was elevated in both frontal lobes and basal ganglia in bipolar patients. In a separate study, CSF glutamate levels were elevated in depressed patients compared with controls [163].

F. Vasopressin

Vasopressin is a peptide hormone cleaved from a pre-prohormone synthesized in the hypothalamus and other brain regions. Its main function is to conserve water and concentrate urine by activation of V_2 receptor on the basolateral surface of the renal conducting duct. High concentrations of vasopressin can also act on the V_1 receptor and cause vasoconstriction. In addition, considerable evidence suggests that vasopressin may play a critical role in learning and memory. Research from many groups demonstrated that vasopressin may also play an important role in the pathophysiology of affective disorders, and contribute to the well-documented hyperactivity of the HPA axis. Plasma vasopressin levels are higher in depressed patients than in controls and also higher in melancholic patients than nonmelancholic patients [164]. Levels of AVP were also positively correlated to severity of psychomotor retardation [165]. Muller recently reported a case of a depressed patient with chronically elevated plasma vasopressin levels due to paraneoplastic vasopressin secretion by an olfactory neuroblastoma [166]. Interestingly, the patient's depressive symptoms were markedly improved after surgical resection of the tumor, and subsequent normalization of plasma vasopressin levels.

G. Substance P

Substance P is a neuropeptide that acts upon the neurokinin-1 (NK-1) receptor. Neurons containing substance P are found in many brain regions that regulate affect, including many of the stress circuits [167]. Preclinical studies indicate that psychological stressors caused rapid downregulation of substance P receptors, presumably due to stress-induced release of substance P [168]. In a recent study, an NK-1 antagonist, MK-869, was shown in a double-blind, controlled study to possess antidepressant properties [168]. MK-869 was equivalent in antidepressant effect to paroxetine. Although these findings need to be replicated, they hypothesized that increased substance P availability in CNS may be related to depression, whereas decreased substance P availability may contribute to mania. Lithium and carbamazepine, when administered chronically, cause an increase of substance P concentrations in the striatum, nucleus accumbens, and frontal cortex of rat brain, suggesting that substance P may play a role in the action of mood stabilizers [169,170].

H. Somatostatin

Somatostatin is a hypothalamic tetradecapeptide noted previously to be involved in the regulation of growth hormone release, and perhaps in the regulation of the HPA axis. Somatostatin has been shown to regulate affect, sleep, ingestive behavior, locomotor activity, memory, and cognition. Its role in mood disorders has been supported by the reports of decreased CSF concentrations of somatostatin in depressed patients [171–173]. In Rubinow's seminal study, 49 bipolar and unipolar depressed patients matched with 49 normal controls were found to have a significant reduction in CSF somatostatin levels [174]. The values during depression were significantly lower than in the improved state. In manic patients, a markedly elevation of CSF somatostatin was reported [175]. Treatment with carbamazepine significantly reduces CSF somatostatin [174] whereas nimodipine (a calcium channel blocker, perhaps effective in treating some rapidly cycling affective disorders) was found to increase CSF somatostatin levels [176]. Alterations in CSF somatostatin concentrations are not specific to mood disorders. Other neuropsychiatric disorders also show such changes: decreased levels in schizophrenia, Alzheimer's disease, Parkinson's disease, and multiple sclerosis; increased levels in post-traumatic stress disorder, compression injuries, meningitis, and the encephalopathies.

VI. CONCLUSION

It is clear that patients with bipolar and unipolar affective disorders share several biological findings but also exhibit a number of differences. The above discussion reviewed such differences based on recent advances in neurobiology, endocrinology, and immunology research. Clearly, advances in molecular biology, brain imaging, and psychopharmacology, as well as novel genetic discoveries, will allow unprecedented advances in a field that has unfortunately languished over the past two decades—namely, the pathophysiology of bipolar disorder. Surely more effective treatment strategies will come available with the further understanding of the pathophysiology of these devastating mood disorders.

REFERENCES

1. FC Raadsheer, WJ Hoogendijk, FC Stam, FJ Tilders, DF Swaab. Increased numbers of corticotropin-releasing hormone expressing neurons in the hypothalamic paraventricular nucleus of depressed patients. Neuroendocrinology 60:436–444, 1994.
2. FC Raadsheer, JJ van Heerikhuize, PJ Lucassen, WJ Hoogendijk, FJ Tilders, DF Swaab. Corticotropin-releasing hormone mRNA levels in the paraventricular nucleus of patients with Alzheimer's disease and depression. Am J Psychiatry 152:1372–1376, 1995.
3. CB Nemeroff, G Bissette, H Akil, M Fink. Neuropeptide concentrations in the cerebrospinal fluid of depressed patients treated with electroconvulsive therapy. Corticotrophin-releasing factor, beta-endorphin and somatostatin. Br J Psychiatry 158:59–63, 1991.
4. MD De Bellis, TD Geracioti Jr, M Altemus, MA Kling. Cerebrospinal fluid monoamine metabolites in fluoxetine-treated patients with major depression

and in healthy volunteers. Biol Psychiatry 33:636–641, 1993.
5. RR Krishnan, AA Maltbie, JR Davidson. Abnormal cortisol suppression in bipolar patients with simultaneous manic and depressive symptoms. Am J Psychiatry 140:203–205, 1983.
6. DL Evans, CB Nemeroff. The dexamethasone suppression test in mixed bipolar disorder. Am J Psychiatry 140:615–617, 1983.
7. JD Amsterdam, DL Marinelli, P Arger, A Winokur. Assessment of adrenal gland volume by computed tomography in depressed patients and healthy volunteers: a pilot study. Psychiatry Res 21:189–197, 1987.
8. PW Gold, G Chrousos, C Kellner, R Post, A Roy, P Augerinos, H Schulte, E Oldfield, DL Loriaux. Psychiatric implications of basic and clinical studies with corticotropin-releasing factor. Am J Psychiatry 141:619–627, 1984.
9. PW Gold, DL Loriaux, A Roy, MA Kling, JR Calabrese, CH Kellner, LK Nieman, RM Post, D Pickar, W Gallucci, Responses to corticotropin-releasing hormone in the hypercortisolism of depression and Cushing's disease. Pathophysiologic and diagnostic implications. New Engl J Med 314:1329–1335, 1986.
10. F Holsboer, D Haack, A Gerken, P Vecsei. Plasma dexamethasone concentrations and differential suppression response of cortisol and corticosterone in depressives and controls. Biol Psychiatry 19:281–291, 1984.
11. RG Kathol, RS Jaeckle, JF Lopez, WH Meller. Consistent reduction of ACTH responses to stimulation with CRH, vasopressin and hypoglycaemia in patients with major depression. Br J Psychiatry 155:468–478, 1989.
12. EA Young, SJ Watson, J Kotun, RF Haskett, L Grunhaus, V Murphy-Weinberg, W Vale, J Rivier, H Akil. Beta-lipotropin-beta-endorphin response to low-dose ovine corticotropin releasing factor in endogenous depression. Preliminary studies. Arch Gen Psychiatry 47:449–457, 1990.
13. JK Rybakowski, K Twardowska. The dexamethasone/corticotropin-releasing hormone test in depression in bipolar and unipolar affective illness. J Psychiatr Res 33:363–370, 1999.
14. E Vieta, MJ Martinez-De-Osaba, F Colom, A Martinez-Aran, A Benabarre, C Gasto. Enhanced corticotropin response to corticotropin-releasing hormone as a predictor of mania in euthymic bipolar patients. Psychol Med 29:971–978, 1999.
15. JH Thakore, TG Dinan. Blunted dexamethasone-induced growth hormone responses in acute mania. Psychoneuroendocrinology 21:695–701, 1996.
16. AC Swann, PE Stokes, R Casper, SK Secunda, CL Bowden, N Berman, MM Katz, E Robins. Hypothalamic-pituitary-adrenocortical function in mixed and pure mania. Acta Psychiatr Scand 85:270–274, 1992.
17. CB Nemeroff, JS Simon, JJ Haggerty, DL Evans. Antithyroid antibodies in depressed patients. Am J Psychiatry 142:840–843, 1985.
18. JJ Haggerty Jr, JS Simon, DL Evans, CB Nemeroff. Relationship of serum TSH concentration and antithyroid antibodies to diagnosis and DST response in psychiatric inpatients. Am J Psychiatry 144:1491–1493, 1987.
19. CM Pariante, CB Nemeroff, AH Miller, A.H. Hormone regulation of behavior. In: DL Dunner, ed. Current Psychiatry Therapy II. Philadelphia: W.B. Saunders, 1997, pp 44–51.
20. CM Banki, G Bissette, M Arato, CB Nemeroff. Elevation of immunoreactive CSF TRH in depressed patients. Am J Psychiatry 145:1526–1531, 1988.
21. C Kirkegaard, J Faber, L Hummer, P Rogowski. Increased levels of TRH in cerebrospinal fluid from patients with endogenous depression. Psychoneuroendocrinology 4:227–235, 1979.
22. JA Hatterer, J Herbert, C Hidaka, SP Roose, JM Gorman. CSF transthyretin in patients with depression. Am J Psychiatry 150:813–815, 1993.
23. GM Sullivan, JA Hatterer, J Herbert, X Chen, SP Roose, E Attia, JJ Mann, LB Marangell, RR Goetz, JM Gorman. Low levels of transthyretin in the CSF of depressed patients. Am J Psychiatry 156:710–715, 1999.
24. KR Krishnan, PM Doraiswamy, SN Lurie, GS Figiel, MM Husain, OB Boyko, EH Ellinwood Jr, CB Nemeroff. Pituitary size in depression. J Clin Endocrinol Metab 72:256–259, 1991.
25. RT Joffe. Refractory depression: treatment strategies, with particular reference to the thyroid axis. J Psychiatry Neurosci 22:327–331, 1997.
26. TK Birkenhager, M Vegt, WA Nolen. An open study of triiodothyronine augmentation of tricyclic antidepressants in inpatients with refractory depression. Pharmacopsychiatry 30:23–26, 1997.
27. CB Nemeroff. Augmentation strategies in patients with refractory depression. Depress Anxiety 4:169–181, 1996.
28. AJ Kastin, RH Ehrensing, DS Schalch, MS Anderson. Improvement in mental depression with decreased thyrotropin response after administration of thyrotropin-releasing hormone. Lancet 2:740–742, 1972.
29. AJ Prange Jr, PP Lara, IC Wilson, LB Alltop, GR Breese. Effects of thyrotropin-releasing hormone in depression. Lancet 2:999–1002, 1972.
30. S Takahashi, H Kondo, M Yoshimura, Y Ochi. Antidepressant effect of thyrotropin-releasing hormone (TRH) and the plasma thyrotropin levels in depression. Folia Psychiatr Neurol Jpn 27:305–314, 1973.

31. DA Sack, SP James, NE Rosenthal, TA Wehr. Deficient nocturnal surge of TSH secretion during sleep and sleep deprivation in rapid-cycling bipolar illness. Psychiatry Res 23:179–191, 1988.
32. E Souetre, E Salvati, TA Wehr, DA Sack, B Krebs, G Darcourt. Twenty-four-hour profiles of body temperature and plasma TSH in bipolar patients during depression and during remission and in normal control subjects. Am J Psychiatry 145:1133–1137, 1988.
33. PT Loosen, AJ Prange, Jr. Serum thyrotropin response to thyrotropin-releasing hormone in psychiatric patients: a review. Am J Psychiatry 139:405–416, 1982.
34. YC Patel, FP Alford, HG Burger. The 24-hour plasma thyrotrophin profile. Clin Sci 43:71–77, 1972.
35. L Vanhaelst, E Van Cauter, JP Degaute, J Golstein. Circadian variations of serum thyrotropin levels in man. J Clin Endocrinol Metab 35:479–482, 1972.
36. F Duval, JP Macher, MC Mokrani. Difference between evening and morning thyrotropin responses to protirelin in major depressive episode. Arch Gen Psychiatry 47:443–448, 1990.
37. J Valle, JL Ayuso-Gutierrez, A Abril, JL Ayuso-Mateos. Evaluation of thyroid function in lithium-naive bipolar patients. Eur Psychiatry 14:341–345, 1999.
38. KD Chang, PE Keck Jr, SP Stanton, SL McElroy, SM Strakowski, TD Geracioti, Jr. Differences in thyroid function between bipolar manic and mixed states. Biol Psychiatry 43:730–733, 1998.
39. LB Marangell, MS George, AM Callahan, TA Ketter, PJ Pazzaglia, TA L'Herrou, GS Leverich, RM Post. Effects of intrathecal thyrotropin-releasing hormone (protirelin) in refractory depressed patients. Arch Gen Psychiatry 54:214–222, 1997.
40. MS Bauer, PC Whybrow. Rapid cycling bipolar affective disorder. II. Treatment of refractory rapid cycling with high-dose levothyroxine: a preliminary study. Arch Gen Psychiatry 47:435–440, 1990.
41. MA Frye, KD Denicoff, AL Bryan, EE Smith-Jackson, SO Ali, D Luckenbaugh, GS Leverich, RM Post. Association between lower serum free T4 and greater mood instability and depression in lithium-maintained bipolar patients. Am J Psychiatry 156:1909–1914, 1999.
42. JJ Schildkraut. The catecholamine hypothesis of affective disorders: a review of supporting evidence. Am J Psychiatry 122:509–22, 1965.
43. J Mendlewicz, P Linkowski, M Kerkhofs, D Desmedt, J Golstein, G Copinschi, E Van Cauter. Diurnal hypersecretion of growth hormone in depression. J Clin Endocrinol Metab 60:505–512, 1985.
44. F Contreras, MA Navarro, JM Menchon, P Rosel, J Serrallonga, F Perez-Arnau, M Urretavizcaya, J Vallejo. Growth hormone response to growth hormone releasing hormone in non-delusional and delusional depression and healthy controls. Psychol Med 26:301–307, 1996.
45. KP Lesch, G Laux, A Erb, H Pfuller, H Beckmann. Attenuated growth hormone response to growth hormone-releasing hormone in major depressive disorder. Biol Psychiatry 22:1495–1499, 1987.
46. KP Lesch, G Laux, H Pfuller, A Erb, H Beckmann. Growth hormone (GH) response to GH-releasing hormone in depression. J Clin Endocrinol Metab 65:1278–1281, 1987.
47. SC Risch. Growth hormone-releasing factor and growth hormone. In: CB Nemeroff, ed. Neuropeptides and Psychiatric Disorders. Washington: American Psychiatric Press, 1991, pp 93–108.
48. SS Skare, MW Dysken, CJ Billington. A review of GHRH stimulation test in psychiatry. Biol Psychiatry 36:249–265, 1994.
49. DS Charney, GR Heninger, DE Sternberg, KM Hafstad, S Giddings, DH Landis. Adrenergic receptor sensitivity in depression. Effects of clonidine in depressed patients and healthy subjects. Arch Gen Psychiatry 39:290–294, 1982.
50. SA Checkley, AP Slade, E Shur. Growth hormone and other responses to clonidine in patients with endogenous depression. Br J Psychiatry 138:51–55, 1981.
51. N Matussek, M Ackenheil, H Hippius, F Muller, HT Schroder, H Schultes, B Wasilewski. Effect of clonidine on growth hormone release in psychiatric patients and controls. Psychiatry Res 2:25–36, 1980.
52. LJ Siever, TW Uhde, EK Silberman, DC Jimerson, JA Aloi, RM Post, DL Murphy. Growth hormone response to clonidine as a probe of noradrenergic receptor responsiveness in affective disorder patients and controls. Psychiatry Res 6:171–183, 1982.
53. JD Amsterdam, G Maislin. Hormonal responses during insulin-induced hypoglycemia in manic-depressed, unipolar depressed, and healthy control subjects. J Clin Endocrinol Metab 73:541–548, 1991.
54. H Agren, G Lundqvist. Low levels of somatostatin in human CSF mark depressive episodes. Psychoneuroendocrinology 9:233–248, 1984.
55. TG Dinan, LN Yatham, V O'Keane, S Barry. Blunting of noradrenergic-stimulated growth hormone release in mania. Am J Psychiatry 148:936–938, 1991.
56. IS Shiah, LN Yatham, RW Lam, EM Tam, AP Zis. Growth hormone response to baclofen in patients with mania: a pilot study. Psychopharmacology 147:280–284, 1999.
57. LN Yatham, AP Zis, RW Lam, E Tam, IS Shiah. Sumatriptan-induced growth hormone release in patients with major depression, mania, and normal

controls. Neuropsychopharmacology 17:258–263, 1997.
58. B Weber, S Lewicka, M Deuschle, M Colla, I Heuser. Testosterone, androstenedione and dihydrotestosterone concentrations are elevated in female patients with major depression. Psychoneuroendocrinology 25:765–771, 2000.
59. W Baischer, G Koinig, B Hartmann, J Huber, G Langer. Hypothalamic-pituitary-gonadal axis in depressed premenopausal women: elevated blood testosterone concentrations compared to normal controls. Psychoneuroendocrinology 20:553–559, 1995.
60. U Schweiger, M Deuschle, B Weber, A Korner, CH Lammers, J Schmider, U Gotthardt, I Heuser. Testosterone, gonadotropin, and cortisol secretion in male patients with major depression. Psychosom Med 61:292–296, 1999.
61. JK Warnock, JC Bundren. Anxiety and mood disorders associated with gonadotropin-releasing hormone agonist therapy. Psychopharmacol Bull 33:311–316, 1997.
62. JK Warnock, JC Bundren, DW Morris. Sertraline in the treatment of depression associated with gonadotropin-releasing hormone agonist therapy. Biol Psychiatry 43:464–465, 1998.
63. JK Warnock, JC Bundren, DW Morris. Depressive symptoms associated with gonadotropin-releasing hormone agonists. Depress Anxiety 7:171–177, 1998.
64. LJ Whalley, JE Christie, J Bennie, H Dick, J Sloan-Murphy, G Fink. Elevated plasma luteinizing hormone concentrations, cryptorchidism and mania. Psychoneuroendocrinology 12:73–77, 1987.
65. LJ Whalley, S Kutcher, DH Blackwood, J Bennie, H Dick, G Fink. Increased plasma LH in manic-depressive illness: evidence of a state-independent abnormality. Br J Psychiatry 150:682–684, 1987.
66. E Young, A Korszun. Psychoneuroendocrinology of depression. Hypothalamic-pituitary-gonadal axis. Psychiatr Clin North Am 21:309–323, 1998.
67. R Ader, N Cohen, D Felten. eds. Psychoneuroimmunology II. New York: Academic Press, 1991.
68. AJ Dunn. Interaction between the nervous system and the immune system: implications for psychopharmacology. In: FE Bloom, D.J. Kupfer, eds. Psychopharmacology: The Fourth Generation of Progress. New York: Raven Press, 1995, pp 719–731.
69. AH Miller, RL Spencer. Immune system and central nervous system interactios. In: HI Kaplan, BJ Saddock, eds. Comprehensive Textbook of Psychiatry. Baltimore: Williams & Wilkins, 1995, pp 112–127.
70. DL Felten, SY Felten. Immune interactions with specific neural structures. Brain Behav Immun 1:279–283, 1987.
71. M Irwin, RL Hauger, L Jones, M Provencio, KT Britton. Sympathetic nervous system mediates central corticotropin-releasing factor induced suppression of natural killer cytotoxicity. J Pharmacol Exp Ther 255:101–107, 1990.
72. RW Bartrop, E Luckhurst, L Lazarus, LG Kiloh, R Penny. Depressed lymphocyte function after bereavement. Lancet 1:834–836, 1977.
73. SJ Schleifer, SE Keller, M Camerino, JC Thornton, M Stein. Suppression of lymphocyte stimulation following bereavement. JAMA 250:374–377, 1983.
74. R Glaser, GR Pearson, JF Jones, J Hillhouse, S Kennedy, HY Mao, JK Kiecolt-Glaser. Stress-related activation of Epstein-Barr virus. Brain Behav Immun 5:219–232, 1991.
75. R Glaser, JK Kiecolt-Glaser, RH Bonneau, W Malarkey, S Kennedy, J Hughes. Stress-induced modulation of the immune response to recombinant hepatitis B vaccine. Psychosom Med 54:22–29, 1992.
76. JK Kiecolt-Glaser, R Glaser, S Gravenstein, WB Malarkey, J Sheridan. Chronic stress alters the immune response to influenza virus vaccine in older adults. Proc Natl Acad Sci USA 93:3043–3047, 1996.
77. JK Kiecolt-Glaser, R Glaser, EC Shuttleworth, CS Dyer, P Ogrocki, CE Speicher. Chronic stress and immunity in family caregivers of Alzheimer's disease victims. Psychosom Med 49:523–535, 1987.
78. JK Kiecolt-Glaser, PT Marucha, WB Malarkey, AM Mercado, R Glaser. Slowing of wound healing by psychological stress. Lancet 346:1194–1196, 1995.
79. Z Kronfol, J Silva Jr, J Greden, S Dembinski, R Gardner, B Carroll. Impaired lymphocyte function in depressive illness. Life Sci 33:241–247, 1983.
80. SJ Schleifer, SE Keller, AT Meyerson, MJ Raskin, KL Davis, M Stein. Lymphocyte function in major depressive disorder. Arch Gen Psychiatry 41:484–486, 1984.
81. TB Herbert, S Cohen. Depression and immunity: a meta-analytic review. Psychol Bull 113:472–486, 1993.
82. G Gatti, R Cavallo, ML Sartori, R Carignola, R Masera, D Delponte, A Salvadori, A Angeli. Circadian variations of interferon-induced enhancement of human natural killer (NK) cell activity. Cancer Detect Prev 12:431–438, 1988.
83. JM Petitto, JD Folds, H Ozer, D Quade, DL Evans. Abnormal diurnal variation in circulating natural killer cell phenotypes and cytotoxic activity in major depression. Am J Psychiatry 149:694–696, 1992.
84. MG Frank, SE Hendricks, DR Johnson, JL Wieseler, WJ Burke. Antidepressants augment natural killer cell activity: in vivo and in vitro. Neuropsychobiology 39:18–24, 1999.
85. A Ballin, V Gershon, A Tanay, J Brener, A Weizman, D Meytes. The antidepressant fluvoxa-

86. A Mizruchin, I Gold, I Krasnov, G Livshitz, R Shahin, AI Kook. Comparison of the effects of dopaminergic and serotonergic activity in the CNS on the activity of the immune system. J Neuroimmunol 101:201–204, 1999.
87. SY Tsai, KP Chen, YY Yang, CC Chen, JC Lee, VK Singh, SJ Leu. Activation of indices of cell-mediated immunity in bipolar mania. Biol Psychiatry 45:989–994, 1999.
88. MH Rapaport, L Guylai, P Whybrow. Immune parameters in rapid cycling bipolar patients before and after lithium treatment. J Psychiatry Res 33:335–340, 1999.
89. MH Rapaport. Immune parameters in euthymic bipolar patients and normal volunteers. J Affect Disord 32:149–156, 1994.
90. RP Schleimer, HN Claman, A Oronsky. eds. Antiinflammatory Steroid Action, Basic and Clinical Aspects. San Diego: Academic Press, 1989.
91. D Mason. Genetic variation in the stress response: susceptibility to experimental allergic encephalomyelitis and implications for human inflammatory disease. Immunol Today 12:57–60, 1991.
92. TR Mosmann, RL Coffman. TH1 and TH2 cells: different patterns of lymphokine secretion lead to different functional properties. Annu Rev Immunol 7:145–173, 1989.
93. MP Stenzel-Poore, JE Duncan, MB Rittenberg, AC Bakke, SC Heinrichs. CRH overproduction in transgenic mice: behavioral and immune system modulation. Ann NY Acad Sci 780:36–48, 1996.
94. MS Labeur, E Arzt, GJ Wiegers, F Holsboer, JM Reul. Long-term intracerebroventricular corticotropin-releasing hormone administration induces distinct changes in rat splenocyte activation and cytokine expression. Endocrinology 136:2678–2688, 1995.
95. HM Schulte, CM Bamberger, H Elsen, G Herrmann, AM Bamberger, J Barth. Systemic interleukin-1 alpha and interleukin-2 secretion in response to acute stress and to corticotropin-releasing hormone in humans. Eur J Clin Invest 24:773–777, 1994.
96. NJ Rothwell, G Luheshi. Pharmacology of interleukin-1 actions in the brain. Adv Pharmacol 25:1–20, 1994.
97. JR Bethea, IY Chung, SM Sparacio, GY Gillespie, EN Benveniste. Interleukin-1 beta induction of tumor necrosis factor-alpha gene expression in human astroglioma cells. J Neuroimmunol 36:179–191, 1992.
98. DJ Tweardy, PL Mott, EW Glazer. Monokine modulation of human astroglial cell production of granulocyte colony-stimulating factor and granulocyte-macrophage colony-stimulating factor. I. Effects of IL-1 alpha and IL-beta. J Immunol 144:2233–2241, 1990.
99. AJ Dunn, J Wang. Cytokine effects on CNS biogenic amines. Neuroimmunomodulation 2:319–328, 1995.
100. SM MohanKumar, PS MohanKumar, SK Quadri. Specificity of interleukin-1beta-induced changes in monoamine concentrations in hypothalamic nuclei: blockade by interleukin-1 receptor antagonist. Brain Res Bull 47:29–34, 1998.
101. HW Clement, J Buschmann, S Rex, C Grote, C Opper, D Gemsa, W Wesemann. Effects of interferon-gamma, interleukin-1 beta, and tumor necrosis factor-alpha on the serotonin metabolism in the nucleus raphe dorsalis of the rat. J Neural Transm (Budapest) 104:981–991, 1997.
102. R Sapolsky, C Rivier, G Yamamoto, P Plotsky, W Vale. Interleukin-1 stimulates the secretion of hypothalamic corticotropin-releasing factor. Science 238:522–524, 1987.
103. EW Bernton, JE Beach, JW Holaday, RC Smallridge, HG Fein. Release of multiple hormones by a direct action of interleukin-1 on pituitary cells. Science 238:519–521, 1987.
104. HO Besedovsky, A del Rey, I Klusman, H Furukawa, G Monge Arditi, A Kabiersch. Cytokines as modulators of the hypothalamus-pituitary-adrenal axis. J Steroid Biochem Mol Biol 40:613–618, 1991.
105. M Maes, E Bosmans, HY Meltzer, S Scharpe, E Suy. Interleukin-1 beta: a putative mediator of HPA axis hyperactivity in major depression? Am J Psychiatry 150:1189–1193, 1993.
106. M Maes, HY Meltzer, E Bosmans, R Bergmans, E Vandoolaeghe, R Ranjan, R Desnyder. Increased plasma concentrations of interleukin-6, soluble interleukin-6, soluble interleukin-2 and transferrin receptor in major depression. J Affect Disord 34:301–309, 1995.
107. M Maes, S Scharpe, HY Meltzer, E Bosmans, E Suy, J Calabrese, P Cosyns. Relationships between interleukin-6 activity, acute phase proteins, and function of the hypothalamic-pituitary-adrenal axis in severe depression. Psychiatry Res 49:11–27, 1993.
108. J Levine, Y Barak, KN Chengappa, A Rapoport, M Rebey, V Barak. Cerebrospinal cytokine levels in patients with acute depression. Neuropsychobiology 40:171–176, 1999.
109. M Maes, E Bosmans, J Calabrese, R Smith, HY Meltzer. Interleukin-2 and interleukin-6 in schizophrenia and mania: effects of neuroleptics and mood stabilizers. J Psychiatry Res 29:141–152, 1995.
110. EC Borden, D Parkinson. A perspective on the clinical effectiveness and tolerance of interferon-alpha. Semin Oncol 25:3–8, 1998.

111. AD Valentine, CA Meyers, MA Kling, E Richelson, P Hauser. Mood and cognitive side effects of interferon-alpha therapy. Semin Oncol 25:39–47, 1998.
112. S Kent, RM Bluthe, KW Kelley, R Dantzer. Sickness behavior as a new target for drug development. Trends Pharmacol Sci 13:24–28, 1992.
113. DL Musselman, DH Lawson, JF Gumnick, AK Manatunga, S Penna, RS Goodkin, K Greiner, CB Nemeroff, AH Miller. Paroxetine for the prevention of depression induced by high-dose interferon alfa. N Engl J Med 344:961–966, 2001.
114. I Iancu, A Sverdlik, PN Dannon, E Lepkifker. Bipolar disorder associated with interferon-alpha treatment. Postgrad Med J 73:834–835, 1997.
115. D Strite, AD Valentine, CA Meyers. Manic episodes in two patients treated with interferon alpha. J Neuropsychiatry Clin Neurosci 9:273–276, 1997.
116. B Carpiniello, MG Orru, A Baita, CM Pariante, G Farci. Mania induced by withdrawal of treatment with interferon alfa [letter]. Arch Gen Psychiatry 55:88–89, 1998.
117. D Kingsley. Interferon-alpha induced 'tertiary mania'. Hosp Med 60:381–382, 1999.
118. DB Greenberg, E Jonasch, MA Gadd, BF Ryan, JR Everett, AJ Sober, MA Mihm, KK Tanabe, M Ott, FG Haluska. Adjuvant therapy of melanoma with interferon-alpha-2b is associated with mania and bipolar syndromes. Cancer 89:356–362, 2000.
119. RJ Wyatt, B Portnoy, DJ Kupfer, F Snyder, K Engelman. Resting plasma catecholamine concentrations in patients with depression and anxiety. Arch Gen Psychiatry 24:65–70, 1971.
120. A Roy, D Pickar, J De Jong, F Karoum, M Linnoila. Norepinephrine and its metabolites in cerebrospinal fluid, plasma, and urine. Relationship to hypothalamic-pituitary-adrenal axis function in depression. Arch Gen Psychiatry 45:849–857, 1988.
121. RC Veith, N Lewis, OA Linares, RF Barnes, MA Raskind, EC Villacres, MM Murburg, EA Ashleigh, S Castillo, ER Peskind. Sympathetic nervous system activity in major depression. Basal and desipramine-induced alterations in plasma norepinephrine kinetics. Arch Gen Psychiatry 51:411–422, 1994.
122. SH Koslow, JW Maas, CL Bowden, JM Davis, I Hanin, J Javaid. CSF and urinary biogenic amines and metabolites in depression and mania. A controlled, univariate analysis. Arch Gen Psychiatry 40:999–1010, 1983.
123. CL Bowden, S Koslow, JW Maas, J Davis, DL Garver, I Hanin. Changes in urinary catecholamines and their metabolites in depressed patients treated with amitriptyline or imipramine. J Psychiatr Res 21:111–128, 1987.
124. AF Schatzberg, JA Samson, KL Bloomingdale, PJ Orsulak, B Gerson, PP Kizuka, JO Cole, JJ Schildkraut. Toward a biochemical classification of depressive disorders. X. Urinary catecholamines, their metabolites, and D-type scores in subgroups of depressive disorders [published erratum appears in Arch Gen Psychiatry 1989;46(9):860]. Arch Gen Psychiatry 46:260–268, 1989.
125. A Roy, DC Jimerson, D Pickar. Plasma MHPG in depressive disorders and relationship to the dexamethasone suppression test. Am J Psychiatry 143:846–851, 1986.
126. M Maj, MG Ariano, F Arena, D Kemali. Plasma cortisol, catecholamine and cyclic AMP levels, response to dexamethasone suppression test and platelet MAO activity in manic-depressive patients. A longitudinal study. Neuropsychobiology 11:168–173, 1984.
127. AC Swann, F Petty, CL Bowden, SC Dilsaver, JR Calabrese, DD Morris. Mania: gender, transmitter function, and response to treatment. Psychiatry Res 88:55–61, 1999.
128. TG Johnston, CB Kelly, MR Stevenson, SJ Cooper. Plasma norepinephrine and prediction of outcome in major depressive disorder. Biol Psychiatry 46:1253–1258, 1999.
129. M Asberg, P Thoren, L Traskman, L Bertilsson, V Ringberger. "Serotonin depression"—a biochemical subgroup within the affective disorders? Science 191:478–480, 1976.
130. RD Gibbons, JM Davis. Consistent evidence for a biological subtype of depression characterized by low CSF monoamine levels. Acta Psychiatr Scand 74:8–12, 1986.
131. A Roy, J De Jong, M Linnoila. Cerebrospinal fluid monoamine metabolites and suicidal behavior in depressed patients. A 5-year follow-up study. Arch Gen Psychiatry 46:609–612, 1989.
132. L Traskman-Bendz, C Alling, L Oreland, G Regnell, E Vinge, R Ohman. Prediction of suicidal behavior from biologic tests. J Clin Psychopharmacol 12:21S–26S, 1992.
133. PL Delgado, HL Miller, RM Salomon, J Licinio, JH Krystal, FA Moreno, GR Heninger, DS Charney. Tryptophan-depletion challenge in depressed patients treated with desipramine or fluoxetine: implications for the role of serotonin in the mechanism of antidepressant action. Biol Psychiatry 46:212–220, 1999.
134. A Biegon, N Essar, M Israeli, A Elizur, S Bruch, AA Bar-Nathan. Serotonin 5-HT2 receptor binding on blood platelets as a state dependent marker in major affective disorder. Psychopharmacology (Berl) 102:73–75, 1990.
135. IS Shiah, HC Ko, JF Lee, RB Lu. Platelet 5-HT and plasma MHPG levels in patients with bipolar I and bipolar II depressions and normal controls. J Affect Disord 52:101–110, 1999.

136. M Leboyer, P Quintin, P Manivet, O Varoquaux, JF Allilaire, JM Launay. Decreased serotonin transporter binding in unaffected relatives of manic depressive patients. Biol Psychiatry 46:1703–1706, 1999.
137. RT Malison, LH Price, R Berman, CH van Dyck, GH Pelton, L Carpenter, G Sanacora, MJ Owens, CB Nemeroff, N Rajeevan, RM Baldwin, JP Seibyl, RB Innis, DS Charney. Reduced brain serotonin transporter availability in major depression as measured by [^{123}I]-2 beta-carbomethoxy-3 beta-(4-iodophenyl)tropane and single photon emission computed tomography. Biol Psychiatry 44:1090–1098, 1998.
138. A Roy, D Pickar, M Linnoila, AR Doran, P Ninan, SM Paul. Cerebrospinal fluid monoamine and monoamine metabolite concentrations in melancholia. Psychiatry Res 15:281–292, 1985.
139. A Roy, F Karoum, S Pollack. Marked reduction in indexes of dopamine metabolism among patients with depression who attempt suicide. Arch Gen Psychiatry 49:447–450, 1992.
140. PL Reddy, S Khanna, MN Subhash, SM Channabasavanna, BS Rao. CSF amine metabolites in depression. Biol Psychiatry 31:112–118, 1992.
141. AS Brown, S Gershon. Dopamine and depression. J Neural Transm Gen Sect 91:75–109, 1993.
142. P Willner. Dopamine and depression: a review of recent evidence. II. Theoretical approaches. Brain Res 287:225–236, 1983.
143. P Willner. Dopamine and depression: a review of recent evidence. III. The effects of antidepressant treatments. Brain Res 287:237–246, 1983.
144. P Willner. Dopamine and depression: a review of recent evidence. I. Empirical studies. Brain Res 287:211–224, 1983.
145. ML Johnson, MD Roberts, AR Ross, CM Witten. Methylphenidate in stroke patients with depression. Am J Phys Med Rehabil 71:239–241, 1992.
146. LW Lazarus, PJ Moberg, PR Langsley, VR Lingam. Methylphenidate and nortriptyline in the treatment of poststroke depression: a retrospective comparison. Arch Phys Med Rehabil 75:403–406, 1994.
147. LW Lazarus, DR Winemiller, VR Lingam, I Neyman, C Hartman, M Abassian, U Kartan, L Groves, J Fawcett. Efficacy and side effects of methylphenidate for poststroke depression. J Clin Psychiatry 53:447–449, 1992.
148. MH Corrigan, AQ Denahan, CE Wright, RJ Ragual, DL Evans. Comparison of pramipexole, fluoxetine, and placebo in patients with major depression. Depress Anxiety 11:58–65, 2000.
149. G Lambert, M Johansson, H Agren, P Friberg. Reduced brain norepinephrine and dopamine release in treatment-refractory depressive illness: evidence in support of the catecholamine hypothesis of mood disorders. Arch Gen Psychiatry 57:787–793, 2000.
150. A Anand, P Verhoeff, N Seneca, SS Zoghbi, JP Seibyl, DS Charney, RB Innis. Brain SPECT imaging of amphetamine-induced dopamine release in euthymic bipolar disorder patients. Am J Psychiatry 157:1108–1114, 2000.
151. IS Shiah, LN Yatham. GABA function in mood disorders: an update and critical review. Life Sci 63:1289–1303, 1998.
152. BI Gold, MB Bowers Jr, RH Roth, DW Sweeney. GABA levels in CSF of patients with psychiatric disorders. Am J Psychiatry 137:362–364, 1980.
153. F Petty, MA Schlesser. Plasma GABA in affective illness. A preliminary investigation. J Affect Disord 3:339–343, 1981.
154. F Petty, AD Sherman. Plasma GABA levels in psychiatric illness. J Affect Disord 6:131–138, 1984.
155. G Sanacora, GF Mason, DL Rothman, KL Behar, F Hyder, OA Petroff, RM Berman, DS Charney, JH Krystal. Reduced cortical gamma-aminobutyric acid levels in depressed patients determined by proton magnetic resonance spectroscopy. Arch Gen Psychiatry 56:1043–1047, 1999.
156. R Bernasconi. The GABA hypothesis of affective illness: influence of clinically effective antimanic drugs on GABA turnover. In Basic Mechanism in the Action of Lithium. Amsterdam: Excerpta Medica, 1981.
157. N Motohashi, K Ikawa, T Kariya. GABAB receptors are up-regulated by chronic treatment with lithium or carbamazepine. GABA hypothesis of affective disorders? Eur J Pharmacol 166:95–99, 1989.
158. N Motohashi. GABA receptor alterations after chronic lithium administration. Comparison with carbamazepine and sodium valproate. Prog Neuropsychopharmacol Biol Psychiatry 16:571–579, 1992.
159. RM Post, TA Ketter, RT Joffe, KL Kramlinger. Lack of beneficial effects of l-baclofen in affective disorder. Int Clin Psychopharmacol 6:197–207, 1991.
160. RM Berman, A Cappiello, A Anand, DA Oren, GR Heninger, DS Charney, JH Krystal. Antidepressant effects of ketamine in depressed patients. Biol Psychiatry 47:351–354, 2000.
161. DP Auer, B Putz, E Kraft, B Lipinski, J Schill, F Holsboer. Reduced glutamate in the anterior cingulate cortex in depression: an in vivo proton magnetic resonance spectroscopy study. Biol Psychiatry 47:305–313, 2000.
162. M Castillo, L Kwock, H Courvoisie, SR Hooper. Proton MR spectroscopy in children with bipolar affective disorder: preliminary observations. Am J Neuroradiol 21:832–838, 2000.
163. J Levine, K Panchalingam, A Rapoport, S Gershon, RJ McClure, JW Pettegrew. Increased cerebrospinal

fluid glutamine levels in depressed patients. Biol Psychiatry 47:586–593, 2000.
164. L van Londen, JG Goekoop, GM van Kempen, AC Frankhuijzen-Sierevogel, VM Wiegant, EA van der Velde, D De Wied. Plasma levels of arginine vasopressin elevated in patients with major depression. Neuropsychopharmacology 17:284–292, 1997.
165. L van Londen, GA Kerkhof, F van den Berg, JG Goekoop, KH Zwinderman, AC Frankhuijzen-Sierevogel, VM Wiegant, D de Wied. Plasma arginine vasopressin and motor activity in major depression. Biol Psychiatry 43:196–204, 1998.
166. MB Muller, R Landgraf, MF Keck. Vasopressin, major depression, and hypothalamic-pituitary-adrenocortical desensitization. Biol Psychiatry 48:330–333, 2000.
167. T Hokfelt, M-N Castel, P Morino, X Zhang, A Dangerlind. General overview of neuropeptides. In: FE Blook, DJ Kupfer, ed. Psychopharmacology: The Fourth Generation of Progress. New York: Raven Press, 1995, pp 483–492.
168. MS Kramer, N Cutler, J Feighner, R Shrivastava, J Carman, JJ Sramek, SA Reines, G Liu, D Snavely, E Wyatt-Knowles, JJ Hale, SG Mills, M MacCoss, CJ Swain, T Harrison, RG Hill, F Hefti, EM Scolnick, MA Cascieri, GG Chicchi, S Sadowski, AR Williams, L Hewson, D Smith, NM Rupniak. Distinct mechanism for antidepressant activity by blockade of central substance P receptors. Science 281:1640–1645, 1998.
169. JS Hong, HA Tilson, K Yoshikawa. Effects of lithium and haloperidol administration on the rat brain levels of substance P. J Pharmacol Exp Ther 224:590–593, 1983.
170. H Mitsushio, M Takashima, N Mataga, M Toru. Effects of chronic treatment with trihexyphenidyl and carbamazepine alone or in combination with haloperidol on substance P content in rat brain: a possible implication of substance P in affective disorders. J Pharmacol Exp Ther 245:982–989, 1988.
171. RH Gerner, T Yamada. Altered neuropeptide concentrations in cerebrospinal fluid of psychiatric patients. Brain Res 238:298–302, 1982.
172. DR Rubinow, PW Gold, RM Post, JC Ballenger, R Cowdry, J Bollinger, S Reichlin. CSF somatostatin in affective illness. Arch Gen Psychiatry 40:409–412, 1983.
173. G Bissette, E Widerlov, H Walleus, I Karlsson, K Eklund, A Forsman, CB Nemeroff. Alterations in cerebrospinal fluid concentrations of somatostatin-like immunoreactivity in neuropsychiatric disorders. Arch Gen Psychiatry 43:1148–1151, 1986.
174. DR Rubinow. Cerebrospinal fluid somatostatin and psychiatric illness. Biol Psychiatry 21:341–365, 1986.
175. RP Sharma, G Bissette, PG Janicak, JM Davis, CB Nemeroff. Elevation of CSF somatostatin concentrations in mania. Am J Psychiatry 152:1807–1809, 1995.
176. PJ Pazzaglia, MS George, RM Post, DR Rubinow, CL Davis. Nimodipine increases CSF somatostatin in affectively ill patients. Neuropsychopharmacology 13:75–83, 1995.

29

Neurobiology of Obsessive-Compulsive Disorder

BAVANISHA VYTHILINGUM
University of Stellenbosch, Cape Town, South Africa

DAN J. STEIN
University of Stellenbosch, Cape Town, South Africa, and University of Gainesville, Gainesville, Florida, U.S.A.

I. INTRODUCTION

Obsessive-compulsive disorder (OCD), thought to be the fourth most common psychiatric disorder [1], is one of the most incisive exemplars of how a disorder that was once viewed as secondary to unconscious conflict is now known to be the result of specific neuropathological processes. Recent research has shown that OCD is mediated by specific abnormalities in both neuroanatomical and neurochemical systems. Current theories of the neurobiology of OCD can be divided into those emphasizing the role of dysfunction of specific corticostriatal pathways (neuroanatomical models of OCD) and those emphasizing the role of dysfunction in the serotonergic and to a lesser extent dopaminergic systems (neurochemical models of OCD).

II. NEUROANATOMICAL MODELS OF OCD

The current neuroanatomical model of OCD emphasizes the role of corticostriatothalamocortical (CSTC) circuitry. Alexander et al. [2,3], described multiple, parallel segregated circuits, which project from the cortex to corresponding striatal subterritories, from there to the basal ganglia, and via the thalamus back to the prefrontal regions from which they originated. To understand a CSTC model of OCD, it is necessary to first understand the relevant normal neuroanatomy.

A. Relevant Normal Neuroanatomy

1. Prefrontal Cortex

The prefrontal cortex is responsible for several cognitive functions, including response inhibition and planning, organizing, controlling, and verifying operations [4]. The prefrontal cortex can be subdivided in several functional subterritories: the dorsolateral prefrontal cortex which subserves memory, learning, and other executive functions, the posteromedial orbitofrontal cortex, a component of the paralimbic system, which plays a role in mediating affective and motivational functions [5]; and the anterior and lateral orbitofrontal cortex, which acts as an intermediary between the lateral prefrontal and posteromedial orbitofrontal zones.

2. Paralimbic System

This is an area of cortex which forms a functional link between other areas of cortex and the limbic system proper. It includes the posteromedial orbitofrontal cortex, cingulate, anterior temporal, parahippocampal, and insular cortex [5]. This system is believed to be important in mediating intense emotional states; in particular, it has been implicated in anxiety [6] and in the modulation of autonomic effects associated with intense anxiety [5].

3. Striatum

The striatum is composed of the caudate nucleus, putamen, and nucleus accumbens. Recent work has shown that it not only modulates motor functions, but cognitive and affective functions as well [7]. It has been theorized that the function of a healthy striatum is to process information automatically, without conscious representation. Hence a healthy striatum could be seen to act as a filter at the level of the thalamus, ensuring that stereotyped processes can be carried out with reaching consciousness.

4. Corticostriatothalamocortical Circuits

CSTC circuits can be divided in two major branches: the corticothalamic branch, and the corticostriatothalamic branch. The corticothalamic branch is a reciprocal monosynaptic communication between the cortex and the thalamus that mediates consciously accessible and consciously mediated information. The corticostriatothalamic branch modulates transmission at the level of the thalamus and, as discussed earlier, is involved in the regulation of information reaching consciousness. Modern imaging studies confirm the role of CSTC circuitry in OCD.

B. Structural Studies

Several volumetric studies of the caudate have shown structural abnormalities. The nature of the abnormalities described has been inconsistent. Scarone et al. [8] in a mixed-gender cohort found increased right caudate volume in the OCD group, whereas Robinson et al. [9], also studying a mixed gender cohort, found bilaterally decreased volumes in the OCD group. In an all-female cohort, Jenike et al. [10] found rightward shift in caudate volume as well as a trend toward overall reduced caudate volume. However Stein et al. [11] found no change in caudate volume between patients with OCD and a control group. It is possible that caudate volume changes over time, with increased volume in the aftermath of streptococcal infection [12], and later shrinkage.

Volumetric changes in the orbital frontal and anterior cingulate regions have been less well studied. Of three studies reported so far, only one [13] found structural abnormalities (reduced bilateral orbital frontal and amygdala volumes). More impressive evidence for involvement of these structures has been provided by functional imaging studies (see below).

White matter reductions in OCD have been reported and a subsequent replication study confirmed overall white matter reduction but increased opercular volume, which correlated with both severity of OCD and nonverbal immediate memory [14].

Studies using magnetic resonance spectroscopy (MRS) have also demonstrated striatal abnormalities. Two studies have found decreased N-acetyl-aspartate (NAA) levels in the striatum [15,16], suggesting decreased density of healthy neurons in this region. Furthermore, one of these studies failed to find significant differences in striatal volumes [16], underscoring the purported greater sensitivity of MRS-NAA over current morphometric MRI methods.

Rosenberg's group has also demonstrated abnormalities in a pediatric population. Decreased NAA levels were found in right and left medial thalami, with the decreased levels in the left medial thalamus correlating with increased severity of disease [17]. In addition, caudate glutamatergic levels were found to be increased in children with OCD [18], but this was found to normalize after treatment with paroxetine, perhaps suggesting that paroxetine treatment is mediated by a serotonergically modulated reduction in frontostriatal glutamatergic concentration.

C. Functional Studies

Neutral state studies have implicated hyperactivity in the prefrontal cortex and, less consistently, striatal and cingulate involvement [19–25]. Pre/posttreatment studies also point to involvement of these areas. Decreased activity after medication was found in the medial frontal cortex [26] and orbitofrontal cortex [23,27], with one study correlating treatment response to activity in the right frontal cortex. Changes in the caudate and cingulum have also been reported [23].

Interestingly, Baxter et al. found decreased right caudate activity in a group receiving medication as well as a different group receiving behavior therapy [28]. This was subsequently replicated in a second study of behavior therapy, which also confirmed a correlation between orbitofrontal and caudate activity pretreatment that disappeared posttreatment [29]. These studies confirm that effective treatment of

OCD, whether pharmacotherapeutic or psychotherapeutic in nature, is associated with reduced activity in the orbitofrontal cortex, caudate, or cingulate cortex; i.e., effective treatment of OCD is associated with changes in CSTC circuits.

These results may suggest that behavioral and pharmacotherapeutic modalities work via a specific therapeutic mechanism of action. However, Brody et al. [30] found differing patterns of cerebral metabolism in patients who responded to behavior therapy than in those who responded to fluoxetine, with higher normalized metabolism in the left orbitofrontal cortex being associated with good outcome in the behavior therapy group but worse outcome in the fluoxetine group. Furthermore, thalamic volumes normalize after treatment with paroxetine but not behavior therapy [31]. It may be that the changes observed represent the differences between a symptomatic and symptom-free brain rather than any therapeutic mechanism of action.

Why should dysfunction in CSTC circuits lead to OCD symptoms? There is mounting evidence that striatal function is associated with the development, maintenance, and selection of motoric cognitive and procedural strategies; this has been variously described as "habit system," "response set," and "procedural mobilization." Thus, it may be argued that striatal lesions can lead to the inappropriate release of genetically programmed sequences (such as hand-washing, hoarding, etc.).

The "striatal topography model," an early heuristic model [32], postulated that different circuits may be involved in the mediation of different kinds of OCD symptoms. Accordingly, the cognitive symptoms of OCD are mediated by the caudate, motoric symptoms by the putamen, and affective symptoms by paralimbic CSTC circuits. More recent evidence shows involvement of a range of CSTC circuits in OCD; nevertheless, it may still be suggested that projections to specific fields or cells mediate different kinds of OCD symptoms.

Rauch has suggested that failure of thalamic filtering of information may be a key element in producing the intrusive phenomena that are a hallmark of OCD [33]. Information can be processed in two ways—explicitly (i.e., consciously), and implicitly (i.e., unconsciously)—with implicit operations being primarily processed via corticostriatal systems. Rauch postulates that in OCD, pathology in the corticostriatal pathways may allow this information to gain access to consciousness, presenting as intrusive phenomena. Indeed, his team has shown that the striatum is usually recruited during an implicit sequence learning task, but that in patients with OCD, this fails to occur; instead, medial temporal structures, usually associated with conscious information processing, are recruited [33,34].

In this model repetitive behaviours (compulsions and tics) are viewed as compensatory mechanisms, possibly serving to recruit viable corticostriatalthalamic circuits, thereby facilitating filtering at the level of the thalamus. The repetitions required would reflect the inefficiency of such mechanisms. This is also consistent with clinical observation that patients often suddenly no longer experience the urge to perform a behavior—"as if a switch were turned off." Presumably, once sufficient repetitions have been performed, a threshold level of filtering is reached and the intrusive stimuli no longer reach consciousness. Rauch et al. have also demonstrated in functional imaging studies a characteristic pattern of thalamic deactivation with striatal recruitment [35].

III. AUTOIMMUNE PATHOLOGY IN OCD

Sydenham's chorea is a manifestation of acute rheumatic fever that is often accompanied by neuropsychiatric symptoms, including symptoms of OCD. In a series of landmark studies [36,37], Swedo and colleagues confirmed these earlier observations and also showed that OCD symptoms often preceded motor manifestations of the disease. Follow-up of children with OCD [38] demonstrated that a subgroup had OCD symptoms of abrupt onset, and showed exacerbations that often were associated with demonstrable group A β-hemolytic streptococcus infection. In addition, a subset of children with OCD have antineuronal antibodies.

Together, these finding have led to the designation of Pediatric Autoimmune Neuropsychiatric Disorders Associated with Streptococcal infections (PANDAS) [38]. Specific criteria include (1) presence of OCD and/or a tic disorder, (2) prepubertal onset, (3) episodic course of symptom severity, (4) association with group A β-hemolytic streptococcus infection, and (5) association with neurologic abnormalities.

Autoimmune basal ganglia damage has been identified as an important pathogenic mechanism in Sydenham's chorea [39]. It is thought that basal ganglia damage is mediated by antineuronal antibodies that occur as a part of an autoimmune response to group A β-hemolytic streptococcal infection. In addition acute changes in striatal volume parallel the clinical course of PANDAS [40]. These findings therefore strengthen the case for striatal damage as a pathogenic mechanism for OCD.

The B-lymphocyte antigen D8/17 has been identified as a possible marker for susceptibility to rheumatic fever, occurring in 100% of rheumatic fever sufferers [41], with significantly higher expression in the rheumatic fever patients than in either unaffected first-degree relatives or normal controls. As increased D8/17 has not been reported in post streptococcal glomerulonephritis, it may indicate specific vulnerability to developing rheumatic fever and related complications. Elevated D8/17 expression has been described in patients with childhood-onset OCD, Tourette's syndrome, and autism, but not in trichotillomania [42–46].

The role of autoimmune pathology in adult OCD remains less well known. A few studies, however, suggest that in some adults, autoimmune pathology may play a role in the development of OCD. Bodner et al. [47] describe the case of a 25-year-old male who developed OCD after an episode of severe, antibiotic-resistant pharyngitis. Apart from age, he fulfilled all criteria for PANDAS. Lougee et al. [48] also report that rates of OCD and tic disorders in first-degree relatives of pediatric probands with PANDAS are higher than those of the general population. The exact role of autoimmune pathology in the development of adult OCD, however, is still uncertain.

The possibility of an autoimmune mechanism in the pathogenesis of OCD suggests that immunological therapies may represent a new treatment modality. However, results of trials using antibiotic prophylaxis and plasmapheresis have so far shown mixed results [49,50], and more work in is needed in this area.

IV. NEUROCHEMISTRY AND NEUROPHARMACOLOGY

A number of neurotransmitter systems appear to play a role in mediating OCD symptoms. These include serotonin, dopamine, and neuropeptide systems.

A. Serotonin and OCD

It was the observation that serotonergic reuptake inhibitors (SRIs) were more effective in alleviating the symptoms of OCD, that first prompted a serotonergic hypothesis of OCD [51,52]. The mechanism of action of SRIs in OCD is not yet fully elucidated—whether they work by correcting some fundamental abnormality or whether they modulate an intact system to compensate for underlying abnormalities in OCD is not yet known. One postulated mechanism of action of the SRIs is that by blocking the reuptake pump, they lead to increased synaptic serotonin and a resultant increased stimulation of the postsynaptic $5HT_2$ and $5HT_{1A}$ receptors. However, inhibition of the reuptake pump occurs in 24 h whereas clinical improvement may only be seen 8–12 weeks later. One possible explanation is that the delay may represent the time needed to desensitize the autoreceptor.

An interesting set of preclinical studies has found that in order to desensitize the $5HT_{1D}$ autoreceptor in orbitofrontal cortex, the administration of relatively high doses of SRIs for relatively long periods is required (low doses, short duration, and ECT do not have an effect) [53]. Furthermore, Mansari et al. [54] showed that changes in serotonergic transmission occurred more quickly in the lateral frontal cortex than the medial frontal cortex following SRI administration. This work is reminiscent of clinical findings in OCD, where it is observed that up to 12 weeks of treatment at higher doses is needed to produce a therapeutic response, and that depressive symptoms tend to remit earlier than OCD symptoms. It also corresponds with current models which postulate the lateral frontal cortex to be important in depression and the medial frontal (or orbitofrontal) cortex to be important in the pathophysiology of OCD. Together, these findings suggest that this receptor may therefore have a particularly important role in the pathogenesis of OCD.

There is also work suggesting that $5HT_2$ receptors are important in OCD. Case reports suggest that certain hallucinogens (psilocybin and LSD), which are potent stimulators of the $5HT_{2A}$ and $5HT_{2C}$ receptors, can decrease OCD symptoms [55]. Conversely, administration of ritanserin, a $5HT_2$ antagonist, results in the exacerbation of OCD symptoms [56]. Arguably, enhancement of neurotransmission through $5HT_{2A}$ or $5HT_{2C}$ receptors may be a common pathway for drugs with therapeutic effect in OCD.

Studies of indirect measures of central serotonergic function (such as platelet receptor binding and CSF concentrations of 5HT metabolites) in OCD have been inconsistent. In addition, these measures are not necessarily accurate representations of serotonergic function within the brain. There is somewhat more consistency in studies of serotonergic agonists; OCD symptoms are exacerbated by mCPP (a $5HT_{1A}$ and $5HT_{2C}$ agonist) [57–59] and sumatriptan (a $5HT_{1D}$ agonist) [60]. Administration of sumatriptan during functional imaging demonstrated a significant association between symptom exacerbation and decreased frontal activity, arguably consistent with a role for the $5HT_{1D}$ receptor in OCD [60]. Nevertheless, findings with both mCPP [61–63] and sumatriptan [64] have not always been consistent, and sumatriptan has poor blood-brain barrier penetration, so additional work in this area remains necessary.

B. Dopaminergic Systems and OCD

Preclinical studies demonstrate that stereotypic behavior can be elicited by the administration of dopamine agonists, and decreased by dopamine blockers. Similarly, stereotypic, repetitive behaviors have been described in stimulant abusers [65,66]. Furthermore, cocaine, a dopamine reuptake blocker, has been reported to exacerbate symptoms in patients with OCD and to induce obsessive-compulsive behavior in subjects with a family but not personal history of OCD.

Tourette's syndrome (TS) is a disorder for which a dopaminergic basis is well elucidated. For example, the principal dopamine metabolite homovanillic acid (HVA) is decreased in the CSF of patients with TS [67], and dopamine blockers are a standard form of treatment in TS. Recent imaging studies have demonstrated a significant increase in the number of striatal presynaptic dopamine carrier sites in the caudate and putamen in TS patients [68–70]. Overlap between TS and OCD has been well documented, further pointing to a dopaminergic basis for OCD.

Pharmacologic studies in OCD support a potential role for the dopamine system. Forty percent to 60% of patients with OCD are treatment resistant, and patients with comorbid tics are particularly likely not to respond to SRIs [71]. However, augmentation of SRIs with dopamine blockers has been shown effective in both open [72,73] and controlled trials [71,74]. Typical neuroleptics are particularly effective in OCD patients with comorbid tics [71], while the atypicals appear useful in OCD patients both with and without tics [74].

C. Neuropeptides and OCD

Preclinical evidence has linked neuropeptides to repetitive behavior in animals, and initial clinical investigations in OCD patients suggest that they may play a role in modulation of the disorder. Neuropeptides implicated in OCD include arginine vasopressin (AVP), oxytocin, adrenocorticotropic hormone (ACTH), corticotropin-releasing factor (CRF), somatostatin, and the opioid system.

In animals, AVP is associated with enhancement of memory acquisition and retrieval and with grooming behaviors. Grooming behaviors in animals are often viewed as analogous to human washing and cleaning behavior, and excessive grooming is often viewed as an animal correlate of a washing or cleaning compulsion. AVP may also inhibit extinction, decreasing the likelihood of changing a behavioral pattern once it has been established. It can thus be seen that AVP is a likely candidate for involvement in the pathogenesis of OCD. Studies in humans, however, have been inconsistent. One study found that OCD patients had significantly elevated basal levels of AVP and secreted more AVP into plasma in response to hypertonic saline [75]. However, this has not been replicated [76]. Nevertheless, in children and adolescents with OCD, a negative correlation between symptom severity and AVP levels was found [77].

As with AVP, oxytocin administration in animals is associated with changes in grooming behavior, with marked increases in grooming. Oxytocin has also been shown to induce maternal behavior in female rats, but only in animals primed with estrogen [78]. Elevated levels of oxytocin (and estrogen) may be postulated to induce OCD symptoms in a vulnerable subgroup of women, explaining the increased risk for development of OCD in the pregnancy and puerperium, and the higher incidence of washing and cleaning compulsions in this subgroup of patients. Higher CSF oxytocin levels have been found in adult patients with no family or personal history of tic disorders, and oxytocin levels were significantly correlated with Y-BOCS scores [79]. In children, the AVP/oxytocin ratio was negatively correlated with symptom severity [77]. Administration of oxytocin to adults with OCD, however, has had no consistent therapeutic effect [80].

ACTH and CRF are both noted to increase self grooming in animals. In humans, both basal plasma ACTH and the increase following CRF administration was found to be less in adults with OCD than controls [81]. Studies of CRF levels have been inconsistent, with initial reports of elevated CRF in OCD patients not confirmed in replication studies. In children, no correlation has been found between CSF, ACTH, or CRF levels and symptom severity [77]. As both ACTH and CRF are released in response to stress, it is possible that any elevations found may be a nonspecific response to the stress of a chronic illness.

In animals, somatostatin delays the extinction of active and passive avoidance behaviors (which may be similar to the persistent repetition of OCD) and can also produce stereotypic behaviors [82,83]. Studies of both adults and children with OCD have found higher CSF somatostatin as compared to healthy adults and conduct-disordered children [84,85].

Opioids mediate reward signals and it has been postulated that they may be involved in mechanisms that signal successful task completion. Deficiencies in these mechanisms may potentially explain the "self-doubt" experienced by many patients with OCD. OCD patients have elevated serum antibodies for the dynorphin precursor prodynorphin [86]. In Tourette's syndrome, CSF dynorphin was found to correlate with OCD (but not tic) symptom severity [87]. However, no correlation was found between dynorphin levels and symptom severity in children with OCD. Furthermore, challenges with opioid antagonists in OCD have produced inconsistent results [88,89].

In summary, preclinical evidence suggests that various neuropeptides may play a role in the pathogenesis of OCD. While the evidence for neuropeptides inducing OCD-like behaviors in animals is fairly robust, studies in humans have produced less convincing results. Differences between results in adult and pediatric populations suggest that developmental factors impact the functioning of the different neuropeptides. Further studies are warranted to fully elucidate the role of these peptides in OCD.

V. CONCLUSION

In the last two decades significant strides have been made in our understanding of the pathogenesis of OCD. We now know that it is a disorder mediated by specific neuroanatomic and neurochemical mechanisms. Furthermore, we have translated our improved understanding of the neurobiology of OCD into several effective therapeutic modalities. However, there are still gaps in our understanding of OCD. The challenge now is to bridge these gaps and to develop new therapeutic modalities so that we may even more effectively treat this fascinating and complex disorder.

REFERENCES

1. Karno M, Goldin JM, Sorenson SB, Burnom A. The epidemiology of obsessive compulsive disorder in five US communities. Arch Gen Psychiatry 45:1094–1099, 1988.
2. Alexander GE, DeLong MR, Strick PL. Parallel organization of functionally segregated circuits linking basal ganglia and cortex. Annu Rev Neurosci 9:357–381, 1986
3. Alexander GE, Crutcher MD, Delong MR. Basal ganglia-thalamocortical circuits: parallel substrates for motor, oculomotor, "prefrontal", and "limbic" functions. Prog Brain Res 85:119–146, 1990.
4. Otto 1990.
5. Mesulam MM. Patterns in behavioral neuroanatomy: association areas, the limbic system and hemispheric specialization. In: Mesulam MM, ed. Principles of Behavioral Neurology. Philadelphia: FA Davis, 1985.
6. Rauch SL, Shin LM. Functional neuroimaging studies in posttraumatic stress disorder. Ann NY Acad Sci 821:83–98, 1997.
7. Houk JC, Wise SP. Distributed modular architectures linking basal ganglia, cerebellum, and cerebral cortex: their role in planning and controlling action. Cereb Cortex 5(2):95–110, 1995.
8. Scarone S, Colombo C, Livian S, Abbruzzcse M, Ronchi P, Locatelli M, et al. Increased right caudate nucleus size in obsessive-compulsive disorder: detection with magnetic resonance imaging. Psychiatry Res 45(2):115–121, 1992.
9. Robinson D, Wu H, Munne RA, Ashtari M, Alvir JM, Lerner G, et al. Reduced caudate nucleus volume in obsessive-compulsive disorder. Arch Gen Psychiatry 52(5):393–398, 1995.
10. Jenike MA, Breiter HC, Baer L, Kennedy DN, Savage CR, Olivares MJ, et al. Cerebral structural abnormalities in obsessive-compulsive disorder. A quantitative morphometric magnetic resonance imaging study. Arch Gen Psychiatry 53(7):625–632, 1996.
11. Stein DJ, Hollander E, Chan S, DeCaria CM, Hilal S, Liebowitz MR. Computerized tomography and soft signs in obsessive-compulsive disorder. Psychiatry Res 50:143–150, 1993.
12. Giedd JN, Rapoport JL, Garvey MA, Perlmutter S, Swedo SE. MRI assessment of children with obsessive-compulsive disorder or tics associated with streptococcal infection. Am J Psychiatry 157(2):281–283, 2000.
13. Szeszko PR, Robinson D, Alvir, JMJ, et al. Orbital frontal and amygdala volume reductions in obsessive-compulsive disorder. Arch Gen Psychiatry 56:913–919, 1999.
14. Jenike MA, Breiter HC, Baer L, et al. Cerebral structural abnormalities in obsessive-compulsive disorder. A quantitative morphometric magnetic resonance imaging study. Arch Gen Psychiatry 53(7):625–632, 1996.
15. Ebert D, Speck O, Konig A, et al. ^{1}H-magnetic resonance spectroscopy in obsessive-compulsive disorder: evidence for neuronal loss in the cingulate gyrus and the right striatum. Psychiatry Res 74(3):173–176, 1997.
16. Bartha R, Stein MB, Williamson PC, et al. A short echo ^{1}H spectroscopy and volumetric study MRI study of the corpus striatum in patients with obsessive-compulsive disorder and comparison subjects. Am J Psychiatry 155(11): 1584–1591, 1998.
17. Fitzgerald KD, Moore GJ, Paulson LA, et al. Proton spectroscopic imaging of the thalamus in treatment-naïve pediatric obsessive compulsive disorder. Biol Psychiatry 47(3):174–182, 2000.

18. Rosenberg DR, MacMaster FP, Keshavan MS, et al. Decrease in caudate glutamatergic concentrations in pediatric obsessive-compulsive disorder patients taking paroxetine. J Am Acad Child Adolesc Psychiatry 39 (9): 1096–1103, 2000.
19. Baxter L, Schwartz J, Mazziotta J, et al. Cerebral glucose metabolic rates in non-depressed patients with obsessive-compulsive disorder. Am J Psychiatry 145:1560–1563, 1988.
20. Swedo SE, Shapiro MB, Grady CL, et al. Cerebral glucose metabolism in childhood-onset obsessive-compulsive disorder, Arch Gen Psychiatry 46:518–523, 1989.
21. Perani D, Colombo C, Bressi S, et al. FDG PET study in obsessive compulsive disorder: a clinical metabolic correlation study after treatment. Br J Psychiatry 166:244–250, 1995.
22. Nordahl TE, Benkelfat C, Semple W, et al. Cerebral glucose metabolic rates in obsessive-compulsive disorder. Neuropsychopharmacology 2:23–28, 1989.
23. Benkelfat C, Nordahl TE, Semple WE, et al. Local cerebral glucose metabolic rate in obsessive-compulsive disorder: patients treated with clomipramine. Arch Gen Psychiatry 47:840–848, 1990.
24. Machlin SR, Harris GJ, Pearlson GD, et al. Elevated medial-frontal cerebral blood flow in obsessive compulsive patients: a SPECT study. Am J Psychiatry 148:1240–1242, 1991.
25. Rubin RT, Villaneuva-Myer J, Ananth J, et al. Regional xenon-133 cerebral blood flow and cerebral technetium-99m HMPAO uptake in unmedicated patients with obsessive-compulsive disorder and matched normal control subjects. Arch Gen Psychiatry 49:695–702, 1992.
26. Hoehn-Saric R, Pearlson GD, Harris GJ, et al. Effects of fluoxetine on regional cerebral blood flow in obsessive compulsive patients. Am J Psychiatry 148:1243–1245, 1991.
27. Swedo SE, Pietrini P, Leonard HL, et al. Cerebral glucose metabolism in childhood onset obsessive-compulsive disorder: revisualization during pharmacotherapy. Arch Gen Psychiatry 49:609–694, 1992.
28. Baxter LR Jr, Schwartz JM, Bergman KS, et al. Caudate glucose metabolic rate changes with both drug and behavior therapy for obsessive-compulsive disorder. Arch Gen Psychiatry 49:681–689, 1992.
29. Schwartz JM, Stoessel PW, Baxter LR, et al. Systematic changes in cerebral glucose metabolic rate after successful behavior modification.
30. Brody AL Saxena S, Schwartz JM, Stoessel PW, Maidment K, Phelps ME, Baxter LR Jr. FDG- PET predictor of response to behavioral therapy and pharmacotherapy in obsessive compulsive disorder. Psychiatry Res 84(1): 1–6, 1998.
31. Rosenberg DR, Benazon NR, Gilbert A, et al. Thalamic volume in pediatric obsessive-compulsive disorder patients before and after behavioral therapy. Biol Psychiatry 48(4):294–300, 2000.
32. Baxter LR, Schwartz JM, Guze BH, et al. Neuroimaging in obsessive-compulsive disorder: seeking the mediating neuroanatomy. In: Obsessive Compulsive Disorder: Theory and Management, 2nd ed. eds Jenike MA, Baer L, Minichiello WE. Chicago: Year Book Publishers, 1990, pp 167–188.
33. Rauch SL, Savage CR, Alpert NM, et al. A PET investigation of implicit and explicit sequence learning. Hum Brain Mapping 3:271–286, 1995.
34. Rauch SL, Savage CR, Alpert NM, et al. Probing striatal function in obsessive compulsive disorder: A PET study of implicit sequence learning. J Neuropsychiatry 9:568–573, 1997.
35. Rauch SL, Whalen PJ, Curran T, et al. Thalamic deactivation during early implicit sequence learning: a functional MRI study. NeuroReport 9:865–870, 1998.
36. Swedo SE, Rapoport JL, Cheslow DL, et al. High prevalence of obsessive-compulsive symptoms in patients with Sydenham's chorea. Am J Psychiatry 146:246–249, 1989.
37. Swedo SE, Leonard HL, Schapiro MB, et al. Sydenham's chorea: physical and psychological symptoms of St Vitus' dance. Pediatrics 91:706–713, 1993.
38. Swedo SE, Leonard HL, Garvey M, et al. Pediatric autoimmune neuropsychiatric disorders associated with streptococcal infections: clinical description of the first 50 cases. Am J Psychiatry 155:264–271, 1998.
39. Husby G, Van de Rijn, Zabriskie JB, et al. Antibodies reacting with cytoplasm of subthalamic and caudate nuclei neurons in chorea and rheumatic fever. J Exp Med 144:1094–1110, 1976.
40. Gibofsky A, Khanna A, Suh E, Zabriskie JB. The genetics of rheumatic fever: relationship to streptococcal infection and autoimmune disease. J Rheumatol Suppl 30:1–5, 1991.
41. Khanna AK, Buskirk DR, Williams RC Jr, Gibofsky A, Crow MK, Menon A, Fotino M, Reid HM, Poon-King T, Rubinstein P. Presence of a non-HLA B cell antigen in rheumatic fever patients and their families defined by a monoclonal antibody. J Clin Invest 83(5):1710–1171, 1989.
42. Chapman F, Visvanathan K, Carreno-Manjarrez R, Zabriskie JB. A flow cytometric assay for D8/17 B cell marker in patients with Tourette's syndrome and obsessive compulsive disorder. J Immunol Methods 219(1–2):181–186, 1998.
43. Murphy TK, Goodman WK, Fudge MW, Williams RC Jr, Ayoub EM, Dalal M, Lewis MH, Zabriskie JB. B lymphocyte antigen D8/17: a peripheral marker for childhood-onset obsessive-compulsive disorder and Tourette's syndrome. Am J Psychiatry 154:402–404, 1997.
44. Swedo SE, Leonard HL, Mittleman BB, Allen AJ, Rapoport JL, Dow SP, Kanter ME, Chapman F,

Zabriskie JB. Identification of children with pediatric autoimmune neuropsychiatric disorders associated with streptococcal infections by a marker associated with rheumatic fever. Am J Psychiatry 154:110–112, 1997.

45. Swedo SE, Leonard HL. Trichotillomania: a obsessive compulsive spectrum disorder? Psychiat Clin North Am 15(4):777–790, 1992.

46. Stein DJ, Wessels C, Carr J, Hawkridge S, Bouwer C, Kalis N. Hair-pulling in a patient with Sydenham's chorea. Am J Psychiatry 154:1320, 1997.

47. Bodner SM, Morshed SA, Peterson BS. The question of PANDAS in adults. Biol Psychiatry 49(9): 807–810, 2001.

48. Lougee L, Perlmutter SJ, Nicolson R, Garvey MA, Swedo SE. Psychiatric disorders in first-degree relatives of children with pediatric autoimmune neuropsychiatric disorders associated with streptococcal infections (PANDAS). J Am Acad Child Adolesc Psychiatry 39(9):1120–1126, 2000.

49. Garvey MA, Perlmutter SJ, Allen AJ, Hamburger S, Lougee L, Leonard HL, et al. A pilot study of penicillin prophylaxis for neuropsychiatric exacerbations triggered by streptococcal infections. Biol Psychiatry 45(12):1564–1571, 1999.

50. Giedd JN, Rapoport JL, Leonard HL, Richter D, Swedo SE. Case study: acute basal ganglia enlargement and obsessive-compulsive symptoms in an adolescent boy. J Am Acad Child Adolesc Psychiatry 35(7):913–915, 1996.

51. Fernandez-Cordoba E, Lopez-Ibor AJ. La monocloimipramina en enfermos psyquiatricos resistentes a otros tratamientos. Acta Luso-Esp Neurol Psiquiatr Ciene Afines 26:119–147, 1967.

52. Greist JH, Jefferson JW, Kobak KA, et al. Efficacy and tolerability of serotonin transport inhibitors in obsessive-compulsive disorder: meta-analysis. Arch Gen Psychiatry 52:53–60, 1995.

53. Zohar J, Insel TR. Obsessive-compulsive disorder: psychobiological approaches to diagnosis, treatment, and pathophysiology. Biol Psychiatry 22:667–687, 1987.

54. Mansari ME, Bouchard C, Blier P. Alteration of serotonin release in the guinea pig orbito-frontal cortex by selective serotonin reuptake inhibitors: relevance to treatment of obsessive-compulsive disorder. Neuropsychopharmacology 13:117–127, 1995.

55. Delgado PL, Morena FA. Hallucinogens, serotonin and obsessive-compulsive disorder. J Psychoac Drugs 30(4):359–366, 1998.

56. Ergovesi S, Ronchi P, Smeraldi E. 5HT2 receptor and fluvoxamine effect in obsessive compulsive disorder. Hum Psychopharmacol 7:287–289, 1992.

57. Zohar J, Mueller EA, Insel TR, Zohar-Kadouch RC, Murphy DL. Serotonergic responsivity in obsessive-compulsive disorder. Comparison of patients and healthy controls. Arch Gen Psychiatry 44(11):946–951, 1987.

58. Hollander E, De Caria C, Gully R, et al. Effects of chronic fluoxetine treatment on behavioral and neuroendrocrine responses to meta-chlorophenylpiperazine in obsessive-compulsive disorder. Psychiatry Res 36(1):1–17, 1991.

59. Piggot TA, Hill JL, Grady TA, et al. A comparison of the behavioral effects of oral versus intravenous mCPP administration in OCD patients and the effect of metergoline prior to i.v. mCPP. Biol Psychiatry 33(1):3–14, 1993.

60. Stein DJ, Van Heerden B, Wessels CJ, et al. Single photon emission computed tomography of the brain with Tc-99m HMPAO during sumatriptan challenge in obsessive-compulsive disorder: investigating the functional role of the serotonin auto-receptor. Prog Neuropsychopharmacol Biol Psychiatry 23(6):1079–1099.

61. Hott Pian KL, Westenberg HG, den Boer JA, et al. Effects of meta-chlorophenylpiperazine on cerebral blood flow in obsessive-compulsive disorder and controls. Biol Psychiatry 44(5):367–370, 1998.

62. Goodman WK, McDougle CJ, Price LH, et al. m-Chlorophenylpiperazine in patients with obsessive-compulsive disorder: absence of symptom exacerbation. Biol Psychiatry 38(3):138–149, 1995.

63. Charney DS, Goodman WK, Price LH, et al. Serotonin function in obsessive-compulsive disorder. A comparison of the effects of tryptophan and m-chlorophenylpiperazine in patients and healthy subjects. Arch Gen Psychiatry (2):177–185, 1988.

64. Pian KL, Westenberg HG, van Megen HJ, den Boer JA. Sumatriptan (5-HT1D receptor agonist) does not exacerbate symptoms in obsessive-compulsive disorder. Psychopharmacology (Berl) 140(3):365–370, 1998.

65. Ellinwood EH Jr. Amphetamine psychosis I: description of the individuals and process. J Nerv Ment Dis 144:273–283, 1967.

66. Schiorring E. Changes in individual and social behavior induced by amphetamine and related compounds in monkeys and man. Behavior 43:481–521, 1975.

67. McDougle CJ, Goodman WK, Delgado PL, et al. Pathophysiology of obsessive compulsive disorder [letter]. Am J Psychiatry 146:1350–1351, 1989.

68. Singer HS, Hahn IH, Moran TH. Abnormal dopamine uptake sites in postmortem striatum from patients with Tourette's syndrome. Ann Neurol 30:558–562, 1991.

69. Malison RT, McDougle CJ, van Dyck CH, et al. [^{123}I]B-CIT SPECT imaging of striatal dopamine binding in Tourette's disorder. Am J Psychiatry 152:1359–1361, 1995.

70. Wolf SS, Jones DW, Knable MB, et al. Tourette syndrome: prediction of phenotypic variation in monozygotic twins by caudate nucleus D2 receptor binding. Science 273:1225–1227, 1996.

71. McDougle CJ, Goodman WK, Leckman JK, et al. Haloperidol addition in fluvoxamine-refractory obses-

sive-compulsive disorder: adouble placebo controlled study in patients with and without tics. Arch Gen Psychiatry 51:302–308, 1994.
72. Jacobsen FM. Risperidone in the treatment of affective illness and obsessive compulsive disorder. J Clin Psychiatry 56:413–429, 1995.
73. Stein DJ, Bouwer C, et al. Risperidone augmentation of serotonin reuptake inhibitors in obsessive-compulsive and related disorders. J Clin Psychiatry 58(3):119–122, 1997.
74. McDougle CJ, Epperson CN, Pelton GH, Wasylink S, Price LH. A double-blind, placebo-controlled study of risperidone addition in serotonin reuptake inhibitor-refractory obsessive-compulsive disorder. Arch Gen Psychiatry. 57(8):794–801, 2000.
75. Altemus M, Piggot T, Kalogeras KT, et al. Abnormalities in the regulation of vasopressin and corticotropin releasing factor secretion in obsessive-compulsive disorder. Arch Gen Psychiatry 49:9–20, 1992.
76. Leckman JF, Goodman WK, North WG, et al. Elevated cerebrospinal fluid levels of oxytocin in obsessive-compulsive disorder. Comparison with Tourette's syndrome and healthy controls. Arch Gen Psychiatry 51(10):782–792, 1994.
77. Swedo SE, Leonard HL, Kruesi MJ, et al. Cerebrospinal fluid neurochemistry in children and adolescents with obsessive-compulsive disorder. Arch Gen Psychiatry 49:29–36, 1992.
78. Insel TR. Oxytocin—a neuropeptide for affiliation: evidence from behavioral, receptor sutoradiographic, and comparative studies. Psychoneuroendocrinology 17(1):3–35, 1992.
79. Leckman JF, North W, Price LH, et al. Elevated levels of CSF oxytocin in obsessive-compulsive disorder patients without a personal or family history of tics. Arch Gen Psychiatry 51:782–792, 1994.
80. Epperson CN, McDougle CJ, Price LH. Intranasal oxytocin in obsessive-compulsive disorder. Biol Psychiatry 40:547–549. 1996.
81. Bailly D, Servant D, Dewailly D, et al. Corticotropin releasing factor stimulation test in obsessive compulsive disorder. Biol Psychiatry 35:143–146, 1994.
82. Vecsei L, Bollok L, Penke B, et al. Somatostatin and (D-Trp8, D-Cys14) somastatin delay extinction and reverse electroconvulsive shock-induced amnesia in rats. Psychoneuroendocrinology 11:111–115, 1986.
83. Vecsei L, Widerlov E. Effects of intracerebroventricularly administered somatostatin on passive avoidance, shuttlebox and openfield activity in rats. Neuropeptides 12:237–242, 1988.
84. Altemus M, Piggot T, L'Heureux, et al. CSF somatostatin in obsessive compulsive disorder. Am J Psychiatry 150: 460–464, 1993.
85. Kruesi MJP, Swedo S, Leonard H, et al. CSF somastatin in childhood psychiatric disorders: a preliminary investigation. Psychiatr Res 33:277–284, 1990.
86. Roy BF, Benkelfat C, Hill JL, et al. Serum antibody for somatostatin-14 and prodynorphin in 209–240 in patients with obsessive compulsive disorder, schizophrenia, Alzheimer's disease, multiple sclerosis, and advanced HIV infection. Biol Psychiatry 35:335–344, 1994.
87. Leckman JF, Riddle MA, Berrettini WH, et al. Elevated CSF dynorphin A[1–8] in Tourette's syndrome. Life Sci 43:2015–2033, 1988.
88. Insel TR, Pickar D. Naloxone administration in obsessive-compulsive disorder: report of 2 cases. Am J Psychiatry 140:1219–1220, 1983.
89. Keuler DJ, Altemus M, Michelson D, et al. Behavioral effects of naloxone infusion in obsessive-compulsive disorder. Biol Psychiatry 40:154–156, 1996.

30

Neurobiology of Panic Disorder

SANJAY J. MATHEW and JACK M. GORMAN
Columbia University and New York State Psychiatric Institute, New York, New York, U.S.A.

JEREMY D. COPLAN
SUNY Health Science Center at Brooklyn, and New York State Psychiatric Institute, New York, New York, U.S.A.

I. INTRODUCTION

Panic disorder (PD) is a common and disabling illness, with a reported lifetime prevalence of 1.5–3.5% [1,2]. Women are affected about twice as often as men, and the disorder is most common in the ages 30–44 [3]. PD is frequently comorbid with mood disorders and the other anxiety disorders, and, in terms of severity, approximately one-third of patients report poor physical and emotional health, rates comparable with those for major depression [2]. At the same time, there is accumulating evidence that PD has a distinct neurobiology from the other anxiety disorders as well as the mood disorders. Panic may also differ from a normal fear reaction [4], defined by Walter Cannon as a biologically disposed alarm reaction to perceived threat that mobilizes the organism for action [5].

The occurrence of *unexpected* and *spontaneous* panic attacks is required for the diagnosis of panic disorder; however, individuals with PD may report *situationally bound* panic attacks as well. Besides recurrent unexpected panic attacks, sequelae of the attack are necessary for diagnosis, which might include anticipatory anxiety about having another attack, phobic avoidance of situations associated with the panic attack, and worry about the implications of the attack or its consequences (e.g., losing control, having a heart attack, "going crazy"). Agoraphobia (a fear of circumstances in which escape or getting help is limited) occurs in ~ 30% of patients with PD, and is generally associated with a worse prognosis [6].

This chapter begins with a synopsis of neurodevelopmental issues relevant to understanding the relationship between childhood anxiety disorders and adult PD. Characterizing the ontogeny of psychobiological alterations throughout development is potentially important for the early identification and treatment of at-risk children. Accordingly, this article attempts to build the case that there likely exist distinct genetically mediated trait markers for PD beginning in childhood that are chronic and persistent even after effective treatment and disease remission. The trait markers span the gamut of areas investigated biologically in PD, including respiratory, cardiovascular, neuroendocrine, genetic, and neuroanatomic systems.

A growing body of evidence implicates hypothalamic-pituitary-adrenal (HPA) axis overdrive as an influential factor in the pathophysiology of a significant portion of adult mood and anxiety disorders [7]. As an example of the developmental complexity in the search for trait markers, we examine in children the interrelationships between HPA axis and another area extensively investigated, ventilatory regulation. Second, we continue with an analysis of this interrelationship in adults, as well as examining evidence for traitlike respiratory irregularities in adults with PD. Selected reviews of neurotransmitter systems that have been extensively investigated (norepinephrine, glutamate/GABA, serotonin) in PD, all of which have marked dynamic interactions with HPA axis, are then presented.

Candidates for neuronal modulation of the varied cortical, subcortical, and brainstem circuits implicated in PD are most likely found in multiple brain regions. In moving away from the single-locus hypothesis, dynamic interactions of multiple brain regions over time are likely important. In this light, pertinent recent findings in neuroimaging and genetics are then discussed. Finally, we present several areas of research requiring future investigation.

II. NEURODEVELOPMENTAL STUDIES AS A MEANS TO IDENTIFY TRAIT MARKERS OF PANIC DISORDER

Detailed childhood and adolescent histories in adult PD patients often reveal the presence of significant premorbid anxiety, manifesting as separation anxiety disorder, isolated panic attacks, or overanxious disorder [8–11]. Even in those adult patients with PD without overt childhood symptoms, biological trait markers for the illness can manifest before the presence of any overt symptoms. Only recently has work begun to probe the biological substrates of these childhood variants of PD [12–14].

A heightened response to carbon dioxide (CO_2) inhalation (a so-called CO_2 hypersensitivity) has been identified in adults with PD [15,16], in related conditions such as isolated panic attacks [16,17], and in non-ill first-degree relatives of patients with PD [18,19]. CO_2 hypersensitivity appears to be specific for PD and premenstrual dysphoric disorder, as compared with major depression, which appears to be insensitive to CO_2 inhalation [20].

Pine et al. [12] showed that CO_2 hypersensitivity was also found in children with separation anxiety disorder (and to a lesser degree in generalized anxiety disorder), while absent in social phobia. Using the same pediatric cohort, our group demonstrated a significant relation between HPA axis activation and susceptibility to ventilatory-based laboratory-induced panic using CO_2 inhalation [14]. In striking resemblance in adults with PD [21], elevations of salivary cortisol concentrations taken immediately prior to a standard CO_2 inhalation procedure were associated with increased rates of CO_2-induced panic. Subjective anticipatory anxiety and HPA axis activation, but not anxiety disorder diagnosis, were the most significant predictors of CO_2-induced panic in this pediatric sample [14].

Also as seen with adults [22], the CO_2 challenge itself had little effect on salivary cortisol values, suggesting that certain mechanisms for "suppression" of the HPA axis [23] may already be in place in childhood [14]. These preliminary reports are suggestive of a pathophysiological link between ventilatory disturbances and HPA axis from childhood into adulthood.

One implication of these reports is that children undergoing CO_2 challenge who display anticipatory anxiety, HPA axis activation and CO_2 hypersensitivity should likely be observed for the development of PD. CO_2 hypersensitivity might thus represent one important biological trait marker of familial vulnerability to panic disorder.

III. BIOLOGICAL SYSTEMS OPERATIVE IN ADULT PANIC DISORDER

In early investigations, Klein and Fink noted the effectiveness of imipramine hydrochloride in aborting spontaneous panic, but not chronic anxiety or agoraphobic avoidance [24]. Spontaneous panic was further distinguished biologically from fear, which did not respond to antidepressant treatment and is not marked by dyspnea [see 4 for review]. Since these early suggestions of distinct biological findings in panic, numerous investigations have further attempted to discriminate the core neurobiological features of PD. In this section we will focus on three areas extensively studied—respiratory physiology, HPA axis functioning, and the noradrenergic (NE) system—to delineate specific abnormalities unique to PD.

A. Respiratory Physiology in Panic Disorder

The unique clinical finding of dyspnea in patients with PD, compared with other anxiety disorders as well as normal fearful reactions to danger, has prompted numerous investigations into the role of respiratory regulation in PD. A prominent theory of pathophysiology is Klein's false suffocation alarm hypothesis [4], which suggests a respiratory control center abnormality in patients with PD. The suffocation alarm system posits an evolutionarily derived set point subject to various influences, which can be triggered by increasing levels of brain lactate and blood CO_2 [4].

Another prominent view is that respiratory stimulation such as with CO_2 challenge could act as a nonspecific stimulus that activates an overly sensitive neuroanatomical anxiety network in patients with PD [25]. The nonspecific stimulus notion is concordant with cognitive theories of panic and might explain in part the efficacy of cognitive-behavioral therapy for PD [26].

Several lines of evidence suggest that perhaps neither theory—suffocation alarm or cognitive catastrophe—is sufficient by itself to explain particular respiratory findings in PD. A recent study in fact found no difference in minute ventilation (MV) response to CO_2 inhalation–induced panic or in formal CO_2 sensitivity between patients with PD and other groups [27]. This study showed that once a panic attack is triggered, MV and respiratory rate increase regardless of diagnosis, and the physiological features of the panic attack itself appeared similar across groups [27]. A generalized fear response involving the amygdala and limbic regions, thought to be abnormally sensitive in PD, was proposed [27]. Based on the neural circuit that subserves conditioned fear in rodents, Gorman et al. have hypothesized that an overactive central nucleus of the amygdala, which has caudal projections to respiratory brain stem sites such as the parabrachial nucleus, might result in dysregulated breathing patterns in certain patients with PD [28]. Contrary to earlier reports, this study suggests that there might not be any fundamental abnormality in an adult panic patient's ventilatory physiology [27], but rather that the primary abnormalities likely involve central fear pathways.

Central pathways might be responsible for the increased baseline respiratory variability observed in PD. A recent report found that PD patients had greater tidal volume irregularity as well as elevated frequency compared to controls at baseline, which was primarily attributable to a sighing pattern of breathing [29]. The irregular breathing patterns were essentially stable over time and were, surprisingly, independent of doxapram (a respiratory stimulant)-induced panic or cognitive manipulation [29]. Similarly, our group recently confirmed that PD patients show increased baseline variability in tidal volume and minute ventilation compared to normal controls and major depressives [30]. The increased variability at baseline was predictive of subsequent vulnerability to CO_2-induced panic [30].

As noted above, respiratory variability manifesting as sighing appears to be a cardinal feature of panic, and has been an area of recent research interest as a potential trait marker for the illness. Sighing, defined as breaths with twice the size of a person's average resting tidal volume, abruptly lowers PCO_2 and is believed to relieve respiratory distress. Klein has argued that the sighing observed in PD patients may represent a compensatory mechanism to keep PCO_2 below a depressed suffocation alarm threshold [4].

Preliminary studies support the specificity of sighing in PD versus both social phobia [31] and generalized anxiety disorder [32]. Sighing occurs in PD patients even when not exposed to immediate anxiety provocation, suggestive of a traitlike characteristic [33]. PD patients seem to not only have more frequent sighs, but the magnitude of sighs are greater than controls. Presigh PCO_2 levels also return to baseline slower, suggesting either deficits in peripheral chemoreceptor compensation or an adaptive maintenance hyperventilation [33].

At the same time, there is evidence that some sighs are independent of peripheral chemoreceptor and PCO_2 effects [29], and could be centrally mediated. Central mediation of respiratory function is suggested by inputs from brain regions beyond brainstem respiratory control centers, such as the hippocampus [34], paraventricular hypothalamus [35], and the central nucleus of the amygdala (CeN) [36], structures integral to the anxiety neurocircuitry described in Gorman's hypothesis.

In summary, there are numerous unanswered questions regarding the role of respiration in panic, although the unique relationship is increasingly evident. While there is longitudinal evidence of respiratory variability and irregular breathing patterns that might be operative in the familial transmission of PD [12,16,30,37,38], there are contradictory conclusions when examining the CO_2 challenge literature. As noted by Roy-Byrne, the most important weakness in the CO_2 paradigm is its probable lack of neuroanatomic specificity, potentially limiting its usefulness as an endophenotypic trait marker [25]. More recent investigations suggest that the breath-by-breath variation in tidal volume manifested as sighing may provide a robust and fairly stable marker for PD [29,33].

Intimately related to the respiratory physiological abnormalities are the cardiovascular findings in panic disorder, which are briefly reviewed herein [see 39 for review]. Patients have shown faster heart rates in baseline laboratory measures, and tachycardia is a prominent feature of panic attacks [40]. More recent findings, however, suggest that there is not consistent evidence for baseline elevations in heart rate and blood pressure in PD [41].

Findings from the Epidemiological Catchment Area (ECA) study demonstrated that PD patients were at greater risk of high blood pressure, myocardial infarction, and stroke than were to subjects with no psychiatric disorder [42]. This association has been explained by a decreased cardiac vagal tone or an increased cardiac sympathetic responsiveness, both of which are associated with increased cardiovascular mortality [43]. It is known that PD patients have reduced parasympathetic innervation to the heart compared with control adults [44,45], and display reduced heart period variability (HPV) in some studies [44,46], another risk factor for proarrhythmic cardiac events.

Yeragani [45] showed that PD patients have increased adrenergic and decreased cholinergic responsiveness by an analysis of power spectrum. Alterations in central cholinergic activity in PD was also recently suggested in a study in which biperden, a centrally active muscarinic antagonist, blocked the response to CO_2 challenge in 12 patients [47]. Thus, while brainstem cholinergic neurons appear to play a role in modulating CO_2-induced panic, the precise role of cholinergic systems in PD itself is unclear.

In conclusion, the findings in HPV, autonomic, and cardiovascular regulation in PD require further investigation until its full consideration as a biological trait marker. Where the heart might in fact have the most relevance for PD is in the production of atrial natriuretic peptide (ANP), which was found to inhibit CCK-4-induced increases in corticotropin and cortisol levels in a recent study [48]. Further, ANP inhibited sympathetic stimulation in PD patients and controls [48]. A greater understanding of the role of this peptide as a modulator among the heart, hypothalamus and brainstem sites in anxiety conditions is necessary.

B. HPA Axis

PD has generally been distinguished from two comorbid conditions, major depression and post-traumatic stress disorder (PTSD), by its relative lack of persistent elevation of hypothalamic corticotropin-releasing factor (CRF) and adrenal cortisol dysregulation [49], although there are inconsistencies in studies examining these systems. CRF has emerged as a neurotransmitter/neuropeptide that plays a critical role in stress and stress-related disorders [50]. Recent data of cortisol regulation suggest a reexamination of the role of the HPA axis in PD.

Early evidence for dysregulation of CRF systems focused on the blunted ACTH response to CRF stimulation in panic patients compared to controls [51,52], a finding contradicted in a later study with a small sample size [53]. In fact, the preponderance of early studies investigating the discrete panic attack itself showed a curious lack of activation of a corticoid response in both normal controls and PD patients, both in naturalistic and laboratory settings [see 4 for review]. In a more recent, 24-h study of ACTH and cortisol secretion in PD, patients had increased overnight plasma cortisol secretion and greater amplitude of ultradian secretory episodes [54], although the findings could be attributed to anticipatory anxiety.

More recent work has focused on salivary cortisol and has contradicted earlier reports of suppressed HPA axis activity. Salivary cortisol might represent a better measure of HPA axis activity than plasma values in that it highly correlates with free plasma cortisol [55], the biologically active component. Salivary cortisol levels were found to be elevated following spontaneous panic attacks in a naturalistic setting [56]. Increased salivary cortisol could of course reflect increased stressful experiences during an attack, and might not suggest an underlying dysregulation of the HPA axis. However, Bandelow's group further noted that basal levels of total plasma, plasma-free cortisols, and salivary cortisols were all significantly elevated in PD patients compared to controls [57]. The major limitation of the salivary cortisol reports, however, is that the distinction between anticipatory anxiety and panic cannot be made from the study design.

In our analysis of 170 PD patients undergoing lactate infusions at our center, the strongest predictors of lactate-induced panic, prior to infusion, were fear and the combined or "interactive" effect of high cortisol and low pCO_2 [21]. We also examined blood cortisol responses to CO_2-induced panic. Cortisol levels did not increase and actually decreased significantly in 10 panicking subjects with PD, while in a separate study no reductions were noted after CO_2 inhalation in normals and nonpanicking PD patients [22].

We have hypothesized that the psychological, neuroendocrinological, and ventilatory interactions observed in the above studies could be explained by a CRF-mediated amygdaloid complex overactivation interacting with the following brain regions: (1) reciprocal cortical areas (cognitive misappraisal of fear); (2) the paraventricular nucleus (PVN) of the hypothalamus (cortisol response); and (3) the nucleus parabrachialis in the medulla (hyperventilation-induced low pCO_2) [58]. Thus, dysregulated HPA axis function might represent another trait marker of vulnerability to panic disorder, although current laboratory assessments have notable methodological limitations in differentiating the endocrine response in panic versus anticipatory anxiety.

C. The Noradrenergic System in Panic Disorder

Exploring functional linkages between the noradrenergic (NE)/locus ceruleus (LC) systems and relevant systems such as HPA axis, and other neurotransmitter systems, might further illustrate underlying neurobiological mechanisms of PD, given the prominence of hyperadrenergic symptoms in panic attacks (e.g., tachycardia, increased diastolic blood pressure, diaphoresis). Anatomically, there are important connections between the LC and the amygdala mediated by CRF-secreting neurons. The LC contains the highest concentration of NE cell bodies in the brain and sends numerous efferent projections to regions important in fear responses [for review, see 59].

Several other neurotransmitter systems appear to play an important interactive effect on LC functioning, including glutamatergic systems. The medullary nucleus paragigantocellularis (NPGi) sends excitatory input via glutamatergic receptors to the LC, suggesting an important link between glutamate and noradrenergic systems [60]. Given the neuroanatomical efferents to the LC, we hypothesized that chronic attenuation of glutamatergic transmission with the novel metabotropic glutamate (mGlu2/3) agonist LY354740 would blunt both HPA axis and LC responsivity in nonhuman primates [61]. We found that chronic treatment (6 weeks) with a functional glutamate antagonist did indeed reduce baseline cortisol levels, but failed to attenuate yohimbine (an alpha-2 adrenergic antagonist) challenge-induced plasma 3-methoxy-4-hydroxyphenylglycol (MHPG) levels [61].

In a prior clinical study, we had demonstrated that clonidine (an alpha-2 adrenergic agonist) induced greater decreases in MHPG and serum cortisol in PD patients versus control subjects, an effect which persisted even with effective treatment with fluoxetine [62]. In contrast to controls, PD patients demonstrated an "uncoupling" of the NE system and the HPA axis, meaning a lack of the typical correlation between MHPG and cortisol. Treatment with the glutamate antagonist in the nonhuman primate study selectively "uncoupled" the two systems, protecting the HPA axis, while retaining LC responsivity. Thus,

LY354740's ability to modulate the HPA axis suggests a potential therapeutic action in stress-related conditions such as PD, and its effect on LC functioning as evidenced by the yohimbine-induced MHPG response is potentially important in understanding the role of glutamatergic neurotransmission on noradrenergic function.

Pharmacological probes employing clonidine and yohimbine have provided the most useful clinical data linking NE and the HPA axis. One of the most replicated findings in PD is the blunted growth hormone (GH) response to clonidine challenge, which results in less sedation, a greater hypotensive response, and a disproportionate reduction in plasma MHPG in patients compared to controls [63–65]. Limitations of this finding, however, are both its nonspecificity to PD and its ambiguous pathophysiological significance, in that the blunted GH response might represent an intrinsic alpha-2 receptor abnormality, or a dysregulation of other afferent neuronal systems (such as CRF) affecting this receptor. Regarding the latter possibility, we recently found that adversely reared nonhuman primates with relatively high CRF concentrations exhibited relatively diminished GH responses to clonidine [66]. These data raise the possibility that reductions of GH response to clonidine may relate, in part, to trait-like increases of CNS CRF activity [66].

Yohimbine challenge, which is accompanied by increased serum MHPG, cortisol, and cardiovascular responses, elicits high rates of panic attacks in PD patients (~54%) [67]. A series of studies have revealed that the group of PD patients who experienced panic attacks with yohimbine had significantly greater increases in plasma MHPG following yohimbine than healthy subjects or PD patients who did not experience panic attacks, although these findings have not been consistently replicated [reviewed in 67].

Although much has been written about noradrenergic mechanisms in PD, the centrality of the NE system in the pathogenesis of panic anxiety has come into question. First, there is inconsistent evidence for increases in measures of NE function during provocative challenge with "respiratory" panicogens such as lactate, CO_2, and doxapram [4,68,69]. Further, there is supportive evidence that the LC/NE system might actually be more important in modulating arousal and anticipatory anxiety (by LC activation of amygdalohippocampal structures) than in mediating panic attacks themselves [69,70]. See **Figure 1** for a review of noradrenergic pathways in PD.

In summary, the study of ventilatory physiology, HPA axis, and the NE system has been useful in lending direction for the identification of endophenotypic trait markers of the illness. Some of the inconsistencies in the literature might reflect differences in subject illness severity or clinical characteristics; for example, Abelson's finding of increased nocturnal cortisol [54] was most evident in patients recruited from clinical settings versus those responding to advertisement. Some inconsistencies might reflect failure to distinguish among normal fear reactions, panic disorder, anticipatory anxiety, and generalized anxiety.

Despite the inconsistencies, tentative conclusions can be made. First, during anticipatory anxiety, such as is observed in PD subjects prior to lactate infusion, increased cortisol secretion coupled with hypocapnia is the profile most strongly predictive of subsequent panic. Second, during the panic attack itself, cortisol appears suppressed. The recent findings of elevated salivary cortisol levels require refinement in methodology to distinguish between anticipatory anxiety and panic. Finally, patients with PD appear to have increased within-subject noradrenergic volatility during clonidine challenge [71], which is in accordance with the increased variability in baseline ventilatory measures reported.

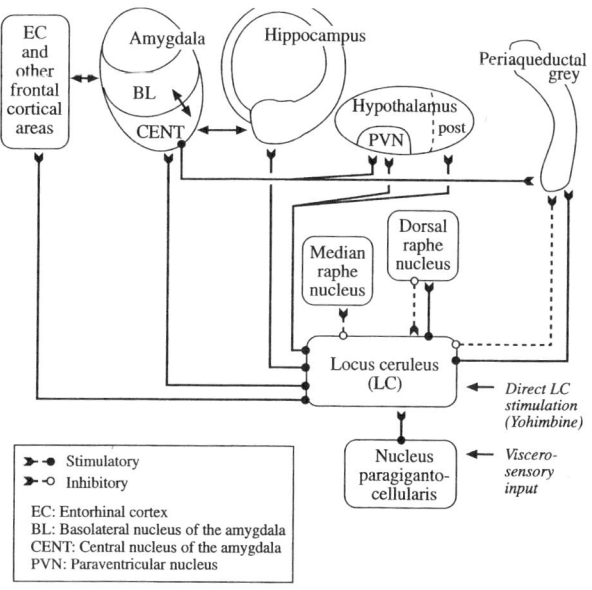

Figure 1 Noradrenergic pathways in panic disorder. (From Ref. 131.)

D. GABA/Glutamate Systems in Panic Disorder: Potential Markers for Assessment of Early Environmental Influences on Stress Response

The benzodiazepines remain very useful drugs for certain patients with PD, suggesting a role for the inhibitory neurotransmitter GABA in the pathophysiology of PD. There is evidence that the benzodiazepines, which potentiate synaptic actions of GABA, exert their anxiolytic effects at critical sites such as CRF neurons within the amygdala and the ascending noradrenergic systems [72]. A series of investigations strongly suggest that the CRF system is in fact a principal target for the anxiolytic effects of benzodiazepines [73,74]. Additionally, there is evidence of frontal cortex involvement as a target site for benzodiazepines. Antidepressants, which are recognized as clinically useful in treating PD, also interact with the GABA(A) receptor complex and enhance its function [75,76]. Of course, none of the preclinical investigations discussed above are specific for PD. Indeed, in certain subsets of patients, such as those with prominent dyspnea, benzodiazepines might fare poorly, as imipramine has been shown to be more effective than alprazolam in these patients [77].

Preclinically, a series of studies by Meaney's group have found that repeated periods of prolonged maternal separation resulted in decreased $GABA_A$ receptor binding, as well as diminished central benzodiazepine (BZ) receptor levels [72]. The potential relevance to PD stems from the observed epidemiological association between early maternal death and agoraphobia with panic attacks, as well as parental separation or divorce, findings specific for PD among the anxiety disorders [78].

Although the clinical studies of PD have yet to directly demonstrate decreased central BZ receptor levels as seen in Meaney's work in rodents, several human studies are highly suggestive of such. A positron emission tomography (PET) study in unmedicated patients with a history of PD revealed a significant decrease in brain BZ receptor levels using the flumazenil ligand [79], with a striking decrease in right orbitofrontal cortex and right insula. Another group more recently reported a decrease in left hippocampal and precuneus BZ receptor binding in a SPECT study, which was hypothesized to be due to changes in GABA-ergic transmission or to endogenous BZ compounds [80]. Notably, PD patients who panicked at the time of the scan had a decrease in prefrontal cortex BZ receptor binding compared to patients who did not panic [80], suggesting differences between state and trait-related panic anxiety.

Compared to the GABA/BZ system, much less attention has been given to the major excitatory amino acid, glutamate, in PD, although there is accumulating evidence that it plays a role in modulating stress responses. Rodent models indicate that prefrontal cortical efferents, either directly or via thalamic nuclei efferents, utilize the glutamatergic system as a primary source for neuronal stimulation of the "fear" neurocircuitry, which originates from the central nucleus of the amygdala and bed nucleus of the stria terminalis [81]. Stressful situations faced by a person with PD or other anxiety states might stimulate glutamate release in hippocampal [82] and other brain regions. In this light, agents that attenuate glutamatergic neurotransmission should reduce anxiety levels, as well as the concomitant biochemical alterations associated with stress [see 83 for review of glutamate-HPA axis interactions].

Thus, the balance between GABA and glutamate systems can be potentially disrupted with early environmental stressors, which may be associated with the development of PD in adulthood [84]. We have shown that subtle disruptions in the maternal-infant interaction results in CRF overexpression in bonnet macaques [85]; this in turn could result in alterations in other systems relevant to stress, anxiety and PD, such as the GABA/glutamate and LC/NE systems. Again, the specificity to PD is lacking in these models, an important limitation in their overall applicability.

IV. SSRI THERAPY AND PATHOPHYSIOLOGY

The use of antidepressants, particularly the SSRIs, has supplanted the long-term use of benzodiazepines in PD, and the former are now considered the first-line treatments. Questions remain as to why the SSRIs are beneficial in PD, what subtypes of patients are most likely to improve with the SSRIs, and what the role of serotonin in this disorder is. Effective treatments for PD, such as the SSRIs, might work by downregulation of overactive HPA/LC-NE systems. Indeed, our group demonstrated that after 12 weeks of treatment with fluoxetine, PD patients responding to treatment showed a decrease in plasma MHPG volatility during clonidine administration [71]. By having a noradrenergic-stabilizing effect, SSRIs would have a therapeutic role in decreasing symptoms associated with panic attacks such as tachycardia and increased diastolic blood pressure.

Other serotonergic projections of potential therapeutic relevance in PD include the projection of the raphe neurons to the periacqueductal gray region of the midbrain, which is important in defense/escape behaviors [86]. SSRIs, by inhibiting the periacqueductal gray region, might allow a disinhibition of the avoidance behaviors seen with panickers. Another important target for the SSRIs attenuates the hypothalamic release of CRF [87], which, as discussed above, appears to play a role in the mediation of fear in preclinical models. Regarding serotonin receptors, recent serotonergic challenge data postulate an increased sensitivity of central 5HT2C receptors and decreased responsiveness of 5HT1A receptors in panic, although replication is needed [88].

Finally, SSRIs might be effective in aborting panic attacks by a direct modulatory effect on the central nucleus of the amygdala. Stutzmann and Ledoux [89] have shown that 5HT inhibits excitatory glutamatergic inputs from thalamus and cortex at the lateral nucleus of the amygdala. An increase in 5HT with chronic SSRI use might prevent amygdaloid activation, as the amygdala is known to receive dense serotonergic input from raphe nuclei. So in effect, SSRIs might ultimately work in PD by attenuating glutamatergic hyperactivity at the level of the amygdala, as well as in other areas of excessive release in stress, such as the hippocampus, thalamus, and anterior cingulate, although this hypothesis remains to be tested.

We conclude that serotonergic abnormalities are unlikely the primary cause of PD, although antidepressants with serotonin activity are effective. SSRIs remain effective treatments for PD probably by diminishing the activity of brainstem centers that receive input from the amygdala and control autonomic and neuroendocrine response during attacks.

V. NEUROIMAGING STUDIES

A comprehensive review of the neuroimaging literature in PD is beyond the scope of this chapter [see 90]; herein we identify several key findings in the clinical literature. In general, PD patients do not differ from controls in cerebral blood flow (CBF) measures at baseline, but show different blood flow patterns when given panicogenic stimuli. PET and SPECT studies have found regional abnormalities in metabolism and blood flow in limbic structures, including hippocampus, parahippocampus, and temporal lobe [91–

94]. The studies measuring cerebral blood flow in PD, however, have methological limitations [28], including the fact that PD patients hyperventilate when anxious, and the resultant hypocapnia-induced vasoconstriction might obsure results by counteracting expected increases in blood flow.

There is accumulating evidence that PD patients are more sensitive to the vasoconstrictive effects of hyperventilation-induced hypocapnia than comparison subjects [28]. When controlling for level of hypocapnia, as measured by the end tidal CO_2 level, PD patients who hyperventilated during [^{133}Xe]-SPECT scans showed significantly greater decreases in CBF than normal controls [28]. A transcranial Doppler ultrasonography study similarly showed that patients with PD had greater reduction in basilar artery flow rates after hyperventilation than normal controls [95]. The implication from these studies is that patients with PD display greater cerebral vessel vasoconstriction, independent of degree of hyperventilation and hypocapnia. These findings might account for the development of neurological symptoms during certain panic attacks, such as dizziness, lightheadedness, and aura-like symptoms.

Several factors might explain these findings. First, the noradrenergic system activation observed in panickers might be contributory. It is known that noradrenergic fibers innervate cerebral blood vessels and cause vasoconstriction [96]. During periods of hyperventilation, increased LC discharge stemming from a hyperadrenergic state might cause a NE-mediated vasoconstrictive pattern observed in CBF studies [97]. Another explanation for the vasoconstrictive pattern in PD is the role of the parabrachial nucleus, a medullary structure that has been shown to cause cerebral vasoconstriction when stimulated [98]. The anatomical route is via the rostral serotonergic raphe nuclei, which relay information from the brainstem parabrachial nucleus (adjacent to the pontine locus ceruleus) to the cerebral cortex. Hyperventilation in a PET or SPECT study might produce symptoms reminiscent of a panic attack and trigger an amygdala-centered fear network, leading to increased activity in parabrachial nucleus sites, which then in turn mediates the vasoconstrictive effects seen in PD [28]. Another relevant brainstem nucleus is the nucleus tractus solitarius. In rats, stimulation with microinjection of L-glutamate causes vasoconstriction and a decrease in CBF. The NTS has afferents from the lungs and may be stimulated by hyperventilation, which we have observed to be increased in PD patients. Thus, increased stimulation of these various brainstem nuclei involved in the vasoconstrictive process might explain some of the CBF findings in PD. See **Figure 2** for a review of key neuroanatomical pathways in PD.

Besides CBF abnormalities, neuroimaging studies have explored anatomical morphometric volumes in PD. Unlike those observed in major depression and PTSD, patients with PD do not appear to have volumetric deficits in hippocampus [99]. In a quantitative MRI study, patients with PD displayed decreased overall temporal lobe volumes bilaterally compared with normal controls [99], a finding consistent with prior MRI studies. Previous MRI studies [100,101] showing asymmetric temporal lobe atrophy and larger dilatation of the temporal horn of the lateral ventricle were limited by the the use of qualitative MR measures. The pathophysiological significance of the reduction in the temporal lobe volume in the absence of hippocampal volume reduction is unclear, as are the CBF studies documenting alterations in hippocampal and adjacent cortex (parahippocampus) structures. Further prospective MRI studies are indicated to determine whether decreased temporal lobe volumes are a risk factor for panic disorder, a consequence of severity and duration of the illness or both.

VI. GENETIC CONSIDERATIONS AND ROLE OF COMORBIDITY

The struggle to identify biological trait markers for panic disorder likely reflects the complex genetic heterogeneity of the illness. This section briefly highlights important genetic considerations in PD [see 102 for a comprehensive review].

Family studies, while unable to differentiate between genetic and environmental influences, have shown that PD rates are substantially elevated over the base rate in the population if one has a first-degree relative with PD [103]. Twin studies that compare the rate of PD between monozygotic (MZ) and dizygotic (DZ) twins are useful for identifying genetic factors if the rate of monozygotic concordance is much higher than dizygotic rates. Although there is a higher concordance rate for PD in monozygotic than in dizygotic twins, the ranges observed (14–31%) are unimpressively low [104–106].

Genetic factors also likely play a limited role in the etiology of sporadic panic attacks, as suggested by Perna et al.'s twin study comparing the MZ/DZ ratio of PD with sporadic attacks [107]. They found no significant difference in concordance rates of sporadic

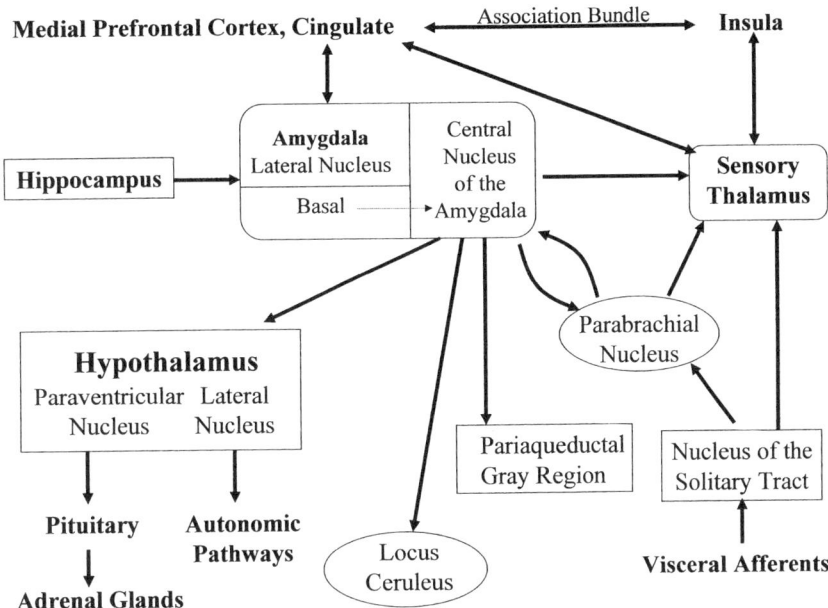

Figure 2 Viscerosensory information is conveyed to the amygdala by two major pathways: downstream, from the nucleus of the solitary tract via the parabrachial nucleus or the sensory thalamus; and upstream, from the primary viscerosensory cortices and via corticothalamic relays allowing for higher-level neurocognitive processing and modulation of sensory information. Contextual information is stored in memory in the hippocampus and conveyed directly to the amygdala. Major efferent pathways of the amygdala relevant to anxiety include the following: the locus ceruleus (increases norepinephrine release, which contributes to physiologic and behavioral arousal), the periaqueductal gray region (results in defensive behaviors and postural freezing), the hypothalamic paraventricular nucleus (activates the hypothalamic-pituitary-adrenal axis, releasing adrenocorticoids), the hypothalamic lateral nucleus (activates the sympathetic nervous system), and the parabrachial nucleus (influences respiratory rate and timing). (From Ref. 28.)

panic attacks between MZ and DZ twins, while there was a highly significant difference seen in PD (73% vs. 0%) [107]. Certainly classical Mendelian genetics does not provide an ideal model for PD.

Linkage studies investigating candidate genes thus far have yielded many negative results. These negative studies have included investigations of genes coding for the GABA(A) receptor, adrenergic receptor, pro-opiomelanocortin, serotonin transporter [108], and most recently, the CCK and CCK B receptor [109], and dopamine receptor and transporter [110]. Association studies exploring candidate genes have also yielded many negative results, notably the functional promoter polymorphism of the serotonin transporter [111], a finding consistent with the negative results in the linkage study.

A recent genomewide screen, however, yielded evidence for linkage with a marker on chromosome 20p [112]. Data from the same pedigrees, examining the parent of origin effect, suggest that the 2:1 increased female ratio observed in PD might be hereditary [113]. As has been noted in schizophrenia [114], a single major locus model for PD is improbable, and a complex inheritance model is likely. The genetics of PD is likely further complicated by incomplete penetrance and pleiotropy (e.g., a single genotype with multiple expressed phenotypes), as is discussed below.

A. Comorbid Medical Conditions and Preliminary Evidence for a Genetic Panic "Syndrome"

While there are often no physical abnormalities found on examination, there is an overrepresentation of several medical conditions in patients with PD. Recent data have emerged suggesting a panic disorder "syndrome," linked to chromosome 13, involving clustering of several medical illnesses such as bladder/kidney problems, mitral valve prolapse (MVP), serious headaches, and thyroid problems [115]. Our group's and others' clinical observations have suggested further clustering of medical disorders such as fibromyalgia, irritable bowel syndrome, chronic fatigue syndrome, asthma, joint hypermobility, and sinusitis/rhinitis in panic disorder patients [116–118]. These associations might lend support to the notion of pleiotropy playing a role in PD. The assumption of this work is that a candidate gene for the panic syndrome should be expressed in the various organs affected: kidney, thyroid, gut, heart, cerebral blood vessels, and of course, brain.

In this theory, a putative genetic change could give rise to dysfunction at several additional autonomically regulated sites [115]. Notably, autonomic mechanisms appear to be prominent factors in headaches, disorders of bladder contractility, and MVP. Another common pathophysiologic mechanism underlying some panic spectrum illnesses appears to be abnormalities in psychoimmune function. Regarding the panic-fibromyalgia link, a report by Klein [119] indicated elevations of antibodies to serotonin and gangliosides in patients with primary fibromyalgia. Given the putative role of serotonin in panic disorder [120], we measured plasma levels of antiserotonin and serotonin anti-idiotypic antibodies in PD patients and healthy controls, and found only the anti-idiotypic antibodies to be significantly elevated [121]. This preliminary report suggests that interruption of 5HT neurotransmission through autoimmune mechanisms may be significant in certain patients with PD [121]. Coupled with reports of elevations of plasma interleukin-1β in panic disorder [122], these data raise the possibility of psychoimmune dysfunction in panic spectrum illnesses, notably sinusitis/rhinitis, fibromyalgia, chronic fatigue syndrome, and Hashimoto's thyroiditis.

In accordance with the extended panic "syndrome" concept, there is evidence that effective antipanic treatments might ameliorate symptoms in the related medical disorders as well. For example, a resolution of MVP per echocardiogram criterion was observed following effective antipanic treatment [123]. Tricyclic antidepressants (TCAs) have long been used as effective migraine prophylaxis, and the SSRIs and TCAs have been used clinically with utility for irritable bowel syndrome.

In conclusion, genetic factors undoubtedly play a major role in the etiology of PD, although the specific mechanisms are unknown. A major challenge in future investigations will be the development and identification of valid and reliable "endophenotypes" based on potential biological markers of the illness (**Table 1**).

Table 1 Candidates for Biological Markers in Panic Disorder

Carbon dioxide hypersensitivity/respiratory dysregulation on CO_2 challenge
Increased respiratory variability at baseline marked by prominent sighing responses
Reduced heart period variability
HPA axis activity dysregulation
Noradrenergic system volatility
Decreased temporal lobe volume
Treatment responsivity to antidepressants vs. benzodiazepines (pharmacogenomics)
Chromosome 13 cluster illnesses

VII. CONCLUSIONS AND FUTURE DIRECTIONS

The search for biological trait markers in PD has been fraught with difficulty. This article has attempted to outline some of the important investigations in that search over the past four decades. Several areas requiring future research are addressed.

First, in the realm of experimental therapeutics, there is clearly a need for more effective treatments, as well as clearer delineation of treatment response by panic subtype. Experimental agents showing promise in paniclike models in rodents include the group II metabotropic receptor agonist LY354740 [124] and drugs acting at the neuropeptide receptors, including neuropeptide-Y agonists and neurokinin substance P antagonists [125]. Other new classes of drugs being studied include the benzodiazepine partial agonists abecarnil and pagoclone, and agents modulating the HPA axis such as CRF antagonists. Regarding subtype and treatment response, further cluster analyses investigating dyspneic versus nondyspneic PD treatment response are warranted.

Second, imaging studies represent an area of enormous potential. The preliminary findings of reduced temporal volumes in PD need to be replicated as well as investigations in other relevant anxiety neurocircuitry structures, such as the amygdala. A neurodevelopmental perspective on PD would mandate longitudinal prospective MRI studies beginning in childhood to assess what is a risk factor for the illness and what is a consequence. DeBellis [126] showed that children and adolescents with GAD had significantly larger right and total amygdala volumes than matched controls. Given the potential role of amygdaloid projections in the pathogenesis of panic disorder, this type of study, employing both functional and morphometric components, would be illuminating.

PET and SPECT imaging studies in PD have relatively neglected serotonin and norepinephrine receptors and transporters sites that might be important in the pathophysiology of the disorder. Since chronic SSRI administration is the treatment of choice for both depression and PD, and presumably desensitizes presynaptic somatodendritic 5HT1A autoreceptors [127], it would be intriguing to investigate 5HT1A receptor function in PD. Serotonin-1A receptor binding potential (BP) was found to be abnormally decreased in the depressed phase of familial mood disorders [128,129]; this finding merits investigation in PD.

A potential use of magnetic resonance spectroscopy (MRS) is to assess 5HT-glutamate interactions in vivo. This interaction has been explored in pediatric OCD, as effective treatment with paroxetine attenuated the "Glx" (consisting of glutamate-glutamine-GABA) signal in the caudate in effectively treated patients [130]. Future investigations of this kind in PD would lend credence to the notion of the SSRIs attenuating a hyperglutamatergic state.

Finally, although researchers have productively utilized preclinical models such as conditioned fear in rodents to provide explanatory hypotheses for PD, there is no current animal model for panic that has been capable of generating the signature spontaneous panic attack. As these models provide the basis for much of our thinking about clinical conditions, the development of more realistic models of the disorder continues to pose a major challenge.

REFERENCES

1. WW Eaton, RC Kessler, HU Wittchen, WJ Magee. Panic and panic disorder in the United States. Am J Psychiatry 151:413–420, 1994.
2. JS Markowitz, MM Weissman, R Ouellette, JD Lish, GL Klerman. Quality of life in panic disorder. Arch Gen Psychiatry 46:984–992, 1989.
3. MM Weissman. The epidemiology and genetics of panic disorder. Clin Neuropharmacol 15(suppl 1, pt A):18A–19A, 1992.
4. DF Klein. False suffocation alarms, spontaneous panics, and related conditions: an integrative hypothesis. Arch Gen Psychiatry 50:306–317, 1993.
5. WB Cannon. Bodily Changes in Pain, Hunger, Fear and Rage: An Account of Recent Researches Into the Function of Emotional Excitement, 2nd ed. New York: D. Appleton, 1929.
6. N Shinoda, K Kodama, T Sakamoto, N Yamanouchi, T Takahashi, S OkNoda, N Komatsu, T Sato. Predictors of 1-year outcome for patients with panic disorder. Compr Psychiatry 40(1):39–43, 1999.
7. C Heim, DJ Newport, S Heit, YP Graham, M Wilcox, R Bonsall, AH Miller, CB Nemeroff. Pituitary-adrenal and autonomic responses to stress in women after sexual and physical abuse in childhood. JAMA 284:592–597, 2000.
8. DS Pine, P Cohen, D Gurley, JS Brook, Y Ma. The risk for early-adulthood anxiety and depressive disorders in adolescents with anxiety and depressive disorders. Arch Gen Psychiatry 55:56–64, 1998.
9. RG Klein. Is panic disorder associated with childhood separation anxiety disorder? Clin Neuropharmacol 18(suppl 2):S7–S14, 1995.
10. MH Pollack, MW Otto, S Sabatino, D Majcher, JJ Worthington, ET McArdle, JF Rosenbaum. Relationship of childhood anxiety to adult panic disorder: correlates and influence on course. Am J Psychiatry 153:376–381, 1996.
11. PM Keyl, MW Eaton. Risk factors for the onset of panic disorder and other panic attacks in a prospective, population-based study. Am J Epidemiol 131:301–311, 1990.
12. DS Pine, RG Klein, JD Coplan, LA Papp, CW Hoven, J Martinez, P Kovalenko, DJ Mandell, D Moreau, DF Klein, JM Gorman. Differential carbon dioxide sensitivity in childhood anxiety disorders and nonill comparison group. Arch Gen Psychiatry 57:960–967, 2000.
13. DS Pine, JD Coplan, LA Papp, RG Klein, JM Martinez, P Kovalenko, N Tancer, D Moreau, ES Dummit 3rd, D Shaffer, DF Klein, JM Gorman. Ventilatory physiology of children and adolescents with anxiety disorders. Arch Gen Psychiatry 55:123–129, 1998.
14. JD Coplan, D Moreau, F Chaput, JM Martinez, CW Hoven, DJ Mandell, JM Gorman, DS Pine. Salivary cortisol concentrations before and following carbon-dioxide inhalations in children. (Manuscript under review, 2001.)
15. JM Gorman, MR Fyer, R Goetz, J Askanazi, MR Liebowitz, AJ Fyer, J Denny, DF Klein. Ventilatory physiology of patients with panic disorder. Arch Gen Psychiatry 45:31–39, 1988.
16. LA Papp, JM Martinez, DF Klein, JD Coplan, RG Norman, R Cole, MJ de Jesus, D Ross, R Goetz, JM Gorman. Respiratory psychophysiology of panic disorder: three respiratory challenges in 98 subjects. Am J Psychiatry 154:1557–1565, 1997.
17. LA Papp, DF Klein, JM Gorman. Carbon dioxide hypersensitivity, hyperventilation and panic disorder. Am J Psychiatry 150:1149–1157, 1993.

18. W Coryell. Hypersensitivity to carbon dioxide as a disease-specific trait marker. Biol Psychiatry 41:259–263, 1997.
19. G Perna, S Cocchi, A Bertani, C Arancio, L Bellodi. Sensitivity to 35% CO_2 in healthy first-degree relatives of patients with panic disorder. Am J Psychiatry 152:623–625, 1995.
20. JM Kent, LA Papp, JM Martinez, ST Browne, JD Coplan, DF Klein, JM Gorman. Specificity of panic response to CO2 inhalation in panic disorder: a comparison with major depression and premenstrual dysphoric disorder. Am J Psychiatry 158:58–67, 2001.
21. JD Coplan, R Goetz, DF Klein, LA Papp, AJ Fyer, MR Liebowitz, SO Davies, JM Gorman. Plasma cortisol concentrations preceding lactate-induced panic. Psychological, biochemical and physiological correlates. Arch Gen Psychiatry 55(2):130–136, 1998.
22. SS Sinha, JD Coplan, DS Pine, JA Martinez, DF Klein, JM Gorman. Panic induced by carbon dioxide inhalation and lack of hypothalamic-pituitary-adrenal axis activation. Psychiatry Res 86 (2):93–98, 1999.
23. M Kellner, L Herzog, A Yassouridis, F Holsboer, K Wiedemann. Possible role of atrial natriuretic hormone in pituitary-adrenocortical unresponsiveness in lactate-induced panic. Am J Psychiatry 152:1365–1367, 1995.
24. DF Klein, M Fink. Psychiatric reaction patterns to imipramine. Am J Psychiatry 119:432–438, 1962.
25. P Roy-Byrne, MB Stein. Inspiring panic. Arch Gen Psychiatry 58:123–124, 2001.
26. DM Clark. Cognitive mediation of panic attacks induced by biological challenge tests. Adv Behav Res Ther 15:75–84, 1993.
27. JM Gorman, J Kent, J Martinez, S Browne, J Coplan, LA Papp. Physiologic changes during carbon dioxide inhalation in patients with panic disorder, major depression and premenstrual dysphoric disorder: evidence for a central fear mechanism. Arch Gen Psychiatry 2001.
28. JM Gorman, JM Kent, GM Sullivan, JD Coplan. Neuroanatomical hypothesis of panic disorder, revised. Am J Psychiatry 157:493–505, 2000.
29. JL Abelson, JG Weg, RM Nesse, GC Curtis. Persistent respiratory irregularity in patients with panic disorder. Biol Psychiatry 49:588–595, 2001.
30. JM Martinez, JD Coplan, ST Browne, LA Papp, JM Kent, GM Sullivan, M Kleber, AJ Fyer, DF Klein, JM Gorman. Respiratory variability in panic disorder. Depress Anxiety (in press).
31. Wilhelm FH, Gerlach AL, Roth WT. Slow recovery from voluntary hyperventilation in panic disorder. Psychosom Med (in press).
32. Wilhelm FH, Trabert W, Roth WT. Physiological instability in panic disorder and generalized anxiety disorder. Biol Psychiatry 49:596–605, 2001.
33. Wilhelm FH, Trabert W, Roth WT. Characteristics of sighing in panic disorder. Biol Psychiatry 49:606–614, 2001.
34. RM Harper, GR Poe, DM Rector, MP Kristensen. Relationships between hippocampal activity and breathing patterns. Neurosci Biobehav Rev 22:233–236, 1998.
35. Kristensen MP, GR Poe, DM Rector, RM Harper. Activity changes of the cat paraventricular hypothalamus during phasic respiratory events. Neuroscience 80:811–819, 1997.
36. JX Zhang, RM Harper, HF Ni. Cryogenic blockade of the central nucleus of the amygdala attenuates aversively conditioned blood pressure and respiratory responses. Brain Res 386:136–145, 1986.
37. Stein MB, TW Millar, DK Larsen, MH Kryger. Irregular breathing patterns during sleep in patients with panic disorder. Am J Psychiatry 152:1168–1173, 1995.
38. W Coryell, A Fyer, D Pine, J Martinez, S Arndt. Aberrant respiratory sensitivity to CO_2 as a trait of familial panic disorder. Biol Psychiatry 49:582–587, 2001.
39. JM Gorman, RP Sloan. Heart rate variability in depressive and anxiety disorders. Am Heart J 140:S77–S83, 2000.
40. MR Liebowitz, JM Gorman, AJ Fyer, M Levitt, D Dillon, G Levy, IL Appleby, S Anderson, M Palij, SO Davies, DF Klein. Lactate provocation of panic attacks II: Biochemical and physiological findings. Arch Gen Psychiatry 42:709–71, 1985
41. D Wilkinson, JM Thompson, GW Lambert, GL Jennings, RG Schwarz, D Jefferys, AG Turner, MD Esler. Sympathetic activity in patients with panic disorder at rest, under laboratory mental stress, and during panic attacks. Arch Gen Psychiatry 55:511–520, 1998.
42. MM Weissman, JS Markowitz, R Ouellete, S Greenwald, JP Kahn. Panic disorder and cardiovascular/cerebrovascular problems: results from a community survey. Am J Psychiatry 147:1504–1508, 1990.
43. JT Bigger, JL Fleiss, RC Steinman, LM Rolnitzky, RE Kleiger, JN Rottman. Frequency domain measures of heart period variability and mortality after myocardial infarction. Circulation 85:164–171, 1992.
44. E Klein, E Cnaani, T Harel, S Braun, SA Ben-Haim. Altered heart rate variability in panic disorder patients. Biol Psychiatry 37:18–24, 1995.
45. VK Yeragani, R Pohl, R Berger, R Balon, C Ramesh, D Glitz, K Srinivasan, P Weinberg. Decreased heart rate variability in panic disorder patients: a study of power-spectral analysis of heart rate. Psychiatry Res 46:89–103, 1993.

46. VK Yeragani, E Sobolewski, G Igel, C Johnson, VC Jampala, J Kay, N Hillman, S Yeragani, S Vempati. Decreased heart-period variability in patients with panic disorder: a study of Holter ECG records. Psychiatry Res 78:89–99, 1998.
47. M Battaglia, S Bertella, A Ogliari, L Bellodi, E Smeraldi. Modulation by muscarinic antagonists of the response to carbon dioxide challenge in panic disorder. Arch Gen Psychiatry 58:114–119, 2001.
48. K Wiedemann, H Jahn, A Yassouridis, M Kellner. Anxiolytic effects of atrial natriuretic peptide on cholecystokinin tetrapeptide-induced panic attacks. Arch Gen Psychiatry 58:371–377, 2001.
49. J Jolkkonen, U Lepola, G Bissette, C Nemeroff, P Riekkinen. CSF corticotropin-releasing factor is not affected in panic disorder. Biol Psychiatry 33(2):136–138, 1993.
50. F Holsboer. The corticosteroid receptor hypothesis of depression. Neuropsychopharmacology 23:477–501, 2000.
51. PP Roy-Byrne, TW Uhde, RM Post, W Gallucci, GP Chrousos, PW Gold. The corticotropin-releasing hormone stimulation test in patients with panic disorder. Am J Psychiatry 143:896–899, 1986.
52. U Von Bardeleben, F Holsboer. Human corticotropin releasing hormone: clinical studies in patients with affective disorders, alcoholism, panic disorder and in normal controls. Prog Neuropsychopharmacol Biol Psychiatry 12:S165–S187, 1988.
53. MH Rapoport, SC Risch, S Golshan, JC Gillin. Neuroendocrine effects of ovine corticotropin-releasing hormone in panic disorder patients. Biol Psychiatry 26:344–348, 1989.
54. JL Abelson, GC Curtis. Hypothalamic-pituitary-adrenal axis activity in panic disorder. Arch Gen Psychiatry 53:323–332, 1996.
55. RF Vining, RA McGinley, JJ Maksvytis, KY Ho. Salivary cortisol: a better measure of adrenal cortical function than serum cortisol. Ann Clin Biochem 20:329–335, 1983.
56. B Bandelow, D Wedekind, J Pauls, A Broocks, G Hajak, E Ruther. Salivary cortisol in panic attacks. Am J Psychiatry 157:454–456, 2000.
57. D Wedekind, B Bandelow, A Broocks, G Hajak, E Ruther. Salivary, total plasma and plasma free cortisol in panic disorder. J Neural Transm 107(7):831–837, 2000.
58. JD Coplan, GM Sullivan, JM Gorman. The psychoneuroendocrinology of panic disorder: a linkage to ventilatory pathophysiology. In: L Bellodi, G Perna, eds. The Panic Respiration Connection. Milan: Sergraf, 1998, pp 95–110.
59. GM Sullivan, JD Coplan, JM Kent, JM Gorman. The noradrenergic system in pathological anxiety: a focus on panic with relevance to generalized anxiety and phobias. Biol Psychiatry 46:1205–1218, 1999.
60. J Vandergriff, K Rasmussen. The selective mGlu2/3 receptor agonist LY354740 attenuates morphine-withdrawal-induced activation of locus ceruleus. Neuropharmacology 38:217–222, 1999.
61. JD Coplan, SJ Mathew, ELP Smith, RC Trost, BA Scharf, JM Gorman, J Martinez, JA Monn, DD Schoepp, LA Rosenblum. Effects of LY354740, a novel glutamatergic metabotropic agonist, on nonhuman primate hypothalamic-pituitary adrenal function. CNS Spectrums (in press).
62. JD Coplan, D Pine, L Papp, J Martinez, T Cooper, LA Rosenblum, JM Gorman. Uncoupling of the noradrenergic-hypothalamic-pituitary-adrenal axis in panic disorder patients. Neuropsychopharmacology 13:65–73, 1995.
63. JD Coplan, LA Papp, J Martinez, D Pine, LA Rosenblum, T Cooper, MR Liebowitz, JM Gorman. Persistence of blunted human growth hormone response to clonidine in fluoxetine-treated patients with panic disorder. Am J Psychiatry 152:619–622, 1995.
64. T Uhde, RT Joffe, DC Jimerson, RM Post. Normal urinary free cortisol and plasma MHPG in panic disorder: clinical and theoretical implications. Biol Psychiatry 23:575–585, 1988.
65. DJ Nutt. Altered alpha2-adrenoceptor sensitivity in panic disorder. Arch Gen Psychiatry 46:165–169, 1989.
66. JD Coplan, EL Smith, RC Trost, BA Scharf, M Altemus, L Bjornson, MJ Owens, JM Gorman, CB Nemeroff, LA Rosenblum. Growth hormone response to clonidine in adversely reared young adult primates:relationship to serial cerebrospinal fluid corticotropin-releasing factor concentrations. Psychiatry Res 95 (2):93–102, 2000.
67. JD Coplan, DF Klein. Pharmacological probes in panic disorder. In: HGM Westenberg, JA Den Boer, DL Murphy, eds. Advances in the Neurobiology of Anxiety Disorders. New York: John Wiley & Sons, 1996, pp 173–196.
68. RB Lydiard, JC Ballenger, MT Laraia, et al. Effects of chronic alprazolam and imipramine treatment on catacholamine function in patients with agoraphobia with panic attacks or agoraphobia. In: JC Ballenger, ed. Clinical Aspects of Panic Disorder. New York: Wiley-Liss, 1990, pp 239–249.
69. JM Gorman, MR Liebowitz, AF Fyer, J Stein. A neuroanatomical hypothesis for panic disorder. Am J Psychiatry 146:148–161, 1989.
70. G Grove, JD Coplan, E Hollander. The neuroanatomy of 5-HT regulation and panic disorder. J Neuropsychiatry Clin Neurosci 9:198–207, 1997.

71. JD Coplan, L Papp, DS Pine, J Martinez, TB Cooper, LA Rosenblum, DF Klein, JM Gorman. Clinical improvement with fluoxetine therapy normalizes noradrenergic function in patients with panic disorder. Arch Gen Psychiatry 54:643–648, 1997.
72. C Caldji, D Francis, S Sharma, PM Plotsky, MJ Meaney. The effects of early rearing environment on the development of $GABA_A$ and central benzodiazepine receptor levels and novelty-induced fearfulness in the rat. Neuropsychopharmacology 22:219–229, 2000.
73. SF den Boer, JL Katz, RJ Valentino. Common mechanism underlying the proconflict effects of corticotropin-releasing factor, a benzodiazepine inverse agonist and electric footshock. J Pharmacol Exp Ther 262:335–342, 1992.
74. MJ Owens, MA Vargas, DL Knight, CB Nemeroff. The effects of alprazolam on corticotropin-releasing factor neurons in the rat brain: acute time course, chronic treatment and abrupt withdrawal. J Pharmacol Exp Ther 258:349–356, 1991.
75. M Matsubara, S Suzuki, K Miura, M Terashima, S Sugita, H Kimura, S Hatsuda, T Mori, H Murakami, T Hayashi, T Ohta, M Ohara. Electrophysiologic analysis of antidepressant drug effects on the GABA (A) receptor complex based upon antagonist-induced encephalographic power spectrum changes. Neuropsychobiology 42 (3):149–157, 2000.
76. G Tunnicliff, NL Schindler, GJ Crites, R Goldenberg, A Yochum, E Malatynska. The GABA (A) receptor complex as a target for fluoxetine action. Neurochem Res 24 (10):1271–1276, 1999.
77. AC Briggs, DD Stretch, S Brandon. Subtyping of panic disorder by symptom profile. Br J Psychiatry 163:201–209, 1993.
78. JL Tweed, VJ Schoenbach, LK George, DG Blazer. The effects of childhood parental death and divorce on six-month history of anxiety disorders. Br J Psychiatry 154:823–828, 1989.
79. AL Malizia, VJ Cunningham, CJ Bell, PF Liddle, T Jones, DJ Nutt. Decreased brain $GABA_A$-benzodiazepine receptor binding in panic disorder. Arch Gen Psychiatry 55:715–720, 1998.
80. JD Bremner, RB Innis, T White, M Fujita, D Silbersweig, AW Goddard, L Staib, E Stern, A Cappiello, S Woods, R Baldwin, DS Charney. SPECT [I-123] iomezenil measurement of the benzodiazepine receptor in panic disorder. Biol Psychiatry 47 (2):96–106, 2000.
81. J LeDoux:. Fear and the brain: where have we been, and where are we going? Biol Psychiatry 44 (12):1229–1238, 1998.
82. B Moghaddam, M Bolinao, B Stein-Behrens, R Sapolsky. Glucocorticoids mediate the stress induced extracellular accumulation in the hippocampus. J Neurochem 63:596–602, 1994.
83. SJ Mathew, JD Coplan, ELP Smith, D Schoepp, LA Rosenblum, JM Gorman. Glutamate-HPA axis interactions: implications for mood and anxiety disorders. CNS Spectrums (in press).
84. N Horesh, M Amir, P Kedem, Y Goldberger, M Kotler. Life events in childhood, adolescence and adulthood and the relationship to panic disorder. Acta Psychiatr Scand 96:373–378, 1997.
85. JD Coplan, MW Andrews, LA Rosenblum, MJ Owens, JM Gorman, CB Nemeroff. Increased cerebrospinal fluid CRF concentration in adult nonhuman primates previously exposed to adverse experiences as infants. Proc Natl Acad Sci USA 93:1619–1623, 1996.
86. JFW Deakin, F Graeff. 5-HT and mechanisms of defence. J Psychopharmacol 5:305–315, 1991.
87. LS Brady, PW Gold, M Herkenham, AB Lynn, HJ Whitfield J. The antidepressants fluoxetine, idazoxan and phenelzine alter corticotropin-releasing hormone and tyrosine hydroxylase mRNA levels in rat brain: therapeutic implications. Brain Res 572:117–125, 1992.
88. A Broocks, B Bandelow, A George, C Jestrabeck, M Opitz, U Bartmann, CH Gleiter, I Meineke, IS Roed, E Ruther, G Hajak. Increased psychological responses and divergent neuroendocrine responses to m-CPP and ipsapirone in patients with panic disorder. Int Clin Psychopharmacol 15(3):153–161, 2000.
89. GE Stutzmann, JE Ledoux. GABAergic antagonists block the inhibitory effects of serotonin in the lateral amygdala: a mechanism for modulation of sensory inputs related to fear conditioning. J Neurosci 19:RC8, 1999.
90. JM Kent, GM Sullivan, SL Rauch. The neurobiology of fear: relevance to panic disorder and posttraumatic stress disorder. Psychiatr Ann 30(12):733–742, 2000.
91. A Bisaga, J Katz, A Antonini, E Wright, C Margouleff, J Gorman, D Eidelberg. Cerebral glucose metabolism in women with panic disorder. Am J Psychiatry 155:1178–1183, 1998.
92. E Reiman, M Raichle, E Robins, F Butler, P Herscovitch, P Fox, J Perlmutter. The application of positron emission tomography to the study of panic disorder. Am J Psychiatry 143:469–477, 1986.
93. M De Cristofaro, A Sessarego, A Pupi, F Biondi, C Faravelli. Brain perfusion abnormalities in drug-naïve, lactate-sensitive panic patients: a SPECT study. Biol Psychiatry 33:505–512, 1993.
94. TE Nordahl, WE Semple, M Gross, TA Mellman, MB Stein, P Goyer, AC King, P Goyer, AC King, TW Uhde, RM Cohen. Cerebral glucose metabolic differences in patients with panic disorder. Neuropsychopharmacology 3:261–271, 1990.
95. S Ball, A Shekhar. Basilar artery response to hyperventilation in panic disorder. Am J Psychiatry 154(11):1603–1604, 1997.

96. RN Kalaria, CA Stockmeier, SI Harik. Brain microvessels are innervated by locus ceruleus noradrenergic neurons. Neurosci Lett 97:203–208, 1989.
97. RJ Mathew. Sympathetic control of cerebral circulation: relevance to psychiatry. Biol Psychiatry 37(5):283–285, 1995.
98. S Marovitch, C Iadecola, DA Ruggiero, DJ Reis. Widespread reductions in cerebral blood flow and metabolism elicited by electrical stimulation of the parabrachial nucleus in the rat. Brain Res 314:283–296, 1985.
99. M Vythilingam, EA Anderson, A Goddard, SW Woods, LH Staib, DS Charney, JD Bremner. Temporal lobe volume in panic disorder—a quantitative magnetic resonance imaging study. Psychiatry Res: Neuroimag Sec 99:75–82, 2000.
100. A Ontiveros, R Fontaine, G Breton, R Elie, S Fontaine, R Dery. Correlation of severity of panic disorder and neuroanatomical changes on magnetic resonance imaging. J Neuropsychiatry Clin Neurosci 1:404–408, 1989.
101. R Fontaine, G Breton, R Dery, S Fontaine, R Elie. Temporal lobe abnormalities in panic disorder: an MRI study. Biol Psychiatry 27:304–310, 1990.
102. OA van den Heuvel, BJM van de Wetering, DJ Veltman, DL Pauls. Genetic studies of panic disorder: a review. J Clin Psychiatry 61:756–766, 2000.
103. MM Weissman, P Wickramaratne, PB Adams, JD Lish, E Horwath, D Charney, SW Woods, E Leeman, E Frosch. The relationship between panic disorder and major depression: a new family study. Arch Gen Psychiatry 50:767–780, 1993.
104. S Togersen. Genetic factors in anxiety disorders. Arch Gen Psychiatry 40:1085–1089, 1983.
105. KS Kendler, MC Neale, RC Kessler, AC Heath, LJ Eaves. Panic disorder in women: a population-based twin study. Psychol Med 23:397–406, 1993.
106. I Skre, S Onstad, S Togersen, S Lygren, E Kringlen. A twin study of DSM-III-R anxiety disorders. Acta Psychiatr Scand 88:85–92, 1993.
107. G Perna, D Caldirola, C Arancio, L Bellodi. Panic attacks: a twin study. Psychiatry Res 66:69–71, 1997.
108. SP Hamilton, GA Heiman, F Haghighi, S Mick, DF Klein, SE Hodge, MM Weissman, AJ Fyer, JA Knowles. Lack of genetic linkage or association between a functional serotonin transporter polymorphism and panic disorder. Psychiatr Genet 9(1):1–6, 1999.
109. SP Hamilton, SL Slager, L Helleby, GA Heiman, DF Klein, SE Hodge, MM Weissman, AJ Fyer, JA Knowles. No association or linkage between polymorphisms in the genes encoding cholecystokinin and the cholecystokinin B receptor and panic disorder. Mol Psychiatry 6(1):59–65, 2001.
110. SP Hamilton, F Haghighi, GA Heiman, DF Klein, SE Hodge, AJ Fyer, MM Weissman, JA Knowles. Investigation of dopamine receptor (DRD4) and dopamine transporter (DAT) polymorphisms for genetic linkage or association to panic disorder. Am J Med Genet 96(3):324–330, 2000.
111. J Deckert, M Catalano, A Heils, et al. Functional promotor polymorphism of the human serotonin transporter: lack of association with panic disorder. Psychiatr Genet 7:45–47, 1997.
112. JA Knowles, AJ Fyer, VJ Vieland, MM Weissman, SE Hodge, GA Heiman, F Haghighi, GM de Jesus, H Rassnick, X Preud'homme-Rivelli, Austin, J Cunjak, S Mick, LD Fine, KA Woodley, K Das, W Maier, PB Adams, NB Freimer, DF Klein, TC Gilliam. Results of a genome-wide genetic screen for panic disorder. Am J Med Genet 81:139–147, 1998.
113. F Haghighi, AJ Fyer, MM Weissman, JA Knowles, SE Hodge. Parent-of-origin effect in panic disorder. Am J Med Genet 88:131–135, 1999
114. GD Pearlson. Neurobiology of schizophrenia. Ann Neurol 48:556–566, 2000.
115. MM Weissman, AJ Fyer, F Haghighi, G Heiman, Z Deng, R Hen, SE Hodge, JA Knowles. Potential panic disorder syndrome: clinical and genetic linkage evidence. Am J Med Genet 96 (1):24–35, 2000.
116. A Bulbena, JC Duro, M Porta, R Martin-Santos, A Mateo, L Molina, R Vallescar, J Vallejo. Anxiety disorders in the joint hypermobility syndrome. Psychiatry Res 46 (1):59–68, 1993.
117. AJ Gruber, JI Hudson, HG Pope Jr. The management of treatment-resistant depression in disorders on the interface of psychiatry and medicine. Fibromyalgia, chronic fatigue syndrome, migraine, irritable bowel syndrome, atypical facial pain, and premenstrual dysphoric disorder. Psychiatr Clin North America 19 (2):351–369,1996.
118. TS Zaubler, W Katon. Panic disorder and medical comorbidity: a review of the medical and psychiatric literature. Bull Menninger Clin 60(2 suppl A):A12–A38, 1996.
119. R Klein, M Bansch, PA Berg. Clinical relevance of antibodies against serotonin and gangliosides in patients with primary fibromyalgia syndrome. Psychoneuroendocrinology 17(6):593–598, 1992.
120. JD Coplan, JM Gorman, DF Klein. Serotonin-related function in panic disorder: a critical overview. Neuropsychopharmacology 6(3):189–200, 1992.
121. JD Coplan, H Tamir, D Calaprice, M DeJesus, M de al Nuez, D Pine, LA Papp, DF Klein, JM Gorman. Plasma anti-serotonin and serotonin anti-idiotypic antibodies are elevated in panic disorder. Neuropsychopharmacology 20(4):386–391, 1999.
122. F Brambilla, L Bellodi, G Perna, M Battaglia, G Sciuto, G Diaferia, F Petraglia, A Panerai, P Sacerdote. Plasma interleukin-1 beta concentrations in panic disorder. Neuropsychobiology 26(1–2):12–22, 1994.

123. JD Coplan, LA Papp, DL King, JM Gorman. Amelioration of mitral valve prolapse after treatment for panic disorder. Am J Psychiatry 149:1587–1588, 1992.
124. A Shekhar, SR Keim. LY354740, a potent group II metabotropic glutamate receptor agonist prevents lactate-induced panic-like response in panic-prone rats. Neuropharmacology 39:1139–1146, 2000.
125. G Griebel. Is there a future for neuropeptide receptor ligands in the treatment of anxiety disorders? Pharmacol Ther 82:1–61, 1999.
126. MD De Bellis, BJ Casey, RE Dahl, B Birmaher, DE Williamson, KM Thomas, DA Axelson, K Frustaci, AM Boring, J Hall, ND Ryan. A pilot study of amygdala volumes in pediatric generalized anxiety disorder. Biol Psychiatry 48:51–57, 2000.
127. Y Chaput, C deMontigny, P Blier. Presynaptic and postsynaptic modifications of the serotonin system by long-term administration of antidepressant treatments: an in vivo electrophysiologic study in the rat. Neuropsychopharmacology 5:219–229, 1991.
128. PA Sargent, KH Kjaer, CJ Bench, EA Rabiner, C Messa, J Meyer, RN Gunn, PM Grasby, PJ Cowen. Brain sertonin$_{1A}$ receptor binding measured by positron emission tomography with [^{11}C]Way-100635. Arch Gen Psychiatry 57:174–180, 2000.
129. WC Drevets, E Frank, JC Price, DJ Kupfer, D Holt, PJ Greer, Y Huang, C Gautier, C Mathis. PET imaging of serotonin 1A receptor binding in depression. Biol Psychiatry 46:1375–1387, 1999.
130. DR Rosenberg, FP MacMaster, MS Keshavan, KD Fitzgerald, CM Stewart, GJ Moore. Decrease in caudate glutamatergic concentrations in pediatric obsessive compulsive disorder patients taking paroxetine. J Am Acad Child Adolesc Psychiatry 39(9):1096–103, 2000.
131. JD Coplan, RB Lydiard. Brain circuits in panic disorder. Biol Psychiatry 44:1264–1276, 1998.

31

Neurobiology of Posttraumatic Stress Disorder Across the Life Cycle

MICHAEL D. DE BELLIS
Duke University Medical Center, Durham, North Carolina, U.S.A.

I. POSTTRAUMATIC STRESS DISORDER

As described in the Diagnostic and Statistical Manual of Mental Disorders: Fourth Edition Text Revision (DSM-IV-TR), the essential feature (criterion A) of posttraumatic stress disorder (PTSD) is exposure to an extreme traumatic stressor in which the person experienced, witnessed, or was confronted with an event or events that involved actual or threatened death or serious injury, or a threat to the physical integrity of self or others; and responded with intense fear, helplessness, horror, or, in children, disorganized or agitated behaviors [1]. The DSM-IV-TR diagnosis of PTSD is made when criterion A is experienced and when three clusters of categorical symptoms are present for > 1 month after the traumatic event(s): (1) intrusive reexperiencing of the trauma(s) (criterion B); (2) persistent avoidance of stimuli associated with the trauma(s) (criterion C); and (3) persistent symptoms of increased physiological arousal (criterion D).

Cluster B reexperiencing and intrusive symptoms can best be conceptualized as a classically conditioned response. An external or internal conditioned stimulus (e.g., the traumatic reminder) activates unwanted and distressful recurrent and intrusive memories of the traumatic experience(s) (e.g., the unconditioned stimulus). Intrusive phenomena take the form of distressing intrusions such as nightmares or night terrors, dissociative flashback episodes, and psychological distress and physical reactivity on exposure to traumatic reminders. In young children, these intrusive thoughts may be part of repetitive play or trauma-specific reenactment(s) or compulsive rituals. Cluster C symptoms represent both avoidant and dissociative behaviors and can be thought of as ways to control painful and distressing reexperiencing of symptoms. These include efforts to avoid thoughts, feelings, conversations, activities, places, people, and memories associated with the trauma; amnesia for the trauma; diminished interest in others; feelings of detachment from others; a restricted range of affect; and a sense of a foreshortened future. Cluster D hyperarousal symptoms consist of persistent symptoms of increased physiological arousal. These include difficulty falling or staying asleep, irritable mood or angry outbursts, difficulty concentrating, hypervigilance, and exaggerated startle response. PTSD symptoms are thought to be mediated by dysregulation of the neurobiologic stress systems which mediate the fear or anxiety response.

II. EPIDEMIOLOGY OF PTSD

PTSD is a serious and debilitating chronic mental illness with enormous societal costs [2]. Traditionally,

PTSD was primarily identified in male soldiers and combat veterans. However, PTSD may arise from a variety of traumatic events in both males and females throughout the life cycle. The diagnostic picture of PTSD in children is similar to that in adults [3,4], with the exception of children < 4 years where more objective criteria based on observable behaviors are warranted [5]. Children are more vulnerable to develop PTSD as they are more likely to be diagnosed with PTSD, once traumatized, than their adult counterparts [6]. According to the National Co-Morbidity Survey, the estimated lifetime prevalence of PTSD in persons aged 15–54 years is 7.8% [7]. The National Co-Morbidity Survey reported a lifetime history of at least one other Axis I disorder (i.e., mood, other anxiety, and substance use disorders) in 88.3% of men and in 79% of women with PTSD. In contrast to adult PTSD research, there are no epidemiological studies and hence no published community lifetime prevalence rates for PTSD in children or adolescents to date [8]. However, PTSD lifetime prevalence rates for children and adolescents are thought to be similar to or even higher than those of adults. Hence, a recent community sample estimated a DSM-III-R PTSD prevalence rate by use of the NIMH Diagnostic Interview Schedule Version III-R (DIS-III-R) of 6.3% in adolescents [9]. PTSD in childhood is also associated with high rates of comorbid mood and other anxiety disorders [10,11]. High rates of comorbid mood, other anxiety disorders, and substance use disorders are seen in adolescents with PTSD [9,12,13]. Furthermore, even if childhood trauma does not result in childhood PTSD, it increases the risk for adult PTSD [14] and adult psychiatric illness [15].

III. IMPORTANT CLINICAL FACTORS ASSOCIATED WITH PTSD

The PTSD trauma may have interpersonal origins if the cause of the trauma is of human design. Examples of this include military combat, violent personal assault (i.e., child abuse, kidnapping, incarceration as a prisoner of war, mugging, rape, robbery, terrorist attack, or torture), and witnessing domestic or community violence. The trauma may be of noninterpersonal origin such as experiences of natural or human-caused disaster(s) (i.e., floods, earthquakes, hurricanes), diagnosis with a life-threatening illness, and/or an accident. War experiences, child abuse, and domestic and/or community violence may be the most common causes of interpersonal trauma-related PTSD. This type of PTSD is thought to cause more severe and long-lasting symptoms. The DSM-IV-TR states that the following constellation of symptoms occurs more commonly in association with an interpersonal stressor: anxiety, a loss of previously sustained beliefs, depression, dissociation, feeling permanently damaged, hostility, hopelessness, self-destructive and impulsive behaviors, somatization, shame, and personality and relational disturbances, and an increased risk for substance abuse/dependence [1]. Another way of looking at this clinical picture is PTSD with comorbidity or the concept of Disorders of Extreme Stress (DESNOS) [16].

A review of the longitudinal course of PTSD suggested that PTSD symptoms are common within the first month of a trauma. These symptoms may be a normal response to severe stress as these symptoms usually fade within 3 months [17]. However, certain risk factors increase the probability that an individual will develop PTSD after a trauma. These factors are divided into three categories: factors prior to; factors relating to; and factors following the traumatic experience(s). Factors that increase the risks of having PTSD prior to the traumatic experience include a prior history of poor social support and adverse life events, parental poverty, prior history of childhood maltreatment, poor family functioning, familial/genetic family history of psychiatric disorders, introversion or extreme behavioral inhibition, being female, and poor health and prior mental illness [18]. Of these, genetics and the trauma experience may play a critical role. In a twin study, True et al. [19] found that genetic factors accounted for 13–30% of the variance in the reexperiencing cluster, 30–34% in the avoidance cluster, and 28–32% in the arousal cluster of PTSD symptoms in Vietnam veterans with combat-related PTSD. While symptoms in the reexperiencing cluster and one symptom in the avoidance and numbing cluster were strongly associated with trauma exposure, shared environment did not contribute to the development of the disorder. Risk factors for PTSD associated with the trauma are the degree of trauma exposure and an individual's subjective sense of danger, and other related traumatic events [20]. Chronicity of psychiatric impairment from PTSD also increases with the dose of traumatic exposure [20]. Risk factors associated with PTSD after the trauma include lack of social supports, continued negative life events, and lack of posttrauma interventions [20]. Thus, effective clinical intervention posttrauma may alleviate the disability and chronicity associated with PTSD.

Consequently, PTSD may be regarded as a complex environmentally-induced psychiatric disorder on both descriptive and neurobiologic levels. We will review the neurobiology of PTSD, one of four diagnoses (acute stress disorder, reactive attachment disorder of infancy or early childhood, and adjustment disorder[s]) in the DSM-IV-TR in which an identified stressor precipitated the onset of a mental illness, and the one which has been the most extensively studied.

IV. NEUROBIOLOGY OF TRAUMA: AN OVERVIEW

The essential feature of a criterion A trauma is to cause overwhelming fear or anxiety. Cannon, in 1929, was the first to demonstrate the "fight or flight" reaction in response to life-threatening stress [21]. He showed that physical and emotional stress triggered the same response from an organism. This response involves activation of the peripheral sympathetic nervous system (SNS), a division of the autonomic nervous system. Hans Selye then studied the effects of chronic stress on the hypothalamic-pituitary-adrenal (HPA) axis and the immune system and postulated the idea of "homeostatic balance." Selye said that successful coping to traumatic stress is followed by a restoration of homeostatic balance and unsuccessful adaptation may result in significant deviations from this normative balance [22]. McEwen went further to call this latter balance "allostatis," an equilibrium that places severe strain on an organism and may be impossible to sustain indefinitely [23].

Contemporary theories of the neurobiology of stress and PTSD have been extensively reviewed [24]. PTSD symptoms are thought to be mediated by dysregulation of biological stress systems, e.g., the neural circuits and neurotransmitter and neuroendocrine stress systems, which mediate the fear or anxiety response. The main physiological mechanisms for coping with trauma are the neurotransmitter systems, the neuroendocrine systems, and the immune systems. These systems are interconnected at many levels to coordinate the individual's responses and adaptations to acute and chronic environmental stressors. In this chapter, we will focus on the neurobiology of trauma and its relationship to the neurobiology of PTSD. We will pay particular attention to the neurobiological stress systems that can help inform us about the symptom profile and the psychopharmacology of PTSD.

Trauma is perceived by afferent sensory inputs through our senses of sight, hearing, and/or touch. Traumatic reminders (i.e., the sight of a gun, a city street, or the face of a perpetrator) can lead to PTSD reexperiencing and intrusive symptoms through the learning mechanisms of classical conditioning. The initial fear response is thought to be associated to the original fear-producing stimuli or stressors (unconditioned stimuli), whereas anxiety is thought to be associated with the conditioned stimuli or traumatic reminders. These fear-associated sensory inputs are relayed through the dorsal thalamus and to primary sensory cortical brain regions (i.e., occipital [vision], temporal [auditory], postcentral gyrus [tactile]). Olfaction is relayed directly to the amygdala and entorhinal cortex. Primary sensory brain regions, in turn, project to the lateral and basolateral nuclei of the amygdala, a part of the brain's limbic or emotional system. Information from the lateral and basolateral nuclei of the amygdala project of the central nucleus of the amygdala. The central nucleus of the amygdala has direct projections to a variety of anatomical areas that are important in fear- or anxiety-related behaviors [25,26]. The most important of these neuroconnections include projections to the locus ceruleus and the preoptic area of the hypothalamus, the bed nucleus of the stria terminalis, and the paraventricular nucleus and lateral nucleus in the hypothalamus, which are involved in SNS and limbic-hypothalamic-pituitary-adrenal (LHPA) axis activation. These neuroconnections also include important projections to: the ventral tegmental area, which is responsible for increases in prefrontal cortical dopamine activity during stress; the parabrachial nucleus, which is responsible for increased respiration during an anxiety or stress reaction; the central gray, which is involved in conditioned fear, freezing, and stress-induced analgesia; the nucleus reticularis pontis caudalis, which is involved in the fear potentiation of the startle reflex; the dorsal motor nucleus of the vagus, nucleus of the solitary tract, and ventrolateral medulla, which are involved with stress-induced modulation of heart rate and blood pressure; and the trigeminal and facial nerve which are involved in the facial expressions of fear (Fig. 1).

V. AMYGDALA AND PTSD

In preclinical studies, electrical stimulation of the amygdaloid region of animals is associated with fearful behaviors, including increases in heart rate, blood pressure, freezing, activation of fear-related facial movements, and increases in plasma corticosteroid levels. Amygdala lesions reduce these fearful behaviors and emotional reactivity, and interfere with the acquisition

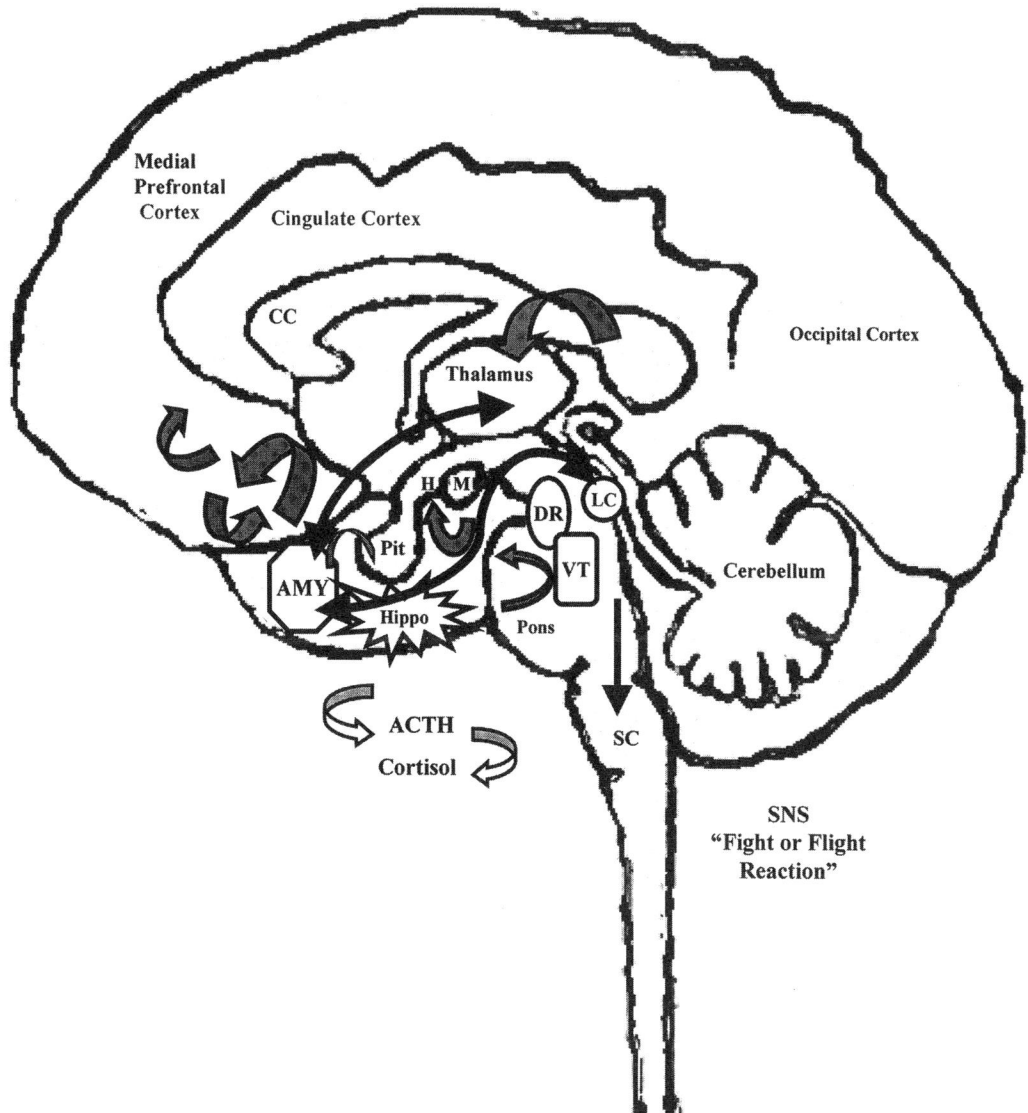

Figure 1 An overview of the neurobiology of the traumatic stress response. PTSD symptoms are thought to be mediated by dysregulation of the neural circuits and neuroendocrine stress systems which mediate fear or anxiety responses. Trauma is perceived by afferent sensory inputs through our senses of sight, hearing, and/or touch. The initial fear response is thought to be associated to the original fear producing stimuli or stressors (unconditioned stimuli), whereas PTSD symptoms are thought to be associated with the conditioned stimuli or traumatic reminders. These fear-associated sensory inputs are relayed through the dorsal thalamus and to primary sensory cortical brain regions. Primary sensory brain regions, in turn, project back to the thalamus and to the lateral and basolateral nuclei of the amygdala, a part of the brain's limbic or emotional system. Information from the lateral and basolateral nuclei of the amygdala project to the central nucleus of the amygdala (AMY) which is responsible for activating the fear response and involved in emotional memory. The central nucleus of the amygdala has direct projections to the locus ceruleus (LC) and the hypothalamus (H), which are involved in SNS ("fight or flight") activation and limbic-hypothalamic-pituitary (Pit)-adrenal (LHPA) axis (increased ACTH and cortisol) activation. The central nucleus of the amygdala also has important projections to the ventral tegmental (VT) area, which is responsible for increases in prefrontal cortical dopamine activity during stress. During stress, the prefrontal cortex and the central and basolateral nuclei of the amygdala receive serotonergic inputs from the dorsal and median raphe nuclei in the brainstem. The hippocampus has important connections with the prefrontal cortex and amygdala, and also plays an important role in short-term memory and in assigning significance to events within space and time. CC, corpus callosum; DR, dorsal raphe nucleus; Hippo, hippocampus; M, mammillary bodies; SC, spinal cord.

of conditioned fear and the rise in plasma corticosteroid levels [for review see 25].

In human studies, electrical stimulation of the amygdaloid region of patients undergoing surgery for temporal lobe epilepsy is associated with complex fear states involving palpitation, mydriasis, pallor, and fear-related thoughts [for review see 27]. Children and adults who have a history of temporal lobe epilepsy or status epilepticus, with amygdala involvement, have ictal fear [28]. Results from a recent positron emission tomography (PET) study showed that during a modified Stroop task, bilateral amygdala activation was significantly greater during color naming of threat words than during color naming of neutral words in healthy subjects [29]. Moreover, results from recent functional magnetic resonance imaging (MRI) investigations showed activation in the amygdala during viewing of masked fearful faces [30] and in the amygdala/periamygaloid cortex during both conditioned fear acquisition and extinction in healthy subjects [31].

PTSD may be the result of hyperresponsivity of the central amygdala, which may mediate stimulus-bound fears or traumatic reminders and cluster B reexperiencing and intrusive symptoms. PTSD may also be the result of hyperresponsivity of amygdala projections, which may mediate trauma-related autonomic SNS hyperactivity and cluster D hyperarousal symptoms. For example, another PET study has implicated activation of the right amygdala in traumatic autobiographical memories [32]. Bilateral amygdaloid complex damage in humans is associated with loss of enhanced recall of emotionally aversive memories [33]. Furthermore, results from a recent functional MRI investigation showed that PTSD patients demonstrated exaggerated amygdala responses during viewing of general nontraumatic negative stimuli (i.e., masked fearful faces) [34]. The amygdala serves to enhance declarative memory for emotionally arousing and fearful events [for review see 35] and for the identification and recognition of emotion in human faces [36]. This process may be exaggerated in PTSD. Failures of the inhibitory influences of the medial prefrontal cortex may also contribute to amygdala hyperreactivity.

VI. MEDIAL PREFRONTAL CORTEX AND PTSD

Stress activates noradrenergic, serotonergic, and dopaminergic neurons in the prefrontal cortex. The anterior cingulate cortex, a region of the medial prefrontal cortex, is involved in the extinction of conditioned fear responses and is implicated in the pathophysiology of PTSD [for review see 37]. The anterior cingulate region is part of an executive attention system, as it is activated during decision making and novel or dangerous situations [38]. Since intrusive thoughts of trauma (danger) and poor concentration are core symptoms of PTSD, anterior cingulate integrity may be affected in PTSD. LeDoux has shown that medial prefrontal cortex may inhibit activation of the amygdala and its related nuclei and circuitry [for review see 26].

Recent neuroimaging studies provide evidence for medial prefrontal and anterior cingulate dysfunction in adult PTSD. PET investigations comparing women who had been sexually abused as children and who had PTSD with women with similar history who did not have PTSD found a lower level of anterior cingulate blood flow during traumatic script-driven imagery [39] and during memories of sexual abuse [40]. A lower level of anterior cingulate blood flow has also been seen in Vietnam combat veterans with PTSD compared to those without PTSD during exposure to combat-related traumatic stimuli [41]. In these studies, subjects with PTSD activated the amygdala, while subjects without PTSD did not show the same degree of limbic activation.

PET investigations are not feasible in developing children. However, magnetic resonance spectroscopy can be used to further study the in vivo neurochemistry of trauma associated neurobiological alterations in the brains of living children. The N-acetyl signal in the proton (^{1}H) spectrum mainly comprises of N-acetylaspartate (NAA) and is considered to be a marker of neural integrity. Decreased NAA concentrations are associated with increased metabolism and loss of neurons [for review see 42]. A preliminary investigation suggested that maltreated children and adolescents with PTSD have lower NAA/creatine ratios than sociodemographically matched controls [43]. These findings were suggestive of neuronal loss in the anterior cingulate region of the medial prefrontal cortex and were not specific to gender. Neuronal loss in the anterior cingulate of pediatric PTSD patients agrees with the recent adult neuroimaging studies, which provide evidence for medial prefrontal and anterior cingulate dysfunction in adult PTSD.

Exposure to mild to moderate uncontrollable stress impairs prefrontal cortical function in studies of humans and animals [for review see 44]. This impairment may be norepinephrine and dopamine mediated [for review see 45]. Thus, PTSD symptoms may represent dysfunction in the inhibitory influences of the medial prefrontal cortex on amygdala hyperreactivity. Thus, dysfunction of the anterior cingulate cortex, which is involved in the extinction of conditioned fear responses, may be implicated in the pathophysiology of both adult and pediatric PTSD.

VII. DOPAMINE SYSTEM AND PTSD

Dopaminergic innervations of the prefrontal cortex originate from neurons of the substantia nigra and the retrorubral field in the ventral midbrain [for review see 46]. These mesencephalon brain regions receive inputs from the prefrontal cortex, ventral pallidum, lateral hypothalamus, and dorsal raphe nucleus. The dopaminergic inputs to the medial prefrontal cortex appear to be particularly sensitive to stress. An increase in the firing rate of mesoprefrontal cortical dopamine neurons inhibit the activity of prefrontal pyramidal cells by exerting a modulatory role over excitatory afferents to the prefrontal cortex. Dopamine neurons also inhibit prefrontal pyramidal cell activity indirectly by enhancing the release of the inhibitory neurotransmitter gamma-aminobutyric acid (GABA) from interneurons. Mild stressors (i.e., novel environment) which do not activate the locus ceruleus, SNS or the LHPA axis (see below) appear to selectively activate the dopaminergic innervations of the mesencephalon, the amygdala, and the prefrontal cortex. Enhanced dopamine prefrontal cortical function in response to stress may reflect the heightened attention or cognitive processes needed to cope with the stressor [47].

However, dopaminergic innervations of the prefrontal cortex block the stress-induced excitatory glutamatergic inputs onto prefrontal pyramidal cells [46]. These excitatory glutamatergic inputs from the prefrontal cortex originate in the basolateral amygdala. Gutamatergic inputs feedback to and activate the mesoprefrontal cortical dopamine neurons located in the ventral tegmental areas. Thus, excitatory glutamatergic efferents from the prefrontal cortex to mesoprefrontal cortical dopamine neurons further inhibit prefrontal activity by stimulating dopaminergic innervations of the prefrontal cortex. This process may result in more prefrontal cortical dopamine than is functionally necessary and thus may impair prefrontal cortical function. Thus, it has been suggested that some functional defect in cortical dopamine systems occur in PTSD (i.e., less dopamine-induced inhibition of orbital and medial prefrontal excitatory glutamatergic inputs). This deficit may lead a traumatized person with an inability to cope with the trauma [46].

Higher concentrations of urinary dopamine and its metabolite homovanillic acid were found in patients with combat-related PTSD [48], in sexually abused girls [49], and in abused male and female prepubertal children with PTSD [50]. Urinary dopamine was positively associated with overall severity of PTSD symptoms, particularly symptoms of intrusive flashbacks, avoidance, and hyperarousal in adult PTSD [48] and avoidant and dissociative symptoms in abused children with PTSD [50]. Findings of higher urinary dopamine concentrations may reflect higher central dopamine activity resulting in hypervigilance and paranoia in PTSD patients. Although a functional defect in cortical dopamine regulation may occur in PTSD, to date, dopamine function has not been extensively studied in PTSD.

VIII. LOCUS CERULEUS AND PTSD

Stress, particularly unpredictable and uncontrollable stress, is known to increase responsiveness of the central amygdala and the locus ceruleus to excitatory stimulation [51]. The locus ceruleus is the major norepinephrine-containing nucleus in the brain. Increased responsiveness of these locus ceruleus neurons, in turn, increases norepinephrine turnover in specific brain regions (locus ceruleus, hypothalamus, hippocampus, amygdala, and prefrontal cortex). These brain regions are associated with regulation of stress reactions, memory, and emotion in experimental animals [52]. Traumatic stress also results in simultaneous activation of another very basic and ancient cell body, the paragigantocellularis. It and the nucleus tractus solitarius in the brainstem receive inputs from visceral organs. The paragigantocellularis is reciprocally connected to the locus ceruleus, but also controls and activates the SNS causing the biologic changes of the fight-or-flight reaction, or of life-saving responses to acute threats [53]. Direct and indirect effects of the flight-or-flight reaction include: increased heart rate; increased blood pressure; dilated pupils; sweating; inhibition of renal sodium excretion; redistribution of the blood to the heart, brain, and skeletal muscle and away from skin, gut, and kidneys; enhanced blood coagulation by increasing platelet aggregability; increased glycogenolysis; and increased metabolic rate and alertness. Activation of the locus ceruleus results in activation of the LHPA axis via indirect connections through the amygdala.

In adult PTSD, it is hypothesized that the locus ceruleus/SNS/catecholamine system and LHPA axis responses to stress become maladaptive, causing long-term negative consequences [for review see 54]. Results from adult combat-related PTSD studies suggest that there is increased sensitivity of the locus ceruleus/SNS/catecholamine system that is most clearly evident under experimental conditions of stress or challenge. These findings include increased heart rate, systolic blood pressure, skin conductance, and other SNS responses to adrenergic or traumatic reminder challenge compared to healthy combat or noncombat controls. Although most baseline studies of single or multiple time point plasma catecholamines found no significant differences between adult PTSD and controls, elevated levels of catecholamines (i.e., norepinephrine, epinephrine, and dopamine) were found in 24-hr urinary excretions in three of five studies. Single time point measures of catecholamines and cortisol may not provide an accurate measure of baseline functioning because these neurotransmitters have circadian influences (i.e., a 24-hr diurnal rhythm), and the stress of a single-stick venipuncture may result in elevations of cortisol and catecholamine concentration alone, obscuring any baseline differences. Cortisol, which reflects LHPA axis activity, and essentially all catecholamines and their metabolites, which reflect SNS activity, are excreted into urine [55,56]. Rather than randomly timed urine measures, timed 24-hr measures of urinary free cortisol (UFC) and catecholamine concentrations are a better way to noninvasively evaluate for alterations in baseline activity of the LHPA axis and the locus ceruleus/SNS/catecholamine system. Thus, in adult PTSD, elevated 24-hr urinary excretion of catecholamines provides evidence of an increase in baseline functioning of the catecholamine system. Combat-related PTSD is consistently associated with hyperactivity of the locus ceruleus/SNS, and increases in circulating catecholamines. Combat-related PTSD is associated with increased heart rate, systolic blood pressure, skin conductance, and other sympathetic nervous system responses to adrenergic or traumatic reminder challenge [reviewed by 54,57,58], decreased sleep latency and efficiency [59], and elevated 24-hr urinary excretion of catecholamines [48,60].

However, the limited data published to date in traumatized children suggest that the locus ceruleus/SNS/catecholamine system is dysregulated in traumatized children who may suffer from depressive and PTSD symptoms but who may or may not have a diagnosis of PTSD. Findings of elevated baseline 24-hr urinary catecholamine concentrations were seen: (1) in male children who suffer from severe clinical depression and had a history of parental neglect [61]; (2) in a pilot study of sexually abused girls, 58% of whom had histories of severely depressed mood with suicidal behavior (but only one of whom had PTSD) [49]; and (3) in male and female children with abuse-related PTSD [50]. Furthermore, decreased platelet alpha$_2$-adrenergic receptors and increased heart rate following orthostatic challenge were found in physically and sexually abused children with PTSD, suggesting an enhancement of SNS tone in childhood PTSD [62]. An increase in baseline functioning of the locus ceruleus/SNS/catecholamine system in childhood PTSD is also provided by two separate, open-label treatment trials of the medications clonidine (a central alpha$_2$-adrenergic partial agonist) and propranolol (a beta-adrenergic antagonist), both of which dampen catecholamine transmission. Clonidine treatment was associated with general clinical improvement and decreases in the arousal cluster of PTSD symptoms and basal heart rate [62]. Propranolol treatment was associated with decreases in aggressive behaviors and insomnia [63].

IX. LHPA AXIS AND PTSD

Direct projections of the central nucleus of the amygdala to the paraventricular nucleus of the hypothalamus cause increases in secretion of corticotropin-releasing hormone (CRH) and activation of the LHPA axis [64]. CRH has important neurotransmitter and neuroendocrine effects. When given centrally to experimental animals, CRH promotes hypercortisolism, stimulates the SNS, and causes behavioral activation and intense arousal which are independent of its neuroendocrine effects of adrenocorticotropin (ACTH) and glucocorticoid secretion [65,66]. Consequently, CRH cell bodies and receptors are located in the amygdala as well as throughout the brain. Activation of these receptors is responsible for this behavioral activation. Activation of the locus ceruleus/SNS/catecholamine system and CRH results in animal behaviors consistent with anxiety, hyperarousal, and hypervigilance, which are the core symptoms of PTSD.

The important neuroendocrine functions of CRH include activation of the LHPA axis by stimulating the pituitary to secrete ACTH. Plasma ACTH in turn stimulates adrenal secretion of glucocorticoids or cortisol, which causes increases in gluconeogenesis, inhibition of growth and reproductive systems, and containment of the inflammatory response [for review see 55]. These functions enhance survival during a life threat. Functionally, CRH and the locus ceruleus/SNS/catecholamine system seem to participate in a positive, reverberatory feedback loop. Amygdala lesions will disrupt some of these stress effects.

Unlike the increased sensitivity to stress of the locus ceruleus/SNS/catecholamine system seen in adult PTSD, results from baseline and challenge studies of the LHPA axis appear to show that this system functions in a more complicated manner. In adult combat-related PTSD, elevated levels of central CRH were found [67,68]. Infusion studies of metyrapone, which blocks the conversion of 11-deoxycortisol to cortisol and allows for the direct measure of pituitary release of ACTH, suggest that there is downregulation of anterior pituitary CRH receptors presumably secondary to elevated central CRH and enhanced negative feedback inhibition of the pituitary for cortisol [69]. Further evidence for enhanced negative feedback inhibition includes findings of increased number of glucocorticoid receptors on lymphocytes presumably secondary to decreased circulating cortisol [70], suppression of cortisol with low-dose dexamethasone [71], and lower 24-hr UFC concentrations in three of four studies of adult combat-related PTSD compared with controls [48,72,73]. Low 24-hr UFC levels were also found in one study of male and female adults with PTSD who survived the Holocaust during childhood compared to survivors without PTSD [74]. In two other studies, 24-hour UFC concentrations were higher in male combat veterans with PTSD than in combat veterans without PTSD [75] and in women with PTSD secondary to childhood sexual abuse compared to women abused as children without PTSD and healthy nonabused controls [76].

Results from investigations of the LHPA axis and childhood trauma are similar to those of adult studies in that the data also suggest that the LHPA axis functions in a complex manner. These discrepant findings may be related to a mechanism called "priming" or sensitization in which responses to repeated stress increase in magnitude. A possible long-term consequence of the trauma experience may be to prime the LHPA axis so that ACTH and cortisol secretion are set at lower 24-hr levels [50]. Priming may occur as a reflection of chronic compensatory adaptation of the LHPA axis long after trauma exposure. LHPA axis regulation is affected by other hormones that are stress mediated such as arginine vasopressin and the catecholamines, both of which act synergistically with CRH [55]. A "primed system" will "hyper"-respond during an acute stress. Thus when a new emotional stressor is experienced, LHPA axis functioning will be enhanced (i.e., higher ACTH and higher 24-hr UFC concentrations in response to stress). Since the adult PTSD studies focus on past trauma, the latter hypothesis may best explain the data in childhood PTSD studies. For example, results fall into a predictable pattern when addressed as a reflection of a chronic compensatory adaptation of the LHPA axis long after trauma exposure. This compensatory adaptation may involve the "priming" mechanism.

In studies of children undergoing current adversity, evidence of elevations of cortisol or ACTH and priming are seen. For example, augmented mean morning serial plasma cortisol levels were found in sexually abused girls recruited within 6 months of disclosure compared with nonabused, sociodemographically matched controls. This suggests morning hypersecretion of cortisol in sexually abused girls [77]. Medically healthy, clinically referred prepubertal medication-naive abused children with chronic PTSD studied within a year of disclosure PTSD excreted significantly greater concentrations of 24-hr UFC than nontraumatized healthy controls [50]. Maltreated young children with major depression failed to show the expected diurnal decrease in cortisol secretion from morning to afternoon, suggesting higher baseline cortisol activity in these young children [78,79]. Increased ACTH response to human CRH, but normal cortisol secretion in maltreated prepubertal depressed children undergoing current psychosocial adversity compared to depressed children with prior histories of maltreatment, depressed nonabused children, and healthy children, were reported [80]. This last finding may be related to priming.

In studies of children with past trauma, chronic compensatory adaptation of the LHPA axis is seen. Attenuated plasma ACTH responses to ovine CRH in sexually abused girls studied several years after abuse disclosure were reported [81]. The abused subjects had histories of severely depressed mood with suicidal behavior, but only one had a diagnosis of PTSD. The abused girls exhibited reduced evening basal, ovine CRH-stimulated, and time-integrated total plasma ACTH concentrations compared with controls. Plasma total and free cortisol responses to ovine CRH stimulation did not differ between the two groups. Thus, sexually abused girls manifest a dysregulatory disorder of the LHPA axis, associated with hyporesponsiveness of the pituitary to exogenous CRH and normal overall cortisol secretion to CRH challenge. CRH hypersecretion may have led to an adaptive downregulation of CRH receptors in the anterior pituitary, which is similar to the mechanism suggested in adult PTSD [67,68]. Furthermore, adults with combat-related PTSD also showed a blunted plasma ACTH responses to ovine CRH [82]. Armenian adolescents who lived close to the epicenter of the 1988 earthquake and experienced a significant direct threat to life had greater PTSD and comorbid depressive symptoms, lower baseline mean salivary cortisol levels, and greater afternoon suppression of cortisol by dexamethasone 5 years after exposure, when compared to Armenian adolescents who lived 20 miles from the epicenter [83]. These results are similar to the LHPA axis findings in adult PTSD. These studies show that traumatic experiences throughout the life cycle are associated with profound changes in the dynamics of the LHPA axis. These changes may contribute to PTSD symptoms.

X. HIPPOCAMPUS AND PTSD

Elevated levels of glucocorticoids during traumatic stress may have neurotoxic effects and lead to learning and concentration impairments secondary to damage to the brain's hippocampi [84], a principal neural target tissue of glucocorticoids [85]. The hippocampus has important connections with the prefrontal cortex and also plays an important role in short-term memory and in assigning significance to events within space and time. The hippocampus also has important connections to the amygdala, which, as discussed above, is involved in emotional memory. Elevated levels of cortisol may have neurotoxic effects on the hippocampus through the N-methyl-D-aspartate (NMDA) excitotoxicity [86]. Hippocampal degeneration was noted in monkeys after sustained social stress [87]. Smaller hippocampal volumes were reported in adults with Cushing's syndrome [88], combat veterans with PTSD [89,90], adult PTSD secondary to child abuse [91], and female adult survivors of childhood sexual abuse [92]. However, pediatric PTSD was not associated with the predicted decrease in hippocampal volume [93]. Subcortical gray matter structures which include the limbic system (septal area, hippocampus, amygdala) actually show an increase in volume during adolescence [94]. This increase may "mask" any effects of traumatic stress in maltreated children with PTSD.

However, the results of a pilot longitudinal study of hippocampal volumes in pediatric maltreatment-related PTSD do not support a role for neurodevelopmental stunting by cortisol as a possible explanation for the differences in hippocampal findings between children and adults with PTSD [95]. High rates of comorbid lifetime alcohol dependence were seen in the adult PTSD MRI studies. Although these investigators attempted to control for lifetime alcohol consumption, these studies may not have controlled for adolescent-onset alcohol abuse. Results from animal studies show that the hippocampus is susceptible to the effects of chronic alcohol administration [96]. The additional negative impact of excessive alcohol consumption on the regulation of NMDA receptors [97] in persons with trauma history may lead to more profound excitotoxic neuronal damage in alcoholic adults comorbid for PTSD. Psychiatric comorbidity for alcohol and substance abuse/dependence in adult PTSD subjects, especially during adolescence [98], may have contributed to smaller hippocampal findings in adult PTSD.

XI. SEROTONIN SYSTEM AND PTSD

The serotonin system is a stress response system that may activate both anxiogenic and anxiolytic pathways. Serotonin is regarded as a master control neurotransmitter of complex neuronal communication [99]. The prefrontal cortex and the central and basolateral nuclei of the amygdala receive serotonergic inputs from the dorsal and median raphe nuclei in the brainstem. In primate studies of chronic stress, serotonin levels decrease in the prefrontal cortex [100]. In animal studies of unpredictable and uncontrollable stress (e.g., inescapable shock, restraint stress), serotonin turnover increases and serotonin levels decrease in the amygdala, medial prefrontal cortex, nucleus accumbens, and lateral hypothalamus. This process depletes serotonin and results in "learned helplessness" [101]. Drugs that increase brain serotonin (serotonin agonists) prevent some of these behavioral changes. Compared with controls, paroxetine binding (a measure of serotonin uptake) was significantly decreased in the platelets [102] and in platelet-poor plasma [103] of male combat veterans with PTSD.

Serotonin plays important roles in compulsive behaviors and the regulation of emotions (mood) and behavior (aggression, impulsivity). Serotonin is also implicated in major depression, impulsivity, and suicidal behaviors. Low serotonin function is associated with suicidal and aggressive behaviors in adults, children, and adolescents [for review see 104,105]. PTSD cluster B reexperiencing and intrusive symptoms most closely resemble another psychiatric disorder, obsessive-compulsive disorder, which is characterized by intrusive and recurrent and persistent thoughts, impulses or images and is a disorder of serotonin regulation [for review see 106]. Because of serotonin's interdependence with the noradrenergic system [107], another stress response system that is involved in the psychobiology of adult and child mood disorders, dysregulation of serotonin may not only play a major role in cluster B symptoms but also may also increase the risk for comorbid major depression in PTSD. Consequently, it was shown that the onset of major depression is markedly increased for trauma-exposed persons who suffer from PTSD, but not in trauma-exposed persons who did not suffer from PTSD [108]. Thus, PTSD may lead to major depression and be influenced by common genetic vulnerabilities to serotonin dysregulation and trauma related factors as discussed above.

Recently, clinical studies have demonstrated strong support for the efficacy of the serotonin reuptake inhibitor antidepressant and anti-obsessive-compulsive disorder medications sertraline [109] and fluoxetine [110] in adult PTSD. Practice parameters for the treatment of pediatric PTSD, published by the American Academy of Child and Adolescent Psychiatry, state that selective serotonin reuptake inhibitors are the first-line medication treatment for child and adolescent PTSD, particularly PTSD comorbid with major depression [111].

XII. BENZODIAZEPINE RECEPTOR SYSTEM AND PTSD

Benzodiazepine receptors are functionally linked to inhibitory neurotransmitter GABA and are found in cortical gray matter. These binding sites are part of the same macromolecular complex and regulate GABA type A receptors to prolong and potentiate synaptic actions of the GABA inhibitory neurotransmitter systems. This system downregulates the locus ceruleus and cortical dopamine activity [112]. Animals exposed to experimental stress develop decreases in benzodiazepine receptor binding in the frontal cortex [113]. Decreases in benzodiazepine receptor binding have been demonstrated in the genetically fearful strain of Maudsley rats [114]. One can speculate that decreases in benzodiazepine receptor binding may initially be adaptive in an acutely stressful situation. However, a chronic decrease in benzodiazepine receptor activity could contribute to the cluster D hyperarousal symptoms seen in PTSD patients.

XIII. ENDOGENOUS OPIATE SYSTEM AND PTSD

Exposure to stress causes an increase in endogenous opiates and contributes to the development of stress-induced analgesia to pain [115]. Opiates also decrease the firing rate of locus ceruleus neurons and dampen down the stress response. Vietnam veterans with PTSD have reduced pain sensitivity during exposure to traumatic reminders of war [115]. This analgesia is reversible with the opiate antagonist naloxone [116]. Beta endorphin levels have been found to be higher in CSF [117] and lower in the plasma [118] of PTSD patients. Thus lower levels of endogenous opiates may contribute to PTSD cluster C avoidance and numbing symptoms or lower levels may contribute to PTSD cluster D hyperarousal symptoms. Endogenous opiate systems have not been studied in traumatized children and but may be contributory to the constricted affect and high incidence of self injury reported in maltreated children and in adults who have experienced maltreatment as children [119].

XIV. TRAUMA, PTSD, AND PHYSICAL HEALTH

An extensive review of the literature [120] indicates that PTSD promotes poor health (i.e., hypertension, atherosclerotic heart disease, gastrointestinal disorders, increased susceptibility to infections) through a complex interaction among excessive SNS activity, LHPA axis dysregulation, and negative life style choices. For example, increased rates of cardiovascular and gastrointestinal disorders were observed in World War II prisoners of war [121]. Chronic activation of the locus ceruleus/SNS/catecholamine system can lead to increased vulnerability to hypertension, atherosclerotic heart disease, peptic ulcer disorders, and immune dysfunction. Self-medication of PTSD symptoms can lead to alcohol and other substance abuse/dependence, which have independent adverse effects on physical health. A variety of stressors, including psychological stress, have been shown to modify measures of the immune system in experimental animals and humans. As discussed below, chronic stress has been shown to impair immune function and may also impair hypothalamic-pituitary-thyroid (HPT) axis regulation.

XV. IMMUNE SYSTEM AND PTSD

The central nervous system signals to the immune system are mediated by the LHPA axis and the sympathetic division of the autonomic nervous system. As early as 1936, Selye showed that restraining rats produced involution of the thymus and stress-induced lymphopenia [122]. An extensive review of the literature on the effects of stress on cellular immune response in animals concluded that a variety of acute and chronic stressors, such as inescapable noise, social isolation, and uncontrollable shock, are associated with suppression of immune responses [123]. Stressed animals are at significantly greater risk for development of infections, tumors, and death after experimentally induced immune (antigenic) challenge. Emotional or physical stress causes elevation of plasma cortisol which generally exerts immunosuppressive and antiinflammatory effects on circulating blood lymphocytes [124]. Activation of the SNS and peripheral catecholamines mediates suppression of the cellular immune response of cells located in physiological compartments such as suppression of splenic natural killer (NK) cell activity. Norepinephrine, the major neurotransmitter of the sympathetic nervous system, has a complex role in the modulation of the immune response, facilitating certain immunologic responses while inhibiting others. Stressful life events have been shown to suppress immune responses in humans [123]. Bereavement, sleep deprivation, job loss, and medical school final examinations have been associated with decreased lymphocyte proliferation to mitogenic stimulation, decreased NK cell activity, decreased phagocytosis, decreased interferon production, decreased salivary IgA, increased antibody titers to herpes virus, and decreased helper and suppressor T-cell percentages and helper-to-suppressor ratios.

In the last decade, scientific interest in trauma, PTSD, and immune function has increased and with somewhat contradictory results. Vietnam veterans with PTSD showed decreased NK cell activity in response to in vitro methionine-enkephalin challenge compared with healthy volunteers [125]. Victims of Hurricane Andrew with PTSD showed lower NK cell cytotoxicity than did community volunteers without PTSD [126]. However, studies have also found elevated rates of NK activity in PTSD patients [127] and in women displaced by war [128]. Other studies have shown that PTSD patients with a history of childhood sexual abuse exhibit chronic immune activation [129]. Vietnam veterans with PTSD showed clinically elevated leukocyte, total T-cell counts, and highly sensitized T-cell lymphocytes [130]. These findings may lead to and have been associated with autoimmune diseases. In children, a significantly higher incidence of plasma antinuclear antibody titers was seen in sexually abused girls when compared with the frequency of positive antinuclear antibody titers in a sample of adult healthy women [131]. One may speculate that the severe stress of sexual abuse may lead to suppression of the mechanisms (T-suppressor cells) that actively suppress the autoantibody-producing lymphocytes (B-lymphocytes) and may thus increase the incidence of positive antinuclear antibody titers in these sexually abused girls. Decreased NK cell activity can lead to increased rates of infection and initiation and progression of cancers. Enhanced NK activity may be associated with the high rates of substance abuse in PTSD patients, and is related to enhanced immune surveillance. Highly sensitized T-cell lymphocytes and suppression of T-suppressor cells may lead to an increased incidence of autoimmune diseases in traumatized persons. Thus, these studies show that traumatic experiences throughout the life cycle are associated with profound changes in the immune system. Immune dysregulation may lead to the increase in reported rates of poor health in victims of PTSD.

XVI. TRAUMA, THE HPT AXIS, AND PTSD

Preclinical investigations have shown that acute stress leads to activation of the locus ceruleus noradrenergic neurons and results in direct stimulation of hypothalamic thyrotropin-releasing hormone (TRH)-secreting neurons [132]. TRH stimulates secretion of thyroid-stimulating hormone (TSH), which in turn stimulates the thyroid gland to secrete thyroid hormone. Additionally, during acute stress, direct stimulation by norepinephrine through postganglionic sympathetic innervation of the thyroid gland and by plasma epinephrine also stimulates release and increased synthesis of thyroid hormone through cyclic adenosine monophosphate (cAMP) production [133]. Thyroid hormone is responsible for the regulation of metabolism. During an episode of acute stress, the increased metabolic rate provides "emergency" energy. Thyroid hormones are also necessary for the normal growth and differentiation of brain neurons and glial cells throughout fetal, child, and adolescent development [134]. Thyroid hormone inhibits TSH release. Chronic TRH secretion secondary to prolonged stress may not cause sustained TSH secretion because of downregulation of pituitary TRH receptors. Thus, chronic stress is associated with decreased production of TSH and inhibition of the conversion of thyroxine to the more biologically active tri-iodothyronine in peripheral tissues. This mechanism would serve to conserve energy during chronic stress, and is seen in chronic medical illnesses.

There are few human studies of the association of stress and/or adult PTSD and the HTP axis. Elevated levels of total and free triiodothyronine (T_3)- and thyroxine (T_4)-binding globulin were demonstrated in male combat veterans with combat-related PTSD [135]. These findings were not those classic hyperthyroidism or liver disease, but correlated with overall PTSD symptoms, especially those of hyperarousal. There were no significant differences between the TSH responses of adults male combat veterans with PTSD and controls to TRH stimulation in another study [136]. However, this study was confounded by the fact that 6 of the 11 subjects were taking psychotropic medications, and there was a wide variation of individual responses [136]. In a pilot study of traumatized children, thyroid function tests did not differ between sexually abused and control girls [131]. However, chronic stress such as childhood maltreatment may lead to physiologically normal central suppression of the HPT axis. Because lower TSH can result in a reduced set point for metabolic rate, we speculate that lower TSH may contribute to the higher rates of obesity reported in women with a history of sexual abuse [137]. We also speculate that suppression of the HPT axis secondary to chronic stresses of childhood maltreatment may lead to profound changes in brain development and possibly decreased intelligence.

XVII. SUMMARY

In this chapter, evidence supporting that chronic hyperresponsivity of the amygdala, prefrontal cortical dysfunction, chronic activation of the locus ceruleus/SNS/catecholamine system, and dysregulation of the LHPA axis associated with trauma may be responsible for PTSD symptoms. The functional interconnections of these neurobiological stress systems may also influence other neurotransmitter and neuroendocrine systems. These changes may be adaptive [for review see 55]. However, in PTSD, the responses of these neurobiological stress systems become maladaptive. These maladaptive changes may also cause adverse cardiac changes and suppression of immune function in adults. In the adult brain, alterations of locus ceruleus/SNS/catecholamine system and the LHPA may result in sensitization of mature structures. However, in the developing brain, elevated levels of catecholamines and cortisol may lead to adverse brain development through the mechanisms of accelerated loss (or metabolism) of neurons, delays in myelination, abnormalities in developmentally appropriate pruning, and/or by inhibiting neurogenesis [for review see 138]. Evidence of adverse brain development (i.e., smaller cerebral volumes and corpus callosum areas) were seen in maltreated children and adolescents with abused-related PTSD [93]. It is highly probable that many of the acute and chronic symptoms associated with traumatic child maltreatment arise in conjunction with disturbances and dysregulation of these systems. Consequently, evidence of chronic activation of these neurobiological stress systems is seen in victims of PTSD throughout the life cycle. As was reviewed throughout this chapter, preliminary research and clinical data show that dysregulated neurobiological stress systems can be treated with antianxiety and antidepressant medications and psychosocial interventions.

ACKNOWLEDGMENTS

This work was supported by NIMH grant 5 K08 MHO1324-02 (Principal Investigator: Michael D. De Bellis, M.D.) and by 1995 and 1998 NARSAD Young Investigator Awards (Principal Investigator: Michael D. De Bellis, M.D.).

REFERENCES

1. American Psychiatric Association. Diagnostic and Statistical Manual of Mental Disorders: Fourth Edition Text Revision. Washington: American Psychiatric Press, 2000, pp 424-432.
2. Kessler RC. Posttraumatic stress disorder: the burden to the individual and to society. J Clin Psychiatry 2000; 61(suppl 5):4–12.
3. Pynoos RS, Eth S, eds. Witnessing Acts of Personal Violence. Washington: American Psychiatric Press, 1985.
4. De Bellis MD. Posttraumatic stress disorder and acute stress disorder. In: Handbook of Prevention and Treatment with Children and Adolescents, eds Ammerman RT, Hersen M. New York: John Wiley & Sons, 1997, pp 455–494.
5. Scheeringa MS, Zeanah CH, Drell MJ, Larrieu JA. Two approaches to the diagnosis of posttraumatic stress disorder in infancy and early childhood. J Am Acad Child Adolesc Psychiatry 1995; 34:191–200.
6. Fletcher KE. Childhood posttraumatic stress disorder. In Child Psychopathology, eds Mash EJ, Barkley RA. New York: Guilford Publications, 1996, pp 242–276.
7. Kessler RC, Sonnega A, Bromet E, Hughes M, Nelson CB. Posttraumatic stress disorder in the national comorbidity survey. Arch Gen Psychiatry 1995; 52:1048–1060.

8. Amaya-Jackson L, March JS. Posttraumatic stress disorder. In: Anxiety Disorders in Children and Adolescents, ed March JS. New York: Guilford Press, 1995, pp 276–300.
9. Giaconia RM, Reinherz HZ, Silverman AB, Pakiz B, Frost AK, Cohen E. Trauma and posttraumatic stress disorder in a community population of older adolescents. J Am Acad Child Adolesc Psychiatry 1995; 34:1369–1380.
10. March JS, Amaya-Jackson L, Terry R, Costanzo P. Posttraumatic symptomatology in children and adolescents after an industrial fire. J Am Acad Child Adolesc Psychiatry 1997; 36(8):1080–1088.
11. Pynoos RS, Steinberg AM, Wraith R. A developmental model of childhood traumatic stress. In: Developmental Psychopathology, eds Cicchetti D, Cohen DJ. New York, John Wiley & Sons, 1995, pp 72–95.
12. Clark DB, Lesnick L, Hegedus A. Trauma and other stressors in adolescent alcohol dependence and abuse. J Am Acad Child Adolesc Psychiatry 1997; 36:1744–1751.
13. Deykin EY, Buka SL. Prevalence and risk factors for posttraumatic stress disorder among chemically dependent adolescents. Am J Psychiatry 1997; 154:752–757.
14. Widom CS. Posttraumatic stress disorder in abused and neglected children grown up. Am J Psychiatry 1999; 156:1223–1229.
15. Davidson S, Smith R. Traumatic experiences in psychiatric outpatients. J Trauma Stress 1990; 3:459–475.
16. Herman JL. Sequelae of prolonged and repeated trauma: evidence for a complex posttraumatic syndrome (DESNOS). In: Posttraumatic Stress Disorder: DSM-IV and Beyond, eds Davidson JRT, Foa EB. Washington: Am Psychiatric Press, 1993, pp 213–228.
17. Blank AS. The longitudinal course of posttraumatic stress disorder. In: Posttraumatic Stress Disorder: DSM-IV and Beyond, eds JRT Davidson, EB Foa. Washington: Am Psychiatric Press, 1993, pp 3–22.
18. Davidson JRT, Fairbank JA. The epidemiology of posttraumatic stress disorder. In: Posttraumatic Stress Disorder: DSM-IV and Beyond, eds Davidson JRT, Foa EB. Washington: American Psychiatric Press, 1993, pp 147–169.
19. True WR, Rice J, Eisen SA, Heath AC, Goldberg J, Lyons MJ, Nowak J. A twin study of genetic and environmental contributions to liability for posttraumatic stress symptoms. Arch Gen Psychiatry 1993; 50:257–264.
20. Pynoos RS, Nader K. Mental health disturbances in children exposed to disaster: Prevention intervention strategies. In: Preventing Mental Health Disturbances in Childhood, eds Goldston S, Yager J, Heinicke C, Pynoos RS. Washington; American Psychiatric Press, 1990, pp 211–233.
21. Cannon WB. The wisdom of the body. Physiol Rev 1929; 9:399–431.
22. Selye H. Homeostasis and heterostasis. Perspec Biol Med 1973; 16:441–445.
23. McEwen BS. Adrenal steroid action on brain: dissecting the fine line between protection and damage. In: Neurobiological and Clinical Consequences of Stress, eds Friedman MJ, Charney DS, Deutch AY. Philadelphia: Lippincott-Raven, 1995, pp 135–147.
24. Friedman MJ, Charney DS, Deutch AY. Neurobiological and Clinical Consequences of Stress. Philadelphia: Lippincott-Raven, 1995.
25. Davis M. Neurobiology of fear responses: the role of the amygdala. J Neuropsychiatry Clin Neurosci 1997; 9:382–402.
26. LeDoux J. Fear and the brain: where have we been, and where are we going? Biol Psychiatry 1998; 44:1229–1238.
27. Gloor P. Role of the amygdala in temporal lobe epilepsy. In: The Amygdala: Neurobiological Aspects of Emotion, Memory and Mental Dysfunction, ed Aggleton JP. New York: Wiley-Liss, 1992, pp 339–352.
28. Cendes F, Andermann F, Gloor P, Gambardella A, Lopes-Cendes I, Watson C, Evans A, Carpenter S, Olivier A. Relationship between atrophy of the amygdala and ictal fear in temporal lobe epilepsy. Brain 1994; 117:739–746.
29. Isenberg N, Silbersweig D, Engelien A, Emmerich S, Malavade K, Beattie B, Leon AC, Stern E. Linguistic threat activates the human amygdala. Proc Nat Acad Sci USA 1999; 96:10456–10459.
30. Whalen PJ, Rauch SL, Etcoff NL, McInerney SC, Lee MB, Jenike MA. Masked presentations of emotional facial expressions modulate amygdala activity without explicit knowledge. J Neurosci 1998; 18:411–418.
31. LaBar KS, Gatenby JC, Gore JC, LeDoux JE, Phelps EA. Human amygdala activation during conditioned fear acquisition and extinction: a mixed-trial fMRI study. Neuron 1998; 20:937–945.
32. Rauch SL, Van der Kolk BA, Fisler RE, Alpert NM, Orr SP, Savage CR, Fischman AJ, Jenike MA, Pitman RK. A symptom provocation study of posttraumatic stress disorder using positron emission tomography and script-driven imagery. Arch Gen Psychiatry 1996; 53:380–387.
33. Cahill L, Babinsky R, Markowitsch HJ, McGaugh JL. The amygdala and emotional memory. Nature 1995; 377:295–296.
34. Rauch SL, Whalen PJ, Shin LM, McInerney SC, Macklin ML, Lasko NB, Orr SP, Pitman RK. Exaggerated amygdala response to masked facial sti-

muli in posttraumatic stress disorder: a functional MRI study. Biol Psychiatry 2000; 47:769–776.
35. Cahill L, McGaugh JL. Mechanisms of emotional arousal and lasting declarative memory. Trends Neurosci 1998; 21:294–299.
36. Adolphs R, Tranel D, Damasio H, Damasio AR. Fear and the human amygdala. J Neurosci 1995; 15:5879–5891.
37. Hamner MB, Lorberbaum JP, George MS. Potential role of the anterior cingulate cortex in PTSD: review and hypothesis. Depress Anxiety 1999; 9:1–14.
38. Posner MI, Petersen SE. The attention system of the human brain. Ann Review Neurosci 1990; 13:25–42.
39. Shin LM, McNally RJ, Kosslyn SM, Thompson WL, Rauch SL, Alpert NM, Metzger LJ, Lasko NB, Orr SP, Pitman RK. Regional cerebral blood flow during script-imagery in childhood sexual abuse-related PTSD: a PET investigation. Am J Psychiatry 1999; 156:575–584.
40. Bremner JD, Narayan M, Staib L, Southwick SM, McGlashan T, Charney DS. Neural correlates of memories of childhood sexual abuse in women with and without posttraumatic stress disorder. Am J Psychiatry 1999; 156:1787–1795.
41. Bremner JD, Staib L, Kaloupek D, Southwick SM, Soufer R, Charney DS. Neural correlates of exposure to traumatic pictures and sound in Vietnam combat veterans with and without posttraumatic stress disorder: a positron emission tomography study. Biol Psychiatry 1999; 45:806–816.
42. Prichard JW. MRS of the brain-prospects for clinical application. In: MR Spectroscopy: Clinical Applications and Techniques, eds Young IR, Charles HC. London: Livery House, 1996, pp 1–25.
43. De Bellis MD, Keshavan MS, Spencer S, Hall J. N-acetylaspartate concentration in the anterior cingulate in maltreated children and adolescents with PTSD. Am J Psychiatry 2000; 157:1175–1177.
44. Arnsten AFT, Goldman-Rakic PS. Noise stress impairs cortical function: evidence for a hyperdopaminergic mechanism. 1998; 55:362–368.
45. Arnsten AFT. The biology of being frazzled. Science 1998; 1711–1712.
46. Deutch AY, Young CD. A model of the stress-induced activation of prefrontal cortical dopamine systems. In: Neurobiological and Clinical Consequences of Stress: From Normal Adaptation to Post-traumatic Stress Disorder, eds Friedman MJ, Charney DS, Deutch AY. Philadelphia: Lippincott-Raven, 1995, pp 163–175.
47. Bertolucchi-D'Angio M, Serrano A, Scatton B. Involvement of mesocorticolimbic dopaminergic systems in emotional states. Prog Brain Res 1990; 85:405–416.
48. Yehuda R, Southwick S, Giller EL, Ma X, Mason JW. Urinary catecholamine excretion and severity of PTSD symptoms in Vietnam combat veterans. J Nerv Ment Dis 1992; 180:321–325.
49. De Bellis MD, Lefter L, Trickett PK, Putnam FW. Urinary catecholamine excretion in sexually abused girls. J Am Acad Child Adolesc Psychiatry 1994; 33:320–327.
50. De Bellis MD, Baum A, Birmaher B, Keshavan M, Eccard CH, Boring AM, Jenkins FJ, Ryan ND. A.E. Bennett Research Award. Developmental traumatology. Part I: Biological stress systems. Biol Psychiatry 1999; 45:1259–1270.
51. Simson PE, Weiss JM. Altered activity of the locus coeruleus in an animal model of depression. Neuropsychopharmacology 1988; 1:287–295.
52. Tsuda A, Tanaka M. Differential changes in noradrenaline turnover in specific regions of rat brain produced by controllable and uncontrollable shocks. Behav Neurosci 1985; 99:802–807.
53. Aston-Jones G, Shipley MT, Chouvet G, Ennis M, VanBockstaele EJ, Pieribone V, Shiekhatter R. Afferent regulation of locus coeruleus neurons: anatomy, physiology, and pharmacology. Prog Brain Res 1991; 88:47–75.
54. Southwick SM, Yehuda R, Morgan CA. Clinical studies of neurotransmitter alterations in post-traumatic stress disorder. In: Neurobiological and Clinical Consequences of Stress: From Normal Adaptation to Post-traumatic Stress Disorder, eds Friedman MJ, Charney DS, Deutch AY. Philadelphia: Lippincott-Raven, 1995, pp 335–349.
55. Chrousos GP, Gold PW. The concepts of stress and stress system disorders: overview of physical and behavioral homeostasis. JAMA 1992; 267:1244–1252.
56. Maas JW, Koslow SII, Davis J, Katz M, Frazer A, Bowden CL, Berman N, Gibbons R, Stokes P, Landis DH. Catecholamine metabolism and disposition in healthy and depressed subjects. Arch Gen Psychiatry 1987; 44:337–344.
57. Charney DS, Deutch AY, Krystal JH, Southwick SM, Davis M. Psychobiological mechanisms of post-traumatic stress disorder. Arch Gen Psychiatry 1993; 50:294–305.
58. Pitman PK. Biological findings in posttraumatic stress disorder: implications for DSM-IV classification. In: Posttraumatic Stress Disorder: DSM-IV and Beyond, eds Davidson JRT, Foa EB. Washington: American Psychiatric Press, 1993, pp 173–189.
59. Ross RJ, Ball WA, Sullivan KA, Caroff SN. Sleep disturbance as the hallmark of posttraumatic stress disorder. Am J Psychiatry 1989; 146:697–707.
60. Kosten TR, Mason JW, Giller EL, Ostroff RB, Harkness L. Sustained urinary norepinephrine and epinephrine elevation in posttraumatic stress disorder. Psychoneuroendocrinology 1987; 12:13–20.

61. Queiroz EA, Lombardi AB, Santos Furtado CRH, Peixoto CCD, Soares TA, Z.L. F, Basques JC, M.L.M. F, Lippi JRS. Biochemical correlate of depression in children. Arq Neuro-Psiquiat 1991; 49(4):418–425.
62. Perry BD. Neurobiological sequelae of childhood trauma: PTSD in children. In: Catecholamine Function in Posttraumatic Stress Disorder: Emerging Concepts, ed Murburg M. Washington: American Psychiatric Press, 1994, pp 233–255.
63. Famularo R, Kinsherff R, Fenton T. Propranolol treatment for childhood posttraumatic stress disorder, acute type. Am J Dis Child 1988; 142:1244–1247.
64. De Kloet R, Vreugdenhil E, Oitzl MS, Joes A. Brain corticosteroid receptor balance in health and disease. Endocr Rev 1998; 19:269–301.
65. Elkabir DR, Wyatt ME, Vellucci SV, Herbert J. The effects of separate or combined infusions of CSF corticotrophin-releasing factor and vasopressin either intraventricularly or into the amygdala on aggressive and investigative behaviour in the rat. Regul Peptides 1990; 28:199–214.
66. Koob GF, Bloom FE. Corticotropin-releasing factor and behavior. Fed Proc 1985; 44:259–253.
67. Baker DG, West SA, Nicholson WE, Ekhator NN, Kasckow JW, Hill KK, Bruce AB, Orth DN, Geracioti TD Jr. Serial CSF corticotropin-releasing hormone levels and adrenocortical activity in combat veterans with posttraumatic stress disorder. Am J Psychiatry 1999; 156:585–588.
68. Bremner JD, Licinio J, Darnell A, Krystal JH, Owens MJ, Southwick SM, Nemeroff CB, Charney DS. Elevated CSF corticotropin-releasing factor concentrations in posttraumatic stress disorder. Am J Psychiatry 1997; 154:624–629.
69. Yehuda R, Levengood RA, Schmeidler J, Wilson S, Guo LS, Gerber D. Increased pituitary activation following metyrapone administration in post-traumatic stress disorder. Psychoneuroendocrinology 1996; 21:1–16.
70. Yehuda R, Lowy MT, Southwick SM, Shaffer D, Giller ELJ. Lymphocyte glucocorticoid receptor number in posttraumatic stress disorder. Am J Psychiatry, 1991; 148:499–504.
71. Yehuda R, Southwick SM, Krystal JH, Bremner D, Charney DS, Mason JW. Enhanced suppression of cortisol following dexamethasone administration in posttraumatic stress disorder. Am J Psychiatry 1993; 150:83–86.
72. Mason JW, Giller EL, Kosten TR, Ostroff RB, Podd L. Urinary-free cortisol levels in post-traumatic stress disorder patients. J Nerv Ment Dis 1986; 174:145–159.
73. Yehuda R, Southwick S, Giller EL, Ma X, Mason JW. Low urinary cortisol excretion in PTSD. J Nerv Ment Dis 1991; 178:366–369.
74. Yehuda R, Kahana B, Binder-Brynes K, Southwick S, Mason JW, Giller EL. Low urinary cortisol excretion in Holocaust survivors with posttraumatic stress disorder. Am J Psychiatry 1995; 152:982–986.
75. Pitman PK, Orr SP. Twenty-four hour cortisol and catecholamine excretion in combat-related posttraumatic stress disorder. Biol Psychiatry 1990; 27:245–247.
76. Lemieux AM, Coe CL. Abuse-related posttraumatic stress disorder: evidence for chronic neuroendocrine activation in women. Psychosom Med 1995; 57:105–115.
77. Putnam FW, Trickett PK, Helmers K, Dorn L, Everett B. Cortisol abnormalities in sexually abused girls. In: 144th Annual Meeting Program. Washington: Am Psychiatric Press, 1991, p 107.
78. Hart J, Gunnar M, Cicchetti D. Altered neuroendocrine activity in maltreated children related to symptoms of depression. Dev Psychopathol 1996; 8:201–214.
79. Kaufman J. Depressive disorders in maltreated children. J Am Acad Child Adolesc Psychiatry 1991; 30:257–265.
80. Kaufman J, Birmaher B, Perel J, Dahl RE, Moreci P, Nelson B, Wells W, Ryan N. The corticotropin-releasing hormone challenge in depressed abused, depressed nonabused, and normal control children. Biol Psychiatry 1997; 42:669–679.
81. De Bellis MD, Chrousos GP, Dorn LD, Burke L, Helmers K, Kling MA, Trickett PK, Putnam FW. Hypothalamic-pituitary-adrenal axis dysregulation in sexually abused girls. J Clin Endocrinol Metab 1994; 78:249–255.
82. Smith MA, Ritchie JC, Kudler H, Lipper S, Chappell P, Nemeroff CB. The corticotropin-releasing hormone test in patients with posttraumatic stress disorder. Biol Psychiatry 1989; 26:349–355.
83. Goenjian AK, Yehuda R, Pynoos RS, Steinberg AM, Tashjian M, Yang RK, Najarian LM, Fairbanks LA. Basal cortisol, dexamethasone suppression of cortisol, and MHPG in adolescents after the 1988 earthquake in Armenia. Am J Psychiatry 1996; 153:929–934.
84. Edwards E, Harkins K, Wright G, Menn F. Effects of bilateral adrenalectomy on the induction of learned helplessness. Behav Neuropsychopharmacol 1990; 3:109–114.
85. Sapolsky RM. Glucocorticoids and hippocampal atrophy in neuropsychiatric disorders. Arch Gen Psychiatry 2000; 57:925–935.
86. Armanini MP, Hutchins C, Stein BA, Sapolsky RM. Glucocorticoid endangerment of hippocampal neurons is NMDA-receptor dependent. Brain Res 1990; 532:7–12.
87. Uno H, Tarara R, Else J, Suleman MA, Sapolsky RM. Hippocampal damage associated with pro-

longed and fatal stress in primates. J Neurosci 1989; 9:1705–1711.
88. Starkman MN, Gebarksi SS, Berent S, Schteingart DE. Hippocampal formation volume, memory dysfunction, and cortisol levels in patients with Cushing's syndrome. Biol Psychiatry 1992; 32:756–765.
89. Bremner JD, Randall P, Scott TM, Bronen RA, Southwick SM, Seibyl JP, Delaney RC, McCarthy G, Charney DS, Innis RB. MRI-based measurement of hippocampal volume in patients with combat-related posttraumatic stress disorder. Am J Psychiatry 1995; 152:973–981.
90. Gurvits TV, Shenton ME, Hokama H, Ohta H, Lasko NB, Gilbertson MW, Orr SP, Kikinis R, Jolesz FA, McCarley RW, Pitman RK. Magnetic resonance imaging study of hippocampal volume in chronic, combat-related posttraumatic stress disorder. Biol Psychiatry 1996; 40:1091–1099.
91. Bremner JD, Randall P, Vermetten E, Staib L, Bronen RA, Mazure C, Capelli S, McCarthy G, Innis RB, Charney DS. Magnetic resonance imaging-based measurement of hippocampal volume in posttraumatic stress disorder related to childhood physical and sexual abuse—a preliminary report. Biol Psychiatry 1997; 41:23–32.
92. Stein MB, Koverola C, Hanna C, Torchia MG, McClarty B. Hippocampal volume in women victimized by childhood sexual abuse. Psychol Med 1997; 27:1–9.
93. De Bellis MD, Keshavan M, Clark DB, Casey BJ, Giedd J, Boring AM, Frustaci K, Ryan ND. A.E. Bennett Research Award. Developmental traumatology. Part II: Brain development. Biol Psychiatry 1999; 45:1271–1284.
94. Jernigan TL, Sowell ER. Magnetic resonance imaging studies of the developing brain. In: Neurodevelopment & Adult Psychopathology, eds Keshavan MS, Murray RM. Cambridge: Cambridge University Press, 1997, pp 63–70.
95. De Bellis MD, Hall J, Boring AM, Frustaci K, Moritz G. A pilot longitudinal study of hippocampal volumes in pediatric maltreatment-related posttraumatic stress disorder. Biol Psychiatry 2001 (in press).
96. Lescaudron L, Jaffard R, Verna A. Modification in the number and morphology of dendritic spines resulting from chronic ethanol consumption and withdrawal: a Golgi study in the mouse anterior and posterior hippocampus. Exp Neurol 1989; 106:156–163.
97. Breese CR, Freedman R, Leonard SS. Glutamate receptor subtype expression in human postmortem brain tissue from schizophrenics and alcohol abusers. Brain Res 1995; 674:82–90.
98. De Bellis MD, Clark DB, Beers SR, Soloff P, Boring AM, Hall J, Kersh A, Keshavan MS. Hippocampal volume in adolescent onset alcohol use disorders. Am J Psychiatry 2000; 157:737–744.
99. Lesch KP, Moessner R. Genetically driven variation in serotonin update: is there a link to affective spectrum, neurodevelopmental and neurodegenerative disorders? Biol Psychiatry 1998; 44:179–192.
100. Fontenot MB, Kaplan JR, Manuck SB, Arango V, Mann JJ. Long-term effects of chronic social stress on serotonergic indices in the prefrontal cortex of adult male cynomolgus macaques. Brain Res 1995; 705:105–108.
101. Petty F, Kramer GL, Wu J. Serotonergic modulation of learned helplessness. Ann NY Acad Sci 1997; 821:538–541.
102. Arora RC, Fichtner CG, O'Connor F, Crayton JW. Paraoxetine binding in the blood platelets of posttraumatic stress disorder patients. Life Sci 1993; 53:919–928.
103. Spivak B, Vered Y, Graff E, Blum I, Mester R, Weizman A. Low platelet-poor plasma concentrations of serotonin in patients with combat-related posttraumatic stress disorder. Biol Psychiatry 1999; 45:840–845.
104. Benkelfat C. Serotonergic mechanisms in psychiatric disorders: new research tools, new ideas. Int Clin Psychopharmacol 1993; 8(suppl 2):53–56.
105. Siever L, Trestman RL. The serotonin system and aggressive personality disorder. Int Clin Psychopharmacol 1993; 8(suppl 2):33–40.
106. Rosenberg DR, Keshavan MS. A.E. Bennett Research Award. Toward a neurodevelopmental model of obsessive-compulsive disorder. Biol Psychiatry 1998; 43:623–640.
107. Sulser F. Serotonin-norepinephrine receptor interactions in the brain: implications for the pharmacology and pathophysiology of affective disorders. J Clin Psychiatry 1987; 3:12–18.
108. Breslau N, Davis GC, Peterson E, Schultz LR. A second look at comorbidity in victims of trauma: the posttraumatic stress disorder–major depression connection. Biol Psychiatry 2000:902–909.
109. Brady K, Pearlstein T, Asnis GM, Baker D, Rothbaum B, Sikes CR, Farfel GM. Efficacy and safety of sertraline treatment of posttraumatic stress disorder: a randomized controlled trial. JAMA 2000; 283:1837–1844.
110. Van der Kolk BA, Dreyfuss D, Michaels M, Shera D, Berkowitz R, Fisler R, Saxe G. Fluoxetine in posttraumatic stress disorder. J Clin Psychiatry 1994; 55:517–522.
111. Cohen JA, Work Group on Quality Issues: Practice parameters for the assessment and treatment of children and adolescents with posttraumatic stress

112. Friedman MJ, Southwick SM. Toward psychopharmacology for post-traumatic stress disorder. In: Neurobiological and Clinical Consequences of Stress: From Normal Adaptation to Post-traumatic Stress Disorder, eds Friedman MJ, Charney DS, Deutch AY. Philadelphia: Lippincott-Raven, 1995, pp 465–481.
113. Weizman R, Weizman A, Kook KA, Vocci F, Deutsch SI, Paul SM. Repeated swim stress alters brain benzodiazepine receptors measured in vivo. J Pharmacol Exp Ther 1989; 249:701–707.
114. Robertson HA, Martin IL, Candy JM. Differences in benzodiazepine receptor binding in Maudsley-reactive and non-reactive rats. Eur J Pharmacol 1978; 50:455–457.
115. Van der Kolk BA, Greenberg MS, Orr SP, Pitman RK. Endogenous opioids, stress induced analgesia, and posttraumatic stress disorder. Psychopharmacol Bull 1989; 25:417–421.
116. Pitman PK, Van der Kolk BA, Orr SP, Greenberg MS. Naloxone-reversible analgesic response to combat-related stimuli in posttraumatic stress disorder. Arch Gen Psychiatry 1990; 47:541–544.
117. Baker DG, West SA, Orth DN, Hill KK, Nicholson WE, Ekhator NN, Bruce AB, Wortman MD, Keck PE, Geracioti TD Jr. Cerebrospinal fluid and plasma beta endorphin in combat veterans with posttraumatic stress disorder. Psychoneuroendocrinology 1997; 22:517–529.
118. Hoffman L, Watsgon PD, Wilson G, Montgomery J. Low plasma beta endorphin in posttraumatic stress disorder. Aust NZ J Psychiatry 1989; 23:268–273.
119. Van der Kolk BA, Perry JC, Herman JL. Childhood origins of self-destructive behavior. Am J Psychiatry 1991; 148:1665–1671.
120. Friedman MJ, Schurr PP. The relationship between trauma, post-traumatic stress disorder, and physical health. In: Neurobiological and Clinical Consequences of Stress: From Normal Adaptation to Post-traumatic Stress Disorder, eds Friedman MJ, Charney DS, Deutch AY. Philadelphia: Lippincott-Raven, 1995, pp 507–524.
121. Beebe GW. Follow-up studies of World War II and Korean war prisoners: II. Morbidity, disability, and maladjustments. Am J Epidemiol 1975; 101:400–422.
122. Selye H. A syndrome produced by diverse nocuous agents. Nature 1936; 138:32.
123. Weiss JM, Sundar S. Effects of stress on cellular immune responses in animals. In: Review of Psychiatry, eds Tasman A, Riba MB. Washington: Am Psychiatric Press, 1992, pp 145–168.
124. Bellinger DL, Felten SY, Felten DL. Neural-immune interactions. In: Review of Psychiatry, eds Tasman A, Riba MB. Washington: Am Psychiatric Press, 1992, pp 127–144.
125. Mosnaim AD, Wolf ME, Maturana P, Mosnaim G, Puente J, Kucuk O, Gilman-Sachs A: In vitro studies of natural killer cell activity in post traumatic stress disorder patients: response to methionine-enkephalin challenge. Immunopharmacology 1993; 25:107–116.
126. Ironson G, Wynings C, Schneiderman N, Baum A, Rodriguez M, Greenwood D, Benight C, Antoni M, LaPerriere A, Huang HS, Klimas N, Fletcher MA. Posttraumatic stress symptoms, intrusive thoughts, loss, and immune function after Hurricane Andrew. Psychosom Med 1997; 59:128–141.
127. Laudenslager ML, Aasal R, Adler L, Berger CL, Montgomery PT, Sandberg E, Wahlberg LJ, Wilkins RT, Zweig L, Reite ML. Elevated cytotoxicity in combat veterans with long-term post-traumatic stress disorder: preliminary observations. Brain Behav Immun 1998; 12:74–79.
128. Sabioncello A, Kocijan-Hercigonja D, Rabati S, Tomasi J, Jeren T, Matijevi L, Rijavec M, Dekaris D. Immune, endocrine, and psychological responses in civilians displaced by war. Psychosom Med 2000; 62:502–508.
129. Wilson SN, Van der Kolk B, Burbridge J, Fisler R, Kradin R. Phenotype of blood lymphocytes in PTSD suggests chronic immune activation. Psychosomatics 1999; 40:222–225.
130. Boscarino JA, Chang J. Higher abnormal leukocyte and lymphocyte counts 20 years after exposure to severe stress: research and clinical implications. Psychosom Med 1999; 61:378–386.
131. De Bellis MD, Burke L, Trickett PK, Putnam FW. Antinuclear antibodies and thyroid function in sexually abused girls. J Trauma Stress 1996; 9:369–378.
132. Gillette GM, Garbutt JC, Prange AJ. Anxiety and the thyroid axis. In: Handbook of Anxiety, eds Burrows GD, Roth M, Noyes R. New York: Elsevier, 1990, pp 365–379.
133. Delange F. Thyroid hormones: biochemistry and physiology. In: Pediatric Endocrinology: Physiology, Pathophysiology, and Clinical Aspects, eds Bertrand J, Rappaport R, Sizonenko PC. Baltimore: Williams & Wilkins, 1993, pp 242–252.
134. Czernichow P. Thyrotropin and thyroid hormones. In: Pediatric Endocrinology: Physiology, Pathophysiology, and Clinical Aspects, eds Bertrand J, Rappaport R, Sizonenko PC. Baltimore: Williams & Wilkins, 1993, pp 79–88.
135. Mason J, Southwick SM, Yehuda R, Wang S, Riney S, Bremner D, Johnson D, Lubin H, Blake D, Zhou G, Gusman F, Charney DS. Elevation of serum free triiodothyronine, total triiodothyronine, thyroxine-binding globulin, and total thyroxine levels in com-

bat-related posttraumatic stress disorder. Arch Gen Psychiatry 1994; 51:629–641.

136. Kosten TR, Wahby V, Giller E Jr., Mason J. The dexamethasone suppression test and thyrotropin-releasing hormone stimulation test in posttraumatic stress disorder. Biol Psychiatry 1990; 28:657–664.

137. Felitti VJ, Anda RF, Nordenberg D, Williamson DF, Spitz AM, Edwards V, Koss MP, Marks JS. Relationship of childhood abuse and household dysfunction to many of the leading causes if death in adults. Am J Prev Med 1998; 14:245–258.

138. De Bellis MD. Developmental traumatology: the psychobiological development of maltreated children and its implications for research, treatment, and policy. Dev Psychopathol 2001; 13:539–564.

32

Genetics of Panic Disorder, Social Phobia, and Agoraphobia

JOEL GELERNTER
Yale University School of Medicine, New Haven, and Veterans Administration Medical Center, West Haven, Connecticut, U.S.A.

MURRAY B. STEIN
University of California, San Diego, La Jolla, and Veterans Affairs San Diego Healthcare System, San Diego, California, U.S.A.

I. INTRODUCTION

The genetic influences on behavior are now widely appreciated, and there has been widespread interest in identifying risk loci (or specific genes that influence risk) for a range of psychiatric illnesses and behaviors, including schizophrenia, bipolar affective disorder, alcohol dependence, and drug dependence. Anxiety disorders are heritable as well, although the best available data indicate that the contribution of genetic factors to risk of illness tends to be somewhat lower than that for the disorders enumerated above. We will concentrate in this chapter on the genetics of panic disorder (PD), social phobia (SocP), and agoraphobia (AgP).

No specific genes that contribute to the causation of these disorders (taken as broad diagnoses) have been identified, nor are the locations of any such genes known. Knowledge of the specifics of the genetic bases of these behaviors will inevitably lead to improved understanding of disease physiology, improved treatments, and better prevention. We discuss here (1) the clinical genetic data that establish that these particular anxiety disorders are both familial and genetically influenced, (2) strategies that can be used to identify specific genes that influence risk of illness, and (3) molecular studies with the goal of identifying risk loci.

II. CLINICAL GENETICS OF PANIC DISORDER, SOCIAL PHOBIA, AND AGORAPHOBIA

A. Epidemiology and Comorbidity

Panic disorder (PD) and agoraphobia (AgP) are common anxiety disorders that often co-occur. PD is characterized by recurrent panic attacks that include both somatic (e.g., palpitations, sweating, shortness of breath) and psychological (e.g., fear of losing control, fear of dying) symptoms. AgP is characterized by fear and avoidance of certain situations from which escape might be difficult (e.g., crowds, standing in line, bridges or tunnels). It is common, but not invariant, for agoraphobia to develop in the course of PD. Results from the (United States) National Comorbidity Study showed lifetime prevalence of DSM-III-R-defined [1] PD was 3.5%, and lifetime prevalence of DSM-III-R AgP without PD was 5.3% [2]. Wittchen et al. [3] studied the relationship of agoraphobia and PD in a German sample. In this sample, lifetime prevalence of DSM-IV-defined PD was 1.6% (0.8% with and 0.8% without agoraphobia), and lifetime prevalence of AgP was 8.5%. These findings confirm that although PD and AgP are frequently comorbid, there are indeed cases of isolated AgP that occur in the general population.

Social phobia (SocP) is characterized by fear (and, in many cases, avoidance) of situations where an individual is subject to the scrutiny of others; in such situations, the individuals fears that they will say or do something that will result in embarrassment or humiliation, and/or that others will see that they are anxious. SocP shows lifetime prevalence of 13.3% and is thus very common [4]. It is thought that there may be subtypes of SocP, distinguishable on the basis of the extent of the social fears; DSM-IV refers to a "generalized" subtype in which most social situations are avoided [5]. The delineation and, indeed, the existence of SocP subtypes remains controversial [6], although a consensus seems to be emerging that persons with multiple social fears are distinct from those with public-speaking-only fears [7,8].

These anxiety disorders can be disabling, and frequently result in reduced quality of life [9]. All three disorders show considerable female predominance [2]. All three disorders also show frequent co-occurrence, beyond the comorbidity of PD and AgP, as described above. In the National Comorbidity Survey subjects with SocP had a 23.3% rate of AgP, a 37.6% rate of simple phobia, and a 10.9% rate of PD [10].

B. Twin and Family Studies; Heritability

Twin studies (in females) suggest that the heritability of PD is ~ 32–46% [11]. The best relevant heritability data for AgP and SocP come from two reports based on population-based studies of female and male twins, respectively (where heritabilities for animal phobia, blood/injury phobia, and situational phobia were also considered) [12,13]. Estimated heritabilities (with correction for unreliability) for AgP and SocP in women were 61–67% and 50–51%, respectively. For men a^2 for the best-fit model for fears and phobias were 43% and 24% for AgP and SocP, respectively [13]. Multivariate analyses, conducted separately in men and women, revealed common genetic factors as well as genetic factors specific to each phobic subtype. It can be concluded from these studies that genes play a moderate role in the etiology of phobias. These studies did not attempt to clarify the genetic relationship of the phobic disorders with panic disorder, although an earlier study suggested that genetic risk factors may be shared between PD and AgP [11]. This remains an area in need of further research, as it impacts directly upon phenotype delineation for family and genetic studies of PD and AgP [14].

Many family studies of PD [for review, see 14] have demonstrated that the rate of PD is increased among first-degree relatives of PD probands. In comparison, there are very few reports of rates of AgP in relatives of agoraphobic probands (without panic). One study [15] considered diagnoses in relatives of subjects with AgP alone, and concluded that AgP is, in effect, a severe form of PD. However, their data are also consistent with specific coaggregation for each diagnosis; AgP was seen more frequently in relatives of subjects with AgP than in relatives of subjects with PD (11.6% vs. 1.9%), whereas PD was more common in relatives of subjects with PD than in relatives of subjects with AgP (17.3% vs. 8.3%).

SocP may be genetically related to PD, with a rate of 5.7% in relatives of probands with PD but without depression, compared to 1.6% in relatives of normal controls [16]. Several family studies demonstrate that SocP aggregates in families of SocP probands [17,18]. Stein et al. [19] showed a greatly increased risk of generalized SocP in relatives of generalized SocP probands compared to relatives of controls (26.4% vs. 2.7%), in a direct-interview family study. In that study, avoidant personality disorder was found exclusively in relatives of generalized SocP probands, consistent with the growing consensus that avoidant personality disorder may be better thought of as a severe form of SocP [20].

C. Biological Markers in Family Studies

Patients with PD frequently experience panic attacks when they inhale CO_2-enriched air [for a review of this topic see 21]; they do so at a rate that exceeds that of healthy control subjects. This pattern of response is also seen in first-degree relatives of patients with PD, and has been suggested as a means of identifying a genetically homogenous subtype of PD [22]. It is unclear whether this response is "biologically" or "psychologically" based (i.e., it may be a manifestation of the tendency to fear physical sensations, which itself has shown to be moderately heritable [23]), but in either case, this approach to phenotype delineation is promising and deserves further study.

D. Investigating Mode of Inheritance Through Segregation Analysis

Early segregation analyses suggested that PD inheritance is consistent with a single major locus dominant model [24,25]. Hopper et al. [26], in an analysis of data from a large family study, demonstrated vertical transmission of PD, although they also found evidence for a sibship environment component. The data established increased incidence of PD in relatives of PD patients [27,28] and supported a genetic distinction between PD and GAD. Based on pedigree segregation analysis, Pauls et al. [29] and then Crowe et al. [28] proposed specific genetic models for PD. Although single major-locus autosomal-dominant transmission of PD was consistent with segregation analyses, it became clear later that mode of transmission and pattern of inheritance could not be established unambiguously [26,30]. Vieland et al. [30] reported similar support for dominant and recessive models. Overall, the data strongly support a genetic contribution to the development of PD, but do not consistently identify a mode of inheritance [28–30]. Some recent data support a parent-of-origin effect [31]. At this point it is well accepted that PD is a genetically complex disorder; i.e., it is influenced by multiple genes and does not in general follow a simple Mendelian mode of inheritance. We are not aware of any segregation studies in AgP or SocP.

III. STRATEGIES TO IDENTIFY RISK LOCI

The most important classes of study used to identify risk loci are linkage (which relies on observation of cotransmission of genetic markers with the phenotype of interest within families) and association (which relies on observation of identical-by-state marker alleles in sets of subjects with the phenotype of interest compared with subjects without the phenotype of interest). (Specifics may be found in many textbooks and chapters, e.g., Gelernter [32].)

Risch [33] showed that power for detecting linkage depends primarily on the risk ratio characterizing a given trait, the recombination fraction, 2, and informativeness of the markers studied. For sib pairs, 8_s is the probability of observing the phenotype (here, PD) in sibs of affected individuals compared to unrelated population individuals. Smoller and Tsuang [14] estimated 8_s for PD as 5–10 (compared to 10 for schizophrenia and bipolar disorder, 2–4 for migraine, and 2–3 for major depression [14]). This places PD in a range where linkage studies should clearly be usable to identify risk loci.

Genome scan linkage provides the most general solution for identification of risk loci. Linkage analysis in families has therefore been the preferred initial approach to mapping genes, when appropriate family materials are available. Linkage provides a general solution to the problem of localization of genetic susceptibility loci, a solution that does not depend on any prior knowledge other than that the phenotype studied has at least a partially genetic basis (for model-free analyses: NPL analysis) and sometimes an idea of how the disorder is transmitted (for model-based analyses: LOD score analysis).

However, linkage only provides a general location for a risk locus, and therefore a follow-up strategy for positional cloning (i.e., identify the specific genetic variants that give rise to the phenotype) that relies on linkage disequilibrium (LD) (nonrandom association of alleles are two genetic loci, which is important for genetic association) rather than linkage is likely to be necessary. It has also been argued [e.g., 34,35] that LD is, potentially, a very efficient strategy for identifying genes influencing risk for complex disorders. LD methods therefore provide an approach complementary to linkage for gene identification. Genetic association studies may help identify genes that are either important in increasing liability for psychiatric illness or for affecting certain phenotypes within these illnesses. Samples for case control association studies are composed of unrelated individuals. Difference in allele frequency between cases and controls might be attributable to a relationship between the variant studied (or another variant in LD with it) and the phenotype, or to population subdivision (or stratification). Population stratification is a frequent cause of false-positive results in association studies, and is thought to be a major reason for the frequent failures to replicate observed for studies using this general design.

Population stratification can be addressed either through use of family-controlled designs such as HRR and TDT, or through correction of stratification in a case control context. The haplotype relative risk (HRR) method [36,37], a family-based genetic association method using subjects and their parents, compares allele frequency in a set of ill subjects with the set of nontransmitted parental alleles. The transmission/disequilibrium test (TDT) [38], which uses parent offspring trios, uses parents heterozygous for the disease associated marker and considers observed transmission vs. nontransmission of the alleles at a locus to affected offspring compared to the expected transmission frequency (i.e., 50%). While the family-controlled methods require specialized sample collection, correction of stratification can be accomplished with a standard case control sample. The method proposed by Pritchard et al. [39,40] has just been applied successfully for a study mapping variation in flowering time in maize [41]; although this is a plant study, it provides an important proof of principle for the method and is likely to be followed by many studies of similar design in man. Devlin and Roeder [42] also presented a solution to the problem of stratification for case control studies, the "genomic control" method. Success in application of these methods requires either (1) direct testing of candidate variants, or (2) the existence of sufficient linkage disequilibrium (LD; nonrandom association of alleles at different closely mapped loci) across the genome to be able to detect signal indirectly via LD.

IV. MOLECULAR STUDIES

A. Candidate Gene Studies

Numerous candidate gene linkage and association studies have been published for PD. Crowe et al. [43,44] tested a variety of classical genetic markers for linkage in PD families without identifying a significant linkage. Candidate gene studies have likewise failed to demonstrate significant linkage signals: Mutchler et al. [45] studied tyrosine hydroxylase; Wang et al. [46] evaluated the α1, two α2, β1, and β2 adrenergic receptor loci; Schmidt et al. [47] studied the GABA β1 receptor; Crowe et al. [48] studied 8 $GABA_A$ receptor subunit genes. Ohara et al. [49] studied the 5HT1Dα and 5HT1Dβ (HTR1B) genes by direct sequencing in 20 Japanese PD patients and controls. A single report [50] suggests possible association between adenosine 2A receptor gene ($A_{2A}R$) variants and PD. Kato et al. [51] identified a missense mutation in the cholecystokinin B receptor (CCKRB) gene that was not significantly associated with PD nor linked in a small number of informative pedigrees. Wang et al. [52] studied a polymorphism in the cholecystokinin promoter (CCK-36C/T) and reported possible LD with PD, depending on disease model; their linkage study was uninformative. Kennedy et al. [53] supported genetic association between CCKRB and PD [54]; however, Hamilton et al. [55] found neither association nor linkage of CCKRB to PD, using a different polymorphism. Gelernter et al. [56], discussed below, found "suggestive" linkage. Consistent with the notion that genetic variation in the CCK neurotransmitter system may affect risk for PD, Hattori et al. [57] reported an association between CCK alleles and haplotypes and PD in a Japanese population. Gelernter et al. [56] studied a different CCK polymorphism in their European-American PD linkage series and did not find evidence for linkage, but this could be attributable to the difference in the populations studied. Hamilton et al. [58] did not provide significant support for linkage or association between PD and either the D4 dopamine receptor gene (DRD4) or the dopamine transporter protein (DRD4).

In the only SocP linkage study to date, Stein et al. [59] failed to find evidence for linkage to either the serotonin transporter or the 5HT2A receptor in families ascertained for generalized SocP.

B. Genome Scan Studies

There have been three full genome scans for PD (each with approximately 10 centiMorgan resolution) [56,60,61] and one "targeted" genome screen with favored chromosomal regions selected based on mouse QTL studies [62]. Knowles et al. [60] published the first complete genome scan for PD, with up to 23 families, and observed six LOD scores between 1.0 and 2.0; two were under a dominant model, on chromosomes 1p and 20p, and four under a recessive model, on chromosomes 7p, 17p, 20q, and X/Y. There were no LOD scores >2. Crowe et al. [61] published the second full genome scan for PD, also with 23 families, reporting results of pairwise LOD score analyses and multipoint NPL analyses. They identified two LOD scores >2.0, both on chromosome 7, and several LOD scores between 1 and 2. Gelernter et al. [56] published a genome scan of 20 families segregating both PD and agoraphobia, and included analyses (multipoint parametric and NPL) of each of these phenotypes taken separately. They reported two regions meeting criteria for "suggestive" linkage with PD with LOD score >2, one of which, on chromosome 1, coincided with a region previously implicated [61] with a LOD score >1. The other "suggestive" linkage was observed at the CCK-b receptor locus (CCKBR). (CCKBR was one of eight candidate genes these authors added to their full genome scan.) This finding is of particular interest in light of previous positive associations observed both for CCKBR [53] and CCK [57], although there is also a report to the contrary [55]. The cholecystokinin neurotransmitter system is thought to be of importance for anxiety. Cholecystokinin tetrapeptide (CCK-4) induces panic, and does so at much higher rates in subjects with PD than in control subjects [63]; these effects are reduced by a cholecystokinin receptor antagonist [64]. Notably, there were regions of possible linkage in common between each set of studies [discussed in 61 and 56].

Smoller et al. [62] reported results of a targeted genome screen for PD and "anxiety disorder proneness" in a single large extended pedigree. They chose regions for study based on results of mouse quantitative trait locus (QTL) studies that identified regions with anxiety-related QTLs; they concentrated on regions in the human genome homologous to regions where mouse QTLs were mapped. Their two strongest results were on chromosome 12q13 for PD/agoraphobia (NPL 4.96, $P = 0.006$) and on chromosome 10q (dominance model) for anxiety proneness (LOD score, 2.38). While this is a very appealing approach, its utility depends on both the comparability of the mouse phenotypes to the human phenotypes, and on the genesis of those phenotypes not just through similar pathophysiology but through similar genetic mechanisms.

Gelernter et al. [56] also completed a full genome scan for agoraphobia. No regions meeting criteria for "suggestive" linkage were identified—the highest LOD score observed over the whole series was 1.8. However, one individual family generated an NPL score of 10.01 ($P = .0039$) and LOD score 2.10. Although this could represent a chance occurrence, it could also represent a genetically distinct subtype of agoraphobia.

Finally, Weissman et al. [65] described a possible PD syndrome, characterized by combinations of PD, kidney or bladder problems, severe headaches, thyroid abnormalities, and mitral valve prolapse. Their clinical sample included those reported by Knowles et al. [60] plus additional families. When their analysis was restricted to families where the putative syndrome was present, they identified a chromosomal region with significant linkage—LOD score 4.2—on chromosome 13. With this very intriguing finding, the authors demonstrate the merit of careful clinical observation in the identification of a PD subset that could be more genetically homogeneous; if confirmed, it is likely to lead to important insights into the pathophysiology of PD.

In addition to these studies of Axis I anxiety disorder diagnoses, there have been numerous studies of anxiety as a personality trait, not necessarily in the pathological range. Notable among these are candidate gene studies of the serotonin transporter protein SLC6A4. Lesch et al. [66] reported that a functional polymorphism at this locus is linked to the personality traits of anxiety and neuroticism. There have been many studies since then addressing this issue, and the results have been quite inconsistent; however, a consensus seems to be emerging that this is a true relationship in some, but not all, populations [67].

C. Possible Insights from Medical Illness

In other areas of psychiatric genetics research, important clues about psychiatric illness have come from study of medical syndromes that include psychiatric symptoms. For example, velocardiofacial syndrome (VCSF) is a common chromosome 22 deletion syndrome. There are an increased rate of psychotic symptoms in patients with VCFS [68] and an increased rate of chromosome 22 deletion in patients with schizophrenia [69]. This overlap identifies a subgroup of schizophrenia. Several studies have suggested that autism is associated with elevated rates in relatives of psychiatric disorders such as social phobia, as well as anxiety-related personality traits [70,71]. The eventual delineation of genes for autism may help identify genes for these associated mental disorders.

Similarly, numerous other medical genetic disorders are characterized by anxiety, in addition to medical, symptoms, and study of these may lead to insight into the pathophysiology and genetics of anxiety disorders. For example, anxiety disorders including panic (as well as other psychiatric disorders) have been reported to occur at increased frequency in Wolfram syndrome heterozygotes [72], and a particular tuberous sclerosis mutation has been associated with anxiety symptoms in the context of otherwise mild phenotypic manifestations [73]. The presence of particular medical symptoms in families has been used to identify a putative subtype of panic disorder, as described earlier in this chapter [65]. That such syndromes are not identified readily may reflect the phenomenon that psychiatric symptoms are often not assessed systematically in the description of genetic syndromes.

V. DISCUSSION

Identifying those genes that influence risk for anxiety disorders would be expected to result in improved understanding of the pathophysiology of the illness and, eventually, improvements in prevention and in treatment. Anxiety disorders are common, cause high morbidity, and are often disabling. Biological aspects of illness could be strictly defined, leading to improved understanding of nonbiological factors as well.

Another use of linkage is for research on the correlates of diagnosis. As stated by Kendler et al. [74:374] in the context of a discussion of genetic epidemiology, "although most nosologists agree that diagnoses should ultimately be based on etiologic characteristics, this has, with minor exceptions, been an unattainable goal in psychiatry." Since each separate linked marker presumably represents a different disease-related variant and a separate etiology, one would expect that differences may be found in course and treatment response in the separately linked forms of a disorder. Identification of linked markers, or genes influencing illness or treatment response, may therefore be expected to lead to improved diagnosis (with attendant improvements in knowledge of prognosis for different forms of disease) and improved clinical care.

PD and agoraphobia have often been conceptualized clinically as parts of a severity continuum, with agoraphobia tending to occur as a response to situational panic attacks, with increasing severity and generalization of the disorder. As discussed by Gelernter et al. [56], the epidemiological data are generally not consistent with this model. The complex web of comorbidity between the major anxiety disorders is a complicating factor for gene identification.

The genetic factors contributing to risk for different anxiety phenotypes are very likely a combination of risk factors that are common to more than one diagnosis (e.g., a gene with an allelic variant that increase risk both for agoraphobia and for PD, separately or together), factors that are relatively specific to one disorder (e.g., a gene that increases risk for social phobia but that does not affect risk for PD), and factors that affect risk to a set of disorders differentially (e.g., a gene that quadruples risk for PD, triples risk for agoraphobia, and doubles risk for social phobia). Each successful identification of a particular risk allele holds the potential of simplifying the remainder of the genetic picture a little, thereby leading to identification of additional risk loci.

Indeed, some researchers have suggested that the DSM-IV approach to the taxonomy of mood and anxiety disorders falls short of explaining the most commonly occurring patterns of symptom aggregation [75,76]. These researchers have suggested that future studies may benefit from considering these alternative phenotypic possibilities. To accomplish this goal, future "diagnostic" efforts in family and genetic studies will need to structure their information gathering to permit collection of information at the symptom level, thereby enabling the reconstruction of DSM as well as identification of more novel syndromes.

It must also be considered that anxiety disorders may not be inherited at any all-or-none "syndrome" level, and that efforts to exclusively identify individuals on the basis of being "affected" or not may be insufficient. Stein et al. [77], for example, showed that a host of anxiety-related traits are elevated in family members of probands with generalized social phobia. Smoller and colleagues have also noted the potential utility of the measurement of quantitative traits (e.g., behavioral inhibition, a risk factor for the development of anxiety disorders) in genetic studies of anxiety disorders [78]. This approach may help identify genes that increase risk for a variety of anxiety disorders.

There is no published linkage study of a "DSM" anxiety disorder with significant support for a particular linkage. This can be taken as an indication of insufficient power in the face of inheritance that is more complex than was anticipated. The quite considerable overlap in regions of interest between published studies should be taken as encouraging. However, Weissman et al. [65] did report significant evidence of linkage for a panic disorder subsyndrome. This very interesting finding may point the way toward identification of genetically (and therefore biologically) more homogeneous subjects of PD patients, an event that would have important implications for the understanding of pathophysiology and possibly for treatment. Replication of this result is therefore important.

Few family or genetic studies in anxiety disorders have included children, presumably because of the increased complexity inherent in administering age-appropriate assessments. However, it is becoming clear that children with certain anxiety-related disorders have increased rates of anxiety disorders in their families. For example, children with separation anxiety disorder have increased rates of panic disorder and/or agoraphobia in their parents [79], and selectively mute children have increased familial rates of social phobia [80]. These early-onset manifestations of anxiety may denote a more severe familial form of the illness, and should therefore be more extensively studied. The inclusion of children in future family and genetics studies is therefore highly recommended.

Finally, published results for the anxiety disorders should be considered with the understanding that there has been much less study of these disorders than of other psychiatric disorders such as schizophrenia and bipolar affective disorders. The latter two disorders both show higher heritability than any anxiety disorder, and both are considered more important from a public health standpoint. Still, we are hopeful that in the future larger studies of the genetics of anxiety disorders will be initiated, and that if they are, specific genes that increase risk for these disorders will be identified unambiguously.

ACKNOWLEDGMENTS

This work was supported in part by funds from the U.S. Department of Veterans Affairs (the VA Medical Research Program, and the VA Connecticut-Massachusetts Mental Illness Research, Education and Clinical Center (MIRECC)), and NIMH grant K02-MH01387.

REFERENCES

1. American Psychiatric Association. Diagnostic & Statistical Manual for Mental Disorders (DSM), 3rd ed, revised. 1987. Washington: American Psychiatric Press.
2. Kessler RC, McGonagle KA, Zhao S, Nelson CB, Hughes M, Eshleman S, Wittchen H-U, Kendler KS. Lifetime and 12-month prevalence of psychiatric disorders in the United States: results from the National Comorbidity Survey. Arch Gen Psychiatry. 1994;51:8–19.
3. Wittchen H-U, Reed V, Kessler RC. The relationship of agoraphobia and panic in a community sample of adolescents and young adults. Arch Gen Psychiatry. 1998;55:1017–1024.
4. Kessler RC, Stein MB, Berglund PA. Social phobia subtypes in the National Comorbidity Survey. Am J Psychiatry. 1998;155:613–619.
5. American Psychiatric Association. Diagnostic & Statistical Manual for Mental Disorders (DSM), 4th ed. 1994. Washington: American Psychiatric Press.
6. Stein MB, Torgrud LJ, Walker JR. Social phobia symptoms, subtypes and severity: findings from a community survey. Arch Gen Psychiatry. 2000;57:1046–1052.
7. Eng W, Heimberg RG, Coles ME, Schneier FR, Liebowitz MR. An empirical approach to subtype identification in individuals with social phobia. Psychol Med. 2000;30:1345–1357.
8. Furmark T, Tillfors M, Stattin H, Ekselius L, Fredrikson M. Social phobia subtypes in the general population revealed by cluster analysis. Psychol Med. 2000;30:1335–1344.
9. Mendlowicz MV, Stein MB. Quality of life in individuals with anxiety disorders. Am J Psychiatry. 2000;157:669–682.
10. Magee WJ, Eaton WW, Wittchen H-U, McGonagle KA, Kessler RC. Agoraphobia, simple phobia, and social phobia in the National Comorbidity Survey. Arch Gen Psychiatry. 1996;53:159–168.
11. Kendler KS, Neale MC, Kessler RC, Heath AC, Eaves LJ. Panic disorder in women: A population-based twin study. Psychol Med. 1993;20:581–590.
12. Kendler KS, Karkowski LM, Prescott CA. Fears and phobias: reliability and heritability. Psychol Med. 1999;29:539–553.
13. Kendler KS, Myers J, Prescott CA, Neale MC. The genetic epidemiology of irrational fears and phobias in men. Arch Gen Psychiatry. 2001;58:257–265.
14. Smoller JW, Tsuang MT. Panic and phobic anxiety: defining phenotypes for genetic studies. Am J Psychiatry. 1998;155:1152–1162.
15. Noyes RJ, Crowe RR, Harris EL, Hamra BJ, McChesney CM, Chaudhry DR. Relationship between panic disorder and agoraphobia: a family study. Arch Gen Psychiatry. 1986;43:227–232.
16. Goldstein RB, Weissman MM, Adams PB, Horwath E, Lish JD, Charney D, Woods SW, Sobin C, Wickramaratne PJ. Psychiatric disorders in relatives of probands with panic disorder and/or major depression. Arch Gen Psychiatry. 1994;51:383–394.
17. Reich JH, Yates W. Family history of psychiatric disorders in social phobia. Compr Psychiatry. 1988;29:72–75.
18. Fyer AJ, Mannuzza S, Chapman TF, Liebowitz M, Klein DF. A direct-interview family study of social phobia. Arch Gen Psychiatry. 1993;50:286–293.
19. Stein MB, Chartier MJ, Hazen AL, Kozak MV, Tancer ME, Lander S, Chubaty D, Furer P, Walker JR. A direct-interview family study of generalized social phobia. Am J Psychiatry. 1998;155:90–97.
20. Chavira DA, Stein MB. Phenomenology and epidemiology of social phobia. In: Stein DJ, Hollander E, eds. *American Psychiatric Press Textbook of Anxiety Disorders*. Washington: American Psychiatric Press (in press).
21. Stein MB, Rapee RM. Anxiety sensitivity: is it all in the head? In: Taylor S, ed. *Anxiety Sensitivity: Theory, Research and Treatment of the Fear of Anxiety*. Mahwah, NJ: Lawrence Erlbaum Associates, 1998:199–215.
22. Cavallini MC, Perna G, Caldirola D, Bellodi L. A segregation study of panic disorder in families of panic patients responsive to the 35% CO_2 challenge. Biol Psychiatry. 1999;46:815–820.
23. Stein MB, Jang KL, Livesley WJ. Heritability of anxiety sensitivity: a twin study. Am J Psychiatry. 1999;156:246–251.
24. Pauls DL, Crowe RR, Noyes RJ. Distribution of ancestral secondary cases in anxiety neurosis (letter). J Affect Disord. 1979;1:287–290.
25. Pauls DL, Noyes RJ, Crowe RR. The familial prevalence in second-degree relatives of patients with

anxiety neurosis (panic disorder). J Affect Disord. 1979;1:279–285.
26. Hopper JL, Judd FK, Derrick PL, et al. A family study of panic disorder: reanalysis using a regressive logistic model that incorporates a sibship environment. Genet Epidemiol. 1990;7:151–161.
27. Harris EL, Noyes RJ, Crowe RR, Chaudhry DR. Family study of agoraphobia. Arch Gen Psychiatry. 1983;40:1061–1064.
28. Crowe RR, Noyes RJ, Pauls DL, Slymen D. A family study of panic disorder. Arch Gen Psychiatry. 1983;40:1065–1069.
29. Pauls DL, Bucher KD, Crowe RR, Noyes RJ. A genetic study of panic disorder pedigrees. Am J Hum Genet. 1980;32:639–644.
30. Vieland VJ, Goodman DW, Chapman T, Fyer AJ. A new segregation analysis of panic disorder. Am J Med Genet, 1996;67:146–153.
31. Haghighi F, Fyer AJ, Weissman MM, Knowles JA, Hodge SE. Parent-of-origin effect in panic disorder. Am J Med Genet (Neuropsychol Genet). 1999;88:131–135.
32. Gelernter J. Clinical molecular genetics of psychiatric illness. In: Charney DS, Nestler EJ, Bunney BS, eds. *Neurobiological Foundation of Mental Illness*. Oxford: Oxford University Press; 1999:108–120.
33. Risch N. Linkage strategies for genetically complex traits. II. The power of affected relatives pairs. Am J Hum Genet. 1990;46:229–241.
34. Risch N, Merikangas KR. The future of genetic studies of complex human disorders. Science. 1996;273:1516–1617.
35. Camp NJ. Genomewide transmission/disequilibrium testing—consideration of the genotypic relative risks at disease loci. Am J Hum Genet. 1997;61:1424–1430.
36. Falk CT, Rubinstein P. Haplotype relative risks: an easy reliable way to construct a proper control sample for risk calculations. Ann Hum Genet. 1987;51:227–233.
37. Terwilliger JD, Ott J. A haplotype-based 'Haplotype Relative Risk' approach to detecting allelic associations. Hum Hered. 1992;42:337–346.
38. Spielman RS, McGinnis RE, Ewens WJ. Transmission test for linkage disequilibrium: the insulin gene region and insulin-dependent diabetes mellitus (IDDM). Am J Hum Genet. 1993;52:506–516.
39. Pritchard JK, Stephens M, Rosenberg NA, Donnely P. Association mapping in structured populations. Am J Hum Genet. 2000;67:170–181.
40. Pritchard JK, Stephens M, Donnely P. Inference of population structure using multilocus genotype data. Genetics. 2000;155:945–959.
41. Thornsberry JM, Goodman MM, Doebley J, Kresovich S, Nielsen D, Buckler ESIV. Dwarf8 polymorphisms associate with variation in flowering time. Nat Genet. 2001;28:286–289.
42. Devlin B, Roeder K. Genomic control for association studies. Biometrics. 1999;55:997–1004.
43. Crowe RR, Noyes RJ, Wilson AF, et al. A linkage study of panic disorder. Arch Gen Psychiatry. 1987;44:933–937.
44. Crowe RR, Noyes RJ, Samuelson S, et al. Close linkage between panic disorder and α-haptoglobin excluded in 10 families. Arch Gen Psychiatry. 1990;47:377–380.
45. Mutchler K, Crowe RR, Noyes RJ, Wesner R. Exclusion of the tyrosine hydroxylase gene in 14 panic disorder pedigrees. Am J Psychiatry. 1990;147:1367–1369.
46. Wang ZW, Crowe RR, Noyes RJ. Adrenergic receptor genes as candidate genes for panic disorder: a linkage study. Am J Psychiatry. 1992;149:470–474.
47. Schmidt SM, Zoega T, Crowe RR. Excluding linkage between panic disorder and the gamma-aminobutyric acid beta 1 receptor locus in five Icelandic pedigrees. Acta Psychiatr Scand. 1993;88:225–228.
48. Crowe RR, Wang Z, Noyes RJJ, Albrecht BE, Darlison MG, Bailey ME, Johnson KJ, Zoega T. Candidate gene study of eight $GABA_A$ receptor subunits in panic disorder. Am J Psychiatry. 1997;154:1096–1100.
49. Ohara K, Xie D-W, Ishigaki T, Deng Z-L, Nakamura Y, Suzuki Y, Miyasato K. The genes encoding the $5HT_{1Da}$ and $5HT_{1Db}$ receptors are unchanged in patients with panic disorder. Biol Psychiatry. 1996;39:5–10.
50. Deckert J, Nöthen MM, Franke P, Delmo C, Fritze J, Knapp M, Maier W, Beckmann H, Propping P. Systematic mutation screening and association study of the A1 and A2a adenosine receptor genes in panic disorder suggest a contribution of the A2a gene to the development of disease. Mol Psychiatry. 1998;3:81–85.
51. Kato T, Wang ZW, Zoega T, Crowe RR. Missense mutation of the cholecystokinin B receptor gene: lack of association with panic disorder. Am J Med Genet (Neuropsychol Genet). 1996;67:401–405.
52. Wang Z, Valdes J, Noyes RJ, Zoega T, Crowe RR. Possible association of a cholecystokinin promoter polymorphism (CCK_{-36CT}) with panic disorder. Am J Med Genet (Neuropsychol Genet). 1998;81:228–234.
53. Kennedy JL, Bradwejn J, Koszycki D, King N, Crowe RR, Vincent J, Fourie O. Investigation of cholecystokinin system genes in panic disorder. Mol Psychiatry. 1999;4:284–285.
54. Paterson AD, Sunohara GA, Kennedy JL. Dopamine D4 receptor gene: novelty or nonsense? Neuropsychopharmacology. 1999;21:3–16.
55. Hamilton SP, Slager SL, Helleby L, Heiman GA, Klein DF, Hodge SE, Weissman MM, Fyer AJ, Knowles JA. No association or linkage between polymorphisms in the genes encoding cholecystokinin and

56. Gelernter J, Bonvicini KA, Page G, Woods SW, Goddard AW, Kruger S, Pauls DL, Goodson S. Linkage genome scan for loci predisposing to panic disorder or agoraphobia. Am J Med Genet (Neuropsychol Genet). 2001; 105:548–557.
57. Hattori E, Ebihara M, Yamada K, Ohba H, Shibuya H, Yoshikawa T. Identification of a compound short tandem repeat stretch in the 5′-upstream region of the cholecystokinin gene, and its association with panic disorder but not with schizophrenia. Mol Psychiatry. 2001;6:465–470.
58. Hamilton SP, Haghighi F, Heiman GA, Klein DF, Hodge SE, Fyer AJ, Weissman MM, Knowles JA. Investigation of dopamine receptor (DRD4) and dopamine transporter (DAT) polymorphisms for genetic linkage or association to panic disorder. Am J Med Genet (Neuropsychol Genet). 2000;96:324–330.
59. Stein MB, Chartier MJ, Kozak MV, Hazen AL, King N, Kennedy JL. Genetic linkage to the serotonin transporter and 5HT2A receptor excluded in generalized social phobia. Psychiatry Res. 1998;81:283–291.
60. Knowles JA, Fyer AJ, Vieland VJ, Weissman MM, Hodge SE, Heiman GA, Haghighi F, De Jesus GM, Rassnick H, Preud'homme-Rivelli X, Austin T, Cunjack J, Mick S, Fine JD, Woodley KA, Das K, Maier W, Adams PB, Freimer NB, Klein DF, Gilliam TC. Results of a genome-wide genetic screen for panic disorder. Am J Med Genet (Neuropsychol Genet). 1998;81:139–147.
61. Crowe RR, Goedken R, Samuelson S, Wilson R, Nelson J, Noyes RJJ. Genomewide survey of panic disorder. Am J Med Genet (Neuropsychol Genet). 2001;105:105–109.
62. Smoller JW, Acierno JS Jr, Rosenbaum JF, Biederman J, Pollack MH, Meminger SR, Pava JA, Chadwick LH, White C, Bulzacchelli M, Slaugenhaupt SA. Targeted genome screen of panic disorder and anxiety disorder proneness using homology to murine QTL regions. Am J Med Genet (Neuropsychol Genet). 2001;105:195–206.
63. Bradwejn J, Koszycki D, Shriqui C. Enhanced sensitivity to cholecystokinin tetrapeptide in panic disorder. Clinical and behavioral findings. Arch Gen Psychiatry. 1991;48:603–610.
64. Bradwejn J, Koszycki D, Couetoux du Tertre A, van Megen H, den Boer J, Westenberg H. The panicogenic effects of cholecystokinin-tetrapeptide are antagonized by L-365,260, a central cholecystokinin receptor antagonist, in patients with panic disorder. Arch Gen Psychiatry. 1994;51:486–493.
65. Weissman MM, Fyer AJ, Haghighi F, Heiman G, Deng Z, Hen R, Hodge SE, Knowles JA. Potential panic disorder syndrome: cinical and genetic linkage evidence. Am J Med Genet (Neuropsychol Genet). 2000;96:24–35.
66. Lesch K-P, Bengel D, Heils A, Sabol SA, Greenberg BD, Petri S, Benjamin J, Müller CR, Hamer DH, Murphy DL. Association of anxiety-related traits with a polymorphism in the serotonin transporter gene regulatory region. Science. 1996;274:1527–1531.
67. Greenberg BD, Li Q, Lucas FR, Hu S, Sirota LA, Benjamin J, Lesch K-P, Hamer DH, Murphy DL. Association between the serotonin transporter promoter polymorphism and personality traits in a primarily female population sample. Am J Med Genet (Neuropsychol Genet). 2000;96:202–216.
68. Pulver AE, Nestadt G, Goldberg R, Shprintzen RJ, Lamacz M, Wolyniec PS, Morrow B, Karayiorgou M, Antonarakis SE, Housman DE, Kucherlapati R. Psychotic illness in patients diagnosed with velo-cardio-facial syndrome and their relatives. J Nerv Ment Dis. 1994;182:476–478.
69. Karayiorgou M, Morris MA, Morrow B, Shprintzen RJ, Goldberg R, Borrow J, Gos A, Nestadt G, Wolyniec PS, Lasseter VK, Eisen H, Childs B, Kazazian HH, Kucherlapati R, Antonarakis SE, Pulver AE, Housman DE. Schizophrenia susceptibility associated with interstitial deletions of chromosome 22q11. Proc Natl Acad Sci USA. 1995;92:7612–7616.
70. Smalley SL, McCracken J, Tanguay P. Autism, affective disorders, and social phobia. Am J Med Gen. 1995;60:19–26.
71. Murphy M, Bolton PF, Pickles A, Fombonne E, Piven J, Rutter M. Personality traits of the relatives of autistic probands. Psychol Med. 2000;30:1411–1424.
72. Swift RG, Polymeropoulos MH, Torres R, Swift M. Predisposition of Wolfram syndrome heterozygotes to psychiatric illness. Mol Psychiatry. 1998;3:86–91.
73. Khare L, Strizheva GD, Bailey JN, Au K-S, Northrup H, Smith M, Smalley SL, Henske EP. A novel missense mutation in the GTPase activating protein homology region of TSC2 in two large families with tuberous sclerosis complex. J Med Genet. 2001;38:347–349.
74. Kendler KS, Kessler RC, Walters EE, Maclean C, Neale MC, Heath AC, Eaves LJ. Stressful life events, genetic liability, and onset of an episode of major depression in women. Am J Psychiatry. 1995;152:833–842.
75. Krueger RF. The structure of mental disorders. Arch Gen Psychiatry. 1999;56:921–926.
76. Vollebergh WAM, Iedema J, Bijil RV, de Graaf R, Smit F, Ormel J. The structure and stability of common mental disorders: the NEMESIS study. Arch Gen Psychiatry. 2001;58:597–603.

77. Stein MB, Jang KL, Livesley WJ. Heritability of social-anxiety related concerns and personality characteristics: A twin study. (submitted for publication). 2001.
78. Smoller JW, Rosenbaum JF, Biederman J, et al. Genetic association analysis of behavioral inhibition using candidate loci from mouse models. Am J Med Genet (Neuropsychol Genet). 2001;105:226–235.
79. Martin C, Cabrol S, Bouvard MP, Lepine JP, Mouren-Siméoni MC. Anxiety and depressive disorders in fathers and mothers of anxious school-refusing children. J Am Acad Child Adolesc Psychiatry. 1999;38:916–922.
80. Dummit ESI, Klein RG, Tancer NK, Asche B, Martin J, Fairbank JA. Systematic assessment of 50 children with selective mutism. J Am Acad Child Adolesc Psychiatry. 1997;36:653–660.

33

Imaging Brain Structure and Function in Aging and Alzheimer's Disease

VICENTE IBÁÑEZ
University of Geneva, Geneva, Switzerland

STANLEY I. RAPOPORT
National Institute on Aging, National Institutes of Health, Bethesda, Maryland, U.S.A

I. INTRODUCTION

A. Definition of Healthy Aging

An increase in life expectancy in industrialized countries has been accompanied by an increased prevalence of dementia, particularly of Alzheimer's disease (AD). Indeed, it has been asked, "If we live long enough, will we all be demented?" [1,2]. AD contributes to marked functional as well as social and economic burdens in the later years of life. Distinguishing AD in its early stages from the aging process has become an important imperative in medicine, as it might allow initiating treatment before irreversible neuronal and functional losses occur [3,4]. New methods for in vivo structural and functional imaging of brain provide promise for distinguishing AD from brain aging, for the differential diagnosis of AD, and for evaluating therapeutic efficacy as AD progresses.

Confusion exists, however, about the distinction between "healthy" and "normal" brain aging. The distinction has changed over the years, as more sophisticated noninvasive in vivo techniques (e.g., computer assisted tomography [CT], magnetic resonance imaging [MRI], single-photon emission computed tomography [SPECT], noninvasive angiography) have been developed to identify underlying brain structural and functional deficits, or disease states that may affect brain. Normal aging might be considered in epidemiological terms, referring to aging changes that occur generally in a population that is not overtly demented or has overt strokes. In contrast, healthy aging refers to brain age changes in a population in which functional or structural brain pathology and underlying

Abbreviations: AD, Alzheimer's disease; AIR, automated image registration; CMRglc, global cerebral metabolic rate for glucose; CSF, cerebrospinal fluid; CT, computer assisted tomography; DG, 2-fluoro-2-deoxy-D-glucose; MRI, magnetic resonance imaging; PET, positron emission tomography; PVE, partial volume effect; rCBF, regional cerebral blood flow; rCMRglc, regional cerebral metabolic rate for glucose; rCMRO$_2$, regional cerebral metabolic rate for oxygen; rOEF, regional oxygen extraction fraction; SPECT, single-photon emission computed tomography; SPM, statistical parametric mapping.

disease states have been excluded by the newer techniques [5,6]. It now is recognized that hypertension and other cardiac abnormalities, trauma, diabetes, vitamin B_{12} deficiency, and thyroid disease, for example, can contribute to brain defects in the elderly [7–12].

B. Characterization of Brain Aging and AD

Brain adaptive changes occur during human aging, because the senescent nervous system can undergo significant neuroplastic changes. Neuroplasticity has been demonstrated at the level of cellular and macroscopic neuroanatomy [13–17], at the biochemical level [18], and when measuring metabolism and function by in vivo imaging [19]. Although marked neuronal loss in the cortex had been thought to accompany human aging, recent studies suggest that neuronal loss, while present, is not dramatic [20]. Some cortical pyramidal neurons decline in size, and their synapse density falls. For example, in the hippocampal formation, decreases of the dendritic tree have been observed in the very old [21,22], and reduced synaptic density in the frontal lobe has been reported [23,24]. However, the dendritic tree also may be increased in the senescent brain [15,21], consistent with neuroplastic compensation.

Brain aging may be associated with losses in certain neurotransmitter systems. Neuronal loss in the substantia nigra can be substantial and be accompanied by decreased striatal dopamine uptake and fewer dopaminergic D_1 receptors in prefrontal cortex and striatum. These changes are considered responsible for some motor and cognitive age declines [25,26]. Cholinergic dysfunction has been proposed to explain memory changes with aging [27,28], and cholinergic therapy has been shown to enhance timing of memory performance in brain [29].

Some cognitive features, referred to as "fluid intelligence" and including perceptual speed, memory span, and associative memory, usually decline with age, whereas others, referred to as "crystallized intelligence," including verbal comprehension, general information, and arithmetic skills, may remain intact [30]. This suggests that a large part of cognitive processing, related to ability to cope with the environment, is preserved in healthy older people [31]. Language can be affected but not consistently [32,33]. Declines have been reported in memory storage [34] and in some components of working memory [35,36]. Some reductions in memory test scores have been described as "age-associated memory impairment," others as a pathological "mild cognitive impairment" [37–40].

Overt dementia affects about 6–8% of individuals older than 65 years of age; AD contributes to two-thirds of these cases and is frequently associated with the pathology of vascular dementia [41,42]. AD is a slowly progressive neurodegenerative disease in which memory declines in the presence of normal vigilance [8], but changes in attention, language, or visual abilities, or neuropsychiatric disturbances, also can be presenting features [43–45]. Individual rates of general cognitive decline can vary widely among AD patients [46]. With disease progression in usual cases, problems of language, calculation, visuospatial function, and praxis become evident, and memory loss is accentuated [47]. Using the Mini-Mental State Examination, the stages of dementia in AD can be classified as mild (score 30–21), moderate (20–11) or severe (10–0) [48]. Neuropsychiatric disturbances such as depression, agitation, delusions, and hallucinations may occur at any time during the illness, but they are most frequent at late stages [43,45,49].

Using NINCDS-ADRDA or other criteria, AD can be diagnosed in life with an accuracy of 80–90% [50–52]. A "definite" diagnosis, however, requires histopathological demonstration of large numbers of senile (neuritic) plaques and neurofibrillary tangles within the brain on biopsy or postmortem [53]. Neuronal and synaptic losses are quite significant [54–57]. Markers of all neurotransmitter systems are affected, but particularly those of the cholinergic system [58–60].

Neuropathology in AD is most severe in association neocortex, cingulate cortex, corticobasolateral nucleus of amygdaloid complex, entorhinal cortex, and posterior hippocampus, as well as in certain neurotransmitter specific nuclei connected to these regions (substantia nigra, nucleus basalis of Meynert). These compose a "telencephalic association system" that, comparative studies indicate, expanded and differentiated during primate, but particularly, during human evolution. That AD pathology is fully evident only in the human brain, and that in vivo imaging shows earliest metabolic changes in brain association neocortex (see below), suggest that AD is a phylogenic disease which was introduced during primate evolution [61–66].

C. In Vivo Imaging Techniques

In vivo brain imaging can help in the early diagnosis of AD, in distinguishing AD from healthy aging [67–72], and in characterizing AD in individual subjects in relation to cognitive changes and perhaps therapy [73–76]. Structural imaging techniques include CT and MRI. Functional methods include positron emission tomography (PET), SPECT, magnetic resonance spectroscopy (MRS), and functional magnetic resonance imaging (fMRI) [77]. PET and SPECT both depend on gamma ray emission, but PET has higher sensitivity and spatial resolution than SPECT and is not subject to inhomogeneities that prevent absolute quantification of regional radioactivity [75,78,79].

Data obtained using CT or MRI can be used to calculate volumes or areas of specific brain regions, and the fractional contributions of white matter, gray matter, and cerebrospinal fluid (CSF) to these volumes (segmentation analysis) [80–84]. Evidence obtained in this way indicates that aging is accompanied by volume losses in certain brain structures, including the basal ganglia and thalamus, accompanied by increased ventricular and intrasulcal CSF spaces [85–95]. But age differences in volumes of some structures (e.g., temporal lobe) are not always found [96]. Furthermore, cross-sectional values for regional brain or CSF volumes in mildly and moderately demented AD patients can overlap with values in age-matched controls, limiting their utility for diagnosis. On the other hand, serial longitudinal measurements and discriminant analysis of data can better distinguish AD from the aging process [86,97–99]. In AD, volume changes are more severe and they progress at faster rates than in age-matched controls.

PET allows measuring regional cerebral metabolic rates for glucose (rCMRglc) and for oxygen (rCMRO$_2$), receptor densities and binding constants, regional cerebral blood flow (rCBF), and the regional oxygen extraction fraction (rOEF), depending on the radiotracer employed. Many PET studies have described metabolic and flow changes with brain aging [reviewed by 75,100–102]. Health status was ignored in many studies, although the critical importance of health status was clearly demonstrated in early studies of global brain metabolism and flow using an inert gas, nitrous oxide (NO) [7,103]. These studies showed that certain disease conditions (e.g., hypertension, organic brain disease, arteriosclerosis) reduced brain flow and metabolism and should be excluded in studies of "healthy" aging.

Additionally, PET-derived metabolic or flow rates usually are calculated per volume element (voxel) within a brain image. The voxel may contain white matter, gray matter, and cerebrospinal fluid (CSF). The CSF fraction can alter the estimate of tissue radioactivity within the volume by producing a "partial voluming effect" (PVE). Furthermore, if the CSF fraction were to increase with age or disease, owing to tissue loss (atrophy), a calculated decline in metabolism or flow per *volume* brain might reflect increased CSF alone, as metabolism or flow per *gram* brain may not change. Thus, methods must be employed to correct for the PVE if we wish to understand intrinsic metabolic or flow changes in brain tissue.

Reviews of PET studies that ignored the PVE can be found elsewhere [75, 100–102]. Some few PET studies of aging have tried to correct flow or metabolism measurements for brain atrophy, when using approximation methods [82,104]. We will emphasize in this review only PET studies done in the resting state in nonhypertensive healthy subjects, particularly the studies that corrected for the PVE exactly. Exact PVE-corrected PET shows no statistically significant age difference in rCMRglc, whereas in AD the pattern of regional brain hypometabolism is the same whether or not an exact PVE correction is performed.

II. EXPLORING BRAIN FUNCTION

A. Relations of Cerebral Blood Flow, Metabolism, and Functional Activity

The brain produces the energy necessary for its functioning by oxidizing glucose. Although the adult human brain constitutes 2% of body weight, it consumes ∼ 20% of the glucose consumed by the body as a whole [105]. Energy is produced in the form of ATP by glycolysis but mainly by oxidative metabolism within mitochondria. ATP is required for active ion transport for synthesis of proteins and other products and for maintaining dynamic metabolism of brain lipids [105–107]. It has long been recognized, therefore, that regional brain functional activity can be examined by measuring regional brain metabolism or the rCBF which is coupled to metabolism [108–111].

One hypothesis regarding brain energy consumption derives from studies of cultured astrocytes exposed to glutamate [112,113]. According to this interpretation, glutamate, the main excitatory amino acid neurotransmitter in brain, is released into the synaptic cleft during neuronal activity and binds to postsynaptic receptors. The glutamate is then transported to neighboring astrocytes where it stimulates incorporation of glucose into astrocytic end feet. The glucose is converted to lactate, then is returned to synaptic terminals for conversion to pyruvate, a substrate for oxidative phosphorylation and ATP formation. The glutamate in the astrocytes uses two ATPs to produce glutamine and reestablish the Na$^+$ gradient across the astrocyte membrane.

B. Positron Emission Tomography (PET)

PET can image regional functional activity by quantifying rCMRglc, rCMRO$_2$, or rCBF. The PET method involves the intravenous injection of a radiotracer that can be utilized for one of these parameters, quantifying its incorporation into brain with a scanner, then fitting time-variant brain and blood data to equations derived from representative models. The injected radiotracer contains positron-emitting isotopes that have short radioactive half-lives (minutes to hours), including ^{15}O, ^{11}C, ^{18}F, and ^{13}N. Positrons (particles with same mass as an electron but positively charged) interact (undergo annihilation) with electrons to release a pair of photons at 180° to each other. Their location in brain can be identified by coincidence counting with a scanner.

A labeled molecule is injected intravenously into a subject whose head is positioned within a circular array of detectors. Each detector, consisting of a crystal scintillator and a photomultiplier, transforms the gamma rays produced by annihilation into an electric current. Depending on their array, PET devices can acquire signals in two or three dimensions [114,115]. Algorithms are used to construct activity images (emission scans) from accumulated counts. The images are composed of volumes or "voxels" of radioactivity. To convert volume images (radioactivity/mL) to "intrinsic" tissue images (radioactivity/g tissue), it is necessary to submit the data to an exact PVE correction (see below).

After the tracer is injected, serial scans are acquired (dynamic frames) to reconstruct regional tissue time-activity curves. Brain radioactivity will depend on the arterial input function, the ability of the tracer to cross the blood-brain barrier (extraction), and its distribution in different brain compartments (blood, extracellular, intracellular, metabolic, bound). Differential equations derived from compartmental models are fitted to the data to estimate appropriate kinetic constants, using iterative techniques such as the Marquardt algorithm [116]. Regional blood volume normally is taken as 4% of brain volume.

C. Cerebral Blood Flow

Delivery of a highly diffusible tracer from blood to brain will depend on rCBF [117] and tracer extraction by brain [118]. The most common technique to measure rCBF with PET involves the intravenous injection of labeled water (H$_2$^{15}O) and the application of a two-compartment model to estimate two constants (Fig. 1) [117,119–121]. K$_1$ is related to rCBF and the extraction

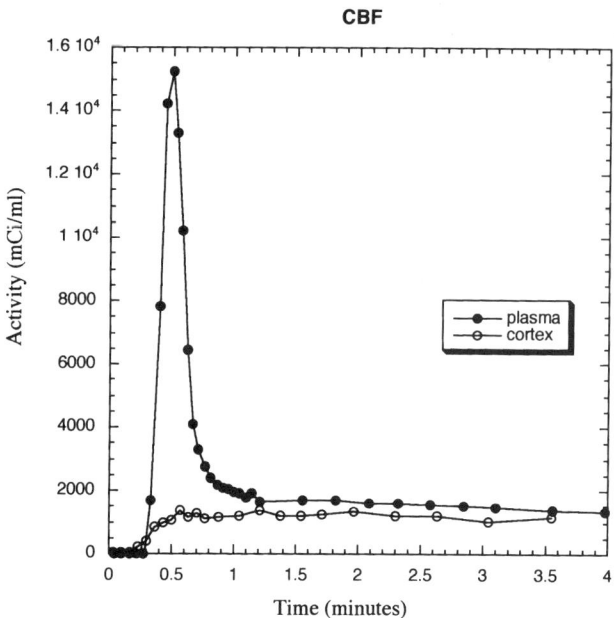

Figure 1 Cerebral blood flow model. The differential equation of the model is: $dCp/dt = K_1 Cp - k_2 Ct$, where $K_1 = F E = F(1 - e^{-PS/F})$; $k_2 = K_1/V_d$. F, cerebral blood flow; E, extraction fraction; V$_d$, volume of distribution of H$_2$^{15}O at equilibrium; Ct, concentration H$_2$^{15}O measured with PET in brain; Cp, arterial blood concentration of H$_2$^{15}O. E is directly related to regional capillary permeability-surface area product, PS. The distribution volume is defined as the equilibrium ratio of tracer in tissue to tracer in blood.

fraction, k$_2$ to back-diffusion of H$_2$^{15}O from brain to blood. rCBF can range from 50–100 mL/min/100 mL tissue in gray matter to 15–40 mL/min/100 mL tissue in white matter. rCBF is nearly linearly related to PET activity counts [122], so some researchers use only tissue counts due to ^{15}O-labeled water to assess relative rCBF differences within brain.

D. Deoxyglucose Model

To measure rCMRglc, a tracer analog of glucose, [^{18}F]2-fluoro-2-deoxy-D-glucose ([^{18}F]DG), is injected intravenously [111,123]. Like glucose, [^{18}F]DG is transported across the blood-brain barrier by a monosaccharide carrier mechanism [118] and then is rapidly phosphorylated by brain hexokinase to [^{18}F]DG-6-phosphate. Unlike glucose-6-phosphate, [^{18}F]DG-6-phosphate cannot undergo glycolysis and thus accumulates in brain [124]. A small amount, however, may be hydrolyzed back to [^{18}F]DG by glucose-6-phosphatase.

The [^{18}F]DG model used by us is presented in Figure 2 [123]. It has four rate constants. K_1 and k_2 have been discussed with regard to rCBF (see above); k_3 represents the fraction of [^{18}F]DG converted to [^{18}F]DG-6-phosphate per unit time; k_4, the fraction of [^{18}F]DG-6-phosphate hydrolyzed back to [^{18}F]DG per unit time. PET images are analyzed using a modification of the operational equation of Sokoloff [111,125], with a lumped constant of 0.42.

III. IMAGE PROCESSING OF PET DATA

A. Talairach Space

Differences between mean values of rCBF or rCMRglc can be determined using region of interest (ROI) or voxel-by-voxel comparisons. With the latter method, image processing must be performed. This consists of image registration and transformation into stereotactic space, followed by statistical analysis to assess statistical significance of mean differences.

To compare experimental conditions, therefore, effects of head motion must be reduced by aligning PET scans in the subject's brain space. This is done by matching landmarks or surface characteristics directly in different scans [126,127], or by employing an automated image registration (AIR) algorithm [128,129]. The common "Talairach space" is a published stereotactic atlas of a human brain [130]. Its origin is at the anterior commissure (x = 0, y = 0, z = 0), and its x-z planes are parallel to the plane of the anterior and posterior commissure. Registration uses a 12-parameter affine transformation and rescaling along the x, y, and z axes defined by landmarks of the Talairach space. Nonlinear algorithms for spatial transformation are also available [131].

B. Statistical Parametric Mapping

A widely used image registration procedure is statistical parametric mapping (SPM) [131–134]. In addition to realigning scans, SPM can normalize PET scans into

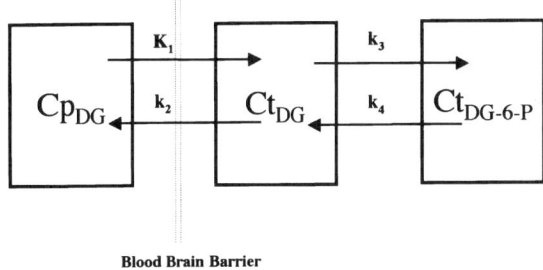

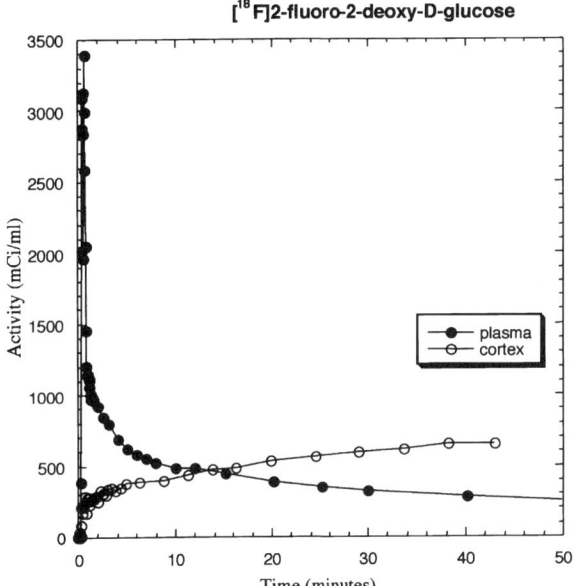

Figure 2 Deoxyglucose model. The differential equations of the model are: $dCt_{DG}/dt = K_1Cp_{DG} - k_2Ct_{DG} - k_3Ct_{DG} + k_4Ct_{DG-6-P}$; $dCt_{DG-6-P}/dt = k_3Ct_{DG} - k4Ct_{DG-6-P}$; $d(Ct_{DG} + Ct_{DG-6-P})/dt = K_1Cp_{DG} - k_2Ct_{DG}$. To calculate the regional cerebral metabolic rate for glucose: $rCMRglc = (C_PG/LC)(K_1k_3/(k_2 + k_3))$, Ct_{DG} is the concentration of the [^{18}F]2-fluoro-2-deoxy-D-glucose; Ct_{DG-6-P} is the concentration of the tracer [^{18}F]2-fluoro-2-deoxy-D-glucose-6-phosphate; $Ct_{DG} + Ct_{DG-6-P}$ is the total tissue tracer concentration as measured with PET; Cp_{DG} is the arterial blood plasma concentration of [^{18}F]2-fluoro-2-deoxy-D-glucose; C_{PG} is the arterial blood concentration of glucose; LC is the lumped constant.

Talairach space and perform statistical comparisons for different conditions (rest vs. task) or different groups for the same condition (patients vs. controls). SPM can test for significant differences between voxels by taking into account existing correlations between voxels (smoothness of image) using the theory of Gaussian random fields. A t value is calculated and substituted at the site of the compared voxels to obtain an image of t-statistics, the SPM(t) map. Because of the few degrees of freedom due to the limited number of scans in a PET study, the SPM(t) map does not have a Gaussian distribution. The t value for each voxel is therefore transformed into a Z value to obtain an SPM(z) map, which is more appropriate for Gaussian fields statistics. Voxels with Z values above a significance threshold are characterized by their number and/or intensity (maximal value of Z to reach threshold). A 2D analysis of PET data (suprathreshold ellipsoid) can then be used to find the number of expected foci above a given threshold. Alternatively, the Euler characteristic (the number of blobs minus the number of holes) [135] can be used to detect the number of significant foci and then do a 3D analysis. A probability, corrected for multiple comparisons, is calculated from parameters such as smoothness of the SPM map, volume, and dimension of the map [131,135]. To apply Gaussian random field theory to PET images, voxel size should be made small relative to smoothness of the field by smoothing PET images in the three spatial coordinates. Dimensions of the PET image should be greater than the smoothness of the field.

C. Correcting for the Partial Volume Effect (PVE)

Calculated differences in PET-derived mean rCMRglc or rCBF may not reflect actual differences per gram tissue, but only measured differences in radioactivity per volume PET image, if attention is not paid to atrophy correction. This is because of the PVE (see above). If a group mean difference were solely a consequence of atrophy, it should become insignificant after a PVE correction. If not, it should remain statistically significant even after the correction [83].

To correct PET rCMRglc data for the PVE, the MRI of each subject's skull is stripped (removed) manually from his brain MRI image. Edited images are then segmented into gray matter, white matter, and CSF, using an algorithm accounting for random noise and magnetic field inhomogeneities [84]. Gray plus white matter excluding CSF is defined as brain tissue (Fig. 3), and CSF radioactivity is taken as 0. Coregistration of the subject's MRI to his PET scan is performed with AIR software. PET metabolic values are corrected for the PVE using an algorithm that considers dispersion due to the point-spread function of the PET system (Fig. 3) [83,136–138]. SPM then is used to assess significance of differences between the groups, before and after correction for the PVE, using a voxel-based analysis [137].

IV. BRAIN METABOLISM AND AGING

A. Prior Studies Without an Atrophy Correction

The literature abounds with contradictory conclusions regarding age differences in brain metabolism or rCBF [100,102,139]. Different health selection criteria likely contributed to some of the reported differences, as age-related diseases can by themselves reduce flow and metabolism and cause atrophy [7,11,12]. Different sensory conditions during PET also may have contributed. Visual contrast sensitivity, auditory acuity, and other sensory modalities decline with age [140–142]. Auditory or visual stimulation can produce widespread cortical metabolic increases [143,144]. Thus, PET studies not performed in the "resting state" when visual and auditory inputs are reduced may reflect age differences in sensory input rather than intrinsic brain differences. A few investigators have paid attention to both health status and resting state in PET aging studies [5,100,104]. Using a high-resolution PET camera, the best conclusion from these studies is that statistically significant declines in (non-PVE-corrected) rCMRglc or global CMRglc of the order of 12% can be demonstrated between the ages of 20 and 70 in healthy subjects [100].

Ignoring health status and/or resting state in cross-sectional studies, Martin et al. [145] found no age difference in global CBF but decreased rCBF in some regions, including the anterior and posterior cingulate cortex. Marchal et al. [146] and Burns and Tyrell [147] reported age-reduced rCMRO$_2$ in some cortical regions. Additionally, decreases in rCMRglc with age were reported in frontal, parietal, and temporal cortical regions [145,148–152]. Declines on the order of 6% per decade, between 20 and 70 years of age, have been reported for rCMRO$_2$ and rCMRglc [146,153].

B. Atrophy-Corrected rCMRglc Is Age Invariant

The question remains whether even the small, 10–12% age declines in atrophy-uncorrected rCMRglc or CMRglc, noted in healthy subjects studied in the resting state with a high-resolution camera [100], represented actual declines per gram tissue or reflected age-related brain atrophy. If calculated decreases are solely a consequence of atrophy, they should become insignificant after a PVE correction. If they are real, they should remain statistically significant even after the correction. To test this question, we used PET to quantify

Brain Structure and Function in Aging

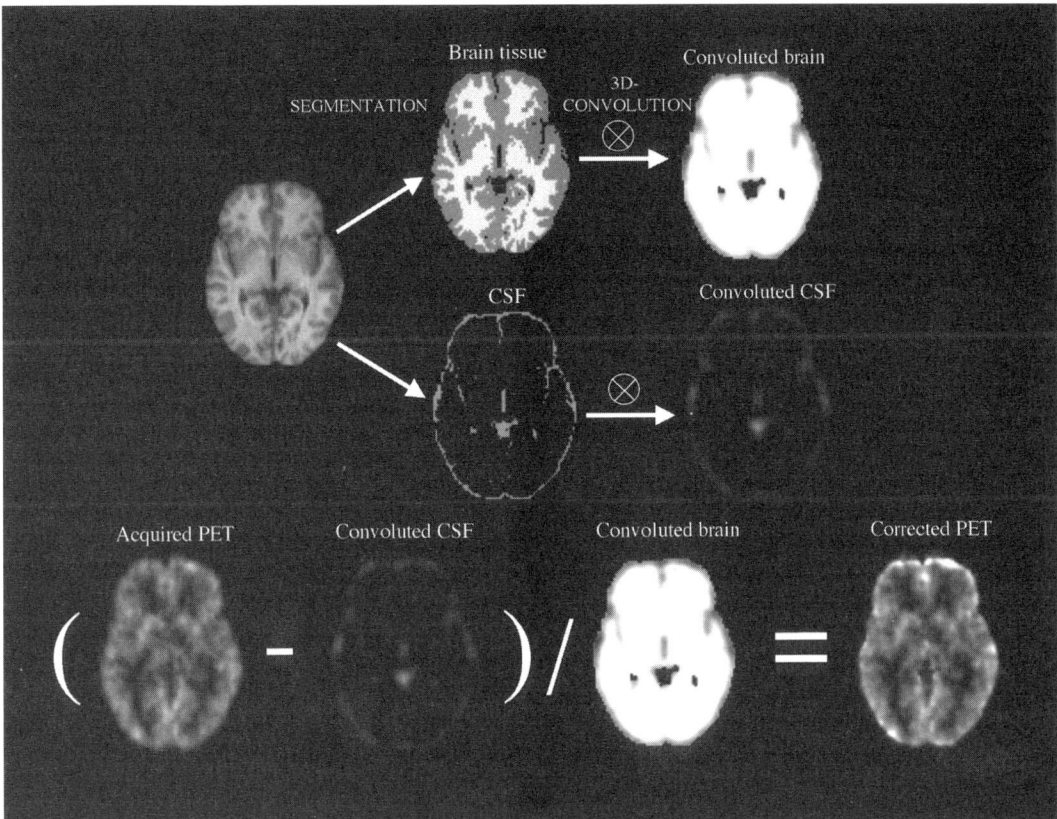

Figure 3 Algorithm for the partial volume effect (PVE) correction on voxel-by-voxel basis. To correct the rCMRglc PET image for the PVE, the MRI image first is segmented into brain tissue (gray and white matter) and CSF. A 3D convolution is applied to a binary image of brain tissue. The 3D convolution also can be applied to CSF image where all pixels have the average value of CSF radioactivity measured on the PET image. The convoluted CSF image is subtracted from the acquired PET image and the result is divided by the convoluted brain image to obtain the atrophy-corrected PET image. If the CSF average activity is considered negligible (0), the atrophy correction is achieved by directly dividing the acquired PET image by the convoluted brain image.

rCMRglc in healthy subjects studied in the resting state, when the data were analyzed with or without the PVE correction described in Section III.C [154].

Thirty healthy adults whose eyes were covered and ears plugged with cotton were screened to exclude hypertension and other conditions that might contribute to brain disease [154]. They were divided into a young group (11 men, aged 22–34) and an old group (13 men, 6 women, aged 55–84). Their cognitive integrity was assured by a normal Mini Mental State Examination score [48] and by normal scores on additional psychometric tests. rCMRglc was measured with a PC-2048 scanner (Scanditronix, Uppsala, Sweden), using arterial sampling. PET images were analyzed using a modification of the operational equation of Sokoloff [111,125] and a lumped constant of 0.42.

The PVE correction was performed as described in Section II.C. Gray plus white matter excluding CSF was defined as brain tissue (Fig. 3), and CSF radioactivity was taken as 0. PET values were corrected for the PVE using an algorithm that considers dispersion due to the point spread function of the PET system (Fig. 3). Examples of PVE-corrected scans from a control subject and an AD patient are presented in Figure 4.

SPM was used to assess statistically significant differences before and after correction for the PVE, using a voxel-by-voxel analysis [137]. Without the PVE correction, mean global CMRglc (in units of mg/100 mL brain/min) did not differ significantly between the old (8.02 ± 1.22 SD) and young (8.68 ± 1.30 SD) groups. After the correction, the difference (in mg/100 g brain/min) remained statistically insignificant (9.11 ± 1.39

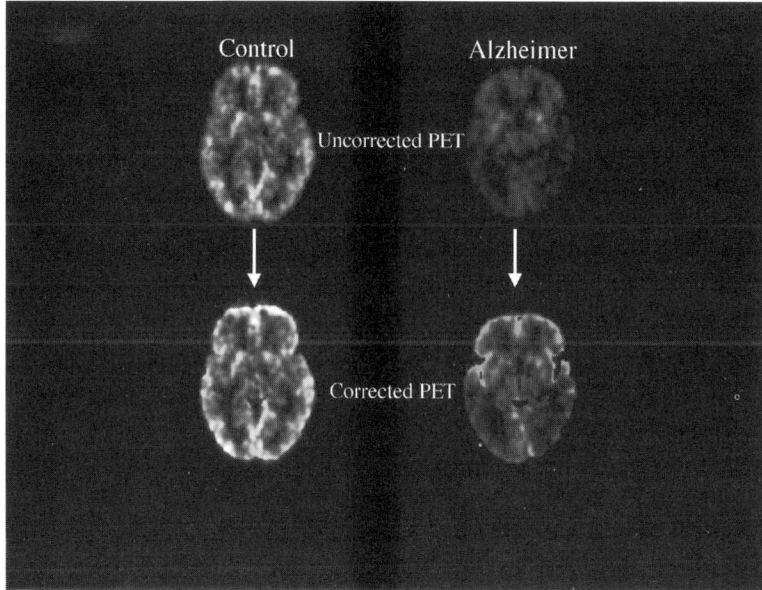

Figure 4 Example of partial volume correction for a control subject and an AD patient. The correction of metabolic values is greater over frontal areas than parietal areas in both subjects.

for the old group; 9.63 ± 1.51 for the young group). On the other hand, without the PVE correction, rCMRglc was decreased significantly in the older group in the left and right anterior insula close to the lateral prefrontal cortex, left supratemporal gyrus, and anterior cingulate cortex, regions close to CSF spaces and thus most susceptible to a PVE. After the correction, rCMRglc was significantly less in the old than in the young group only in the cingulate cortex (Fig. 5). Even the significance of this difference disappeared when men only were compared in both groups. In another study, a reduced uncorrected global CBF in older subjects was shown to be largely, although not entirely, due to atrophy [155]. Together, these analyses suggest that reported age declines in rCMRglc in healthy subjects, if uncorrected for the PVE, do not reflect intrinsic reductions in glucose metabolism per gram brain, but only the effect of tissue loss (atrophy).

V. BRAIN METABOLISM AND AD

A. Brain Pathology, Function, and Structure in AD

Numerous cross-sectional PET studies have been performed on AD patients; many are summarized in detail elsewhere [75]. The different data were obtained with scanners differing in anatomic resolution (full width/half maximum (FWHM) of line spread function), sensitivity, or attenuation correction. Patients also differed with regard to dementia severity and scanning conditions, and, like the controls, had different levels of medical screening. Despite these differences, the overall picture is remarkably consistent. Metabolic and flow reductions in AD occur throughout the neocortex, more so in association than in primary sensorimotor neocortical areas. Reductions are more severe in relation to dementia severity, ranging from about 17% in the prefrontal association cortex of mildly demented patients to about 54% in the parietal association cortex of severely demented patients.

An informative study with a high-resolution multi-slice PET scanner (Scanditronix PC 1024–7B, 6 mm in-plane and 10 mm axial resolution) was performed in the resting state on 47 carefully screened AD patients of differing dementia severity, compared with 30 controls [156]. With the exception of the caudate nucleus, mean values for rCMRglc, even in mildly demented AD patients, were significantly less than control means. At each level of dementia severity [48], rCMRglc was lower in association than primary neocortices or subcortical nuclei. rCMRglc in association neocortex in mildly demented subjects was 74–86% of the control value, whereas it was 87% in the primary neocortex and 90–93% in the subcortical nuclei.

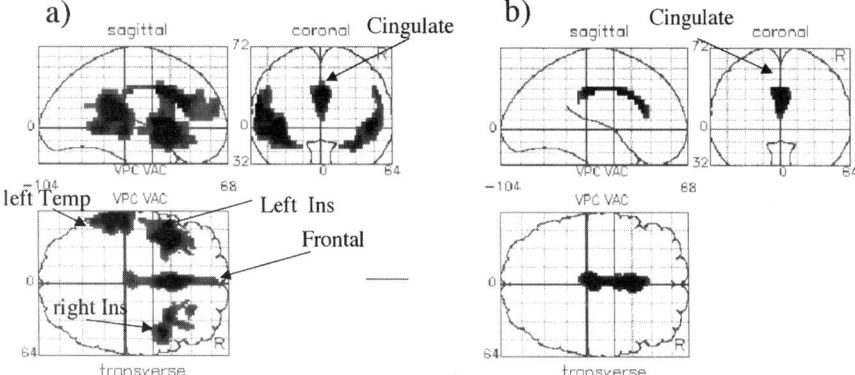

Figure 5 Statistical parametric mapping of significant metabolic differences between old and young healthy subjects. (a) Before a correction for atrophy, rCMRglc is significantly reduced in the older compared with young controls in temporal, frontal, insula, and cingulate cortical regions. (b) After the correction, only the cingulate cortex had significantly reduced metabolism in the older subjects. The statistical threshold level was set to a Z value of 2.3 corrected for multiple comparisons.

Selective vulnerability of association compared with primary neocortex in life agrees with evidence of greater neuropathology in association areas postmortem [61,63,64], supporting the notion of an evolution-related selective neurodegeneration (see above) [61,62,157].

In moderately to severely demented AD patients, hypometabolic patterns correspond to specific patterns of behavioral or cognitive abnormalities, consistent with principles of behavioral neurology [44]. In mildly demented patients, PET measurements can be more sensitive to cortical dysfunction than can cognitive tests. In such patients or in subjects genetically at risk for AD, cortical hemispheric metabolic asymmetries may exist in the absence of visuospatial or language deficits [74,158]. Presenting hemispheric asymmetries predict with statistical significance the cognitive deficits that appear 1-3 years later in individual patients. Thus, patients with worse left- than right-sided rCMRglc develop worse language than visuospatial performance, and vice versa. In moderately demented subjects, on the other hand, worse language performance correlates with lower left-sided metabolism, worse visuospatial performance with lower right-sided metabolism. Regional reductions in rCMRglc in severely demented subjects correlate with the extent of neurofibrillary tangles and synaptic loss on postmortem examination [55,64].

PET alone cannot reliably distinguish AD from vascular dementia [75]. Both syndromes demonstrate progressive reductions in metabolism and flow in relation to dementia severity [159], as well as heterogeneous cognitive and metabolic deficits. Large asymmetric deficits that correspond to CT or MRI abnormalities, or metabolic reductions in the basal ganglia or thalamus, suggest vascular dementia, whereas sparing of primary compared with association neocortex suggests AD (see above) [160]. However, AD appears not to be accompanied by an elevated rOEF, whereas rOEF can be elevated in vascular dementia [161–164].

B. Alzheimer Pattern of Brain Hypometabolism

Early attempts have been made to correct PET data obtained on AD patients for atrophy. The correction itself, based on CT, was found to be greater in patients than in age-matched controls (17% vs. 9%), consistent with more atrophy in patients [148]. The product of global CMRglc and MRI-derived whole-brain volume was noted to be less in patients than in controls [82]. Using the MRI-generated PVE correction described in Section III.C, cortex-to-cerebellum ratios were noted to be less in the temporal, parietal, and frontal regions of eight AD patients compared with 10 controls [137].

We recently estimated the effect of a PVE correction on rCMRglc in 15 otherwise healthy AD patients (68.9 ± 11.1 years; 10 men, 5 women) and 19 healthy age-matched controls (69.7 ± 7.6 years; 13 men, 6 women) [83], using the procedure of Section III.C. Before a PVE correction, mean global CMRglc was reduced significantly in the patients compared with controls. The correction caused mean global CMRglc to rise by 19.4% in the AD group and by 11.9% in controls, without changing the statistical significance of the difference between the means. A greater percent PVE correction in AD is consistent with greater atrophy in AD patients.

Additionally, before a PVE correction, mean rCMRglc in the inferior parietal cortex, lateral temporal cortex bilaterally, posterior cingulate, and the precuneus was significantly less in AD than control subjects (Fig. 6). After the correction, mean metabolic rates in these areas remained significantly less than control means, although the differences were quantitatively less than before the correction (Fig. 6). The overall pattern of hypometabolism conformed to reported hypometabolic patterns in brains in which atrophy correction was not performed [156,158,165–167].

Neuronal loss has been found in postmortem hippocampus from AD patients [168,169], but we could not demonstrate with PET significantly decreased hippocampal rCMRglc after the PVE correction. Other investigators did not find metabolic abnormalities in the AD hippocampus, even without a PVE correction [170,171].

VI. CONCLUSIONS

A. Atrophy Corrected Metabolism (per gram brain)

rCMRglc, corrected for atrophy (in units of mg/100 g brain/min) and determined with PET in healthy subjects in the resting state, does not decline with age.

Thus, the many age differences reported in the absence of a PVE correction most likely did not represent intrinsic reductions in brain rCMRglc. In contrast, both PVE-uncorrected and corrected values for rCMRglc are reduced in patients with AD, and the pattern of the reductions does not differ between the two analyses.

Age invariance of PVE-corrected rCMRglc, in the face of age-related cerebral atrophy (see above) and cognitive decline [172], clearly indicates that rCMRglc alone does not represent the entire picture of brain functional activity. Cognitive processes actually depend on the "integrated" activity of extended and overlapping groups of brain regions or networks [173–177]. This integrated activity can be represented by the matrix of statistically significant correlation coefficients between PET-derived values for rCMRglc [174]. The number of such significant correlations has been shown to be lower in healthy elderly than in young subjects [178–180]. Additional multivariate methods, including path analysis, can be used to examine network integrated activity in aging and AD [181].

That a PVE correction did not disturb the hypometabolic pattern in AD demonstrates that reductions in rCMRglc represent intrinsic metabolic defects per gram tissue. The reductions are accompanied by marked disruption of the correlation matrix relating regional values of rCMRglc, suggesting network disconnection and dysfunction [182–184]. In the late stages of AD, they correlate on a regional basis with

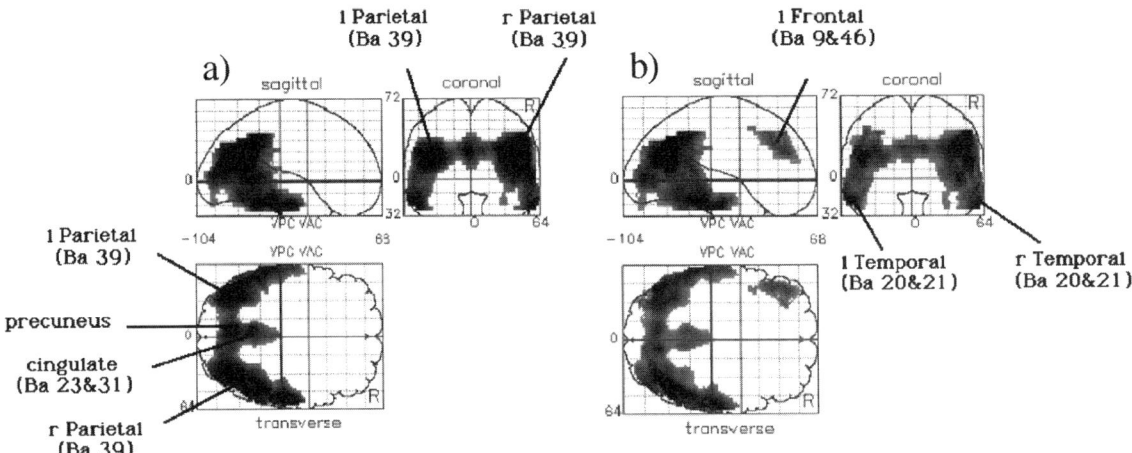

Figure 6 Statistical parametric mapping showing hypometabolic regions in AD compared to control subjects. Same threshold level as Figure 5. (a) Before atrophy correction, rCMRglc is decreased significantly in posterior parietal and temporal regions bilaterally, as well as posterior cuneate. (b) After correction, the pattern of hypometabolism is unchanged except for the left frontal region, which now shows reduced rCMRglc in AD patients. (From Ref. 83.)

postmortem neurofibrillary tangle densities and synaptic losses [55,64].

B. Discriminant Analysis

A diagnosis of AD in a subject with only a memory complaint may be provided by applying a discriminant analysis with multiple regression to PET metabolic data. This statistical procedure constructs a linear combination of observed variables to best describe group differences and to classify group membership of any individual [185]. It affords a probabilistic statement regarding the likelihood of a single scan or other data set being similar to datasets from controls compared with diagnosed AD patients. A discriminant function, derived from values of $rCMR_{glc}$ in diagnosed AD patients and controls, classified subjects with 87% accuracy. The function then identified as "pathological" an apparently normal PET scan from an at-risk subject; 1 year later, a second scan and the appearance of dementia confirmed the AD diagnosis [67]. The same function later correctly classified 10 older demented Down's syndrome subjects as having AD, as well as two of four older, nondemented subjects known to be at risk for AD [186,187]. The potential of discriminant functions can be enhanced by adding genetic, anatomic, or CSF measurements to PET measurements [188,189].

C. Activation PET for Aging and AD: Parametric Stress Tests

In view of postmortem evidence for synaptic and neurotransmitter losses in AD, and for changes albeit less with aging, PET and possibly fMRI might be employed with pharmacological or functional activation to characterize synaptic integrity and signal transduction in aging with early diagnosis, identifying genetically at-risk patients, and understanding disease progression, and evaluating drug efficacy in AD [29,76,190,191]. In such "stress" activation tests, furthermore, varying the stimulus "parameter" may provide much more information than simply choosing one rest and one stimulus condition [190,191]. As with resting PET studies, however, it is not known whether a lack of correction for atrophy impacted on published results and conclusions of prior activation studies. It is likely that a correction for atrophy would decrease variability at areas of activation and therefore help to better detect significant signaling differences. Clearly, future work is necessary to examine this issue.

In one "parametric" activation study, goggles were used to administer alternating patterned light flashes at frequencies of 0–14 Hz to AD patients and age-matched controls. PET and $H_2^{15}O$ were used to quantify rCBF at each frequency [191,192]. rCBF was activated by the patterned flashes in many cortical areas in control subjects, in relation to stimulus frequency. Compared to control responses, rCBF responses were reduced in prima (striate) and extrastriate visual cortical areas in mildly demented AD patients, and more so in moderately demented patients. Another PET study showed that rCBF activation and performance on a memory task in controls subjects could be modified by giving the anticholinesterase physostigmine, suggesting a way to examine declining cholinergic integrity in aging and AD [29].

A lack of responsiveness to cholinergic or other neurotransmitter therapies in AD may be related to signaling failure at the level of G-proteins or the signaling enzymes phospholipase C, adenylate cyclase, or phospholipase A_2 [193,194]. Postmortem studies suggest disturbed G-protein and signaling enzymes in the AD brain [195–198]. A new method, using [1-^{11}C]arachidonate acid with PET, shows promise for examining the phospholipase A_2-mediated release of the second messenger arachidonic acid in response to appropriate transmitter agonists [199–201]. Other methods to examine signaling beyond the receptor should be explored as well.

REFERENCES

1. DA Drachman. If we live long enough, will we all be demented? Neurology 44:1563–1565, 1994.
2. BA Yankner. A century of cognitive decline. Nature 404(6774):125, 2000.
3. L Berg. Does Alzheimer's disease represent an exaggeration of normal aging? Arch Neurol 42:737–739, 1985.
4. MJ West, PD Coleman, DG Flood, JC Troncoso. Differences in the pattern of hippocampal neuronal loss in normal aging and Alzheimer's disease. Lancet 344:769–772, 1994.
5. R Duara, C Grady, J Haxby, D Ingvar, L Sokoloff, RA Margolin, RG Manning, NR Cutler, SI Rapoport. Human brain glucose utilization and cognitive function in relation to age. Ann Neurol 16:702–713, 1984.
6. CL Grady, SI Rapoport. Cerebral metabolism in aging and dementia. In: Handbook of Mental Health and Aging (eds J Birren, RB Stone, GD Cohen). New York: Academic Press, 1992, pp 201–228.
7. DK Dastur, MH Lane, DB Hansen, SS Kety, RN Butler, S Perlin, L Sokoloff. Effects of aging on cere-

bral circulation and metabolism in man. In: Human Aging—A Biological and Behavioral Study. (eds JE Birren, RN Butler, SW Greenhouse, L Sokoloff, MR Yarrow). DHEW publication No. 986. Bethesda, MD: U.S. Dept. Health, Education and Welfare, Public Health Service, 1963, pp 59–76.
8. R Katzman. The prevalence and malignancy of Alzheimer disease: a major killer. Arch Neurol 33:217–218, 1976.
9. JL Cummings, DF Benson. Dementia: A Clinical Approach. Boston, Butterworths, 1983.
10. DK Dastur. Cerebral blood flow and metabolism in normal human aging, pathological aging, and senile dementia. J Cereb Blood Flow Metab 5:1–9, 1985.
11. JA Salerno, DGM Murphy, B Horwitz, C DeCarli, JV Haxby, SI Rapoport, MB Schapiro. Brain atrophy in hypertension. A volumetric magnetic resonance imaging study. Hypertension 20:340–348, 1992.
12. JA Salerno, MJ Mentis, A Gonzalez-Aviles, C Grady, E Wagner, MB Schapiro, SI Rapoport. Brain metabolic function in older men with chronic essential hypertension. J Gerontol 50:M147-M154, 1995.
13. SM Aamodt, M Constantine-Paton. The role of neural activity in synaptic development and its implications for adult brain function. Adv Neurol 79:133–144, 1999.
14. JM Long, PR Mouton, M Jucker, DK Ingram. What counts in brain aging? Design-based stereological analysis of cell number. J Gerontol Biol Sci Med Sci 54:B407-B417, 1999.
15. PD Coleman, DG Flood. Neuron numbers and dendritic extent in normal aging and Alzheimer's disease. Neurobiol Aging 8:521–545, 1987.
16. I Adams. Plasticity of the synaptic contact zone following loss of synapses in the cerebral cortex of aging humans. Brain Res 424:343–351, 1987.
17. K Hatanpää, KR Isaacs, T Shirao, DR Brady, SI Rapoport. Loss of brain synaptic proteins regulating plasticity in human aging and Alzheimer's disease. J Neuropathol Exp Neurol 58:637–643, 1999.
18. CE Finch, RE Tanzi. Genetics of aging. Science 278:407–411, 1997.
19. B Horwitz. Neuroplasticity and the progression of Alzheimer's disease. Int J Neurosci 41:1–14, 1988.
20. JH Morrison, PR Hof. Life and death of neurons in the aging brain. Science 278:412–419, 1997.
21. DG Flood, M Guarnaccia, PD Coleman. Dendritic extent in human CA2-3 hippocampal pyramidal neurons in normal aging and senile dementia. Brain Res 409(1):88–96, 1987.
22. DG Flood, SJ Buell, CH Defiore, GJ Horwitz, PD Coleman. Age-related dendritic growth in dentate gyrus of human brain is followed by regression in the 'oldest old.' Brain Res 345:366–3688, 1985.
23. PR Huttenlocher. Synaptic density in human frontal cortex—developmental changes and effects of aging. Brain Res 163:195–205, 1979.
24. E Masliah, M Mallory, L Hansen, R DeTeresa, RD Terry. Quantitative synaptic alterations in the human neocortex during normal aging. Neurology 43:192–197, 1993.
25. J de Keyser, G Ebinger, G Vauquelin. Age-related changes in the human nigrostriatal dopaminergic system. Ann Neurol 27:157–161, 1990.
26. N Kemppainen, H Ruottinen, K Nagren, JO Rinne. PET shows that striatal dopamine D1 and D2 receptors are differentially affected in AD. Neurology 55:205–259, 2000.
27. RT Bartus, RL Dean, B Beer, AS Lippa. The cholinergic hypothesis of geriatric memory dysfunction. Science 217:408–414, 1982.
28. JR Atack, C May, JA Kaye, AD Kay, SI Rapoport. Cerebrospinal fluid cholinesterases in aging and in dementia of the Alzheimer type. Ann Neurol 23:161–167, 1988.
29. ML Furey, P Pietrini, JV Haxby, E Alexander, HC Lee, J Van Meter, CL Grady, U Shetty, SI Rapoport, MB Schapiro, U Freo. Cholinergic stimulation alters performance and task specific regional cerebral blood flow during working memory. Proc Natl Acad Sci USA 94:6512–6516, 1997.
30. JL Horn. Psychometric studies of aging and intelligence. In: Aging, Vol 2 (eds. S Gershon, A Raskin). New York: Raven Press, 1975, pp 19–23.
31. H Creasey, SI Rapoport. The aging human brain. Ann Neurol 17:2–10, 1985.
32. RR McCrae, D Arenberg, PT Costa. Declines in divergent thinking with age: cross-sectional, longitudinal, and cross-sequential analyses. Psychol Aging 2:130–137, 1987.
33. E LaBarge, D Edwards, JW Knesevich. Performance of normal elderly on the Boston Naming Test. Brain Lang 27:380–384, 1986.
34. PW Foos, L Wright. Adult age differences in the storage of information in working memory. Exp Aging Res 18:51–57, 1992.
35. R Dolman, EA Roy, PT Dimeck, CR Hall. Age, gesture span, and dissociations among component subsystems of working memory. Brain Cogn 43:164–168, 2000.
36. P Chiappe, L Hasher, LS Siegel. Working memory, inhibitory control, and reading disability. Mem Cogn 28:8–17, 2000.
37. T Crook, RT Bartus, SH Ferris, P Whitehouse, GD Cohen, S Gershon. Age-associated memory impairment: Proposed diagnostic criteria and measures of clinical change. Report of a National Institute of Mental Health Work Group. Dev Neuropsychol 2:261–276, 1986.
38. GE Smith, RJ Ivnik, RC Petersen, JF Malec, E Kokmen, E Tangalos. Age-associated memory impairment diagnoses: problems of reliability and concerns for terminology. Psychol Aging 6:551–558, 1991.

39. JR Youngjohn, TH Crook 3rd. Stability of everyday memory in age-associated memory impairment: a longitudinal study. Neuropsychology 7:406–416, 1993.
40. T Hanninen, H Soininen. Age-associated memory impairment. Normal aging or warning of dementia? Drugs Aging 11:480–489, 1997.
41. V Hachinski. Preventable senility: a call for action against the vascular dementias. Lancet 340:645–648, 1992.
42. I Skoog, A Wallin, P Fredman, C Hesse, O Aevarsson, I Karlsson, CG Gottfries, K Blennow. A population study on brain blood-brain barrier function in 85 year olds: relation to Alzheimer's disease and vascular dementia. Neurology 50:966–971, 1998.
43. A Burns, R Jacoby, R Levy. Psychiatric phenomena in Alzheimer's disease. IV. Disorders of behaviour. Br J Psychiatry 157:86–94, 1990.
44. CL Grady, JV Haxby, MB Schapiro, A Gonzalez-Aviles, A Kumar, MJ Ball, L Heston, SI Rapoport. Subgroups in dementia of the Alzheimer type identified using positron emission tomography. J Neuropsychiatry Clin Neurosci 2:373–384, 1990.
45. J Rosen, GS Zubenko. Emergence of psychosis and depression in the longitudinal evaluation of Alzheimer's disease. Biol Psychiatry 29:224–232, 1991.
46. JV Haxby, K Raffaele, J Gillette, MB Schapiro, SI Rapoport. Individual trajectories of cognitive decline in patients with dementia of the Alzheimer type. J Clin Exp Neuropsychol 14:575–592, 1992.
47. J Victoroff, WJ Mack, SA Lyness, HC Chui. Multicenter clinicopathological correlation in dementia. Am J Psychiatry 152:1476–1484, 1995.
48. MF Folstein, SE Folstein, PR McHugh. Mini Mental State. A practical method for grading the cognitive state of patients for the clinician. J Psychiatr Res 12:189–198, 1975.
49. WC Drevets, EH Rubin. Psychotic symptoms and the longitudinal course of senile dementia of the Alzheimer type. Biol Psychiatry 25:39–48, 1989.
50. CL Joachim, JH Morris, DJ Selkoe. Clinically diagnosed Alzheimer's disease: autopsy results in 150 cases. Ann Neurol 24:50–56, 1988.
51. JC Morris, DW McKeel, K Fulling, RM Torrak, L Berg. Validation of clinical diagnostic criteria for Alzheimer's disease. Ann Neurol 24:17–22, 1988.
52. D Galasko, LA Hansen, R Katzman, W Wiederholt, E Masliah, R Terry, LR Hill, P Lessin, LJ Thal. Clinical-neuropathological correlations in Alzheimer's disease and related dementias. Arch Neurol 51:888–895, 1994.
53. G McKhann, D Drachman, M Folstein, R Katzman, D Price, EM Stadlan. Clinical diagnosis of Alzheimer's disease: report of the NINCDS-ADRDA work group under the auspices of Department of Health and Human Services task force on Alzheimer's disease. Neurology 34:939–944, 1984.
54. CQ Mountjoy, M Roth, NJ Evans, HA Evans. Cortical neuronal counts in normal elderly controls and demented patients. Neurobiol Aging 4:1–11, 1983.
55. RD Terry, E Masliah, DP Salmon, N Butters, R DeTeresa, R Hill, LA Hansen, R Katzman. Physical basis of cognitive alterations in Alzheimer's disease: synapse loss is the major correlate of cognitive impairment. Ann Neurol 30:572–580, 1991.
56. ST DeKosky, SW Scheff. Synapse loss in frontal cortex biopsies in Alzheimer's disease: correlation with cognitive severity. Ann Neurol 27:457–464, 1990.
57. ST DeKosky, SW Scheff, SD Styren. Structural correlates of cognition in dementia: quantification of synapse loss. Neurodegeneration 5:417–421, 1996.
58. CM Yates, J Simpson, A Gordon, AFJ Maloney, Y Allison, IM Richie, A Urquhart. Catecholamines and cholinergic enzymes in pre-senile and senile Alzheimer-type dementia and Down's syndrome. Brain Res 280:119–126, 1983.
59. PJ Whitehouse. Neurotransmitter receptor alterations in Alzheimer's disease: a review. Alzheimer Dis Assoc Disord 1:9–18, 1987.
60. JA Kaye, C May, E Daly, JR Atack, E Daly, DL Sweeney, MF Beal, S Kaufman, S Milstien, RP Friedland, SI Rapoport. Cerebrospinal fluid monoamine markers are decreased in dementia of the Alzheimer type with extrapyramidal features. Neurology 38:554–557, 1988.
61. SI Rapoport. Brain evolution and Alzheimer's disease. Rev Neurol (Paris) 144:79–90, 1988.
62. SI Rapoport. Integrated phylogeny of the primate brain, with special reference to humans and their diseases. Brain Res Rev 15:267–294, 1990.
63. DA Lewis, MJ Campbell, RD Terry, JH Morrison. Laminar and regional distributions of neurofibrillary tangles and neuritic plaques in Alzheimer's disease: a quantitative study of visual and auditory cortices. J Neurosci 7:1799–1808, 1987.
64. CS DeCarli, JR Atack, MJ Ball, JA Kaye, CL Grady, P Fewster, KD Pettigrew, SI Rapoport, MB Schapiro. Post-mortem regional neurofibrillary tangle densities but not senile plaque densities are related to regional cerebral metabolic rates for glucose during life in Alzheimer's disease patients. Neurodegeneration 1:113–121, 1992.
65. H Braak, E Braak, J Bohl. Staging of Alzheimer-related cortical destruction. Eur Neurol 33:403–408, 1993.
66. H Braak, E Braak, J Bohl, H Bratzke. Evolution of Alzheimer's disease related cortical lesions. J Neural Transm Suppl 54:97–106, 1998.
67. P Pietrini, NP Azari, CL Grady, JA Salerno, A Gonzales-Aviles, LL Heston, KD Pettigrew, B Horwitz, JV Haxby, MB Schapiro. Pattern of cerebral metabolic interactions in a subject with isolated am-

nesia at risk for Alzheimer's disease: a longitudinal evaluation. Dementia 4:94–101, 1993.
68. GW Small, JC Mazziotta, MT Collins, LR Baxter, ME Phelps, MA Mandelkern, A Kaplan, A La Rue, CF Adamson, L Chang, BH Guze, EH Corder, AM Saunders, JL Haines, MA Pericak-Vance, AD Roses. Apolipoprotein E type 4 allele and cerebral glucose metabolism in relatives at risk for familial Alzheimer disease. JAMA 273:942–947, 1995.
69. GW Small, LM Ercoli, DHS Silverman, S-C Huang, S Komo, SY Bookheimer, H Lavretsky, K Miller, P Siddarth, JC Mazziotta, S Saxena, HM Wu, MS Mega, JL Cummings, AM Saunders, MA Pericak-Vance, AD Roses, JR Barrio, ME Phelps. Cerebral metabolic and cognitive decline in persons at genetic risk for Alzheimer's disease. Proc Natl Acad Sci USA 97:6037–6042, 2000.
70. EM Reiman, A Uecker, RJ Caselli, S Lewis, D Bandy, MJ de Leon, S De Santi, A Convit, D Osborne, A Weaver, SN Thibodeau. Hippocampal volumes in cognitively normal persons at genetic risk for Alzheimer's disease. Ann Neurol 44:288–291, 1998.
71. EM Reiman, RJ Caselli, LS Yun, K Chen, D Bandy, S Minoshima, SN Thibodeau, D Osborne. Preclinical evidence of Alzheimer's disease in persons homozygous for the e4 allele for apolipoprotein E. N Engl J Med 334:752–758, 1996.
72. AM Kennedy, RSJ Frackowiak, SK Newman, PM Bloomfield, J Seaward, P Roques, G Lewington, VJ Cunningham, MN Rossor. Deficits in cerebral glucose metabolism demonstrated by positron emission tomography in individuals at risk of familial Alzheimer's disease. Neurosci Lett 186:17–20, 1995.
73. CL Grady, JV Haxby, B Horwitz, M Sundaram, G Berg, M Schapiro, RP Friedland, SI Rapoport. Longitudinal study of the early neuropsychological and cerebral metabolic changes in dementia of the Alzheimer type. J Clin Exp Neuropsychol 10:576–596, 1988.
74. JV Haxby, CL Grady, E Koss, B Horwitz, L Heston, M Schapiro, RP Friedland, SI Rapoport. Longitudinal study of cerebral metabolic asymmetries and associated neuropsychological patterns in early dementia of the Alzheimer type. Arch Neurol 47:753–760, 1990.
75. SI Rapoport. Anatomic and functional brain imaging in Alzheimer's disease. In: Psychopharmacology: The Fourth Generation of Progress (eds. FE Bloom, DJ Kupfer). New York: Raven, 1985, pp 1401–1415.
76. SI Rapoport. Functional brain imaging to identify affected subjects genetically at risk for Alzheimer's disease. Proc Natl Acad Sci USA 97:5696–5698, 2000.
77. CT Moonen, PC van Zijl, JA Frank, D Le Bihan, ED Becker. Functional magnetic resonance imaging in medicine and physiology. Science 250(4977):53–61, 1990.
78. RP Friedland, WJ Jagust. Positron and single photon emission tomography in the differential diagnosis of dementia. In: Positron Emission Tomography in Dementia. Frontiers of Clinical Neuroscience, Vol 10 (ed R Duara). New York: Wiley-Liss, 1990, pp 161–177.
79. BL Holman, JS Nagel, KA Johnson, TC Hill. Imaging dementia with SPECT. Ann NY Acad Sci 620:165–174, 1991.
80. JM DeLeo, M Schwartz, H Creasey, N Cutler, SI Rapoport. Computer-assisted categorization of brain computerized tomography pixels into cerebrospinal fluid, white matter, and gray matter. Comput Biomed Res 18:79–88, 1985.
81. CC Meltzer, JP Leal, HS Mayberg, HJ Wagner, JJ Frost. Correction of PET data for partial volume effects in human cerebral cortex by MR imaging. J Comput Assist Tomogr 14:561–570, 1990.
82. A Alavi, AB Newberg, E Souder, JA Berlin. Quantitative analysis of PET and MRI data in normal aging and Alzheimer's disease: atrophy weighted total brain metabolism and absolute whole brain metabolism as reliable discriminators. J Nucl Med 34:1681–1687, 1993.
83. V Ibáñez, P Pietrini, GE Alexander, ML Furey, D Teichberg, JC Rajapakse, SI Rapoport, MB Schapiro, B Horwitz. Regional glucose metabolic abnormalities are not the result of atrophy in Alzheimer's disease. Neurology 50:1585–1593, 1998.
84. JC Rajapakse, JN Giedd, SI Rapoport. Statistical approach to segmentation of single channel cerebral MR images. IEEE Trans Med Imaging 16:176–186, 1997.
85. H Creasey, SI Rapoport. Use of quantitative transverse tomography (CT) to evaluate brain and cerebrospinal fluid dimensions in healthy men in relation to age. Maladies Medicaments/Drugs Diseases 1:181–185, 1984.
86. JA Kaye, C DeCarli, JS Luxenberg, SI Rapoport. The significance of age-related enlargement of the cerebral ventricles in healthy men and women measured by quantitative computed x-ray tomography. J Am Geriatr Soc 40:225–231, 1992.
87. DG Murphy, C DeCarli, AR McIntosh, E Daly, MJ Mentis, P Pietrini, J Szczepanik, MB Schapiro, CL Grady, B Horwitz, SI Rapoport. Sex differences in human brain morphometry and metabolism: an in vivo quantitative magnetic resonance imaging and positron emission tomography study on the effect of aging. Arch Gen Psychiatry 53:585–594, 1996.
88. CE Coffey, WE Wilkinson, IA Parashos, SA Soady, RJ Sullivan, LJ Patterson, GS Figiel, MC Webb, CE Spritzer, WT Djang. Quantitative cerebral anatomy of the aging human brain: a cross-sectional study using

magnetic resonance imaging. Neurology 42:527–536, 1992.

89. C DeCarli, DG Murphy, M Tranh, CL Grady, JV Haxby, JA Gillette, JA Salerno, J Gonzalez-Aviles, B Horwitz, SI Rapoport, MB Schapiro. The effect of white matter hyperintensity volume on brain structure, cognitive performance and cerebral metabolism of glucose in very healthy adults. Neurology 45:2077–2084, 1995.

90. AL Foundas, D Zipin, CA Browning. Age-related changes of the insular cortex and lateral ventricles: conventional MRI volumetric measures. J Neuroimaging 8:216–221, 1998.

91. JA Kaye, T Swihart, D Howieson, A Dame, MM Moore, T Karnos, R Camicioli, M Ball, B Oken, G Sexton. Volume loss of the hippocampus and temporal lobe in healthy elderly persons destined to develop dementia. Neurology 48:1297–1304, 1997.

92. F Fazekas, A Alavi, JB Chawluk, RA Zimmerman, D Hackney, L Bilaniuk, M Rosen, WM Alves, HI Hurtig, DG Jamieson. Comparison of CT, MR, and PET in Alzheimer's dementia and normal aging. J Nucl Med 30:1607–1615, 1989.

93. TL Jernigan, DP Salmon, N Butters, JR Hesselink. Cerebral structure on MRI. Part II. Specific changes in Alzheimer's and Huntington's diseases. Biol Psychiatry 29:68–81, 1991.

94. H Rusinek, MJ de Leon, AE George, LA Stylopoulos, R Chandra, G Smith, T Rand, M Mourino, H Kowalski. Alzheimer disease: measuring loss of cerebral gray matter with MR imaging [see comments]. Radiology 178:109–114, 1991.

95. DGM Murphy, CD DeCarli, E Daly, JA Gillette, AR McIntosh, JV Haxby, D Teichberg, MB Schapiro, SI Rapoport, B Horwitz. Volumetric magnetic resonance imaging in men with dementia of the Alzheimer type: correlations with disease severity. Biol Psychiatry 34:612–621, 1993.

96. C DeCarli, DG Murphy, JA Gillette, JV Haxby, D Teichberg, MB Schapiro, B Horwitz. Lack of age-related differences in temporal lobe volume of very healthy adults. AJNR Am J Neuroradiol 15:689–696, 1994.

97. JS Luxenberg, JV Haxby, H Creasey, M Sundaram, SI Rapoport. Rate of ventricular enlargement in dementia of the Alzheimer type correlates with rate of neuropsychological deterioration. Neurology 37:1135–1140, 1987.

98. A Dani, P Pietrini, M Furey, AR McIntosh, CL Grady, B Horwitz, U Freo, GE Alexander, MB Schapiro. Brain cognition and metabolism in Down syndrome adults in association with development of dementia. NeuroReport 7:2933–2936, 1996.

99. MJ De Leon, A Convit, S DeSanti, M Bobinski, AE George, HM Wisniewski, H Rusinek, R Carroll, LA Saint Louis. Contribution of structural neuroimaging to the early diagnosis of Alzheimer's disease. Int Psychogeriatr 9(suppl 1):183–190, 1997.

100. CL Grady, SI Rapoport. Cerebral metabolism in aging and dementia. In: Handbook of Mental Health and Aging (eds J Birren, RB Stone, GD Cohen). New York: Academic Press, 1992, pp 201–228.

101. P Pietrini, SJ Teipel, P Bartenstein, SI Rapoport, H-J Möller, H Hampel. PET and the effects of aging and neurodegeneration on brain function: basic principles. Drugs New Perspect 11:161–168, 1998.

102. P Pietrini, SI Rapoport. Cerebral blood flow and glucose metabolism in healthy human aging assessed by functional brain imaging. In: Textbook of Geriatric Neuropsychiatry, 2nd ed. (eds. CE Coffey, JL Cummings). Washington: American Psychiatric Press, 2000, pp. 239–266.

103. SS Kety, CF Schmidt. The determination of cerebral blood flow in man by the use of nitrous oxide in low concentration. Am J Physiol 145:53–66, 1944.

104. NL Schlageter, B Horwitz, H Creasey, R Carson, R Duara, GW Berg, SI Rapoport. Relation of measured brain glucose utilization and cerebral atrophy in man. J Neurol Neurosurg Psychiatry 50:779–785, 1987.

105. L Sokoloff. The action of drugs on the cerebral circulation. Pharmacol Rev 11:1–85, 1959.

106. OH Lowry. Energy metabolism in brain and its control. In: Brain Work, Alfred Benzon Symposium VIII (eds. DH Ingvar, NA Lassen). New York: Academic Press, 1975, pp 48–64.

107. AD Purdon, SI Rapoport. Energy requirements for two aspects of phospholipid metabolism in mammalian brain. Biochem J 335:313–318, 1998.

108. CS Roy, CS Sherrington. On the regulation of the blood supply of the brain. J Physiol (Lond) 11:85–105, 1890.

109. SS Kety, CF Schmidt. The nitrous oxide method for the quantitative determination of cerebral blood flow in man: theory, procedure, and normal values. J Clin Invest 27:476–483, 1948.

110. M Reivich. Blood flow metabolism couple in brain. Res Publ Assoc Res Nerv Ment Dis 53:125–140, 1974.

111. L Sokoloff, M Reivich, C Kennedy, MH Des Rosiers, CS Patlak, KD Pettigrew, O Sakurada, M Shinohara. The [^{14}C]deoxyglucose method for the measurement of local cerebral glucose utilization: theory, procedure, and normal values in the conscious and anesthetized albino rat. J Neurochem 28:897–916, 1977.

112. PJ Magistretti, L Pellerin, DL Rothman, RG Shulman. Energy on demand. Science 283:496–497, 1999.

113. L Pellerin, PJ Magistretti. Glutamate uptake into astrocytes stimulates aerobic glycolysis: a mechanism coupling neuronal activity to glucose utilization. Proc Natl Acad Sci USA 91:10625–10629, 1994.

114. DL Bailey, MP Miller, TJ Spinks, PM Bloomfield, L Livieratos, HE Young, T Jones. Experience with fully

3D PET and implications for future high-resolution 3D tomographs. Phys Med Biol 43:777–786, 1998.
115. DW Townsend, M Defrise, A Geissbuhler, TJ Spinks, DL Bailey, MC Gilardi, T Jones. Normalization and reconstruction of PET data acquired by a multi-ring camera with septa retracted. Med Prog Technol 17:223–228, 1991.
116. D Marquardt. An algorithm for least squares estimation of nonlinear parameters. J Soc Ind Appl Math 11:431–441, 1963.
117. SS Kety. Basic principles for the quantitative estimation of regional cerebral blood flow. Res Publ Assoc Res Nerv Ment Dis 63:1–7, 1985.
118. SI Rapoport. Blood-Brain Barrier in Physiology and Medicine. New York: Raven Press, 1976.
119. I Kanno, AA Lammertsma, JD Heather, JM Gibbs, CG Rhodes, JC Clark, T Jones. Measurement of cerebral blood flow using bolus inhalation of $C^{15}O_2$ and positron emission tomography: description of the method and its comparison with the $C^{15}O_2$ continuous inhalation method. J Cereb Blood Flow Metab 4:224–234, 1984.
120. AA Lammertsma, RJ Wise, TC Cox, DG Thomas, T Jones. Measurement of blood flow, oxygen utilization, oxygen extraction ratio, and fractional blood volume in human brain tumours and surrounding oedematous tissue. Br J Radiol 58:725–734, 1985.
121. P Herscovitch, J Markham, ME Raichle. Brain blood flow measured with intravenous O-15 water. I. Theory and error analysis. J Nucl Med 24:782–789, 1983.
122. PT Fox, MA Mintun. Noninvasive functional brain mapping by change distribution analysis of averaged PET images of H_2 $_{(15)}O$ tissue activity. J Nucl Med 30:141–49, 1989.
123. ME Phelps, SC Huang, EJ Hoffman, MS Selin, L Sokoloff, DE Kuhl. Tomographic measurement of local glucose metabolic rate in humans with (F-18)2-fluoro-2-deoxy-D-glucose: validation of method. Ann Neurol 6:371–388, 1979.
124. DD Clarke, L Sokoloff. Circulation and energy metabolism of the brain. In: Basic Neurochemistry: Molecular, Cellular and Medical Aspects (eds GJ Siegel, BW Agranoff, RW Albers, SK Fisher, MD Uhler). Philadelphia: Lippincott-Raven, 1999.
125. RA Brooks. Alternative formula for glucose utilization using labeled deoxyglucose. J Nucl Med 23:538–539, 1982.
126. AC Evans, S Marrett, J Torrescorzo, S Ku, L Collins. Anatomical-functional correlative analysis of the human brain using three dimensional imaging systems. SPIE Med Imag III: Image Proc 1092:264–274, 1989.
127. CA Pelizzari, GT Chen, DR Spelbring, RR Weichselbaum, CT Chen. Accurate three-dimensional registration of CT, PET, and/or MR images of the brain. J Comput Assist Tomogr 13:20–26, 1989.
128. RP Woods, JC Mazziotta, SR Cherry. MRI-PET registration with automated algorithm. J Comp Assist Tomogr 17:536–546, 1993.
129. RP Woods, JC Mazziotta. A rapid automated algorithm for accurately aligning and reslicing positron emission tomography images. J Comput Assist Tomogr 16:620–633, 1992.
130. J Talairach, P Tournoux. Coplanar stereotaxic atlas of the human brain. Stuttgart: Thieme, 1988.
131. KJ Friston, CD Frith, PF Liddle, RSJ Frackowiak. Comparing functional (PET) images: the assessment of significant change. J Cereb Blood Flow Metab 11:690–699, 1991.
132. KJ Friston, J Ashburner, CD Frith, J-B Poline, JD Heather, RSJ Frackowiak. Spatial registration and normalization images. Hum Brain Mapping 3:165–189, 1995.
133. KJ Friston, CD Frith, PF Liddle, AA Lammertsma, RD Dolan, RSJ Frackowiak. The relationship between local and global changes in PET scans. J Cereb Blood Flow Metab 10:458–466, 1990.
134. KJ Friston, KJ Worsley, RSJ Frackowiak, JC Mazziotta, AC Evans. Assessing the significance of focal activations using their spatial extent. Hum Brain Mapping 1:210–220, 1994.
135. KJ Worsley, AC Evans, S Marrett, P Neelin. A three-dimensional statistical analysis for CBF activation studies in human brain. J Cereb Blood Flow Metab 12:900–918, 1992.
136. TO Videen, JS Perlmutter, MA Mintun, ME Raichle. Regional correction of positron emission tomography data for the effects of cerebral atrophy. J Cereb Blood Flow Metab 8:662–670, 1988.
137. CC Meltzer, JK Zubieta, J Brandt, LE Tune, HS Mayberg, JJ Frost. Regional hypometabolism in Alzheimer's disease as measured by positron emission tomography after correction for effects of partial volume. Neurology 47:465–461, 1996.
138. HW Müller-Gärtner, JM Links, JL Prince, RN Bryan, E McVeigh, JP Leal, C Davatzikos, JJ Frost. Measurement of radiotracer concentration in brain gray matter using positron emission tomography: MRI-based correction for partial volume effects. J Cereb Blood Flow Metab 12:571–583, 1992.
139. P Pietrini, SI Rapoport. Functional neuroimaging: positron-emission tomography in the study of cerebral blood flow and glucose utilization in human subjects at different ages. In: Textbook of Geriatric Neuropsychiatry. Chapter 10 (eds CE Coffey, JL Cummings, MR Lovell, GD Perlson). Washington: American Psychiatric Press, 1994, pp 195–214.
140. JF Corso. Auditory perception and communication. In: Handbook of the Psychology of Aging (eds JE Birren, KW Schaie). New York: Van Nostrand Reinhold, 1997, pp 535–553.

141. JL Fozzard, E Wolf, B Bell, RA McFarland, S Podolsky. Visual perception and communication. In: Handbook of the Psychology of Aging (eds JE Birren, KW Schaie). New York: Van Nostrand Reinhold, 1977, pp. 497–534.
142. W Lehnert, H Wuensche. Das Electroretinogramm in verschiedenen Lebensaltern. Graef Arch Clin Exp Ophthalmol 170:147–155, 1966.
143. ME Phelps, JC Mazziotta, DE Kuhl, M Nuwer, J Packwood, J Metter, J Engel Jr. Tomographic mapping of human cerebral metabolism: visual stimulation and deprivation. Neurology 31:517–529, 1981.
144. JC Mazziotta, ME Phelps, RE Carson, DE Kuhl. Tomographic mapping of human cerebral metabolism: auditory stimulation. Neurology 32:921–937, 1982.
145. AJ Martin, KJ Friston, JG Colebatch, RS Frackowiak. Decreases in regional cerebral blood flow with normal aging. J Cereb Blood Flow Metab 11:684–689, 1991.
146. G Marchal, P Rioux, MC Petit-Taboue, G Sette, JM Travere, C Le Poec, P Courtheoux, JM Derlon, JC Baron. Regional cerebral oxygen consumption, blood flow, and blood volume in healthy human aging. Arch Neurol 49:1013–1020, 1992.
147. A Burns, P Tyrrell. Association of age with regional cerebral oxygen utilization: a positron emission tomography study. Age Ageing 21:316–320, 1992.
148. JB Chawluk, A Alavi, R Dann, HI Hurtig, S Bais, MJ Kushner, RA Zimmerman, M Reivich. Positron emission tomography in aging and dementia: effect of cerebral atrophy. J Nucl Med 28:431–437, 1987.
149. JM Hoffman, BH Guze, LR Baxter, JC Mazziotta, ME Phelps. [^{18}F]Fluorodeoxyglucose (FDG) and positron emission tomography (PET) in aging and dementia. A decade of studies. Eur Neurol 29(suppl 3):16–24, 1989.
150. P Pantano, JC Baron, P Lebrun-Grandie, N Duquesnoy, MG Bousser, D Comar. Regional cerebral blood flow and oxygen consumption in human aging. Stroke 15:645–641, 1984.
151. JR Moeller, T Ishikawa, V Dhawan, P Spetsieris, F Mandel, GE Alexander, CL Grady, P Pietrini, D Eidelberg. The metabolic topography of normal aging. J Cereb Blood Flow Metab 16:385–398, 1996.
152. S De Santi, MJ de Leon, A Convit, C Tarshish, H Rusinek, WH Tsui, E Sinaiko, GJ Wang, E Bartlet, N Volkow. Age-related changes in brain. II. Positron emission tomography of frontal and temporal lobe glucose metabolism in normal subjects. Psychiatr Q 66:357–370, 1995.
153. MC Petit-Taboue, B Landeau, JF Desson, B Desgranges, JC Baron. Effects of healthy aging on the regional cerebral metabolic rate of glucose assess with statistical parametric mapping. Neuroimage 7:176–184, 1998.
154. V Ibáñez, P Pietrini, GE Alexander, P Millet, AL Bokde, D Teichberg, MB Schapiro, B Horwitz, SI Rapoport. Different patterns of age-related metabolic brain changes during healthy aging and AD, using atrophy correction. Neurology 56(suppl 3):A373, 2001.
155. CC Meltzer, MN Cantwell, PJ Greer, D Ben-Eliezer, G Smith, G Frank, WH Kaye, PR Houck, JC Price. Does cerebral blood flow decline in healthy aging? A PET study with partial-volume correction. J Nucl Med 41:1842–1848, 2000.
156. A Kumar, MB Schapiro, C Grady, JV Haxby, E Wagner, JA Salerno, RP Friedland, SI Rapoport. High-resolution PET studies in Alzheimer's disease. Neuropsychopharmacology 4:35–46, 1991.
157. SI Rapoport. Hypothesis: Alzheimer's disease is a phylogenic disease. Med Hypoth 29:147–150, 1989.
158. JV Haxby, CL Grady, R Duara, N Schlageter, G Berg, SI Rapoport. Neocortical metabolic abnormalities precede nonmemory cognitive deficits in early Alzheimer's-type dementia. Arch Neurol 43:882–885, 1986.
159. RSJ Frackowiak, C Pozzilli, NJ Legg, GH Du Boulay, J Marshall, GL Lenzi, T Jones. Regional cerebral oxygen supply and utilization in dementia. A clinical and physiological study with oxygen-15 and positron tomography. Brain 104:753–778, 1981.
160. DF Benson, DE Kuhl, RA Hawkins, ME Phelps, JL Cummings, SY Tsai. The fluorodeoxyglucose ^{18}F scan in Alzheimer's disease and multi-infarct dementia. Arch Neurol 40:711–714, 1983.
161. H Yao, S Sadoshima, S Ibayashi, Y Kuwabara, Y Ichiya, M Fujishima. Leukoaraiosis and dementia in hypertensive patients. Stroke 23:1673–1677, 1992.
162. K Ishii, H Kitagaki, M Kono, E Mori. Decreased medial temporal oxygen metabolism in Alzheimer's disease is shown by PET. J Nucl Med 37:1159–1164, 1996.
163. S Yamaji, K Ishii, M Sasaki, T Imamura, H Kitagaki, S Sakamoto, E Mori. Changes in cerebral blood flow and oxygen metabolism related to magnetic resonance imaging white matter hyperintensities in Alzheimer's disease. J Nucl Med 38:1471–1474, 1997.
164. K Nagata, H Maruya, H Yuya, H Terashi, Y Mito, H Kato, M Sato, Y Satoh, Y Watahiki, Y Hirata, E Yokoyama, J Hatazawa. Can PET data differentiate Alzheimer's disease from vascular dementia? Ann NY Acad Sci 903:252–261, 2000.
165. K Herholz. FDG PET and differential diagnosis of dementia. Alzheimer Dis Assoc Disord 9:6–16, 1995.
166. RP Friedland, WJ Jagust, RH Huesman, E Koss, B Knittel, CA Mathis, BA Ober, BM Mazoyer, TF Budingher. Regional cerebral glucose transport and utilization in Alzheimer's disease. Neurology 39:1427–1434, 1989.

167. R Duara, C Grady, J Haxby, M Sundaram, NR Cutler, L Heston, A Moore, N Schlageter, S Larson, SI Rapoport. Positron emission tomography in Alzheimer's disease. Neurology 36:879–887, 1986.
168. MJ Ball. Neuronal loss, neurofibrillary tangles and granulovascular degeneration in the hippocampus with aging and dementia. Acta Neuropathol (Berl) 37:111–118, 1977.
169. BT Hyman, GW Van Hoesen, AR Damasio, CL Barnes. Alzheimer's disease: cell-specific pathology isolates the hippocampal formation. Science 225:1168–1170, 1984.
170. H Fukuyama, K Harada, H Yamauchi, T Miyoshi, S Yamaguchi, J Kimura, M Kameyama, M Senda, Y Yonekura, J Konishi. Coronal reconstruction images of glucose metabolism in Alzheimer's disease. J Neurol Sci 106:128–134, 1991.
171. WJ Jagust. Functional imaging patterns in Alzheimer's disease. Relationships to neurobiology. Ann NY Acad Sci 777:30–36, 1996.
172. E Koss, JV Haxby, CS DeCarli, MB Schapiro, RP Friedland, SI Rapoport. Patterns of performance preservation and loss in healthy aging. Dev Neuropsychol 7:99–113, 1991.
173. AR Luria. The Working Brain. An Introduction to Neuropsychology. New York: Basic Books, 1973.
174. B Horwitz. Functional neural systems analyzed by use of interregional correlations of glucose metabolism. In: Visuomotor Coordination (eds J-P Ewert, MA Arbib). New York: Plenum Press, 1989, pp 873–892.
175. MM Mesulam. Large-scale neurocognitive networks and distributed processing for attention, language, and memory. Ann Neurol 28:597–613, 1990.
176. AR Damasio, D Tranel, H Damasio. Face agnosia and the neural substrates of memory. Annu Rev Neurosci 13:89–109, 1990.
177. A Berardi, JV Haxby, CL Grady, SI Rapoport. Asymmetries of brain glucose metabolism and memory in the healthy elderly. Dev Neuropsychol 7:87–97, 1991.
178. NP Azari, SI Rapoport, CL Grady, MB Schapiro, JA Salerno, A Gonzalez-Aviles, B Horwitz. Interregional correlations of resting cerebral glucose metabolism in old and young women. Brain Res 589:279–290, 1992.
179. B Horwitz, R Duara, SI Rapoport. Age differences in intercorrelations between regional cerebral metabolic rates for glucose. Ann Neurol 19:60–67, 1986.
180. SI Rapoport, B Horwitz. Use of positron emission tomography to study patterns of brain metabolism in relation to age and disease: a correlation matrix approach. In: Regulatory Mechanisms of Neuron to Vessel Communication in the Brain, Vol 33. Berlin: Springer-Verlag, 1989, pp 393–410.
181. B Horwitz, AR McIntosh, JV Haxby, CL Grady. Network analysis of brain cognitive function using metabolic and blood flow data. Behav Brain Res 66:187–193, 1995.
182. SI Rapoport, B Horwitz, JV Haxby, CL Grady. Alzheimer's disease: metabolic uncoupling of associative brain regions. Can J Neurol Sci 13:540–545, 1986.
183. B Horwitz, CL Grady, NL Schlageter, R Duara, SI Rapoport. Intercorrelations of regional cerebral glucose metabolic rates in Alzheimer's disease. Brain Res 407:294–306, 1987.
184. JH Morrison, PR Hof, MJ Campbell, AD DeLima, T Voigt, C Bouras, K Cox, WG Young. Cellular pathology in Alzheimer's Disease: implications for cortico-cortical disconnection and differential vulnerability. In: Imaging, Cerebral Topography and Alzheimer's Disease, Research and Perspectives in Alzheimer's Disease (eds SI Rapoport, H Petit, D Leys, Y Christen). Berlin: Springer-Verlag, 1990, pp 19–40.
185. CM Clark, W Ammann, WR Martin, P Ty, MR Hayden. The FDG/PET methodology for early detection of disease onset: a statistical model. J Cereb Blood Flow Metab 11:A96–A102, 1991.
186. DM Mann, PO Yates, B Marcyniuk. Alzheimer's presenile dementia, senile dementia of Alzheimer type and Down's syndrome in middle age form an age related continuum of pathological changes. Neuropathol Appl Neurobiol 10:185–207, 1984.
187. NP Azari, KD Pettigrew, P Pietrini, B Horwitz, MB Schapiro. Detection of an Alzheimer disease pattern of cerebral metabolism in Down syndrome. Dementia 5:69–78, 1994.
188. C DeCarli, DGM Murphy, AR McIntosh, D Teichberg, MB Schapiro, B Horwitz. Discriminant analysis of MRI measures as a method to determine the presence of dementia of the Alzheimer type in males and females. Psychiatry Res 57:119–130, 1995.
189. H Hampel, SJ Teipel, F Padberg, A Haslinger, M Riemenschneider, MJ Schwarz, HU Kotter, M Scheloske, K Buch, S Stubner, R Dukoff, R Lasser, N Muller, T Sunderland, SI Rapoport, HJ Moller. Discriminant power of combined cerebrospinal fluid tau protein and of the soluble interleukin-6 receptor complex in the diagnosis of Alzheimer's disease. Brain Res 823:104–112, 1999.
190. SI Rapoport, CL Grady. Parametric in vivo brain imaging during activation to examine pathological mechanisms of functional failure in Alzheimer disease. Int J Neurosci 70:39–56, 1993.
191. MJ Mentis, B Horwitz, CL Grady, GE Alexander, JW VanMeter, JM Maisog, P Pietrini, MB Schapiro, SI Rapoport. Visual cortical dysfunction in Alzheimer's disease evaluated with a temporally graded "stress test" during PET. Am J Psychiatry 153:32–40, 1996.
192. MJ Mentis, GE Alexander, J Krasuski, P Pietrini, ML Furey, MB Schapiro, SI Rapoport. Increasing required neural response to expose abnormal brain function in mild versus moderate or severe Alzheimer's disease:

PET study using parametric visual stimulation. Am J Psychiatry 155:785–794, 1998.
193. J Axelrod. Phospholipase A2 and G proteins. Trends Neurosci 18:64–65, 1995.
194. JR Cooper, FE Bloom, RH Roth. The Biochemical Basis of Neuropharmacology. Oxford: Oxford University Press, 1996.
195. G Ferrari-DiLeo, DC Mash, DD Flynn. Attenuation of muscarinic receptor–G-protein interaction in Alzheimer disease. Mol Chem Neuropathol 24:69–91, 1995.
196. S Shimohama, Y Homma, S Fujimoto, T Suenaga, T Taniguchi, W Araki, Y Yamaoka, H Matsushima, T Takenawa, J Kimura. Aberrant accumulation of phospholipase C in Alzheimer brains. Neurobiol Aging 13(suppl 1):S59, 1992.
197. AA Farooqui, LA Horrocks. Plasmalogen selective phospholipase A2 and its involvement in Alzheimer's disease. Biochem Soc Trans 26:243–246, 1998.
198. BM Ross, A Moszczynska, J Erlich, SJ Kish. Phospholipid-metabolizing enzymes in Alzheimer's disease: increased lysophospholipid acyltransferase activity and decreased phospholipase A2 activity. J Neurochem 70:786–793, 1998.
199. SI Rapoport, D Purdon, HU Shetty, E Grange, Q Smith, C Jones, MCJ Chang. In vivo imaging of fatty acid incorporation into brain to examine signal transduction and neuroplasticity involving phospholipids. Ann NY Acad Sci 820:56–74, 1997.
200. MCJ Chang, T Arai, LM Freed, S Wakabayashi, MA Channing, BB Dunn, MG Der, JM Bell, T Sasaki, P Herscovitch, WC Eckelman, SI Rapoport. Brain incorporation of [1-^{11}C]-arachidonate in normocapnic and hypercapnic monkeys, measured with positron emission tomography. Brain Res 755:74–83, 1997.
201. SI Rapoport, MC Chang, K Connolly, D Kessler, A Bokde, RE Carson, P Herscovitch, M Channing, WC Eckelman. In vivo imaging of phospholipase A2-mediated signaling in human brain using [^{11}C]arachidonic acid and positron emission tomography (PET). J Neurochem 74:S21, 2000.

34

Brain Imaging in Dementia

FRANCESCA MAPUA FILBEY, ROBERT COHEN, and TREY SUNDERLAND
National Institute of Mental Health, Bethesda, Maryland, U.S.A.

I. INTRODUCTION

The diagnosis of "probable" or "possible" Alzheimer's disease (AD) according to the National Institute for Neurological and Communicative Disorders and Stroke and the Alzheimer's Disorders Association (NINCDS/ADRDA) [McKhann et al. 1984] is made clinically and can only be verified by neuropathological examination of brain tissue. Thus, one of the primary goals of brain imaging is to detect and identify dementia whether before onset or as early as possible in vivo to increase therapeutic gain (i.e., begin treatment as early as possible). The incorporation of both structural and functional neuroimaging techniques with traditional clinical tools (e.g., standard history, mental state examinations, neurological exam, etc.) has already made not only diagnosing, but also prognosing of dementia disorders more realistic. A study in 1997 revealed that diagnostic accuracy was improved by neuroimaging methods, changing clinical diagnosis by as much as 19–28% and management by 15% (Chui and Zhang 1997). In a recent review of the use of neuroimaging in clinical settings, Cummings (2000) concluded that neuroimaging increases diagnostic accuracy and should be considered a part of routine dementia assessment. At present, diagnostic tools such as the California Alzheimer's Disease Diagnostic and Treatment Centers (CAD-DTC) [Chui 1992] and the National Institute of Neurological Disorders and Stroke and the Association *Internationale pour la Recherche et l'Enseignement en Neurosciences* (NINDS-AIREN) [Roman et al. 1993] rely on neuroimaging. This is a tremendous advance for as recently as five years ago, neuroimaging was not even included in the consensus recommendations for the diagnostic evaluation of a potential Alzheimer's patient [Small et al. 1997]. What follows is a brief introduction to the variety of neuroimaging techniques currently available to diagnosticians and researchers alike.

A. Structural Brain Imaging

Since the mid-1970s, structural neuroimaging particularly computer tomography (CT) and magnetic resonance imaging (MRI) have made significant contributions to the evaluation of dementia. CT and MRI are helpful in identifying combined cerebrovascular and degenerative diseases, in addition to being able to facilitate the discrimination between the overlapping symptom profiles [Cummings 2000]. CT is particularly good at detecting vascular lesions (e.g., acute intracerebral hemorrhage and tumors with little water content such as meningiomas) with accuracy rates of diagnosing AD reported as high as 91.5% [Willmer et al. 1993]. It is less expensive and more widely available than MRI, and can be used with subjects despite the presence of ferromagnetic materials that might be contained in cardiac pacemakers, intracranial aneurysm clips, or metal fragments in eyes, etc. MRI scans, however, have much higher spatial and anatomical resolution than CT providing greater soft tissue contrast and definition. MRI also allows imaging in multiple planes and does not involve radiation. Moreover, MRI is better at defining brain morphology, shows increased sensitivity to white matter and vascular pathology, and can easily be repeated over time.

In recent years, the developments of semi-automated techniques and volumetric magnetic resonance (MR) sequences have provided more quantitative and reliable measurement of structural brain changes. One such technique used by Jernigan and colleagues [1991a,b] measures computer-defined blocks of tissue in a reproducible manner. Other developments include observer-independent, fully automated techniques such as computer-generated segmentation. These computerized MRI segmentation techniques help differentiate the signal intensity of the brain from the cerebrospinal fluid (CSF), but there is still a great deal of variability with this technique in research settings. Some researchers have developed pulse sequences that are designed to estimate specifically the differences in tissue relaxation times [Kohn et al. 1991; Rusinek et al. 1991]. A third approach, used by Jack and colleagues (1992), involves observer-defined anatomic boundaries referred to as regions of interest (ROI) that are then summated for volumetric measurements. With this MR-based volumetric technique, the authors were able to focus selectively on those anatomic regions known to be involved in memory function and in the neuropathology of AD (i.e., hippocampal formation and anterior temporal lobe). The reliability of this technique was shown by repeated measures testing, and accuracy was evidenced by correlations with phantoms of known volume [Jack et al. 1990]. This approach has great promise and is an area of intense research interest.

B. Functional Brain Imaging

In recent years, functional neuroimaging has added new dimensions to studies of dementia. With use of positron emission tomography (PET), single-photon emission computer tomography (SPECT), magnetic resonance spectroscopy (MRS), and functional magnetic resonance imaging (fMRI), researchers have been able to investigate neural function in vivo. Functional brain imaging provides quantitative estimates of brain physiology such as cerebral blood flow, glucose metabolism, receptor binding kinetics, and neurotransmitter distribution. Thus, functional neuroimaging techniques may allow for the detection of subtle pathological changes that may predate the onset of dementia and structural changes.

In PET imaging, radiopharmaceuticals are synthesized with positron-emitting isotopes in order to provide insight into the metabolic, physiologic, and receptor processes. One widely used functional imaging technique in dementia uses the tracer [^{18}F]fluorodeoxyglucose (FDG) to determine glucose metabolism by PET scan (FDG-PET). Another technique uses $H_2^{15}O$ as the tracer to measure regional cerebral blood flow (rCBF) with PET. Unfortunately, PET has limited spatial resolution, which affects image quality and changes the apparent size of small anatomic structures. In addition, the requirement of applying mathematical models to convert scan data into measurements of relevant physiological processes, introduces further restrictions.

Interpretation of PET results in dementia is based on several methods. Although some investigators use the visual assessment of color-coded images, others prefer to more directly control for the variation in global cerebral metabolism among individuals. An integrated approach has been to create a color-coded image based on the ratio between regional cerebral metabolic rate for glucose (rCMRglu) and the global cerebral metabolic rate for glucose (gCMRglu) for the whole brain, providing a comparable index of metabolism at any given brain region for each subject. Over the past few years, however, more complex metabolic ratios have been proposed. For example, in a multicenter study, it was found that a composite ratio of rCMRglu of regions most typically affected over rCMRglu of regions least typically affected resulted in a 95.8% diagnostic accuracy when groups of clinically diagnosed AD patients were compared to controls [Herholz et al. 1993]. Sensitivity of PET has been reported to be as great as 92% with specificity as high as 88% [Powers et al. 1992].

Like PET, SPECT imaging also uses radiopharmaceuticals to generate images reflecting function or biochemistry. Compared to PET, SPECT uses direct photon-emitting isotopes rather than relying upon the interaction of an emitted positron with an electron in the surrounding tissue to generate two photons. However, in general, the relatively lower energy of SPECT tracers results in longer imaging times to acquire adequate counts and lower spatial resolution than PET. The most frequently used radiopharmaceuticals in dementia research are technetium-99m (^{99m}Tc) for labeling neurotransmitter ligands, and iodine-123 (^{123}I) for perfusion imaging. For example, Jobst [1998] tested the diagnostic value of [^{99cm}Tc]hexamethylpropylene amine oxime (HMPAO) SPECT on 104 patients with dementia and found that SPECT perfusion imaging was 83% accurate in assessing diagnoses (compared to 80% by CT scanning of temporal lobe). SPECT is considered safe, relatively easy to operate, well tolerated by patients, and inexpensive.

Functional brain imaging studies have also utilized MRS. MRS is used to measure biochemical and physiological changes in the brain that may indicate subtle changes before significant structural changes. The use of MRS in the neuropsychiatric population to assess neuronal loss is not yet as established as PET. Like with other neuroimaging techniques in dementia, an important question is how researchers handle atrophy differences in their AD versus control populations. Studies that have applied MRS in dementia have commonly utilized N-acetyl aspartate (NAA) and choline-containing compounds. Unlike PET, MRS does not use ionizing radiation and thus can be applied serially to patients. However, studies have found it more difficult to do in vivo MRS of the medial temporal lobes—an area of particular importance to dementia. MR spectroscopic imaging or MRSI is an MRS method that samples multiple areas of the brain at the same time unlike conventional MRS that employs a single-voxel method. MRSI has the advantage of sampling larger portions of the brain, and characteristic patterns of abnormal metabolism can thus be mapped. The disadvantage of MRSI is the relatively longer time requirement.

Functional magnetic resonance imaging (fMRI) is a functional brain imaging technique that can be applied in a variety of ways to yield information relevant to AD. Magnetic susceptibility measures reflecting regional cerebral blood volumes (rCBV) have been reported to closely correlate with FDG-PET (i.e., $r = .58$) [Gonzalez et al. 1995]. A concordance test of fMRI, rCBV, and PET in evaluating AD classification revealed a rate of 78% in a study of 10 patients. Compared to PET and SPECT, fMRI has superior spatial resolution and avoids the practical problems and safety concerns associated with radioactive isotope use. A type of fMRI called magnetic susceptibility (MS) contrast MRI uses contrast agents, e.g., lanthanide chelates that produce a change in MRI signal as they perfuse or enter tissue. Findings using this technique are similar to those of PET and SPECT with respect to AD. Another fMRI technique is blood oxygen level–dependent (BOLD) imaging. Because oxygenated and deoxygenated hemoglobin have different paramagnetic properties, changes in regional blood flow (rCBF) that produce changes in oxygenated and deoxygenated hemoglobin concentrations can be measured as changes in the proton relaxation properties of nearby tissue. BOLD is usually used in task activation studies designed to study changes in rCBF in response to tasks. Although BOLD techniques have been able to provide insight into the underlying neural mechanisms of symptoms, such as visual hallucinations in dementia, its usefulness in clinical diagnostic settings has yet to be determined. Enthusiasm for its clinical use is dampened by the knowledge that accurate application of the BOLD technique requires the full cooperation of patients with regard to both task performance and head movement restriction.

In this chapter, progress of brain imaging methods applied to various dementia syndromes are discussed as well as the clinical implications of these developments.

II. ALZHEIMER'S DISEASE

AD is the most common form of dementia, affecting 2–4 million people in the United States. Its diagnosis is based on the determination of an insidious onset and progression of symptoms in at least two out of five cognitive domains that interfere with normal functioning [American Psychiatric Association 1994]. In the best clinical setting, the diagnosis of AD is made with 85% accuracy, with postmortem examination providing the only definitive diagnosis. Clearly, there is a need for improved diagnostic accuracy with neuroimaging likely to play an increasingly important role in the early detection and prognosis of AD.

A. Structural Brain Imaging

Structurally, AD and normal control groups are distinguished by ventricular enlargement and cortical atrophy. For instance, using a combination of ventricular size and cortical atrophy, Jacoby and Levy [1980] correctly classified 80% of subjects. Additionally, longitudinal studies demonstrate an increased rate of ventricular size enlargement (i.e., $\sim 9\%$ compared to 2%) and cortical atrophy in AD compared to controls [Burns et al. 1991a; de Leon et al. 1989]. At present, there is no consensus as to whether cortical atrophy or ventricular size is the better measure for AD. However, the absence of correlation between these two measurements suggests that each is likely to contribute to diagnostic CT discrimination. Several studies have found that cognitive correlates of the two measures overlap, e.g., global rating of dementia, age [Ford and Winter 1981], memory [Albert et al. 1984; Bigler et al. 1985], Mini-Mental State Examination (MMSE), Cambridge Cognitive Examination (CAMCOG) [Burns et al. 1991b; Forstl et al. 1991].

A limitation of the diagnostic utility of structural brain imaging methods (i.e., CT and MRI) is in the overlap between AD and normal aging as well as other disorders. Specifically, in cross-sectional studies, sulcal widening and ventricular enlargement have also been noted in normal aging and in late-life schizophrenia and depressive disorders [DeCarli et al. 1990; Earnest et al. 1979; Pearlson et al. 1991]. Various methods have been used to improve diagnostic accuracy of CT, e.g., qualitative measures; quantitative linear, area, and volumetric assessments. Qualitative ratings of temporal lobe atrophy, e.g., sylvian fissure, temporal horn, and temporal sulcus and width of the suprasellar cistern, have been shown to differentiate AD from normal aging. These ratings are taken from images acquired with a scan angle parallel to or as much as 20° cephalic to the canthomeatal line [Davis et al. 1994]. Nonetheless, there is considerable variability across studies as measurement techniques differ from one research facility to another.

Linear measurements on axial images, although less reliable than volumetric techniques, have also been used in AD. It has been found that ROI measurements based on thin-section coronal T1-weighted images can detect volume loss in the anterior part of the temporal lobe and hippocampus [Jack et al. 1992]. Other studies utilizing linear measurements have shown that with 90% specificity, the entorhinal cortex (95% sensitivity) and temporal cortex (63% sensitivity), followed by enlargement of the temporal horn (56% sensitivity) and atrophy of hippocampal formation (41% sensitivity), best distinguished AD from normal controls [Erkinjuntti et al. 1993].

Quantitative volumetric MR studies indicate greater CSF volume, smaller brain volume, and greater atrophy in AD than age-matched normal controls [Jernigan et al. 1991a,b]. In a review of specificity and sensitivity of these various measures, it was found that specificity is consistent across measures while sensitivity improves with greater detail of analysis [DeCarli 2001; DeCarli et al. 1990].

The early contributions of sMRI to the diagnosis of AD are primarily related to establishing that MRI provided a better method than CT for measuring brain atrophy. Using sMRI, Duara and colleagues (1989) concluded that the decline in cerebral volume in AD mostly reflects a decrease in cerebral gray matter and a concomitant increase in CSF in cerebral sulci, lateral ventricles, third ventricles, and temporal horns. In general, the decline in brain volume is correlated to global measures of disease severity. More recently, the use of visual analysis of structural damage through MRI has been complemented by the quantitative method of magnetization transfer (MT) imaging. MT imaging is based on interactions between immobile protons and free protons of tissue [Balaban and Ceckler 1992]. The MT ratio is derived from the macromolecular concentration and exchange rates characteristic of the different underlying histologic structures of the brain. Thus, a decreased MT ratio suggests the presence of gliosis and neuronal loss.

In one of the first studies to utilize this technique in dementia, Hanyu and colleagues [2000] investigated the difference in hippocampal MT ratios between patients with AD, vascular dementia (VaD), and normal controls. Their results showed that the MT ratios of patients with AD differed from the normal controls whereas the VaD patients were similar to the normal controls [Hanyu et al. 2000].

Temporal lobe atrophy has been consistently reported in AD and may be the pathognomonic neural abnormality of the disease with high specificity for AD when compared to normal controls [Jobst et al. 1992b; O'Brien et al. 1997; Smith et al. 1999b; Wilcock 1983]. Unfortunately, there are difficulties in viewing medial temporal structures on typical CT scans due to artifacts; thus, measures of the suprasellar cistern have been used as an indirect measurement of medial temporal atrophy [LeMay et al. 1986; Pearlson et al. 1991]. LeMay and colleagues [1986] demonstrated that suprasellar measures could be used to classify patients with AD and normal controls with a high degree of accuracy. Four methods of measuring the suprasellar cistern (SSC) that have shown high reliability in distinguishing AD from normal controls are the SSC area ratio, the hexagonal area ratio, the width ratio, and perceptual rating [Aylward et al. 1991].

Improved diagnostic accuracy for AD can also be achieved by obtaining CT slices oriented along the axis of the temporal lobes [Jobst et al. 1992a,b]. Using this method, Jobst and colleagues [1992b] correctly classified 92% of patients with AD and found that the narrowest thickness of the medial temporal lobe was ~ 50% thinner in AD. Combining this approach with temporoparietal hypoperfusion as measured by SPECT increased specificity (90% sensitivity and 97% specificity) in this study. However, Lavenu and colleagues [1997] failed to replicate these findings, reporting a diagnostic accuracy rate (correct assessments out of total number of assessments) of only 68%.

Of the medial temporal lobe structures, hippocampal volumes have been studied most extensively in AD. In general, sensitivity and specificity increases with age- and gender-corrected hippocampal volume data. For example, in a study of patients in the prodromal phase of AD, sMRI measurements of the entorhinal cortex, the banks of the superior temporal sulcus, and the anterior cingulate were found to be the most useful in predicting the status of subjects three years after testing [Killiany et al. 2000]. Increasing hippocampal atrophy may also be an early sign of AD [Convit et al. 1997; Fox et al. 1996; Laakso et al. 1995]. Fox and colleagues [1996] performed serial MRI scans on five members of an early-onset familial AD pedigree with the 717 valine-to-glycine mutation in the amyloid precursor protein (APP). After a 2-year interscan interval, two of the five at-risk members who developed AD had a 20% hippocampal volume loss and notable hippocampal asymmetry prior to their development of overt symptoms [Fox et al. 1996].

In cross-sectional studies, hippocampal volume atrophy has been found to correlate with hypometabolism in ipsilateral posterior association cortices, i.e., temporal and angular gyri, suggesting that cortical hypometabolism in AD could be the result of the loss of hippocampal-cortical projections [Jobst et al. 1992a; Meguro et al. 2001]. Alternatively, a loss of intracortical projecting neocortical pyramidal neurons reflected in smaller corpus callosum sizes might contribute to cortical hypometabolism in AD [Teipel et al. 2002]. Yamauchi and colleagues [2000] demonstrated that the ratio of the posterior corpus callosum to skull area was significantly smaller in AD patients than in normal controls. Furthermore, this ratio distinguished AD from other dementias such as frontotemporal dementia (FTD) and progressive supranuclear palsy (PSP) [Yamauchi et al. 2000].

Through cross-sectional studies, hippocampal volume loss has also been found to correlate with cognitive deficits, particularly memory disorders [Deweer et al. 1995; Laakso et al. 1995; O'Brien et al. 1997]. In a study by Deweer and colleagues [1995], 18 AD patients were given a battery of neuropsychological tests including dementia rating scales—MMSE, Mattis Dementia Rating Scale (DRS); and tests of memory function—Wechsler Memory Scale (WMS), California Verbal Learning Test (CVLT), and the Buschke test. Of the hippocampal formation, amygdala, and caudate nucleus volumetric measures, only hippocampal volume measures were correlated with the memory variables [Deweer et al. 1995]. These findings are consistent with (1) the role of the hippocampus in memory function, and (2) the specificity of AD memory deficits to hippocampal abnormalities. In a study by Stout and colleagues [1999], however, impairment in the CVLT was related not only to the medial temporal lobe volume, but also to thalamic volumes.

Of note, in the presence of an illness with progressive regional volume losses, hypometabolism and memory failure, associations between regional volumes, regional hypometabolism, and task performance in AD patients cannot be accepted as proof of causation.

B. Functional Brain Imaging

The most consistently reported PET findings in AD are reductions (30–70%) in regional cerebral glucose metabolism (rCMRglu) and regional cerebral blood flow (rCBF) in the parietal and temporal associate cortices, often bilaterally [Benson et al. 1983; Frackowiak et al. 1981; Friedland et al. 1984]. Less severe cortical metabolic abnormalities may appear even in the preclinical stages, i.e., prior to the onset of measurable cognitive disturbance, of AD [Haxby et al. 1985; Reiman et al. 1996; Small et al. 1995, 1999a]. Temporoparietal metabolic asymmetry has also been found with left hypometabolism more pronounced than right hypometabolism [Loewenstein et al. 1989]. Correlations of PET-rCBF with language tasks have provided additional support for the notion of greater left hemisphere than right hemisphere abnormalities in AD [Rossor et al. 1982; Seltzer and Sherwin 1983], as AD patients with greater language deficits have been found to have more pronounced left frontotemporal asymmetry [Haxby et al. 1985; Haxby and Rapoport 1985; Loewenstein et al. 1989].

Prominent reductions in rCMRglu have also been noted in the paralimbic areas of the orbitofrontal cortex and the anterior cingulate. To a lesser extent, abnormalities in rCBF and oxidative metabolism have been found in the frontal association cortices of severely demented patients [Frackowiak et al. 1981]. In general, areas less affected include the sensorimotor and visual cortices, basal ganglia, and cerebellum [Benson et al. 1983; Frackowiak et al. 1981].

Although atrophy accounts for part of these early findings, it is unlikely that abnormalities are due solely to atrophy [Ibanez et al. 1998; Meltzer et al. 1996]. In the early stages of AD, a variable regional pattern is superimposed on the global decline in metabolic rate such that there is a match between types of behavioral change and the regions most affected [Haxby and Rapoport 1986]. For example, rCMRglu of temporoparietal regions, with or without atrophy correction, was found to be correlated with neuropsychological data [Slansky et al. 1995].

Activation studies have also been performed in attempts to increase sensitivity and specificity of PET studies in AD patients. For instance, deficits in task-relevant brain areas were reported in AD during divided and sustained attention [Johannsen et al. 1999], continuous visual recognition task [Kessler et al. 1991], and a temporally graded visual stimulation task [Mentis et al. 1996]. During a face-matching task, it was found that AD patients were able to activate the visual association areas equally as well as healthy controls despite decreased functional activity at rest [Grady et al. 1993]. Of note, the AD patients recruited brain areas such as the frontal cortex that were not found activated in the normal controls. The authors posit that the recruitment of additional areas of brain activation in AD is a result of the greater effort required for AD patients to perform the task.

fMRI has recently been utilized to examine the effects of cerebral atrophy on the BOLD signal. A BOLD study was performed on eight patients with AD while they performed a semantic task known to activate the left inferior frontal and left superior temporal gyri. Unlike the 16 control subjects, the AD patients showed a significantly positive correlation between clusters of brain activation and measures of local atrophy in the left inferior frontal gyrus, but not in the left superior temporal gyrus. The authors suggested that the association between atrophy and activation in the left inferior frontal gyrus might reflect a compensatory mechanism [Johnson et al. 2000]. Additionally, diminished entorhinal activation was also found in some of the patients with mild cognitive impairment, suggesting that functional abnormalities in the entorhinal cortex during task studies might be an early sign of AD [Small et al. 1999]. Diminished activation in mid- and posterior inferotemporal regions have also been observed during visual naming and letter fluency tasks in individuals at risk for AD [Smith et al. 1999a].

Holman and colleagues [1992b] determined the probability of diagnosing AD using SPECT. The results indicated the following probabilities: 19% for patients with memory loss and normal SPECT perfusion patterns; 82% for patients with abnormal perfusion patterns and memory loss, 77% for patients with abnormal bilateral temporoparietal deficiency; 43% for patients with confined frontal region deficiencies; and 0% for patients with small perfusion abnormalities confined to the cortex. Despite expectations that rCBF reductions using SPECT will be found in the temporoparietal regions in AD, its sensitivity and specificity remain unclear. For instance, Weiner and colleagues [1993] found this expected pattern in only 28% of AD patients. However, SPECT-determined reduction in CBF has been shown to occur in the absence of substantial atrophy in the same region [Wyper et al. 1993]. Thus, reduced rCBF found using SPECT can be utilized as a preclinical predictor of the development of AD [Johnson et al. 1998]. Johnson and colleagues [1998] found that lower rCBF was more prominent in the hippocampal-amygdaloid complex, the anterior and posterior cingulate, and the anterior thalamus of those who later developed AD, with a predictive capacity at 83%. Selective hippocampal uptake deficit in AD by SPECT has been reported with variable degrees of frontal, temporal, and parietal deficits [Villa et al. 1995]. Other studies, however, have suggested that hippocampal perfusion is maintained in mild to moderate AD [Ishii et al. 1998].

Functional neuroimaging has also provided neurotransmitter-dependent measures in AD. Presynaptic cholinergic terminal densities (PCTD) have been mapped in vivo using [^{123}I]Iodobenzovesamicol. In contrast to normal aging that has a 3.7% decline in PCTD per decade, PET studies have found that early-onset AD is associated with an approximately 30% PCTD decline throughout the cortex including the hippocampus. Using the muscarinic receptor binding tracer [^{123}I] dexetimide, Claus and colleagues [1997] found a reduction in temporoparietal binding of the tracer in early AD, whereas benzodiazepine receptors appear to be relatively preserved despite the presence of decreased rCBF [Kitamura et al. 1996]. Using radiolabelled acetylcholine analogues such as N-[^{11}C]methylpiperidin-4-yl propionate ([^{11}C]PMP) in vivo findings have reported a decrease of 30–40% in the temporoparietal areas of AD [Kuhl et al. 1999). Others have also found reductions of acetylcholinesterase in the temporal cortex (31%), parietal cortex (38%), and primary sensory cortex (20–25%) in AD [Iyo et al. 1997). However, controversy about how early in the course of AD cholinergic neuron loss occurs suggests the possibility that the above in vivo imaging approaches to the cholinergic system may not prove valuable for early AD diagnosis.

Loss of serotonin has also been evidenced by PET studies using the tracer [^{18}F]setoperone and [^{18}F]altanserin [Blin et al. 1993; Meltzer et al. 1999]. Meltzer and colleagues [1999] reported decrements in serotonin-2A-receptor avidity in AD in the anterior cingulate, prefrontal, and sensorimotor cortices. Decrements in the dopaminergic pathways of AD have also been found. A reduction of 20% in the uptake of the dopamine reuptake ligand [^{11}C]β-DFT has been reported in the putamen and caudate in AD [Rinne et al. 1998]. [^{123}I]β-CIT, a dopamine transporter ligand, has been used with SPECT to distinguish AD patients from dementia with Lewy bodies (DLB) patients. In one study, it was found that the striatal/

cerebellar ratio of [^{123}I]β-CIT was 5.5 in AD compared to 2.1 in the DLB patients 18 hr after tracer injection [Donnemiller et al. 1997], suggesting a relative preservation of dopamine transporter sites in the striatum in AD compared to DLB patients.

Recent developments in radiotracers have also made it possible to measure amyloid plaques and neurofibrillary tangles in vivo. PET and SPECT methods have been proposed using labeled analogs of fluorescent dyes that stain amyloid in postmortem tissue [Klunk et al, 2001; Shoghi-Jadid et al, 2002; Zhuang et al, 2001]. For example, in a PET study by Barrio and colleagues [1999] using the radiotracer 2-(I-{6-[2-[^{18}F]fluoroethyl)-(methyl)-amino]-2-napthyl}ethylene) malononitrile ([^{18}F]FDDNP), [^{18}F]FDDNP was found to have slower clearance in patients with AD than normal controls. Furthermore, greater accumulation of [^{18}F]FDDNP was found in the hippocampal region even in patients with mild AD, suggesting the presence of amyloid plaques. Postmortem studies later confirmed [^{18}F]FDDNP binding to amyloid plaques. Although promising, the sensitivity and selectivity of this and the other proposed tracers of AD are yet to be established.

Studies of brain energy metabolism have also been investigated using MRS in AD. To date, the existence of energy deficits in AD have been inconsistent. In general, many report little or no metabolite changes (i.e., *myo*-inositol and NAA) in AD and argue against the utility of MRS as an early diagnostic tool for AD [Bottomley et al. 1992; Miatto et al. 1986; Murphy et al. 1993; Stoppe et al. 2000]. However, others report differences in AD (e.g., nucleoside triphosphate, phosphocreatine, inorganic phosphate) when compared to normal controls [Brown et al. 1989]. For instance, Huang and colleagues [2001] found increased levels of total creatine (Cr), *myo*-inositol (mI), and reduced levels of NAA in the occipital and parietal regions of AD patients. Interestingly, in patients with mild AD, only Cr and mI but not NAA concentration abnormalities were found [Huang et al. 2001]. High levels of Cr and mI can be indicators of gliosis; thus, detection via MRS in mild AD may not directly reflect neuronal loss. However, caution in interpreting MRS data is required, as the field generally lacks standardization of techniques across research labs, particularly in the way brain atrophy is handled in the analysis.

C. Brain Imaging and Genotyping

The influence of genetics is also of great interest in the neuroimaging field. For instance, known to infer an increased risk for the development of AD, the ε4 allele of apolipoprotein E (ApoE) has also, in some studies, been found to be associated with a more rapid cognitive decline with age in community-dwelling individuals [Roses et al. 1996; Jonker et al. 1998]. In a cross-sectional study of AD by Geroldi [1999], the presence of the APOE ε4 allele was associated with smaller volumes of the hippocampus, entorhinal cortex, and anterior temporal lobe.

In a longitudinal study, an increased rate of hippocampal volume loss not associated with memory changes was found in a group of healthy women in their sixth decade of life with a single APOE ε4 allele [Cohen et al. 2001]. Although cognitive details were not provided, a similar association of increased hippocampal atrophy and the APOE ε4 allele was observed in an older group that consisted almost exclusively of men, half of whom were homozygotes for the APOE ε4 allele, in the Baltimore Longitudinal Study of Aging [Moffat et al. 2000]. Similarly, PET studies of nondemented individuals with either one or two APOE ε4 alleles have shown these people to have lower metabolism in the parietal lobe, and posterior cingulate and prefrontal cortices, and on longitudinal study to have an enhanced metabolic decline in areas that include the posterior cingulate, parietal, and lateral temporal lobes [Reiman et al. 1996, 2001; Small et al. 1995, 2000; Smith et al. 1999a].

On the other hand, some studies have shown that persons without dementia who carry the ε4 allele have more widespread brain activation than noncarriers in regions required for memory, possibly because they require greater cognitive effort to complete the tasks presented to them. This was illustrated by Burggren and colleagues [2002], who showed that additional cognitive effort in those at risk for AD is specific to encoding episodic memory, and cannot be attributed to task difficulty. Clearly, this is a rapidly emerging field that requires much greater study.

III. VASCULAR DEMENTIA

Vascular dementia (VaD) may account for 90% of all non-AD dementias. VaD has been reported to be the second leading cause of dementia with prevalence rates of 14–47% [Bobek-Billewicz et al. 2001]. As the clinical picture of VaD is heterogeneous, so are the underlying neural changes. In general, the regional deficits depend on the location of the lesion. The use of brain imaging techniques in detecting patterns of underlying brain abnormalities characteristic of VaD has advanced the understanding of the nature of VaD. The diagnosis of VaD (as opposed to AD) depends on the presence of periventricular hyperintensity, subcortical lesions (e.g., thalamus), cortical infarcts (e.g., cerebellum), and basal ganglia lacunar infarcts [Pantano et al. 1999]. By definition, the lesions that lead to VaD are heterogeneous and sometimes overlapping; thus, the associated neuroimaging results are also heterogeneous.

A. Structural Brain Imaging

Volumetric studies have shown that VaD is often associated with smaller temporal lobes, amygdala, and hippocampal volumes compared to age-matched controls [Barber et al. 2000; Bobek-Billewicz et al. 2001]. These reductions, particularly in the hippocampus and gray matter, have been noted to correlate with severity of cognitive impairment [Fein et al. 2000]. In contrast to stroke-related dementia, some studies have shown that cortical and total white matter lesion area accurately classified VaD patients, suggesting that the cortical lesions that develop after a stroke are responsible for the dementia [Liu et al. 1992].

In an attempt to find a differential MRI profile for VaD, Schmidt [1992] delineated abnormalities that appeared more prevalent in patients with VaD than AD and healthy individuals, controlling for similarities in age and dementia severity and duration. These abnormalities included: (1) basal ganglionic/thalamic hyperintense foci; (2) thromboembolic infarctions; (3) confluent white matter; and (4) irregular periventricular hyperintensities. However, it was noted that extent of atrophy was not different between the two dementia groups [Schmidt 1992].

B. Functional Brain Imaging

Because of the variability in the location and extent of damage to tissues and type of blood vessels involved in VaD, it is not surprising that rCBF and metabolic findings are found to differ among the subtypes of VaD. For example, SPECT studies have revealed heterogeneous and irregular patterns in patients with VaD [Talbot et al. 1998]. In patients with VaD due to large infarcts, regional cerebral blood flow (rCBF) and regional metabolic rate for oxygen (rCMRO$_2$) have been reported to be equally decreased in all regions, whereas in patients with VaD due to lacunes and white matter changes, only a moderate loss of vasoreactivity in response to acetazolamide was found [De Reuck et al. 1998, 1999]. Furthermore, periventricular white matter changes and thalamic lacunes, postulated to increase susceptibility to dementia, have been shown to be associated with a more profound reduction in rCBF in the cerebral cortex [Kawamura et al. 1991].

In an early attempt to elucidate the mechanisms of CBF reductions found in VaD, Frackowiack and colleagues [1981] investigated CBF and cerebral oxygen utilization in a group of patients with VaD using $^{15}O_2$ PET. They found that CBF and mean cerebral oxygen utilization correlated negatively with severity of dementia. It was also noted that oxygen utilization was most impaired in the parietal lobe [Frackowiak et al. 1981]. These findings were replicated by Mielke and colleagues [1992], who showed that severity of dementia was associated with reduced glucose metabolic in the temperoparietal and frontal association cortex and the basal ganglia, thalamus, and cerebellum of VaD patients.

Comparing VaD patients to normal controls and stroke patients using a new PET tracer that mimics calcium influx in the ischemic tissue called cobalt-55 chloride (^{55}Co) PET (^{55}Co corresponds to the inflammatory response and to the severity of the ischemic damage shortly after a stroke), De Reuck and colleagues [2001] found that in VaD ^{55}Co uptake was significantly increased in the cerebral white matter, coinciding with the increased lucency scores observed on CT scan and indicative of recent damage. The absence of increased ^{55}Co uptake in the cerebral cortex and deep gray nuclei was consistent with the presence of old and stable lesions, believed to no longer contribute significantly to the progression of cognitive impairment in VaD patients [De Reuck et al. 2001]. In short, white matter changes (WMC) may progress independently from cortical infarcts and lacunes, and it is possible that a certain threshold of damage must be reached in the cerebral white matter before cognitive impairment appears [De Reuck et al. 2001].

In general, defects found using PET or SPECT are larger than those seen on structural imaging studies, providing further support for the use of functional brain imaging techniques for the early detection of vascular dementia [Seiderer et al. 1989].

C. White Matter Changes

White matter changes (WMC) are generally divided into those immediately adjacent to the ventricles (periventricular hyperintensities) and those located in the deep white matter. White matter lesions are signaled by reduced attenuation or leukoaraiosis on CT scanning or areas of increased intensity on proton density and T2-weighted MRI or fluid-attenuated inversion recovery (FLAIR). WMC has been associated with advanced age, stroke risk factors, focal neurological deficits, impaired cognition, and cerebral hypoperfusion in areas supplied by deep penetrating arteries [Inzitari 2000; Mathews et al. 1992]. Previous literature posits that the presence of significant WMC can predict the development of VaD [Inzitari 2000].

Studies have attempted to localize the area of white matter hyperintensities in VaD. Using magnetization transfer measurement ratios, Tanabe and colleagues [1999] found that pathologic changes in vascular dementia are most severe in the periventricular white matter. They made comparisons of white matter signal hyperintensities location and size between subcortical ischemic vascular dementia and normal controls, and found that the patients had reduced periventricular white matter signal hyperintensities [Tanabe et al. 1999]. Compared to AD, Wahlund and colleagues [1994] found that the regional distribution of WMC was greater in the posterior regions and right hemisphere of the brain in VaD.

Researchers have also investigated the relationship of severity of WMC and cerebral blood flow in patients with VaD. One study using computerized densitometric measurements of white matter and xenon CT measurements of local cerebral blood flow found the ratio of frontal WMC area to total area of parenchyma was increased and the local cerebral blood flow reduced in 35 patients with VaD compared to 16 age-matched controls [Kawamura et al. 1991]. Additionally, multivariate regression analysis showed that the severity of WMC correlated with blood flow reductions in the putamen and thalamus. The authors suggested two possible explanations for the findings: (1) abnormal perfusion by deep penetrating arteries may contribute to the pathogenesis of WMC, or (2) perfusion of deep gray matter structures is reduced secondary to diaschisis or reduced metabolic demand, and thus WMC is associated with disruption of pathways between cortical and subcortical gray matter [Kawamura et al. 1991].

D. Distinguishing Vascular Dementia from Alzheimer's Disease

Because the considerable overlap between the behavioral and cognitive manifestations of VaD and AD can lead to differential diagnostic problems, brain imaging studies have sought to find diagnostically useful characteristic patterns in VaD and AD patients. Pantel and colleagues [1998], using analysis of covariance, were unable to find any global or regional cerebral volume differences between patients with VaD and AD. The authors posited that the similarities between the two groups are reflective of the vulnerability of the neuronal structures as opposed to specificity of disease pathology [Pantel et al. 1998]. In a unique study using a central rating system, Scheltens and Kittner [2000] performed ratings on CT and MRI scans in 486 patients diagnosed with AD and 440 people diagnosed with VaD from multiple international centers. They found that VaD was associated with deep white matter hyperintensities and medial temporal atrophy. These changes, however, were also found present in the group of AD patients. The contribution that variability in concepts applied to each dementia group (i.e., NINCDS/ADRDA for AD group and NINDS/AIREN for VaD group) made to their failure to discriminate the two patient groups is difficult to assess.

Progressive brain atrophy has also been utilized to differentiate VaD from AD. Using serial MRI, O'Brien and colleagues [2001] found no significant difference between VaD and AD, although both groups had significantly greater rates of atrophy than did the normal controls. Furthermore, the authors found that the rate of atrophy was positively correlated with severity of cognitive impairment [O'Brien et al. 2001].

Perfusion and metabolic studies have also been used to characterize VaD and AD. Unlike AD, patterns of perfusion and metabolism in VaD are highly heterogeneous owing to the marked variability in pathology (e.g., multi-infarct, atherosclerosis, myeloproliferative disorders, CADASIL, hemorrhagic infarcts). Marked reductions have been observed in the frontal, temporal, and parietal lobes [Mielke and Heiss 1998; Mielke et al. 1996; Sabri et al. 1999]. However, in a comparative PET study, Nagata and colleagues [2000] found that, unlike the well-reported hypoperfusion and hypometabolism in the temporoparietal region in AD, VaD was associated with a reduction of cerebral blood flow and energy metabolism, mostly in the frontal lobe [Nagata et al. 2000]. In addition to regional differences, composite patterns, such as contrast between association areas and subcortical regions [Mielke and Heiss 1998] and parietal-cerebellar ratio [Kuhl 1985], have also been reported to be lower in AD than VaD. Given the overlap in the histopathologies of AD and VD the difficulties in distinguishing these two disorders prior to postmortem is not surprising.

IV. DEMENTIA WITH LEWY BODIES (DLB)

The presence of Lewy bodies is the cardinal feature of DLB that distinguishes it from AD, although DLB overlaps with AD in symptom profile and in some of its neuropathology (i.e., β-amyloidosis, plaques, acetylcholine depletion).

A. Structural Brain Imaging

Structural brain imaging studies have suggested that neural abnormalities in DLB include ventricular enlargement, periventricular and white matter hyperintensities, and reductions in temporal and hippocampal volume [Barber et al. 1999b, 2000]. However, compared to AD, DLB has been reported to have relative preservation of both temporal lobes and hippocampus [Barber et al. 2000] that parallels the findings of relatively preserved memory functions in DLB [Barber et al. 1999b]. Although some postmortem studies have reported greater frontal atrophy in DLB than in AD, these findings have failed to be replicated by antemortem MRI studies where diagnostic distinctions were made on clinical grounds [Barber et al. 2000; Harvey et al. 1999]. Compared to VaD, no apparent volumetric differences or rate of atrophy have been reported for DLB [Barber et al. 2000; O'Brien et al. 2001]. DLB has been reported to have a mean rate of atrophy of 1.4% per year that correlated with increasing severity of cognitive impairment [O'Brien et al. 2001].

B. Functional Brain Imaging

Although several studies in DLB suggest that the occipital lobe is relatively spared, DLB has been associated with occipital hypoperfusion as demonstrated by PET and SPECT [Ishii et al. 1999; Lobotesis et al. 2001; Middelkoop et al. 2001]. In a relatively large study with 23 patients with DLB and 50 patients with AD, occipital hypoperfusion in DLB was reported not only when compared to age-matched control subjects, but also when compared to the AD patients who were matched for severity of impairment [Lobotesis et al. 2001]. Similar findings have been reported by others despite smaller sample sizes [Okamura et al. 2001; Imamura et al. 2001]. Further, Imamura and colleagues [2001] reported that the medial and lateral occipital rCMRglc reduction is present in both DLB with and without parkinsonism. Hence, occipital hypometabolism appears to be a robust phenomenon in DLB.

Blood flow reductions in the occipital cortex may [Howard et al. 1997] or may not [Lobotesis et al. 2001] be associated with visual hallucinations, a pathognomonic feature of DLB. Of note, in the first study to investigate volumetric measurements of the occipital area in DLB, structural abnormalities were not found nor were correlations between occipital volume and visual hallucinations or cognitive functioning despite blood flow and metabolic abnormalities in the same patients [Middelkoop et al. 2001]. Occipital cholinergic loss, white matter changes [Middelkoop et al. 2001], and pathological processes in the brainstem or basal forebrain structures [Imamura et al. 2001] have been offered as explanations for the presence of hypoperfusion and hypometabolism in the absence of structural changes in the occipital cortex of DLB.

More recently, a reduction in presynaptic nigrostriatal dopaminergic function in the striatum in DLB has been found using ^{18}F-fluoroDOPA-PET (F-DOPA-PET) [Hu et al. 2000]. FDOPA-PET distinguished DLB from AD with 86% sensitivity and 100% specificity. Furthermore, the rate of FDOPA uptake in the caudate nucleus was found to be the best discriminator with a rate of 100% for specificity (71% sensitivity) [Hu et al. 2000]. These results support the neuropathological findings of loss of neurons in the substantia nigra and depletion of striatal dopamine in DLB. Thus, the authors posit that FDOPA-PET may be a useful tool for distinguishing DLB from AD.

V. FRONTOTEMPORAL DEMENTIA (FTD)

FTD has several etiologies including Pick's disease, motor neuron dementia (MND), and progressive subcortical gliosis. As suggested by name, FTD is associated with abnormalities of the frontal and temporal cortices. This pattern of atrophy has been associated with predominant white matter changes as shown by Larsson and colleagues [2001].

A. Structural Brain Imaging

In comparison with AD, FTD is generally associated with greater frontal atrophy, which is variable among the subtypes of FTD [Chan et al. 2001]. Additionally, compared to AD, FTD has less atrophy in the hippocampal formation and is also reported to have a qualitatively different pattern, i.e., predominantly in the anterior hippocampus [Laakso et al. 2000]. However, some have shown that FTD has equally great entorhinal cortex atrophy as AD [Frisoni et al. 1996; 1999].

Using automated hemispheric surface display of MRI images, Kitagaki and colleagues [1998] noted that the mean hemispheric-to-intracranial volume ratio in patients with FTD (56.2%) was significantly smaller than the ratio in the control subjects (66.0%). Additionally, it was found that asymmetry of hemispheric volume was significantly larger in the FTD group than in the AD and control groups. The authors posited that FTD is characterized by a more widespread cortical atrophy with asymmetric frontal and anterior temporal atrophy that distinguishes it from AD [Kitagaki et al. 1998]. Thus, although whole-brain rate of atrophy cannot distinguish FTD from AD, markedly different patterns of regional atrophy have been found between the two groups.

Atrophy of the corpus callosum has also been reported in FTD. For example, Yamauchi and colleagues [2000] reported that the anterior quarter callosal/skull area ratio in a group of patients with FTD was significantly smaller than in patients with AD and PSP and in normal controls. These findings suggest a differential pattern of corpus callosum atrophy in FTD compared to normal controls and other dementias. Corpus callosum atrophy may reflect the pathological changes in the cerebral cortex.

B. Functional Brain Imaging

Functional brain imaging has also revealed predominant frontal perfusion abnormalities that have been found present prior to symptoms of structural atrophy. For example, in a SPECT study using ^{99m}Tc-HMPAO, bilateral frontal hypoperfusion corresponding with frontal gliosis and neuronal loss in the absence of plaques or tangles were found in a group of seven patients with FTD [Read et al. 1995]. The same was also reported in patients with normal levels of CSF β-amyloid and tau-protein and atypical FTD neuropsychological profiles in an FDG-PET study [Jauss et al. 2001]. In distinguishing FTD from AD, studies have suggested that the use of calculated ratios can be more sensitive, e.g., parietal and frontal cortices CBF [Miller et al. 1991]. Others have found that the anterior/posterior CBF ratio (e.g., <0.89) correctly identified FTD patients from AD patients [Graff-Radford et al. 1995; Julin et al. 1995]. Overall, greater frontal cortex changes in FTD than other brain regions particularly temporoparietal-occipital regions can discriminate FTD as a patient group from AD in functional brain imaging studies [Charpentier et al. 2000].

Nevertheless, temporal abnormalities are observed in functional imaging studies. For example, in the study by Miller and colleagues [1991], SPECT revealed both frontal and temporal hypoperfusion in patients with FTD with the selectivity of neuropsychological impairments corresponding with their SPECT abnormalities. Specifically, performance of the patients during the frontal and memory tasks was impaired while attention, language, and visuospatial skills appeared to be preserved [Miller et al. 1991].

Functional brain imaging has also revealed abnormalities in the neural connections between the frontal and subcortical regions in FTD. For instance, using FDG-PET, Garraux and colleagues [1999] found that compared to normal controls, FTD patients had reduced glucose metabolism in the dorsolateral and ventrolateral prefrontal cortices and frontopolar and anterior cingulate regions, in addition to bilateral anterior temporal, right inferior parietal, and bilateral striatal regions. Compared to patients with PSP, FTD patients had greater striatofrontal metabolic impairment than PSP [Garraux et al. 1999]. Thus, metabolic impairment was found present in distinct subcorticocortical networks in FTD.

MRS studies have also reported biochemical frontal abnormalities in FTD. For example, Ernst and colleagues [1997] found reduced N-acetyl compounds (−28%) and glutamate plus glutamine (−16%) in FTD patients, possibly the result of neuronal loss. In contrast, AD patients showed significant abnormalities in the temporoparietal region, but not in the frontal region. With use of linear discriminant analysis, 92% of the FTD patients were correctly differentiated from the AD patients and control subjects using this method [Ernst et al. 1997].

Although working with a relatively small sample, Gregory and colleagues [1999] investigated the diagnostic capabilities of structural (i.e., MRI) and functional (i.e., HMPOA-SPECT) brain imaging methods in two male patients with FTD [Gregory et al. 1999]. They reported that neither technique was sensitive to the early changes of FTD, especially in those occurring in the ventromedial frontal cortex. Although typical changes of FTD were found during subsequent assessments (i.e., ~ 3–5 years later), neither frontal atrophy nor frontal hypoperfusion was found during the patients" initial assessments. The authors concluded that initial findings of normal MRI or SPECT cannot exclude the diagnosis of FTD, as typical pathophysiological signs may appear in follow-up assessments [Gregory et al. 1999].

VI. MIXED AND OTHER DEMENTIA DISORDERS

A. Huntington's Disease (HD)

Of the subcortical dementias, HD has probably received the most attention. Thus far, the most robust finding in HD is basal ganglia (i.e., putamen, caudate, and thalamus) atrophy, which has been found present in as early as preclinical stages [Brooker et al. 1991; De la Monte et al. 1988; Halliday et al. 1998]. For example, decreased size of the caudate nucleus, particularly the head of the caudate nucleus (HCN), has been reported to be of diagnostic value in differentiating HD from normal controls [Culjkovic et al. 1999; Roth et al. 1996]. More recently, studies have also suggested continued atrophy in HD, particularly in the frontal lobes [Aylward et al. 1998]. For instance, Aylward and colleagues [1998] reported that frontal lobe atrophy rates correlated positively with severity of HD. The authors found that patients who were mildly affected had frontal lobe volumes identical to those of normal controls despite abnormalities in the basal ganglia, while those who were moderately affected had reductions in total frontal lobe volume (17%) and frontal white matter volume (28%) that were significantly different from controls [Aylward et al. 1998]. Other structural abnormalities include decreased thalamic and medial temporal volumes [Jernigan et al. 1991b] and increased hyperintense signals in the striatum [Oliva et al. 1993]. These findings complement diminished metabolic activity of the corpus striatum as observed on PET for added diagnostic specificity [Brooker et al. 1991].

FDG-PET has been shown to be more sensitive than structural brain imaging methods in characterizing the pattern of abnormalities in HD. PET has demonstrated striatal hypometabolism, particularly of the caudate nucleus, in early HD, in preclinical HD [Kuhl et al. 1984], and even in patients with preservation of the caudate nucleus [Garnett et al. 1984]. Similarly, total absence of perfusion has also been reported in 21 patients with HD despite lack of complete atrophy of the structure in some of the patients as measured by CT [Deisenhammer et al. 1989]. Furthermore, abnormalities in HD have been shown to correlate significantly with cognitive impairment—e.g., caudate atrophy and the MMSE [Tanahashi et al. 1985], basal ganglia atrophy and memory tasks, particularly during encoding [Brandt et al. 1995], caudate atrophy, frontal atrophy, and atrophy of the left (but not the right) sylvian cistern and memory tasks [Starkstein et al. 1992].

In a coupled FDG-PET and fMRI study of a patient with HD with dementia, discrepancies between the two methods were reported. Using FDG-PET, the parietal areas showed extensive atrophy and reduced resting rCMRglu. The behavior response data indicated that the patient performed with similar accuracy but with longer response time in a visuospatial task compared with healthy control subjects. However, fMRI BOLD signal in these areas showed greater task-dependent activation in the HD patient than in the control group. The authors postulate that the increased activation found in the HD patients reflects the higher neuronal effort, as evidenced by the longer reaction times, necessary to reach a similar degree of accuracy as in control subjects. These findings indicate that fMRI may be used as a tool for the "assessment of functionality of morphologically abnormal cortex and for the investigation of compensatory resource allocation in neurodegenerative disorders" [Dierks et al. 1999].

Brain imaging findings have also been correlated with findings from molecular genetic studies [Halliday et al. 1998]. For example, Hayden and colleagues [1987] studied individuals at risk for HD using a polymorphic human linked DNA marker (D4S10) and PET. Their findings indicated that the at-risk HD subjects had reduced rCMRglu in the caudate compared to the controls [Hayden et al. 1987]. SPECT studies have also been performed in at-risk subjects. These studies suggest reductions in glucose metabolism in the caudate nucleus and [^{123}I]Iodobenzamide (IBZM) dopamine D2 receptor striatum-to-frontal cortex ratio and perfusion ratios (HMPAO), in addition to rCBF changes in subjects at risk [Ichise et al. 1993; Tanahashi et al. 1985].

Of four diagnostic tools for HD—neurological examination, PET measurement of glucose metabolism, CT measurement of caudate size, and genetic testing at the polymorphic DNA loci D4S10, D4S43, and D4S125—Grafton and colleagues [1990] reported that PET measurements of caudate metabolism best predicted HD in 54 at-risk individuals with a sensitivity of 75%. The authors propose that abnormalities of cerebral metabolism precede clinical or structural abnormalities in those at risk for HD.

B. Progressive Supranuclear Palsy (PSP)—The Steele-Richardson-Olszewski Syndrome

PSP is the second most common form of degenerative parkinsonism. Genetic studies posit that PSP is a recessive disorder in linkage disequilibrium with the tau gene. Neuropathology studies provide further evidence for this linkage by showing that the accumulation of cortical tau contributes to the pathology of PSP. In a study by Bigio and colleagues [1999], it was found that higher levels of cortical tau correlated with cognitive impairment in PSP.

PSP neuropathological changes usually involve the enlargement of the aqueduct of Sylvius, third and fourth ventricles, and atrophy of globus pallidus or subthalamic nucleus. MR findings provide further support for this neuropathologic profile. These include focal midbrain atrophy with enlargement of the cerebral aqueduct, quadrigeminal plate cistern, and posterior third ventricle [Savoiardo et al. 1989]. A major interest in the brain imaging of PSP are the causes of subcortical abnormalities. Midbrain atrophy is characteristic of PSP in the majority of cases, and is often found in the absence of cortical abnormalities. Common abnormalities found using brain imaging techniques include brainstem and basal ganglia atrophy [Savoiardo et al. 1989]. Hypointensities of the basal ganglia and midbrain have also been reported [Savoiardo et al. 1989]. Hanyu and colleagues [2001] found significantly lower MTR in the subcortical gray matter, including the putamen, globus pallidus and thalamus, and subcortical white matter in patients with PSP that distinguished them from patients with PDD [Hanyu et al. 2001]. Others, however, found decreases in the areas of the globus pallidus and thalamus in the absence of changes in the caudate nucleus and putamen [Mann et al. 1993]. In an analysis of covariance, Yamauchi and colleagues [2000] found that the ratio of middle-anterior quarter area over total skull area in PSP was significantly smaller than the ratios in FTD, AD, and normal controls.

PET studies in PSP have also shown reduced frontal metabolic rates with frontal hypometabolism correlating with subsequent neuropsychological tests, particularly tests of executive functioning [Blin et al. 1990; D'Antona et al. 1985]. Using FDG-PET, Garraux and colleagues [1999] found abnormal correlations between the metabolic rates of the midbrain tegmentum and cerebellar, temporal, and pallidal regions and frontal cortex in PSP, suggesting to the investigators that the abnormal hypometabolism of the frontal cortex in PSP might be the result of a loss of subcortical afferents to the prefrontal cortex.

Salmon and colleagues [1996], using neuropsychological and neuroimaging measures, reported that early neuropsychological testing in a patient with a clinical pattern consistent with PSP revealed frontal lobe dysfunction. Although sMRI scans were unremarkable, statistical parametric mapping analysis of fMRI scans revealed a highly significant metabolic impairment in the anterior cingulate gyrus, further substantiating that subcorticofrontal dementia might be a key feature in PSP [Salmon et al. 1996].

C. Corticobasal Degeneration (CBGD)

CBGD is characterized by extrapyramidal symptoms, progressive unilateral rigidity, and laterized cortical abnormalities. Although not always present, structural neuroimaging in CBGD has found slight asymmetry and atrophy, usually in the frontal and parietal areas, often in the perirolandic gyri [Frasson et al. 1998]. Others have reported involvement of the basal ganglia, thalamus, substantia nigra, and cerebellum to various degrees [Jellinger 1996; Oyanagi et al. 2001]. PET studies have also reported glucose metabolic asymmetry in the parietal lobe and thalamus compared to normal controls and patients with PD [Eidelberg et al. 1991].

In a study using both structural (MRI) and functional imaging (FDG-PET) in three patients with CBGD, Frasson and colleagues [1998] found cortical dilatation of the frontal and perirolandic regions, and asymmetrical frontal and parietal cortices and basal ganglia. Further, the authors noted that the functional neuroimaging findings correlated well with the neuropsychological features of CBGD [Frasson et al. 1998]. These findings of marked asymmetry were later replicated by a study using MRI, SPECT, and FDG-PET [Koide et al. 1995]. In this latter study, MRI showed asymmetric cortical atrophy, especially in the parietal cortex. SPECT revealed asymmetric reduction of parietal cerebral blood flow that coincided with the MRI findings. Lastly, the FDG-PET also showed significant asymmetric rCMRglu reductions (~10%) in the lateral frontal cortex, lateral posterior frontal cortex, and primary motor and sensory cortex [Koide et al. 1995].

D. Parkinson's Disease with Dementia (PDD)

Dementia in those with Parkinson's disease occurs in 15–40% cases. Not only is PDD associated with the neuropathological changes of Parkinson's disease, but also those of AD. Variations in brain imaging findings in PDD are due to the heterogeneous clinical presentations of the disease. Nondemented PD is associated with frontal lobe dysfunction. PDD can coexist with AD and with LBD. PDD is secondary to cortical and subcortical changes rather than nigral striatal changes of Parkinson's disease. Using MTR to indicate neuronal loss, it has been reported that patients with PDD has significantly lower MTR in the subcortical white matter, including the frontal white matter and the genu of the corpus callosum, than the controls [Hanyu et al. 2001].

As with DLB, the cardinal feature of PDD is the presence of Lewy bodies. Despite the fact that Lewy bodies seldom affect the occipital lobes, like DLB, PDD has been associated with hypoperfusion and hypometabolism in the occipital region [Bohnen et al. 1999]. It has been posited that the occipital abnormalities of PDD might be due to the nigostriatal degeneration that is associated with the movement disorders [Bohnen et al. 1999]. Alternatively, an abnormality in cholinergic innervation may be responsible for the blood flow and metabolism changes in the occipital region of PDD, as decreases in presynaptic choline binding in the occipital cortex have also been shown in individuals with PDD [Kuhl et al. 1996].

Of note, a study by Sasaki and colleagues [1992] found contradictory results in the occipital cortex of patients with PDD. They studied five patients with PDD, nine patients with PD without dementia, and five normal controls using PET. They reported that the most significant decrease in glucose metabolism in PDD was found in the angular gyrus (49.7% of the normal controls) while the glucose metabolism in the cingulate, pre- and postcentral, occipital, and subcortical regions were relatively spared (62.1–85.5% of the normal controls) [Sasaki et al. 1992]. Others have also shown that compared to AD, PDD has the same pattern of temporal parietal hypometabolism [Peppard et al. 1992]. PET imaging in PDD using presynaptic dopaminergic ligands such as F-dopa have provided great insight to the abnormalities of dopaminergic functions associated with PDD. For example, studies with F-dopa have shown correlated reduction in F-dopa uptake with neuronal cell loss in PDD [Eidelberg 1992].

E. Creutzfeld-Jakob Disease (CJD)

Although varying degrees of atrophy or focal lesions can be present in CJD, CT scans can also appear normal. MRI scans, however, consistently show hyperintense signals in the basal ganglia on T2 and proton density images and bilateral thalamic lesions. In a single case study reported by Hutzelmann and Biederer [1998], MRI scans were performed on a 75-year-old woman over a 4-month period for diagnostic purposes. Progressive cortical atrophy in addition to signal hyperintensities in the caudate nuclei and putamen was found. CJD was later confirmed by neuropathology.

Diffuse, multifocal metabolic deficits described as appearing "moth-eaten'" are also commonly found in CJD [Read et al. 1995]. For example, in a case study of a 72-year-old man with confirmed CJD at autopsy, FDG-PET confirmed hypometabolism in the posterior frontal, parietal, Sylvian, and temporal regions [Matochik et al. 1995]. In three CJD cases, Salmon and colleagues [1994] found three underlying patterns of cortical hypometabolism: temporoparietal, frontal, and temporoparietal and diffuse cortical. Using SPECT, Cohen and colleagues [1989] found perfusion abnormalities in the left frontal and right temporoparietal areas in a patient whose CT scan was found to be "normal." SPECT also predicted the underlying pathology in two patients with CJD studied by Read and colleagues [1995]—irregular and diffuse hypoperfusion. Thus, SPECT provides information with sensitivity and specificity that may not be apparent in structural brain imaging.

F. Multisystem Atrophy (MSA)

MSA is a term used to describe three conditions with overlapping symptoms. In general, the three clinical presentations of MSA—olivopontocerebellar atrophy, striatonigral degeneration, and the Shy-Drager syndrome—are associated with glial cytoplasmic inclusions [Lantos and Papp 1994]. Besides the hallmark neural pathology of inclusions, both structural and functional brain imaging techniques have contributed to further characterizing neural abnormalities in MSA. sMRI studies suggest pontocerebellar and putamenal hyperintensities on T2-weighted images regardless of MSA type [Schulz et al. 1994].

In a study by Schrag and colleagues [1998], the clinical utility of MRI was investigated. The authors blindly rated MRI scans of 44 patients with multiple system atrophy and 45 control subjects. The 0.5 T and 1.5 T scans had high specificity for putaminal atrophy, a hyperintense putaminal rim, and infratentorial signal change, but low sensitivities—73% on 0.5 T acquired scans and 88% on 1.5 T acquired scans. Furthermore, any of the MRI abnormalities led to a positive predictive value of 93% on the 0.5 T scanner, and 85% on the 1.5 T scanner for MSA [Schrag et al. 1998]. These findings illustrate the diagnostic utility of MRI methods in MSA.

G. HIV-Related Dementia (HRD)

Neuronal damage in HRD is due to the neurotoxic effects of HIV-infected lymphocytes, macrophages, and microglia. Structural imaging studies in HRD have shown increased ventricle size, decreased gray and white matter volumes, and signal abnormalities in both subcortical and cortical regions [Aylward et al. 1993; Jernigan et al. 1993; Raininko et al. 1992]. Volumetric reductions related to HIV have been reported to be regional, particularly in the temporal limbic cortex, cerebral white matter, and caudate nucleus, and correlated to severity of HIV infection [Heindel et al. 1994; Jernigan et al. 1993].

In an effort to delineate progressive cerebral atrophy in the disease stages of HRD, Stout and colleagues [1998] compared multiple serial MRI scans of HIV-infected males classified in the three stages (A, B, C) according to the Centers for Disease Control and Prevention (CDC). They discovered that the rate of cortical atrophy was greater in stage A and stage C subjects than in normal controls [Stout et al. 1998]. Rate of subcortical atrophy as measured by value change was only greater in stage C subjects compared to normal controls. These findings are consistent with the hypothesis that HIV-related abnormalities are present in the asymptomatic stage A individuals. Additionally, this study suggests greater rate of cortical atrophy, particularly in the gray matter of the caudate nucleus, in the early (stage A) and late (stage C) stages of the disease [Stout et al. 1998].

Functional brain imaging such as PET and SPECT has shown hypometabolism in white and subcortical gray matter with greater defects in the frontal lobes associated with HIV infection [Holman et al. 1992; Masdeu et al. 1991; Rosci et al. 1992]. Furthermore, Kuni and colleagues [1991] found that the degree of basal ganglia abnormalities was correlated with the severity of neuropsychological impairment. Some suggest that functional brain imaging abnormalities are present prior to onset of neuropsychological deficits and can be used to detect early signs of AIDS-related dementia [Rosci et al. 1992]. For instance, using SPECT, Rosci and colleagues [1992] showed perfusion abnormalities in 79% of asymptomatic HIV-infected patients. Interestingly, Holman and colleagues [1992] found that AIDS dementia complex and cocaine-related changes were associated with similar perfusion abnormalities. Both groups showed indistinguishable perfusion patterns that revealed defects in the frontal, temporal, and parietal lobes [Holman et al. 1992]. MRS has also shown decreased levels of NAA in the early stages of HIV infection and prior to abnormalities found by structural neuroimaging. A decreased level of the metabolite NAA may be an indicator of neuronal damage. As expected, many studies have demonstrated a greater NAA reduction in HIV patients with dementia than those without [Kuni et al. 1991; Menon et al. 1992].

As extensive and severe as the metabolic abnormalities of HIV dementia can be, using serial FDG-PET scans before and after 3′-azido-2′, 3′-dideoxythymidine (AZT, zidovudine) therapy, Brunetti and colleagues [1989] found the abnormalities to be at least partially reversible in all four patients studied, and the focal abnormalities in two completely eliminated. While these findings have yet to be replicated, they illustrate the added value of FDG-PET in monitoring metabolic improvement in response to therapy.

To evaluate the neural correlates of attention and working memory deficits in patients with HIV, Chang and colleagues [2001] performed fMRI on 11 patients with HIV and compared their performance with seronegative subjects. Patients with HIV showed greater BOLD activation in the parietal and frontal regions compared to the control group despite similar performance on the tasks as measured by reaction time and rate of accuracy. The authors posit that greater attentional modulation of the neural circuits and greater use of brain reserve occurs in HIV-infected individuals. Thus, attention deficits found in patients with HIV may be the result of excessive attentional modulation due to frontostriatal brain dysfunction [Chang et al. 2001].

VII. CONCLUSIONS

In summary, recent neuroimaging literature indicates:

1. Earliest structural AD abnormalities are found in the medial temporal lobes where neuritic plaques, neurofibrillary tangles are found at the earliest stages of the disease, and functional abnormalities may first appear in paralimbic areas such as the posterior cingulate.

2. VaD is associated with periventricular and white matter hyperintensities, subcortical infarcts, and lesions.

3. FTD shows frontotemporal atrophy corresponding to spongiosis and gliosis with or without neuronal inclusions (i.e., Pick bodies) and ballooned cells.

4. Dementia related to Lewy bodies (i.e., PDD, LBD) shows similar temporoparietal pattern to AD.

5. PSP mainly involves the subcortical areas, which affect the prefrontal cortex.

6. Dementia from neuronal diseases such as CJD present widespread abnormalities including cortical and subcortical meatabolic changes, while MSA reveal abnormalities in the brainstem and cerebellum corresponding to the ubiquitous neuronal and oligodendroglial inclusions mainly in the brainstem and cerebellum.

7. In neurodegenerative disorders (i.e., HD, CBGD, PSP) involvement of the basal ganglia, degeneration of striatofrontal and hippocampal region are found.

8. HIV-related dementia results in widespread gray and white matter abnormalities (see Table 1) [Jellinger 1996].

Since the mid-1970s, brain imaging techniques have contributed significantly to the body of knowledge and understanding of dementia disorders (see Table 2). What research has shown is that brain imaging continues to play an important role in the evaluation and treatment of dementia. Recent studies have verified the utility of PET in the diagnosis and prognosis of dementia [Brunetti et al. 1989; Silverman et al. 2002; Small et al. 2000]. For example, in a 2-year longitudinal PET study by Small and colleagues [2000], a 4% left posterior cingulate metabolic decline and a 5% inferior parietal and lateral temporal region metabolic decline were observed in patients with AD. The authors also suggest that metabolic rates measured by PET can be a means for response monitoring in pharmacologic trials [Small et al. 2000]. In addition, Silverman and colleagues [2002] examined the costs (measured in dollars) and benefits (measured in number of accurate diagnoses) of PET against the traditional clinical approach in assessing early AD. Results indicated that PET incurred lower costs per correct diagnosis. The savings were based in part on a 15% improvement in the accuracy of diagnosis when using PET in addition to the traditional method and the benefits of therapy decreasing with the advance of AD. These benefits are likely to increase as better treatments become available because of the likelihood that treatments will slow or prevent further progression of the disease, but are unlikely to substantially reverse damage already incurred.

Table 1 Key Areas of Brain Imaging Abnormalities in the Dementia Syndromes

Disorder	Key Regions
Alzheimer's disease	Sulci, temporal horns, third ventricle, mesencephalic cisterns abnormalities on CT and MRI
	Medial temporal lobe structural and functional abnormalities on MRI, PET, SPECT, and MRS
Vascular dementia	Cerebral white matter hyperintensities on CT and MRI scans
	Increased basal ganglia, thalamus, pons on CT and MRI
Frontotemporal dementia	Frontotemporal abnormalities on MRI, PET, and SPECT
	Corpus callosum atrophy on MRI
Lewy body dementia	Occipital hypoperfusion on PET and SPECT
Huntington's disease	Basal ganglia (i.e., caudate nucleus) abnormalities on CT, MRI, and PET
Progressive supranuclear palsy	Subcortical abnormalities on MRI
	Frontal lobe abnormalities on PET and fMRI
Corticobasal degeneration	Lateralized frontal, parietal, and basal ganglia abnormalities on MRI, PET, and SPECT
Parkinson's disease with dementia	Frontal lobe abnormalities on MRI
	Occipital lobe hypoperfusion and hypometabolism on PET
Creutzfeld-Jakob disease	Basal ganglia abnormalities on MRI scans
	Temporoparietal functional abnormalities on PET and SPECT
Multisystem atrophy	Brainstem and cerebellum abnormalities on MRI
HIV-related dementia	Widespread white and gray matter abnormalities on MRI, PET and SPECT
	Subcortical and cortical regions abnormalities on MRI, PET, SPECT, and MRS

Table 2 Potential Clinical Contributions of Brain Imaging Techniques

Diagnosis	Early diagnosis before symptoms appear/screening
	Exclusion of other causes of dementia
	Confirmation of disorder
Treatment	Development of novel pharmacological interventions
	Dose titration
	Evidence of therapeutic efficacy

In addition to the direct clinical relevance of brain imaging techniques, an important contribution has been in the availability of neuroanatomical data for associations with other areas of relevance, e.g., genetics, neuropsychological measures. For instance, as noted earlier, there are substantial data suggesting that ApoE ε4 status has an influence on hippocampal volumes [Bookheimer et al. 2000; Lehtovirta et al. 1995]. Of note, factors such as ApoE ε4 status and estrogen replacement or vascular risk factors have not been shown to consistently influence either cross-sectional or longitudinal measures of temporal lobe or whole-brain volumes [Barber et al. 1999a; Jack et al. 1998a,b; Lehtovirta et al. 1995; Tanaka et al. 1998]. Thus, genetics alone is deemed insufficient to predict neuropathology and therefore is likely to be insufficient in predicting neuroimaging findings [Bird et al. 1999].

To date, associations between brain imaging findings and cognitive function have been inconsistent. For instance, the relationship of WMC to function remains unknown. Wahlund and colleagues [1994] reported no significant correlations between severity of WMC and cognitive impairment as measured by the MMSE; therefore, the authors concluded that white matter hyperintensities were not related to the degree of global cognitive decline in dementia.

To conclude, brain imaging techniques reveal that many dementia syndromes are superimposed with AD pathology and overlaps exist between the syndromes (see Table 2). For instance, periventricular and white matter hyperintensities are found in DLB, AD, and VaD [Snowdon et al. 1997]. However, with brain imaging studies, the detection of differential patterns of neural abnormalities between syndromes is possible. For instance, Yamauchi and colleagues [2000] found that although atrophy of the corpus calossum is not specific to any dementia disorder, such as AD, PSP, and FTD, differential patterns of atrophy exist that could differentiate between the syndromes.

The failure of studies to delineate discriminatory features between dementia syndromes may possibly be attributed to diagnostic misclassification of diseases or to small numbers within a sample. There is also evidence for the lack of specificity of single cross-sectional measurements as opposed to longitudinal measurements. Lastly, measures of sensitivity and specificity are highly sensitive to the stage of the dementia disorder. Future studies will benefit not only from the contributions of brain imaging methods, but also from combining clinical, genetic, cognitive, and neuropathologic studies with imaging studies to fully elucidate the mechanisms and neurobiological changes that underlie dementia; also, further investigation is required not only in differentiating between diseases but also in determining the causative role of neural abnormalities in the development of dementia symptoms.

REFERENCES

Akanuma J, Saito N, Aoki M, et al. Chorea with prominent spasticity associated with an expansion of the CAG trinucleotide repeat in the IT15 gene: a case report. Rinsho Shinkeigaku (1995) 35(11):1253–1255.

Albert M, Naeser MA, Levine HL, et al. Ventricular size in patients with presenile dementia of the Alzheimer's type. Arch Neurol (1984) 41(12):1258–1263.

American Psychiatric Association. Diagnostic and Statistical Manual of Mental Disorders—Fourth Edition (DSM-IV). Washington: American Psychiatric Association, 1994.

Aylward EH, Anderson NB, Bylsma FW, et al. Frontal lobe volume in patients with Huntington's disease. Neurology (1998) 50(1):252–258.

Aylward EH, Henderer JD, McArthur JC, et al. Reduced basal ganglia volume in HIV-1-associated dementia: results from quantitative neuroimaging. Neurology (1993) 43(10):2099–2104.

Aylward EH, Karagiozis H, Pearlson G., et al. Suprasellar cistern measures as a reflection of dementia in Alzheimer's disease but not Huntington's disease. J Psychiatr Res (1991) 25(1–2):31–47.

Balaban RS, and Ceckler TL Magnetization transfer contrast in magnetic resonance imaging. Magn Reson Q (1992) 8(2):116–137.

Barber R, Ballard C, McKeith IG, et al. MRI volumetric study of dementia with Lewy bodies: a comparison with AD and vascular dementia. Neurology (2000) 54(6):1304–1309.

Barber R, Gholkar A, Scheltens P, et al. Apolipoprotein E epsilon4 allele, temporal lobe atrophy, and white matter lesions in late-life dementias. Arch Neurol (1999a) 56(8):961–965.

Barber R and O'Brien J. Structural and functional magnetic resonance imaging (MRI). In: O'Brien J., Ames D., Burns A., eds. Dementia. London: Arnold (2000).

Barber R, Scheltens P, Gholkar A, et al. White matter lesions on magnetic resonance imaging in dementia with Lewy bodies, Alzheimer's disease, vascular dementia, and normal aging. J Neurol Neurosurg Psychiatry (1999b) 67(1):66–72.

Barboriak DP, Provenzale JM, and Boyko OB. MR diagnosis of Creutzfeldt-Jakob disease: significance of high signal intensity of the basal ganglia. AJR (1994) 162(1):137–140.

Barrio JR, Huang SC, Cole G, et al. PET imaging of tangles and plaques in Alzheimer disease with a highly hydrophobic probe. J Labelled Cpd Radiopharm (1999) 42(suppl 1):5194–5195.

Benson DF, Kuhl DE, Hawkins RA, et al. The fluorodeoxyglucose 18F scan in Alzheimer's disease and multi-infarct dementia. Arch Neurol (1983) 40(12):711–714.

Bigler ED, Hubler DW, Cullum CM, et al. Intellectual and memory impairment in dementia. Computerized axial tomography volume correlations. J Nerv Ment Dis (1985) 173(6):347–352.

Bird TD, Nochlin D, Poorkaj P, et al. A clinical pathological comparison of three families with frontotemporal dementia and identical mutations in the tau gene (P301L). Brain (1999) 122(Pt 4):741–756.

Blin J, Baron JC, Dubois B, et al. Loss of brain 5-HT2 receptors in Alzheimer's disease. In vivo assessment with positron emission tomography and [^{18}F]setoperone. Brain (1993) 116(Pt 3):497–510.

Blin J, Baron JC, Dubois B, et al. Positron emission tomography study in progressive supranuclear palsy. Brain hypometabolic pattern and clinicometabolic correlations. Arch Neurol (1990) 47(7):747–752.

Bobek-Billewicz B, Dziewiatkowski J, and Hermann M. Magnetic resonance volumetric study of the temporal lobe structures in ischaemic vascular dementia. Folia Neuropathol (2001) 39(1):15–18.

Bohnen NI, Minoshima S, Giordani B, et al. Motor correlates of occipital glucose hypometabolism in Parkinson's disease without dementia. Neurology (1999) 52(3):541–546.

Bookheimer SY, Strojwas MH, Cohen MS, et al. Patterns of brain activation in people at risk for Alzheimer's disease. N Engl J Med (2000) 343(7):450–456.

Bottomley PA, Cousins JP, Pendrey DL, et al. Alzheimer dementia: quantification of energy metabolism and mobile phosphoesters with P-31 NMR spectroscopy. Radiology (1992) 183(3):695–699.

Brandt J, Bylsma FW, Aylward EH, et al. Impaired source memory in Huntington's disease and its relation to basal ganglia atrophy. J Clin Exp Neuropsychol (1995) 17(6):868–877.

Brooker AE, Dougherty DS, Love KF, et al. Neuropsychological, neurological, and MRI correlates of dementia in advanced Huntington's disease: a single case study. Percept Mot Skills (1991) 72(3 Pt 2):1363–1374.

Brown GG, Levine SR, Gorell JM, et al. In vivo ^{31}P NMR profiles of Alzheimer's disease and multiple subcortical infarct dementia. Neurology (1989) 39(11):1423–1427.

Brunetti A, Berg G, Di Chiro G, et al. Reversal of brain metabolic abnormalities following treatment of AIDS dementia complex with 3′-azido-2′,3′-dideoxythymidine (AZT, zidovudine): a PET-FDG study. J Nucl Med (1989) 30(5):581–590.

Burggren AC, Small GW, Sabb FW, et al. Specificity of brain activation patterns in people at genetic risk for Alzheimer disease. Am J Geriatr Psychiatry (2002) 10(1):44–51.

Burns A, Jacoby R, and Levy R. Computed tomography in Alzheimer's disease: a longitudinal study. Biol Psychiatry (1991a) 29(4):383–390.

Burns A, Jacoby R, Philpot M, et al. Computerised tomography in Alzheimer's disease. Methods of scan analysis, comparison with normal controls, and clinical/radiological associations. Br J Psychiatry (1991b) 159:609–614.

Cardebat D, Demonet JF, Puel M, et al. Brain correlates of memory processes in patients with dementia of Alzheimer's type: a SPECT activation study. J Cereb Blood Flow Metab (1998) 18(4):457–462.

Chabriat H, Levasseur M, Vidailhet M, et al. In-vivo SPECT imaging of D2 receptor with iodine-iodolisuride: results in supranuclear palsy. J Nucl Med (1992) 33(8):1481–1485.

Chan D, Fox NC, Jenkins R, et al. Rates of global and regional cerebral atrophy in AD and frontotemporal dementia. Neurology (2001) 57(10):1756–1763.

Chang L, Speck O, Miller EN, et al. Neural correlates of attention and working memory deficits in HIV patients. Neurology (2001) 57(6):1001–1007.

Charpentier P, Lavenu I, Defebvre L, et al. Alzheimer's disease and frontotemporal dementia are differentiated by discriminant analysis applied to (99m)Tc HmPAO SPECT data. J Neurol Neurosurg Psychiatry (2000) 69(5):661–663.

Chui H and Zhang Q. Evaluation of dementia: a systematic study of the usefulness of the American Academy of Neurology's practice parameters. Neurology (1997) 49(4):925–935.

Cohen RM, Andreason PJ, and Sunderland T. The ratio of mesial to neocortical temporal lobe blood flow as a predictor of dementia. J Am Geriatr Soc (1997) 45(3):329–333.

Cohen RM, Small C, Lalonde F, et al. Effect of apolipoprotein E genotype on hippocampal volume loss in aging healthy women. Neurology (2001) 57(12):2223–2228.

Convit A, De Leon MJ, Tarshish C, et al. Specific hippocampal volume reductions in individuals at risk for Alzheimer's disease. Neurobiol Aging (1997) 18(2):131–138.

Culjkovic B, Stojkovic O, Vojvodic N, et al. Correlation between triplet repeat expansion and computed tomography measures of caudate nuclei atrophy in Huntington's disease. J Neurol (1999) 246(11):1090–1093.

Cummings JL. Neuroimaging in the dementia assessment: is it necessary? J Am Geriatr Soc (2000) 48(10):1345–1346.

D'Antona R, Baron JC, Samson Y, et al. Subcortical dementia. Frontal cortex hypometabolism detected by positron tomography in patients with progressive supranuclear palsy. Brain (1985) 108(Pt 3):785–799.

Davis PC, Mirra SS, and Alazraki N. The brain in older persons with and without dementia: findings on MR, PET, and SPECT images. AJR (1994) 162(6):1267–1278.

De la Monte SM, Vonsattel JP, and Richardson EP Jr. Morphometric demonstration of atrophic changes in the cerebral cortex, white matter, and neostriatum in Huntington's disease. J Neuropathol Exp Neurol (1988) 47(5):516–525.

De Leon MJ, George AE, Reisberg B, et al. Alzheimer's disease: longitudinal CT studies of ventricular change. AJR (1989) 152(6):1257–1262.

De Reuck J, Decoo D, Hasenbroekx MC, et al. Acetazolamide vasoreactivity in vascular dementia: a positron emission tomographic study. Eur Neurol (1999) 41(1):31–36.

De Reuck J, Decoo D, Marchau M, et al. Positron emission tomography in vascular dementia. J Neurol Sci (1998) 154(1):55–61.

De Reuck J, Santens P, Strijckmans K, et al. Cobalt-55 positron emission tomography in vascular dementia: significance of white matter changes. J Neurol Sci (2001) 193(1):1–6.

DeCarli C. The role of neuroimaging in dementia. Clin Geriatr Med (2001) 17(2):255–279.

DeCarli C, Kaye JA, Horwitz B, et al. Critical analysis of the use of computer-assisted transverse axial tomography to study human brain in aging and dementia of the Alzheimer type. Neurology (1990) 40(6):872–883.

Deisenhammer E, Reisecker F, Leblhuber F, et al. Single-photon emission-computed tomography in the differential diagnosis of dementia. Dtsch Med Wochenschr (1989) 114(43):1639–1644.

Deweer B, Lehericy S, Pillon B, et al. Memory disorders in probable Alzheimer's disease: the role of hippocampal atrophy as shown with MRI. J Neurol Neurosurg Psychiatry (1995) 58(5):590–597.

Dierks T, Linden DE, Hertel A, et al. Multimodal imaging of residual function and compensatory resource allocation in cortical atrophy: a case study of parietal lobe function in a patient with Huntington's disease. Psychiatry Res (1999) 90(1):67–75.

Donnemiller E, Heilmann J, Wenning GK, et al. Brain perfusion scintigraphy with 99mTc-HMPAO or 99mTc-ECD and 123I- beta-CIT single-photon emission tomography in dementia of the Alzheimer-type and diffuse Lewy body disease. Eur J Nucl Med (1997) 24(3):320–325.

Duara R, Barker W, Loewenstein D, et al. Sensitivity and specificity of positron emission tomography and magnetic resonance imaging studies in Alzheimer's disease and multi- infarct dementia. Eur Neurol (1989) 29(suppl 3):9–15.

Earnest MP, Heaton RK, Wilkinson WE, et al. Cortical atrophy, ventricular enlargement and intellectual impairment in the aged. Neurology (1979) 29(8):1138–1143.

Eidelberg D. Positron emission tomography studies in parkinsonism. Neurol Clin (1992) 10(2):421–433.

Eidelberg D, Dhawan V, Moeller JR, et al. The metabolic landscape of cortico-basal ganglionic degeneration: regional asymmetries studied with positron emission tomography. J Neurol Neurosurg Psychiatry (1991) 54(10):856–862.

Erkinjuntti T, Lee DH, Gao F, et al. Temporal lobe atrophy on magnetic resonance imaging in the diagnosis of early Alzheimer's disease. Arch Neurol (1993) 50(3):305–310.

Ernst T, Chang L, Melchor R, et al. Frontotemporal dementia and early Alzheimer disease: differentiation with frontal lobe H-1 MR spectroscopy. Radiology (1997) 203(3):829–836.

Fein G, Di Sclafani V, Tanabe J, et al. Hippocampal and cortical atrophy predict dementia in subcortical ischemic vascular disease. Neurology (2000) 55(11):1626–1635.

Ford CV and Winter J Computerized axial tomograms and dementia in elderly patients. J Gerontol (1981) 36(2):164–169.

Forstl H, Burns A, Jacoby R, et al. Neuroanatomical correlates of clinical misidentification and misperception in senile dementia of the Alzheimer type. J Clin Psychiatry (1991) 52(6):268–271.

Fox NC, Warrington EK, Stevens JM, et al. Atrophy of the hippocampal formation in early familial Alzheimer's disease. A longitudinal MRI study of at-risk members of a family with an amyloid precursor protein 717Val-Gly mutation. Ann NY Acad Sci (1996) 777:226–232.

Frackowiak RS, Pozzilli C, Legg NJ, et al. Regional cerebral oxygen supply and utilization in dementia. A clinical and physiological study with oxygen-15 and positron tomography. Brain (1981) 104(Pt 4):753–778.

Frasson E, Moretto G, Beltramello A, et al. Neuropsychological and neuroimaging correlates in corticobasal degeneration. Ital J Neurol Sci (1998) 19(5):321–328.

Friedland RP, Budinger TF, Brant-Zawadzki M, et al. The diagnosis of Alzheimer-type dementia. A preliminary comparison of positron emission tomography and proton magnetic resonance. JAMA (1984) 252(19):2750–2752.

Friedland RP, Kalaria R, Berridge M, et al. Neuroimaging of vessel amyloid in Alzheimer's disease. Ann NY Acad Sci (1997) 826:242–247.

Frisoni GB, Beltramello A, Geroldi C, et al. Brain atrophy in frontotemporal dementia. J Neurol Neurosurg Psychiatry (1996) 61(2):157–165.

Frisoni GB, Bianchetti A, Trabucchi M, et al. The added value of neuroimaging for diagnosing dementia. AJNR Am J Neuroradiol (1999) 20(5):947–949.

Garnett ES, Firnau G, Nahmias C, et al. Reduced striatal glucose consumption and prolonged reaction time are early features in Huntington's disease. J Neurol Sci (1984) 65(2):231–237.

Garraux G, Salmon E, Degueldre C, et al. Comparison of impaired subcortico-frontal metabolic networks in normal aging, subcortico-frontal dementia, and cortical frontal dementia. Neuroimage (1999) 10(2):149–162.

Gonzalez RG, Fischman AJ, Guimaraes AR, et al. Functional MR in the evaluation of dementia: correlation of abnormal dynamic cerebral blood volume measurements with changes in cerebral metabolism on positron emission tomography with fludeoxyglucose F 18. AJNR Am J Neuroradiol (1995) 16(9):1763–1770.

Grady CL, Haxby JV, Horwitz B, et al. Activation of cerebral blood flow during a visuoperceptual task in patients with Alzheimer-type dementia. Neurobiol Aging (1993) 14(1):35–44.

Graff-Radford NR, Russell JW, and Rezai K. Frontal degenerative dementia and neuroimaging. Adv Neurol (1995) 66:37–47.

Grafton ST, Mazziotta JC, Pahl JJ, et al. A comparison of neurological, metabolic, structural, and genetic evaluations in persons at risk for Huntington's disease. Ann Neurol (1990) 28(5):614–621.

Gregory CA, Serra-Mestres J, and Hodges JR. Early diagnosis of the frontal variant of frontotemporal dementia: how sensitive are standard neuroimaging and neuropsychologic tests? Neuropsychiatry Neuropsychol Behav Neurol (1999) 12(2):128–135.

Halliday GM, McRitchie DA, Macdonald V, et al. Regional specificity of brain atrophy in Huntington's disease. Exp Neurol (1998) 154(2):663–672.

Hanyu H, Asano T, Iwamoto T, et al. Magnetization transfer measurements of the hippocampus in patients with Alzheimer's disease, vascular dementia, and other types of dementia. AJNR Am J Neuroradiol (2000) 21(7):1235–1242.

Hanyu H, Asano T, Sakurai H, et al. Magnetisation transfer measurements of the subcortical grey and white matter in Parkinson's disease with and without dementia and in progressive supranuclear palsy. Neuroradiology (2001) 43(7):542–546.

Harvey GT, Hughes J, McKeith IG, et al. Magnetic resonance imaging differences between dementia with Lewy bodies and Alzheimer's disease: a pilot study. Psychol Med (1999) 29(1):181–187.

Haxby JV Duara R, Grady CL, et al. Relations between neuropsychological and cerebral metabolic asymmetries in early Alzheimer's disease. J Cereb Blood Flow Metab (1985) 5(2):193–200.

Haxby JV and Rapoport SI. Asymmetry of brain metabolism and cognitive function. Geriatr Nurs (1985) 6(4):200–203.

Haxby JV and Rapoport SI. Abnormalities of regional brain metabolism in Alzheimer's disease and their relation to functional impairment. Prog Neuropsychopharmacol Biol Psychiatry (1986) 10(3–5):427–438.

Hayden MR, Hewitt J, Stoessl AJ, et al. The combined use of positron emission tomography and DNA polymorphisms for preclinical detection of Huntington's disease. Neurology (1987) 37(9):1441–1447.

Heindel WC, Jernigan TL, Archibald SL, et al. The relationship of quantitative brain magnetic resonance imaging measures to neuropathologic indexes of human immunodeficiency virus infection. Arch Neurol (1994) 51(11):1129–1135.

Herholz K, Perani D, Salmon E, et al. Comparability of FDG PET studies in probable Alzheimer's disease. J Nucl Med (1993) 34(9):1460–1466.

Holman BL, Garada B, Johnson KA, et al. A comparison of brain perfusion SPECT in cocaine abuse and AIDS dementia complex. J Nucl Med (1992) 33(7):1312–1315.

Howard R, David A, Woodruff P, et al. Seeing visual hallucinations with functional magnetic resonance imaging. Dement Geriatr Cogn Disord (1997) 8(2):73–77.

Hu XS, Okamura N, Arai H, et al. ^{18}F-fluorodopa PET study of striatal dopamine uptake in the diagnosis of dementia with Lewy bodies. Neurology (2000) 55(10):1575–1577.

Huang W, Alexander GE, Chang L, et al. Brain metabolite concentration and dementia severity in Alzheimer's disease: a (^{1})H MRS study. Neurology (2001) 57(4):626–632.

Hutzelmann A and Biederer J. MRI follow-up in a case of clinically diagnosed Creutzfeld-Jakob disease. Eur Radiol (1998) 8(3):421–423.

Ibanez V, Pietrini P, Alexander GE, et al. Regional glucose metabolic abnormalities are not the result of atrophy in Alzheimer's disease. Neurology (1998) 50(6):1585–1593.

Ichise M, Toyama H, Fornazzari L, et al. Iodine-123-IBZM dopamine D2 receptor and technetium-99m-HMPAO brain perfusion SPECT in the evaluation of patients with and subjects at risk for Huntington's disease. J Nucl Med (1993) 34(8):1274–1281.

Imamura T, Ishii K, Hirono N, et al. Occipital glucose metabolism in dementia with Lewy bodies with and without parkinsonism: a study using positron emission tomography. Dement Geriatr Cogn Disord (2001) 12(3):194–197.

Inzitari D. Age-related white matter changes and cognitive impairment. Ann Neurol (2000) 47(2):141–143.

Ishii K, Sasaki M, Yamaji S, et al. Paradoxical hippocampus perfusion in mild-to-moderate Alzheimer's disease. J Nucl Med (1998) 39(2):293–298.

Ishii K, Yamaji S, Kitagaki H, et al. Regional cerebral blood flow difference between dementia with Lewy bodies and AD. Neurology (1999) 53(2):413–416.

Ishiwata A, Kitamura S, Nagazumi A, et al. Cerebral blood flow of patients with age-associated memory impairment and the early stage of Alzheimer's disease. A study by SPECT using the ARG method. Nippon Ika Daigaku Zasshi (1998) 65(2):140–147.

Iyo M, Namba H, Fukushi K, et al. Measurement of acetylcholinesterase by positron emission tomography in the brains of healthy controls and patients with Alzheimer's disease. Lancet (1997) 349(9068):1805–1809.

Jack CR Jr, Bentley MD, Twomey CK, et al. MR imaging-based volume measurements of the hippocampal formation and anterior temporal lobe: validation studies. Radiology (1990) 176(1):205–209.

Jack CR Jr, Petersen RC, O'Brien PC, et al. MR-based hippocampal volumetry in the diagnosis of Alzheimer's disease. Neurology (1992) 42(1):183–188.

Jack CR Jr, Petersen RC, Xu Y, et al. Rate of medial temporal lobe atrophy in typical aging and Alzheimer's disease. Neurology (1998a) 51(4):993–999.

Jack CR Jr, Petersen RC, Xu YC, et al. Hippocampal atrophy and apolipoprotein E genotype are independently associated with Alzheimer's disease. Ann Neurol (1998b) 43(3):303–310.

Jauss M, Herholz K, Kracht L, et al. Frontotemporal dementia: clinical, neuroimaging, and molecular biological findings in 6 patients. Eur Arch Psychiatry Clin Neurosci (2001) 251(5):225–331.

Jellinger KA. Structural basis of dementia in neurodegenerative disorders. J Neural Transm Suppl (1996) 47:1–29.

Jernigan TL, Archibald S, Hesselink JR, et al. Magnetic resonance imaging morphometric analysis of cerebral volume loss in human immunodeficiency virus infection. The HNRC Group. Arch Neurol (1993) 50(3):250–255.

Jernigan TL, Archibald SL, Berhow MT, et al. Cerebral structure on MRI. Localization of age-related changes. Biol Psychiatry (1991a) 29(1):55–67.

Jernigan TL, Salmon DP, Butters N, et al. Cerebral structure on MRI. Specific changes in Alzheimer's and Huntington's diseases. Biol Psychiatry (1991b) 29(1):68–81.

Jobst KA, Smith AD, Barker CS, et al. Association of atrophy of the medial temporal lobe with reduced blood flow in the posterior parietotemporal cortex in patients with a clinical and pathological diagnosis of Alzheimer's disease. J Neurol Neurosurg Psychiatry (1992a) 55(3):190–194.

Jobst KA, Smith AD, Szatmari M, et al. Detection in life of confirmed Alzheimer's disease using a simple measurement of medial temporal lobe atrophy by computed tomography. Lancet (1992b) 340(8829):1179–1183.

Johannsen P, Jakobsen J, Bruhn P, et al. Cortical responses to sustained and divided attention in Alzheimer's disease. Neuroimage (1999) 10(3 Pt 1):269–281.

Johnson KA, Jones K, Holman BL, et al. Preclinical prediction of Alzheimer's disease using SPECT. Neurology (1998) 50(6):1563–1571.

Johnson SC, Saykin AJ, Baxter LC, et al. The relationship between fMRI activation and cerebral atrophy: comparison of normal aging and alzheimer disease. Neuroimage (2000) 11(3):179–187.

Jonker C, Schmand B, Lindeboom J, et al. Association between apolipoprotein E epsilon4 and the rate of cognitive decline in community-dwelling elderly individuals with and without dementia. Arch Neurol (1998) 55(8):1065–1069.

Julin P, Wahlund LO, Basun H, et al. Clinical diagnosis of frontal lobe dementia and Alzheimer's disease: relation to cerebral perfusion, brain atrophy and electroencephalography. Dementia (1995) 6(3):142–147.

Kawamura J, Meyer JS, Terayama Y, et al. Leukoaraiosis correlates with cerebral hypoperfusion in vascular dementia. Stroke (1991) 22(5):609–614.

Kessler J, Herholz K, Grond M, et al. Impaired metabolic activation in Alzheimer's disease: a PET study during continuous visual recognition. Neuropsychologia (1991) 29(3):229–243.

Killiany RJ, Gomez-Isla T, Moss M, et al. Use of structural magnetic resonance imaging to predict who will get Alzheimer's disease. Ann Neurol (2000) 47(4):430–439.

Kitagaki H, Mori E, Yamaji S, et al. Frontotemporal dementia and Alzheimer disease: evaluation of cortical atrophy with automated hemispheric surface display generated with MR images. Radiology (1998) 208(2):431–439.

Kitamura S, Koshi Y, Komiyama T, et al. Benzodiazepine receptor and cerebral blood flow in early Alzheimer's disease—SPECT study using ^{123}I-iomazenil and ^{123}I-IMP]. Kaku Igaku (1996) 33(1):49–56.

Klunk WE, Wang Y, Huang GF, et al. Uncharged thioflavin-T derivatives bind to amyloid-beta protein with high affinity and readily enter the brain. Life Sci (2001) 69(13):1471–1484.

Kohn MI, Tanna NK, Herman GT, et al. Analysis of brain and cerebrospinal fluid volumes with MR imaging. Part I. Methods, reliability, and validation. Radiology (1991) 178(1):115–122.

Koide T, Hozumi I, Souma Y, et al. Three cases of clinically diagnosed corticobasal degeneration—neuroimaging studies with MRI, SPECT and PET. Rinsho Shinkeigaku (1995) 35(11):1184–1190.

Kuhl D, Metter E, Benson F, et al. Similarities of cerebral glucose metabolism in Alzheimer's and Parkinson's dementia. J Cereb Blood Flow Metab (1985) 5:169–170.

Kuhl DE, Koeppe RA, Minoshima S, et al. In vivo mapping of cerebral acetylcholinesterase activity in aging and Alzheimer's disease. Neurology (1999) 52(4):691–699.

Kuhl DE, Metter EJ, Riege WH, et al. Patterns of cerebral glucose utilization in Parkinson's disease and Huntington's disease. Ann Neurol (1984) 15(suppl): S119–S125.

Kuhl DE, Minoshima S, Fessler JA, et al. In vivo mapping of cholinergic terminals in normal aging, Alzheimer's disease, and Parkinson's disease. Ann Neurol (1996) 40(3):399–410.

Kuni CC, Rhame FS, Meier MJ, et al. Quantitative I-123-IMP brain SPECT and neuropsychological testing in AIDS dementia. Clin Nucl Med (1991) 16(3):174–177.

Kurihara A and Pardridge WM Abeta(1–40) peptide radiopharmaceuticals for brain amyloid imaging: (^{111})In chelation, conjugation to poly(ethylene glycol)-biotin linkers, and autoradiography with Alzheimer's disease brain sections. Bioconjug Chem (2000) 11(3):380–386.

Laakso MP, Frisoni GB, Kononen M, et al. Hippocampus and entorhinal cortex in frontotemporal dementia and Alzheimer's disease: a morphometric MRI study. Biol Psychiatry (2000) 47(12):1056–1063.

Laakso MP, Soininen H, Partanen K, et al. Volumes of hippocampus, amygdala and frontal lobes in the MRI-based diagnosis of early Alzheimer's disease: correlation with memory functions. J Neural Transm Park Dis Dement Sect (1995) 9(1):73–86.

Lantos PL, and Papp MI. Cellular pathology of multiple system atrophy: a review. J Neurol Neurosurg Psychiatry (1994) 57(2):129–133.

Lehtovirta M, Laakso MP, Soininen H, et al. Volumes of hippocampus, amygdala and frontal lobe in Alzheimer patients with different apolipoprotein E genotypes. Neuroscience (1995) 67(1):65–72.

LeMay M, Stafford JL, Sandor T, et al. Statistical assessment of perceptual CT scan ratings in patients with Alzheimer type dementia. J Comput Assist Tomogr (1986) 10(5):802–809.

Liu CK, Miller BL, Cummings JL, et al. A quantitative MRI study of vascular dementia. Neurology (1992) 42(1):138–143.

Lobotesis K, Fenwick JD, Phipps A, et al. Occipital hypoperfusion on SPECT in dementia with Lewy bodies but not AD. Neurology (2001) 56(5):643–649.

Loewenstein DA, Barker WW, Chang JY, et al. Predominant left hemisphere metabolic dysfunction in dementia. Arch Neurol (1989) 46(2):146–152.

Mann DM, Oliver R, and Snowden JS. The topographic distribution of brain atrophy in Huntington's disease and progressive supranuclear palsy. Acta Neuropathol (1993) 85(5):553–559.

Masdeu JC, Yudd A, Van Heertum RL, et al. Single-photon emission computed tomography in human immunodeficiency virus encephalopathy: a preliminary report. J Nucl Med (1991) 32(8):1471–1475.

Mathews VP, Candy EJ, and Bryan RN. Imaging of neurodegenerative diseases. Curr Opin Radiol (1992) 4(1):89–94.

Matochik JA, Molchan SE, Zametkin AJ, et al. Regional cerebral glucose metabolism in autopsy-confirmed Creutzfeldt-Jakob disease. Acta Neurol Scand (1995) 91(2):153–157.

Meguro K, LeMestric C, Landeau B, et al. Relations between hypometabolism in the posterior association neocortex and hippocampal atrophy in Alzheimer's disease: a PET/MRI correlative study. J Neurol Neurosurg Psychiatry (2001) 71(3):315–321.

Meltzer CC, Price JC, Mathis CA, et al. PET imaging of serotonin type 2A receptors in late-life neuropsychiatric disorders. Am J Psychiatry (1999) 156(12):1871–1878.

Meltzer CC, Zubieta JK, Brandt J, et al. Regional hypometabolism in Alzheimer's disease as measured by positron emission tomography after correction for effects of partial volume averaging. Neurology (1996) 47(2):454–461.

Menon DK, Ainsworth JG, Cox IJ, et al. Proton MR spectroscopy of the brain in AIDS dementia complex. J Comput Assist Tomogr (1992) 16(4):538–542.

Mentis MJ, Horwitz B, Grady CL, et al. Visual cortical dysfunction in Alzheimer's disease evaluated with a temporally graded "stress test" during PET. Am J Psychiatry (1996) 153(1):32–40.

Miatto O, Gonzalez RG, Buonanno F, et al. In vitro ^{31}P NMR spectroscopy detects altered phospholipid metabolism in Alzheimer's disease. Can J Neurol Sci (1986) 13(4 suppl):535–539.

Middelkoop HA, Van der Flier WM, Burton EJ, et al. Dementia with Lewy bodies and AD are not associated with occipital lobe atrophy on MRI. Neurology (2001) 57(11):2117–2120.

Mielke R and Heiss WD. Positron emission tomography for diagnosis of Alzheimer's disease and vascular dementia. J Neural Transm Suppl (1998) 53:237–250.

Mielke R, Kessler J, Szelies B, et al. Vascular dementia: perfusional and metabolic disturbances and effects of therapy. J Neural Transm Suppl (1996) 47:183–191.

Miller BL, Cummings JL, Villanueva-Meyer J., et al. Frontal lobe degeneration: clinical, neuropsychological, and SPECT characteristics. Neurology (1991) 41(9):1374–1382.

Moffat SD, Zonderman AB, Harman SM, et al. The relationship between longitudinal declines in dehydroepiandrosterone sulfate concentrations and cognitive performance in older men. Arch Intern Med (2000) 160(14):2193–2198.

Murphy DG, DeCarli CD, Daly E, et al. Volumetric magnetic resonance imaging in men with dementia of the

Alzheimer type: correlations with disease severity. Biol Psychiatry (1993) 34(9):612–621.

Nagata K, Maruya H, Yuya H, et al. Can PET data differentiate Alzheimer's disease from vascular dementia? Ann NY Acad Sci (2000) 903:252–261.

O'Brien JT, Desmond P, Ames D, et al. Temporal lobe magnetic resonance imaging can differentiate Alzheimer's disease from normal ageing, depression, vascular dementia and other causes of cognitive impairment. Psychol Med (1997) 27(6):1267–1275.

O'Brien JT, Paling S, Barber R, et al. Progressive brain atrophy on serial MRI in dementia with Lewy bodies, AD, and vascular dementia. Neurology (2001) 56(10):1386–1388.

Okamura N, Arai H, Higuchi M, et al. [^{18}F]FDG-PET study in dementia with Lewy bodies and Alzheimer's disease. Prog Neuropsychopharmacol Biol Psychiatry (2001) 25(2):447–456.

Oliva D., Carella F., Savoiardo M., et al. Clinical and magnetic resonance features of the classic and akinetic-rigid variants of Huntington's disease. Arch Neurol (1993) 50(1):17–19.

Pantano P, Caramia F, and Pierallini A. The role of MRI in dementia. Ital J Neurol Sci (1999) 20(5):S250–S253.

Pantel J, Schroder J, Essig M, et al. In vivo quantification of brain volumes in subcortical vascular dementia and Alzheimer's disease. An MRI-based study. Dement Geriatr Cogn Disord (1998) 9(6):309–316.

Pearlson GD, Rabins PV, and Burns A. Centrum semiovale white matter CT changes associated with normal ageing, Alzheimer's disease and late life depression with and without reversible dementia. Psychol Med (1991) 21(2):321–328.

Peppard RF, Martin WR, Carr GD, et al. Cerebral glucose metabolism in Parkinson's disease with and without dementia. Arch Neurol (1992) 49(12):1262–1268.

Powers WJ, Perlmutter JS, Videen TO, et al. Blinded clinical evaluation of positron emission tomography for diagnosis of probable Alzheimer's disease. Neurology (1992) 42(4):765–770.

Raininko R, Elovaara I, Virta A, et al. Radiological study of the brain at various stages of human immunodeficiency virus infection: early development of brain atrophy. Neuroradiology (1992) 34(3):190–196.

Read SL, Miller BL, Mena I, et al. SPECT in dementia: clinical and pathological correlation. J Am Geriatr Soc (1995) 43(11):1243–1247.

Reiman EM, Caselli RJ, Yun LS, et al. Preclinical evidence of Alzheimer's disease in persons homozygous for the epsilon 4 allele for apolipoprotein E. N Engl J Med (1996) 334(12):752–758.

Rinne JO, Sahlberg N, Ruottinen H, et al. Striatal uptake of the dopamine reuptake ligand [^{11}C]beta-CFT is reduced in Alzheimer's disease assessed by positron emission tomography. Neurology (1998) 50(1):152–156.

Rosci MA, Pigorini F, Bernabei A, et al. Methods for detecting early signs of AIDS dementia complex in asymptomatic HIV-1-infected subjects. AIDS (1992) 6(11):1309–1316.

Roses AD. Apolipoprotein E alleles as risk factors in Alzheimer's disease. Annu Rev Med (1996) 47:387–400.

Rossor MN, Garrett NJ, Johnson AL, et al. A post-mortem study of the cholinergic and GABA systems in senile dementia. Brain (1982) 105(Pt 2):313–330.

Roth J, Havrdova E, Stikova V, et al. The CT image of atrophy of the head of the caudate nucleus in Huntington's chorea. Cas Lek Cesk (1996) 135(9):277–279.

Rusinek H, De Leon MJ, George AE, et al. Alzheimer disease: measuring loss of cerebral gray matter with MR imaging. Radiology (1991) 178(1):109–114.

Sabri O, Ringelstein EB, Hellwig D, et al. Neuropsychological impairment correlates with hypoperfusion and hypometabolism but not with severity of white matter lesions on MRI in patients with cerebral microangiopathy. Stroke (1999) 30(3):556–566.

Salmon E, Meulemans T, van der Linden M, et al. Anterior cingulate dysfunction in presenile dementia due to progressive supranuclear palsy. Acta Neurol Belg (1996) 96(3):247–253.

Sasaki M, Ichiya Y, Hosokawa S, et al. Regional cerebral glucose metabolism in patients with Parkinson's disease with or without dementia. Ann Nucl Med (1992) 6(4):241–246.

Savoiardo M, Strada L, Girotti F, et al. MR imaging in progressive supranuclear palsy and Shy-Drager syndrome. J Comput Assist Tomogr (1989) 13(4):555–560.

Scheltens P and Korf ES. Contribution of neuroimaging in the diagnosis of Alzheimer's disease and other dementias. Curr Opin Neurol (2000) 13(4):391–396.

Schmidt R. Comparison of magnetic resonance imaging in Alzheimer's disease, vascular dementia and normal aging. Eur Neurol (1992) 32(3):164–169.

Schrag A, Kingsley D, Phatouros C, et al. Clinical usefulness of magnetic resonance imaging in multiple system atrophy. J Neurol Neurosurg Psychiatry (1998) 65(1):65–71.

Schulz JB, Klockgether T, Petersen D, et al. Multiple system atrophy: natural history, MRI morphology, and dopamine receptor imaging with 123IBZM-SPECT. J Neurol Neurosurg Psychiatry (1994) 57(9):1047–1056.

Seiderer M, Krappel W, Moser E, et al. Detection and quantification of chronic cerebrovascular disease: comparison of MR imaging, SPECT, and CT. Radiology (1989) 170(2):545–548.

Seltzer B and Sherwin I. A comparison of clinical features in early- and late-onset primary degenerative dementia. One entity or two? Arch Neurol (1983) 40(3):143–146.

Shoghi-Jadid K, Small GW, Agdeppa ED, et al. Localization of neurofibrillary tangles and beta-amyloid plaques in the brains of living patients with Alzheimer disease. Am J Geriatr Psychiatry 2002; 10(1):24–35.

Silverman DH, Gambhir SS, Huang HW, et al. Evaluating early dementia with and without assessment of regional cerebral metabolism by PET: a comparison of predicted costs and benefits. J Nucl Med (2002) 43(2):253–266.

Slansky I., Herholz K, Pietrzyk U, et al. Cognitive impairment in Alzheimer's disease correlates with ventricular width and atrophy-corrected cortical glucose metabolism. Neuroradiology (1995) 37(4):270–277.

Small GW, Ercoli LM, Silverman DH, et al. Cerebral metabolic and cognitive decline in persons at genetic risk for Alzheimer's disease. Proc Natl Acad Sci USA (2000) 97(11):6037–6042.

Small GW, Mazziotta JC, Collins MT, et al. Apolipoprotein E type 4 allele and cerebral glucose metabolism in relatives at risk for familial Alzheimer disease. JAMA (1995) 273(12):942–947.

Small SA, Perera GM, De la Paz R, et al. Differential regional dysfunction of the hippocampal formation among elderly with memory decline and Alzheimer's disease. Ann Neurol (1999) 45(4):466–472.

Smith CD, Andersen AH, Kryscio RJ, et al. Altered brain activation in cognitively intact individuals at high risk for Alzheimer's disease. Neurology (1999a) 53(7):1391–1396.

Smith CD, Malcein M, Meurer K, et al. MRI temporal lobe volume measures and neuropsychologic function in Alzheimer's disease. J Neuroimaging (1999b) 9(1):2–9.

Snowdon DA, Greiner LH, Mortimer JA, et al. Brain infarction and the clinical expression of Alzheimer disease. The Nun Study. JAMA (1997) 277(10):813–817.

Starkstein SE, Brandt J, Bylsma F, et al. Neuropsychological correlates of brain atrophy in Huntington's disease: a magnetic resonance imaging study. Neuroradiology (1992) 34(6):487–489.

Stoppe G, Bruhn H, Pouwels PJ, et al. Alzheimer disease: absolute quantification of cerebral metabolites in vivo using localized proton magnetic resonance spectroscopy. Alzheimer Dis Assoc Disord (2000) 14(2):112–119.

Stout JC, Ellis RJ, Jernigan TL, et al. Progressive cerebral volume loss in human immunodeficiency virus infection: a longitudinal volumetric magnetic resonance imaging study. HIV Neurobehavioral Research Center Group. Arch Neurol (1998) 55(2):161–168.

Talbot PR, Lloyd JJ, Snowden JS, et al. A clinical role for ^{99m}Tc-HMPAO SPECT in the investigation of dementia? J Neurol Neurosurg Psychiatry (1998) 64(3):306–313.

Tanabe JL, Ezekiel F, Jagust WJ, et al. Magnetization transfer ratio of white matter hyperintensities in subcortical ischemic vascular dementia. AJNR Am J Neuroradiol (1999) 20(5):839–844.

Tanahashi N, Meyer JS, Ishikawa Y, et al. Cerebral blood flow and cognitive testing correlate in Huntington's disease. Arch Neurol (1985) 42(12):1169–1175.

Tanaka S, Kawamata J, Shimohama S, et al. Inferior temporal lobe atrophy and APOE genotypes in Alzheimer's disease. X-ray computed tomography, magnetic resonance imaging and Xe-133 SPECT studies. Dement Geriatr Cogn Disord (1998) 9(2):90–98.

Teipel SJ, Bayer W, Alexander GE, et al. Progression of corpus callosum atrophy in Alzheimer disease. Arch Neurol (2002) 59(2):243–248.

Villa G, Cappa A, Tavolozza M, et al. Neuropsychological tests and [^{99m}Tc]HM PAO SPECT in the diagnosis of Alzheimer's dementia. J Neurol (1995) 242(6):359–366.

Volkow ND, Ding YS, Fowler JS, et al. Imaging brain cholinergic activity with positron emission tomography: its role in the evaluation of cholinergic treatments in Alzheimer's dementia. Biol Psychiatry (2001) 49(3):211–220.

Wilcock GK. The temporal lobe in dementia of Alzheimer's type. Gerontology (1983) 29(5):320–324.

Willmer J, Carruthers A, Guzman DA, et al. The usefulness of CT scanning in diagnosing dementia of the Alzheimer type. Can J Neurol Sci (1993) 20(3):210–216.

Wolfe N, Reed BR, Eberling JL, et al. Temporal lobe perfusion on single photon emission computed tomography predicts the rate of cognitive decline in Alzheimer's disease. Arch Neurol (1995) 52(3):257–262.

Wyper D, Teasdale E, Patterson J, et al. Abnormalities in rCBF and computed tomography in patients with Alzheimer's disease and in controls. Br J Radiol (1993) 66(781):23–27.

Yamauchi H, Fukuyama H, Nagahama Y, et al. Comparison of the pattern of atrophy of the corpus callosum in frontotemporal dementia, progressive supranuclear palsy, and Alzheimer's disease. J Neurol Neurosurg Psychiatry (2000) 69(5):623–629.

Zhuang ZP, Kung MP, Hou C, et al. IBOX(2-(4′-dimethylaminophenyl)-6-iodobenzoxazole): a ligand for imaging amyloid plaques in the brain. Nucl Med Biol 2001; 28(8):887–894.

35

Genetics of Alzheimer's Disease

M. ILYAS KAMBOH
Western Psychiatric Institute and Clinic, University of Pittsburgh School of Medicine, Pittsburgh, Pennsylvania, U.S.A.

I. INTRODUCTION

Alzheimer's disease (AD) is a complex multifactorial neurodegenerative disease and a leading cause of dementia among elderly people. About 5% of the people aged 65 or above are affected with AD, and the prevalence rises steeply to 19% after age 75 and to 47% after age 85 [1]. Currently there are approximately > 4 million AD cases in the United States and ~12–14 million worldwide. Owing to its long clinical course, AD is a major public health problem. The average life expectancy after diagnosis is 8–10 years, though the disease can last for up to 20 years. The estimated annual cost for caring of one AD patient in the United States ranges from about $18,000 for a patient with mild AD, to $30,000 for a patient with moderate AD, up to $36,000 for a patient with severe AD; this translates into a hefty total annual cost of > $50 billion [2]. Approximately 360,000 incidence cases occur each year [3], and this number is increasing as the population ages and life expectancy increases. Currently ~ 35 million Americans are age 65 and older, and the Bureau of the Census estimates that this number will double by the year 2030 and exceeds 80 million in 2050. Furthermore, the 85 and older group, in which almost 50% of the people are affected with some form of dementia, is one of the fastest-growing segments of the U.S. population [4]. Currently ~ 4 million Americans are in this group, which is expected to double by the year 2030 and quadruple by the year 2050. Because of this alarming increase in the elderly population and with the possibility that the bulk of this elderly population will suffer from AD, it is essential to devise effective preventive measures soon to curb the disease. Up until a decade ago the understanding of the causes of AD were either lacking or limited. Although we still do not understand the exact underlying cause of AD, the combined research findings from genetic, molecular, and functional studies over the past few years have been illuminating, and now we are closer than ever in establishing the molecular and biochemical basis of the disease.

Alzheimer's disease is characterized by two main pathological hallmarks—the presence of extracellular neuritic plaques, and the occurrence of intracellular neurofibrillary tangles. The main culprit in neuritic plaques is a small fragment of 39–42 amino acid (aa) residue, called amyloid β-peptide (Aβ). It is believed that Aβ peptides, especially the 42-aa fragment, form fibrils by self-aggregation and then they clump into plaques in AD brains. Neurofibrillary tangles are made up of a highly phosphorylated protein, called tau. The normal function of tau is to bind and stabilize the microtubule assembly in the cytoplasm. However, the hyperphosphorylated tau clumps into tangles and causes the microtubules to destabilize and eventually collapse in the neurons of AD patients. Whether plaques or tangles are the primary lesion in AD is still a matter of debate, although most AD researchers believe that Aβ is the primary culprit and that other events are a consequence of amyloid deposition. Genetic findings in conjunction with biochemical data also support the latter hypothesis.

Because of variation in age at onset, AD is categorized into early- (<60 years age) and late- (≥60 years age) onset forms. There are two types of AD: familial AD (FAD), which runs in families, and sporadic AD, in which no obvious family history is present. Sporadic AD, especially late-onset, accounts for ~ 90% of all patients. Early-onset AD, which is usually familial, follows an autosomal-dominant inheritance pattern, where a mutation in a single gene can cause the disease. On the other hand, late-onset AD does not show a clear mode of inheritance, as it is caused by a complex gene-environment interaction. This chapter summarizes the up-to-date advances made in the molecular genetics of early-onset and late-onset AD.

II. EARLY-ONSET ALZHEIMER'S DISEASE

To date three genes—amyloid precursor protein (APP) on chromosome 21 [5], presenilin (PS)-1 on chromosome 14 [6], and PS-2 on chromosome 1 [7,8]—have been linked to FAD (Table 1). Mutations in the APP, PS-1, and PS-2 genes account for ~ 50% of early-onset AD, with the main contribution from the PS-1 gene. Altogether, mutations in these genes explain <2% of all AD cases, young and old.

A. Amyloid Precursor Protein (APP) Gene

The APP gene, with 19 exons, codes for a transmembrane protein, ranging in size from 677 to 770 aa due to alternative splicing. The longest isoform (APP-770) consists of an amino terminal domain of 699 aa in the extracellular region, a short transmembrane region of 24 aa, and 47 aa carboxyl-terminal tail in the cytoplasm. Aβ, a small fragment of 39–43 aa, which is encoded by parts of exon 16 and 17 [9], is derived from APP by alternative processing. The Aβ sequence begins 99 aa from the carboxyl-terminal (at position 672 in APP-770), which spans 28 aa in the extracellular domain and extends to the first 11–15 hydrophobic residues in the transmembrane region [10,11]. The APP undergoes three alternative steps of proteolytic cleavages within or the surrounding sequence of Aβ to generate either nonamyloidogenic or amyloidogenic peptides (Fig. 1). In the nonamyloidogenic pathway, a putative α-secretase enzyme cleaves the APP between residues 16 and 17 (after residue 687) within the Aβ sequence to generate the secreted long amino-terminal of APP, called α-APP and a membrane-bound 83aa long fragment called C83. Subsequently the membrane-bound carboxyl-terminal (C83) is cleaved by a putative γ-secretase after the end of the Aβ sequence to generate a harmless 3-kDa peptide fragment, called p3. In the amyloidogenic pathway, another enzyme called β-secretase [12] first cleaves APP at the beginning of the Aβ sequence (after residue 671) and generates a membrane-bound 99-aa-long fragment called C99, which is subsequently cut by γ-secretase at the end of the Aβ sequence to release a series of 4-kDa 39 to 43-aa-long intact fragments of Aβ. Under normal circumstances most of the generated Aβ are 39 to 40-aa-long fragments, which appear to be harmless. However, ~ 10% of the Aβ are 42 aa or longer, which are considered to be neurotoxic and they are involved in forming neuritic plaques in AD brains [13].

The mutations in the APP gene causing early-onset FAD are rare and account for <1% of FAD cases [14]. However, all pathogenic APP mutations are clustered in or around the Aβ sequence close to the β-secretase (codons 670/671), α-secretase (codons 692 and 693) and γ-secretase (codons 716 and 717) sites, and they are associated with elevated production of either total Aβ or Aβ$_{42}$.

B. Presenilin (PS-1 and PS-2) Genes

The PS-1 and PS-2 are integral membrane proteins which share a significant structural homology [15,16]. Each gene consists of a total of 13 exons with 10 exons coding for the 467-aa-long PS-1 protein and 448-aa-long PS-2 protein. The proposed eight or more hydrophobic domains of presenilins are inserted in the cell membranes of mainly endoplasmic reticulum, the Golgi apparatus, and the perinuclear envelope. The amino and carboxyl terminals, along with a hydrophilic domain between the 6th and 7th transmembrane

Table 1 Genes (Autosomal-Dominant) in Early-Onset Alzheimer's Disease

Gene	Chromosome	Reference
APP	21q21.2	Goate et al. [5]
PS-1	14q24.3	Sherrington et al. [6]
PS-2	1q41	Levy-Lahad et al. [7]
		Rogaeva et al. (8)

Genetics of Alzheimer's Disease

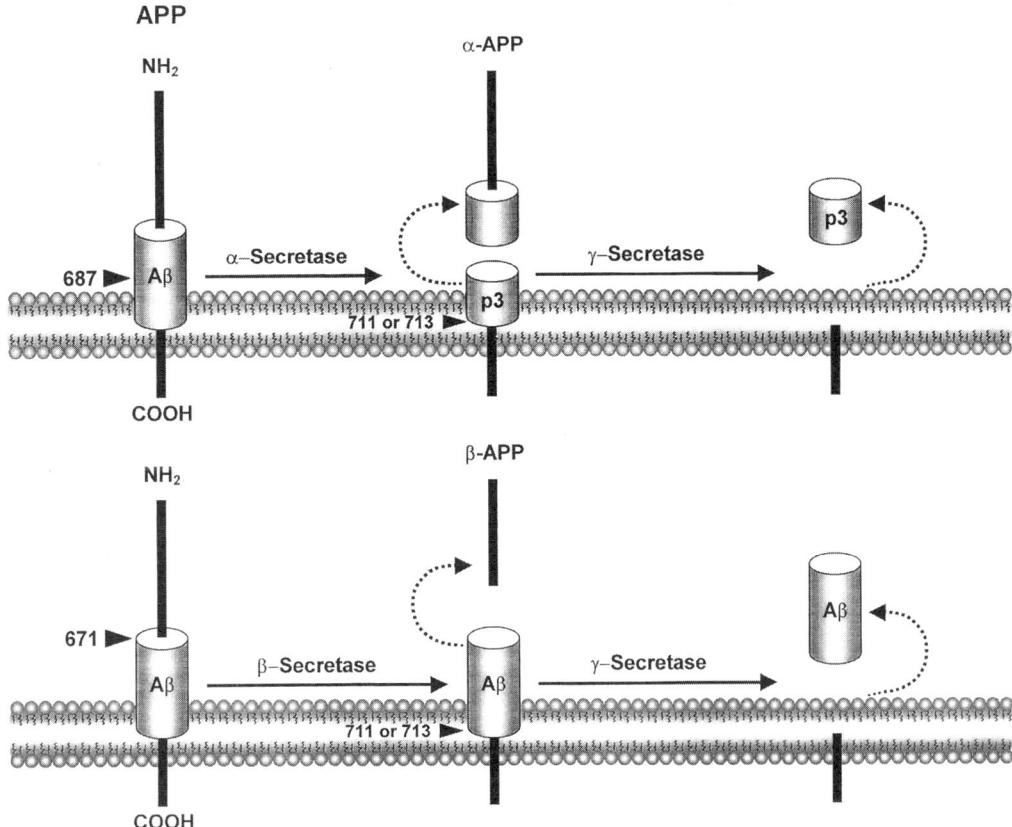

Figure 1 Processing of APP by α, β, and γ secretases. In the nonamyloidogenic pathway (top), an α-secretase enzyme cleaves within the Aβ sequence (boxed) after residue 687 (arrowhead) and releases the large secreted NH$_2$-terminal of APP, called α-APP and leaves behind the membrane-bound 83-residue carboxyl-terminal, which is subsequently cleaved by γ-secretase at residues 711 or 713 to release the harmless p3 peptide. In the amyloidogenic pathway (bottom), a β-secretase cuts at the start of the Aβ sequence after residue 671, which results in the generation of a truncated APP, called β-APP and the retention of a membrane-bound 99-residue carboxyl-terminal, which is subsequently cleaved by γ-secretase at residues 711 or 713 outside the Aβ sequence to generate various forms of Aβ having 40–42 aa.

domains, are protruded into the cytoplasm. Only very small amounts of the PS-1 and PS-2 holoproteins (full-length intact proteins) exist in in vivo. PS-1 and PS-2 are proteolytically cleaved by a yet to be discovered esterase between the transmembrane domains 6 and 7, leading to a membrane-attached ~30-kDa amino-terminal and ~20-kDa carboxyl-terminal fragments, both of which are required for presenilins to be functionally active. Although the exact function of presenilins is not yet fully elucidated, strong evidence indicates that they regulate the processing of APP. Based on the evidence that PS-1-deficient mice lack γ-secretase activity [17], it has been proposed that either presenilins are themselves γ-secretases or they modulate the activities of γ-secretases.

To date > 70 different missense mutations and two splicing defect mutations have been identified in the PS-1 gene, and they explain the bulk of FAD cases [18]. Only two FAD mutations in the PS-2 gene have been identified: one in the Volga German families, and one in an Italian family [7,8]. Two additional PS-2 mutations have been identified in sporadic Dutch and Spanish cases [19,20]. Altogether the PS-2 gene explains <1% of FAD cases. Similar to the APP mutations, all presenilin mutations in FAD are associated with abnormal processing of APP, which leads to the overproduction of Aβ_{42}. These data strongly suggest that these genes operate through a common biochemical pathway.

III. LATE-ONSET ALZHEIMER'S DISEASE

The late-onset form of the disease is much more common and far more complex than early-onset AD. As compared to early-onset AD, which usually follows an autosomal-dominant inheritance pattern, the late-onset AD does not show a clear mode of inheritance, as it is probably polygenic. To delineate the genetic architecture of late-onset AD, two approaches have been and are being used to identify the risk genes: linkage studies on multiplex families or affected sib-pairs using whole-genome scans, and association studies on case control cohorts using candidate genes or genes surrounding the linkage peak areas identified in linkage studies. Table 2 provides a summary of genes in late-onset AD implicated by linkage [21–28] and association [29–48] studies. As the results of most association studies have been inconsistent, the following sections are devoted to discussion of linkage studies and the results of association of only those candidate genes that reside around the areas identified in linkage studies.

A. Chromosome 19 and the Apolipoprotein E Gene

In 1991 the evidence of linkage for late-onset AD was reported to chromosome 19q13 [21]. Subsequent asso-

Table 2 Susceptibility Genes in Late-Onset Alzheimer's Disease

Gene	Chromosome	Reference
Linkage Studies		
(APOE)	19q13	Pericak-Vance et al. [21]
?	12p, 12q	Pericak-Vance et al. [22]
		Rogaeva et al. [23]
		Wu et al. [24]
		Kehoe et al. [25]
?	10q	Bertman et al. [26]
		Myers et al. [27]
?	9p, 9q	Kehoe et al. [25]
		Pericak-Vance et al. [28]
Association Studies		
IL-1A	2q13	Nicoll et al. [29]
IL-1B	2q13	Grimaldi et al. [30]
BCHE-K	3q26.1	Lehmann et al. [31]
NACP/α-synuclein	4q21.3	Xia et al. [32]
HLA-DR	6p21.3	Curran et al. [33]
IL-6	7p15.3	Papassotiropoulous et al. [34]
NOS3	7q35	Dahiyat et al. [35]
VLDLR	9p24	Okuizumi et al. [36]
Fe65 (APBB1)	11p15	Hu et al. [37]
CTSD	11p15	Papassotiropoulous et al. [38]
A2M	12p13.2	Blacker et al. [39]
LRP1	12q13	Lendon et al. [40]
ACT	14q32.1	Kamboh et al. [41]
PS-1	14q24	Wragg et al. [42]
ACE	17q23	Kehoe et al. [43]
MPO	17q23	Reynolds et al. [44]
Tau	17q21.1	Bullido et al. [45]
APOE	19q13.2	Strittmatter et al. [46]
CST3	20p11.21	Crawford et al. [47]
mtDNA	M	Hutchin and Cortopassi [48]

ciation studies identified the apolipoprotein E (APOE) gene, which also maps to 19q13, as a strong susceptibility marker for late-onset AD [46,49]. The APOE gene, which is closely linked with three other members of the apolipoprotein gene family—APOC1, APOC2, and APOC4 on chromosome 19q13.2—is genetically polymorphic with the occurrence of three common alleles, designated *APOE*2*, *APOE*3*, and *APOE*4*. The three alleles differ from each other by missense mutations at either codon 112 or codon 158 in exon 3 (Fig. 2). *APOE*3* is the wild-type allele, which has cysteine at position 112 and arginine at position 158. The *APOE*2* allele codes for cysteine at both positions, while the *APOE*4* allele codes for arginine at both positions. The frequencies of the three alleles differ significantly among the three major racial groups [50]. Among white populations the average frequencies of the *APOE*2* and *APOE*4* alleles are ~ 8% and 14%, respectively. However, the respective frequencies are ~ 4% and 25% among blacks, and 7% and 9% among Asians. Several case control studies conducted since 1993 have established that the frequency of the *APOE*4* is significantly higher, while the frequency of the *APOE*2* allele is significantly lower among AD cases than controls. In a meta analysis involving 5939 AD cases and 8746 controls from 40 studies, comprising U.S. whites, U.S. blacks, Hispanics, and Japanese [51], it was established that the *APOE*4* allele was a significant risk factor in all populations and the *APOE*2* allele was protective mainly in U.S. whites and Japanese (Table 3). The frequency of the *APOE*4* allele was about threefold higher and the frequency of the *APOE*2* allele was twofold lower in U.S. white and Japanese AD cases than their respective controls. However, the meta-analysis revealed that the association of the *APOE*4* allele with AD is weaker in U.S. blacks and Hispanics, where its frequency was only 1.7-fold higher in AD cases than controls in both racial groups. Similarly the *APOE*2*-associated protective effect observed in U.S. whites and Japanese was absent in U.S. blacks and Hispanics. The AD risk associated with the *APOE*4* allele was dose related in most populations, except in Hispanics. In the meta-analysis, the respective odds ratios (OR) associated with the 3/4 genotype (one copy of the *APOE*4* allele) and 4/4 genotype (two copies of the *APOE*4* allele), were 2.7 and 12.5 in U.S. whites, 1.1 and 5.7 in U.S. blacks, 2.2 and 2.2 in Hispanics, and 5.6 and 33.1 in Japanese. The weaker association of the *APOE*4* allele with AD in U.S. blacks and Hispanics could be due to relatively smaller sample sizes in these two groups. Alternatively, other yet to be identified genetic and environmental factors in these groups may modify the risk of AD.

Despite the robust association of the *APOE*4* allele with AD, the *APOE*4* allele is neither necessary nor required for the development of AD. This suggests that the *APOE*4* allele is a susceptibility marker, which in conjunction with other genetic and/or environmental factors can increase the risk of AD. The exact mechanism by which the *APOE*4* allele increases the risk of AD is not clear. The pos-

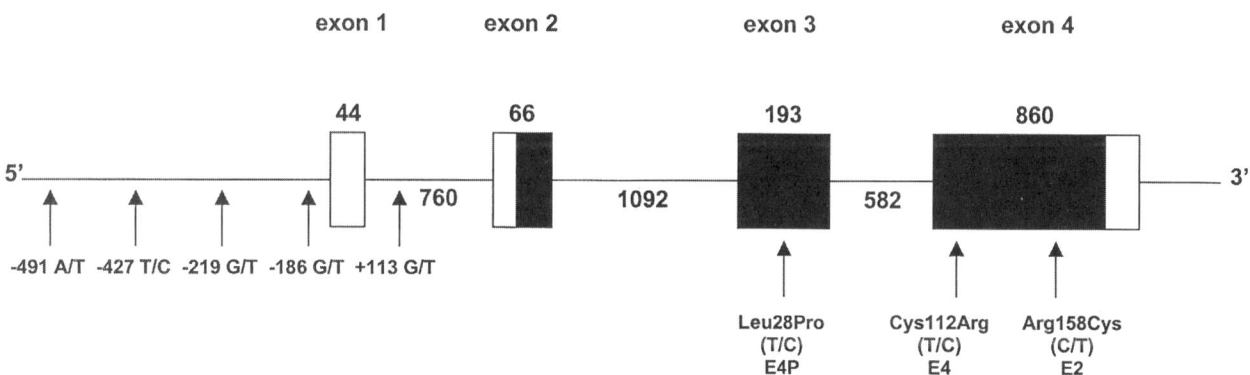

Figure 2 Structure of the APOE gene showing exons (solid boxes, coding regions; blank boxes, noncoding regions), intron and 5′ and 3′ regions (lines). The positions of polymorphic sites along with amino acids and nucleotide substitutions and APOE forms (E2, E4, E4P) in exon 3 and 4 are shown by arrows. The five polymorphic sites in the APOE regulatory region (5′ and intron 1) are also indicated by arrows. The sizes of exons are given in base pairs (bp) above each exon, the sizes of introns (bp) are given below each intron.

Table 3 Percentage of APOE Genotype and Allele Frequencies in AD Cases and Controls in Different Racial Groups from a Meta-Analysis

	U.S. Whites		U.S. Blacks		U.S. Hispanics		Japanese	
	Cases (n=5107)	Controls (n=6262)	Cases (n=235)	Controls (n=240)	Cases (n=261)	Controls (n=267)	Cases (n=336)	Controls (n=1977)
Genotype								
2/2	0.2	0.8	1.7	0.8	0.4	0.4	0.3	0.4
2/3	4.8	12.7	9.8	12.9	9.6	12.0	3.9	6.9
2/4	2.6	2.6	2.1	2.1	2.3	0.8	0.9	0.8
3/3	36.4	60.9	36.2	50.4	54.4	67.4	49.1	75.7
3/4	41.1	21.2	37.9	31.8	30.7	17.6	36.9	15.5
4/4	14.8	1.8	12.3	2.1	2.7	1.9	8.9	0.8
Allele								
E*2	3.9	8.4	7.7	8.3	6.3	6.7	2.7	4.2
E*3	59.4	77.9	59.1	72.7	74.5	82.3	69.5	86.9
E*4	36.7	13.7	32.2	19.0	19.2	11.0	27.8	8.9

Source: Ref. 51.

sibility that the *APOE*4* allele may be in linkage disequilibrium with a nearby functional mutation exists, but a substantial amount of biochemical data suggest that the polymorphism by itself could be functional. APOE binds to Aβ and tau, which are major components of amyloid plaques and neurofibrillary tangles, respectively. As compared to the E3 isoform, the E4 isoform binds to Aβ more rapidly [46], promotes Aβ monofibril formation more efficiently [52–54], and leads to a higher Aβ plaque burden [55]. APOE binds to the low-density lipoprotein–related receptor protein (LRP1), and it mediates the clearance of Aβ through this receptor in the brain. It has been proposed that the *APOE*4* allele is associated with impaired clearance of the APOE-Aβ complexes as compared to the *APOE*3* allele [56,57]. APOE is also involved in neuronal repair and remodeling and it has been shown that as compared to the *APOE*3* allele, the *APOE*4* allele is associated with inhibition of neurite growth and destabilizing microtubule assembly [58,59]. There is also isoform-specific binding of APOE with tau, the protein which stabilizes microtubules. Tau binds to E3 but not to the E4 isoform and this isoform-specific binding difference may lead to the formation of neurofibrillary tangles [60]. APOE has also been shown to have anti-oxidant activity, with *APOE*2* allele the most effective, *APOE*3* moderately effective, and *APOE*4* allele the least effective [61].

The APOE isoform-specific differences seen in in vitro studies have also been confirmed in in vivo studies in transgenic mice. APOE-null mice have shown age-related neurodegeneration of synaptodendritic connections [62]. However, APOE-null mice expressing either *APOE*3* and *APOE*4* have shown that while *APOE*3* prevents the APOE-null-induced, age-dependent neurodegeneration, the *APOE*4* does not [63]. Furthermore, compared to *APOE*3*, the *APOE*4* expression in the brains of APOE-null mice is associated with impaired ability to perform a water maze task [64]. These data strongly suggest that APOE may directly affect the risk of AD and that this affect is modulated by APOE genetic variation at codons 112 and 158 (E2/E3/E4 polymorphism).

In addition to the *APOE*4* allele, several polymorphisms in the transcriptional regulatory region of APOE have been identified, which alone or in combination with *APOE*4* can modify the risk of AD. These polymorphic sites include, −491 A/T, 427 T/C, 219 G/T, 186 G/T, and +113 C/G [65–67] (see Fig. 1). The −491 A/T site has been found to be associated with the risk of AD in several [68–72], but not in all studies [70,73,74]. The association studies for the −427 T/C site are also equivocal [66–69]. The 186 G/T and +113 C/G polymorphic sites have also been found to be associated with the risk of AD [65,67,69]. In one study [67], the −491T and +113G alleles were associated with a protective effect, but the −427T and

−186T alleles were associated with an increased risk of AD, and these associations were independent of the known (E2/E3/E4) polymorphism [67,68].

Recently, we have also identified a unique Leu28Pro mutation, which is associated with AD risk [75]. The Leu28Pro mutation was found to be strongly associated with the *APOE*4* allele and therefore we called it as *APOE*4 Pittsburgh* (*APOE*4P*). In 1118 AD cases, the carrier frequency of the E4P mutation was 2.4% compared to 0.2% observed in 1123 controls. The age, sex, and *APOE*4* adjusted OR associated with the *APOE*4P* mutation was 5.3, indicating that its effect is independent of the *APOE*4* allele. We also found that the risk associated with the combination of the *APOE*4/APOE*4P* was about five times the risk associated with just the *APOE*4* allele. The functional significance of the E4P mutation is not yet known.

B. Chromosome 12 Gene

In addition to the APOE susceptibility gene on chromosome 19, the first evidence that additional susceptibility genes exist for late-onset AD came in 1997 when Pericak-Vance et al. [22] presented statistical evidence of a putative risk gene on chromosome 12 in a linkage analysis on 54 pedigrees. A maximum LOD score (MLS) of 3.9 was observed near D12S1042 (12 p11–12) (Table 4) in 27 families that lacked the *APOE*4* allele, suggesting that the chromosome 12 gene explains the risk of AD in non-*APOE*4* carriers. Subsequently, several linkage studies have replicated the original findings, but they don't agree on the location of the risk gene. In 53 families, Rogaeva et al. [23] implicated a broad region of ∼ 50 cM, covering both the short and long arms of chromosome 12. However, the strongest evidence for the putative gene was found near D12S96, which is on the long arm of chromosome 12 near the LRP1 gene (discussed later) in families carrying the *APOE*4* allele (Table 4). On the other hand, in a linkage study of 230 families, Wu et al. [24] found no evidence for linkage in the two regions implicated by Pericak-Vance et al. [22] and Rogaeva et al. [23]. Wu et al. [24] rather found evidence for the existence of a locus with a smaller effect in non-*APOE*4* families near D12S98, which is close to the α2-macroglobulin (A2M) gene (discussed later), but > 20 cM proximal from the 12p11–12 region implicated by Pericak-Vance et al. [22]. The same group also found the evidence of the susceptibility locus among non-*APOE*4* carriers near A2M in 292 affected sib pairs [25].

The apparent discrepancies between studies about the location of the susceptibility locus could be due

Table 4 Summary of Linkage Studies on Chromosome 12

Location (in cM)	Marker	Gene	Reference
12p			
20	D12S1695		
25	D12S358	(A2M)[a]	Wu et al. [24]
26	D12S98	(OLR1)	Kehoe et al. [25]
36	D12S373		
42	D12S1688		
44	D12S1057		Pericak-Vance et al. [22]
49	D12S1042		Scott et al. [76]
12q			
56	D12S1090		
63	D12S1701		
68	D12S390		
68	D12S96	(LRP1)	Rogaeva et al. [23]
68	D12S398	(LBP-1c/CP2/LSF)	Scott et al. [76]
72	D12S1632		
76	D12S75		

[a]Locations of the genes are approximate relative to the positions of the markers.

to several factors, including among others, diagnostic criteria (inclusion of clinically or autopsy-assessed cases), phenotypic heterogeneity in the disease (inclusion of pure AD cases and/or AD cases with additional diagnoses, e.g., Lewy bodies), sibship size and nature of samples (multiplex families or affected sibling pairs), sample heterogeneity, and analytical methods employed. Another possibility is that there are two loci within the vicinity of about 50-cM region on chromosome 12, each with a modest effect. In an attempt to address the issue of genetic and phenotypic heterogeneity in AD families that might influence the linkage analysis, Pericak-Vance and colleagues screened their original 54 families [22] for additional markers by weighing the results by clinical and neuropathologic factors, family size, and APOE genotype [76]. Upon considering all possible affected sibpairs per nuclear familiy, Scott et al. [76] obtained a peek MLS at the same position (12p11–12, between D12S1057 and D12S1042) they originally reported [22]. However, the magnitude and location of the MLS changed ~ 25 cM distal (between D12S398 and D12S1632 on 12q) from the original location when different weighting schemes were used to control for the number of affected sib pairs in each family (Table 4). Scott et al. [76] also found that much of the evidence of linkage on chromosome 12 came from families that either lacked APOE*4 or had Lewy bodies (LB) and predicted that the putative gene may lie in the ~30-cM region between D12S1057 and D12S1632, which contain both the overall linkage peak at 12q (near D12S1632) and linkage peak specific to LB families at 12p (near D12S1057).

Two candidate genes on chromosome 12, A2M and LRP1, which encompass the same regions where linkage studies indicate the presence of AD risk genes, have been examined extensively in association studies. A2M is a major serum protease inhibitor and can bind a variety of foreign proteins [77]. A2M is upregulated in the brain during injury [78]. In AD patients, A2M has been localized immunochemically to senile plaques [79]. In vitro, A2M binds to and attenuates the propensity of Aβ peptide of forming neurotoxic fibrils [80,81]. LRP1 is a cell receptor that binds to APOE, A2M, and APP [57,79,82], and thus it may affect the risk of AD.

Two common A2M polymorphisms, an intronic deletion/insertion and Ile1000Val, have been described. The first involves a pentanucleotide deletion 5' splice site of exon II of bait region (exon 18) [83]; the second is an isoleucine to valine substitution in exon 24 near the thiolester site of the gene [84].

Blacker et al. [39] first reported the association of the deletion/insertion polymorphism with late-onset AD in a family-based case control study. Since then the association between this polymorphism and late-onset AD has been investigated extensively, with variable results. Some studies have confirmed that the A2M intronic polymorphism confers an increased risk [85–87] even in age-dependent manner [88], but other studies have failed to replicate such an association [89–94]. Association studies of the Ile1000Val polymorphism have been equally conflicting. Some studies have found a positive association with the A/A genotype (Ile) and AD; the effect of the A allele was stronger among non-APOE*4 carriers [86]. However, Liao et al [85] found an increased risk of AD with the G allele (Val). The OR for AD associated with the GG genotype was 1.8, and it increased to 9.7 in combination with APOE*4 [85]. However, other groups found no association between the risk of AD and the Ile1000Val polymorphism [95–98]. A meta-analysis of these two polymorphisms has also failed to show a significant association among whites, but a suggestive association with the deletion/insertion polymorphism was observed among Asian populations [99].

In view of these inconsistent results, possible explanations are as follows:

1. The A2M polymorphisms may be a stronger risk factor in familial AD cases, as observed by Blacker at al. [39], than in sporadic AD cases.
2. The genetic associations may reflect linkage with another mutation or polymorphism either in the A2M gene itself or in a nearby gene on chromosome 12.
3. The A2M polymorphisms are associated with AD in some populations because of an interactive effect with other susceptibility gene(s) or environmental factor(s) present in some, but not in other populations.
4. The reported association of the A2M polymorphisms represents a chance observation.

Two polymorphisms in the LRP1 gene, a tetranucleotide (TTTC), repeat in the 5' region and a same-sense mutation (C → T) in exon 3, and have been investigated in relation to the risk of AD, but the results are conflicting. For the tetranucleotide repeat polymorphism, some groups found an association of AD with the long (91 bp) repeat allele [100,101], others with the short (87 bp) repeat allele [40], but other groups found no association with either of the repeat alleles [102,103]. Similar results have been reported for the exon 3 polymorphism, in which some groups reported an association [103,104], but others did not [105]. Even the originally reported association in Kamboh et al.'s data [103] disappeared when the sample size was increased (unpublished data). In addition to these two variable sites, 46 more mutations have been identified by sequencing all 89 exons of LRP1 and their intron-exon boundaries [106]. Of the total 48 mutations, only one changes amino acid at position 216 (Ala → Val). An investigation of this mutation in 670 controls and 648 AD cases revealed that the carrier frequency of the Val216 allele was significantly lower in AD cases than controls (2.9% vs. 5.2%) with an OR of 0.55 [107]. Furthermore, this polymorphism was not in linkage disequilibrium with the other two polymorphisms, suggesting that a relatively uncommon polymorphism at position 216 confers a protective effect against the risk of AD. The role of 45 other new polymorphisms in relation to the AD risk has not been reported, and nor has the promoter region of the LRP1 gene been explored for functional mutations.

Recently a gene coding for transcription factor LBP-1c/CP2/LSF, which is located close to the LRP1 gene (∼6 cM), has been shown to modify the risk of AD in three samples [108]. The A allele of a G → A polymorphism in 3′UTR was found to confer a protection against the risk of AD in the French (OR = 0.48) and British (OR = 0.46) samples, and a similar but nonsignificant trend was observed in the American sample (OR = 0.87). The report also found that the protective effect of the A allele was significant only in AD patients <70 years old. The authors suggested that the age-dependent effect may explain why the effect of the A allele was not significant in the American sample, which was older than the other two samples. In a large sample of U.S. whites (553 AD cases, 510 controls), we have confirmed the protective effect of the A allele (OR = 0.65), but it was not age dependent (Luedecking, DeKosky, Kamboh, unpublished data). The transcription factor LBP-1c/CP2/LSF is a potential candidate gene for AD, as it affects the expression of A2M [109] and interacts with the Fe65 protein that appears to control the expression of APP [110]. Additional case control studies in different population groups may help to delineate the role of this marker in the etiology of AD.

C. Chromosome 10 Gene

A genomewide scan of 292 affected sibpairs with late-onset AD identified a candidate region on chromosome 10q with a MLS of 2.48 [25]. Using an expanded number of affected sib pairs (n = 429), the same research group reported an MLS of 3.83 close to the D10S1225 marker at 81 cM [27]. A linkage analysis on five late-onset AD families with extremely high plasma Aβ levels also found a MLS of 3.93 at 81 cM, close to D10S1225 [111]. However, a linkage analysis of 435 multiplex late-onset AD families with the D10S1225 marker showed no significant linkage, but rather a susceptibility locus was identified about 30 cM distal to D10S1225 at 115 cM close to D10S583 [26]. An association study between the D10S583 marker and AD suggests that the putative AD locus may reside in the 10q region. In this region a candidate gene coding for insulin-degrading enzyme (IDE) resides, which degrades Aβ in neurons and microglia. Direct association studies between the IDE gene and AD patients may help to identify the role of IDE in the etiology of AD.

The presence of a susceptibility locus on the short arm of chromosome 10 has also been suggested, as indicated by a moderate MLS of >1 (1.04 using dominant model and 1.22 using recessive model) close to D10S1426 (10p11.23) in autopsy-confirmed AD families, but not in clinically assessed AD families [28]. Additional support for a putative risk gene on 10p was provided by a separate genomewide scan in a case control study [112], which revealed that a 234-bp allele of D10S1423, located on 10p13, was a significant risk factor for AD. The frequency of the 234-bp allele was significantly higher in 100 autopsy-confirmed AD cases than in 100 controls (29% vs. 15%). Further evidence that the 234-bp allele may be in linkage disequilibrium with a functional locus on the short arm of chromosome 10 was provided by a significant association of the 234 bp allele with reduced levels of dopamine in all the six cortical regions examined, including middle frontal cortex, superior temporal cortex, inferior parietal cortex, occipital cortex, entorhinal cortex of the hippocampus, and cerebellar cortex [113]. Furthermore, the 234-bp allele carriers had high concentrations of cortical norepinephrine. Taking these data together, it appears that chromosome 10 may harbor two putative functional genes, one on the short arm and one on the long arm.

D. Chromosome 9 Gene

A genomewide scan with 292 affected sibpairs identified two peaks with MLS >1, one on the short arm of chromosome 9 (close to D9S171 in the p21 region) and one on the long arm of chromosome 9 (close to D9S176 in the q22 region) [25]. Similar results were obtained in a separate genomewide scan of 466 families with 730 affected sib pairs [28], which identified one peak at 9p22.1 close to D9S741 and the other at 9q34.2 near D9S1818. Interestingly, the 4.31 MLS observed in autopsy-confirmed cases in the 9p22.1 region was the highest ever seen in a genomewide scan for AD, suggesting that this region harbors a risk gene of major effect. The gene coding for very low density lipoprotein receptor (VLDLR), which is located in this region on the 9p24 band [114,115], is a possible candidate for AD, as this is a receptor for APOE [116]. A triplet (CGG) repeat polymorphism in the 5' UTR region of the VLDLR gene was reported to be a significant risk factor for AD in a Japanese sample [36]. The same authors also found a stronger immunoreactivity of VLDLR in hippocampal neurons of AD patients than in hippocampal neuron of controls, indicating a possible involvement of VLDLR in the pathogenesis of AD. However, the correlation of immunoreactivity with AD was independent of the triplet repeat polymorphism, suggesting that the triplet repeat polymorphism does not directly affect the risk of AD, but rather it could be in linkage disequilibrium with a functional mutation. Subsequent association studies of this polymorphism with AD in Japanese [117], Caucasians [118–121] and Chinese [122], however, failed to confirm the original association. Linkage analysis on 53 late-onset AD families also excluded at least 13 cM on either side of the VLDLR gene [118]. However, a recent linkage analysis on a large number of families by the latter group has implicated the same broad region at 9p22 being a strong candidate to harbor a putative risk gene [28]. A fine mapping of this region by single nucleotide polymorphisms (SNPs) may help to identify the putative risk gene(s).

IV. CONCLUSIONS

Genetic discoveries made in conjunction with biochemical findings over the past decade or so have significantly advanced our understanding about the possible causes of AD. To date the mutations identified in three causative genes for early-onset AD—APP, PS-1, and PS-2—and a susceptibility gene for late-onset APOE, point out a common biochemical pathway, which affects the processing of APP and leads to the production of elevated levels of $A\beta_{42}$. This provides a promising target to design effective drugs that could either block the production of $A\beta$ by inhibiting the β- or γ-secretases, restrict $A\beta$ accumulation or accelerate its breakdown in the brain. In animal models of AD, it has been shown that the accumulation of $A\beta$ contributes to learning and memory defects in mice [123–125], but the phenotype can be rescued by either immunization [124] or vaccination [125] with $A\beta$ peptide. The long-term effects of $A\beta$ vaccination in mice and whether this therapy will be beneficial in humans await more research and data.

Although we have come a long way in understanding the genetic basis of AD, more research needs to be done and additional discoveries need to be made to identify the unknown risk genes for AD. The three genes identified in early-onset AD explain only 50% of such cases, and the APOE gene likewise explains only 50% of the risk in late-onset AD cases. Compared to the deterministic nature of the mutations in the APP, PS-1, and PS-2 genes for early-onset AD, the relationship of the *APOE*4* allele (and yet to be discovered additional mutations) with late-onset AD is not as straightforward, because the late-onset form is much more complex. Like all other multifactorial diseases, where both genetic and environmental factors are involved in the etiology of the AD, it is envisioned that multiple genes, each with a small but cumulative effect, would explain the genetic basis for late-onset AD.

ACKNOWLEDGMENTS

This work was supported by NIH grants AG13672 and AG05133. The excellent clerical assistance of Ms. Noel Eisel is greatly appreciated.

REFERENCES

1. DA Evans, HH Funkenstein, MS Albert, PA Scherr, NR Cook, MJ Chown, LE Hebert, CH Hennekens, JO Taylor. Prevalence of Alzheimer's disease in a community population of older persons: higher than previously reported. JAMA 262:2551–2556, 1989.
2. J Leon, CK Cheng, PJ Neumann. Alzheimer's disease care: costs and potential savings. Health Affairs 17:206–216, 1998.
3. R Brookmeyer, S Gray, C Kawas. Projections of Alzheimer's disease in the United States and the public impact of delaying disease onset. Am J Public Health 88:1337–1342, 1998.
4. National Institute on Aging. Progress Report on Alzheimer's Disease. Silver Spring, MD: National Institutes of Health, 1999.
5. AM Goate, M-C Chartier-Harlin, MC Mullan, J Brown, F Crawford, L Fidani, L Giuffra, A Haynes, N Irving, L James, R Mant, P Newton, K

Rooke, P Roques, C Talbot, M Pericak-Vance, A Roses, R Williamson, MR Rosser, MJ Owen, J Hardy. Segregation of a missense mutation in the amyloid precursor protein gene with familial Alzheimer's disease. Nature 349:704–706, 1991.

6. R Sherrington, EI Rogaev, Y Liang, EA Rogaeva, G Levesque, M Ikeda, H Chi, C Lin, G Li, K Holman, T Tsuda, L Mar, J-F Foncin, AC Bruni, MP Montesi, S Sorbi, I Rainero, L Pinessi, L Nee, I Chumakov, D Pollen, A Brookes, P Sanseau, RJ Polinsky, W Wasco, HAR Da Silva, JL Haines, MA Pericak-Vance, RE Tanzi, AD Roses, PE Fraser, JM Rommens, PH St George-Hyslop. Cloning of a gene bearing missense mutations in early-onset familial Alzheimer's disease. Nature 375:754–760, 1995.

7. E Levy-Lahad, W Wasco, P Poorkaj, DM Romano, J Oshima, WH Pettingell, CE Yu, PD Jondro, SD Schmidt, K Wang, AC Crowley, F Ying-Hui, SY Guenette, D Galas, E Nemens, EM Wijsman, TD Bird, GD Schellenberg, RE Tanzi. Candidate gene for the chromosome 1 familial Alzheimer's disease locus. Science 269:973–977, 1995.

8. EI Rogaeva, R Sherrington, EA Rogaeva, G Levesque, M Ikeda, Y Liang, H Chi, C Lin, K Holman, T Tsuda, YT Mar, L Sorbi, S NacMias, S Piacentini, L Amaducci, I Chumakov, D Cohen, L Lannfelt, PE Fraser, JM Rommens, PH St George-Hyslop. Familial Alzheimer's disease in kindreds with missense mutations in a gene on chromosome 1 related to the Alzheimer's disease type 3 gene. Nature 376:775–778, 1995.

9. HG Lemaire, JM Salbaum, G Multhaup, J Kang RM Bayney, A Unterbeck, K Beyreuther, B Muller-Hill. The preA4 695 precursor protein of Alzheimer's disease A4 amyloid is encoded by 16 exons. Nucl Acids Res 17:517–522, 1989.

10. SS Sisodia, EH Koo, K Beyreuther, A Unterbeck, DL Price. Evidence that β-amyloid protein in Alzheimer's disease is not derived by normal processing. Science 248:492–495, 1990.

11. M Shoji, TE Golde, J Ghiso, TT Cheung, S Estus, LM Shaffer, X-D Cai, DM McKay, R Tinter, B Frangione, SG Younkin. Production of the Alzheimer amyloid β protein by normal proteolytic processing. Science 258:126–129, 1992.

12. R Vassar, BD Bennett, S Babu-Khan, S Kahn, EA Mendiaz, P Denis, DB Teplow, S Ross, P Amarante, R Loeloff, Y Luo, S Fisher, J Fuller, S Edenson, J Lile, MA Jarosinski, AL Biere, E Curran, T Burgess, J-C Louis, F Collins, J Treanor, G Rogers, M Citron. Beta-secretase cleavage of Alzheimer's amyloid precursor protein by the transmembrane aspartic protease BACE. Science 286:735–741, 1999.

13. PH St George-Hyslop. Molecular genetics of Alzheimer's disease. Biol Psychiatry 47:183–199, 2000.

14. DJ Selkoe. Amyloid β-protein and the genetics of Alzheimer's disease. J Biol Chem 271:18295–18298, 1996.

15. M Hutton, J Hardy. The presenilins and Alzheimer's disease. Hum Mol Genet 6:1639–1646, 1997.

16. C Haass, B De Strooper. The presenilins in Alzheimer's disease—proteolysis holds the key. Science 286:916–919, 1999.

17. B De Strooper, P Saftig, K Craessaerts, H Vanderstichele, G Guhde, W Annaert, K von Figura, F van Leuven. Deficiency of presenilin-1 inhibits the normal cleavage of amyloid precursor protein. Nature 391:387–390, 1998.

18. A Tandon, E Rogaeva, M Mullan, PH St George-Hyslop. Molecular genetics of Alzheimer's disease: the role of β-amyloid and the presenilins. Curr Opin Neurol 13:377–384, 2000.

19. M Cruts, CM van Duijn, H Backhovens, M van den Broeck, A Wehnert, S Serneels, R Sherrington, M Hutton, J Hardy, PH St. George-Hyslop, A Hofman, C van Broeckhoven. Estimation of the genetic contribution of presenilin-1 and -2 mutations in a population-based study of presenile Alzheimer's disease. Hum Mol Genet 7:43–51, 1998.

20. E Levy-Lahad, D Tsuang, TD Bird. Recent advances in the genetics of Alzheimer's disease. J Geriatr Psychiatry Neurol 11:42–54, 1998.

21. MA Pericak-Vance, JL Bebout, PC Gaskell Jr, LA Yamaoka, WY Hung, MJ Alberts, AP Walker, RJ Bartlett, CA Haynes, KA Welsh, NL Earl, A Heyman, CM Clark, AD Roses. Linkage studies in familial Alzheimer's disease: evidence of chromosome 19 linkage. Am J Hum Genet 48:1034–1050, 1991.

22. MA Pericak-Vance, MP Bass, LH Yamaoka, PC Gaskell, WK Scott, HA Terwedow, MM Menold, PM Conneally, GW Small, JM Vance, AM Saunders, AD Roses, JL Haines. Complete genomic screen in late-onset familial Alzheimer disease. Evidence for a new locus on chromosome 12. JAMA 278:1237–1241, 1997.

23. E Rogaeva, S Prekumar, Y Song, S Sorbi, N Brindle, A Paterson, R Duara, G Levesque, G Yu, M Nishimura, M Ikeda, C O'Toole, T Kawarai, R Jorge, D Vilarino, AC Bruni, LA Farrer, PH St George-Hyslop. Evidence for an Alzheimer's disease susceptibility locus on chromosome 12 and for further locus heterogeneity. JAMA 280:614–618, 1998.

24. WS Wu, P Holmans, W Wavrant-DeVrièze, S Shears, P Kehoe, R Crook, J Booth, N Williams, J Pérez-Tur, K Roehl, I Fenton, M-C Chartier-Harlin, S Lovestone, J Williams, M Hutton, J Hardy, MJ Owen, A Goate. Genetic studies on chromosome 12 in late-onset Alzheimer's disease. JAMA 280:619–622, 1998.

25. P Kehoe, F Wavrant-DeVrièze, R Crook, WS Wu, P Holmans, I Fenton, G Spurlock, N Norton, H

Williams, N Williams, S Lovestone, J Pérez-Tur, M Hulton, M-C Chartier-Harlin, S Shears, K Roehl, J Booth, WV Voorst, D Ramic, J Williams, A Goate, J Hardy, MJ Owen. A full genome scan for late-onset Alzheimer's disease. Hum Mol Genet 8:237–245, 1999.

26. L Bertram, D Blacker, K Mullin, D Keeney, J Jones, S Basu, S Yhu, MG McInnis, RCP Go, K Vekrellis, D Selkoe, AJ Saunders, RE Tanzi. Evidence for genetic linkage of Alzheimer's disease to chromosome 10q. Science 290:2302–2303, 2000.

27. A Myers, P Holmans, H Marshall, J Kwon, D Meyer, D Ramic, S Shears, J Booth, F Wavrant-DeVrièze, R Crook, M Hamshere, R Abraham, N Turnstall, F Rice, S Carty, S Lillystone, P Kehoe, V Rudrasingham, L Jones, S Lovestone, J Pérez-Tur, J Williams, MJ Owen, J Hardy, AM Goate. Susceptibility locus for Alzheimer's disease on chromosome 10. Science 290:2304–2305, 2000.

28. MA Pericak-Vance, J Grubber, LR Bailey, D Hedges, S West, L Santoro, B Kemmerer, JL Hall, AM Saunders, AD Roses, GW Small, WK Scott, PM Conneally, JM Vance, JL Haines. Identification of novel genes in late-onset Alzheimer's disease. Exp Gerontol 35:1343–1352, 2000.

29. JAR Nicoll, RE Mrak, DI Graham, J Stewart, G Wilcock, S MacGowan, MM Esiri, LS Murray, D Dewar, S Love, T Moss, WST Griffin. Association of interleukin-1 gene polymorphisms with Alzheimer's disease. Ann Neurol 47:365–368, 2000.

30. LME Grimaldi, VM Casadei, C Ferri, F Veglia, F Licastro, G Annoni, I Biunno, G De Bellis, S Sorbi, C Mariani, N Canal, WST Griffin, M Franceshi. Association of early-onset Alzheimer's disease with an interleukin-1α gene polymorphism. Ann Neurol 47:361–365, 2000.

31. DJ Lehmann, C Johnston, AD Smith. Synergy between the genes for butyrylcholinesterase K variant and apolipoprotein E4 in late-onset confirmed Alzheimer's disease. Hum Mol Genet 6:1933–1936, 1997.

32. Y Xia, R da Silva, BL Rosi, LH Yamaoka, JB Rimmler, MA Pericak-Vance, AD Roses, X Chen, E Masliah, R DeTeresa, A Iwai, M Sundsmo, RG Thomas, CR Hofstetter, E Gregory, LA Hanson, R Katzman, LJ Thal, T Saitoh. Genetic studies in Alzheimer's disease with an NACP/alpha-synuclein polymorphism. Ann Neurol 40:207–215, 1996.

33. M Curran, D Middleton, J Edwardson, R Perry, I McKeith, C Morris, D Neill. HLA-DR antigens associated with major genetic risk for late-onset Alzheimer's disease. Neuroreport 8:1467–1469, 1997.

34. A Papassotiropoulos, M Bagli, F Jessen, TA Bayer, W Maier, ML Rao, R Heun. A genetic variation of the inflammatory cytokine interleukin-6 delays the initial onset and reduces the risk for sporadic Alzheimer's disease. Ann Neurol 45:666–668, 1999.

35. M Dahiyat, A Cumming, C Harrington, C Wischik, J Xuereb, F Corrigan, G Breen, D Shaw, D St Clair. Association between Alzheimer's disease and the NOS3 gene. Ann Neurol 46:664–667, 1999.

36. K Okuizumi, O Onodera, Y Namba, K Ikeda, T Yamamoto, K Seki, A Ueki, S Nanko, H Tanaka, H Takahashi, K Oyanagi, H Mizusawa, I Kanazawa, S Tsuji. Genetic association of the very low density lipoprotein (VLDLR) receptor gene with sporadic Alzheimer's disease. Nat Genet 11:207–209, 1995.

37. Q Hu, WA Kukull, SL Bressler, MD Gray, JA Cam, EB Larson, GM Martin, SS Deeb. The human FE65 gene: genomic structure and an intronic biallelic polymorphism associated with sporadic dementia of the Alzheimer type. Hum Genet. 103:295–303, 1998.

38. A Papassotiropoulos, M Bagli, O Feder, F Jessen, W Maier, ML Rao, M Ludwig, SG Schwab, R Heun. Genetic polymorphism of cathepsin D is strongly associated with the risk for developing sporadic Alzheimer's disease. Neurosci Lett 262:171–174, 1999.

39. D Blacker, MA Wilcox, NM Laird, L Rodes, SM Horvath, RC Go, R Perry, B Watson Jr, SS Bassett, MG McInnis, MS Albert, BT Hyman, RE Tanzi. Alpha-2-macroglobulin is genetically associated with Alzheimer disease. Nat Genet 19:357–360, 1998.

40. CL Lendon, CJ Talbot, NJ Craddock, SW Han, M Wragg, JC Morris, AM Goate. Genetic association studies between dementia of the Alzheimer's type and three receptors for apolipoprotein E in a Caucasian population. Neurosci Lett 222:187–190, 1997.

41. MI Kamboh, DK Sanghera, RE Ferrell, ST DeKosky. APOE*4-associated Alzheimer's disease risk is modified by α1-antichymotrypsin polymorphism. Nat Genet 10:486–488, 1995.

42. M Wragg, M Hutton, C Talbot. Genetic association between intronic polymorphism in presenilin-1 gene and late-onset Alzheimer's disease. Alzheimer's Disease Collaborative Group. Lancet 347:509–512, 1996.

43. PG Kehoe, C Russ, S McIlory, H Williams, P Holmans, C Holmes, D Liolitsa, D Vahidassr, J Powell, B McGleenon, M Liddell, R Plomin, K Dynan, N Williams, J Neal, NJ Cairns, G Wilcock, P Passmore, S Lovestone, J Williams, MJ Owen. Variation in DCP1, encoding ACE, is associated with susceptibility to Alzheimer's disease. Nat Genet 21:71–72, 1999.

44. WF Reynolds, J Rhees, D Maciejewski, T Paladino, H Sieburg, RA Maki, E Masliah. Myeloperoxidase

polymorphism is associated with gender specific risk for Alzheimer's disease. Exp Neurol 155:31–41, 1999.

45. MJ Bullido, J Aldudo, A Frank, F Coria, J Avila, F Valdivieso. A polymorphism in the tau gene associated with risk for Alzheimer's disease. Neurosci Lett 278:49–52, 2000.

46. WJ Strittmatter, AM Saunders, D Schmechel, PH St George-Hyslop, MA Pericak-Vance, J Enghild, GS Salvesen, AD Roses. Apolipoprotein E: high-avidity binding to β-amyloid and increased frequency of type 4 allele in late-onset familial Alzheimer's disease. Proc Natl Acad Sci USA 90:1977–1981, 1993.

47. FC Crawford, MJ Freeman, JA Schinka, LI Abdullah, M Gold, R Hartman, K Krivian, MD Morris, D Richards, R Duara, R Anaud, MJ Mullan. A polymorphism in the cystatin C gene is a novel risk factor for late-onset Alzheimer's disease. Neurology 55:763–768, 2000.

48. T Hutchin, G Cortopassi. A mitochondrial DNA clone is associated with increased risk for Alzheimer's disease. Proc Natl Acad Sci USA 92:6892–6895, 1995.

49. AM Saunders, WJ Strittmatter, D Schmechel, PH St George-Hyslop, MA Pericak-Vance, SH Joo, BL Rosi, JF Gusella, DR Crapper-MacLachlan, MJ Alberts, C Hulette, B Crain, D Goldberger, AD Roses. Association of apolipoprotein E allele ε4 with late-onset familial and sporadic Alzheimer's disease. Neurology 43:1467–1472, 1993.

50. MI Kamboh. Apolipoprotein E polymorphism and susceptibility to Alzheimer's disease. Hum Biol 67:195–215, 1995.

51. LA Farrer, LA Cupples, JL Haines, B Hyman, WA Kukull, R Mayeux, RH Myers, MA Pericak-Vance, N Risch, CM van Duijn. Effects of age, sex, and ethnicity on the association between apolipoprotein E genotype and Alzheimer disease. A meta-analysis. APOE and Alzheimer Disease Meta Analysis Consortium. JAMA 278:1349–1356, 1997.

52. DA Sanan, KH Weisgraber, ST Russell, RW Mahley, D Huang, A Saunders, D Schmechel, T Wisniewski, B Frangione, AD Roses, WJ Strittmatter. Apolipoprotein E associates with β-amyloid peptide of Alzheimer's disease form novel monofibrils. Isoform apoE4 associates more efficiently than apoE3. J Clin Invest 94:860–869, 1994.

53. J Ma, A Yee, HB Brewer Jr, S Das, H Potter. Amyloid-associated proteins α1-antichymotrypsin and apolipoprotein E promote assembly of Alzheimer β-protein into filaments. Nature 372:92–94, 1994.

54. T Wisniewski, EM Castano, A Golabek, T Vogel, B Frangione. Acceleration of Alzheimer's fibril formation by apolipoprotein E in vitro. Am J Pathol 145:1030–1035, 1994.

55. DE Schmechel, AM Saunders, WJ Strittmatter, BJ Crain, CM Hulette, SH Joo, MA Pericak-Vance, D Goldberg, AD Roses. Increased amyloid beta-peptide deposition in cerebral cortex as a consequence of apolipoprotein E genotype in late-onset Alzheimer's disease. Proc Natl Acad Sci USA 90:9649–9653, 1993.

56. GW Rebeck, JS Reiter, DK Strickland, B Thyman. Apolipoprotein E in sporadic Alzheimer's disease: allelic variation in receptor interactions. Neuron 11:575–580, 1993.

57. M Kounnas, R Moir, W Rebeck, A Bush, S Argraves, R Tanzi, B Hyman, D Strickland. LDL receptor related protein, a multifunctional apoE receptor, binds secreted β-amyloid precursor protein and mediates its degradation. Cell 82:331–340, 1995.

58. BP Nathan, S Bellosta, DA Sana, KH Weisgraber, RW Mahley, RE Pitas. Differential effects of apolipoproteins E3 and E4 on neuronal growth in vitro. Science 264:850–852, 1994.

59. BP Nathan, KC Chang, S Bellosta, E Brisch, G Nianfeng, RW Mahley, RE Pitas. The inhibitory effect of apolipoprotein E4 on neurite outgrowth is associated with microtubule depolymerization. J Biol Chem 270:19791–19799, 1995.

60. WJ Strittmatter, KH Weisgraber, M Goedert, AM Saunders, D Huang, EH Corder, LM Dong, R Jakes, MJ Alberts, JR Gilbert, SH Han, C Hulette, G Einstein, DE Schmechal, MA Pericak-Vance, AD Roses. Hypothesis: microtubule instability and paired helical filament formation in the Alzheimer's disease brain are related to apolipoprotein E genotype. Exp Neurol 125:163–171, 1994.

61. M Miyata, JD Smith. Apolipoprotein E allele-specific antioxidant activity and effects on cytoxicity by oxidative insults and β-amyloid peptides. Nat Genet 14:55–61, 1996.

62. E Masliah, M Mallory, N Ge, M Alford, I Veinbergs, AD Roses. Neurodegeneration in the central nervous system of apoE-deficient mice. Exp Neurol 136:107–122, 1995.

63. RW Mahley, Y Huang. Apolipoprotein E: from atherosclerosis to Alzheimer's disease and beyond. Curr Opin Lipidol 10:207–217, 1999.

64. J Raber, D Wong, M Buttini, M Orth, S Bellosta, RE Pitas, R Mahley, L Mucke. Isoform-specific effects of human apolipoprotein E on brain function revealed in apoE knockout mice: increased susceptibility of females. Proc Natl Acad Sci USA 95:10914–10919, 1998.

65. S Mui, M Briggs, H Chung, RB Wallace, T Gomez-Isla, GW Rebeck, BT Hyman. A newly identified polymorphism in the apolipoprotein E enhancer gene region is associated with Alzheimer's disease and strongly with the ε4 allele. Neurology 47:196–201, 1996.

66. MJ Artiga, MJ Bullido, I Sastre, M Recuero, MA Garcia, J Aldudo, J Vázquez, F Valdivieso. Allelic polymorphisms in the transcriptional regulatory region of apolipoprotein E gene. FEBS Lett 421:105–108, 1998.
67. J-C Lambert, C Berr, F Pasquier, A Delacourte, B Frigard, D Cottel, J Pérez-Tur, V Mouroux, M Mohr, D Cécyre, D Galasko, C Lendon, J Poirier, J Hardy, D Mann, P Amouyel, M-C Chartier-Harlin. Pronounced impact of Th1/E47cs mutation compared with −491 A/T mutation on neural APOE gene expression and risk of developing Alzheimer's disease. Hum Mol Genet 7:1511–1516, 1998.
68. MJ Bullido, MJ Artiga, M Recuero, I Sastre, MA García, J Aldudo, C Leridon, SW Han, JC Morris, A Frank, J Vázquez, A Goate, F Valdivieso. A polymorphism in the regulatory region of APOE associated with risk for Alzheimer's dementia. Nat Genet 18:69–71, 1998.
69. J-C Lambert, F Pasquier, D Cottel, B Frigard, P Amouyel, M-C Chartier-Harlin. A new polymorphism in the APOE promoter associated with risk of developing Alzheimer's disease. Hum Mol Genet 7:533–540, 1998.
70. G Roks, M Cruts, NJ Bullido, H Backhovens, MJ Artiga, A Hofman, F Valdivieso, F van Broeckhoven, CM van Duijn. The −491 A/T polymorphism in the regulatory region of the apolipoprotein E gene and early-onset Alzheimer's disease. Neurosci Lett 258:65–68, 1998.
71. T Town, D Paris, D Fallin, R Duarra, W Barker, M Gold, F Crawford, M Mullan. The −491 A/T apolipoprotein E promoter polymorphism association with Alzheimer's disease: independent risk and linkage disequilibrium with the known APOE polymorphism. Neurosci Lett 252:95–98, 1998.
72. ARH Ahmed, SH MacGowan, D Culpan, RW Jones, GK Wilcock. The −491 A/T polymorphism of the apolipoprotein E gene is associated with the apoE ε4 allele and Alzheimer's disease. Neurosci Lett 263:217–219, 1999.
73. Y-Q Song, E Rogaeva, S Premkumar, N Brindle, T Kawarai, AN Orlacchio, G Yu, G Levesque, M Nishimura, M Ikeda, Y Pei, C O'Toole, R Duara, W Barker, S Sorbi, M Freedman, L Farrer, P St George-Hyslop. Absence of association between Alzheimer disease and the −491 regulatory region polymorphism of APOE. Neurosci Lett 250:189–192, 1998.
74. H Toji, H Maruyama, K Sasaki, S Nakamura, H Kawakami. Apolipoprotein E promoter polymorphism and sporadic Alzheimer's disease in a Japanese population. Neurosci Lett 259:56–58, 1999.
75. MI Kamboh, CE Aston, J Perez-Tur, E Kohmen, RE Ferrell, J Hardy, ST DeKosky. A novel mutation in the apolipoprotein E gene (APOE*4 Pittsburgh) is associated with the risk of late-onset Alzheimer's disease. Neurosci Lett 263:129–132, 1999.
76. WK Scott, JM Grubber, PM Conneally, GW Small, CM Hulette, CK Rosenberg, AM Saunders, AD Roses, MA Pericak-Vance. Fine mapping of the chromosome 12 late-onset Alzheimer's disease locus. Potential genetic and phenotypic heterogeneity. Am J Hum Genet 66:922–932, 2000.
77. W Borth. Alpha-2-macroglobulin, a multifunctional binding protein with targeting characteristics. FASEB J 6:3345–3353, 1992.
78. S Strauss, J Bauer, U Ganter, U Jonas, M Berger, B Volk. Detection of interleukin-6 and alpha 2-macroglobulin immunoreactivity in cortex and hippocampus of Alzheimer's disease patients. Lab Invest 66:223–230, 1992.
79. GW Rebeck, SD Harr, DK Strickland, BT Hyman. Multiple, diverse senile plaque-associated proteins are ligands of an apolipoprotein E receptor, the alpha 2-macroglobulin receptor/low-density-lipoprotein receptor-related protein. Ann Neurol 37:211–217, 1995.
80. Y Du, KR Bales, RC Dodel, X Liu, MA Glinn, JW Horn, SP Little, SM Paul. Alpha-2-macroglobulin attenuates beta-amyloid peptide 1–40 fibril formation and associated neurotoxicity of cultured fetal rat cortical neurons. J Neurochem 70:1182–1188, 1998.
81. SR Hughes, O Khorkova, S Goyal, J Knaeblein, J Heroux, NG Riedel, S Sahasrabudhe. α2-Macroglobulin associates with beta-amyloid peptide and prevents fibril formation. Proc Natl Acad Sci USA 95:3275–3280, 1998.
82. U Beisiegel, W Weber, G Ihrke, J Herz, K Stanely. The LDL-receptor-related protein LRP, is an apolipoprotein E binding protein. Nature 341:162–164, 1989.
83. G Matthijs, P Marynen. A deletion polymorphism in the human alpha-2-macroglobulin (A2M) gene. Nucl Acids Res 19:5102, 1991.
84. W Poller, JP Faber, G Klobeck, K Olek. Cloning of the human alpha 2-macroglobulin gene and detection of mutations in two functional domains: the bait region and the thiolester site. Hum Genet 88:313–319, 1992.
85. A Liao, RM Nitsch, SM Greenberg, U Finckh, D Blacker, M Albert, GW Rebeck, T Gomez-Isla, A Clatworthy, G Binetti, C Hock, T Mueller-Thomsen, U Mann, K Zuchowski, U Beisiegel, H Staehelin, JH Growdon, RE Tanzi, BT Hyman. Genetic association of an α2-macroglobulin (Val1000Ile) polymorphism and Alzheimer's disease. Hum Mol Genet 7:1953–1956, 1998.
86. L Myllykangas, T Polvikoski, R Sulkava, A Verkkoniemi, R Crook, PJ Tienari, AK Pusa, L Niinisto, P O'Brien, K Kontula, J Hardy, M Haltia, J Perez-Tur. Genetic association of α2-macroglobulin

with Alzheimer's disease in a Finnish elderly population. Ann Neurol 46:382–390, 1999.

87. RC Dodel, Y Du, KR Bales, F Gao, B Eastwood, B Glazier, R Zimmer, B Cordell, A Hakek, R Evans, D Gallagher-Thompson, LW Thompson, JR Tinklenberg, A Pfefferbaum, EV Sullivan, J Yesavage, L Alstiel, T Gasser, MR Farlow, GM Murphy, SM Paul. Alpha-2-macroglobulin and the risk of Alzheimer's disease. Neurology 54:438–442, 2000.

88. 88.V Alvarez, R Alvarez, CH Lahoz, C Martinez, J Pena, LM Guisasola, J Salas-Puig, G Moris, D Uria, BB Menes, R Ribacoba, JA Vidal, JM Sanchez, E Coto. Association between an α2-macroglobulin DNA polymorphism and late-onset Alzheimer's disease. Biochem Biophys Res Commun 264:48–50, 1999.

89. L Chen, L Baum, HK Ng, LY Chan, I Sastre, MJ Artiga, F Valdivieso, MJ Bullido, HF Chiu, CP Pang. Apolipoprotein E promoter and α2-macroglobulin polymorphisms are not genetically associated with Chinese late onset Alzheimer's disease. Neurosci Lett 269:173–177, 1999.

90. DJ Dow, N Lindsey, NJ Cairns, C Brayne, D Robinson, FA Huppert, ES Paykel, J Xuereb, G Wilcock, JL Whittaker, DC Rubinsztein. α2-Macroglobulin polymorphism and Alzheimer disease risk in the UK. Nat Genet 22:16–17, 1999.

91. EA Rogaeva, S Premkumar, J Grubber, L Serneels, WK Scott, T Kawarai, Y Song, DL Hill, SM Abou-Donia, ER Martin, JJ Vance, G Yu, A Orlacchio, Y Pei, M Nishimura, A Supala, B Roberge, AM Saunders, AD Roses, D Schmechel, A Crane-Gatherum, S Sorbi, A Bruni, GW Small, MA Pericak-Vance. An α2-Macroglobulin insertion-deletion polymorphism in Alzheimer disease. Nat Genet 22:19–22, 1999.

92. V Rudrasingham, F Wavrant-DeVrieze, JC Lambert, S Chakraverty, P Kehoe, R Crook, P Amouyel, W Wu, F Rice, J Perez-Tur, B Frigard, JC Morris, S Carty, R Petersen, D Cottel, N Tunstall, P Holmans, S Lovestone, MC Chartier-Harlin, A Goate, J Hardy, MJ Owen, J Williams. α2-Macroglobulin gene and Alzheimer disease. Nat Genet 22:17–19, 1999.

93. AB Singleton, AM Gibson, IG McKeith, CA Ballard, RH Perry, PG Ince, JA Edwardson, CM Morris. α2-Macroglobulin polymorphisms in Alzheimer's disease and dementia with Lewy bodies. Neuroreport 10:1507–1510, 1999.

94. X Wang, EK Luedecking, RL Minster, M Ganguli, ST DeKosky, MI Kamboh. Lack of association between the α2-macroglobulin polymorphisms and Alzheimer's disease. Hum Genet 108:105–108, 2001.

95. F Crawford, T Town, M Freeman, J Schinka, M Gold, R Duara, M Mullan. The alpha-2 macroglobulin gene is not associated with Alzheimer's disease in a case-control sample. Neurosci Lett 270:133–136, 1999.

96. SN Romas, R Mayeux, D Rabinowitz, MX Tang, HR Zadroga, R Lantigua, M Medrano, B Tycko, JA Knowles. The deletion polymorphism and Val1000Ile in alpha-2 marcroglobulin and Alzheimer disease in Caribbean Hispanics. Neurosci Lett 279:133–136, 2000.

97. N Shibata, T Ohnuma, T Takahashi, E Ohtsuka, A Ueki, M Nagao, H Arai. No genetic association between alpha-2 macroglobulin I1000V polymorphism and Japanese sporadic Alzheimer's disease. Neurosci Lett 290:154–156, 2000.

98. F Wavrant-DeVrieze, V Rudrasingham, JC Lambert, S Chakraverty, P Kehoe, R Crook, P Amouyel, W Wu, P Holmans, F Rice, J Pérez-Tur, B Frigard, JC Morris, S Carty, D Cottel, N Tunstall, S Lovestone, RC Petersen, MC Chartier-Harlin, A Goate, MJ Owen, J Williams, J Hardy. No association between the alpha-2-macroglobulin I1000V polymorphism and Alzheimer's disease. Neurosci Lett 262:137–139, 1999.

99. MN Kostner, B Dermaut, M Cruts, JJ Houwing-Duistermaat, G Roks, J Tol, A Ott, A Hofman, G Munteanm, MMB Breteler, CM van Duijn, C van Broeckhoven. The α2-macroglobulin gene in AD. A population-based study and meta analysis. Neurology 55:678–684, 2000.

100. F Wavrant-DeVrieze, J Perez-Tur, J-C Lambert, B Frigard, F Pasquier, A Delacourte, P Amouyel, J Hardy, M-C Chartier-Harlin. Association between the low-density lipoprotein receptor–related protein (LRP) and Alzheimer's disease. Neurosci Lett 227:68–70, 1997.

101. J-C Lambert, M-C Chartier-Harlin, D Cottle, F Richard, E Neuman, D Guez, S Legrain, C Berr, P Amouyel, N Helbecque. Is the LDL receptor-related protein involved in Alzheimer's disease? Neurogenetics 2:109–113, 1999.

102. D Fallin, A Hundtz, T Town, AC Gauslett, R Duara, W Barker, F Crawford, N Mullan. No association between low-density lipoprotein receptor–related protein (LRP) gene and late-onset Alzheimer's disease in a community-based sample. Neurosci Lett 233:145–147, 1997.

103. MI Kamboh, RE Ferrell, ST DeKosky. Genetic association studies between Alzheimer's disease and two polymorphisms in the low-density lipoprotein receptor–related protein gene. Neurosci Lett 244:65–68, 1998.

104. DE Kang, T Saitoh, X Chen, Y Xia. Genetic association of the low-density lipoprotein receptor–related protein gene (LRP), an apolipoprotein E receptor, with late-onset Alzheimer's disease. Neurology 49:56–61, 1997.

105. U Beffert, C Arguin, J Poirier. The polymorphism in exon 3 of the low-density lipoprotein receptor–related protein gene is weakly associated with Alzheimer's disease. Neurosci Lett 259:29–32, 1999.
106. F Van Leuven, L Stas, E Thiry, B Nelissen, Y Miyake. Strategy to sequence the 89 exons of the human LRP1 gene coding for the lipoprotein receptor-related protein: identification of one expressed mutation among 48 polymorphisms. Genomics 52:138–144, 1998.
107. F Wavrant-DeVrièze, J-C Lambert, L Stas, R Crook, D Cottel, F Pasquier, B Frigard, M Lambrechts, E Thiry, P Amouyel, J Pérez-Tur, M-C Chartier-Harlin, J Hardy, F Van Leuven. Association between coding variability in the LRP gene and the risk of late-onset Alzheimer's disease. Hum Genet 104:432–434, 1999.
108. J-C Lambert, L Goumidi, F Wavrant-DeVrièze, B Frigard, JM Harris, A Cummings, J Coates, F Pasquier, D Cottel, M Gaillac, D St. Clar, DMA Mann, J Hardy, CL Lendon, P Amouyel, M-C Chartier-Harlin. The transcriptional factor *LBP-1c/CP2/LSF* gene on chromosome 12 is a genetic determinant of Alzheimer's disease. Hum Mol Genet 9:2275–2280, 2000.
109. Z Bing, SA Reddy, Y Ren, J Qin, WS Liao. Purification and characterization of the serum amyloid A3 enhancer factor. J Biol Chem 274:24649–24656, 1999.
110. N Zambrano, G Minopoli, P de Candia, T Russo. The Fe65 adaptor protein interacts through its PID1 domain with the transcription factor CP2/LSF/LBP1. J Biol Chem 273:20128–20133, 1998.
111. N Ertekin-Taner, N Graff-Radford, LH Youkin, C Eckman, M Baker, J Adamson, J Ronald, J Blangero, M Hutton, SG Youkin. Linkage of plasma $A\beta_{42}$ to a quantitative locus on chromosome 10 in late-onset Alzheimer's disease pedigrees. Science 290:2303–2304, 2000.
112. GS Zubenko, HB Hughes, JS Stiffler, MR Hurtt, BB Kaplan. A genome survey for novel Alzheimer's disease risk loci results at 10 cM resolution. Genomics 50:121–128, 1998.
113. GS Zubenko, HB Hughes III, JS Stiffler. Clinical and neurobiological correlates to D10S1423 genotype in Alzheimer's disease. Biol Psychiatry 46:740–749, 1999.
114. K Oka, K-W Tzung, M Sullivan, E Lindsay, A Baldini, L Chan. Human very-low-density lipoprotein receptor complementary DNA and deduced amino acid sequence and localization of its gene (VLDL-R) to chromosome band 9p24 by fluorescence in situ hybridization. Genomics 20:298–300, 1994.
115. J Sakai, A Hoshino, S Takahashi, Y Miura, H Ishii, H Suzuki, Y Kawarabayas, T Yamamoto. Structure, chromosome location, and expression of the human very-low-density lipoprotein receptor gene. J Biol Chem 269:2173–2182, 1994.
116. S Takahashi, K Oida, M Ookubo, J Suzuki, M Kohno, T Murase, T Yamamoto, T Nakai. Very-low density lipoprotein receptor binds apolipoprotein E 2/2 as well as apolipoprotein E 3/3. FEBS Lett 386:197–200, 1996.
117. T Arinami, K Takekoshi, H Yanagi, M Hamamoto, H Hamaguchi. The 5-repeat allele in the very-low-density lipoprotein receptor gene polymorphism is not increased in sporadic Alzheimer's disease in Japanese. Neurology 47:1349–1350.
118. ML Pritchard, AM Saunders, PC Gaskell, GW Small, PM Conneally, B Rosi, LH Yamaoka, AD Roses, JL Haines, Pericak-Vance MA. No association between very-low-density lipoprotein receptor (VLDL-R) and Alzheimer's disease in American Caucasians. Neurosci Lett 209:105–108, 1996.
119. K Okuizumi K, Onodera O, K Seki, H Tanaka, Y Namba, K Ikeda, AM Saunders, MA Pericak-Vance, AD Roses, S Tsuji. Lack of association of very low density lipoprotein receptor gene polymorphism with Caucasian Alzheimer's disease. Ann Neurol 40:251–254, 1996.
120. H Chung, CT Roberts, S Greenberg, GW Rebeck, R Christie, R Wallace, HJ Jacob, BT Hyman. Lack of association of trinucleotide repeat polymorphism in the very-low-density lipoprotein receptor gene with Alzheimer's disease. Ann Neurol 39:800–803, 1996.
121. D Fallin, AC Gauntlett, P Scibelli, X Cai, R Duara, M Gold, F Crawford, M Mullan. No association between the very-low-density lipoprotein receptor gene and late-onset Alzheimer's disease nor interaction with the apolipoprotein E gene in population-based and clinical samples. Genet Epidemiol 14:299–305, 1997.
122. L Chen, L Baum, HK Ng, YS Chan, YT Mak, J Woo, H Chiu, CP Pang. No association between very-low-density lipoprotein receptor (VLDL-R) and late-onset Alzheimer's disease in Hong Kong Chinese. Neurosci Lett 241:33–36, 1998.
123. G Chen, KS Chen, J Knox, J Inglis, A Bernard, SJ Martin, A Justice, L McConlogue, D Games, SB Freidman, RGM Morris. A learning deficit related to age and β-amyloid plaques in a mouse model of Alzheimer's disease. Nature 408:975–979, 2000.
124. C Janus, J Pearson, J McLaurin, PM Mathews, Y Jiang, SD Schmidt, MA Chishti, P Horne, D Heslin, J French, HTJ Mount, RA Nixon, M Mercken, C Bergeron, PE Fraser, PH St George-Hyslop, D Westaway. $A\beta$ Peptide immunization reduced behavioral impairment and plaques in a model of Alzheimer's disease. Nature 408:979–982, 2000.
125. D Morgan, DM Diamond, PE Gottschall, KE Uger, C Dickey, J Hardy, K Duff, P Jantzen, G DiCarlo, D Wilcock, K Conner, J Hatcher, C Hope, M Gordon, GM Arendash. $A\beta$ Peptide vaccination prevents memory loss in an animal model of Alzheimer's disease. Nature 408:982–985, 2000.

36

Neurobiology of Alzheimer's Disease

OSCAR L. LOPEZ and STEVEN T. DeKOSKY
Western Psychiatric Institute and Clinic, University of Pittsburgh School of Medicine, Pittsburgh, Pensylvannia, U.S.A.

STEVEN T. DeKOSKY
University of Pittsburgh School of Medicine, Pittsburgh, Pennsylvania, U.S.A.

I. INTRODUCTION

Alzheimer's disease (AD) is the most frequent form of dementia in the adult. The incidence and prevalence of AD rise with increasing age, especially over 65. The incidence of AD ranges from 1% to 4% per year, rising by half decade from its lowest levels between ages 65 and 70 to rates that may approach 4% per year over the age of 85 [1]. Although the prevalence of AD has been a subject of discussion [2], most of the studies have found that the incidence of AD doubles every 4.3 to 5.7 years of age [1]. In general, estimates range from 3% in individuals between the ages of 65 and 75 to 47% in those over the age of 85 [3]. Because the U.S. population of individuals age 65 or older will triple over the next 50 years, the incidence and prevalence of AD will increase, as well. Data are similar for other Western countries. Therefore, AD and related dementias will constitute a significant burden for physicians, public health planners, and society as a whole.

We have witnessed significant advances in the understanding of the pathophysiology of AD in the past several years. These have provided researchers with models that can test therapeutic strategies for the disease. In general, the deficits in AD can be divided into two general categories: those associated with neurotransmitter metabolism deficits, and those associated with structural loss of brain tissue. In this chapter we will present the fundamental pathobiology of the disorder.

II. SELECTIVE VULNERABILITY AND DISRUPTION OF NORMAL NEURAL CIRCUITRY

The cognitive manifestations of AD are secondary to a disruption of normal neural brain circuits. Specific memory circuits are among the earliest and most vulnerable structures to AD pathology [4–6]. Studies examining very early changes in the brains of patients with either early or incipient (presymptomatic) AD indicate that the earliest changes occur in layer II neurons on the entorhinal cortex (paralimbic structure) of the temporal lobe, and subsequently in the hippocampus itself (limbic structure) [7–9]. The hippocampus does not have direct connections with other cortical areas; its cortical inputs are originated in the entorhinal cortex. Therefore, all connections between the hippocampus and primary and multimodal association cortical areas are channeled through the entorhinal cortex. Similarly, the cortical information processed by the hippocampus (mainly from areas CA1, prosubiculum, and subiculum) is later channeled back to the entorhinal cortex, orbitofronatal cortex, cygulate gyrus, retrospennial cortex, amygdala, and mammillary bodies. The hippocampus has also afferent and efferent connections with the hypothalamus. The initial damage of AD pathology to the entorhinal cortex deprives the hippocampus of cortical input, and damage to CA1 and subiculum affects hippocampal outflow [10,11].

In its progressive stages, AD pathology is densely concentrated in limbic and paralimbic areas, followed by multimodal association areas, with a relative preservation of primary motor and sensory cortices, cerebellum, and many parts of brainstem [7,12,13]. The distribution of AD pathology is associated with decreased dendritic extent, and synapse and neuronal loss [14,15]. This leads to a disconnection of multiple association areas, which reflects the global cognitive impairment that AD patients develop during their illness. Interestingly, in some cases, the initial clinical manifestations of AD start with cognitive symptoms ascribed to the occipital-parietal regions [16] or to the prefrontal cortex [17]. The factors that precipitate the onset of AD pathology in regions other than in the medial temporal lobe are unknown, but may follow circuitry or connectivity of limbic and association cortices.

III. STRUCTURAL ABNORMALITIES

The neuropathological diagnostic hallmarks of AD are the presence of senile (neuritic) plaques (NP), neurofibrillary tangles (NFT), synapse loss, and neuronal cell loss. Large neurons are more affected than small ones. The brains of AD patients can also have other lesions, such as granulovacuolar degeneration, Hirano bodies, and Lewy bodies [18] (Table 1).

A. Amyloid Metabolism

NP localized in the neuropil are composed of deposits of β amyloid (Aβ), which appears to be the major contributor to AD pathology [19]. There are several types of NP, and it is thought that they represent maturational stages of a single pathological process. The gradual deposition of Aβ first constitutes a diffuse plaque, and later the amyloid transforms into fibrils. The "mature" NP is formed by Aβ and dystrophic neurites, which may represent neuronal tissue damaged by the deposition of Aβ (Fig. 1) and the subsequent inflammatory reaction that occurs. Amyloid deposits are also observed in the walls of cerebral blood vessels of all AD patients. The severity of this vascular process ranges from minimal amounts of amyloid to massive deposits that can obliterate the architecture of the vessels (cerebral amyloid angiopathy) [20].

Because accumulation of β amyloid in the brain has been considered the central pathological event in AD, there have been considerable efforts to understand both the normal and abnormal metabolism of amyloid in the human brain. The amyloid precursor protein (APP) is a transmembrane s protein, with a short carboxyl tail in the intracellular space, an intramembranous section, and a substantial extracellular portion. In the normal amyloid metabolism, an enzyme cuts the extracellular portion of the molecule at a site close to the membrane surface, producing a long protein, composed of a long, entirely extracellular portion of the molecule. This compound is known as soluble APP alpha. Because this molecule is extracellular, it is "secreted" to the extracellular space when it is cut. The enzyme that performs this action has not been definitely identified but is termed the alpha secretase since it results in secretion of APP alpha (Fig. 2).

Table 1 Structural Changes in Alzheimer's disease Brain

Areas of neuronal loss	Structural lesions	
	Specific	Nonspecific
Large cortical neurons	Neuritic plaques	Hirano bodies
Amygdala	Neurofibrillary tangles	Granulovacuolar degeneration
Hippocampus	Amyloid deposition	Lewy bodies
Entorhinal cortex	Inflammation	
Basal forebrain cholinergic nuclei	Neuropil threads	
Locus ceruleus		
Dorsal raphe nuclei		

Neurobiology of Alzheimer's Disease

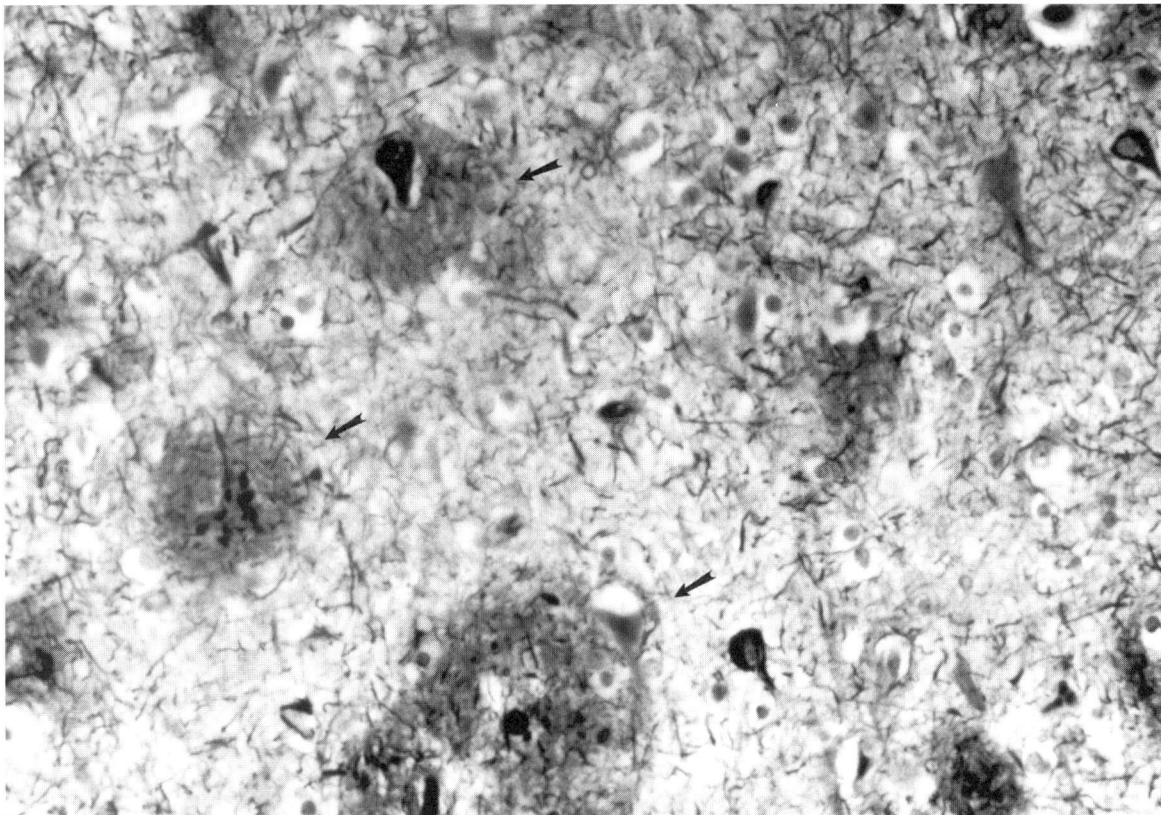

Figure 1 Arrows show "mature" neuritic plaques in the hippocampus of a patient with Alzheimer's disease.

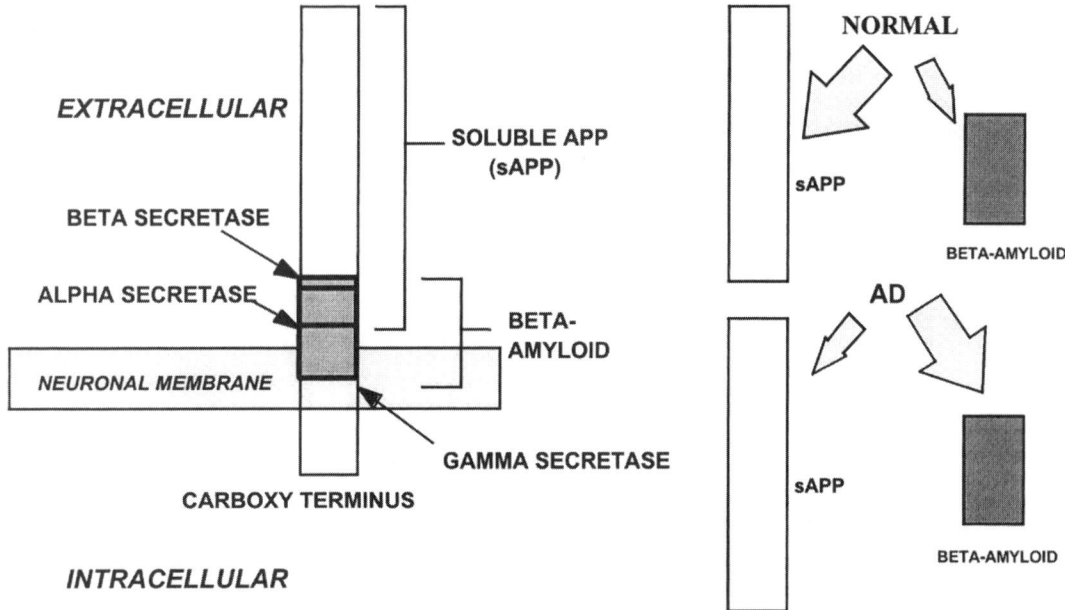

Figure 2 Metabolism of amyloid precursor protein (APP). Normal metabolism results in alpha-secretase cutting the APP full-length molecule at a site just above the surface of the neuronal membrane, resulting in a long extracellular molecule called soluble APP. In Alzheimer's disease two other enzymes, beta-secretase and gamma-secretase, severe the molecule at different sites, resulting in the beta-amyloid fragment that is deposited in amyloid plaques in Alzheimer's disease. Beta-secretase is a newly discovered enzyme. Gamma-secretase appears to either be or be closely associated with the membrane protein presenilin 1, which when mutated causes autosomal-dominant Alzheimer's disease (Adaped from DeKosky ST; American Academy of Neurology.)

The normal APP metabolism is considered non-amyloidogenic because the clevage impedes the formation of AB peptides. The other pathways involve the formation of large amounts of a molecular fragment termed the β fragment (Aβ), in either a 1-40 or 1-42 amino acid length, which are deposited in specific cerebral regions. Aβ consists of a portion of the APP molecule which begins at a location which is normally within the transmembrane portion of the molecule and ends at an extracellular site distal to the α secretase site. Normal processing of the APP molecule by the α secretase would make it impossible to generate any of the "beta fragments" which accumulate in AD. The secretase which makes the more distal cut in the APP molecule to produce Aβ is called the β secretase [19], and the one that makes the cut in the putative intramembranous portion is termed gamma secretase [19]. The β secretase, was initially identified in 1999 [21,22], it is a membrane-bound aspartyl protease. Selkoe [23] has suggested that gamma secretase, which is still unidentified, is presenilin 1 (PS1), and when mutated can produce increase amounts of Aβ, and consequently AD.

The major change in AD is a shift to the production of β fragments, and perhaps sAPP metabolism. The initial deposition in AD appears to be the 1-42 polypeptide length fragment. By contrast, deposition of the 1-40 amino acid fragment appears to be more associated with the NP, and with the inflammatory reaction [24–26].

B. Inflammatory Reaction and Amyloid Deposition

One of the most interesting observations in AD pathology has been the possible role that inflammatory processes play in the formation of the NP. Activated microglia often surround NP, especially in the limbic and paralimbic areas, but not in less vulnerable areas, such as the primary sensory motor cortex, cerebellum, and brainstem. It is believed that amyloid proteins can initiate the inflammatory response around the NP through different mechanisms: (1) via activation of the RAGE receptor; (2) via activation of the CD40 receptor; or (3) via perioxisome proliferator-activated receptor gamma [27–29].

Inflammatory markers have also been observed in the NP, such as α-1-antichymotrypsin, and α-2-macroglobulin, and interleukins, which are found in the activated microglia [30–32]. This inflammatory process contributes to neuronal death through the formation of free radicals, oxidative stress, and altering the calcium homeostasis.

C. Neurofibrillary Tangles

NFT appear to form early in the course of disease in the perirhinal and entorhinal regions, and from there, they spread throughout the mesial temporal lobe and then up into the neocortex [7,33,34] (Fig. 3). NFT can also be seen in normal aging, and up to 80% of normal elderly will develop some neurofibrillary tangles in the entorhinal cortical regions by their ninth decade [18]. However, in patients with AD, there is widespread NP formation associated with the NFT, even in the early stages. Some authors have suggested that deposits of NP would accelerate the formation of NFT [33], and recent data from studies conducted in double mutant mice (tau/APP) suggest that NP, or the presence of Aβ, can influence the formation of NFT [35].

The initiating event for formation of NFT is not completely understood. NFT are intracellular deposits of cytoskeletal elements in the cytoplasm, and are formed of paired helical filaments. There are protein changes in the filament structures in neurons that form a "pre-NFT" condition, which can be detected with immunocytochemical staining of neurons in the regions that are predisposed to developing NFT [36]. The major component of the NFT is abnormally phosphorylated tau proteins. These microtubule-associated proteins can also be present in the neuropil threads, and represent a neurodegenerative process. NFT alters the intraneuronal transport of cellular components, by displacing intracytoplasmic elements, disrupting exodendritic transport, and eventually leading to neuronal death [37,38] (Fig. 3). However, it is important to note that NFT are also observed in other neurodegenerative diseases (e.g., progressive supranuclear palsy, corticobasal degeneration, frontotemporal dementia) [39]. In addition, mutations in the tau protein gene are not associated with AD, but with frontotemporal lobe dementia or progressive supranuclear palsy [40,41]. In these disorders, the deposition of cellular NFT may be in a different neuronal distribution than AD, accounting for the different phenotypes.

D. Synapse Loss

Synaptic integrity is essential for maintaining intellectual functions. There is still debate about the extent of age-related synapse loss, but this is not thought to sig-

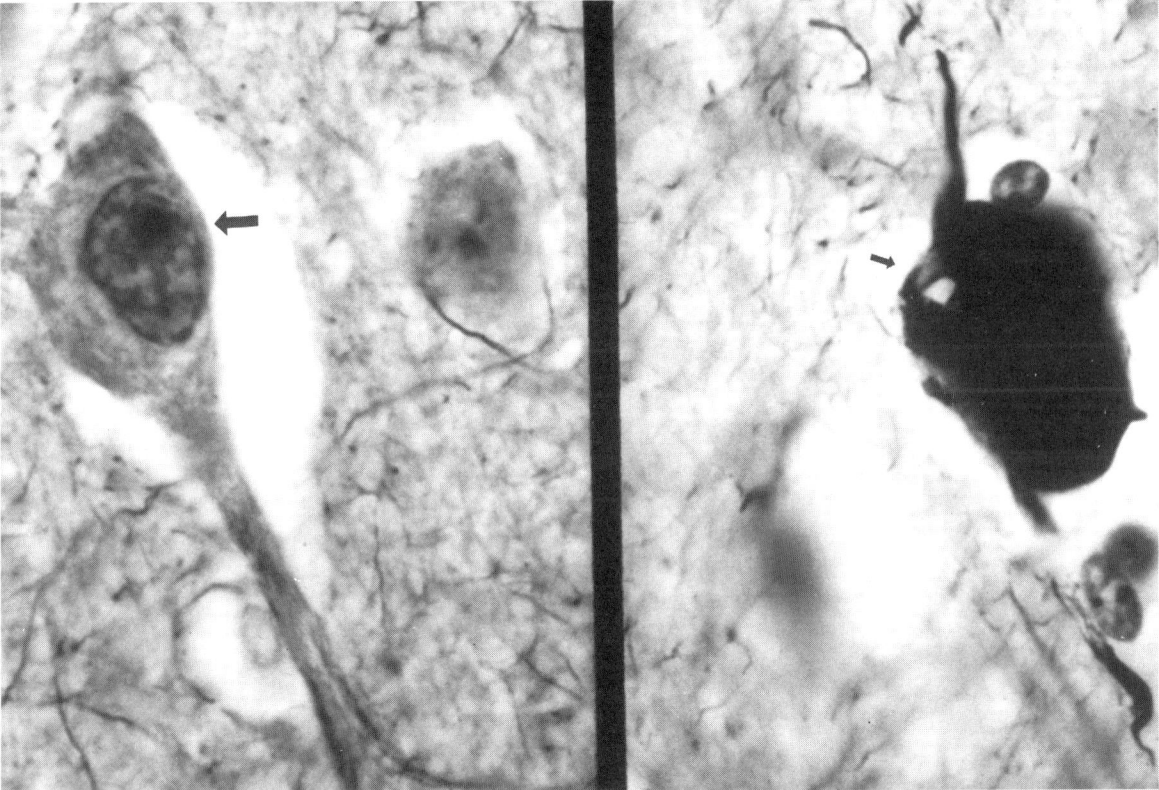

Figure 3 The large arrow (left) shows a normal neuron and the small arrow (right) shows neurofibrillary tangles.

nificantly affect cortical-cortical connectivity [42]. However, synapse loss is significant in the regions of the brain affected by the pathology of AD [14,43,44], and it is the strongest structural correlate of dementia severity as shown in cortical biopsy samples [43]. Quantitation of synaptic proteins such as the vesicular protein synaptophysin also correlates with severity of dementia [45]. The pathological mechanisms that lead to synapse damage and disappearance are not well understood. It is possible that synaptic loss is caused by neuronal death, the dying back of axonal arbors as cytoskeletal aberrations disrupt axonal flow, or direct toxicity to the synaptic bouton by endogenous neurotoxins.

E. Neuropil Threads

The significance of the neuropil threads and dystrophic neurites is not clear. It has been suggested that they represent aberrant sprouting neurites secondary to a neurodegenerative process [46]. The number of neuropil threads increases with the number of NFT, and inmunohistochemical studies have shown antitau and antiubiquitin reactivity [47].

F. Hirano Bodies

Hirano bodies are not specific to AD, and can be found in normal aging and in several neurodegenerative disorders. Indeed, they were first described in the Guam-Parkinson-dementia complex [48]. Electron microscopy studies showed that they are formed by longitudinal or crossed rows of filaments [49,50]. It appears that the Hirano bodies represent less specific protein components of the neurofilaments, while the NFT represent neuronal microtubular proteins.

G. Granulovacuolar Degeneration

As with Hirano bodies, granulovacuolar degeneration can be present in normal aging as well as in other neurorodegenerative disorders [51]. They are localized in the cytoplasm of hippocampal pyramidal cells [52], and inmunohistological reactivity studies have revealed microtubular neurofilaments in these structures [53]. Their significance remains unclear.

H. Lewy Bodies

Lewy bodies (LB) are intracytoplasmatic neuronal inclusions, and are formed by altered neurofilaments, microtubular, and paired helical filament epitopes, suggesting a disrupted neurofilament metabolism or transportation. It is believed that early studies underreported the presence of LB in dementia syndromes because of the difficulty of detecting LB with routine H&E staining. New techniques using antiubiquitin antibodies or alpha-synuclein antibodies have brought to light the importance and frequency of these lesions in dementia. Alpha-synuclein, a component of the Lewy body, is a protein that can be found at axon terminals or synapses. A dementia syndrome has been described associated with the presence of brainstem, diencephalic, and cortical LB [54–56]. Clinically, the most common symptomatology associated with this dementia with LB (DLB) is the presence of fluctuating cognition with pronounced variations in alertness, visual hallucinations, and extrapyramidal signs [57]. However, most cases with DLB have concomitant AD pathology, and those with pure DLB, without NP and NFT, are less frequent [58]. Neuropathological series have found that up to 60% of the patients with AD can have LB in the amygdala, and 50% in the neocortex and brainstem [59].

IV. PATHOLOGICAL DIAGNOSIS OF ALZHEIMER'S DISEASE

Because AD is a clinicopathological syndrome, there has been a significant debate over the years to define how many NFT and NP are necessary to confirm the diagnosis of AD. The first quantitative guidelines for the neuropathological diagnosis of AD were proposed by the National Institute on Aging in 1985 [60]. These criteria were based on the count of NP/mm^3. For patients age 50–65, it was required the presence of at least $8 NP/mm^3$; for patients age 66–75, $10 NP/mm^3$; and for patients age 75 or older, $16 NP/mm^3$. These criteria were criticized because they were based solely on the neuropathological characteristics of the patients and did not take into account the presence of dementia. Therefore, nondemented individuals with high NP counts could be neuropathologically diagnosed as having AD—high sensitivity with low specificity.

In 1991, the Consortium to Establish a Registry for Alzheimer's Disease (CERAD) proposed a semiquantitative assessment of NP according to the age of the patient, and took into account the presence of clinical dementia [61]. These criteria did not consider the presence of NFT essential for the diagnosis of AD, although they provided guidelines for the NFT severity grading and classification. The CERAD neuropathological criteria classify patients based on the level of clinicopathological certainty as possible, probable, and definite. Thus, a subject with no evidence of dementia during life, who had abundant NP and NFT at autopsy, could only have a possible AD diagnosis by the CERAD criteria.

In 1991, Braak and Braak proposed a neuropathological staging of AD based on the amyloid deposition and NFT [34]. However, these authors found that NP and amyloid deposition had great inter- and intrasubject variability, and had limited value for consistent neuropathological staging. By contrast, they found that the presence of NFT followed a specific hierarchical evolutionary pattern, starting in the entorhinal area and extending to other cortical areas. Therefore, Braak and Braak classified the distribution of NFT in six stages (I–VI), starting with the enthorinal stages (grade I–II), and extending to limbic (stages III–V) and neocortical (stages V–VI) stages [34]. Retrospective analyses have shown that subjects in stages III–IV had cognitive deficits, although there are not many strong studies correlating cognitive status with Braak and Braak staging. In 1997, the National Institute on Aging and the Nancy and Ronald Reagan Institute of the U.S. Alzheimer's Association suggested that the routine postmortem diagnosis of AD should be done using a combination of NP and NFT assessments. Therefore, the pathological diagnosis of AD should be based on the semiquantitative assessment of NP proposed by the CERAD and the Braak & Braak NFT staging [62]. Because of the significant variability of AD pathology, these guidelines recommended that the diagnosis of AD be based on the certainty of its presence as high, intermediate, and low.

V. THE SEARCH FOR BIOMARKERS

The definite diagnosis of AD is still done at autopsy. Many researchers have search for in vivo biomarkers that can confirm the clinical diagnosis before death, and even before symptom manifestation. Most of the studies searching for biomarkers have focused on the presence of different subproducts of the AD pathology in the cerebrospinal fluid (CSF), such as β amyloid (1-42) [63] tau proteins [64], and neural thread proteins (AD7C-NTP) [65]. The identification of proteins associated with AD metabolic processes may provide information about the presence and staging of the disease. It has been shown that there is a decreased CSF β amyloid level, possibly due to its accelerated deposition in the neuropil. There are increased levels of CSF tau and thread proteins, due to neuronal death, with subsequent release of microfilaments. Therefore, it was suggested that a combination of both, β amyloid and tau levels (low β amyloid with high tau levels) could increase the sensitivity and specificity for the diagnosis of AD [66]. CSF assessments of these two compounds are commercially available, and are based on probabilities; there is no clear-cut point for the markers or their ratio. Other proposed peripheral biomarkers include APP platelet isoforms [67] and urine AD7C-NTP levels [68]. Interestingly, high plasmatic levels of β amyloid have been identified in groups of AD patients, and these appear to be elevated before AD is clinically evident [69]. The clinical utility of this finding is not yet shown, since there is a wide variability.

VI. APOPTOSIS AND NEURONAL DEATH IN ALZHEIMER'S DISEASE

One of the end products of the cascade of neuropathology is programmed cell death, or apoptosis. There are now significant data suggesting that apoptosis occurs in AD brain, and amyloid deposits play a key role in this process [70,71]. The pathway to apoptosis is complex and multifactorial, and it appears to start at the level of synapses and dendites [72]. Lipton has suggested that there is a common final pathway in neurodegenerative disorders that leads to neuronal death [73]. Neurotoxic substances can elicit an overactivation of channels permeable to calciun ions, especially those operated by the N-methyl-D-aspartate receptor, which is a glutamate receptor that mediates excitatory neurotransmission. The overstimulation of this receptor results in an excessive influx of calcium, leading to neuronal death. This leads to increased release of glutamate, and the cycle continues, resulting in nonreversible neuronal damage. Others have suggested that altered, or the loss of, calcium-binding proteins, calbindin-D28k, can increase the intracellular calcium leading to neuronal death [74]. Indeed, experimental studies have shown that calbindin-D28k can "protect" neurons from amyloid toxicity [75].

VII. NEUROTRANSMITTER ABNORMALITIES

A. Acetylcholine

The first neurotransmitter defect discovered in AD was that of acetylcholine (ACh) [76]. Because cholinergic function is required for short-term memory function, it was initially felt that the cholinergic deficit in AD was responsible for much of the short-term memory deficit in the disease. Cholinergic neurons are localized in the basal forebrain, and they have been divided into groups based on their location and target areas. The hippocampal area receives cholinergic afferents from the neurons of the medial septum (cholinergic group 1 [Ch1]) and from the vertical limb of diagonal band of Broca (Ch2). The olfactory bulb receives afferents from Ch3 neurons, and the neocortex and amygdala from the nucleus basalis of Meynert (Ch4) neurons [77]. The highest density of cholinergic innervation can be found in the limbic areas (hippocampus and amygdala) and paralimbic areas, followed by unimodal and multimodal association areas. The primary visual area receives the lowest density of cholinergic fibers.

In AD, there is a loss of many cholinergic neurons, especially those located in the nucleus basalis of Meynert [78], as well as a decrease of choline acetyl transferase activity (CHAT) [79–82]. CHAT is mainly located in presynaptic cholinergic axons of the human cortex. This led to the cholinergic hypothesis of AD, which suggested that the loss of cognitive function, especially memory, was caused by the loss of cholinergic input [83]. This hypothesis has served as the model for the development of current symptomatic medications for AD. The use of acetylcholinesterase inhibitors can prolong the half-life of ACh at the synapse.

More recently, evidence has emerged to indicate that significant losses in the cholinergic system do not occur as early in the course of disease as initially thought. The first studies of cholinergic enzymes and cells in AD brain were done in autopsy cases with severe, end-stage disease. New studies of individuals dying at earlier stages indicate that cholinergic neurons, especially those of the more anterior regions (Ch1 and Ch2), are spared until later in the disease [84], and levels of the enzyme ChAT were spared in the cortex and hippocampus in mild to moderate AD at autopsy [85–88], not descending to very low levels until the disease had reached severe clinical impairment. Thus, the early memory changes in AD may be related more to disruption of entorhinal pathways to the hippocampus rather than drastic loss of ChAT activity.

1. Cholinergic Receptors

ACh receptors have been divided in two types based on their phamacological properties: muscarinic and nicotinic. Muscarinic receptors are involved in the action of ACh in glands and smooth muscle, and are blocked by atropine. Nicotinic receptors stimulate postganglionic neurons, and are localized at the neuromuscular junction and between neurons. Both nicotinic and muscarinic receptors are found in large numbers in the CNS [89]. In AD, the number of brain muscarinic receptors (m1–m5) appear to remain stable [90,91], although in some cases a 20–30% reduction has been found [92,93]. This loss appeared to be at expenses of the m1 and m2 subtype, while the m3 and m4 subtypes remained stable [94]. However, some studies have found an abnormal coupling between muscarinic receptors and G proteins, suggesting an altered signal transduction after the receptor stimulation [95].

By contrast, nicotinic receptors, which are present on the presynaptic and postsynaptic side, appear to be diminished, and may decrease early in the disease [96]. Both neuroradiological and neuropathological studies have shown that the number of nicotinic receptors is reduced in AD patients [97]. Marutle and colleagues found that the number of nicotinic receptors was more accentuated in familial cases (−73% −89%) than in sporadic AD (−37% −57%) [98]. However, some studies have found the α4, but not the α3 or α7, nicotinic receptor subtypes were diminished in AD [99].

Interestingly, positron emission tomography (PET) studies have shown that long-term exposure to cholinesterase inhibitors (i.e., tacrine) can increase the number of nicotinic receptors in AD patients [100,101]. This was interpreted as a result of elevated acetyl cholinesterase gene expression. In addition, it was thought that cholinesterase inhibitors, the major therapy currently available for AD, might have a direct allosteric activation on these receptors, which results in increase ACh release [102]. Therefore, these medications may increase the amount of ACh at the synapse by hydrolysis inhibition and by presynaptic allosteric activation of the nicotinic receptor [103].

2. Relationship Between Structural Lesions and Cholinergic Innervation

Correlations between global cognitive state (i.e., overall severity of dementia) and brain structure changes have always indicated a stronger correlation with synapse number or cortical neuron number than with markers of cholinergic neurotransmission. For example, correlations of global cognitive measures (e.g., Mini-Mental State Examination) with cortical synapse counts yield a correlation of nearly 0.8, and a similar high correlation is obtained for counts of large neurons in the cortex. By contrast, correlations between cognitive measures and ChAT in general are much lower, on the order of 0.3 or 0.4 [14,44,104].

Whether neuronal loss in the basal forebrain (Ch4) and subsequent anterograde degeneration are the main cause of cortical deposits of NP in AD, or these cortical deposits initiate a retrograde degeneration, and eventually, neuronal loss in the basal forebrain is still unknown. Because some studies found a negative correlation between between ChAT activity and density of NP, it has been suggested that cortical NP are caused by degeneration of cholinergic neurons [105,106]. However, studies that examined the relationship between NP and cholinergic fibers found a low association, on the order of −0.4 to −0.5 [78]. By contrast, it appears to be a higher correlation between NFT and cholinergic fibers (0.52–0.79) [107,108]. Some studies have found a greater correlation between neuronal loss in the basal forebrain (Ch4) and NP [109] and NFT [110] in cortical related areas compared with other cortical unrelated areas. These possible interrelationships remain to be elucidated, and will require more studies on individuals who die at an earlier stage of the disease.

3. β Amyloid Proteins and Cholinergic Neurons

Experimental studies have suggested the β amyloid exerts a neurotoxic effect on neurons and can induce or unhance the formation of NFT [111]. Indeed, recent studies conducted in transgenic mice showed that APP can modulate NFT formation [35]. The soluble form of β amyloid, which is the one produced normally in the brain, can cause a reduced ACh synthesis under experimental conditions [111,112]. In addition, there are several lines of research that suggested that β amyloid can affect the cholinergic receptors. The brains of patients with the Swedish APP 670/671 mutation, which is localized in the chromosome 21, have a greater loss of nicotinic receptors than those with sporadic AD (see above).

B. Other Neurotransmitters

1. Serotonin

The dorsal raphe nuclei of the brainstem are the major source of serotonin (5-hydroxytryptamine [5HT]) in the brain, and they usually contain deposits of NFT in AD [113,114]. These patients also have neuronal loss in the dorsal raphe nuclei [115–117], loss of serotonergic terminals in the neocortex [118], and decreased concentrations of 5HT and of its major metabolite 5-hidroxyindol acetic acid (5HAA) in the brain, especially in the temporal lobes [119,120]. However, the neuronal loss is relatively small compared to that suffered by cholinergic neurons in the basal forebrain. Serotonergic system dysfunction has been associated with psychiatric symptomatology in AD (e.g., anxiety, depression, psychosis, sleep disturbances) [for review see 121].

2. Noradrenaline

The major source of CNS noradrenaline (NA) is the locus ceruleus (LC) in the the midbrain. As occurs with the dorsal raphe nuclei, the LC also has deposits of NFT in AD patients. However, the LC has a greater neuronal loss, in the range of 40–80% [115,122, 123–128]. The loss is greater in its anterodorsal aspects, which project to the cerebral cortex, than in the ventral area, which project to subcortical regions [124,125]. In addition, decreased levels of NA, and of its synthetic enzyme dopamine-β-hydroxilase have been found in the neocortex in the range of 10–30% [122–124]. The most important neurobehavioral symptom associated with NA dysfunction in AD is depression. Several neuropathological studies have shown that there is a loss of 50% or more of LC neurons of AD patients with depression [113,126–127].

3. Dopamine

There is little or no loss of pigmented neurons of the substantia nigra (SN) and ventral tegmental area (VTA), as well as little NFT accumulation in the SN of AD patients [115,129,130]. Levels of cortical dopamine (DA) and its metabolite homovallinic acid remain within the normal range in AD [131,132]. However, some studies have found that there is more pronounced neuronal loss in the regions of the VTA that project to the neocortex, and higher NFT in the neurons of the substantia nigra that project to the striatum [133]. The relationship between DA system change and DLB, alone or associated with AD, remains under study.

4. Glutamate

Abnormal glutamate activity, an exitatory neurotransmitter, and dysregulation of glutamate receptors can cause neuronal damage, and eventually neuronal death. Therefore, it was hypothesized that such mechanism can play a role in AD. Indeed, large pyramidal cells of the cortex and hippocampus utilize glutamate and have abundant glutamate receptors [134]. In addition, some studies have found altered cortical glutamate receptor structure [135,136], and glutamate depletion in the hippocampal perforant pathway zone [137] in AD patients. By contrast, other studies have not found abnormal glutamate receptors in AD [138]. There is no evidence of glutamate abnormality, other than the loss of the large neurons that use glutamate as a neurotransmitter.

5. Gamma-Aminobutyric Acid

Some studies have found decreased gamma-aminobutiric acid (GABA) levels [139], an inhibitory neurotransmitter, in the brain of AD patients, while others have not found changes compared to controls. There are no data indicating a relationship between cognitive deficits and GABA levels. The GABA neurons project from the striatum to the globus pallidus and from the olivary nucleus to the vestibular nucleus [140,141]. It has an important role in the modulation of other neurotransmitters, especially serotonin, and dopamine [141]. Therefore, it is possible that GAB-Aergic neurons play a role in the etiology of behavioral manifestations of AD rather than in its cognitive symptoms.

6. Peptides Neurotransmitters

A number of peptide neurotransmitters are reported altered in AD, such as corticotrophin-releasing factor (CRF), somatostatin, and neuropeptide Y [see 142 for review]. The loss of the small interneurons that utilize these neurotransmitters, or downregulation of their function in response to diminished neural activity, may account for such findings. The relationship between neuropeptides and clinical manifestation of AD is unknown. Negative correlation between neuropeptides and behavioral manifestations of AD have been reported [143,144].

VIII. PATHOLOGICAL CORRELATES OF MILD COGNITIVE IMPAIRMENT

The term mild cognitive impairment (MCI) defines a condition or state that can progress to AD [145]. The most-studied form of MCI is that of an isolated amnestic disorder, or difficulty with short-term memory. Case control studies in a number of Alzheimer's disease research centers have indicated an increased rate of clinical "conversion" of these cases to Alzheimer's disease, averaging ~ 15% of cases per year. This is in comparison to "conversion" rates from 1–3% or 4% per year (depending on age) of normal subjects to AD. Thus MCI appears to be a risk state for the development of AD [145,146]. However, it is important to note that even well-characterized MCI patients sometimes do not progress to AD, or they can improve over time [147]. Because most of the patients who come to autopsy are in late stages of AD, it has been difficult to identify the neuropathological characteristics associated with this syndrome, although studies are beginning to appear that helps define the neuropathological underpinnings.

Neuroradiological studies have found that MCI patients with small hippocampal size are at greater risk of developing AD [148], while others have found that these patients also have more widespread atrophy, involving the cyngulate gyrus, and the temporoparietal cortex [149]. Neuropathological studies have shown that MCI patients have NP and NFT widely distributed in the neocortex and limbic areas, while normal elderly subjects had NFT localized in the hippocampus and parahipocampal areas [33]. Neocortical inflammatory processes can also be seen in MCI patients [150]. This suggests that the neuropathological process associated with AD starts several years before the patients develop MCI.

Recent studies have found that MCI patients have normal levels of ChAT in a variety of brain regions, with NFT and NP in medial temporal areas [85,88,151]. This does not mean that the cholinergic function is normal, but does indicate that the structures of the cholinergic system are preserved further into the disease course than previously thought.

IX. CONCLUSIONS

We have made significant advances in understanding both the clinical manifestations and pathobiological underpinnings of AD. Over the past years we have been gradually understanding that AD pathology is not distributed randomly. It appears to have a characteristic pattern that affects mainly limbic and cortical–cortical connectivity, and the subcortical nuclei with dense connections with the neocortex. Loss of cholinergic innervation of the cerebral cortex is the central neurochemical event in AD. However, the mechanisms of specific vulnerability of the cholinergic system to AD pathology are unknown. In spite of the complexity of the neuropathological mechanisms involved in the etiology of AD, scientists are gradually finding clues for its treatment. The availability of cholinesterase inhibitors has been a major step forward in this respect. Nevertheless, after reviewing the magnitude of the changes that the brain suffers during the course of disease, we expect that their effects to be modest. New understanding of the pathology specific to AD, especially that of amyloid metabolism, offers significant hope that we can intervene in this neurodegenerative disorder. Given the epidemiological data that suggest an epidemic of AD over the next 30 years, our continued studies of the pathological changes and increased use of animal models to accelerate efforts at developing treatments will hopefully allow us to win the race.

ACKNOWLEDGMENTS

Prepared with support from Grants AG 05133, AG 14449 and AG 13672 from the National Institute of Aging. We thank Dr. Julio Martinez for the neuropathological figures.

REFERENCES

1. Jorm AF, Jolley D. The incidence of dementia: a meta-analysis. Neurology 1998;51(3):728–733.
2. Corrada M, Brookmeyer R, Kawas C. Sources of variability in prevalence rates of Alzheimer's disease. Int J Epidemiol 1998;24:1000–1005.
3. Evans DA, Funkenstein HH, Alberts MS. Prevalence of Alzheimer's disease in a community population of older persons: higher than previously reported. JAMA 1989;262(18):2551–2556.
4. Hyman BT, Van Hoesen GW, Kromer LJ, Damasio AR. Perforant pathway changes and the memory impairment of Alzheimer's disease. Ann Neurol 1986;20:472–481.
5. Hyman BT, Van Hoesen GW, Damasio AR. Alzheimer's disease: cell specific pathology isolates the hippocampal formation. Science 1984;225:1168–1170.
6. Hof PR, Morrison JH. The cellular basis of cortical disconnection in Alzheimer disease and related dementing conditions. In: Terry RD, Katzman R, Bick KL, Sisodia SS, eds. Alzheimer Disease, 2nd ed. Philadelphia: Lippincott Williams & Wilkins; 1999.

7. Delacourte A, David JP, Sergeant N, et al. The biochemical pathway of neurofibrillary degeneration in aging and Alzheimer's disease. Neurology 1999; 52:1158–1165.
8. Mann DM, Marcyniuk B, Yates PO, Neary D, Snowden JS. The progression of the pathological changes of Alzheimer's disease in frontal and temporal neocortex examined both at biopsy and at autopsy. Neuropathol Appl Neurobiol 1988; 14:177–195.
9. Price JL, Ko AI, Wade MJ, Tsou SK, McKeel DW, Morris JC. Neuron number in the entorhinal cortex and CAI in preclinical Alzheimer's disease. Arch Neurol 2001;58:1395–1402.
10. Van Hoesen GW, Mesulam MM, Haaxma R. Temporal cortical projections to the olfactory tubercle in the rh monkey. Brain Res 1976; 109(2):375–381.
11. Van Hoesen GW, Hyman BT. Hippocampal formation: anatomy and the patterns of patholog Alzheimer's disease. Brain Res 1990;83:445–457.
12. Pearson RCA, Esiri MM, Hiorns RW, Wilcock GK, Powell TPS. Anatomical correlates of the distribution of the pathological changes in the neocortex in Alzheimer's disease. Proc Nat Acad Sci. USA 1985;82:4531–4534.
13. Hof PR, Cox K, Morrison JH. Quantitative analysis of a vulnerable subset of pyramidal neurons in Alzheimer's Disease. I. Superior frontal and inferior temporal cortex. J Comp Neurol 1990;301:44–54.
14. Scheff SW, DeKosky ST, Price DA. Quantitative assessment of cortical synaptic density in Alzheimer's disease. Neurobiol Aging 1990;11:29–37.
15. Gomez-Isla T, Hollister R, West H, Mui S, Growdom JH, Petersen RC. Neuronal loss correlates with but exceeds neurofibrillary tangles in Alzheimer's disease. Ann Neurol 1997;41:17–24.
16. Hof PR, Archin N, Osmand AP, et al. Posterior cortical atrophy in Alzheimer's disease: analysis of a new case and re-evaluation of a historical report. Acta Neuropathol (Berl) 1993;86(3):215–223.
17. Johnson JK, Head E, Kim R, Starr A, Cotman CW. Clinical and pathological evidence for a frontal variant of Alzheimer disease. Arch Neurol 1999;56(10):1233–1239.
18. Terry RD, Masliah E, Hansen LA. The neuropathology of Alzheimer disease and the structural basis of its cognitive alterations. In: Terry RD, Katzman R, Bick KL, Sisodia SS, eds. Alzheimer Disease, 2nd ed. Philadelphia: Lippincott Williams & Wilkins; 1999:187–206.
19. Selkoe DJ. Alzheimer's disease: a central role for the amyloid. J Neuropathol Exp Neurol 1994;53:438–447.
20. Lopez OL, Claassen D. Cerebral amyloid angiopathy in Alzheimer's disease: clinicopathological correlations. Dementia 1991;2:285–290.
21. Yan R, Bienkowski MJ, Shuck ME, Miao H, Tory MC, Pauley AM. Membrane-anchored aspartyl protease with Alzheimer's disease beta-secretase activity. Nature 1999;402:533–537.
22. Vassar R, Bennet BD, Babu-Khan S, Kahn S, Mendiaz EA, Denis P. Beta-secretase cleavage of Alzheimer's amyloid precursor protein by the transmembrane aspartic protease BACE. Science 1999;286(5440):735–741.
23. Selkoe DJ. Alzheimer's disease: genotypes, pehotype, and treatments. Science 1997;275:630–631.
24. Mann DMA, Ivatsubo T, Cairns NJ, Lantis PL, Nochlin D, Sumi SM. Amyloid beta protein deposition in chromosome 14-linked Alzheimer disease: predominance of A eta 42(43). Ann Neurol 1996;40:149–156.
25. Iwatsubo T, Odaka A, Suzuki N, Mizusawa H, Nukina N, Ihara Y. Visualization of A-beta-42(43) and A-beta-40 in senile plaques with end specific A-beta monoclonals: evidence that an initially deposited species as A-beta-42(43). Neuron 1994;13:45–53.
26. Citron M, Diehl TS, Gordon G, Biere AL, Seubert P, Selkoe DJ. Evidence that the 42- and 40-amino acid forms of amyloid protein are generated from the beta-amyloid precursor protein by different protease activities. Proc Natl Acad Sci USA 1996;93:13170–13175.
27. Yan SD, Chen X, Fu J. RAGE and amyloid-8 peptide neurotoxicity in Alzheimer's disease. Nature 1996;382:685–691.
28. Rogers J, Luber-Narod J, Styren SD, Civin WH. Expression of immune system associated antigens by cells of the human central nervous system: relationship to the pathology of Alzheimer's disease. Neurobiol Aging 1988;9:339-349.
29. Tan J, Town T, Paris D, Mori T, Suo Z, Crawford F. Microglial activation resulting from CD40-CD40L interaction after beta-amyloid stimulation. Science 1999;286:2352–2355.
30. Mrak RE, Sheng JG, Griffin WST. Glial cytokines in Alzheimer's disease: review and pathogenic implications. Hum Pathol 1995;26:816–823.
31. McGeer PL, Rogers J, McGeer EG. Neuroimmune mechanisms in Alzheimer's disease patients. Alzheimer Dis Assoc Disord 1994;8:149–158.
32. Griffin WST, Stanley LC, Ling C, White L, Macleod V, Perrot LJ. Brain interleukin 1 and S-100 immunoreactivity are elevated in Down syndrome and Alzheimer's disease. Proc Natl Acad Sci USA 1989;86:7611–7615.
33. Price JL, Morris JC. Tangles and plaques in nondemented aging and "preclinical" Alzheimer's disease. Ann Neurol 1999;45(3):358–368.
34. Braak H, Braak E. Neuropathological staging of Alzheimer-related changes. Acta Neuropathol 1991;82:239–259.

35. Lewis J, Dickson DW, Lin WL, et al. Enhanced neurofibrillary degeneration in transgenic mice expressing mutant tau and APP. Science 2001;293(5534):1487–1491.
36. Ohtsubo K, Izumiyama N, Shimada H, Tachikawa T, Nakamua H. Three-dimensional structure of Alzheimer's neurofibrillary tangles of the aged human brain revealed by the quick-freeze, deep-etch and replica method. Neuropathology 1990;79:480–485.
37. Terry RD. The fine structure of neurofibrillary tangles in Alzheimer's disease. J Neuropathol Exp Neurol 1963;22:629–642.
38. Brion JP, Passrererio H, Nunez J. Immunological detectionof tau protein in neurofibrillary tangles of Alzheimer's disease. Arch Biol 1985;96:229–235.
39. Lee VM-L, Goedert M, Trojanowski JQ. Neurodegenerative tauopathies. Annu Rev Neurosci 2001;24:1121–1159.
40. Conrad C, Andreadis CC, Trojanowski JQ, Dickson DW, Kang D, Chen X. Genetic evidence for the involvement of tau in progressive supranuclear palsy. Ann Neurol 1997;41:277–281.
41. Spillantini MG, Bird TD, Ghetti B. Frontotemporal dementia and parkinsonism linked to chromosome 17: a new Group of tauopathies. Brain Pathol 1998;8:387–402.
42. Jahn R, Schiebler W, Quinent C, Greengard P. A 38,000 dalton membrane protein (p38) present in synaptic vesicles. Proc Natl Acad Sci USA 1985;82:4137–4141.
43. DeKosky ST, Scheff SW. Synapse loss in frontal cortex biopsies in Alzheimer's disease: correlations with cognitive severity. Ann Neurol 1990;27:457–464.
44. Zhan S, Beyreuther K, Schmitt H. Quantitative assessment of the synaptophysin immuno-reactivity of the cortical neuropil in various neurodegenerative disorders with dementia. Dementia 1993;4:66–74.
45. Masliah E, Terry RD, Alford M, DeTeresa R, Hansen LA. Cortical and subcortical patterns of synaptophysinlike immunoreactivity in Alzheimer's disease. Am J Pathol 1991;138:235–246.
46. Masliah E, Ellisman M, Carragher B. Three-dimensional analysis of the relationship between synaptic pathology and neuropil threads in Alzheimer's disease. J Neuropathol Exp Neurol 1992;51:404–414.
47. Perry G, Kawai M, Tabaton M. Neuropil threads of Alzheimer's disease show a marked alteration of the normal cytoskeleton. J Neurosci 1991;11:1748–1755.
48. Hirano A, Dembitzer HM, Kurland LT, Zimmerman HM. The fine structure of some intraganglionic alterations, neurofibrillary tangles, granulovacuolar bodies and rod-like structures as seen in Guam amyotrophic lateral sclerosis and parkinsonism-dementia complex. J Neuropathol Exp Neurol 1986;27:167–182.
49. Goldman JE. The association of actin with Hirano bodies. J Neuropathol Exp Neurol 1983;42:146–152.
50. Galloway PG, Perry G, Kosik KS, Gambetti P. Hirano bodies contain tau protein. Brain Res 1987;403:337–340.
51. Ball MJ, Lo P. Granulovacuolar degeneration in the aging brain and in dementia. J Neuropathol Exp Neurol 1977;36:474–487.
52. Price DL, Altschuler RJ, Struble RG, Casanova MF, Cork LC, Murphy DB. Sequestration of tubulin in neurons in Alzheimer's disease. Brain Res 1986;385:305–310.
53. Dickson DW, Ksiezak-Reding H, Davies P, Yen SH. A monoclonal antibody that recognizes a phosphorylated epitope in Alzheimer neurofibrillary tangles, neurofilaments, and tau proteins immunostains granulo-vacuolar degeneration. Acta Neuropathol 1987;73:254–258.
54. Kosaka K. Diffuse Lewy body disease in Japan. J Neurol 1990;237:197–204.
55. Perry RH, Irving D, Blessed G, Perry EK, Fairbairn AF. Clinically and pathologically distinct form of dementia in the elderly. Lancet 1989;1:166.
56. Hansen L, Salmon D, Galasko D, et al. The Lewy body variant of Alzheimer's disease: a clinical and pathologic entity. Neurology 1990;40(1):1–8.
57. McKeith IG, Galasko D, Kosaka K, et al. Consensus guidelines for the clinical and pathologic diagnosis of dementia with Lewy bodies (DLB): report on the consortium on DLB international workshop. Neurology 1996;47:1113–1124.
58. Hansen LA. The Lewy body variant of Alzheimer disease. J Neural Transm Suppl 1997;51:83–93.
59. Hamilton RL. Lewy bodies in Alzheimer's disease: a neuropathological review of 145 cases using alpha-synuclein immunohistochemistry. Brain Pathol 2000;10:378–384.
60. Khachaturian Z. Diagnosis of Alzheimer's disease. Arch Neurol 1985;42:1097–1105.
61. Mirra SS, Hart MN, Terry RD. Making the diagnosis of Alzheimer's disease: a primer for practicing pathologists. Arch Pathol Lab Med 1993;117:132–144.
62. National Institute on Aging. Consensus recommendations for the postmortem diagnosis of Alzheimer's disease. National Institute on Aging and Reagan Institute Working Group on Diagnostic Criteria for the Neuropathological Assessment of Alzheimer's Disease. Neurobiol Aging 1997;18(suppl 4):S1–S2.
63. Galasko D. Cerebrospinal fluid levels of A beta 42 and tau: potential markers of Alzheimer's disease. J Neural Transm Suppl 1998;53:209–221.
64. Kurz A, Riemenschneider M, Buch K, et al. Tau protein in cerebrospinal fluid is significantly increased at the earliest clinical stage of Alzheimer's disease. Alzheimer Dis Assoc Disord 1998;12(4):372–377.

65. De La Monte SM, Carlson RI, Brown NV, Wands JR. Profiles of neuronal thread protein expression in Alzheimer's disease. J Neuropathol Exp Neurol 1996;55(10):1038–1050.
66. Galasko D, Chang L, Motter R, et al. High cerebrospinal fluid tau and low amyloid beta42 levels in the clinical diagnosis of Alzheimer disease and relation to apolipoprotein E genotype. Arch Neurol 1998;55(7):937–945.
67. DiLuca M, Pastorino L, Bianchetti A, et al. Differential level of platelet amyloid beta precursor protein isoforms: an early marker for Alzheimer disease. Arch Neurol 1998;55(9):1195–1200.
68. Ghanbari H, Ghanbari K, Behesti I, Munzar M, Vasauskas A, Averback P. Biochemical assay for AD7C-NTP in urine as an Alzheimer's disease marker. J Clin Lab Anal 1998;12(5):285–288.
69. Mayeux R, Tang MX, Jacobs DM, et al. Plasma amyloid beta peptide 1-42 and incipient Alzheimer disease. Ann Neurol 1999;46:412–416.
70. Cotman CW, Anderson AJ. A potential role for apoptosis in neurodegeneration and Alzheimer's disease. Mol Neurobiol 1995;10(1):19–45.
71. LaFerla FM, Tinkle BT, Bieberich CJ, Haudenschild CC, Jay G. The Alzheimer's A beta peptide induces neurodegeneration and apoptotic cell death in transgenic mice. Nat Genet 1995;9(1):21–30.
72. Mattson MP, Partin J, Begley JG. Amyloid Beta-peptide induces apoptosis-related events in synapses and dendrites. Brain Res 1998;807(1-2):167–176.
73. Lipton SA, Rosenberg PA. Excitatory amino acids as a final common pathway for neurologic disorders. N Engl J Med 1994;330:613–622.
74. Selden N, Geula C, Hersh L, Mesulam MM. Human striatum: chemoarchitecture of the caudate nucleus, putamen and ventral striatum in health and Alzheimer's disease. Neuroscience 1994;3:621–636.
75. Guo Q, Christakos S, Robinson S, Mattson MP. Calbindin D28k blocks the proapoptotic actions of mutant presinilin 1: reduced oxidative stress and preserved nitochondrial function. Proc Natl Acad Sci USA 1998;95(6):3227–3232.
76. Whitehouse P, Price DL, Clark AW, Coyle JT, DeLong MR. Alzheimer's disease: evidence from selective loss of cholinergic neurons in the nucleus basalis. Ann Neurol 1981;10:122–126.
77. Mesulam M-M. Structure and function of cholinergic pathways in the cerebral cortex, limbic system, basal ganglia, and thalamus of the human brain. In: Bloom FE, Kupfer DJ, eds. Psychopharmacology: The Fourth Generation of Progress. New York: Raven Press; 1995:135–146.
78. Geula C, Mesulam M-M. Cortical cholinergic fibers in aging and Alzheimer's disease: a morphometric study. Neuroscience 1989;33:469–481.
79. Warach S, Lettigrew LC, Dashe JF, et al. effect of citicoline on ischemic lesions as measured by diffusion-weighted magnetic resonance imaging. Citicoline 010 Investigators. Ann Neurol 2000;48(5):713–722.
80. Rao AM, Hatcher JF, Dempsey RJ. Lipid alterations in transient forebrain ischemia: possible new mechanisms of CDP-choline neuroprotection. J Neurochem 2000;75(6):2528–2535.
81. Perry EK, Perry RH, Blessed G, Tomlinson BE. Necropsy evidence of central cholinergic deficits in senile dementia. Lancet 1977;1.
82. Baskin DS, Browning JL, Pirozzolo FJ, Korporaal S, Baskin JA, Appel SH. Brain choline acetyltransferase and mental function in Alzheimer disease. Arch Neurol 1999;56:1121–1123.
83. Bartus RT. On neurodegenerative diseases, models, and treatment strategies: lessons learned and lessons forgotten a generation following the cholinergic hypothesis. Exp Neurol 2000;163(2):495–529.
84. Kordower JH, Chu Y, Stebbins GT, et al. Loss and atrophy of layer II entorhinal cortex neurons in elderly people with mild cognitive impairment. Ann Neurol 2001;49(2):202–213.
85. Davis KL, Mohs RC, Marin D, et al. Cholinergic markers in elderly patients with early signs of Alzheimer's disease. JAMA 1999;281(15):1433–1434.
86. DeKosky ST, Ikonomovic MD, Paulin ME, et al. Cognitive, cholinergic, and neuropathologic changes in normal aging, mild cognitive impairment, and mild Alzheimer's disease (abstract). Neurology 2000;54(suppl 3):A78.
87. Tiraboschi P, Hansen LA, Alford M, Masliah E, Thal LJ, Corey-Bloom R. The decline in synapses and cholinergic activity is asynchronous in Alzheimer's disease. Neurology 2000;55(9):1278–1283.
88. Gilmor ML, Erickson JD, Varoqui H, et al. Preservation of nucleus basalis neurons containing choline acetyltransferase and the vesicular acetylcholine transporter in the elderly with mild cognitive impairment and early Alzheimer's disease. J Comp Neurol 1999;411(4):693–704.
89. Schroder H, Zilles K, Luiten PGM, Strosberg AD, Aghchi A. Human cortical neurons contain both nicotinic and muscarinic acetylcholine receptors: an immunocytochemical double-labeling study. Synapse 1989;4:319–326.
90. Araujo DM, Lapchak PA, Robitaille Y, Quirion R. Differential alteration of various cholinergic markers in cortical and subcortical regions of human brain in Alzheimer's disease. J Neuroschem 1988;50:1914–1923.
91. DeKosky ST, Scheff SW, Markesbery WR. Laminar organization of cholinergic circuits in human frontal cortex in Alzheimer's disease and aging. Neurology 1985;35:1425–1431.

92. Nordber A, Alafuzoff I, Winblad B. Nicotinic and muscarinic subtypes in the human brain change with aging and dementia. J Neurosci Res 1992;31:103–111.
93. Probst A, Cortes R, Ulrich J. Differential modification of muscarinic cholinergic receptors in the hippocampus of patients with Alzheimer's disease: an autoradiographic study. Brain Res 1988;150:190–201.
94. Flynn DD, Ferrari-DiLeo G, Levey AI, Mash DC. Differential alterations in muscarinic receptor subtypes in Alzheimer's disease: implcations for cholinergic-based therapies. Life Sci 1995;56(11-12):869–876.
95. Ferrari-DiLeo G, Mash DC, Flynn DD. Attenuation of muscarinic receptor-G-protein interaction in Alzheimer's disease. Mol Chem Neuropathol 1995;24(1):69–91.
96. Nordberg A. Nicotonic receptor abnormalities of Alzheimer's disease: therapeutic implications. Biol Psychiatry 2001;49:200–210.
97. Paterson D, Nordberg A. Neural nicotinic receptors in the human brain. Prog Neurobiol 2000;61:75–111.
98. Marutle A, Warpman U, Bognanovic N, Lannfelt L, Nordberg A. Neuronal nicotinic receptor deficits in Alzheimer patients with the swedish amyloid precursor 670/671 mutation. J Neurochem 1999;72:1161–1169.
99. Martin-Ruiz CM, Molnar E, Lee M, et al. Alpha4 but not alpha3 and alpha7 nicotinic acetylcholine receptor subunits are lost from the temporal cortex in Alzheimer's disease. J Neurochem 1999;73:1635–1640.
100. Nordberg A, Amberla K, Shigeta M, Lundqvist H, Viitanen M, Hellstrom-Lindahl E. Long-term tactine treatment in three mild Alzheimer patients: effects on nicotinic receptors, cerebral blood flow, glucose metabolism, EEG and cognitive abilities. Alzheimer Dis Assoc Disord 1998;12:228–237.
101. Nordberg A, Lilja A, Lundqvist H, Hartvig P, Amberla K, Viitanen M. Tacrine restores cholinergic nicotinic receptors and glucose metabolism in Alzheimer patients as visualized by positron emission tomography. Neurobiol Aging 1992;13:747–758.
102. Maelicke A, Schrattenholtz A, Storch A, et al. Noncompetitive agonism at nicotinic acetylcholine receptors; functional significance for CNS signal transduction. J Recept Signal Transduct Res 1995;15(1–4):333–353.
103. Maelicke A, Schrattenholz A, Samochocki M, Radina M, Albuquerque T. Allosterically potentiating ligands of nicotinic receptors as a treatment strategy for Alzheimer's disease. Behav Brain Res 2000;113(1–2):199–206.
104. Hamos JE, DeGennaro LJ, Drachman DA. Synaptic loss in Alzheimer's disease and other dementias. Neurol 1989;39:355–361.
105. McGeer PL, McGeer EG, Suzuki J, Dolman CE, Nagai T. Aging, Alzheimer's disease, and the cholinergic system of the basal forebrain. Neurology 1984;34:741–745.
106. Beach TG, McGeer EG. Senile plaques, amyloid beta-protein, and acetylcholinesterase fibers: laminar distributors in Alzheimer's disease striate cortex. Acta Neuropathol 1992;83:292–299.
107. Ransmayr G, Cervera P, Hirsch EC, Berger W, Fischer W, Agid Y. Alzheimer's disease: is the decrease of cholinergic innervation of the hippocampus related to intrinsic hippocampal pathology? Neuroscience 1992;47:843–851.
108. Zubenko GS, Moosey J, Martinez AJ, Rao GR, Kopp U, Hanin JA. A brain regional analysis of morphometric and cholinergic abnormalities in Alzheimer's disease. Arch Neurol 1989;46:634–638.
109. Arendt T, Taubert G, Bigl V, Arendt A. Amyloid deposition in the nucleus basalis of Meynert complex, a topographic marker for degenerating cell clusters in Alzheimer's disease. Acta Neuropathol 1988;75:226–232.
110. Mann DMA, Yates PO, Marcyniuk B. Correlation between senile plaque and neurofibrillary tangle counts in cerebral cortex and neuronal counts in cortex and subcortical structures in Alzheimer's disease. Neurosci Lett 1985;56:51–55.
111. Harkany T, De Jong GI, Soos K, Penke B, Luiten PG, Gulya K. Beta-amyloid (1-42) affects cholinergic but not parvalbumin-containing neurons in the septal complex of the rat. Brain Res 1995;698:270–274.
112. Harkany T, Lengyel Z, Soos K, Penke B, Luiten PG, Gulya K. Cholinotoxic effects of beta-amyloid (1-42) peptide on cortical projections of the rat nucleus basalis magnocellularis. Brain Res 1995;695:71–75.
113. Zweig R, Ross C, Hedreen JC. The neuropathology of aminergic nuclei in Alzheimer's disease. Ann Neurol 1988;24(2):233–242.
114. Halliday GM, McCann HL, Pamphliett R. Brain stem serotonin-synthesizing neurons in Alzheimer's disease: a clinicopathological correlation. Acta Neuropathol 1992;84:638–650.
115. Mann DMA, Lincoln J, Yates PO, Stamp JE, Toper S. Changes in the monoamine containing neurons of the human CNS in senile dementia. Br J Psychiatry 1980;136:533–541.
116. Yamamoto T, Hirano A. Nucleus raphe dorsalis in Alzheimer's disease: neurofibrillary tangles and loss of large neurons. Ann Neurol 1985;17:573–577.
117. Cross AJ, Crow TJ, Ferrier IN. Serotonin receptor changes in dementia of the Alzheimer type. J Neurochem 1984;43:1574–1581.
118. Bowen DM, Allen SJ, Benton JS. Biochemical assessment of serotonergic and cholinergic dysfunction and cerebral atrophy in Alzheimer's disease. J Neurochem 1983;41:266–272.

119. Palmer AM, Stratmann GC, Procter AW, Bowen DM. Possible neurotransmitter basis of behavioral changes in Alzheimer's disease. 1988;23:616–620.
120. Mann DMA, Yates PO. Serotonic nerve cells in Alzheimer's disease. J Neurol Neurosurg Psychiatry 1983;46:96–98.
121. Lanctot KL, Herrmann N, Mazzotta P. Role of serotonin in the behavioral and psychological symptoms of dementia. J Neuropsychiatry Clin Neurosci 2001;13:5–21.
122. Palmer AM, Francis PT, Bowen DM. Catechlaminergic neurones assessed antemortem in Alzhiemer's disease. Brain Res 1987;414:365–375.
123. Chan-Palay V, Asan E. Alterations in catecholamine neurons of the locus coeruleus in senile dementia of the Alzheimer type and in Parkinson's disease with and without dementia and depression. J Comp Neurol 1989;287(3):373–392.
124. Marcyniuk B, Mann DMA, Yates PO. The topography of cell loss from locus coeruleus in Alzheimer's disease. J Neurol Sci 1986;76:335–345.
125. Bondareff W, Mountjoy CQ, Roth M. Selective loss of neurones of origin of adrenergic projection to cerebral cortex (nucleus locus coeruleus) in senile dementia. Lancet 1981;1(8223):783–784.
126. Zubenko G, Moossy J. Major depression in primary dementia: clinical and neuropathological correlates. Arch Neurol 1988;45:1182–1186.
127. Forstl H, Burns A, Luthert P, Cairns N, Lantos P, Levy R. Clinical and neuropathological correlates of depression in Alzheimer's disease. Psychol Med 1992;22:877–884.
128. Chan-Palay V. Depression and dementia in Parkinson's disease: catecholamine changes in the locus coeruleus—basis for therapy. Dementia 1991;2:7–17.
129. Rinne JO, Rummukainen J, Paljarvi L, Sako E, Molsa P, Rinne UK. Neuronal loss in the substantia nigra in patients with Alzheimer's disease and Parkinson's disease in relation to extrapyramidal symptoms and dementia. Prog Clin Biol Res 1989;317:325–332.
130. Victoroff J, Zarow C, Mack WJ, Hsu E, Chui HC. Physical aggression is associated with preservation of substantia nigra pars compacta in Alzheimer's disease. Arch Neurol 1996;53:428–434.
131. Ebinger G, Bruyland M, Martin JJ. Distribution of biogenic amines and their catabolies in brains from patients with Alzheimer's disease. J Neurol Sci 1987;77:267–283.
132. Curcio CA, Kemper T. Nucleus raphe dorsalis in dementia of the Alzheimer type: neurofibrillary changes and neuronal packing density. J Neuropathol Exp Neurol 1984;43:359–368.
133. Mann DMA, Yates PO, Marcyniuk B. Dopaminergic neurotransmitter systems in Alzheimer's disease and in Down's syndrome at middle-age. J Neurol Neurosurg Psychiatry 1987;50:341–344.
134. Proctor AW, Palmer AM, Francis PT, Lowe SL, Neary D, Murphy E. Evidence of glutamatergic denervation and possible abnormal metabolism in Alzheimer's disease. J Neurochem 1988;50:790–802.
135. Chalmers DT, Dewar D, Graham DI, Brooks DN, McCulloch J. Differential alterations of cortical glutamatergic binding sites in senile dementia of the Alzheimer type. Proc Natl Acad Sci USA 1990;87(4):1352–1356.
136. Ikonomovic MD, Mizukami K, Warde D, et al. Distribution of glutamate receptor subunit NMDAR1 in the hippocampus of normal elderly and patients with Alzheimer's disease. Exp Neurol 1999;160(1):194–204.
137. Hyman BT, Van Hoesen GW, Damasio AR. Alzheimer's disease: glutamate depletion in the hippocampal perforant pathway zone. Ann Neurol 1987;22(1):37–40.
138. Palmer AM. Excitatory amino acid neurons and receptors in Alzheimer's disease. In: Kozikowski AP, Barrionuevo G, eds. Neurobiology of the NMDA Receptor: From Chemistry to Clinic. New York: VCH Publishers; 1991:203–237.
139. Lowe SL, Francis PT, Procter AW. Gamma-aminobutyric acid concentration in brain tissue at two stages of Alzheimer's disease. Brain 1988;111(pt 4):785–799.
140. Guidotti I, Corda MC, Wise BC. GABAergic synapses: supramolecular organization and biochemical regulation. Neuropharmacology 1983;22:1471–1479.
141. Zorumski CF, Isenberg KE. Insights into the structure and function of GABA-benzodiazepine receptors: ion channels and psychiatry. Am J Psychiatry 1991;148:162–173.
142. Gottfries CG, Frederiksen SO, Heilig M. Neuropeptides and Alzheimer's disease. Eur Neuropsychopharmacol 1995;5:491–500.
143. Minthon L, Edvinsson L, Gustafson L. Correlation between clinical characteristics and cerebrospinal fluid neuropeptide Y levels in dementia of the Alzheimer type and frontotemporal dementia. Alzheimer Dis Assoc Disord 1996;10:197–203.
144. Minthon L, Edvinsson L, Gustafson L. Somatostatin and neuropeptide Y in cerebrospinal fluid correlations with severity of disease and clinical signs in Alzheimer's disease and frontotemporal dementia. Dement Geriatr Cogn Disord 1997;8:232–239.
145. Petersen RC, Smith GE, Waring SC, Ivnik RJ, Tangalos EG, Kokmen E. Mild cognitive impairment: clinical characterization and outcome. Arch Neurol 1999;56:303–308.

146. Morris JC, Storandt M, Miller JP, et al. Mild cognitive impairment represents early-stage Alzheimer disease. Arch Neurol 2001;58:397–405.
147. Miceli G, Colosimo C, Daniele A, Marra C, Perani D, Fazio E. Isolated amnesia with slow onset and stable course, without ensuing dementia: MRI and PET data and a six-year neuropsychological follow-up. Dementia 1996;7(2):104–110.
148. Jack CR, Petersen RC, Xu YC, et al. Prediction of AD aith MRI-based hippocampal volume in mild cognitive impairment. Neurology 1999;52(7):1397–1403.
149. Fox NC, Crum WR, Scahill RI, Stevens JM, Janssen JC, Rossor MN. Imaging of onset and progression of Alzheimer's disease with voxel-compression mapping of serial magnetic resonance images. Lancet 2001;358:201–205.
150. Cagnin A, Brooks DJ, Kennedy AM, et al. In vivo measurement of activated microglia in dementia. Lancet 2001;358:461–467.
151. DeKosky ST, Ikonomovic MD, Styren SD, Paulin M, Wisniewski S, Cochran E. Cortical and hippocampal ChAT activity in normal aging, mild cognitive impairment, and mild Alzheimer's disease. Soc Neurosci 1999;25:2117.

37

Psychiatric Comorbidity
Implications for Treatment and Clinical Research

JACK R. CORNELIUS, IHSAN M. SALLOUM, OSCAR G. BUKSTEIN, and DUNCAN B. CLARK
Western Psychiatric Institute and Clinic, University of Pittsburgh School of Medicine, Pittsburgh, Pennsylvania, U.S.A.

I. INTRODUCTION

Patients commonly demonstrate comorbidities involving psychiatric disorders in combination with alcohol use disorder (AUD) and other substance use disorders (SUDs). The results of two recent large community surveys emphasize the prevalence of comorbid psychiatric and substance use disorders, the Epidemiologic Catchment Area (ECA) study [1], and the National Comorbidity Survey (NCS) [2]. Data from the ECA study showed that U.S. population lifetime prevalence rates were 22.5% for any non-substance-abuse mental disorder, 13.5% for alcohol dependence abuse, and 6.1% for other drug dependence abuse. Among those with a mental disorder, the odds ratio of having some addictive disorder was 2.7, with a lifetime prevalence of 29%. Conversely, among those with an alcohol use disorder, 37% had a comorbid mental disorder. Comorbidity was particularly prevalent among individuals treated in speciality mental health and addictive disorder clinical settings [1]. Data from NCS study demonstrated that the vast majority of lifetime disorders (79%) was comorbid disorders [2], and that the comorbidity was more highly concentrated than previously recognized in roughly one-sixth of the population who had a history of three or more comorbid disorders. Data from that study also demonstrated that many more Americans age 15–54 have been affected by dependence on psychoactive substances than by other non-substance-related psychiatric disturbance [3], which may help explain the prevalence of comorbid substance use disorders among those with psychiatric disorders. However, despite the prevalence and adverse consequences of comorbidity among individuals with psychiatric disorders in combination with AUDs and other SUDs, little research has been devoted to the study of pharmacological agents or other treatments that might decrease these problems [4,5]. Consequently, a number of large gaps in knowledge continue to exist involving the treatment of alcoholics with comorbid disorders.

This chapter will review comorbidity involving psychiatric disorders in combination with alcohol or other substance use disorders, and the implications of this comorbidity for treatment and clinical research. Because of space limitations, this chapter will address only the most common comorbid conditions. This chapter will focus more on alcohol use disorders than on other nonalcohol substance use disorders, since most of the studies involving comorbid populations have involved alcohol use disorders. Also, this chapter will focus primarily on pharmacologic treatments of comorbidity rather than psychological treatments, since most of the treatment studies involving these comorbid populations have involved medication trials.

II. COMORBIDITY INVOLVING SUD AND MAJOR DEPRESSION

Because of their relatively high overall lifetime prevalence and frequent association with SUDs in the literature, the affective disorders will be considered in greater detail in this manuscript than other comorbid disorders. The National Comorbidity Survey (NCS) data demonstrated that the most common psychiatric disorders were major depression (17%) and alcohol dependence (14%) [2,6]. Data from the NCS showed that the risk factors for comorbid depression were different from those of major depression without comorbid substance use disorders ("pure depression"). For example, comorbid depression was more strongly associated with younger age, lower level of education, lower income, and African-American ethnicity [7]. Data from the NCS also showed that most cases of lifetime major depressive disorder are secondary, in that they occur in people with a prior history of another DSM disorder [8]. Helzer and Pryzbeck [9] reported a significant association between depressive disorders and alcohol use disorders in data from the ECA study, which shows that these disorders tend to co-occur significantly more often than would be expected by chance alone. Perhaps reflecting this particularly prevalent comorbidity, more treatment studies have been conducted involving AUDS with affective disorders than with any other class of comorbid disorder.

A few recent well-controlled studies have been conducted evaluating the efficacy of tricyclic antidepressants (TCAs) in individuals with comorbid major depressive disorder and alcohol use disorders. McGrath and colleagues [10] studied the TCA imipramine versus placebo in 69 alcoholics with primary depression. They found that treatment with imipramine was associated with improvement in depression, but no overall effect on drinking outcome was observed. A study by Powell and colleagues [11] of nortriptyline showed no significant improvement versus placebo for either the depressive symptoms or the drinking of their depressed alcoholics. Mason and colleagues [12] conducted a study of 71 patients with primary alcohol dependence, 28 of whom had major depression secondary to alcoholism. They found final HAM-D scores of desipramine patients to be significantly decreased relative to those of placebo patients, with baseline HAM-D as the covariate. Survival curves demonstrated a significant difference between placebo and desipramine in time to relapse, favoring the desipramine group. There were more relapses on placebo than on desipramine among depressed patients (40% vs. 8%) and among nondepressed patients (27% vs. 14%), but these rates did not reach statistical significance. These findings suggested that desipramine is efficacious in treating the depressive symptoms of alcoholics with secondary major depression, and that a statistically significant increase in length of abstinence is noted among those with comorbid depression. However, the use of desipramine to reduce relapse in nondepressed alcoholics was not supported. The authors of that article suggested that selective serotonergic reuptake inhibitor (SSRI) antidepressants might have certain advantages over tricyclic antidepressants, such as greater tolerability and lower toxicity in overdose.

To date, only a few double-blind, placebo-controlled studies have evaluated the efficacy of SRI antidepressants in individuals with comorbid alcohol dependence and major depression. These studies follow from the work of Naranjo and colleagues [13] involving flexitime in nondepressed alcohol abusers. One such study [14] evaluated the SRI flexitime in 51 severely depressed subjects with comorbid major depression and alcohol dependence, many of whom demonstrated suicidal additions at baseline. In that study, fluoxetine demonstrated efficacy versus placebo for decreasing both the drinking and the depressive symptoms of this population. However, the authors cautioned that it was unclear to what extent these results generalized to the treatment of less severely depressed and less suicidal alcoholics with major depression or to alcoholics with other, less serious depressive disorders. The beneficial effects associated with fluoxetine treatment persisted at a 1-year follow-up evaluation [15]. Kernels and colleagues [16] conducted a trial of fluoxetine to prevent relapse in 101 alcoholics, 14 of whom demonstrated a current major depression. The study demonstrated that fluoxetine is not of use for relapse prevention with mild to moderate alcohol dependence and no comorbid depression. The authors also concluded that in alcoholics with major depression, the medication might reduce depressive symptoms. The authors recommended that subsequent studies with the fluoxetine should focus on more severely alcohol-dependent subjects or those with comorbid depression.

One study to date has assessed the efficiency of the SSRI medication sertraline in depressed alcoholics [17]. That study involved 36 subjects who remained in an intensive day program throughout the study. The results of that study demonstrated efficacy for sertraline versus placebo for decreasing the depressive symptoms of depressed alcoholics. However, the effects of sertraline on the drinking of this population could not be adequately assessed, because their treatment setting precluded them from drinking.

III. COMORBIDITY INVOLVING SUDS AND BIPOLAR DISORDER

In both the ECA study and the NCS study, bipolar disorder has been shown to have a particularly high rate of co-occurrence with AUDs and other SUDs. In the ECA study, the odds of having a bipolar disorder were five times greater if one had an AUD than if one did not have an AUD [1]. In the NCS study, the odds of having a diagnosis of alcohol dependence were 12 times greater among those with a bipolar disorder than among those without a bipolar disorder, which was the highest odds ratio noted for any Axis I disorder [6]. Thus, bipolar disorder appears to be more strongly associated with comorbid disorders than is unipolar major depressive disorder. Also, comorbidity among persons with bipolar disorder has been shown to be associated with the development of cycle acceleration and more severe episodes over time [18].

Despite increased awareness in recent years of the common co-occurrence and serious consequences of bipolar disorder in combination with SUDs, no double-blind studies have addressed the efficacy of any medication in this dual-diagnosis population [19]. Patients with AUDs are generally excluded form clinical trials of psychotropic medications in an effort to reduce sources of bias. Lithium carbonate, the current treatment of choice in the acute and prophylactic treatment of bipolar disorder among nonalcoholics, presents a number of difficulties when used in bipolar alcoholics [19]. For example, lithium may exacerbate the central nervous system effects of ethanol. Alcoholism also may worsen the prognosis of bipolar disorder [19].

Even though no double-blind trials to date have evaluated the efficacy of lithium carbonate in bipolar alcoholics, several trials involving lithium have been conducted involving alcoholics with unipolar depression and alcoholics without an affective disorder. Fawcett et al. [20] conducted a double-blind, placebo-controlled trial of lithium in a study group that included both depressed and nondepressed alcoholics. That study found no effects of lithium on the abstinence rates of depressed or nondepressed alcoholics. Dorus and colleagues [21] conducted a multisite double-blind, placebo-controlled trial in a study sample that included both depressed and nondepressed alcoholic veterans. That study found no efficacy for lithium for any outcome measure in either the depressed or nondepressed alcoholics. Thus, lithium appears not to demonstrate efficacy in treating alcoholics with unipolar depression or alcoholics with no affective disorder.

The anticonvulsant medications carbamazepine and valproate have recently demonstrated efficacy in the treatment of bipolar disorder among nonalcoholics, including the demonstration of efficacy among subtypes of bipolar disorder that are less responsive to lithium carbonate, such as rapid cycling, mixed, or dysphoric mania [22]. Both controlled and uncontrolled clinical trials report that valproate is effective in acute and prophylactic treatment of mania in subjects who could not tolerate or had a poor response to lithium [23–28]. A recent multisite placebo-controlled study reported valproate to be as effective as lithium and more effective than placebo in acute mania [28]. However, to date, no double-blind trials of carbamazepine or valproate have been conducted in patients with comorbid bipolar disorder and an AUD [29].

IV. COMORBIDITY INVOLVING SUDS AND ANXIETY DISORDERS

According to the National Comorbidity Survey [2], one in every four Americans reports a history of at least one anxiety disorder, making anxiety disorders roughly equivalent in prevalence to substance use disorders. That study also reported that anxiety disorders, as a group, are considerably more likely to occur in the 12 months before the interview (17%) than either substance use disorders (11%) or affective disorders (11%). The prevalence of other NCS disorders was quite low. In that study, 61% of women and 36% of men with any lifetime anxiety disorder reported a lifetime diagnosis of alcohol dependence, and these disorders were significantly correlated with each other. However, despite the prevalence of these disorders, only one pharmacological agent, buspirone, has been evaluated in clinical studies with alcoholics suffering anxiety disorders.

Buspirone is a partial 5HT1A agonist. Studies involving busiprone in alcoholics are based on the hypothesis that alteration in central nervous system serotonin function can predispose individuals to relapse [30].

This hypothesis, in turn, is based on the apparent link between low serotonin turnover rate and increased alcohol consumption [30]. To date, four clinical studies involving buspirone have been conducted involving patients with an anxiety disorder and alcohol dependence, and two other double-blind placebo-controlled studies involving buspirone have been conducted involving alcoholics with no comorbid anxiety disorder.

In the first of these studies involving patients with anxiety disorders and alcohol dependence (anxious alcoholics), Bruno [31] studied patients with mild to moderate alcohol abuse and mild to moderate anxiety in an 8-week trial. That research group found that patients in the buspirone group experienced a lower dropout rate, less craving, and a reduction in alcohol consumption, depression, anxiety, and global psychopathology. Tollefson and colleagues [32] studied anxious alcoholic outpatients who had already abstained from alcohol for 30–90 days. The buspirone group in that study exhibited a greater reduction in anxiety, a greater global reduction in drinking, a fewer number of days of desiring alcohol, and a better retention in treatment than the placebo group. Malcolm and colleagues [33] studied a group of anxious alcoholics who had been detoxified in a veterans' hospital and who subsequently had been followed for 6 months as outpatients. That research group found no therapeutic efficacy for busiprone for decreasing anxiety or for prolonging the maintenance of abstinence. Kranzler and colleagues [34] conducted a randomized 12-week, placebo-controlled study of buspirone in 61 anxious alcoholics who were able to stop drinking for 7 days as outpatients. They found that buspirone treatment was associated with a greater reduction in level of anxiety, a slower return to heavy alcohol consumption, a greater retention in the trial, and a lesser number of drinking days during a 6-month follow-up period. In summary, three of the four studies in this area demonstrated efficacy for buspirone for treating anxious alcoholics, while one did not. These findings suggest that buspirone is probably of benefit in the treatment of at least some anxious alcoholics.

The first controlled study of buspirone in nonanxious alcoholics was conducted by Malec et al. [35]. That group failed to find a reduction in alcohol consumption among alcoholics who were followed for 12 weeks. Similarly, George and colleagues [30] found that treatment with buspirone did not increase the days to relapse in their sample of nonanxious alcoholics. These findings suggest that buspirone is probably not of benefit in treating alcoholics who do not display comorbid anxiety.

Other classes of pharmacotherpeutic agents have of course been studied for the treatment of anxiety disorders in patients without comorbid substance use disorders, such as TCAs, SSRI antidepressants, MAO inhibitors, and benzodiazepines [36]. However, to date none of these classes of medications have been studied in patients with anxiety disorders and comorbid alcohol or substance use disorders [5]. Consequently, the efficacy of these medications in this comorbid population remains unclear.

V. COMORBIDITY INVOLVING SUDS AND PSYCHOTIC DISORDERS

The ECA study [1] reported that schizophrenia has a prevalence rate of only 3.8% among those with AUDs, but that this disorder is seen three times more often among alcoholics than among nonalcoholics. Conversely, the prevalence of any AUD among schizophrenics is 34%, suggesting that comorbid alcohol disorders are a common problem among schizophrenics. To date, no controlled pharmacotherapy trials have been conducted in patients with comorbid schizophrenia and a substance or alcohol use disorder, so the efficacy of various medications in this population remains unclear. However, it has been reported that disulfiram should be used with caution in this dual-diagnosis population, since it may increase central levels of dopamine by blocking dopamine B-hydroxylase and thereby exacerbate psychosis [37].

VI. COMORBIDITY INVOLVING NONALCOHOL SUDS

Few papers have been published dealing with the pharmacotherapy of patients demonstrating a substance use disorder other than alcohol abuse or dependence in combination with a comorbid psychiatric disorder. Batki and colleagues [38] conducted a fluoxetine study in a sample of 16 patients who displayed cocaine dependence and opioid dependence who were participating in methadone maintenance. Most of the subjects in that study also had a lifetime history of major depression, heavy alcohol use, and HIV-positive blood tests. Both cocaine use and cocaine craving significantly decreased during the course of the study, and both depressive symptoms and anxiety symptoms significantly improved as well. In another study involving fluoxetine, a secondary data analysis was conducted

23. R. Brown. U.S. experience with valproate in manic depressive illness: a multicenter trial. J Clin Psychiatry 50(suppl):13–16, 1989.
24. RH Gerner, A Stanton. Algorithm for patient management of acute manic states: lithium, valproate or carbamazepine? J Clin Psychopharmacol 12(suppl 1):57S–63S, 1992.
25. JR Calabrese, PJ Markovitz, SE Kimmel, SC Wagner. Spectrum of efficacy of valproate in 78 rapid-cycling bipolar patients. J Clin Psychopharmacol 12(suppl 1):53S–56S, 1992.
26. SG Hayes. Long-term valproate prophylaxis in refractory affective disorders. Ann Clin Psychiatry 4:55–63, 1992.
27. HG Pope, SL McElroy, PE Keck, JI Hudson. Valproate in the treatment of acute mania: a placebo-controlled study. Arch Gen Psychiatry 48:62–68, 1991.
28. CL Bowden, AM Brugger, AC Suann, JR Calabrese, PG Janicak, F Petty, SC Dilsaver, JM Savis, AJ Rush, JG Smally, ES Garza-Trevino, C Risch, PJ Goodnick, DD Morris. Efficacy of divalproex vs. lithium and placebo in the treatment of mania. JAMA 271:918–924, 1994.
29. KT Brady, SC Sonne, R Anton, JC Ballenger. Valproate in the treatment of acute bipolar affective episodes complicated by substance abuse: a pilot study. J Clin Psychiatry 56:118–121, 1995.
30. DT George, R Rawlings, MJ Eckardt, MJ Phillips, SE Shoaf, M Linnoila. Buspirone treatment of alcoholism: age of onset and cerebrospinal fluid 5-hydroxyindolacetic acid and homovanillic acid concentrations, but not medication treatment, predict return to drinking. Alcohol Clin Exper Res 23:272–278, 1999.
31. F Bruno. Buspirone treatment of alcoholic patients. Psychopathology 22:49–59, 1989.
32. GD Tollefson, J Montague-Clouse, SL Tollefson. Treatment of comorbid generalized anxiety in a recently detoxified alcoholic population with a selective serotonergic drug (buspirone). J Clin Psychopharmacol 12:19–26, 1992.
33. R Malcolm, RF Anton, CL Randall, A Johnston, K Brady, A Thevos. A placebo-controlled trial of buspirone in anxious inpatient alcoholics. Alcohol Clin Exp Res 16:1007–1013, 1992.
34. HR Kranzler, JA Burleson, FK Del Boca, TF Babor, P Korner, J Brown, M Bohn. Buspirone treatment of anxious alcoholics. Arch Gen Psychiatry 51:720–731, 1994.
35. E Malec, T Malec, MA Gagne, M Dongier. Buspirone in the treatment of alcohol dependence: a placebo-controlled trial. Alcohol Clin Exp Res 20:307–312, 1996.
36. RB Lydiard, PP Roy-Byrne, JC Ballenger. Recent advances in the psychopharmacological treatment of anxiety disorders. Hosp Commun Psychiatry 39:1157–1165, 1988.
37. JN Wilkins. Pharmacotherapy of schizophrenia patients with comorbid substance abuse. Schizophr Bull 23:215–228, 1997.
38. SL Batki, LB Manfredi, P Jacob, RT Jones. Fluoxetine for cocaine dependence in methadone maintenance: quantitative plasma and urine cocaine benzoylecgonine concentrations. J Clin Psychopharmacol 13:243–250, 1993.
39. JR Cornelius, IM Salloum, ME Thase, RF Haskett, DC Daley, A Jones-Barlock, C Upsher, JM Perel. Fluoxetine versus placebo in depressed alcoholic cocaine abusers. Psychopharmacol Bull 34:117–121, 1998.
40. JR Cornelius, IM Salloum, RF Haskett, JG Ehler, PJ Jarrett, ME Thase, JM Perel. Fluoxetine versus placebo for the marijuana use of depressed alcoholics. Addict Behav 24:111–114, 1999.
41. RZ Litten, JP Allen. Pharmacotherapies for alcoholism: promising agents and clinical issues. Alcohol Clin Exper Res 15:620–633, 1991.
42. RZ Litten, J Allen, J Fertig. Pharmacotherapies for alcohol problems: a review of research with focus on developments since 1991. Alcohol Clin Exper Res 20:859–876, 1996.
43. RZ Litten, J Fertig. International update: new findings on promising medications. Alcohol Clin Exp Res 20(suppl):216A–218A, 1986.
44. JR Cornelius, H Fabrega, PJ Maher, A Jones-Barlock, IM Salloum, RF Ulrich, JE Mezzich. Age effects on the clinical presentation of alcoholics at a psychiatric hospital. Compr Psychiatry 38:213–217, 1997.
45. RZ Litten, JP Allen. Pharmacologic treatment of alcoholics with collateral depression: issues and future directions. Psychopharmacol Bull 34:107–110, 1998.
46. CA King, MW Naylor, EM Hill, BN Shain, JF Greden. Dysthymia characteristic of heavy alcohol use in depressed adolescents. Biol Psychiatry 33:210–212, 1993.
47. B Geller, TB Cooper, K Sun, B Zimmerman, J Frazier, M Williams, J Heath. Double-blind and placebo-controlled study of lithium for adolescent bipolar disorders with secondary substance dependence. J Am Acad Child Adolesc Psychiatry 37:171–178, 1998.
48. K Brady, T Pearlstein, G Asnis, D Baker, B. Rothbaum, C Sikes, G Farfel. Efficacy and safety of sertraline treatment of posttraumatic stress disorder: a randomized controlled trial. JAMA 283:1837–1844, 2000.
49. IM Salloum, JR Cornelius, JE Mezzich, L Kirisci, DC Daley, CR Spotts, A Zuckoff. Characterizing female bipolar alcoholic patients presenting for initial evaluation. Addict Behav 26:341–348, 2001.

50. SG Simpson, JR Depaulo. Fluoxetine treatment of bipolar II depression. J Clin Psychopharmacol 11:52–54, 1991.
51. KT Brady, P Halligan, RJ Malcolm. Dual diagnosis. In: M Galanter, HD Kleber, eds. Textbook of Substance Abuse Treatment, 2nd ed. Washington; American Psychiatric Press, 1999, pp 475–483.
52. OG Bukstein, LJ Glancy, Y Kaminer. Comorbidity of substance abuse and other psychiatric disorders in adolescents. Am J Psychiatry 146:1131–1141, 1989.
53. JR Cornelius, K Lynch, CS Martin, MD Cornelius, DB Clark. Clinical correlates of heavy tobacco use among adolescents. Addict Behav 26:273–277, 2001.
54. JR Cornelius, KA Perkins, IM Salloum, ME Thase, HB Moss. Fluoxetine versus placebo to decrease the smoking of depressed alcoholic patients. J Clin Psychopharmacol 19:181–184, 1999.
55. JR Cornelius, DB Clark, IM Salloum, OG Bukstein, TM Kelly. Management of suicidal behavior in alcoholism. Clin Neurosci Res 1:381–386, 2001
56. JR Cornelius, IM Salloum, MD Cornelius, JM Perel, ME Thase, JG Ehler, JJ Mann. Fluoxetine trial in suicidal depressed alcoholics. Psychopharmacol Bull 29:195–199, 1993.
57. JR Cornelius, IM Salloum, JE Mezzich, ME Cornelius, H Fabrega, JG Ehler, RF Ulrich, ME Thase, JJ Mann. Disproportionate suicidality in patients with comorbid major depression and alcoholism. Am J Psychiatry 152:358–364, 1995.
58. IM Salloum, DC Daley, JR Cornelius, ME Thase, L Kirisci. Disproportionate lethality in psychiatric patients with alcohol and cocaine co-abuse. Am J Psychiatry 153:953–955, 1996.
59. JR Cornelius, IM Salloum, NL Day, ME Thase, JJ Mann. Patterns of suicidality and alcohol use in alcoholics with major depression. Alcohol Clin Exp Res 20:1451–1455, 1996.
60. JR Cornelius, IM Salloum, K Lynch, DB Clark, JJ Mann. Treating the substance-abusing suicidal patient. Ann NY Acad Sci 932:78–93, 2001.
61. JR Cornelius, ME Thase, IM Salloum, MD Cornelius, A Black, JJ Mann. Cocaine use associated with increased suicidal behavior in depressed alcoholics. Addict Behav 23:119–121, 1998.
62. IM Salloum, JR Cornelius, DC Daley, ME Thase. The utility of diazepam loading in the treatment of alcohol withdrawal among psychiatric inpatients. Psychopharmacol Bull 31:305–310, 1995.
63. RZ Litten, JP Allen. Medications for alcohol, illicit drug, and tobacco dependence: an update of research findings. J Subst Abuse Treat 16:105–112, 1999.
64. DB Clark, N Pollock, OG Bukstein, AC Mezzich, JT Bromberger, JE Donovan. Gender and comorbid psychopathology in adolescents with alcohol dependence. J Am Acad Child Adolesc Psychiatry 36:1195–1203, 1997.
65. DB Clark, AM Parker, KG Lynch. Psychopathology and substance-related problems during early adolescence: a survival analysis. J Clin Child Psychol 28:333–341, 1999.
66. JR Cornelius, OG Bukstein, B Birmaher, IM Salloum, KG Lynch, NK Pollock, S Gershon, DB Clark. Fluoxetine in adolescents with major depression and an alcohol use disorder: An open label trial. Addict Behav 26:735–739, 2001.
67. GJ Emslie, AJ Rush, WA Weinberg, RA Kowatch, CW Hughes, T Carmody, J Rintelmann. A double-blind, randomized, placebo-controlled trial of fluoxetine in children and adolescents with depression. Arch Gen Psychiatry 54:1031–1037, 1997.
68. CS Martin, NA Kaczynski, SA Maisto, OG Bukstein, HB Moss. Patterns of DSM-IV alcohol abuse and dependence symptoms in adolescent drinkers. J Stud Alcohol 56:672–680, 1995.
69. RD Riggs, SK Mikulich, LM Coffman, TJ Crowley. Fluoxetine in drug-dependent delinquents with major depression: an open trial. J Child Adolesc Psychopharmacol 7:97–95, 1997.
70. B Vitiello, PS Jensen. Medication development and testing in children and adolescents. Arch Gen Psychiatry 54:871–876, 1997.
71. SS O'Malley, KM Carroll. Psychotherapeutic considerations in pharmacological trials. Alcohol Clin Exp Res 20:17A–22A, 1996.
72. FM Paille, JD Guelfi, AC Perkins, RJ Royer, L Steru, P Parot. Double-blind randomized multicenter trial of acamprosate in maintaining abstinence from alcohol. Alcohol Alcohol 30:239–247, 1995.
73. IM Salloum, HB Moss, DC Daley, JR Cornelius, L Kirisci, M Al-Maalouf. Problem awareness and treatment readiness in dual diagnosis patients. Am J Addict 7:35-42, 1998.
74. JR Volpicelli, AI Alterman, M Hayashida, CP O'Brien. Naltrexone in the treatment of alcohol dependence. Arch Gen Psychiatry 49:876–880, 1992.
75. JR Cornelius, PJ Jarrett, ME Thase, H Fabrega, GL Haas, A Jones-Barlock, JE Mezzich, RF Ulrich. Gender effects on the clinical presentation of alcoholics at a psychiatric hospital. Compr Psychiatry 36:1–7, 1995.
76. JR Cornelius, H Fabrega, MD Cornelius, JE Mezzich, PJ Maher, IM Salloum, ME Thase, RF Ulrich. Racial effects on the clinical presentation of alcoholics at a psychiatric hospital. Compr Psychiatry 37:102-108, 1996.
77. AT McLellan, L Luborsky, GE Woody, CP O'Brien, KA Drule. Predicting response to alcohol and drug abuse treatments. Arch Gen Psychiatry 40:620–625, 1983.
78. EV Nunes, PF McGrath, FM Quitkin, JW Stewart, L Goehl, K Ocepek-Welikson. Predictors of antide-

pressant response in depressed alcoholic patients. Am J Addict 5:308–312, 1996.

79. Project MATCH Research Group. Matching alcoholism treatments to client heterogeneity: Project MATCH three-year drinking outcomes. Alcohol Clin Exp Res 22:1300–1311, 1998.

80. JR Cornelius, J Pringle, J Jernigan, L Kirisci, DB Clark. Correlates of mental health service utilization and unmet need among a sample of male adolescents. Addict Behav 26:11–19, 2001.

81. IM Salloum, JR Cornelius, ME Thase, DC Daley, L Kirisci, C Spotts. Naltrexone utility in depressed alcoholics. Psychopharmacol Bull 34:111–115, 1998.

enjoyable or less meaningful in its absence. The emotional attachment that alcoholics feel toward alcohol should not be underestimated, and its strength is dramatically demonstrated when they continue to drink in the face of life-threatening liver or heart disease. It is unclear whether the attraction to alcohol is based primarily on its rewarding qualities or its ability to reverse unpleasant mood associated with abstinence. In either event, clinicians are challenged by the alcoholic's inexorable tendency to drink regardless of adverse life consequences, past promises, and logical considerations. Their loss of control over alcohol intake is not particularly amenable to rational approaches, presumably because it results from the disruption of limbic regions that mediate motivation and reward.

Craving is an essential feature of alcoholism that serves to perpetuate the addiction through negative reinforcement. Alcohol is thought to produce craving by dysregulating brain centers that mediate survival-related drives, and specific regions of activation during craving induced by alcohol cues have been demonstrated with brain imaging studies [4]. While talking therapy can reduce craving, the high rate of recidivism with alcoholism demonstrates the intrinsic difficulty of treating a biological phenomenon with psychological treatments alone. Through conditioning, environmental stimuli associated with alcohol consumption gain the ability to generate intense craving in alcoholics. Many environmental stimuli that are very difficult to avoid, such as restaurants, social events, and advertisements depicting alcohol, can trigger cue-induced craving. Elucidating neuronal mechanisms of cue-induced craving may identify pharmacological treatments for this important negative reinforcer.

Alcoholism is often perpetuated by denial, a cardinal feature of the disorder. Denial shields alcoholics from gaining insight into their problem even when it is obvious to most external observers. Denial and motivation for sobriety tend to be inversely related, and many alcoholics drink without concern until reality shatters their denial system and forces them to reconsider their predicament. Job loss, family turmoil, divorce, legal charges, and medical problems may surprise alcoholics who were otherwise oblivious to the adverse effects of their drinking. Alcoholism is associated with reduced metabolism in the frontal cortex that may contribute to these deficits in executive function and logical decision making. A final clinical aspect of alcoholism is that of progression, or the tendency for alcohol use and alcohol-related problems to worsen over time. An interesting aspect of progression is seen when recovering alcoholics relapse after long periods of sobriety, and then promptly resort to the same patterns of alcoholism that predated their abstinence. The mechanism of progression is not understood, but the persistent vulnerability of alcoholics may involve changes in brain pathways leading to a permanent proneness to relapse.

III. BIOLOGICAL FEATURES OF ALCOHOLISM

The biological effects of alcohol are influenced by hereditary factors and vary greatly across individuals. It has been estimated that children of alcoholics have a fivefold greater chance of developing the disease than those lacking a family history [5], even after being adopted away [6]. In fact, genetic variables are thought to explain between 40% and 60% of the risk of developing alcoholism [7], and polymorphism affecting the metabolism, rewarding, and aversive qualities of alcohol may account for much of this influence. For instance, Asians are thought to have lower rates of alcoholism because they frequently experience flushing and anxiety after drinking. This reaction results from the buildup of acetaldehyde, a toxic metabolite of alcohol that is normally inactivated by the enzyme aldehyde dehydrogenase. Asians commonly inherit an allele that codes for an inefficient form of aldehyde dehydrogenase, leading to the reaction described above. Conversely, an inherited tolerance to aversive intoxication effects of alcohol is associated with an increased risk of developing the disorder [8]. Furthermore, individuals with a family history of alcoholism show an enhanced release of β-endorphin after drinking and may therefore experience a greater intensity of alcohol-induced euphoria [9]. Numerous genes undoubtedly contribute to risk, although genetic vulnerability neither predetermines the development of alcoholism nor serves as a prerequisite for the disease.

Subsequent sections of this chapter will review the acute and chronic actions of alcohol in the brain. Because they often reflect compensatory mechanisms, chronic neuroadaptations to alcohol tend to be opposite to the acute effects of this drug. For instance, the acute administration of alcohol enhances GABA and dopamine (DA) neurotransmission, both of which are reduced after chronic exposure. Similarly, alcohol initially inhibits glutamate neurotransmission, while repeated doses of alcohol enhance excitatory glutamatergic neurotransmission, contributing to many of the clinical signs and symptoms of alcohol withdrawal.

Similar opposite effects may also occur in endogenous opioid peptide (EOP) systems that are initially activated by alcohol. The linkage of neurotransmitter function with subjective states such as alcohol intoxication and alcohol withdrawal is remarkable and provides biological insight into important clinical phenomena of alcoholism.

This chapter will focus on the neurotransmitter actions of alcohol that occur in specific regions of the brain. Unlike most addictive agents, which attach tightly to specific membrane-bound receptors, alcohol exerts its actions on several neurotransmitter systems through nonspecific and poorly understood mechanisms. The major systems affected by alcohol include GABA, glutamate, EOP, DA, and serotonin-containing neurons that not only comprise the reward centers but also mediate numerous functions that are entirely unrelated to reward. For instance, alcohol-induced ataxia is mediated by GABA neurons in the cerebellum that are unrelated to alcohol reward. On the other hand, GABA-containing neurons found in key anatomical sites such as the nucleus accumbens (NAc) and the central nucleus of the amygdala are intimately involved in alcohol reward and the mechanisms of addiction. Interestingly, many GABA-containing neurons that comprise the reward centers also produce endogenous opioids and express EOP receptor types [10]. Because localization is essential in the neurobiology of alcoholism, the next section will review the anatomy and circuitry of brain reward regions.

IV. REWARD CENTERS

Addictive agents such as alcohol are thought to produce reward by activating brain centers that have evolved to ensure survival. In fact, the potential lethality of alcohol may derive in part from its disruption of survival-related systems in the brain. Brain regions that normally mediate the natural drive states of hunger and libido are presumably recruited during alcohol craving, explaining its potency as a negative reinforcer. Specific anatomical regions and neuronal circuits comprising the reward centers have been studied extensively and include the NAc and amygdala (extended amygdala), the DA-containing ventral tegmentum (VTA), the lateral hypothalamus, and the medial prefrontal cortex (PFC). Reward circuitry may be viewed as the anatomical substrate of alcoholism, much as the liver is the organ of involvement in cirrhosis.

Mesocorticolimbic DA neurons in the VTA, also termed the A10 region, play a critical role in appetitive and consummatory reward. These cell bodies comprise ~85% of VTA neurons and engage in baseline pacemaker activity at rest and characteristic burst firing when activated. DA burst firing occurs with the consumption of food [11] and fluid [12], as well as during sexual activity [13]. VTA burst firing also occurs after animals are exposed to appetitive cues, such as the sight or smell of food, or the presence of a mating opportunity [14]. DA release thus reinforces the consumption and procurement of survival-related goals, and provides the vigilance, psychomotor activation, and motivational drive that are characteristic of mesocorticolimbic arousal. Satiety does not appear to be associated with DA firing but may result from opioid receptor activation that punctuates survival-related behavior through a DA-independent reward mechanism [15]. As we will discuss, alcohol acutely stimulates both DA and EOP release, resulting in enhanced neurotransmission through both systems [16].

The VTA sends major projections to the NAc and the amygdala, the medial prefrontal and anterior cingulate cortex, and other targets such as the EOP-rich ventral pallidum. The A10 DA-containing neurons are often classified as either mesolimbic or mesocortical, and a recent study has clarified that subpopulations of DA neurons project specifically to either limbic or cortical regions [17] (Fig. 1). The shell of the NAc, also termed the universal addiction site, receives a large bundle of mesolimbic projections that release DA in response to all known addictive drugs, including alcohol, cocaine, amphetamine, heroin, marijuana, phencyclidine (PCP), and nicotine [18]. The release of DA into the NAc may thus be viewed as a neurochemical signature of drug reward. DA release into the NAc shell is a result of VTA burst firing, as seen with food consumption and sexual activity, demonstrating that natural reward centers are recruited during alcohol intoxication.

The universal addiction site comprises medium-size spiny cells that have very interesting characteristics. These NAc neurons utilize GABA as their primary neurotransmitter, but also synthesize enkephalin and dynorphin. GABA-containing neurons in the central nucleus of the amygdala and the bed nucleus of the stria terminalis share embryological and cytoarchitectural features with medium-size spiny cells in the NAc, and these three structures comprise the extended amygdala [19]. The extended amygdala forms reciprocal connections with the frontal cortex, hippocampus, midbrain, mediodorsal thalamus, and hypothalamus and is conceptualized to be a system of forebrain circuitry that mediates emotional, motor, visceral, and

Neurobiology of Alcoholism

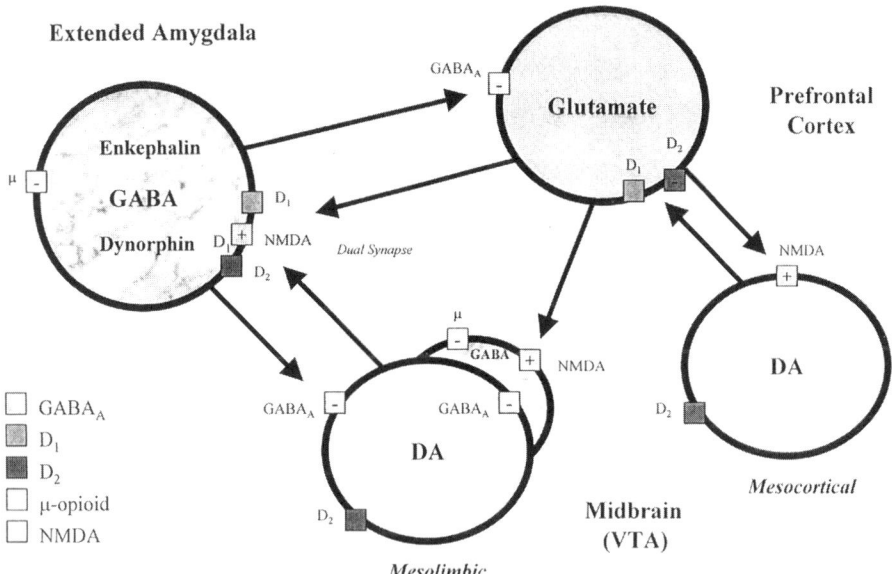

Figure 1 **Brain pathways involved in alcoholism.** $GABA_A$ and DA neurotransmission are enhanced by alcohol while NMDA neurotransmission is attenuated. Opposite effects occur with chronic alcohol exposure, including DA depletion. $5HT_3$ neurotransmission is increased by alcohol. EOP and GABA neurotransmitters colocalize in the NAc and the extended amygdala. Glutamatergic projections form the PFC form dual synapses with DA projections on GABA/EOP target neurons. Hypothalamic cell bodies release β-endorphin in the NAc and VTA. Stimulation of μ and δ opioid and DA receptors contributes to alcohol reward.

hormonal responses to the environment. EOP involvement in the extended amygdala is very pronounced. As with cells in the shell of the NAc, neurons in the central nucleus of the amygdala and stria terminalis contain GABA, synthesize endogenous opioids [20], and express EOP receptors [21].

In the NAc, there is evidence that separate populations of medium-size spiny cells contain either enkephalin or dynorphin, with the dynorphin-containing GABA/EOP neuron typically expressing D_1 receptors and enkephalin-containing neuron expressing D_2 membrane receptors [10]. Dynorphin and enkephalin regulate the VTA in opposite directions. Dynorphin inhibits DA release and has aversive qualities, whereas enkephalin releases DA and is rewarding [10]. This dichotomy is important because animal studies demonstrate enkephalin release with alcohol administration [22] and dynorphin release during the aversive state of alcohol withdrawal [23]. Dynorphin-containing axons tend to be long and project to distant κ-opioid receptors, while shorter enkephalin-containing fibers activate δ and μ opioid receptors. That the universal addiction site (NAc) and other elements of the extended amygdala are rich in opioid receptors and endogenous opioids is noteworthy and has important implications with respect to alcoholism.

GABA/EOP neurons in the extended amygdala express DA receptors that mediate mesolimbic DA neurotransmission. As a matter of review, there are five known types of DA receptors that are usually classified as the D_1 family (including D_1 and D_5 receptors) or the D_2 family (including D_2, D_3, and D_4 receptors) that are grouped on the basis of homologous residue sequences. D_1 and D_2 receptor families often affect neuronal function in opposite directions, as evidenced by their actions on second-messenger systems. D_1 receptors increase cAMP formation by activating the excitatory G-protein (G_s) whereas D_2 receptors inhibit cAMP formation by activating the inhibitory G-protein (G_i). D_2 receptor polymorphism may affect the risk of developing alcoholism [24].

The effect of DA release on GABA/EOP firing rates is very complicated. While D_2 activation tends be inhibitory, D_1 receptor activation can either increase or decrease neuronal firing of GABA/EOP neurons, depending on their preexisting state. When these NAc neurons are in the "down" state they are further inhibited by D_1 activation, while those in the "up" state they are further excited [25]. Therefore, modulatory DA projections to GABA/EOP-containing neurons can either excite or inhibit neuronal firing, and has the effect of increasing the signal-to-noise ratio. In addition, DA modulation tends to occur in concert with excitatory glutamate projections. DA and glutamate axons actually form dual-synapses on GABA/EOP-containing neurons in the NAc [26] (Fig. 1), creating an interesting convergence of DA, glutamate, GABA, and EOP neurons, all of which are strongly implicated in alcohol reward and alcohol dependence.

Reciprocal fibers from GABA/EOP-containing neurons project to the VTA and provide tonic inhibition by stimulating GABA receptors that are located on DA neurons. Regulation is also furnished by serotonin axons arising in the raphe nucleus that project to the VTA and the NAc. These projections probably mediate serotonergic influences on reward circuitry that affect the risk and development of alcoholism. Inhibitory GABA-containing interneurons in VTA, and those projecting from the extended amygdala, express μ opioid receptors on their neuronal membranes. The stimulation of these μ receptors hyperpolarizes GABA neurons, thereby releasing DA neurons from tonic GABA inhibition (Fig. 1). Opioid receptors found in the extended amygdala and VTA are thought to play an essential role in the rewarding properties of alcohol [27].

The amygdala has been implicated in reward-related memory and the recognition of emotionally relevant stimuli. The central nucleus of the amygdala is populated by GABA/EOP-containing neurons [28] and is clearly involved in alcohol reward and alcohol withdrawal. This region of the extended amygdala shares attributes with the NAc, and is distinct from the basolateral nucleus of the amygdala that is composed primarily of quasi-cortical glutamate-containing neurons. The microinjection of GABA$_A$ antagonists directly into the central nucleus of the amygdala reduces lever pressing for alcohol [29], suggesting a role for GABA$_A$ neurotransmission in alcohol reward. Injection of EOP antagonists into the central nucleus also suppresses alcohol self-administration, further indicating this structure's importance in alcohol reward. The central nucleus of the amygdala also produces corticotropin-releasing factor (CRF) which is released in response to stress and anxiety. CRF functions as a centrally acting peptide and activates the hypothalamic-pituitary-adrenal (HPA) axis, releasing cortisol and other stress hormones into the bloodstream. CRF levels are elevated during alcohol withdrawal and during withdrawal from cocaine, opiates, and marijuana. Interesting, CRF antagonists injected directly into the central nucleus of the amygdala attenuate symptoms of alcohol withdrawal [18], including withdrawal seizures [30].

Projections from the frontal cortex and the hippocampus to reward circuitry is provided by glutamate-containing pyramidal cells. These neurons, along with glutamate projections from the basolateral amygdala and thalamus, activate excitatory NMDA, AMPA, and KA glutamate receptors that are located on DA and GABA/EOP neurons (Fig. 1). When activated, the glutamate receptors open gated ion channels that allow positively charged Ca^{2+} and Na^+ ions to travel down their concentration gradients into signal-receiving neurons, resulting in neuronal excitation. Alcohol interferes with this process through the allosteric blockade of NMDA neurotransmission, thereby inhibiting frontal lobe projections to the extended amygdala and other limbic structures. This effect is interesting in light of the notorious disinhibition of frontal lobe functions by alcohol, such as executive decision making and impulse control. Similarly, the disruption of memory during alcohol intoxication (including "blackouts") may result from NMDA blockade in the hippocampus. Although alcohol acutely blocks NMDA neurotransmission, chronic alcohol exposure increases the number of NMDA receptors.

The PFC also sends excitatory axons to the VTA that stimulate NMDA receptors located on the cell bodies of DA neurons that are exclusively mesocortical [17]. The medial forebrain bundle conveys this glutamatergic projection to the VTA, along with reciprocal DA fibers, forming a circuit that has been extensively studied and implicated in reward, working memory, goal-directed behavior, and schizophrenia [31]. Mesolimbic DA neurons that project to the NAc and form the "reward circuit" do not receive glutamate fibers from the PFC (Fig. 1). However, GABA-containing neurons in the VTA do receive glutamate projections and could mediate cortical suppression of reward circuitry [17]. NMDA blockade by alcohol undermines cortical influence and may play a role in certain intoxicating effects of alcohol.

GABA/EOP cells in the NAc are outflow neurons, capable of sending long projections to distant brain regions that complete several multisynaptic loops of the reward circuitry. These axons exert inhibitory effects on target neurons through the activation of GABA (GABA$_A$ and GABA$_B$) receptors, and also release endogenous opioids. Alcohol enhances the sensitivity GABA$_A$ receptors to GABA, thereby increasing inhibitory neurotransmission in these circuits. Direct projections from the NAc extend to the lateral hypothalamus and preoptic areas, EOP-rich regions that are strongly implicated in consummatory reward associated with feeding, drinking, and sexual activity. Hypothalamic cell bodies in the nucleus arcuatus send β-endorphin-containing axons, in turn, to the NAc, the VTA, and many cerebral and limbic regions [27]. Indirect outflow from the NAc projects to the ventral pallidum, a relay structure that is also implicated in motivation, drug-seeking behavior, and the processing of reward information through opioid modulation [32]. The ventral pallidum, in turn, projects through thalamic nuclei to the frontal lobe, including the PFC and the anterior cingulate.

The pallidal-thalamocortical pathway has been termed the "motive circuit" and is strongly implicated in drug craving. Positron emission tomography (PET) measurements in normal subjects demonstrate that alcohol-induced euphoria correlates with cerebral metabolic inhibition [33]. Also, alcoholics show reduced blood flow at baseline in the left orbitofrontal cortex and prefrontal cortex [34], which is positively correlated with the duration and severity of alcohol dependence [35]. It is unclear whether hypofrontality precedes or results from alcohol exposure. Individuals with a family history of alcoholism experience a more rapid inhibition of prefrontal regions by alcohol, suggesting a genetic influence [36]. Although orbitofrontal and cingulate metabolic inhibition can be protracted [37], hypofrontality may result in part from alcohol exposure because it varies with severity and can eventually disappear with abstinence [38]. The effect of hypofrontality on frontal lobe function is not known, but this alteration could underlie some of the clinical characteristics of alcoholics, including denial, impaired judgment, and the inability to control limbic impulses.

This discussion of brain reward centers is by no means exhaustive, and is meant to provide some anatomical familiarity with neurotransmitter systems that are involved in alcoholism. As we will discuss in the following sections, alcohol exerts significant actions, acutely and chronically, on this interconnected network of pleasure circuitry. Ultimately, a more refined understanding of neuronal mechanism involved in alcoholism should uncover effective therapeutic agents, as exemplified by the discovery of naltrexone. In addition, delineating the biological basis of alcoholism should undermine the still popular notion that alcoholics are weak or morally challenged, rather than suffering from a brain disorder. The next sections will focus on the major neurotransmitter actions of alcohol and review the compelling evidence that the neurobiology of alcoholism involves the dysregulation of reward centers in the brain.

V. GABA

It is well established that alcohol facilitates GABA-mediated neurotransmission in most brain regions, an action that contributes to many of its depressant effects. GABA receptors are ubiquitous in the brain, perhaps explaining why imaging studies show marked suppression of whole-brain and regional metabolism after alcohol administration. GABA-ergic effects of alcohol are mediated primarily by $GABA_A$ receptors, a heterogeneous family of ligand-gated ion channels that constitute the primary GABA receptor group [39]. However, alcohol also increases neurotransmission through the $GABA_B$ receptor [40], a metabotropic complex that is linked to the Gi-protein, as are μ opioid and D_2 receptors. $GABA_B$ stimulation lowers cAMP levels within signal-receiving neurons [41], an interesting effect that has been linked to drug reward [42]. The $GABA_A$ receptor is an integrated complex of five protein molecules that spans the neuronal membrane, forming a channel at the center that is specifically permeable to Cl^- ions. This protein complex varies in composition across different brain regions, perhaps explaining differential sensitivity to alcohol. Receptor activation by GABA increases the flow of negatively charged Cl^- ions into signal-receiving neurons, causing hyperpolarization and neuronal inhibition.

While it is known that benzodiazepines and barbiturates bind α and γ subunits the $GABA_A$ receptor (that are separate and distinct from the GABA-binding site) [43], the precise mechanism by which alcohol enhances $GABA_A$ neurotransmission is a matter of debate. It has been hypothesized that alcohol produces allosteric modulation of $GABA_A$ receptors by either binding hydrophobic regions of the protein complex or changing the surrounding lipid environment. This latter explanation might explain why alcohol affects several ligand and voltage-gated ion channels. In either case, increased $GABA_A$ neurotransmission occurs and is specifically responsible for some of the intoxicating effects of alcohol, such as ataxia and sedation [18].

In addition to extraneuronal receptor binding sites, the $GABA_A$ receptor has important intracellular binding regions that are regulated by phosphorylation. In fact, a number of studies suggest that the action of alcohol requires $GABA_A$ receptor phosphorylation by protein kinase C (PKC) enzymes. This conclusion is based on studies demonstrating that PKC knockout mice do not display enhancement of GABA$_A$ neurotransmission by alcohol, and have reduced behavioral effects after alcohol administration [44]. Furthermore, agents that increase protein phosphorylation within neurons, such as β-adrenergic receptor agonists (which stimulate PKC), enhance the effect of alcohol on GABA neurotransmission [45,46]. GABA$_B$ stimulation also facilitates the effect of alcohol on GABA$_A$ neurotransmission [47].

There is compelling evidence that alcohol tolerance is mediated by compensatory changes involving the GABA$_A$ receptor. After repeated doses, there develops a marked reduction in the ability of alcohol to enhance GABA$_A$ neurotransmission, as measured by Cl$^-$ conductance through GABA$_A$-gated ion channels. GABA$_A$ downregulation results from a reduction in GABA$_A$ receptor density [48]. Several studies have reported decreased levels of the GABA$_A$ α_1 subunit after chronic alcohol exposure, and reduced synthesis of the receptor complex is also suggested by altered gene expression of GABA$_A$ subunits (Table 2). A reduction in the number of GABA$_A$ receptors reduces the effect of alcohol on this system, contributing to alcohol tolerance. Benzodiazepines and barbiturates produce a similar downregulation of the GABA$_A$ receptor with repeated administration [49], explaining why alcoholics develop cross-tolerance to these agents. Therefore, while alcohol enhances GABA$_A$ neurotransmission, this effect is reduced as these receptors disappear, leading to the acquisition of tolerance.

Reduced GABA$_A$ neurotransmission may also contribute to alcohol withdrawal, and a reduction of inhibitory neurotransmission could explain the overall neuronal excitability and convulsant vulnerability of this syndrome. Animals bred to experience severe alcohol withdrawal show linkage of this trait to genes encoding GABA$_A$ α_1, α_6, and γ_2 subunits by quantitative trait analyses [50]. Bicuculline, a GABA$_A$ antagonist, is much more likely to induce seizures during alcohol withdrawal, presumably owing to reduced GABA tone [51]. Furthermore, alcohol-withdrawal seizures respond to anticonvulsants that enhance GABA function. Indeed, both alcohol withdrawal symptoms and withdrawal-related seizures can be prevented by the administration of benzodiazepines or barbiturates, which increase GABA$_A$ neurotransmission. Therefore, the inhibition of GABA$_A$ neurotransmission by repeated alcohol administration contributes to both alcohol tolerance and withdrawal symptoms.

GABA function is also implicated in an individual's susceptibility for developing alcoholism. One imaging study of subjects with a significant family history of alcoholism found evidence of reduced GABA$_A$ function [52]. Another study reported low levels of GABA benzodiazepine (GABA$_A$) receptor in certain brain regions of abstinent alcoholics [53], representing either a genetic predisposition or an alcohol-induced effect. These findings are consistent with a classic study showing reduced physiological response to alcohol in sons of alcoholics who later develop alcoholism [8]. An inherited deficit of GABA$_A$ function may be associated with the development of alcoholism because it might allow a greater consumption of alcohol owing to fewer aversive intoxication effects.

GABA$_A$ receptor function may be linked to alcohol reward because sons of alcoholics have enhanced mood effects in response to benzodiazepines [36,54]. Since benzodiazepines are similar in action to alcohol, preference for these agents may correlate with preference for alcohol. Regional GABA$_A$ alterations in the extended amygdala may be associated with alcohol reward, as evidenced by the finding that alcohol-preferring rats have increased GABA-containing terminals in the NAc but show no differences in other regions [55]. Also, GABA$_A$ antagonists applied directly into the central nucleus of the amygdala reduce alcohol self-administration [29]. Since GABA$_A$ receptors are found throughout the brain and have varying composition, depending on their location, the significance of GABA$_A$ receptor findings within discrete regions of the extended amygdala is unclear.

Additional information regarding the role of the GABA$_A$ receptor in alcohol dependence is furnished by studies on allopregnanolone. Allopregnanolone is a metabolite of progesterone that binds the GABA$_A$ receptor complex and powerfully augments Cl$^-$ conductance. This leads to the enhancement of GABA$_A$ function and may explain the anticonvulsant action of allopregnanolone when administered during alcohol withdrawal [56]. Since alcohol withdrawal is also associated with reduced levels of allopregnanolone, a protective role for this hormone has been proposed [56]. This and other actions of allopregnanolone may contribute to gender differences in alcoholism.

It can be concluded that alcohol acutely enhances GABA$_A$ neurotransmission through an allosteric mechanism. A number of studies suggest that this acute action on GABA$_A$ receptors is associated with the more aversive intoxicating effects of alcohol, such as ataxia and sedation. Genetic studies also suggest that polymorphism for the GABA$_A$ receptor can affect alcohol intake. The response of the GABA$_A$ receptor to repeated administration of alcohol warrants particular emphasis. Since disruption in GABA neurotransmission can lead to either seizures or coma, this system displays homeostatic responses to exogenous influences such as alcohol exposure. Compelling evidence suggests that GABA$_A$ downregulation is an important compensatory response to GABA$_A$ enhancement by alcohol. This response results in tolerance and the alcohol withdrawal syndrome.

VI. GLUTAMATE

Glutamate, the principal excitatory neurotransmitter in the brain, is released in regions that mediate drug reward and dependence. Cortical glutamatergic cell bodies in the frontal cortex and hippocampus are implicated in many essential functions relating to addiction, including executive decision making, reward, learning, and memory. The glutamate system is associated with three known receptor families (termed NMDA, AMPA, and KA) that excite target neurons by increasing the conductance of positively charged ions. AMPA and KA receptors gate Na$^+$-specific ion channels, while NMDA receptors gate both Na$^+$ and Ca^{2+} ion channels. NMDA receptors are best activated in the presence of Mg^{2+} ions and glycine, and generally require some prior depolarization of the membrane by adjacent KA or AMPA receptors. This produces a delayed onset of NMDA excitation that may be conducive to certain neural functions such as memory.

Alcohol interferes with signal transmission through the NMDA receptor, reducing the flow of Ca^{2+} and Na$^+$ through NMDA-gated ion channels in the presence of glutamate. This action reduces excitatory neurotransmission in the brain [57] and thereby compounds inhibitory GABA$_A$ effects of alcohol. The mechanism by which alcohol diminishes NMDA sensitivity to glutamate may involve presynaptic GABA$_B$ receptors because the action is eliminated by GABA$_B$ antagonists [40]. NMDA blockade has been shown to vary linearly with aversive intoxicating effects of alcohol [57].

Repeated alcohol administration upregulates the NMDA receptor, producing an increased number of binding sites and increasing excitatory neurotransmission [58]. This action appears to represent a compensatory response to NMDA blockade by alcohol, similar to that seen with the GABA$_A$ complex. NMDA supersensitivity with chronic alcohol exposure involves increased synthesis of the receptor protein, as evidenced by elevated mRNA levels for various subunits [59], and this neuroadaptation normalizes with the abatement of withdrawal symptoms [60]. During withdrawal, increased glutamate has been measured in the NAc, hippocampus, and striatum, with levels exceeding 250% of baseline [61]. The combination of NMDA supersensitivity and elevated glutamate levels produces profound neuronal activation which is mechanistically linked to alcohol withdrawal. In fact, NMDA antagonists are capable of reversing alcohol withdrawal [61]. NMDA perturbations associated with alcohol dependence may be reversed by acamprosate, a partial NMDA agonist [62]. Studied extensively in Europe on > 3000 patients, acamprosate has been found to enhance abstinence [63] and normalize glutamate overactivity during alcohol withdrawal [64].

Alcohol also affects nongated voltage-sensitive Ca^{2+} channels. These channels become increasingly permeable to Ca^{2+} as the neuron begins to depolarize, speeding up the process that generates an action potential. Calcium channel blockers, such as dihydropyridine (DHP), are widely prescribed in the treatment of hypertension and cardiac illness and produce their therapeutic effects by antagonizing voltage-sensitive Ca^{2+} channels. Interestingly, chronic alcohol administration has been shown to increase the number of DHP-binding sites by $\sim$ 50%, contributing further to neuronal excitability during alcohol withdrawal [65]. In fact, mice bred specifically to experience severe alcohol withdrawal show a greater increase in DHP-binding sites. The role of voltage-sensitive Ca^{2+} channels in alcohol withdrawal has led to the consideration of calcium channel blockers as a treatment for this condition.

A final consideration regarding glutamate systems and alcoholism is that of glutamate toxicity, a cause of neuronal death secondary to the toxic effects of excessive Ca^{2+} influx. Excessive levels of intraneuronal Ca^{2+} can result from the upregulation of NMDA receptors and voltage-sensitive Ca^{2+} channels, both known consequences of chronic alcohol exposure. It has been suggested that glutamate toxicity is more likely to occur with a binge pattern of drinking because episodic high levels of alcohol alternate with abstinence [66]. Alcohol-induced activation of the HPA [67] may also contribute to glutamate toxicity since glucocorticoids augment Ca^{2+} conductance through NMDA-gated ion channels [68]. Glutamate toxicity is thought to be the cause of alcohol-related brain toxicity, such as that seen with delirium tremens, Wernicke-Korsakoff syndrome [69], dementia, and fetal alcohol syndrome [70].

The full implications of glutamate toxicity in alcoholism are potentially far-reaching. Aside from its proposed involvement in severe forms of neurotoxicity, glutamate toxicity could contribute to more subtle impairment of cortical function, which is evident on imaging studies. A number of these studies report reduced frontal-lobe metabolism in chronic alcoholics, affecting the prefrontal cortex, orbitofrontal cortex, and the anterior cingulate regions. Hypofrontality in alcoholics could result from glutamate toxicity and contribute to phenomena indicative of poor executive function such as denial, difficulty suppressing destructive impulses, and maladaptive decision-making capabilities. Hypofrontality in alcoholics could also explain, to some extent, the notorious ineffectiveness of logical treatment recommendations in the clinical setting.

VII. SEROTONIN

Serotonin pathways, known to influence emotion, motivation, and attention, have also been implicated in the neurobiology of alcoholism [18]. Serotonin cell bodies located in the raphe nuclei and hypothalamus modulate brain reward through projections to the VTA, amygdala, NAc, and other crucial reward regions. Animal studies generally show that manipulations of serotonin neurotransmission have an inverse effect on alcohol intake [71]. For instance, serotonin depletion increases alcohol self-administration while serotonin enhancement reduces alcohol intake [72]. In animal studies, the acute administration of alcohol releases brain serotonin and specifically elevates serotonin levels in the NAc [73]. Similarly, human subjects show increased levels of serotonin metabolites in the blood and urine after alcohol administration [71]. The ability of alcohol to release serotonin is diminished with repeated administration [74] and may represent a significant neuroadaptation in the development of alcohol dependence.

Serotonin receptors are linked to G-proteins that activate second messenger cascades and alter ion channels, causing multiple effects on neuronal function and gene expression. These receptors are dense in limbic regions, and $5HT_3$ receptors are found on the terminals of mesocorticolimbic DA neurons. Alcohol enhances $5HT_3$ neurotransmission through an allosteric receptor action [75], an effect that would be expected to release DA from NAc terminals. Furthermore, with repeated administration of alcohol, the $5HT_3$ receptor is upregulated [74], perhaps to compensate for reductions in alcohol-induced serotonin release noted above. Some studies suggest that EOP release with alcohol administration, thought to underlie alcohol reward, may be a consequence of $5HT_3$ activation. Serotonin agonists increase levels of β-endorphin [76], and a recent study demonstrated that serotonin, applied directly into the NAc, produced a 190% increase in β-endorphin [77]. This may explain findings that alcohol-induced positive mood effects can be blocked by administration of ondansetron, a $5HT_3$ antagonist [78]. These data suggest that serotonin release may contribute to alcohol reward by activating the endogenous opioid systems through the $5HT_3$ receptor.

Table 2 Summary of Acute and Chronic Effects of Alcohol in Animals and Humans

	Acute	Chronic
Animals	Increased $GABA_A$ neurotransmission Decreased NMDA neurotransmission DA release and burst firing Acute reversal of DA depletion β-Endorphin and enkephalin release Serotonin release (NAc) Increased $5HT_3$ neurotransmission Brain reward by alcohol (lever pressing)	Decreased $GABA_A$ neurotransmission Increased NMDA neurotransmission DA depletion and reduced firing Chronic worsening of DA depletion Decreased β-endorphin levels Reduced serotonin release after alcohol $5HT_3$ upregulation Reduction in brain reward (ICSS Increased CRF levels
Humans	Increased β-endorphin release Metabolic suppression ($GABA_A$ effect) Serotonin release	Decreased β-endorphin levels Low levels of $GABA_A$ receptor (imaging) Serotonin deficiency

Genetic studies further link alcoholism with serotonin mechanisms. Alcohol-preferring rats have a number of serotonin abnormalities, including lower brain content of serotonin, fewer receptor sites, and a reduced number of immunostained serotonin fibers [73]. In addition, alcohol-preferring rats have fewer serotonin cell bodies and reduced serotonin levels in the NAc [71]. Conversely, mice bred to overexpress 5HT$_3$ receptors are very sensitive to the intoxicating effects of alcohol, and show reduced consumption [79]. There is evidence that a subgroup of alcoholics have constitutionally low levels of serotonin as well as early onset, a positive family history of alcoholism, and antisocial behaviors [1,71,80]. These alcoholics have reduced CSF concentrations of 5-hydroxyindoleascetic acid (5HIAA), consistent with reduced brain levels of serotonin [71]. Serotonin deficiency states could result from polymorphism affecting the synthetic enzyme of serotonin, tryptophan hydroxylase, which has been associated with alcoholism, suicidality, and impulsivity [81]. Since alcohol releases serotonin, individuals with inherited reductions of serotonin function may be predisposed to using alcohol as a means of achieving balance [82].

Serotonin pathways may also influence alcohol reward through DA mechanisms. The application of a 5HT$_3$ selective agonist into the NAc produces a 1000% rise in DA levels [83], thought to be mediated by 5HT$_3$ receptors located on the terminals of mesolimbic DA neurons [84]. Also, pretreatment with a 5HT$_3$ antagonist prevents the ability of alcohol to release DA into the NAc [73], similar to the ability of opioid antagonists to block alcohol-induced DA release [16]. Serotonin has also been reported to enhance DA release by alcohol through 5HT$_2$ receptor activation [85].

Although serotonin systems are clearly involved in the neurobiology of alcoholism, and their pharmacological manipulation can alter alcohol intake by laboratory animals, clinical trials with serotonin agents have yielded inconsistent results in alcoholics. There is some evidence that a subgroup of alcoholics with serotonin deficiency may benefit from serotonin agonists, such as selective serotonin reuptake inhibitor (SSRI) agents [63]. Ondansetron, a 5HT$_3$ antagonist, may be effective in a subgroup of alcoholics, but requires further study [78]. It appears that serotonin affects alcohol reward indirectly, by facilitating either the release of endogenous opioids or the release of DA after alcohol administration. This indirect effect may explain the modest action of serotonergic agents in the clinical setting.

VIII. DOPAMINE

Mesocorticolimbic DA neurons are intrinsically involved in natural reward states, and are directly and indirectly activated by alcohol. Alcohol increases the release, synthesis, and turnover of DA, and numerous animal studies have implicated this system in the neurobiology of alcoholism [48]. Rats bred to prefer alcohol show enhanced DA release after alcohol, while D$_2$ knockout rats (rats genetically lacking D$_2$ receptors) show aversion to alcohol (Table 3). Biological impairment of D$_2$ receptors in the NAc of rats with antisense oligodeoxynucleotide sharply reduces alcohol intake [86], again suggesting a role for the D$_2$ receptor in alcohol reward. Disassociated DA neurons from the VTA show robust firing when bathed in alcohol [87]. Since this effect is independent of neuronal interconnections, it demonstrates the ability of alcohol to directly stimulate DA neurons. In addition, the systemic administration of alcohol releases DA into the NAc and other regions of the extended amygdala [88]. Therefore, it is tempting to conclude that DA activation contributes significantly to alcohol reward. However, a number of animal studies link the rewarding properties of alcohol more to EOP receptor activation, as will be discussed.

DA neurotransmission has not been established to be essential to the rewarding action of alcohol. DA antagonists administered systemically or applied directly into reward centers do not consistently alter lever pressing for alcohol [48], and show no effect in some studies [72]. Furthermore, the destruction of mesolimbic DA neurons projecting to the NAc fails to alter the acquisition or maintenance of alcohol self-administration [72], strongly suggesting a DA-independent mechanism in the rewarding action of alcohol. Another study reported that the chemical ablation of DA projections to all regions of the extended amygdala failed to alter alcohol self-administration [89], again suggesting that while DA release occurs during alcohol ingestion, it is not a critical mechanism for alcohol reward. In fact, the ability of alcohol to release DA into the NAc can be completely blocked by naltrindole, a δ opioid antagonist [16], strongly implicating the involvement of EOP neurotransmission in the mechanism of alcohol reward.

As seen with other addictive substances, chronic exposure to alcohol produces functional inhibition of DA pathways. Repeated alcohol administration results in decreased DA release [88] and an inhibition of DA neuronal firing [90]. The latter effect was found to be associated with dramatic reductions in DA outflow that persisted well past the period of alcohol withdrawal. It has been suggested that DA depletion is a clinically significant phenomenon in alcoholism, contributing to craving and hedonic inhibition in alcoholics [91]. An animal model of hedonic function has been developed that utilizes intracranial self-stimulation (ICSS), in which electrical current is delivered into DA-containing regions of the reward centers. Chronic exposure to alcohol increases the threshold of electrical current that is required for ICSS [92], indicating a reduction of hedonic tone that is thought to result from DA depletion. Given the important role of mesocorticolimbic neurons in orchestrating natural reward states, and the action of alcohol on reward thresholds, it is a reasonable hypothesis that DA depletion by alcohol might have an adverse effect on human hedonic function. This could explain the high prevalence of depression and suicide in alcoholics, and the dysphoria commonly experienced with abstinence. Therefore, the link between DA depletion and craving, first proposed with cocaine [93], may also hold with alcohol. Interestingly, DA depletion is acutely reversed by the administration of alcohol [90], and drinking may relieve craving through a DA mechanism. In effect, alcohol may be consumed to temporarily correct the very imbalance it produces. DA depletion by alcohol, measured through microdialysis in the NAc, can also be reversed by the administration of an NMDA antagonist [94]. NMDA antagonism may release DA by suppressing GABA/EOP reciprocals to the VTA. D_2 receptor agonists, such as bromocriptine, have not been found to be particularly effective in alcoholics. However, the dysregulation of mesocorticolimbic neurons by alcohol may be too profound to be reversed by mere DA receptor stimulation.

IX. OPIOIDS

Endogenous opioids in the brain are classified as endorphins, enkephalins, and dynorphins, with each class derived from a distinct precursor molecule. These molecules are cleaved by peptidases and then modified through the addition of various chemical groups, creating many representatives of each of the three classes in the brain. Enkephalin-containing neurons tend to have short axons while those that synthesize β-endorphin and dynorphin have longer axons and project to more distant brain regions. Several brain areas that form part of the reward circuitry, such as the extended amygdala and the hypothalamus, are populated by opioid-containing cell bodies. The pituitary and adrenal glands also synthesize endogenous opioids that are released in response to stress and a number of physiological conditions. Three opioid receptor families (μ, δ, and κ) have been identified,

Table 3 Summary of Effects of Alcohol in Alcohol-Craving Animals, Animals Bred with Specific Traits, and Nonalcoholic Humans with a Positive Family History of Alcoholism

Genetic predisposition	Alcohol effect
Alcohol-craving **animals**	Increased β-endorphin release after alcohol
	Increased μ opioid receptor density
	Decreased κ opioid receptor density
	Decreased serotonin function
	Enhanced DA release after alcohol
	Decreased GABA response to alcohol
D2 knockout rats	Reduced alcohol self-administration
Rats bred for enhanced withdrawal	Genes encode GABA$_A$ receptor complex are affected
	Greater number of Ca^{2+}-binding sites
Excessive 5HT$_3$ sites	Reduced alcohol consumption
Alcohol noncraving	Increased dynorphin levels in the NAc
Nonalcoholic **humans** (family history of alcoholism)	Enhanced β-endorphin release by alcohol
	Low baseline β-endorphin levels
	Serotonin deficiency (reduced CSF 5HIAA)
	Increased rewarding effects of benzodiazepines
	Reduced intoxicating effects from alcohol
	Reduced GABA$_A$ function

sequenced, and cloned. Their activation produces hyperpolarization, primarily by increasing K^+ conductance, thereby reducing the firing rate and neurotransmitter release of the signal-receiving neuron. As with DA receptors, EOP receptors are coupled to G-proteins that produce sustained changes in target cells, including altered gene expression through second-messenger cascades.

The involvement of EOP systems in alcohol reward is based on several lines of research. Animals bred to prefer alcohol have alterations in EOP function, including increased β-endorphin release in the hypothalamus after alcohol administration [95]. Alcohol preferring rats have been reported to show high levels of EOP-related mRNA in the hypothalamus, prefrontal cortex, and mediodorsal nucleus of the thalamus [96]. This study also reported increased μ opioid receptor density in the NAc and PFC, and decreased κ opioid receptor density in these animals. Alcohol-non-preferring animals have increased NAc dynorphin levels [97]. It is also possible that alcohol increases the expression of δ receptors and affects binding properties of other EOP receptors in the brain [27]. In a number of animal studies, alcohol administration increases levels of β-endorphin and enkephalin in the brain while alcohol withdrawal is associated with decreased EOP brain levels [22]. β-Endorphin elevations after alcohol are specifically seen in discrete reward regions of the hypothalamus [98], VTA, and NAc [99]. It is important to note that β-endorphin-deficient rats continue to self-administer alcohol, suggesting that this substance does not exclusively produce alcohol reward [100]. The importance of μ opioid receptor activation as a mechanism for alcohol reward is underscored by the fact that alcohol consumption in alcohol-preferring rats is persistently reduced after inactivating μ opioid receptors in the NAc [86].

Human studies also implicate EOP systems in the neurobiology of alcoholism. Direct measurements of β-endorphin in the cerebrospinal fluid of alcoholics show increased levels after alcohol intake and decreased levels during alcohol withdrawal [48,101]. Reduced levels of plasma β-endorphin are found in chronic alcoholics tested several hours after their last drink [102]. Low baseline β-endorphin levels may be inherited. Subjects with a family history of alcoholism have low baseline β-endorphin levels and display a 170% rise after alcohol, as compared to an absence of β-endorphin release in subjects without a family history [9]. This study indicates the ability of alcohol to normalize low β-endorphin levels in subjects with genetic loading for alcoholism. Also consistent with an inherited EOP-related vulnerability is the finding that polymorphism of the μ-opiate receptor may contribute to alcoholism [103]. In addition, the ACTH response to naltrexone is consistent with β-endorphin deficiency in alcoholics and in nonalcoholics with genetic loading for the disorder [103]. That β-endorphin may be deficient in these individuals is interesting, especially in light of the fact that alcohol acutely releases β-endorphin. Reversal of an EOP deficit, either due to genetic or alcohol-induced mechanisms, could be a significant factor in the neurobiology of alcoholism. Additionally, the surge of β-endorphin seen in alcoholics and individuals with genetic predisposition may reflect enhanced euphoria, comparable to the action of an exogenous opiate. After receiving doses of alcohol in a laboratory setting, nonalcoholic volunteers with a family history of alcoholism experience more euphoria than do those without a family history of the disorder [104]. Furthermore, the euphoria experienced by subjects in this study was blocked by naltrexone, strongly suggesting an opioid mechanism. It stands to reason that individuals experiencing enhanced reward from alcohol would be more vulnerable to alcoholism.

Additional evidence of EOP involvement in alcohol reward is provided by numerous animal studies showing that opioid antagonists reduce alcohol consumption in animals [10,103]. Nonspecific opioid antagonists such as naltrexone, and those specific for μ and δ receptors, clearly reduce alcohol intake in a number of paradigms. Conversely, low doses of opioid agonists increase alcohol consumption [105] owing to a priming effect, although high doses of opiates replace alcohol consumption [27]. Opioid antagonists also reduce alcohol intake when administered directly into the central nucleus of the amygdala [10], specifically implicating this component of the extended amygdala in alcohol reward [48].

Given the evidence for EOP involvement in alcohol reward and the ability of opioid antagonists to reduce alcohol intake by animals, naltrexone was investigated in alcoholics [106,107]. Nearly all controlled clinical trials conclude that naltrexone reduces alcohol intake and prevents full relapse in subjects who resume drinking [106,108,109]. Naltrexone may also ameliorate craving [110] and diminish the pleasurable effects of alcohol [111], presumably by interfering with opioid mediated mechanisms. Studies with naltrexone were so conclusive that it was approved by the Food and Drug Administration in 1994 as a treatment for alcoholism. It is possible that naltrexone may be particularly effective for patients with a family history of alcoholism, or individuals who show enhanced release of β-endorphin after alcohol administration. Unfortunately, the clinical use of naltrexone has not been widely adopted by practitioners, and poor adherence remains an impediment to its effectiveness.

The role that EOP systems play in the acquisition and perpetuation of alcohol dependence requires further clarification and additional research. While genetic factors may influence EOP function and predispose some individuals to alcoholism, the repeated administration of alcohol may also produce significant EOP neuroadaptations. For instance, rats undergoing alcohol withdrawal have increased NAc levels of prodynorphin mRNA in conjunction with robust dynorphin release [23]. This finding is interesting in light of the fact that enkephalin and dynorphin have opposite regulatory actions on mesolimbic DA neurons. While alcohol reward is associated with the stimulation of μ and δ opioid receptors by enkephalin and β-endorphin, alcohol withdrawal (and perhaps craving) is associated with the stimulation of κ opioid receptors with dynorphin. Dynorphin-containing neurons in the striatum may represent a separate population of GABA/EOP cells that specifically express D_1 receptors and mediate compensatory actions in response to excessive DA stimulation [10]. Dynorphin inhibits DA activity and produces aversion, perhaps as a result of this action. Since naltrexone antagonizes κ opioid receptors, in addition to μ and δ opioid receptors, its efficacy against craving and relapse may result, in part, from the reversal of dynorphin overactivity. More research is required to determine how chronic alcohol exposure affects EOP and DA neuromodulator systems, and how their dysregulation affects rewarding and aversive states associated with alcohol intake.

X. CONCLUSIONS

This chapter has reviewed the neurobiology of alcoholism with a focus on neurotransmitter systems that are involved in the rewarding and aversive effects of alcohol. Rewarding and aversive states represent positive and negative reinforcers that drive alcohol addiction, particularly in genetically vulnerable individuals. Research into brain reward centers has provided significant insight into the mechanisms of alcohol reward and chronic neuroadaptations that lead to tolerance, withdrawal, and altered hedonic function. Tolerance and withdrawal involve compensatory changes in the balance of excitatory and inhibitory neurotransmission and become unopposed by alcohol after its abrupt discontinuation. Although alcohol withdrawal can be serious and even life-threatening, it responds very well to an appropriate and timely detoxification regimen. Less treatable are the persistent craving and dysphoria that are often reported by alcoholics who are attempting to achieve sobriety. This chapter has presented evidence that altered hedonic function by chronic alcohol exposure involves the dysregulation DA and EOP neuromodulator systems. These reward-related neuromodulators are intensely regulated by GABA, glutamate, and serotonin circuits which are extensively interconnected and integrated. Improving our understanding of the actions of alcohol on these complicated neuronal systems should identify pharmacological strategies to ameliorate aversive states associated with alcohol abstinence and thereby enhance recovery from this prevalent disorder.

The neurobiology of alcoholism supports many clinical strategies currently employed in the treatment of this disorder. The notion that alcoholics should strive for total sobriety is supported by the fact that repeated alcohol administration produces opposite effects on neurotransmitter systems. These compensatory actions produce brain imbalances that are temporarily normalized by alcohol, but then exacerbated. Examples of this vicious cycle include the actions of alcohol on the $GABA_A$ and NMDA receptor complexes, and on EOP and DA function. Also, common actions by all substances of abuse, such as the release of DA into the NAc, provide a scientific basis for the established clinical principle that alcoholics attempting sobriety should avoid using all addictive agents, including benzodiazepines and barbiturates, which actually have similar allosteric actions on $GABA_A$ receptors. Denial, often attributed merely to the alcoholic's strong wish to continue drinking, could have a basis in hypofrontality, which would explain its tenacity in the clinical setting. Finally, the prudence of avoiding "people, places, and things" associated with alcohol use is illustrated by studies showing limbic activation during cue-induced craving for alcohol. Given its biological basis, alcoholism should be viewed as a brain disease rather than a character weakness, and alcoholics should have the same access to treatment that has become the right of patients suffering from any medical illness.

REFERENCES

1. Fils-Aime ML, Eckardt MJ, George DT, Brown GL, Mefford I, Linnoila M. Early-onset alcoholics have lower cerebrospinal fluid 5-hydroxyindoleacetic acid

1. levels than late-onset alcoholics. Arch Gen Psychiatry 1996; 53(3):211–216.
2. Mendelson JH, Mello NK. Medical progress. Biologic concomitants of alcoholism. N Engl J Med 1979; 301(17):912–921.
3. Ballenger JC, Post RM. Kindling as a model for alcohol withdrawal syndromes. Br J Psychiatry 1978; 133:1–14.
4. Modell JG, Mountz JM. Focal cerebral blood flow change during craving for alcohol measured by SPECT. J Neuropsychiatry Clin Neurosci 1995; 7(1):15–22.
5. Midanik L. Familial alcoholism and problem drinking in a national drinking practices survey. Addict Behav 1983; 8(2):133–141.
6. Goodwin DW. Alcoholism and heredity. A review and hypothesis. Arch Gen Psychiatry 1979; 36(1):57–61.
7. Schuckit MA. Genetics of the risk for alcoholism. Am J Addict 2000; 9(2):103–112.
8. Schuckit MA. Low level of response to alcohol as a predictor of future alcoholism. Am J Psychiatry 1994; 151(2):184–189.
9. Gianoulakis C, Angelogianni P, Meaney M, Thavundayil J, Tawar V. Endorphins in individuals with high and low risk for development of alcoholism. In Opioids, Bulimia, and Alcohol Abuse and Alcoholism, ed. Reid LD. Berlin; Springer, 1990, pp 229–246.
10. Akil H, Owens C, Gutstein H, Taylor L, Curran E, Watson S. Endogenous opioids: overview and current issues. Drug Alcohol Depend 1998; 51(1-2):127–140.
11. Bassareo V, Di Chiara G. Modulation of feeding-induced activation of mesolimbic dopamine transmission by appetitive stimuli and its relation to motivational state. Eur J Neurosci 1999; 11(12):4389–4397.
12. Alheid GF, McDermott L, Kelly J, Halaris A, Grossman SP. Deficits in food and water intake after knife cuts that deplete striatal DA or hypothalamic NE in rats. Pharmacol Biochem Behav 1977; 6(3):273–287.
13. Van Furth WR, Van Ree JM. Sexual motivation: involvement of endogenous opioids in the ventral tegmental area. Brain Res 1996; 729(1):20–28.
14. Schultz W, Dayan P, Montague PR. A neural substrate of prediction and reward. Science 1997; 275(5306):1593–1599.
15. Dackis CA, O'Brien CP. The neurobiology of addiction. In Diseases of the Nervous System, eds Asbury A, Goadsby PJ, McArthur J. Cambridge: University Press (in press).
16. Acquas E, Meloni M, Di Chiara G. Blockade of delta-opioid receptors in the nucleus accumbens prevents ethanol-induced stimulation of dopamine release. Eur J Pharmacol 1993; 230(2):239–241.
17. Carr DB, Sesack SR. Projections from the rat prefrontal cortex to the ventral tegmental area: target specificity in the synaptic associations with mesoaccumbens and mesocortical neurons. J Neurosci 2000; 20(10):3864–3873.
18. Koob GF, Sanna PP, Bloom FE. Neuroscience of addiction. Neuron 1998; 21(3):467–476.
19. Heimer L, Alheid GF. Piecing together the puzzle of basal forebrain anatomy. Adv Exp Med Biol 1991; 295:1–42.
20. Day HE, Curran EJ, Watson SJ Jr, Akil H. Distinct neurochemical populations in the rat central nucleus of the amygdala and bed nucleus of the stria terminalis: evidence for their selective activation by interleukin-1beta. J Comp Neurol 1999; 413(1):113–128.
21. Walker JR, Ahmed SH, Gracy KN, Koob GF. Microinjections of an opiate receptor antagonist into the bed nucleus of the stria terminalis suppress heroin self-administration in dependent rats. Brain Res 2000; 854(1-2):85–92.
22. Ulm RR, Volpicelli JR, Volpicelli LA. Opiates and alcohol self-administration in animals. J Clin Psychiatry 1995; 56(suppl 7):5–14.
23. Przewlocka B, Turchan J, Lason W, Przewlocki R. Ethanol withdrawal enhances the prodynorphin system activity in the rat nucleus accumbens. Neurosci Lett 1997; 238(1-2):13–16.
24. Hill SY, Zezza N, Wipprecht G, Xu J, Neiswanger K. Linkage studies of D2 and D4 receptor genes and alcoholism. Am J Med Genet 1999; 88(6):676–685.
25. Hernandez-Lopez S, Bargas J, Surmeier DJ, Reyes A, Galarraga E. D1 receptor activation enhances evoked discharge in neostriatal medium spiny neurons by modulating an L-type Ca^{2+} conductance. J Neurosci 1997; 17(9):3334–3342.
26. Sesack SR, Pickel VM. In the rat medial nucleus accumbens, hippocampal and catecholaminergic terminals converge on spiny neurons and are in apposition to each other. Brain Res 1990; 527(2):266–279.
27. Herz A. Endogenous opioid systems and alcohol addiction. Psychopharmacology (Berl) 1997; 129(2):99–111.
28. Johnson LR, Aylward RL, Hussain Z, Totterdell S. Input from the amygdala to the rat nucleus accumbens: its relationship with tyrosine hydroxylase immunoreactivity and identified neurons. Neuroscience 1994; 61(4):851–865.
29. Hyytia P, Koob GF. GABAA receptor antagonism in the extended amygdala decreases ethanol self-administration in rats. Eur J Pharmacol 1995; 283(1-3):151–159.
30. Roberts AJ, Keith LD. Corticosteroids enhance convulsion susceptibility via central mineralocorticoid receptors. Psychoneuroendocrinology 1995; 20(8):891–902.

31. Durstewitz D, Seamans JK, Sejnowski TJ. Dopamine-mediated stabilization of delay-period activity in a network model of prefrontal cortex. J Neurophysiol 2000; 83(3):1733–1750.
32. Napier TC, Mitrovic I. Opioid modulation of ventral pallidal inputs. Ann NY Acad Sci 1999; 877:176–201.
33. De Wit H, Metz J, Wagner N, Cooper M. Behavioral and subjective effects of ethanol: relationship to cerebral metabolism using PET. Alcohol Clin Exp Res 1990; 14(3):482–489.
34. Catafau AM, Etcheberrigaray A, Perez de los Cobos J, Estorch M, Guardia J, Flotats A, Berna L, Mari C, Casas M, Carrio I. Regional cerebral blood flow changes in chronic alcoholic patients induced by naltrexone challenge during detoxification. J Nucl Med 1999; 40(1):19–24.
35. Mathew RJ, Wilson WH. Substance abuse and cerebral blood flow. Am J Psychiatry 1991; 148(3):292–305.
36. Streeter CC, Ciraulo DA, Harris GJ, Kaufman MJ, Lewis RF, Knapp CM, Ciraulo AM, Maas LC, Ungeheuer M, Szulewski S, Renshaw PF. Functional magnetic resonance imaging of alprazolam-induced changes in humans with familial alcoholism. Psychiatry Res 1998; 82(2):69–82.
37. Volkow ND, Wang GJ, Overall JE, Hitzemann R, Fowler JS, Pappas N, Frecska E, Piscani K. Regional brain metabolic response to lorazepam in alcoholics during early and late alcohol detoxification. Alcohol Clin Exp Res 1997; 21(7):1278–1284.
38. Volkow ND, Wang GJ, Hitzemann R, Fowler JS, Overall JE, Burr G, Wolf AP. Recovery of brain glucose metabolism in detoxified alcoholics. Am J Psychiatry 1994; 151(2):178–183.
39. McKernan RM, Whiting PJ. Which GABAA-receptor subtypes really occur in the brain? [see comments]. Trends Neurosci 1996; 19(4):139–143.
40. Steffensen SC, Nie Z, Criado JR, Siggins GR. Ethanol inhibition of N-methyl-D-aspartate responses involves presynaptic gamma-aminobutyric acid(B) receptors. J Pharmacol Exp Ther 2000; 294(2):637–647.
41. Odagaki Y, Nishi N, Koyama T. Functional coupling of GABA(B) receptors with G proteins that are sensitive to N-ethylmaleimide treatment, suramin, and benzalkonium chloride in rat cerebral cortical membranes. J Neural Transm 2000; 107(10):1101–1116.
42. Self DW, Genova LM, Hope BT, Barnhart WJ, Spencer JJ, Nestler EJ. Involvement of cAMP-dependent protein kinase in the nucleus accumbens in cocaine self-administration and relapse of cocaine-seeking behavior. J Neurosci 1998; 18(5):1848–1859.
43. Harris RA, Mihic SJ, Valenzuela CF. Alcohol and benzodiazepines: recent mechanistic studies. Drug Alcohol Depend 1998; 51(1-2):155–164.
44. Mihic S, Harris R. GABA and the GABA$_A$ receptor. Alcohol Health Res World 1997; 21(2):127–131.
45. Freund RK, Palmer MR. Beta adrenergic sensitization of gamma-aminobutyric acid receptors to ethanol involves a cyclic AMP/protein kinase A second-messenger mechanism. J Pharmacol Exp Ther 1997; 280(3):1192–1200.
46. Weiner JL, Valenzuela CF, Watson PL, Frazier CJ, Dunwiddie TV. Elevation of basal protein kinase C activity increases ethanol sensitivity of GABA(A) receptors in rat hippocampal CA1 pyramidal neurons. J Neurochem 1997; 68(5):1949–1959.
47. Yang X, Criswell HE, Breese GR. Ethanol modulation of gamma-aminobutyric acid (GABA)-mediated inhibition of cerebellar Purkinje neurons: relationship to GABAb receptor input. Alcohol Clin Exp Res 2000; 24(5):682–690.
48. Koob GF, Weiss F. Neuropharmacology of cocaine and ethanol dependence. Recent Dev Alcohol 1992; 10:201–233.
49. Buck KJ. Molecular genetic analysis of the role of GABAergic systems in the behavioral and cellular actions of alcohol. Behav Genet 1996; 26(3):313–323.
50. Buck KJ, Metten P, Belknap JK, Crabbe JC. Quantitative trait loci involved in genetic predisposition to acute alcohol withdrawal in mice. J Neurosci 1997; 17(10):3946–3955.
51. Morrow AL. Regulation of GABAA receptor function and gene expression in the central nervous system. Int Rev Neurobiol 1995; 38:1–41.
52. Volkow ND, Wang GJ, Begleiter H, Hitzemann R, Pappas N, Burr G, Pascani K, Wong C, Fowler JS, Wolf AP. Regional brain metabolic response to lorazepam in subjects at risk for alcoholism. Alcohol Clin Exp Res 1995; 19(2):510–516.
53. Lingford-Hughes AR, Acton PD, Gacinovic S, Suckling J, Busatto GF, Boddington SJ, Bullmore E, Woodruff PW, Costa DC, Pilowsky LS, Ell PJ, Marshall EJ, Kerwin RW. Reduced levels of GABA-benzodiazepine receptor in alcohol dependency in the absence of grey matter atrophy. Br J Psychiatry 1998; 173:116–122.
54. Cowley DS, Roy-Byrne PP, Godon C, Greenblatt DJ, Ries R, Walker RD, Samson HH, Hommer DW. Response to diazepam in sons of alcoholics. Alcohol Clin Exp Res 1992; 16(6):1057–1063.
55. Hwang BH, Lumeng L, Wu JY, Li TK. Increased number of GABAergic terminals in the nucleus accumbens is associated with alcohol preference in rats. Alcohol Clin Exp Res 1990; 14(4):503–507.
56. Romeo E, Brancati A, De Lorenzo A, Fucci P, Furnari C, Pompili E, Sasso GF, Spalletta G, Troisi A, Pasini A. Marked decrease of plasma neuroactive steroids during alcohol withdrawal. Clin Neuropharmacol 1996; 19(4):366–369.

57. Lovinger DM, White G, Weight FF. Ethanol inhibits NMDA-activated ion current in hippocampal neurons. Science 1989; 243(4899):1721–1724.
58. Trujillo KA, Akil H. Excitatory amino acids and drugs of abuse: a role for N-methyl-D-aspartate receptors in drug tolerance, sensitization and physical dependence. Drug Alcohol Depend 1995; 38(2):139–154.
59. Follesa P, Ticku MK. Chronic ethanol treatment differentially regulates NMDA receptor subunit mRNA expression in rat brain. Brain Res Mol Brain Res 1995; 29(1):99–106.
60. Fitzgerald LW, Nestler EJ. Molecular and cellular adaptations in signal transduction pathways following ethanol exposure. Clin Neurosci 1995; 3(3):165–173.
61. Rossetti ZL, Carboni S. Ethanol withdrawal is associated with increased extracellular glutamate in the rat striatum. Eur J Pharmacol 1995; 283(1-3):177–183.
62. Al Qatari M, Bouchenafa O, Littleton J. Mechanism of action of acamprosate. II. Ethanol dependence modifies effects of acamprosate on NMDA receptor binding in membranes from rat cerebral cortex. Alcohol Clin Exp Res 1998; 22(4):810–814.
63. Kranzler HR. Pharmacotherapy of alcoholism: gaps in knowledge and opportunities for research. Alcohol Alcohol 2000; 35(6):537–547.
64. Dahchour A, De Witte P, Bolo N, Nedelec JF, Muzet M, Durbin P, Macher JP. Central effects of acamprosate. 1. Acamprosate blocks the glutamate increase in the nucleus accumbens microdialysate in ethanol withdrawn rats. Psychiatry Res 1998; 82(2):107–114.
65. Little HJ. The role of neuronal calcium channels in dependence on ethanol and other sedatives/hypnotics. Pharmacol Ther 1991; 50(3):347–365.
66. Hunt WA. Are binge drinkers more at risk of developing brain damage? Alcohol 1993; 10(6):559–561.
67. Costa A, Bono G, Martignoni E, Merlo P, Sances G, Nappi G. An assessment of hypothalamo-pituitary-adrenal axis functioning in non-depressed, early abstinent alcoholics. Psychoneuroendocrinology 1996; 21(3):263–275.
68. Armanini MP, Hutchins C, Stein BA, Sapolsky RM. Glucocorticoid endangerment of hippocampal neurons is NMDA-receptor dependent. Brain Res 1990; 532(1-2):7–12.
69. Tsai G, Gastfriend DR, Coyle JT. The glutamatergic basis of human alcoholism [see comments]. Am J Psychiatry 1995; 152(3):332–340.
70. Savage DD, Queen SA, Sanchez CF, Paxton LL, Mahoney JC, Goodlett CR, West JR. Prenatal ethanol exposure during the last third of gestation in rat reduces hippocampal NMDA agonist binding site density in 45-day-old offspring. Alcohol 1992; 9(1):37–41.
71. LeMarquand D, Pihl RO, Benkelfat C. Serotonin and alcohol intake, abuse, and dependence: clinical evidence. Biol Psychiatry 1994; 36(5):326–337.
72. Lyness WH, Smith FL. Influence of dopaminergic and serotonergic neurons on intravenous ethanol self-administration in the rat. Pharmacol Biochem Behav 1992; 42(1):187–192.
73. McBride WJ, Murphy JM, Gatto GJ, Levy AD, Yoshimoto K, Lumeng L, Li TK. CNS mechanisms of alcohol self-administration. Alcohol Alcohol Suppl 1993; 2:463–467.
74. Yoshimoto K, Yayama K, Sorimachi Y, Tani J, Ogata M, Nishimura A, Yoshida T, Ueda S, Komura S. Possibility of 5-HT3 receptor involvement in alcohol dependence: a microdialysis study of nucleus accumbens dopamine and serotonin release in rats with chronic alcohol consumption. Alcohol Clin Exp Res 1996; 20(9 suppl):311A–319A.
75. Lovinger DM. 5-HT3 receptors and the neural actions of alcohols: an increasingly exciting topic. Neurochem Int 1999; 35(2):125–130.
76. Bagdy G, Calogero AE, Szemeredi K, Gomez MT, Murphy DL, Chrousos GP, Gold PW. Beta-endorphin responses to different serotonin agonists: involvement of corticotropin-releasing hormone, vasopressin and direct pituitary action. Brain Res 1990; 537(1–2):227–232.
77. Zangen A, Nakash R, Yadid G. Serotonin-mediated increases in the extracellular levels of beta-endorphin in the arcuate nucleus and nucleus accumbens: a microdialysis study. J Neurochem 1999; 73(6):2569–2574.
78. Johnson BA, Ait-Daoud N, Prihoda TJ. Combining ondansetron and naltrexone effectively treats biologically predisposed alcoholics: from hypotheses to preliminary clinical evidence. Alcohol Clin Exp Res 2000; 24(5):737–742.
79. Engel SR, Allan AM. 5-HT3 receptor over-expression enhances ethanol sensitivity in mice. Psychopharmacology (Berl) 1999; 144(4):411–415.
80. Pettinati HM. Use of serotonin selective pharmacotherapy in the treatment of alcohol dependence. Alcohol Clin Exp Res 1996; 20(7 suppl):23A–29A.
81. Virkkunen M, Goldman D, Nielsen DA, Linnoila M. Low brain serotonin turnover rate (low CSF 5-HIAA) and impulsive violence. J Psychiatry Neurosci 1995; 20(4):271–275.
82. Heinz A, Higley JD, Gorey JG, Saunders RC, Jones DW, Hommer D, Zajicek K, Suomi SJ, Lesch KP, Weinberger DR, Linnoila M. In vivo association between alcohol intoxication, aggression, and serotonin transporter availability in nonhuman primates. Am J Psychiatry 1998; 155(8):1023–1028.
83. Campbell AD, McBride WJ. Serotonin-3 receptor and ethanol-stimulated dopamine release in the

nucleus accumbens. Pharmacol Biochem Behav 1995; 51(4):835–842.
84. Kilpatrick GJ, Hagan RM, Gale JD. 5-HT3 and 5-HT4 receptors in terminal regions of the mesolimbic system. Behav Brain Res 1996; 73(1–2):11–13.
85. Brodie MS, Trifunovic RD, Shefner SA. Serotonin potentiates ethanol-induced excitation of ventral tegmental area neurons in brain slices from three different rat strains. J Pharmacol Exp Ther 1995; 273(3):1139–1146.
86. Myers RD, Robinson DE. Mmu and D2 receptor antisense oligonucleotides injected in nucleus accumbens suppress high alcohol intake in genetic drinking HEP rats. Alcohol 1999; 18(2–3):225–233.
87. Brodie MS, Pesold C, Appel SB. Ethanol directly excites dopaminergic ventral tegmental area reward neurons. Alcohol Clin Exp Res 1999; 23(11):1848–1852.
88. Weiss F, Parsons LH, Schulteis G, Hyytia P, Lorang MT, Bloom FE, Koob GF. Ethanol self-administration restores withdrawal-associated deficiencies in accumbal dopamine and 5-hydroxytryptamine release in dependent rats. J Neurosci 1996; 16(10):3474–3485.
89. Rassnick S, Stinus L, Koob GF. The effects of 6-hydroxydopamine lesions of the nucleus accumbens and the mesolimbic dopamine system on oral self-administration of ethanol in the rat. Brain Res 1993; 623(1):16–24.
90. Diana M, Pistis M, Muntoni A, Gessa G. Mesolimbic dopaminergic reduction outlasts ethanol withdrawal syndrome: evidence of protracted abstinence. Neuroscience 1996; 71(2):411–415.
91. Wise RA. Neurobiology of addiction. Curr Opin Neurobiol 1996; 6(2):243–251.
92. Koob GF, Nestler EJ. The neurobiology of drug addiction. J Neuropsychiatry Clin Neurosci 1997; 9(3):482–497.
93. Dackis CA, Gold MS. New concepts in cocaine addiction: the dopamine depletion hypothesis. Neurosci Biobehav Rev 1985; 9(3):469–477.
94. Rossetti ZL, Hmaidan Y, Gessa GL. Marked inhibition of mesolimbic dopamine release: a common feature of ethanol, morphine, cocaine and amphetamine abstinence in rats. Eur J Pharmacol 1992; 221(2–3):227–234.
95. De Waele JP, Papachristou DN, Gianoulakis C. The alcohol-preferring C57BL/6 mice present an enhanced sensitivity of the hypothalamic beta-endorphin system to ethanol than the alcohol-avoiding DBA/2 mice. J Pharmacol Exp Ther 1992; 261(2):788–794.
96. Marinelli PW, Kiianmaa K, Gianoulakis C. Opioid propeptide mRNA content and receptor density in the brains of AA and ANA rats. Life Sci 2000; 66(20):1915–1927.
97. Terenius L. Reward and its control by dynorphin peptides. EXS 1994; 71:9–17.
98. Popp RL, Erickson CK. The effect of an acute ethanol exposure on the rat brain POMC opiopeptide system. Alcohol 1998; 16(2):139–148.
99. Rasmussen DD, Bryant CA, Boldt BM, Colasurdo EA, Levin N, Wilkinson CW. Acute alcohol effects on opiomelanocortinergic regulation. Alcohol Clin Exp Res 1998; 22(4):789–801.
100. Grahame NJ, Low MJ, Cunningham CL. Intravenous self-administration of ethanol in beta-endorphin-deficient mice. Alcohol Clin Exp Res 1998; 22(5):1093–1098.
101. Genazzani AR, Nappi G, Facchinetti F, Mazzella GL, Parrini D, Sinforiani E, Petraglia F, Savoldi F. Central deficiency of beta-endorphin in alcohol addicts. J Clin Endocrinol Metab 1982; 55(3):583–586.
102. Vescovi PP, Coiro V, Volpi R, Giannini A, Passeri M. Plasma beta-endorphin, but not met-enkephalin levels are abnormal in chronic alcoholics. Alcohol Alcohol 1992; 27(5):471–475.
103. Vaccarino AL, Kastin AJ. Endogenous opiates: 1999. Peptides 2000; 21(12):1975–2034.
104. King AC, Volpicelli JR, Frazer A, O'Brien CP. Effect of naltrexone on subjective alcohol response in subjects at high and low risk for future alcohol dependence. Psychopharmacology (Berl) 1997; 129(1):15–22.
105. Volpicelli JR, Berg BJ, Watson NT. Opioid mediation of alcohol self-administration: pre-clinical studies. In: The Pharmacology of Alcohol Abuse, ed. Kranzler. Berlin; Springer-Verlag, 1995, pp 169–184.
106. Volpicelli JR, Alterman AI, Hayashida M, O'Brien CP. Naltrexone in the treatment of alcohol dependence [see comments]. Arch Gen Psychiatry 1992; 49(11):876–880.
107. O'Malley SS, Jaffe AJ, Chang G, Schottenfeld RS, Meyer RE, Rounsaville B. Naltrexone and coping skills therapy for alcohol dependence. A controlled study. Arch Gen Psychiatry 1992; 49(11):881–887.
108. O'Brien CP, Volpicelli LA, Volpicelli JR. Naltrexone in the treatment of alcoholism: a clinical review. Alcohol 1996; 13(1):35–39.
109. O'Brien CP, McKay JR. Pharmacological treatments of substance use disorders. In: A Guide to Treatments That Work, eds. Nathan PE, Gorman JM. New York; Oxford University Press, 1998, pp 127–155.
110. Volpicelli JR, Clay KL, Watson NT, O'Brien CP. Naltrexone in the treatment of alcoholism: predicting response to naltrexone. J Clin Psychiatry 1995; 56(suppl 7):39–44.
111. Volpicelli JR, Watson NT, King AC, Sherman CE, O'Brien CP. Effect of naltrexone on alcohol "high" in alcoholics. Am J Psychiatry 1995; 152(4):613–615.

39

Biological Basis of Drug Addiction

TONY P. GEORGE
Yale University School of Medicine, New Haven, Connecticut, U.S.A.

I. INTRODUCTION

Drug abuse and dependence constitute a major public health problem in the United States. The consequences of licit (e.g., alcohol and nicotine) and illicit (e.g., cocaine, heroin, marijuana, phencyclidine) drug use leads to significant medical morbidity, mortality, and health care expenditure, and contributes to significant personal, family, and social misfortune. It is estimated that drug addiction costs U.S. society ~ $67 billion each year in terms of crime, lost job productivity, and other social problems [1]. However, drug addiction continues to be both underrecognized and undertreated by primary care physicians and psychiatrists. This is particularly unfortunate since there are several very effective treatments for alcohol, opioid, and nicotine dependence disorders, especially when combined with appropriate psychosocial interventions (e.g., Alcoholics Anonymous, drug counseling, smoking cessation counseling). The belief among health care providers that drug addiction is a "moral failing" or "bad habit" is, unfortunately, still a common one, and it is well appreciated that many physicians (including psychiatrists) take a stance of "therapeutic nihilism" with respect to treatment of individuals with drug addiction. However, there is increasing evidence that addictive disorders have a strong biological basis, and this knowledge will most likely lead to effective treatments for all addictive disorders, including those that do not currently have effective pharmacotherapies such as cocaine and methamphetamine addiction [2]. The purpose of this chapter is to delineate the biological underpinnings of drug addiction, and to describe current and future biological treatment approaches for these disorders based on such knowledge.

II. DEFINITIONS: DRUG ABUSE, DEPENDENCE AND ADDICTION:

It is important to clearly define common terms that are used to describe drug-seeking behaviors, and the functional consequences of drug misuse syndromes, since these terms have specific connotations, and should not be used interchangeably. Drug *abuse*, according to the DSM-IV [3], refers use of a psychoactive substance that leads to impairment of social and/or occupational functioning as evidenced by one of: (1) use of the drug under **h**azardous circumstances (e.g., driving a car); (2) drug use leads to neglect of **e**xternal obligations (e.g., intoxicated and then forgets to pick up their child from daycare); (3) **l**egal problems arising from drug use (e.g., driving under the influence [DUI] conviction); (4) inter**p**ersonal problems related to persistent drug use (e.g., loss of job, divorce). The above-referred pneumonic ("**h-e-l-p**") is useful for remembering the four components that contribute to the diagnosis of drug *abuse* disorders. In contrast, drug *dependence* describes a constellation physiological adaptations (e.g., tolerance and withdrawal) and functional consequences of such physiological adaptation (drug taken in larger amounts, and for longer than intended, social and occupation activities impaired by drug use). It is important to note that the terms abuse and dependence are not mutually exclusive when describing drug use disorders, and it is possibly to be diagnosed with one, both, or neither diagnosis when classifying drug use. Finally, drug *addiction* refers to compulsive drug-seeking, loss of control, and the adverse social and occupational consequences related to use of drugs of abuse.

III. NEURAL SUBSTRATES OF DRUG ADDICTION

A. Summary of Receptor Site(s) of Action of Drugs of Abuse

Table 1 describes the major classes of drugs of abuse, their purported site(s) of action at the molecular level, and the endogenous neurotransmitters that appear to mediate their actions. One common mechanism of all addictive drugs is their ability to increase dopamine (DA) release and turnover in the mesolimbic ("reward") pathway (Fig. 1). In fact, there is increasing evidence for afferent regulation of mesolimbic DA neurons by most other major central neurotransmitter systems including serotonin, GABA, glutamate, endogenous opioid peptide, and nicotinic cholinergic systems [2].

B. Mesolimbic DA System

A number of studies over the past 25 years have suggested that mesolimbic DA neurons, which project from the ventral tegmental area (VTA) in the midbrain to the anterior forebrain nucleus accumbens (NAS) mediate the reinforcing effects of drugs of abuse (Fig. 1). This is suggested by experiments involving lesions to the VTA by mechanical (e.g., electrolytic), chemical (6-hydroxydopamine, kainic acid) methods that have implicated the involvement of this pathway in drug reward [4]. However, the normal function of the mesolimbic DA system seems to relate to forming relevant associations between salient and arousing chemical and behavioral stimuli (e.g., food, sex, stress) and internal rewarding or aversive states.

Thus, this system helps the organism acquire behaviors reinforced by both natural rewards and drug stimuli. It is thought that the activity of mesolimbic DA neurons normally habituates with repeated exposure [5,6]. However, drugs of abuse abort this habituation leading to a change in the set point of the mesolimbic DA system [7], which may underlie addictive behaviors.

C. Endogenous Opioid Peptide Reward Pathways

There is increasing evidence for afferent regulation of mesolimbic DA pathways by EOP systems. In addition, it appears that μ- and κ-opioid systems have opposing actions on mesolimbic DA neurons, with stimulation of μ-receptors (in the VTA) increasing DA release, and stimulation of κ-receptors (in the NAS) inhibiting DA release [8]. There is good neuroanatomic and function evidence for this interaction of opioid and DA systems at the level of the VTA [9]. In addition, recent studies suggest that EOP regulation of central DA pathways extends to tuberoinfundibular [10] and mesocortical DA pathways [11].

Besides mediating the reinforcing effects of opioid drugs, there is evidence from preclinical and clinical studies for EOP involvement in the reinforcing actions of other drugs of abuse, including alcohol [12–14], cocaine [15,16], methamphetamine [17], and nicotine [11,12]. These effects may ultimately be mediated through the DA reward system, given the afferent regulation of these DA neurons by opioidergic systems.

D. Hypothalamic-Pituitary-Adrenal (HPA) Axis

Evidence from animal and human studies indicates that environmental stress appears to be an important factor in drug relapse, and successful drug addiction treatment involves helping patients cope and address life stressors that inexorably lead to relapse. Numerous preclinical studies have documented that physical (e.g., footshock, restraint stress) and psychological (e.g., cue-induced) stressors can cause drug use reinstatement [16], and that stressors can lead to drug craving behaviors in human addicts [18]. In fact, increased cortisol (or corticosterone in rats) levels are known to potentiate the mesolimbic DA system, and may be a basis for stress-induced drug craving [16].

Table 1 Site(s) of Action of Various Drugs of Abuse and Neurotransmitters Implicated in Their Actions[a]

Drug	Site of action	Endogenous neurotransmitter systems	Pharmacologic treatments
Alcohol/sedatives	Nonspecific membrane effects NMDA receptors (noncompetitive site) GABAa receptors (chloride channels) Voltage-dependent calcium channels	Glutamate GABA Dopamine Serotonin Endogenous opioids	Disulfiram Naltrexone Acamprosate SSRIs
Cocaine	Dopamine transporter (DAT) Norephinephrine transporter (NET) Serotonin transporter (SERT)	Dopamine Norephinephrine Serotonin GABA Glutamate Endogenous opioids	No proven pharmacotherapy Desipramine (and other TCAs) Dopamine Agonists, Disulfiram
Opioids	μ-Opioid receptors (e.g., morphine, heroin)	Endogenous opioids Dopamine Glutamate	Methadone Clonidine Naltrexone Buprenorphine
Marijuana	Cannabinoid (CB1, CB2) receptors	Anandamide Dopamine Endogenous opioids	No proven pharmacotherapy
Nicotine (tobacco)	Nicotinic acetylcholine receptors ? Monoamine oxidase (A/B isoforms)	Acetylcholine Dopamine Serotonin Norephinephrine GABA Glutamate Endogenous opioids	Nicotine Replacement (patch, gum, inhaler, spray) Sustained-Release Bupropion
Amphetamine	Vesicular monoamine transporter (VMAT) Monoamine transporter (DA, 5HT, NE)	Dopamine Serotonin Norepinephrine	No proven pharmacotherapy
Phencyclidine	NMDA receptors Dopamine transporter (DAT)	Glutamate Dopamine	No proven pharmacotherapy
MDMA (Ectasy)	Serotonin transporter (SERT) Serotonin synthesis	Serotonin	No proven pharmacotherapy

[a] Examples of pharmacological agents which have been devised for use in the treatment of these drug abuse disorders are also given.

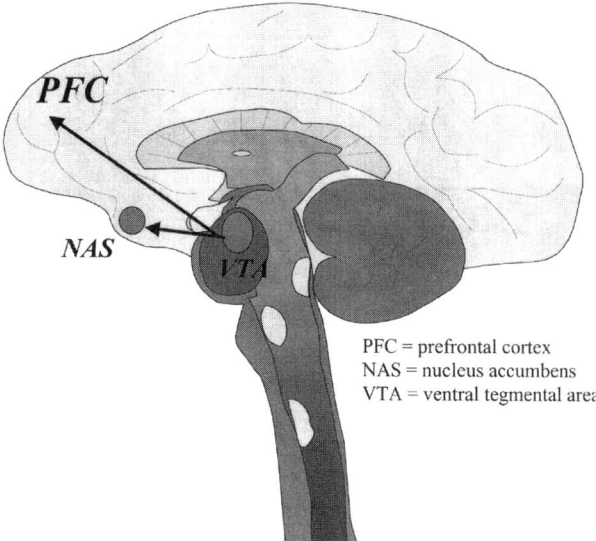

Figure 1 Mesolimbic dopamine ("reward") pathways. The dopaminergic projections from the ventral tegmental area (VTA) to the nucleus accumbens (NAS) and prefrontal cortex (PFC) are diagrammed.

E. Pharmacokinetics of Addictive Drugs: Implications for Drug Reward

There is substantial evidence that the rewarding effects of drugs of abuse correlate with how much drug gets into the brain and how quickly the drug reaches the brain. That is, in pharmacokinetic studies, both the drug level obtained and the rate of rise (e.g., ascending portion of curve) are important factors in predicting drug "liking" and "rewarding" effects. An example of cocaine pharmacokinetics with administration of cocaine by various routes, as assessed by plasma cocaine levels (in arbitrary units) over time after cocaine administration [19], is presented in Figure 2.

Oral cocaine (A) administration (e.g., chewing coca leaves) leads to very slow absorption of cocaine hydrochloride, which is a charged molecule that does not easily cross the mucous membranes. Consequently, the reported drug "high" is modest. Intranasal (i.e., snorted) cocaine (B) has a slightly faster rate of absorption and therefore produces more drug "high" than orally ingested cocaine. Finally, intravenous and freebase (crack) uses of cocaine (C) have much faster rates of absorption (in the first case due to an intravenous bolus of cocaine which gets to the brain in large amounts; in the second case because freebase cocaine is more membrane permeable and is rapidly absorbed through the pulmonary circulation and into the brain), which correlate with a profoundly enhanced cocaine "high" compared to oral and intranasal routes. Interestingly, in controlled animal studies, the correlations between plasma levels of cocaine and reinforcing effects are not exact, and this may relate to differential tolerance with intravenous versus oral administration and differences in metabolite profiles produced by these two routes of cocaine administration [20].

IV. BIOLOGICAL THEORIES TO EXPLAIN COMPULSIVE DRUG USE

There are several current and seemingly contradictory theories regarding the development of compulsive drug-seeking behavior and ultimately drug addiction [4,7,21–23]. Several aspects of these theories are compatible with the clinical course of addictive disorders, and the disagreements between the theories relate to the complexities of drug addiction and the biochemical, neuroendocrine behavioral models in preclinical studies on which these theories are based.

A. Allostatic Dysregulation Model

This theory of drug addiction has been proposed by Koob and LeMoal [7,21]. Allostasis refers to the counteradaptive changes in brain function induced by

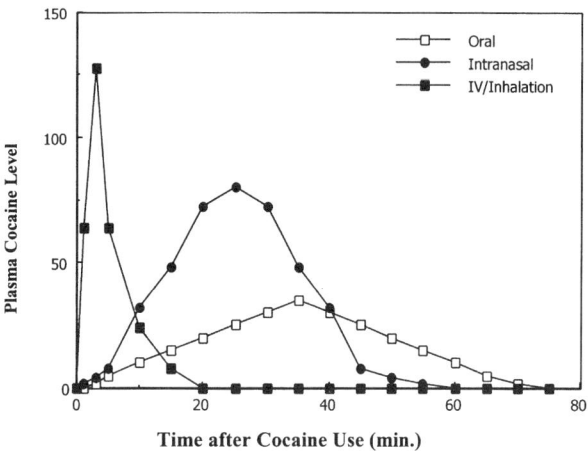

Figure 2 Pharmacokinetics of cocaine administration by three routes. The plasma concentrations of cocaine (in arbitrary units) produced by three routes of cocaine administration (oral, intranasal, and intravenous/inhalation) are depicted. The rewarding effects of cocaine and other drugs of abuse relate to how rapidly the drug enters the brain, which directly correlates with plasma drug levels.

chronic drug administration, such that there is a chronic deviation of the brain reward "set point," which relates to reward circuit dysregulation. The brain circuits involved are presumably in the corticostriatothalamic loop [24]. They describe a cycle of "spiraling distress" whereby alternating binge intoxication (with resultant drug tolerance) and negative affect associated with acute drug withdrawal leads to adaptive changes in brain reward mechanisms (e.g., the mesolimbic dopamine pathway, endogenous opioid systems) that consequently produce compensatory compulsive drug-seeking behavior, leading to the classical impairments in social and occupational functioning that constitutes drug addiction. Environmental stressors are seen as an important cofactor in both initiation and perpetuation of this cycle, presumably through alterations in HPA axis function [16]. As such, this view focuses on the positive (drug-liking) and negative (drug withdrawal) aspects of drug addiction, which are both processes that occur in the short term and lead to a dysregulation of "hedonic homeostasis."

B. Incentive-Sensitization Model

This theory, proposed by Berridge and Robinson [22], purports that like the allostatic model, chronic drug use leads to changes in reward system function, such that an addict becomes sensitized to drug use, but that these brain systems do not mediate euphoric effects of drug use (e.g., drug liking) but mediate a specific component of drug reward ("drug wanting"), which they refer to as "incentive salience." This view of drug addiction, in contrast, is not based on short-term drug reward and withdrawal syndromes to explain the process of addictive behaviors, and may in fact be compatible with the observations that many drug users who achieve initial abstinence often relapse to drug use in the context of exposure to environmental cues that potentiate drug "wanting," which is dissociable from drug "liking" [22]. Experimental support for the "incentive sensitization" model comes from recent functional neuroimaging studies in cocaine addicts [25] which demonstrated that the nucleus accumbens showed increases in blood flow (activation) during craving for cocaine, and not during acute intravenous administration.

C. Phasic/Tonic DA Release Model

This model of drug addiction, posited by Grace [23], was first formulated in the context of understanding how dysregulated dopamine dynamics may mediate the symptoms of schizophrenia [26]. It suggests that the mesolimbocortical dopamine system is dysregulated by chronic drug administration and that this dysregulation leads to drug addiction. Functionally, mesolimbic DA neurons have two types of activity: (1) tonic DA release, which is mediated by cortical glutamatergic afferents that ensures an appropriate basal level of mesolimbic DA activity; and (2) phasic DA release, which refers to evoked DA release, and is typically the type of DA activity stimulated by drugs of abuse like cocaine, amphetamine, and nicotine that leads to a large increase in synaptic DA levels. Of note, mesolimbic DA neurons have release-inhibiting preterminal DA autoreceptors (D_2) that normally function to shut down mesolimbic DA neuron function when synaptic DA levels are excessive. With chronic drug exposure, tonic DA levels would be expected to rise, causing enhanced presynaptic DA autoreceptor stimulation, thus inhibiting mesolimbic DA neuron activity. Accordingly, the experience drug user will take drugs to offset this dysregulation in tonic DA release in an attempt to augment the diminished phasic DA release that is counteracted by increased tonic DA levels. This model assumes that the mesolimbic DA system is the unitary biological substrate of drug addiction, and is similar in concept to the allostatic state proposed by Koob and LeMoal [7,21].

D. Cognitive Deficits Model

The prefrontal cortex is important in regulation of judgment, planning, and other executive functions, and it sends inhibitory projections to subcortical areas, which include the mesolimbic DA reward pathway. This model posits that: (1) individuals who develop addictive disorders have preexisting cognitive (e.g., prefrontal cortical) deficits that predispose them to impulsivity and compulsive drug-seeking behavior [27,28]; and (2) continued drug use further worsens the severity of these deficits through chronic and repeated insults to the prefrontal cortex [24]. For example, it is known that cocaine addicts have cerebral cortical perfusion deficits [28]. Such abnormalities in the "frontostriatal loop" are believed to contribute to impulsivity, compulsive drug-seeking behavior, and loss of behavioral control, which are associated with frontal cortical cognitive deficits and may explain the increasing severity of drug addiction with chronic and persistent drug use, especially in individuals with known deficits in PFC function (e.g., schizophrenia, antisocial personality disorder).

V. MECHANISMS OF ADDICTIVE DRUG ACTION

A. Cocaine and Psychostimulants

The monoamine transporter proteins, which act as a reuptake mechanism for terminating synaptic monoaminergic neurotransmission, are the primary site(s) of cocaine's action in the brain. Cocaine inhibits the reuptake of monoamine transmitters, in the order: dopamine (DA) > norepinephrine (NE) > serotonin (5-hydroxytryptamine; 5HT). Accordingly, cocaine administration leads to a massive elevation of synaptic monoamine levels [29]. DA is thought to be the most important neurotransmitter relevant to the reinforcing effects of cocaine, and DA agonists and antagonists have been tested as potential pharmacotherapies based on this putative mechanism. With repeated cocaine administration, a constellation of changes in brain function are induced, including in levels of postsynaptic receptors (e.g., downregulation of DA-D_2 receptors) and in second-messenger systems (e.g., cyclic-AMP response element binding protein [CREB], neurotrophins, [30]), which may explain some of the long-term clinical effects of chronic cocaine administration such as tolerance, withdrawal, and sensitization [31].

Psychostimulants (including methamphetamine, methyphenidate, and congeners) work primarily by releasing monoamines (DA, NE, 5HT) from presynaptic nerve terminals by two mechanisms: (1) blocking the vesicular monoamine transporter (VMAT), which sequesters monoamines in presynaptic vesicles, leading to increased levels of presynaptic free monoamines; and (2) reversing transport through monoamine transporter proteins (probably a consequence of #1). This leads to massive elevation of synaptic monoamine levels, the most important being DA. While the molecular mechanisms of psychostimulant drugs other than cocaine have received less study, there appear to be similar chronic adaptations in neural systems involved [22,32].

B. Alcohol and Sedative Hypnotic Drugs

A discussion of the mechanisms of action of alcohol is given in Chapter 38 ("Biological Basis of Alcoholism"). Sedative-hypnotic agents like barbiturates (e.g., phenobarbital, secobarbital) appear to work through mechanisms in common with alcohol, including facilitation of $GABA_A$-linked chloride ion transients (leading to target membrane hyperpolarization and reduced firing rates). The role of GABA-ergic and glutamatergic systems in mediating the effects of sedative-hypnotic drugs is becoming clearer [7], especially in light of the observation that benzodiazepines and related agents inhibit mesolimbic DA release (through stimulation of GABA-ergic afferent inputs onto these DA neurons).

C. Nicotine and Tobacco

Nicotine is the primary constituent of tobacco products that appears to be responsible for the reinforcing effects of tobacco use [33]. The most common method of nicotine delivery is through smoking cigarettes. The primary site of action of nicotine is the nicotinic acetylcholine receptor (nAChR). The nAChR is a heteromeric ion channel complex that is composed of combinations of two α (α2-9) and three β (β2-4) subunits, with the α4β2 nAChR being the predominant subunit complex in human brain [34]. The main ions that permeate this channel are sodium (Na^+) and calcium (Ca^{2+}), leading to neuronal membrane depolarization. Autoradiographic and immunocytochemical studies have demonstrated that nAChRs are located presynaptically on numerous neurotransmitter secreting neurons [34,35], including those for DA, NE, 5HT, GABA, glutamate, and EOPs, and stimulation of these receptors by nicotine leads to release of these transmitters. In contrast to other agonist drugs, after nicotine stimulates the nAChR, the receptor desensitizes almost immediately, and this progresses to nAChR inactivation. With repeated nicotine administration (as is the case with habitual smoking), this leads to a compensatory upregulation of nAChRs, known as the "paradoxical upregulation" of nAChRs by nicotine. This phenomenon may explain why dependent smokers find that the most satisfying cigarette of the day is the first one, and why nicotine cravings and withdrawals are so intense in the majority of dependent smokers. Animal models of nicotine dependence suggest that it takes 2–3 weeks for upregulated nAChR levels to return to normal after cessation of nicotine administration. Such a change in nAChR number and function is consistent with an allostatic alteration in these systems induced by repeated nicotine administration [7,21].

There is recent evidence from in vitro and positron emission tomography (PET) studies to suggest that an unidentified component of tobacco smoke (not nicotine) inhibits monoamine oxidase A (5HT) and B (DA, NE) isoforms, which are responsible for the degradation of monoamines. This additional action of tobacco may contribute to its psychopharmacologic properties [36,37].

D. Opioids

All opioid drugs work through agonism at the μ-opioid receptor, at which the enkephalin subclass of endogenous opioid peptides (EOPs) are the endogenous neurotransmitters for these receptor systems. Full μ-receptor agonist drugs include morphine, heroin (a morphine pro-drug), oxycodone, and methadone, and binding of opioid drugs to the μ-receptor leads to activation of cAMP systems and inhibition of an outwardly rectifying K^+ current, leading the membrane hyperpolarization [31,32]. Most addictive opioids are short acting (e.g., morphine, heroin, oxycodone), and long-acting preparations (e.g., methadone) have been used to treat opioid addiction using long-term maintenance (e.g., methadone maintenance). Most recently, partial μ-receptor agonists (mixed agonist-antagonists) such as buprenorphine (which also has κ-antagonist properties, which presumably augments mesolimbic DA function) have shown effectiveness for the treatment of opioid dependence and addiction. In addition, there is good evidence that long-acting μ-opioid antagonists (e.g., naltrexone) can be useful as a relapse prevention pharmacotherapy for opioid dependence.

E. Cannabinoids

Cannabinoids are plant alkaloids (from *Cannabis sativa*) with well-described euphoric, sedating, analgesic, antiemetic, and appetite-stimulating properties. In 1990, several groups cloned brain cannabinoid receptors which bound with high affinity to delta^9-tetrahydrocannabinol (THC), the principal psychoactive component of marijuana and related preparations. It was later shown that a condensation product of two constituents of lipid membranes, arachidonic acid and ethanolamine, known as anandamide (arachidonylethanolamine), was the endogenous ligand for the cannabinoid receptor [38]. There is evidence for two distinct subtypes of cannabinoid receptor, designated CB_1 and CB_2 [39]. CB receptors are G-protein-coupled receptors. The exact physiological functions of CB receptors are not known, though a recent study with CB_1 transgenic mice (with "knockout" of the CB_1 receptor) demonstrated an attenuated morphine withdrawal behavioral syndrome [40]. There is strong evidence that cannabinoid administration increases, and cannabinoid abstinence decreases, mesolimbic DA release [41], suggesting that mesolimbic DA systems subserve the reinforcing effects of cannabinoids.

F. Phencyclidine (PCP):

Also known as angeldust, PCP is an arylcyclohexylamine which has well-described psychotomimetic properties. In healthy human subjects, its produces a constellation of cognitive and clinical symptoms which resemble a schizophrenic psychosis [42], and produces cognitive deficits similar to those present in schizophrenic patients when repeatedly administered to nonhuman primates and rats [24,43]. PCP binds to the NMDA receptor complex at its noncompetitive (ion channel) site. It closely resembles the actions of ketamine, a dissociative anesthetic and veterinary tranquilizer, which produces similar effects in human subjects. At higher concentration, PCP is known to inhibit the DAT, which could contribute to its propensity to lead to positive symptoms of psychosis such as delusions, hallucinations and thought disorder. It is chemically similar to ketamine ("Special K"), a frequently abused psychotogenic and recreational drug.

G. Methylenedioxymethamphetamine (MDMA; Ecstasy)

MDMA is a psychedelic drug which is a derivative of methamphetamine that has become frequently abused by young adults, particularly at "rave" parties [44]. Typical single doses of MDMA are 100–200 mg, and it produces a "rush" similar to methamphetamine lasting 3–4 hours and feelings of "connectedness," tranquility, apathy, and alterations in time perception. While not well studied, there may be a withdrawal syndrome associated with MDMA cessation in chronic users which resembles psychostimulant abstinence. Its mechanism involves indirect 5HT agonist activity by potentiation of 5HT release and through 5HT reuptake blockade. Further, there is evidence that it inhibits the synthesis of 5HT and that it may be toxic to serotonergic neurons. It has been associated with a posthallucinogen perception disorder reminiscent of that observed with LSD, and with serotonin syndrome, because of excessive central serotonergic activity. At present, no specific pharmacologic treatment exists for MDMA abuse.

VI. CLINICAL ASSESSMENT OF THE DRUG-ADDICTED INDIVIDUAL: IMPLICATIONS FOR PHARMACOTHERAPY OF ADDICTIVE DISORDERS

The emerging biological knowledge about drug addictions has had profound implications for our treatment approaches to addictive disorders. In this section, I will briefly discuss available pharmacotherapies for addictive disorders, including opioid, nicotine, and cocaine (stimulant) addiction. Subsequently, I will describe a general approach to the assessment and treatment of individuals with addictive disorders in three specific populations: the monodrug user; the polydrug user; and the drug user with a comorbid psychiatric disorder(s).

A. Specific Pharmacotherapies for Addictive Disorders

1. Pharmacotherapy of Opioid Dependence

Methadone (Including LAAM).

This full μ-opioid receptor agonist has become the mainstay of opioid maintenance treatment in the United States [45]. The pioneering studies of Dole and Nyswander established its efficacy as a treatment for opioid addiction in the 1960s [16]. The drug is classified as a schedule II controlled substance by the Drug Enforcement Agency (DEA), and can only be administered in federally sponsored methadone programs which require careful monitoring of patients and weekly drug counseling [46]. The half-life of the drug is 24–36 hr in patients without hepatic disease, and methadone is primarily metabolized by the CYP 3A4 system. Patients beginning treatment are generally started on a daily dose of 20–30 mg/day, with weekly dose increases of 5–10 mg/day until a dose of 60–100 mg/day is achieved, that produces full suppression of opioid craving symptoms and resultant opioid-free urine toxicology [46]. Patients generally stay on methadone for 6 months to 3 years, although it is still common for some patients to receive lifelong methadone maintenance. A longer-acting derivative of methadone (L-alpha-acetomethadol; LAAM) is also FDA approved, and because of its long half-life (48–72 hr) can be given three times per week.

Naltrexone (Trexan)

Naltrexone is a long-acting (half-life ~ 24 hr) congener of naloxone, the short-acting (half-life ~ 0.5 hr) μ-opioid receptor antagonist. It is generally given to opioid-dependent individuals who have been successfully detoxified from opioids; in opioid-dependent patients, administration will produce the rapid onset of the opioid withdrawal syndrome. It is typically started at 12.5–25 mg/day once daily with food, and titrated to a dose of 50–100 mg/day. Nausea and gastric irritation are common side effects. Liver function tests should be obtained at baseline prior to initiation of treatment since naltrexone is associated with elevation of transaminases and, rarely hepatotoxicity, necessitating periodic monitoring of liver function [47]. In addition, naltrexone (ReVia) was approved in 1992 for the treatment of alcohol dependence [13,14].

Buprenorphine (Subutex)

Buprenorphine is a partial μ-opioid receptor agonist and κ-antagonist which is expected to be approved for the treatment of opioid dependence in 2001. Several recent clinical trials have established its safety and efficacy (comparable to methadone) in opioid-dependent patients [48,49]. Because of its partial agonist properties, it appears to be safer in drug overdoses, and since it has a half-life of 36 hr, it can be given three times per week. Because of its safety and convenience of dosing, it may be useful for the treatment of opioid addiction in primary care settings, which is especially helpful since most opioid addicts have significant medical problems (e.g., hepatitis B/C, HIV). Buprenorphine will be available in 4- and 8-mg tablets, and as a combination tablet with naloxone (Suboxone; to reduce illegal diversion of the medication) it is also likely to be approved by the FDA by the end of 2001. The daily maintenance dose of buprenorphine is 24–36 mg/day.

2. Pharmacotherapy of Nicotine Dependence

Nicotine Replacement Therapies (NRTs)

The best studied of the pharmacological treatments for tobacco addiction are the nicotine replacement therapies (NRTs), which include the nicotine gum, nicotine patch, nicotine nasal spray, and nicotine inhaler [33,50,51]. The more slowly absorbed formulations (gum and patch) appear to be helpful to alleviate nicotine withdrawal symptoms, and the faster-absorbed preparations (nasal spray and inhaler) appear to better substitute for the rewarding effects of cigarettes. The smoking cessation rates at the end of treatment are typically 50–70%, and 30–40% of subjects remained abstinent at 6- and 12-month follow-up assessments [52]. The gum and patch are available over the counter (OTC), but the nasal spray and inhaler are prescription drugs. Unfortunately, the cost of these preparations ($25–35/week) are prohibitive for many smokers who want to quit, and the prescription preparations are often not covered by health insurance [52].

Sustained-Release Bupropion

Bupropion is a heterocyclic antidepressant agent which was approved by the FDA for the treatment of depression (Wellbutrin) in the late 1980s. Several clinical studies in the early 1990s documented than it could reduce smoking [53–55], and the drug was approved as a treatment for nicotine dependence by the FDA in 1997 as Zyban. The initial dose is 150 mg PO QD, and the dose is increased to 150 mg PO BID (300 mg/day) by the second week of treatment; patients are encouraged to try to quit smoking when they reach the 300 mg/day dose. Treatment with Zyban is recommended for 6–12 weeks. Smoking cessation rates with Zyban are typically higher than for the nicotine patch, but are reduced after the medication is discontinued [54], and there appears to be a modest (but nonsignificant) improvement in quit rates when Zyban is combined with the nicotine patch [56]. A history of seizures is a contraindication for the use of this drug.

Other Promising Agents for the Treatment of Nicotine Addiction

Other, nonapproved agents which may be useful for the treatment of nicotine addiction include clonidine [57,58]; an α2 agonist which may reduce withdrawal symptoms]; buspirone [59], a 5HT1$_a$ agonist and anxiolytic agent; nortriptyline [60], a tricyclic antidepressant; moclobemide [61], a monoamine oxidase A inhibitor; and the combination of nicotine patch and mecamylamine, a high-affinity nicotinic receptor antagonist [62,63].

3. *Pharmacotherapy of Cocaine (Stimulant) Dependence*

Desipramine and Other Tricyclic Antidepressants (TCAs)

Desipramine hydrochloride (DMI) is the best-studied TCA, and several early studies (particularly those which used open-label designs [64]), and three placebo-controlled studies at Yale [65,66], found that DMI was efficacious for reducing cocaine use in cocaine-dependent subjects. However, the results of subsequent placebo-controlled studies, including those at other sites, have been equivocal, and based on a meta-analysis of the initial six placebo-controlled trials, the efficacy of DMI for cocaine addiction treatment has been questioned [67]. Similar equivocal findings have been reported with imipramine [68] for both cocaine and methamphetamine addiction. However, DMI and other TCAs may have some benefit in cocaine-addicted individuals with a history of depression [69].

Selective Serotonin Reuptake Inhibitors (SSRIs)

There is little evidence that SSRI drugs are effective treatments for cocaine dependence [70], except perhaps in individuals with comorbid major depressive symptoms.

Dopaminergic Agonists and Antagonists

Amantadine and bromocriptine have shown limited success [71,72], but dopamine D$_2$ antagonists (chlorpromazine, haloperidol) have not [73]. D$_1$ agonists have looked promising in animal self-administration studies [32] and in human cuereactivity studies [74], but preliminary clinical trials have not been encouraging. Bupropion, a catecholamine reuptake inhibitor, and mazindol, a selective dopamine reuptake inhibitor, have also not shown efficacy in cocaine pharmacotherapy trials [75,76].

Disulfiram

Disulfiram, best known as an aldehyde dehydrogenase inhibitor used in the treatment of alcohol dependence, has been shown in three studies at Yale University to have efficacy for the treatment of cocaine addiction [65,66,77]. Its mechanism of action appears to be independent of effects in reducing comorbid alcohol use [66], and it may act through increasing plasma cocaine levels by inhibiting plasma esterases which metabolize [78], and inhibition of the dopamine-β-hydroxylase (DBH), the enzyme that converts dopamine to norepinephrine, thus presumably increasing synaptic DA levels, which are thought to be depleted in chronic cocaine users. The drug is associated with some toxicity (e.g., transaminase elevations, psychotic reaction) and with severe reactions when combined with alcohol, so widespread use for the treatment of cocaine addiction may be limited.

B. Approach to the Addicted Individual

1. The Monodrug User

The approach to the monodrug using patients entails selecting an effective agent for the treatment of the single addictive disorder. Such effective treatments are available for opioid dependence (e.g., methadone, buprenorphine), alcohol dependence (e.g., disulfiram and naltrexone), and tobacco (nicotine replacement therapies, sustained-release bupropion), but not as yet for cocaine or other psychostimulants. The effectiveness of these pharmacotherapies has been reviewed elsewhere, and is greatly enhanced by the patient's motivation to quit using drugs at the beginning of treatment [79,80], though effective addiction pharmacotherapies can often be helpful in those individuals without substantial motivation to quit (e.g., the individual who just wants to take a pill, rather than do behavioral treatment). With respect to pharmacotherapies, one must strive to use the safest agent available (minimal side effects) balanced with one that will have treatment effectiveness. Accordingly, in an opioid-dependent patient who is noncompliant with treatment and at risk for drug overdose, treatment with buprenorphine (which can be given three times daily and has minimal overdose potential) might be preferable to methadone (daily administration, high risk of overdose) treatment. Use of structured assessment scales like the Addiction Severity Index (ASI [81]) provides multimodal assessment of preexisting functional impairment prior to drug treatment, and can provide individualized information that can be used to tailor treatments (e.g., treatment matching).

2. The Polydrug User

Similarly, any effective pharmacotherapy(ies) for the individual drug abused may be helpful, but targeting only one drug of abuse in a polysubstance abuser is often likely to fail since the use of one drug of abuse can condition use of another (e.g., a cocaine user who also injects heroin and drinks alcohol during cocaine binges may promote cocaine craving after initial abstinence if he uses heroin or alcohol). Furthermore, the severity of addiction is likely to be higher in the polydrug abuser and these patients are more likely to have concurrent (chronic) mental and medical illness [82] and therefore to have poor treatment outcomes. In general, if one of the drugs of abuse has a defined pharmacotherapy (e.g., heroin), then a specific treatment can be initiated (e.g., methadone, naltrexone) and this addiction stabilized, prior to addressing abuse of a substance that does not have a well-established pharmacotherapy (e.g., concurrent cocaine dependence in a methadone-maintained individual).

3. The Drug User with Psychiatric Comorbidity

The psychiatric drug abuser poses considerable diagnostic and therapeutic challenges for clinicians, and the therapeutic approach taken with these "dually diagnosed" individuals is often colored by the treatment philosophy of the treating clinician (e.g., mental health versus addictions treatment provider). Accordingly, mental health clinicians tend to underemphasize (or ignore) substance abuse treatment in their psychiatric patients, and primary substance abuse providers tend to overlook psychiatric issues in their patients [83]. Given the typical fragmentation of mental health and addictions treatment in most health care systems, these individuals often "fall between the cracks," and in many cases this is related to their low motivation to receive treatment [84], which is frequently related to a lack of insight into the severity of their combined mental health and addiction problems. Nonetheless, in cases where individuals may be self-medicating psychiatric symptoms with substances of abuse (e.g., the depressed cocaine user), pharmacotherapies directed at the underlying psychiatric disorder may be useful. For example, it has been shown that the tricyclic antidepressant desipramine, which may have some efficacy in the pharmacotherapy of cocaine dependence, may be especially effective in depressed cocaine addicts [69]. Furthermore, individuals with schizophrenia may use nicotine to alleviate clinical (e.g., negative symptoms, extrapyramidal side effects) and cognitive (e.g., working memory, attentional) deficits associated with this illness [53,85]. There is evidence that the atypical antipsychotic drug clozapine [86–88] can reduce smoking and that clozapine and other atypical antipsychotic drugs such as risperidone and olanzapine can increase smoking cessation rates in combination with the nicotine transdermal patch, compared to typical antipsychotic agents (e.g., haloperidol, chlorpromazine) [89]. Methods that increase compliance with pharmacotherapies, like using medications with minimal side effects (e.g., SSRIs vs. TCAs in substance-abusing depressed patients; atypical antipsychotic drugs in drug-abusing schizophrenics), medications that can be given once daily, or by injection on a monthly or bimonthly basis (e.g., haloperidol and fluphenazine decanoate, respectively), and those with low overdose potential (e.g., anticonvulsant mood stabilizer [e.g., sodium valproate or gabapentin] vs. lithium in a substance abuser with bipolar disorder) are all strategies to deliver more effective and tolerable treatment in dually diagnosed individuals. More research is needed on the efficacy of substance abuse pharmacotherapies in psychiatric populations, but conducting such research is difficult owing to the poor compliance of dually diagnosed subjects with the study interventions, and the high subject attrition rates in these trials. Nonetheless, conducting research in dually diagnosed subjects will yield important new information which can guide clinicians as to what pharmacological and behavioral interventions are useful and practical in this challenging patient population.

VII. TREATMENT OPTIMIZATION: COMBINATION OF BIOLOGICAL AND PSYCHOSOCIAL (BEHAVIORAL) TREATMENT OF ADDICTIVE DISORDERS

Use of substance abuse pharmacotherapies is most effective when combined with standardized psychosocial (behavioral) treatments for these disorders [90]. For individuals who are attempting abstinence initiation (e.g., trying to stop using drugs), the motivational enhancement therapies, which encourage individuals to make the choice to become abstinent for their own reasons, are the psychosocial therapy of choice. Individuals who have stopped using drugs and who want to maintain their sobriety from drug use are best treated with the relapse prevention therapies, a derivative of cognitive-behavioral therapies, which emphasize strategies for avoiding cues that promote drug relapse (people, places, and things associated previously with their drug use). Several studies have reported an interaction between pharmacotherapeutic and psychotherapeutic interventions [60,90]. In fact, in federally funded methadone maintenance programs, drug counseling is a mandatory part of treatment with methadone [46].

VIII. CONCLUSIONS

There is increasing preclinical and clinical evidence for a biological basis to addictive disorders, which should lead to a new era of innovative and effective pharmacotherapies for addictive disorders. Addictive disorders should be considered as chronic medical disorders like hypertension, schizophrenia, and diabetes [1], given the long-term nature of these disorders, frequent symptom relapse, need for extended treatment, and absence of any "cure" for these disorders. The common biological system that appears to be involved in the pathophysiology of all addictive disorders is the mesolimbic dopamine (DA) system, but other neural pathways including the endogenous opioid peptide systems and the HPA axis are probably of relevance to several addictive drugs, including opioids, alcohol, cocaine, and nicotine. Treatments for these addictive disorders are increasing with the emerging knowledge of the biological basis of addiction, but one glaring deficit is the absence of an effective pharmacotherapy for cocaine dependence and other illicit psychostimulant addictions. The effective use of any such pharmacotherapy for addictive disorders will necessitate combination with effective psychosocial treatments for addiction, especially given the complex biological, psychological, and social aspects of addictive illnesses.

ACKNOWLEDGMENTS

Supported in part by grants P50-DA-12762 (PI: T.R. Kosten), P50-DA-13334 (PI: S.S. O'Malley) and R01-DA-14039 (to T.P.G.) from the National Institute on Drug Abuse (NIDA), the VISN 1 Mental Illness Research, Education and Clinical Center (MIRECC) of the Department of Veterans Affairs and a Wodecroft Foundation Young Investigator Award from the National Alliance for Research on Schizophrenia and Depression (NARSAD) to T.P.G. The helpful comments of Thomas R. Kosten, M.D. and Richard S. Schottenfeld, M.D. on the manuscript are gratefully acknowledged.

REFERENCES

1. McLellan AT, Lewis DC, O'Brien CP, Kleber HD. Drug dependence, a chronic medical illness:

Implications for treatment, insurance and outcomes evaluation. JAMA 2000;284:1689–1695.
2. O'Brien CP. A range of research-based pharmacotherapies for addiction. Science 1997;287:66–70.
3. Frances A, Pincus HA, First MB. Diagnostic and Statistical Manual of Mental Disorders, 4th ed (DSM-IV). Washington; American Psychiatric Association, 1994:886.
4. Wise RA. Drug-activation of brain reward pathways. Drug Alcohol Depend 1998;51:13–22.
5. Spanagel R, Weiss F. The dopamine hypothesis of reward: past and current status. Trends Neurosci 1999;22:521–527.
6. Horvitz JC. Mesolimbocortical and nigrostriatal dopamine responses to salient non-reward events. Neuroscience 2000;96:651–656.
7. Koob GF, Le Moal M. Drug addiction, dysregulation of reward, and allostasis. Neuropsychopharmacology 2001;24:97–129.
8. Spanagel R. Modulation of drug-induced sensitization process by endogenous opioid systems. Behav Brain Res 1995;70:37–49.
9. Sesack SR, Pickel VM. Dual ultrastructural localization of enkephalin and tyrosine hydroxylase immunoreactivity in the rat ventral tegmental area: multiple substrates for opiate-dopamine interactions. J Neurosci 1992;12:1335–1350.
10. Shieh K-R, Pan J-T. Nicotinic control of tuberoinfundibular dopaminergic neuron activity and prolactin secretion: diurnal rhythm and involvement of endogenous opiatergic system. Brain Res 1997;756:266–272.
11. George TP, Verrico CD, Xu L, Roth, RH. Effects of repeated nicotine administration and footshock stress on rat mesoprefrontal dopamine systems: evidence for opioid mechanisms. Neuropsychopharmacology 2000;23(1):79–88.
12. Krishnan-Sarin S, Rosen MI, O'Malley SS. Evidence for an opioid component in nicotine dependence. Arch. Gen. Psychiatry 1999;56:663–668.
13. O'Malley SS, Jaffe AJ, Chang G, Schottenfeld RS, Meyer RE, Rounsaville B. Naltrexone and coping skills therapy for alcohol dependence: a controlled study. Arch. Gen. Psychiatry 1992;49:881–887.
14. Volpicelli JR, Alterman AI, Hayashida M, O'Brien CP. Naltrexone in the treatment of alcohol dependence. Arch Gen Psychiatry 1992;49:876–880.
15. Spangler R, Zhou Y, Schussman SD, Ho A, Kreek MJ. Prodynorphin, proenkephalin and kappa opioid receptor mRNA responses to acute "binge" cocaine. Mol Brain Res 1997;44:139–142.
16. Kreek MJ, Koob GF. Drug dependence: stress and dysregulation of brain reward pathways. Drug Alcohol Depend 1998;51:23–47.
17. Masukawa Y, Suzuki T, Misawa M. Differential modification of the rewarding effects of methamphetamine and cocaine by opioids and antihistamines. Psychopharmacology 1993;111:139–143.
18. Shaham Y, Erb S, Stewart J. Stress-induced relapse to heroin and cocaine seeking in rats: a review. Brain Res Rev 2000;33:13–33.
19. Cone EJ, Kumor K, Thompson LK, Sherer M. Correlation of saliva cocaine levels with plasma levels and with pharmacologic effects after intravenous cocaine administration in human subjects. J Anal Toxicol 1988;12:200–206.
20. Ma F, Falk JL, Lau CE. Cocaine pharmacodynamics after intravenous and oral administration in rats: relation to pharmacokinetics. Psychopharmacology 1999;144:323–332.
21. Koob GF, Le Moal M. Drug abuse: hedonic homeostasis dysregulation. Science 1997;278:52–58.
22. Robinson TE, Berridge KC. The psychology and neurobiology of addiction: an incentive-sensitization view. Addiction 2000;95(suppl 2):S91–S117.
23. Grace AA. The tonic/phasic model of dopamine system regulation and its implications for understanding alcohol and stimulant craving. Addiction 2000;95(suppl 2):S119–S128.
24. Jentsch JD, Taylor JR. Impulsivity resulting from frontostriatal dysfunction in drug abuse: implications for the control of behavior by reward-related stimuli. Psychopharmacology 1999;146:373–390.
25. Breiter HC, Gollub RL, Weisskoff RM, et al. Acute effects of cocaine on human brain activity and emotion. Neuron 1997;19:591–611.
26. Grace AA. Cortical regulation of subcortical dopamine systems and its possible relevance to schizophrenia. J Neural Transm 1993;91:111–134.
27. Bolla KI, Funderburk FR, Cadet JL. Differential effects of cocaine and cocaine alcohol on neurocognitive performance. Neurology 2000;54:2285–2292.
28. Kosten TR. Pharmacotherapy of cerebral ischemia in cocaine dependence. Drug Alcohol Depend 1998;49:133–144.
29. Mendelson JH, Mello NK. Management of cocaine abuse and dependence. N Engl J Med 1996;334:965–972.
30. Horger BA, Iyasere CA, Berhow MT, Messer CJ, Nestler EJ, Taylor JR. Enhancement of locomotor activity and conditioned reward to cocaine by brain-derived neurotrophic factor. J Neurosci 1999;19:4110–4122.
31. Nestler EJ. Genes and addiction. Nat Genet 2000;26:277–281.
32. Self DW, Nestler EJ. Relapse to drug-seeking: neural and molecular mechanisms. Drug Alcohol Depend 1998;51:49–60.
33. Balfour DJK, Fagerstrom KO. Pharmacology of nicotine and its therapeutic use in smoking cessation and neurodegenerative disorders. Pharmacol Ther 1996;72:51–81.

34. Picciotto MR, Caldarone BJ, King SL, Zachariou V. Nicotinic receptors in the brain: links between molecular biology and behavior. Neuropsychopharmacology 2000;22:451–465.
35. Clarke PBS, Fu DS, Jakubovic A, Fibiger HC. Evidence that mesolimbic dopamine activation underlies the locomotor stimulant action on nicotine in rats. J Pharmacol Exp Ther 1988;246:701–708.
36. Fowler JS, Volkow ND, Wang G-J, et al. Inhibition of monoamine oxidase B in the brains of smokers. Nature 1996;379:733–736.
37. Fowler JS, Volkow ND, Wang G-J, et al. Brain monoamine oxidase A: inhibition by cigarette smoke. Proc Natl Acad Sci USA 1996;93:14065–14069.
38. Devane WA, Hanus L, Breuer A, et al. Isolation and structure of a brain constituent that binds to the cannabinoid receptor. Science 1992;258:1882–1884.
39. Pertwee R. Pharmacology of cannabinoid receptor ligands. Curr Med Chem 1999;6:635–664.
40. Ledent C, Valverde O, Cossu G. Unresponsiveness to cannabinoids and reduced addictive effects of opiates in CB1 receptor knockout mice. Science 1999;283:401–404.
41. Tanda G, Loddo P, Di Chiara G. Dependence of mesolimbic dopamine transmission on delta9-tetrahydrocannabinol. Eur J Phamracol 1999;376:23–26.
42. Krystal JH, Karper LP, Seibyl JP, et al. Subanesthetic effects of the non-competitive NMDA antagonist, ketamine in humans: psychotomimetic, perceptual, cognitive and neuroendocrine responses. Arch Gen Psychiatry 1994;51:199–214.
43. Jentsch JD, Redmond DE Jr, Elsworth JD, Taylor JR, Youngren KD, Roth RH. Enduring cognitive deficits and cortical dopamine dysfunction in monkeys after long-term administration of phencyclidine. Science 1997;277:953–955.
44. McCann UD, Eligulashvili V, Ricaurte GA. (+/−)-3,4-Methylenedioxymethamphetamine ("Ectasy")-induced serotonin neurotoxicity: clinical studies. Neuropsychobiology 2000;42:11–16.
45. O'Connor PG, Fiellin DA. Pharmacologic treatment of heroin-dependent patients. Ann Intern Med 2000;133:40–54.
46. Judd LL, Attkissoon C, Berrettini W, et al. Effective medical treatment of opiate addiction. JAMA 1998;280:1936–1943
47. Verebey KG, Mule SJ. Naltrexone (Trexan): a review of hepatotoxicity issues. NIDA Res Monogr 1986;67:73–81.
48. Ling W, Charuvastra C, Collins JF, et al. Buprenorphine maintenance treatment of opiate dependence: a multicenter, randomized clinical trial. Addiction 1998;93:475–486.
49. Schottenfeld RS, Pakes JR, Oliveto A, Zeidonis D, Kosten TR. Buprenorphine versus methadone maintenance treatment for concurrent opioid dependence and cocaine abuse. Arch Gen Psychiatry 1997;54:713–720.
50. Hughes JR. The future of smoking cessation therapy in the United States. Addiction 1996;91(12):1797–1802.
51. Ziedonis DM, Wyatt SA, George TP. Current issues in nicotine dependence and treatment. In: New Treatments in Chemical Addictions, eds TR Kosten, EF McCance-Katz. Washington: American Psychiatric Press, 1998;1–34.
52. Hughes JR, Goldstein MG, Hurt RD, Shiffman S. Recent advances in the pharmacotherapy of smoking. JAMA 1999;281:72–76.
53. Ziedonis DM, George TP. Schizophrenia and nicotine use: report of a pilot smoking cessation program and review of neurobiological and clinical issues. Schizophr Bull 1997;23(2):247–254.
54. Hurt RD, Sachs DPL, Glover ED, et al. A comparison of sustained-release bupropion and placebo for smoking cessation. N Engl J Med 1997;337:1195–1202.
55. Ferry LH, Burchette RJ. Efficacy of bupropion for smoking cessation in non-depressed smokers. J Addict Dis 1994;13:249.
56. Jorenby DE, Leischow SJ, Nides MA, et al. A controlled trial of sustained-release bupropion, a nicotine patch, or both for smoking cessation. N Engl J Med 1999;340:685–691.
57. Glassman AH, Stetner F, Walsh BT, et al. Heavy smokers, smoking cessation, and clonidine. JAMA 1988;259:2863–2866.
58. Glassman AH, Covey LS, Dalack GW, et al. Smoking cessation, clonidine, and vulnerability to nicotine among dependent smokers. Clin Pharmacol Ther 1993;54(6):670–679.
59. Cinciripini PM. A placebo-controlled evaluation of the effects of buspirone on smoking cessation: differences between high- and low-anxiety smokers. J Clin Psychopharmacol 1995;15:182–191.
60. Hall SM, Reus VI, Munoz RF, et al. Nortriptyline and cognitive-behavioral therapy in the treatment of cigarette smoking. Arch Gen Psychiatry 1998;55:683–690.
61. Berlin I, Said S, Spreux-Varoquaux O, et al. A reversible monoamine oxidase A inhibitor (moclobemide) facilitates smoking cessation and abstinence in heavy, dependent smokers. Clin Pharmacol Ther 1995;58:444–452.
62. Rose JE, Behm FM, Westman EC, Levin ED, Stein RM, Ripka GV. Mecamylamine combined with nicotine skin patch facilitates smoking cessation beyond nicotine patch treatment alone. Clin Pharmacol Ther 1994;56(1):86–99.
63. Rose JE, Behm FM, Westman EC. Nicotine-mecamylamine treatment for smoking cessation: the role of

64. Gawin FH, Kleber HD. Cocaine abuse treatment: Open pilot trial with desipramine and lithium carbonate. Arch Gen Psychiatry 1984;41:903–910.
65. Carroll KM, Nich C, Ball SA, McCance E, Rounsaville BJ. Treatment of cocaine and alcohol dependence with psychotherapy and disulfiram. Addiction 1998;93:713–728.
66. George TP, Chawarski MC, Pakes J, Carroll KM, Kosten TR, Schottenfeld RS. Disulfiram versus placebo for cocaine dependence in buprenorphine-maintained subjects: a preliminary study. Biol Psychiatry 2000;47:1080–1086.
67. Levin FR, Lehman AF. Meta-analysis of desipramine as an adjunct in the treatment of cocaine addiction. J Clin Psychopharmacol 1991;11:374–383.
68. Galloway GP, Newmeyer J, Knapp T, et al. Imipramine for the treatment of cocaine and methamphetamine dependence. J Addict Dis 1994;13:201–208.
69. Ziedonis DM, Kosten TR. Depression as a prognostic factor for pharmacological treatment of cocaine dependence. Psychopharmacol Bull 1991;27:337–343.
70. Grabowski J, Rhoades H, Elk R, et al. Fluoxetine is ineffective for treatment of cocaine dependence or concurrent opioid and cocaine dependence. Two placebo-controlled, double-blind trials. J Clin Psychopharmacol 1995;15:163–178.
71. Gawin FR, Morgan C, Kosten TR, et al. Double-blind evaluation of the effect of acute amantadine on cocaine craving. Psychopharmacology 1989;97:402–407.
72. Kosten TR, Morgan CM, Falcione J, Schottenfeld RS. Pharmacotherapy for cocaine-abusing methadone-maintained patients using amantadine or desipramine. Arch Gen Psychiatry 1992;49:894–898.
73. Warner EA, Kosten TR, O'Connor PG. Pharmacotherapy for opioid and cocaine abuse. Med Clin North Am 1997;81:909–925.
74. Haney M, Collins ED, Ward AS, Foltin RW, Fischman MW. Effect of a selective dopamine D1 agonist (ABT-431) on smoked cocaine self-administration in humans. Psychopharmacology 1999;143:102–110.
75. Stine SM, Krystal JH, Kosten TR, Charney DS. Mazindol treatment of cocaine dependence. Drug Alcohol Depend 1995;39:245–252.
76. Margolin A, Kosten TR, Avants SK, et al. A multicenter trial of bupropion for cocaine dependence in methadone-maintained patients. Drug Alcohol Depend 1995;40:125–131.
77. Petrakis IL, Carroll KM, Nich C, et al. Disulfiram treatment for cocaine dependence in methadone-maintained opioid addicts. Addiction 2000;95:219–228.
78. McCance-Katz EF, Kosten TR, Jatlow PI. Disulfiram effects on acute cocaine administration. Drug Alcohol Depend 1998;57:27–39.
79. Miller WR, Rollnick S. Motivational Interviewing. New York: Guilford Press, 1991.
80. Prochaska JO, DiClemente CC. Stages and processes of self-change of smoking: Toward an integrative model of change. J Consult Clin Psychol 1983;51(3):390–395.
81. McLellan AT, Kuschner T, Metzger H, et al. The fifth edition of the addiction severity index. J Subst Abuse Treatment 1992;8:199–213.
82. George TP, Krystal JH. Comorbidity of psychiatric and substance abuse disorders. Curr Opin Psychiatry 2000;13:327–331.
83. Drake RE, Mercer-McFadden C, Mueser KT, McHugo GJ, Bond GR. Review of integrated mental health and substance abuse treatment for patients with dual disorders. Schizophr Bull 1998;24:589–608.
84. Ziedonis DM, Trudeau K. Motivation to quit using substances among individuals with schizophrenia: implications for a motivation-based treatment model. Schizophr Bull 1997;23(2):229–238.
85. Dalack GW, Healy DJ, Meador-Woodruff JH. Nicotine dependence and schizophrenia: clinical phenomenon and laboratory findings. Am J Psychiatry 1998;155:1490–1501.
86. George TP, Sernyak MJ, Ziedonis DM, Woods SW. Effects of clozapine on smoking in chronic schizophrenic outpatients. J Clin Psychiatry 1995;56(8):344–346.
87. McEvoy JP, Freudenreich O, Wilson WH. Smoking and therapeutic response to clozapine in patients with schizophrenia. Biol Psychiatry 1999;46:125–129.
88. McEvoy J, Freudenreich O, McGee M, VanderZwaag C, Levin E, Rose J. Clozapine decreases smoking in patients with chronic schizophrenia. Biol Psychiatry 1995;37:550–552.
89. George TP, Zeidonis DM, Feingold A, et al. Nicotine transdermal patch and atypical antipsychotic medications for smoking cessation in schizophrenia. Am J Psychiatry 2000;157(11):1835–1842.
90. Carroll KM. Manual-guided psychosocial treatment: a new virtual requirement for pharmacotherapy trials? Arch Gen Psychiatry 1997;54:923–928.

40

Neuroimaging Abnormalities in Drug Addiction and Alcoholism

WYNNE K. SCHIFFER, DOUGLAS A. MARSTELLER, and STEPHEN L. DEWEY
Brookhaven National Laboratory, Upton, New York, U.S.A.

I. INTRODUCTION

Although the theoretical premise of positron emission tomography (PET) research has remained largely the same over the past two decades, advances in chemistry and PET instrumentation coupled with a detailed examination of the biochemistry of new radiotracers have allowed PET to be applied to new areas of biology and medicine. The basis for the PET method is the use of tracer kinetics in the study of human biochemistry and physiology in vivo. Thus, any PET study involves a multiplicity of processes which together result in the PET image and the pharmacokinetics that define that image. PET studies allow us to observe, noninvasively, the morphology associated with addiction both in terms of physiology and function. In this, PET is not used to define a biochemical pathway in a single cell, and it does not compete with the elegant basic work or the structure and function of single cells or small groups of cells. By the same token, and this is one of the great powers of PET, the ability to assay the dynamic activity of a large aggregate of cells in vivo, especially the human brain, involving systems with numerous complex interactions in quantitative terms, is unique to PET.

As a whole, neurochemical imaging studies of addiction and the addictive process have three main goals, which are integrated into the overall clinical application of treatment and prevention. One is to determine the actions of these drugs on the brain, with the hopes of clarifying those actions that contribute to the rewarding or reinforcing processes of drug dependence. This is critical both to the development of treatment options and to potential hereditary effects produced by prolonged drug exposure. The second objective, then, is to elucidate the physiological nature of drug vulnerability, such that an increased susceptibility to drug dependence might be expressed by different physiological markers or functional responses to rewarding drugs. For example, chronic drug abusers might express an increased number of receptors compared to healthy controls, which might subsequently alter the neurochemical and behavioral response of these patients to drug therapies targeting other symptoms (like anxiety). Finally, given the subtle plasticity of the brain and the vulnerability of neural systems to chronic drug exposure, it is likely that prolonged drug abuse produces physiological and functional changes that may possess hereditary significance. Given that PET can measure both neurophysiology and neurochemical function, the third objective is to use our understanding of drug mechanisms and drug effects to locate and protect vulnerable populations.

PET can be used to label proteins of physiological relevance, such as receptors, transporters, and enzymes in the human brain, as well as to provide an indirect index of synaptic neurotransmitter activity in the living system. These studies also allow an evaluation of the relationship between the kinetics of an abused drug in the brain and the temporal relationship to its behavioral effects (Fig. 1). PET radiotracers are chemically similar to the endogenous compounds whose actions they probe and possess similar pharmacological profiles to many drugs under investigation. To date, methamphetamine [Nakamura et al. 1996, 1997), nicotine [Nyback et al. 1994], opiates [Hartvig et al. 1984], cocaine [Fowler et al. 1989], and methylphenidate [Ding et al. 1994] have been successfully labeled. Thus, some radiotracers probe biochemical and physiological changes directly, while others provide an indirect mechanism of what we believe a drug action is in the brain. Studies exploring the pharmacologic activity of marijuana use a labeled compound that mimics the activity of what we believe to be an endogenous ligand for the cannabinoid receptor [Gatley et al. 1998]. PET is uniquely suited to simultaneously manipulate and measure synaptic neurotransmitter responsiveness in the living brain. This approach can be used to assess the functional integrity of neurotransmitter systems and the multiple mechanisms of drug action. In this, the development of radiotracers for studying various systems remains one of the major thrusts of PET research. At this point, a broad spectrum of radiotracers has been developed and applied to the study of the brain with a special focus on drug mechanisms and the physiological changes associated with drug addiction.

This chapter will begin with a brief overview of current philosophies regarding the nature of drug reward and drug abuse as they relate to possible physiological adaptations in the addicted patient. In the next section, we provide a summary of findings in our laboratory and others using carbon-11-labeled cocaine to examine both drug mechanism and physiological changes specific to psychostimulant abuse. Since the development of [^{11}C]cocaine provided the impetus for quantitative methods that are widely applied today, we will briefly discuss issues related to the application of these methods. This will be followed by sections describing the status of other labeled drugs of abuse, and what they have contributed to our understanding of the addicted brain. A discussion of the use of PET to develop various treatments for addiction will be included following that, and the chapter will conclude with a section on the challenges facing the development of appropriate pharmacotherapies for addiction given the altered physiological states associated with chronic drug abuse or vulnerability to drug abuse.

II. UNDERSTANDING DRUG DEPENDENCE

All drugs of abuse initially interact with specific receptor or reuptake proteins, which, depending on the pharmacokinetic and pharmacodynamic properties of the drug, produce a chain of events that activates a central reward system in the brain. Given that drugs with different mechanisms can produce similar rewarding behaviors, it follows that the mechanism of the drug per se might not be responsible for drug dependence and that subsequent physiological adaptations might extend beyond the site of action of the drug in question. Neural circuits within the mesolimbic/mesocortical system have been identified that mediate the acute reinforcing effects of most abused drugs [Koob 1992]. In particular, dopaminergic neurotransmitter systems in the striatum (including the nucleus accumbens; NAc, which is the ventral striatum), ventral tegmental area (VTA) and prefrontal cortex appear sensitive to addictive compounds, since lesions to any one of these areas reduces drug self-administration or drug-seeking behaviors [Roberts and Koob 1982]. Further, the addictive liability of many abused drugs appears to be a function of the magnitude to which they increase dopamine activity in these regions [Di Chiara and Imperato 1988; Di Chiara et al. 1999].

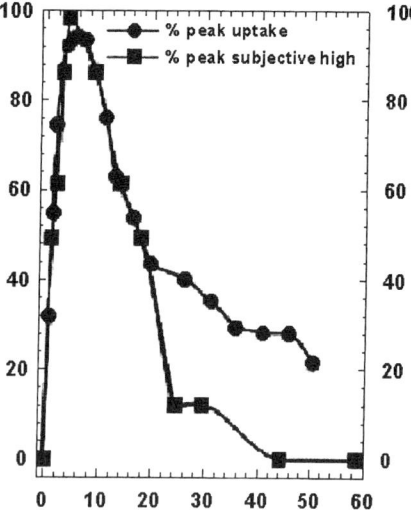

Figure 1 Time activity curves for [^{11}C]cocaine in the striatum plotted alongside the temporal course for the self reported "high" induced by intravenous cocaine administration. Measures are shown as percentage change from peak response. (From Volkow et al. 1995.)

Since the dopamine system appears fundamental to addiction, many PET studies have focused on physiological and functional alterations within this system. It is important to clarify the different ways in which PET is used to study these adaptations. First, PET studies exploring physiological alterations in the brain typically employ radiotracers with a high affinity for a given dopamine receptor (either presynaptic dopamine transporters, DAT, or postsynaptic D_2 receptors). This ensures that the binding of the radiotracer will not be influenced by changes in synaptic dopamine, since presumably they are both competing for the same receptor site [Seeman et al. 1989]. Second, PET studies exploring dynamic fluctuations in radiotracer concentrations use radiotracers with a moderate receptor affinity, comparable to or lower than that of dopamine itself. The theory behind this approach is that radiotracers which compete equally with dopamine for a given receptor site are sensitive to changes in synaptic dopamine concentrations [Dewey et al. 1993]. For example, increases in synaptic dopamine have repeatedly demonstrated the ability to reduce the binding of the moderate-affinity D_2 radiotracer, [^{11}C]raclopride [Dewey et al. 1993, 1999; Endres et al. 1997; Smith et al. 1998; Volkow et al. 1999]. The reverse holds true for decreases in synaptic dopamine, such that drugs which inhibit dopaminergic systems increase the binding of [^{11}C]raclopride [Dewey et al. 1992, 1995; Ginovart et al. 1997; Hietala et al. 1997]. This allows quantification of changes in the releasable pool of dopamine resulting from chronic drug abuse, such that chronic exposure to a psychostimulant might diminish the dopaminergic response to a drug challenge, without affecting receptor number.

In humans, both the effects of drug intake on emotional variables and the motivation for drug seeking usually, initially, depend on psychological variables (i.e., stress) and individual differences in sensitivity and response. For example, PET studies with the high-affinity dopamine D_2 receptor ligand [^{18}F]N-methylspiroperidol and indices of glucose metabolic activity with [^{18}F]DG suggest that a disruption of mesocortical dopamine systems from chronic cocaine use leads to abnormal glucose metabolic activity in terminal, primarily cortical, areas [Fowler and Volkow 1994]. Dysregulation of these frontal regions in cocaine addicts might favor the emergence of behaviors associated with addiction, such as the loss of control leading to compulsive drug-taking behavior. Thus, the central reward system of the brain appears to integrate individual variables and to adjust drug seeking and drug taking accordingly.

Under healthy conditions, the dopaminergic reward system is regulated by several physiological mechanisms that remain sensitive to pharmacologic, environmental, and behavioral interventions [Deutch et al. 1990; Dewey et al. 1991; Innis et al. 1992]. Although the initial effects of rewarding drugs on the brain are related to alterations within the dopaminergic system, it is likely that the development of drug dependence is also a function of the ability of dopamine to modulate or be modulated by other neurotransmitter systems. Serotonin, GABA, glutamate, and dopamine neurotransmitter systems are continually interacting to maintain a level of functional homeostasis, such that changes in one system may be compensated for by endogenous alterations in a related system. In turn, each of these neurotransmitter systems plays a specific role in mediating behaviors associated with drug dependence like craving, stress, or withdrawal. Thus, although addiction has been classically attributed to isolated changes in the dopamine system, each of these systems is most likely modified during the development of dependence, and they appear to remain sensitive to future perturbations.

For example, cocaine produces a large influx in synaptic dopamine concentrations by blocking dopamine reuptake in the striatal region of the brain. The expression of dopamine-mediated behaviors requires the activation of GABA pathways [Scheel-Kruger 1986], which are therefore a particularly susceptible target for cocaine's effects. Further, repeated overstimulation of dopaminergic systems by chronic cocaine use might alter the responsivity of the GABA system to a perturbation of the dopaminergic system. Consistent with this hypothesis, studies in our laboratory have demonstrated that cocaine-dependent subjects have an enhanced metabolic response to a drug targeting the GABA system [Volkow et al. 1998]. In addition, there appear to be significant reductions in striatal dopamine D_2 receptors in cocaine dependent subjects that persist long after detoxification [Volkow et al. 1990, 1993]. Taken together, these findings suggest an involvement of GABA in the dopamine abnormalities characteristic of chronic cocaine abuse.

III. PET STUDIES OF DRUG MECHANISM AND THE ADDICTED BRAIN

PET is uniquely suited to simultaneously manipulate and measure changes in synaptic neurotransmitter responsiveness or physiology in the living brain. This approach can be used to assess the functional integrity of neurotransmitter systems and the multiple mechanisms of drug action. In this, the development of radiotracers for studying various systems remains one of the major thrusts of PET research. At this point, a broad spectrum of radiotracers has been developed and applied to the study of the brain with a special focus on drug mechanisms and the physiological changes associated with drug addiction.

A. PET Studies of Cocaine Addiction

Cocaine possesses a reward value such that laboratory animals, given free access, will self-administer until death [Koob and Bloom 1988]. This phenomenon distinguishes cocaine from other drugs of abuse, since most are not self-administered at the expense of self-preservation. In humans, cocaine is one of the most widely abused drugs [Gawin and Ellinwood 1988], and it is also associated with major medical problems like myocardial infarction, seizures, and psychosis [Johanson and Fischman 1989]. Acute cocaine administration increases subcortical dopamine levels by blocking the dopamine transporter (DAT), preventing reuptake and subsequent catabolism [Reith 1988]. Studies in primates revealed that the binding of [^{11}C]cocaine in the striatum is reduced by prior treatment with nomifensine, a drug that binds to DAT sites, supporting in vitro evidence that cocaine binding occurs to a site associated with the DAT [Fowler et al. 1989]. When animals were pretreated with other drugs that inhibit norepinephrine and serotonin transporters, [^{11}C]cocaine binding was not altered [Volkow et al. 1995b]. These studies are consistent with the notion that while the mechanisms for cocaine's reinforcing properties are complex, they primarily involve the brain dopamine system [Ritz et al. 1987]. Given that PET measures the regional distribution and kinetics of radioisotopes in tissues of living subjects [Mullani and Volkow 1992], it has been used to address these measurements with respect to cocaine's behavioral and toxic effects.

The ability of PET to measure sequential changes in the distribution of positron labeled compounds makes it an ideal technique to investigate the binding characteristics of psychoactive drugs in vivo. From studies using [^{11}C]cocaine, several observations have revealed significant biological characteristics that relate to its abuse liability. First, pharmacokinetic PET investigations of [^{11}C]cocaine in the brain indicate maximal uptake in the striatum. Figure 2 presents the radioactivity distribution in the human brain (Fig. 2a), the nonhuman primate brain (b), and the rodent brain

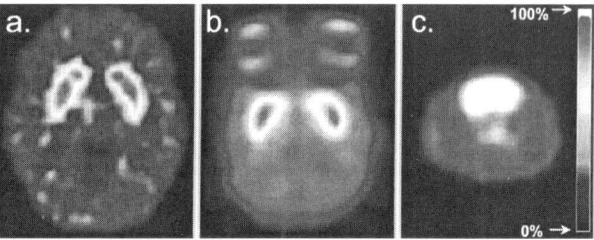

Figure 2 Radioactivity distribution of [^{11}C]cocaine in the human brain (a), the primate brain (female *Papio anubis* baboon (b), and the rodent brain (c). The color scale has been normalized to the injected dose of [^{11}C]cocaine.

(c) measured with PET. Figure 3a presents these temporal dynamics in the primate striatum and cerebellum, where the intensity and duration of [^{11}C]cocaine binding are clearly greater in the striatum. This information has been used to demonstrate that the dose of cocaine typically used by cocaine addicts ($\sim$ 25–50 mg/kg IV) [Verebey and Gold 1988] occupies roughly 63% of DAT high-affinity sites [Volkow et al. 1996a], although given considerations of pharmacokinetics, these occupancies might be underestimated. Second, these studies demonstrate that the uptake kinetics of cocaine are very rapid, with a peak concentration at 4–8 min after injection. Previous studies suggest that the rate of change at which total DAT occupancy is achieved will affect the intensity of cocaine's effects [Pettit and Justice 1991; Volkow et al. 1995a]. When compared with the DAT inhibitor, methylphenidate (Ritalin), which is much less addictive and clears from the brain at a much slower rate than cocaine, it appears that pharmacokinetics play a critical role in the addictive liability of abused substances [Volkow et al. 1995a]. Thus, while the relationship of DAT blockade to euphoria can be estimated, it is likely that higher doses will achieve total blockade faster, and will also maintain this blockade for a longer period of time [Volkow et al. 1995a]. In this, analysis of the pharmacokinetic behavior of cocaine in the human brain reveals that it is not only an affinity for the DAT that makes cocaine uniquely addictive, but also its fast uptake.

These studies are critically dependent on the modeling parameters used to estimate change in radiotracer distribution over time. Studies with [^{11}C]cocaine initiated the development of a graphical method for the calculation of binding potential from time-activity curves and radiotracer plasma concentrations [Logan et al. 1990]. In going from the labeled compound to the

Neuroimaging Abnormalities

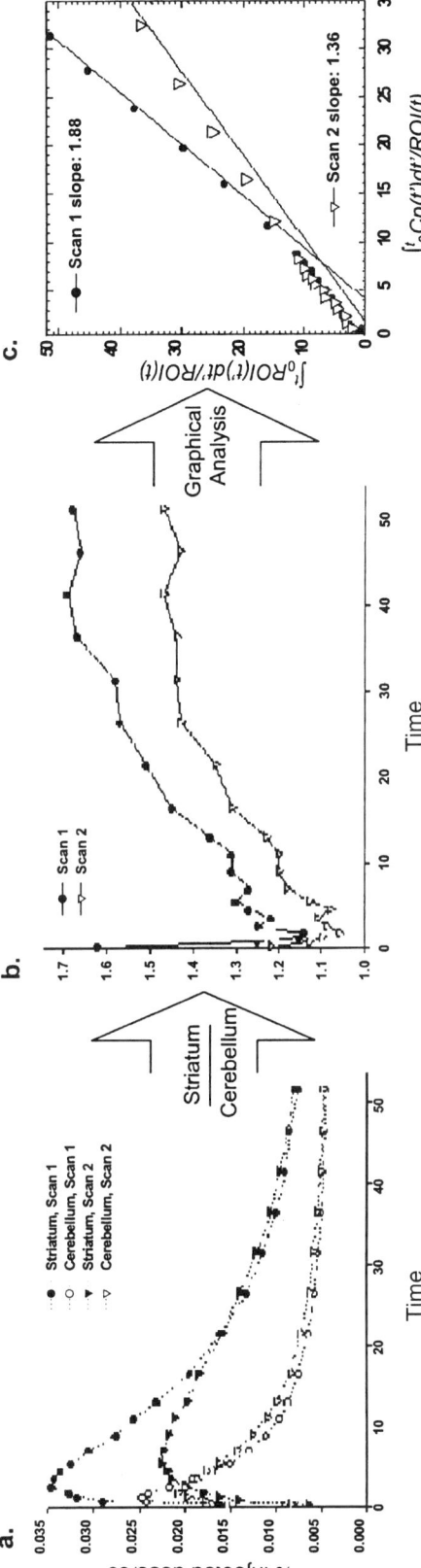

Figure 3 Strategy for graphical analysis from the time activity curves corrected for plasma concentrations of [^{11}C]cocaine (a), followed by conversion to striatum over cerebellum ratio of [^{11}C]cocaine (b), converted to a Logan plot for graphical analysis. Data are given as baseline scan (scan 1, circles) and challenge scan (scan 2, triangles). For the challenge scan, phencyclidine (PCP) was co-injected with [^{11}C]cocaine, and the decrease in [^{11}C]cocaine binding most likely represents direct competition from PCP for dopamine transporter (DAT) sites (c).

biochemical basis of the PET image, we enter an area which is the heart of the PET method and one which is far beyond the scope of this chapter. Mechanistic information must be derived from in vivo PET studies where kinetic radiotracer effects and pharmacokinetics must be estimated from mathematical models. One method, described below, is generally suited to tracers characterized by rapid pharmacokinetic profiles and is also widely applied to PET studies assessing either regional or drug-induced changes in brain pharmacodynamics. For this reason, it is critical to the interpretation of PET studies to understand the parameters used to quantitate the data, especially where measures of change over time are fundamental to the outcome of a given experiment.

3. Graphical Analysis of PET Data

A Logan plot, describing functions of time relative to tissue and plasma concentrations of the radiotracer gives a reliable index of the binding potential (affinity for and density of DAT sites). This is critical to the interpretation of any studies using radiotracers with fast kinetic profiles. Figure 3 demonstrates the analytical procedure through which regionally specific temporal dynamics are used to calculate the binding potential of [^{11}C]cocaine. For comparison, data from animals given phencyclidine (PCP) which has an affinity for the DAT similar to cocaine, are also presented. In these studies, animals were given a baseline [^{11}C]cocaine scan followed by administration of saline or PCP, immediately prior to a second [^{11}C]cocaine scan.

These data indicate that that there is a linear relationship between radiotracer tissue concentration and plasma volume. Linearity is expressed as the slope, which corresponds to the steady state space of the radiotracer (distribution volume; DV). The ratio of distribution volumes in a receptor/transporter-rich region to that in a receptor/transporter-poor region (Fig. 3b, c) is called the distribution volume ratio (DVR) and is related to the apparent binding potential. Usually, at least with ligands for D$_2$ receptors and DAT sites, the receptor rich region comprises the striatum while the receptor poor region consists of cerebellar areas. Binding potential is fundamental to the interpretation of PET studies, and is defined as B_{max}/K_d, where B_{max} is the number of binding sites and K_d^{-1} represents the binding affinity [Mintun et al. 1984]. This graphical method has been applied to the given PET study in Figure 3c, which represents a typical Logan plot. The graphical analysis allows a measure of change over time that incorporates both the intensity and duration of radiotracer binding, such that subsequent comparisons can be made with related variables.

The DAT, located on the presynaptic terminal of the dopamine neuron, is an important subject of research not only because it is linked to the addictive properties of cocaine but also because it is a marker for the integrity of the dopamine neuron. DAT sites appear to be related to neuronal mass and thus these tracers have been of particular value in monitoring the progress of neurodegenerative processes secondary to chronic drug abuse. For example, a logical prediction would be that through prolonged targeting of the DAT protein, chronic cocaine abuse induces compensatory alterations in the physiology and function of these sites. [^{11}C]Cocaine was used to evaluate the DAT in 12 detoxified cocaine abusers with 20 age-matched controls who had never used cocaine [Volkow et al. 1996d]. Cocaine abusers had significantly lower global radiotracer uptake in the striatum compared to control subjects; however, they also had less uptake in the cerebellum. As a result, their DVR was not significantly different. However, since neither current nor detoxified cocaine abusers demonstrated the typical age-related decline in DAT characteristic of healthy populations [Wang et al. 1997a], it might be that excessive blockade of the DAT induces some neuroprotection, although this merits further investigation.

B. PET Studies of Simultaneous Cocaine/Alcohol Abuse

A significant medical issue in cocaine abuse is the documented increased risk in toxicity when cocaine and alcohol are used in combination. In fact, the concurrent use of cocaine and alcohol confers an 18-fold increase in the risk of sudden death relative to the use of cocaine alone [Rose et al. 1990]. It has been proposed that cocaethylene, an enzyme formed by the reaction of cocaine with alcohol in the presence of liver esterases found in the blood and other organs of postmortem polydrug abusers [Hearn et al. 1991a, b), might be toxic. However, PET studies with [^{11}C]cocaethylene demonstrated this is unlikely [Fowler et al. 1992b]. Alternatively, since the combined use of cocaine and alcohol is one of the most frequent patterns of polydrug use, it is possible that alcohol changes the pharmacokinetics of cocaine in the brain and in the heart. Since later studies used concurrent [^{11}C]cocaine and alcohol administration to demonstrate that the pharmacokinetics of cocaine were not changed by alcohol administration [Fowler et al. 1992a], this is also unlikely. These PET studies are consistent with the notion that the direct effects of cocaine and alcohol contribute to the fatality of the combination, rather than their metabolic interaction. Cocaine abusers express a blunted response to alcohol in limbic regions and in cortical regions connected to limbic areas, which might be a result of tolerance from prolonged cocaine exposure [Volkow et al. 2000]. Similarly, PET studies of alcoholics indicate significant reductions in D_2 receptors (postsynaptic marker) but not in DAT availability (presynaptic marker) when compared with nonalcoholics [Hietala et al. 1994; Volkow et al. 1996c)].

C. PET Studies of Methamphetamine Abuse

Methamphetamine is a popular and highly addictive drug of abuse that has raised concerns because it is neurotoxic to dopamine terminals in animal studies [Villemagne et al. 1998]. While the mechanisms of methamphetamine are unclear, it appears to increase the synthesis of dopamine [Schmidt et al. 1985]. PET studies using radiotracers with a high affinity for the DAT have demonstrated significant reductions in DAT density in methamphetamine abusers [McCann et al. 1998; Villemagne et al. 1998; Volkow et al. 2001]. These studies suggest loss of DAT or loss of dopamine terminals, and raise the possibility that as this population ages, they may be at increased risk for the development of parkinsonism or neuropsychiatric conditions associated with diminished activity of dopamine neurons [McCann et al. 1998]. Moreover, reduced DAT density in the caudate/putamen and nucleus accumbens has been associated with the duration of methamphetamine use, and closely related to the severity of persistent psychiatric symptoms [Sekine et al. 2001]. These studies also suggest that even if methamphetamine use ceases, DAT reduction may be prolonged [Melega et al. 1997; Sekine et al. 2001]. Although a neuroprotective phenomenon provides a salient explanation for findings in cocaine abusers, more studies are needed to rule out sampling effects as well as confounding variables like cigarette smoking.

D. PET Studies of Nicotine Abuse

In spite of the fact that there are 45 million cigarette smokers in the United States and there are 400,000 deaths per year associated with smoking, surprisingly little is known about the neurochemical actions of tobacco smoke on the human brain. Imaging studies have been summarized in a recent book [Domino 1995]. Nicotine stimulates nicotinic acetylcholine receptors, which in turn are thought to stimulate dopaminergic transmission [Clarke et al. 1988]. The pharmacokinetics of inhaled nicotine have been measured using [^{11}C]nicotine [Bergstrom et al. 1995], and acute administration of intravenous nicotine has been reported to reduce brain metabolism [Stapleton et al. 1993].

Recently, monoamine oxidase A and B (MAO A and B) have been examined in the human brain (Fowler et al. 1996a, b). MAO breaks down neurotransmitter amines like dopamine, serotonin, and norepinephrine, as well as amines from exogenous sources. It occurs in two subtypes, MAO A and MAO B, which can be imaged in vivo using [^{11}C]clorgyline and [^{11}C]L-deprenyl, respectively. It has been proposed that MAO is one of the molecular targets proposed to link smoking and depression [Berlin et al. 1995; Yu et al. 1988], due to the antidepressant properties of MAO inhibitors. Since the antidepressant effects of the nonselective MAO inhibitors are generally attributed to the inhibition of MAO A [Caldecott-Hazard and Schneider 1992], it is possible that depressed smokers are self-medicating an overactive MAO A system.

[^{11}C]L-Deprenyl is a labeled version of the MAO B inhibitor drug L-deprenyl. Both clorgyline and L-deprenyl act through irreversible mechanisms, so when they are labeled with ^{11}C, they provide the opportunity to visualize enzymatic activity in vivo and to study the pharmacodynamics of MAO. PET studies indicate that smokers have a 28% reduction in MAO A [Fowler et al. 1996b] and a 40% reduction in MAO B, relative to age-matched nonsmokers [Fowler et al. 1996a]. Since MAO inhibition is associated with enhanced activity of dopaminergic systems, this reduction may account for the reduced rate of Parkinson's disease in smokers [Newhouse and Hughes 1991]. Further, these findings indicate that smoking-induced changes in MAO activity may also contribute to some of the features of smoking epidemiology, including high rates of smoking in people with psychiatric disorders like depression and schizophrenia, or polydrug abuse. There is evidence that smokers are self-medicating in the case of certain psychiatric disorders and that they use smoking to reduce anxiety and to increase alertness and cognition [Levin et al. 1996; Newhouse and Hughes 1991].

E. PET Studies of Opiate Abuse

Morphine and related drugs activate G-protein-coupled receptors whose physiological ligands are peptides. Three classes of opioid receptors, each comprising two or more subtypes, are generally recognized, termed mu (μ), delta (δ) and kappa (κ) receptors. μ-Opioid receptors appear to be the major targets involved in drug dependence. [^{11}C]carfentanil [Saji et al. 1992], a tracer which binds selectively to the μ-opiate system, has been shown to concentrate in regions of the brain such as the basal ganglia and the thalamus, which contain high levels of μ-opiate receptors [Frost et al. 1985]. Its uptake can be reduced by pretreatment with nalaxone, an opiate antagonist [Lee et al. 1988]. In addition, the opioid antagonist [^{11}C]diprenorphine has also been labeled for PET studies. However, [^{11}C]diprenorphine labels other opiate receptor subtypes in addition to the μ-opioid sites selectively labeled by [^{11}C]carfentanil, thus limiting its usefulness in defining abnormalities of specific opiate receptor subtypes in various diseases [Frost et al. 1990].

Stabilized heroin addicts treated with effective doses of methadone have markedly reduced drug craving; reduction or elimination of heroin use; normalized stress-responsive hypothalamic-pituitary-adrenal, reproductive, and gastrointestinal function; and marked improvement in immune function and normal responses to pain, all of which are physiological indices modulated in part by endogenous and exogenous opioids directed at the μ-opiate receptors and, in some cases, the κ-opioid systems. In a PET study using the μ- and κ-opioid receptor antagonist [^{18}F]cyclofoxy, recovering heroin addicts on maintenance methadone therapy demonstrated altered receptor binding in the thalamus, amygdala, caudate, anterior cingulate cortex, and putamen when compared with healthy controls [Kling et al. 2000]. This finding agrees with prior studies of glucose metabolism in healthy controls given an acute dose of fentanyl [Firestone et al. 1996] or morphine [London et al. 1990]. Although the differences in radiotracer binding may be related to receptor occupancy with methadone, this study suggests that significant numbers of opioid receptors may be available to function normally, despite chronic blockade of the opiate system [Kling et al. 2000].

Inasmuch as dopamine plays a role in opiate withdrawal and dependence, chronic opiate exposure might alter the dopaminergic system in a manner to that demonstrated by cocaine and methamphetamine. [^{11}C]raclopride has been used to measure D_2 receptor availability in opiate-dependent subjects at baseline, and then again during naloxone-precipitated withdrawal [Wang et al. 1997b]. Because [^{11}C]raclopride is sensitive to changes in endogenous dopamine [Dewey et al. 1993], this strategy enabled us to test whether we could document in humans dopaminergic reductions reported in animal models of opiate withdrawal. Although there were decreases in D_2 receptors in opiate-dependent subjects, there were no significant changes in striatal DA concentration during acute withdrawal. PET investigations in our own laboratory have demonstrated that the addictive liability of opiate drugs is associated with increased dopamine activity in the striatum of primates (unpublished results), consistent with in vivo microdialysis studies [Leone et al. 1991; Pothos et al. 1991; Rada et al. 1991].

F. PET Studies of Phencyclidine (PCP) and Ketamine ("Special K") Abuse

PCP and related dissociative anesthetics act by antagonizing the NMDA glutamate receptor. Although they are widely used as anesthetic drugs for children and animals, PCP has been a widely abused substance for over two decades, and ketamine is now in fashion. The use of PET to study PCP abuse is very preliminary. The uptake of [^{11}C]ketamine in primates, like cocaine, is very rapid in the striatum [Shiue et al. 1997]. A single report done in a group of PCP abusers who were studied with [^{18}F]FDG indicated that, when compared with normal controls, PCP abusers demonstrate diminished glucose metabolism in frontal cortical areas, striatum, and thalamus [Wu et al. 1991b]. This is consistent with the applicability of NMDA antagonists as models of schizophrenia, since schizophrenic patients demonstrate a similar regional glucose pattern [Wolkin et al. 1985; Wu et al. 1991a], and stabilized schizophrenic patients given the NMDA antagonist ketamine experience an exacerbation of symptoms identical in content to those exhibited prior to clinical stabilization [Lahti et al. 1995]. Primate PET studies in our own laboratory have demonstrated that PCP and ketamine might share with cocaine the ability to block DAT proteins, thus increasing mesolimbic dopamine activity and producing a rewarding response in addition to a dissociative state. We used [^{11}C]cocaine in both pretreatment and coadministration paradigms to demonstrate that the increases in subcortical dopamine produced by PCP in a related study (measured with [^{11}C]raclopride) can be attributed to occupancy of DAT sites (Fig. 3).

G. PET Studies of Marijuana Abuse

Marijuana is the most widely used illegal drug of abuse in the United States [Goodman and Gilman 1990]. Although the mechanisms by which Δ^9-tetrahydrocannabinol (THC; the main psychoactive substance in marijuana) exerts its psychoactive effects are still not known, they may occur through an interaction of THC with regionally localized receptor sites in the human brain [Howlett 1990]. Attempts to investigate THC in the living brain with PET by labeling it with a positron emitter have been unsuccessful because of the highly lipophilic nature of THC. This was also a limitation for $(-)$-5-^{18}F-Δ^8-THC, an analog of Δ^9-THC, which was labeled with fluorine-18 but did not show specific binding [Charalambous et al. 1991]. Although a promising alternative may be the use of THC antagonists with high receptor affinities [Gatley et al. 1996, 1997, 1998], this issue has yet to be resolved. Thus, imaging studies of chronic marijuana users have concentrated on the measurement of the effect of THC intoxication on cerebral blood flow and metabolism. For example, acute marijuana administration has been reported to decrease blood flow in subjects who were not experienced marijuana smokers, and to increase it in subjects who were experienced marijuana smokers [Mathew et al. 1997]. Chronic marijuana users demonstrated a temporary reduction in cerebral blood flow that reverted to normal with abstinence [Mathew et al. 1992, 1999] however, the measurement of the effects of THC and marijuana on blood flow may be confounded by the vasoactive properties of THC [Nahas 1986].

Since measures of brain glucose activity using [^{18}F]DG are insensitive to fluctuations in blood flow [Sokoloff et al. 1977], the acute effects of THC could be measured without confounding vasoactive effects. PET studies have been performed in nonabusing controls as well as in marijuana abusers, in which subjects received a baseline PET scan with [^{18}F]DG and a second scan after intravenous administration of THC. Though the whole-brain metabolic response to the effects of THC was variable among individuals, there appeared to be a consistent pattern of cerebellar activation paralleling the high cerebellar concentration of THC receptors [Volkow et al. 1996b]. Since the cerebellum is involved in motor coordination, proprioception, and learning, activation of the cerebellum by THC could explain the disruption of motor coordination and proprioception during THC intoxication.

H. PET Studies of Inhalant Abuse

While the rate of inhalant abuse continues to rise in this country, it remains one of the least-studied and least-discussed groups of abused substances [Brouette and Anton 2001]. Three groups of inhalants have demonstrated significant abuse liability in humans, especially children and adolescents: volatile solvents, nitrous oxide, and nitrites, among which glues, paints, and aerosol propellants are the most commonly abused [Howard et al. 2001; Howard and Jenson 1999; Kurtzman et al. 2001]. Recent studies suggest the existence of overlapping molecular sites of action for ethanol, inhalants, and volatile anesthetics like PCP on glycine receptors, and illustrate the feasibility of pharmacological antagonism of the effects of these drugs [Beckstead et al. 2001]. Since organic solvents have been implicated in a number of neuropsychiatric disturbances, neuroleptics have typically been used to treat inhalant abuse [Hernandez-Avila et al. 1998; Misra et al. 1999]. In a recent study, Tc-99m-hexamethylpropyleneamine oxime (Tc-99m-HMPAO) brain SPECT scans along with psychiatric and biochemical tests were performed in 10 inhalant-dependent patients ranging from 16 to 18 years of age [Kucuk et al. 2000]. This study found that prolonged exposure to inhalants produced significant abnormalities in brain SPECT images, including hypo- and hyperperfusion in primarily temporal and parietal regions, respectively, demonstrated by nonhomogeneous radiotracer uptake.

Direct assessment of the mechanism of action of solvents is often difficult to validate since these drugs are absent of the typical receptor binding kinetics of most abused drugs. Instead, organic solvents, like alcohol, have been classically related to a more generalized alteration in neuronal membrane function [Kurtzman et al. 2001]. Recent studies in our laboratory have demonstrated that toluene, which is found in adhesives, spray paint, glues, and paint thinners, possesses a regionally specific binding profile influencing in subcortical and cerebellar areas (Fig. 4). PET investigations of dopaminergic activity in patients receiving an acute dose of toluene demonstrated no significant effects of the drug on dopamine synthesis or postsynaptic receptor activity [Edling et al. 1997; Hageman et al. 1999]. This is especially perplexing in light of the moderate therapeutic efficacy of dopamine receptor antagonists in the treatment of inhalant abuse [Hernandez-Avila et al. 1998; Misra et al. 1999].

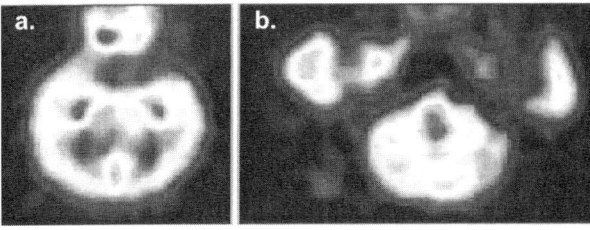

Figure 4 Radioactivity distribution of [¹¹C]toluene in the primate brain, with (a) representing distribution at the striatal level and (b) representing radioactivity distribution at the level of the cerebellum. The color scale has been normalized to the injected dose of [¹¹C]toluene.

I. PET Studies of Alcohol Abuse

The neurochemical mechanisms by which alcohol produces its psychoactive effects, as well as the changes in the brain accompanying chronic alcohol abuse, are not well understood. In nonalcoholic people, alcohol decreases occipital and temporal cortex metabolism, producing a metabolic response similar to the benzodiazepine lorazepam [Wang et al. 2000]. These findings agree with evidence demonstrating alcohol and benzodiazepines share a binding site on the GABA-benzodiazepine receptor complex [Bosio et al. 1982; Burch and Ticku 1980; Hemmingsen et al. 1982; Ticku 1983; Ticku et al. 1983; Ticku and Davis 1981]. Neuroimaging studies using the benzodiazepine receptor ligands [¹¹C]flumazenil or [¹²³I]iomazenil indicate that alcoholic patients express altered numbers of benzodiazepine receptors comared with healthy controls [Abi-Dargham et al. 1998; Litton et al. 1993]. Specifically, the DVR was significantly lower in several cortical regions and the cerebellum of alcoholic subjects compared to healthy comparison subjects. These results suggest either a toxic effect of alcoholism on benzodiazepine receptors or a vulnerability factor for developing alcoholism. In fact, children of alcoholics given lorazepam demonstrate a metabolic response similar to alcoholic patients, as well as a diminished sensitivity to both lorazepam and alcohol [Volkow et al. 1995c].

Dopaminergic systems are also altered in alcoholic patients. PET studies with [¹¹C]raclopride demonstrate reductions in dopamine D_2 receptors in alcoholics relative to controls, which persisted over a 1- to 68-week detoxification period [Hietala et al. 1994]. DAT availability in alcoholics using the high affinity ligand, [¹²³I]-β-CIT, was increased in violent and decreased in nonviolent alcoholic patients as compared to nonalcoholic controls [Tiihonen et al. 1995]. Studies measuring D_2 receptors and DAT sites in alcoholic patients either report decreases in DAT sites but no difference in D_2 receptors [Repo et al. 1999], or decreases in D_2 receptors but not DAT sites [Volkow et al. 1996c]. Changes in DAT sites and D_2 receptors must be considered in light of the fact that dopamine transporters reflect dopamine neuron integrity, whereas dopamine receptors occur mainly on GABA-ergic neurons. In the absence of neurological impairment, [¹⁸F]DG PET studies in alcoholic patients express abnormalities in frontal metabolism with [Volkow et al. 1992; Wik et al. 1988], consistent with studies of blood flow using xenon inhalation techniques [Mathew and Wilson 1986].

J. Conclusions

The above studies illustrate the use of PET in investigating the mechanisms of toxicity of drugs of abuse, as well as changes in brain chemistry that may account for the addictive actions of these drugs in the human brain. Although these studies remain preliminary, they have already documented neurochemical changes in the brains of individuals addicted to drugs, and provided a target for pharmacological intervention. Given the importance of radiotracer development in the advancement and application of neuroimaging techniques to the study of addiction, it is safe to say that basic research in labeling biomolecules with positron emitters has shaped the PET field as we know it today. Studies using carbon-11-labeled compounds can thus make significant contributions to our awareness of the many physiological and cognitive effects produced by chronic exposure to a number of different compounds [for review, see Kling et al. 2000; Sadzot et al. 1990; Sekine et al. 2001; Weinstein et al. 1998]. It is clear from studies presented above that PET has provided invaluable information on the addicted human brain that may be useful for developing new treatment strategies for addiction.

IV. USING PET TO DEVELOP A TREATMENT FOR SUBSTANCE ABUSE

PET provides an ideal technique to probe a specific drug mechanism, and we have been able to use this technology to advance our understanding of the fundamental changes in neural activity and structure associated with chronic drug abuse. However, the development and clinical implementation of an adequate therapy for addiction is not commensurate with our understanding of the neurochemical mechanisms of drugs of abuse. Given that prolonged exposure to drugs of abuse produces abnormalities in brain structure and function, potential pharmacotherapies that produce one response in the normal brain might produce quite another in an environment altered by prolonged drug exposure. The observation that chronic drug abuse produces changes in the dynamics of the dopamine system has provided an impetus for the development of many strategies targeting this system to weaken the initial stimulatory effects of rewarding drugs [O'Brien 1997]. It is possible that the most effective of these therapies might not act on dopaminergic systems directly, but on systems functionally related to dopamine. Thus, drugs that are already used in altered neural environments might prove more favorable to those experimental compounds which as of yet have no clinical target.

For over a decade, we have been using PET and in vivo microdialysis techniques to study neurotransmitter interactions in the human, nonhuman primate and rodent brain [for review, see Schloesser et al. 1996]. The sensitivity of PET for detecting alterations in labeled D_2 radiotracer binding (i.e., [^{11}C]raclopride or [^{18}F]NMSP) has been demonstrated by pharmacologic agents that selectively increase or decrease synaptic dopamine concentrations by neurochemically different mechanisms like DAT blockade or increased synthesis of dopamine [Dewey et al. 1991, 1993; Innis et al. 1992). These findings suggest that this experimental approach is well suited for studies designed to investigate disease states that begin with, or result from, a loss in the ability to adequately regulate synaptic dopamine activity.

The potential for PET paradigms clearly extends beyond the ability to measure changes in a single neurotransmitter system after a specific challenge. Studies in our laboratory [Dewey et al. 1988, 1990] and others [Hietala et al. 1997] have been exploring pharmacologic interventions outside the dopaminergic system that might subsequently inhibit the dopaminergic response to psychostimulants and other abused drugs. These studies are based on the premise that neurotransmitter systems do not work in isolation, and that healthy brain function depends on the ability of the system to maintain a functional state of homeostasis across a network of interacting neurotransmitter systems. In this, the inability of a specific neurotransmitter to be regulated by other etiologically relevant, and functionally linked systems, underlies the characteristic addictive state of tolerance and insensitivity. This, then, is indicative of a lack of plasticity or an inability to respond to previously stimulating doses of the addictive compound. For example, the diminished euphoria experienced by chronic cocaine abusers over time may be related to other factors such as the integrity of other neurotransmitter systems that remain functionally linked to dopamine. Consequently, measuring the responsiveness of a specific neurotransmitter to a pharmacologic challenge may be more revealing than measuring changes in the more inherent static properties of these systems.

Dopaminergic homeostasis is primarily maintained by the activity of excitatory amino acid (EAA) and inhibitory GABA-ergic systems [Kalivas 1993]. Thus, these neurotransmitters become promising targets to alter the functional homeostasis of the dopamine system, and in this, the responsivity of this system to a pharmacologic perturbation. Under the hypothesis that either a priori diminishing EAA neurochemical stimulation of dopamine or augmenting inhibitory GABA-ergic control over dopamine will reduce the reward-associated response to a drug challenge, our research team and others have been aggressively exploring the potential of these agents as therapies for drug abuse. However, while rodent and nonhuman primate studies suggest that antagonizing EAA glutamate receptors directly may reduce the dopaminergic response to drugs of abuse [Li et al. 1999, 2000; Wolf 1998], glutamate receptor antagonists are known to produce psychosis [Javitt and Zukin 1991]. The GABA-ergic system thus provides a more feasible approach to indirectly modulate the dopaminergic response to drugs of abuse. Since PET provides the most clinically relevant technique to explore the effects of drugs of abuse, we have relied largely on PET data to guide further behavioral and in vivo techniques.

Our initial studies of GABA-ergic modulation of dopamine activity focused on the interaction between the anticonvulsant drug, γ-vinyl GABA (vigabatrin, GVG, Sabril) and the dopaminergic response to psychostimulants [Dewey et al. 1992, 1997, 1998, 1999; Kushner et al. 1997b; Morgan and Dewey 1998]. GVG is a widely prescribed anticonvulsant with a particular mechanism of action designed specifically to act indirectly on GABA-ergic systems [Jung et al. 1977] in neurochemical environments altered by disease. Through irreversible inhibition of the enzyme responsible for the catabolism of GABA, GABA-transaminase (GABA-T), GVG increases GABA concentrations in both vesicular and cytosolic pools [Petroff and Rothman 1998]. Recent evidence suggests that the ability of GVG to increase cytosolic pools of GABA may contribute to its promise as a therapy for addiction. Drugs that depress dopaminergic function usually produce concomitant reductions in locomotor behavior [Swerdlow et al. 1986]. However, recent studies suggest that increases in cytosolic pools of GABA produced by GVG are only released in response to abnormal stimulation of the dopaminergic system [Jackson et al. 2000; Wu et al. 2001], such that normal locomotor activity and "natural" rewarding effects may be spared. This may explain findings suggesting that GVG does not diminish locomotor activity at clinically relevant doses [Bevins et al. 2001; Dewey et al. 1997; Stromberg et al. 2001]. Further, because the mechanism of GVG is through irreversible inhibition, the time required between doses depends on the ability of the system to synthesize new stores of GABA-T, implying that minimal dosing schedules might provide prolonged protection of dopaminergic systems. In this, the potential for pharmacologic tolerance within GABA-ergic systems is greatly reduced [Jung et al. 1977]. Moreover, rodent studies using prolonged GVG treatment have demonstrated no tolerance within related dopaminergic systems [Gardner et al. 1983; but see Neal and Shah 1990]. In addition to these mechanistic advantages, increasing GABA activity as a general strategy has demonstrated remarkable success in both behavioral and neurochemical paradigms [Roberts and Brebner 2000].

Inasmuch as the dopaminergic response to abused drugs diminishes the addictive liability of these drugs, PET studies are ideal for assessing the impact of potential therapies on the dopaminergic response to psychostimulants or other abused drugs. The success of indirect modulation of dopaminergic activity by augmenting inhibitory GABA-ergic tone is inherent in the many behavioral paradigms in animals demonstrating GVGs potential as a pharmacotherapy for addiction. GVG reduces the dopaminergic response to cocaine [Dewey et al. 1998], nicotine [Dewey et al. 1999], heroin (unpublished observations), PCP [Schiffer et al. 2000], and a cocaine/heroin combination (speedball) [Gerasimov and Dewey 1999] in rodents and non-human primates. Concomitantly, GVG reduces the effects of cocaine-induced brain reward stimulation [Kushner et al. 1997b] and cocaine self-administration [Kushner et al. 1997a], without affecting the reward associated with food [Kushner et al. 1997a] or water [Buckett 1981; Stromberg et al. 2001] intake. In addition, GVG reduces indices of craving and drug-seeking behavior to cocaine [Dewey et al. 1998], nicotine [Dewey et al. 1999], and heroin [Paul et al. 2001], as assessed by the conditioned place preference paradigm.

Although animal models are typically designed to evaluate those factors maintaining drug-seeking behavior, little effort has been directed at developing animal models of polydrug use. However, evidence presented in Stromberg et al. [2001] suggests that it is possible to develop a successful model of cocaine/alcohol abuse. The clinical relevance of this issue, described above, along with the ability of GVG to modulate concurrent cocaine/alcohol intake [Stromberg et al. 2001], increases the promise of this strategy to treat drug abuse.

V. SUMMARY OF FINDINGS AND THE STATUS OF TREATMENT OPTIONS

PET has made significant contributions to the development of several approaches for diminishing the initial dopamine-related reward produced by drugs of abuse. Strategies either directly interfere with the mechanism of a rewarding drug or indirectly approach the reward-related response from a different neurochemical perspective. Although, at present, the National Institute of Drug Abuse has > 30 compounds under preclinical investigation, several factors impede the clinical application of such therapies. Primarily, given the close ties between the mesolimbic dopamine system and locomotor activity, many drugs that appear to reduce the locomotor-activating properties of drugs of abuse merely inhibit the functioning of the basal ganglia and other systems related to movement. An example of this is the GABA-ergic compound baclofen, which reduces dopamine activity and self-administration of psychostimulants [Roberts and Brebner 2000], but does not affect the subjective euphoria of cocaine in humans [Ling et al. 1998] or animal models [Munzar et al. 2000]. One conclusion is that, by diminishing global motor activity, baclofen also diminishes the actual act of drug self-administration in animals [Munzar et al. 2000]. Second, given a central reward system, antagonism of this entirety would also antagonize reward induced by "natural" appetitive events, such that these drugs would not be well tolerated in humans. Finally, since a great deal of drug addiction per se incorporates psychosocial variables, it is unlikely that isolating pharmacological targets alone will prove successful in the treatment of drug dependence.

One should perhaps separate research with PET and what it can tell us about the brain and the use of PET as a clinical tool. Clinical PET, to some the end result of PET research, is no more than the routine application of PET methods which prove clinically useful and can be converted to routine procedures, whether this be the reading of a PET scan generated by a specific labeled probe or a quantitative number reflecting a particular condition generated by mathematical modeling of PET data. There is little argument that simplification of kinetic models in interpreting PET is necessary for a clinical environment. The PET image itself, produced by a particular radiopharmaceutical, e.g., an [^{11}C]raclopride image, is already being used today in a purely clinical context. The outlook is particularly bright for methods of assessing physiologic vulnerability toward addiction, patients at risk in the case of hereditary factors which have not yet presented clinical symptoms, and the quantification of an addicted state relative to the potential for pharmacotherapeutic treatment.

REFERENCES

1. Abi-Dargham A, Krystal JH, Anjilvel S, Scanley BE, Zoghbi S, Baldwin RM, Rajeevan N, Ellis S, Petrakis IL, Seibyl JP, Charney DS, Laruelle M, Innis RB (1998) Alterations of benzodiazepine receptors in type II alcoholic subjects measured with SPECT and [^{123}I]iomazenil. Am J Psychiatry 155:1550–1555.
2. Beckstead MJ, Phelan R, Mihic SJ (2001) Antagonism of inhalant and volatile anesthetic enhancement of glycine receptor function. J Biol Chem 276:24959-24964.
3. Bergstrom M, Nordberg A, Lunell E, Antoni G, Langstrom B (1995) Regional deposition of inhaled ^{11}C-nicotine vapor in the human airway as visualized by positron emission tomography. Clin Pharmacol Ther 57:309–317.
4. Berlin I, Said S, Spreux-Varoquaux O, Launay JM, Olivares R, Millet V, Lecrubier Y, Puech AJ (1995) A reversible monoamine oxidase A inhibitor (moclobemide) facilitates smoking cessation and abstinence in heavy, dependent smokers. Clin Pharmacol Ther 58:444–452.
5. Bevins RA, Besheer J, Pickett KS (2001) Nicotine-conditioned locomotor activity in rats: dopaminergic and GABAergic influences on conditioned expression. Pharmacol Biochem Behav 68:135–145.
6. Bosio A, Lucchi L, Spano PF, Trabucchi M (1982) Central toxic effects of chronic ethanol treatment: actions on GABA and benzodiazepine recognition sites. Toxicol Lett 13:99–103.
7. Brouette T, Anton R (2001) Clinical review of inhalants. Am J Addict 10:79–94.
8. Buckett WR (1981) The influence of a GABA transaminase inhibitor, gamma-vinyl GABA, on voluntary morphine consumption in the rat. Psychopharmacology (Berl) 75:214–216.
9. Burch TP, Ticku MK (1980) Ethanol enhances [^{3}H]diazepam binding at the benzodiazepine-GABA-receptor-ionophore complex. Eur J Pharmacol 67:325–326.
10. Caldecott-Hazard S, Schneider LS (1992) Clinical and biochemical aspects of depressive disorders: III. Treatment and controversies. Synapse 10:141–168.
11. Charalambous A, Marciniak G, Shiue CY, Dewey SL, Schlyer DJ, Wolf AP, Makriyannis A (1991) PET studies in the primate brain and biodistribution in mice using (−)-5′-^{18}F-delta 8-THC. Pharmacol Biochem Behav 40:503–507.
12. Clarke PB, Fu DS, Jakubovic A, Fibiger HC (1988) Evidence that mesolimbic dopaminergic activation underlies the locomotor stimulant action of nicotine in rats. J Pharmacol Exp Ther 246:701–708.
13. Deutch AY, Clark WA, Roth RH (1990) Prefrontal cortical dopamine depletion enhances the responsiveness of mesolimbic dopamine neurons to stress. Brain Res 521:311–315.
14. Dewey SL, Brodie JD, Fowler JS, MacGregor RR, Schlyer DJ, King PT, Alexoff DL, Volkow ND, Shiue CY, Wolf AP (1990) Positron emission tomography (PET) studies of dopaminergic/cholinergic interactions in the baboon brain. Synapse 6:321–327.
15. Dewey SL, Brodie JD, Gerasimov M, Horan B, Gardner EL, Ashby CRJ (1999) A pharmacologic strategy for the treatment of nicotine addiction. Synapse 31:76–86.
16. Dewey SL, Chaurasia CS, Chen CE, Volkow ND, Clarkson FA, Porter SP, Straughter-Moore RM, Alexoff DL, Tedeschi D, Russo NB, Fowler JS, Brodie JD (1997) GABAergic attenuation of cocaine-induced dopamine release and locomotor activity. Synapse 25:393–398.
17. Dewey SL, Logan J, Wolf AP, Brodie JD, Angrist B, Fowler JS, Volkow ND (1991) Amphetamine induced decreases in (^{18}F)-N-methylspiroperidol binding in the baboon brain using positron emission tomography (PET). Synapse 7:324–327.
18. Dewey SL, Morgan AE, Ashby CR, Jr., Horan B, Kushner SA, Logan J, Volkow ND, Fowler JS, Gardner EL, Brodie JD (1998) A novel strategy for the treatment of cocaine addiction. Synapse 30:119–129.
19. Dewey SL, Smith GS, Logan J, Alexoff D, Ding YS, King P, Pappas N, Brodie JD, Ashby CRJ (1995) Serotonergic modulation of striatal dopamine measured with positron emission tomography (PET) and in vivo microdialysis. J Neurosci 15:821–829.
20. Dewey SL, Smith GS, Logan J, Brodie JD, Fowler JS, Wolf AP (1993) Striatal binding of the PET ligand ^{11}C-raclopride is altered by drugs that modify synaptic dopamine levels. Synapse 13:350–356.

21. Dewey SL, Smith GS, Logan J, Brodie JD, Yu DW, Ferrieri RA, King PT, MacGregor RR, Martin TP, Wolf AP (1992) GABAergic inhibition of endogenous dopamine release measured in vivo with ^{11}C-raclopride and positron emission tomography. J Neurosci 12:3773–3780.
22. Dewey SL, Wolf AP, Fowler JS, Brodie JD, Shiue C-Y, Alavi A, Hiesiger E, Schlyer D, Volkow N, Raulli R, Christman D (1988) The effects of central cholinergic blockage on [^{18}F]-N-methylspiroperidol binding in the human brain using PET. XVIth C.I.N.P. Congress 96:162.
23. Di Chiara G, Imperato A (1988) Drugs of abuse preferentially stimulate dopamine release in the mesolimbic system of freely moving rats. Proc Natl Acad Sci USA 85:5274–5278.
24. Di Chiara G, Tanda G, Bassareo V, Pontieri F, Acquas E, Fenu S, Cadoni C, Carboni E (1999) Drug addiction as a disorder of associative learning. Role of nucleus accumbens shell/extended amygdala dopamine. Ann NY Acad Sci 877:461–485.
25. Ding YS, Fowler JS, Volkow ND, Gatley SJ, Logan J, Dewey SL, Alexoff D, Fazzini E, Wolf AP (1994) Pharmacokinetics and in vivo specificity of [^{11}C]dl-threo-methylphenidate for the presynaptic dopaminergic neuron. Synapse 18:152–160.
26. Domino EF (1995) Brain Imaging of Nicotine and Tobacco Smoking. Ann Arbor: NPP Books.
27. Edling C, Hellman B, Arvidson B, Johansson G, Andersson J, Hartvig P, Valind S, Langstrom B (1997) Positron emission tomography studies of healthy volunteers—no effects on the dopamine terminals and synthesis after short-term exposure to toluene. Hum Exp Toxicol 16:171–176.
28. Endres CJ, Kolachana BS, Saunders RC, Su T, Weinberger D, Breier A, Eckelman WC, Carson RE (1997) Kinetic modeling of [^{11}C]raclopride: combined PET-microdialysis studies. J Cereb Blood Flow Metab 17:932–942.
29. Firestone LL, Gyulai F, Mintun M, Adler LJ, Urso K, Winter PM (1996) Human brain activity response to fentanyl imaged by positron emission tomography. Anesth Analg 82:1247–1251.
30. Fowler JS, Volkow ND (1994) Multi-tracer PET studies of cocaine pharmacokinetics and pharmacodynamics. Med Chem Res 5:193–207.
31. Fowler JS, Volkow ND, Logan J, MacGregor RR, Wang GJ, Wolf AP (1992a) Alcohol intoxication does not change [^{11}C]cocaine pharmacokinetics in human brain and heart. Synapse 12:228–235.
32. Fowler JS, Volkow ND, MacGregor RR, Logan J, Dewey SL, Gatley SJ, Wolf AP (1992b) Comparative PET studies of the kinetics and distribution of cocaine and cocaethylene in baboon brain. Synapse 12:220–227.
33. Fowler JS, Volkow ND, Wang GJ, Pappas N, Logan J, MacGregor R, Alexoff D, Shea C, Schlyer D, Wolf AP, Warner D, Zezulkova I, Cilento R (1996a) Inhibition of monoamine oxidase B in the brains of smokers. Nature 379:733–736.
34. Fowler JS, Volkow ND, Wang GJ, Pappas N, Logan J, Shea C, Alexoff D, MacGregor RR, Schlyer DJ, Zezulkova I, Wolf AP (1996b) Brain monoamine oxidase A inhibition in cigarette smokers. Proc Nat Acad Sci USA 93:14065–14069.
35. Fowler JS, Volkow ND, Wolf AP, Dewey SL, Schlyer DJ, Macgregor RR, Hitzemann R, Logan J, Bendriem B, Gatley SJ (1989) Mapping cocaine binding sites in human and baboon brain in vivo. Synapse 4:371–377.
36. Frost JJ, Mayberg HS, Sadzot B, Dannals RF, Lever JR, Ravert HT, Wilson AA, Wagner HN Jr, Links JM (1990) Comparison of [^{11}C]diprenorphine and [^{11}C]carfentanil binding to opiate receptors in humans by positron emission tomography. J Cereb Blood Flow Metab 10: 484–492.
37. Frost JJ, Wagner HNJ, Dannals RF, Ravert HT, Links JM, Wilson AA, Burns HD, Wong DF, McPherson RW, Rosenbaum AE (1985) Imaging opiate receptors in the human brain by positron tomography. J Comput Assist Tomogr 9:231–236.
38. Gardner CR, Mallorga P, Klein J, Huot-Olivier S, Palfreyman MG (1983) Chronic elevation of brain GABA by gamma-vinyl GABA treatment does not alter the sensitivity of GABAergic or dopaminergic receptors in rat CNS. Psychopharmacology 79:130–136.
39. Gatley SJ, Gifford AN, Volkow ND, Lan R, Makriyannis A (1996) ^{123}I-labeled AM251: a radioiodinated ligand which binds in vivo to mouse brain cannabinoid CB1 receptors. Eur J Pharmacol 307:331–338.
40. Gatley SJ, Lan R, Pyatt B, Gifford AN, Volkow ND, Makriyannis A (1997) Binding of the non-classical cannabinoid CP 55,940, and the diarylpyrazole AM251 to rodent brain cannabinoid receptors. Life Sci 61:PL191–197.
41. Gatley SJ, Lan R, Volkow ND, Pappas N, King P, Wong CT, Gifford AN, Pyatt B, Dewey SL, Makriyannis A (1998) Imaging the brain marijuana receptor: development of a radioligand that binds to cannabinoid CB1 receptors in vivo. J Neurochem 70:417–423.
42. Gawin FH, Ellinwood EH Jr (1988) Cocaine and other stimulants. Actions, abuse, and treatment. N Engl J Med 318: 1173–1782.
43. Gerasimov MR, Dewey SL (1999) Gamma-vinyl gamma-aminobutyric acid attenuates the synergistic elevations of nucleus accumbens dopamine produced by a cocaine/heroin (speedball) challenge. Eur J Pharmacol 380:1–4.

44. Ginovart N, Farde L, Halldin C, Swahn CG (1997) Effect of reserpine-induced depletion of synaptic dopamine on [^{11}C]raclopride binding to D2-dopamine receptors in the monkey brain. Synapse 25:321–325.
45. Goodman LS, Gilman A (1990) The Pharmacological Basis of Therapeutics, 8th ed. New York: Pergamon Press.
46. Hageman G, Van der Hoek J, Van Hout M, Van der Laan G, Steur EJ, De Bruin W, Herholz K (1999) Parkinsonism, pyramidal signs, polyneuropathy, and cognitive decline after long-term occupational solvent exposure. J Neurol 246:198–206.
47. Hartvig P, Bergstrom K, Lindberg B, Lundberg PO, Lundqvist H, Langstrom B, Svard H, Rane A (1984) Kinetics of ^{11}C-labeled opiates in the brain of rhesus monkeys. J Pharmacol Exp Ther 230:250–255.
48. Hearn WL, Flynn DD, Hime GW, Rose S, Cofino JC, Mantero-Atienza E, Wetli CV, Mash DC (1991a) Cocaethylene: a unique cocaine metabolite displays high affinity for the dopamine transporter. J Neurochem 56:698–701.
49. Hearn WL, Rose S, Wagner J, Ciarleglio A, Mash DC (1991b) Cocaethylene is more potent than cocaine in mediating lethality. Pharmacol Biochem Behav 39:531–533.
50. Hemmingsen R, Braestrup C, Nielsen M, Barry DI (1982) The benzodiazepine/GABA receptor complex during severe ethanol intoxication and withdrawal in the rat. Acta Psychiatr Scand 65:120–126.
51. Hernandez-Avila CA, Ortega-Soto HA, Jasso A, Hasfura-Buenaga CA, Kranzler HR (1998) Treatment of inhalant-induced psychotic disorder with carbamazepine versus haloperidol. Psychiatr Serv 49:812–815.
52. Hietala J, Kuoppamaki M, Nagren K, Lehikoinen P, Syvalahti E (1997) Effects of lorazepam administration on striatal dopamine D2 receptor binding characteristics in man—a positron emission tomography study. Psychopharmacology 132:361–365.
53. Hietala J, West C, Syvalahti E, Nagren K, Lehikoinen P, Sonninen P, Ruotsalainen U (1994) Striatal D2 dopamine receptor binding characteristics in vivo in patients with alcohol dependence. Psychopharmacology (Berl) 116:285–290.
54. Howard MO, Cottler LB, Compton WM, Ben-Abdallah A (2001) Diagnostic concordance of DSM-III-R, DSM-IV, and ICD-10 inhalant use disorders. Drug Alcohol Depend 61: 223-228.
55. Howard MO, Jenson JM (1999) Inhalant use among antisocial youth: prevalence and correlates. Addict Behav 24:59–74.
56. Howlett AC (1990) Reverse pharmacology applied to the cannabinoid receptor. Trends Pharmacol Sci 11:395–397.
57. Innis RB, Malison RT, al-Tikriti M, Hoffer PB, Sybirska EH, Seibyl JP, Zoghbi SS, Baldwin RM, Laruelle M, Smith EO (1992) Amphetamine-stimulated dopamine release competes in vivo for [^{123}I]IBZM binding to the D2 receptor in nonhuman primates. Synapse 10:177–184.
58. Jackson MF, Esplin B, Capek R (2000) Reversal of the activity-dependent suppression of GABA-mediated inhibition in hippocampal slices from gamma-vinyl GABA (vigabatrin)- pretreated rats. Neuropharmacology 39:65–74.
59. Javitt DC, Zukin SR (1991) Recent advances in the phencyclidine model of schizophrenia. Am J Psychiatry 148:1301–1308.
60. Johanson CE, Fischman MW (1989) The pharmacology of cocaine related to its abuse. Pharmacol Rev 41:3–52.
61. Jung MJ, Lippert B, Metcalf BW, Bohlen P, Schechter PJ (1977) Gamma-vinyl GABA (4-amino-hex-5-enoic acid), a new selective irreversible inhibitor of GABA-T: effects on brain GABA metabolism in mice. J Neurochem 29:797–802.
62. Kalivas PW (1993) Neurotransmitter regulation of dopamine neurons in the ventral tegmental area. Brain Res Rev 18:75–113.
63. Kling MA, Carson RE, Borg L, Zametkin A, Matochik JA, Schluger J, Herscovitch P, Rice KC, Ho A, Eckelman WC, Kreek MJ (2000) Opioid receptor imaging with positron emission tomography and [(^{18})F]cyclofoxy in long-term, methadone-treated former heroin addicts. J Pharmacol Exp Ther 295:1070–1076.
64. Koob GF (1992) Neural mechanisms of drug reinforcement. Annals NY Acad Sci 654:171–191.
65. Koob GF, Bloom FE (1988) Cellular and molecular mechanisms of drug dependence. Science 242:715–723.
66. Kucuk NO, Kilic EO, Ibis E, Aysev A, Gencoglu EA, Aras G, Soylu A, Erbay G (2000) Brain SPECT findings in long-term inhalant abuse. Nucl Med Commun 21:769–773.
67. Kurtzman TL, Otsuka KN, Wahl RA (2001) Inhalant abuse by adolescents. J Adolesc Health 28:170–180.
68. Kushner SA, Dewey SL, Kornetsky C (1997a) Comparison of the effects of vigabatrin on cocaine self-administration and food reinforcement. Soc Neurosc Abstr 23:1942.
69. Kushner SA, Dewey SL, Kornetsky C (1997b) Gamma-vinyl GABA attenuates cocaine-induced lowering of brain stimulation reward thresholds. Psychopharmacology 133:383–388.
70. Lahti AC, Koffel B, LaPorte D, Tamminga CA (1995) Subanesthetic doses of ketamine stimulate psychosis in schizophrenia. Neuropsychopharmacology 13:9–19.
71. Lee MC, Wagner HN Jr, Tanada S, Frost JJ, Bice AN, Dannals RF (1988) Duration of occupancy of opiate receptors by naltrexone. J Nucl Med 29:1207–1211.

72. Leone P, Pocock D, Wise RA (1991) Morphine-dopamine interaction: ventral tegmental morphine increases nucleus accumbens dopamine release. Pharmacol Biochem Behav 39:469–472.
73. Levin ED, Wilson W, Rose JE, McEvoy J (1996) Nicotine-haloperidol interactions and cognitive performance in schizophrenics. Neuropsychopharmacology 15:429–436.
74. Li Y, Hu XT, Berney TG, Vartanian AJ, Stine CD, Wolf ME, White FJ (1999) Both glutamate receptor antagonists and prefrontal cortex lesions prevent induction of cocaine sensitization and associated neuroadaptations. Synapse 34:169–180.
75. Li Y, White FJ, Wolf ME (2000) Pharmacological reversal of behavioral and cellular indices of cocaine sensitization in the rat. Psychopharmacology (Berl) 151:175–183.
76. Ling W, Shoptaw S, Majewska D (1998) Baclofen as a cocaine anti-craving medication: a preliminary clinical study. Neuropsychopharmacology 18:403–404.
77. Litton JE, Neiman J, Pauli S, Farde L, Hindmarsh T, Halldin C, Sedvall G (1993) PET analysis of [^{11}C]flumazenil binding to benzodiazepine receptors in chronic alcohol-dependent men and healthy controls. Psychiatry Res 50:1–13.
78. Logan J, Fowler JS, Volkow ND, Wolf AP, Dewey SL, Schlyer DJ, MacGregor RR, Hitzemann R, Bendriem B, Gatley SJ (1990) Graphical analysis of reversible radioligand binding from time-activity measurements applied to [N-^{11}C-methyl]-(−)-cocaine PET studies in human subjects. J Cereb Blood Flow Metab 10:740–747.
79. London ED, Broussolle EP, Links JM, Wong DF, Cascella NG, Dannals RF, Sano M, Herning R, Snyder FR, Rippetoe LR (1990) Morphine-induced metabolic changes in human brain. Studies with positron emission tomography and [fluorine 18]fluorodeoxyglucose. Arch Gen Psychiatry 47:73–81.
80. Mathew RJ, Wilson WH (1986) Regional cerebral blood flow changes associated with ethanol intoxication. Stroke 17:1156–1159.
81. Mathew RJ, Wilson WH, Chiu NY, Turkington TG, Degrado TR, Coleman RE (1999) Regional cerebral blood flow and depersonalization after tetrahydrocannabinol administration. Acta Psychiatr Scand 100:67–75.
82. Mathew RJ, Wilson WH, Coleman RE, Turkington TG, DeGrado TR (1997) Marijuana intoxication and brain activation in marijuana smokers. Life Sci 60:2075–2089.
83. Mathew RJ, Wilson WH, Humphreys DF, Lowe JV, Wiethe KE (1992) Regional cerebral blood flow after marijuana smoking. J Cereb Blood Flow Metab 12:750–758.
84. McCann UD, Wong DF, Yokoi F, Villemagne V, Dannals RF, Ricaurte GA (1998) Reduced striatal dopamine transporter density in abstinent methamphetamine and methcathinone users: evidence from positron emission tomography studies with [^{11}C]WIN-35,428. J Neurosci 18:8417–8422.
85. Melega WP, Raleigh MJ, Stout DB, Lacan G, Huang SC, Phelps ME (1997) Recovery of striatal dopamine function after acute amphetamine- and methamphetamine-induced neurotoxicity in the vervet monkey. Brain Res 766:113–120.
86. Mintun MA, Raichle ME, Kilbourn MR, Wooten GF, Welch MJ (1984) A quantitative model for the in vivo assessment of drug binding sites with positron emission tomography. Ann Neurol 15:217–227.
87. Misra LK, Kofoed L, Fuller W (1999) Treatment of inhalant abuse with risperidone. J Clin Psychiatry 60:620.
88. Morgan AE, Dewey SL (1998) Effects of pharmacologic increases in brain GABA levels on cocaine-induced changes in extracellular dopamine. Synapse 28:60–65.
89. Mullani NA, Volkow ND (1992) Positron emission tomography instrumentation: a review and update. Am J Physiol Imaging 7:121–135.
90. Munzar P, Kutkat SW, Miller CR, Goldberg SR (2000) Failure of baclofen to modulate discriminative-stimulus effects of cocaine or methamphetamine in rats. Eur J Pharmacol 408:169–174.
91. Nahas GG (1986) Cannabis: toxicological properties and epidemiological aspects. Med J Aust 145:82–87.
92. Nakamura H, Hishinuma T, Tomioka Y, Ido T, Iwata R, Funaki Y, Itoh M, Fujiwara T, Yanai K, Sato M, Numachi Y, Yoshida S, Mizugaki M (1996) Positron emission tomography study of the alterations in brain distribution of [^{11}C]methamphetamine in methamphetamine-sensitized dog. Ann NY Acad Sci 801:401–408.
93. Nakamura H, Hishinuma T, Tomioka Y, Ishiwata S, Ido T, Iwata R, Funaki Y, Itoh M, Fujiwara T, Yanai K, Sato M, Numachi Y, Yoshida S, Mizugaki M (1997) Effects of haloperidol and cocaine pretreatments on brain distribution and kinetics of [^{11}C]methamphetamine in methamphetamine sensitized dog: application of PET to drug pharmacokinetic study. Nucl Med Biol 24:165–169.
94. Neal MJ, Shah MA (1990) Development of tolerance to the effects of vigabatrin (gamma-vinyl-GABA) on GABA release from rat cerebral cortex, spinal cord and retina. Br J Pharmacol 100:324–328.
95. Newhouse PA, Hughes JR (1991) The role of nicotine and nicotinic mechanisms in neuropsychiatric disease. Br J Addict 86:521–526.
96. Nyback H, Halldin C, Ahlin A, Curvall M, Eriksson L (1994) PET studies of the uptake of (S)- and (R)-[^{11}C]nicotine in the human brain: difficulties in visualizing specific receptor binding in vivo. Psychopharmacology (Berl) 115:31–36.

97. O'Brien CP (1997) A range of research-based pharmacotherapies for addiction. Science 278:66–70.
98. Paul M, Dewey SL, Gardner EL, Brodie JD, Ashby CR Jr (2001) Gamma-vinyl GABA (GVG) blocks expression of the conditioned place preference response to heroin in rats. Synapse 41:219–220.
99. Petroff OA, Rothman DL (1998) Measuring human brain GABA in vivo: effects of GABA-transaminase inhibition with vigabatrin. Mol Neurobiol 16:97–121.
100. Pettit HO, Justice JB Jr (1991) Effect of dose on cocaine self-administration behavior and dopamine levels in the nucleus accumbens. Brain Res 539:94–102.
101. Pothos E, Rada P, Mark GP, Hoebel BG (1991) Dopamine microdialysis in the nucleus accumbens during acute and chronic morphine, naloxone-precipitated withdrawal and clonidine treatment. Brain Res 566:348–350.
102. Rada P, Mark GP, Pothos E, Hoebel BG (1991) Systemic morphine simultaneously decreases extracellular acetylcholine and increases dopamine in the nucleus accumbens of freely moving rats. Neuropharmacology 30:1133–1136.
103. Reith ME (1988) Cocaine receptors on monoamine transporters and sodium channels. NIDA Res Monogr 88:23–43.
104. Repo E, Kuikka JT, Bergstrom KA, Karhu J, Hiltunen J, Tiihonen J (1999) Dopamine transporter and D2-receptor density in late-onset alcoholism. Psychopharmacology (Berl) 147:314–318.
105. Ritz MC, Lamb RJ, Goldberg SR, Kuhar MJ (1987) Cocaine receptors on dopamine transporters are related to self- administration of cocaine. Science 237:1219–1223.
106. Roberts DC, Brebner K (2000) GABA modulation of cocaine self-administration. Ann NY Acad Sci 909:145–158.
107. Roberts DC, Koob GF (1982) Disruption of cocaine self-administration following 6-hydroxydopamine lesions of the ventral tegmental area in rats. Pharmacol, Biochem Behav 17:901–904.
108. Rose S, Hearn W, Hime GW, Wetli CV, Ruttenber AI, Mash DC (1990) Cocaine and cocaethylene concentrations in human postmortem cerebral cortex. Soc Neurosci Abstr 11(6):16.
109. Sadzot B, Mayberg HS, Frost JJ (1990) Imaging opiate receptors in the human brain with positron emission tomography. Potential applications for drug addiction research. Acta Psychiatr Belg 90:9–19.
110. Saji H, Tsutsumi D, Magata Y, Iida Y, Konishi J, Yokoyama A (1992) Preparation and biodistribution in mice of [^{11}C]carfentanil: a radiopharmaceutical for studying brain mu-opioid receptors by positron emission tomography. Ann Nucl Med 6:63–67.
111. Scheel-Kruger J (1986) Dopamine-GABA interactions: evidence that GABA transmits, modulates and mediates dopaminergic functions in the basal ganglia and the limbic system. Acta Neurol Scand Suppl 107:1–54.
112. Schiffer WK, Gerasimov MR, Marsteller DA, Hofmann LC, Brodie JD, Alexoff D, Dewey S (2001) Gamma-vinyl GABA differentially modulates NMDA antagonist induced increases in mesocortical versus mesolimbic dopamine activity. Neuropsychopharmacology 25:704–712.
113. Schloesser R, Simkowitz P, Bartlett EJ, Wolkin A, Smith GS, Dewey SL, Brodie JD (1996) The study of neurotransmitter interactions using positron emission tomography and functional coupling. Clin Neuropharmacol 19:371–389.
114. Schmidt CJ, Ritter JK, Sonsalla PK, Hanson GR, Gibb JW (1985) Role of dopamine in the neurotoxic effects of methamphetamine. J Pharmacol Exp Ther 233:539–544.
115. Seeman P, Guan HC, Niznik HB (1989) Endogenous dopamine lowers the dopamine D2 receptor density as measured by [^{3}H]raclopride: implications for positron emission tomography of the human brain. Synapse 3:96–97.
116. Sekine Y, Iyo M, Ouchi Y, Matsunaga T, Tsukada H, Okada H, Yoshikawa E, Futatsubashi M, Takei N, Mori N (2001) Methamphetamine-related psychiatric symptoms and reduced brain dopamine transporters studied with PET. Am J Psychiatry 158:1206–1214.
117. Shiue CY, Vallabhahosula S, Wolf AP, Dewey SL, Fowler JS, Schlyer DJ, Arnett CD, Zhou YG (1997) Carbon-11 labelled ketamine-synthesis, distribution in mice and PET studies in baboons. Nucl Med Biol 24:145–150.
118. Smith GS, Schloesser R, Brodie JD, Dewey SL, Logan J, Vitkun SA, Simkowitz P, Hurley A, Cooper T, Volkow ND, Cancro R (1998) Glutamate modulation of dopamine measured in vivo with positron emission tomography (PET) and ^{11}C-raclopride in normal human subjects. Neuropsychopharmacology 18:18–25.
119. Sokoloff L, Reivich M, Kennedy C, Des Rosiers MH, Patlak CS, Pettigrew KD, Sakurada O, Shinohara M (1977) The [^{14}C]deoxyglucose method for the measurement of local cerebral glucose utilization: theory, procedure, and normal values in the conscious and anesthetized albino rat. J Neurochem 28:897–916.
120. Stapleton JM, Henningfield JE, Wong DF, Phillips RL, Grayson RF, Dannals RF, London ED (1993) Nicotine reduces cerebral glucose utilizaiton in humans. In: NIDA Research Monograph. Washington: DHHS.
121. Stromberg MF, Mackler SA, Volpicelli JR, O'Brien CP, Dewey SL (2001) The effect of gamma-vinyl-GABA on the consumption of concurrently available oral cocaine and ethanol in the rat. Pharmacol Biochem Behav 68:291–299.

122. Swerdlow NR, Vaccarino FJ, Amalric M, Koob GF (1986) The neural substrates for the motor-activating properties of psychostimulants: a review of recent findings. Pharmacol Biochem Behav 25:233–248.
123. Ticku MK (1983) Benzodiazepine-GABA receptor-ionophore complex. Current concepts. Neuropharmacology 22:1459–1470.
124. Ticku MK, Burch TP, Davis WC (1983) The interactions of ethanol with the benzodiazepine-GABA receptor-ionophore complex. Pharmacol Biochem Behav 18(Suppl 1):15–18.
125. Ticku MK, Davis WC (1981) Evidence that ethanol and pentobarbital enhance [^{3}H]diazepam binding at the benzodiazepine-GABA receptor-ionophore complex indirectly. Eur J Pharmacol 71:521–522.
126. Tiihonen J, Kuikka J, Bergstrom K, Hakola P, Karhu J, Ryynanen OP, Fohr J (1995) Altered striatal dopamine re-uptake site densities in habitually violent and non-violent alcoholics. Nat Med 1:654–657.
127. Verebey K, Gold MS (1988) From coca leaves to crack: the effects of dose and routes of administration in abuse liability. Psychiatr Ann 18:513–520.
128. Villemagne V, Yuan J, Wong DF, Dannals RF, Hatzidimitriou G, Mathews WB, Ravert HT, Musachio J, McCann UD, Ricaurte GA (1998) Brain dopamine neurotoxicity in baboons treated with doses of methamphetamine comparable to those recreationally abused by humans: evidence from [^{11}C]WIN-35,428 positron emission tomography studies and direct in vitro determinations. J Neurosci 18:419–427.
129. Volkow ND, Chang L, Wang GJ, Fowler JS, Leonido-Yee M, Franceschi D, Sedler MJ, Gatley SJ, Hitzemann R, Ding YS, Logan J, Wong C, Miller EN (2001) Association of dopamine transporter reduction with psychomotor impairment in methamphetamine abusers. Am J Psychiatry 158:377–382.
130. Volkow ND, Ding YS, Fowler JS, Wang GJ, Logan J, Gatley JS, Dewey S, Ashby C, Liebermann J, Hitzemann R (1995a) Is methylphenidate like cocaine? Studies on their pharmacokinetics and distribution in the human brain. Arch Gen Psychiatry 52:456–463.
131. Volkow ND, Fowler JS, Gatley SJ, Dewey SL, Wang GJ, Logan J, Ding YS, Franceschi D, Gifford A, Morgan A, Pappas N, King P (1999) Comparable changes in synaptic dopamine induced by methylphenidate and by cocaine in the baboon brain. Synapse 31:59–66.
132. Volkow ND, Fowler JS, Logan J, Gatley SJ, Dewey SL, MacGregor RR, Schlyer DJ, Pappas N, King P, Wang GJ (1995b) Carbon-11-cocaine binding compared at subpharmacological and pharmacological doses: a PET study. J Nucl Med 36:1289–1297.
133. Volkow ND, Fowler JS, Wang GJ, Hitzemann R, Logan J, Schlyer DJ, Dewey SL, Wolf AP (1993) Decreased dopamine D2 receptor availability is associated with reduced frontal metabolism in cocaine abusers. Synapse 14:169–177.
134. Volkow ND, Fowler JS, Wolf AP, Schlyer D, Shiue CY, Alpert R, Dewey SL, Logan J, Bendriem B, Christman D (1990) Effects of chronic cocaine abuse on postsynaptic dopamine receptors. Am J Psychiatry 147:719–724.
135. Volkow ND, Gatley SJ, Fowler JS, Logan J, Fischman M, Gifford AN, Pappas N, King P, Vitkun S, Ding YS, Wang GJ (1996a) Cocaine doses equivalent to those abused by humans occupy most of the dopamine transporters. Synapse 24:399–402.
136. Volkow ND, Gillespie H, Mullani N, Tancredi L, Grant C, Valentine A, Hollister L (1996b) Brain glucose metabolism in chronic marijuana users at baseline and during marijuana intoxication. Psychiatry Res 67:29–38.
137. Volkow ND, Hitzemann R, Wang GJ, Fowler JS, Burr G, Pascani K, Dewey SL, Wolf AP (1992) Decreased brain metabolism in neurologically intact healthy alcoholics. Am J Psychiatry 149:1016–1022.
138. Volkow ND, Wang GJ, Begleiter H, Hitzemann R, Pappas N, Burr G, Pascani K, Wong C, Fowler JS, Wolf AP (1995c) Regional brain metabolic response to lorazepam in subjects at risk for alcoholism. Alcohol, Clin Exp Res 19:510–516.
139. Volkow ND, Wang GJ, Fowler JS, Franceschi D, Thanos PK, Wong C, Gatley SJ, Ding YS, Molina P, Schlyer D, Alexoff D, Hitzemann R, Pappas N (2000) Cocaine abusers show a blunted response to alcohol intoxication in limbic brain regions. Life Sci 66:PL161–167.
140. Volkow ND, Wang GJ, Fowler JS, Hitzemann R, Gatley SJ, Dewey SS, Pappas N (1998) Enhanced sensitivity to benzodiazepines in active cocaine-abusing subjects: a PET study. Am J Psychiatry 155:200–206.
141. Volkow ND, Wang GJ, Fowler JS, Logan J, Hitzemann R, Ding YS, Pappas N, Shea C, Piscani K (1996c) Decreases in dopamine receptors but not in dopamine transporters in alcoholics. Alcohol, Clin Exp Res 20:1594–1598.
142. Volkow ND, Wang GJ, Fowler JS, Logan J, Hitzemannn R, Gatley SJ, MacGregor RR, Wolf AP (1996d) Cocaine uptake is decreased in the brain of detoxified cocaine abusers. Neuropsychopharmacology 14:159–168.
143. Wang GJ, Volkow ND, Fowler JS, Fischman M, Foltin R, Abumrad NN, Logan J, Pappas NR (1997a) Cocaine abusers do not show loss of dopamine transporters with age. Life Sci 61:1059–1065.

144. Wang GJ, Volkow ND, Fowler JS, Logan J, Abumrad NN, Hitzemann RJ, Pappas NS, Pascani K (1997b) Dopamine D_2 receptor availability in opiate-dependent subjects before and after naloxone-precipitated withdrawal. Neuropsychopharmacology 16:174–182.
145. Wang GJ, Volkow ND, Franceschi D, Fowler JS, Thanos PK, Scherbaum N, Pappas N, Wong CT, Hitzemann RJ, Felder CA (2000) Regional brain metabolism during alcohol intoxication. Alcohol Clin Exp Res 24:822–829.
146. Weinstein A, Feldtkeller B, Malizia A, Wilson S, Bailey J, Nutt DJ (1998) Integrating the cognitive and physiological aspects of craving. J Psychopharmacol 12:31–38.
147. Wik G, Borg S, Sjogren I, Wiesel FA, Blomqvist G, Borg J, Greitz T, Nyback H, Sedvall G, Stone-Elander S (1988) PET determination of regional cerebral glucose metabolism in alcohol-dependent men and healthy controls using ^{11}C-glucose. Acta Psychiatr Scand 78:234–241.
148. Wolf ME (1998) The role of excitatory amino acids in behavioral sensitization to psychomotor stimulants. Prog Neurobiol 54:679–720.
149. Wolkin A, Jaeger J, Brodie JD, Wolf AP, Fowler J, Rotrosen J, Gomez-Mont F, Cancro R (1985) Persistence of cerebral metabolic abnormalities in chronic schizophrenia as determined by positron emission tomography. Am J Psychiatry 142:564–571.
150. Wu JC, Buchsbaum MS, Bunney WE (1991a) Positron emission tomography study of phencyclidine users as a possible drug model of schizophrenia. Yakubutsu Seishin Kodo 11:47–48.
151. Wu JC, Buchsbaum MS, Potkin SG, Wolf MJ, Bunney WE (1991b) Positron emission tomography study of phencyclidine users. Schizophr Res 4:415.
152. Wu Y, Wang W, Richerson GB (2001) GABA transaminase inhibition induces spontaneous and enhances depolarization-evoked GABA efflux via reversal of the GABA transporter. J Neurosci 21:2630–2639.
153. Yu PH, Durden DA, Davis BA, Boulton AA (1988) Interaction of biogenic amines with components of cigarette smoke. Formation of cyanomethylamine derivatives. Biochem Pharmacol 37:3729–3734.

41

Genetics of Addictive Disorders

TATIANA FOROUD and JOHN I. NURNBERGER, JR.
Indiana University School of Medicine, Indianapolis, Indiana, U.S.A.

I. INTRODUCTION

Alcoholism is a chronic or intermittent condition characterized by loss of control over drinking. It typically begins in adolescence or young adulthood and may be associated with medical, social, or legal sequelae at any stage. One of the most consistent observations in all epidemiologic studies of alcohol consumption is that women drink less than men [1,2]. Estimates of prevalence vary, but the condition may affect 5–10% of the male population and 1–3% of the females in many Western societies. Recent data suggest that prevalence may be increasing in younger cohorts [3] in the United States. There are ∼20 million Americans who have serious drinking problems.

While alcohol remains the most commonly used drug in the United States, there is substantial use of other drugs, including tobacco, cocaine, amphetamines, and marijuana. About 5–10% of the U.S. population, or 10–25 million Americans, meet diagnostic criteria for nonalcohol substance dependence at some point in their lives. Uniformly, rates are at least two to three times greater in males than in females. Use of illicit drugs contributed to ∼20,000 deaths in 1990, the most common causes of death including overdose, suicide, homicide, motor vehicle accident injury, HIV infection, pneumonia, hepatitis, and endocarditis [4].

II. GENETIC ASPECTS OF ALCOHOLISM

A. Family Studies

Review of family studies has concluded that there is a concentration of alcoholics in the families of alcoholic probands [5,6]. Cotton reports an overall prevalence of 27.0% alcoholism in fathers of alcoholics and of 4.9% in mothers; 30.8% of alcoholics had at least one alcoholic parent. The same preponderance of alcoholism was not seen in the parents of comparison groups of patients with other psychiatric disorders. The studies of nonpsychiatric controls reviewed in the same study show a rate of 5.2% in fathers and 1.2% in mothers.

A notable family study reported by Cloninger et al. [7] included 365 first-degree relatives of alcoholics selected from consecutive admissions to St. Louis hospitals. The particular question addressed was whether the predominance of males among alcoholic relatives of alcoholic probands was due to familial or nonfamilial factors. If it takes greater familial "loading" for a woman to become alcoholic, then it would be expected that there would be more alcoholic relatives of a female alcoholic than of a male alcoholic. If nonfamilial factors are responsible, then the risk in relatives should be comparable and independent of the sex of the proband. This latter was found to be the case. The authors suggested, therefore, that women do not become alcoholic as often as men because women are not "allowed" to drink as often or as much. An implication is that while the predisposition to alcoholism is largely genetic, the manifestation of the illness is dependent upon continued heavy drinking, which in itself is largely socioculturally conditioned.

This is consistent with the study of grandsons of alcoholics by Kaij and Dock [8]; in that study, the rate of alcoholism in the sons of daughters of alcoholics was equivalent to the rate of alcoholism in the sons of sons of alcoholics, suggesting that the daughters passed on the genetic predisposition to alcoholism even though they did not manifest the illness themselves. Recent data from a multicenter study of the genetics of alcoholism show familial aggregation among female relatives of alcoholics as well as male relatives [9].

Hill and Yuan [10] examined a sample of children and adolescents between the ages of 8 and 18. These individuals came from either high-density multigenerational alcoholic families or from families without any history of alcoholism in first- or second-degree relatives. They found that the offspring from high-density families began drinking at a significantly earlier age than the individuals from low-risk families and tended to drink more heavily. Recently, Dawson [11] also found that a positive family history of alcoholism was associated with earlier initiation of alcohol drinking.

B. Twin Studies

Twin studies have consistently found significant heritability of drinking behavior. The Finnish twin study of Partanen [12] included interview data on 902 male twins between 28 and 37 years of age. Heritability, or that proportion of the variance in a trait due to genetic factors, was estimated to be 0.39 for the phenotype defined as the frequency of drinking and 0.36 for the amount of alcohol consumed per session. A second Finnish study by Kaprio et al. [13] included data on several thousand pairs of twins in the state twin registry. Overall heritability for total alcohol consumption was 0.37 in males and 0.25 in females. Clifford et al. [14] report a study in which 572 twin families from the Institute of Psychiatry register were examined. Additive genetic factors were found to account for 37% of the variance in alcohol consumption among drinkers when pedigree data were considered together with twin data and the effect of shared environment on twin concordance is taken into account. The critical data from these three large twin studies are strikingly similar, at least in males.

Twin studies of alcoholism itself have also generally shown significant heritability. Kaij [15] studied registration of twin subjects at the Swedish County Temperance Boards. Such registration implies that a complaint was made about a person's behavior while drinking, either by the police or a third party. This would not generally include alcoholics who were socially isolated, though they might be significantly impaired. The registration information was followed up with personal interviews of probands and cotwins. In a total of 205 twin pairs, probandwise concordance was 54.2% in monozygotic (MZ) and 31.5% in dizygotic (DZ) twins ($P < .01$). Concordance rates in MZ twins increased with the severity of the disturbance. A reanalysis of these data by Gottesman and Carey [16] shows heritability to vary from 0.42 to 0.98, with the more serious forms of alcoholism being more heritable.

Hrubec and Omenn [17] examined medical records of 15,924 veteran male twin pairs in the National Academy of Sciences/National Research Council Twin Registry. Concordance for alcoholism was higher among MZ (82/312 = 26.3%) than among DZ twins (56/472 = 11.9%). Concordance for medical consequences of alcoholism (alcoholic psychosis, liver cirrhosis) is higher than that expected on the basis of concordance for alcoholism alone; that is, there is reason to postulate independent heritable effects that lead some alcoholics to manifest psychosis or cirrhosis while others do not. However, a recent reanalysis of these twin data supports a more important role for vulnerability factors for alcoholism per se in cirrhosis risk [18].

Kendler et al. [19] conducted a population-based study of female twin pairs from the Virginia twin registry. Personal interviews were completed on 1033 of 1176 pairs. MZ concordance rates varied from 26% to 47% (narrow to broad definition of alcoholism) while DZ concordance rates ranged from 12% to 32%. The heritability was estimated to be between 50% and 61%. This suggests substantial genetic influence in alcoholism in women in the populations studied. Subsequent studies by Prescott et al. [20] found that the genetic sources of vulnerability in males and females were partially, although not completely, overlapping.

C. Adoption Studies

Adoption studies have generally shown a relationship between alcohol problems in an adoptee and such problems in biologic relatives. Goodwin et al. [21] compared 55 adopted-away male children of an alcoholic parent with 78 adoptees without an alcoholic parent. The groups were matched by age, sex, and time of adoption. The principal finding was that 18% of the proband group were alcoholic compared with 5% of the controls ($P < .02$). This pattern does not hold true for adoptees designated as "problem drinkers" or "heavy drinkers." There is no difference between groups if these categories are considered separately or if they are combined with the alcoholic group. It is only alcoholism itself that was heritable, with alcoholism defined as the presence of heavy drinking consisting of either 1 year of daily drinking with six or more drinks at least twice a month, or six or more drinks at least once a week for over a year. In addition, individuals also had problems in three out of the following four groups: (1) disapproval of drinking by friends, parents, wife; (2) trouble at job because of drinking, traffic arrests, or other police problem; (3) frequent blackouts, tremor, or serious withdrawal symptoms; (4) loss of control or repeated morning drinking. This result is consistent with Kaij's finding [15] that heritability increases with the severity of the disorder.

Goodwin also compared adopted-away sons of alcoholics with sons of alcoholics raised by the alcoholic parent [22], and found no differences. Twenty-five percent of the adopted sons became alcoholic compared with 17% of nonadopted sons. The sample sizes in each group were relatively small, with only 20 and 30 individuals, respectively. Additional studies in daughters of alcoholics did not show evidence for a heritable predisposition to alcoholism in women. These studies did show an increase in depression among daughters of alcoholic fathers, but only if the alcoholic father raised the daughter. This increase was not observed if the daughter was adopted away from the biological environment. These results are an apparent demonstration of an environmental cause of depression or perhaps a genetic-environmental interaction [22].

Bohman [23] used state registers in Stockholm to study 2324 adoptees born in that city between 1930 and 1949. Male adoptees whose fathers abused alcohol (excluding those who were also sociopathic) were more likely to be alcoholic themselves (39.4% vs. 13.6%; $P < .01$) compared with adoptees without an alcoholic (or sociopathic) father. The findings were similar, though not significant, for male adoptees with an alcoholic biologic mother. Cloninger et al. [24] then reanalyzed Bohman's dataset, and postulated a familial distinction of alcoholics: the milieu-limited (type I) and male-limited (type II) groups. Type I alcoholics (as defined in Cloninger [25]) usually have onset after age 25, manifest problems with loss of control, and have a great deal of guilt and fear about alcohol use. Type II alcoholics are primarily males and have onset before age 25, are unable to abstain from alcohol, and have fights and arrests when drinking, but less frequently show loss of control and guilt and fear about alcohol use. Cloninger reanalyzed the Stockholm adoption data using these specific categories. This analysis showed that type I alcoholics were significantly increased in prevalence only among those adoptees with both genetic and environmental risk factors (alcoholism in both biologic and adoptive parents). Type I was the most common type of alcoholism, however, being present in 4.3% of the controls with no risk factors. Type II alcoholism was present in only 1.9% of the controls but 16.9–17.9% of adoptees with genetic risk factors, whereas the presence or absence of environmental risk factors (alcoholism in adoptive parents) did not appear to make a difference.

Cloninger has further integrated these concepts with a personality typology based on behavioral and neurochemical data. The type I alcoholics, he theorizes, show low novelty seeking, high harm avoidance, and high reward dependence. The Type II alcoholics show high novelty seeking, low harm avoidance, and low reward dependence. As part of a more extensive, neurochemically based theory of personality, Cloninger associates novelty-seeking traits with dopamine pathways in the brain, harm avoidance with serotonin systems, and reward dependence with norepinephrine systems [25,26].

The Bohman-Cloninger analysis of the Stockholm sample is the largest adoption study in the field of alcoholism. However, the quality of the initial information (based on population registers) may not have been as complete as that gathered by Goodwin and colleagues, who performed personal interviews on the adoptees. Cloninger states that the population registers can identify ~ 70% of alcoholics, without a bias for type I or type II, but it is not clear that there might not be a bias for the unregistered 30% of alcoholics to be found preferentially in one or another of the adoptee groups. However, the two studies reach essentially the same conclusion, heritable factors are important in the development of alcoholism in at least a subpopulation of heavy-drinking men.

A variant on the usual adoption study format was reported by Schuckit et al. [27], who studied a population of half-siblings of alcoholic probands.

Half-siblings with an alcoholic biologic parent had a high risk for alcoholism (46–50%) whether or not they were raised with an alcoholic parent figure. Those without an alcoholic biologic parent had a lower risk, regardless of environmental variables considered.

D. Disorders Possibly Genetically Related to Alcoholism

Winokur et al. [28] reported an increased prevalence of depression in the female relatives of alcoholics roughly comparable to the increased prevalence of alcoholism in male relatives. This was not found in the adoption study of Goodwin et al. [29] except in daughters brought up in the home of the alcoholic father; this may mean that the incidence of affective disorder and alcoholism in the same families may be related to environmental rather than genetic factors. A later study by Winokur and Coryell [30], showing increased alcoholism in the relatives of female depressive probands but not male depressive probands, is also compatible with that explanation. Some family studies in this area show an increase in risk for alcoholism in relatives of depressive probands, as well as an increase in depression in relatives of alcoholics; however, many other studies do not show this pattern [see review, 31].

It is clear that alcoholics themselves have an increased lifetime risk for depression [31]. The comorbidity between bipolar illness and alcoholism is particularly evident. If family studies are performed starting with probands with both disorders, then both disorders are found in relatives [32]. But family studies starting with bipolar probands or unipolar probands without alcoholism do not usually show an increase in alcoholism in relatives [33]. Similarly, family studies of primary alcoholics do not generally show an increase in relatives with major depression [31]. There may be some forms of illness that result from shared vulnerability factors. Recent studies suggest that comorbid disorders, including features of alcoholism and affective illness, may themselves run in families [34]. Bohman et al. [35] and Cloninger et al. [36] have observed that adopted-away daughters of type II (male-limited) alcoholics manifest no increase in alcoholism but do show an increase in somatization disorder.

A major question is the relationship of alcoholism to sociopathy. Is there a genetic predisposition that may manifest as alcoholism in some and antisocial personality or criminality in others? The summaries of family studies by Goodwin [6] and Cotton [5] conclude that there is evidence for an increase in sociopathy in relatives of alcoholics in a number of family studies. The Swedish adoptee population studied by Bohman [23] showed a relationship between alcoholism and criminality in individual adoptees and their biologic fathers; however, this association was not demonstrated within the families. Thus, adoptees registered for alcohol abuse alone did not show an excess of criminality in relatives, and adoptees registered for criminality alone did not show an excess of alcoholism in relatives. Adoptees registered for both showed an excess of alcoholism only in relatives, but no more than adoptees registered for alcoholism alone. In the adoption data of Goodwin et al. [21], antisocial personality is not more common in adopted-away sons of biologic fathers with alcoholism. In the adoption study of Cadoret et al. [37], significant relationships were observed between alcoholism in adoptees and alcoholism in biologic relatives, and also between sociopathy in adoptees and sociopathy in biologic relatives. This relationship was not observed for alcoholism in adoptees and sociopathy in biologic relatives, or vice versa; however, there were nonsignificant trends, suggesting that a larger study might also show a positive relationship. Cadoret et al. summarize data from adoption studies of antisocial personality, also leading to the conclusion that the disorders are separable. It is not possible to conclude at this time that a single genetic predisposing factor may be manifest as either alcoholism or sociopathy. However, some sociopathic alcoholics may transmit both alcoholism and sociopathy as part of the same syndrome.

A series of studies have shown an increased prevalence of alcoholism in parents of children with hyperactivity. Earls et al. [38] report an increase in DSM-III behavior disorder in general (attention deficit disorder with hyperactivity, oppositional disorder, and conduct disorder) in offspring of alcoholic parents. The risk was greater for offspring of two alcoholic parents than for those of one alcoholic parent.

Merikangas et al. [39] examined a series of 165 probands selected for alcoholism and/or anxiety disorder and compared them with a sample of 61 unaffected controls. First-degree relatives of the probands completed a structured diagnostic interview. In this sample, rates of alcoholism were higher among relatives of the alcoholic probands, regardless of the presence or absence of anxiety disorder in the proband, as compared with the relatives of controls. There was also a twofold increase in the risk of anxiety disorder among the relatives of the probands with anxiety. The rate of comorbidity of alcohol dependence and anxiety disorders was higher among female relatives than among male relatives of alcoholic probands.

III. GENETIC ASPECTS OF DRUG ABUSE

There is a growing body of evidence confirming the familial aggregation of drug abuse. Numerous family history studies and systematic family studies of substance abusers in treatment settings [40–46] reveal a significantly increased risk of drug abuse among relatives of the addicted proband when compared to population estimates. In the first controlled family study of drug use disorders, Merikangas et al. [47] reported a strong familial aggregation of drug use disorders in families. The lifetime prevalence of drug disorders in the first-degree relatives of probands with drug abuse was 17.7% compared to 4.9% in relatives of unaffected controls, yielding a population relative risk of $\sim$ 3.6.

Several twin studies have provided evidence that genetic factors play a major role in the familial aggregation of substance use and abuse with heritability estimated between 30% and 80 [48–53]. In the first study, using diagnostic criteria for drug abuse and dependence, Pickens et al. [51] reported far greater heritability for drug dependence than for abuse. In the largest twin study to date, Tsuang et al. [53] found that substance abuse in general was highly heritable, and that the contribution of genetic factors was more significant for frequent use or abuse than for nonproblematic use. Grove et al.'s [50] study of a small set of MZ twins who were reared apart yielded significant estimates of heritability for drug-related problems (0.45).

The prevalence of drug abuse is far greater among males than females, with approximately fourfold greater rates of drug disorders among males. There is some evidence in the literature that the genetic factors underlying drug disorders in women differ from those in men. The twin study of Pickens et al. [51] suggested that whereas drug disorders in males are attributable to both common genes and common environmental factors, unique environmental factors play a major role in drug disorders in women (e.g., events specific to each person, but not to family members). Subsequent analyses of these twin data [54] suggested that heritability for substance abuse was much greater (heritability = 0.73) for males with early age of onset, compared to males with later onset (heritability = 0.30) or females (heritability = 0.0). The results of some family studies suggest that the relatives of female drug abusers have an elevated risk of drug disorders compared to male drug abusers, thereby suggesting that females may manifest a more severe form of drug abuse than males or may have greater accumulation of underlying genetic and environmental risk factors for drug abuse [47].

The classic adoption studies of Cadoret [55] and Cadoret et al. [56,57], which employed an optimal study paradigm for discriminating the joint influence of genetic and environmental factors, have been highly informative in elucidating the role of genetic factors in the development of drug use and abuse in a U.S. sample. The results of their studies revealed the importance of the role of genetic factors in the development of drug disorders, with a far greater impact on the transition from drug use to abuse than on drug use itself.

Most studies have consistently reported a higher concordance rate for cigarette smoking among MZ than among DZ twins. The mean heritability estimate for tobacco use is 53%, although there is a wide range of reported estimates, from 28 to 84% [58–62]. Family studies have also found an increased risk of nicotine dependence among siblings of individuals who are nicotine dependent, with recurrence risk estimates of 2.1–3.5, depending on the instrument used to evaluate nicotine dependence [63]. Studies have found that genetic factors play a role not only in the initiation of smoking, but also contribute to the age of onset of smoking, the number of cigarettes smoked per day, and the persistence and intensity of smoking [60,64].

IV. FAMILIAL RELATIONSHIPS BETWEEN ALCOHOLISM AND DRUG ABUSE

Among alcohol-dependent individuals, the rate of other mental disorders has been estimated to be as high as 47%, with a substantial proportion of this comorbidity due to other drug dependencies [65,66]. Family history of alcoholism contributes to an increased risk of drug use. In a sample of male college students, McCaul and colleagues [67] found the greatest level of alcohol and drug use among the students with a high density of alcoholism in their families. Intermediate levels of alcohol and drug use were noted among those students with lower rates of alcoholism and the least amount of alcohol and drug use among those students without a family history of alcoholism. Studies among opiate-dependent individuals have found an increased rate of alcoholism among relatives, even after controlling for the presence of alcoholism in the proband [46]. Cadoret et al. [56,68] also found higher rates of drug and alcohol use among male adoptees with an alcoholic parent as compared to those whose biological parents were not alcoholics; the same effect was not observed in a sample of female adoptees [57].

These results suggest that a general predisposition for addictive disorders might be inherited [62,69,50], although other studies have not supported this conclusion [40]. Support for this hypothesis was found in a large sample of World War I male veteran twins where the development of both heavy alcohol use and smoking was found to be due to both unique and shared genetic factors [62]. Analyses of a sample of Vietnam veteran twins found substantial genetic correlation between nicotine and alcohol dependence among middle aged male twins [61], suggesting a common genetic susceptibility to both dependencies. Kendler et al. [69] also found that common familial factors predispose to alcohol abuse/dependence and drug abuse/dependence.

In a large study designed to address the contribution of genetic factors to substance use disorders, Merikangas et al. [47] identified a sample of 299 probands with drug (nonalcohol) dependence or alcohol dependence. Among the 149 individuals with non-alcohol drug dependence were probands with opioid, cocaine, and cannabis dependence. In addition, a sample of 61 control probands without any lifetime history of any diagnosis in DSM-III-R was also ascertained. Individuals and their first-degree relatives completed a structured diagnostic interview to identify any drug dependencies. There was an eightfold increased risk of drug and alcohol disorders among relatives of probands with drug disorders across a wide range of specific substances (including opioids, cocaine, marijuana, and sedatives) as compared with that of relatives of controls. There was also a sixfold increase in drug or alcohol disorders among relatives of the alcoholic probands, although this effect was largely due to the increase in alcoholism among the relatives of the alcoholic probands. The findings from Merikangas et al. [47] suggest that there may be some specificity in the familial aggregation of the predominant drug disorder with increasing rates of more "serious" drug disorders among probands with more "serious" substance disorders. Specifically, rates of opioid disorders were highest among probands with opioid dependence as compared with probands with marijuana dependence.

V. STUDIES TO IDENTIFY GENES UNDERLYING ALCOHOLISM SUSCEPTIBILITY

These and other studies suggest that, rather than being a disorder due to a single gene, alcoholism is more likely a complex genetic disorder resulting from the action of multiple, possibly interacting, genes, as well as environmental factors. In the search for such genes, researchers have pursued a two-pronged strategy. Some investigators have focused on the evaluation of the role of known functionally polymorphic genes with alcoholism while others have used anonymous markers distributed throughout the genome to detect linkage of alcoholism susceptibility to chromosomal regions wherein such genes might reside.

A. Candidate Gene Studies

Efforts to identify the genetic loci underlying alcoholism susceptibility in human subjects have primarily relied on the evaluation of candidate genes, but the only consistently replicated findings are those involving the protective effects of certain functional polymorphisms of the alcohol metabolizing enzymes alcohol dehydrogenase (ADH) and the mitochondrial aldehyde dehydrogenase (ALDH2) [70–76]. Most ingested alcohol is metabolized to acetaldehyde by ADH and by microsomal cytochrome P450IIE1 (CYP2E1) present in the liver. The acetaldehyde is in turn metabolized to acetate by ALDH.

Alcohol dehydrogenase exists as a polygene family on chromosome 4 consisting of seven genes two of which, *ADH2* and *ADH3*, are functionally polymorphic. The *ADH2* gene encodes the β subunit of the dimeric enzyme, and there are polymorphic forms called β_1, β_2, and β_3. They differ by single nucleotide exchanges and one amino acid differences. The enzyme variants, however, are quite different in catalytic properties. The enzyme with the β_1 subunit has low activity and high affinity for ethanol, whereas the β_2 and the β_3 forms have higher activity and lower affinity for ethanol. The prevalence of the variant enzyme forms varies in different ethnic populations. Among Caucasians, 95% have the β_1 enzyme form, while in the Pacific rim Asian populations, such as Chinese, Japanese, and Korean, 90% have the β_2 form. Among Africans and African-Americans, 24% have the β_3 form. There is another ADH, *ADH3*, which is also functionally polymorphic, and encodes the γ-subunits; however, the two forms differ only twofold in their activity. Ninety percent of Asians have the γ_1 form and 50% of Caucasians have the γ_2 form.

Aldehyde dehydrogenases (ALDH) are found in the cytosol and mitochondria of liver cells. The mitochondrial form is called ALDH2 and has the highest affinity for acetaldehyde and is the enzyme most responsible for acetaldehyde oxidation. The form that is found in most populations around the world is a highly active enzyme, encoded by the *ALDH2*1* allele. Among Asians, especially the Chinese, Japanese, and Koreans, a high prevalence of a variant form, *ALDH2*2*, has been observed, which encodes a protein subunit that confers very low or absent activity to the tetrameric enzyme. Individuals who are homozygous for the *ALDH2*2* allele have virtually no enzyme activity in the liver, while those who are heterozygous have considerably lower activity than *ALDH2*1* homozygotes. Therefore, the *ALDH2*2* allele is functionally dominant.

Studies have consistently demonstrated that functional polymorphisms in the ADH and ALDH2 enzymes in Asian populations [70–76] result in lower risks for alcoholism. The *ALDH2*2* allele remains the single most powerful known genetic factor that reduces alcohol consumption. Individuals with this allele have elevated levels of acetaldehyde and experience a flushing reaction after drinking even small amounts of alcohol [77]. This reaction, similar to the alcohol-disulfiram reaction, is aversive, thereby discouraging alcohol ingestion. The *ADH2*2* allele, which codes for the β_2 subunit, has also been shown to be at lower frequency among alcoholics than in the general population, supporting a protective effect [70]. Recently, Neumark and colleagues [78] found that the *ADH2*2* allele was present in about 20% of individuals of Jewish ancestry, and those individuals with the *ADH2*2* allele had lower peak weekly alcohol intake than individuals without the allele. No association of the microsomal P450IIE1 (CYP2E1) polymorphism with alcoholism has been found.

The dopamine D2 receptor (*DRD2*) gene on chromosome 11 is considered a candidate for involvement in alcoholism as well as the personality trait of novelty seeking and central nervous system reward [79,80]. It has been studied extensively by a number of research groups following the report of an association between the TaqI-A1 polymorphism in the *DRD2* gene and alcoholism [81]. A number of positive reports [82–87] and many more negative reports have appeared [88–102]. The bulk of evidence does not favor a major role in alcoholism vulnerability for DRD2 at this time, but a minor role can not be excluded.

The serotonin transporter gene (*HTT*) has also been actively studied as a candidate gene for alcoholism due to the numerous roles of serotonin as a neurotransmitter. A functional polymorphism (5HTTLPR) was reported in the *HTT* promoter, with the two common alleles resulting in either a long, 528-bp allele or a short, 484-bp allele [103]. The short allele was initially reported to be associated with an increase in anxiety-related traits, including harm avoidance [104]. This finding was not confirmed following examination in another study population [105]. A recent population-based association study found the phenotype of severe alcoholism, marked by withdrawal seizure or delirium, to be associated with the 5HTTLPR promoter polymorphism, with alcoholics having an excess of the shorter allele as compared to population controls [106]. However, this finding was not confirmed in a large sample of alcoholic families using a more powerful, family-based association analysis [107].

B. Family-Based Linkage Studies

To more efficiently identify genetic loci contributing to alcoholism susceptibility, recent studies have focused on a genomewide approach, which would allow novel genetic loci to be identified. After the collection of extended pedigrees with multiple members diagnosed with alcoholism, genetic analysis techniques can be employed to evaluate the evidence for linkage throughout the genome. Such a strategy was employed by the Collaborative Study of the Genetics of Alcoholism (COGA) which ascertained, evaluated, and genotyped 105 pedigrees as part of an initial genome screen [75,108]. The initial linkage analyses used only one definition of alcoholism with individuals defined as affected if they fulfilled criteria for alcoholism based on DSM-III-R and Feighner criteria (termed "COGA" criteria). Using 382 affected sibling pairs, regions on chromosomes 1, 2, and 7 were identified as harboring genes that predispose an individual to alcoholism [108]. The most significant finding of the study was on chromosome 7, with a LOD score of 3.5 near the marker D7S1793. On chromosome 1, a peak LOD score of 2.9 was found near the marker D1S1588. A second locus on chromosome 1, ~60 cm from the initial linkage finding, had a LOD score of 1.6. A LOD score of 1.8 was found on chromosome 2, near the marker D2S1790.

Additional analyses using individuals without a diagnosis of alcoholism, who were part of families with multiple alcoholic members, supported a protective locus on chromosome 4 near the *ADH* genes.

Linkage to chromosome 4 was particularly interesting since the COGA sample has few Asian families, but rather consists primarily of non-Hispanic Caucasian and African-American families. This linkage result on chromosome 4 suggests that the protective effects of *ADH* might not be limited to the Asian population.

Subsequently, linkage analyses were completed in a replication dataset of 157 pedigrees ascertained and evaluated using criteria identical to those used in the initial sample [109]. Genetic analyses of affected sibling pairs supported linkage to chromosome 1 (LOD = 1.6) in the replication dataset as well as in a combined analysis of the two samples (LOD = 2.6). Evidence of linkage to chromosome 7 increased in the combined data (LOD = 2.9). The LOD score on chromosome 2 in the initial dataset increased following genotyping of additional markers; however, combined analyses of the two datasets resulted in overall lower LOD scores (LOD = 1.8) on chromosome 2. A new finding of linkage to chromosome 3 was identified in the replication data set (LOD = 3.4). Thus, analyses of a second large sample of alcoholic families provided further evidence of genetic susceptibility loci on chromosomes 1 and 7. Genetic analyses also identified possible susceptibility loci on chromosomes 2 and 3 that require further confirmation.

A genome screen has also been completed in a sample of alcoholics from a southwestern American Indian population [110], which is likely to be genetically more homogeneous than a sample of U.S. Caucasian families. Linkages to chromosomes 4 and 11 were reported. Further analyses of a chromosome 11 candidate gene, tyrosine hydroxylase, supported linkage of this locus in a sample of Finnish offenders with alcoholism and comorbid antisocial personality [111].

Another approach to the identification of genes contributing to alcoholism is to identify novel phenotypes that may have greater genetic contribution and may reduce genetic heterogeneity. A study by Kendler et al. [112] found a genetic correlation of 0.4–0.6 between major depression and alcoholism. Based on these data, a novel phenotype was developed in the COGA sample in which individuals were considered affected if they had either alcoholism (both DSM-III-R alcohol dependence and alcoholism by Feighner criteria) or depression (either DSM-III-R major depression or depressive syndrome). Using this phenotype, strong evidence of linkage was observed on chromosome 1 with a LOD score of 5.12 in the same region previously reported linked to alcoholism alone in this sample [34, 113]. Importantly, using the phenotype of alcoholism or depression, the strength of the linkage finding increased both in terms of the LOD score and the proportion of alleles shared identical by descent.

VI. STUDIES TO IDENTIFY GENES UNDERLYING DRUG DEPENDENCE

A. Candidate Genes for Drug Dependence

Because of the convincing evidence [53,39] regarding the specificity of the familial aggregation of opioid dependence, the genes encoding key proteins in central nervous system opioid systems have been given extensive study as plausible candidate susceptibility genes. In the coding region of the mu opioid receptor gene (OPRM1), two relatively frequent amino acid substitutions have been identified, an A6V substitution [114], and an N40D substitution [115,116]. The A6V variant has been reported by Berrettini et al. [114] and by Bond et al. [116] to be marginally overrepresented among opioid-dependent individuals ($P = .05$ in each study). A common exon 1 SNP variant of the OPRM1, N40D, increases the affinity by severalfold of a POMC gene product, beta-endorphin, for the OPRM1 receptor [116]. Since POMC is an endogenous ligand of the OPRM1 receptor, this finding raises the possibility that variation in POMC expression may be important for the risk to opioid dependence in the presence of the OPRM1 N40D polymorphism. Additional studies by Kranzler et al. [117] reported minimal evidence for association of substance abuse with a microsatellite polymorphism located near OPRM1. Not all studies have confirmed an association between OPRM1 and opioid dependence [118].

For the delta-opioid receptor gene (OPRD1), there is a common, silent coding SNP (C → T at bp 307) which has been found to be associated with opioid dependence using a case-control design. A follow-up study in a larger sample found no evidence for association of the OPRD1 gene with opioid dependence [119]. Gelernter and Kranzler [120] performed a family-based association study of the OPRD1 SNP in a sample of 72 opioid-dependent kindreds and found evidence for an association with opioid dependence, but no evidence for an association with cocaine dependence or alcoholism.

There are several reports of association between opioid or cocaine dependence and nonfunctional variants of the *DRD2* gene [96,121,122]. O'Hara et al. [96] reported an association between *DRD2* and polysubstance dependence among Caucasian, but not African-

American individuals. Noble et al. [121] also observed this association in a group of Caucasian cocaine dependent individuals. Berrettini and Persico [122] confirmed the observation of O'Hara et al. [96] that there was no association for opioid or cocaine dependence among African-Americans.

The D4 dopamine receptor gene (*DRD4*) is characterized by one to eight copies of a 48-bp imperfect exonic repeat [123]. The number of repeats determines the affinity with which some ligands bind DRD4 [124]. Novelty-seeking behavior [125–127] has been associated with larger alleles (seven copies) of the 48-bp repeat in *DRD4*. Elevated scores in novelty-seeking behavior may be characteristic of cocaine- and opioid-dependent persons [128,129]. There is a reported association of this *DRD4* polymorphism with opioid dependence [130], but this has not been confirmed by Franke et al. [119], who studied > 800 persons, using both case control and trio designs.

B. Genetic Studies of Nicotine Use

Only a few studies have attempted to elucidate the genes contributing to the underlying genetic susceptibility to tobacco use. Recently, Spitz and colleagues [131] reported an association with *DRD2* among individuals who had ever smoked, defined as > 100 cigarettes in their lifetime. The initial study reported an increased frequency of the A1 allele, either in the homozygous or heterozygous state, among individuals who smoked. A similar association had been previously reported [83,86]. However, a larger study, utilizing a family-based association method, did not find evidence of an association of the *DRD2* alleles among individuals who had ever smoked, were habitual smokers or even individuals who were habitual smokers and alcohol dependent [132].

Only one genome screen has been reported to date to identify genetic loci underlying nicotine dependence. Using a sample from New Zealand, Straub and colleagues [133] reported linkage to several chromosomal regions with modest results. To further examine these regions, a second sample collected in the United States was analyzed, and consistent, though still modest, evidence of linkage was found on chromosomes 17 and 18.

VII. ETIOLOGIC MARKER STUDIES

Major areas of concentration in the search for a potential biologic trait marker of alcoholism include (1) EEG and evoked potentials before and after alcohol, (2) psychologic/psychophysiologic measures, and (3) behavioral and neuroendocrine responses to alcohol.

A poorly synchronized resting EEG (lower alpha) has been thought to be related to a predisposition for alcoholism [134]. Change in alpha rhythm following alcohol is more concordant in MZ than DZ twins, as are multiple other EEG parameters [135,136]. A relationship was found between resting EEG of the unselected twins and drinking behavior, with less alpha in the twins who drank more. In subsequent work, Propping et al. [137] found that relatives of alcoholics with poorly synchronized resting EEGs demonstrated the same characteristic themselves. Change in alpha rhythm following alcohol was also found to differentiate young adult subjects at high risk for alcoholism from controls [138].

Measurements of event-related potentials (ERP) have shown decreased amplitude of the P300 wave following visual stimuli in 7- to 13-year-old sons of alcoholics compared to controls [139], lessening the likelihood of previous alcohol exposure. Similar findings using an auditory stimulus had been reported in an older group (age 21–26) both before and after alcohol administration [140]. These findings have been confirmed in other populations, including the families from the Collaborative Study on the Genetics of Alcoholism (COGA) [141]. Hill et al. [142] found a significant increase in P300 latency in adolescent and adult relatives of alcoholics compared to controls. The EEG/ERP area remains one of the more promising in the field of pathophysiologic markers for alcoholism.

In a study by Tarter et al. [143], sons of alcoholics performed more poorly than sons of nonalcoholics on 8 out of a series of 47 neuropsychological measurements. The authors discuss possible explanations including physical abuse by the father, psychiatric illness in the mother, and perinatal injury, as well as predisposition to alcoholism. Other investigators have not found such deficits, suggesting that they may not be a general feature of alcoholic populations [144]. A number of investigators report increased static ataxia in children of alcoholics [see summary in Hill et al., 145]. Finn and Pihl [146,147] have demonstrated increased cardiovascular reaction to unavoidable shock in sons of alcoholics, especially those with multigenerational family histories of alcoholism. Hill et al. [148] have found increases in the MMPI psychopathic deviance scale in alcoholics, and some evidence indicates this may be predictive of alcoholism. Von Knorring et al. [149] found increases in a personality factor related to impulsivity, sensation seeking, and psychopathy in type II alcoholics compared with controls.

Schuckit [150–152] has studied behavioral and neuroendocrine responses to alcohol administration in a series of high-risk populations; offspring of alcoholics displayed less subjective intoxication than controls. A follow-up study by Schuckit and Smith [153] shows that decreased subjective intoxication is correlated with later development of alcoholism in sons of alcoholics. Using a 12-item questionnaire that measures an individuals level of response to alcoholism, the Self Rating of the Effects of Alcohol (SRE) instrument, data from 745 individuals from COGA was used to identify chromosomal regions linked to an individual's level of response to ethanol [154]. From these data, several chromosomal regions were identified which appear to contribute to this phenotype. In particular, the region on chromosome 1 that is linked to a low level of response to alcohol is also linked in the same sample to alcohol dependence [108,109].

VIII. ANIMAL MODELS OF ADDICTIVE DISORDERS

The use of animal models with similar or related behaviors may provide important genetic clues that will improve the efficiency of identifying genes underlying human addictions. Well-characterized animal lines with phenotypes related to certain aspects of human addictive behaviors can be used as an approach to study more homogeneous populations in which isolation of candidate regions and loci should be faster and more efficient. Most mouse studies have utilized B6 and D2 progenitors and a variety of breeding schemes. Unique quantitative trait loci (QTLs) have been identified in each experiment, but there are some consistent linkage findings that appear to replicate across these studies. While definitive QTL identification is certainly not yet available, several chromosomal regions show great promise for gene identification, especially murine chromosome 2 [155–160]. Selective breeding based on the phenotype of high and low alcohol consumption has resulted in the development of selected rat lines. Genome screen studies using the inbred alcohol-preferring (P) and alcohol-nonpreferring (NP) rat lines have resulted in strong evidence of linkage to rat chromosome 4, in the region near the neuropeptide Y gene [161].

The use of animal models has also proven to be successful in the identification of QTL contributing to the observed differences among the B6 and D2 mice in oral voluntary morphine consumption. Two major loci have been identified [162]. A locus on proximal murine chromosome 10 [162] explained ~50% of the genetic variance in morphine consumption. Subsequently, the murine OPRM1 gene was localized to this interval [163–165]. Two groups of investigators have produced OPRM1 knockout mice [166,167]. These mice are indifferent to the analgesic and rewarding properties of morphine, suggesting that these opioid effects are mediated mostly through OPRM1. The second major locus that was identified was on mouse chromosome 6.

IX. SUMMARY

There is substantial evidence that genetic factors play a major role in the susceptibility to alcohol, opiate, and other drug abuse as well as nicotine use. Studies of extended pedigrees suggest that there may be a subset of genetic loci that nonspecifically increase the predisposition to various addictions. Ongoing studies have also identified chromosomal regions that may harbor susceptibility loci influencing addiction to specific drugs.

ACKNOWLEDGMENTS

This work was supported by U.S. Public Service grants AA10707, AA08403, and AA00285.

REFERENCES

1. LT Midanik, WB Clark. The demographic distribution of US drinking patterns in 1990: description and trends from 1984. Am J Public Health 84:1218–1222, 1994.
2. DA Dawson, L Archer. Gender differences in alcohol consumption: effects of measurement. Br J Addict 87:119–123, 1992.
3. KC Burke, JD Burke Jr, DS Rae, DA Regier. Comparing age at onset of major depression and other psychiatric disorders by birth cohorts in five US community populations. Arch Gen Psychiatry 48:789–795, 1991.
4. JM McGinnis, WH Foege. Actual causes of death in the United States. JAMA 270:2207–2212, 1993.
5. N Cotton. The familial incidence of alcoholism. J Stud Alcohol 40:89–116, 1979.
6. DW Goodwin. Is alcoholism hereditary? A review and critique. Arch Gen Psychiatry 25:545–549, 1971.
7. CR Cloninger, KO Christiansen, T Reich, II Gottesman. Implications of sex differences in the

prevalences of antisocial personality, alcoholism, and criminality for familial transmission. Arch Gen Psychiatry 35:941–951, 1978.
8. L Kaij, J Dock. Grandsons of alcoholics. A test of sex-linked transmission of alcohol abuse. Arch Gen Psychiatry 32:1379–1381, 1975.
9. T Reich. Presented at the Park City (IL) Molecular Psychiatry Meeting, 1997.
10. SY Hill, H Yuan. Familial density of alcoholism and onset of adolescent drinking. J Stud Alcohol 60:7–17, 1999.
11. DA Dawson. The link between family history and early onset alcoholism: earlier initiation of drinking or more rapid development of dependence? J Stud Alcohol 61:637–646, 2000.
12. J Partanen, K Bruun, T Markkanen. Inheritance of Drinking Behavior; A Study on Intelligence, Personality, and Use of Alcohol of Adult Twins. Helsinki: Finnish Foundation for Alcohol Studies, 1966.
13. J Kaprio, M Koskenvuo, H Langinvainio, K Romanov, S Sarna, RJ Rose. Genetic influences on use and abuse of alcohol: a study of 5638 adult Finnish twin brothers. Alcohol Clin Exp Res 11:349–356, 1987.
14. CA Clifford, JL Hopper, DW Fulker, RM Murray. A genetic and environmental analysis of a twin family study of alcohol use, anxiety, and depression. Genet Epidemiol 1:63–79, 1984.
15. L Kaij. Alcoholism in twins: studies on the etiology and sequels of abuse of alcohol. Stockholm: Almqvist & Wiksell, 1960.
16. II Gottesman, G Carey. Extracting meaning and direction from twin data. Psychiatr Dev 1:35–50, 1983.
17. Z Hrubec, GS Omenn. Evidence of genetic predisposition to alcoholic cirrhosis and psychosis: twin concordances for alcoholism and its biological end points by zygosity among male veterans. Alcohol Clin Exp Res 5:207–215, 1981.
18. T Reed, WF Page, RJ Viken, JC Christian. Genetic predisposition to organ-specific endpoints of alcoholism. Alcohol Clin Exp Res 20:1528–1533, 1996.
19. KS Kendler, AC Heath, MC Neale, RC Kessler, LJ Eaves. A population-based twin study of alcoholism in women. JAMA 268:1877–1882, 1992.
20. CA Prescott, SH Aggen, KS Kendler. Sex differences in the sources of genetic liability to alcohol abuse and dependence in a population-based sample of U.S. twins. Alcohol Clin Exp Res 23:1136–1144, 1999.
21. DW Goodwin, F Schulsinger, L Hermansen, S Guze, G Winokur. Alcohol problems in adoptees raised apart from alcoholic biological parents. Arch Gen Psychiatry 28:238–243, 1973.
22. DW Goodwin, F Schulsinger, N Moller, L Hermansen, G Winokur, SB Guze. Drinking problems in adopted and nonadopted sons of alcoholics. Arch Gen Psychiatry 31:164–169, 1974.

23. M Bohman. Some genetic aspects of alcoholism and criminality. A population of adoptees. Arch Gen Psychiatry 35:269–276, 1978.
24. CR Cloninger, M Bohman, S Sigvardsson. Inheritance of alcohol abuse. Cross-fostering analysis of adopted men. Arch Gen Psychiatry 38:861–868, 1981.
25. CR Cloninger. A systematic method for clinical description and classification of personality variants. A proposal. Arch Gen Psychiatry 44:573–588, 1987.
26. CR Cloninger. A unified biosocial theory of personality and its role in the development of anxiety states. Psychiatr Dev 4:167–226, 1986.
27. MA Schuckit, DA Goodwin, G Winokur. A study of alcoholism in half siblings. Am J Psychiatry 128:1132–1136, 1972.
28. G Winokur, T Reich, J Rimmer, FN Pitts, Jr. Alcoholism. 3. Diagnosis and familial psychiatric illness in 259 alcoholic probands. Arch Gen Psychiatry 23:104–111, 1970.
29. DW Goodwin, F Schulsinger, J Knop, S Mednick, SB Guze. Alcoholism and depression in adopted-out daughters of alcoholics. Arch Gen Psychiatry 34:751–755, 1977.
30. G Winokur, W Coryell. Familial alcoholism in primary unipolar major depressive disorder. Am J Psychiatry 148:184–188, 1991.
31. KR Merikangas, CS Gelernter. Comorbidity for alcoholism and depression. Psychiatr Clin North Am 13:613–632, 1990.
32. JR Morrison. The family histories of manic-depressive patients with and without alcoholism. J Nerv Ment Dis 160:227–229, 1975.
33. ES Gershon, J Hamovit, JJ Guroff, E Dibble, JF Leckman, W Sceery, SD Targum, JI Nurnberger Jr, LR Goldin, WE Bunney Jr. A family study of schizoaffective, bipolar I, bipolar II, unipolar, and normal control probands. Arch Gen Psychiatry 39:1157–1167, 1982.
34. JI Nurnberger Jr, T Foroud, L Flury, J Su, ET Meyer, K Hu, R Crowe, H Edenberg, A Goate, L Bierut, T Reich, M Schuckit, W Reich. Evidence for a locus on chromosome 1 that influences vulnerability to alcoholism and affective disorder. Am J Psychiatry 158:718–724, 2001.
35. M Bohman, CR Cloninger, AL von Knorring, S Sigvardsson. An adoption study of somatoform disorders. III. Cross-fostering analysis and genetic relationship to alcoholism and criminality. Arch Gen Psychiatry 41:872–878, 1984.
36. CR Cloninger, S Sigvardsson, SB Gilligan, AL von Knorring, T Reich, M Bohman. Genetic heterogeneity and the classification of alcoholism. Adv Alcohol Subst Abuse 7:3–16, 1988.
37. RJ Cadoret, TW O'Gorman, E Troughton, E Heywood. Alcoholism and antisocial personality.

Interrelationships, genetic and environmental factors. Arch Gen Psychiatry 42:161–167, 1985.
38. F Earls, W Reich, KG Jung, CR Cloninger. Psychopathology in children of alcoholic and antisocial parents. Alcohol Clin Exp Res 12:481–487, 1988.
39. KR Merikangas, DE Stevens, B Fenton, M Stolar, S O'Malley, SW Woods, N Risch. Co-morbidity and familial aggregation of alcoholism and anxiety disorders. Psychol Med 28:773–788, 1998.
40. SY Hill, CR Cloninger, FR Ayre. Independent familial transmission of alcoholism and opiate abuse. Alcohol Clin Exp Res 1:335–342, 1977.
41. JL Croughan. The contributions of family studies to understanding drug abuse In: LN Robins, ed. Studying Drug Abuse. New Brunswick, NJ: Rutgers University Press, 1985.
42. J Gfroerer. Correlation between drug use by teenagers and drug use by older family members. Am J Drug Alcohol Abuse 13:95–108, 1987.
43. WH Meller, R Rinehart, RJ Cadoret, E Troughton. Specific familial transmission in substance abuse. Int J Addict 23:1029–1039, 1988.
44. SM Mirin, RD Weiss, J Michael, ML Griffin. Psychopathology in substance abusers: diagnosis and treatment. Am J Drug Alcohol Abuse 14:139–157, 1988.
45. SM Mirin, RD Weiss, ML Griffin, JL Michael. Psychopathology in drug abusers and their families. Compr Psychiatry 32:36–51, 1991.
46. BJ Rounsaville, TR Kosten, MM Weissman, B Prusoff, D Pauls, SF Anton, K Merikangas. Psychiatric disorders in relatives of probands with opiate addiction. Arch Gen Psychiatry 48:33–42, 1991.
47. KR Merikangas, M Stolar, DE Stevens, J Goulet, MA Preisig, B Fenton, H Zhang, SS O'Malley, BJ Rounsaville. Familial transmission of substance use disorders. Arch Gen Psychiatry 55:973–979, 1998.
48. MB van den Bree, EO Johnson, MC Neale, RW Pickens. Genetic and environmental influences on drug use and abuse/dependence in male and female twins. Drug Alcohol Depend 52:231–241, 1998.
49. KL Jang, WJ Livesley, PA Vernon. Alcohol and drug problems: a multivariate behavioural genetic analysis of co-morbidity. Addiction 90:1213–1221, 1995.
50. WM Grove, ED Eckert, L Heston, TJ Bouchard, Jr., N Segal, DT Lykken. Heritability of substance abuse and antisocial behavior: a study of monozygotic twins reared apart. Biol Psychiatry 27:1293–1304, 1990.
51. RW Pickens, DS Svikis, M McGue, DT Lykken, LL Heston, PJ Clayton. Heterogeneity in the inheritance of alcoholism. A study of male and female twins. Arch Gen Psychiatry 48:19–28, 1991.
52. MT Tsuang, MJ Lyons, SA Eisen, J Goldberg, W True, N Lin, JM Meyer, R Toomey, SV Faraone, L Eaves. Genetic influences on DSM-III-R drug abuse and dependence: a study of 3,372 twin pairs. Am J Med Genet 67:473–477, 1996.
53. MT Tsuang, MJ Lyons, JM Meyer, T Doyle, SA Eisen, J Goldberg, W True, N Lin, R Toomey, L Eaves. Co-occurrence of abuse of different drugs in men: the role of drug-specific and shared vulnerabilities. Arch Gen Psychiatry 55:967–972, 1998.
54. M McGue, RW Pickens, DS Svikis. Sex and age effects on the inheritance of alcohol problems: a twin study. J Abnorm Psychol 101:3–17, 1992.
55. RJ Cadoret. Genetic and environmental factors in initiation of drug use and the transition to abuse. In: MD Glantz, RW Pickens, eds. Vulnerability to Drug Abuse. Washington: American Psychological Association, 1992, pp 99–113.
56. RJ Cadoret, E Troughton, TW O'Gorman, E Heywood. An adoption study of genetic and environmental factors in drug abuse. Arch Gen Psychiatry 43:1131–1136, 1986.
57. RJ Cadoret, WR Yates, E Troughton, G Woodworth, MA Stewart. An adoption study of drug abuse/dependency in females. Compr Psychiatry 37:88–94, 1996.
58. JR Hughes. Genetics of smoking: A brief review. Behav Ther 17:335–345, 1986.
59. GE Swan, D Carmelli, RH Rosenman, RR Fabsitz, JC Christian. Smoking and alcohol consumption in adult male twins: genetic heritability and shared environmental influences. J Subst Abuse 2:39–50, 1990.
60. D Carmelli, GE Swan, D Robinette, R Fabsitz. Genetic influence on smoking—a study of male twins. N Engl J Med 327:829–833, 1992.
61. WR True, H Xian, JF Scherrer, PA Madden, KK Bucholz, AC Heath, SA Eisen, MJ Lyons, J Goldberg, M Tsuang. Common genetic vulnerability for nicotine and alcohol dependence in men. Arch Gen Psychiatry 56:655–661, 1999.
62. GE Swan, D Carmelli, LR Cardon. Heavy consumption of cigarettes, alcohol and coffee in male twins. J Stud Alcohol 58:182–190, 1997.
63. T Niu, C Chen, J Ni, B Wang, Z Fang, H Shao, X Xu. Nicotine dependence and its familial aggregation in Chinese. Int J Epidemiol 29:248–252, 2000.
64. AC Heath, NG Martin. Genetic models for the natural history of smoking: evidence for a genetic influence on smoking persistence. Addict Behav 18:19–34, 1993.
65. JE Helzer, TR Pryzbeck. The co-occurrence of alcoholism with other psychiatric disorders in the general population and its impact on treatment. J Stud Alcohol 49:219–224, 1988.

66. RC Kessler, RM Crum, LA Warner, CB Nelson, J Schulenberg, JC Anthony. Lifetime co-occurrence of DSM-III-R alcohol abuse and dependence with other psychiatric disorders in the National Comorbidity Survey. Arch Gen Psychiatry 54:313–321, 1997.
67. ME McCaul, JS Turkkan, DS Svikis, GE Bigelow, CC Cromwell. Alcohol and drug use by college males as a function of family alcoholism history. Alcohol Clin Exp Res 14:467–471, 1990.
68. RJ Cadoret, WR Yates, E Troughton, G Woodworth, MA Stewart. Adoption study demonstrating two genetic pathways to drug abuse. Arch Gen Psychiatry 52:42–52, 1995.
69. KS Kendler, CG Davis, RC Kessler. The familial aggregation of common psychiatric and substance use disorders in the National Comorbidity Survey: a family history study. Br J Psychiatry 170:541–548, 1997.
70. HR Thomasson, HJ Edenberg, DW Crabb, XL Mai, RE Jerome, TK Li, SP Wang, YT Lin, RB Ly, SJ Yin. Alcohol and aldehyde dehydrogenase genotypes and alcoholism in Chinese men. Am J Hum Genet 48:677–681, 1991.
71. S Higuchi, S Matsushita, H Amazeki, T Kinoshita, S Takagi, H Kono. Aldehyde dehydrogenase genotypes in Japanese alcoholics. Lancet 343:741–742, 1994.
72. F Tanaka, Y Shiratori, O Yokosuka, F Imazeki, Y Tsukada, M Omata. High incidence of ADH2*1/ALDH2*1 genes among Japanese alcohol dependents and patients with alcoholic liver disease. Hepatology 23:234–239, 1996.
73. Y Maezawa, M Yamauchi, G Toda, H Suzuki, S Sakurai. Alcohol metabolizing enzyme polymorphisms and alcoholism in Japan. Alcohol, Clin Exp Res 19:951–954, 1995.
74. K Nakamura, K Iwahashi, Y Matsuo, R Miyatake, Y Ichikawa, H Suwaki. Characteristics of Japanese alcoholics with the atypical aldehyde dehydrogenase 2*2. I. A comparison of the genotypes of ALDH2, ADH2, ADH3, and cytochrome P-4502E1 between alcoholics and nonalcoholics. Alcohol, Clin Exp Res 20:52–55, 1996.
75. WJ Chen, EW Loh, YPP Hsu, CC Chen, JM Yu, ATA Cheng. Alcohol-metabolizing genes and alcoholism among Taiwanese Han men: independent effect of ADH2, ADH3 and ALDH2. Br J Psychiatry 168:762–767, 1996.
76. YC Shen, JH Fan, HJ Edenberg, TK Li, YH Cui, YF Wang, CH Tian, CF Zhou, RL Zhou, J Wang, ZL Zhao, GY Xia. Polymorphism of ADH and ALDH genes among four ethnic groups in China and effects upon the risk for alcoholism. Alcohol Clin Exp Res 21:1272–1277, 1997.
77. DW Crabb. Ethanol oxidizing enzymes: roles in alcohol metabolism and alcoholic liver disease. Prog Liver Dis 13:151–172, 1995.
78. YD Neumark, Y Friedlander, HR Thomasson, TK Li. Association of the ADH2*2 allele with reduced ethanol consumption in Jewish men in Israel: a pilot study. J Stud Alcohol 59:133–139, 1998.
79. CR Cloninger. Neurogenetic adaptive mechanisms in alcoholism. Science 236:410–416, 1987.
80. RA Wise, PP Rompre. Brain dopamine and reward. Annu Rev Psychol 40:191–225, 1989.
81. K Blum, E Noble, P Sheridan, A Montgomery, T Ritchie, P Jagadeeswaran, H Nogami, A Briggs, J Cohn. Allelic association of human dopamine D2 receptor gene in alcoholism. JAMA 263:2055–2060, 1990.
82. K Blum, EP Noble, PJ Sheridan, O Finley, A Montgomery, T Ritchie, T Ozkaragoz, RJ Fitch, F Sadlack, D Sheffield. Association of the A1 allele of the D2 dopamine receptor gene with severe alcoholism. Alcohol 8:409–416, 1991.
83. DE Comings, BG Comings, D Muhleman, G Dietz, B Shahbahrami, D Tast, E Knell, P Kocsis, R Baumgarten, BW Kovacs. The dopamine D2 receptor locus as a modifying gene in neuropsychiatric disorders. JAMA 266:1793–1800, 1991.
84. A Parsian, RD Todd, EJ Devor, KL O'Malley, BK Suarez, T Reich, CR Cloninger. Alcoholism and alleles of the human D2 dopamine receptor locus. Studies of association and linkage. Arch Gen Psychiatry 1991 Jul 48:655–663, 1991.
85. S Amadeo, M Abbar, ML Fourcade, G Waksman, MG Leroux, A Madec, M Selin, JC Champiat, A Brethome, Y Leclaire, D Castelnau, J Benisse, J Mallet. D2 dopamine receptor gene and alcoholism. J Psychiatr Res 27:173–179, 1993.
86. EP Noble, K Syndulko, RJ Fitch, T Ritchie, MC Bohlman, P Guth, PJ Sheridan, A Montgomery, C Heinzmann, RS Sparkes. D2 dopamine receptor TaqI A alleles in medically ill alcoholic and nonalcoholic patients. Alcohol Alcohol 29:729–744, 1994.
87. K Neiswanger, SY Hill, BB Kaplan. Association and linkage studies of the TAQI A1 allele at the dopamine D2 receptor gene in samples of female and male alcoholics. Am J Med Genet 60:261–271, 1995.
88. AM Bolos, M Dean, S Lucas-Derse, M Ramsburg, GL Brown, D Goldman. Population and pedigree studies reveal a lack of association between the dopamine D2 receptor gene and alcoholism. JAMA 264:3156–3160, 1991.
89. J Gelertner, S O'Malley, N Risch, HR Kranzler, J Krystal, K Merikangas, JL Kennedy, KK Kidd. No association between an allele at the D2 dopamine receptor gene (DRD2) and alcoholism. JAMA 266:1801–1807, 1991.

90. S Schwab, M Soyka, M Niederecker, M Ackenheil, J Scherer, DB Wildenauer. Allele association of human dopamine D2-receptor DNA polymorphism ruled out in 45 alcoholics. Am J Hum Genet 49:1991.
91. BL Cook, ZW Wang, RR Crowe, R Hauser, M Freimer. Alcoholism and the D2 receptor gene. Alcohol, Clin Exp Res 16:806–809, 1992.
92. D Goldman, M Dean, GL Brown, AM Bolos, R Tokola, M Virkkunen, M Linnoila. D2 dopamine receptor genotype and cerebrospinal fluid homovanillic acid, 5-hydroxyindoleacetic acid and 3-methyl-4-hydroxyphenylglycol in alcoholics in Finland and the United States. Acta Psychiatr Scand 86:351–357, 1992.
93. E Turner, J Ewing, P Shilling, TL Smith, M Irwin, M Schuckit, JR Kelsoe. Lack of association between an RFLP near the D2 dopamine receptor gene and severe alcoholism. Biol Psychiatry 31:285–290, 1992.
94. T Arinami, M Itokawa, T Komiyama, H Mitsushio, H Mori, H Mifune, H Hamaguchi. Association between severity of alcoholism and the A1 allele of the dopamine D2 receptor gene TaqIA RFLP in Japanese. Biol Psychiatry 33:108–114, 1993.
95. D Goldman, GL Brown, B Albaugh, R Robin, S Goodson, M Trunzo, L Akhtar, S Lucas-Derse, J Long, M Linnoila, M Dean. DRD2 dopamine receptor genotype linkage disequilibrium, and alcoholism in American Indians and other populations. Alcohol Clin Exp Res 17:199–204, 1993.
96. BF O'Hara, SS Smith, G Bird, AM Persico, BK Suarez, GR Cutting, GR Uhl. Dopamine D2 receptor RFLPs, haplotypes and their association with substance use in black and Caucasian research volunteers. Hum Hered 43:209–218, 1993.
97. A Parsian, BK Suarez, B Tabakoff, P Hoffman, L Ovchinnikova, L Fisher, CR Cloninger. Monoamine oxidases and alcoholism: studies in unrelated alcoholics, normal controls and alcoholic families. Alcohol; Alcohol 2:45–49, 1994.
98. T Sander, H Harms, J Podschus, U Finckh, B Nickel, A Rolfs, H Rommelspacher, LG Schmidt. Dopamine D1, D2 and D3 receptor genes in alcohol dependence. Psychiatr Genet 5:171–176, 1995.
99. RB Lu, HC Ko, FM Chang, CM Castiglione, G Schoolfield, AJ Pakstis, JR Kidd, KK Kidd. No association between alcoholism and multiple polymorphisms at the dopamine D2 receptor gene (DRD2) in three distinct Taiwanese populations. Biol Psychiatry 39:419–429, 1996.
100. CH Chen, SH Chien, HG Hwu. Lack of association between TaqI A1 allele of dopamine D2 receptor gene and alcohol-use in Atayal natives of Taiwan. Am J Med Genet 67:488–490, 1996.
101. D Goldman, M Urbanek, D Guenther, R Robin, JC Long. Linkage and association of a functional DRD2 variant [Ser311Cys] and DRD2 markers to alcoholism, substance abuse and schizophrenia in southwestern American Indians. Am J Med Genet 74:386–394, 1997.
102. HJ Edenberg, T Foroud, DL Koller, A Goate, J Rice, P VanErdewegh, T Reich, CR Cloninger, JI Nurnberger, M Kowalczuk, B Wu, TK Li, PM Conneally, JA Tischfield, W Wu, S Shears, R Crowe, V Hesselbrock, M Schucket, B Porjesz, H Begleiter. A family-based analysis of the association of the dopamine D2 receptor (DRD2) with alcoholism. Alcohol Clin Exp Res 22:505–512, 1998.
103. A Heils, A Teufel, S Petri, G Stober, P Riederer, D Bengel, KP Lesch. Allelic variation of human serotonin transporter gene expression. J Neurochem 66:2621–2624, 1996.
104. KP Lesch, D Bengel, A Heils, SZ Sabol, BD Greenberg, S Petri, J Benjamin, CR Muller, DH Hamer, DL Murphy. Association of anxiety-related traits with a polymorphism in the serotonin transporter gene regulatory region. Science 274:1527–1531, 1996.
105. RP Ebstein, I Gritsenko, L Nemanov, A Frisch, Y Osher, RH Belmaker. No association between the serotonin transporter gene regulatory region polymorphism and the Tridimensional Personality Questionnaire (TPQ) temperament of harm avoidance. Mol Psychiatry 2:224–226, 1997.
106. T Sander, H Harms, KP Lesch, P Dufeu, S Kuhn, M Hoehe, H Rommelspacher, LG Schmidt. Association analysis of a regulatory variation of the serotonin transporter gene with severe alcohol dependence. Alcohol Clin Exp Res 21:1356–1359, 1997.
107. HJ Edenberg, J Reynolds, DL Koller, H Begleiter, KK Bucholz, PM Conneally, R Crowe, A Goate, V Hesselbrock, TK Li, JI Nurnberger Jr, B Porjesz, T Reich, JP Rice, M Schuckit, JA Tischfield, T Foroud. A family-based analysis of whether the functional promoter alleles of the serotonin transporter gene HTT affect the risk for alcohol dependence. Alcohol Clin Exp Res 22:1080–1085, 1998.
108. T Reich, HJ Edenberg, A Goate, JT Williams, JP Rice, P Van Eerdewegh, T Foroud, V Hesselbrock, MA Schuckit, K Bucholz, B Porjesz, TK Li, PM Conneally, JI Nurnberger Jr, JA Tischfield, RR Crowe, CR Cloninger, W Wu, S Shears, K Carr, C Crose, C Willig, H Begleiter. Genome-wide search for genes affecting the risk for alcohol dependence. Am J Med Genet 81:207–215, 1998.
109. T Foroud, HJ Edenberg, A Goate, J Rice, L Flury, DL Koller, LJ Bierut, PM Conneally, JI Nurnberger Jr, KK Bucholz, TK Li, V Hesselbrock, R Crowe, M Schuckit, B Porjesz, H Begleiter, T Reich. Alcoholism susceptibility loci: confirmation studies in a replicate sample and further mapping. Alcohol Clin Exp Res 24:933–945, 2000.

110. JC Long, WC Knowler, RL Hanson, RW Robin, M Urbanek, E Moore, PH Bennett, D Goldman. Evidence for genetic linkage to alcohol dependence on chromosomes 4 and 11 from an autosome-wide scan in an American Indian population. Am J Med Genet 81:216–221, 1998.

111. DA Nielsen, M Virkkunen, J Lappalainen, M Eggert, GL Brown, JC Long, D Goldman, M Linnoila. A tryptophan hydroxylase gene marker for suicidality and alcoholism. Arch Gen Psychiatry 55:593–602, 1998.

112. KS Kendler, AC Heath, MC Neale, RC Kessler, LJ Eaves. Alcoholism and major depression in women. A twin study of the causes of comorbidity. Arch Gen Psychiatry 50:690–698, 1993.

113. VM Hesselbrock, T Foroud, H Edenberg, JI Nurnberger Jr, T Reich, JP Rice. Genetics and alcoholism: the COGA project. In: DP Agarwal, HK Seitz, eds. Alcohol in Health and Disease. New York: Marcel Dekker, 2001, pp 103–124.

114. WH Berrettini, MR Hoehe, TN Ferraro, PA DeMaria, E Gottheil. Human mu opioid receptor gene polymorphisms and vulnerability to substance abuse. Addict Biol 2:303–308, 1997.

115. AW Bergen, J Kokoszka, R Peterson, JC Long, M Virkkunen, M Linnoila, D Goldman. Mu opioid receptor gene variants: lack of association with alcohol dependence. Mol Psychiatry 2:490–494, 1997.

116. C Bond, KS LaForge, M Tian, D Melia, S Zhang, L Borg, J Gong, J Schluger, JA Strong, SM Leal, JA Tischfield, MJ Kreek, L Yu. Single-nucleotide polymorphism in the human mu opioid receptor gene alters beta-endorphin binding and activity: possible implications for opiate addiction. Proc Natl Acad Sci USA 95:9608–9613, 1998.

117. HR Kranzler, J Gelernter, S O'Malley, CA Hernandez-Avila, D Kaufman. Association of alcohol or other drug dependence with alleles of the mu opioid receptor gene (OPRM1). Alcohol Clin Exp Res 22:1359–1362, 1998.

118. J Gelernter, H Kranzler, J Cubells. Genetics of two mu opioid receptor gene (OPRM1) exon I polymorphisms: population studies, and allele frequencies in alcohol- and drug-dependent subjects. Mol Psychiatry 4:476–483, 1999.

119. P Franke, MM Nothen, T Wang, M Knapp, D Lichtermann, H Neidt, T Sander, P Propping, W Maier. DRD4 exon III VNTR polymorphism-susceptibility factor for heroin dependence? Results of a case-control and a family-based association approach. Mol Psychiatry 5:101–104, 2000.

120. J Gelernter, HR Kranzler. Variant detection at the delta opioid receptor (OPRD1) locus and population genetics of a novel variant affecting protein sequence. Hum Genet 107:86–88, 2000.

121. EP Noble, K Blum, ME Khalsa, T Ritchie, A Montgomery, RC Wood, RJ Fitch, T Ozkaragoz, PJ Sheridan, MD Anglin. Allelic association of the D2 dopamine receptor gene with cocaine dependence. Drug Alcohol Depend 33:271–285, 1993.

122. WH Berrettini, AM Persico. Dopamine D2 receptor gene polymorphisms and vulnerability to substance abuse in African Americans. Biol Psychiatry 40:144–147, 1996.

123. JB Lichter, CL Barr, JL Kennedy, HH Van Tol, KK Kidd, KJ Livak. A hypervariable segment in the human dopamine receptor D4 (DRD4) gene. Hum Mol Genet 2:767–773, 1993.

124. HH Van Tol, CM Wu, HC Guan, K Ohara, JR Bunzow, O Civelli, J Kennedy, P Seeman, HB Niznik, V Jovanovic. Multiple dopamine D4 receptor variants in the human population. Nature 358:149–152, 1992.

125. J Benjamin, L Li, C Patterson, BD Greenberg, DL Murphy, DH Hamer. Population and familial association between the D4 dopamine receptor gene and measures of novelty seeking. Nat Genet 12:81–84, 1996.

126. RP Ebstein, O Novick, R Umansky, B Priel, Y Osher, D Blaine, ER Bennett, L Nemanov, M Katz, RH Belmaker. Dopamine D4 receptor (D4DR) exon III polymorphism associated with the human personality trait of novelty seeking. Nat Genet 12:78–80, 1996.

127. RP Ebstein, L Nemanov, I Klotz, I Gritsenko, RH Belmaker. Additional evidence for an association between the dopamine D4 receptor (D4DR) exon III repeat polymorphism and the human personality trait of novelty seeking. Mol Psychiatry 2:472–477, 1997.

128. PA Compton, MD Anglin, ME Khalsa-Denison, A Paredes. The D2 dopamine receptor gene, addiction, and personality: clinical correlates in cocaine abusers. Biol Psychiatry 39:302–304, 1996.

129. M Vukov, N Baba-Milkic, D Lecic, S Mijalkovic, J Marinkovic. Personality dimensions of opiate addicts. Acta Psychiatr Scand 91:103–107, 1995.

130. M Kotler, H Cohen, R Segman, I Gritsenko, L Nemanov, B Lerer, I Kramer, M Zer-Zion, I Kletz, RP Ebstein. Excess dopamine D4 receptor (D4DR) exon III seven repeat allele in opioid-dependent subjects. Mol Psychiatry 2:251–254, 1997.

131. MR Spitz, H Shi, F Yang, KS Hudmon, H Jiang, RM Chamberlain, CI Amos, Y Wan, P Cinciripini, WK Hong, X Wu. Case-control study of the D2 dopamine receptor gene and smoking status in lung cancer patients. J Natl Cancer Inst 90:358–363, 1998.

132. LJ Bierut, JP Rice, HJ Edenberg, A Goate, T Foroud, CR Cloninger, H Begleiter, PM Conneally, RR Crowe, V Hesselbrock, TK Li, JI Nurnberger Jr, B Porjesz, MA Schuckit, T Reich. Family-based study of the association of the dopamine D2 receptor

gene (DRD2) with habitual smoking. Am J Med Genet 90:299–302, 2000.
133. RE Straub, PF Sullivan, Y Ma, MV Myakishev, C Harris-Kerr, B Wormley, B Kadambi, H Sadek, MA Silverman, BT Webb, MC Neale, CM Bulik, PR Joyce, KS Kendler. Susceptibility genes for nicotine dependence: a genome scan and followup in an independent sample suggest that regions on chromosomes 2, 4, 10, 16, 17 and 18 merit further study. Mol Psychiatry 4:129–144, 1999.
134. P Naitoh. The value of electroencephalography in alcoholism. Ann NY Acad Sci 215:303–320, 1973.
135. P Propping. Genetic control of ethanol action on the central nervous system. An EEG study in twins. Hum Genet 35:309–334, 1977.
136. P Propping. Alcohol and alcoholism. Hum Genet Suppl 91–99, 1978.
137. P Propping, J Kruger, N Mark. Genetic disposition to alcoholism. An EEG study in alcoholics and their relatives. Hum Genet 59:51–59, 1981.
138. VE Pollock, J Volavka, DW Goodwin, SA Mednick, WF Gabrielli, J Knop, F Schulsinger. The EEG after alcohol administration in men at risk for alcoholism. Arch Gen Psychiatry 40:857–861, 1983.
139. H Begleiter, B Porjesz, B Bihari, B Kissin. Event-related brain potentials in boys at risk for alcoholism. Science 225:1493–1496, 1984.
140. R Elmasian, H Neville, D Woods, M Schuckit, F Bloom. Event-related brain potentials are different in individuals at high and low risk for developing alcoholism. Proc Natl Acad Sci USA 79:7900–7903, 1982.
141. B Porjesz, H Begleiter, A Litke, L Bauer, S Kuperman, S O'Connor, J Rohrbaugh. Visual P3 as a potential phenotypic marker for alcoholism: evidence from the COGA national project In: C Ogura, Y Koga, Shimokochi M., eds. Recent Advances in Event-Related Brain Potential Research. Amsterdam: Elsevier, 1996, pp 539–549.
142. SY Hill, C Aston, B Rabin. Suggestive evidence of genetic linkage between alcoholism and the MNS blood group. Alcohol Clin Exp Res 12:811–814, 1988.
143. RE Tarter, AM Hegedus, G Goldstein, C Shelly, AI Alterman. Adolescent sons of alcoholics: neuropsychological and personality characteristics. Alcohol Clin Exp Res 8:216–222, 1984.
144. MA Schuckit, N Butters, L Lyn, M Irwin. Neuropsychologic deficits and the risk for alcoholism. Neuropsychopharmacology 1:45–53, 1987.
145. SY Hill, J Armstrong, SR Steinhauer, T Baughman, J Zubin. Static ataxia as a psychobiological marker for alcoholism. Alcohol Clin Exp Res 11:345–348, 1987.
146. PR Finn, RO Pihl. Men at high risk for alcoholism: the effect of alcohol on cardiovascular response to unavoidable shock. J Abnorm Psychol 96:230–236, 1987.
147. PR Finn, RO Pihl. Risk for alcoholism: a comparison between two different groups of sons of alcoholics on cardiovascular reactivity and sensitivity to alcohol. Alcohol Clin Exp Res 12:742–747, 1988.
148. SY Hill, SR Steinhauer, J Zubin. Biological markers for alcoholism: a vulnerability model conceptualization. Nebr Symp Motiv 34:207–256, 1986.
149. L von Knorring, AL von Knorring, L Smigan, U Lindberg, M Edholm. Personality traits in subtypes of alcoholics. J Stud Alcohol 48:523–527, 1987.
150. MA Schuckit. Self-rating of alcohol intoxication by young men with and without family histories of alcoholism. J Stud Alcohol 41:242–249, 1980.
151. MA Schuckit. Subjective responses to alcohol in sons of alcoholics and control subjects. Arch Gen Psychiatry 41:879–884, 1984.
152. MA Schuckit. Genetics and the risk for alcoholism. JAMA 254:2614–2617, 1985.
153. MA Schuckit, TL Smith. An 8-year follow-up of 450 sons of alcoholic and control subjects. Arch Gen Psychiatry 53:202–210, 1996.
154. MA Schuckit, HJ Edenberg, J Kalmijn, L Flury, TL Smith, T Reich, L Bierut, A Goate, T Foroud. A genome-wide search for genes that relate to a low level of response to alcohol. Alcohol Clin Exp Res 25:323–329, 2001.
155. TJ Phillips, JC Crabbe, P Metten, JK Belknap. Localization of genes affecting alcohol drinking in mice. Alcohol Clin Exp Res 18:931–941, 1994.
156. JK Belknap, SP Richards, LA O'Toole, ML Helms, TJ Phillips. Short-term selective breeding as a tool for QTL mapping: ethanol preference drinking in mice. Behav Genet 27:55–66, 1997.
157. TJ Phillips, JK Belknap, KJ Buck, CL Cunningham. Genes on mouse chromosomes 2 and 9 determine variation in ethanol consumption. Mamm Genome 9:936–941, 1998.
158. LA Rodriguez, R Plomin, DA Blizard, BC Jones, GE McClearn. Alcohol acceptance, preference, and sensitivity in mice. II. Quantitative trait loci mapping analysis using BXD recombinant inbred strains. Alcohol Clin Exp Res 19:367–373, 1995.
159. LM Tarantino, GE McClearn, LA Rodriguez, R Plomin. Confirmation of quantitative trait loci for alcohol preference in mice. Alcohol Clin Exp Res 22:1099–1105, 1998.
160. JA Melo, J Shendure, K Pociask, LM Silver. Identification of sex-specific quantitative trait loci controlling alcohol preference in C57BL/ 6 mice. Nat Genet 13:147–153, 1996.
161. LG Carr, T Foroud, P Bice, T Gobbett, J Ivashina, H Edenberg, L Lumeng, TK Li. A quantitative trait locus for alcohol consumption in selectively bred rat lines. Alcohol Clin Exp Res 22:884–887, 1998.

162. WH Berrettini, TN Ferraro, RC Alexander, AM Buchberg, WH Vogel. Quantitative trait loci mapping of three loci controlling morphine preference using inbred mouse strains. Nat Genet 7:54–58, 1994.
163. CA Kozak, J Filie, MC Adamson, Y Chen, L Yu. Murine chromosomal location of the mu and kappa opioid receptor genes. Genomics 21:659–661, 1994.
164. B Giros, M Pohl, JM Rochelle, MF Seldin. Chromosomal localization of opioid peptide and receptor genes in the mouse. Life Sci 56:L369–L375, 1995.
165. DL Kaufman, DE Keith Jr, B Anton, J Tian, K Magendzo, D Newman, TH Tran, DS Lee, C Wen, YR Xia. Characterization of the murine mu opioid receptor gene. J Biol Chem 270:15877–15883, 1995.
166. HW Matthes, R Maldonado, F Simonin, O Valverde, S Slowe, I Kitchen, K Befort, A Dierich, M Le Meur, P Dolle, E Tzavara, J Hanoune, BP Roques, BL Kieffer. Loss of morphine-induced analgesia, reward effect and withdrawal symptoms in mice lacking the mu-opioid-receptor gene. Nature 383:819–823, 1996.
167. I Sora, N Takahashi, M Funada, H Ujike, RS Revay, DM Donovan, LL Miner, GR Uhl. Opiate receptor knockout mice define mu receptor roles in endogenous nociceptive responses and morphine-induced analgesia. Proc Natl Acad Sci USA 94:1544–1549, 1997.

42

Biological Basis of Eating Disorders

WALTER H. KAYE and NICOLE C. BARBARICH
Western Psychiatric Institute and Clinic, University of Pittsburgh School of Medicine, Pittsburgh, Pennsylvania, U.S.A.

I. INTRODUCTION

Anorexia nervosa (AN) and bulimia nervosa (BN) are disorders characterized by abnormal patterns of feeding behavior and weight regulation, with disturbances in perceptions and attitudes toward shape and weight [1]. The characteristic feature of AN is an inexplicable fear of weight gain and an unrelenting obsession with fatness even in the face of increasing cachexia. In BN, the onset of binge eating usually emerges after a period of dieting, which may or may not have been associated with weight loss. In addition, binge eating is followed by the use of inappropriate behaviors such as self-induced vomiting; misuse of laxatives, diuretics, or enemas; excessive exercise; or fasting as a means of compensation for the excess food ingested. Although individuals with BN are typically at a normal body weight, some 25–30% presenting to treatment centers have a prior history of AN.

In certain respects, both diagnostic labels are misleading. In AN, weight loss is rarely associated with a true loss of appetite, but rather a volitional, and more often than not, ego syntonic resistance to feeding drives with an eventual preoccupation with food and eating rituals to the point of obsession [2]. In addition, binge eating in BN is not associated with a primary pathological increase of appetite. Individuals with BN have a seemingly relentless drive to restrain their food intake, an extreme fear of weight gain, and often a distorted view of their actual body shape. Loss of control over food intake usually occurs intermittently and typically only some time after the onset of dieting behavior [2]. Episodes of binge eating also develop in a significant proportion of people with AN [3], whereas a smaller percentage of those with BN will eventually develop AN [4]. Considering that restrained eating behavior and dysfunctional cognitions relating weight and shape to self-concept are shared by patients with both of these syndromes, and that transitions between AN and BN occur in many, it has been argued that AN and BN share at least some risk and liability factors.

The etiology of eating disorders is still unknown; however, it seems clear that multiple factors may be linked to the pathogenesis of AN and BN, with current research focused on identifying the relative pathophysiological contributions of genetic, biological, psychological, and social factors [2]. While it has been argued that cultural attitudes toward standards of physical attractiveness have relevance to the psychopathology of eating disorders, it is unlikely that cultural influences in pathogenesis are very prominent. For one thing, dieting behavior and drive for thinness are quite commonplace in industrialized countries throughout the world, yet AN and BN affect only an estimated 0.3–0.7% and 1.7–2.5%, respectively, of females in the general population. Moreover, numerous clear descriptions of AN date back to the middle of the 19th century [5] suggests that factors other than a cultural emphasis on thinness play an etiologic role. In addition, these syndromes, particularly in the case of AN, have a relatively stereotypic clinical presentation, sex distribution, and age of onset, which provides support for the possibility of some biologic vulnerability to the disorders. This chapter provides a brief overview of the illness phenomenology and behavioral traits characteristic of AN and BN. Current knowledge of the potential etiological significance of genetic and neurobiological risk and vulnerability factors in the development of AN and BN is also discussed.

II. ILLNESS PHENOMENOLOGY AND COURSE

A. Phenomenology

Variations in feeding behaviors have been used to distinguish individuals with AN into two meaningful diagnostic subgroups that differ in other psychopathological characteristics. In the restricting subtype of AN, weight loss and an ongoing malnourished state are accomplished primarily through unremitting food avoidance and/or excessive exercise. In the binge-eating/purging subtype of AN, there is comparable weight loss and malnutrition, yet the course of illness is marked by supervening episodes of binge eating, usually followed by inappropriate compensatory behaviors such as self-induced vomiting or laxative abuse. Compared to the restricting subtype of AN, individuals with the binge-eating/purging subtype are also more likely to exhibit histories of behavioral dyscontrol, substance abuse, and overt family conflict. Marked perfectionism, conformity, obsessionality, constriction of affect and emotional expressiveness, and reduced social spontaneity are personality traits that are particularly common in individuals with AN. These traits appear to be premorbid and persist even after long-term weight restoration, indicating the presence of disturbances that are not merely the result of acute malnutrition and disordered eating behavior [6,7].

Although many individuals with BN aspire to ideal weights far below the range of normalcy for their age and height, most remain at normal body weight. The core features of BN include repeated episodes of binge eating followed by inappropriate compensatory behaviors including self-induced vomiting, laxative abuse, or pathologically extreme exercise, as well as abnormal concerns with shape and weight. The DSM-IV [1] has specified two distinct subgroups of BN to distinguish between those individuals who engage in self-induced vomiting or abuse of laxatives, diuretics, or enemas (purging type), and those who exhibit other forms of compensatory behaviors such as fasting or excessive exercise (nonpurging type).

Beyond these diagnostic categories, it has been proposed [8] that there are two clinically divergent subgroups of individuals with BN differing significantly in psychopathological characteristics: a multi-impulsive type, in whom BN occurs in conjunction with more pervasive difficulties in behavioral self-regulation and affective instability; and a second type, whose distinguishing features include self-effacing behaviors, dependence on external rewards, and extreme compliance. Individuals with BN of the multi-impulsive type are far more likely to have histories of substance abuse and display other impulse control problems such as shoplifting and self-injurious behaviors. Considering these differences, it has been postulated that multi-impulsive-type BN individuals rely on binge eating and purging as a means of regulating intolerable states of tension, anger, and fragmentation. In contrast, individuals with the latter type of BN may have binge episodes precipitated through dietary restraint with compensatory behaviors maintained through reduction of guilty feelings associated with fears of weight gain.

B. Course

The mean age of onset of AN is 17 years, with some data suggesting bimodal peaks at ages of 14 and 18 years [1]. Although childhood onset of AN has been reported, it is not clear whether prepubertal onset of the illness confers a less ominous prognosis. Recovery from AN tends to be protracted, but studies of long-term outcome reveal a highly variable course: roughly 50% of individuals will eventually have reasonably complete resolution of the illness, whereas another 30% will have lingering residual features that fluctuate in severity long into adulthood. In 10% of individuals, AN will pursue a chronic, unremitting course, and the remaining 10% of those affected will eventually die from the disease.

Compared to AN, the age of onset of BN is more variable, with most cases developing during the period from middle to late adolescence through the mid-20s [9]. It is usually precipitated by dieting and weight loss, yet it can occur in the absence of apparent dietary restraint. There is considerable variation among individuals in the frequency of binge episodes, their duration, and the amount of food consumed during any one episode. Follow-up studies of clinic samples 5–10 years after presentation showed a 50% rate of recovery while nearly 20% continued to meet full criteria for BN [9]. Following onset, severity of disturbed eating behavior will fluctuate over the course of several years in a high percentage of clinic cases. Approximately 30% of women who had been in remission experienced relapse into bulimic symptoms, although the risk of relapse appeared to decline 4 years after presentation [9].

III. BEHAVIORAL TRAITS

Eating disorders are associated with a number of psychological symptoms aside from pathological eating behaviors. Recent studies in AN [10–12] have consistently found elevated scores of harm avoidance (the tendency to inhibit behavior to avoid punishment) and persistence (perseverance without intermittent reinforcement). In addition, decreased scores have been reported on measures of novelty seeking (behavioral activation to pursue rewards), self-directedness (the degree to which the self is viewed as autonomous and integrated), and cooperativeness (the degree to which the self is viewed as a part of society) [10,11]. Personality styles of women with AN are characterized by marked rigidity, overcontrol, obsessionality, and perfectionism [7,13]. Studies in BN have reported increased scores on measures of impulsivity, disorganization, and affective lability [14].

Additional psychological disturbances in AN and BN include depression, anxiety, substance abuse, and personality disorders. Theories regarding a shared vulnerability between AN and obsessive compulsive disorder have also received a substantial amount of attention [15,16]. A major methodological issue in the study of these disorders is determining whether such symptoms are a consequence or a potential cause of pathological feeding behavior and malnutrition. Owing to the young age of onset and difficulty in premorbid identification of people who will develop an eating disorder (ED), it is impractical to study AN and BN prospectively. Instead, subjects can be studied after long-term recovery under the assumption that in the absence of confounding nutritional influences, persistent psychobiological abnormalities might be trait related and potentially contribute to the pathogenesis of the disorder. While the definition of recovery from an ED has not been formalized, the limited number of studies that have investigated people who have recovered from an ED tend to include people formerly ill with AN after they were at a stable and healthy body weight for months or years and had not been malnourished or engaged in pathologic eating behavior during that period of recovery. In studies of BN, investigators tend to include subjects who have been abstinent from binging and purging for months or years. In addition, some studies have included criteria of normal menstrual cycles and a minimal duration of recovery, such as 1 year, for inclusion in the study.

Studies have reported that women who were long-term recovered from AN had a persistence of obsessional behaviors as well as inflexible thinking, restraint in emotional expression, and a high degree of self- and impulse control [6,7,17,18]. In addition, they have social introversion, overly compliant behavior, limited social spontaneity, and greater risk and harm avoidance. In terms of core ED symptoms, individuals who are long-term recovered from AN had residual disturbances, such as ineffectiveness, a drive for thinness, and significant psychopathology related to eating habits. Similarly, individuals who have recovered from BN continue to be overly concerned with body shape and weight, and have abnormal eating behaviors and dysphoric mood [19–23]. Both recovered AN and BN women have increased scores on measures of perfectionism with the need for symmetry and ordering/arranging as their most common obsessional target symptoms.

Overall, these residual behaviors can be characterized as overconcerns with body image and thinness; obsessionality with symmetry, exactness, and perfectionism; and dysphoric/negative affect. Pathological eating behavior and malnutrition during the acute phase of syndromes appear to exaggerate the magnitude of these concerns. Thus, while target symptoms are the same in both ill and recovered individuals, the intensity of the symptoms is greater during the acute illness. The persistence of these symptoms after recovery raises the possibility that the disturbances are premorbid traits that contribute to the pathogenesis of AN and BN.

IV. FAMILY/GENETICS

Despite the lack of empirical evidence, traditional theories of etiology have often viewed eating disorders as sociocultural in origin. However, emerging evidence suggests that both AN and BN are familial, and that clustering of the disorders in families may result from genetic transmission of risk. Family studies provide guidance as to whether a disorder is possibly genetic by establishing whether it clusters among biologically related individuals. Results from the largest and most systematic studies suggest a 7- to 12-fold increase in the prevalence of AN and BN in relatives of eating-disordered probands compared to controls [24,25]. However, given that first-degree relatives share genes and environment, these studies are unable to definitively differentiate genetic versus environmental causes for the familial clusters.

In contrast, twin studies are able to provide a better estimate of genetic versus environmental effects of a disorder by comparing similarities for a trait between identical (monozygotic; MZ) and fraternal (dizygotic; DZ) twins. Data from a large epidemiological sample of twins obtained via the Virginia Twin Registry [26,27] found evidence for a strong association between AN and BN. The cotwin of a twin affected with AN was 2.6 times more likely to have a lifetime diagnosis of BN compared to the cotwins of unaffected twins. There are several reports of greater pairwise concordance rates of eating disorders in MZ than in DZ twin pairs [28,29]. Studies reported that 58–76% of the variance in AN [30,31] and 54–83% of the variance in BN [26,32] can be accounted for by genetic factors. These heritability estimates are similar to those found in other psychiatric disorders, such as schizophrenia and bipolar disorder, suggesting that eating disorders may be as genetically influenced as disorders traditionally viewed as biological.

Several family and twin studies have examined the covariation between eating disorders and a range of other psychiatric conditions that occur with comorbidity in AN and BN individuals [see reviews, 24,33]. Studies of AN probands have yielded familial risk estimates in the range of 7–25% for major affective disorder, with relative risk estimates in studies employing normal controls in the range of 2.1–3.4. Similar studies of BN probands have shown, with rare exception, that their first-degree relatives are several times more likely to develop affective disorders than relatives of control subjects. Most studies considering the effects of proband comorbidity on familial risk have shown that affective illness is more likely to be transmitted by probands with the same diagnostic comorbidity. In short, although AN and BN often co-occur with major mood disorders, particularly unipolar depression, the two conditions do not appear to express a single, shared transmitted liability.

Evidence from family studies suggests a relatively low prevalence of substance abuse disorders among relatives of restricting-type AN probands. These rates are elevated in relatives of probands with BN. However, recent studies have consistently shown [34,35] that the genetic variation influencing susceptibility to alcoholism was independent of those genetic factors underlying risk to BN. Tentative evidence of independent familial transmission of obsessive-compulsive disorders (OCD) and AN and BN have been reported. However, preliminary data from other investigators suggest a common familial transmission of AN and obsessive-compulsive personality disorder (OCPD), suggesting the existence of a broad, genetically influenced phenotype with core features of rigid perfectionism and propensity for extreme behavioral constraint. Consequently, in spite of the formidable challenges encountered in the biological study of malnourished individuals, efforts to better understand the pathophysiology of AN and BN continue to have clinical and heuristic value.

V. NEUROTRANSMITTER

The role of biological determinants in the etiology of AN has been proposed for the past 60 years [5]. An increased knowledge of the neurotransmitter modulation of appetitive behaviors has raised the question whether some disturbance of neurotransmitter function causes AN and/or BN [36–38]. Although it is possible that the monoamine disturbances found in patients with eating disorders could be a consequence of dietary abnormalities, it is equally important to consider that these disturbances may be premorbid traits that contribute to a vulnerability to develop AN or BN. To understand the relative effects of starvation and malnutrition, individuals are studied while symptomatic and after recovery.

A. Serotonin

There has been substantial interest in the role that serotonin (5HT) may play in AN and BN. In part this is related to evidence that has found alterations in the metabolism of 5HT both during the acute phase of eating disorders and after long-term recovery. These disturbances are of particular interest to eating disorders since 5HT has been implicated in a wide number of systems including feeding, mood, impulse regulation, anxiety, and obsessionality.

Serotonin is a neurotransmitter that is widely distributed in the brain. It is synthesized from its amino acid precursor tryptophan (TRP), which is taken up by the brain and hydroxylated by the enzyme tryptophan-5-hydroxylase [39]. The product of this reaction, 5-

hydroxytryptophan, is then decarboxylated by the aromatic amino acid decarboxylase to the compound 5-hydroxytryptamine. Monoamine oxidase further metabolizes 5HT to the metabolite product known as 5-hydroxyindoleacetic acid (5HIAA), which may be measured as a means of assessing serotonin turnover or metabolism [39].

Measuring the concentration of 5HIAA in cerebrospinal fluid (CSF) provides an index of presynaptic activity in serotonergic pathways [40] and has been utilized as a measure of 5HT metabolism in a number of psychiatric disorders. Diminished 5HT function is associated with an impulsive-aggressive behavioral style [41], and low concentrations of CSF 5HIAA are associated with a significant increase in aggressive behavior and suicide risk [42,43]. It has been argued that the region-specific increase in $5HT_2$ receptors in the brains of suicide victims may be increased in number secondary to decreased 5HT and/or 5HIAA levels. Therefore, decreased 5HT neurotransmission as a function of impulsivity has important implications for studying patients with AN since the core symptoms of the disorder are typically at the opposite extreme.

During the acute phase of the illness, individuals with AN have a significant reduction in basal levels of CSF 5HIAA compared to healthy controls [44]. In addition, a blunted plasma prolactin response to drugs with serotonin activity and reduced ^{3}H-imipramine binding suggests reduced serotonergic activity in underweight AN, although these findings may be secondary to reductions in dietary supplies of the amino acid precursor TRP. In contrast, CSF 5HIAA activity in long-term weight recovered AN was reported to be significantly elevated, which may be correlated with the persistent behavioral traits characteristic of the disorder [45]. In particular, evidence suggests a possible association between the overly inhibited, anxious, and obsessional behavior of individuals recovered from AN with increased levels of 5HT activity.

Several recent studies have reported alterations in binding of $5HT_{1A}$ and $5HT_{2A}$ receptors in AN. Frank [46] reported an association between increased frontal-limbic-temporal postsynaptic $5HT_{1A}$ receptor binding and the anxious, harm-avoidant traits characteristic of AN. In particular, high correlations were found between anxiety or harm avoidance and binding in the medial temporal region of the brain, which includes the structural center responsible for the modulation of anxiety.

Considerable evidence also exists for a disturbance of serotonin regulation in BN. During the acute phase, individuals with BN have a blunted prolactin response to 5HT receptor agonists m-chlorophenylpiperazine (m-CPP), 5-hydroxytryptophan, and dl-fenfluramine, and an enhanced migrainelike headache response to m-CPP challenges [47,48]. In addition, similar to individuals with AN, women with long-term recovery from BN have elevated levels of CSF 5HIAA and a dysphoric response to m-CPP administration [22].

The relative contribution of a disturbance in 5HT function to specific human behaviors remains indeterminate. Serotonin has been postulated to contribute to temperament or personality traits, such as harm avoidance [49] and behavioral inhibition [50], or to categorical dimensions such as OCD [51], anxiety and fear [52], and depression [53], as well as satiety for food consumption. It is possible that separate components of 5HT neuronal systems (i.e., different pathways, receptors) are coded for specific behaviors. However, that may not be consistent with the neurophysiology of serotonin neuronal function. All of the monoamine neuronal systems, including 5HT, have a diffuse, widespread distribution and, it can be argued, have a threshold function for information processing, independent of specific behaviors. According to Spoont [54], 5HT regulates or stabilizes the flow of information through a neural system. 5HT neuronal activity prevents overshoot of other neurotransmitter systems and thus attenuates signal amplitude. In addition, it controls the sensitivity of the system to perturbations by new stimuli entering the system. Decreased 5HT neurotransmission would impair the ability of neural networks to maintain the integrity of signal flow pattern. This would result in increased switching, unstable, amplified signal passage, and impulsive, exaggerated stimulus reactivity. In contrast, with increased 5HT neurotransmission, the brain would be insensitive to new stimuli entering the brain, and there might be redundant signal propagation or maintenance of prepotent response patterns.

One point of interest in studying 5HT in eating disorders is that since the enzyme tryptophan hydroxylase is not normally saturated by TRP, the rate of 5HT synthesis can be influenced by changes in brain TRP concentration [55]. This concentration is dependent on the plasma concentration of TRP, in addition to the ratio of TRP to other large neutral amino acids (LNAA) with which it competes for uptake [56]. Since TRP is an essential amino acid that must be obtained through the diet, one important factor in determining the relative concentration of TRP available for 5HT synthesis is dietary intake. Numerous studies on dieting in healthy individuals have reported a decrease in plasma TRP after short-term food restriction [57]. In addition, a marked increase in prolactin response was found following intravenous administration of L-tryptophan in dieting women, but not men [58]. This finding has important implications for studying possible biological risk factors for AN, since approximately 90–95% of AN individuals are women [1].

In most people, food restriction is not an inherently reinforcing behavior. However, persistent dieting to the point of starvation raises the possibility that food restriction might have some benefit for people with AN. A recent study [59] found that the ratio of TRP to other LNAAs was significantly decreased in AN patients. Since starvation decreases the levels of TRP through a reduction in dietary TRP, less precursor is available for 5HT synthesis. Based on premorbid rates of anxiety, it has been argued [60] that patients with AN may initially have higher levels of 5HT in the synapse which contributes to a dysphoric state. Through dieting, the levels of TRP decrease leading to smaller amounts of the amino acid available for 5HT synthesis. Since less 5HT is available in the synapse, anxiety diminishes and mood in AN patients is elevated. A recent study supports the theory that a diet-induced reduction of TRP is associated with decreased anxiety in people with AN [60]. Based on this evidence, alterations in dietary TRP levels may represent a mechanism through which patients with AN attempt to regulate a dysphoric mood.

BN, a more common eating disorder, may be the prototypic expression of a disturbance of 5HT activity which contributes to the pathogenesis of eating disorders. Clinically, people with BN have extremes of eating and behavior. They tend to either diet or overeat, with infrequent consumption of normal meals. Behaviorally, they tend to fluctuate between minimization and inhibition of mood states and extremes of mood and catastrophic overconcerns. These clinical observations, coupled with data from studies in ill and recovered BN, lead to the speculation that the 5HT system in people with BN is inherently unstable and poorly modulated. Certain traits, such as restricted eating and high harm avoidance, perfectionism, and exactness, appear consistent with increased 5HT transmission in the nondieting state. In contrast, a diet-induced reduction in synaptic 5HT release could result in a reduction of behavioral inhibition and might, in turn, lead to extremes of unstable mood and binge eating. It is possible that people with such an inherent modulatory defect in 5HT function may be prone to develop BN. They cannot respond appropriately and precisely to stress or stimuli, or modulate their affective states owing to their modulatory 5HT defect. They may learn that extremes of dietary intake, by effects on plasma TRP, are a means by which they can crudely modulate their brain 5HT functional activity. Several investigators [47,61] have proposed a model in which individuals with BN may restrict eating or overeat as a means of self-modulating 5HT activity. Dieting or binge episodes could alter the TRP/LNAA ratio in plasma, which in turn alters TRP availability to the brain changing 5HT synthesis and release [62]. Tryptophan depletion causes ill BN women to have an increase in labile and dysphoric mood and overeat compared to control women [63]. These changes in mood and feeding behavior support the possibility that individuals with BN have a fragile and dysregulated serotonin system that is vulnerable to dietary manipulations.

The possibility of a common vulnerability for AN and BN may seem counterintuitive given the differences in 5HT disturbances and feeding behavior in these disorders. However, recent studies suggest that AN and BN have a shared etiologic vulnerability. There is a familial aggregation of a range of eating disorders in relatives of probands with either AN or BN, and these two disorders are highly comorbid in twin studies. Both disorders respond to serotonin-specific medications, and both disorders have high levels of harm avoidance [12,18,64,65], a personality trait hypothesized to be related to increased serotonin activity. These data raise the possibility that a disturbance of 5HT activity may create a vulnerability for the expression of a cluster of symptoms that are common to both AN and BN. Other factors independent of a vulnerability for the development of eating disorder may contribute to the development of eating disorder subgroups. For example, people with restrictor-type AN have extraordinary self-restraint and self-control. The risk for obsessive-compulsive personality disorder is elevated only in this subgroup and in their families and shows a shared transmission with restrictor-type AN [24]. In other words, an additional vulnerability for behavioral overcontrol and rigid and inflexible mood states, combined with a vulnerability for an eating disorder, may result in restrictor-type AN.

Overall, the evidence for a disturbance of serotonin presented above suggests a differential response for individuals with AN and BN. It appears that manipulations which decrease 5HT levels, such as the serotonin agonist m-CPP, produce euphoria in individuals recovered from AN and dysphoria in BN. Challenges such as ATD which lower plasma tryptophan levels, and consequently brain 5HT synthesis, decrease anxiety in both ill and recovered AN and increase depression and eating-disordered symptoms in BN. Thus, although a disturbance of 5HT is apparent in both AN and BN and the specific mechanism appears to be fundamentally different between syndromes, it is possible that a predisposition to a disturbance of 5HT creates a vulnerability for the expression of a cluster of symptoms common to both AN and BN.

B. Dopamine

Additional evidence has been reported for a disturbance of dopaminergic function in patients with eating disorders. Dopamine neuronal function has been associated with motor activity, reward, and novelty seeking. In a recent study, women who were recovered from restricting-type AN had significantly lower levels of CSF HVA than women who were recovered from BN [66]. Thus, altered dopamine activity could potentially account for some behavioral traits characteristic of AN.

VI. CONCLUSION

Phenomenological and etiologic research of AN and BN has found that eating disorders are characterized by protracted courses of illness, a persistence of psychological disturbances after recovery, and significant genetic contributions to their development and maintenance. Emerging evidence also raises the possibility that a disturbance of serotonergic activity may create a vulnerability for the expression of a cluster of symptoms that are common to both AN and BN. However, to what extent abnormalities detected are consequences of pathological eating behavior, malnutrition, or premorbid traits remains somewhat speculative. Clearly, some of the atypicalities in monoaminergic function in eating disorders are state dependent; however, given the effects of these systems on mood, anxiety, memory organization, and body physiology, they may well have significant pathogenic influence, both sustaining and exacerbating certain psychological and cognitive elements of these syndromes. Future research should continue to explore the biological and genetic underpinnings of these disorders to develop more effective approaches to prevention and treatment.

REFERENCES

1. American Psychiatric Association. Diagnostic and Statistical Manual of Mental Disorders. Washington: American Psychiatric Association, 1994.
2. U Schweiger, M Fichter. Eating disorders: clinical presentation, classification and etiologic models. In: DC Jimerson, WH Kaye, eds. Balliere's Clinical Psychiatry. London: Balliere's Tindall, 1997, pp 199–216.
3. KA Halmi, E Eckert, P Marchi, V Sampugnaro, R Apple, J Cohen. Comorbidity of psychiatric diagnoses in anorexia nervosa [see comments]. Arch Gen Psychiatry 48:712–718, 1991.
4. LKG Hsu, TA Sobkiewicz. Bulimia nervosa: a four- to six-year follow-up study. Psychol Med 19:1035–1038, 1989.
5. J Treasure, I Campbell. The case for biology in the aetiology of anorexia nervosa [editorial]. Psychol Med 24:3–8, 1994.
6. NM Srinivasagam, WH Kaye, KH Plotnicov, C Greeno, TE Weltzin, R Rao. Persistent perfectionism, symmetry, and exactness after long-term recovery from anorexia nervosa. Am J Psychiatry 152:1630–1634, 1995.
7. M Strober. Personality and symptomatological features in young, nonchronic anorexia nervosa patients. J Psychosom Res 24:353–359, 1980.
8. K Vitousek, F Manke. Personality variables and disorders in anorexia nervosa and bulimia nervosa. J Abnorm Psychol 103:137–147, 1994.
9. PK Keel, JE Mitchell. Outcome in bulimia nervosa. Am J Psychiatry 154:313–321, 1997.
10. KL Klump, CM Bulik, C Pollice, KA Halmi, MM Fichter, WH Berrettini, B Devlin, M Strober, A Kaplan, DB Woodside, J Treasure, M Shabbout, LR Lilenfeld, KH Plotnicov, WH Kaye. Temperament and character in women with anorexia nervosa. J Nerv Ment Dis 188:559–567, 2000.
11. EI Kleifield, S Sunday, S Hurt, KA Halmi. The Tridimensional Personality Questionnaire: an exploration of personality traits in eating disorders. J Psychiat Res 28:413–423, 1994.
12. TD Brewerton, LD Hand, ER Bishop, Jr. The Tridimensional Personality Questionnaire in eating disorder patients. Int J Eat Disord 14:213–218, 1993.
13. PJ Beumont, GC George, DE Smart. "Dieters" and "vomiters and purgers" in anorexia nervosa. Psychol Med 6:617–622, 1976.
14. RC Casper, D Hedeker, JF McClough. Personality dimensions in eating disorders and their relevance for subtyping. J Am Acad Child Adolesc Psychiatry 31:830–840, 1992.
15. WH Kaye. Anorexia and bulimia nervosa, obsessional behavior, and serotonin. In: WH Kaye, DC Jimerson, eds. Eating Disorders. London: Balliere's Tindell, 1997, pp 319–337.
16. N Barbarich. Is there a common mechanism of serotonin dysregulation in anorexia nervosa and obsessive compulsive disorder? (In Press.)

17. RC Casper. Personality features of women with good outcome from restricting anorexia nervosa. Psychosom Med 52:156–170, 1990.
18. AM O'Dwyer, JV Lucey, GF Russell. Serotonin activity in anorexia nervosa after long-term weight restoration: response to D-fenfluramine challenge. Psychol Med 26:353–359, 1996.
19. S Collings, M King. Ten-year follow-up of 50 patients with bulimia nervosa. Br J Psychiatry 164:80–87, 1994.
20. BA Fallon, BT Walsh, C Sadik, JB Saoud, V Lukasik. Outcome and clinical course in inpatient bulimic women: a 2- to 9-year follow-up study. J Clin Psychiatry 52:272–278, 1991.
21. E Johnson-Sabine, D Reiss, D Dayson. Bulimia nervosa: a 5-year follow-up study. Psychol Med 22:951–959, 1992.
22. WH Kaye, CG Greeno, H Moss, J Fernstrom, M Fernstrom, LR Lilenfeld, TE Weltzin, JJ Mann. Alterations in serotonin activity and psychiatric symptomatology after recovery from bulimia nervosa. Arch Gen Psychiatry 55:927–935, 1998.
23. CE Norring, SS Sohlberg. Outcome, recovery, relapse and mortality across six years in patients with clinical eating disorders. Acta Psychiatr Scand 87:437–444, 1993.
24. LR Lilenfeld, WH Kaye, CG Greeno, KR Merikangas, K Plotnicov, C Pollice, R Rao, M Strober, CM Bulik, L Nagy. A controlled family study of anorexia nervosa and bulimia nervosa: psychiatric disorders in first-degree relatives and effects of proband comorbidity. Arch Gen Psychiatry 55:603–610, 1998.
25. M Strober, R Freeman, C Lampert, J Diamond, W Kaye. Controlled family study of anorexia nervosa and bulimia nervosa: evidence of shared liability and transmission of partial syndromes. Am J Psychiatry 157:393–401, 2000.
26. KS Kendler, C MacLean, M Neale, R Kessler, A Heath, L Eaves. The genetic epidemiology of bulimia nervosa. Am J Psychiatry 148:1627–1637, 1991.
27. EE Walters, KS Kendler. Anorexia nervosa and anorexic-like syndromes in a population-based female twin sample. Am J Psychiatry 152:64–71, 1995.
28. AJ Holland, A Hall, R Murray, GF Russell, AH Crisp. Anorexia nervosa: a study of 34 twin pairs and one set of triplets. Br J Psychiatry 145:414–419, 1984.
29. AJ Holland, N Sicotte, J Treasure. Anorexia nervosa: evidence for a genetic basis. J Psychosom Res 32:561–571, 1988.
30. KL Klump, KB Miller, PK Keel, M McGue, WG Iacono. Genetic and environmental influences on anorexia nervosa syndromes in a population-based twin sample. Psychol Med 31:737–740, 2001.
31. TD Wade, CM Bulik, M Neale, KS Kendler. Anorexia nervosa and major depression: shared genetic and environmental risk factors. Am J Psychiatry 157:469–471, 2000.
32. CM Bulik, PF Sullivan, KS Kendler. Heritability of binge-eating and broadly defined bulimia nervosa. Biol Psychiatry 44:1210–1218, 1998.
33. M Strober. Family-genetic studies of eating disorders. J Clin Psychiatry 52 (suppl)9–12, 1991.
34. WH Kaye, LR Lilenfeld, K Plotnicov, KR Merikangas, L Nagy, M Strober, CM Bulik, H Moss, CG Greeno. Bulimia nervosa and substance dependence: association and family transmission. Alcohol Clin Exp Res 20:878–881, 1996.
35. MA Schuckit, JE Tipp, RM Anthenelli, KK Bucholz, VM Hesselbrock, JI Nurnberger Jr. Anorexia nervosa and bulimia nervosa in alcohol-dependent men and women and their relatives. Am J Psychiatry 153:74–82, 1996.
36. M Fava, PM Copeland, U Schweiger, DB Herzog. Neurochemical abnormalities of anorexia nervosa and bulimia nervosa. Am J Psychiatry 146:963–971, 1989.
37. SF Leibowitz. Brain monoamines and peptides: role in the control of eating behavior. Fed Proc 45:1396–1403, 1986.
38. JE Morley, JE Blundell. The neurobiological basis of eating disorders: some formulations. Biol Psychiatry 23:53–78, 1988.
39. F Petty, LL Davis, D Kabel, GL Kramer. Serotonin dysfunction disorders: a behavioral neurochemistry perspective. J Clin Psychiatry 57(suppl 8):11–16, 1996.
40. DC Jimerson, MD Lesem, AP Hegg, TD Brewerton. Serotonin in human eating disorders. Ann NY Acad Sci 600:532–544, 1990.
41. EF Coccaro, ME Berman, RJ Kavoussi, RL Hauger. Relationship of prolactin response to d-fenfluramine to behavioral and questionnaire assessments of aggression in personality-disordered men [see comments]. Biol Psychiatry 40:157–64, 1996.
42. KR Jamison. Night Falls Fast. New York: Vintage Books, 1999.
43. GL Brown, MH Ebert, PF Goyer, DC Jimerson, WJ Klein, WE Bunney, FK Goodwin. Aggression, suicide, and serotonin: relationships to CSF amine metabolites. Am J Psychiatry 139:741–746, 1982.
44. WH Kaye, MH Ebert, M Raleigh, R Lake. Abnormalities in CNS monoamine metabolism in anorexia nervosa. Arch Gen Psychiatry 41:350–355, 1984.
45. WH Kaye, HE Gwirtsman, DT George, MH Ebert. Altered serotonin activity in anorexia nervosa after long-term weight restoration. Does elevated cerebrospinal fluid 5-hydroxyindoleacetic acid level correlate with rigid and obsessive behavior? Arch Gen Psychiatry 48:556–562, 1991.
46. WH Kaye, GK Frank, CC Meltzer, JC Price, WC Drevets, CA Mathis. Enhanced pre- and postsynaptic 5HT1A receptor binding after recovery from anorexia nervosa: relationship to anxiety and harm avoidance. (Submitted.)

47. DC Jimerson, MD Lesem, WH Kaye, TD Brewerton. Low serotonin and dopamine metabolite concentrations in cerebrospinal fluid from bulimic patients with frequent binge episodes. Arch Gen Psychiatry 49:132–138, 1992.
48. TD Brewerton, DL Murphy, EA Mueller, DC Jimerson. Induction of migrainelike headaches by the serotonin agonist m- chlorophenylpiperazine. Clin Pharmacol Ther 43:605–609, 1988.
49. CR Cloninger. A systematic method for clinical description and classification of personality variants. A proposal. Arch Gen Psychiatry 44:573–588, 1987.
50. P Soubrie. Reconciling the role of central serotonin neuroses in human and animal behavior. Behav Brain Sci 9:319–363, 1986.
51. LC Barr, WK Goodman, LH Price, CJ McDougle, DS Charney. The serotonin hypothesis of obsessive compulsive disorder: implications of pharmacologic challenge studies. J Clin Psychiatry 53(suppl):17–28, 1992.
52. DS Charney, SW Woods, JH Krystal, GR Heninger. Serotonin function and human anxiety disorders. Ann NY Acad Sci 600:558–572, 1990.
53. DG Grahame-Smith. Serotonin in affective disorders. Int Clin Psychopharmacol 6(suppl 4):5–13, 1992.
54. MR Spoont. Modulatory role of serotonin in neural information processing: implications for human psychopathology. Psychol Bull 112:330–350, 1992.
55. JD Fernstrom, RJ Wurtman. Brain serotonin content: physiological dependence on plasma tryptophan levels. Science 173:149–152, 1971.
56. JD Fernstrom, RJ Wurtman. Brain serotonin content: physiological regulation by plasma neutral amino acids. Science 178:414–416, 1972.
57. IM Anderson, M Parry-Billings, EA Newsholme, CG Fairburn, PJ Cowen. Dieting reduces plasma tryptophan and alters brain 5HT function in women. Psychol Med 20:785–791, 1990.
58. GM Goodwin, CG Fairburn, PJ Cowen. The effects of dieting and weight loss on neuroendocrine responses to tryptophan, clonidine, and apomorphine in volunteers. Important implications for neuroendocrine investigations in depression. Arch Gen Psychiatry 44:952–957, 1987.
59. A Favaro, L Caregaro, AB Burlina, P Santonastaso. Tryptophan levels, excessive exercise, and nutritional status in anorexia nervosa. Psychosom Med 62:535–538, 2000.
60. WH Kaye, NC Barbarich, K Putnam, KA Gendall, J Fernstrom, M Fernstrom, CW McConaha, A Kishore. Anxiolytic effects of acute tryptophan depletion (ATD) in anorexia nervosa. (In Press).
61. WH Kaye, HE Gwirtsman, DT George, DC Jimerson, MH Ebert. CSF 5-HIAA concentrations in anorexia nervosa: reduced values in underweight subjects normalize after weight gain. Biol Psychiatry 23:102–105, 1988.
62. JD Fernstrom, DV Faller. Neutral amino acids in the brain: changes in response to food ingestion. J Neurochem 30:1531–1538, 1978.
63. TE Weltzin, JD Fernstrom, C McConaha, WH Kaye. Acute tryptophan depletion in bulimia: effects on large neutral amino acids. Biol Psychiatry 35:388–397, 1994.
64. CM Bulik, PF Sullivan, TE Weltzin, WH Kaye. Temperament in eating disorders. Int J Eat Disord 17:251–261, 1995.
65. EI Kleifield, S Sunday, S Hurt. Psychometric validation of the Tridimensional Personality Questionnaire: application to subgroups of eating disorders. Compr Psychiatry 34:249–253, 1993.
66. WH Kaye, GK Frank, C McConaha. Altered dopamine activity after recovery from restricting-type anorexia nervosa. Neuropsychopharmacology 21:503–506, 1999.

43

Biological Basis of Personality Disorders

CUNEYT ISCAN
University of Massachusetts Medical School, Worcester, Massachusetts, U.S.A.

CHARLOTTE L. ALLPORT and KENNETH R. SILK
University of Michigan Health System, Ann Arbor, Michigan, U.S.A.

I. OVERVIEW

As we move beyond the 1990s, past the decade of the brain and into a new millennium, there has been an exponential increase in knowledge into understanding the biological basis of human psychology and behavior. Freud's original concept of the biological basis of behavior, expressed in the "Project" [1] at the close of the 19th century, may become reality in the early parts of the 21st century. Yet to achieve complete understanding the task before us remains enormous.

As we continue research into understanding the etiology of psychiatric disorders, the complexity of the human brain and behavior demands integrating different theoretical approaches and applying reductionism whenever necessary without losing perspective. Our current level of knowledge in the area of behavioral sciences compels us to bring together data at many levels of analysis. Those data include molecular genetics, neurochemistry, neurophysiology, cognitive science, and developmental psychology/psychopathology [2]. We now appear to possess the technology and the means to improve upon the technology to provide ever more sophisticated data from these fields that will facilitate our understanding of behavior at the molecular level.

Prior to the 1980s, most explorations into the cause of personality disorders were relegated to the area of psychological theories [3]. These theoretical propositions were based on appreciating fully the developing individual in his/her environment and the reaction of that individual to interpersonal experiences [4,5]. While it was believed that axis I disorders would eventually be found to have significant etiologic roots in biologic predispositions and mechanisms, personality disorders were viewed as resulting primarily as a response to external factors [3]. These assumptions with respect to differences between DSM axes in the importance of the role of biology in etiology and treatment persisted despite evidence and argument to the contrary [6].

Papers published in the late 1980s and early 1990s proposed biologic theories for explaining some of the underlying pathologic processes found in personality disorders [7], and there was a growing body of empirical research to begin to support some of the biologic theories. The early biological theories and studies focused on comparisons between a specific personality disorder with what was thought to be a near-neighbor axis I disorder, e.g., borderline personality disorder (BPD) and mood disorders, specifically major affective disorder and currently bipolar II disorder, cyclothymic disorder, or posttraumatic stress disorder (PTSD); schizotypal personality disorder (SPD) and schizophrenia; avoidant personality disorder and social phobia; histrionic personality disorder and somatization disorder; paranoid personality disorder and delusional disorder or schizophrenia, paranoid type. Early biological studies in BPD focused on biologic indices such as the dexamethasone suppression test (DST) or time of onset of REM sleep to try to discover similarities and differences that might help delineate more carefully the relationship between these BPD patients and patients with mood disorders [8–12]. While there were a decent number of studies in these areas, these studies failed to produce consistent results to support strongly the axis I–axis II spectrum hypothesis or to distinguish clearly the axis II disorder as a separate biological entity from the putative axis I disorder [7].

The interest in studying the similarities and differences between a specific personality disorder and a near-neighbor axis I disorder waned to be replaced by an interest in studying the biological underpinnings of the personality and personality disorders in general. Researchers began to look at types of behaviors or traits that were thought to cut across a number of personality disorders and the biological mechanisms that might be responsible or related to these behaviors or traits. These "second-generation" biological studies looked across personality disorders in contrast to earlier studies that tried to compare a specific axis I disorder with a specific axis II disorder [7]. Any given dimension of psychopathology can be disturbed in different degrees of severity across many of the personality disorders. Studying these dimensions has led to new research methodologies that have expanded our appreciation of the role of biology in the personality disorders. Most of the studies that have been done in recent years focused on this biological dimensional approach. The only exception to this generalization is SPD. There is considerable amount of research, especially in the area of neuroimaging, targeted to appreciating the specific link between schizophrenia, SPD in particular, and cluster A personality disorders in general.

Several dimensional classifications have been put forth in recent years in an attempt to define a "phenotype" or trait which not only will appropriately reflect an underlying biological mechanism but also will hopefully provide us with a link to causality. These classification systems or dimensional models include Cloninger's [13] seven-factor model of personality, Siever and Davis's [14] four-dimensional psychobiological model, the five-factor model of Costa and McCrae [15], and Livesley's [16] studies that employ factor analysis to define dimensional traits to be researched biologically.

Understanding personality in a dimensional framework is a long-standing practice in the field of psychology, and two traditional domains of the personality have been defined as temperament and character [13,17]. Temperament refers to inborn and constitutional differences in the automatic responses of individuals to emotional or affect-laden stimuli; these responses are fortified under the influence of associative conditioning. Character and its corresponding traits are reflections of differences in early learning and self-teaching about life that stem from intuition and are shaped and modified by the learning individuals have absorbed from parents and important others [18]. Cloninger [13] conceptualizes temperament as involving individual differences in habit learning whereas character involves differences in higher cognitive processing. This conceptualization proposes a higher level of organization in terms of brain functions and aims to sort out the biological foundations of the personality. According to this perspective, character development is defined along the lines of abstract symbolic processes that are most highly developed in humans and include self-directed behavior, empathic social cooperation, and creative symbolic invention. These dimensions call for higher brain functions in the prefrontal and frontal brain regions, whereas temperament is defined along the lines of habit learning which does not utilize the cerebral neocortex and is well developed at an early age in almost all vertebrates. Based on this model, Cloninger et al. [17] defined four dimensions under temperament (harm avoidance, novelty seeking, reward dependence, and persistence) and three dimensions under character (self-directedness, cooperativeness, and self-transcendence).

Siever and Davis [14] have proposed a "psychobiological model" based on four dimensions: cognitive/perceptual organization, impulsivity/aggression, affective instability, and anxiety/inhibition. According to their model, core features of clusters of axis I disorders reflect disturbances in fundamental psychobiological dimensions: cognitive/perceptual organization disturbances and schizophrenic disorders; impulsivity/aggression and impulse control and perhaps conduct disorders; affective instability and major affective disorders; and anxiety/inhibition and anxiety disorders. Based on these dimensions, Siever and Davis [14] classify odd cluster (cluster A) axis II disorders as being linked to schizophrenia through disturbances along a dimension in the area of cognitive/perceptual organization. Using the same reasoning, they link impulsivity/aggression and affective instability to the dramatic cluster (cluster B) as well as to axis I disorders of impulsivity and affective lability, and anxiety/inhibition to cluster C (anxious cluster) as well as to axis I disorders of anxiety and inhibition.

Costa and McCrae's five-factor model of personality proposes five dimensions: neuroticism (versus emotional stability) (N), extraversion (E), openness to experience (O), agreeableness (A), and conscientiousness (i.e., disciplined adherence to goals, and strict adherence to principles) (C). Much work, particularly in the field of psychology, has been forth to explain this particular model further [19].

Studies that have been done in the area of personality disorders can be categorized in several ways. We have chosen to organize this chapter around the different methodological (and technological) ways in which researchers are exploring the biology of personality disorders and the data that have been gleaned from these studies. Thus we have organized this chapter around (1) neurotransmitter functions, (2) family-genetic techniques, and (3) neuroimaging techniques that study structural alterations in the brain and functionally assess brain activity via measurements of blood flow or metabolic activity with certain cognitive tasks. We will also discuss briefly the research on life events (trauma, especially childhood abuse and early development/attachment) and the possible alterations in the central nervous system's functioning as a result of trauma.

II. NEUROTRANSMITTER STUDIES

As stated above, early research into the biology of personality disorders focused on comparisons, particularly with respect to neurotransmitters and neurotransmitter function, between a specific personality disorder with what was thought to be a near-neighbor axis I disorder. Current trends in biologic research on personality disorders have now moved from exploring what particular substrate might be disturbed in a particular personality disorder to the idea of which neurotransmitter might be most closely related to a particular behavioral manifestation of a certain dimension of psychopathology that reveals itself as disturbed across a number of personality disorders [4].

The most heavily researched neurotransmitter with regard to personality and personality disorders is 5HT (serotonin). Over the course of more than two decades, research in this area has continually supported a strong role for 5HT in aggression and impulsivity [20]. These studies repeatedly reveal that 5HT levels are inversely related to aggression and impulsivity. The first evidence of an inverse relationship in humans between 5HT and aggression was reported by Asberg et al. [21]. Dysfunction in the 5HT system has been associated with self-directed and non-self-directed impulsive aggression. Evidence for this association continues to emerge from studies of violent suicide attempters and of individuals who had committed violent acts [22]. In a study of violent offenders, Linnoila et al. [23] found that cerebral spinal fluid (CSF) 5HIAA (a metabolite of 5HT) levels were significantly lower in violent offenders who committed impulsive crimes but not in violent offenders who committed premeditated crimes. A decrease in CSF 5HIAA level was noted among people who had murdered their own children [24].

Pharmacologic challenge studies also support this inverse relationship between 5HT levels and impulsive aggression. In pharmacological challenge studies, a physiological response (hormonal-prolactin, cortisol, thermal changes, blood pressure, heart rate) is monitored after an agent that stimulates a specific neurotransmitter system (in this instance the serotonergic system) is administered to the subjects. A variety of 5HT pharmacological challenge studies have been performed in subjects with personality disorders. Most common agents that have been used for this purpose are the 5HT-releasing agent and reuptake inhibitor d,l-fenfluramine (d,l-FEN), the direct 5HT agonist meta-chlorophenylpiperazine (m-CPP), and ipsapirone (IPS), which is a potent 5HT-1A agonist. In a comprehensive review [20], Coccaro summarized six studies using the prolactin response to d,l-FEN. These studies reveal a blunted prolactin response of 5HT to the d,l-FEN challenge (infusion) in subjects with personality disorders who engage in some sort of self-mutilative or suicidal behavior. A recent study revealed blunted prolactin response to d-fenfluramine in depressed patients who had made suicide attempts. Furthermore, there was a negative correlation between change in prolactin levels and lethality of suicide attempts [25]. Blunted prolactin response to d-fenfluramine has correlated with aggression in personality-disordered patients as well [20].

Other pharmacologic challenge studies have been done with ipsapirone (IPS), a 5HT-1A agonist. IPS has been shown to be a useful probe of serotonin function in normal subjects. IPS acts both pre- and post-synaptically, and the response to IPS has been shown to be blunted in unipolar depressed patients. Other studies, however, reveal a blunted response to IPS associated with self-reported aggression. In an IPS challenge study by Reynolds et al. [26], subjects with BPD were compared with normal controls. There was an inverse correlation between the physiologic response to IPS and impulsivity, whereas cortisol response to IPS was correlated positively with scores of depression. Again, then, we find an inverse relationship between concentration of 5HT and aggression, in particular, impulsive aggression.

Other neurotransmitters of interest are norepinephrine, dopamine, acetylcholine, gamma-aminobutyric acid (GABA), and arginine vasopressin (AVP). Based on animal studies that suggested a positive correlation between aggression and CSF vasopressin level, Coccaro et al. [27] found in humans that central AVP levels correlated positively with life history of aggression and inversely with the prolactin response to fenfluramine. It is possible that central AVP plays role in aggression independent of the serotonin system or by interacting with it [27].

Diminished activity in the GABA-minergic pathways has been proposed as playing a role in affective instability especially in patients with cluster B personality disorders [22]. GABA may have a damping effect that is triggered as a response to rapid surges of strong affect. Affective instability appears to show some response to anticonvulsants that are now used as mood stabilizers. Some anticonvulsant drugs are known to increase the GABA-minergic transmission [28].

Acetylcholine is another neurotransmitter that probably plays some role in affective instability. Limbic structures that are implicated in emotion regulation, such as the amygdala, hippocampus, and cingulate cortex, have rich cholinergic innervation [22]. Based on observations that depressive symptoms can be generated by the administration of cholinomimetics such as arecholine and physostigmine [29], similar studies have been performed with patients with personality disorders. In a study by Steinberg et al. [30], subjects with BPD responded to intravenous physostigmine infusion with a shift into depressive affect that was significantly more rapid in onset, greater in intensity, and more persistent than the response of healthy controls. The rapid shift in mood correlated with clinical measures of affective instability.

The catecholamines (dopamine and norepinephrine) have not received as much attention and interest from personality disorders researchers as has serotonin. The norepinephrine (noradrenergic) system (NE) is believed to modulate arousal and reactivity to the environment through the locus ceruleus. NE is thought to play a role in heightened reactivity to environmental stimuli and contributes to affective instability in people with BPD [20]. The behavioral correlates of dopamine fall into two main areas: schizotypy and aggression. Coccaro reports at least two studies that support a positive correlation between schizotypy and higher CSF homovanillic acid (HVA, a dopamine metabolite) concentrations [20]. Cloninger [13], in his seven-factor model, has proposed that dopamine would be the principal neuromodulator for the novelty-seeking dimension, including thrill-seeking behavior, extravagant spending, binge eating, sexual hedonism, and substance abuse. According to this model, harm avoidance is associated with GABA and serotonin (dorsal raphe), reward dependence with norepinephrine and serotonin (medial raphe), and persistence with glutamate and serotonin (dorsal raphe).

Another neurotransmitter system that has drawn interest because of its possible relationship to behavior found in personality disorders, particularly self-injurious behavior (SIB), is the opioid or endorphin system [31]. SIB is a common phenomenon in the cluster B group and especially in BPD. One model proposes that SIB is a result of a state of pain insensitivity and sensory depression that stem from a physiological (congenital) excess of B-endorphin or another endogenous opioid. Then SIB could be driven by an addiction to a relative excess of opioid activity. The individual goes through adaptive changes and becomes tolerant to high levels of circulating opioid transmitters, and experiences shortages if endogenous opioid levels fall, which in turn reinforces the SIB behavior. According to the model proposed by Sandman et al. [32] congenital conditions could result in a permanent upregulation of opiate receptors. A permanent upregulation of opiate receptors may have diverse effects with an elevation in pain threshold as one of the consequences. Based on this model, opiate blockers (e.g., naloxone and naltrexone) may attenuate SIB by making these behaviors more painful (aversive conditioning).

Opiate peptides also affect the catecholamine systems. Although opiates exert an inhibitory effect on catecholamine systems, they potentiate dopaminergic neuron-firing rates in the hippocampus. Stein and Belluzi [33] suggest that increased dopaminergic firing may be responsible for reinforcement of the behavior that would be consistent with the "addiction" model. Another model proposes that a birth defect results in permanent attenuation of b-endorphin release that may ultimately result in a need to perform behaviors that stimulate endogenous opioid release.

Though not a neurotransmitter, cholesterol along with its level in the blood and its relationship to aggression has also been studied. There is a possible interconnection among serum cholesterol levels, central serotonergic activity and impulsive-aggressive behavior. In a study by Novotny et al. [34], a trend toward an inverse correlation between serum cholesterol levels and prolactin response to fenfluramine was found. Another study also supports the association between low plasma cholesterol, low blood serotonin concentrations, and a history of violent suicide attempts in psychiatric inpatients [35]. In one study, patients with BPD were found to have significantly lower serum cholesterol levels than patients with other personality disorders [36].

While the above summarizes studies done with some neurotransmitters that are currently thought to play a role in some of the dimensions of psychopathology discussed above, it is important to keep in mind that more than 70 neurotransmitters have been identified to date [37]. The role of most of these endogenous substrates in brain neurochemistry and function remains a mystery to be disentangled in future studies.

III. FAMILY-GENETIC STUDIES IN PD

Psychiatric genetics involves a variety of research strategies, from family studies focusing on the increased frequency of certain disorders among family members on one end of the spectrum to studies on a molecular level on the other end of the spectrum. These latter studies are designed to look at certain gene loci and polymorphism at these loci and the relationship between the polymorphism and certain behaviors or phenotypic expressions or endophenotypes. Endophenotypes are phenotypic traits that are believed to be "closer" to the genes, and it is these endophenotypes that affect susceptibility to disease. For example, genes causing high cholesterol levels predispose the individual to myocardial infarction. Hence high cholesterol level can be considered an endophenotype enabling a closer link between the gene (high cholesterol) and the phenotypic trait (myocardial infarction).

Advances in neuroscience combined with a better understanding of changes that occur on a molecular level allow us to speculate about gene-environment interaction and to appreciate the reciprocity that occurs between genes and environment since there are data to suggest that environment affects genes and alters the expression of genes [2,4,38,39]. This interaction hypothesis of mutual effects of genes and environment on each other should lead one to be cautious in interpreting studies of genes on a molecular level, because a particular gene may not necessarily reflect the inheritability of a specific trait since environmental factors have the potential to impinge on genes or gene expression.

Studies of genes pose other problems. Genes function at a molecular level, and there are several levels in the hierarchy of the functioning of the behavior of the organism. Thus, traits and behavior are complex constructs, and most likely what we see and measure in terms of behavior both clinically and in the laboratory may be far too distant from genes in this hierarchy [2] to draw immediate conclusions or to conclude direct relationships. Keeping these possible drawbacks in mind, we will examine the major findings in this area beginning with the family studies.

Family studies in personality disorders can be categorized as studies done in probands with personality disorders, where personality disorders can be viewed as variants of axis I disorders or personality disorders are an extreme variant of a personality trait [40]. Family-genetic studies in probands with personality disorders are very limited. Antisocial personality disorder (ASPD) is the most-studied personality disorder in this group. Adoption studies suggest that criminal behavior in biological parents is associated with criminality and ASPD in adopted-away children. ASPD has also been proposed as a variant of substance abuse disorder based on adoption and family studies showing excess risk for ASPD among biological relatives of probands with substance abuse [41]. Studies that look at the coaggregation of certain personality disorders and axis I disorders in certain families (particularly cluster A disorders and schizophrenia) support only SPD and ASPD as sharing familial and genetic risk factors with specific axis I disorders (schizophrenia and substance-related disorders, respectively) [40]. This does not mean that other axis II disorders do not share "risk" factors with other axis I disorders; it means that at the moment we only have evidence related to SPD and ASPD.

Family studies in the area of cluster A personality disorders focus on a possible genetic link between schizophrenia and SPD. In the famous Copenhagen adoption studies, Kety et al. [42,43] looked at mental illnesses in the biological and adoptive families of adoptees with schizophrenia. Adopted-away children of subjects with schizophrenia had a higher incidence of SPD. Kendler and Gruenberg [44] reported a similar finding in another Danish adoption study involving schizophrenia. Future studies in this area are necessary to shed light on which features (formal thought disorder, affective flattening, idiosyncrasies in social interactions, etc.) of these disorders are genetically more transmissible or heritable than others.

It is too early to say to what extent genes play a role in BPD, but because personality traits generally show a substantial genetic influence, there should certainly be aspects or symptoms of BPD for which this holds true. BPD reflects the interactional complexity between environmental conditions and genetic predisposition [45]. Only one study of BPD inheritance using twin methodology has been published. In a Norwegian sample of seven MZ and 18 DZ twin pairs, BPD was found to have zero concordance in MZ and 11% concordance in DZ twins. Although this study might seem to suggest that environmental factors are of greater importance than genetic factors, the sample size is too small to make real conclusions. Additional studies both large and small are needed to reach firmer conclusions about the relationship of genetic features and functions on the symptoms of BPD [46].

What is transmitted between generations in borderline patients has been a question that has interested researchers for more than a decade. Some studies have suggested that it is the affective component (affective lability, propensity to major affective episodes) that is transmitted; other studies suggest it is impulsive aggression that is transmitted, and still other suggest the borderline "syndrome" itself [38,47–49]. Studies of twins reared apart using the five-factor model showed that neuroticism, to a lesser extent conscientiousness, and to a moderate degree agreeableness, are influenced by genes [50].

On a molecular level, genes related to serotonin synthesis and metabolism have been of interest to researchers. The serotonin-related gene best studied for its relationship to impulsive aggressive behavior is the gene coding for tryptophan hydroxylase (TPH), the first enzyme involved in the synthesis of serotonin [51]. A polymorphism on chromosome 11 coding for TPH has been identified, and the two alleles have been designated L and U. In a Finnish cohort of violent offenders, the L allele was associated with reduced CSF 5HIAA concentrations and a history of suicide attempts [52]. A recent study with a nonpatient sample revealed individual differences in aggressive disposition associated with an intronic polymorphism of the TPH gene [53]. Other studies involving this polymorphism reveal that the LL genotype appears to be associated with significantly higher total scores on the Buss-Durkee hostility inventory when compared with UL or UU genotypes [51,54].

Other genetic loci have been studied that target receptors and neurotransmitters that are thought to be involved in behavior related to personality psychopathology. These loci are serotonin receptor 1B (HTR1B) genotype, serotonin receptor 2A (HTR2A) genotype, serotonin transporter (SLC6A4), and D4 dopamine receptor gene (DRD4).

Preliminary studies suggest a relationship between HTR1B genotype and suicide attempts and between HTR2A genotype and suicidality and self-mutilation. The serotonin 1B receptor gene has also been studied for its association with alcoholism and aggression. Antisocial alcohol consumption and antisocial behavior showed significant evidence of linkage to this gene's polymorphism [55]. Also, a polymorphism at the serotonin 1B locus reveals a significant relationship between the presence of the HincII(−) allele and positive measures of aggression in patients with personality disorders. Though the results are not always consistent across different studies, these preliminary studies do point to the fact that allelic variability or polymorphisms in serotonin related genes are probably associated with impulsive aggression [56]. This is logical because, as reviewed above, known clinical and laboratory work has repeatedly shown a relationship between low levels of circulating serotonin and impulsive aggression as well as blunted 5HT responses among impulsive and aggressive patients when challenged with pharmacologically active agents that should provoke substantial release of serotonin or serotonin-related compounds.

Another gene implicated in susceptibility to impulsive aggression is the gene coding for the serotonin transporter, SLC6A4. A polymorphism in the promoter region of the serotonin transporter was also found to be associated with a high degree of harm avoidance [57]. Sander et al.'s [58] study in "dissocial alcoholics" revealed an association between S allele of the 5′ regulatory SLC6A4 polymorphism that confers susceptibility to a temperamental profile of high novelty seeking and low harm avoidance [58].

Additional studies of gene polymorphisms reveal other interesting relationships between specific genes and behavior often seen in personality disorder patients. A preliminary study suggests a linear relationship between harm avoidance and the presence of the S allele for a polymorphism in the serotonin transporter. The association between novelty seeking and DRD4 polymorphisms has also been studied with some preliminary and at this point controversial findings [59]. Despite the elegance of these studies, research in this area is in its very early phase. Obviously, as more data accumulate, we will be able to define more specific relationships.

IV. NEUROIMAGING STUDIES

Neuroimaging methodologies offer the opportunity first to identify structural alterations in the brain that may be associated with certain dimensions or traits in personality disorders and, second, to assess brain activity functionally via measurements of blood flow or metabolic activity [51]. Continued technological advances enable better visualization of the brain structures and functionality in different brain areas. Computed tomography (CT) and magnetic resonance imaging (MRI) enable observation of the brain structures. Positron emission tomography (PET), single-positron emission computed tomography (SPECT), and functional magnetic resonance imaging (fMRI) enable the visualization of regional patterns of brain activation during different tasks or emotional states.

In recent years, neuroimaging studies in the area of personality disorders focused on structural differences, comparing regional brain size and activity between normal subjects and people with personality disorders and particular personality dimensions. Functional neuroimaging has allowed the study of changes in brain activity associated with specific cognitive and emotional tasks. This techonology should enable us to pursue certain positive findings (impulsivity and serotonergic system, antisocial personality disorder and prefrontal cortex dysfunction, and proposed similarities between schizophrenia and SPD). Most of the neuroimaging studies in recent years have focused on SPD. There are several studies in ASPD and BPD.

One area of focus in neuroimaging studies is impulsivity and aggression. From a neuroanatomic viewpoint, aggression and impulsivity have been thought to reside primarily in the frontal cortex. The prototype for frontal lobe activity and aggression is railroad worker Phineas Cage, who in the 1800s sustained an injury to his frontal cortex and subsequently underwent personality changes with increased aggressiveness and impulsivity [60]. PET studies in murderers revealed decreased use of glucose in prefrontal cortical areas, but the decrease in glucose use was found among impulsive murderers and not among murderers who planned the crime [61]. Goyer et al. [62] found decreased rates of glucose metabolism in BPD patients when compared with controls. In a fenfluramine mediated PET study, subjects with BPD had diminished response to serotonergic stimulation in areas of prefrontal cortex [63]. In an MRI study in subjects with BPD, Lyoo et al. [64] showed decreased frontal lobe volume. Raine et al. [65] studied gray and white matter volumes in the prefrontal cortex in subjects with antisocial personality disorder (ASPD). The ASPD group showed an 11% reduction in prefrontal gray matter volume in the absence of ostensible brain lesions, and also reduced autonomic activity during stress. The researchers conclude that this prefrontal deficit may underlie the low arousal, poor fear conditioning, lack of conscience, and decision-making deficits. Thus, overall, studies support the relationship between decreased metabolic activity and decreased volume and increased impulsivity and aggression.

Biologic research in the area of SPD appears to be targeting two purposes. A better understanding of the differences and similarities between the SPD and schizophrenia holds the hope of disentangling the multiple pathophysiologic pathways to schizophrenia. Considering both SPD and schizophrenia as two phenotypic expressions (i.e., clinical expressions) of the same core pathology has led to studies to try to answer the fundamental question of what causes the difference in the expression. The second purpose of research in this area would be to understand better the core features in SPD, namely cognitive impairment and social deficits and/or eccentricity, as a dimension of personality.

SPD patients, like schizophrenic patients, demonstrate volume reductions in temporal cortex and thalamus that are associated with severity of social deficits and cognitive impairment [66]. A recent study supports larger brain CSF volumes in subjects with SPD [67]. Overall, findings from the neuroimaging studies in SPD are consistent with decreased volume in frontal and temporal regions (especially superior temporal lobe reduction), decreased posterior corpus callosum size, and some evidence for the involvement of thalamus and putamen. In most of the studies, individuals with SPD fall in the gray area between patients with schizophrenia and normal controls. This finding lends support to the long-standing hypothesis that SPD is a "mild" or "subclinical" expression of the pathology underlying schizophrenia.

Pharmacological and/or cognitive activation techniques during functional brain imaging will most likely lead to more sophisticated studies in the future. This should eventually provide more interesting results about brain activity and functions of certain areas in the brain [68].

V. LIFE EVENTS AND BIOLOGY

The nature-nurture debate into the etiology of psychiatric disorders has been a long-standing one with little resolution. Based on early observations that childhood abuse and early emotional trauma were present in the histories of individuals who were diagnosed with personality disorders (especially cluster B disorders), studies have been conducted to shed light on the role of life events, upbringing, and early trauma in the etiology of personality disorders. These studies supported a higher incidence of early-childhood trauma. Childhood sexual abuse and neglect in childhood have been found to be significantly higher in patients with BPD [69–71]. These findings have led to hypotheses such as BPD being a form of PTSD, specifically a chronic PTSD [72].

It appears that patients with BPD may experience a range of different types of abuse that could all be categorized under the umbrella of childhood trauma. Figueroa and Silk [73] reviewed the biological underpinnings of BPD while attempting to integrate the biology of stress and trauma. According to McEwen [74] there is a point at which stress is reversible, but prolonged exposure to stress can produce permanent changes in the biochemistry of the brain. It becomes clear that significant traumatic experiences can be an influencing factor in our biological makeup.

According to van der Kolk [75], Nigg et al. [76], and Sabo [77], childhood abuse and neglect are significant trauma for a developing child, particularly if they are ongoing. Caregivers who are supposed to protect become dangerous and threatening, and this then affects attachment to others and other aspects of object relations [75,76]. Sabo adds: "Early childhood experience, including separation/neglect and trauma, may contribute to alterations in neurotransmission for BPD patients. Thus the constitutional vulnerability in BPD patients could derive from genetic or environmental experiences early in development" [77, p 62].

The biological changes in these patients cause a broad array of problems. The effects of prolonged stress produce changes in the neurochemistry of the brain; the effects of an overwhelming and inescapable trauma probably affect the brain in many of the same ways:

> Autonomic activation is necessary to cope with the major stress, so a diminished capacity to activate appropriated autonomic stress reactions causes impaired physiological adaptation to stress. In many traumatized people this adaptive mechanism has been disturbed by the trauma; they continue to respond even to minor stimuli with an intensity appropriate to emergency situations [78, p 66].

Trauma and stress, then, certainly can lead to difficulties in attachment. Studies done based on attachment theory seem to open new avenues in understanding the underlying biological vulnerabilities in individuals and the closely interwoven dance between the environment and the evolving or shaping brain in its early developmental stages. Fonagy et al. [79] emphasize the importance of reflective function in the infant and the mother, defined as the capacity to reflect on one's own mental state. They describe the person with BPD as someone who has likely been a victim of childhood trauma, who has low reflective functioning, and who has a preoccupied attachment style. In that study, parents who rated high in reflective function were about four times more likely to have children with secure attachment than parents who rated low in reflective function. Yet despite having parents who had high ratings in the reflective functioning scale, some children had insecure attachment, indicating that they were innately more vulnerable to psychopathology [18,79]. It thus appears that it is impossible to ignore the complex two-way interaction between life events/environment and the individual's genetic makeup or constitutional predispositions. The role of the attachment process and the initial phases of infant-mother interaction in shaping and/or affecting permanently the limbic system and higher cortical areas (prefrontal and fontal cortex) is a fertile area that awaits further studies.

VI. FREUD'S PROJECT: BIOLOGY AND ITS CLINICAL IMPLICATIONS

To return to where we began, we look to Freud's "Project," which predicted a biological or neurological underpinning to all mental processes. Yet through most of this century, the followers of Freud turned away from consideration of biological mechanisms and paid most attention to the psychotherapeutic process, particularly the psychoanalytic process. Yet today we are beginning to appreciate that psychotherapy and the changes that occur in psychotherapy appear to have biological ramifications as well [80,81], and that the symptom picture attributed to object relations deformities in personality disordered patients is a combination of biological predispositions and parental rearing or reaction to these dispositions [18,82,83]. Therapies can focus on the biological issues within the context of psychodynamic understanding, a process which is evident in the work of Kernberg et al.'s [18] Transference Focused Therapy and its spotlight on attachment and the biology of attachment and aggression and its impact on the early developmental stages. This can also be seen in the psychodynamic work of Fonagy as well [79,84]. A better understanding of underlying biological mechanisms can help the clinician, the patient, and the family to consider the vulnerabilities without being critical or judgmental. Thus, as more data accumulates from "biological" laboratories as well as from consulting rooms, we should be able to refine our links from the biology behind personality traits to the clinical picture and behavioral symptoms. This increased knowledge should help us better organize our clinical approach in working with patients who suffer from personality disorders.

This idea of considering biology in psychotherapeutic work can be found in Linehan's Dialectical Behavior Therapy (DBT) [85]. DBT has gained significant popular support over the past decade, particularly in the treatment of BPD, and it is one of the few forms of psychotherapeutic intervention that has been empirically studied, though recently Bateman and Fonagy [84] have begun to systematically study their intervention. DBT integrates proposed underlying biological vulnerabilities—namely, affective instability, impulsivity, and stress intolerance—in BPD with behavioral strategies designed to help the patient modify disordered behavior resulting from these vulnerabilities. One of the significant advantages of DBT theory is that it incorporates both aspects of constitution (predisposition) and environment in defining the etiology of BPD [77,82]. It also correlates symptoms with the growing knowledge of the biology of the personality disorders. The five key areas of dysfunction that Linehan identifies are emotion, interpersonal, self-, behavior, and cognitive dysregulation. Table 1 presents the key areas of each dysfunction with the possible corresponding underlying biological dysfunction. This model allows the clinician to define a patient's symptoms, then, in terms of both its biological basis and the behavioral components or clinical symptoms that these deficits produce.

Referring to a patient's symptoms as evolving from a biological basis helps a patient to consider her illness in terms of deficits that can be compensated for by learning new skills and behavioral adaptations. It also helps a clinician in using pharmacological interventions. This process can be compared to the situation in a patient with diabetes who must learn new behaviors around types and timing of food intake as well as use (at times) of medication to compensate for the lack of insulin production. The skills training manual for DBT presents skills that address these deficits or dysfunctions and helps patients to view their illness from a more empowering stance, as opposed to the role of victim [86].

The most immediate result of these biological studies would be a more rational and biologically informed approach to the psychopharmacological treatment of patients with personality disorders as well as better biological information to pursue the development of new medications. While most of our current pharmacological treatment of the personality disorders remains essentially empirical, there have recently been developed for BPD a series of pharma-

Table 1 DBT Identified Areas of Dysregulation and Possible Underlying Biology

Dialectical behavior therapy	Proposed biological dysregulation
Emotion dysregulation	
Affective instability	Serotonin leading to impulsivity
Anger	Acetylinecholine leading to rapid-onset affective states
	GABA leading to lack of inhibitory actions
Interpersonal dysregulation	Dopamine and norepinephrine leading to increased reactivity to environment including to people
Self-dysregulation	Genetic factors
	Emotional dysregulation leading to a lack of consistent self
Behavior dysregulation	Genetic as in high novelty seeking or low harm avoidance
Parasuicidal behavior	Serotonin; opioids and endorphin system
Impulsive behavior	
Cognitive dysregulation	Dopamine
Irrational thoughts	
Paranoid ideation	

cologic algorithms that may ultimately be able to provide us with a better and more organized approach to our current empirical one [87].

Hopefully, then, the study of the biology of the personality and its disorders allows the clinician to construct an understanding of the sufferings and difficulties of the patient with more empathy and less stigma, both of which are needed in the treatment of these difficult conditions. This would allow a true synthesis to occur in the treatment of these patients, a synthesis of psychodynamically informed sociotherapies [45,82] with behavioral therapies and techniques that improve daily coping and functioning accompanied by medication to reduce immediate biological risk. A full, thoughtful synthetic approach can be achieved when psychoeducational elements, designed to inform patient and family, are added to the above strategies and interventions [45,88].

REFERENCES

1. S Freud. Project for a scientific psychology (1950[1895]). In: J Strachey, ed. The Standard Edition of the Complete Psychological Works of Sigmund Freud, Vol. 1. London: Hogarth Press, 1966, pp 281–397.
2. J Paris. The classification of personality disorders should be rooted in biology. J Personality Disord 14(2):127–136, 2000.
3. KR Silk. Foreword. In: KR Silk, ed. Biology of Personality Disorders. Washington: American Psychiatric Press, 1998, pp xiii–xx.
4. KR Silk. Overview of biological factors. Psychiatr Clin North Am 23(1): 61–75, 2000.
5. JF Clarkin, MF Lenzenweger, eds. Major Theories of Personality Disorders. New York: Guilford Press, 1996.
6. JG Gunderson, WS Pollack. Conceptual risks of Axis I-II division. In: H Klar, LJ Siever, eds. Biological Response Styles: Clinical Implications. Washington: American Psychiatric Press, 1985, pp 81–95.
7. KR Silk. From first- to second-generation studies of borderline personality disorder. In: KR Silk, ed. Biological and Neurobehavioral Studies of Borderline Personality Disorder. Washington: American Psychiatric Press, 1994, pp xvii–xxix.
8. HS Akiskal, BI Yerevanian, GC Davis. The nosologic status of borderline personality: clinical and polysomnographic study. Am J Psychiatry 142:192–198, 1985.
9. HW Lahmeyer, E Val, M Gaviria, RB Prasad, GN Pandey, P Rodgers, MA Weiler, EG Altman. EEG sleep, lithium transport, dexamethasone suppression and monoamine oxidase activity in borderline personality disorder. Psychiatry Res 25:19–30, 1988.
10. CF Reynolds, PH Soloff, DJ Kupfer, LC Taska, K Restifo, PA Coble, ME McNamara. Depression in borderline patients: a prospective EEG sleep study. Psychiatry Res 14:1–15, 1985.
11. PH Soloff, A George, R Nathan. Dexamethasone suppression test in patients with borderline personality disorder. Am J Psychiatry 139:1621–1622, 1982.
12. HA Sternbach, J Fleming, I Extein, AL Pottash, MS Gold. The dexamethasone suppression and thyrotropin-releasing hormone tests in depressed borderline patients. Psychoneuroendocrinology 8:459–462, 1983.
13. CR Cloninger. The genetics and psychobiology of the seven-factor model of personality. In: KR Silk, ed. Biology of Personality Disorders. Washington: American Psychiatric Press, 1998, pp 63–92.
14. LJ Siever, KL Davis. A psychobiological perspective on the personality disorders. Am J Psychiatry 148:12, 1991.
15. RR McCrae, PT Costa Jr. Validation of the five-factor model of personality across instruments and observers. J Pers Soc Psychol 52(1):81–90, 1987.
16. JW Livesley, KL Jang. Toward an empirically based classification of personality disorder. J Pers Disord 14(2):137–151, 2000.
17. CR Cloninger, DM Svrakic, TR Pryzbeck. A psychobiological model of temperament and character. Arch Gen Psychiatr 50:975–990, 1993.
18. HW Koenigsberg, OF Kernberg, MH Stone, AH Appelbaum, FE Yeomans, D Diamond. Borderline Patients: Extending the Limits of Treatability. New York: Basic Books, 2000.
19. PT Costa Jr, TA Widiger, eds. Personality Disorders and the Five-Factor Model of Personality. 1st ed. Washington: American Psychological Association, 1994.
20. EF Coccaro. Neurotransmitter function in personality disorders, In: KR Silk, ed. Biology of Personality Disorders. Washington: American Psychiatric Press, 1998, pp 1–25.
21. M Asberg, L Traksman, P Thoren. 5HIAA in the cerebrospinal fluid: a biochemical suicide predictor? Arch Gen Psychiatry 33:1193–1197, 1976.
22. IG Gurvits, HW Koenigsberg, LJ Siever. Neurotransmitter dysfunction in patients with borderline personality disorder. Psychiatr Clin North Am 23(1):27–40, 2000.
23. M Linnoila, M Virkkunen, M Scheinin, A Nuutila, R Rimon, FK Goodwin. Low cerebrospinal fluid 5-hydroxyindolacetic acid concentration differentiates impulsive from non-impulsive behavior. Life Sci 33:2609–2614, 1983.
24. L Lindberg, M Asberg, M Sunquist-Stensman. 5HIAA levels in attempted suicides who have killed their children. Lancet 2:928, 1984
25. H Correa, F Duval, MC Mokrani, MA Crocq, P Bailey, TS Diep, JP Macher. Prolactin response to d-

25. fenfluramine and suicidal behavior in depression. Biol Psychiatry 45(8S):62S, 1999.
26. D Reynolds, V Mitropoulou, AS New, LJ Siever. Ipsapirone (IPS) as a serotonergic probe in personality disorder patients. Biol Psychiatry 47(8S):144S, 2000.
27. EF Coccaro, RJ Kavoussi, RL Hauger, TB Cooper, CF Ferris. Cerebrospinal fluid vasopressin levels correlate with aggression and serotonin function in personality disordered subjects. Arch Gen Psychiatry 55:708-714, 1998.
28. RL Macdonald, LJ Greenfield Jr. Mechanisms of action of new antiepileptic drugs. Curr Opin Neurol 10(2):121–128, 1997.
29. DS Janowsky, MK El-Yousef, JM Davis. Acetylcholine and depression. Psychosom Med 36:248–257,1974.
30. BJ Steinberg, R Trestman, V Mitropoulou, M Serby, J Silverman, E Coccaro, S Weston, M de Vegvar, LJ Siever. Depressive response to physostigmine challenge in borderline personality disorder patients. Neuropsychopharmacology 17:264–273,1997.
31. RM Winchel, M Stanley. Self-injurious behavior and the biology of self-mutilation. Am J Psychiatry 148:306–317, 1991.
32. CA Sandman, AJ Kastin. Neuropeptide modulation of development and behavior. In: S Deutch, A Weisman, R Weisman. eds. Application of Basic Neuroscience to Child Psychiatry. New York: Plenum, 1990, pp 101–124.
33. L Stein, JD Belluzi. Cellular investigations of behavioral reinforcement. Neurosci Biobehav Rev 13: 69–80, 1989.
34. S Novotny, A New, E Sevin, A Callahan, LJ Siever. Serum cholesterol and impulsive aggressive behavior in personality disorder patients. Biol Psychiatry 43(8S):51S, 1998.
35. ML Rao, A Papassotiropoulos, B Hawellek, C Frahnert. Suicidal psychiatric inpatients have low plasma cholesterol and low blood serotonin. Biol Psychiatry 43(8S):105S, 1998.
36. AS New, EM Sevin, V Mitropoulou, D Reynolds, SI Novotny, A Callahan, RL Trestman, LJ Siever. Serum cholesterol and impulsivity in personality disorders. Psychiatry Res 85:145–50, 1999.
37. SH Preskorn, The human genome project and drug discovery in psychiatry. J Psychiatr Pract 7:133–137, 2001.
38. JM Silverman, L Pinkham, T Horvath, EF Coccaro, H Klar, S Schear, S Apter, M Davidson, RC Mohs, LJ Siever. Affective and impulsive personality disorder traits in the relatives of patients with borderline personality disorder. Am J Psychiatry 148:1378–1385, 1991.
39. D Reiss, R Plomin, EM Hetherington. Genetics and psychiatry: an unheralded window on the environment. Am J Psychiatry 148:283–291,1991.
40. W Maier, P Franke, B Hawellek. Special feature: family-genetic research strategies for personality disorders. J Pers Disord 12(3):262–276,1998.
41. RJ Cadoret, M Stewart. An adoption study of attention deficit/hyperactivity/aggression and their relationship to adult antisocial behavior. Compr Psychiatry 32:73–82, 1991.
42. SS Kety, D Rosenthal, PH Wender, F Schulsinger. The types and prevalence of mental illness in the biological families of adopted schizophrenics. J Clin Res 6:345–362, 1968.
43. SS Kety, PH Wender, B Jacobsen, LJ Ingraham, L Jansson, B Faber, DK Kinney. Mental illness in the biological and adoptive relatives of schizophrenic adoptees: replication of the Copenhagen study in the rest of Denmark. Arch Gen Psychiatry 51:442–455, 1994.
44. KS Kendler, AM Gruenberg. An independent analysis of the Danish adoption study of schizophrenia. Arch Gen Psychiatry 41:555–564, 1984.
45. JG Gunderson. Borderline Personality Disorder: A Clinical Guide. Washington: American Psychiatric Publishing, 2001.
46. S Torgersen. Genetics of patients with BPD. Psychiatr Clin North Am 23(1):1–9, 2000.
47. AW Loranger, JH Oldham, EH Tulis EH. Familial transmission of DSM-III borderline personality disorder. Arch Gen Psychiatr 39:795–799, 1982.
48. EF Coccaro, S Bergeman, GE McClearn. Heritability of irritable impulsiveness: a study of twins reared together and apart. Psychiatry Res 48:229–242, 1993.
49. EF Coccaro, J Silverman, HM Klar, TB Horvath, LJ Siever. Familial correlates of reduced central serotonergic function in patients with personality disorders. Arch Gen Psychiatry 51:318–324, 1994.
50. S Torgersen. The genetic transmission of borderline personality features displays multidimensionality. Presented at the 31st Annual Meeting of the American College of Neuropharmacology, San Juan, Puerto Rico, 1992.
51. LJ Siever, AS New, R Kirrane, S Novotny, H Koenigsberg, R Grossman. New biological research strategies for personality disorders. In: KR Silk, ed. Biology of Personality Disorders. Washington: American Psychiatric Press, 1998, pp 27–61.
52. DA Nielsen, D Goldman, M Virkkunen, R Tokola, R Rawlings, M Linnoila. Suicidality and 5HIAA concentration associated with a tryptophan hydroxylase polymorphism. Arch Gen Psychiatry 51:34–38, 1994.
53. SB Manuck, JD Flory, RE Ferrell, KM Dent, JJ Mann, MF Muldoon. Aggression and anger-related traits associated with a polymorphism of the tryptophan hydroxylase gene. Biol Psychiatry 45:603–614, 1999.
54. AS New, J Gelernter, V Mitropoulo, LJ Siever. Serotonin related genotype and impulsive aggression. Biol Psychiatry 45(8S):120S, 1999.

55. J Lappalainen, JC Long, M Eggert, RW Robin, GL Brown, H Naukkarinen, M Virkkunen, M Linnoila, D Goldman. Linkage of antisocial alcoholism to the serotonin 5HT1B receptor gene in 2 populations. Arch Gen Psychiatry 55:989–994, 1998.
56. AS New, M Goodman, V Mitropoulou, HW Koenigsberg, LJ Siever. Serotonin related genes and impulsive aggression in personality disorders. Biol Psychiatry 47(8S):118S, 2000.
57. K Lesch, D Bengel, A Heils, SZ Sabol, BD Greenberg, S Petri, J Benjamin, CR Muller, DH Hamer, DL Murphy. Association of anxiety related traits with a polymorphism in the serotonin transporter gene regulatory region. Science 274:1527–1531,1996.
58. T Sander, H Harms, P Dufeu, S Kuhn, M Hoehe, KP Lesch, H Rommelspacher, LG Schmidt. Serotonin transporter gene variants in alcohol-dependent subjects with dissocial personality disorder. Biol Psychiatry 43:908–912, 1998.
59. J Gelernter, H Kranzler, E Coccaro, L Siever, A New, CL Mulgrew. D4 dopamine receptor (DRD4) alleles and novelty seeking in substance-dependent, personality disorder, and control subjects. Am J Hum Genet 61:1144–1152, 1997.
60. H Damasio, T Grabowski, R Frank, MA Galaburda, AR Damasio. The return of Phineas Gage: clues about the brain from the skull of a famous patient. Science 264:1102–1105, 1994.
61. Raine A, Meloy JR, Bihrle S, Stoddard J, LaCasse, Buchsbaum MS. Reduced prefrontal and increased subcortical brain functioning assessed using positron emission tomography in predatory and affective murderers. Behav Sci Law 16:319–332, 1998.
62. PF Goyer, PJ Andreason, WE Semple, AH Clayton, AC King, BA Compton-Toth, SC Schulz, RM Cohen. Positron-emission tomography and personality disorders. Neuropsychopharmology 10:21–28,1994.
63. PH Soloff, CC Meltzer, PJ Gree, D Constantine, T Kelly. A fenfluramine mediated PET study of borderline personality disorder. Biol Psychiatry 45(8S):113S, 1999.
64. IK Lyoo, MH Han, DY Cho. A brain MRI study in subjects with borderline personality disorder. J Affect Disord 50:235–43, 1998.
65. A Raine, T Lencz, S Bihrle, L LaCasse, P Colletti. Reduced prefrontal gray matter volume and reduced autonomic activity in antisocial personality disorder. Arch Gen Psychiatry 57:119–127, 2000.
66. LJ Siever. Psychosis and spectrum endophenotypes in schizotypal personality disorder. Biol Psychiatry 45(8S):7S, 1999.
67. CC Dickey, ME Shenton, Y Hirayasu, I Fischer, MM Voglmaier, MA Niznikiewicz, LJ Seidman, S Fraone, RW McCarley. Large CSF volume not attributable to ventricular volume in schizotypal personality disorder. Am J Psychiatry 157:48–54, 2000.
68. PF Goyer, PE Konicki, SC Schulz. Brain imaging in personality disorders. In: KR Silk, ed. Biological and Neurobehavioral Studies of Borderline Personality Disorder. Washington: American Psychiatric Press, 1994, pp 109–127.
69. JL Herman, JC Perry, BA van der Kolk. Childhood trauma in borderline personality disorder. Am J Psychiatry 146:490–495, 1989.
70. MC Zanarini, AA Williams, RE Lewis, RD Reich, SC Vera, MF Marino, A Levin, L Yong, FR Frankenburg. Reported pathological childhood experiences associated with the development of borderline personality disorder. Am J Psychiatry 145:1101–1106, 1997.
71. MC Zanarini. Childhood experiences associated with the development of borderline personality disorder. Psychiatr Clin North Am 23(1):89–101, 2000.
72. JL Herman, BA van der Kolk. Traumatic antecedents of borderline personality disorder. In: BA van der Kolk, ed. Psychological Trauma. Washington: American Psychiatric Press, 1987, pp 111–126.
73. E Figueroa, KR Silk. Biological implications of childhood sexual abuse in borderline personality disorder. J Pers Disord 11:71–92, 1997.
74. BS McEwen, E Stellar. Stress and the individual mechanisms leading to disease. Arch Intern Med 153:2093–2101, 1993.
75. BA van der kolk. The separation cry and the trauma response: developmental issues in the psychobiology of attachment and separation. In: BA van der Kolk, ed. Psychological Trauma. Washington: American Psychiatric Press, 1987, pp 31–62.
76. JT Nigg, NE Lohr, D Westen, LJ Gold, KR Silk. Malevolent object representations in borderline personality disorder and major depression. J Abnorm Psychol 101:61–67,1992.
77. A Sabo. Etiological significance of associations between childhood trauma and adult psychopathology. J Pers Disord 11:50–70, 1997.
78. BA van der Kolk, MS Greenberg. The psychobiology of the trauma response: hyperarousal, constriction, and addiction to traumatic reexposure. In: BA van der Kolk, ed. Psychological Trauma. Washington: American Psychiatric Press, 1987, pp 63–87.
79. P Fonagy, M Target, G Gergely. Attachment and borderline personality disorder. Psychiatr Clin North Am 23(1):103–122, 2000.
80. PS Wong, E Bernat, S Bunce, H Shevrin. Brain indices of nonconscious associative learning. Conscious Cogn 6:519–544, 1997.
81. JM Schwartz, PW Stoessel, LR Baxter Jr, KM Martin, ME Phelps. Systematic changes in cerebral glucose metabolic rate after successful behavior modification treatment of obsessive-compulsive disorder. Arch Gen Psychiatry 53:109–113, 1996.
82. J Paris. Significance of biological research for a biopsychosocial model of the personality disorders. In:

KR Silk, ed. Biology of Personality Disorders. Washington: American Psychiatric Press, 1998, pp 129–150.
83. M Rutter. Temperament, personality, and personality development. Br J Psychiatry 150:443–448, 1987.
84. A Bateman, P Fonagy. Treatment of borderline personality disorder with psychoanalytically oriented partial hospitalization: an 18-month follow-up. Am J Psychiatry 158:36–42, 2001.
85. MM Linehan. Cognitive-Behavioral Treatment of Borderline Personality Disorder. New York Guilford: 1993.
86. MM Linehan. Skill Training Manual for Treating Borderline Personality Disorder. New York: Guilford, 1993.
87. PH Soloff. Psychopharmacology of borderline personality disorder. Psychiatr Clin North Am 23(1):169–192, 2000.
88. WJ Livesley. A practical approach to the treatment of patients with borderline personality disorder. Psychiatr Clin North Am 23(1):211–232, 2000.

44

Iatrogenic Sexual Dysfunction

MARLENE P. FREEMAN and ALAN J. GELENBERG
University of Arizona College of Medicine, Tucson, Arizona, U.S.A.

I. INTRODUCTION

Sexual dysfunction, usually defined by subjective dissatisfaction, is common in the general population and even more in psychiatric patients. Sexual dysfunction may involve any aspect of normal sexual function, including desire, arousal, and orgasm. Causes of sexual dysfunction include psychiatric disorders, nonpsychiatric causes (including medical conditions), and medications [1]. With many psychotropic medications, men and women often experience sexual side effects. Arousal may be affected, with women having decreased vaginal lubrication, and men erectile dysfunction. Orgasmic problems, including inhibition or delay, occur in both males and females, with men experiencing ejaculatory dysfunction. Menses and fertility also can be disturbed.

Since the etiology of sexual dysfunction may be complicated, clinicians need to assess baseline sexual function, as well as incorporating a sexual and reproductive history into routine psychiatric evaluation. Many patients are hesitant to discuss sex, or may not realize its relevance. So it is imperative that psychiatrists regularly inquire nonjudgmentally about sexual symptoms and side effects.

Many psychotropic medications impact sexual function. However, the study of iatrogenic sexual dysfunction has been historically limited, as formal screening for sexual function has not typically been incorporated into psychiatric research methodology. Analyses from clinical trials reveals that the incidence of sexual side effects is higher in studies which included systematic inquiries about sexual dysfunction, rather than those that rely on spontaneous patient reports [2]. Sexual side effects often interfere with quality of life, and, if unaddressed, may affect compliance.

In this chapter, sexual dysfunction associated with different classes of psychotropic medications will be addressed and mechanisms for sexual side effects discussed. Finally, we present treatment options for iatrogenic sexual dysfunction.

II. ANTIDEPRESSANTS AND SEXUAL DYSFUNCTION

Dissatisfaction with sex is a frequent complaint. The most common symptoms in community surveys are low libido (34%) and orgasmic dysfunction (24%) in women, and premature ejaculation (29%), inhibition of orgasm (10%), and erectile dysfunction (10%) in men [3]. Mathew and Weinman [4] reported higher rates of sexual dysfunction in depressed men: decreased libido (31%), erectile dysfunction (35%), and delayed ejaculation (47%) versus nondepressed controls (6%, 0%, 6% respectively). Sexual dysfunction due to major depression might be more common than the sexual side effects caused by medication. In one study, more than half of both female and male patients said that depression had negatively affected their sexual function, whereas only 14% of females and 26% of males had sexual side effects with clomipramine [5].

Sexual dysfunction from antidepressants is well documented. Tricyclic antidepressants (TCAs) and monoamine oxidase inhibitors (MAOIs) cause sexual side effects. Harrison et al. [6] conducted a double-blind study of the effects of imipramine, phenelzine, and placebo on sexual function in depressed outpatients, assessed before and 6 weeks after treatment. Both drugs were associated with a significantly greater incidence of sexual side effects than placebo. Dysfunction of orgasm and ejaculation occurred more often than erectile dysfunction, and men had more sexual side effects than women. The degree of a TCAs' effect on serotonergic neurotransmission may determine its impact on sexual dysfunction. Tricyclics with greater impact on serotonin reuptake blockade, such as clomipramine and imipramine, seem to cause more sexual dysfunction. Some patients who have had anorgasmia with imipramine improved when switched to desipramine [7,8]. In another study, clomipramine caused sexual side effects in as many as 14% of females and 26% of males [9].

Moclobemide, a reversible monoamine oxidase A inhibitor (RIMA) not approved for use in the United States, may be associated with fewer sexual side effects. No difference was found in response to a sexual function questionnaire between subjects who received either moclobemide, 300 mg/day, or placebo (N = 60) in a 3-week trial [10]. Sexual side effects with moclobemide may differ between men and women. Kennedy et al. [11] found that while women reported significantly more sexual dysfunction with selective serotonin reuptake inhibitors (SSRIs) than with moclobemide, rates of sexual dysfunction between the drugs did not differ in men.

The underlying psychiatric disorder may affect these side effects. In a naturalistic study of patients with panic disorder, rates of sexual impairment with tricyclics and SSRIs were 56.6% and 45%, respectively, higher than most reports of antidepressant-induced sexual side effects [12]. As over half of the patients also met criteria for another mental illness, the presence of more than one diagnosis, or the diagnosis of panic disorder itself, might have contributed to high rates of sexual dysfunction.

Although trazodone has a well-known side effect of priapism, other types of sexual dysfunction may occur with its use. Ejaculatory inhibition has been reported [13], and trazodone might decrease pathological sexual behavior. Decreased exhibitionism occurred in a male patient taking trazodone [14].

Some new antidepressants may be less likely to produce sexual side effects. Segraves et al. [15] conducted a double-blind comparison of sustained-release bupropion and sertraline in depression. Subjects were in stable relationships and had normal sexual functioning. Efficacy was comparable, but patients who received bupropion experienced less sexual dysfunction: only 15% in men and 7% in women, significantly less than with sertraline. Coleman and colleages [16] found similar results with sustained-release bupropion versus sertraline. Anecdotes, however, suggest some patients may have sexual dysfunction with bupropion [17].

Mirtazapine also appears to cause a lower incidence of sexual side effects. Boyarsky et al. [18] treated male and female patients with depression with open-label mirtazapine; sexual function measured by the Arizona Sexual Experiences Scale (ASEX) improved significantly with treatment. Also, patients who have experienced sexual side effects during treatment with SSRIs may benefit from treatment with mirtazapine instead. Koutouvidis et al. [19] reported on 11 patients who had poor compliance while receiving treatment with SSRIs due to sexual dysfunction. When treated with open-label mirtazapine, all experienced improvement in depressive symptoms without sexual side effects. Also, Gelenberg and colleagues [20] treated 19 patients with mirtazapine who had experienced remission from depression and SSRI-induced sexual dysfunction. When mirtazapine was substituted for the SSRI, 11 (58%) had return of normal sexual function with mirtazapine treatment, and all maintained remission from depression. Nonetheless, a case has been reported of sexual dysfunction associated with the use of mirtazapine [21].

Nefazodone is another new antidepressant that may produce low rates of sexual dysfunction. When 681 outpatients with chronic major depressive disorder were randomized to 12 weeks of nefazodone, cognitive behavioral therapy, or the combination, sexual function in males and females improved across all groups as depression improved [22]. In another study, Ferguson et al. [23] randomly assigned 105 patients with sertraline-induced sexual dysfunction to receive either nefazodone or sertraline. After 8 weeks, sexual dysfunction reemerged only 26% in the nefazodone group, compared with 76% of those treated with sertraline.

While SSRIs have been mostly associated with decreased libido and sexual function, some patients may experience heightened sexual parameters. Paradoxical sexual excitement has been reported. Morris [24] reported a case in which a patient treated with fluoxetine had an intermittent and dose-dependent increase in sexual stimulation. Elmore and Quattlebaum [25] similarly described two cases of women treated with SSRIs who experienced undesirable sexual arousal and one who experienced had sexual desire, arousal, and hypersexuality. Also, SSRIs benefit men with premature ejaculation and paraphilias [26,27].

III. ANXIOLYTICS AND SEXUAL DYSFUNCTION

In an open-label study of buspirone in patients with generalized anxiety disorder, Othmer and Othmer [28] noted improved sexual function in eight of nine patients, all but one of whom had experienced sexual dysfunction at study entry. Patients were treated for 4 weeks after washout of other medications, with an average buspirone dose of 45 mg/day. The investigators acknowledged that improved sexual function may have resulted from the discontinuation of other medications.

Benzodiazepines, including alprazolam, chlordiazepoxide, diazepam, and clonazepam, have been reported to cause sexual dysfunction [28–35]. Concomitant benzodiazapine use was associated with greater sexual dysfunction than the use of lithium alone or with other medications in bipolar patients [36]. The risk of sexual dysfunction with benzodiazepines appears to be lower than with SSRIs.

IV. ANTIPSYCHOTICS AND SEXUAL DYSFUNCTION

As with depression, sexual dysfunction may result from the disorder of schizophrenia and may precede treatment with antipsychotic medications [37,38]. Possible mechanisms include hormonal or neurologic abnormalities or social awkwardness. Sexual side effects are common with older (typical) antipsychotic medications. Sexual side effects are estimated to occur in 30–60% of both men and women taking typical antipsychotics and may include erectile and ejaculatory dysfunction, decreased libido, orgasmic dysfunction, and menstrual disturbances [39]. In men, the most prevalent sexual side effects of antipsychotics are erectile and ejaculatory dysfunction [40]. While all typical antipsychotics may be associated with sexual dysfunction, it is most prevalent with the use of thioridazine, which causes high rates of retrograde ejaculation [41]. Sexual side effects have been reported to differing degrees with virtually all typical antipsychotics [42,43]. Priapism also has been reported and may require emergency surgical intervention [44,45].

Menstrual irregularities, including amenorrhea, are common in women receiving treatment with traditional neuroleptics, presumably related to elevated levels of prolactin. In one random sampling of outpatients with schizophrenia, more men than women reported sexual dysfunction while receiving treatment with neuroleptics (54% vs. 30%), yet 91% of women reported menstrual changes while receiving treatment with neuroleptics [46]. Hence, in women, neuroleptics may impact fertility as well as sexual function.

Aizenberg et al. [47] conducted a pilot study in which eight male patients with schizophrenia experienced ejaculatory dysfunction and decreased sexual satisfaction while taking thioridazine. The addition of low-dose imipramine, 25–50 mg qhs, resulted in resolution of sexual side effects in four patients (50%) and partial improvement in one other.

Except for risperidone, the newer antipsychotic medications have been associated with less hyperprolactinemia than the older antipsychotics and have also been associated with less sexual dysfunction [48]. Standard doses of clozapine and quetiapine do not seem to cause hyperprolactinemia, and normal menstrual function has returned in women switched from typical antipsychotics to clozapine [49,50]. Switching to clozapine also has been associated with improved libido, possibly as a result of successful treatment of negative side effects [51]. Between increased libido and fertility, the risk of pregnancy rises when a woman is switched from a traditional antipsychotic to an atypical. Lack of elevation of serum prolactin with clozapine has been demonstrated also in the pediatric population [52]. Switching patients from traditional neuroleptics to clozapine has resulted in lowering of serum prolactin levels [53]. However, in a prospective systematic study of side effects, no significant differences in sexual side effects were found between patients receiving haloperidol and patients receiving clozapine during the first 6 weeks of treatment [54]. Sexual side effects with clozapine treatment decreased with longer duration of treatment. Sexual side effects significantly decreased in men from 53% (first 6 weeks) to 22.2% (18 weeks), and in women from 23% to 0%, respectively.

Risperidone, on the other hand, seems to increase prolactin levels. Breier et al. [55] conducted a 6-week double-blind, parallel-group comparison of risperidone and clozapine in patients previously treated with fluphenazine. Patients receiving clozapine had decreases in plasma prolactin, but those who took risperidone had increases. The investigators did not report sexual side effects during the trial. Markianos et al. [56] also reported increases in prolactin levels in patients switched from treatment with a traditional antipsychotic to risperidone. Kapur et al. [57] have suggested that since prolactin elevation is related to the extent of D2 receptor occupancy, increases in prolactin with risperidone and other medications may be related to dosage. The clinical relevance of risperidone-induced prolactin increases is unclear. Guille et al. [58] reported that in patients with bipolar disorder treated with atypicals, including risperidone, retrospective chart reviews ($N = 42$) failed to elicit prolactin-related side effects. However, Kim et al. [59] described five cases which risperidone treatment was associated with elevated serum prolactin levels and amenorrhea, and Popli et al. [60] reported a case of risperidone-induced galactorhea. Kleinberg et al. [61] analyzed data from all randomized, double-blind studies of risperidone in patients with schizophrenia to assess the relationship between risperidone, serum prolactin levels, and clinical sequelae. Dose-related increases in prolactin levels were observed in both men and women. In male patients, the incidence of adverse events associated with hyperprolactinemia (including erectile dysfunction, ejaculatory dysfunction, gynecomastia, and decreased libido) was positively correlated with risperidone dose, but this was not demonstrated in female patients. While related to risperidone dose, adverse effects in men were not related to prolactin level. Also, at risperidone dose of 4–10 mg, adverse events were not experienced at significantly higher rates than seen with placebo. Risperidone-induced sexual side effects reported by Montejo et al. [62] reversed when patients were switched to treatment with olanzapine.

Olanzapine may produce less hyperprolactinemia and associated effects than risperidone. David et al. [63] found that patients switched from haloperidol to olanzapine had decreases in serum prolactin, although serum prolactin was moderately elevated by olanzapine in general. They found that prolactin was more strongly elevated by risperidone than by haloperidol or olanzapine. Wudarsky et al. [64] also reported prolactin elevation occurring in pediatric patients with olanzapine, but at rates lower than with haloperidol.

Antipsychotics may cause sexual dysfunction through a variety of mechanisms. They obviously affect central neurotransmission, but they may also act by interfering at a peripheral level—e.g., through blockade of cholinergic and alpha-adrenergic receptors [65]. Thioridazine's calcium channel antagonist activity could impact sexual function [66]. Alpha-adrenergic receptors are important in sexual function in the autonomic nerous system, with the parasympathetic system responsible for arousal and erection, and the sympathetic responsible for ejaculation and orgasm. Antipsychotics' influence on hormones, particularly by increasing prolactin levels via blockade of pituitary dopamine receptors, also may account for sexual dysfunction [67]. Sequellae of increased prolactin levels can include galactorrhea, breast tenderness, ejaculatory and orgasmic disturbances, and menstrual irregularities. Ghadirian et al. [68] found that in a random sample of outpatients with schizophrenia, sexual dysfunction was more strongly associated with high prolactin levels in men than in women.

Androgens also can be affected by antipsychotics. Haloperidol decreases serum testosterone levels in male rats [69]. A patient experienced sexual dysfunction, lowered testosterone levels, and hyperprolactinemia during risperidone treatment [70]. Hyperprolactimemia may also decrease estrogen levels in reproductive-age women [71].

V. MOOD STABILIZERS AND SEXUAL DYSFUNCTION

It is unclear whether lithium influences sexual function. In a study of sexual function in euthymic male patients ($N = 35$) with bipolar or schizoaffective disorder who were treated with lithium monotherapy, Aizenberg et al. [72] administered a questionnaire of sexual function. Most frequently reported were reduction in sexual thoughts (22.9%), diminished waking erection (17.1%), and loss of erection during coitus (20%). Thirty-one percent reported sexual dysfunction on at least two items, but overall patients reported a high degree of sexual satisfaction. Lithium levels were not related to sexual function. Additionally, cases of decreased libido and erectile dysfunction have been attributed to lithium [73]. However, Ghadirian et al. [74] studied sexual function using a self-rated scale in 104 outpatients with bipolar disorder. Concomitant benzodiazepine use was associated with sexual dysfunction. Sexual dysfunction was more commonly reported with patients treated with a combination of lithium and benzodiazepines (49%) than those treated with either lithium alone (14%) or lithium with other concomitant drugs (17%). Lithium treatment may increase serotonergic neurotransmission [75], possibly accounting for some sexual side effects.

Less evidence is documented regarding carbamazepine and sexual function. A case has been reported in which a man developed ejaculatory and orgasmic dysfunction after beginning treatment with carbamazepine for trigeminal neuralgia [76]. When carbamazepine was discontinued, sexual function returned to baseline. Anticonvulsants are often utilized to treat bipolar disorder. Sex hormone binding globulin (SHBG) increases during pharmacotherapy with carbamazepine, and acute decreases in free and total testosterone levels have occurred with initiation of carbamazepine treatment [77]. Free testosterone may be decreased as a result of the induction of hepatic synthesis of SHBG [78], but the clinical importance of this is not clear, and there are few data on the impact of anticonvulsants on sexual function in psychiatric patients.

Valproate, although not implicated in sexual dysfunction, may possibly interfere with endocrine function, such as increased androgen levels and polycystic ovarian syndrome (PCOS) [79]. While the question of valproate's role in the development of PCOS in psychiatric patients is controversial, elevation of androgens could theoretically protect against sexual side effects of concomitant psychotropic medications. Also, there are three cases of men with epilepsy and erectile dysfunction whose sexual function improved when they were started on lamotrigine [80].

VI. STRATEGIES TO TREAT PSYCHOTROPIC-INDUCED SEXUAL DYSFUNCTION

Sometimes lowering the dose of a drug may reverse or improve sexual dysfunction [81,82]. However, many patients need to discontinue a drug to reverse sexual side effects. Taking a 3-day "drug holiday," an interruption in use of medication, improved SSRI-induced sexual function in approximately half of patients, with improved orgasmic function, sexual satisfaction, and libido [83]. Drug holidays work better with shorter half-life SSRIs, sertraline and paroxetine, than fluoxetine. The addition of or switching to a different medication with less sexual dysfunction is an alternative strategy.

VII. PHARMACOTHERAPY FOR SEXUAL DYSFUNCTION

(Please see Table 1 at the end of this section.)

A. Buspirone

Buspirone, a partial 5-hydroxytryptamine-1A (5HT1A) agonist, has shown some benefit in treating antidepressant sexual side effects. For example, Othmer and Othmer [84] conducted an open-label study of buspirone for sexual function in patients with generalized anxiety disorder. All but one had complained of sexual dysfunction from other medications. Patients were treated with buspirone, average 45 mg/day, after a washout of other psychotropic medications. After 1 month, eight of nine men and women returned to normal sexual function, without correlation with reduction in anxiety. In another study, patients with depression who had previously failed to respond to an SSRI were treated with added buspirone, up to 60 mg/day, or placebo in double-blind fashion [85]. There were no differences in antidepressant response between buspirone and placebo, but of 119 patients, 39.5% had SSRI-related sexual dysfunction prior to study entry. Significantly more patients in the buspirone group reported remittance of sexual dysfunction than in the placebo group. Improved sexual function occurred within the first week of treatment and was more pronounced in women than men, with benefits in both libido and orgasmic function. In a negative study, Michaelson et al. [86] conducted a double-blind, placebo-controlled trial of buspirone, amantadine, and placebo in women who had been successfully treated with fluoxetine but had experienced fluoxetine-associated sexual dysfunction. All groups reported improved sexual function, highlighting the importance of including placebo groups in such studies.

B. Bupropion

Bupropion has been associated less with sexual dysfunction than other antidepressants [87,88]. As a result, clinicians often augment with or switch to bupropion from an SRI when sexual side effects have occurred. Additionally, Clayton et al. [89]) conducted an 8-week study of patients ($N = 11$) who had had depression successfully treated with SSRIs but experienced sexual dysfunction. For each patient, the SSRI was tapered as open-label treatment with sustained-release bupropion was initiated. Overall, patients experienced improved sexual function, with no significant change in depressive symptoms. However, five patients dropped out of the study, likely owing to a discontinuation syndrome secondary to tapering the SSRI. Of the dropouts, most reported symptoms associated with SSRI discontinuation syndrome—including agitation, gastrointestinal distress, sweating, flushing, headache, dizziness, and dysphoria. Gitlin et al. [90] also demonstrated improvement in SSRI-associated sexual dysfunction with the addition of open-label bupropion (150–300 mg/day). However, Ashton et al. [91] did not find that SSRI-associated sexual dysfunction improved significantly more with bupropion, 150 mg/day, than with placebo in a double-blind trial.

C. Mirtazapine

Substituting mirtazepine may be an effective strategy for treating SRI-induced sexual dysfunction. As previously mentioned, Gelenberg and colleagues [92] treated patients experiencing SSRI-induced sexual dysfunction with mirtazapine. Eleven (58%) had return of normal sexual function with mirtazapine treatment, and all maintained remission from depression.

D. Cyproheptadine

Cyproheptadine, an antiserotonergic and antihistaminergic agent, has been used adjunctively to treat SSRI-induced sexual dysfunction. In some case cyproheptadine, 4–12 mg, is used PRN 1–2 h before sexual activity [93–95], while others employ daily dosing, 12–16 mg [96–98].

In a single case, single-blind crossover study, a woman with sexual dysfunction induced by imipramine took cyptroheptadine, diphenhydramine, or placebo 2 h before intercourse, then recorded the ease of achieving orgasm [99]. She reached orgasm 40% of the time with cyproheptadine 4 mg, which was significantly more effective than diphenhydramine and nonsignificantly more effective than placebo.

Sedation is common in patients receiving cyproheptadine for sexual side effects [100]. However, more serious side effects have been reported. Goldbloom and Kennedy [101] reported the reversal of therapeutic effects of fluoxetine in two patients with bulimia who were treated with cyproheptadine 4–8 mg/day for sexual dysfunction. Bulimic symptoms subsided after cyproheptadine was discontinued. Price and Grunhaus [102] described a man with increased depressive symptoms and the emergence of suicidal ideation after he started cyproheptadine for clomipramine-induced anorgasmia [102]. Feder [103] also found diminished antidepressant efficacy when cyproheptadine was used either daily or PRN for SSRI-induced sexual dysfunction. While there are positive reports on cyproheptadine for sexual dysfunction associated with MAOIs [104,105], Kahn [106] wrote of one patient experienced visual hallucinations, fear, and irritability when 2 mg QHS was added to his medication regimen; symptoms resolved with the discontinuation of cyproheptadine.

E. Mianserin

Another serotonin antagonist, the ICA mianserin, has been tried as an antidote for SRI-induced sexual dysfunction. Aizenberg et al. [107] added mianserin 15 mg to 15 male patients with SRI-induced sexual side effects for 4 weeks. Patients generally experienced improved orgasmic function and sexual satisfaction, with marked improvement in sexual function in nine of 15, partial improvement in two, and no improvement in four. In an open-label trial of mianserin, 15 mg/day for 3 weeks, two-thirds of women with SRI-induced sexual side effects ($N = 16$) reported significant improvement in sexual function, with no major adverse effects or psychiatric decompensation [108].

F. Amantadine

Amantadine, a dopamine agonist, has been used to counteract SSRI-induced sexual side effects. Balon [109] described a woman whose fluoxetine-associated anorgasmia improved with amantadine, 100 mg PRN 5–6 h before sex. Prior to the PRN use, she was treated with 100 mg BID, which resulted in anxiety. Balogh et al. [110] reported on seven patients who experienced fluoxetine-induced anorgasmia. Of the four men and three women who were treated with amantadine, 100 mg QD or BID, all but one man and one woman had resolution of anorgasmia. In a randomized, placebo-controlled study for the treatment of fluoxetine-associated sexual dysfunction in women, Michaelson et al. [111] administered either amantadine, buspirone, or placebo for 8 weeks. Patients who received amantadine had greater improvements in energy, while all groups reported improvement in sexual function.

G. Yohimbine

Adjunctive yohimbine is another strategy to combat psychotropic-induced sexual dysfunction. Yohimbine is an indole alkaloid from the bark of the yohimbine tree, with alpha-2 adrenoceptor antagonist activity, central blockade of alpha-2 receptors, and noradrenergic activity [112]. In a meta-analysis of all placebo-controlled trials of erectile dysfunction (not specifically related to psychotropic use), yohimbine has been shown to be superior to placebo and well tolerated in doses of 5–10 mg TID [113]. Jacobsen [114] reported an open trial of yohimbine, 5.4 mg TID for at least 3 weeks for fluoxetine-induced sexual dysfunction. Eight of nine patients had improved sexual function with yohimbine, although five had side effects, leading to discontinuation in two. Side effects included nausea, anxiety, insomnia, and urinary frequency.

In a double-blind placebo-controlled crossover study, a patient who had previously not responded to cyproheptadine had successful treatment of clomipramine-induced anorgasmia with yohimbine [115]. Initially the patient experienced headache with yohimbine, which subsided after he received several doses. While 10 mg yohimbine 90 min before sex resulted in restoration of orgasmic function after each administration, 15 mg resulted in premature ejaculation. After placebo the patient experienced orgasm only one of seven times.

Segraves [116] reported successful treatment of all of 10 cases of SSRI-induced anorgasmia with yohimbine, 5.4 mg 1–2 h prior to sexual intercourse. Similarly, Hollander and McCarley [117] reported that yohimbine, 5.4–10.8 mg 2–4 h before sex, successfully counteracted SSRI-induced anorgasmia in five of six patients. Investigators found that if the dosage was too low, patients experienced no results, but if too high, patients complained of feeling "wired or wound up," and insomia, fatigue, anxiety, and excessive sweating.

Yohimbine has also been combined with trazodone for sexual dysfunction [118]. Fifty-five male patients were diagnosed with at least 3 months of psychogenic erectile dysfunction, determined after physical examinations, laboratory analyses, Doppler sonography of the cavernosal arteries, and polysomnographic recording of nocturnal erections. Each patient underwent two courses of treatment, 8 weeks with a combination of yohimbine (5mg TID) and trazodone (50 mg/day), then 8 weeks of placebo. Partial and complete response to placebo totaled 22%, compared with 71% with the yohimbine-trazodone combination. The study was complicated by the use of both yohimbine and trazodone, which is a triazolopyridine derivative and influences alpha-adrenergic and dopamine function. However, since trazodone alone was no more effective than placebo for erectile dysfunction in another double-blind study [119], the benefits were likely due to yohimbine.

H. Stimulants

Stimulants may be beneficial in treating sexual side effects of psychotropics. Bartlik et al. [120] reported on five cases in which either methylphenidate, 15–25 mg or 5–10 mg PRN ~1h prior to sex, or dextroamphetamine, 5 mg 1 h before sex, reversed sexual side effects in patients treated with SSRIs.

I. Sidenafil

Sildenafil appears to be a useful antidote. It is a phosphodiesterase-5 (PDE-5) inhibitor, and affects the corpus cavernosum and systemic vasculature. Fava et al. [121] conducted an open trial of sildenafil in nine men and five women, 12 of whom were being treated with SSRIs, and two of whom were receiving mirtazapine. After 4 weeks, patients experienced statistically significant improvement in sexual functioning, measured by the Arizona Sexual Experiences Scale (ASEX). Both men and women reported improvements in libido, arousal, orgasm, and sexual satisfaction, and men reported improved erectile function. Efficacy is also supported by a case report of a woman with fluoxetine-induced sexual dysfunction, successfully treated with sildenafil 50 mg 1 h prior to sexual intercourse [122]. She experienced return of normal arousal and orgasm in seven of seven trials. She had not responded to cyproheptadine and buproprion, and had only partial response to dextroamphetamine in previous trials to counteract the sexual side effects. In a larger report of cases, Salerian et al. [123] described 92 patients (31 women and 61 men) with psychotropic-induced sexual dysfunction, treated with sildenafil. Significant improvement was noted with all classes of psychotropic medications, and men and women responded equally well to sildenafil. Nurnberg et al. [124] conducted a double-blind placebo-controlled trial of sildenafil 50–100 mg for SRI-induced sexual dysfunction in 90 men. Sildenafil resulted in significantly greater improvements in erectile and orgasmic function, intercourse satisfaction, and overall satisfaction than placebo. Open-label extension in nonresponders also demonstrated the efficacy of sildenafil in SRI-associated sexual dysfunction.

A case has also been reported of a male patient with schizoaffective disorder who experienced erectile dysfunction induced by haloperidol, successfully treated with sildenafil 50 mg PRN [125]. The patient did not experience any side effects secondary to the use of sildenafil.

While most evidence suggests that sildenafil is a safe medication, it is contraindicated in patients taking organic nitrates, as synergistic decreases in arterial pressure have been demonstrated to occur [126].

J. Ginkgo Biloba

Ginkgo biloba has been used to treat antidepressant-associated sexual dysfunction. Cohen and Bartlik [127] reported on an open trial of ginkgo biloba 60–240 QD in patients experiencing sexual dysfunction while being treated with antidepressants. They found a positive effect on all four phases of the sexual response cycle: desire, excitement, orgasm, resolution. In that trial, women (n = 33) responded better than men (n = 30), 91% vs. 76%. Some patients experienced gastrointestinal side effects, headache, and general CNS activation. In a letter critical of that trial, Balon [128] expressed concern over lack of pretreatment evaluation prior to starting antidepressant treatment, and inconsistencies of data interpretation and reporting of side effects. A case report supports a possible role for gingko biloba extract in the treatment of a woman with fluoxetine-induced sexual dysfunction [129]. However, in another open trial, Ashton et al. [130] treated 22 consecutive patients with SSRI-induced sexual dysfunction for 1 month with ginkgo biloba 300 mg TID. They found little improvement in sexual function, with only three patients (13.6%) reporting at least partial improvement.

K. Ginseng

Ginseng is another potential treatment for sexual dysfunction, but data are lacking in the treatment of psychotropic-associated sexual dysfunction. In a study of male patients with erectile dysfunction, 90 patients were randomized to receive Korean red ginseng, trazodone, or placebo [131]. With ginseng, patients experienced significant increases in sexual satisfaction, libido, and penile rigidity. The overall efficacy was 60% for ginseng, 30% each for placebo and trazodone. While this study was not specific for the treatment of iatrogenic sexual dysfunction, results merit further study.

VI. CONCLUSIONS

Sexual side effects are common with many psychotropic medications. Clinicians must actively inquire about sexual function in order to make accurate assessments. Women in particular may be reticent on this topic.

Baseline assessments of sexual function are necessary to determine whether or not sexual dysfunction is attributable to medication. Psychiatric and medical disorders can impact sexual function, independent of medication. A medical differential diagnosis and use of a standardized scale, such as the ASEX, may be helpful.

Several mechanisms could account for iatrogenic sexual dysfunction from psychotropic medications. Sites of action leading to side effects may be central or peripheral. Several neurotransmitter systems are likely involved. Medications that increase serotonergic activity and/or decrease noradrenergic or dopaminergic activity have been implicated in sexual dysfunction. Increased dopaminergic activity in the medial preoptic area has been associated with increased sexual activity, and the administration of serotonin in this area may cause decreased sexual activity [132]. More specifically, activation of 5HT2 receptors can inhibit dopaminergic activity, and some antidotes for sexual dysfunction increase noradrenergic transmission by inhibition of autoreceptors.

Hormones might be involved in the etiology of iatrogenic sexual dysfunction. Increased prolactin from antipsychotics can produce clinically troublesome side effects. Older antipsychotic medications tend to increase prolactin levels. Atypicals, with the exception of risperidone, do so to a lesser degree.

Testosterone might mediate psychotropic-induced sexual dysfunction. Animal models have demonstrated suppression of serum gonadal steroids with serotonin reuptake inhibitors [133]. A case report has demonstrated the occurrence of low testosterone levels in a patient during treatment with venlafaxine; the testosterone level increased after the venlafaxine was discontinued [134]. Testosterone has been traditionally thought of as a male hormone. Low levels of testosterone have been associated with sexual dysfunction in men, and testosterone supplementation has been demonstrated to improve sexual function in hypogonadal men [135,136]. Testosterone deficiency in women also has been associated with decreased libido and sexual responsiveness [137]. Combination hormonal replacement, using both estradiol and testosterone, results in greater improvement in sexual function than estrogen therapy alone in postmenopausal women [138]. Androgens increase sexual desire and arousal in women after surgical menopause [139,140]. Testosterone increases sexual desire in premenopausal women also [141].

As the neurobiological basis for mental illnesses becomes better understood, we should be able to

Table 1 Pharmacotherapy for Iatrogenic Sexual Dysfunction

Treatment for sexual dysfunction	Dosages reported	Supporting data	Mechanism of action? Other comments
Buspirone	45–60 mg/d	Double-blind, placebo-controlled; open label	Serotonergic blockade, enhancement of dopaminergic noradrenergic activity
Cyproheptadine	4–12 mg PRN 1–2 h before sexual activity	Open label; case reports	Serotonergic blockade; may interfere with efficacy of SRIs
Amantadine	100–200 mg/d	Case reports suppose use, one double-blind trial showed improvement but not significantly different from placebo group	Dopamine agonist
Yohimbine	5–10 mg PRN 2–4 h before sexual intercourse or 5 mg TID	Open label, case reports; double-blind data not specific for antidepressant-induced sexual dysfunction	Increases noradrenergic activity
Sildenafil	5–100 mg PRN 1 h before sexual intercourse	Double-blind, open label, case reports	Inhibition of phosphodiesterase-5
Bupropion	150–300 mg/d	Double-blind, open label	Increased dopaminergic activity
Gingko biloba	60–240 mg/d	Open label	Unknown
Mianserin	15 mg/d	Open label	Serotonin antagonism
Methylphenidate	15–25 mg; 25 mg/d; 5 mg 45 min prior to sexual activity (PRN); 5–10 mg methylphenidate PRN 1 h prior	Case reports	Increased dopaminergic activity
Dextroamphetamine	5 mg PRN 1 h before sexual activity	Case reports	Increased dopaminergic activity

develop more rational pharmacotherapies with fewer side effects. Currently, choosing from our arsenal of psychotropic mediations involves balancing benefits with unwanted effects, including sexual dysfunction. We have described strategies to treat sexual dysfunction, but most importantly, clinicians must discuss sexual function with their patients openly and consider the impact of psychotropic medications on this important aspect of their lives.

REFERENCES

1. Hirschfeld RMA. Care of the sexually active depressed patient. J Clin Psychiatry 1999; 60:32–35.
2. Michaels KB. Problems assessing nonserious adverse drug reactions: antidepressant drug therapy and sexual dysfunction. Pharmacotherapy 1999; 19:424–429.
3. Laumann EO, Gagnon JH, Michel RT, et al. The social organization of sexuality: sexual practices in the United states. London: University of Chicago Press; 1994:368–375.
4. Mathew RJ, Weinman ML. Sexual dysfunctions in depression. Arch Sex Behav 1982; 11:323–328.
5. Beaumont G. Sexual side-effects of clomipramine (Anafranil). J Int Med Res 1977; 5:37–44.
6. Harrison WM, Rabkin JG, Ehrhardt AA, Stewart JW, McGrath PJ, Ross D, Quitkin FM. Effects of antidepressant medication on sexual function: a controlled study. J Clin Psychopharmacol 1986; 6:144–149.
7. Sovner R. Anorgasmia associated with imipramine but not desipramine: case report. J Clin Psychiatry 1983; 44:345–346.
8. Steele TE, Howell EF. Cyproheptadine for imipramine-induced anorgasmia. J Clin Psychopharmacol 1986; 6:326–327.
9. Beaumont G. Sexual side-effects of clomipramine (Anafranil). J Int Med Res 1977; 5:37–44.
10. Kennedy SH, Ralevski E, Davis C, Neitzert C. The effects of moclobemide on sexual desire and function in healthy volunteers. Eur Neuropsychopharmacol 1996; 6:177–181.

11. Kennedy SH, Eisfeld BS, Dickens SE, Bacchiochi JR, Bagby M. Antidepressant-induced sexual dysfunction during treatment with moclobemide, paroxetine, sertraline, and venlafaxine. J Clin Psychiatry 2000; 61:276–281.
12. Toni C, Perugi G, Frare F, Mata B, Vitale B, Mengali F, Recchia M, Serra G, Akiskal HS. A prospective naturalistic study of 326 panic-agorabic patients treated with antidepressants. Pharmacopsychiatry 2000; 33:121–131.
13. Jones SD. Ejaculatory inhibition with trazodone. J Clin Psychopharmacol 1984; 4:279–281.
14. Terao T, Nakamura J. Exhibitionism and low-dose trazodone treatment. Hum Psychopharmacol Clin Exp 2000; 15:347–349.
15. Segraves RT, Kavoussi R, Hughes AR, Batey SR, Johnston JA, Donahue R, Ascher JA. Evaluation of sexual functioning in depressed outpatients: a double-blind comparison of sustained-release bupropion and sertraline treatment.
16. Coleman CC, Cunningham LA, Foster VJ, Batey SR, Donahue RM, Houser TL, Ascher JA. Sexual dysfunction associated with the treatment of depression: a placebo-controlled comparison of bupropion sustained release and sertraline treatment. Ann Clin Psychiatry 1999; 11:205–215.
17. Ramasubbu R. Bupropion treatment-related sexual side effects: a case report. Can J Psychiatry 2000; 45:200.
18. Boyarsky BK, Haque W, Rouleau MR, Hirschfeld RMA. Sexual function in depressed outpatients taking mirtazapine. Depress Anxiety 1999; 9:175–179.
19. Koutouvidis N, Pratikakis M, Fotiadou A. The use of mirtazapine in a group of 11 patients following poor compliance to selective serotonin reuptake inhibitor treatment due to sexual dysfunction. Int Clin Psychopharmacol 1999; 14:253–255.
20. Gelenberg AJ, laukes C, McGaheuy C, Okayli G, Moreno F, Zentner L, Delgado P. Mirtazapine substitution in SSRI-induced sexual dysfunction. J Clin Psychiatry 2000; 61:356–360.
21. Berigan TR, Harazin JS. Sexual dysfunction associated with mirtazapine: a case report. J Clin Psychiatry 1998; 59:319–320.
22. Zajecka J, Dunner DL, Hirschfeld RMA, Kornstein SG, Ninan P, Rush AJ, Trivedi MH, Gelenberg AJ, Thase ME, Borian FE. Sexual function and satisfaction in the treatment of chronic major depression with nefazodone, CBAS-psychotherapy and their combination. ACNP Annual Meeting, December 10–14, 2000; San Juan, Puerto Rico.
23. Ferguson JM, Shrivastava R, Stahl SM, Hartford J, Borian F, Ieni J, McQuade RD, Jody D. Reemergence of sexual dysfunction in patients with major depressive disorder: double-blind comparison of nefazodone and sertraline. J Clin Psychiatry 2001; 62:24–29.
24. Morris PL. Fluoxetine and orgasmic sexual experiences. Int J Psychiatry Med 1991; 21:379–382.
25. Elmore JL, Quattlebaum JT. Female sexual simulation during antidepressant treatment. Pharmacotherapy 1997; 17:612–616.
26. Balon R. Antidepressants in the treatment of premature ejaculation. J Sex Marital Ther 1996; 22:85–96.
27. Kafka MP, Hennen J. Psychostimulant augmentation during treatment with selective serotonin reuptake inhibitors in men with paraphilias and paraphilia-related disorders: a case series. J Clin Psychiatry 2000; 61:664–670.
28. Othmer E, Othmer SC. Effect of buspirone on sexual dysfunction in patients with generalized anxiety disorder. J Clin Psychiatry 1987; 48:201–203.
29. Sangal R. Inhibited female orgasm as a side effect of alprazolam. Am J Psychiatry 1985; 142:1223–1224.
30. Hughes JM. Failure to ejaculate with chlordiazepoxide. Am J Psychiatry 1984; 121:610–611.
31. Cohen LS, Rosenbaum JF. Clonazepam: new uses and potential problems. J Clin Psychiatry 1987; 48:50–56.
32. Munjack DJ, Crocker B. Alprazolam-induced ejaculatory inhibition. J Clin Psychopharmacol 196; 6:57–58.
33. Balon R, Ramesh C, Pohl R. Sexual dysfunction associated with diazepam but not with clonazepam. Can J Psychiatry 1989; 34:947–948.
34. Uhde TW, Tancer ME, Shea CA. Sexual dysfunction related to alprazolam treatment of social phobia. Am J Psychiatry 1988; 145:531–532.
35. Khandelwal SK. Complete loss of libido with short-term use of lorazepam. Am J Psychiatry 1988; 145:1313–1314.
36. Ghardirian AM, Annable L, Belanger MC. Lithium, benzodiazepines, and sexual function in bipolar patients. Am J Psychiatry 1992; 149:801–805.
37. Friedman S, Harrison G. Sexual histories, attitudes, and behavior of schizophrenic and normal women. Arch Sex Behav 1984; 14:555–567.
38. Aizenberg D, Zemishlany Z, Dorfman-Etrog P, Weizman A. Sexual dysfunction in male schizophrenic patients. J Clin Psychiatry 1995; 56:137–141.
39. Sullivan G, Lukoff D. Sexual side effects of antipsychotic medication: evaluation and interventions. Hosp Community Psychiatry 1990; 41:1238–1241.
40. Mitchell JE, Popkin MK. Antipsychotic drug therapy and sexual dysfunction in men. Am J Psychiatry 1982; 139:633–637.
41. Hansen TE, Casey DE, Hoffman WF. Neuroleptic intolerance. Schizophren Bull 197; 23:567–582.
42. Greenberg HR. Inhibition of ejaculation by chlorpromazine. J Nerv Ment Dis 1971; 152:364–366.

43. Ananth J. Impotence associated with pimozide. Am J Psychiatry 1982; 139:1374.
44. Mitchell JE, Popkin MK. Antipsychotic drug therapy and sexual dysfunction in men. Am J Psychiatry 1982; 139:633–637.
45. Griffith SR, Zil JS. Priapism in a patient receiving antipsychotic therapy. Psychosomatics 1984; 25:629–631.
46. Ghadirian AM, Chouinard G, Annable L. Sexual dysfunction and plasma prolactin level in neuroleptic-treated schizophrenic outpatients. J Nerv Ment Dis 1982; 170:463–367.
47. Aizenberg D, Shiloh R, Zemishlany Z, Weizman A. Low-dose imipramine for thioridazine-induced male orgasmic disorder. J Sex Marital Ther 1996; 22:225–229.
48. Dickson RA, Seeman MV, Corenblum B. Hormonal side effects in women: typical versus atypical antipsychotic treatment. J Clin Psychiatry 2000; 61:10–15.
49. Breier AF, Malhotra AK, Tung-Ping Su, Pinals DA, Elman I, Adler CM, Lafargue T, Clifton A, Pickar D. Clozapine and risperidone in chronic schizophrenia: effects on symptoms, parkinsonian side effects, and neuroendocrine response. Am J Psychiatry 1999; 156:294–298.
50. Small JG, Hirsch SR, Arvanitis LA, Miller BG, Link CG. Quetiapine in patients with schizophrenia. A high- and low-dose double-blind comparison with placebo. Seroquel Study Group. Arch Gen Psychiatry 1997; 54:549–557.
51. Collaborative Working Group on Clinical Trial Evaluations. Adverse effects of the atypical antipsychotics. J Clin Psychiatry 1998; 59:17–22.
52. Wudarsky M, Nicolson R, Hamburger SD, Sechler L, Gochman P, Bedwell J, Lenane MC, Rapoport JL. Elevated prolactin in pediatric patients on typical and atypical antipsychotics. J Child Adolesc Psychopharmacol 1999; 9:239–245.
53. Hatzimanolis J, Lykouras L, Markianos M, Oulis P. Neurochemical variables in schizophrenic patients during switching from neuroleptics to clozapine. Prog Neuopsychopharmacol Biol Psychiatry 1998; 22:1077–1085.
54. Hummer MH, Kemmler G, Kurz M, Kurzthaler I, Oberbauer H, Fleischhacker WW. Sexual disturbances during clozapine and haloperidol treatment for schizophrenia. Am J Psychiatry 1999; 156:631–633.
55. Breier AF, Malhotra AK, Tung-Ping Su, Pinals DA, Elman I, Adler CM, Lafargue T, Clifton A, Pickar D. Clozapine and risperidone in chronic schizophrenia: effects on symptoms, parkinsonian side effects, and neuroendocrine response. Am J Psychiatry 1999; 156:294–298.
56. Markianos M, Hatzimanolis J, Lykouras L. Dopamine receptor responsivity in schizophrenic patients before and after switch from haloperidol to risperidone. Psychiatry Res 1999; 89:115–122.
57. Kapur S, Zipursky RB, Remington G. Clinical and theoretical implications of 5-HT2 and D2 receptor occupancy of clozapine, risperidone, and olanzapine in schizophrenia. Am J Psychiatry 199; 156:286–293.
58. Guille C, Sachs GS, Ghaemi SN. A naturalistic comparison of clozapine, risperidone, and olanzapine in the treatment of bipolar disorder. J Clin Psychiatry 2000; 61:638–642.
59. Kim YK, Kim L, Lee MS. Risperidone and associated amenorrhea: a report of 5 cases. J Clin Psychiatry 19999; 60:315–317.
60. Popli A, Gupta S, Rangwani SR. Risperidone-induced galactorrhea associated with a prolactin elevation. Ann Clin Psychiatry 1998; 10:31–33.
61. Kleinberg DL, Davis JM, De Coster R, Van Baelen B, Brecher M. Prolactin levels and adverse events in patients treated with risperidone. J Clin Psychopharmacol 1999; 19:57–61.
62. Montejo A, Llorca G, Izquierdo J. Switching to olanzapine in patients with antipsychotic-induced sexual dysfunction: a prospective and naturalistic study. In: New Research Report 696 of the American Psychiatric Association Annual Meeting; May 13–18, 2000; Chicago.
63. David SR, Taylor CC, Kinon BJ, Breier A. The effects of olanzapine, risperidone, and haloperidol on plasma prolactin levels in patients with schizophrenia. Clin Ther 2000; 22:10885-1096.
64. Wudarsky M, Nicolson R, Hamburger SD, Spechler L, Gochman P, Bedwell J, Lenane MC, Rapoport JL. Elevated prolactin in pediatric patients on typical and atypical antipsychotics. J Child Adolesc Psychopharmacol 1999; 9:239–245.
65. Ghadirian AM, Chouinard G, Annable L. Sexual dysfunction and plasma prolactin levels in neuroleptic-treated schizophrenic outpatients. J Nerv Ment Dis 1982; 170:463–467.
66. Gould RJ, Murphy KM, Reynolds IJ, Snyder SH. Calcium channel blockade: possible explanation for thioridazine's peripheral side effects. Am J Psychiatry 1984; 141:352–357.
67. Horowitz JD, Goble AJ. Drugs and impaired male sexual dysfunction. Drugs 1979; 18:206–217.
68. Ghadirian AM, Chouinard G, Annable L. Sexual dysfunction and plasma prolactin levels in neuroleptic-treated schizophrenic outpatients. J Nerv Ment Dis 1982; 170:463–467.
69. Okonmah AD, Bradshaw WG, Couceyro P, Soliman KF. The effect of neuroleptic drugs on serum testosterone levels in the male rat. Gen Pharmacol 1986; 17:235–238.
70. Dickson RA, Glazer WM. Hyperprolactinemia and male sexual dysfunction. J Clin Psychiatry 1999; 60:125.

71. Dickson RA, Seeman MV, Corenblum B. Hormonal side effects in women: typical versus atypical antipsychotic treatment. J Clin Psychiatry 2000; 61:10–15.
72. Aizenberg D, Sigler M, Zemishlani Z, Weizman A. Lithium and male sexual function in affective patients. Clin Neuropharmacol 1996; 19:515–519.
73. Blay SL, Ferraz MP, Calil HM. Lithium-induced male sexual impairment: two case reports. J Clin Psychiatry 1982; 43:497–498.
74. Ghardirian AM, Annable L, Belanger MC. Lithium, benzodiazepines, and sexual function in bipolar patients. Am J Psychiatry 1992; 149:801–805.
75. Price LH, Charney DS, Delgado PL, Heninger GR. Lithium treatment and serotonergic function. Arch Gen Psychiatry 1989; 46:13–19.
76. Stephens LJ, Hines JEW, McNicholas TA Carbamazepine-related ejaculatory failure. Br J Urol 1997; 79:485.
77. Connel JMC, Rapeport WG, Beastall GH, Brodie MJ. Changes in circulating androgens during short term carbamazepine therapy. Br J Clin Pharmacol 1984; 17:347–351.
78. Brunet M, Rodamilans M, Martinez-Osaba J, Santamaria J, To-Figueras J, Torra M, Corbella J, Rivera F. Pharmacol Toxicol 1995; 76:1371–1375.
79. Isojarvi JI, Laatikainen TJ, Pakarinen AJ, Juntunen KTS, Myllyla VV. Polycystic ovaries and hyperandrogenism in women taking valproate for epilepsy. N Engl J Med 1993; 39:383–1388.
80. Husain AM, Carwile ST, Miller PP, Radtke RA. Improved sexual function in three men taking lamotrigine for epilepsy. South Med J 2000; 93:335–336.
81. Jacobsen FM. Fluoxetine-induced sexual dysfunction and an open trial of yohimbine. J Clin Psychiatry 1992; 53:119–122.
82. Labbate LA. Sex and serotonin reuptake inhibitor antidepressants. Psychiatr Ann 999; 29:571–579.
83. Rothchild AJ. Selective serotonin reuptake inhibitor-induced sexual dysfunction: efficacy of a drug holiday. Am J Psychiatry 1995; 152:1514–1516.
84. Othmer E, Othmer SC. Effect of buspirone on sexual dysfunction in patients with generalized anxiety disorder. J Clin Psychiatry 1987; 48:201–203.
85. Landen M, Eriksson E, Agren H, Fahlen T. Effect of busipirone on sexual dysfunction in depressed patients treated with selective serotonin reuptake inhibitors. J Clin Psychopharmacol 1999; 19:268–271.
86. Michaelson D, Bancroft J, Targum S, Kim Y, Tepner R. Female sexual dysfunction associated with antidepressant administration: a randomized, placebo-controlled study of pharmacologic intervention. Am J Psychiatry 2000; 157:239–243.
87. Segraves RT, Kavoussi R, Hughes AR, Batey SR, Johnston JA, Donahue R, Ascher JA. Evaluation of sexual functioning in depressed outpatients: a double-blind comparison of sustained-release bupropion and sertraline treatment. J Clin Psychopharmacol 2000; 20:122–128.
88. Coleman CC, Cunningham LA, Foster VJ, Batey SR, Donahue RM, Houser TL, Ascher JA. Sexual dysfunction associated with the treatment of depression: a placebo-controlled comparison of bupropion sustained release and sertraline treatment. Ann Clin Psychiatry 1999; 11:205–215.
89. Clayton AH, McGarvey EL, Abouesh A, Pinkerton R. Substitution of SSRI with bupropion sustained-release following SSRI-induced sexual dysfunction. J Clin Psychiatry 2001; 62:185–190.
90. Gitlin M, Suri R, Altshuler L, et al. Bupropion as a treatment for SSRI-induced sexual side effects. In: New Research Report 617 of the American Psychiatric Association Annual Meeting; May 13–18, 2000; Chicago.
91. Ashton A, Massant P, Gupta S, et al. Bupropion sustained release for SSRI-induced sexual dysfunction: a randomized, double-blind, placebo-controlled parallel group study. In: New Research Report 617 of the American Psychiatric Association Annual Meeting; May 13–18, 2000; Chicago.
92. Gelenberg AJ, Laukes C, McGaheuy C, Okayli G, Moreno F, Zentner L, Delgado P. Mirtazapine substitution in SSRI-induced sexual dysfunction. J Clin Psychiatry 2000; 61:346–360.
93. McCormick S, Olin J, Brotman AW. Reversal of fluoxetine-induced anorgasmia by cyproheptadine in two patients. J Clin Psychiatry 1990; 51:383–384.
94. Lauerma H. Successful treatment of citalopram-induced anorgasmia by cyproheptadine. Acta Psychiatr Scand 1996; 93:69–70.
95. Aizenberg D, Zemishlany Z, Weizman A. Cyproheptadine treatment of sexual dysfunction induced by serotonin reuptake inhibitors. Clin Neuropharmacol 1995; 18:320–324.
96. McCormick S, Olin J, Brotman AW. Reversal of fluoxetine-induced anorgasmia by cyproheptadine in two patients. J Clin Psychiatry 1990; 51:383–384.
97. Cohen AJ. Fluoxetine-induced yawning and anorgasmia reversed by cyproheptadine treatment. J Clin Psychiatry 1992; 53:174.
98. Lauerma H. Successful treatment of citalopram-induced anorgasmia by cyproheptadine. Acta Psychiatr Scand 1996; 93:69–70.
99. Steele TE, Howell EF. Cyproheptadine for imipramine-induced anorgasmia. J Clin Psychopharmacol 1986; 6:326–327.
100. Aizenberg D, Zemishlany Z, Weizman A. Cyproheptadine treatment of sexual dysfunction induced by serotonin reuptake inhibitors. Clin Neuropharmacol 1995; 18:320–324.
101. Goldbloom DS, Kennedy SH. Adverse interaction of fluoxetine and cyproheptadine in two patients with bulimia nervosa. J Clin Psychiatry 1991; 52:261–262.

102. Price J, Grunhaus LJ. Treatment of clomipramine-induced anorgasmia with yohimbine: a case report. J Clin Psychiatry 1990; 51:32–33.
103. Feder R. Reversal of antidepressant activity of fluoxetine by cyproheptadine in three patients. J Clin Psychiatry 1991; 52:163–164.
104. Decastro RM. Reversal of MAOI-induced anorgasmia with cyproheptadine. Am J Psychiatry 1985; 142:783.
105. Riley AJ, Riley EJ. Cyproheptadine and antidepressant induced anorgasmia. Br J Psychiatry 1986; 142:217–218.
106. Kahn DA. Possible toxic interaction between cyproheptadine and phenelzine. Am J Psychiatry 1987; 144:1242–1243.
107. Aizenberg D, Gur S, Zemishlany Z, Granek M, Jeczmien P, Weizman A. Mianserin, a 5-HT2a/2c and alpha 2 antagonist, in the treatment of sexual dysfunction introduced by serotonin reuptake inhibitors. Clin Neuropharmacol 1997; 20:210–214.
108. Aizenberg D, Naor S, Zemishlany Z, Weizman A. The serotonin antagonist mianserin for treatment of serotonin reuptake inhibitor-induced sexual dysfunction in women: an open-label add-on study. Clin Neuropharmacol 1999; 22:347–350.
109. Balon R. Intermittent amantadine for fluoxetine-induced anorgasmia. J Sex Marital Ther 1996; 22:290–292.
110. Balogh S, Hendricks SE, Kang J. Treatment of fluoxetine-induced anorgasmia with amantadine. J Clin Psychiatry 1992; 53:212–213.
111. Michaelson D, Bancroft J, Targum S, Kim Y, Tepner R. Female sexual dysfunction associated with antidepressant administration: a randomized, placebo-controlled study of pharmacologic intervention. Am J Psychiatry 2000; 157:239–243.
112. Montorsi F, Strambi LF, Guazzoni G, Galli L, Barbieri L, Rigatti P, Pizzini G, Miani A. Effect of yohimbine-trazodone on psychogenic impotence: a randomized, double-blind, placebo-controlled study. Urology 1994; 44:732–736.
113. Ernst E, Pittler MH. Yohimbine for erectile dysfunction: a systematic review and meta-analysis of randomized clinical trials. J Urol 1998; 159:433–436.
114. Jacobsen FM. Fluoxetine-induced sexual dysfunction and an open trial of yohimbine. J Clin Psychiatry 1992; 53:119–122.
115. Price J, Grunhaus LJ. Treatment of clomipramine-induced anorgasmia with yohimbine: a case report. J Clin Psychiatry 1990; 51:32–33.
116. Segraves RT. Treatment of drug-induced anorgasmia. Br J Psychiatry 1994; 165:554.
117. Hollander E, McCarley A. Yohimbine treatment of sexual side effects induced by serotonin re-uptake blockers. J Clin Psychiatry 1992; 53:207–209.
118. Montorsi F, Strambi LF, Guazzoni G, Galli L, Barbieri L, Rigatti P, Pizzini G, Miani A. Effect of yohimbine-trazodone on psychogenic impotence: a randomized, double-blind, placebo-controlled study. Urology 1994; 44:732–736.
119. Costabile RA, Spevak M. Oral trazodone is not effective therapy for erectile dysfunction: a double-blind placebo controlled trial. J Urol 1999; 161:1819–1822.
120. Bartlik BD, Kaplan OP, Kaplan HS. psychostimulants apparent reverse sexual dysfunction secondary to selective serotonin re-uptake inhibitors. J Sex Marital Ther 1995; 21:264–271.
121. Fava M, Rankin MA, Alpert JE, Nierenberg AA, Worthington JJ. An open trial of oral sildenafil in antidepressant-induced sexual dysfunction. Psychother Psychosom 1998; 67:328–331.
122. Shen WW, Urosevich Z, Clayton DO. Sildenafil in the treatment of female sexual dysfunction induced by selective serotonin reuptake inhibitors. J Reprod Med 199; 44:535–542.
123. Salerian AJ, Deibler WE, Vittone BJ, Popowitz Geyer A, Drell L, Mirmirani N, Mirczak JA, Byrd W, Tunick SB, Wax M, Fleisher S. Sildenafil for psychotropic-induced sexual dysfunction in 31 women and 61 men. J Sex Marital Ther 2000; 26:133–140.
124. Nurnberg HG, Harrison WM, Wohlhuter CM, Siegel RL, Hensley PL, Lauriello J, Gelenberg AJ, Fava M, Stecher VJ. Sildenafil citrate for the treatment of sexual dysfunction associated with serotonergic reuptake inhibitors (Submitted as an abstract for the APA Annual Meeting, 2001; New Orleans, LA.)
125. Lare SB, Labbate LA, Sildenafil and erectile dysfunction. Am J Psychiatry 2000; 157:2055–2056.
126. Kloner RA. Cardiovascular risk and sildenafil. Am J Cardiol 2000; 86:57–61.
127. Cohen AJ, Bartlik B. Ginkgo biloba for antidepressant-induced sexual dysfunction. J Sex Marital Ther 1998; 24:139–143.
128. Balon R. Ginkgo biloba for antidepressant-induced sexual dysfunction? Sex Marital Ther 1999; 23:1–2.
129. Ellison JM, DeLuca P. Fluoxetine-induced genital anesthesia relieved by ginkgo biloba extract. J Clin Psychiatry 1998; 59:199–200.
130. Ashton AK, Ahrens K, Gupta S, Masand PS. Antidepressant-induced sexual dysfunction and ginkgo biloba. Am J Psychiatry 2000; 157:836.
131. Choi HK, Seong DH, Rha KH. Clinical efficacy of Korean red ginseng for erectile dysfunction. Int J Impot Res 1995; 7:181–186.
132. Alcantara AG. A possible dopaminergic mechanism in the serotonergic antidepressant-induced sexual dysfunctions. J Sex Marital Ther 1999; 25:125–129.

133. Rehavi M, Attali G, Gil-Ad I, Weizman A. Suppression of swerum gonadal steroids in rats by chronic treatment with dopamine and serotonin reuptake inhibitors Eur Neuropsychopharmacol 2000; 10:145–150.
134. Bell S, Shipman M. Reduced testosterone level in a venlafaxine treated patient. Ann Clin Psychiatry 2000; 12:171–173.
135. Wang C, Swedloff RS, Iranmanesh A, Dobs A, Snyder PJ, Cunningham G, Matsumoto AM, Weber T, Berman N. Transdermal testosterone gel improves sexual function, mood, muscle strength, and body composition parameters in hypogonadal men. Testosterone Gel Study Group. J Clin Endocrinol Metab 2000; 85:2839–2853.
136. McClellan KJ, Goa KL. Transdermal testosterone. Drugs 1998; 55:253–258.
137. Kaplan HS, Owett T. The female androgen deficiency syndrome. J Sex Marital Ther 1993; 19:3–24.
138. Davis SR, McCloud P, Strauss BJ, Burger H. Testosterone enhances estradiol's effects on postmenopausal bone density and sexuality. Maturitas 1995; 21:227–236.
139. Sherwin BB, Gelfand MM, Brender W. Androgen enhances sexual motivation in females: a prospective, crossover study of sex steroid administration in the surgical menopause. Psychosom Med 1985; 47:339–351.
140. Shifren JL, Braunstein GD, Simon JA, Casson PR, Buster JE, Redmond GP, Burki RE, Ginsburg ES, Rosen RC, Leiblum SR, Caramelli KE, Mazer NA. Transdermal testosterone treatment in women with impaired sexual function after oophorectomy. N Engl J Med 2000; 343:682–688.
141. Tuiten A, Van Honk J, Koppeschaar H, Bernaards C, Thijssen J, Verbaten R. Time course of effects of testosterone administration on sexual arousal in women. Arch Gen Psychiatry 2000; 57:149–153.

45

Neurobiology of Violence and Aggression

MICHAEL S. McCLOSKEY, ROYCE J. LEE, and EMIL F. COCCARO
University of Chicago, Chicago, Illinois, U.S.A.

I. INTRODUCTION

Aggression, defined as a verbal or physical act with the intent to cause emotional, psychological, or physical harm, is ubiquitous. Individuals are continually exposed, directly or indirectly, to the aggressive acts of others. Not surprisingly, violence, typically conceptualized as physical aggression with injurious intent, has become increasingly endemic in American society. Estimates suggest that upwards of 10,000 violent crimes are committed in America each day [1], with this number representing only a proportion of the more severe acts of aggression. The effects of aggression have cost our society billions of dollars, to say nothing of the human cost. Accordingly, the importance of determining factors that contribute to aggressive behavior in order to better predict and prevent such behavior cannot be overstated.

Aggression has multiple forms. It may be culturally sanctioned, premeditated, or impulsive. Culturally sanctioned aggression, as its name suggests, pertains to aggressive behavior that is viewed as acceptable and often necessary by the society in which the individual lives. The use of force to protect oneself, one's family, or one's country from imminent harm are examples of culturally sanctioned aggression, and these behaviors are not generally seen as being pathological. In contrast, premeditated or "instrumental" aggression is planned aggressive behavior used to obtain a specific goal that is typically not culturally sanctioned. Premeditated behavior may occur in the absence of significant anger or hostility, and is under the person's volitional control. Impulsive aggression is similar to premeditated aggression in that is often seen as pathological. However, unlike premeditated aggression, impulsive aggression is usually unplanned, accompanied by feelings of anger and hostility, and often described by the individual as being beyond their control.

Just as there are multiple forms of aggression, there are also multiple factors that influence ones decision to engage (or not engage) in aggressive behavior. Cultural norms, economic factors, past aggressive experiences, and parental modeling are but of few of the environmental influences that help determine one's propensity for aggression [2]. A growing body of literature suggests that neurobiological factors [3] also affect one's tendency to behave aggressively, and that pathological aggression may reflect in part a neurobiological abnormality. This chapter will examine research aimed at identifying the neurobiological substrates that underlie aggression and violence.

II. NEUROCHEMICAL CORRELATES OF AGGRESSION

A. Serotonin

Serotonin (5HT) is the neurotransmitter most often associated with aggression, particularly impulsive aggression. Early research by Sheard et al. [4] found that compared to placebo, treatment with lithium resulted in a reduction of impulsive aggression among prison inmates. It was hypothesized that the 5HT-enhancing properties of lithium were responsible for the decrease in aggression. This finding coincided with Asberg et al.'s [5] study showing that among depressed individuals, lower lumbar cerebral spinal fluid (CSF) 5-hydroxyindoleacetic acid (5HIAA) levels correlated with violent suicide attempts and completed suicide. Additional research on personality disordered adults [6,7] showed that frequency of aggression and past suicidal behavior were each inversely related with CSF-5HIAA levels, formalizing the trivariate relationship between aggression, suicidal behavior and reduced CSF-5HIAA.

Linnoila et al. [8] hypothesized the trivariate relationship between aggression, suicidal behavior, and reduced 5HT was mediated by impulsivity. In a study of violent criminals, they found that violent offenders whose crimes were "impulsive" (i.e., not an a priori plan) showed significantly lower CSF-5HIAA levels than violent offenders whose crimes were premeditated. Violent criminals with a history of attempted suicide had the lowest CSF-5HIAA levels. Other studies of violent offenders by Lidberg et al. [9] and Virkkunen et al. [10] obtained similar results. Furthermore, Virkkunen et al. [11–13] extended these findings by showing that individuals who engaged in acts of impulsive fire setting also had CSF-5HIAA levels that resembled those of impulsive offenders and were significantly reduced compared to healthy controls. These results have been paralleled by research on CSF-5HIAA and impulsive aggression among primates [14,15].

More recent research suggests the relationship between impulsive aggression and reduced CSF-5HIAA is not as clear as was originally believed. A number of studies have failed to produce the hypothesized relationship between reduced CSF-5HIAA and increased aggression [16–20]. A meta-analysis [21] also failed to link aggression and reduced CSF-5HIAA. Negative findings such as these have led some to suggest that the evidence for the role of 5HT in aggression is more equivocal than originally believed [22]. Others have noted that the failed replications were on populations with less severe forms of aggression (e.g., personality disorder populations or healthy volunteers), and have suggested that reduced CSF-5HIAA levels may only be related to severe levels of aggressive behavior. An alternative hypothesis by Coccaro [23] is that increased 5HT, which was found in a number of the failed replications, may also lead to decreased 5HT receptor responsiveness via a compensatory reduction in postsynaptic 5HT function. Concerns about the sensitivity and interpretability of CSF-5HIAA among individuals exhibiting less severe forms of aggressive behavior fostered the development of alternative methodologies to examine 5HT function, including neuropharmacological challenges.

Fenfluramine is a challenge agent that, for most adults, leads to a robust activation of 5HT. This in turn results in the release of prolactin [24], which can be measured in the blood. The specific 5HT receptors believed to be activated by fenfluramine are the 5HT2c and possibly the 5HT2a receptors [25,26]. 5HT1a receptors do not appear to be involved in the fenfluramine induced prolactin response [27], though they may still have some involvement with aggression [28–30]. Thus, differences in prolactin response to fenfluramine indicate a role not only for serotonin, but for specific 5HT receptor sites.

Using 60 mg of d,l-fenfluramine as the challenge agent, Coccaro et al. [31,32] found an inverse correlation between prolactin response and history of impulsive aggression among personality-disordered individuals. Furthermore, an inverse correlation was also found between prolactin response and past suicidal behavior across both mood- and personality-disordered participants. No relationship between impulsive aggression and prolactin response was found for mood-disordered patients. The authors felt this last finding was consistent with animal research showing that reduced NE levels (common among mood-disordered individuals) partially inhibits the aggression-facilitating effects of 5HT [33].

The relationship between blunted prolactin response and increased history of aggression has been replicated in studies using personality-disordered subjects [27,34–36], alcoholic subjects [37,38], sociopaths [39], and healthy volunteers [40]. A reduced prolactin response has also been found among individuals with histories of suicidal and other self-injurious behaviors [41]. However, some populations have not shown the predicted relationship between prolactin response and history of aggressive behavior. Both Fishbein et al. [42] and Bernstein and Handlesman [43] found a positive relationship between prolactin response to fenfluramine and past instances of aggression among nonalcoholic drug abusers. The reason for these findings is unclear. One speculation is that the habitual drug abuse may have sufficiently altered the neurochemistry of the brain to modify the relationship between 5HT indices and impulsive aggression.

Neuropharmacological 5HT challenges using children as subjects has also yielded inconsistent results, with some studies showing prolactin response positively correlating with aggression [44,45], one study showing an inverse correlation between prolactin response and aggression [46], and other studies showing no significant relationship between the two [47,48]. Again, the reason for the disparity is unclear. It is possible that systems that regulate 5HT's effect on aggression are not fully developed in prepubescent children. However, this is only speculative. More research is needed to elucidate the relationship between 5HT and aggression among both children and adult substance abusers.

The majority of findings from the neuropharmacological challenges support the conceptualization that reduced 5HT activity is associated with increased aggression. In contrast, results from CSF-HIAA studies were equivocal. To resolve this discrepancy, Coccaro et al. [20] examined prolactin responses to d,l-fenfluramine and m-CPP (a 5HT2 agonist) in addition to measuring basal CSF-5HIAA levels in personality-disordered subjects. Results indicated that prolactin response to d,l-fenfluramine and m-CPP were each inversely correlated with history of aggression. However, basal CSF-5HIAA levels did not correlate with aggression, and inversely correlated with prolactin response to d,l-fenfluramine. This suggests that receptor sensitivity rather than basal CSF-5HIAA levels may be key in modulating aggression, particularly among individuals without acts of severe aggression.

Most studies of aggression, including the majority of studies cited in this chapter, rely on self-report questionnaires and/or interviews to provide an index of aggression. Retrospective self-report measures are subject to multiple sources of error including social desirability, over- or underreporting, lying, and response set issues [49], and thus may not provide a valid estimate of aggression. Fortunately, behavioral measures of aggression exist that provide a directly observable sample of aggressive responding. The two most commonly used laboratory measures of aggression are the Point Subtraction Aggression Paradigm [50] and the Taylor Aggression Paradigm [51]. Both occur in the context of a (faux) social interaction, and use provocation as a means to elicit aggression. The PSAP operationalizes aggression as the number of times a participant chooses a response, which he believes will to cause his opponent to lose money. The TAP operationalizes aggression as the level of electrical shock administered to an opponent. Both measures have been shown to correlate highly with aggressive behavior in naturalistic settings [52].

Laboratory measures of aggression have generally supported the hypothesis that 5HT functioning modulates aggressive behavior. Studies using healthy volunteers showed that short-term reduction in brain 5HT via dietary tryptophan depletion resulted in increased aggressive responding on laboratory aggression measures, whereas dietary tryptophan supplementation had an inhibiting effect on aggression [53–56]. Acute increase of 5HT levels through the use of the 5HT agonists d,lfenfluramine [29], eltoprazine [57], and paroxetine [58] also resulted in a reduction in aggressive responding on laboratory aggression tasks compared to placebo. These results support the CSF-5HIAA and neuropharmacological challenge studies implicating 5HT in the regulation of aggression. Furthermore, they suggest that the use of medications that increase 5HT (e.g., lithium, SSRIs) may be beneficial in reducing aggressive behavior.

Lithium was the first psychotropic agent to have empirically supported antiaggressive properties, showing that it reduced impulsive (but not premeditated) aggression among prison inmates [4]. These findings have been replicated and extended to children with conduct disorder, and other mentally ill populations [59,60]. It has been hypothesized that lithium enhances 5HT function [61], though other studies suggest that 5HT may not be responsible for lithium's antiaggressive effects [62].

Selective serotonin reuptake inhibitors (SSRIs), the first line of treatment for most forms of unipolar depression, are believed to exert their effect by increasing the levels of 5HT in the synaptic terminals, resulting in increased 5HT functioning. As SSRIs predominantly affect 5HT, they should theoretically be effective in treating individuals with recurrent impulsive aggression. Controlled studies using personality-disordered patients with a history of impulsive aggression [63], borderline personality-disordered patients [64], depressed patients with a history of anger attacks [65], and adults with autism [66] all have shown reduced physical and/or verbal aggression in response to SSRIs as compared to placebo. Furthermore, a number of atypical antipsychotics that are believed to affect 5HT2 receptors have been found to reduce aggressive behavior over and above their palliative effects on psychotic symptoms [67–70].

B. Other Neurotransmitters

Compared to 5HT, few studies have examined the role of norepinephrine (NE) and dopamine (DA) in the expression of aggressive behaviors. Some animal research has suggested that increased NE facilitates aggression [71]. One of the earliest studies in neurotransmitter function and aggression [6] found that history of aggressive behavior positively correlated with the CSF-MHPG, the major metabolite of NE. Though the magnitude of this relationship was very small in comparison to the variance accounted for by CSF-5HIAA, it still suggest that NE may have at a minimum an auxiliary role in the regulation of aggressive behavior. Other studies using CSF-MHPG [11], NE plasma concentrations [34], and NE neuropharmacological challenges [72] have also suggested a relationship between increased NE and increased impulsive aggression and irritability, though failed attempts at replication have also occurred [12,13].

Additional evidence indicates that NE facilitates aggression comes from pharmacological trials, which have shown that beta-noradrenergic blockers propanolol or nadolol reduce aggressive behavior in patients with traumatic brain injuries [73,74], dementia [75], and chronic psychiatric inpatients [76–78]. The role of NE in aggression has yet to be fully determined, though the current findings suggest that NE may serve a supportive function in the regulation of aggression.

Research evaluating the role of DA in the regulation of aggression has also been lacking. The few studies that examined DA and aggression have yielded inconsistent results. Some studies have documented an inverse relationship between aggression and level of homovanillic acid (HVA) in the CSF among violent offenders [12], individuals with antisocial personality disorder [8], and abstinent alcoholics and healthy volunteers [79]. However, other studies were unable to find any relationship between CSF-HVA and aggression [6,11]. Adding to the confusion, it has been postulated that the significant findings were secondary to 5HT's regulation of both aggression and CSF-HVA [80]. However, this is still a matter of debate [81], and the role of DA in the expression of aggression remains undefined.

C. Neuropeptides and Neurosteroids

Neuropeptides and neurosteroids have multiple functions in the central nervous system (CNS). They may act as neurohormones, as neuromodulators, or even as neurotransmitters alone or in conjunction with other neurotransmitters. Because of their role in, among other things, social behavior, sexual behavior, stress, and pain, they are of interest in studies of aggression.

Vasopressin is a neuropeptide that has been shown to facilitate aggressive behavior in lower animals [82]. Among humans the evidence mixed. Coccaro et al. [83] found that increased levels of CSF vasopressin positively correlated with past aggressive behaviors in a sample of personality-disordered men. In contrast, Virkkunen et al. [13] found no difference in CSF vasopressin levels among impulsive and nonimpulsive violent offenders. Coccaro et al. [83] suggested the inconsistency between his finding and those of Virkkunen et al. [13] may be a function of the different populations sampled. Without additional research, any conclusions are speculative.

Increased levels of endogenous opiates have been linked to aggressive and self-aggressive behavior. Suicide victims have been found to have increased mu-opioid receptors [84], circulating metenkephalin levels have correlated with acts of self-aggressive behaviors [85], and opiate blockers appear to reduce self-aggression [86]. Participants receiving oral morphine also showed increased aggressive behavior when compared to a participant's receiving placebo [87], and increased levels of CSF opiate binding proteins were found among healthy volunteers with higher levels of "assaultiveness" [88].

Testosterone levels have often been associated with increased aggression [89], particularly in men [90]. Plasma testosterone levels have been reported to be higher in populations characterized by aggressive behavior. Alcoholic men with a history of domestic violence were found to have higher levels of plasma testosterone than a comparison group that did not engage in domestic violence [91].

There may be an interaction between testosterone level and type of aggression. One study found that CSF free testosterone was related to aggression only among criminal offenders who exhibit both violent behaviors that are both antisocial and impulsive [13]. Anecdotal reports have suggested that ingestion of exogenous testosterone produces an increase in impulsive violence. Unfortunately, no controlled studies have been able to experimentally examine this relationship.

Cortisol is believed to be associated with decreased aggression, though the actual evidence appears mixed. Cortisol has been negatively correlated with testosterone in healthy volunteers [92]. Furthermore, plasma cortisol was decreased among alcoholics with a history of repeated domestic violence [91], and decreased levels of free cortisol were also found among a group of antisocial violent offenders [93]. However, the same study found that cortisol levels were unrelated to non-antisocial aggression. Nonhuman primate studies have actually shown increased cortisol levels in association with aggressive competition for alpha status. Furthermore, studies of children have shown that both increased [94] and decreased [95] cortisol levels were associated with aggressive or disruptive behavior.

D. Cholesterol

Decreased cholesterol has been implicated in the facilitation of impulsive aggressive and self-aggressive behaviors. Virkkunen [96,97] demonstrated that impulsive violent offenders have reduced levels of serum cholesterol. These results were also extended to include individuals with a history of suicidal behavior [98–101]. A meta-analysis of cholesterol reducing agents associated them with increased likelihood of death as a result violence or suicide [102]. One study did find that among adolescents admitted to a psychiatric inpatient unit, serum cholesterol was positively correlated suicidal ideation [103]. Despite this contradictory finding, the majority of evidence reviewed seems to favor an inverse relationship between aggression/self-aggression and serum cholesterol.

E. Neurochemical Correlates of Aggression: Summary

Serotonin has been hypothesized to exhibit inhibitory control over aggressive impulses. The studies reviewed generally support this hypothesis. Aggression is associated with blunted responses to 5HT challenges and, at least among the very violent, decreased CSF-5HIAA levels. Laboratory measures show increased aggression in response to 5HT deprivation and reduced aggression in response to use of SSRIs or tryptophan loading, and controlled studies indicate that SSRIs have also been successfully used to treat pathological aggression. Pharmacological challenges and clinical drug trials suggest that NE may also affect aggression by facilitating its expression.

Among the other neurochemicals reviewed, endogenous opiates have been found to facilitate aggressive behavior. Testosterone has also been associated with increased aggression, particularly in men who demonstrate antisocial and impulsive violence. In contrast, serum cholesterol levels were inversely related to aggression. Once some of the neurotransmitters and other neuromodulaters associated with the regulation of aggression have been identified, emphasis can switch to locating the cortical and subcortical structures where these neurochemicals exert their effect.

III. NEUROANATOMICAL CORRELATES OF AGGRESSION

Neuropsychological and neuroimaging studies suggest that a number of specific brain structures are involved in the regulation of aggressive behavior. Among these, the prefrontal cortex area, including the orbitofrontal and ventral medial cortex, appears to be of particular importance. Research has also implicated the temporal cortex, cingulate cortex, and amygdala in the regulation of aggression.

A. Prefrontal Cortex

The prefrontal and orbitofrontal cortex has been associated with the modulation of aggressive impulses since the case of Phineas Gage [104]. Since then numerous clinical studies have found an association between lesions in the prefrontal-orbitofrontal cortex and dysregulation of aggressive impulses [e.g., 105–109]. Neurologic patients with orbitofrontal cortex damage also show irritability and aggressiveness [110,111]. The orbitofrontal cortex is also involved in olfactory identification, and it was recently shown that combat veterans diagnosed with PTSD were less proficient at olfactory identification than a combat-exposed control group [112], suggesting involvement of the orbitofrontal cortex in PTSD, a disorder often accompanied by anger dyscontrol. PET studies have shown reduced metabolic activity in the prefrontal-orbitofrontal cortex of violent criminals [113,114], and among personality-disordered individuals, regional glucose metabolism to the orbitofrontal cortex was negatively correlated with life history of aggression.

B. Amygdala

The amygdala is involved with evaluations of potential threat [115]. Stimulation of the amygdala has been associated with aggressive attacks in both humans and animals [116], and amygdalotomy has been found to reduce aggressive attacks among patients with intractable aggression [117]. Rich connections exist between the amygdala and prefrontal cortex. It has been suggested that one way in which the prefrontal cortex may modulate aggression is via inhibition of the amygdala. No direct imaging studies of the amygdala have been performed. However, Raine et al.'s [118] PET study of murderers found both reduced glucose metabolism in the prefrontal cortex and increased glucose metabolism in subcortical areas, which could include the amygdala.

C. Temporal Lobe

Temporal lobe dysfunction has also been linked to aggression. Aggressive outbursts have been associated with seizure activity among patients with temporal lobe epilepsy [119]. Temporal lobe lesions have also been associated with violent behavior in criminal [120,121] and noncriminal [122] populations. Furthermore, PET studies have repeatedly shown reduced metabolic activity in the temporal lobes for psychiatric patients with recurrent acts of violence [123,124]. One study also showed that temporal lobe metabolic activity was inversely correlated with life history of aggression among personality-disordered patients [125].

D. Brain Structures and 5HT

Prefrontal, temporal, and limbic structures all appear to play a role in the regulation of aggression. All of these areas are heavily innervated by 5HT neurons, suggesting that decreased 5HT transmissions in these areas are largely responsible for the biological component of aggression dysregulation. There is empirical support for this theory. Siever et al. [126] compared brain metabolic activity of personality-disordered patients with impulsive aggression to nonaggressive controls after administration of d,l-fenfluramine. Compared to the control group, individuals with impulsive aggression showed reduced cerebral glucose metabolism in the orbitofrontal, ventral medial, and cingulate cortex. Both groups showed increased metabolic activity in the inferior parietal lobe in response to the neuropharmacological challenge, suggesting some structural specificity for reduced 5HT in aggressive individuals. These results were replicated comparing a sample of patients with borderline personality disorder to normal controls [127].

E. Neuroanatomical Correlates of Aggression: Summary

Neuroanatomical findings suggest that areas of the brain richly innervated with 5HT neurons (e.g., the orbitofrontal cortex, limbic cortex, temporal lobe) appear to regulate aggression. This is consistent with the neurobiological research showing a primary role for 5HT in the regulation of aggression. If abnormalities in 5HT functioning in temporal, limbic, and/or prefrontal cortex contribute to pathological aggression, the question remains to what extent are these abnormalities are heritable, developmental, or acquired.

IV. GENETIC STUDIES OF AGGRESSION

As stated earlier, aggression is a complex, multidetermined behavior whose expression is likely affected by numerous environmental and biological factors, as well as the exponential interactions between the two. Behavioral genetic studies are useful in that they provide a rough estimate of the extent to which inherited biological factors may influence expression of a behavior.

A. Twin Studies

Twins studies examine the relative concordance rates of monozygotic (MZ) and dizygotic (DZ) siblings in the expression of a behavior to estimate the heritability for that behavior. Twin studies have generally yielded variable results ranging from findings that genetic influences account for close to 50% of the variance in aggression [128,129], to failing to find a significant increase in the concordance of MZ twins as compared to DZ twins for aggressive behavior [130,131].

One study that examined aggression amongst a population of male twins found that the heritability of aggression is a function of the type and severity of the aggressive acts committed [132]. Life history of verbal aggression, often considered a milder form of aggression was shown to have a heritability estimate of 28%. In contrast, life history of direct physical aggression (e.g., fist fights) had a heritability estimate of 47%. This suggests that tendencies toward physical aggression may be significantly influenced by biological factors, whereas verbal outbursts are less so.

B. Molecular Genetics

Evidence for abnormalities at the gene level which could transmit traits of increased aggression has been somewhat confusing. The most studied DNA polymorphism is within the noncoding region of the tryptophan hydroxylase (TPH) gene. TPH is the rate-limiting enzyme in the synthesis of serotonin, putatively involved in the expression and regulation of impulsive aggression. Nielson et al. [133] reported that impulsive violent offenders with one or two copies of the TPH "L" allele had significantly lower CSF concentrations of CSF 5HIAA than to impulsive violent offenders with two copies of the "U" allele. The "L" allele in impulsive and nonimpulsive violent offenders was associated with a greater frequency of past suicide attempt (LL 65% vs. LU 53% vs. UU 17%, $P < .02$). In fact, almost all of the offenders who attempted suicide had either the LL or UL genotype, independent of CSF 5HIAA levels. TPH genotype was not associated with psychiatric diagnosis such as affective or anxiety disorders. Although Nielsen et al. [134] replicated his finding in a study of 804 Finnish alcoholic offenders, and there has been an independent replication by New [41], there have been nonreplicating studies published as well [135–137], correlating the more common U allele with suicidality and/or aggression or not finding a correlation [Coccaro, unpublished data]. The reason for these failures to replicate the original findings may be related to the fact that the polymorphism is on the noncoding region of the TPH gene. Hence, it may be in linkage dysequilibrium with an unknown polymorphism in some study populations, but not in others [138]. An association between antisocial alcoholism and the C allele biallelic polymorphism of the 5HT-1d-beta receptor has been found [139]. Antisocial alcoholism is alcohol abuse along with antisocial personality disorder or intermittent explosive disorder. Violence in schizophrenics has been associated with a "low-activity" allele of a biallelic polymorphism for COMT in schizophrenics by Strous [140] with replication by Lachman [141].

C. Genetic Studies of Aggression: Summary

Though results are inconsistent, is appears that ~ 30–50% of variance in aggressive behavior may be attributable to biogenetic factors, with more severe forms of aggression having a stronger heritability. Future advances in molecular genetics may lead to the identification of specific combination of genes that account for these biogenetic factors.

V. CONCLUSIONS

Findings from neurobiological studies have increasingly implicated serotonin in the regulation of aggressive behavior. Data from CSF studies, neuropharmacological challenges, 5HT depletion studies, and controlled pharmacological treatment trials, all provide evidence that decreased levels of 5HT is associated with increased acts of aggression, especially impulsive aggression. Decreased 5HT receptor responsivity may also be implicated in pathological aggression. Finally, neuroanatomical research data suggest 5HT exhibits its antiaggressive effects via synapses in the orbitofrontal, prefrontal, temporal, and limbic cortex. Information about the role of other neurochemicals is still limited, but evidence is emerging that other neurotransmitters and modulators may also assist in the regulation of aggression.

REFERENCES

1. Reiss AJ, Miczek KA, Roth JA. Understanding and Preventing Violence, Vol. 2. Biobehavioral Influences. Washington: National Academy Press, 1994.
2. Haapasalo J, Tremblay R. Physically aggressive boys from ages 6 to 12: family background, parenting behavior, and prediction of delinquency. J Consult Clin Psychol 1994; 62(5):1044–1052.
3. Coccaro EF. Intermittent explosive disorder. Curr Psychiatry Rep 2000; 2:67–71.
4. Sheard M, Manini J, Bridges C, Wapner A. The effect of lithium on impulsive aggressive behavior in man. Am J Psychiatry 1976; 133:1409–1413.
5. Asberg M, Traksman L, Thoren P. 5HIAA in the cerebrospinal fluid: a biochemical suicide predictor? Arch Gen Psychiatry 1976; 33:1193–1197.
6. Brown GL, Goodwin FK, Ballenger JC, Goyer PF, Major LF. Aggression in human correlates with cerebrospinal fluid amine metabolites. Psychiatry Res 1979; 1:131–139.
7. Brown GL, Ebert MH, Goyer PF, et al. Aggression, suicide, and serotonin: relationships to CSF amine metabolites. Am J Psychiatry 1982; 139:741–746.
8. Linnoila M, Virkkunen M, Scheinin M, Nuutila A, Rimon R, Goodwin FK. Low cerebrospinal fluid 5-hydroxylndolacetic acid concentration differentiates impulsive from nonimpulsive violent behavior. Life Sci 1983; 33:2609–2614.

9. Lidberg L, Tuck JR, Asberg M, Scalia-Tomba GP, Bertilsson L. Homicide, suicide and CSF 5HIAA. Acta Psychiatr Scand 1985; 71:230–236.
10. Virkkunen M, Goldman D, Linnoila M. Serotonin in alcoholic violent offenders. Ciba Found Symp 1996; 194:168–177.
11. Virkkunen M, Nuutila A, Goodwin FK, Linnoila M. Cerebrospinal fluid monoamine metabolite levels in male arsonists [published erratum appears in Arch Gen Psychiatry 1989; 46(10):960]. Arch Gen Psychiatry 1987; 44:241–247.
12. Virkkunen M, De Jong J, Bartko J, Linnoila M. Psychobiological concomitants of history of suicide attempts among violent offenders and impulsive fire setters [published erratum appears in Arch Gen Psychiatry 1989; 46(10):913]. Arch Gen Psychiatry 1989; 46:604–606.
13. Virkkunen M, Rawlings R, Tokola R, Poland RE, Guidotti A, Ncmcroff C, Bissette G, Kalogeras K, Karonen SL, Linnoila M. CSF biochemistries, glucose metabolism, and diurnal activity rhythms in alcoholic, violent offenders, fire setters, and healthy volunteers. Arch Gen Psychiatry 1994; 51:20–27.
14. Higley JD, Mehlman PT, Taub DM, Higley SB, Suomi SJ, Vickers JH, Linnoila M. Cerebrospinal fluid monoamine and adrenal correlates of aggression in free-ranging rhesus monkeys [published erratum appears in Arch Gen Psychiatry 1992; 49(10):773]. Arch Gen Psychiatry 1992; 49:436–441.
15. Westergaard GC, Suomi SJ, Higley JD, Mehlman PT. CSF 5HIAA and aggression in female macaque monkeys: species and interindividual differences. Psychopharmacology 1999; 146:440–44.
16. Gardner DL, Lucas PB, Cowdry RW. CSF metabolites in borderline personality disorder compared with normal controls. Biol Psychiatry 1990; 28:247–254.
17. Castellanos FX, Elia J, Kreusi MJP, Gulotta CS, Mefford IN, Potter WZ, Ritchie GF, Rapoport JL. Cerebrospinal fluid monoamine metabolites in boys with attention deficit hyperactivity disorder. Psychiatry Res 1994; 52:305–316.
18. Moller SE, Mortensen EL, Breum L, Alling C, Larsen OG, Boge-Rasmussen T, Jensen C, Bennicke K. Aggression and personality: association with amino acids and monoamine metabolites. Psychol Med 1996; 26:323–331.
19. Coccaro EF, Kavoussi RJ, Trestman RL, Gabriel SM, Cooper TB, Siever LJ. Serotonin function in personality and mood disorder: intercorrelations among central indices and aggressiveness. Psychiatry Res 1997; 73:1–14.
20. Coccaro EF, Kavoussi RJ, Cooper TB, Hauger RL. Central serotonin and aggression: inverse relationship with prolactin response to d-fenfluramine, but not with CSF 5HIAA concentration in human subjects. Am J Psychiatry 1997; 154:1430–1435.
21. Balaban E, Alper JS, Kasamon YL. Mean genes and the biology of aggression: a critical review of recent animal and human research. J Neurogenet 1996; 11:1–43.
22. Berman ME, Tracy JI, Coccaro EF. The serotonin hypothesis of aggression revisited. Clin Psychol Rev 1997; 17(6):651–665.
23. Coccaro EF. Neurotransmitter correlates of impulsive aggression in humans. Ann NY Acad Sci 1996; 794:82–89.
24. Quattrone A, Tedeschi G, Aguglia U, Scopacasa F, Direnzo GF, Annunziato L. Prolactin secretion in man: a useful tool to evaluate the activity of drugs on central 5-hydroxytryptaminergic neurons. Studies with fenfluramine. Br J Clin Pharmacol 1983; 16:471–475.
25. Coccaro EF, Kavoussi RJ, Oakes M, Cooper TB, Hauger R. 5HT2a/2c receptor blockade by amesergide fully attenuates prolactin response to d-fenfluramine challenge in physically healthy human subjects. Psychopharmacology (Berl) 1996; 126:24–30.
26. Albinsson A, Palazidou E, Stephenson J, Andersson G. Involvement of the 5HT-2 receptor in the 5HT receptor-mediated stimulation of prolactin release. Eur J Pharmacol 1994; 251:157–161.
27. Park SBG, Cowen PJ. Effect of pindolol on the prolactin response to d-fenfluramine. Psychopharmacology 1995; 118:471–474.
28. Coccaro EF, Gabriel S, Siever LJ. Buspirone challenge: preliminary evidence for a role for 5HT-1a receptors in impulsive aggressive behavior in humans. Psychopharmacol Bull 1990; 26:393–405.
29. Cherek DR, Moeller FG, Khan-Dawwod F, Swann A, Lane SD. Prolactin response to buspirone was reduced in violent compared to non-violent parolees. Psychopharmacology 1999; 142:144–148.
30. Coccaro EF, Kavoussi RJ, Hauger RL. Physiologic responses to d-fenfluramine and ipsapirone challenge correlate with indices of aggression in males with personality disorder. Int Clin Psychopharmacol 1995; 10:177–180.
31. Coccaro EF, Kavoussi RJ, Trestman RL, Gabriel SM, Cooper TB, Siever LJ. Serotonin function in personality and mood disorder: intercorrelations among central indices and aggressiveness. Psychiatry Res 1997; 73:1–14.
32. Coccaro EF, Siever LJ, Klar HM, Maurer G, Cochrane K, Mohs RC, Davis KL. Serotonergic studies in affective and personality disorder: correlates with suicidal and impulsive aggressive behavior. Arch Gen Psychiatry 1989; 46:587–599.
33. Hodge GK, Butcher LL. Catecholamine correlates of isolation-induced aggression in mice. Eu J Pharmacol 1975; 31:81–93.
34. Siever L, Trestman RL. The serotonin system and aggressive personality disorder. Int Clin Psychopharmacol 1993; 8(suppl 2):33–39.

35. Stein D, Trestman RL, Mitropoulou V. Impulsivity and serotonergic function in compulsive personality disorder. J Neuropsychiatry Clin Neurosci 1996; 8:393–398.
36. Coccaro EF, Berman ME, Kavoussi RJ, Hauger RL. Relationship of prolactin response to d-fenfluramine to behavioral and questionnaire assessments of aggression in personality-disordered men. Biol Psychiatry 1996; 40:157–164.
37. Moss HB, Yao JK, Panzak GL. Serotonergic responsivity and behavioral dimensions in antisocial personality disorder with substance abuse. Biol Psychiatry 1990; 28:325–338.
38. Handlesman L, Holloway K, Kahn RS, et al. Hostility is associated with a low prolactin response to meta-chlorophenylpiperazine in abstinent alcoholics. Alcohol Clin Exp Res 1996; 20:824–829.
39. O'Keane V, Loloney E, O'Neil H, O'Connor A, Smith C, Dinam TB. Blunted prolactin responses to d-fenfluramine challenge in sociopathy: evidence for subsensitivity of central serotonergic function. Br J Psychiatry 1992; 160:643–646.
40. Manuck SB, Flory JD, McCaffery JM, Matthews KA, Mann JJ, Muldoon MF. Aggression, impulsivity, and central nervous system serotonergic responsivity in a nonpatient sample. Neurpsychopharmacology 1998;19:287–299.
41. New AS, Trestman RL, Mitropoulou V, Benishay DS, Coccaro E, Silverman J, Siever LJ. Serotonergic function and self-injurious behavior in personality disorder patients. Psychiatry Res 1997; 69:17–26.
42. Fishbein DH, Lozovsky D, Jaffe JH. Impulsivity, aggression, and neuroendocrine responses to serotonergic stimulation in substance abusers. Biol Psychiatry 1989; 25:1049–1066.
43. Bernstein DP, Handlesman L. The neurobiology of substance abuse and personality disorders. In: Ratey JJ, ed. Neuropsychiatry of Behavior Disorders. Cambridge: Blackwell Scientific Publications 1995:120–148.
44. Halperin JM, Sharma V, Siever LJ, Schwartz ST, Matier K, Wornell G, Newcorn JH. Serotonergic function in aggressive and nonaggressive boys with attention deficit hyperactivity disorder. Am J Psychiatry 1994; 151:243–248.
45. Pine DS, Coplan JD, Wasserman GA et al. Neuroendocrine response to d,l-fenfluramine challenge in boys: associations with aggressive behavior and adverse rearing. Arch Gen Psychiatry 1997; 54:839–846.
46. Donovan AM, Halperin JM, Newcorn, Sharma V. Thermal response to serotonergic challenge and aggression in attention-deficit hyperactivity disorder children. J Child Adolesc Psychopharmacol 1999; 9:85–91.
47. Stoff DM, Pastiempo AP, Yeung JH, Cooper TB, Bridger WH, Rabinovich H. Neuroendocrine responses to challenge with d,l-fenfluramine and aggression in disruptive behavior disorders of children and adolescents. Psychiatry Res 1992; 43:263–276.
48. Halperin JM, Newcorn JH, Schwartz ST, et al. Age-related changes in the association between serotonergic function and aggression in boys with ADHD. Biol Psychiatry 1997; 41:682–689.
49. Piedmont RL, McCrae RR, Riemann R, Angleitner A. On the invalidity of validity scales: evidence from self-reports and observer ratings in volunteer samples. J Pers Soc Psychol 2000; 78:582–593.
50. Cherek DR, Moeller G, Schnapp W, Dougherty DM. Studies of violent and non-violent male parolees. I. Laboratory and psychometric measurements of aggression. Biol Psychiatry 1997; 41:514–522.
51. Taylor SP. Aggressive behavior and physiological arousal as a function of provocation and the tendency to inhibit aggression. J Pers 1967; 35:297–310.
52. Anderson CA., Bushman, BJ. External validity of "trivial" experiments: the case of laboratory aggression. Rev Gen Psychol 1997; 1(1):19–41.
53. Pihl R-O, Young S, Harden P, Plotnick S, Chamberlain B, Ervin FR. Acute effect of altered tryptophan levels and alcohol on aggression in normal human males. Psychopharmacology 1995; 119:353–360.
54. Cleare AJ, Bond AJ. The effect of tryptophan depletion and enhancement on subjective and behavioural aggression in normal male subjects. Psychopharmacology 1995; 118:72–81.
55. Moeller FG, Dougherty DM, Swann AC, et al. Tryptophan depletion and aggressive responding in healthy males. Psychopharmacology 1996; 126:97–103.
56. Dougherty DM, Bjork JM, Marsh DM, Moeller FG. Influence of trait hostility on tryptophan depletion-induced laboratory aggression. Psychiatry Res 1999; 88:227–232.
57. Cherek DR, Spiga R, Creson DL. Acute effects of eltoprazine on aggressive and point-maintained responding of normal male participants: phase I study. Exp Clin Psychopharmacol 1995; 3:287–293.
58. McCloskey M, Berman M, Posey P, Crawford V. Coccaro E. Experimental investigation of the serotonin hypothesis of aggression. Convention of the International Society for Aggression Research, Mahwah, NJ, June 1998.
59. Campbell M, Adams PB, Small AM, et al. Lithium in hospitalized aggressive children with conduct disorder: a double-blind and placebo-controlled study. J Am Acad Child Adolesc Psychiatry 1995; 34:445–453.

60. Craft M, Ismail IA, Krishnamurti D, et al. Lithium in the treatment of aggression in mentally handicapped patients. A double-blind trial. Br J Psychiatry 1987; 150:685–689.
61. McCance SL, Cohen PR, Cowen PR. Lithium increases 5HT mediated prolactin release. Psychopharmacology 1989; 99:276–281.
62. Hughes JH, Dunne F, Young AH. Effects of acute tryptophan depletion on mood and suicidal ideation in bipolar patients symptomatically stable on lithium. Br J Psychiatry 2000; 177:447–451.
63. Coccaro EF, Kavoussi RJ. Fluoxetine and impulsive aggressive behavior in personality disordered subjects. Arch Gen Psychiatry 1997; 54:1081–1088.
64. Salzman C, Wolfson AN, Schatzberg A, et al. Effect of fluoxetine on anger in symptomatic volunteers with borderline personality disorder. J Clin Psychopharmacol 1995; 15:23–29.
65. Fava M, Rosenbaum JF, Pava JA, McCarthy MK, Steingard RJ, Bouffides E. Anger attacks in unipolar depression. Part 1. Clinical correlates and response to fluoxetine treatment. Am J Psychiatry 1993; 150:1158–1163.
66. McDougle CJ, Naylor ST, Cohen DJ, et al. A double-blind, placebo-controlled study of fluoxatine in adults with autistic disorder. Arch Gen Psychiatry 1996; 53:1001–1008.
67. Buckley P, Bartell J, Donenwirth K, et al. Violence and schizophrenia: clozapine as a specific antiaggressive agent. Bull Am Acad Psychiatry Law 1995; 23:607–611.
68. Rabinowitz J, Avnon M, Rosenberg V. Effect of clozapine on physical and verbal aggression. Schizophr Res 1996; 22:249–255.
69. Ratey JJ, Leveroni C, Kilmer D, et al. The effects of clozapine on severely aggressive psychiatric inpatients in a state hospital. J Clin Psychiatry 1993; 54:219–223.
70. Czobor P, Volavka J, Meibach RC. Effect of risperidone on hostility in schizophrenia J Clin Psychopharmacol 1995; 15:243–249.
71. Barrett JA, Edinger H, Siegel A. Intrahypothalamic injections of norepinephrine facilitate feline affective aggression via alpha-2 adrenoceptors. Brain Res 1990; 525:285–293.
72. Coccaro EF, Lawrence T, Trestman R, Gabriel S, Klar HM, Siever L. Growth hormone responses to intravenous clonidine challenge correlates with behavioral irritability in psychiatric patients and in healthy volunteers. Psychiatry Res 1991; 39:129–139.
73. Yudofsky S, Williams D, Gorman J. Propranolol in the treatment of rage and violent behavior in patients with chronic brain syndromes. Am J Psychiatry 1981; 138:218–220.
74. Brooke MM, Patterson DR, Questad KA. The treatment of agitation during initial hospitalization after traumatic brain injury. Arch Phys Med Rehabil 1992; 73:917–921.
75. Shankle WR, Nielson KA, Cotman CW. Low-dose propranolol reduces aggression and agitation resembling that associated with orbitofrontal dysfunction in elderly demented patients. Alzheimer Dis Assoc Disord 1995; 9:233–237.
76. Sorgi PJ, Ratey JJ, Polakoff S. Beta adrenergic blockers for the control of aggressive behaviors in patients with chronic schizophrenia. Am J Psychiatry 1986; 143:775–776.
77. Ratey JJ, Sorgi P, O'Driscoll GA, et al. Nadolol to treat aggression and psychiatric symptomatology in chronic psychiatric inpatients: a double-blind, placebo-controlled study. J Clin Psychiatry 1992; 53:41–46.
78. Kravitz HM, Haywood TW, Kelly J, et al. Medroxyprogesterone treatment for paraphiliacs. Bull Am Acad Psychiatry Law 1995; 23:19–33.
79. Limson R, Goldman D, Roy A, Lamparski D, Ravitz B, Adinoff B, Linnoila M. Personality and cerebrospinal fluid monoamine metabolites in alcoholics and controls. Arch Gen Psychiatry 1991; 48:437–441.
80. Agren H, Mefford IN, Rudorfer MV, et al. Interacting neurotransmitter systems: a non-experimental approach to the 5HIAA-HVA correlation in human CSF. J Psychiatr Res 1986; 20:175–193.
81. Kuikka JT, Tiihonen J, Bergstrom KA, et al. Abnormal structure of human striatal dopamine re-uptake sites in habitually violent alcoholic offenders: a fractal analysis. Neurosci Lett 1998; 253(3):195–197.
82. Ferris CF, Delville Y, Irvin RW, Potegal M. Septo-hypothalamic organization of a stereotyped behavior controlled by vasopressin in golden hamsters. Physiol Behav 1994; 55:755–759.
83. Coccaro EF, Kavoussi RJ, Hauger RL, Cooper TB, Ferris CF Cerebrospinal fluid vasopressin: correlates with aggression and serotonin function in personality disordered subjects. Arch Gen Psychiatry 1998; 55:708–714.
84. Gross-Isseroff R, Dillon KA, Israeli M, et al. Regionally selective increases in mu opioid receptor density in the brains of suicide victims. Brain Res 1990; 530:312–316.
85. Coid J, Allolio B, Rees LH. Raised plasma metenkephalin in patients who habitually mutilate themselves. Lancet 1983; 2:545–546.
86. Sandman CA, Barron JL, Colman H. An orally administered opiate blocker, naltrexone, attenuates self-injurious behavior Am J Ment Retard 1990; 95(1):93–102.
87. Berman M, Taylor S, Marged B. Morphine and human aggression. Addict Behav 1993; 18(3):263–268.

88. Post RM, Pickar D, Ballenger JC, Naber D, Rubinow DR. Endogenous opiates in cerebrospinal fluid: relationship to mood and anxiety. In: Post RM, Ballenger JC eds. Neurobiology of Mood Disorders. Baltimore: Williams and Wilkins, 1984:356–368.
89. Archer J. The influence of testosterone on human aggression. Br J Psychology 1991; 82:1–28.
90. Moffitt T, Caspi A, Fawcett P, Brammer GL, Raleigh M., Yuwiler A, Silva P. Whole blood serotonin and family background relate to male violence. In: Raine A, Brennan PA, Farrington DP, Mednick SA, eds. Biosocial Bases of Violence. New York: Plenum Press, 1997:223–229.
91. Bergman B, Brismar B. Characteristics of imprisoned wife-beaters. Forens Sci Int 1994; 65(3):157–167.
92. Essman WB. Drug effects upon aggressive behavior. In: Valzelli I, Morgese I, eds. Aggression and Violence: A Psychobiological and Clinical Approach. Milan: Edizioni Saint Vincent, 1981:150–175.
93. Virkkunen M. Urinary free cortisol secretion in habitually violent offenders. Acta Psychiatr Scand 1985; 72:40–44.
94. Dettling AC, Gunnar MR, Donzella B. Cortisol levels of young children in full-day childcare centers: relations with age and temperament. Psychoneuroendocrinology 1999; 24(5):19–36.
95. McBurnett K, Lahey BB, Rathouz PJ, et al. Low salivary cortisol and persistent aggression in boys referred for disruptive behavior. Arch Gen Psychiatry 2000; 57(1)38–43.
96. Virkkunen M. Serum cholesterol in antisocial personality disorder. Neuropsychobiology 1979; 5:27–32.
97. Virkkunen M. Serum cholesterol in levels in homicidal offenders. A low cholesterol level is connected with a habitually violent tendency under the influence of alcohol. Neuropsychobiology 1983; 10:65–69.
98. Goier, JA, Marzuk PM, Leon AC, et al. Low serum cholesterol and attempted suicide. Am J Psychiatry 1996; 152:419–423.
99. Zureik M, Courbon D, Ducimetiere P. Serum cholesterol concentration and death from suicide in men: Paris prospective study I. BMJ 1996; 313:649–651.
100. Maes M, Sharpe P, D'Hondt P, et al. Biochemical metabolic and immune correlates of seasonal variation in violent suicide: a chronoepidemiologic study. Eur Psychiatry 1996; 11:21–33.
101. Kunugi H, Takei N, Aoki H, et al. Low serum cholesterol in suicide attempters. Biol Psychiatry 1997; 41(2):196–200.
102. Muldoon MF, Manuck SB, Matthews KA. Lowering cholesterol concentrations and mortality: a quantitative review of primary prevention trials [see comments]. BMJ 1990; 301:309–314.
103. WHO European Collaborative Group. European collaborative trial multi-factorial prevention of coronary heart disease. Final report on the 6-year results. Lancet 1986; 1:869–872.
104. Damasio H, Grabowski T, Frank R, et al. The return of Phineas Gage: clues about the brain from the skull of a famous patient. Science 1994; 264:1102–1105.
105. Damasio AR, Van Hoesen GW. Emotional disturbances associated with focal lesions of the limbic frontal lobe. In: Heilman KM, Satz P, eds. Neuropsychology of Human Emotion. New York: Guilford Press, 1983.
106. Grafman J, Vance S, Wingartner H, Salazar A, Amin D. The effects of lateralized frontal lesions on mood regulation. Brain 1986; 109:1127–1148.
107. Grafman J, Schwab K, Warden D, Pridgen A, Brown H, Salazar A. Frontal lobe injuries, violence, and aggression: a report of the Vietnam Head Injury Study. Neurology 1996; 4:1231–1238.
108. Volvaka J. Neurological, neuropsychological, and electrophysiological correlates of violent behavior. Neurobiology of Violence, Washington DC: American Psychiatric Press, 1995:77–122.
109. Anderson SW, Bechara A, Damasio H, et al. Impairment of social and moral behavior related to early damage in human prefrontal cortex. Nat Neurosci 1999; 2(11):1032–1037.
110. Weiger WA, Bear DM. An approach to the neurology of aggression. J Psychiatr Press 1988; 22:85–88.
111. Miller BL, Darby A, Benson DF, et al. Aggressive, socially disruptive and antisocial behaviour associated with fronto-temporal dementia. Br J Psychiatry 1997; 170:150–154.
112. Vasterling JJ, Brailey K, Sutker PB. Olfactory identification combat-related posttraumatic stress disorder. J Trauma Stress 2000; 13:241–253.
113. Raine A, Buchsbaum M, Stanley J, et al. Selective reductions in prefrontal glucose metabolism in murderers. Biol Psychiatry 1994; 36(6):365-373.
114. Raine A, Stoddard J, Bihrle S, Buchsbaum M. Prefrontal glucose deficits in murderers lacking psychosocial deprivation. Neuropsychiatry Neuropsychol Behav Neurol 1998; 11(1):1–7.
115. Adolphs R, Tranel D, Damasio AR. The human amygdala in social judgment. Nature 1998; 393:470–474.
116. Gregg TR, Siegel A. Brain structures and neurotransmitters regulating aggression in cats: implications for human aggression. Prog Neuropsychopharmacol Biol Psychiatry 2001; 25:91–140.
117. Lee GP, Bechara A, Adolphs R, et al. Clinical and physiological effects of sterotaxic bilateral amygdalotomy for intractable aggression. J Neuropsychiatry Clin Neurosci 1998; 10(4):413–420.

118. Raine A, Buchsbaum M, LaCasse L. Brain abnormalities in murderers indicated by positron emission tomography. Biol Psychiatry 1997; 42:495–508.
119. DeVinsky O, Bear D. Varieties of aggressive behavior in temporal lobe epilepsy. Am J Psychiatry 1984; 141:651–656.
120. Tonkonogy JM. Violence and temporal lobe lesion: head CT and MRI data. J Neuropsychiatry 1991; 3(2):189–196.
121. Tonkonogy JM, Geller JL. Hypothalamic lesions and intermittent explosive disorder. J Neuropsychiatry Clin Neurosci 1992; 4(1):45–50.
122. Martinius J. Homicide of an aggressive adolescent boy with right temporal lesion: a case report. Neurosci Biobehav Rev 1983; 7(3):419–422.
123. Volkow ND, Tancredi LR. Neural substrates of violent behavior: a preliminary study with positron emission tomography. Br J Psychiatry 1987; 151:668–673.
124. Volkow ND, Tancredi LR, Grant C, et al. Brain glucose metabolism in violent psychiatric patients: a preliminary study. Psychiatry Res 1995; 61(4):243–253.
125. Goyer PF, Andreason PJ, Semple WE, et al. Positron-emission-tomography and personality disorders. Neuropsychopharmacology 1994; 10(1):21–28.
126. Siever LJ, Buchsbaum MS, New AS, Spiegel-Cohen J, Wei T, Hazlett EA, Sevin E, Nunn M, Mitropoulou V. d,l-Fenfluramine response in impulsive personality disorder assessed with [^{18}F]fluorodeoxyglucose positron emission tomography. Neuropsychopharmacology 1999; 20:413–423.
127. Soloff PH, Meltzer CC, Greer PJ, Constantine D, Kelly TM. A fenfluramine-activated FDG-PET study of borderline personality disorder. Biol Psychiatry 2000; 47:540–547.
128. Tellegen A, Lykken DT, Bouchard TJ, Wilcox KJ, Segal NL, Rich S. Personality similarity in twins reared apart and together. J Pers Soc Psychol 1988; 54:1031–1039.
129. Rushton JP, Fulker DW, Neale MC, Nias DKB, Eysenk HJ. Altruism and aggression: the heritability of individual differences. J Pers Soc Psychol 1986; 50:1192–1198.
130. Vanderberg SG. The heredity abilities study: heredity components in a psychological test battery Am J Hum Genet 1962; 14:220–237.
131. Plomin R, Foch TT, Rowe DC. Bobo clown aggression in childhood: environment, not genes. J Res Pers 1981; 15:331–342.
132. Coccaro EF, Bergeman CS, Kavoussi RJ, Seroczynski AD. Heritability of aggression and irritability: a twin study of the Buss-Durkee aggression scales in adult male subjects. Biol Psychiatry 1997; 41:273–284.
133. Nielsen DA, Goldman D, Virkkunen M, Tokola R, Rawlings R, Linnoila M. Suicidality and 5-hydroxyindoleacetic acid concentration associated with a tryptophan hydroxylase polymorphism. Arch Gen Psychiatry 1994; 51:34–38.
134. Nielsen DA, Virkkunen M, Lappalainen J, Eggert M, Brown GL, Long JC, Goldman D, Linnoila M. A tryptophan hydroxylase gene marker for suicidality and alcoholism. Arch Gen Psychiatry 1998; 55:593–602.
135. Buresi C. Association between suicide attempt and the tryptophan hydroxylase (TPH) gene. Am J Hum Genet 1997; 61:A270.
136. Mann JJ, Malone KM, Nielsen DA, Goldman D, Erdos J, Gelernter J. Possible association of a polymorphism of the tryptophan hydroxylase gene with suicidal behavior in depressed patients. Am J Psychiatry 1997; 154:1451–1453.
137. Manuck SB, Flory JD, McCaffery JM, Matthews KA, Mann JJ, Muldoon MF. Aggression, impulsivity, and central nervous system serotonergic responsivity in a nonpatient sample. Neuropsychopharmacology 1998; 19:287–299.
138. Coccaro E, McNamee B. Biology of agresssion: relevance to crime. In: Skodol AE, ed. Psychopathology and Violent Crime. Washington: American Psychiatric Press, 1998:99–128.
139. Lappalainen J, Long JC, Eggert M, Ozaki N, Robin RW, Brown GL, Naukkarinen H, Virkkunen M, Linnoila M, Goldman D. Linkage of antisocial alcoholism to the serotonin 5HT1B receptor gene in 2 populations. Arch Gen Psychiatry 1998; 55:989–994.
140. Strous RD, Bark N, Parsia SS, Volavka J, Lachman HM. Analysis of a functional catechol-O-methyltransferase gene polymorphism in schizophrenia: evidence for association with aggressive and antisocial behavior. Psychiatry Res 1997; 69:71–77.
141. Lachman HM, Nolan KA, Mohr P, Saito T, Volavka J. Association between catechol O-methyltransferase genotype and violence in schizophrenia and schizoaffective disorder. Am J Psychiatry 1998; 155:835–837.

46

Pathological Gambling
Clinical Aspects and Neurobiology

MARC N. POTENZA
Yale University School of Medicine, New Haven, Connecticut, U.S.A.

I. INTRODUCTION

Gambling is a human behavior that has persisted throughout millennia and been documented in diverse cultures. Early records document gambling in ancient Egyptian, Japanese, and Persian societies [1,2], and similarly early accounts can be found of problematic gambling behaviors [3]. For example, in the Mahabharat, a central book of Hinduism, one character is described as gambling away his kingdom and his wife [4]. Historically, gambling has gone through periods of expansion and restriction. For example, in the 1700s and 1800s, it was not uncommon for public works (construction of bridges, roads, schools, hospitals, or churches) to be financed in part through lotteries or for travelers to resort in large, elegant European casinos [2]. In contrast, in the early 1900s, many forms of gambling were illegal or largely restricted in the United States.

Throughout these periods, although gambling was generally considered a moral vice, it remained a popular activity within the general population. Over the past several decades, many regions of the world, including the United States, have witnessed a rapid growth in legalized gambling. The introduction of state lotteries in New Hampshire in 1964 has been followed by a progressive growth in state-run and interstate lotteries such as Powerball [5]. A growth in casinos has been witnessed following the passing of legislature such as the Indian Gaming Regulatory Act in 1988 and that allowing for the introduction of riverboat casinos on the Mississippi in 1989 [5,6]. From 1976 to 1997, legalized gambling revenues in the United States have increased 1600% [6–8], and gambling ventures currently gross more than the motion picture, music, and theme park industries combined ($50 billion in 1998, with predictions of further increased growth in the near future) [5,8]. With the growth in legalized gambling there has been a concurrent increase in the prevalence rates of individuals with gambling disorders [9]. As such, there exists an increasing need for understanding the spectrum of gambling behaviors, the biological processes underlying the behaviors, the potential for associated adverse health consequences, and the ways in which prevention and treatment efforts can be utilized to promote improved clinical care [10].

II. DEFINTIONS

A. Gambling

Gambling by definition is placing something of value at risk in the hopes of gaining something of greater value. Gambling, like many routine daily processes, involves decision making based on the assessment of risk and reward. The centrality of risk- and reward-based decision-making processes to gambling might in part explain its persistence throughout time. In most forms of gambling, the risked item is money, and traditional forms of gambling include wagering on lotteries, card games, horse and dog racing, sports, and slot machines. Newer forms of gambling, such as Internet gambling, appear to be growing in popularity, with current estimates suggesting Internet gambling revenues to reach $2.3 billion by the end of 2001 [11]. Internet gambling might present an increase risk for abuse given the ready access, rapidity of action, ability to be used in isolation, and difficulties in regulating usage.

B. Problem Gambling and Pathological Gambling

Excessive gambling has been described by multiple terms including compulsive, addictive, or disordered gambling. Only in 1980 was a gambling-related disorder, pathological gambling (PG), introduced into the Diagnostic and Statistical Manual of Mental Disorders (DSM) [12]. The diagnostic criteria have undergone several revisions since their original inclusion, and a current listing is included in Table 1 [13]. The criteria for PG are similar to those for substance dependence, and include features of diminished control over the self-destructive behavior, aspects of tolerance and withdrawal, and interference in major areas of life functioning due to the behavior.

1. Prevalence Rates of Problem Gambling and PG

Although the majority of people gamble, a relatively small proportion develops problems with gambling. For example, 86% of the general population is thought to have engaged in traditional forms of gambling at some point in their lives [6]. In contrast, a meta-analysis of prevalence studies performed in North America over the past several decades estimates lifetime rates of problem and PG of 3.85% and 1.60%, respectively [9]. The same study found more recent studies generating higher estimates, suggesting an increase in the number of individuals with problem and PG concurrent with the increase in access to legalized gambling [9]. Consistently higher lifetime prevalence rates of problem gambling (9.45%) and PG (3.88%) have been found in adolescents and young adults, data which in

Table 1 Diagnostic Criteria for Pathological Gambling

A. Persistent and recurrent maladaptive gambling behavior as indicated by five (or more) of the following:
(1) is preoccupied with gambling (e.g., preoccupied with reliving past gambling experiences, handicapping or planning the next venture, or thinking of ways to get money with which to gamble)
(2) needs to gamble with increasing amounts of money in order to achieve the desired excitement
(3) has repeated unsuccessful efforts to control, cut back, or stop gambling
(4) is restless or irritable when attempting to cut down or stop gambling
(5) gambles as a way of escaping from problems or of relieving a dysphoric mood (e.g., feelings of helplessness, guilt, anxiety, depression)
(6) after losing money gambling, often returns another day to get even ("chasing" after one's losses)
(7) lies to family members, therapist, or others to conceal the extent of involvement with gambling
(8) has committed illegal acts such as forgery, fraud, theft, or embezzlement to finance gambling
(9) has jeopardized or lost a significant relationship, job, or educational or career opportunity because of gambling
(10) relies on others to provide money to relieve a desperate financial situation caused by gambling

B. The gambling behavior is not better accounted for by a Manic Episode

Source: Ref. 13.

conjunction with the adult rates are consistent with a cohort effect [9].

2. Comorbidities

PG is often observed in setting of other mental health disorders [14–16]. High rates of comorbidity between substance use disorders (SUDs) and PG have been described, with individuals with SUDs reported as having 4- to 10-fold higher rates of PG (rates of 5–15%, depending on the substance and the study) [14,17–19]. Studies have also revealed high rates of SUDs in groups of individuals with PG; e.g., rates of alcohol abuse or dependence have been found in the range of 45–55% [20,21], and nicotine dependence in the range of 70% [14]. Given the phenomenological similarities and the high rates of comorbidity between SUDs and PG, PG has been described as "an addiction without the drug" [22]. Emerging data suggest common genetic factors contributing to the development of PG and certain SUDs, suggesting in part a common etiology [23,24].

PG also shares comorbidities with non-substance-related mental health disorders. Some studies suggest high rates of attention deficit and bipolar disorder in individuals with PG [14,25–27]. Studies of the relationship between obsessive-compulsive disorder (OCD) and PG have been mixed, with some studies reporting elevated rates [21,28] but most larger studies reporting nonelevated or low rates [15,29,30]. Data from the St. Louis Epidemiologic Catchment Area Study found problem gamblers as compared with nongamblers to have elevated odds ratios for major depression (3.3; 95% confidence interval [CI] 1.6, 6.8), schizophrenia (3.5; CI 1.3, 9.7), phobias (2.3; CI 1.2, 4.3), somatization syndrome (3.0; CI 1.6, 5.8), and antisocial personality disorder (6.1; CI 3.2, 11.6) [15]. The study also provided additional data on the relationship between problem gambling and SUDs, with problem gamblers as compared with nongamblers reported as having elevated odds ratios for alcohol use (7.2; CI 2.3, 23.0), alcohol abuse/dependence (3.3; CI 1.9, 5.6), nicotine use (2.6; CI 1.6, 4.4), and nicotine dependence (2.1; CI 1.1, 3.8) [15]. Recreational gamblers as compared with nongamblers were also observed to have elevated odds ratios for psychiatric disorders and related behaviors, including major depression (1.7; CI 1.1, 2.6), dysthymia (1.8; CI 1.0, 3.0), "somatization syndrome" (1.7; CI 1.1, 2.8), antisocial personality disorder (2.3; CI 1.6, 3.4), alcohol use (3.9; CI 2.4, 6.3), alcohol abuse/dependence (1.9; CI 1.3, 2.7), nicotine use (1.9; CI 1.6, 2.4), and nicotine dependence (1.3; CI 1.0, 1.7) [15]. These and other data support the notion that gambling behaviors can be conceptualized along a spectrum ranging from nongambling to recreational to problem to pathological gambling [6,9,23,24]. A need exists for naturalistic studies to identify the course over time of gambling behaviors within individuals and their movement from one group to another, as well as for better identifying and defining the health and disease factors associated with the respective patterns of gambling [31].

3. High-Risk Groups

As described above, (1) adolescents and young adults and (2) individuals with SUDs represent two high-risk groups for developing problem or PG. Given the comorbidities detailed above, individuals with other specific mental health disorders (e.g., depression, schizophrenia, anxiety disorders, antisocial personality disorder) likely also represent high-risk groups. Males also represent a high-risk group, with most studies reporting an $\sim 2:1$ male:female ratio [32]. Nonetheless, given the recent increase in accessibility to legalized gambling, particularly forms which appear more problematic for women (e.g., slot machines), the male:female ratio may diminish in the near future [32].

Studies have suggested that minority groups, particularly African-Americans, represent a high-risk group for PG [15,16]. For example, African-Americans comprised 31.0% of the group of problem gamblers as compared with 15.2% of the recreational and 21.4% of the nongamblers in the St. Louis Epidemiologic Catchment Study [15]. Limited data exist examining carefully the gambling patterns of other racial and ethnic groups, although it has been suggested that Hispanic, Asian-American, and Native American groups might be at elevated risk for developing problem or PG [16]. Data support the notion that lower socioeconomic status is associated with higher rates of problem and PG [16]. However, given the complex relationship between socioeconomic status and race and ethnicity and the limited data currently available, more work needs to be done in this area to clarify the relationship [16]. As with other potential at-risk populations, more research is needed to investigate whether older adults might represent a high-risk group, particularly as there has been an increase in the gambling rates of older adult Americans in the past 25 years: lifetime gambling rates in adults 65 years of age or older have risen from 35% in 1975 to 80% in 1998, and past-year rates from 23% in 1975 to 50% in 1998 [6].

III. CONCEPTUALIZATION AND CLASSIFICATION OF PG

The two most prominent theories regarding the conceptualization of PG describe the disorder as: (1) an addiction without the drug-bearing similarities to SUDs; or (2) a disorder lying along an impulsive/compulsive spectrum [22,33,34]. These classifications are not mutually exclusive, and there exist data to support each view [10,22]. PG is currently included in the DSM-IV-TR in the category of Impulse Control Disorders Not Elsewhere Classified with such disorders as pyromania, intermittent explosive disorder, trichotillomania, and kleptomania [13]. Additional non-substance-related disorders that share similar features but are either formally included in DSM-IV-TR or are classified elsewhere have been grouped with PG and include compulsive buying, compulsive sexual behaviors, and compulsive computer use [35]. These disorders share a difficulty in controlling impulse to engage in a behavior which, although often hedonic in nature at some point in the disorder, ultimately leads to interference in major areas of life functioning. Neurobiological similarities appear to explain some of the common elements among these disorders [35].

IV. NEUROBIOLOGY

A. Serotonin Systems

1. Neurochemical Studies

Serotonin (5HT) is arguably the most widely-implicated neurotransmitter system in impulse control. A role for 5HT in PG and other impulse control disorders has been suggested, particularly in behavioral initiation and cessation [35,36]. Low levels of the 5HT metabolite 5-hydroxyindoleacetic acid (5-HIAA) have been observed in multiple groups of individuals with poor impulse control, including those attempting suicide, alcoholic criminals, and fire setters [37–41]. In a study of ten males with PG, Nordin and Eklundh observed decreased cerebrospinal fluid (CSF) levels of 5-HIAA when correcting for CSF flow parameters [42].

2. Pharmacological Challenge Studies

Additional support for a role for 5HT in PG comes from pharmacological challenge studies. A study using the 5HT and norepinephrine transporter inhibitor clomipramine (CMI) at a dose thought to preferentially target the 5HT transporter has been performed [43]. PG as compared with control subjects demonstrated lower prolactin levels at baseline and exhibited significantly blunted prolactin increases 60 min following CMI administration [43]. The blunted prolactin response raises the possibility of diminished 5HT transporter binding in individuals with PG. An independent challenge study employed the agent meta-chlorophenylpiperazine (m-CPP), which was administered to 10 males with PG and 10 healthy male control subjects [44]. A metabolite of the antidepressant trazodone and a partial $5HT_1$ and $5HT_2$ receptor agonist, m-CPP binds with high affinity to $5HT_{1A}$, $5HT_{1D}$, $5HT_{2A}$, $5HT_{2C}$, and $5HT_3$ receptors, and has particularly high affinity for $5HT_{2C}$ receptors [45–47]. $5HT_{2C}$ receptors are localized to brain regions including the cortex and caudate and have been implicated in mediating aspects of mood, anxiety, appetite, behavior (including sexual activity), and neuroendocrine function [48,49]. Individuals with PG as compared with controls were more likely to report a euphoric effect or "high" following m-CPP administration, a finding which has been described in other individuals with disorders or behaviors characterized by impaired impulse control—e.g., antisocial personality disorder [50], borderline personality disorder [51], trichotrillomania [52], and alcohol abuse/dependence [53]. In addition, the group of individuals with PG as compared with the controls exhibited an increase in prolactin levels following m-CPP administration, and greater prolactin increases correlated with increasing gambling severity [44].

3. Genetic Studies

Genetic studies support the notion that 5HT systems might be involved in mediating the pathophysiology of PG [24,54,55]. One report did not find a statistically significant association between PG and allelic variants of the tryptophan 2,3-dioxygenase gene, whose gene product regulates 5HT metabolism [54]. A variant of the 5HT transporter (5HTT) promoter region [56] has been associated with altered protein expression [57] and was previously implicated in anxiety [57] and depression [58]. Specifically, individuals with at least one copy of the short variant, associated with decreased protein levels, have been found to have higher measures of anxiety or depression [57,58]. An increased association between the short (less functional) variant and PG in the group of males but not females studied has been reported, with increasing association observed with increasing severity of PG [59]. These findings further support a role for 5HT dysregulation in PG, and suggest the direct target of 5HT reuptake inhibitors (SRIs), drugs with apparent efficacy in the treatment of PG (see below, Sec. V.C.1), might be differentially regulated in certain groups with PG. Further studies are warranted to replicate and extend these findings.

4. Monoamine Oxidase Studies

Additional support for a role for 5HT in PG comes from studies of monoamine oxidase (MAO) function. The MAOs, subtypes MAO_A and MAO_B, are enzymes responsible for metabolizing 5HT, norepinephrine (NE), and dopamine (DA) [60]. Peripheral MAO derived from platelets is of the MAO_B subtype and has been suggested to be an indicator of 5HT function [61,62], although MAO_B also binds with high affinity to and catabolizes DA [60]. Low levels of platelet MAO activity have been found in association with impulsive behaviors (e.g., suicidality and alcohol abuse) [63,64], high levels of sensation seeking [65–67], and disorders involving impaired impulse control, including eating disorders [68]. Low platelet MAO activity has also been observed in males with PG, although no clear pattern of a relationship between MAO levels and measures of sensation seeking emerged [69,70]. Additionally, an association between an MAO$_A$ gene polymorphism and PG in males has been reported [71].

B. Dopamine Systems

1. Neurochemical Studies

The neurochemical dopamine has been widely implicated in mediating rewarding and reinforcing behaviors. In particular, the mesocorticolimbic dopamine pathway, extending from the ventral tegmental area in the midbrain to the nucleus accumbens in the ventral striatum with additional neuronal connections to cortical and subcortical brain areas, is thought to underlie many aspects of the initiation and maintenance of self-administration of drugs with addictive potential [72–74]. A role for dopamine in the rewarding and reinforcing aspects of PG has been proposed [44,75]. One study consistent with such a relationship, published by Bergh et al. [76], reported decreased levels of ceberospinal fluid levels of dopamine and elevated ceberospinal fluid levels of the dopamine metabolites 3,4-dihydroxyphenylacetic acid (DOPAC) and homovanilic acid (HVA) in males with PG. The authors concluded these findings to be consistent with an increased rate of dopamine neurotransmission, although more recently the same group did not find decreased HVA levels when correcting for CSF flow rate [42].

A separate study investigated peripheral levels of DA under gambling conditions [77]. Plasma levels of dopamine were measured when playing Pachinko, and following a winning streak or machine payout described as a "Fever," six males who were regular Pachinko players were found to have elevated levels of DA. It was suggested that the DA changes may be related to the motivational processes underlying repeated Pachinko playing.

2. Neuroimaging Studies

One study investigated the role of the mesocorticolimbic dopamine system in video tank game in which participants were paid increasing amounts of money depending upon the skill level reached [78]. Positron emission tomography (PET) studies using ^{11}C-labeled raclopride, a ligand with high affinity for D$_2$-like dopamine receptors (D2Rs), found decreased levels of striatal binding in eight male subjects playing the tank videogame as compared to when they viewed a gray screen image [78]. The authors concluded the observed 13% reduction in ^{11}C-raclopride signal during the gaming condition is consistent with at least a twofold increase in levels of extracellular dopamine [78]. As the game involved increasing monetary reward associated with each skill level reached during the video game, the paradigm is similar but not identical to actual gambling.

Another gambling-related study of healthy subjects involved a paradigm in which subjects viewed a spinner which would ultimately land on one of three varying, seemingly random outcomes, each associated with a specific monetary reward or punishment (79). As assessed by blood oxygen level dependent (BOLD) functional magnetic resonance imaging (fMRI), individuals exhibited changes in brain activity in specific brain circuitry (e.g., in DA pathways originating in the ventral tegmental area and projecting to the nucleus accumbens, orbitofrontal cortex, amygdala, sublenticular extended amygdala, and hypothalamus) in anticipation of and response to rewarding and punishing outcomes [79]. These findings suggest similar brain circuitry as being involved in processing monetary rewards and punishments as are activated in response to cocaine [80]. Additionally, preliminary findings suggest abnormal function of similar limbic and cortical brain regions as mediating gambling urges in subjects with PG to those involved in cocaine cravings in subjects with cocaine dependence [81,82]. Together, these findings further support a relationship between the SUDs and PG, perhaps as mediated by abnormalities in functioning of neural pathways involved in the assessment of the risks of potential reward and punishment associated with specific behaviors [83].

An independent study investigated for specific dopamine and 5HT abnormalities in individuals with PG [84]. Using PET, the researchers found decreased striatal binding in PG subjects of ^{11}C-n-methylspiperone, a ligand with high affinity for D2Rs and 5HT$_{2A}$ and 5HT$_{2C}$ receptors [85]. The striatal signal, corresponding to D2R-receptor occupancy, could be explained by multiple, nonmutually exclusive possibilities including decreased numbers of available D2Rs, decreased affinity of D2Rs for the tracer, or increased synaptic concentrations of dopamine.

3. Genetics Studies

Genetic studies also suggest a role for dopamine systems in PG. A study was performed investigating the D_2A1 allelic variant of the D2R, an allele previously reported by the same research group to be implicated in multiple compulsive/addictive behaviors such as cocaine and other drug abuse, compulsive eating, and smoking [86,87]. In a group of 171 Caucasians with PG, 50.9% carried the D_2A1 allele as compared with 25.9% of the control group (odds ratio [OR] = 2.96; $P < 0000001$) [88]. Gambling severity was also found to correlate with an increased likelihood of carrying the D_2A1 allele, and the group of individuals without compared to those with a history of a major depressive episode were more likely to carry the D_2A1 allele [88]. This latter finding suggests differences in underlying motivations for gambling and comorbidity may be important factors in relation to the genetics of PG. The authors have postulated a reward deficiency theory based on their findings [86,87], although additional studies appear warranted to more precisely identify specific genetic factors contributing to the pathophysiology of PG and related disorders.

Associations of polymorphic variants of the D_1, D_3, and D_4 dopamine receptors with PG have also been explored [54,89,90]. The frequency of the Dde I allele of the D_1 dopamine receptor (D1R) has been reported to be significantly higher than controls in each of three groups: pathological gamblers, tobacco smokers, and Tourette's syndrome probands [89]. A negative association for heterozygosity at the Dde I polymorphism was observed for all three disease groups. Given the roles of the D1R and D2R in modulating rewarding/reinforcing behaviors [91], the authors proposed heterosis as an reason for the distribution of the genetic variants of the D2R and D1R in PG [90]. Heterosis, with regard to populations, refers to a situation where the progeny (hybrid) has a significantly greater effect on phenotype than either parental strain (e.g., certain hybrid strains of corn exhibiting increased vigor) [90].

Allelic variants of the dopamine D_4 receptor (D4R) have been described which differ in the number of 48-base-pair (BP) nucleotide repeats and generate proteins with functional differences, a finding which lends support to the idea that the allelic variants might contribute directly to differences in D4R function and human behavior [92]. These allelic variants have been implicated in some studies of novelty-seeking behavior [93,94] but not others [95–98]. One group reported a significant positive association between PG and the longest allele of the D4R (D7), with a stronger association observed in the female group and a nonsignificant relationship seen in the male group [99]. An independent group found no significant association between the D7 allele carriers and PG, although a significant positive association was found with regard to the number of individuals with a high number of 48-BP repeats [5–8] and PG [90]. The second group also reported an increase in heterozygosity at the D4R allele in association with PG, invoking the notion of heterosis. Discrepancies in the findings of the two groups might be explained by genetic heterogeneity, or by the fact that the genetic contributions from these loci might be only modest or additive. Comings et al also described a decrease in heterozygosity of the Msc I allele of the D3 dopamine receptor individually in groups with PG or Tourette's syndrome [54]. Together, the findings from association studies support a potential role for dopamine receptor allelic variants in PG; however, further studies are warranted to replicate the findings, identify specific functional correlates to the genetic findings, and clarify the relationship to the underlying pathophysiology of PG.

C. Norepinephrine Systems

1. Neurochemical Studies

Norepinephrine has been hypothesized as mediating aspects of arousal, attention and sensation seeking in individuals with PG [44,100–102]. In support of this notion, male subjects with PG were found to have higher cerebrospinal fluid levels of the norepinephrine metabolite 4-hydroxy-3-methoxyphenyl glycol (HMPG) and higher urinary measures of norepinephrine [100]. Scores of extraversion were found to correlate positively and significantly with cerebrospinal fluid and plasma levels of HMPG, urinary measures of vanilylmandelic acid (VMA), and the sum of urinary levels of norepinephrine and norepinephrine metabolites [101]. Increased cerebrospinal fluid levels of NE and HMPG were also found in an independent group of males with PG [76], although a subsequent report from the same research team reported findings of decreased HMPG in males with PG when correcting for cerebrospinal fluid flow [42].

2. Neurochemical Studies and Stress

A study of male Pachinko players found changes in norepinephrine during gambling [77]. Blood levels of norepinephrine were found to increase from baseline over time during Pachinko play, with statistically significant changes noted at the onset and end of the machine payout period. Levels of norepinephrine remained significantly elevated 30 min following the end of payout periods. Alterations in heart rate, a physiological measurement associated with arousal and noradrenergic activity, was also observed, with peak heart rate measured at the onset of payout. Changes in immune function, including alterations in levels of T-cells and natural killer cells, were noted concurrently [77]. Consistent with these findings, two independent groups found physiological changes in association with gambling. Meyer et al. [103] described elevated heart rate and salivary measures of cortisol persisting over a several hour period of gambling in males who gambled regularly on casino blackjack. Schmitt et al. [104] described higher epinephrine and cortisol levels and blood pressure differences approaching statistical significance in Aboriginal individuals on days in which gambling behavior was concentrated. Together, these findings suggest that alteration in norepinephrine and related stress-response pathways might explain some of the pathophysiology associated with PG [105].

D. Opioid Systems

A role for endogenous opioids in PG has been investigated given: (1) their mediation of levels of pleasure; (2) modulation of mesocorticolimbic dopamine activity via gamma-aminobutyric acid (GABA) input to dopamine neurons in the VTA; and (3) efficacy of the μ-opioid receptor antagonist naltrexone in targeting urges/cravings in alcohol and opioid dependence [106–109]. Blood levels of beta-endorphins, endogenous agonists for the μ-opioid receptor, were found to become elevated during Pachinko play, peaking during the period of machine payout [77]. Recent pharmacological investigations into the potential of naltrexone in the treatment of PG further substantiate a role for opioid systems in PG (see below, Sec. V.C.2) [110–113].

E. Genetic Studies

Historically, twin studies, allowing for comparison of rates of disorders in monozygotic (MZ) and dizygotic (DZ) twins, have been informative in investigating for genetic influences. Twin studies investigating disordered gambling behaviors have recently been published [23,24,114,115]. One study observed significantly greater rates of similarities in male MZ as compared with male DZ twins with regard to participation in past-year high-action forms of gambling (e.g., casino cards, lottery, or gambling machine) [114]. No statistically significant differences were observed in the two groups of males with regard to measures of low action forms of gambling or in female MZ versus DZ groups with regard to past-year participation in either high- or low-action forms gambling [114]. The VietNam Era Twin Registry has served as the basis for several additional investigations into the heretibility of gambling disorders in a large group of male MZ ($n = 1869$ pairs) and DZ ($n = 1490$ pairs) twins [23,24,115]. The authors found that faimilial factors accounted for ~50% of the liability to report one or two symptoms of PG, and that familial factors (genetic and/or environmental) explained ~60% of the liability for reporting three or four symptoms [24,115]. The results are comparable to findings derived from the same sample for the heritability of drug use disorders, with 34% and 28% of the variance accounted for by genetic and shared environmental factors, respectively [116]. Additional analyses on the same dataset suggest significant shared proportion of genetic factors, accounting for 12–20% of the variance, contributing to the development of gambling and alcohol use problems [23]. These estimates are similar to those for the shared genetic contributions for marijuana and alcohol use disorders, and less than those for shared genetic contributions for nicotine and alcohol use disorders [23]. Additional analyses suggest that the high rates of comorbidity for PG, antisocial personality disorder, and conduct disorder to be determined largely by genetic factors, with between 61% and 86% of the variance for these behaviors to be determined by shared genetic factors [24]. Together, these findings support significant roles for genetic and common and unique environmental factors in the development of PG, and suggest both common and unique elements for the development of PG and other psychiatric disorders like alcohol dependence, conduct disorder and antisocial personality disorder.

V. TREATMENT

A. Self-Help

Arguably the most widespread form of help over the past several decades for individuals with problem or pathological gambling has been Gamblers Anonymous (GA). GA, founded in 1957, is based on the 12-step principles originally developed for Alcoholics Anonymous and currently has chapters throughout the world. Although reported to be effec-

tive and life-saving for many individuals, GA's efficacy in general has not been systematically explored in detail. One study reported that only 8% of patients entering GA remained at 1 year, with the majority leaving after one or two meetings [117], findings not dissimilar from structured investigations of other self-help programs [118]. Further information regarding GA can be obtained by telephone at 1-800-266-1908 or on the internet at
http://www.gamblersanonymous.org.

B. Behavioral Treatments

Although behavioral treatments for PG have been explored for many decades with varying degrees of success, few well-controlled studies of significant magnitude have been performed to date [119]. One group has reported positive outcomes using imaginal desensitization, with individuals randomly assigned to that treatment reporting less gambling and fewer urges to gamble at 1 month and up to 9 years after treatment as compared with individuals assigned to aversion therapy [120–122]. Given the relatively small sample size (20 subjects) and inpatient population used in the study, further investigations are warranted to confirm and extend these results.

Several groups have been examining the applicability of cognitive behavioral therapy to PG [119]. Gambling-related interventions focusing on skills training, cognitive restructuring, problem solving, and relapse prevention were reported to be helpful in an initial study of three subjects, and a more extensive trial found the active treatment superior to wait-list control in reducing gambling and increasing perceptions of control over the behavior [123,124]. In a majority of cases, gains were maintained one year after treatment in the actively treated group. Although promising, the study included only a total of 29 subjects. Currently, a large scale controlled trial of cognitive behavioral therapy for PG is being conducted with promising initial findings [119].

C. Pharmacotherapies

3. SSRIs

Given the efficacy of serotonin reuptake inhibitors (SRIs) in targeting obsessive-compulsive behaviors in obsessive compulsive disorder [125] and the data supporting 5HT dysregulation in PG (see above, Secs. IV.A.1–4), trials of SRIs in the treatment of individuals with PG have been undertaken. A double-blind, placebo-controlled, crossover case study of clomipramine was described [126]. Although only minimal improvement was observed after 10 weeks of placebo treatment, gambling behavior was discontinued at week 3 with abstinence from gambling persisting at 38 weeks following initiation of active drug at 25 mg/day with an increase up to 175 mg/day [126]. Increased irritability observed during treatment was effectively treated with a temporary decrease in dose.

As selective SRIs (SSRIs) are often better tolerated than nonselective SRIs, many recent studies have examined the tolerability and efficacy of SSRIs in the treatment of PG [112]. A single-blind crossover study of the SSRI fluvoxamine has been reported [127]. Sixteen subjects entered the 16-week trial (8-week placebo lead-in, 8-week active), and seven of 10 completers were determined to be responders by scores on the Clinical Global Impression score for gambling severity (PG-CGI) and PG modification of the Yale-Brown Obsessive-Compulsive Scale (PG-YBOCS) [127]. The medication was well tolerated, and the average dose for completers was 220 mg/day at endpoint, with responders receiving a slightly lower average dose of 207 mg/day. Two of the three completers who were deemed nonresponders had histories of cyclothymia, suggesting that individuals with comorbid cycling mood disorders may respond preferentially to alternative pharmacotherapies (see below, Sec. V.C.3).

More recently, randomized, double-blind, placebo-controlled studies have been performed for two SSRIs: fluvoxamine and paroxetine (Table 2) [112]. Hollander and colleagues [128] have recently performed a randomized double-blind, placebo-controlled 16-week crossover study of fluvoxamine in the treatment of PG. Fifteen subjects with PG were enrolled, and 10 participants (all male) completed the study. Study drug dosing was initiated at 50 mg/day, increased incrementally to 150 mg/day, and adjusted based on clinical response and drug tolerance, with a maximum of 250 mg/day and a minimum of 100 mg/day. Mean endpoint dose of fluvoxamine was 195 ± 50 mg/day. Adverse effects were minimal, and active drug was found to be superior to placebo, as measured by PG-CGI and PG-YBOCS scores, in reducing gambling and related symptomatology. However, there was a significant placebo response observed. Both groups (those receiving active medication and those receiving placebo) showed improvement during the first 8 weeks of the study regardless of group assignment, and the most significant difference in response was observed at the end of the second 8-week block. These findings suggest acute trials of longer duration than 8 weeks might be impor-

Table 2 Major Placebo-Controlled, Double-Blind Drug Trials in the Treatment of PG

Category	Reference	Drug	Sample size	Duration	Average Dose, mg/day	Outcome
SSRIs	Hollander, et al. 2000	Fluovoxamine (Luvox)	15 Subjects enrolled, 10 completed (10 male)	16 weeks (crossover design, 8 weeks each of active/placebo) with initial 1-week placebo lead-in	> 195	7 of 10 Completers determined to be responders by PG-CGI and PG-YBOCS scores; fluvoxamine superior to placebo, particularly at end of 16 weeks of treatment
	Kim and Grant 2000	Paroxetine (Paxil)	41 Subjects (20 paroxetine, 21 placebo)	8 weeks with 1-week placebo lead-in	51	Paroxetine group significantly improved as compared with placebo as determined by CGI, G-SAS
Opioid antagonists	Kim et al. 2001	Naltrexone (ReVia)	89 Subjects enrolled, 45 completed (20 naltrexone, 25 placebo)	12 weeks with 1-week placebo lead-in	188	Naltrexone group significantly improved as compared with placebo as determined by CGI, G-SAS; risk of LFT abnormalities with analgesics

Legend: PG-CGI = Clinical Global Impression Scale for Gambling Behavior; PG-YBOCS = Yale-Brown Obsessive Compulsive Scale Modified for Pathological Gambling; CGI = Clinical Global Impression Scale; G-SAS = Gambling Symptom Assessment Scale; LFT = Liver Function Test.

tant in distinguishing responses to active drug as compared with placebo, and indicate that open-label trials, such as those reported for fluoxetine and citalopram, should be interpreted cautiously in this patient population [129,130].

A longer-term, placebo-controlled trial of fluvoxamine in the treatment of PG has been performed by an independent group [131]. Patients were treated for 6 months with placebo or fluvoxamine at 200 mg/day, and outcome was measured by quantification of time and money spent on gambling. Although the authors found no statistically significant differences in response rates to placebo as compared with active drug for the overall sample, they described fluvoxamine as being superior to placebo for the male and younger-age pathological gamblers. However, the large proportion of individuals for whom follow-up was not available significantly limits the interpretation of the data, which suggests that long-term compliance with drug treatment may be a concern for the PG patient population.

The findings of a recent parallel-group, 8-week (following 1 week single-blind placebo lead-in), flexible dosage, randomized, placebo-controlled, double-blind trial of paroxetine are the basis of the first multicenter drug treatment trial for individuals with PG [112]. Dosing, initiated at 20 mg/day, was adjusted up to 60 mg/day as clinically indicated. Forty-one patients with PG completed the study (20 paroxetine, 21 placebo), with a significant proportion dropping out of treatment. Adverse effects were mild in nature (mainly headache, fatigue, and dry mouth) and were observed with greater frequency in the paroxetine-treated group (2.3 treatment-emergent symptoms per patient in the paroxetine group as compared with 1.2 in the placebo). Outcome as measured by scores on the patient- and clinician-rated CGI and the Gambling Symptom Assessment Scale (G-SAS) showed paroxetine to be superior to placebo.

Together, the initial findings from studies of SSRIs suggest that they are well tolerated and efficacious drugs in the treatment of PG. Larger-scale (e.g., multicenter), placebo-controlled trials of these drugs are necessary to confirm and extend these initial results and better define the short- and long-term efficacies and tolerabilities of the SSRIs in specific groups of individuals with PG, particularly those with co-occurring disorders.

2. Opioid Antagonists

Naltrexone, a mu-opioid antagonist, has FDA approval for the treatment of alcohol dependence and opiate dependence. Case reports of individuals with PG treated with naltrexone suggested a role for the drug in PG [110,111]. Recently, a randomized, flexible-dosage, double-blind, placebo-controlled study of naltrexone was performed [113]. The trial was of 12 weeks duration (1 week placebo lead-in followed by an 11-week treatment phase), and 89 subjects were enrolled and 45 completed week 6 or later (20 naltrexone, 25 placebo). Average end-of-study dosages of naltrexone were 187.50 ± 96.45 mg/day and 243.18 ± 31.98 mg/day for the active drug and placebo groups, respectively. Approximately one-quarter of the group receiving naltrexone experienced increased liver function enzyme elevations, a finding that appeared most frequently in individuals taking concurrent nonsteroidal anti-inflammatory drugs. Statistically significant improvement as measured by the patient-rated and clinician-rated CGIs, and the G-SAS was observed in the active drug as compared with the placebo group. Although encouraging, the clinical potential of naltrexone in the treatment of PG requires further study to determine better the long-term clinical efficacy and tolerability given the short-term nature of the study, high doses of naltrexone used, and increased rate of liver function abnormalities observed in the present study.

3. Mood Stabilizers

Given that mood lability is not infrequently observed in individuals with PG and that a history of cyclothymia may be related to poor outcome with SSRI treatment (see above), the use of mood stabilizers in the treatment of individuals with PG has been described. Lithium, a salt with mood-stabilizing properties believed to modulate 5HT systems [132], has been examined in the treatment of PG [133]. Open-label treatment of three males with PG and comorbid cycling mood disorders with lithium at daily doses up to 1800 mg/day was found to be at least partially effective in controlling gambling, cycling mood, hypomania/mania, and risk-taking behaviors. Many treatment-related factors (specific duration of treatment, structured outcome measures) were not described, and larger controlled studies are being performed to investigate the efficacy and tolerability of lithium in the treatment of individuals with PG and cycling mood disorders [134,135].

A placebo-controlled, double-blind case report trial of carbamazepine in the treatment of a male with PG has been reported [136]. Although no improvement was noted in gambling behavior over a 12-week placebo phase, a decease in gambling behavior was observed 2 weeks into active treatment with carbemazepine, with gains maintained at 30 months. The drug was introduced at 200 mg/day and increased to 600 mg/day (reaching blood levels of 4.8–9.5 μg/mL). Additional larger studies are needed to confirm these findings. Studies of valproic acid in the treatment of PG are also under way [134,135].

4. Atypical Antipsychotics

Limited data are available on the tolerability and efficacy of antipsychotic drugs in the treatment of individuals with PG. One open-label case report found olanzapine administration in conjunction with behavioral intervention targeting gambling behaviors to be effective in decreasing gambling and thought disorder symptoms in an individual with comorbid schizophrenia and PG [137]. However, a larger, placebo-controlled, double-blind study of olanzapine in the treatment of inpatients with PG did not find a difference in outcome in the groups treated with active drug or placebo [138].

D. Future Directions

Although treatment trials to date are limited by small sample sizes and often relatively short durations, encouraging reports of behavioral and pharmacological treatments are emerging. Future efforts should be directed at determining: (1) which treatment strategies will be efficacious and well tolerated over the long term; (2) whether interventions combining behavioral and pharmacological elements will be more effective than either alone; (3) if specific groups of individuals with PG (e.g., those with comorbid disorders, specific age groups, or other typologies [139,140]) might respond preferentially to specific treatment strategies; and (4) whether gambling-specific interventions (e.g., debt restructuring) might represent important therapeutic components.

VI. CONCLUSIONS

As described above (Secs. V.A–D), well-tested, effective, and well-tolerated treatment strategies appear to be emerging. Many areas have professional clinicians and self-help programs available. Currently, suggested interventions for general practitioners or other health care providers include: (1) routine screening for problem gambling and PG; (2) sensitive broaching with the patient of a suspected gambling problem; (3) motivating the patient to contact a self-help group (e.g., GA: 1-800-266-1908 or http://www.gamblersanonymous.org), a local gambling treatment program, and/or a gambling helpline (e.g., National Council on Problem Gambling helpline: 1-800-522-4700 or http://www.ncpgambling.org) to facilitate engagement in locally available gambling treatment; and (4) following up with the patient and gambling treatment facility regarding the status of the patient's gambling problem [10]. The availability of a brief questionnaire for problem gambling and PG, like the CAGE for alcoholism [141], will be helpful in the screening process, and such instruments are under development, testing, and use [105,142,143]. Additionally, help for family members affected by a relative's gambling problems is available (e.g., Gam-Anon: http://gamblersanonymous.org/gamanon.html or 1-718-352-1671), and these interventions can be helpful even in the absence of recovery of the individual with PG.

As the availability of legalized gambling has increased in many areas over the past decade, so have the prevalence rates of problem gambling and PG [9]. As such, there is a growing need for the identification of efficacious, well-tolerated treatments for individuals with gambling disorders. As effective treatments emerge, it will become increasingly important to develop, enact and modify education and prevention strategies in the areas of problem gambling and PG [144].

ACKNOWLEDGMENTS

Supported in part by NIDA grant K12-DA00366, the National Alliance for Research on Schizophrenia and Depression, the National Center for Responsible Gaming, and Women's Health Research at Yale.

REFERENCES

1. CJ France. The gambling impulse Am J Psychology. 13:364–407, 1902.
2. MC McGurrin. Diagnosis and treatment of pathological gambling. In: J Lewis, ed. Addictions: Concepts and Strategies for Treatment. Gaithersburg, MD: Aspen Publishers, 1994.
3. MN Potenza, DS Charney. Pathological gambling: a current perspective. Semin Clin Neuropsychiatry 6:153–154, 2001.
4. Anonymous. Mahabharata. Adiparva. English translation by KM Ganguli. Calcutta and Evanston: Bharata Press and American Theological Library, 1884.

5. KC James. National Gambling Impact Study Commission: Final Report to Congress. http://www.ngisc.gov/reports/fullrpt.html. Accessed Aug. 30, 1999.
6. D Gerstein, J Hoffmann, C Larison, L Engelman, S Murphy, A Palmer, L Chuchro, M Toce, R Johnson, T Buie, MA Hill. Gambling impact and behavior study. National Opinion Research Center, University of Chicago. http://www.norc.uchicago.edu/new/gamb-fin.htm. Accessed March 27, 1999.
7. S Cox, H Lesieur, R Rosenthal, R Volberg. Problem and pathological gambling in America: the national picture. New York: National Council on Problem Gambling, 1997.
8. EM Christiansen. The United States annual gross wager: 1997. International Gambling and Wagering Business, Supplement. August 1998.
9. HJ Shaffer, MN Hall, J Vander Bilt. Estimating the prevalence of disordered gambling behavior in the United States and Canada: a research synthesis. Am J Public Health 89:1369–1376, 1999.
10. MN Potenza, TR Kosten, BJ Rounsaville. Pathological gambling. JAMA 286:141–144, 2001.
11. M Mitka. Win or lose, internet gambling stakes are high. JAMA. 285:1005, 2001.
12. American Psychiatric Association Committee on Nomenclature and Statistics, Diagnostic and Statistical Manual of Mental Disorders, 3rd ed. Washington,: American Psychiatric Association, 1980.
13. American Psychiatric Association Committee on Nomenclature and Statistics. Diagnostic and Statistical Manual of Mental Disorders, 4th ed.—Text Revision). Washington: American Psychiatric Association, 2000.
14. DN Crockford, N el-Guebaly. Psychiatric comorbidity in pathological gambling: a critical review. Can J Psychiatry 43:43–50, 1998.
15. RM Cunningham-Williams, LB Cottler, WM Compton 3rd, EL Spitznagel. Taking chances: problem gamblers and mental health disorders—results from the St. Louis Epidemiologic Catchment Area Study. Am J Public Health 88:1093–1096, 1998.
16. RM Cunningham-Williams, LB Cottler. The epidemilogy of pathological gambling. Semin Clin Neuropsychiatry 6:155–166, 2001.
17. PW Haberman. Drinking and other self-indulgences: complements or counter-attractions? Int J Addict 4:157–167, 1969.
18. MA Steinberg, TA Kosten, BJ Rounsaville. Cocaine abuse and pathological gambling. Am J Addict 1:121–132, 1992.
19. W Feigelman, PH Kleinman, HR Lesieur, RB Millman, ML Lesser. Pathological gambling among methadone patients. Drug Alcohol Depend 39:75–81, 1995.
20. RA McCormick, AM Russo, LF Ramirez, JI Taber. Affective disorders among pathological gamblers seeking treatment. Am J Psychiatry 141:215–218, 1984.
21. RD Linden, HG Pope Jr, JM Jonas. Pathological gambling and major affective disorder: preliminary findings. J Clin Psychiatry 47:201–203, 1986.
22. C Blanco, P Moreyra, EV Nunes, J Saiz-Ruiz, A Ibanez. Pathological gambling: addiction or obsession? Semin Clin Neuropsychiatry 6:167–176, 2001.
23. WS Sultske, S Eisen, WR True, MJ Lyons, J Goldberg, M Tsuang. Common genetic vulnerability for pathological gambling and alcohol dependence in men. Arch Gen Psychiatry 57:666–674, 2000.
24. SA Eisen, WS Slutske, MJ Lyons, J Lassman, H Xian, R Toomey, S Chantarujikapong, MT Tsuang. The genetics of pathological gambling. Semin Clin Neuropsychiatry 6:195–204, 2001.
25. PL Carlton, P Manowitz, H McBride, R Nora, M Swartzburg, L Goldstein, L. Attention deficit disorder and pathological gambling. J Clin Psychiatry 48:487 488, 1987.
26. PL Carlton, P Manowitz. Physiological factors as determinants of pathological gambling. Special Issue: Compulsive gambling: an examination of relevant models. J Gambling Behav 3:274–285, 1988.
27. SM Specker, GA Carlson, GA Christenson, M Marcotte. Impulse control disorders and attention deficit disorder in pathological gamblers. Ann Clin Psychiatry 7:175–179, 1995.
28. RC Bland, SC Newman, H Orn, G Stebelsky. Epidemiology of pathological gambling in Edmonton. Can J Psychiatry 38:108–112, 1993.
29. OJ Bienvenu, JF Samuels, MA Riddle, R Hoehn-Saric, K-Y Liang, BAM Cullen, MA Grados, G Nestadt. The relationship of obsessive-compulsive disorder to possible spectrum disorders: results from a family study. Biol Psychiatry 48:287–293, 2000.
30. E Hollander, DJ Stein, JH Kwon, C Rowland, CM Wong, J Broatch, C Himelin. Psychosocial function and economic costs of obsessive-compulsive disorder. CNS Spectrums 2(10):16–25, 1997.
31. DA Korn, Shaffer HJ. Gambling and the health of the public: adopting a public health perspective. J Gambling Stud 15:289–365, 1999.
32. MN Potenza, MA Steinberg, SD McLaughlin, R Wu, BJ Rounsaville, SS O'Malley. Gender-related differences in the characteristics of problem gamblers using a gambling helpline. Am J Psychiatry 158:1500–1505, 2002.
33. SL McElroy, JI Hudson, HG Pope, PE Keck Jr, HG Aizley. The DSM-III-R impulse control disorders not elsewhere classified: clinical characteristics and relationship to other psychiatric disorders. Am J Psychiatry 149:318–327, 1992.

34. E Hollander, CM Wong. Obsessive-compulsive spectrum disorders. J Clin Psychiatry 56(suppl 4):3–6, 1995.
35. MN Potenza, E Hollander E. Pathological gambling and impulse control disorders. In: J.Coyle, C Nemeroff, D Charney, K Davis, eds. Neuropsychopharmacology: The 5th Generation of Progress. Baltimore: Lippincott Williams and Wilkins 1725–1742, 2002.
36. E Hollander, AJ Buchalter, CM DeCaria. Pathological gambling. Psychiatr Clin North Am 23:629–642, 2000.
37. M Asberg, L Traskman, P Thoren. 5-HIAA in the cerebrospinal fluid: a biochemical predictor. Arch Gen Psychiatry 33:1193–1197, 1976.
38. M Linnoila, M Virkunnen, M Scheinen, A Nuutila, R Rimon, F Goodwin. Low cerebrospinal fluid 5 hydroxy indolacetic acid concentrations differentiates impulsive from non impulsive violent behavior Life Sci. 33:2609–2614, 1983.
39. M Virkunnen, A Nuutila, FK Goodwin, M Linnoila. Cerebrospinal fluid monoamine metabolites in male arsonists. Arch Gen Psychiatry 44:241–247, 1987.
40. M Virkunnen, R Rawlings, R Tokola, R Poland, A Guoidotti, C Nemeroff, G Bissette, K Kalogeras, S-L Karonen, M Linnoila. CSF biochemistries, glucose metabolism, and diurnal activity rhythms in alcoholic violent offenders, fire setters, and healthy volunteers. Arch Gen Psychiatry 51:20–27, 1994.
41. EF Coccaro, LJ Siever, HM Klar, G Maurer, K Cochrane, TB Cooper, RC Mohs, KL Davis. Serotonergic studies in patients with affective and personality disorders: correlates with suicidal and impulsive aggressive behavior. Arch Gen Psychiatry 46:587–599, 1990.
42. C Nordin, T Eklundh. Altered CSF 5-HIAA disposition in pathologic male gamblers. CNS Spectrums 4(12):25–33, 1999.
43. I Moreno, J Saiz-Ruiz, JJ Lopez-Ibor. Serotonin and gambling dependence. Hum Psychopharmacol 6(suppl):9–12, 1991.
44. CM DeCaria, T Begaz, E Hollander. Serotonergic and noradrenergic function in pathological gambling. CNS Spectrums 3(6):38–47, 1998.
45. S Caccia, M Ballabio, R Saminin, MG Zanini, S Garrattini. M-CPP, a central 5-HT agonist, is a metabolite of trazodone. J Pharm Pharmacol 33:477–478, 1981.
46. A Hamik, SJ Peroutka. 1-(m-Chlorophenyl) piperazine (mCPP) interactions with neurotransmitter receptors in the human brain. Biol Psychiatry 25:569–575, 1989.
47. D Hoyer. Functional correlates of serotonin 5-HT1 recognition sites. J Recept Res 8:59–81, 1988.
48. Kennett, G., Curzon, G. Evidence that mCPP may have behavioural effects mediated by the 5HT1C receptor. Br J Pharmacol 94:137–147, 1988.
49. GA Kennett, G Curzon. Evidence that hypophagia induced by mCPP and TFMPP requires 5HT1C and 5HT1B receptors; hypophagia induced by RU 24969 requires only 5HT1B receptors. Psychopharmacology 96:93–100, 1998.
50. HB Moss, JK Yao, GL Panzak. Serotonergic responsivity and behavioral dimensions in antisocial personality associated with substance abuse. Biol Psychiatry 28:325–338, 1990.
51. E Hollander, D Stein, CM DeCaria, L Cohen, JB Saoud, D Kellman, L Rosnick, JM Oldham. Serotonergic sensitivity in borderline personailty disorder: preliminary findings. Am J Psychiatry 151:277–280, 1994.
52. DJ Stein, E Hollander, C DeCaria, L Cohen, D Simeon. Behavioral responses to m-chlorophenyl-piperazine and clonidine in trichotrillomania. J Serotonin Res 4:11–15, 1997.
53. C Benkelfat, DL Murphy, JL Hill, DT George, D Nutt, M Linnoila. Ethanol like properties of the serotonergic partial agonist m-chlorophenylpiperazine in chronic alcoholic patients. Arch Gen Psychiatry 48:383, 1991.
54. DE Comings. The molecular genetics of pathological gambling. CNS Spectrums 3(6):20–37, 1998.
55. I Perez de Castro, A Ibanez, J Saiz-Ruiz, J Fernandez-Piqueras. Genetic contribution to pathological gambling: possible association between a DNA polymorphism at the serotonin transpoter gene (5HTT) and affected men. Pharmacogenetics 9:397–400, 1999.
56. A Heils, A Teufel, S Petri, G Stober, P Riederer, D Bengal, KP Lesch. Allelic variation of human serotonin transporter gene expression. J Neurochem 66:2621–2624, 1996.
57. KP Lesch, D Bengal, A Heils, SZ Sabol, BD Greenberg, S Petri, J Benjamin, CR Muller, DH Hamer, DL Murphy. Association of anxiety-related traits with a polymorphism in the serotonin transporter gene regulatory region. Science 274:1527–1531, 1996.
58. DA Collier, G Stober, T Li, A Heils, M Catalano, D Di Bella, MJ Arranz, RM Murray, HP Vallada, D Bengel, CR Muller, GW Roberts, E Smeraldi, G Kirov, P Sham, KP Lesch. A novel functional polymorphism within the promoter of the serotonin transporter gene: possible role in susceptibility to affective disorders. Mol Psychiatry 1:453–460, 1996.
59. A Ibanez, J Saiz-Ruiz, I Perez De Castro, J Fernandez-Piqueras. Is serotonin transporter gene associated with pathological gambling? American Psychiatric Association Annual Convention. Toronto, Canada, 1998.
60. AY Deutch, RH Roth. Neurochemical systems in the central nervous system. In: DS Charney, EJ Nestler, BS Bunney, eds. Neurobiology of Mental

Illness. New York: Oxford University Press, 1999, pp 10–25.
61. L Oreland, A Wiberg, M Asberg, L Traskman, L Sjostrand, P Thoren, L Bertilsson, G Tybring. Platelet MAO activity and monoamine metabolites in cerebrospinal fluid in depressed and suicidal patients and in healthy controls. Psychiatry Res 4:21–29, 1981.
62. P Levitt, JE Pintar, XO Braekefield. Immunocytochemical demonstration of monoamine oxidase B in brain astrocytes and serotonin neurons. Proc Natl Acad Sci USA 79:6385–6389, 1982.
63. MS Buchsbaum, RJ Haier, DL Murphy. Suicide attempts, platelet monoamine oxidase and the average evoked response. Acta Psychiatr Scand 56:69–79, 1977.
64. L von Knorring, L Oreland, AL von Knorring. Personailty traits and platelet MAO activity in alcohol and drug abusing teenage boys. Acta Psychiatr Scand 75:307–314, 1987.
65. CJ Fowler, L von Knorring, L Oreland. Platelet monoamine activity in sensation seekers. Psychiatry Res 3:273–279, 1980.
66. PB Ward, SV Catts, TR Norman, GD Burrows, N McConaghy. Low platelet monoamine oxidase and sensation seeking in males: an established relationship? Acta Psychiatr Scand 75:86–90, 1987.
67. JL Carrasco, J Saiz-Ruiz, M Diaz-Marsa, J Cesar, JJ Lopez-Ibor. Low platelet monoamine oxidase activity in sensation-seeking bullfighters. CNS Spectrums 4(12):21–24, 1999.
68. J Hallman, E Sakurai, L Oreland. Blood platelet monoamine oxidase activity, serotonin uptake, and release rates in anorexia and bulimia patients and in healthy controls. Acta Psychiatr Scand 81:73–77, 1990.
69. JL Carrasco, J Saiz-Ruiz, E Hollander, J Cesar, JJ Lopez-Ibor Jr. Low platelet monoamine oxidase activity in pathological gambling. Acta Psychiatr Scand 90:427–31, 1994.
70. C Blanco, L Orensanz-Munoz, C Blanco-Jerez, J Saiz-Ruiz. Pathological gambling and platelet MAO activity: a psychobiological study. Am J Psychiatry 153:119–121, 1996.
71. A Ibanez, I Perez de Castro, J Fernandez-Piqueras, C Vlanco, J Saiz-Ruiz. Pathological gambling and DNA polymorphic markers at MAO-A and MAO-B genes. Mol Psychiatry 5:105–109, 2000.
72. GF Koob. Drugs of abuse: anatomy, pharmacology and functions of reward pathways. Trends Pharmacol Sci 13:177–184, 1992.
73. DW Self, EJ Nestler. Molecular mechanisms of drug reinforcement. Annu Rev Neurosci 18:463–495, 1995.
74. GF Koob, EJ Nestler. The neurobiology of drug addiction. J Neuropsychiatry Clin Neurosci 9:482–497, 1997.
75. MN Potenza. The neurobiology of pathological gambling. Semin Clin Neuropsychiatry 6:217–226, 2001.
76. C Bergh, T Eklund, P Sodersten, C Nordin. Altered dopamine function in pathological gambling. Psychol Med 27:473–475, 1997.
77. K Shinohara, A Yanagisawa, Y Kagota, A Gomi, K Nemoto, E Moriya, E Furusawa, K Furuya, K Tersawa. Physiological changes in Pachinko players; beta-endorphin, catecholamines, immune system substances and heart rate. Appl Hum Sci 18:37–42, 1999.
78. MJ Koepp, RN Gunn, AD Lawrence, VJ Cunningham, A Dagher, T Jones, DJ Brooks, CJ Bench, PM Grasby. Evidence for striatal dopamine release during a video game. Nature 393:266–268, 1998.
79. HC Breiter, I Aharon, D Kahneman, A Dale, P Shizgal. Functional imaging of neural responses to expectancy and experience of monetary gains and losses. Neuron 30:619–639, 2001.
80. HC Breiter, RL Gollub, RM Weisskopf, DN Kennedy, N Makris, JD Berke, JM Goodman, HL Kantor, DR Gastfriend, JP Riorden, RT Mathew, BR Rosen, SE Hyman. Acute effects of cocaine on human brain activity and emotion. Neuron 19:591–611, 1997.
81. BE Wexler, CH Gottschalk, RF Fulbright, I Prohovnik, CM Lacadie, BJ Rounsaville, JC Gore. fMRI of cocaine craving. Am J Psychiatry 158:86–95, 2001.
82. MN Potenza, CJ Armentano, MA Steinberg, RK Fulbright, BJ Rounsaville, SS O'Malley, JC Gore, BE Wexler. An fMRI study of gambling urges in individuals with pathological gambling. World Congress of Biological Psychiatry Convention. Berlin, Germany, 2001.
83. A Bechara. Neurobiology of decision-making: risk and reward. Semin Clin Neuropsychiatry 6:205–216, 2001.
84. PF Goyer, WE Semple, L Rugle, R McCormick, C Lewis, S Kowaliw, MS Berridge. Brain blood flow and dopamine receptor PET imaging in pathological gamblers. National Conference on Problem Gambling. Detroit, MI, 1999.
85. S Nyberg, B Eriksson, G Oxenstierna, C Halldin, L Farde. Suggested minimal effective dose of risperidone based on PET-measured D2 and 5-HT2A receptor occupancy in schizophrenic patients. Am J Psychiatry 156:869-875, 1999.
86. K Blum, PJ Sheridan, RC Wood, ER Braverman, T Chen, DE Comings. Dopamine D2 receptor gene variants: association and linkage studies in impulsive-addictive-compulsive behavior. Pharmacogenetics 5:121–141, 1995.
87. K Blum, JG Cull, ER Braverman, DE Comings. Reward deficiency syndrome. Am Sci 84:132–145, 1996.

88. DE Comings, RJ Rosenthal, HR Lesieur, LJ Rugle, D Muhleman, C Chiu, G Dietz, R Gade. A study of the dopamine D2 receptor gene in pathological gambling. Pharmacogenetics 6:223–234, 1996.
89. DE Comings, R Gade, S Wu, C Chiu, G Dietz, D Muhleman, G Saucier, L Ferry, RJ Rosenthal, HR Lesieur, LJ Rugle, P MacMurray. Studies of the potential role of the dopamine D1 receptor gene in addictive behaviors. Mol Psychiatry 2:44–56, 1997.
90. DE Comings, N Gonzalez, S Wu, R Gade, D Muhleman, G Saucier, P Johnson, R Verde, RJ Rosenthal, HR Lesieur, LJ Rugle, WB Miller, JP MacMurray. Studies of the 48 bp repeat polymorphism of the DRD4 gene in impulsive, compulsive, addictive behaviors: Tourette syndrome, ADHD, pathological gambling, and substance abuse. Am J Hum Genet 88:358–368, 1999.
91. DW Self, WJ Barnhart, DA Lehman, EJ Nestler. Opposite modulation of cocaine-seeking behavior by D1- and D2-like dopamine receptor agonists. Science 271:1586–1589, 1996.
92. HH van Tol, CM Wu, HC Guan, K Ohara, JR Bunzow, O Civelli, J Kennedy, P Seeman, HB Niznik, V Jovaovic. Multiple dopamine D4 receptor variants in the human population. Nature 358:149–152, 1992.
93. J Benjamin, C Patterson, BD Greenber, DL Murphy, DH Hamer. Population and familial association between the D4 dopamine receptor and measures of novelty seeking. Nat Genet 12:81–84, 1996.
94. RP Ebstein, O Novick, R Umansky, B Priel, Y Osher, D Blaine, ER Bennett, L Nemanov, M Katz, RH Belmaker. Dopamine D4 receptor (DRD4) exon III polymorphism associated with the human personality trait of novelty seeking. Nat Genet 12:78–80, 1996.
95. AK Malhotra, M Virkunnen, W Rooney, M Eggert, M Linnoila, D Goldman. The association between the dopamine D4 (D4DR) 16 amino acid repeat and novelty seeking. Mol Psychiatry 1:388–391, 1996.
96. J Gelernter, H Kranzler, E Coccaro, L Siever, A New, CL Mulgrew. D4 dopamine-receptor (DRD4) alleles and novelty-seeking in substance-dependent, personality-disorder and control subjects. Am J Hum Genet 61:1144–1152, 1997.
97. EG Jonssen, MM Nothen, JP Gustavson, H Neidt, S Brene, A Tylec, P Propping, GC Sedval. Lack of evidence for allelic association between personality traits and the dopamine D4 receptor gene polymorphisms. Am J Psychiatry 154:697–699, 1997.
98. PF Sullivan, WJ Fifield, MA Kennedy, RT Mulder, JD Sellman, PR Joyce. No association between novelty seeking and the type 4 dopamine receptor gene (DRD4) in two New Zealand samples. Am J Psychiatry 155:98–101, 1998.
99. I Perez de Castro, A Ibanez, P Torres, J Saiz-Ruiz, J Fernandez-Piqueras. Genetic association study between pathological gambling and a functional DNA polymorphism at the D4 receptor gene. Pharmacogenetics 7:345–348, 1997.
100. A Roy, B Adinoff, L Roehrich, D Lamparski, R Custer, V Lorenz, M Barbaccia, A Guidotti, A Costa, M Linnoila. Pathological gambling. A psychobiological study. Arch Gen Psychiatry 45:369–373, 1988.
101. A Roy, J De Jong, M Linnoila. Extraversion in pathological gamblers. Correlates with indexes of noradrenergic function. Arch Gen Psychiatry 46:679–681, 1989.
102. M Zuckerman. Sensation seeking: beyond the optimal level of arousal. Hillsdale, NJ: Lawrence Erlbaum Associates, 1979.
103. G Meyer, BP Hauffa, M Schedlowski, C Pawluk, MA Stadler, MS Exton. Casino gambling increases heart rate and salivary cortisol in regular gamblers. Biol Psychiatry 48:948–953, 2000.
104. LH Schmitt, GA Harrison, RM Spargo. Variation in epinephrine and cortisol excretion rates associated with behavior in an Australian aboriginal community. Am J Phys Anthropol 106:249–253, 1998.
105. MN Potenza, DA Fiellen, GR Heninger, BJ Rounsaville, CM Mazure. Gambling: an addictive behavior with health and primary care implications. J Gen Intern Med (submitted).
106. AG Phillips, FG LePiane. Reinforcing effects of morphine microinjection on to the ventral tegmental area. Pharmacol Biochem Behav 12:965–968, 1980.
107. L von Wolfswinkel, JM van Ree. Effects of morphine and naloxone on thresholds of ventral tegmental electrical self-stimulation. Naunyn Schmiedebergs Arch Pharmacol 330:84–92, 1985.
108. SS O'Malley, AJ Jaffe, G Chang, RS Schottenfeld, RE Meyer, B Rounsaville. Naltrexone and coping skills therapy for alcohol dependence. A controlled study. Arch Gen Psychiatry 49:881–887, 1992.
109. JR Volpicelli, AI Alterman, M Hayashida, CP O'Brien. Naltrexone in the treatment of alcohol dependence [see comments]. Arch Gen Psychiatry 49:876–880, 1992.
110. DN Crockford, N el-Guebaly. Naltrexone in the treatment of pathological gambling and alcohol dependence [letter]. Can J Psychiatry 43:86, 1998.
111. SW Kim. Opioid antagonists in the treatment of impulse-control disorders. J Clin Psychiatry 59:159–164, 1998.
112. SW Kim, J Grant. The psychopharmacology of pathological gambling. Semin Clin Neuropsychiatry 6:184–194, 2001.
113. SW Kim, JE Grant, DE Adson, YC Shin. Double-blind naltrexone and placebo comparison study in the

treatment of pathological gambling. Biol Psychiatry 49:28–35, 2001.
114. KC Winters, T Rich. A twin study of adult gambling behavior. J Gambling Stud 14:213–225, 1998.
115. SA Eisen, N Lin, MJ Lyons, JF Scherrer, K Griffith, WR True, J Goldberg, MT Tsuang. Familial influences on gambling behavior: an analysis of 3359 twin pairs. Addiction 93:1375–1384, 1998.
116. MT Tsuang, MJ Lyons, SA Eisen, J Goldberg, W True, N Lin, JM Meyer, R Toomey, SV Faraone, L Eaves. Genetic influences on DSM-III-R drug abuse and dependence: a study of 3,372 twin pairs. Am J Med Genet 67:473–477, 1996.
117. RM Stewart, RI Brown. An outcome study of Gamblers Anonymous. Br J Psychiatry 152:284–288, 1988.
118. RJ Kownacki, WR Shadish. Does Alcoholics Anonymous work? The results from a meta-analysis of controlled experiments. Subst Use Misuse 34:1897–1916, 1999.
119. NM Petry, JM Roll. A behavioral approach to understanding and treating pathological gambling. Semin Clin Neuropsychiatry 6:177–183, 2001.
120. N McConaghy, MS Armstrong, A Blaszczynski, C Allcock. Controlled comparison of aversive therapy and imaginal desensitization in compulsive gambling. Br J Psychiatry 142:366–372, 1983.
121. A Blaszczynski, N McConaghy, A Frankova. Control versus abstinence in the treatment of pathological gambling: a two to nine year follow-up. Br J Addict 86:299–306, 1991.
122. N McConaghy, A Blaszczynski, A Frankova. Comparison of imaginal desensitisation with other behavioural treatments of pathological gambling: a two- to nine-year follow-up. Br J Psychiatry 159:390–393, 1991.
123. A Bujold, R Ladouceur, C Sylvain, JM Boisvert. Treatment of pathological gamblers: an experimental study. J Behav Ther Exp Psychiatry 25:275–282, 1994.
124. C Sylvain, R Ladouceur, JM Boisvert. Cognitive and behavioral treatment of pathological gambling: a controlled study. J Consult Clin Psychol 65:727–732, 1997.
125. WK Goodman, LH Price, SA Rasmussen, PL Delgado, GR Heninger, DS Charney. Efficacy of fluvoxamine in obsessive-compulsive disorder: a double-blind comparison with placebo. Arch Gen Psychiatry 46:36–43, 1989.
126. E Hollander, M Frenkel, C Decaria, S Trungold, DJ Stein. Treatment of pathological gambling with clomipramine [letter]. Am J Psychiatry 149:710–711, 1992.
127. E Hollander, CM DeCaria, E Mari, CM Wong, S Mosovich, R Grossman, T Begaz. Short-term single-blind fluvoxamine treatment of pathological gambling. Am J Psychiatry 155:1781–1783, 1998.
128. E Hollander, CM DeCaria, JN Finkell, T Begaz, CM Wong, CA Cartwright. A randomized double-blind fluvoxamine/placebo crossover trial in pathological gambling. Biol Psychiatry 47:813–817, 2000.
129. JJ De La Gandara, O Sanz, I Gilaberte. Fluoxetine: open-trial in pathological gambling. American Psychiatric Association Annual Convention. Washington, DC, 1999.
130. M Zimmerman, R Breen. An open-label study of citalopram in the treatment of pathological gambling. 11th International Conference on Gambling and Risk Taking. Las Vegas, NV, 2001.
131. C Blanco-Jerez, E Petkova, A Ibanez, J Saiz-Ruiz. A long-term, double-blind, placebo-controlled study of fluvoxamine for pathological gambling. American Psychiatric Association Annual Convention. Washington, DC, 1999.
132. LH Price, DS Charney, PL Delgado, GR Heninger. Lithium and serotonin function: implications for the serotonin hypothesis of depression. Psychopharmacology 100:3–12, 1990.
133. JA Moskowitz. Lithium and lady luck; use of lithium carbonate in compulsive gambling. NY State J Med 80:785–788, 1980.
134. E Hollander. The aggressive impulsivity spectrum: pathological gambling. American Psychiatric Association Annual Conference. New Orleans, LA, 2001.
135. S Pallanti. Lithium and valproate treatment of pathological gambling: a randomized, single-blind study. 15th National Council on Problem Gambling Conference. Seattle, WA, 2001.
136. R Haller, H Hinterhuber. Treatment of pathological gambling with carbamazepine. Pharmacopsychiatry 27:129, 1994.
137. RA Chambers, MN Potenza. Schizophrenia and pathological gambling [letter]. Am J Psychiatry 158:497–498, 2001.
138. L Rugle. A double-blind, placebo-controlled trial of olanzapine in the treatment of pathological gambling. National Center for Responsible Gaming Conference on Comorbidity. Las Vegas, NV, 2000.
139. MN Potenza, MA Steinberg, SD McLaughlin, R Wu, BJ Rounsaville, SS O'Malley. Illegal behaviors in problem gambling: analysis of data from a gambling helpline. J Am Acad Psychiatry Law 28:389–403, 2000.
140. HR Lesieur. Types, lotteries, and substance abuse among problem gamblers: commentary on "Illegal behaviors in problem gambling: analysis of data from a gambling helpline." J Am Acad Psychiatry Law 28:404–407, 2000.

141. DA Fiellin, Reid MC, O'Connor PG. Screening for alcohol problems in primary care: a systematic review. Arch Intern Med 160:1977–1989, 2000.
142. S Sullivan. Development of the 'Eight' problem gambling screen. Thesis in Dept. Gen Practice Primary Care, Auckland, NZ, 1999.
143. EE Johnson, R Hamer, RM Nora, Rena, B Tan. The Lie/Bet Questionnaire for screening pathological gamblers. Psychol Rep 80:83–88, 1997.
144. MN Potenza. A perspective on future directions in the prevention, treatment and research of pathological gambling. Psychiatr Ann 32:203–207, 2002.

47

Neurobiology of Suicide

LEO SHER and J. JOHN MANN
Columbia University, New York, New York, U.S.A.

I. STRESS-DIATHESIS MODEL OF SUICIDAL BEHAVIOR

There are approximately 30,000 deaths per year by suicide in the United States [1,2]. In 1999, suicide was the eighth leading cause of death, ranking ahead of AIDS and liver and kidney disease [1]. Despite the decrease in the death rates from leading causes such as myocardial infarction and AIDS, rates of suicide have remained stubbornly high.

Suicide is a very extreme type of behavior. We have proposed a stress-diathesis model to explain what is different in people who are at risk for suicide compared to people who are relatively protected [3]. Over the past two decades, there has been increasing evidence that part of diathesis for suicidal behavior has a biological component. The study of neurobiology of suicide can yield new understanding of the diathesis or what contributes to vulnerability for suicide, may eventually assist in improved screening of high-risk patients and permit development of new treatment modalities to prevent suicide. Thus, the neurobiologic studies of risk for suicide, may not only potentially improve identification of patients at high risk for suicide, but also suggest new approaches for therapeutic intervention.

Suicide is usually a complication of a psychiatric disorder, a stressor that is present in > 90% of suicides [1–4]. Suicide is most commonly associated with mood disorders, present in ~ 60% of cases [5–9]. Suicide is also associated with schizophrenia, cluster B type personality disorders, alcoholism, substance abuse, Huntington's disease, and epilepsy [10–22]. The lifetime mortality due to suicide is estimated at ~ 20% for bipolar disorder, 15% for unipolar depression, 10–17% for alcoholism, and 5–10% for personality disorders [10–13]. These numbers apply to sicker patients associated with teaching hospitals. Bostwick and Pankratz [23] recently reported that for affective disorder patients hospitalized without specification of suicidality, the lifetime risk of suicide was 4.0% compared with 0.5% for the nonaffectively ill population. Murphy and Wetzel [24] also calculated a lower suicide rate in alcoholism in general. Nevertheless, the lifetime rates of suicide attempts and suicide are still much higher in these disorders than in the general population.

Most patients with psychiatric disorders do not commit suicide, indicating that other factors influence risk. Suicide attempters have a tendency to make more than one suicide attempt, sometimes with increasing lethality in succeeding attempts [25]. At the same time, other persons with the same level of objective severity of major depression may never make a suicide attempt, suggesting that some individuals have a predisposition to suicidal behavior. Malone et al. [25] reported that most vulnerable individuals with a mood disorder who make a suicide attempt, do so early in the course of illness. Mann [3] has suggested that suicide is not simply a logical response to extreme stress, and proposed a stress-diathesis model of suicidal behavior. Typical stressors associated with suicidal acts include the psychiatric disorder, and often also acute use of alcohol or sedatives that may disinhibit patients, sometimes an acute medical illness especially affecting the CNS, and finally adverse life events.

Mann [3] suggests that the diathesis or predisposition to suicidal behavior is a key element that differentiates psychiatric patients who are at high risk versus those at lower risk. Although the objective severity of the psychiatric illness does not assist greatly in distinguishing patients at high risk for suicide attempt or suicide from those who are at low risk, suicide attempters react differently to the same objectively determined level of severity of depression and life events. Suicide attempters experience more subjective depression, hopelessness, and suicidal ideation than psychiatric controls.

The vulnerability or diathesis for suicidal behavior is influenced by genetic factors [26–28], parenting [29]; medical illness, especially affecting the brain, e.g., epilepsy [20]; migraine [30,31]; Huntington's disease [21,22]; alcoholism and substance abuse [14–19]; and cholesterol level [32–39]. Some of these factors may be interrelated. Diathesis (vulnerability) determines how an individual reacts to a given stressor, and depends on factors that mold personality such as environmental and genetic factors, childhood experiences, etc. The neurobiologic findings can represent a combination of state- and trait-related effects [40]. The trait-related effects may represent the diathesis, whereas the state-dependent effects may reflect acute psychiatric conditions or stressors.

II. GENETIC STUDIES OF SUICIDAL BEHAVIOR

It has long been recognized that psychiatric disorders run in families. In 1621 Robert Burton wrote in his book *The Anatomy of Melancholy* that the "inbred cause of melancholy is our temperature, in whole or part, which we receive from our parent," and "such as the temperature of the father is, such is the son's, and look what disease the father had when he begot him, his son will have after him" [41].

Genetic factors also play an important role in the diathesis for suicidal behavior. Evidence that suicidal behavior has a genetic component comes from different types of studies including studies of families, twin and adoption studies, and molecular genetic research. Genetic studies demonstrate that suicidal behavior has a genetic component that is independent of the genetic component of major psychiatric disorders [26–28,42–44].

A. Family History

Suicidal behavior can be transmitted familially by learning, by genetic transmission, by environmental influences, etc. A number of studies suggest that individuals at risk for suicidal behavior have a higher than statistically expected family history of suicide.

Murphy and Wetzel [45] in their review of existing literature noted that 6–8% of those who attempted suicide have a family history of suicide. Roy [46] also reviewed the literature and found that a family history of suicide was more frequent in the families of suicide victims than controls.

Egeland and Sussex [47] reported on the suicide data obtained from the study of affective disorders among the Older Order Amish community in southeastern Pennsylvania. Twenty-six people committed suicide in this community over the 100 years from 1880 to 1980. Almost three-quarters of the 26 suicide victims were clustered in four family pedigrees, each of which contained a heavy loading for affective disorders and suicide. The converse was not true: there were other family pedigrees with an equally heavy loading for affective disorders but without a single suicide in 100 years. A familial loading for affective disorders was not itself a sufficient predictor for suicide.

Some examples will illustrate the point. Shafii et al. [48] performed psychological autopsies on 20 adolescent suicide victims in Louisville, KY. The authors reported that significantly more of the suicide victims as compared to the controls had a family history of suicide.

Linkowski et al. [49] found that 123 of 713 depressed inpatients (17%) had a first- or second-degree relative who had committed suicide. A family history of suicide increased the probablility of a suicide attempt among the depressed patient, especially the risk for a violent suicide attempt.

Brent et al. [44] conducted a family study of adolescent suicide victims (suicide probands) and community control probands (controls). The rate of suicide attempts was increased in the first-degree relatives of suicide probands compared with the relatives of controls, even after adjusting for differences in rates of probands and familial axis I and II disorders. The authors concluded that liability to suicidal behavior might be familially transmitted as a trait independent of axis I and II disorders.

B. Twin Studies

Twin studies help to address the question of whether suicidal behavior may be genetically transmitted. If suicide is a genetically transmitted behavior, then concordance for suicide should be greater among identical twins (monozygotic, MZ) than fraternal (dizygotic, DZ) twins. Twin studies support the presence of a substantial genetic component in suicidal behavior. Roy [43] reported a much higher concordance rate for MZ twins than for DZ twins (13.2% vs. 0.7%). Roy et al. [27] also found a higher rate of concordance for suicide attempts in MZ compared to DZ twins surviving the cotwin suicide. Roy et al. [27] reported that the rate of concordance for attempted suicide (38%) was higher than for completed suicide (13.2%). This indicates that both attempted and completed suicide are heritable, and that they are both components of the phenotype of suicidal behavior. Statham et al. [50] reported a 23.1 concordance rate for serious suicide attempt in MZ twins, over 17-fold greater risk than in the total sample. The authors reported that the heritability for serious suicide attempts was 55%. Twin studies do not rule out effects of a common environment, and do not explain the basis of the heritability such as psychopathology.

C. Adoption Studies

Adoption studies provide the strongest evidence that there may be a genetic factor for suicide and that it is independent of the genetic transmission of major psychiatric disorders. Schulsinger et al. [28] reported results from an adoption study conducted in Denmark. A screening of the adoption register in Copenhagen for causes of death revealed that 57 adoptees had committed suicide. They were matched with 57 adopted controls for age, sex, social class of the adopting parents, and time spent both with their biological relatives and in institutions before being adopted. Twelve of the 269 biological relatives (4.5%) of the adopted suicides had themselves committed suicide, compared with only 2 of the 269 biological relatives (0.7%) of the adopted controls. This difference was statistically significant even allowing for the transmission of major psychiatric illnesses. None of the adopting relatives of either the suicide adoptee group or the control adoptee group had committed suicide.

The examination of the type of affective disorder suffered by the suicide victim is of particular interest. Wender et al. [51] reported that adoptee suicide victims with the diagnosis of "affect reaction" had significantly more biological relatives who had committed suicide than controls. The diagnosis of affect reaction has been used in Denmark to describe a patient who had mood symptoms accompanying a situational crisis, triggering what may have been an impulsive suicide attempt. Perhaps part of the genetic predisposition to suicide may be related to a tendency for impulsive behavior.

D. Molecular Genetic Research

Molecular genetic analyses attempt to identify the specific alleles which may be responsible for the observed familiality and heritability of phenotype. Two techniques that are usually used to identify genes for complex diseases such as psychiatric disorders are positional cloning (linkage) and case/control association methods using candidate gene markers [52–54]. Both types of study have advantages and disadvantages.

Positional cloning is systematic and allows coverage of the whole genome but is not powerful, whereas association methods are powerful but not systematic. In positional cloning the coinheritance of a disorder and a DNA marker is studied in large families or related pairs. Another key approach is linkage disequilibrium (marker/disease gene association) in populations. With most clinical samples, linkage studies are frequently not very powerful for common complex diseases in which no single gene accounts for much of the variance in vulnerability. However, case/control association methods work on a different principle and do not suffer the same vulnerability. All humans have considerable genetic variation or polymorphism. A gene is called polymorphic if no single form of the gene has an abundance of > 99% in a population [54]. Gene variants, including polymorphisms, are related to the development of diseases which are genetically influenced.

Association studies search for correlations in the population between a DNA marker and a disorder. If persons with a disorder have an increased frequency of a specific allele, or genotype, it may mean that the gene contributes to vulnerability to the disease. The candidate gene approach is frequently used in association studies. When biological investigations have provided some clue as to the possible involvement of known genes, these genes may become candidates for studies. If a biochemical pathway leading to a mental disorder has been identified, proteins that participate in this pathway indicate candidate genes that may give results in association tests.

Most candidate gene studies of suicidal behavior have involved the serotonergic system. Serotonergic neurons are located in the brainstem from where they project to virtually every part of the brain, often modulating neuronal responses to other neurotransmitters [55]. As a result of this widespread projection pattern, serotonin plays a key role in the regulation of many different functions and behaviors. Multiple lines of evidence suggest that major depression and suicidal behavior are independently related to abnormalities in serotonergic system [3,56–58]. There is a serotonergic abnormality that contributes to the diathesis or vulnerability to suicidal acts [3]. The risk for suicidal behavior, aggressive acts, alcoholism, and substance abuse appear to have in part a common underlying genetic or biological predisposition mediated by serotonergic activity [3]. Thus, genes related to serotonergic pathways became a focus of attention of genetic researchers studying mood disorders and suicidal behavior.

1. TPH Gene

Tryptophan hydroxylase (TPH) is the rate-limiting enzyme in serotonin biosynthesis. Several candidate gene studies demonstrated an association between a polymorphism of the TPH gene and suicidal behavior, and there is one positive linkage study [59]. An association between a polymorphism in the TPH gene in intron 7, A779C, and suicidal behavior was first reported by Nielsen et al. [60]. The results of this study were replicated by Nielsen et al. [61] in a larger sample. The L allele (equivalent to the C allele) was found to be more common in the impulsive alcoholic criminal offenders who attempted suicide (LL 72%, UL 59%, and UU 31%). In serious or multiple suicide attempters, this finding was even more striking.

Mann et al. [62] studied the distribution of the same polymorphism in 29 depressed attempters and 22 depressed nonattempters. The U allele was shown to be more common (41% vs. 20%) in attempters than in depressed nonattempters.

Buresi et al. [63] investigated the prevalence of the A218C TPH polymorphism in a large sample of suicide attempters and healthy controls and found that rarer A (or U) allele was more common among the suicide attempters (46.4% vs. 35.7%, $P = .003$). The frequency of A allele was even higher in serious suicide attempters. These results were recently replicated by Persson [64] but not by Bellivier et al. [65], Kunugi et al. [66], or Ono et al. (67). Consistent with the results of Mann et al. [62], Buresi et al. [63], and Persson et al. [64], Manuck et al. [68], and Joensson et al. [69] found lower serotonergic activity to be associated with the U allele. Further studies are necessary to clarify the role of the TPH gene in the etiology of suicidal behavior.

2. 5-HTTLPR Allele in the Serotonin Transporter Gene

A 44–base pair deletion/insertion polymorphism in the 5′ flanking regulatory region of the human 5HTT gene results in differential expression of 5HTT and serotonin reuptake in transformed lymphoblastoma cell lines [70]. The short allele (frequency 0.4 in Caucasians and 0.6 in some Asian populations) has reduced transcriptional efficiency, resulting in decreased 5HTT expression and 5HT reuptake and reduced 5HTT density in vivo in transformed lymphoblastoma cell lines [55]. The short form of the serotonin transporter promoter length repeat polymorphism (5HTTLPR) is associated with 40% fewer binding sites in homozygote (SS) and the heterozygote (SL) than the long form (LL). Mann et al. [58] hypothesized that fewer 5HTT sites on platelets of depressed patients, and fewer 5HTT sites in the prefrontal cortex of suicides, may be the consequence of an association of the short allele with suicide and major depression. In this study postmortem brain samples were genotyped for the 5HTTLPR polymorphism, and 5HTT binding was assayed. The 5HTTLPR was associated with major depression but not with suicide. However, the association was due to a difference in the rate of heterozygotes, and moreover, genotype was not associated with any difference in brain serotonin transporter binding. This finding indicates that the serotonergic transporter binding abnormalities abnormalities in the brain of suicide victims may be related to other genetic variants.

Studies of the association of the 5HTTLPR and mood disorders, alcoholism, and certain personality traits have produced inconsistent results [71–74]. The differences in the number and function of the serotonin transporter may make a contribution to the development of certain psychiatric symptoms and personality traits, but additional are needed to determine whether other promoter alleles contribute to the etiopathogenesis of behavioral disorders.

3. 5-HT1B Gene

Several research groups have reported pathological aggressive behavior and increased alcohol and cocaine intake in 5HT1B receptor gene knockout mice [75–78]. This indicates that functional variants in the 5HT1B gene may contribute to human psychopathologies such as suicide, aggression, major depression, alcoholism, or substance abuse. However, Huang et al. [79] found no association of suicide, major depression, or pathological aggression with 5HT1B genotypes or allelic frequency for two identified polymorphisms in a postmortem study of the 5HT1B binding. The sample size was modest, and Huang et al. [79] could have missed an uncommon association. There was a suggestion of an association between alcoholism and lower 5HT1B binding that is consistent with reports of an association with a 5HT1B polymorphism [80,81].

4. 5HT2A Gene

Zhang et al. [82] studied an association between the 102T/C polymorphism in the 5HT2A receptor gene and suicidal behavior and found a weak association of the TT genotype with suicide attempts in patients with mood disorders. However, Turecki et al. [83] found no association between suicide and the TT genotype. Moreover, Du et al. [84] found an association between suicidal ideations and the CC genotype. The role of 102T/C 5HT2A polymorphism in the etiology of suicidal behavior requires further investigation.

III. IN VIVO BIOCHEMICAL STUDIES

5-Hydroxyindolacetic acid (5HIAA) is the major metabolite of serotonin [85]. A number of research groups studied cerebrospinal fluid (CSF) 5HIAA levels in the CSF of psychiatric patients [85–87]. About two-thirds of the studies that looked at suicide attempters with mood disorders compared with nonattempters with mood disorders found that suicide attempters have lower levels of CSF 5HIAA. However, about one-third of the studies do not confirm this. One of the factors that appears to determine whether or not CSF 5HIAA is low is the lethality or medical severity of the attempt. The more lethal the attempt, the lower the level of CSF 5HIAA [86]. Low CSF 5HIAA is also found in some, but not all, studies of suicide attempters with schizophrenia and personality disorders compared with patients who have the same diagnoses without a history of suicidal behavior [85,88–92]. Thus, it appears that the relationship between low CSF 5HIAA and suicide attempts is independent of the neurobiology of specific psychiatric disorders.

CSF 5HIAA levels can predict future behavior. During the 12 months after hospital discharge, patients who had low levels of CSF 5HIAA had a higher rate of completed suicide than with patients who had higher levels of CSF 5HIAA [93]. Low CSF 5HIAA predicts future suicide attempts and suicide completion in mood disorders [93,94] and schizophrenia [88].

The prolactin response to fenfluramine is another index of serotonergic function [86,87]. Fenfluramine causes the release of serotonin and inhibits serotonin reuptake. A history of a highly lethal suicide attempt is associated with a blunted prolactin response to fenfluramine [95]. Patients with a history of a very lethal suicide attempt have a blunted prolactin response compared with individuals with major depression but no history of a "very lethal" suicide attempt [95], and, like low CSF 5HIAA, a blunted prolactin response to fenfluramine may be a biochemical trait. Both low CSF 5HIAA and a blunted prolactin response are related to severity of lifetime aggression [96,97]. The blunting of serotonergic function is independent of how long ago the suicide attempt occurred [95].

Serotonin is involved in a number of platelet functions [98–100]. Platelet 5HT2A receptor binding is increased in patients with suicidal behavior [98]. Upregulation of 5HT2A receptors on the platelets of suicide attempters correlates with the severity of the most recent suicide attempt [99,100].

In summary, three different indices of serotonergic function correlate with suicidal behavior in patients independent of psychiatric diagnosis: CSF 5HIAA, the prolactin response to fenfluramine, and platelet 5HT2A receptor binding. The results of these studies suggest that there is a link between genetics, serotonergic function, and suicidal behavior.

IV. POSTMORTEM STUDIES

Interpretation of the results of postmortem studies is complicated by the presence of contradictory data, the variety of diagnoses included in samples of suicide victims, and methodological issues, such as postmortem delay [101]. For example, postmortem brain measurements of 5HT and 5HIAA are of limited value because of the rapid drop in the concentration of these compounds after death [102].

A number of research groups have found increased density of postsynaptic serotonin receptors in the cortex and, conversely, fewer postsynaptic serotonin transporter sites [103–107]. Decreased serotonin release is one possible cause of an increase in 5HT2A receptors in the prefrontal cortex of suicide victims. There may be some degree of regional specificity of the correlation between suicidal behavior, fewer serotonin transporter sites, and increased 5HT1A receptors [101]. Brain regions most involved in suicidal behavior are likely to be those areas where the changes in serotonin receptors are greatest in suicide victims.

Considerable evidence suggests that there are alterations in serotonergic and noradrenergic receptor binding in membrane homogenates from the brain of suicide victims [101,106], independent of psychiatric diagnosis. This suggests that there is a biological substrate for the vulnerability to commit suicide. Alterations in binding to the serotonin transporter and the 5HT1A receptor were found primarily in the ventral and ventrolateral prefrontal cortex of suicide victims [101]. The ventral prefrontal cortex is of particular importance in relation to the risk for suicide. This brain region is involved in the executive function of inhibition, and injuries to this area of the brain can result in disinhibition [3]. The ventral prefrontal cortex may mediate an universal restraint mechanism that is suboptimal in some suicidal patients [3].

V. LEVELS OF SERUM CHOLESTEROL AND SUICIDAL BEHAVIOR

Low levels of cholesterol or cholesterol-lowering treatments (particularly diet) increase the probability of suicidal behavior [37]. Cholesterol levels appear to have an effect on behavior involving aggression and suicidality. For example, a 12-year follow-up of a group of men found that that those with cholesterol levels < 160 mg/dL had a greater risk of suicide than those with levels of 160 mg/dL or higher [38]. Lindberg et al. [36] reported that a 7-year follow-up revealed that the relative risk for suicide was higher in men in the lowest cholesterol group compared to those in the highest cholesterol group. Kunugi et al. [39] found that cholesterol levels were significantly lower in suicide attempters when compared with both psychiatric controls and normal controls when sex, age, and psychiatric diagnosis were adjusted for. Kaplan et al. [34,35] reported evidence from nonhuman primates that a low-cholesterol diet was associated with more aggression and lower serotonergic function. It remains to be determined if such a mechanism operates in man and is the pathway whereby cholesterol influences suicide risk.

VI. PSYCHOTROPIC MEDICATIONS AND SUICIDAL BEHAVIOR

Pharmacological treatments of suicidal behavior are based on two assumptions: (1) individuals with behavioral disorders such as depression, anxiety, impulsivity, alcohol or drug abuse or dependency, bipolar disorder, and schizophrenia, are at higher risk for suicidal behavior; and (2) there is a diathesis for suicidal acts related to biochemical alterations in the brain and psychotropic medications may correct these alterations. Based on these assumptions, psychotropic medications should reduce the symptoms that contribute to the expression of suicidal behavior. Mann and Kapur [108] and Baldessarini and Jamison [109] propose that some medications may prevent the onset of suicidal behaviors in at-risk persons. Another consideration is the toxicity of antidepressants after overdose. An American College of Neuropsychopharmacology Task Force suggested that "new generation low-toxicity antidepressants, including selective serotonin reuptake inhibitors, may carry a lower risk for suicide than older tricyclic antidepressants. This possible safety advantage may be a consequence of lower toxicity in the event of drug overdose" [110].

A considerable number of new and effective psychotropic medications have been developed over the past three decades. However, the reduction in suicide rate has been very little [3]. With the exception of lithium, which may be an effective treatment against suicide, little is known about specific contributions of mood-altering treatments to minimize mortality rates in persons with mood disorders. It has been suggested that long-term lithium treatment shows a protective effect against suicidal behavior in major affective disorder including both unipolar and bipolar disorders [111,112].

Isometsa et al. [113] found that only 10–14% of individuals who committed suicide in the context of major depression had received adequate doses of antidepressant treatment. Recently, Oquendo et al. [114] reported that a large majority of the depressed patients with a history of suicide attempts, who were at higher risk for future suicide and suicide attempts, received inadequate treatment. There may be a potential for more effective recognition of psychiatric conditions such as major depression, and the treatment of these conditions with adequate doses of medications in terms of reducing suicide rates. Rutz et al. [115] found that education of primary care physicians in the diagnosis and treatment of depression produced an increase in prescription rates of antidepressants and decrease in suicide rates. Education at regular intervals has the potential for benefit in the diagnosis and treatment of depression, thereby lowering suicide rates.

Rihmer et al. [116] studied the regional distribution of the suicide rate, rate of diagnosed depression, and prevalence of working physicians in Hungary. The authors found a strong and significant positive correlation between the rate of working physicians and the rate of diagnosed depression, and both parameters showed a strong and significant negative correlation with the suicide rate. The more physicians per 100,000 inhabitants, the better the recognition of depression and the lower the suicide rate.

Isacsson et al. [117] reported the low rate of antidepressant use in suicide victims reflected insufficient diagnosis and treatment of depressive disorders. Marzuk et al. [118] reported similar data from a population of suicide victims in New York City. Eighty-four percent of these patients were not taking an antidepressant (or neuroleptic) medication at the time of suicide. More recently, Isacsson [119] reported that an increase in the use of antidepressants correlates with a substantially reduced a suicide rate in Sweden. Meltzer [120] reports that clozapine can reduce suicide by 80–85% in neuroleptic-resistant patients. More widespread treatment of depressed and psychotic patients with antidepressants and atypical antipsychotic medications may be effective in preventing suicide.

VII. FUTURE DIRECTIONS

The fundamental question is how to improve recognition of individuals at high risk for suicide. Clinicians should consider features that reflect the diathesis or predisposition for suicidal behavior [3]. Such characteristics include a past history of suicidal behavior, evidence of impulsive aggression, and suicidal ideation or feelings of hopelessness disproportionate to the objective severity of depression.

Functional brain imaging studies may be able to bridge postmortem brain studies, and in vivo studies involving cerebrospinal fluid and neuroendocrine challenge techniques by allowing quantitative imaging of neurotransmitrers systems in vivo. Positron emission tomography (PET) can be used to study neurotransmitters and neuroreceptors in live subjects. If PET imaging in living patients can detect changes in neuroreceptors that were found in the brain of suicide victims, that may enable physicians to determine whether the biochemical abnormalities detected after death in suicide victims are present in patients who are at risk for suicide. This may create an opportunity for timely therapeutic interventions to prevent suicide.

The advantages of a prospective study of a large number of subjects—imaging the brain, studying polymorphisms in many candidate genes, obtaining detailed clinical information in the living patient, and studying the changes using neuropharmacological challenges—allow determination of the relative importance and interrelationship of clinical, social, and biological risk factors for suicidal behavior.

ACKNOWLEDGEMENTS

This work was partly supported by PHS grants MH62185, MH48514, MH56390, and MH40210.

REFERENCES

1. Maris RW, Berman AL, Silverman MM. Comprehensive Textbook of Suicidology. New York: Guilford Press, 2000.
2. Ghosh TB, Victor BS. Suicide. In: Hales RE, Yudofsky SC, Talbott JA, eds. The American Psychiatric Press Textbook of Psychiatry, 3rd ed. Washington: American Psychiatric Press, 1999, pp 1383–1404.
3. Mann JJ. The neurobiology of suicide. Nat Med 4:25–30, 1998.
4. Suominen K, Henriksson M, Suokas J, Isometsa E, Ostamo A, Lonnqvist J. Mental disorders and comorbidity in attempted suicide. Acta Psychiatr Scand 94: 234–240, 1996.
5. Barraclough B, Bunch J, Nelson B, Sainsbury P. One hundred cases of suicide. Clinical aspects. Br J Psychiatry 125:355–373, 1974.
6. Robins E, Murphy GE, Wilkinson RH Jr, Gassner S, Kayes J. Some clinical considerations in the prevention of suicide based on a study of 134 successful suicides. Am J Public Health 49:888–899, 1979.
7. Rich CL, Fowler RC, Wagner J, Black NA. San Diego suicide study. III. Relationships between diagnoses and stressors. Arch Gen Psychiatry 45:58–592, 1988.
8. Dorpat TL, Ripley HS. A study of suicide in the Seattle area. Compr Psychiatry 1:349–359, 1960.
9. Isometsä E, Henriksson M, Aro H, Heikkinen M, Kuoppasalmi K, Lonnqvist J. Mental disorders in young and middle aged men who commit suicide. BMJ 310:1366–1367, 1995.
10. Jamison KR. Suicide and bipolar disorders. Ann NY Acad Sci 487:301–315, 1986.
11. Johns CA, Stanley M, Stanley B. Suicide in schizophrenia. Ann NY Acad Sci 487:294–300, 1986.

12. Roy A, Linnoila M. Alcoholism and suicide. Suicide Life Threat Behav 16:244–273, 1986.
13. Frances A, Fyer M, Clarkin J. Personality and suicide. Ann NY Acad Sci 487:281–293, 1986.
14. Roy A, Lamparski J, De Jong J, Karoum F, Linnoila M. Cerebrospinal fluid monoamine metabolites in alcoholic patients who attempt suicide. Acta Psychiatr Scand 81:58–61, 1990.
15. Roy A, Lamparski J, De Jong J, Moore V, Linnoila M. Characteristics of alcoholics who attempt suicide. Am J Psychiatry 147:761–765, 1990.
16. Murphy GE. Suicide and substance abuse. Arch Gen Psychiatry 45:593–594, 1988.
17. Murphy GE, Wetzel RD, Robins E, McEvoy L. Multiple risk factors predict suicide in alcoholism. Arch Gen Psychiatry 49:459–463, 1992.
18. Dulit RA, Fyer MR, Haas GL, Sullivan T, Frances AJ. Substance use in borderline personality disorder. Am J Psychiatry 147:1002–1007, 1990.
19. Marzuk PM, Mann JJ. Suicide and substance abuse. Psychiat Ann 18:639–645, 1988.
20. Brent DA. Overrepresentation of epileptics in a consecutive series of suicide attempters seen at a Children's Hospital, 1978–1983. J Am Acad Child Psychiatry 25(2):242–246, 1986.
21. Schoenfeld M, Myers RH, Cupples LA, Berkman B, Sax DS, Clark E. Increased rate of suicide among patients with Huntington's disease. J Neurol Neurosurg Psychiatry 47:1283–1287, 1984.
22. Farrer LA. Suicide and attempted suicide in Huntington disease: implications for preclinical testing of persons at risk. Am J Med Genet 24:305–311, 1986.
23. Bostwick JM, Pankratz VS. Affective disorders and suicide risk: a reexamination. Am J Psychiatry 157:1925–1932, 2000.
24. Murphy GE, Wetzel R. The lifetime risk of suicide in alcoholism. Arch Gen Psychiatry 47:383–392, 1990.
25. Malone KM, Haas GL, Sweeney JA, Mann JJ. Major depression and the risk of attempted suicide. J Affect Disord 34:173–185, 1995.
26. Roy A, Segal Segal NL, Centerwall BS, Robinette CD. Suicide in twins. Arch Gen Psychiatry 48:29–32, 1991.
27. Roy A, Segal NL, Sarchiapone M. Attempted suicide among living co-twins of twin suicide victims. Am J Psychiatry 152:1075–1076, 1995.
28. Schulsinger F, Kety SS, Rosenthal D, Wender PH. A family study of suicide. In: Schou M, Stromgren E, eds. Origin, Prevention and Treatment of Affective Disorders. New York: Academic Press, 1979.
29. Brodsky BS, Malone KM, Ellis SP, Dulit RA, Mann JJ. Characteristics of borderline personality disorder associated with suicidal behavior. Am J Psychiatry 154:1715–1719, 1997.
30. Breslau N. Migraine, suicidal ideation, and suicide attempts. Neurology 42:392–395, 1992.
31. Breslau N, Davis GC, Andreski P. Migraine, psychiatric disorders, and suicide attempts: an epidemiologic study of young adults. Psychiatry Res 37:11–23, 1991.
32. Muldoon MF, Manuck SB, Matthews KA. Lowering cholesterol concentrations and mortality: a quantitative review of primary prevention trials. BMJ 301:309–314, 1990.
33. Muldoon MF, Rossouw JE, Manuck SB, Glueck CJ, Kaplan JR, Kaufmann PG. Low or lowered cholesterol and risk of death from suicide and trauma. Metabolism 42(suppl 1):45–56, 1993.
34. Kaplan JR, Muldoon MF, Manuck SB, Mann JJ. Assessing the observed relationship between low cholesterol and violence-related mortality. Implications for suicide risk. Ann NY Acad Sci 836:57–80, 1997.
35. Kaplan JR, Shively CA, Fontenot MB, Morgan TM, Howell SM, Manuck SB, Muldoon MF, Mann JJ. Demonstration of an association among dietary cholesterol, central serotonergic activity, and social behavior in monkeys. Psychosom Med 56:479–484, 1994.
36. Lindberg G, Larsson G, Setterlind S, Rastam L. Serum lipids and mood in working men and women in Sweden. J Epidemiol Community Health 48:360–363, 1994.
37. Golomb BA. Cholesterol and violence: is there a connection? Ann Intern Med 128:478–87, 1998.
38. Neaton JD, Blackburn H, Jacobs D, Kuller L, Lee DJ, Sherwin R, Shih J, Stamler J, Wentworth D. Serum cholesterol level and mortality findings for men screened in the Multiple Risk Factor Intervention Trial. Arch Intern Med 152:1490–500, 1992.
39. Kunugi H, Takei N, Aoki H, Nanko S. Low serum cholesterol in suicide attempters. Biol Psychiatry 41:196–200, 1997.
40. Mann JJ, Arango V. Integration of neurobiology and psychopathology in a unified model of suicidal behavior. J Clin Psychopharmacol 12(2):2S–7S, 1992.
41. Burton R. The Anatomy of Melancholy. London: JM Dent & Sons, 1932.
42. Roy A. Genetics of suicide. Ann NY Acad Sci 487:97–105, 1986.
43. Roy A. Genetic and biologic risk factors for suicide in depressive disorders. Psychiatr Q 64(4):345–358, 1993.
44. Brent DA, Bridge J, Johnson BA, Connolly J. Suicidal behavior runs in families. A controlled family study of adolescent suicide victims. Arch Gen Psychiatry 53:1145–1152, 1996.
45. Murphy GE, Wetzel RD. Family history of suicidal behavior among suicide attempters. J Nerv Ment Dis 170:86–90, 1982.
46. Roy A. Family history of suicide. Arch Gen Psychiatry 40:971–974, 1983.

47. Egeland JA, Sussex JN. Suicide and family loading for affective disorders. JAMA 254:915–918, 1985.
48. Shafii M, Carrigan S, Whittinghill JR, Derrick A. Psychological autopsy of completed suicide in children and adolescents. Am J Psychiatry 142(9):1061–1064, 1985.
49. Linkowski P, De Maertelaer V, Mendlewicz J. Suicidal behaviour in major depressive illness. Acta Psychiatr Scand 72:233–238, 1985.
50. Statham DJ, Heath AC, Madden PA, Bucholz KK, Bierut L, Dinwiddie SH, Slutske WS, Dunne MP, Martin NG. Suicidal behaviour: an epidemiological and genetic study. Psychol Med 28:839–855, 1998.
51. Wender PH, Kety SS, Rosenthal D, Schulsinger F, Ortmann J, Lunde I. Psychiatric disorders in the biological and adoptive families of adopted individuals with affective disorders. Arch Gen Psychiatry 1986; 43:923–9, 1986.
52. Lathrop GM, Terwilliger JD, Weeks DE. Multifactorial inheritance and genetic analysis of multifactorial disease. In: Rimoin DL, Connor JM, Pyeritz RE, eds. Emery and Rimon's Principle and Practice of Medical Genetics. 3rd ed. New York: Churchill Livingstone, 1996, pp. 1765-1770.
53. Eley TC, Plomin R. Genetic analyses of emotionality. Curr Opin Neurobiol 7:279–284, 1997.
54. Gelertner J. Clinical molecular genetics. In: Charney DS, Nestler EJ, Bunney BS, eds. Neurobiology of Mental Ilness. New York: Oxford University Press, 1999, pp 108–120.
55. Cravchik A, Goldman D. Neurochemical individuality: genetic diversity among human dopamine and serotonin receptors and transporters. Arch Gen Psychiatry 57:1105–1114, 2000.
56. Mann JJ, Stoff DM. A synthesis of current findings regarding neurobiological correlates and treatment of suicidal behavior. Ann NY Acad Sci 836:352–363, 1997.
57. Malone KM, Mann JJ. Serotonin and major depression. In: Mann JJ, Kupfer DJ, eds. Biology of Depressive Disorders, Vol. 3, Part A: A System Perspective. New York: Plenum Press, 1993.
58. Mann JJ, Huang YY, Underwood MD, Kassir SA, Oppenheim S, Kelly TM, Dwork AJ, Arango V. A serotonin transporter gene promoter polymorphism (5-HTTLPR) and prefrontal cortical binding in major depression and suicide. Arch Gen Psychiatry 57:729–738, 2000.
59. Mann JJ, Brent DA, Arango V. The neurobiology and genetics of suicide and attempted suicide: a focus on the serotonergic system. Neuropsychopharmacology 24:467–477, 2001.
60. Nielsen DA, Goldman D, Virkkunen M, Tokola R, Rawlings R, Linnoila M. Suicidality and 5-hydroxyindoleacetic acid concentration associated with a tryptophan hydroxylase polymorphism. Arch Gen Psychiatry 51:34–38, 1994.
61. Nielsen DA, Virkkunen M, Lappalainen J, Eggert M, Brown GL, Long JC, Goldman D, Linnoila M. A tryptophan hydroxylase gene marker for suicidality and alcoholism. Arch Gen Psychiatry 55:593–602, 1998.
62. Mann JJ, Malone KM, Nielsen DA, Goldman D, Erdos J, Gelertner J. Possible association of a polymorphism of the tryptophan hydroxylase gene with suicidal behavior in depressed patients. Am J Psychiatry 154:1451–1453, 1997.
63. Buresi C, Courtet P, Leboyer M, Feingold J, Malafosse A. Association between suicide attempt and the Trytophane Hydroxylase (TPH) gene. In: Forty-Seventh Annual Meeting of the American Society of Human Genetics, Baltimore, MD, October 28–November 1, 1997. (abstracts) Am J Hum Genet 61 Suppl: A270, 1997.
64. Persson M-L. Suicide Attempt and Genes. Psychiatric and Genetic Characteristics of Suicide Attempters. Stockholm: Kongl Karolinska Medico Chirurgiska Institutet, 1999.
65. Bellivier F, Leboyer M, Courtet P, Buresi C, Beaufils B, Samolyk D, Allilaire JF, Feingold J, Mallet J, Malafosse A. Association between the tryptophan hydroxylase gene and manic-depressive illness. Arch Gen Psychiatry 55:33–37, 1998.
66. Kunugi H, Ishida S, Kato T, Sakai T, Tatsumi M, Hirose T, Nanko S. No evidence for an association of polymorphisms of the tryptophan hydroxylase gene with affective disorders or attempted suicide among Japanese patients. Am J Psychiatry 156:774–776, 1999.
67. Ono H, Shirakawa O, Nishiguchi N, Nishimura A, Nushida H, Ueno Y, Maeda K. Tryptophan hydroxylase gene polymorphisms are not associated with suicide. Am J Med Genet 96:861–863, 2000.
68. Manuck SB, Flory JD, Ferrell RE, Dent KM, Mann JJ, Muldoon MF. Aggression and anger-related traits associated with a polymorphism of the tryptophan hydroxylase gene. Biol Psychiatry 45:603–614, 1999.
69. Joensson EG, Goldman D, Spurlock G, Gustavsson JP, Nielsen DA, Linnoila M, Owen MJ, Sedvall GC. Tryptophan hydroxylase and catechol-O-methyltransferase gene polymorphisms: relationships to monoamine metabolite concentrations in CSF of healthy volunteers. Eur Arch Psychiatry Clin Neurosci 247:297–302, 1997.
70. Lesch KP, Bengel D, Heils A, Sabol SZ, Greenberg BD, Petri S, Benjamin J, Muller CR, Hamer DH, Murphy DL. Association of anxiety-related traits with a polymorphism in the serotonin transporter gene regulatory region. Science 274:1527–1531, 1996.

71. Stoltenberg SF, Burmeister M. Recent progress in psychiatric genetics—some hope but no hype. Hum Mol Genet 9:927–935, 2000.
72. Gorwood P, Batel P, Ades J, Hamon M, Boni C. Serotonin transporter gene polymorphisms, alcoholism, and suicidal behavior. Biol Psychiatry 48:259–264, 2000.
73. Greenberg BD, McMahon FJ, Murphy DL. Serotonin transporter candidate gene studies in affective disorders and personality: promises and potential pitfalls. Mol Psychiatry 3:186–189, 1998.
74. Sher L. Psychiatric diagnoses and inconsistent results of association studies in behavioral genetics. Med Hypotheses 54:207–209, 2000.
75. Saudou F, Amara DA, Dierich A, Lemeur M, Ramboz S, Segu L, Buhot M-C, Hen R. Enhanced aggressive behavior in mice lacking 5-HT$_{1B}$ receptor. Science 265:1875–1878, 1994.
76. Crabbe JC, Phillips TJ, Feller DJ, Hen R, Wenger CD, Lessov, CN, Schafer GL. Elevated alcohol consumption in null mutant mice lacking 5-HT$_{1B}$ serotonin receptors. Nat Genet 14:98–101, 1996.
77. Ramboz S, Saudou F, Amara DA, Belzung C, Dierich A, Lemeur M, Segu L, Misslin R, Buhot M-C, Hen R. Behavioral characterization of mice packing the 5-HT$_{1B}$ receptor. NIDA Res Monogr 161:39–57, 1996.
78. Rocha BA, Ator R, Emmett-Oglesby MW, Hen R. Intravenous cocaine self-administration in mice lacking 5HT1B receptors. Pharmacol Biochem Behav 57:407–412, 1997.
79. Huang YY, Grailhe R, Arango V, Hen R, Mann JJ. Relationship of psychopathology to the human serotonin1B genotype and receptor binding kinetics in postmortem brain tissue. Neuropsychopharmacology 21:238–246, 1999.
80. Lappalainen J, Long JC, Eggert M, Ozaki N, Robin RW, Brown GL, Naukkarinen H, Virkkunen M, Linnoila M, Goldman D. Linkage of antisocial alcoholism to the serotonin 5HT1B receptor gene in 2 populations. Arch Gen Psychiatry 55:989–994, 1998.
81. Goldman D, Lappalainen J, Vallejo R, Robin RW, Virkkunen M, Linnoila M, Long J. Linkage of the 5HT1B serotonin receptor to antisocial alcoholism in Finns and Southwestern Indians (abstract). Am J Med Genet 81:479, 1998.
82. Zhang H-Y, Ishigaki T, Tani K, Chen K, Shih JC, Miyasato K, Ohara K. Serotonin$_{2A}$ receptor gene polymorphism in mood disorders. Biol Psychiatry 41:768–773, 1997.
83. Turecki G, Briere R, Dewar K, Antonetti T, Lesage AD, Seguin M, Chawky N, Vanier C, Alda M, Joober R, Benkelfat C, Rouleau GA. Prediction of level of serotonin 2A receptor binding by serotonin receptor 2A genetic variation in postmortem brain samples from subjects who did or did not commit suicide. Am J Psychiatry 156:1456–1458, 1999.
84. Du L, Bakish D, Lapierre YD, Ravindran AV, Hrdina PD. Association of polymorphism of serotonin 2A receptor gene with suicidal ideation in major depressive disorder. Am J Med Genet 96:56–60, 2000.
85. Åsberg M, Nordström P, Träskman-Bendz L. Cerebrospinal fluid studies in suicide. An overview. Ann NY Acad Sci 487:243–255, 1986.
86. Mann JJ, Oquendo M, Underwood MD, Arango V. The neurobiology of suicide risk: a review for the clinician. J Clin Psychiatry 60(uppl 2):7–11, 1999.
87. Oquendo MA, Mann JJ. The biology of impulsivity and suicidality. Psychiatr Clin North Am 23:11–25, 2000.
88. Cooper SJ, Kelly CB, King DJ. 5-Hydroxyindoleacetic acid in cerebrospinal fluid and prediction of suicidal behaviour in schizophrenia. Lancet 340:940–941, 1992.
89. Gardner DL, Lucas PB, Cowdry RW. CSF metabolites in borderline personality disorder compared with normal controls. Biol Psychiatry 28:247–254, 1990.
90. Van Praag HM. CSF 5HIAA and suicide in non-depressed schizophrenics. Lancet ii:977–978, 1983.
91. Ninan PT, Van Kammen DP, Scheinin M, Linnoila M Bunney WE Jr, Goodwin FK. CSF 5-hydroxyindoleacetic acid levels in suicidal schizophrenic patients. Am J Psychiatry 141:566–569, 1984.
92. Drake RE, Gates C, Whitaker A, Cotton PG. Suicide among schizophrenics: a review. Compr Psychiatry 26:90–100, 1985.
93. Nordström P, Samuelsson M, Asberg M, Traskman-Bendz L, Aberg-Wistedt A, Nordin C, Bertilsson L. CSF 5HIAA predicts suicide risk after attempted suicide. Suicide Life Threat Behav 24(1):1–9, 1994.
94. Roy A, De Jong J, Linnoila M. Cerebrospinal fluid monoamine metabolites and suicidal behavior in depressed patients. A 5-year follow-up study. Arch Gen Psychiatry 46:609–612, 1989.
95. Malone KM, Corbitt EM, Li S, Mann JJ. Prolactin response to fenfluramine and suicide attempt lethality in major depression. Br J Psychiatry 168:324–329, 1996.
96. Brown GL, Ebert MH, Goyer PF, Jimerson DC, Klein WJ, Bunney WE, Goodwin FK. Aggression, suicide, and serotonin: relationships to CSF amine metabolites. Am J Psychiatry 139:741–746, 1982.
97. Coccaro EF, Kavoussi RJ, Cooper TB, Hauger RL. Central serotonin activity and aggression: inverse relationship with prolactin response to d-fenfluramine, but not CSF 5HIAA concentration, in human subjects. Am J Psychiatry 154:1430–1435, 1997.
98. Stahl SM. The human platelet. Diagnostic and research tool for the study of biogenic amines in psychiatric and neurologic disorders. Arch Gen Psychiatry 34:509–516, 1977.

99. Pandey GN. Altered serotonin function in suicide. Evidence from platelet and neuroendocrine studies. Ann NY Acad Sci 836:182–183, 1997.
100. Pandey GN, Pandey SC, Janicak PG, Marks RC, Davis JM. Platelet serotonin-2 receptor binding sites in depression and suicide. Biol Psychiatry 28:215–222, 1990.
101. Arango V, Underwood MD, Mann JJ. Postmortem findings in suicide victims: Implications for in vivo imaging studies. Ann NY Acad Sci 836:269–287, 1997.
102. Palmer AM, Lowe SL, Francis PT, Bowen DM. Are post-mortem biochemical studies of human brain worthwhile. Biochem Soc Trans 16:472–475, 1988.
103. Arango V, Ernsberger P, Marzuk PM, Chen J-S, Tierney H, Stanley M, Reis DJ, Mann JJ. Autoradiographic demonstration of increased serotonin 5-HT$_2$ and β-adrenergic receptor binding sites in the brain of suicide victims. Arch Gen Psychiatry 47:1038–1047, 1990.
104. Hrdina PD, Demeter E, Vu TB, Sotonyi P, Palkovits M. 5HT uptake sites and 5HT$_2$ receptors in brain of antidepressant-free suicide victims/depressives: increase in 5-HT$_2$ sites in cortex and amygdala. Brain Res 614:37–44, 1993.
105. Mann JJ, Stanley M, McBride PA, McEwen BS. Increased serotonin$_2$ and β-adrenergic receptor binding in the frontal cortices of suicide victims. Arch Gen Psychiatry 43:954–959, 1986.
106. Mann JJ, Underwood MD, Arango V. Postmortem studies of suicide victims. In: Watson SJ, ed. Biology of Schizophrenia and Affective Disease, 1st ed. Washington: American Psychiatric Press., 1996.
107. Stanley M, Mann JJ. Increased serotonin-2 binding sites in frontal cortex of suicide victims. Lancet i:214–216, 1983.
108. Mann JJ, Kapur S. The emergence of suicidal ideation and behavior during antidepressant pharmacotherapy. Arch Gen Psychiatry 48:1027–1033, 1991.
109. Baldessarini RJ, Jamison KR. Effects of medical interventions on suicidal behavior. Summary and conclusions. J Clin Psychiatry 60(suppl 2):117–122, 1999.
110. Suicidal behavior and psychotropic medication. Accepted as a consensus statement by the ACNP Council, March 2, 1992. Neuropsychopharmacology 8:177–183, 1993.
111. Tondo L, Baldessarini RJ. Reduced suicide risk during lithium maintenance treatment. J Clin Psychiatry 61(suppl 9):97–104, 2000.
112. Coppen A. Lithium in unipolar depression and the prevention of suicide. J Clin Psychiatry 61(suppl 9):52–56, 2000.
113. Isometsä E, Henriksson M, Heikkinen M, Aro H, Lonnqvist J. Suicide and the use of antidepressants. Drug treatment of depression is inadequate. BMJ 308:915, 1994.
114. Oquendo MA, Malone KM, Ellis SP, Sackeim HA, Mann JJ. Inadequacy of antidepressant treatment for patients with major depression who are at risk for suicidal behavior. Am J Psychiatry 156:190–194, 1999.
115. Rutz W, Von Knorring L, Wálinder J. Frequency of suicide on Gotland after systematic postgraduate education of general practitioners. Acta Psychiatr Scand 80:151–154, 1989.
116. Rihmer Z, Rutz W, Barsi J. Suicide rate, prevalence of diagnosed depression and prevalence of working physicians in Hungary. Acta Psychiatr Scand 88:391–394, 1993.
117. Isacsson G, Boëthius G, and Bergman U. Low level of antidepressant prescription for people who later commit suicide: 15 years of experience from a population-based drug database in Sweden. Acta Psychiatr Scand 85:444–448, 1992.
118. Marzuk PM, Tardiff K, Leon AC, Stajic M, Morgan EB, Mann JJ. Prevalence of cocaine use among residents of New York City who committed suicide during a one-year period. Am J Psychiatry 149:371–375, 1992.
119. Isacsson G. Suicide prevention—a medical breakthrough? Acta Psychiatr Scand 102:113–117, 2000.
120. Meltzer HY. Suicide and schizophrenia: clozapine and the InterSePT study. International Clozaril/Leponex Suicide Prevention Trial. J Clin Psychiatry 60(suppl 12):47–50, 1999.

48

Sleep Disorders

ERIC A. NOFZINGER
Western Psychiatric Institute and Clinic, University of Pittsburgh School of Medicine, Pittsburgh, Pennsylvania, U.S.A.

I. INTRODUCTION

A working knowledge of sleep and its various disorders is essential to psychiatric clinical care. Alterations in sleep are among the most common clinical disturbances in a broad range of mental disorders. Sleep disturbances may herald the onset of a new episode of a mental disorder. Misdiagnosis of sleep problems may be a cause of treatment failure in patients with mental disorders. And perhaps, most importantly, disturbances in sleep are among the most troubling symptoms for patients with mental disorders. This chapter will first provide a general overview of normal sleep to provide a context within which to understand sleep alterations in disease states. Then, sleep in neuropsychiatric disorders commonly encountered in a psychiatric practice will be reviewed. Finally, a review of nonpsychiatric general sleep disorders will provide a broader context within which to understand the more specific sleep disorders seen in patients with mental disorders.

II. NORMAL SLEEP

Sleep propensity, or the need for sleep, is lowest shortly after awakening, increases in midafternoon, plateaus across the evening, is greatest during the night, and declines across sleep. Sleep has been subclassified polysomnographically into NREM and REM sleep states based on three measures: (1) electroencephalography (EEG); (2) electromyography (EMG); and (3) electrooculography (EOG). With sleep onset, the EEG frequency slows, the amplitude increases and the EMG decreases. This sleep is classified as NREM stages 1, 2, 3, or 4, which are distinguished by increasing amounts of low-frequency, high-amplitude EEG activity, also known as "delta" activity. Delta sleep decreases across the night. REM sleep follows the first NREM period and is characterized by low-amplitude, mixed high-frequency EEG, the occurrence of intermittent REMs, skeletal muscle atonia, and irregular cardiac and respiratory events. Across the night, brain function oscillates between the globally distinct states of NREM and REM sleep about three or four times, approximately every 90 min. Across successive sleep cycles within a night, stages 3 and 4 sleep decrease, then disappear, while REM sleep and lighter NREM sleep stages increase.

The lower-frequency EEG rhythms in NREM sleep represent widespread thalamocortical electrical oscillations. Slow oscillations in the 1–4 Hz delta range have both cortical and thalamic origins. The higher-frequency EEG rhythms (beta and gamma frequencies, roughly > 20 Hz) can be seen during waking and REM sleep [1–16]. They are associated with increased vigilance. Changes in these oscillations can result from state-dependent changes in modulatory systems such as the brainstem, the hypothalamus, and the basal forebrain. Changes in low- or high-frequency EEG rhythms in neuropsychiatric disorders, may therefore result from functional changes at one or more brain system levels including the cortex, thalamus, and modulatory structures.

Rapid eye movement, or REM sleep, represents a unique state of the central nervous system. Evidence from a variety of approaches suggests that REM sleep is generated at the level of the brainstem. Specifically, the laterodorsal and pedunculopontine tegmental cholinergic nuclei (LDT and PPT) in the pontine reticular formation underlie the phasic and tonic components of REM sleep [17–38]. These brainstem structures are under modulatory influence from other brainstem nuclei, including the noradrenergic locus coeruleus and the serotonergic raphe, as well as forebrain structures such as the amygdala [39–45]. Functional neuroimaging studies show that REM sleep is associated with a relative increase in function in limbic and paralimbic structures in relation to both waking and NREM sleep. Alterations in REM sleep in neuropsychiatric disorders may reflect alterations in limbic and paralimbic function in these diseases.

During NREM sleep, there are decreases in relative brain function in heteromodal association cortical areas in relation to waking [35,46–56]. This includes the prefrontal, parietal and temporal association areas. The thalamus is another region where consistent reductions in relative brain function is found.

III. SLEEP DISORDERS

A. Sleep in Neuropsychiatric Disorders

1. Depression

The majority of patients with mood disorders describe difficulty falling asleep, difficulty staying asleep, and difficulty returning to sleep after early-morning awakenings [57]. Clinically, they report a paradoxical state of physical daytime fatigue, yet with persistent mental activity that makes it difficult for them to fall asleep at night. While insomnia characterizes the melancholia of middle-age and elderly unipolar depression, younger patients and bipolar depressed patients will often describe difficulty getting out of bed in the morning and hypersomnia during the daytime [58].

An extensive literature describes the changes in EEG sleep in patients with depression [59–73]. Measures derived from the EEG sleep recordings that have been found to differ between healthy and depressed subjects include measures of sleep continuity, measures of visually scored EEG sleep stages, and automated measures of characteristics of the EEG waveform across the sleep period such as period amplitude or EEG spectral power measures.

The changes in subjective sleep complaints are paralleled by EEG measures of sleep. These include increases in sleep latency and decreases in sleep continuity. In terms of EEG sleep stages or "sleep architecture," depressed patients often show reduced stages 3 and 4 NREM sleep (also known as "slow-wave sleep" (SWS) because of the presence of slow EEG delta activity during these stages). Several changes in REM sleep have also been noted. These have included an increase in the amount of REM sleep, a shortening of the time to onset of the first REM period of the night, a shortened REM latency, and an increase in the frequency of eye movements within a REM period.

In terms of quantitative EEG changes in sleep, many studies have reported reductions in delta sleep in depression. Increased high-frequency EEG activity has also been reported in depressed patients including alpha and beta. Importantly, sex differences have been found in these abnormalities. Depressed women appear to have relative preservation of delta sleep in relation to depressed men, despite elevations in higher-frequency EEG activity in both groups.

Studies have shown that patients with psychotic depression have particularly severe EEG sleep disturbances and very short REM sleep latencies; that patients with recurrent depression have more severe REM sleep disturbances than patients in their first episode; and that sleep continuity and REM sleep disturbances are more prominent early in the depressive episode than later. Some studies suggest that patients with dysthymia and mania (surprisingly) have EEG sleep disturbances very similar to those observed in major depression.

EEG sleep findings help to inform our understanding of the neurobiology of longitudinal course and treatment outcome in depression. Although severely reduced REM latencies, phasic REM measures, and sleep continuity disturbances generally move toward control values after remission of depression, most sleep measures show high correlations across the course of an episode. Reduced REM latency is associated with increased response rates to pharmacotherapy [74] but not to psychotherapy [75]. Depressed patients with abnormal sleep profiles (reduced REM latency, increased REM density, and poor sleep continuity) are significantly less likely to respond to cognitive behavior therapy and interpersonal therapy than patients with a "normal" profile. Other studies have indicated that reduced REM latency and decreased delta EEG activity are associated with increased likelihood of or decreased time until recurrence of depression in patients treated with medications or psychotherapy [76].

Each of the major neurotransmitter systems that have been shown to modulate the ascending activation of the cortex, i.e., the cholinergic, noradrenergic, and serotonergic systems, have been implicated in the pathophysiology of mood disorders. The role of additional brainstem neurotransmitter systems such as GABA-ergic, nitroxergic, glutamatergic, glycinergic, histaminergic, adenosinergic, dopaminergic, and various peptide systems, such as galanin, orexin, vasoactive intestinal polypeptide, and nerve growth factor in the sleep disturbances in depression, remain to be defined. Nearly all effective antidepressant medications show a pronounced inhibition of REM sleep including a prolongation of the first REM cycle and a reduction in the overall percent of REM sleep (exceptions include nefazadone [77] and bupropion, which do not suppress REM sleep [78,79].

Enhanced cholinergic function concurrent with reduced monoaminergic tone in the central nervous system has been proposed as a pharmacologic model for depression. In an exaggerated sense, the state of REM sleep mimics this formulation, i.e., a cholinergically driven state with reduced firing of noradrenergic and serotonergic neurons. Cholinergic agents such as the muscarinic agonist RS 86, arecoline, physostigmine, and scopolamine produce exaggerated REM sleep effects in depressed patients in comparison with patients with eating disorders, personality disorders, anxiety disorders, and healthy controls [80–82]. These studies suggest that there may be a supersensitivity of the cholinergic system driving REM sleep in mood disorders patients, although an alternative plausible hypothesis is that there may be reduced monoaminergic (5-HT and/or NE) inhibition of the brainstem cholinergic nuclei in mood-disordered patients [81]. Cholinergic activation may also play a role in the hyperactivity in the HPA axis and in the blunting of growth hormone secretion noted in depressed patients across the night, given the influence of cholinergic drugs on HPA activity and GH release [83].

Selective serotonin reuptake inhibitors are known to have prominent REM-suppressing activity, most notably early in the night when enhancements in REM sleep are most often seen in mood-disordered patients [60]. A tryptophan-free diet, which depletes central serotonin activity, is noted to decrease REM latency in healthy controls [84] and in depressed patients [85], and ipsaparone, a 5HT1a agonist, is noted to prolong REM latency in both normal controls and depressed patients [86,87]. Anatomically, 5HT1a receptors have been conceptualized as the limbic receptors given their high densities in the hippocampus, the septum, the amygdala, and cortical paralimbic structures. The action in these structures has been shown to be largely inhibitory (hyperpolarizing). Given the importance of limbic and paralimbic structures in REM sleep modulation, the influence of SSRI medications may be mediated by these limbic receptors. Importantly, in the brainstem LDT, a locus of cholinergic cells identified in the generation of REM sleep, bursting cholinergic neurons are inhibited by the action of 5HT on 5HT1a receptors. Finally, the effects of the 5HT1a antagonist pindolol on EEG sleep in healthy subjects were studied and noted to reduce REM sleep [88]. This was interpreted as supportive of a reduction in raphe serotonergic autoregulation, resulting in increased serotonergic input to pontine cholinergic centers and inhibition of REM sleep.

Given the selective activation of limbic and paralimbic structures during REM sleep in healthy subjects, the study of the functional neuroanatomy during REM sleep in depressed patients may provide clues as to alterations in limbic and paralimbic function related to the pathophysiology of depression. In contrast to healthy controls [12], depressed patients fail to activate anterior paralimbic structures (sub- and pregenual anterior cingulate and medial prefrontal cortices) from waking to REM sleep. In contrast to healthy controls, depressed subjects show large activations in the dorsal tectum (superior colliculus and periaqueductal gray) during REM sleep. Finally, in contrast to controls, depressed subjects activate left sensorimotor cortex, left inferior temporal cortex, left uncal gyrus and amygdala, and left subicular complex during REM sleep. These findings suggest that depressed patients demonstrate uniquely different patterns of activation from waking to REM sleep than do healthy controls. In the context of neuroscience models relating forebrain function during REM sleep to attention, motivation, emotion and memory, these results suggest that prior REM sleep abnormalities in mood-disordered patients therefore likely reflect alterations in limbic and paralimbic forebrain function related to depression.

One study reported on the reversibility of these findings following antidepressant therapy [89]. Depressed patients underwent concurrent EEG sleep studies and [^{18}F]fluoro-2-deoxy-D-glucose ([^{18}F]FDG) positron emission tomography (PET) scans during waking and during their second REM period of sleep before and after treatment with bupropion SR. Bupropion SR treatment did not suppress electrophysiologic measures of REM sleep, nor did it alter an indirect measure of global metabolism during either waking or REM sleep. Bupropion SR treatment reversed the previously observed deficit in anterior cingulate, medial prefrontal cortex, and right anterior insula activation from waking to REM sleep. In secondary analyses, this effect was related to a reduction in waking relative metabolism in these structures following treatment in the absence of a significant effect on REM sleep relative metabolism.

Another study sought to clarify the neurobiological basis of variations in one aspect of central nervous system "arousal" in depression by characterizing the functional neuroanatomic correlates of beta EEG power density during NREM sleep [90]. First, nine healthy ($n = 9$) subjects underwent concurrent EEG sleep studies and [^{18}F]FDG PET scans during their first NREM period of sleep in order to generate hypotheses about specific brain structures that show a relationship between increased beta power and increased relative glucose metabolism. Second, brain structures identified in the healthy subjects were then used as a priori regions of interest in similar analyses from identical studies in 12 depressed subjects. Regions that demonstrated significant correlations between beta power and relative cerebral glucose metabolism in both the healthy and depressed subjects included the ventromedial prefrontal cortex and the right lateral inferior occipital cortex. During a baseline night of sleep, depressed patients demonstrated a trend toward greater beta power in relation to a separate age- and gender-matched healthy control group. In both healthy and depressed subjects, beta power negatively correlated with subjective sleep quality. Finally, in the depressed group, there was a trend for beta power to correlate with an indirect measure of absolute whole-brain metabolism during NREM sleep. This study demonstrated a similar relationship between electrophysiologic arousal and glucose metabolism in the ventromedial prefrontal cortex in depressed and healthy subjects. Given the increased electrophysiological arousal in some depressed patients and the known anatomical relations between the ventromedial prefrontal cortex and brain-activating structures, this study raised the possibility that the ventromedial prefrontal cortex plays a significant role in mediating one aspect of dysfunctional arousal found in severely aroused depressed patients.

Functional neuroimaging of NREM sleep in depressed subjects would be expected to provide evidence regarding the functioning of homeostatic mechanisms in mood-disordered patients since this is a time of nonselective nonactivation of the cortex in which the buildup of a sleep-dependent process, process S, is discharged and during which growth hormone secretion occurs. Ho et al. [91] demonstrated that whole-brain and regional cerebral glucose metabolism was elevated during the first NREM period of the night for depressed men in relation to healthy men. These findings are supportive of a deficiency of hemostatic mechanisms in mood-disordered patients, perhaps secondary to cortical hyperarousal. Clark et al. [92] reported that reductions in delta sleep in depressed patients was associated with reductions in afternoon waking relative and global blood flow. This suggests that the elevations in glucose metabolism during NREM sleep in depressed patients is not related to a waking hypermetabolic state. Studies across waking and NREM sleep are needed to clarify this notion.

Wu et al. [93] characterized the functional neuroanatomic changes following sleep deprivation therapy in depressed patients. They found that depressed patients who demonstrated high pretreatment relative glucose metabolic rates in the medial prefrontal cortex were more likely to respond to sleep deprivation. Further, a reduction in relative metabolism in this region was found following sleep deprivation.

2. Late-Life Depression

Assessments of the timing and quality of NREM and REM sleep cycles through EEG sleep studies have proven to be particularly useful indicators of hemostatic and adaptive physiological processes during successful and pathological aging in humans. In a study of healthy "old old" and "young old," Reynolds et al. [94] reported: (1) a small, age-dependent decrease in slow-wave sleep, in contrast to the stability of REM sleep measures from "young old" to "old old"; (2) much better preservation of slow-wave sleep among aging women than men, particularly in the first NREM period of the night, but no sex-related differences in REM sleep measures; (3) greater stability of sleep maintenance among aging men than among aging women; and (4) longer REM sleep latencies among aging women than men.

In comparison with 20-year-olds, 80-year-olds have significant reductions in both REM sleep percent and REM sleep latency, as well as a slower recovery from the effects of acute sleep loss [95]. The elderly show greater rigidity in sleep patterns, with less intersubject and intrasubject variability in habitual sleep times compared to the young [96]. Therefore, while some loss of REM and slow wave NREM sleep characterize the aging process, successful aging is associated with a relative stability of sleep states over the later years. One explanation for these findings may be some mild losses in both hemostatic adaptive physiological mechanisms which result in NREM and REM sleep decrements, respectively. Alternatively, information processing related to both hemostatic and adaptive behavior may be more stable and efficient in the elderly, especially in those for whom the aging process has been bridged successfully.

EEG sleep studies have also provided insights into the pathophysiology of disorders in which affective adaptation is significantly stressed in late life, i.e., in response to significant losses or in acute depressive episodes. In a study of elderly volunteers who had lost a spouse, Reynolds et al. [97] were able to distinguish EEG sleep changes discriminating subjects who did from those who did not develop an episode of major depression. Bereaved subjects with depression had significantly lower sleep efficiency, more early morning awakening, shorter REM latency, greater REM percent, and lower rates of delta wave generation in the first NREM period, as compared to nondepressed bereaved volunteers. These findings are similar to those of elderly patients with recurrent unipolar depression. In a subsequent longitudinal study of bereaved elders who did not become clinically depressed, only increases in phasic REM activity and density (compared to normal controls) were observed throughout the first 2 years of bereavement [98]. These findings are similar to those of Cartwright [99] for depressed vs. nondepressed divorcing women, suggesting that short REM latency and slow-wave sleep are correlates of depression during stressful life events, while increased REM activity may correlate with successful recovery from stress in the absence of major depression.

3. Schizophrenia

Early sleep EEG studies sought to test the intriguing hypothesis that schizophrenia is a spillover of the dream state into wakefulness. No evidence has accrued to support this hypothesis. However, subtle alterations in architecture of REM sleep may occur. REM latency was found to be decreased in several studies [100]. It has been proposed that this may result from a deficit in SWS in the first NREM period leading to a passive advance, or early onset of the first REM period. An alternative explanation is "REM pressure." However, studies of the amounts of REM sleep have been conflicting with increases, decreases, and no change being found [64,100]. Studies examining treatment-naive schizophrenia patients show no increases in REM sleep [101,102]; the increases in REM sleep observed in previously treated subjects may reflect effects of medication withdrawal, and/or changes related to the acute psychotic state [102]. It is therefore unlikely that the observed decreases in REM latency in some schizophrenia patients result from primary abnormalities in REM sleep.

Slow-wave sleep is of particular interest to schizophrenia because of the implication of the prefrontal cortex in this disorder [103] and in generation of SWS [104]. Several studies have shown a reduction of SWS in schizophrenic patients; SWS deficits have been seen in acute, chronic, and remitted states; and in never-medicated, neuroleptic-treated, and unmedicated patients [100]. Studies that fail to find differences in SWS have generally used conventional visual scoring. Three studies that have quantified sleep EEG parameters have consistently shown reductions in SWS. Ganguli et al. [101] observed no change in visually scored SWS. Instead, drug-naive schizophrenic patients showed a significant reduction in delta wave counts. This suggested that automated counts may be a good marker of SWS deficiency in schizophrenia.

The neurobiological correlates of the psychopathological dimensions are critical for our understanding of the pathophysiology of psychiatric disorders. Research during the past decade has focused increasingly on the positive and negative syndromes, a conceptual distinction of particular importance to pathophysiology of schizophrenia. A number of studies have examined the association between REM sleep parameters and clinical parameters. Tandon et al. [102] reported an inverse association between REM latency and negative symptoms. No association has been seen between sleep abnormalities and depressive symptoms [102] but two studies have shown that increased REM sleep may correlate with suicidal behavior in schizophrenia [105,106].

It is important to understand the longitudinal nature of sleep abnormalities in schizophrenia, in order to elucidate their significance for pathophysiology. Stage 4 does not appear to improve, whereas other sleep stages change following 3–4 weeks of conventional antipsychotic treatment [107]. In a longitudinal study, alterations of SWS appeared to be stable when polysomnographic studies were repeated at 1 year, but the

REM sleep parameters appeared to change. These observations suggest that SWS deficits in schizophrenia might be trait related [108]. Consistent with this view, delta sleep abnormalities have been found to correlate with negative symptoms [101,109–111] and with impaired outcome at 1 and at 2 years [112].

Some evidence, albeit modest, for decreased frontal lobe metabolism has been documented in schizophrenia using a variety of techniques, including PET, single-photon emission computed tomography (SPECT), [^{31}P]MRS, and xenon-133 inhalation technique. It may therefore be instructive to examine SWS deficits in the context of such physiological alterations. An association has been demonstrated between SWS deficits and reduced frontal-lobe membrane phospholipid metabolism as examined by [^{31}P]MRS [113].

4. Alzheimer's Disease

Disturbances in sleep commonly accompany Alzheimer's disease [114]. These disturbances are a significant cause of distress for caregivers, often leading to institutionalization of these patients [115,116]. The changes in sleep often parallel the changes in cognitive function in demented patients [117,118]. Also, daytime agitation has been associated with negative sleep quality at night [119]. A large-scale community-based study of Alzheimer's patients reported that sleeping more than usual and early-morning awakenings were the most common sleep disturbances in noninstitutionalized patients [120]. Night-time awakenings, however, were more disturbing to caregivers. Nighttime awakenings were associated with male gender and greater memory and functional declines. Three groups of subjects were identified in association with nocturnal awakenings: (1) patients with only daytime inactivity; (2) patients with fearfulness, fidgeting, and occasional sadness; and (3) patients with multiple behavioral problems including frequent episodes of sadness, fearfulness, inactivity, fidgeting, and hallucinations.

In terms of sleep laboratory–based evaluations, sleep continuity disturbances in these patients include decreased sleep efficiencies, increased lighter stage 1 NREM sleep, and an increased frequency of arousals and awakenings [121,122]. Sleep architecture abnormalities include decreases in stages 3 and 4 NREM sleep and some reports of decreases in REM sleep [123–131]. Loss of sleep spindling and K complexes have also been noted in dementia. Sleep apnea has been observed in 33–53% of patients with probable Alzheimer's disease [132–140]. It is unclear if there is an increased prevalence of sleep apnea, however, in Alzheimer's patients in relation to age- and gender-matched controls. Nocturnal behavioral disruptions, or "sundowning" episodes are reported commonly in the clinical management of Alzheimer's patients, although specific diagnostic criteria for a sundowning episode have been difficult to define [141–144]. Despite extensive clinical research in this area, the pathophysiology of sundowning, including its relationship with brain mechanisms that control sleep/wake and circadian regulation, remain unclear. Overall, the literature on sleep in Alzheimer's disease suggests that the primary defect in this disease is the more general neurodegenerative changes that lead to the profound cognitive and functional declines of this disease, and that the sleep changes are secondary manifestations of the disorder. If sleep is viewed as generated by core sleep systems that then require an intact neural structure throughout the rest of the brain for expression of behavioral states, then the sleep changes in Alzheimer's disease are most likely related to end-organ failure as opposed to pathology in key sleep or circadian systems themselves.

5. Parkinson's Disease

Light, fragmented sleep occurs frequently in Parkinson's disease patients. Sleep problems have been reported in as many as 74–96% of patients [145–147]. Complaints include frequent awakenings, early awakening, nocturnal cramps or pains, nightmares, vivid dreams, visual hallucinations, vocalizations, somnambulisms, impaired motor function, myoclonic jerks, excessive daytime sleepiness, REM sleep behavior disorder, and sleep-related violence leading to injury [145–163]. These changes may result from the disease itself or to complication from treatment with dopaminergic agents [164–175]. Additionally, depression is common in Parkinson's disease. The sleep disruption may in part be related to this comorbid disorder [147,153,167,176,177].

Sleep architecture abnormalities include increased awakenings and reductions in stages 3 and 4 sleep, REM sleep, and sleep spindles [175,178,179]. Reductions in REM latency have been observed. Increased muscular activity, contractions, and periodic limb movements may prevent SWS and foster light, fragmented sleep. Disorganized respiration is also found [180].

B. Sleep Apnea Syndrome

Sleep apnea syndrome refers to episodes of transient cessation of breathing during sleep (for ≥ 10 sec) that disrupt sleep and thus lead to daytime sleepiness. In most cases, this cessation is related to the occlusion of the pharyngeal airway, and is referred to as *obstructive sleep apnea syndrome*. In other cases, there is abnormal ventilatory effort in the absence of any discrete airway obstruction. This is referred to as *central sleep apnea syndrome*. A third condition, the *upper-airway resistance syndrome* (UARS), consists of increased respiratory effort in the absence of discrete apneic events. This increased effort leads to nonrestorative sleep, which subsequently produces daytime sleepiness.

These syndromes are most commonly found in obese, aging men although they are not restricted to these Pickwickian types. Epidemiologic studies suggest that ~ 4% of men and 2% of women ages 30–60 will meet minimal diagnostic criteria for obstructive sleep apnea syndrome [181,182]. The most common clinical symptoms reported are daytime sleepiness in the presence of sleep-related snoring with occasional pauses in breathing or "gasping" for breath during sleep. Other daytime symptoms include fatigue, morning headaches, and cognitive changes such as reduced concentration and attention. The sleepiness of sleep apnea is differentiated from the sleepiness of narcolepsy by the constant, unrelenting nature of the sleepiness. In narcolepsy, the sleepiness is qualitatively more sudden in onset and offset. The constant sleepiness and fatigue need to be differentiated from similar sleep symptoms in psychiatric patients by the concurrent changes in mood or personality found in psychiatric disorders that are not found in the isolated apneic patient.

The pathophysiology of obstructive sleep apnea syndrome is related to the neuroanatomical factors that maintain airway patency during sleep [183,184]. It is widely accepted that the site of airway obstruction in obstructive sleep apnea syndrome lies in the pharynx. Whether this airway will close during sleep is related to the balance between forces that narrow the airway, such as intrapharyngeal suction during inspiration, and forces that dilate the airway, such as the tone of pharyngeal airway muscles. Anatomical abnormalities in this area are often found in apneic patients related to obesity, enlarged tonsils, and facial bony abnormalities. Additionally, sleep itself is associated with a loss of tone in pharyngeal muscles that maintain the outward pressure necessary for airway patency. Alcohol is often an extrinsic suppressant of pharyngeal muscle tone that exacerbates apnea by reducing the outward pressure on the pharyngeal airway.

Central sleep apnea syndrome refers to the periodic loss of ventilatory effort with associated cessation of breathing during sleep. This is differentiated from obstructive-type apneas in which there is a loss of breathing despite persistent attempts at ventilation. These patients constitute < 10% of apneic patients. The pathogenesis of central sleep apnea is likely diverse given the broad conditions that produce this type of breathing during sleep such as central alveolar hypoventilation, congestive heart failure, nasal obstruction, and dysautonomias. In general, a final common pathway appears to be some disturbance in the respiratory control system that includes sensors for (1) hypoxia and hypercapnia and (2) brainstem and forebrain centers that influence respiratory function in response to metabolic and behavioral demands. Clinically, patients with alveolar hypoventilation present with signs of respiratory failure, whereas nonhypercapnic patients may present with insomnia, normal body habitus, and awakenings with gasping for breath. Diagnosis is definitively made by the use of an esophageal balloon. Treatment for the hypercapnic patient with hypoventilation during waking requires ventilation at night using a nasal mask and a pressure-cycled ventilator. For the nonhypercapnic patient, treatment consists of correcting the underlying problem (e.g., nasal obstruction, congestive heart failure) or watchful waiting, as ~ 20 % may resolve spontaneously. Nasal CPAP can be tried if the patient is obese, snores, and has heart failure. Oxygen administration may be helpful if the apneic events are associated with hypoxemia. If persistent, acetazolamide, a carbonic anhydrase inhibitor, can be attempted.

C. Primary Insomnia

Insomnia is the experience of inadequate or poor quality of sleep and is characterized by one or more of the following: difficulty falling asleep, difficulty maintaining sleep, and/or awakening earlier than one would like. Additionally, patients are bothered by daytime dysfunction that may include fatigue, mood symptoms, and difficulty with cognitive function that requires attention and concentration. Roughly 10% of the adult population will suffer from chronic insomnia, and 30–50% will experience transient insomnia at some point in their lives. Females appear to be more affected across the life span, and the elderly are particularly vulnerable. Consequences of insomnia may include poor daytime performance, an increased likelihood of subsequent development of a mental disorder such as depression or anxiety, and increased medical morbidity and mortality. Insomnia may be classified as either short-term (transient) or long-term (chronic) and as either primary or secondary to another general medical or mental disorder.

Transient insomnias occur in otherwise healthy individuals who revert to normal sleeping as an outcome. These may be related to sleeping in an unfamiliar environment; an environment that is temporarily disrupted by noises, sounds, or temperature changes; the occurrence of a recent life stressor; a change in the timing of bedtime related to travel across time zones or shift work; or acute administration or withdrawal of a medication that affects the sleep/wake cycle. In each case, identification of the etiology is important. Short-term (1–4 weeks) sedative hypnotic use may be indicated. Care should be taken to taper and discontinue this medication following resolution of the acute event to avoid the development of psychological or physiological dependence on a sleeping aid.

Chronic primary insomnias are by definition primary and not secondary to other medical or mental disorders. Other terms that have been used to define this population include psychophysiologic insomnia, sleep state misperception, and idiopathic insomnia. The term psychophysiologic insomnia stems from a psychophysiology literature and suggests that insomnia patients suffer from psychophysiologic "hyperarousal." A vicious cycle of precipitating event, increased arousal, difficulty sleeping, preoccupation with inability to sleep leading to even more arousal, and inability to sleep defines the pathophysiology of these patients. The neurobiology of the concept of "hyperarousal," however, remains poorly defined. In part, the presence of an excessive amount of high-frequency EEG activity within the sleep period is used in support of the concept of hyperarousal. Sleep state misperception refers to the subjective perception of being awake throughout the night, despite the presence of polysomnographically determined sleep. In general, primary insomnia patients tend to underestimate the actual amount of sleep they are getting in a night. These observations raise the likelihood that the sleep that insomniac patients experience may not represent the restorative sleep that noninsomniac patients receive each night. The presence of high-frequency EEG activity within polysomnographically determined sleep may represent a less differentiated behavioral state that includes components of both sleep and wakefulness in the same individual. Idiopathic insomnia refers to insomnia that is not secondary but that does not appear to involve the vicious cycle reported by patients with psychophysiologic insomnia. These individuals may simply have genetically less differentiated sleep that appears less restorative.

Treatment of insomnia is multifaceted and includes behavioral and pharmacological approaches. Historically, there should be no evidence that the insomnia is secondary, and if so, the underlying disorder should be evaluated and treated. Several behavioral strategies are available. Relaxation techniques include progressive muscle relaxation, EMG biofeedback, meditation, and guided imagery. *Stimulus control therapy* follows from a learning model of insomnia. In this model, insomniacs develop negative associations to the bedroom, and the sleeping environment produces increased arousal and subsequent insomnia. Stimulus control instructions include "lie down only when you feel sleepy," "use the bed and bedroom for sleep and sex only," and "get out of bed and go to another room if you are not sleeping." Along with these instructions include prescriptions to maintain the same clock times for going to bed and getting out of bed the next day as well as to avoid daytime napping irrespective of how much sleep had been obtained on the preceding night. *Sleep restriction therapy* refers to restricting the amount of time in bed to the time that a person believes he is actually sleeping. For example, a schedule for someone who believes he is sleeping for 6 h might be midnight to 6 AM; for 4 h from 1 AM to 5 AM; or for 8 h from 10 PM to 6 AM. Along with these instructions include avoidance of daytime napping. This counters the natural tendency of insomniac patients to prolong their times in bed in an effort to obtain more sleep. This is often counterproductive as it lightens the sleep that they do get, increasing the likelihood of middle-of-the-night awakenings and early-morning awakenings. *Cognitive therapy* for insomnia includes questioning erroneous beliefs that an insomniac patient may have regarding the catastrophic consequences of insomnia and beliefs regarding the inadequacy of sleep that he is having. Studies are under way to test the relative merits of each of these treatment methods when used individually or in combination.

D. Narcolepsy

There are two independent clusters of symptoms that may require treatment in narcoleptic patients. The first is daytime sleepiness. Given the severity of the sleepiness, it would be unusual for behavioral interventions to be completely effective. Some patients find that adding periodic, brief daytime naps reduces some of the sleep attacks. Allowing for adequate sleep at night is advised. Occasionally, these patients will demonstrate insomnia, or nightmares that require the use of a sedative hypnotic medication. The primary treatment for the sleepiness, however, consists of the use of either a stimulant medication or a medication that relieves sleepiness. The commonly used stimulants include methylphenidate, dextroamphetamine, and pemoline, in descending order of stimulant potency. Short-acting preparations last ~ 4 h, and longer-acting preparations extend this effect a few hours. Consequently, these medications are often prescribed at least in the morning and around lunchtime. Occasionally, a patient may need a late-afternoon dose if he anticipates being involved in activities during the evening that require his full attention. Often, tolerance to low doses builds, requiring escalation to effective levels. Side effects such as nervousness, affective symptoms, and nocturnal insomnia require monitoring. An alternative medication is modafinil. This medication may reduce the need for sleep and subsequently benefits some narcoleptic patients. Some patients, however, do not obtain full relief of their sleepiness with the use of this medication, or experience adverse effects which require switching to, or adding, a stimulant.

The second cluster of symptoms that requires treatment includes cataplexy, hypnogogic hallucinations, and sleep onset paralysis. Of these, the cataplexy is the most significant symptom clinically, as it is associated with considerable limitation in psychosocial function and potential danger to the individual as a result of personal injury from falls. These symptoms are generally effectively managed with the use of antidepressant agents such as clomipramine, the selective serotonin reuptake inhibitors, or venlafaxine. Dosages that relieve cataplexy are generally lower than those used to treat depression. Tolerance to these agents can develop which may require switching to an alternative agent.

E. Restless Legs Syndrome/Periodic Limb Movement Disorder

The restless legs syndrome (RLS) and periodic limb movement disorder (PLMD) are related sleep disorders. Restless legs refers to a waking complaint that interferes with sleep onset, whereas periodic limb movements are found during sleep and may interfere with restorative sleep. The restless legs complaint is a dysesthesia described as an uncomfortable restless, or creeping and crawling sensation in the lower legs. This sensation is only relieved with vigorous movement of the legs, often requiring the patient to get out of bed. The disorder affects ~ 5–10% of the population, beginning generally in midlife [185]. Periodic limb movements during sleep often occur with restless legs syndrome, but may be found in isolation. In this disorder, stereotypic periodic (every 20–40 sec) limb movements (0.5- to 5-sec extensions of the big toe and dorsiflexions of the ankle are often associated with signs of arousal from sleep, such as K complexes followed by alpha EEG waves. The degree to which PLMD is a disorder that either impairs sleep or that requires intervention remains unclear, however, since ~ 11% of the normal population without sleep complaints, especially the aged, will demonstrate PLMD on polysomnographic assessment.

The pathophysiology of RLS and PLMD has not been well defined. There is evidence to suggest that abnormal dopaminergic function in the CNS may play a role. The efficacy of opiates in the treatment of the disorder suggests a role for the endogenous opiate system. There is also thought to be a role for the spinal cord in RLS, and relations between RLS and peripheral neuropathies have been noted.

Associated medical conditions for RLS include uremia, iron deficiency anemia, peripheral neuropathy, fibromyalgia, magnesium deficiency, rheumatoid arthritis, and posttraumatic stress disorder. Treatments that exacerbate RLS or PLMD include lithium, tricyclic and SSRI medications, and withdrawal from anticonvulsants, benzodiazepines, and barbiturates. Bupropion is one antidepressant that has been associated with a reduction in periodic limb movements, perhaps related to its dopaminergic activity.

The treatment of RLS and PLMD primarily involves dopaminergic agonists. Pramipexole 0.125 mg and pergolide 0.1–0.5 mg QHS are often first-line recommendations. Levodopa/carbidopa 100-25 or 200-50 is also helpful when given at bedtime. The short duration of action of this combination often requires a second, middle-of-the-night dose unless the sustained-release preparation is used. Benzodiazepines and traditional sedative/hypnotics consolidate sleep and may reduce arousals secondary to the PLMD. Opiate medications are very beneficial for the treatment of these disorders, although, given their abuse potential, they should be employed as a last resort. Less consistent information is available to support the use of other agents such as carbamazepine, clonidine, and gabapentin.

F. NREM Parasomnias

Three related sleep disorders, or sleep syndromes, fall into a category of NREM parasomnias: confusional arousals, sleep terrors, and sleepwalking. Each is thought to represent a "disorder of arousal." As a group, these disorders tend to occur normally in children below the age of 5 when behavioral state regulation is not yet well differentiated. There appears to be a genetic tendency for these disorders as a group. Persistence into adulthood is not the norm, but when they do, they can interfere with psychosocial functioning. They each tend to occur out of a deeper NREM sleep stage (slow-wave sleep) early in the night, and each is associated with amnesia for the event.

Confusional arousals refer to periods of partial sleep and partial waking behavior with amnesia for the events on full awakening. The individual will have the appearance of being confused, disoriented with incomplete responsiveness to their surroundings. These episodes may last from a few seconds to a few minutes with return to sleep.

Sleep terrors refers to periods in which the individual seems to be in the midst of a paniclike state with crying out, sitting erect in bed with acute autonomic arousal such as increases in heart rate, respiration, and sweating. No recall of the event is noted.

Sleepwalking refers to the appearance of motoric behavior during sleep that can lead to an individual getting out of bed and walking around his environment. Occasionally, the motoric behavior is isolated to the bed, with uncomplicated, brief, automatic behaviors. At other times, the behavior can be very complex, including walking around the bedroom performing some stereotypic act, or leaving the bedroom and walking around the house. Sleep-related eating episodes are not uncommon. On rare occasions, a sleepwalker may leave his immediate home, walk around in neighborhood, or even drive a car. In general, the individual returns to bed voluntarily, either on completion of the episode or after full awakening from the episode. The individual is often somewhat difficult to arouse and only partially responsive to environmental stimuli. Complete amnesia for the events is most common.

The pathophysiology for all of the confusional arousals is unclear. A strong genetic component is recognized for both sleep terrors and sleepwalking. Aside from this, factors associated with increasing the depth of sleep, such as sleep deprivation, or dissociating sleep, such as acute toxic/metabolic changes, or stressing an individual may increase the likelihood that these episodes will occur in genetically predisposed individuals. Presumably, these episodes occur when there is a dissociation between the brain mechanisms that regulate cortical activation or behavioral arousal and those that regulate motoric behavior. It remains unclear whether there is an association between these events and psychopathology. Any association may simply be related to the observations that mental disorders are themselves associated with disruptions in sleep continuity, factors that would be expected to increase the frequency of such events in susceptible individuals.

The diagnosis of each of these disorders is generally a clinical one. Reports of parasomnias in the first third of the night with specific features as described above support the diagnoses. Polysomnography can be performed, although it is only infrequently helpful given the difficulty of "capturing" one of the episodes in the sleep laboratory. Attempts to precipitate an episode in the lab by forced arousals from delta sleep may aid in diagnosis. In cases where a seizure disorder may be suspected, one or several daytime diagnostic EEGs and a full-scalp EEG during sleep may be performed to detect eleptiform EEG activity.

Treatment of these disorders is largely conservative and educational in nature, informing the patient and his family about sleep and the generally benign longitudinal course of parasomnic behaviors. At the time of occurrence, the individuals should not be disturbed, but rather the parasomnic events should be allowed to self-terminate. Occasionally, forced arousals during an event can precipitate an unconscious aggressive attack. Minimizing sleep deprivation, stressors, and medications or dietary factors that may interfere with sleep integrity (e.g., alcohol, caffeine, antidepressant medications) is recommended. If there is reason to suspect that the behaviors may be interfering with either sleep integrity or with daytime functioning, occasional use of sleep-consolidating medications such as the benzodiazepines may be effective in preventing the escalation of these partial arousals into more complex behaviors during sleep. If an underlying mental disorder is present that appears to be interfering with sleep continuity, this can be referred for appropriate intervention, either psychotherapy or pharmacotherapy with nonalerting antidepressant medications. If there is a history of either self or other injury during the events, steps should be taken to "sleepwalkerproof" the bedroom and surrounding environment. This may include the removal of potentially dangerous objects, locking doors, and separating bed partners from the sleepwalker.

G. Nightmares

The term *nightmare* implies a vivid dream in which something catastrophic or frightening is happening either to the dreamer or to someone else. Often, this term also implies an awakening from the frightening dream in a fearful state. There is no clear distinction, however, between a nightmare and a dream. Nearly everyone has experienced a nightmare, suggesting that this is a normal phenomenon of sleep. In general, the casual occurrence of nightmares does not come to the attention of the medical community, and no interventions are required. Nightmares are more common in childhood than in adulthood and more common in girls than in boys. The prevalence of a nightmare disorder is difficult to define, however, given the difficulty in defining a separate disorder from the more common occurrence of having bad dreams.

The pathophysiology of nightmares is unknown. Human brain imaging studies performed during REM sleep consistently reveal selective activation of anterior limbic and paralimbic structures, regions thought to play a significant role in emotional behavior, although no comparative studies have been performed to differentiate regional cerebral function during REM sleep in healthy subjects versus nightmare-disordered subjects. Elevations in autonomic arousal prior to awakening with a nightmare has been observed. Behavioral studies suggest that individuals with "thin" interpersonal boundaries, defined as more open, sensitive, and vulnerable to intrusions, are more susceptible to nightmares. Numerous drugs that affect sleep, and REM sleep specifically, such as many antidepressant medications, are known to precipitate nightmares. Alcohol withdrawal is particularly associated with bizarre, vivid dreaming. Subjects with post-traumatic stress disorder have recurrent intrusive nightmares related to their traumatic life experience, as part of their diagnostic criteria.

Given the diverse etiologies of nightmares, there is no uniform therapy. Identification and removal of precipitating factors including toxic/metabolic or drug induced are often the simplest treatment. There have been no empirical medication trials to determine the efficacy of any medication treatment for nightmare sufferers, and clinical experience would suggest that response is highly individual. Psychotherapy may be of some benefit in cases where the nightmare appears to reflect an unsuccessful attempt at some type of emotionally adaptive behavior to a stressful life situation.

H. REM Sleep Behavior Disorder

Clinically, REM sleep behavior disorder (RBD) refers to a parasomnia in which there are sleep-related behaviors associated with elaborate dream mentation. Depending on the elaborateness of the behavior and the aggressiveness of the dream, these behaviors can result in accidental self or other injury. In general, the nature of the dream enactments is out of character for the person's waking behavior. Often, the presenting complaint comes from the bed partner, who is concerned about the behaviors, rather than the actual patient, who is often unaware that anything unusual has happened during sleep. The disorder most often occurs in men and is more common in aging.

The pathophysiology of the disorder can best be understood based on an understanding of the normal physiology of REM sleep. REM sleep occurs periodically throughout the night, alternating with NREM sleep in roughly 90-min cycles. During REM sleep the brain is in an active behavioral state in which cerebral metabolism and other signs of cortical activation are comparable to those of waking. Two exceptions include the absence of conscious awareness and the near-complete immobilization of skeletal musculature via an active inhibition of motor activity by pontine centers in the perilocus coeruleus region. These exert an excitatory influence on the reticularis magnocellularis nucleus of the medulla via the lateral tegmentoreticular tract. In turn, this nucleus hyperpolarizes spinal motoneuron postsynaptic membranes via the ventrolateral reticulospinal tract. It is presumed that a defect in some aspect of this REM sleep atonia system is disturbed in patients suffering from REM sleep behavior disorder.

Acute toxic/metabolic RBD has been associated with alcohol and benzodiazepine withdrawal, or an adverse effect associated with administration of tricyclic antidepressants, monoamine oxidase inhibitors, selective serotonin re-uptake inhibitors, and clomipramine. Chronic RBD is either idiopathic (estimated to be $\sim 40\%$) or associated with some form of neurologic insult. These can be from a variety of etiologies including vascular, malignant, infectious, and degenerative. The specific pathology in each case, although presumed to have a final common pathway on the REM sleep atonia system, is not known.

Diagnosis is suspected based on a clinical report of potentially harmful sleep-related behaviors in which there appears to be an acting out of some dream sequence. Diagnosis is confirmed in a polysomnographic study that shows increased tone, or increased twitching in the chin EMG channel. Videotaping sleep-related behaviors is helpful diagnostically when increased movements are seen during a polysomnographically identified REM sleep period.

The most widely supported treatment for RBD is administration of clonazepam, 0.5 mg PO QHS titrating upward to achieve clinical benefit. In general, tolerance is not seen. This medication is reported to be helpful in > 90% of cases. At the present time, clonazepam is approved for the treatment of seizure disorders and panic disorders. A wide variety of case reports exist in which numerous other agents may be helpful, although controlled trials are lacking.

ACKNOWLEDGMENTS

Supported in part by grants MH30915, MH52247, MH37869, MH00295, MH01414, and MH45203 from NIMH, and by the Theodore and Vada Stanley Foundation.

REFERENCES

1. FH Lopes da Silva, A van Rotterdam, W Storm ven Leeuwen, AM Tielen. Dynamic characteristics of visual evoked potentials in the dog. II. Beta frequency selectivity in evoked potentials and background activity. Electroencephalogr Clin Neurophysiol 29:260–268, 1970.
2. M Steriade, F Amzica, D Contreras. Synchronization of fast (30 to 40 Hz) spontaneous cortical rhythms during brain activation. J Neurosci 16:392–417, 1996.
3. M Steriade, D Contreras, F Amzica, I Timofeev. Synchronization of fast (30 to 40 Hz) spontaneous oscillations in intrathalamic and thalamocortical networks. J Neurosci 16:2788–2808, 1996.
4. JJ Bouyer, MF Montaron, P Buser, C Durand, A Rougeul. Effects of mediodorsalis thalamic nucleus lesions on vigilance and attentive behaviour in cats. Behav Brain Res 51:51–60, 1992.
5. JJ Bouyer, MF Montaron, A Rougeul. Fast frontoparietal rhythms during combined focused attentive behaviour and immobility in cat: cortical and thalamic localizations. Electroencephalogr Clin Neurophysiol 51:244–252, 1981.
6. JE Desmedt, C Tomberg. Transient phase-locking of 40-Hz electrical oscillations in prefrontal and parietal human cortex reflects the process of conscious somatic perception. Neurosci Lett 168:126–129, 1994.
7. A Destexhe, D Contreras, M Steriade. Cortically-induced coherence of a thalamic-generated oscillation. Neuroscience 92:427–443, 1999.
8. CH Lamarche, RD Ogilvie. Electrophysiological changes during the sleep onset period of psychophysiological insomniacs, psychiatric insomniacs, and normal sleepers. Sleep 20:724–733, 1997.
9. H Merica, R Blois, JM Gaillard. Spectral characteristics of sleep EEG in chronic insomnia. Eur J Neurosci 10:1826–1834, 1998.
10. VN Murthy, EE Fetz. Oscillatory activity in sensorimotor cortex of awake monkeys: synchronization of local field potentials and relation to behavior. J Neurophysiol 76:3949–3967, 1996.
11. VN Murthy, EE Fetz. Synchronization of neurons during local field potential oscillations in sensorimotor cortex of awake monkeys. J Neurophysiol 76:3968–3982, 1996.
12. EA Nofzinger, TE Nichols, CC Meltzer, J Price, DA Steppe, JM Miewald, DJ Kupfer, RY Moore. Changes in forebrain function from waking to REM sleep in depression: preliminary analyses of [^{18}F]FDG PET studies. Psychiatry Res Neuroimaging 91:59–78, 1999.
13. TW Robbins, BJ Everitt. Arousal systems and attention. In: M Gazzaniga, ed. The Cognitive Neurosciences. Cambridge: MIT Press, 1996, pp 703–720.
14. W Singer, CM Gray. Visual feature integration and the temporal correlation hypothesis. Annu Rev Neurosci 18:555–586, 1995.
15. O Tzischinsky, P Lavie. Melatonin possesses time-dependent hypnotic effects. Sleep 17:638–645, 1994.
16. JK Wyatt, RR Bootzin, JJ Allen, JL Anthony. Mesograde amnesia during the sleep onset transition: replication and electrophysiological correlates. Sleep 20:512–522, 1997.
17. G Aston-Jones, FE Bloom. Activity of norepinephrine-containing locus coeruleus neurons in behaving rats anticipates fluctuations in the sleep-waking cycle. J Neurosci 1:876–886, 1981.
18. S Datta, JM Calvo, J Quattrochi, JA Hobson. Cholinergic microstimulation of the peribrachial nucleus in the cat. I. Immediate and prolonged increases in ponto-geniculo-occipital waves. Arch Ital Biol 130:263–284, 1992.
19. S Datta, D Pare, G Oakson, M Steriade. Thalamic projecting neurons in brainstem cholinergic nuclei increase their firing rates one minute in advance of EEG desynchronization associated with REM sleep. Soc Neurosci Abstr 15:452, 1989. Abstract.
20. JA Hobson, S Datta, JM Calvo, J Quattrochi. Acetylcholine as a brain state regulator: triggering and long-term regulation of REM sleep. Prog Brain Res 98:389–404, 1993.
21. JA Hobson, M Stenade. Neuronal basis of behavioral state control. In: VB Mountcastle, FE Bloom, eds. Handbook of Physiology, Vol. IV. Bethesda: American Physiological Society, 1986, pp 701–823.
22. BL Jacobs, J Heym, ME Trulson. Behavioral and physiological correlates of brain serotonergic unit activity. J Physiol 77:431–436, 1981.
23. BE Jones, M Muhlethaler. Cholinergic and GABAergic neurons of the basal forebrain: role in

24. JM Krueger, F Obal Jr, J Fang. Humoral regulation of physiological sleep: cytokines and GHRH. J Sleep Res 8(suppl 1):53–59, 1999.
25. CA Kushida, RK Zoltoski, JC Gillin. Expression of m2 muscarinic receptor mRNA in rat brain with REM sleep deprivation. Sleep Res 24:37, 1995.
26. JI Luebke, RW Greene, K Semba, A Kamondi, RW McCarley, PB Reiner. Serotonin hyperpolarizes cholinergic low threshold burst neurons in the rat laterodorsal tegmental nucleus in vitro. Proc Natl Acad Sci USA 89:743–747, 1992.
27. PH Luppi, C Peyron, C Rampon, D Gervasoni, B Barbagli, R Boissard, P Fort. Inhibitory mechanisms in the dorsal raphe nucleus and locus coeruleus during sleep. In: R Lydic, HA Baghdoyan, eds. Handbook of Behavioral State Control: Cellular and Molecular Mechanisms. Boca Raton: CRC Press, 1999, pp 195–212.
28. SG Massaquoi, RW McCarley. Extension of the limit cycle reciprocal interaction model of REM cycle control: an integrated sleep control model. J Sleep Res 1:138–143, 1992.
29. RW McCarley, SG Massaquoi. A limit cycle mathematical model of the REM sleep oscillator system. Am J Physiol 251:R1011–R1029, 1986.
30. RW McCarley, JA Hobson. Neuronal excitability modulation over the sleep cycle: a structural and mathematical model. Science 189:58–60, 1975.
31. DJ McGinty, RM Harper. Dorsal raphe neurons: depression of firing during sleep in cats. Brain Res 101:569–575, 1976.
32. K Semba. The mesopontine cholinergic system: a dual role in REM sleep and wakefulness. In: R Lydic, HA Baghdoyan, eds. Handbook of Behavioral State Control: Cellular and Molecular Mechanisms. Boca Raton: CRC Press, 1999, pp 161–180.
33. PJ Shiromani, JC Gillin. Acetylcholine and the regulation of REM sleep: basic mechanisms and clinical implications for affective illness and narcolepsy. Annu Rev Pharmacol Toxicol 27:137–157, 1987.
34. JA Williams, PB Reiner. Noradrenaline hyperpolarizes cholinergic neurons in rat laterodorsal tegmentum in vitro. Soc Neurosci Abstr 18:975, 1992. Abstract.
35. AR Braun, TJ Balkin, NJ Wesenten, RE Carson, M Varga, P Baldwin, S Selbie, G Belenky, P Herscovitch. Regional cerebral blood flow throughout the sleep-wake cycle. An H2(15)O PET study. Brain 120:1173–1197, 1997.
36. BE Jones. Basic mechanisms of sleep-wake states. In: MH Kryger, T Roth, WC Dement, eds. Principles and Practice of Sleep Medicine. Philadelphia: W.B. Saunders, 1994, pp 145–162.
37. EA Nofzinger, MA Mintun, MB Wiseman, DJ Kupfer, RY Moore. Forebrain activation in REM sleep: an FDG PET study. Brain Res 770:192–201, 1997.
38. M Steriade, G Buzsaki. Parallel activation of thalamic and cortical neurons by brainstem and basal forebrain cholinergic systems. In: M Steriade, D Biesold, eds. Brain Cholinergic Systems. New York: Oxford University Press, 1990, pp 3–52.
39. JF Bernard, M Alden, JM Resson. The organization of the efferent projections from the pontine parabrachial area to the amygdaloid complex: a phaseolus vulgaris leucoagglutinin (PHA-L) study in rats. J Comp Neurol 329:201–229, 1993.
40. JM Calvo, K Simon-Arceo. Cholinergic enhancement of REM sleep from sites in the pons and amygdala. In: R Lydic, HA Baghdoyan, eds. Handbook of Behavioral State Control: Cellular and Molecular Mechanisms. Boca Raton: CRC Press, 1999, pp 391–406.
41. AR Morrison, LD Sanford, RJ Ross. Initiation of rapid eye movement sleep: beyond the brainstem. In: BN Mallick, S Inoue, eds. Rapid Eye Movement Sleep. New York: Marcel Dekker, 1999.
42. LD Sanford, SM Tejani-Butt, RJ Ross, AR Morrison. Amygdaloid control of alerting and behavioral arousal in rats: involvement of serotonergic mechanisms. Arch Ital Biol 134:81–99, 1995.
43. LD Sanford, RJ Ross, AR Morrison. Serotonergic mechanisms in the amygdala terminate REM sleep. Sleep Res 24:54, 1995.
44. CB Saper, AD Loewy. Efferent connections of the parabrachial nucleus in the rat. Brain Res 197:291–317, 1980.
45. K Semba, HC Fibiger. Afferent connections of the laterodorsal and the pedunculopontine tegmental nuclei in the rat: a retro and antero-grade transport and immunohistochemical study. J Comp Neurol 323:387–410, 1992.
46. JL Andersson, H Onoe, J Hetta, K Lidstrom, S Valind, A Lilja, A Sundin, KJ Fasth, G Westerberg, JE Broman, Y Watanabe, B Langstrom. Brain networks affected by synchronized sleep visualized by positron emission tomography. J Cereb Blood Flow Metab 18:701–715, 1998.
47. MS Buchsbaum, JC Gillin, J Wu, E Hazlett, N Sicotte, RM DuPont, WE Bunney. Regional cerebral glucose metabolic rate in human sleep assessed by positron emission tomography. Life Sci 45:1349–1356, 1989.
48. G Franck, E Salmon, R Poirrier, B Sadzot, G Franco. Study of regional cerebral glucose metabolism, in man, while awake or asleep, by positron emission

tomography. [In French.] Rev Electroencephalogr Neurophysiol Clin 17:71–77, 1987.
49. WD Heiss, G Pawlik, K Herholz, R Wagner, K Wienhard. Regional cerebral glucose metabolism in man during wakefulness, sleep, and dreaming. Brain Res 327:362–366, 1985.
50. J Hetta, H Onoe, J Andersson, JE Broman, S Valind, A Lilja, A Sundin, K Lindstrom, Y Watanabe, B Langstrom. Cerebral blood flow during sleep. A positron emission tomographic (PET) study of regional changes. Sleep Res 24A:87, 1995. Abstract.
51. N Hofle, T Paus, D Reutens, P Fiset, J Gotman, AC Evans, BE Jones. Regional cerebral blood flow changes as a function of delta and spindle activity during slow wave sleep in humans. J Neurosci 15:4800–4808, 1997.
52. PL Madsen, JF Schmidt, G Wildschiodtz. Cerebral oxygen metabolism and cerebral blood flow in humans during deep and rapid-eye movement sleep. J Appl Physiol 70:2597–2601, 1991.
53. P Maquet, D Divc, E Salmon, B Sadzot, G Franco, R Poirrier, R von Frenckell, G Franck. Cerebral glucose utilization during sleep-wake cycle in man determined by positron emission tomography and [^{18}F]2-fluoro-2-deoxy-D-glucose method. Brain Res 513:136–143, 1990.
54. P Maquet, C Degueldre, G Delfiore, J Aerts, JM Peters, A Luxen, G Franck. Functional neuroanatomy of human slow wave sleep. J Neurosci 17:2807–2812, 1997.
55. EA Nofzinger, DJ Buysse, JM Miewald, CC Meltzer, JC Price, RC Sembrat, H Ombao, CF Reynolds, TH Monk, M Hall, DJ Kupfer, RY Moore. Human regional cerebral glucose metabolism during NREM sleep in relation to waking. Brain 125:1105–1115, 2002.
56. F Sakai, JS Meyer, I Karacan, S Derman, M Yamamoto. Normal human sleep: regional cerebral hemodynamics. Ann Neurol 7:471-478, 1980.
57. DJ Buysse, CF Reynolds, TH Monk, SR Berman, DJ Kupfer. The Pittsburgh Sleep Quality Index (PSQI). A new instrument for psychiatric research and practice. Psychiatry Res 28:193–213, 1989.
58. EA Nofzinger, ME Thase, CF Reynolds, JM Himmelhoch, A Mallinger, P Houck, DJ Kupfer. Hypersomnia in bipolar depression: a comparison with narcolepsy using the multiple sleep latency test. Am J Psychiatry 148:1177–1181, 1991.
59. R Armitage, RF Hoffmann, AJ Rush. Biological rhythm disturbance in depression: temporal coherence of ultradian sleep EEG rhythms. Psychol Med 29:1435–1448, 1999.
60. EA Nofzinger, DJ Buysse, CF Reynolds, DJ Kupfer. Sleep disorders related to another mental disorder (nonsubstance/primary): a DSM-IV literature review [review]. J Clin Psychiatry 54:244–255; discussion 256–259, 1993.

61. R Armitage, HP Roffwarg, AJ Rush, JS Calhoun, DG Purdy, DE Giles. Digital period analysis of sleep EEG in depression. Biol Psychiatry 31:52–68, 1992.
62. R Armitage, A Hudson, M Trivedi, AJ Rush. Sex differences in the distribution of EEG frequencies during sleep: unipolar depressed outpatients. J Affect Disord 34:121–129, 1995.
63. R Armitage, R Hoffmann, M Trivedi, AJ Rush. Sleep macro- and microarchitecture in depression: age and gender effects. Sleep Res 26:283, 1997.
64. RM Benca, WH Obermeyer, RA Thisted, JC Gillin. Sleep and psychiatric disorders: a meta-analysis. Arch Gen Psychiatry 49:651–668, 1992.
65. AA Borbély, I Tobler, M Loepfe, DJ Kupfer, RF Ulrich, V Grochocinski, J Doman, G Matthews. All-night spectral analysis of the sleep EEG in untreated depressives and normal controls. Psychiatry Res 12:27–33, 1984.
66. DJ Buysse, DJ Kupfer, E Frank, TH Monk, A Ritenour. Do EEG sleep studies predict recurrence in depressed patients successfully treated with psychotherapy? Depression 2:105–108, 1994.
67. DJ Kupfer, RF Ulrich, PA Coble, DB Jarrett, V Grochocinski, J Doman, G Matthews, AA Borbély. Application of automated REM and slow wave sleep analysis. I. Normal and depressed subjects. Psychiatry Res 13:325–334, 1984.
68. DJ Kupfer, E Frank, AB McEachran, VJ Grochocinski. Delta sleep ratio: a biological correlate of early recurrence in unipolar affective disorder. Arch Gen Psychiatry 47:1100–1105, 1990.
69. DJ Kupfer, VJ Grochocinski, AB McEachran. Relationship of awakening and delta sleep in depression. Psychiatry Res 19:297–304, 1986.
70. CJ Lauer, D Riemann, M Wiegand, M Berger. From early to late adulthood changes in EEG sleep of depressed patients and healthy volunteers. Biol Psychiatry 29:979–993, 1991.
71. WB Mendelson, DA Sack, SP James, JV Martin, R Wagner, P Garnett, J Milton, TA Wehr. Frequency analysis of the sleep EEG in depression. Psychiatry Res 21:89–94, 1987.
72. CF Reynolds, DJ Kupfer, ME Thase, E Frank, DB Jarrett, PA Coble, CC Hoch, DJ Buysse, AD Simons, PR Houck. Sleep, gender, and depression: an analysis of gender effects on the electroencephalographic sleep of 302 depressed outpatients. Biol Psychiatry 28:673–684, 1990.
73. RH Van den Hoofdakker, DG Beersma. On the contribution of sleep-wake physiology to the explanation and treatment of depression. Psychiatry Res 16:155–163, 1986.
74. AJ Rush, DE Giles, RB Jarrett, F Feldman-Koffler, JR Debus, J Weissenburger, PJ Orsulak, HP Roffwarg. Reduced REM latency predicts response

to tricyclic medication in depressed outpatients. Biol Psychiatry 26:61–72, 1989.
75. RB Jarrett, AJ Rush, M Khatami, HP Roffwarg. Does the pretreatment polysomnogram predict response to cognitive therapy in depressed outpatients? A preliminary report. Psychiatry Res 33:285–299, 1990.
76. DE Giles, RB Jarrett, HP Roffwarg, AJ Rush. Reduced rapid eye movement latency: a predictor of recurrence in depression. Neuropsychopharmacology 1:33–39, 1987.
77. AL Sharpley, AE Walsh, PJ Cowen. Nefazodone—a novel antidepressant—may increase REM sleep. Biol Psychiatry 31:1070–1073, 1992.
78. EA Nofzinger, CF Reynolds, ME Thase, E Frank, JR Jennings, AL Fasiczka, LR Sullivan, DJ Kupfer. REM sleep enhancement by bupropion in depressed men. Am J Psychiatry 152(2):274–276, 1995.
79. EA Nofzinger, A Fasiczka, S Berman, ME Thase. Bupropion SR reduces periodic limb movements that are associated with arousals from sleep in depressed patients with periodic limb movement disorder. J Clin Psychiatry, 61:858–862, 2000.
80. JC Gillin, L Sutton, C Ruiz, J Kelsoe, RM DuPont, D Darko, SC Risch, S Golshan, D Janowsky. The cholinergic rapid eye movement induction test with arecoline in depression. Arch Gen Psychiatry 48:264–270, 1991.
81. D Riemann, F Hohagen, S Krieger, H Gann, WE Muller, R Olbrich, HJ Wark, M Bohus, H Low, M Berger. Cholinergic REM induction test: muscarinic supersensitivity underlies polysomnographic findings in both depression and schizophrenia. J Psychiatr Res 28:195–210, 1994.
82. N Sitaram, AM Moore, JC Gillin. Scopolamine-induced muscarinic supersensitivity in normal man: changes in sleep. Psychiatry Res 1:9–16, 1979.
83. DS Janowsky, SC Risch. Cholinomimetic and anticholinergic drugs used to investigate an acetylcholine hypothesis of affective disorder and stress. Drug Dev Res 4:125–142, 1984.
84. T Bhatti, JC Gillin, S Golshan, C Clark, A Demodena, A Schlosser, S Stahl, J Kelsoe, M Rapaport. The effect of a tryptophan-free amino acid drink on sleep and mood in normal controls. Sleep Res 24:153, 1995.
85. T Bhatti, JC Gillin, E Seifritz, P Moore, C Clark, S Golshan, S Stahl, M Rapaport, J Kelsoe. Effects of a tryptophan-free amino acid drink challenge on normal human sleep electroencephalogram and mood. Biol Psychiatry 43:52–59, 1998.
86. JC Gillin, JW Sohn, SM Stahl, M Lardon, J Kelsoe, M Rapaport, C Ruiz, S Golshan. Ipsapirone, a 5HT1A agonist, suppresses REM sleep equally in unmedicated depressed patients and normal controls. Neuropsychopharmacology 15:109–115, 1996.
87. C Ruiz, S Stahl, T Bhatti, S Golshan, J Sohn, L Sutton, J Kelsoe, M Rapaport, JC Gillin. The effects of ipsapirone on the sleep of patients with affective disorders and normal controls. Sleep Res 24:420, 1995.
88. E Seifritz, SM Stahl, JC Gillin. Human sleep EEG following the 5HT1A antagonist pindolol: possible disinhibition of raphe neuron activity. Brain Res 759:84–91, 1997.
89. EA Nofzinger, S Berman, A Fasiczka, JM Miewald, CC Meltzer, JC Price, RC Sembrat, A Wood, ME Thase. Effects of Bupropion SR on anterior paralimbic function during waking and REM sleep in depression: preliminary findings using [^{18}F]-FDG PET. Psychiatry Res Neuroimaging 106:95–111, 2001.
90. EA Nofzinger, JC Price, CC Meltzer, DJ Buysse, VL Villemagne, JM Miewald, RC Sembrat, DA Steppe, DJ Kupfer. Towards a neurobiology of dysfunctional arousal in depression: the relationship between beta EEG power and regional cerebral glucose metabolism during NREM sleep. Psychiatry Res Neuroimaging 98:71–91, 2000.
91. AP Ho, JC Gillin, MS Buchsbaum, JC Wu, L Abel, WE Bunney. Brain glucose metabolism during non-rapid eye movement sleep in major depression: a positron emission tomography study. Arch Gen Psychiatry 53:645–652, 1996.
92. C Clark, R Dupont, P Lehr, D Yeung, S Halpern, S Golshan, JC Gillin. Is there a relationship between delta sleep at night and afternoon cerebral blood flow, assessed by HMPAO-SPECT in depressed patients and normal control subjects? Preliminary data. Psychiatry Res 84:89–99, 1998.
93. J Wu, MS Buchsbaum, JC Gillin, C Tang, S Cadwell, M Wiegand, A Najafi, E Klein, K Hazen, WE Bunney, JH Fallon, D Keator. Prediction of antidepressant effects of sleep deprivation by metabolic rates in the ventral anterior cingulate and medial prefrontal cortex. Am J Psychiatry 156:1149–1158, 1999.
94. CF Reynolds, TH Monk, CC Hoch, JR Jennings, DJ Buysse, PR Houck, DB Jarrett, DJ Kupfer. Electroencephalographic sleep in the healthy "old old": a comparison with the "young old" in visually scored and automated measures. J Gerontol 46:M39–M46, 1991.
95. CF Reynolds, JR Jennings, CC Hoch, TH Monk, SR Berman, FT Hall, JV Matzzie, DJ Buysse, DJ Kupfer. Daytime sleepiness in the healthy "old old": A comparison with young adults. J Am Geriatr Soc 39:957–962, 1991.
96. TH Monk, CF Reynolds, MA Machen, DJ Kupfer. Daily social rhythms in the elderly and their relation to objectively recorded sleep. Sleep 15:322–329, 1992.
97. CF Reynolds, CC Hoch, DJ Buysse, PR Houck, M Schlernitzauer, E Frank, S Mazumdar, DJ Kupfer. Electroencephalographic sleep in spousal bereave-

ment and bereavement-related depression of late life. Biol Psychiatry 31:69–82, 1992.
98. CF Reynolds, CC Hoch, DJ Buysse, PR Houck, M Schlernitzauer, RE Pasternak, E Frank, S Mazumdar, DJ Kupfer. Sleep after spousal bereavement: a study of recovery from stress. Biol Psychiatry 34:791–797, 1993.
99. RD Cartwright, HM Kravitz, CI Eastman, E Wood. REM latency and the recovery from depression: getting over divorce. Am J Psychiatry 148:1530–1535, 1991.
100. VP Zarcone, KL Benson. Sleep and schizophrenia. In: Principles and Practice of Sleep Medicine Philadelphia: W.B. Saunders, 1994, pp 105–214.
101. R Ganguli, CF Reynolds, DJ Kupfer. Electroencephalographic sleep in young, never medicated schizophrenics. Arch Gen Psychiatry 44:36–44, 1987.
102. R Tandon, JE Shipley, S Taylor, JF Greden, A Eiser, J DeQuardo, J Goodson. Electroencephalographic sleep abnormalities in schizophrenia: relationship to positive/negative symptoms and prior neuroleptic treatment. Arch Gen Psychiatry 49:185–194, 1992.
103. MS Keshavan, S Anderson, JW Pettegrew. Is schizophrenia due to excessive synaptic pruning in prefrontal cortex? The Feinberg hypothesis revisited. J Psychiatr Res 28:239–265, 1994.
104. E Werth, P Achermann, AA Borbely. Fronto-occipital EEG power gradients in human sleep. J Sleep Res 6:102–112, 1997.
105. MS Keshavan, CF Reynolds, D Montrose, J Miewald, C Downs, EM Sabo. Sleep and suicidality in psychotic patients. Acta Psychiatr Scand 89:122–125, 1994.
106. C Lewis, R Tandon, JR Shipley, JR Dequardo, M Gibson, SF Taylor, M Goldman. Biological predictors of suicidality in schizophrenia. Acta Psychiatr Scand 94:416–420, 1996.
107. S Maixner, R Tandon, A Eiser, S Taylor, JR Dequardo, J Shipley. Effects of antipsychotic treatment on polysomnographic measures in schizophrenia: a replication and extension. Am J Psychiatry 155:1600–1602, 1997.
108. MS Keshavan, CF Reynolds, JM Miewald, DM Montrose. A longitudinal study of EEG sleep in schizophrenia. Psychiatry Res 59:203–211, 1996.
109. N Kajimura, M Kato, T Okuma, M Sekimoto, T Watanabe, K Takahashi. Relationship between delta activity during all-night sleep and negative symptoms in schizophrenia: a preliminary study. Biol Psychiatry 39:451–454, 1996.
110. MS Keshavan, CF Reynolds, R Ganguli, GL Haas, J Sweeney, J Miewald, D Montrose. Slow wave sleep and symptomatology in schizophrenia and related psychotic disorders. J Psychiatr Res 29:303–314, 1995.
111. DP Van Kammen, WB van Kammen, J Peters, K Goetz, T Neylan. Decreased slow-wave sleep and enlarged lateral ventricles in schizophrenia. Neuropsychopharmacology 1:265–271, 1988.
112. MS Keshavan, CF Reynolds, J Miewald, D Montrose. Slow-wave sleep deficits and outcome in schizophrenia and schizoaffective disorder. Acta Psychiatr Scand 91:289–292, 1995.
113. MS Keshavan, JW Pettegrew, CF Reynolds, KS Panchalingam, D Montrose, J Miewald, DJ Kupfer. Slow wave sleep deficits in schizophrenia: pathophysiological significance. Psychiatry Res 57:91–100, 1995.
114. DL Bliwise. Dementia. In: MH Kryger, T Roth; WC Dement, eds. Principles and Practice of Sleep Medicine. Philadelphia: W.B. Saunders, 1994, p 790.
115. MC Chenier. Review and analysis of caregiver burden and nursing home placement. Geriatr Nurs 18:121–126, 1997.
116. CP Pollak, D Perlick. Sleep problems and institutionalization of the elderly. J Geriatr Psychiatry Neurol 4:204–210, 1991.
117. DL Bliwise, M Hughes, PM McMahon, N Kutner. Observed sleep/wakefulness and severity of dementia in an Alzheimer's disease special care unit. J Gerontol Ser A Biol Sci Med Sci 50:M303–M306, 1995.
118. K Meguro, M Ueda, I Kobayashi, S Yamaguchi, H Yamazaki, Y Oikawa, Y Kikuchi, H Sasaki. Sleep disturbance in elderly patients with cognitive impairment, decreased daily activity and periventricular white matter lesions. Sleep 18:109-114, 1995.
119. J Cohen-Mansfield, P Werner, L Freedman. Sleep and agitation in agitated nursing home residents: an observational study. Sleep 18:674–680, 1995.
120. SM McCurry, RG Logsdon, L Teri, LE Gibbons, WA Kukull, JD Bowen, WC McCormick, EB Larson. Characteristics of sleep disturbance in community-dwelling Alzheimer's disease patients. J Geriatr Psychiatry Neurol 12:53–59, 1999.
121. R Blois, C Pawlak, JM Rossi. Sleep EEG findings in Alzheimer's and Pick's dementia. In: S Smirne, M Franceschi, L Ferini-Strambi, eds. Sleep and Ageing. Milan: Masson, 1991, pp 65–70.
122. SR Allen, WO Seiler, HB Stahelin, R Spiegel. Seventy-two hour polygraphic and behavioral recordings of wakefulness and sleep in a hospital geriatric unit: comparison between demented and nondemented patients. Sleep 10:143–159, 1987.
123. DL Bliwise, J Tinklenberg, JA Yesavage, H Davies, AM Pursley, DE Petta, L Widrow, C Guilleminault, VP Zarcone, WC Dement. REM latency in Alzheimer's disease. Biol Psychiatry 25:320–328, 1989.
124. I Feinberg, RL Koresko, N Heller. EEG sleep patterns as a function of normal and pathological aging in man. J Psychiatr Res 5:107–144, 1967.

125. RJ Loewenstein, H Weingartner, JC Gillin, W Kaye, M Ebert, WB Mendelson. Disturbances of sleep and cognitive functioning in patients with dementia. Neurobiol Aging 3:371–377, 1982.
126. G Mennuni, MA Petrella, C Masullo. Sleep pattern in Alzheimer's disease/senile dementia of the Alzheimer's type (AD/SDAT). In: S Smirne, M Franceschi, L Ferini-Strambi, eds. Sleep and Ageing. Milan: Masson, 1991, pp 71–74.
127. PN Prinz, PP Vitaliano, MV Vitiello, J Bokan, M Raskind, E Peskind, C Gerber. Sleep, EEG and mental function changes in senile dementia of the Alzheimer's type. Neurobiol Aging 3:361–370, 1982.
128. CF Reynolds, DJ Kupfer, LS Taska, CC Hoch, DG Spiker, DE Sewitch, B Zimmer, RS Marin, JP Nelson, D Martin, R Morycz. EEG sleep in elderly depressed, demented, and healthy subjects. Biol Psychiatry 20:431–442, 1985.
129. CF Reynolds, DJ Kupfer, LS Taska, CC Hoch, DE Sewitch, VJ Grochocinski. Slow wave sleep in elderly depressed, demented, and healthy subjects. Sleep 8(2):155–159, 1985.
130. MV Vitiello, PN Prinz, DE Williams, MS Frommlet, RK Ries. Sleep disturbances in patients with mild stage Alzheimer's disease. J Gerontol 45:M131–M138, 1990.
131. PN Prinz, ER Peskind, PP Vitaliano, MA Raskind, C Eisdorfer, W Zembeuznikov, CJ Gerber. Changes in the sleep and waking EEGs of nondemented and demented elderly subjects. J Am Geriatr Soc 30:86–93, 1982.
132. S Ancoli-Israel, MR Klauber, N Butters, L Parker, DF Kripke. Dementia in institutionalized elderly: relation to sleep apnea. J Am Geriatr Soc 39:258–263, 1991.
133. DL Bliwise. Cognitive function and SDB in aging adults. In: ST Kuna, PM Suratt, JE Remmers, eds. Sleep and Respiration in Aging Adults. New York: Elsevier, 1991.
134. DL Bliwise, JA Yesavage, JR Tinklenberg, WC Dement. Sleep apnea in Alzheimer's disease. Neurobiol Aging 10:343–346, 1989.
135. DL Bliwise. Sleep apnea, dementia and Alzheimer's disease: a mini review. Bull Clin Neurosci 54:123–126, 1989.
136. T Erkinjuntti, M Partinen, R Sulkava, T Telakivi, T Salmi, R Tilvis. Sleep apnea in multiinfarct dementia and Alzheimer's disease. Sleep 10:419–425, 1987.
137. T Erkinjuntti, M Partinen, R Sulkava, H Palomaki, R Tilvis. Snoring and dementia. Age Ageing 16:305–310, 1987.
138. CC Hoch, CF Reynolds, RD Nebes, DJ Kupfer, SR Berman, DW Campbell. Clinical significance of sleep-disordered breathing (SDB) in Alzheimer's disease: preliminary data. J Am Geriatr Soc 37:138–144, 1989.
139. CC Hoch, CF Reynolds, DJ Kupfer, PR Houck, SR Berman, JA Stack. Sleep disordered breathing in normal and pathologic aging. J Clin Psychiatry 47(10):499–503, 1986.
140. RG Smallwood, MV Vitiello, EC Giblin, PN Prinz. Sleep apnea: relationship to age, sex, and Alzheimer's dementia. Sleep 6:16–22, 1983.
141. J Cohen-Mansfield, MS Marx, AS Rosenthal. A description of agitation in a nursing home. J Gerontol 44:M77–M84, 1989.
142. J Cohen-Mansfield, MS Marx, AS Rosenthal. Dementia and agitation in nursing home residents: how are they related? Psychol Aging 5:3–8, 1990.
143. J Cohen-Mansfield, MS Marx. Do past experiences predict agitation in nursing home residents? Int J Aging Hum Dev 28:285–294, 1989.
144. J Cohen-Mansfield, N Billig, S Lipson, AS Rosenthal, LG Pawlson. Medical correlates of agitation in nursing home residents. Gerontology 36:150–158, 1990.
145. AJ Lees, NA Blackburn, VL Campbell. The nighttime problems of Parkinson's disease. Clin Neuropharmacol 11:512–519, 1988.
146. PA Nausieda, WJ Weiner, LR Kaplan, S Weber, HL Klawans. Sleep disruption in the course of chronic levodopa therapy: an early feature of the levodopa psychosis. Clin Neuropharmacol 5:183–194, 1982.
147. E Tandberg, JP Larsen, K Karlsen. A community-based study of sleep disorders in patients with Parkinson's disease. Mov Disord 13:895–899, 1998.
148. SA Factor, T McAlarney, JR Sanchez-Ramos, WJ Weiner. Sleep disorders and sleep effect in Parkinson's disease. Mov Disord 5:280–285, 1990.
149. F Stocchi, L Barbato, G Nordera, A Berardelli, S Ruggieri. Sleep disorders in Parkinson's disease. J Neurol 245:S15–S18, 1998.
150. O Bernath, C Guilleminault. Sleep-related violence, injury, and REM sleep behavior disorder in PD. Neurology 52:1924, 1999.
151. CL Comella, TM Nardine, NJ Diederich, GT Stebbins. Sleep-related violence, injury, and REM sleep behavior disorder in Parkinson's disease. Neurology 51:526–529, 1998.
152. CG Goetz, RS Wilson, CM Tanner, DC Garson. Relationship between pain, depression and sleep alteration in Parkinson's disease. In: MD Yahsand; KJ Bergmann, eds. Advances in Neurology. New York: Raven Press, 1986, pp 345–347.
153. K Karlsen, JP Larsen, E Tandberg, K Jorgensen. Fatigue in patients with Parkinson's disease. Mov Disord 14:237–241, 1999.
154. A Laihinen, J Alihanka, S Raitasuo, UK Rinne. Sleep movements and associated autonomic nervous activities in patients with Parkinson's disease. Acta Neurol Scand 76:64–68, 1987.
155. RP Lesser, S Fahn, SR Snider, LJ Cote, WP Isgreen, RE Barrett. Analysis of the clinical problems in par-

kinsonism and the complications of long-term levodopa therapy. Neurology 29:1253–1260, 1979.

156. AD Lowe. Sleep in Parkinson's disease. J Psychosom Res 44:613–617, 1998.

157. PA Nausieda, CM Tanner, HL Klawans. Serotonergically active agents in levodopa-induced psychiatric toxicity reactions. In: S Fahn, DB Calne, I Shoulson, eds. Advances in Neurology. New York: Raven Press, 1983.

158. EJ Pappert, CG Goetz, FG Niederman, R Raman, S Leurgans. Hallucinations, sleep fragmentation, and altered dream phenomena in Parkinson's disease. Mov Disord 14:117–121, 1999.

159. R Pfeiffer. Optimization of levodopa therapy. Neurology 42:39–43, 1992.

160. DB Rye, LH Johnston, RL Watts, DL Bliwise. Juvenile Parkinson's disease with REM sleep behavior disorder sleepiness, and daytime REM onset. Neurology 53:1868–1870, 1999.

161. JR Sanchez-Ramos, R Ortoll, GW Paulson. Visual hallucinations associated with Parkinson disease [see comments]. Arch Neurol 53:1265–1268, 1996.

162. E Tandberg, JP Larsen, K Karlsen. Excessive daytime sleepiness and sleep benefit in Parkinson's disease: a community-based study. Mov Disord 14:922–927, 1999.

163. CM Tanner, C Vogel, CG Goetz, HL Klawans. Hallucinations in Parkinson's disease: a popular study. Neurology 14:136, 1983. Abstract.

164. JJ Askenasy, MD Yahr. Reversal of sleep disturbance in Parkinson's disease by antiparkinsonian therapy: a preliminary study. Neurology 35:527–532, 1985.

165. JJ Askenasy. Sleep in Parkinson's disease. Acta Neurol Scand 87:167–170, 1993.

166. P Bergonzi, C Chiurulla, D Gambi, G Mennuni, F Pinto. L-dopa plus dopa-decarboxylase inhibitor. Sleep organization in Parkinson's syndrome before and after treatment. Acta Neurol Belg 75:5–10, 1975.

167. J Cummings. Neuropsychiatric complications of drug treatment of Parkinson's disease. In: SJ Huber, JL Cummings, eds. Parkinson's Disease: Neurobehavioral Aspects. New York: Oxford University Press, 1992, pp 313–327.

168. PA Nausieda, R Glantz, S Weber, R Baum, HL Klawans. Psychiatric complications of levodopa therapy of Parkinson's disease. Adv Neurol 40:271–277, 1984.

169. M Novak, CM Shapiro. Drug-induced sleep disturbances. Focus on nonpsychotropic medications. Drug Saf 16:133–149, 1997.

170. JA Saint-Cyr, AE Taylor, AE Lang. Neuropsychological and psychiatric side effects in the treatment of Parkinson's disease. Neurology 43:S47–S52, 1993.

171. HS Schmidt, W Knopp. Sleep in Parkinson's disease: the effect of L-dopa. Psychophysiology 9:88, 1972.

172. B Sharf, C Moskovitz, MD Lupton, HL Klawans. Dream phenomena induced by chronic levodopa therapy. J Neural Transm 43:143–151, 1978.

173. KM Van den, J Jacquy, M Gonce, PP De Deyn. Sustained-release levodopa in parkinsonian patients with nocturnal disabilities. Acta Neurol Belg 93:32–39, 1993.

174. RJ Wyatt, TN Chase, J Scott, F Snyder, K Engleman. Effect of L-dopa on the sleep of man. Nature 228:999–1001, 1970.

175. A Kales, RD Ansel, CH Markham, MB Scharf, TL Tan. Sleep in patients with Parkinson's disease and normal subjects prior to and following levodopa administration. Clin Pharmacol Ther 12:397–406, 1971.

176. CG Goetz, RS Wilson, CM Tanner, DC Garron. Relationships among pain, depression, and sleep alterations in Parkinson's disease. Adv Neurol 45:345–347, 1988.

177. SE Starkstein, TJ Preziosi, RG Robinson. Sleep disorders, pain, and depression in Parkinson's disease. Eur Neurol 31:352–355, 1991.

178. VS Kostic, V Susic, S Przedborski, N Sternic. Sleep EEG in depressed and nondepressed patients with Parkinson's disease. J Neuropsychiatry Clin Neurosci 3:176–179, 1991.

179. RS April. Observations on parkinsonian tremor in all-night sleep. Neurology 16:720–724, 1966.

180. MC Apps, PC Sheaff, DA Ingram, C Kennard, DW Empey. Respiration and sleep in Parkinson's disease. J Neurol Neurosurg Psychiatry 48:1240–1245, 1985.

181. TB Ustun, M Privett, Y Lecrubier, E Weiller, G Simon, A Korten, SS Bassett, W Maier, N Sartorius. Form, frequency and burden of sleep problems in general health care: a report from the WHO Collaborative Study on Psychological Problems in General Health Care. Eur Psychiatry 11:5s–10s, 1996.

182. DE Ford, DB Kamerow. Epidemiologic study of sleep disturbances and psychiatric disorders: an opportunity for prevention. JAMA 262:1479–1484, 1989.

183. DW Hudgel. Mechanisms of obstructive sleep apnea. Chest 101:541–549, 1992.

184. JW Shepard, SE Thawley. Localization of upper airway collapse during sleep in patients with obstructive sleep apnea. Am Rev Respir Dis 141:1350–1355, 1990.

185. KA Ekbom. Restless legs. Acta Med Scand Suppl 158:1–123, 1945.

49

Perspectives in the Pharmacological Treatment of Schizophrenia

LARRY ERESHEFSKY
College of Pharmacy, University of Texas at Austin, Austin, Texas, U.S.A.

I. SCHIZOPHRENIA

Schizophrenia is a chronic and disabling illness, which is usually characterized as a constellation of positive, negative, and cognitive symptoms or deficits (Fig. 1). Above all, schizophrenia is a disorder in which social, occupational, self-care, and interpersonal functions are severely reduced [1]. Schizophrenia is the fourth leading cause of disability worldwide; 60–70% of patients do not marry, 10% commit suicide, and 20–40% of patients make at least one suicide attempt during their illness [1–3]. Patients with schizophrenia have a 20% shorter life expectancy than demographically matched control subjects [4], and the combination of impoverished life styles, medical care, and risk factors including both the illness itself and drug therapy result in a 4.3-fold increased rate of mortality from unnatural causes and 1.6-fold increased rate of mortality due to natural causes [5]. Cigarette smoking, obesity, substance abuse and dependence (especially alcohol), poor diet, and limited access to medical services contribute to the increased mortality rate [6]. However, despite many of the medical management issues facing our patients, we have made tremendous progress in treating this tragic illness. Patients maintained long term on second-generation (or atypical) antipsychotics have recovered function and regained their lives and sense of purpose. We must raise the bar on our standard of care for patients with schizophrenia and make restored function to perform and enjoy life's many facets our "bottom line" [7].

II. INTRODUCTION TO ANTIPSYCHOTIC THERAPY

The serendipitous discovery of neuroleptic medications (from the French *neuroleptique*—meaning to clasp the neuron) revolutionized our treatments for persistent psychotic disorders. The observation that these agents almost invariably induced parkinsonian features, led to simple animal models to screen these putative medications. Antipsychotics were screened using rodent models which included antagonism of amphetamine's excitatory effects and the causation of catalepsy, a form of extrapyramidal disturbance [8–10]. Compounds that did not cause catalepsy in animal models were not considered to be effective antipsychotic agents—e.g., clozapine [11]. The theory for dopamine's primary role in mediating psychosis was supported by the pharmacological and neurochemical characterization of stimulant's effects on behavior, Parkinson's disease and its treatment, and neuroleptic activities in both human and animal models. Although dopamine type 2 receptor (D2) blockade is still a component of all marketed antipsychotic agents' pharma-

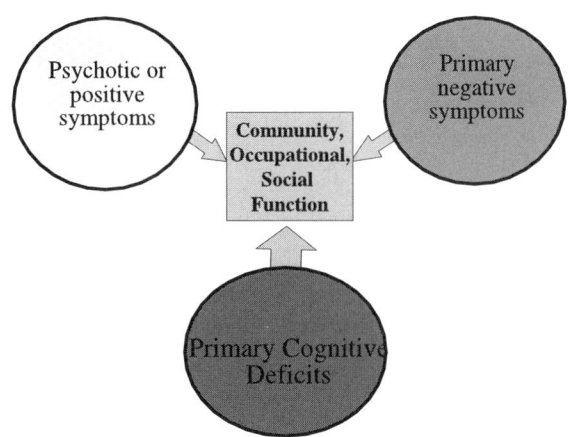

Figure 1 Relationship of symptoms to function in schizophrenia. The relative importance of changes in positive and negative symptoms, and of cognition deficits on functional capacity of patients with schizophrenia, is illustrated by the differently weighted arrows (cognition improvement being the most important predictor of functional change).

cological profiles, the modulation of other biogenic amines, indirect effects on excitatory aminoacids, and possibly peptidergic systems play a role in many second-generation antipsychotic therapies [12–14].

Clozapine's complex pharmacologic profile is illustrated in Figure 2.

Neuroscience insights into brain function and the development of many novel antipsychotics with a wide array of pharmacological effects have led to a dramatic paradigm shift in our conceptualization of schizophrenia and other psychotic disorders [8–10]. Tables 1 and 2 list pharmacological effects of antipsychotic medications, including possible clinical implications and applications for the increasingly diverse selection of drug therapies available for schizophrenia [15–24]. Key pharmacological differences among atypical antipsychotics will be further discussed in this chapter.

III. OLDER TREATMENTS IN THE MANAGEMENT OF SCHIZOPHRENIA

The perceived advantages for the second-generation antipsychotics, e.g., superiority for relieving negative symptoms and their effectiveness in improving several domains of cognitive and social function [25–29], have resulted in the overwhelming majority of patients in the United States receiving these therapies. The goal for rapid calming of agitated or aggressive patients in emergency settings and acute care units poses a chal-

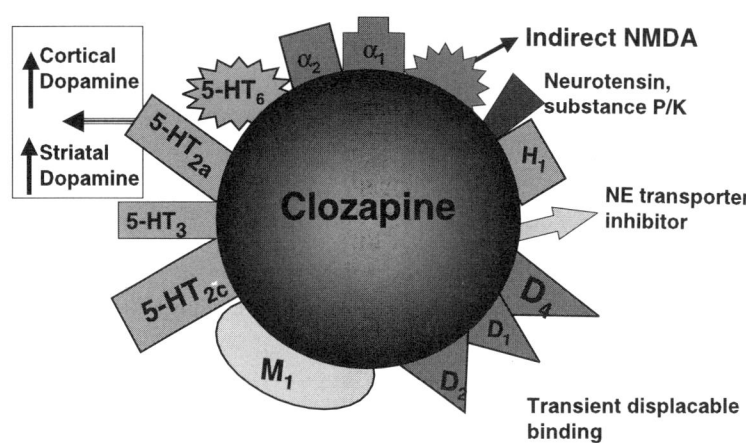

Figure 2 Complex pharmacological profile of clozapine. Clozapine's pharmacologically diverse array of effects is illustrated. Clozapine remains the "gold standard" against which all other medications' efficacies are judged. The unique combination of varied dopaminergic, serotonergic, and adrenergic effects across a wide array of receptor subtypes, along with significant effects on neuropeptide neurotransmission, results in a broad-spectrum medication for patients with persistent, treatment-resistant, psychotic and mood disorders.

Table 1 Antipsychotic Receptor Pharmacology—Relative Effect by Within-Drug in Vitro Receptor Binding

	cis-Thiothixene	Fluphenazine	Haloperidol	Ziprasidone	Risperidone	Loxapine	Chlorpromazine	Olanzapine	Thioridazine	Clozapine	Quetiapine	Iloperidone	Aripiprazole
D1	++++	++++	+	−	−	+++	+++	+++	+++	++	+		−
D2	++++	++++	+++++	++	+++++	+++	+++	++++	+++	++	++	++	++++ p-agonist
D3	nt	nt	+++	+++	+++	nt	nt	++	nt	+	+	nt	++++
D4	nt	nt	+++	++	+++	nt	nt	++++	nt	++	+		++
5HT$_{1a}$	nt	nt	−	+++	+	nt	nt	−	nt	+++	−	nt	+++
5HT$_{1d}$	nt	nt	−	++++	+	nt	nt	+	nt	++++	−	nt	nt
5HT$_{2a}$	+	++	+	++++	+++++	+++	++++	++++	++	++++	++	+++	+++
5HT$_{2c}$	nt	nt	−	+++	++	nt	nt	+++	nt	++++	−	nt	++
5HT$_6$	nt	nt	−	nt	−	nt	nt	++	nt	++	++	nt	nt
5HT$_7$	nt	nt	−	++++	+++	nt	nt		nt	++++	−	nt	nt
Muscarinic M$_1$	−	−	−	−	−	+	++	++++ In vitro ≠ In Vivo	+++	+++++	++	−	−
α$_1$-Adrenoceptor	+++	++	++	+++	+++	++	++++	++	++++	+++++	++++	nt	+
α$_2$-Adrenoceptor	+	−	−	+	++	−	++	+	++	++++	++	nt	nt
H$_1$ histamine	++	+	−	+++	++	+++	++++	++++	+++	+++++	+++	nt	+
Serotonin transport	nt	nt	−	−	−	nt	nt	−	nt	−	−	nt	nt
Norepinephrine transport	nt	nt	−	+++	−	++	nt	+	nt	++	+	nt	nt

− = No effect; + to +++ represent increasing relative effects (though no single study evaluates all drugs in all dimensions); nt = not tabulated in studies.
Source: Ref. 18

Table 2 Receptor Effects and their Possible Consequences on Antipsychotic Efficacy and Side Effects

Receptor	Efficacy	Adverse effects
D2	Reduction in positive symptoms of schizophrenia, relapse prevention	Extrapyramidal side effects, prolactin elevation worsened cognition at high dose, worsened negative symptoms at high dose
D3	Potential alteration in risk of tardive dyskinesia, interacting with genetic polymorphism for D3; possibly enhances efficacy	Unknown
D4	Possible increased dopamine release from neuronal projections to frontal cortex, improving cognition, and reducing negative symptoms	Unknown
5HT$_{1a/d}$ partial agonist/antagonist	Regulation of serotonin release: anxiolytic, antidepressant, and antiaggressive effect	Unknown
5HT$_{2a}$	Modest reductions in positive symptoms, improved cognition and functional status, improved negative symptoms, improved sleep latency, reduced sexual dysfunction	Excessive dosage results in worsening of obsessive compulsive symptoms
5HT$_{2c}$	Minimal effects on positive/negative/cognitive symptoms	Weight gain, possible increased risk of seizures, reduced efficacy
5HT$_6$	Possibly enhances efficacy in parallel to 5HT$_{2a}$ effects	Unknown
5HT$_7$	Possibly enhanced efficacy, especially circadian rhythm disturbances, e.g., sleep.	Unknown
Indirect augmentation of NMDA glutamate	Improved cognition, reduced negative symptoms, and gains in functional status; secondary improvement in positive symptoms	Unknown
Muscarinic M1	Possible indirect neuroprotective effect through glutamatergic system; Reductions in EPS	Dry mouth, constipation, sinus tachycardia, etc.; worsened cognition, sedation and withdrawal upon abrupt discontinuation
Noradrenergic alpha 1	Acute sedating effects may ameliorate aggressive impulses	Orthostatic blood pressure changes, reflex tachycardia, weight gain, nasal congestion
Noradrenergic α_{2c}	Increased dopamine release; improved cognition, reduced negative symptoms, reduced craving for substances of abuse	Tachycardia, tremor, sweating, agitation
Histamine H$_1$	Acute sedating effects may ameliorate aggression and agitation	Weight gain, sedation (may be reduced with chronic dosing)
Serotonin transporter inhibitors (reuptake inhibitors)	Antidepressant and anxiolytic effect; improvement in negative symptoms	Exacerbate EPS, akathisia, alter sleep pattern, cause sexual dysfunction, possibly increase prolactin
Norepinephrine transport inhibitors (reuptake inhibitors)	Antidepressant effect	May increase agitation, insomnia, and restlessness
Neuropeptide effects, Substance P (NK1, NK3), neurotensin, and CRF1 antagonists	Reduce stress mediated brain dysfunction; reduce cortisol and possible midbrain neurotoxicity	Unknown

lenge when using atypical therapies. Rapid calming is not always evident in agitated patients treated with orally administered atypical medications at standard doses. There is a continuing need for intramuscular (IM) therapy using benzodiazepines, e.g., lorazepam, neuroleptics, or combinations of the two, during the crisis management phase for patients with psychotic disorders [30–32]. Second-generation short-acting intramuscular medications are in the final stages of development with olanzapine short-acting intramuscular pending marketing at the time of this chapter's completion (pending resolution of manufacturing issues). Ziprasidone IM is approved as a medication to manage agitation. Ziprasidone IM 20 mg, rapidly reaches peak concentrations within 1-2 h comparable to an 80 mg ziprasidone oral dose and demonstrates comparable efficacy to modest doses of haloperidol, e.g. 5 mg IM. Whether higher doses of second-generation medications are used to facilitate calming of patients, or if they are combined with traditional neuroleptics, it is essential to recognize that these higher doses or combination therapies, driven by health care economic expedience, do not define appropriate maintenance strategies, where monotherapy at standard doses deliver maximal benefit vs. risk [33–35].

Despite the ongoing role for neuroleptic therapy as an emergency intervention in the agitated patient on atypical medications, it is important to remember that when the atypical medications are administered on a subchronic basis, they demonstrate equivalent or superior efficacy in reducing aggressive behavior and positive symptoms [36–38]. The use of adjunctive neuroleptic therapies should therefore be reserved for those patients requiring rapid reductions in these symptoms, or in those in whom there is only partial response despite optimization of the atypical medication's dosage. If neuroleptics are used initially, they should not be continued as long-term therapy; rather, atypical agents should be utilized as front-line therapy. An exception to this would be either a history of treatment resistance to atypical agents with a robust response on neuroleptics, or in those where depot therapy is necessary. Moreover, despite the popularity of benzodiazepines as adjunctive calming agents, they are detrimental to cognitive and memory processes [39]. High-potency neuroleptic antipsychotic agents, when used in the acute setting, are also likely to incur EPS, hence the routine use of prophylactic anticholinergic antiparkinsonian therapies. These antimuscarinic agents also are detrimental for cognitive function [40]. Therefore, management of aggression with an antipsychotic that is less likely to incur EPS is highly desirable.

A. SECOND-GENERATION ANTIPSYCHOTICS

Second-generation antipsychotics are characterized as more complex than high-potency neuroleptics and act beyond the single neurotransmitter focus on dopamine D_2 receptors (Tables 1, 2). The clinical success of the first "atypical" antipsychotic, clozapine, renewed interest in the role of serotonin (5HT) and other neurochemical systems (noradernergic, peptidergic (i.e., neurotensin, substances P and K), and glutamatergic) in schizophrenia [11]. Clozapine is associated with reduced liability for extrapyramidal symptoms (EPS) and is effective in up to 50% of "treatment-resistant" patients. However, adverse effects including agranulocytosis, myocarditis, and seizures limit the widespread use of clozapine, despite its efficacy in treatment-resistant patients. Clozapine is characterized by weak and loose binding activity at D_2 receptors (see below), activity at other dopamine receptors, and potent activity at serotonin $5HT_{2A}$; histaminic; α-adrenergic; and neurotensin (neuropeptide) receptors [41].

B. Dopaminergic System

Many of the effects of antipsychotic medications are tied to their interaction with dopamine neurotransmission in four key brain regions:

1. Mesolimbic system. D2 blockade of the mesolimbic region, including amygdala and hippocampus, is associated with antipsychotic efficacy; all marketed first- and second-generation medications are active in antagonizing the effects of amphetamine or dopamine overactivity.

2. Frontal cortex. Increased dopamine release, mediated by atypical antipsychotics in frontal and prefrontal cortex, leads to improvements in negative symptoms and cognition. In contrast, excessive D2 blockade from high-dose neuroleptic therapy can lead to possible worsening of these symptoms via diminished dopamine firing and release in these brain regions, the result of sustained depolarization blockade.

3. Basal ganglia. Dysregulation resulting from sustained nigral-striatal D2 blocking effects lead to extrapyramidal symptoms, while atypicals reduce the incidence of EPS via a variety of mechanisms including enhanced dopaminergic neuronal firing and release.

4. Turberoinfundibular projections to the pituitary. Antagonism of dopamine's inhibitory effects by potent D2 blockade results in increased pituitary secre-

tion of prolactin [42]. Figure 3 illustrates key dopamine pathways and their significance in the management of patients with psychosis [13].

All antipsychotic drugs have been found, to varying degrees, to antagonize dopamine D2 receptors. Traditional neuroleptic effectiveness has been associated with ~ 65% occupancy of these receptors as demonstrated by positron emission tomography (PET) studies. Usual occupancies at clinically utilized dosages are typically > 75%, a range associated with a high likelihood of EPS. Even at the lower range of occupancies considered effective, the older high-potency neuroleptic drugs maintain a "tight," long-lasting blockade of the receptor, triggering changes in neuronal regulation that lead to dysregulation. Usual conservative doses of neuroleptics are above the threshold for extrapyramidal effects and prolactin elevation. In contrast, clozapine has demonstrated antipsychotic efficacy with only ~ 50–60% occupancy of D2 receptors, even at the highest doses utilized 8–12 h

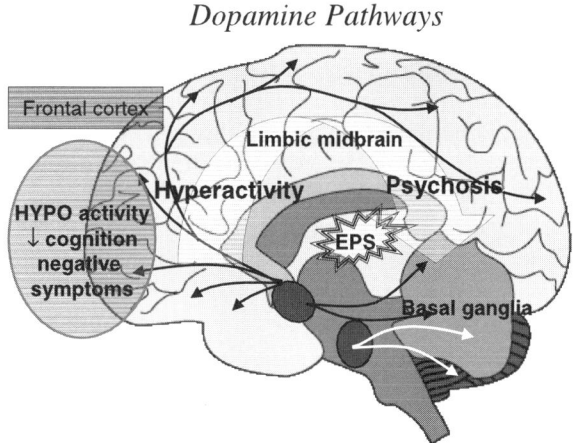

Dopamine Pathways

Figure 3 Dopamine pathways of interest in schizophrenia. The ideal antipsychotic medication for schizophrenia would have three distinct effects in different brain regions of interest. In the basal ganglia, no discernible effect on dopamine neurotransmission is wanted, thereby insuring no EPS. In the limbic midbrain, the classical dopamine hyperactivity (amphetamine) model is still considered applicable to drug mechanism of action, hence the need to block dopamine or counteract its effects. In the frontal cortex and dorsolateral prefrontal cortex, diminished cortical function is thought to result in negative symptoms and reduced cognitive capacity. Increasing cortical function by a variety of mechanisms, including increased dopamine release via $5HT_{2a}$ blockade, D_2 partial agonism and/or $5HT_{1a}$ agonist effects appears to result in improvement in these non-psychotic manifestations of schizophrenia.

postdose, and is associated with very low risk of extrapyramidal side effects and transient, nonsustained hyperprolactinemia. Recent research has refined our awareness of the dopamine D2 receptor system. Work by Kapur and colleagues with 22 patients randomly assigned 2-week low-dose treatment with haloperidol (either 1 or 2.5 mg/d) offers elegant documentation for the threshold of D2 receptor occupancy by antipsychotic: a 65% D2 occupancy is associated with initial efficacy, while prolactin increases already occur at 72% D2 occupancy, and extrapyramidal side effects are observed if D2 occupancy exceeds 75% [41,42].

Atypical antipsychotics continue by a variety of mechanisms to modulate limbic midbrain regions while reducing their deleterious effects on striatal function. Increased cortical function and activity appears to be hallmark of the newer antipsychotics and is probably a result of *non-D2* properties of these medications. Prolactin elevation can occur with those newer agents, e.g., risperidone, which potently block D2 receptors in a sustained, "tight" fashion. At high doses of risperidone, e.g., > 6 mg/day, the magnitude and duration of D2 binding begin to mitigate the benefits of the drug's atypical profile derived principally from serotonin receptor blockade mediated release of dopamine (see the serotonin section). Current treatment guidelines recommend doses of risperidone of ≤ 6 mg/day as optimal [35,36].

The "more complete" atypicality observed with quetiapine and clozapine (freedom from EPS at any dosage used) may be in part be explained by low-affinity occupation ("loose" binding with rapid dissociation) of the D2 receptor [41,43]. Their observations indicate that low-affinity antipsychotics have transient periods of occupancy of D2 receptors paralleling the drug's pharmacokinetics (e.g., blood levels). At maximum concentrations postdose of quetiapine, for instance, higher than previously observed binding of ≥ 70% occurs perhaps accounting for "loose" bound drug's antipsychotic effect. This less sustained D2 occupancy is insufficient to disrupt striatal transmission and precipitate extrapyramidal symptoms. Both clozapine and quetiapine demonstrate D2 receptor occupancy rates in the 60–70% range 2 h postdose, falling to 20–55% at 12–24 h postdose. Prolactin elevations are transient with those drugs, paralleling the time course of significant D2 occupancy, e.g., clozapine and quetiapine. The loose binding associated with quietapine, when coupled with its relatively short half-life, results in rapid receptor dissociation from the D2 receptor, explaining why twice-daily dosing is recommended for acute/initial efficacy, and also explains the need for much higher doses than originally used in the management of acutely psychotic patients, e.g. > 800 mg day.

Olanzapine has attenuated D2 blocking side effects in part due to its intermediate binding for the D2 receptor and due to pharmacological complexity that is most similar to clozapine. Normalization of hyperprolactinemia and related hormonal changes has been reported when patients are switched from neuroleptics or risperidone to olanzapine, clozapine, ziprasidone, or quetiapine [11,44,45]. Seeman and colleagues have suggested that the concept of loose versus tight binding can be used to predict clinical characteristics of antipsychotic medications (Table 3). Ziprasidone is considered intermediate in its binding tightness, as well, based on pilot PET data, with peak occupancies approaching 80% following a 60-mg dose (usually administered BID) and 12-h trough binding < 60%. This rapid fall in occupancy is in part due to ziprasidone's shorter half-life (4–11 h) as well [46].

A novel approach to antipsychotic therapy is the development of D2 partial agonist/antagonist compounds. These partial agonists provide dopaminergic effects in systems where endogenous activity for dopamine is low, and antagonist effects in those areas where dopamine is hyperactive. If the balance point between effects is properly selected, it should be possible to obtain increased dopaminergic function in cortical structures, reduced activity in limbic midbrain regions, and no discernible effects in the striatum. If dopaminergic agonist effects are in excess, then restlessness, insomnia, psychosis, and cardiovascular effects—e.g., hypotension and tachycardia—are observed, while overly potent blockade can lead to hyperprolactinemia, EPS, and tardive dyskinesia risk [47,48]. Of the many dopamine partial agonist medications studied over the past 10 years, aripiprazole (NDA filed with the FDA, Bristol Myer Squibb/Otsuka Pharmaceuticals) seems to best approximate this needed balance [49–51]. [See Table 1 for a summary of receptor pharmacology (51–55).] In addition to partial agonist properties, aripiprazole shares effects on serotonin receptor subtypes, similar to ziprasidone. Aripiprazole is nonsedating and has shown efficacy comparable to risperidone 6 mg/day in short-term, 4-week efficacy trials [50–52]. In contrast to risperidone, prolactin is either lowered or unchanged. Aripiprazole's EPS rate except for akathisia is at a placebo-like level at effective doses.

Looking toward future applications, a specific genetic polymorphism at D2 receptors leads to a significantly lower response rate to neuroleptic therapies. Work by Suzuki et al. [56] suggests that D2 receptor polymorphism (Taq1 A1 vs. A2) may modify D2 occupancy and account for early response rates in a subpopulation with one or two A1 alleles. Although the syndrome of schizophrenia may ultimately be refined into distinct disease states characterized by biological

Table 3 Loose Versus Tight D2 Receptor Binding: Predicted Clinical Implications[a]

	Tight binding (high affinity, long duration)	Intermediate binding	Loose binding (low affinity, short duration
Representative drugs	Haloperidol, risperidone, fluphenazine, chlorpromazine	Ziprasidone, olanzapine, loxapine, (sertindole removed from worldwide markets)	Clozapine, quetiapine (remoxipride removed from worldwide markets)
Dissociation rate from D2	Slow	Intermediate	Fast
EPS and TD risk	High	Moderate to low, dose dependent	Low, dose independent
Hyperprolactinemia	High and sustained	Moderate to low, dose dependent, possibly transient	Low, transient
Rapidity of receptor washout	Weeks to months	Days to weeks	Days
Rapid relapse upon cessation of long term therapy	Low	Low	High
Need for initial divided dosing	Low	Low; except ziprasidone, which has a short half-life	Moderate

[a]Predictions do not take account other relevant pharmacological effects, e.g., $5HT_{2a}$, which modify risk or efficacy parameters.
Source: Ref.

markers that are predictive of disease presentation, genetic evaluations have been inconclusive. In contrast, genetic polymorphisms which appear to predict response and adverse effects from antipsychotic therapy are demonstrating greater initial promise. Such biological markers could inform drug development and drug selection, potentially identifying subpopulations in which a drug's benefits are maximized. Another illustration is the association between the risk of TD from antipsychotics and a specific homozygous D3 receptor polymorphism Ser9Gly. Twenty-two percent to 24% of patients with TD vs. 4–6% in patients without TD have this homozygous polymorphism [57]. Interestingly, newer antipsychotic agents have widely varying D2, D3, and D4 receptor affinities, which deserves further study and might form a basis for selecting a drug with differing side effects potential in subpopulations of patients [58,59]. Lastly, CYP2D6 polymorphisms play a role in risk for TD with phenothiazines and haloperidol.

IV. SEROTONIN

The success of clozapine for treatment-resistant patients also led investigators to seek plausible pharmacologic mechanisms for its atypicality. According to Meltzer and colleagues [60], the central pharmacologic profile for atypicality is a high serotonin $5HT_{2a}/D2$ occupancy ratio resulting in a functional antagonism of D2 blockade-mediated adverse effects in the striatum, as well as beneficial therapeutic effects in mesocortical circuits [60,61]. Refinement of Meltzer's theory has been proposed by Kapur and Remmington [62]: $5HT_2$ occupancy and D2 occupancy as measured by PET are potentially independent (but interacting) dimensions of antipsychotic effect. This model partitions new-generation antipsychotics into three categories (Table 4).

The dopamine neuron's release from serotonergic inhibition by blockade of postsynaptic 5HT2a heteroreceptors leads to increased DA transmission in the striatum (less EPS) and in the cortex (treatment of negative symptoms and improvement in cognitive function) [63]. The density of $5HT_{2a}$ receptors in limbic midbrain is quite low, providing a rationale for the effectiveness of the second-generation drugs to treat, rather than worsen psychosis, while reducing EPS and negative symptoms. Alternatively, inhibition of serotonin firing with reduced serotonin 2 heteroreceptor activation can also increase dopamine transmission in these regions of interest [64]. Changes in serotonin firing rate can be achieved by activating pre- and postsynaptic 5 HT_{1a} receptors. Antipsychotics that act as partial agonists at $5HT_{1a}$ include aripiprazole = ziprasidone > clozapine ≥ quetiapine, and lead to increased dopaminergic release in cortical regions. Additionally, this serotonergic agonist effect when coupled with 5HT2a blockade mimics the antidepressant and anxiolytic actions of many commonly used psychotropics—e.g., SSRIs, nefazodone, and buspirone. The $5HT_{1a}$ partial agonist buspirone is an effective anxiolytic, has been useful in managing aggression, and has been reported to have beneficial effects on symptoms of schizophrenia when used as an adjunct in patients treated with conventional antipsychotics [65].

Several of the newer antipsychotics have nonselective affinity for both $5HT_{2a}$ and $5HT_{2c}$ (clozapine, olanzapine) while others are more selective for $5HT_{2a}$ (risperidone and quetiapine). While there does not appear to be a relationship between 5HT2c affinity and antipsychotic efficacy, there is a possible correlation between activity at this receptor and weight gain [64,65]. The propensity for antipsychotic medications to cause weight gain and possible adverse consequences on glucose and lipid regulation is in part tied to $5HT_{2c}$ and other aspects of serotonin neuromodulation, as well as to H_1 antihistaminic effects and changes in insulin receptor sensitivity and leptin levels. Switching medications in response to significant weight gain should be clinically indicated by a benefit vs. risk assessment. A recent meta-analyses for weight gain

Table 4 Classification of Antipsychotic Drugs by their $5HT_{2a}$ and D2 Receptor Occupancy Characteristics

Combined serotonin $5HT_2$/dopamine D2 threshold model	PET occupancy: high $5HT_2$ (> 80%), high D2 (> 70%)	PET occupancy: high $5HT_2$ (> 80%), intermediate D2 (< 80%)	PET occupancy: high $5HT_2$ (> 80%), low D2 (< 70%)	PET occupancy: low $5HT_2$ (< 80%), low D2 (< 60%)
Antipsychotics	Risperidone Sertindole	Olanzapine Ziprasidone[a]	Clozapine	Quetiapine

[a]Other effects such as serotonin transporter inhibition and $5HT_{1a}$ blockade further modify this drug's profile
Source: Ref. 62.

potential for various antipsychotic medications ranked commonly used medications as follows: clozapine ≥ olanzapine > risperidone > haloperdol ≥ aripiprazole ≥ ziprasidone [66]. A robust patient treatment response should not be sacrificed for potential concerns about weight gain. Overall quality of life may be best served by maintaining the most effective medication. Nondrug interventions to manage weight in responding schizophrenic patients should be considered—e.g., exercise and diet. In patients who have gained significant weight, ongoing monitoring of lipids and fasting glucose are also necessary to forestall the development of dyslipidemia and diabetes mellitus.

Genetic cloning of serotonin receptors has identified additional potential serotonergic targets of antipsychotic drug action. $5HT_6$ receptors pharmacologically resemble $5HT_2$ receptors and $5HT_6$ receptor mRNA is expressed extensively in the striatum. Clozapine and olanzapine have high affinity for the $5HT_6$ receptor which may also contribute to both efficacy and to improved cortical function via excitatory amino acid systems (see below). $5HT_7$ receptor modulation is thought to affect circadian rhythms and may be especially beneficial for patients with insomnia. Ziprasidone and risperidone each have high affinity for the $5HT_7$ receptor with intermediate and no affinity, respectively, for the $5HT_6$ receptor. Clozapine and olanzapine have moderate affinity for $5HT_7$. Activity at one or both of these receptors may account for differential effects seen with some atypical antipsychotics, and could be considered as part of a "multi-dimensional" comparison when deciding upon switching antipsychotic drugs [67].

V. GLUTAMATE EXCITATORY AMINO ACID SYSTEM

N-methyl D-aspartate (NMDA) glutamatergic antagonists such as phencyclidine (PCP) and ketamine can induce a psychosis and altered behavioral/cognitive state that mimics schizophrenia including hallucinations and disturbances of reality testing, autistic preoccupation, memory disturbances, negative symptoms, and reductions in prepulse inhibition (cognitive function) [68–72]. This NMDA hypofunctioning state, characterized by hypofrontality with midbrain overactivity, has been proposed as a model of schizophrenia. This model hypothesizes that hypofunction of the glutamate receptors may be genetically or environmentally mediated early in life, and expressed with maturational changes in the adolescent brain. Hypofunction of the NMDA receptors causes compensatory excessive release of the excitatory neurotransmitters acetylcholine and glutamate in the cerebral cortex. Overstimulation of postsynaptic receptors then causes disturbances of thought and behavior and may also cause excitotoxic damage if exposure is prolonged [73]. This model has been of great heuristic value as it provides a testable hypotheses across a spectrum of investigational technologies. Most of the newer antipsychotic agents by modulating serotonin $5HT_{2a}$ and/or $5HT_6$ receptors appear to normalize and improve glutamate function in a variety of animal and human models for schizophrenia and cognitive function. This is demonstrated in studies using the glutamate antagonist ketamine, and supports a model where glutamatergic receptor hypofunction translates to hypofrontality, cognition deficits, and negative symptoms. Investigations using glycine, an allosteric modulator of the NMDA receptor or d-cycloserine, a full agonist at the glycine site, as augmenting agents for antipsychotics have demonstrated beneficial effects for negative symptoms and cognition, but they do not improve positive symptoms [74–76].

Moreover, clozapine's effects are not augmented by the addition of glycine. This indirect evidence has been interpreted as support for a direct clozapine-mediated effect on NMDA that is not a feature of conventional antipsychotic treatment. Atypical antipsychotics, especially olanzapine, clozapine, and quetiapine, have clearly demonstrated the ability in a dose-related fashion to antagonize the deleterious effects of ketamine administration in either or both animals and patients with schizophrenia, while risperidone does not uniformly cause this effect (low doses protect, high doses do not) [76–78]. Whether clinically meaningful differences in glutamate activity exist among atypical antipsychotics is unclear, but could form the basis for selecting a particular agent when cortical hypofunction, e.g., negative symptoms and cognition deficits dominate the clinical picture.

There does appear to be a significant difference among neuroleptics as a class in comparison to atypical therapies, further reinforcing the preference for the second generation medications [79]. Additional treatment implications arise from the glutamatergic hypothesis including:

1. Genetic linkages to schizophrenia are more likely to be discovered in the genes modulating neuroprotection and neurotoxic processes [80–82].

2. Drug development is being guided in a new and novel direction away from "classical" D2 and $5HT_{2a}$ antagonists [81].

3. Augmentation strategies for partially responding schizophrenics include medications which modulate glutamatergic systems (serine, glycine; see above) as well as anticonvulsants with activity in the excitatory aminoacid systems, e.g., lamotrigine [83].

A. Adrenergic

Side effects mediated by α_1-adrenoceptor antagonism include reductions in blood pressure, with associated orthostatic hypotension and acute sedation. Tachyphylaxis to these effects occurs, so tolerance to orthostasis occurs within a few days, resulting in little need to switch from one therapy to another (except in debilitated or fragile elderly patients). Switching from one α_1 blocking agent to another, in the stable and tolerant patient, is usually uneventful, provided the dose of the current therapy is reduced sufficiently to offset the effects of the new therapy. If an α_1-blocking medication is stopped for more than a week, it is necessary to reinstitute dosage back at the recommended starting dose, since tachyphylaxis abates rapidly following discontinuation of drug [2,8,10,11]. Clozapine, for instance, should be started at 12.5 mg QD or BID, even though maintenance doses as high as 900 mg/day are safely utilized [35].

The α_2-adrenoceptor has been the subject of recent interest as a possible mediator of antipsychotic effect with specific interest focused on the role α_{2C} antagonism plays in augmentation of dopamine output in the cortex [84]. One investigator has demonstrated that administration of an α_2 antagonist (idazoxan) to rats treated with a strong dopamine D_2 antagonists (raclopride) led to increased dopamine release in the prefrontal cortex compared to raclopride alone [85]. In a behavioral model of antipsychotic efficacy, α_2 antagonism resulted in significantly lower doses of raclopride for response than with raclopride alone. The ratio of $\alpha_{2C}/D2$ receptor affinities has been suggested as an important new consideration in identifying drugs with potential atypical properties. Iloperidone (Phase III, Zomaril, Novartis Pharmaceuticals), clozapine, and quetiapine appear to have the greatest selectivity in in vitro receptor antagonist studies [86]. Iloperidone has a prominent effect on dopaminergic neurotransmission via α_{2C}, complementing its favorable impact on negative symptoms and cognition deficits in patients with schizophrenia. Interestingly, it may also stabilize dopamine reward circuits involved in drug "craving," potentially providing clinicians with a new strategy for reducing substance dependence in patients with schizophrenia [87]. Future research is required to clarify the role of the α_2-adrenoceptor subtypes in treating schizophrenia and psychosis (Tables 1, 2).

B. Muscarinic

There is an inverse relationship between affinity for the muscarinic receptors and potential for causing extrapyramidal symptoms. Blockade of muscarinic type 1 (M1) receptors is associated with decreased extrapyramidal side effects with antipsychotic drugs [14]. Blockade of M1 is also associated with anticholinergic side effects typified by classical atropinelike symptoms. More significantly, for patients with schizophrenia, antimuscarinic effects can result in memory disturbances and other cognitive adverse effects (Tables 1, 2). Predicting antipsychotic medications' M1 blockade-induced clinical effects solely by in vitro receptor binding affinity is misleading, since muscarinic effects are modulated by serotonergic and other cholinergic receptors potentially affected by medications. Hence the in vitro M1 potency of olanzapine does not accurately predict clinical side effects. In vivo in patients with schizophrenia it may more potently bind to the M2 receptor, explaining its low anticholinergic side-effects profile [88]. Muscarinic rebound can occur when an antipsychotic agent with M1 antagonist effects is either abruptly discontinued or tapered too quickly. These symptoms include GI cramping, diarrhea, insomnia, nightmares, and nervousness. This is more likely to occur when the antipsychotic being switched to has little or no M1 blocking effects, e.g., risperidone, ziprasidone, or quetiapine. A slower taper of the first agent is warranted.

VI. NEUROPEPTIDES: NEUROTENSIN AND SUBSTANCE P

Neuropeptide systems including neurotensin, enkephalins, and substance P have been implicated in the clinical manifestations of schizophrenia [89–92]. The relevance of these neurotransmitters to the clinical setting and specifically to antipsychotic switching has not been clarified, but future research may identify differential effects for available drugs mediated through one or more of these systems. Neurotensin agonist effects in particular are observed with antipsychotic agents, and appear to be differentially affected by atypical vs. typical antipsychotics. Neurotensin is colocalized on dopaminergic neurons and haloperidol, but not clozapine or olanzapine increase neurotensin concentrations in the striatum, yet both drugs affect nucleus accumbens neurotensin levels [14]. Neurotensin modulators with agonist activity and NK-3 antagonists are in clinical development for schizophrenia, and pivotal trials have demonstrated efficacy and safety. Basic science and behavioral models strongly support neurotensin neurotransmission as a viable target for antipsychotic drug effect [93–96]. Substance P antagonists have been tried in schizophrenia without success [97], but appear to reduce stress reactions under a variety of conditions.

VII. BIOGENIC AMINE TRANSPORTER

The antipsychotic ziprasidone inhibits in vitro both the serotonin and norepinephrine transporter. Ziprasidone's pharmacological similarity to antidepressants may be one of the mechanisms, explaining its beneficial effects on depressive symptoms in double-blind, placebo-controlled studies in schizophrenic patients [98]. Clozapine, olanzapine, and loxapine have moderately potent adrenergic transporter inhibitor effects, potentially contributing to their efficacy for depressive symptoms in patients. Most atypical antipsychotics have demonstrated beneficial effects on mood, but potential significant differences in these effects between various atypical antipsychotics have not been tested in head-to-head clinical trials [99] (Tables 1, 2). However, both clozapine and olanzapine have been demonstrated to reduce the rate of suicide attempts when compared to standard neuroleptic therapy and to risperidone, respectively [100–102].

Comparing and contrasting the pharmacological properties of first- and second-generation agents, and similarly differentiating between atypical therapies, can assist in determining best treatment for the patient. Considerations include potential differences in target symptom responses, risks for adverse effects, and rebound withdrawal reactions upon abrupt discontinuation. Table 2 lists possible clinical consequences of these medications' neurochemistry. These differences can be exploited in both partially responding patients, as well as guide the clinician in selecting a medication likely to reduce adverse effects. These pharmacological differences are consistent with recent treatment guidelines and algorithms on antipsychotic selection [25,26,34,35].

A pharmacologically based evaluation of the atypical agents can facilitate the selection of best therapy for patients with schizophrenia. To illustrate, for negative symptoms, switching from a neuroleptic to an atypical agent, or downward titration of typical antipsychotics toward the lowest possible dose should be considered. In the case of poor or inadequate negative symptom response:

1. Consider if these are primary versus secondary (i.e., adverse drug effect) negative symptoms.
2. Choose a drug that minimizes the impact of EPS (e.g., loose to intermediate D2 binding antagonists, or lower doses of risperidone) which can result in apathy and reduced volition.
3. Select an agent that ameliorates depressive symptoms (i.e., ziprasidone, olanzapine, clozapine) if present.
4. Improve cortical and prefrontal function by selecting a medication which increases dopamine and demonstrates glutamate effects. As discussed above, cortical activation can be accomplished by selecting atypical antipsychotics with $5HT_2$ activity, α_{2c} antagonism (risperidone, clozapine, quetiapine), $5HT_{1a}$ agonist effects (ziprasidone quetiapine), and/or D2 partial agonist effects (aripiprazole).
5. Add an adjunctive drug, with differing pharmacological actions from the antipsychotic being used, that may yield an improvement in negative symptoms [25,26,34,35,99].

These differences between medications provide clinicians and patients with more choices, and increase the chance of finding the right drug for the patient with schizophrenia. Hence, if one drug does not provide the desired benefit for a patient, then switching to another atypical medication is appropriate, and has a good chance of working!

VIII. DOSAGE GUIDANCE

The determination of minimum dosage for drugs with potent D2 receptor antagonist properties is of great interest, though few placebo-controlled trials with fixed-dose paradigms utilize neuroleptic threshold dosing. One recent study incorporated three fixed-dose treatment arms for haloperidol (4, 8, and 16 mg/day) against placebo and sertindole (potent $5HT_{2a}$ antagonist/D2 antagonist withdrawn from testing/marketing in the US due to QTc prolongation and cases of "sudden death"). These doses of haloperidol demonstrated excellent clinical efficacy based on the mean change from baseline on the PANSS. The modest improvements observed in negative symptoms using the SANS, rather than worsening, underscore the need for lower than previously appreciated doses of neuroleptic. However, even at these lower doses, e.g., 4 mg/day of haloperidol, significant extrapyramidal symptoms were present when compared with sertindole [103]. Recently, sertindole has been re-introduced into the european marketplace. Loxapine's intermediate potency for D2 blockade is associated with lower rates of EPS than haloperidol, when utilized in dose ratios of ≤ 10 mg loxapine equivalent to 2 mg haloperidol [104–106]. Moreover, it's possible beneficial effects on negative symptoms via $5HT_{2a}$ blockade deserve further clinical exploration.

The importance of dosage for drugs with 5HT2A/D2 ratios in an intermediate range, e.g., ~ 10–15 as listed in Table 1, is illustrated by two recent comparative trials with risperidone and olanzapine. Risperidone at an average dose of just over 8 mg/day has been demonstrated to have significantly greater EPS (and other adverse effects) when compared in a double-blind trial with olanzapine at an average dose of 18 mg/day [100]. Efficacy as demonstrated by mean change from baseline on the PANSS suggested some advantages for the olanzapine treatment group. In contrast, a different study's results evaluating risperidone at an average dose of 4.8 mg/day demonstrated no statistically significant differences in EPS or response when compared to olanzapine [107]. The nature of clinical trials, including use of placebo controls, and analyses using intent-to-treat with last observation carried forward, leads to a highly conservative approach to ensure rejection of false positive treatment results. However, this leads to distortions in best dosage and in a clear picture of effectiveness in the real world. Table 5 lists recommended dosage ranges from product labeling, and also lists revised dosage ranges based on after-market experience and studies [25,26,34,35,99].

IX. PHARMACOKINETIC AND DRUG INTERACTION CONSIDERATIONS

The pharmacokinetics and drug interaction potential for selected antipsychotics are summarized in Table 6 [108]. In general, half-life is not by itself an important consideration, since plasma concentrations do not always mirror receptor binding, e.g., loose vs. tight binding at D2. However, medications with a short half-life and/or looser D2 binding, e.g., quetiapine, clozapine, and ziprasidone, can require additional care when titrating upward or downward during a transition from one drug to another. Divided daily dosing is recommended during the transition For patients being withdrawn from high-dose neuroleptic therapy longer cross tapers are needed when switching therapies. It may take several weeks or longer to completely wash out the D2 receptor effects and residual EPS. Substituting a weak/loose D2 receptor atypical agent can result in gradual positive symptom worsening over months of time after depot therapy discontinuation as well as withdrawal dyskinesias [109].

Drug interactions from switching are most likely to occur when either haloperidol or phenothiazines are tapered or started (potent CYP2D6 inhibitors). However, since switching entails the gradual decrease in the first drug as the replacement drug is started, drug interactions pose minimal problems. Monitoring for changes in clinical effects and adverse drug effects are necessary whether drug interactions are present or not. Drug interactions can significantly increase or decrease the levels of a drug already titrated to effect resulting in adverse events or treatment failure. Illustrative drug interaction considerations include:

1. Fluvoxamine (to increase levels) with cigarette smoking (to decrease levels) for drugs which are a CYP1A2 substrates (Table 6).
2. Carbamazepine, rifampin, and phenytoin (to decrease levels); or erythromycin, protease inhibitors, grapefruit juice, macrolide antibiotics (erythromycin), and nefazodone (to increase levels) affect drugs metabolized by CYP3A4. Of particular note is the marked sensitivity of quetiapine to CYP3A4 drug interactions explained by its high first-pass metabolism via gut wall.
3. Paroxetine, fluoxetine, haloperidol, and phenothiazines (to increase levels) of drugs metabolized via CYP2D6 (Table 6) [108,110–118].

Drugs with a single identified major metabolic pathway (depicted as +++ in the table) are more sensitive to drug-drug interactions at that metabolic enzyme than those medications which have more than one pathway. For drugs with a major (+++) non-cytochrome P450 metabolic pathway, drug interactions at CYPs are infrequent; i.e., ziprasidone concentrations are only modestly elevated when combined with ketoconazole, due to the major pathway via aldehyde oxidase [119]. Additionally, drugs that have active metabolites of roughly comparable clinical effect are far less likely to undergo significant drug interactions. Risperidone is converted to 9-OH-risperidone, a $5HT_2$ and D2-blocking drug of roughly equivalent effect to the parent drug. Therefore, even though the ratio of risperidone to 9-OH-risperidone dramatically shifts in the presence of an CYP2D6 inhibitor, the sum of the "active moiety" remains constant.

Table 5 Dosing Recommendations in Adults with Schizophrenia

Drug	Label Starting dose	Label maintenance dose	Modified starting dose	Usual dose	Maximum dose
Aripiprazole (Abilitat)	Investigational dosing 15 mg QAM	15–30 mg		20 mg	30 mg
Clozapine (Clozaril, generics)	12.5 mg first dose	200–900 mg/day in divided doses	None	300–400 mg/day in divided doses	900 mg/day in divided doses
Olanzapine (Zyprexa)	10 mg HS	5–20 mg/day	10–30 mg/day; rapid reverse titration in acute settings from 30 mg downward	15–20 mg/day	40 mg/day
Quetiapine (Seroquel)	25 mg BID/TID	150–800 mg/day in divided doses	Inpatient: 50–100 mg BID; rapid titration in acute setting to 400–600 mg/day	400–800 mg/day	≥ 1000 mg/day
Risperidone	1 mg BID	2–16 mg/day	Evaluate 4 mg/day, prior to titrating to 6 mg/day	2–6 mg/day	8 mg/day
Ziprasidone (Geodon)	20 mg BID	40–160 mg/day in divided doses	40 mg BID; rapid titration in acute setting to 120–160 mg/day	80–160 mg	200 mg/day

Table 6 Antipsychotic Pharmacokinetics: Half-Life and Metabolic Pathways

Drug	Half-life (hours)	CYP 1A2	CYP 2C	CYP 2D6	CYP 3A	Other pathways
Haloperidol	14–30	++	—	+(red HL)	+++	Reductase
Clozapine	18–36	+++	+/— (2C9/10)	+/—	++	2E1, FMO
Risperidone	3–4	—	—	+++	—?	
9-OH risperidone	18–36	—	—	—	—	Conjugation
Quetiapine	2–4	—	—	—	+++	20 metabolites
Olanzapine	24–40	+++	+/— (2C19)	+	+/—	FMO Glucuronidation
Ziprasidone	4–10	+	—	—	++	+++ Aldehyde oxidase
Aripiprazole	72	—	—	+++	+++	
Iloperidone	9–22	—	—	+++	++	Reduction; black-oxidation via 2D6?

+++ Major pathway; ++ significant pathway; + minor pathway; +/— possible pathway; — not a pathway; FMO = flavin-containing mono-oxygenase system; CYP = cytochrome P450 (heme-containing mono-oxygenase).

X. REASONS TO SWITCH PATIENTS [18,25,26,34,35,99]

A decision to switch therapy from one antipsychotic to another should be informed by evaluating the available literature for evidence of differential antipsychotic effectiveness, patient safety, medication tolerability, and patient preference. A thorough patient history is essential to identify both potential response patterns and to assess dosage (sensitivity to adverse effects). However, a data-driven approach to decision making is difficult since research lags behind the needs of our patients, and many new therapies have only limited comparative data. As a result, information to guide clinical decisions must be derived in part from an awareness of the more basic sciences: the neurochemistry and pathophysiology for schizophrenia and other persistent psychotic disorders, and pharmacodynamic and pharmacokinetic characteristics of the medications. Best-practice guidelines should be developed based on an evidence-based literature review and use of an expert consensus panel when treatments "beyond" controlled studies are to be considered. This is the approach used in the development of the Texas Medication Algorithm Project: Figure 4 illustrates the current revision of the Texas Implementation of Medication Algorithm's strategies flow sheet http://www.mhmr.state.tx.us/centraloffice/medicaldirector/timascz1algo.pdf) [35]. Failure to respond to one antipsychotic at an appropriate dose and duration should result in the systematic sequential use of other novel antipsychotic therapies. Neuroleptic therapy should be viewed, unless prior history suggests otherwise, as third- to fourth-line therapy, if it is to be tried at all. An exception is in the nonadherent patient where first-generation depot therapy can be necessary, while we await the introduction of long-acting second-generation therapies [120–122]. Moreover, when more than one antipsychotic is considered a comparable choice, then and only then, should cost enter into the decision making process.

XI. POSITIVE SYMPTOMS AND AGGRESSION [18,25,26,34,35,99]

In selecting a new treatment for positive symptoms, numerous pharmacologic approaches are possible. First, maximize current therapy including evaluation of the patient for akathisia and other forms of EPS. If significant EPS is present, increasing the dosage of the current agent is not recommended. If on a neuroleptic agent where plasma concentration monitoring might have meaning, e.g., haloperidol or fluphenazine, then consider an 8- to 12-h postdose level [120–122]. Additionally, consider if impulsive and aggressive symptoms deserve treatment with mood stabilizers or

Pharmacological Treatment of Schizophrenia

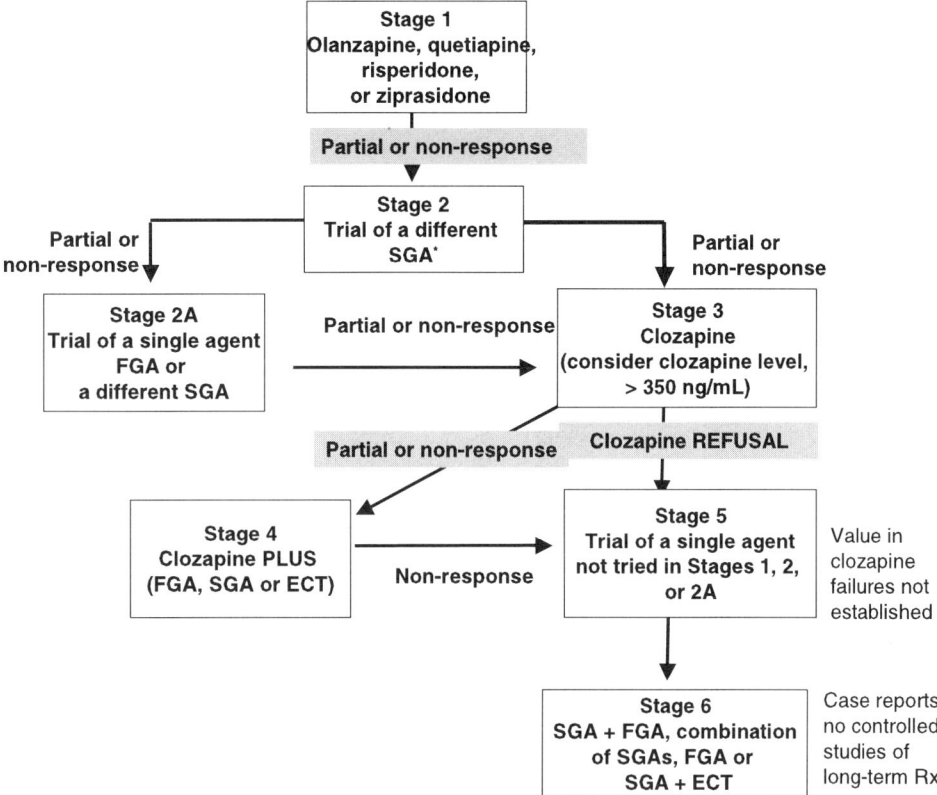

Figure 4 Revised Schizophrenia Texas Medication Algorithm. Revised Texas Medication Algorithm Project, developed by consensus conference for the Texas Implementation of Medication Algorithms. Note that ziprasidone has been added as a first-line second-generation antipsychotic. The role of neuroleptic therapy is relegated to third-line status, while clozapine therapy is recommended following two trials of second-generation antipsychotics of adequate duration and dosage. *Legend*: FGA, first-generation antipsychotic (AP); SGA, second-generation AP.

behavioral therapies. For persistent positive symptoms consider:

1. If currently on neuroleptic therapies, switch to second-generation agents. All of the newer medications demonstrate significant antiaggressive, mood-stabilizing, and antipsychotic effects via D2 and $5HT_{2a}$ blocking effects comparable or superior to neuroleptics.

2. If already on an atypical agent with beneficial effects for symptoms other than the positive ones, then consider increasing the dose of the current therapy (increasing D2 effect), "topping off" with low-dose neuroleptic, or switch to an agent with a more balanced D2/5HT2a effect, e.g., risperidone or loxapine.

3. Choose an agent with activity at $5HT_{1a}$ (clozapine, quetiapine and ziprasidone) potentially useful in diminishing impulsivity and symptoms of anxiety and irritability.

4. Consider the importance of individual drug therapy's unique effects on $5HT_6$, $5HT_7$, neurotensin, substance P, and glycinelike NMDA activity.

5. Use clozapine if at least two other atypical agents have been tried first.

XII. NEGATIVE SYMPTOM [18,25,26,34,35,99]

In general, switching from a typical neuroleptic to an atypical agent, or downward titration of typical antipsychotics toward the lowest possible dose, should be considered. In the case of continuing poor or inadequate response:

1. Consider if these are primary versus secondary (drug ADEs) negative symptoms. Choose a drug that minimizes the impact of EPS (e.g., low/intermediate-

affinity D2 antagonists) and/or ameliorates depressive symptoms (ziprasidone, olanzapine, clozapine).

2. Improve cortical and prefrontal function by increasing dopamine and/or glutamate effects. This can be accomplished by selecting atypical antipsychotics with $5HT_{2a}$ and/or $5HT_6$ activity (increased prefrontal dopamine), α_{2c} antagonism (risperidone, clozapine, quetiapine) and/or $5HT_{1a}$ agonist effects (ziprasidone, quetiapine).

3. Add an adjunctive drug or therapy, with differing pharmacological actions than the antipsychotic being used, that may yield an improvement in negative symptoms (e.g., cycloserine, glycine, SSRIs, bupropion, low-dose psychostimulants, or psychosocial treatment).

XIII. COGNITIVE SYMPTOMS/ DISORGANIZED BEHAVIOR [18,25,26,34,35,63,99]

Atypical antipsychotics are preferred in comparison to conventional agents. In long-term studies of > 3 months and up to 12 months' duration, atypical antipsychotic agents appear to improve cognition and functional attainment of patients, whereas typical neuroleptics demonstrate little to no benefit. Based on empirical data from investigations of cognitive performance in the laboratory in both humans and animals, improvement is probably related to increased dopamine release and/or increased neuronal activity in prefrontal cortex and other mesocortical structures. Choose agents with minimal anticholinergic activity (order of M1 potency: clozapine ≥ low-potency conventionals > olanzapine ≥ quetiapine = risperidone = ziprasidone. Additionally, avoid adjunctive anticholinergics for EPS and benzodiazepines for akathisia, which can worsen cognitive performance. Switch patients to agents with lower EPS potential if abnormal motor function persists. It is also important to note that reducing neuroleptic dosage also appears to improve congnitive test performance.

In many patients an effective therapy, which begins to reduce negative symptoms and improves cognition, can be accompanied with an accompanying worsening in psychic tension, depressive symptoms, insomnia, and even hallucinations. The "awakening" phenomenon, which can sometimes be dramatic in a patient now receiving the "right" therapy, can lead to intense dysphoria as the patient realizes how terrible their life has been, and acknowledges their losses (personal and occupational). Adjunctive psychosocial interventions are a critical part of the successful therapy of patients with schizophrenia [7,123].

XIV. AFFECTIVE SYMPTOMS [18,25,26,34,35,99]

Manic, depressive, or mixed-mood states can be treated either using monotherapy second generation drugs or in combination with mood-stabilizing or antidepressant therapies. Atypical antipsychotic drugs are strongly preferred over typical antipsychotic agents in these patients. Some considerations include:

1. Depressive symptoms are more commonly observed in patients receiving neuroleptics (especially at excessive dose) than with atypical agents. If depressive symptoms are present on risperidone or neuroleptics, consider lowering the dosage prior to switching, since D2 blockade can lead to inadvertent secondary symptoms.

2. Olanzapine and clozapine in monotherapy, and risperidone, quetiapine, and ziprasidone as adjunctive therapies, have all demonstrated utility in acutely manic patients with bipolar affective disorder.

3. Combined $5HT_{2a}$ blockade along with $5HT_{1a}$ agonist effects should result in potent anxiolytic and antidepressant effects.

4. Olanzapine and clozapine have data demonstrating reduced rates of suicide attempts, further illustrating potential benefits on mood.

5. Ziprasidone's significant effects as a dual-mechanism, noradrenergic and serotonergic transporter-importer imparts antidepressant effects at higher doses, e.g., 120–160 mg/day. If manic excitement occurs dosage reduction (20–40 mg/day) is usually sufficient to manage these symptoms.

A. Cardiovascular Safety and Tolerability

The cardiovascular safety of antipsychotics, especially the concerns about cardiac conduction disturbances, leading to torsades de pointes arrhythmias, ventricular fibrillation, and to sudden death, is not new. The rare occurrence of sudden death in patients on sertindole was a reminder of an issue initially raised for low-potency phenothiazine agents such as thioridazine in the 1970s [124–132]. Most antipsychotic therapies appear, at least in vitro, to demonstrate some capacity to block IKr (potassium rectifier fast channel) in the myocardium, potentially causing prolongation of QTc. In June of 1998, the FDA issued to Pfizer Pharmaceuticals a nonapprovable letter for ziprasi-

Pharmacological Treatment of Schizophrenia

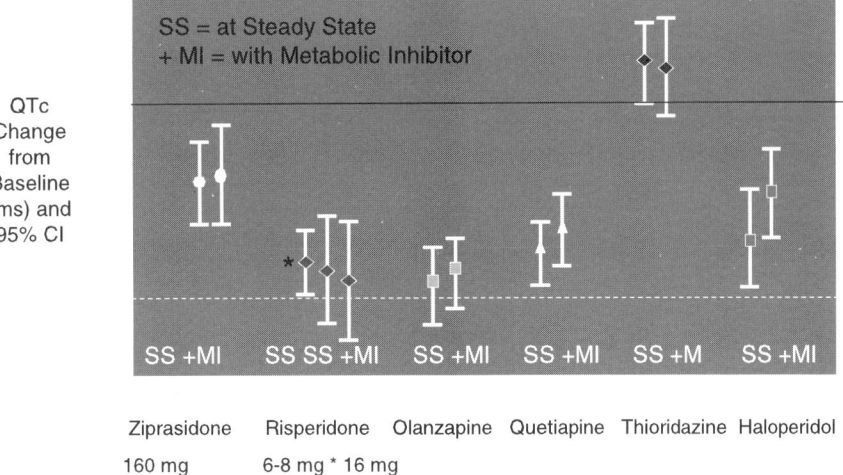

Figure 5 Change in QTc from baseline for various antipsychotic medications. This dose-controlled study utilized normal maximum daily doses of each antipsychotic listed administered to achieve steady state (SS). EKGs were obtained at peak plasma concentration, and the graphic displays the mean change from baseline for QTc along with the 95% confidence intervals (CI). If the CI passes through 0, there is no statistically significant change in QTc. The QTc was calculated, correcting for heart rate, by use of the baseline method = $QT/RR^{0.40}$. Note that the lower CI for thioridazine passes above the upper CI for ziprasidone 160 mg/day. Metabolic inhibitors (MI) were added to each drug at full dosage, and administered until steady state was reachieved. The confidence intervals associated with these observations for each antipsychotic medication's change in QTc represent a worst-case scenario.

done based on "the judgment that ziprasidone prolongs the QTc and that this represents a risk of potentially fatal ventricular arrhythmias that is not outweighed by a demonstrated and sufficient advantage of ziprasidone over already marketed antipsychotics." Haloperidol and droperidol (black box warning recently added to label) also prolong QTc in a concentration-dependent fashion [129,130]. To address these concerns Pfizer conducted an open-label parallel randomized study (#054), as a head-to-head safety evaluation (to maximal doses) against haloperidol (15 mg/day), thioridazine (300 mg/day), olanzapine (20 mg/day), risperidone (16 mg/day), and quetiapine (750 mg/day).

These data were presented at the FDA Psychopharmacological Drugs Advisory Committee Meeting on July 19, 2000 [133] Figure 5 summarizes the data from this seminal evaluation. EKGs were obtained at the time of the presumptive postdose maximum concentration. A metabolic inhibitor phase of the study was employed to ensure the maximal concentrations likely to be observed in real-world practice were evaluated: Ketoconazole (CYP3A4) was added to the quetiapine and ziprasidone treatment arms; paroxetine (CYP2D6) to thioridazine and risperidone treatment arms; and fluvoxamine (CYP 1A2) to olanzapine therapy. Compared to baseline, ziprasidone demonstrated an average 10- to 20-msec prolongation in QTc, depending on the heart rate correction equation utilized. Moreover, although QTc changes with risperidone and olanzapine were basically unchanged from baseline, haloperidol and quetiapine demonstrated significant increases in QTc, though the magnitude of the change was considered not clinically significant.

Thioridazine demonstrated a 30-msec increase in QTc from baseline, prompting a black box warning in labeling, and new contraindications regarding concomitant medications. The label for thioridazine further warns that CYP2D6 inhibitors (e.g., paroxetine and fluoxetine) are contraindicated with this antipsychotic. In the presence of each antipsychotic's specific metabolic inhibitor, the following rank order for mean change from baseline in QTc is reported: Thioridazine (29.6 msec) ≫ Ziprasidone (16.6 msec) ≫ Haloperidol (13 msec) > Quetiapine (8 msec > Olanzapine (3.0 msec) and Risperidone (2.6 msec) [131].

Since marketing, ziprasidone has been used in > 200,000 patients, with 250,000 new prescriptions written through October 2002. No cases of torsades de pointes arrhythmias have been attributed to ziprasidone, and all-cause mortality is no different from that with other second-generation antipsychotic agents. Although use to date cannot preclude a rare but real risk, the magnitude of the risk is now sufficiently low as to justify ziprasidone's use as a front-line agent in the management of schizophrenia [35,134]. In April 2002 (Pfizer Pharmaceuticals, Geodon product labeling), the labeling for ziprasidone was modified to more clearly define potentially dangerous combinations of drugs that might add to the QTc prolongation potential. Significantly, most psychotropics (except thioridazine and mesoridazine) are no longer warned against in combination with ziprasidone.

B. Other Cardiovascular Considerations

1. Weight Gain

Weight gain with atypical antipsychotics is variably observed. As discussed previously, a meta-analysis appears to accurately place the atypicals from least likely weight gain potential, ziprasidone (and also aripiprazole), to olanzapine and clozapine, having the greatest potential [66]. Weight gain itself increases the risk of cardiovascular disease and diabetes mellitus as a primary risk factor. Additionally, weight gain is directly related to changes in lipid regulation leading to hyperlipidemia. The current literature and evaluations of atypical medications in patients cannot determine etiologic sequence of events; rather, there is an interrelationship of these three components of cardiovascular risk [135–138]. In schizophrenia, the prevalence of diabetes is higher, and estimated to be ∼ 9% higher in younger patients receiving atypical antipsychotics than in matched controls [139,140].

Hyperglycemia and an increased rate of diabetes mellitus have been associated with long-term hospitalized patients with psychotic disorders, as well as in patients on traditional neuroleptic agents [141–144]. Despite this apparent disease treatment effect, atypical antipsychotics appear to more frequently, as a class, increase glucose levels and/or insulin concentrations [145–147] and are infrequently associated with diabetic ketoacidosis and hyperosmolar coma [148–152]. Although most cases of diabetes mellitus are associated with weight gain, there have been several incidents of ketoacidosis, hyperosmolar coma, or diabetes mellitus in patients without weight gain. In addition to weight mediated insulin resistance, there is likely to be a more direct effect on insulin responsivity. Whether the insulin resistance causes weight gain, or weight gain precipitates insulin resistance, or both, is unclear. In either case, dyslipidemia is also more frequently associated with atypical antipsychotics, which cause weight gain and insulin resistance [145,153].

2. Glucose Dysregulation

Of the front-line atypical antipsychotics, olanzapine appears to be most frequently implicated in hyperglycemia, increases in plasma insulin concentrations, weight gain, and dyslipidemia. Onset of hyperglycemia occurs typically within 3–6 months [138,150,152–154]. Elevations in glucose and insulin levels normalize after discontinuation of olanzapine, and in part are paralleled by weight loss [151,154,155]. Clozapine is the antipsychotic most associated with causing diabetes. Given the current concerns, it is recommended that baseline laboratory, weight/dietary, and cardiac assessments be made in patients prior to starting any antipsychotic therapies. The EKG can be done one time to rule out rare congenital causes of prolonged QTc in patients aged < 45 years, and repeated only if dizziness or a syncopal episode occurs when on antipsychotic therapy. If weight gain ≥ 7% of body weight occurs, then glucose and lipid monitoring should be instituted every 6 months. A risk-benefit analysis is needed prior to stopping effective treatments in order to reduce the potential adverse consequences associated with diabetes, dyslipidemia, and obesity. If effective treatment is continued, the medical consequences of the medication must be addressed. In the final cost-benefit analysis, the cost of medication, the potential benefits of effective therapy, and the medical monitoring and treatment costs, e.g., lipid-lowering drug therapy, all need to be factored into the ultimate decision [156–158]. In patients at high risk for medical complications from antipsychotic therapies, risperidone or ziprasidone may be preferred over olanzapine. Quetiapine might be an acceptable choice as well, but lags in well-controlled studies evaluating weight gain, lipid effects, and hyperglycemia.

XV. DRUG THERAPY SELECTION VIA GENOTYPING

Selecting therapy by genotyping patients may eventually become commonplace. As previously discussed, the work of Kinon and Lieberman illustrates that D2 receptor polymorphism may predict response to typical neuroleptics [9]. In an evaluation of clozapine and genetic predictors of response, a more complex multifactoral analysis is necessary. Assay of 19 candidate genetic polymorphisms in clozapine responders ($n = 133$) and nonresponders ($n = 67$) was used to identify a combination of genetic features which are predictive of response. These most significant polymorphisms were two $5HT_{2A}$ genotypes: T102/- and His452/His452 associated with good response in 80% of patients while about 50% of nonresponders had this genotype. A more complex model with six allele pairs mapping to four receptor/transmitter systems (5HT$_{2a}$, 5HT$_{2C}$, 5HT transporter and histamine H$_2$ receptors) resulted in 76.7% success in the prediction of clozapine response ($P = .0001$) and a sensitivity of 95% (± 0.04) [159].

XVI. SPECIAL CONSIDERATIONS FOR DEPOT NEUROLEPTICS

The time to steady state for depot medications is based on the rate-limiting absorption half-life rather than the metabolic rate constant. For flupenthixol, fluphenazine, and haloperidol decanoate based on its absorption characteristics, therapy can be administered every 3–4 weeks in the majority of patients [121,160,161]. Taking all depot antipsychotics as a class, if we utilize an average apparent terminal phase half-life of approximately 2–3 weeks, then the time to steady state following repeated injections will be ~ 8–16 weeks. An understanding of the clinical implications resulting from these pharmacokinetic differences between depot and oral therapy is critical for the safe and effective use of these drugs. If depot neuroleptic therapy, i.e., fluphenazine or haloperdol decanoate, is initiated at a clinically effective dosage, e.g. no overlapping therapy is needed, then over the course of repeated injections and several months of time, the concentrations will increase two- to fourfold above these effective levels, resulting in adverse effects and toxicity. Conversely, an initially subtherapeutic dosage of depot antipsychotic, if repeatedly administered over time, will result in concentrations accumulating to steady state, eventually resulting in therapeutic effects. In stable individuals where dosage reductions are desired, 2–3 months should elapse between dosage adjustments to allow sufficient time for Cp to approximate the new steady state. Overly aggressive changes in dosage (either up or down) can result in improper dosage titration. In many chronically ill patients, where a greater delay in pharmacodynamic responsiveness is expected, 4 months or longer may be necessary between dosage changes to optimize the titration of the depot antipsychotic. In chronically medicated, stable patients, dosage intervals as infrequent as 4–6 weeks can be successfully employed for haloperidol decanoate [162].

Tightly bound drugs with long apparent half-lives, e.g., depot neuroleptics such as haloperidol decanoate, can be discontinued abruptly and the replacement medication initiated and titrated upward as the neuroleptic washes out. For haloperidol decanoate, approximately one-half of the drug will wash out in 1 month's time, and a minimum effective dose of the new agent should be administered by the time the next injection would have been administered. It will require up to 4–6 months to completely wash out the depot neuroleptic from systemic circulation. Interestingly, for fluphenazine decanoate, a deep compartment distribution of the drug results in washout times exceeding 6 months, despite a shorter initial terminal half-life than haloperidol decanoate [163].

Atypical antipsychotic therapies in long-acting formulations are finally approaching the marketing stage. Risperidone in a long-acting microspheres formulation (Risperdal Consta, Janssen Pharmaceutica) is closest to marketing [164,165]. Its pharmacokinetics are rate-limited by the slow erosion and disintegration of polylactide-glycolide copolymer microspheres "loaded" with risperidone. The initial dissolution of the microspheres is slow, leading to a latency period of 2–3 weeks until clinically relevant plasma concentrations are detected. Peak concentrations are observed 5–6 weeks after the injection. The dosing interval studied to date is every 2 weeks, and this product, unlike fluphenazine and haloperidol depot preparations, requires the use of overlapping oral risperidone for at least 2 weeks following the first long-acting IM injection. The clinical data and in vitro studies suggest that risperidone concentrations are relatively higher than 9-OH risperidione levels in patients on long-acting therapy. Risperidone penetrates the CNS better and may have slightly greater activity [166]. Olanzapine pamoate, ziprasidone depot, iloperidone microspheres, and 9-hydroxyrisperidone palmitate are other long-acting second-generation antipsychotic therapies now in clinical development.

XVII. CONCLUDING COMMENTS

Disease models for schizophrenia now focus on neurodegenerative changes and functional impairment. New therapies address more directly these deficits by increasing cortical activity via dopaminergic augmentation (by 5HT$_{2a,\ a2c}$, or partial D2 agonism) and indirect effects which enhance glutamate function (antagonism of phencyclidine or ketamine in animal and human evaluations). Treatment to ultimately prevent the prenatal and/or perinatal diathesis by stabilizing excitatory amino acid systems is possible based on animal neurotoxicity and neuroprotection studies.

More immediately, providing the best possible prenatal care for at-risk pregnant women is necessary. Newer therapies for schizophrenia are safe enough to consider as early treatment, e.g., pre-first-break psychosis. Shortening the time of acute psychosis during "first-episode" can also lead to long-term improved prognosis and function, justifying more aggressive identification and treatment of adolescents as they begin to deteriorate into first-break psychosis.

Chronic patients at one point thought to be permanently impaired now have hope for partial to substantial recovery. Improved cognition, self-care, and overall functional capacity occur when second-generation therapies are taken consistently for extended lengths of time. Novel therapies, which more directly prevent stress-mediated neurochemical processes and structural damage, as well as novel treatments designed to increase brain function, are in development, suggesting that the beginning of a new era in the management and treatment of schizophrenia is dawning.

REFERENCES

1. American Psychiatric Association. Diagnostic and Statistical Manual of Mental Disorders. IV-TR, 4th ed. Washington: American Psychiatric Association, 2000.
2. Marken PA, Stanislav SW. Schizophrenia. In: Koada-Kimble MA, Young LY, eds. Applied Therapeutics: The Clinical Use of Drugs, 7th ed. Philadelphia: Lippincott Williams and Wilkins, 2001, Chap 76.
3. Thaker GK, Carpenter WT Jr. Advances in schizophrenia. Nature Med. 2001; 7:667–671.
4. Harris EC, Barraclough B. Excess mortality of mental disorder. Br J Psychiatry 1998; 173:11–53.
5. Newman SC, Bland RC. Mortality in a cohort of patients with schizophrenia: a record linkage study. Can J Psychiatry 1991; 36:239–245.
6. McIntyre RS, McCAnn SM, Kennedy SH. Antipsychotic metabolic effects: weight gain, diabetes mellitus, lipid abnormalities. Can J Psychiatry 2001; 46:273–281.
7. Duckworth K, Nair V, Patel JK. Lost time, found hope and sorrow: the search for self, connection and purpose during "awakenings" on the new antipsychotics. Harv Rev Psychiatry 1997; 5:227–233.
8. Ereshefsky L, Lacombe S. Pharmacological Profile of Risperidone. Can J Psychiatry 1993; 38(suppl 3):S80–S88.
9. Kinon BJ, Lieberman JA. Mechanisms of action of a typical antipsychotic drugs: a critical analysis. Psychopharmacology 1996; 124:2–34.
10. Ereshefsky L, Tran-Johnson T, Watanabe MD. Current concepts in the treatment of schizophrenia: the pathophysiologic basis for atypical antipsychotic efficacy. Clin Pharm 1990; 8:680–707.
11. Ereshefsky L, Watanabe MD, Tran-Johnson T. Clozapine: An atypical antipsychotic. Clin Pharm 1989; 8:691–709.
12. Kane JM. Schizophrenia. N Engl Jr Med. 1996; 334:41–43.
13. Ereshefsky L. Treatment strategies for schizophrenia. Psychiatr Ann 1995; 25(suppl 5):285–296.
14. Arnt J, Skarsfeldt T. Do novel antipsychotics have similar pharmacological characteristics? A review of the evidence. Neuropsychopharmacology 1998; 18:63–101.
15. Roth BL, Craigo SC, Choudhary MS, Uluer A, Monsma FJ Jr, Shen Y, Meltzer HY, Sibley DR. Binding of typical and atypical antipsychotic agents to 5-hydroxytryptamine-6 and 5-hydroxytryptamine-7 receptors. J Pharmacol Exp Ther. 1994; 268:1403–1410.
16. Ellenbroek BA, Lubbers LJ, Cools AR. Activity of "Seroquel" (ICI 204, 636) in animal models for atypical properties of antipsychotics: a comparison with clozapine. Neuropsychopharmacoloy 1996; 15:407–416.
17. Miller AL, Ereshefsky L. Schizophrenia: how should we look at it? J Psychopharmacol 1997:11(suppl 1):21–23.
18. Ereshefsky L, Dugan D. Pharmacokinetic and pharmacodynamic considerations in switching. In: S Marder, ed. Switching Antipsychotic Medication. London: Science Press, 2000, Chap 4.
19. Richelson E. Receptor pharmacology of neuroleptics: relation to clinical effects. J Clin Psychiatry 1999; 60(suppl 10):5–14.
20. Kongasamut S, Roehr JE, Cai J, Hartman HB, Weissensee P, Kerman LL, Tang L, Sandrasagra A. Iloperidone binding to human and rat dopamine and 5HT receptors. Eur J Pharmacol. 1996; 317:417–423.
21. Schotte A, Janssen PF, Gommeren W, Luyten WH, Van Gompel P, Lesage AS, De Loore K, Leysen JE. Risperidone compared with new and reference antipsychotic drugs: in vitro and in vivo receptor binding. Psychopharmacology (Berl) 1996; 124:57–73.
22. Bymaster FP, Calligaro DO, Falcone JF, Marsh RD, Moore NA, Tye NC, Seeman P, Wong DT. Radioreceptor binding profile of the atypical antipsychotic olanzapine. Neuropsychopharmacology 199614:87–96.
23. Simansky KJ, Zorn SH, Schmidt AW, Lebel LA. The unique human receptor binding profile may be related to lack of weight gain with ziprasidone. Presented at the 2000 New Clinical Drug Evaluation Unit, Boca Raton, FL, 2000.

24. Bristol Myers Squibb Inc. Personal communication, 2002.
25. Treatment of schizophrenia 1999. The expert consensus guideline series. J Clin Psychiatry 1999; 60 (suppl 11):3–80.
26. American Psychiatric Association. Practice Guidelines for the Treatment of Patients with Schizophrenia. Am J Psychiatry 1997; 154(suppl 4)1–63.
27. Beasley CM Jr, Tollefson G, Tran P, Satterlee W, Hamilton S. Olanzapine versus placebo and haloperidol: acute phase results of the North American Double-Blind Olanzapine Trial. Neuropsychopharmacology 1996; 14:111–123.
28. Reynolds GP, Czudek C. New approaches to the drug treatment of schizophrenia. Adv Pharmacol. 1995; 32:461–501.
29. Sharma T, Mockler D. The cognitive efficacy of atypical antipsychotics in schizophrenia [review]. J Clin Psychopharmacol 1998; 18(2 suppl 1):12S–19S.
30. Feldman HS. Loxapine succinate as initial treatment of hostile and aggressive schizophrenic criminal offenders. J Clin Pharmacol 1982; 22:366–370.
31. Ward ME, Saklad SR, Ereseh fsky L. Lorazepam in treatment of psychotic agitation. Am J Psychiatry 1986; 143:1195.
32. Ereshefsky L, Richards A. Psychosis. In: Koda-Kimble MA, Young LL, eds. Applied Therapeutics the Clinical Use of Drugs. San Francisco: Applied Therapeutics Press, 1992, Chap 56.
33. Ereshefsky L. pharmacologic and pharmacokinetic considerations in choosing an antipsychotic. J Clin Psychiatry 1999; 60(suppl 10):20–30.
34. Miller AL, Chiles JA, Chiles JK, Crismon ML, Rush AJ, Shon SP. The Texas Medication Algorithm Project (TMAP) schizophrenia algorithms. J Clin Psychiatry 1999; 60(10):649–657.
35. Miller AL, Chiles JA, Chiles, J, Crismon ML. Guidelines for Treating Schizophrenia, Texas Implementation of Medication Algorithms, Physician Procedural Manual. http://www.mhmr.state.tx.us/centraloffice/medicaldirector/timascz-man.pdf, 2002.
36. Cohen SA, Ihrig K, Lott RS, Kerrick JM. Risperidone for aggression and self-injurious behavior in adults with mental retardation. J Autism Dev Disord 1998; 28:229–233.
37. Arvanitis LA, Miller BG. Multiple fixed doses of quetiapine in patients with acute exacerbation of schizophrenia: a comparison with haloperidol and placebo. The Seroquel Trial 13 Study Group. Biol Psychiatry 1997; 42:233–246.
38. Arana GW, Orn A. The use of benzodiazepines for psychotic disorders: a literature review and preliminary clinical findings. Psychopharmacol Bull. 1986; 22:77–87.
39. Tonne U, Hiltunen AJ, Vikander B, Engelbrektsson K, Bergman H, Begman I, Leifman H, Borg S. Neuropsychological changes during steady-state drug use, withdrawal and abstinence in primary benzodiazepine dependent patients. Acta Psychiatr Scand 1995; 91:299–304.
40. Nishiyama K, Sugishita M, Kurisaki H, Sakuta M. Reversible memory disturbances and intelligence impairment induced by long term anticholinergic therapy. Intern Med 1998:37:514–518.
41. Seeman P, Tallerico T. Antipsychotic drugs which elicit little or no parkinsonism bind more loosely than dopamine to brain D2 receptors, yet occupy high levels of these receptors. Mol Psychiatry 1998; 3:123–134.
42. Kapur S, Zipursky R, Jones C, Remmington G, Houle S. Relationship between dopamine D2 occupancy, clinical response, and side-effects: a double-blind PET study of first-episode schizophrenia. Am J Psychiatry 2000; 157:514–520.
43. Kapur S, Zipursky R, Jones C, Shammi CS, Remington G, Seeman P. A positron emission tomography study of quetiapine in schizophrenia: a preliminary finding of an antipsychotic effect with only transiently high dopamine D2 receptor occupancy. Arch Gen Psychiatry 2000; 57:553–559.
44. Kinon BJ, Basson BR, Wang J, Malcolm SK, Stauffer VL. Rapid reduction in hyperprolactinemia with the return of women's menstrual cycles are reported upon switching from conventional antipsychotic drugs or risperidone to other atypical antipsychotics. Abstract at 40th Annual NCDEU Meeting May 30-June 2, 2000, Boca Raton, FL.
45. Seeman P, Tallerico T. Rapid release of antipsychotic drugs from dopamine D2 receptors: an explanation for low receptor occupancy and early clinical relapse upon withdrawal of clozapine or quetiapine. Am J Psychiatry 1999; 156:876–884.
46. Personal communication, Dr. Jeffrey Micelli, Pfizer Research, Groton CT, April 2001.
47. Hall DA, Strange PG. Evidence that antipsychotic drugs are inverse agonists at D2 dopamine receptors. Br J. Pharmacol. 1997; 121:731–736.
48. Tamminga CA. Partial dopamine agonists in the treatment of psychosis. J Neural Transm 2002; 109(suppl 3):411–420.
49. Nakai S, Hirose T, Uwahodo Y, Imaoka T, Okazaki H, Miwa T, Nakai M, Yamada S, Dunn B, Tottori K, Kikuchi T, Altar CA. Catalepsy and striato-limbic dopamine metabolism following chronic aripiprazole, risperidone, and haloperidol. Poster at CINP, Brussels, Belgium, July 2000.
50. Kane J, Ingenito G, Ali M. Efficacy of aripiprazole in psychotic disorders: comparison with haloperidol and placebo. Poster at CINP, Brussels, Belgium, July 2000.

51. NDA filed with the FDA, Bristol Myers Squibb/Otsuka Pharmaceuticals.
52. Kelleher JP, Centorrino F, Albert MJ, Baldessarini RJ. Advances in atypical antipsychotics for the treatment of schizophrenia: new formulations and new agents. CNS Drugs 2002; 16(4):249–261.
53. Lawler CP, Prioleau C, Lewis MM, Mak C, Jiang D, Schetz JA, Gonzalez AM, Sibley DR, Mailman RB. Interactions of the novel antipsychotic aripiprazole (OPC-14597) with dopamine and serotonin receptor subtypes. Neuropsychopharmacology 1999; 20(6):612–627.
54. Stahl SM. Dopamine system stabilizers, aripiprazole, and the next generation of antipsychotics, Part 1. "Goldilocks" actions at dopamine receptors. J Clin Psychiatry 2001; 62(11):841–842.
55. Stahl SM. Dopamine system stabilizers, aripiprazole, and the next generation of antipsychotics, Part 2. Illustrating their mechanism of action. J Clin Psychiatry 2001; 62(suppl 12):923–924.
56. Suzuki A, Mihara K, Kondo T, Tanaka O, Nagashima U, Otani K, Kaneko S. The relationship between dopamine D2 receptor polymorphism at the Taq1 A locus and therapeutic response to nemonapride, a selective dopamine antagonist, in schizophrenic patients. Pharmacogenetics 2000; 10:335–341.
57. Segman R, Neeman T, Heresco-Levy U, Finkel B, Karagichev L, Schlafman M, Dorevitch A, Yakir A, Lerner A, Shelevoy A, Lerer B. Genotypic association between the dopamine D3 receptor and tardive dyskinesia in chronic schizophrenia. Mol Psychiatry 1999; 4:247–253.
58. Lahti RA, Evan DL, Stratman NC, et al. Dopamine D4 vs. D2 receptor selectivity of dopamine receptor antagonists: possible therapeutic implications. Eur J Pharmacol 1993; 236:483–486.
59. Shaikh S, Makoff A, Collier D, et al. Dopamine D4 receptors. Potential therapeutics implications in the treatment of schizophrenia. CNS Drugs 1997; 8:1–11.
60. Meltzer HY, Matsubara S, Lee J-C. Classification of typical and atypical antipsychotic drugs on the basis of dopamine D1, D2 and serotonin 2 pki values. J Pharmacol Exp Ther. 1989; 251:238:246.
61. Stefanski R, Goldberg SR. Serotonin 5HT2 receptor antagonists. Potential in the treatment of psychiatric disorders. CNS Drugs 1997; 7:388–409.
62. Kapur S, Remington G. Serotonin-dopamine interaction and its relevance to schizophrenia. Am J Psychiatry 1996; 153:466–476.
63. Harvey PD, Keefe RSE. Studies of cognitive change in patients with schizophrenia following novel antipsychotic treatment. Am J Psychiatry 2001; 158(suppl 2):176–184.
64. Metzler HY. The role of serotonin in antipsychotic drug action. Neuropsychopharmacology 1999; 21:106S–115S.
65. Simansky KJ, Zorn SH, Schmidt AW. The unique human receptor binding profile may be related to lack of weight gain with ziprasidone. Poster at CINP, Brussels, Belgium, July 2000.
66. Allison DB, Mentore JL, Heo M. Antipsychotic-induced weight gain: a comprehensive research synthesis. Am J Psychiatry 1999; 156:1686–1696.
67. Roth BL, Craigo SC, Choudhary MS, Uluer A, Monsma FJ Jr, Shen Y, Meltzer HY, Sibley DR. Binding of typical and atypical antipsychotic agents to 5-hydroxytryptamine-6 and 5-hydroxytryptamine-7 receptors. J Clin Pharmacol Exp Ther. 1994; 268:1403–1410.
68. Domino EF, Luby ED. Abnormal mental states induced by phencyclidine as a model of schizophrenia. In: Domino EF, ed. PCP (Phencyclidine): Historical and Current Perspectives. Ann Arbor, MI: NPP Books, 1981:400–418.
69. Javitt DC, Zukin SR. Recent advances in the phencyclidine model of schizophrenia. Am J Psychiatry 1991; 148:1301–1308.
70. Krystal JH, Karper LP, Seibyl JP, Freeman GK, Delaney R, Bremner JD, Heninger GR, Bowers MB Jr, Charney DS. Subanesthetic effects of the noncompetitive NMDA antagonist, ketamine, in humans. Psychotomimetic, perceptual, cognitive, and neuroendocrine responses. Arch Gen Psychiatry 1994; 51:199–214.
71. Lahti AC, Holcomb HH, Medoff DR, et al. Ketamine activates psychosis and alters limbic blood flow in schizophrenia. Neuroreport 1995; 6:869–872.
72. Lahti AC, Koffel B, LaPorte D, et al. Subanesthetic doses of ketamine stimulate psychosis in schizophrenia. Neuropsychopharmacology 1995; 13:9–19.
73. Olney JW, Newcomer JW, Farber NB. NMDA receptor hypofunction model of schizophrenia. J Psychiatr Res 1999; 33:523–533.
74. Tsai GE, Yang P, Chung LC, Tsai IC, Tsai CW, Coyle JT. D-serine added to clozapine for the treatment of schizophrenia. Am J Psychiatry 1999; 156:1822–1825.
75. Evins AE, Fitzgerald SM, Wine L, Rosselli R, Goff DC. Placebo-controlled trial of glycine added to clozapine in schizophrenia. Am J Psychiatry 2000; 157:826–828.
76. Tamminga CA. Schizophrenia and glutamatergic transmission. Crit Rev Neurobiol 1998; 12:21–36.
77. Swerdlow NR, Bakshi VP, Geyer MA. Seroquel restores sensorimotor gating in phencyclidine-treated rats. J Pharmacol Exp Ther 1996; 279:1290–1299.
78. Bakshi VP, Geyer MA. Antagonism of phencyclidine-induced deficits in prepulse inhibition by the putative atypical antipsychotic olanzapine. Psychopharmacology 1995; 122:198–201.

79. Goff DC, Hennen J, Lyoo IK, Tsai G, Wald LL, Evins AE, Yurgelun-Todd DA, Renshaw PF. Modulation of brain and serum glutamatergic concentrations following a switch from conventional neuroleptics to olanzapine. Biol Psychiatry 2002; 51(suppl 6):493–497.

80. Begni S, Popoli M, Moraschi S, Bignotti S, Tura GB, Gennarelli M. Association between the ionotropic glutamate receptor kainate 3 (GRIK3) ser310ala polymorphism and schizophrenia. Mol Psychiatry 2002; 7(suppl 4):416–418.

81. Sawa A, Snyder SH. Schizophrenia: diverse approaches to a complex disease. Science 2002; 296(5568):692–695.

82. Schiffer HH. Glutamate receptor genes: susceptibility factors in schizophrenia and depressive disorders? Mol Neurobiol 2002; 25(suppl 2):191–212.

83. Dursun SM, Deakin JF. Augmenting antipsychotic treatment with lamotrigine or topiramate in patients with treatment-resistant schizophrenia: a naturalistic case-series outcome study. J Psychopharmacol 2001; 15(suppl 4):297–301.

84. Richelson E, Souder T. Binding of antipsychotic drugs to human brain receptors focus on newer generation compounds. Life Sci 2000; 68(suppl 1):29–39.

85. Hertel P, Fagerquist MV, Svensson TH. Enhanced cortical dopamine output and antipsychotic-like effects of raclopride by $\alpha 2$ adrenoceptor blockade. *Science* 1999; 286:105–107.

86. Ichikawa J, Meltzer HY. Relationship between dopaminergic and serotonergic neuronal activity in the frontal cortex and the action of typical and atypical antipsychotic drugs. Eur Arch Psychiatry Clin Neurosci 1999; 249(suppl 4):90–98.

87. Jain KK. An assessment of iloperidone for the treatment of schizophrenia. Expert Opin Invest Drugs 2000; 9(suppl 12):2935–2943.

88. Raedler TJ, Knable MB, Jones, DW, Lafargue T, Urbina RA, Egan MF, Pickar D, Weinberger DR. In vivo olanzapine occupancy of muscarinic acetylcholine receptors in patients with schizophrenia. Neuropsychopharmacology 2000; 23(suppl 1):56–68.

89. Tooney PA, Crawter VC, Chahl LA. Increased tachykinin NK(1) receptor immunoreactivity in the prefrontal cortex in schizophrenia. Biol Psychiatry 2001; 49(suppl 6):523–527.

90. Longmore J, Hill RG, Hargreaves RJ. Neurokinin-receptor antagonists: pharmacological tools and therapeutic drugs. Can J Physiol Pharmacol 1997; 75(suppl 6):612–621.

91. Kilts CD. The changing roles and targets for animal models of schizophrenia. Biol Psychiatry 2001; 50(suppl 11):845–855.

92. Rowley M, Bristow LJ, Hutson PH. Current and novel approaches to the drug treatment of schizophrenia. J Med Chem 2001; 44(suppl 4):477–501.

93. Kinkead B, Nemeroff CB. Neurotensin: an endogenous antipsychotic? Curr Opin Pharmacolo 2002; 2(suppl 1):99–103.

94. McMahon BM, Boules M, Warrington L, Richelson E. Neurotensin analogs indications for use as potential antipsychotic compounds. Life Sci 2002; 70(suppl 10):1101–1119.

95. Binder EB, Kinkead B, Owens MJ, Nemeroff CB. Neurotensin and dopamine interactions. Pharmacol Rev 2001; 53(suppl 4):453–486.

96. Binder EB, Kinkead B, Owens MJ, Nemeroff CB. The role of neurotensin in the pathophysiology of schizophrenia and the mechanism of action of antipsychotic drugs. Biol Psychiatry 2001; 50(suppl 11):856–872.

97. Ereshefsky L. Personal communication, July 2000.

98. Seeman P. Atypical antipsychotics: mechanism of action. Can J Psychiatry 2002; 47(suppl 1):27–38.

99. Miller A, Ereshefsky L, Dassori A, Crismon ML. Drug therapy of schizophrenia. In: Dunner ED, Psychiatric Clinics of North America Annual Review of Drug Therapy 2001. Philadelphia: Saunders, 2001.

100. Tran PV, Hamilton SH, Kuntz AJ, Potvin JH, Andersen SW, Beasley C Jr, Tollefson GD. Double blind comparison of olanzapine versus risperidone in the treatment of schizophrenia and other psychotic disorders. J Clin Psychopharmacol 1997; 17:407–418.

101. Sernyak MJ, Desai R, Stolar M, Rosenheck R. Impact of clozapine on completed suicide. Am J Psychiatry 2001; 158(6):931–937.

102. Meltzer HY. Suicide and schizophrenia: clozapine and the InterSePT study. International Clozaril/Leponex Suicide Prevention Trial. J Clin Psychiatry 1999; 60 (suppl 12):47–50.

103. Zimbroff DL, Kane JM, Tamminga CA, Daniel DG, Mack RJ, Wozniak PJ, Sebree TB, Wallin BA, Kashkin KB. Controlled, dose-response study of sertindole and haloperidol in the treatment of schizophrenia. Am J Psychiatry 1997:154:782–791.

104. Selman FB, McClure RF, Helwig H. Loxapine succinate: a double-blind comparison with haloperidol and placebo in acute schizophrenics. Curr Ther Res 1976; 19:645.

105. Dahl SG. Active metabolites of neuroleptic drugs: possible contribution to therapeutic and toxic effects. Ther Drug Monit 1982; 4:33–40.

106. Anon. Loxitane, loxapine succinate. Book from the Medical Advisory Department, Lederle Laboratories, Pearl River, NY, pp 1–95.

107. Conley RR, Mahmoud R. A randomized double-blind study of risperidone and olanzapine in the treatment of schizophrenia or schizoaffective disorder. [erratum appears in Am J Psychiatry 2001; 158(suppl 10):1759.] Am J Psychiatry 2001; 158(suppl 5):765–774.

108. Ereshefsky L. Pharmacokinetics and drug interactions: update for new antipsychotics. J. Clin. Psychiatry 1996; 57(suppl 11):12–25.
109. Ereshefsky L, Toney G, Saklad SR, Anderson C, Seidel D. A loading-dose strategy for converting from oral to depot neuroleptic. Hosp Comm Psychiatry 1993; 44(suppl 12):1155–1161.
110. Schatzberg AF, DeBattista, Ereshefsky L, Overman J. Current psychotropic dosing and monitoring guidelines. Primary Psychiatry 1997; 4(suppl 7):35–63.
111. Ereshefsky L. Antidepressant pharmacodynamics, pharmacokinetics, and drug interactions. Geriatrics 1998; 63(suppl 4):S22–S33.
112. Kidron R, Averbuch I, Klein E, Belmaker RH. Carbamazepine induction reduction of blood levels of haloperidol in chronic schizophrenia. Biol Psychiatry 1985; 20:219–222.
113. Jann MW, Saklad SR, Ereshefsky L, Richards AL, Harrington CA, Davis CM. Effects of smoking on haloperidol and reduced haloperidol plasma concentrations and haloperidol clearance. Psychopharmacology 1986; 90:468–470.
114. Ereshefsky L, Saklad SR, Watanabe MD, Davis CM, Jann MW. Thiothixene pharmacokinetic interactions: a study of hepatic enzyme inducers, clearance inhibitors, and demographic variables. J Clin Psychopharmacol 1991; 11(5):296–301.
115. Ereshefsky L, Jann MW, Saklad SR, Davis C. Bioavailability of psychotropic drugs: historical perspective and pharmacokinetic overview. J Clin Psychiatry 1986; 47:6–15.
116. Jann MW, Ereshefsky L, Saklad SR, Seidel DR, Davis CM, Burch NR, Bowden CL. Effects of carbamazepine on plasma haloperidol levels. J Clin Psychopharmacol 1985; 5:106–109.
117. Ereshefsky L, Dugan D. Review of Pharmacokinetics, Pharmacogenetics, and drug interaction potential of antidepressants: focus on Venlafaxine. Depress Anxiety 2000; 12(suppl 1):30–44.
118. Alfaro CL, Lam YW, Simpson J, Ereshefsky L. CYP2D6 Inhibition by fluoxetine, paroxetine, sertraline, and venlafaxine in a crossover study: intraindividual variability and plasma concentration Correlations. J Clin Pharmacol 2000; 40(1):58–66.
119. Prakash C, Kamel A, Gummerus J, Wilner K. Metabolism and excretion of a new antipsychotic drug, ziprasidone, in humans. Drug Metab Dispos 1997; 25(suppl 7):863–872.
120. Glazer WM, Ereshefsky L. A Pharmacoeconomic model of outpatient antipsychotic therapy in "revolving door" schizophrenic patients. J Clin Psych 1996; 57(suppl 8):337–345.
121. Ereshefsky L, Saklad SR, Jann MW, Davis CM, Richards A, Seidel DR. Future of depot neuroleptic therapy: pharmacokinetic and pharmacodynamic approaches. J Clin Psychiatry 1984; 45:50–59.
122. McCreadie RG, Mackie M, Wiles DH, Jorgensen A, Hansen V, Menzies C. Within-individual variation in steady state plasma levels of different neuroleptics and prolactin. Br J Psychiatry 1984; 144:625–629.
123. Weiden PJ, Aquila R, Emanuel M, Zygmunt A. Long-term considerations after switching antipsychotics. J Clin Psychiatry 1998; 59(suppl 19):36–49.
124. Moore MT, Book MH. Sudden death in phenothiazine therapy. (A clinicopathologic study of 12 cases.) Psychiatric Q 1970; 44(suppl 3):389–402.
125. Chong SA, Mythily, Mahendran R. Cardiac effects of psychotropic drugs. Ann Acad Med Singapore 2001; 30(suppl 6):625–631.
126. Glassman AH, Bigger JT Jr. Antipsychotic drugs: prolonged QTc interval, torsades de pointes, and sudden death. Am J Psychiatry 2001; 158(suppl 11):1774–1782.
127. Buckley NA, Sanders P. Cardiovascular adverse effects of antipsychotic drugs. Drug Safety 2000; 23(suppl 3):215–228.
128. Timell AM. Thioridazine: re-evaluating the risk/benefit equation. Ann Clin Psychiatry 2000; 12(suppl 3):147–151.
129. Droperidol: cardiovascular toxicity and deaths. Can Med Assoc J 2002; 166(suppl 7):932.
130. Lawrence KR, Nasraway SA. Conduction disturbances associated with administration of butyrophenone antipsychotics in the critically ill: a review of the literature. Pharmacotherapy 1997; 17(suppl 3):531–537.
131. Daniel DG, Wozniak P, Mack RJ, McCarthy BG, Sertindole Group. Long-term efficacy and safety comparison of sertindole and haloperidol in the treatment of schizophrenia. Psychopharmacol Bull 1998; 34:61–69.
132. Crumb WJ, Beasley C, Thornton A, Breier A. Cardiac ion channel blocking profile of olanzapine and other antipsychotics. Presented at the 38th American College of Neuropsychopharmacology Annual Meeting, Acapulco, Mexico; Dec 12–16, 1999.
133. Briefing document for Zeldox Capsules (Ziprasidone HCl). FDA Psychopharmacological Drugs Advisory Committee, July 19, 2000.
134. Goodnick PJ. Ziprasidone: profile on safety. Expert Opin Pharmacother 2001; 2(suppl 10):1655–1662.
135. Stamler J, Wentworth D, Neaton JD. Is relationship between serum cholesterol and risk of pre-mature death from coronary heart disease continuous and graded? Findings in 356,222 primary screenees of the Multiple Risk Factor Intervention Trial (MRFIT). JAMA 1986; 256:2823–2828.

136. Sussman N. Review of atypical antipsychotics and weight gain. J Clin Psych 2001; 62(suppl 23);5–12.
137. Wirshing DA. Weight gain associated with novel antipsychotic medications. Prim Psychiatry 2001; 62(suppl 23):39–44.
138. Henderson DC. Clozapine: diabetes mellitus, weight gain, and lipid abnormalities. J Clin Psychiatry 2001; 62(suppl 23):39–44.
139. Mukherjee S. High prevalence of type II diabetes in schizophrenic patients. Schizophr Res 1995; 15:195.
140. Sernyak MJ, Leslie DL, Alarcon RD, Losonczy MF, Rosencheck R. Association of diabetes mellitus with use of atypical neuroleptics in the treatment of schizophrenia. Am J Psychiatry 2002; 159:561–566.
141. Braceland RJ, Meduna LJ, Vaichulis JA. Delayed action of insulin in schizophrenia. Am J Psychiatry 1945; 102:108–110.
142. Freeman H. Resistance to insulin in mentally disturbed soldiers. Arch Neurol Psychiatry 1946; 56:74–78.
143. Kasanin J. The blood sugar curve in mental disease. The dementia praecox groups. *Arch Neurol Psychiatry* 1926; 16:414-419.
144. Wirshing DA, Spellberg BJ, Erhart SM, Marder SR, Wirshing WC. Novel antipsychotics and new onset diabetes. Biol Psychiatry 1998; 44:778–783.
145. Haupt DW, Newcomer JW. Hyperglycemia and antipsychotic medications. J Clin Psychiatry 2001; 62 (suppl 27):15–26; discussion 40–41.
146. Procyshyn RM, Pande S, Tse G. New-onset diabetes mellitus associated with the initiation of quetiapine treatment. Can J Psychiatry 2000; 45(suppl 7):668–669.
147. Wirshing DA, Pierre JM, Eyeler J, Weinbach J, Wirshing WC. Risperdone associated new-onset diabetes. Biol Psychiatry 2001; 50:148–149.
148. Lindenmayer JP, Patel R. Olanzapine-induced ketoacidosis with diabetes mellitus. Am J Psychiatry 1999; 156:1471.
149. Raqucci KR, Wells BJ. Olanzapine-induced diabetic ketoacidosis. Ann Pharmacother. 2001; 35:1556–1558.
150. Ramankutty G. Olanzapine-induced destabilization of diabetes in the absence of weight gain. Acta Psychiatr Scand. 2002; 105:235–236.
151. Rojas P, Arancibia P, Bravo V, Varela S. Diabetes mellitus induced by olanzapine. A case report. Rev Med Chili. 2001; 129:1183–1185.
152. Seaburg HL, McLendon BM, Doraiswarny PM. Olanzapine-associated severe hyperglycemia, ketonuria, and acidosis: case report and review of the literature. Pharmacotherapy 2001; 21:1448–1454.
153. Meyer JM. Novel antipsychotics and severe hyperlipidemia. J Clin Psychopharmacol. 2001; 21:369–374.
154. Bettinger TL, Mendelson SC, Dorson PG, Crismon ML. Olanzapine-induced glucose dysregulation. Ann Pharmacother 2000; 34:865–867.
155. Melkersson K, Hultin AL. Recovery from new-onset diabetes in a schizophrenic man after withdrawal of olanzapine. Psychosomatics 2002; 43:67–70.
156. Muench J, Carey M. Diabetes mellitus associated with atypical antipsychotic medications: new case report and review of the literature. J Am Board Fam Pract. 2001; 14:278–282.
157. Goodnick PJ, Kato MM. Antipsychotic medication: effects on regulation of glucose and lipids. Expert Opin Pharmacother. 2001; 2:1571–1582.
158. Rolka DB, Narayan KM, Thompson TJ, Goldman D, Lindenmayer J, Alich K. Performance of recommended screening tests for undiagnosed diabetes and dysglycemia. Diabetes Care 2001; 24:1899–1903.
159. Arranz MJ, Munro J, Birkett J, Bolonna A, Mancama D, Sodhi M, Lesch KP, Meyer JF, Sham P, Collier DA, Murray RM, Kerwin RW. Pharmacogenetic prediction of clozapine response. Lancet 2000; 355:1615–1616.
160. Jann MW, Ereshefsky L, Saklad SR. Clinical pharmacokinetics of the depot antipsychotics. Clin Pharmacokinet 1985; 10:315–333.
161. Ereshefsky L, Saklad SR, Tran-Johnson T, Toney G, Lyman RC, Davis CM. Kinetics and clinical evaluation of haloperidol decanoate loading dose regimen. Psychopharmacol Bull 1990; 26:108–114.
162. Kane JM, Woerner M, Sarantanos S. Depot neuroleptics: a comparative review of standard, intermediate, and low dose regimens. J Clin Psychiatry 1986; 47 (suppl):30–33.
163. Widstedt B, Wiles D, Jorgensen A. A depot neuroleptic withdrawal study neurological effects. Psychopharmacology 1983; 80:101–105.
164. Kane J et al. Poster presented at APA Institute on Psychiatric Services; Orlando, FL, Oct 10–14, 2001.
165. Rasmussen M, Vermeulen A, Eerdekuns M, et al. IX World Congress of Psychiatry, Hamburg, Germany, Aug 6–11, 1999.
166. Aravagiri M, Yuwiler A, Marder S. Distribution after repeated oral administration of different dose levels of risperidone and 9-hydroxy-risperidone in the brain and other tissues of rat. Psychopharmacology 1998; 139:356–363.

50

Multiple Mechanisms of Lithium Action

ALONA SHALDUBINA, ROBERT H. BELMAKER, and GALILA AGAM
Ben-Gurion University of the Negev, Beer-Sheva, Israel

I. INTRODUCTION

Lithium has therapeutic and prophylactic effects on both the manic and depressive phases of bipolar affective disorder, yet the mechanism of lithium's therapeutic action is not clear. Numerous biochemical effects of lithium have been identified and some of these may be a component of the therapeutic response. One of the current challenges is to distinguish critical effects from the many known biochemical actions of lithium, many of which may contribute to side effects or lead to toxicity [1]. We will summarize six theories of lithium action that have emerged in the last decade.

II. APOPTOSIS PREVENTION

Multiple neuroimaging and postmortem morphology studies have demonstrated reduced brain volume and cell number in mood disorders [2]. These findings may represent neurodevelopmental abnormalities, disease progression, or biochemical changes secondary to changes in neurotransmitter levels in chronic affective disorders [3]. Chronic lithium administration at therapeutically relevant concentrations has been recently found to protect neurons against apoptotic cell death, to prolong cell survival, and to promote growth and regeneration of axons in the mammalian brain [4,5]. Long-term, but not acute, lithium treatment of cultured cerebellar granule cells induces a concentration dependent decrease in mRNA and protein levels of proapoptotic factors p53 and Bax; conversely, mRNA and protein levels of the cytoprotective factor Bcl-2 (B-cell lymphoma/ leukemia-2 protein) are markedly increased [4,6] (Fig. 1).

Manji et al. [7] also demonstrated that chronic lithium treatment robustly increases Bcl-2 level in rat frontal cortex, hippocampus, and striatum. The mechanism of the lithium effect is not known. Manji et al. [7,8] proposed that lithium affects Bcl-2 via alteration of gene expression; however, it is also possible that classic effects of lithium on cyclic AMP or inositol mediate effects on Bcl-2 expression.

Over-expression of Bcl-2 has recently been shown to prolong cell survival and attenuate motor neuron degeneration, and to promote growth and regeneration of axons in the mammalian CNS [5]. Lithium's neuroprotective effect, induced by increasing brain Bcl-2 levels, may be relevant in the long-term treatment of mood disorders for the prevention of neurodegeneration [7,8]. It is hard to understand how Bcl-2 effects could explain lithium's effect on acute mania within 10–21 days, however. Moreover, neuronal cell loss in affective disorder, while possible, is not thought of as a

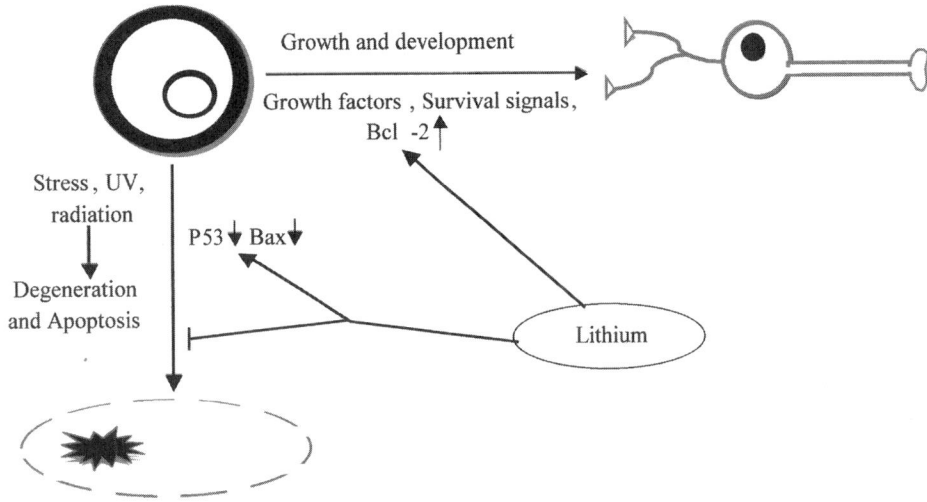

Figure 1 Consequences of Bcl-2 upregulation by lithium.

central feature compared to neurodegenerative disorders where Bcl-2 is usually studied or even compared to schizophrenia.

III. PHOSPHOADENOSINE PHOSPHATE PHOSPHATASE

3′(2′)Phosphoadenosine 5′-phosphate (PAP) phosphatase is a ubiquitous enzyme, highly conserved during evolution [9]. PAP phosphatase specifically catalyzes the hydrolysis of 3′-phosphate from PAP, thereby converting PAP to adenosine 5′-phosphate (AMP) and inorganic phosphate [9,10]. Lithium inhibits PAP phosphatase in an uncompetitive manner well within therapeutic concentrations ($K_i = 0.3$ mM). The human PAP phosphatase (HsPIP) has dual specificity, acting both on PAP and on inositol-1,4-bisphosphate [10,11]. Thus, PAP phosphatase may play a role in inositol recycling and phosphoinositide metabolism [10], and in this sense lithium inhibition of PAP phosphatase may reinforce inositol depletion by inhibition of inositol phosphate dephosphorylation. Lopes-Coronardo et al. [10] have found high PAP phosphatase expression in rat heart, brain, and kidney, but Spiegelberg et al. [11] demonstrated that among human tissues the expression of PAP phosphatase is highest in kidney and lowest in lung and brain. PAP phosphatase activities in rat brain and kidney were recently compared in our lab and were found to have significantly higher activity in brain (1.15 ± 0.15 nmoles/min $\times$ mg protein [SE]) than in kidney (0.51 ± 0.25 [SE]), with no significant difference between frontal cortex and hippocampus or between the medulla and cortex in the kidney. Furthermore, a moderate difference in PAP phosphatase protein levels between postmortem human frontal cortex specimens from bipolar patients versus control subjects were recently observed by Shaltiel et al. [12]. This study was the first to measure PAP phosphatase in tissue derived from bipolar patients. A 24% significantly lower PAP phosphatase protein level in the frontal cortex of bipolar patients vs. normal subjects was observed (two-tailed paired t-test, $t = 2.21$, $P < .05$) [12]. Several other lithium-related biochemical measures in bipolar disorder have been reported to be altered in the direction of their response to lithium treatment, as it was found for PAP phosphatase rather than in the more intuitive opposite direction. For instance, brain inositol is reported to be reduced postmortem [13], although lithium inhibits IMPase. Lithium's effects to counter the underlying abnormality in bipolar illness might involve gene upregulation [14] rather than simply counteracting enzyme expression because of the direct inhibitory effect on the enzyme's activity. The relationship of PAP phosphatase function to brain neurochemistry underlying emotion is not known. The accumulation of PAP upon PAP phosphatase inhibition affects several cellular systems (Fig. 2).

PAP acts as competitive inhibitor of a variety of enzymes that use PAPS (3′-phophoadenosine 5′-phosphosulfate) as sulfate donor, mainly PAPS reductase and sulfotransferases that catalyze sulfation of a large number of substrates [15]. Sulfation plays an impor-

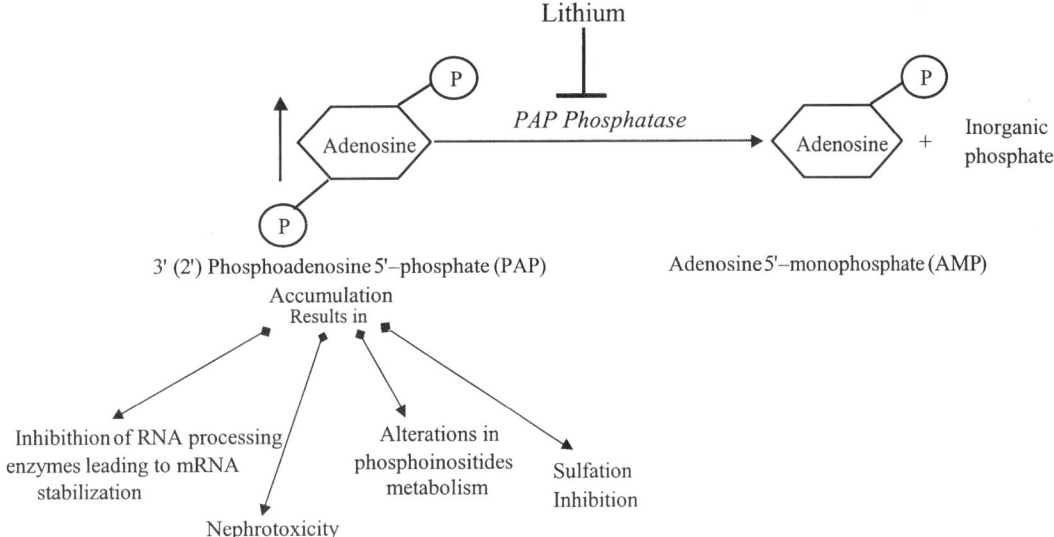

Figure 2 Possible physiological effects of PAP accumulation.

tant role in biotransformation of many exogenous and endogenous compounds, including deactivation of drugs. In addition, some neurosteorids, which can be synthesized de novo in the nervous system, are known to exist not only as free compounds but also as sulfated derivatives. Pharmacological studies indicate that unconjugated and sulfated steroids, such as pregnenolone and pregnenolone sulfate, may have opposite effects on GABA(A) receptors [16]. Thus, pregnenolone acts as a potent positive allosteric modulator of gamma-aminobutyric acid action at GABA(A) receptors, whereas pregnenolone sulfate acts as a potent negative modulator [16]. Recent experiments also suggest that dehydroepiandrosterone and dehydroepiandrosterone sulfate may have distinct effects on growth of neurites from embryonic neocortical neurons in vitro [17]. Thus, regulation of steroid sulfation may have profound behavioral and morphological effects on the nervous system.

In yeast, PAP accumulation interferes with RNA processing enzymes. In particular, two $5' \rightarrow 3'$ exoribonucleases were found to be inhibited, affecting the processing of subspecies of ribosomal RNA and small nucleolar RNA, resulting in inhibition of mRNA turnover [18]. Since Li was found to affect gene expression [8], PAP accumulation due to PAP phosphatase inhibition could represent one of the mechanisms of lithium action. An attractive aspect of the hypothesis is the very low K_i of lithium effect, which would cut off a very large percentage of PAP phosphatase activity during chronic lithium therapy in vivo. It is not clearly related (other than via its secondary effect on inositol polyphosphate phosphatase) to any known signal transduction system. Sulfation per se is perhaps more relevant to solubilization and detoxification in the periphery than to brain function.

IV. THE INOSITOL DEPLETION HYPOTHESIS

A widespread hypothesis explaining lithium's therapeutic and prophylactic effect in affective disorder is that inhibition of inositol monophosphatase impairs the operation of the phosphatidylinositol cycle (PI cycle). The membrane phospholipid, phosphatidylinositol (PI), is sequentially phosphorylated to form phosphatidylinositol bisphosphate (PIP$_2$). Agonist-stimulated phospholipase C (PLC) cleaves PIP$_2$ to two second messengers: inositol 1,4,5-trisphosphate (IP$_3$) and diacylglycerol (DAG). IP$_3$ releases calcium sequestered in endoplasmic reticulum. IP$_3$ may be phosphorylated to form inositol penta- and hexaphosphates, which are subsequently dephosphorylated to inositol monophosphate (IP), which is dephosphorylated by inositol monophosphatase to free inositol. Lithium inhibits the last step in this process. DAG, the second derivative of PIP$_2$ activates protein kinase C. DAG is converted sequentially to cytidine disphosphate—diacyl glycerol (CDP-DG), which is combined with free inositol by PI synthase to re-form PI (Fig. 3).

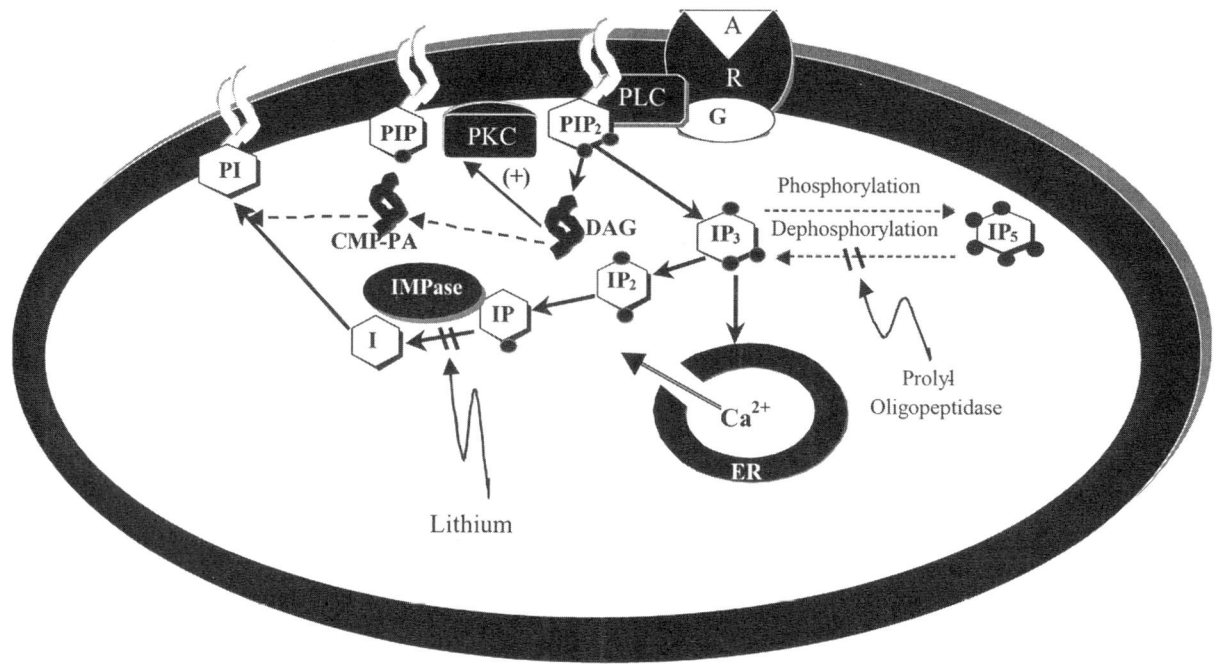

Figure 3 Effect of lithium on the PI cycle.

With discovery of the importance of the cycle as a second-messenger system, the lithium-induced reduction of inositol immediately assumed potential importance as a key mechanism of lithium action [19]. Lithium was first shown to affect the system in 1971, when it was found that lithium decreased free inositol concentrations and increased inositol monophosphate (IP) concentration in brain [20]. Del Rio et al. [21] demonstrated that lithium also reduced intracellular concentration of inositol trisphosphate (IP_3). Hallcher and Sherman [22] showed that lithium at therapeutic doses inhibits bovine brain inositol monophosphatase, thereby explaining the reduction in inositol and accumulation of inositol monophosphate. Inhibition is uncompetitive with a K_i of 0.8 mM, thus within therapeutically effective serum concentrations in the range of 0.5–1.4 mM [22]. Berridge [19] proposed that the Li-induced shortage of inositol in the brain, an organ to which plasmaborne inositol is essentially unavailable, leads to depletion of substrate for phosphatidylinositol resynthesis only in overactive neurons. This theory could explain lithium's specific therapeutic activity in psychopathological states with minimal effects on normal behavior [23].

An intriguing possible interaction with the findings of Maes et al. [24,25], who reported lowered *prolyloligopeptidase* activity during depression but raised during mania, with the PI signal transduction system and lithium's inhibitory effect on IMPase has been suggested by Williams et al. [26]. They have shown that a *Dictyostelium* mutant lacking the prolyl oligopeptidase gene has elevated IP_3 levels, which, apparently, protected it from lithium's interference with cell aggregation during development. IP_3 elevation was found to result from increased dephosphorylation of IP_5 in the mutant [26].

Kofman and Belmaker [27] found that ICV inositol administration reversed a behavioral effect of lithium in rats, supporting the concept that inositol depletion mediated the behavioral effect. However, it has been difficult to demonstrate that lithium in vivo indeed reduces PIP2 concentrations, and some scientists have claimed that, especially in primates, inositol concentrations are in excess of those needed to saturate PI synthase [28]. Belmaker et al. [29] showed that chronic dietary lithium administration, in rats reduced inositol level in hypothalamus by 27%, compared to control group. Furthermore, Moore et al. [30] did find in a small group of patients that 7 days but not 21 days of lithium reduced frontal cortical myoinositol levels in vivo using magnetic resonance spectroscopy. This ambiguity raised the possibility that lithium exerts its effect on inositol monophosphatase at the level of gene expression. To elucidate this supposition, lymphocyte-derived cell lines were treated in vitro with 1 mM lithium. A 40% increase of mRNA levels of one of the two genes coding for inositol monophosphatase was observed [31]. A critical test of the inositol depletion hypothesis will be whether inositol depletion diet in patients augments clinical lithium response [32].

V. LITHIUM AND SEROTONIN

Serotonin (5HT) is released by presynaptic serotonergic neurons and activates specific postsynaptic receptors (mostly $5HT_2$). Serotonin also activates presynaptic autoreceptors ($5HT_{1A}$ or $5HT_{1B}$), which decrease the availability of 5HT by feedback inhibition of serotonin release. The serotonin reuptake channel is another mechanism for regulation of serotonin level in synaptic cleft. This system is a specific target for serotonin-specific reuptake inhibitors.

The use of lithium in combination with antidepressant drugs has been reported to rapidly improve antidepressant response in otherwise treatment-resistant patients [33]. Electrophysiological studies demonstrated that lithium has a capacity to increase the release of 5HT to the synapse, perhaps by inhibiting $5HT_{1A}$ autoreceptors [34]. $5HT_{1A}$ autoreceptors are localized on the soma and dendrites of 5HT neurons and control their firing (Fig. 4).

A very recent finding concerns $5HT_{1B}$ autoreceptors, which are localized on presynaptic neuron terminals and control 5HT release. Activation of the $5HT_{1B}$ autoreceptor decreases release of serotonin to the synaptic cleft. Redrobe and Bourin [35] demonstrated that lithium induced antidepressant effects in the mouse forced swimming test, and this lithium effect was shown to be mediated by $5HT_{1B}$ receptors. Massot et al. [36] demonstrated that lithium, but not other metallic cations, causes specific inhibition of $5HT_{1B}$ receptor binding in membrane preparation. This effect occurs at relevant therapeutic concentrations. The lithium-induced desensitization of $5HT_{1B}$ autoreceptors decreases the efficacy of the negative retrocontrol of 5HT release at neuron terminals, leading to an enhancement of the availability of 5HT in the synaptic cleft. Massot et al. [36] also demonstrated that acute lithium can block $5HT_{1B}$-mediated mouse behavior in vivo and $5HT_{1B}$ inhibition of forskolin-stimulated adenylate cyclase in CHO cell homogenates. Thus, lithium effects on 5HT autoreceptors could be demonstrated at the molecular, physiological, and behavioral levels, which makes for an exciting finding whose replication and extension are worth waiting for. However, it seems to explain mostly lithium's antidepressant effects and it would be hard to connect the above mechanism with its antimanic effects.

VI. EXCITATORY AMINO ACIDS

The possible involvement of glutamate in the mechanism of lithium's therapeutic effect was suggested by Dixon and Hokin [37]. The group was studying the effects of lithium on the PI cycle. Kennedy et al. [38] and Lee et al. [39] found that in the presence of lithium, cholinergic stimulation of rat and mouse cerebral cortex slices resulted in decreased accumulation of IP_3, as would be expected from the inositol depletion hypothesis (see above). However, in guinea pig, rabbit, and rhesus monkey, cerebral cortex slices in the presence of lithium, Dixon et al. [40] and Lee et al. [39] showed

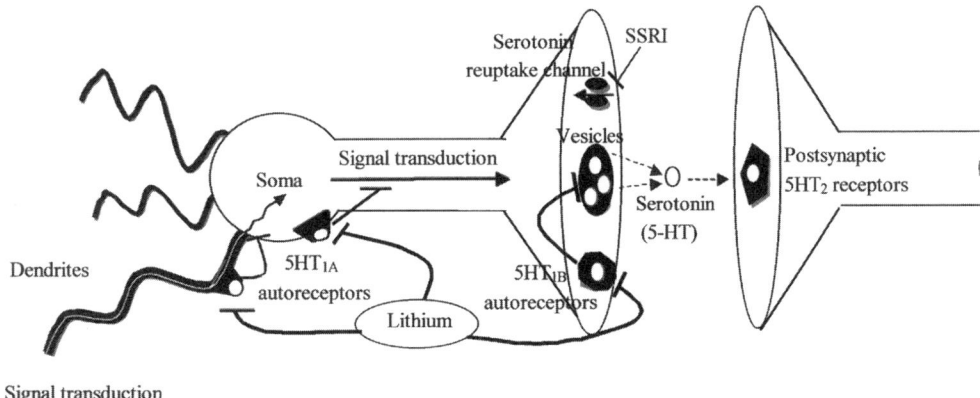

Figure 4 Effect of lithium on 5HT autoreceptors.

increased IP$_3$ accumulation. Species differences in baseline inositol levels were suggested to account for this contrast [39]. Lithium-induced IP$_3$ accumulation in rhesus monkey brain slices was independent of agonist stimulation or inositol supplementation [40]. Involvement of an endogenous neurotransmitter in this lithium effect was postulated, and indeed lithium was found to stimulate glutamate availability in the synaptic cleft [41]. Activation of the N-methyl-D-aspartate (NMDA) receptor by glutamate resulted in IP$_3$ accumulation (Fig. 5).

Lithium-induced glutamate accumulation may be mediated either by increasing its release or by inhibiting its reuptake. Dixon and Hokin [37] examined the effect of lithium administration on the uptake of radioactively labeled glutamate by presynaptic nerve endings in mouse cerebral cortex. Acute lithium inhibited glutamate uptake in a dose-dependent manner, with maximal effect at 20 mM lithium. The maximal lithium effect occurred at very high concentration (20–25 mM) and after a short period of 2 h, and therefore seems to be irrelevant for lithium's therapeutic action, which occurs at lower concentration and after 1–2 weeks of treatment. It may, however, be related to lithium's toxicity. Dixon and Hokin [37] also studied the effect of chronic lithium treatment on glutamate reuptake. Mice were fed lithium-containing chow for 2 weeks, which led to lithium blood levels of 0.7–1.0 mM, and glutamate uptake by cerebrocortical synaptosomes was measured. A small but significant increase of glutamate uptake was obtained. Moreover, lithium also narrowed the range of glutamate uptake (reduced the variance from 0.42 to 0.18), an effect interpreted as stabilization of the uptake and thus perhaps relevant to lithium's mood-stabilizing effect in bipolar disorder [37]. Since glutamate is an excitatory neurotransmitter, upregulation of its uptake may exert an antimanic effect because more glutamate would be removed from the synaptic cleft.

VII. GLYCOGEN SYNTHASE KINASE-3

Glycogen synthase kinase (GSK)-3, first identified in mammals as an inhibitor of glycogen synthase [42], is now known as an ubiquitous, constitutively active, multisubstrate serine/threonine kinase, acting on diverse substrates, including transcription factors, regulatory enzymes, and structural proteins. GSK-3 plays a role in multiple cellular processes, including metabolism, proliferation, differentiation, development, and apoptosis [43,44] (Fig. 6). It is highly abundant in brain tissue and is regulated by inhibition through numerous signal transduction systems [8,45]. Overexpression of GSK-3 to levels 3.5 times that in control (in human neuroblastoma cells) potentiated staurosporine and heat-shock-induced apoptosis [46]. GSK-3 is directly inhibited by lithium at nearly therapeutically relevant concentrations (2.1 ± 0.6 mM) in vitro [47]. Valproic acid, another antibipolar compound, also inhibits GSK-3 [48], strengthening the possibility that this enzyme represents the key site of antibipolar action.

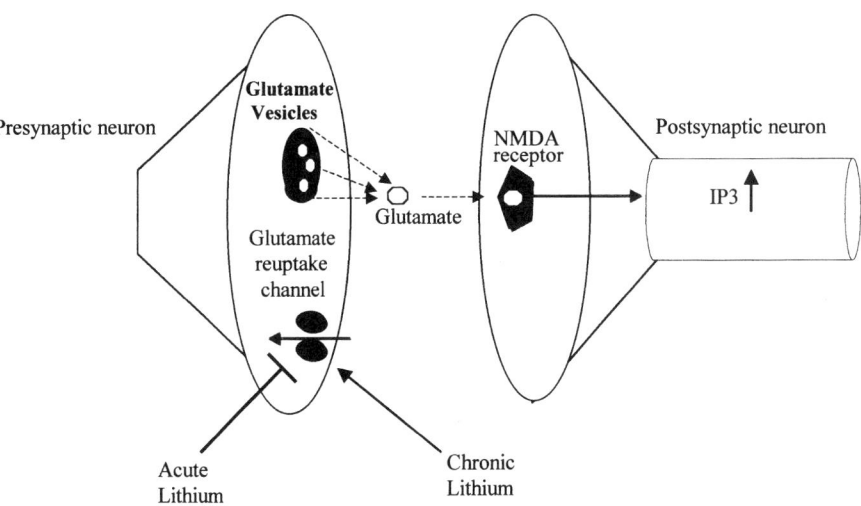

Figure 5 Acute and chronic lithium effect on glutamate neurotransmission.

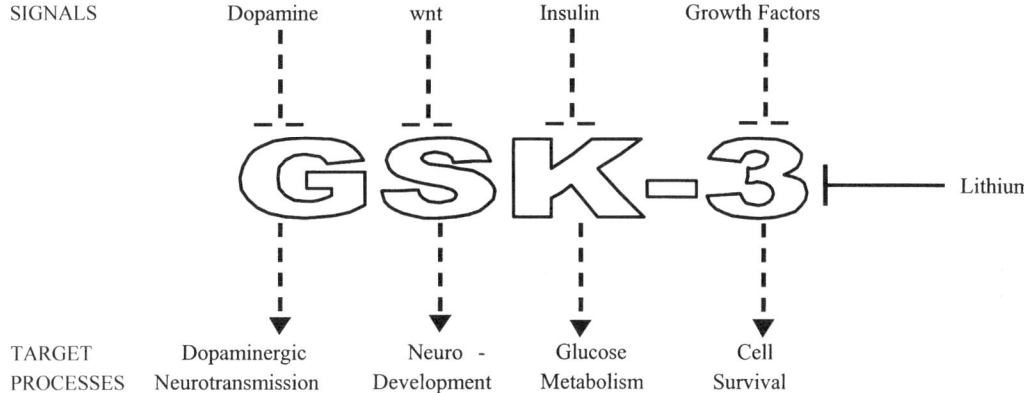

Figure 6 GSK-3 is involved in so many different cascades that it is not possible to draw the usual diagram.

Lithium has a dramatic effect on morphogenesis in the early development of numerous organisms. Klein and Melton [49] presented evidence that inositol monophosphatase inhibition does not explain the teratogenic effect of lithium on development. Lithium teratogenesis in *Xenopus* embryos caused the same effects as activation of Wnt signaling [50,51]. It leads to accumulation of cytosolic β-catenin, which plays a central role in developmental and apoptotic processes by regulation of gene expression [45]. Inhibition of GSK-3 by lithium could explain lithium's ability to mimic Wnt signaling. Because of GSK-3's central role in the cell, it could be an attractive candidate as lithium's target. Apparently, inhibition of GSK-3 by lithium occurs at the top level of its therapeutic range [47], or even higher (H. Eldar, personal communication), suggesting that GSK-3 inhibition could be more relevant to lithium's toxic side effects. However, Ryves and Harwood [52] have recently shown that lithium inhibits GSK-3 by competing with Mg^{2+}. Therefore, this inhibition is dependent on free Mg^{2+} concentration, and the latter is dependent on chelation by ATP. Consequently, given the cellular concentrations of Mg^{2+} and ATP, these authors calculated that lithium's in vivo inhibitory effect on GSK-3 would have a K_i of 0.8 mM or less—well within the therapeutic range. A critical experiment would be to test whether chronic in vivo lithium treatment of rats causes downstream events due to GSK-3 inhibition, such as changes in β-catenin levels.

VIII. CONCLUSIONS

Lithium is a simple ion with numerous biochemical effects. Lithium's clinical effects include prophylaxis of bipolar disorder, antimanic, antidepressant, and antiagressive action; action against migraine and cluster headaches; action in the syndrome of inappropriate secretion of antidiuretic hormone; and alleviation of chemotherapy-induced leukopenia.

"Lumpers" tend to see all or almost all of these clinical effects, or at least the CNS effects, as deriving from a common CNS mechanism. "Occam's razor" would urge that the multiplicity of lithium's biochemical effects be reduced to one true mechanism of clinical action, with other effects being epiphenomena or related to side effects or toxicity. "Clinical splitters," however, see the numerous clinical effects as independent properties of the lithium ion in biology. Biochemical "integrationists" suggest that the multitude of lithium effects together account for its clinical action, and that one biochemical mechanism could not account for even one of lithium's clinical effects.

Critical experiments must be devised to distinguish among these profoundly different and fascinating approaches. For instance, synthetic IMPase inhibitors exist that must be studied for behavioral effects; GSK-3 inhibitors have also been developed [53], and it will be critical to know if they are behaviorally active or only teratogenic. PAP accumulates during lithium administration: it will be important to deliver PAP intracerebroventricularly (perhaps as a penetrable derivative or in liposomes) and to see whether its behavioral effects mimic those of lithium. Bcl-2 knockout mice are available [54]: do they show behavioral effects?

REFERENCES

1. Shaldubina A, Agam G, Belmaker RH. Mechanism of lithium action: state of the art, ten years later. Prog Neuropsychopharmacol Biol Psychiatry 4:855–866, 2001.
2. Drevets WC, Gadde KM, Krishnan KRR Neuroimaging studies of mood disorders in: Neurobiology of Mental Illness. DS Charney, ER Nestler, BS Bunney, eds. New York: Oxford University Press, 1999:394–418.
3. Duman RS, Heninger GR, Nestler EJ. A molecular and cellular theory of depression. Arch Gen Psychiaty 54:597–606, 1997.
4. Chen G, Zeng WZ, Yuan PX, Huang LD, Jiang YM, Zhao ZH, Manji HK. The mood-stabilizing agents lithium and valproate robustly increase the levels of the neuroprotective protein bcl-2 in the CNS. J Neurochem 72:879–882, 1999.
5. Chen DF, Schneider GE, Martinou JC, Tonegava S. Bcl-2 promotes regeneration of severed axons in mammalian CNS. Nature 385:434–439, 1997.
6. Chen RW, Chuang DM. Long term lithium treatment suppresses p53 and Bax expression but increases Bcl-2 expression. J Biol Chem 274:6039–6042, 1999.
7. Manji HK, Moore GJ, Chen G. Lithium up-regulates the cytoprotective protein Bcl-2 in the CNS in vivo: a role for neurotrophic and neuroprotective effects in manic depressive illness. J Clin Psychiatry 61(suppl 9):82–96, 2000.
8. Manji HK, Moore GJ, Chen G. Lithium at 50: have the neuroprotective effects of this unique cation been overlooked? Biol Psychiatry 46:929–940, 1999.
9. Yenush L, Bellés JM, López-Coronado JM, Gil-Mascarell R, Serrano R, Rodríguez PL. A novel target of lithium therapy. FEBS Lett 467:321–325, 2000.
10. López-Coronado JM, Bellés JM, Lesage F, Serrano R, Rodríguez PL. A novel mammalian lithium-sensitive enzyme with a dual enzymatic activity, 3′-phosphoadenosine 5′-phosphate phosphatase and inositol-polyphosphate 1-phosphatase J Biol Chem 274:16034–16039, 1999.
11. Spiegelberg BD, Xiong JP, Smith JJ, Gu RF, York JD. Cloning and characterization of mammalian lithium-sensitive bisphosphate 3′-nucleotidase inhibited by inositol 1,4-bisphosphate. J Biol Chem 274: 13619–13628, 1999.
12. Shaltiel G, Belmaker RH, Agam G. 3′(2′)-phosphoadenosine 5′-phosphate phosphatase is reduced in postmortem frontal cortex of bipolar patients. Biopolar Disord 4:302–306, 2002.
13. Shimon H, Agam G, Belmaker RH, Hyde TM, Kleinman JE. Reduced frontal cortex inositol levels in postmortem brain of suicide victims and patients with bipolar disorder. Am J Psychiatry 154:1148–1150, 1997.
14. Ikonomov OC, Manji HK. Molecular mechanisms underlying mood stabilization in manic-depressive illness: the phenotype challenge. Am J Psychiatry 156(10):1506–1514, 1999.
15. Klassen CD and Boles JW. The importance of 3′-phosphoadenosine 5′ phosphosulphate (PAPS) in the regulaton of sulfation. FASEB J 11: 404–417, 1997.
16. El Etr M, Akwa Y, Robel P, Baulieu EE. Opposing effects of different steroid sulfates on GABAA receptor-mediated chloride uptake. Brain Res 790(1–2):334–338, 1998.
17. Compagnone NA, Mellon SH. Dehydroepiandrosterone: a potential signalling molecule for neocortical organization during development. Proc Natl Acad Sci USA 95(8):4678–4683, 1998.
18. Dichtl B, Stevens A, Tollervey D. Lithium toxicity in yeast is due to the inhibition of RNA processing enzymes. EMBO J 16:7184–7195, 1997.
19. Berridge MJ. Phosphoinositides and signal transduction. Rev Clin Basic Pharm 5(Suppl):5S–13S, 1985.
20. Allison JH, Stewart MA Reduced brain inositol in lithium treated rats. Nat New Biol 233:267–268, 1971.
21. Del Rio E, Shinomura T, Van der Kaay J, Nicholls DG, Downes CP. Disruption by lithium of phosphoinositide signalling in cerebellar granule cells in primary culture. J Neurochem 4:1662–1669, 1998.
22. Hallcher LM, Sherman WR. The effect of lithium ion and other agents on the activity of myo-inositol-1-phosphatase from bovine brain. J Biol Chem 255:10896–10901, 1980.
23. Belmaker RH, Bersudsky Y, Agam G, Levine J, Kofman O How does lithium work on manic depression? Clinical and psychological correlates of the inositol theory. Annu Rev Med 47: 47–56, 1996.
24. Maes M, Goossens F, Scharpe S, Calabrese J, Desnyder R, Meltzer HY. Alterations in plasma prolyl endopeptidase activity in depression, mania, and schizophrenia: effects of antidepressants, mood stabilizers, and antipsychotic drugs. Psychiatry Res 58(3):217–225, 1995.
25. Maes M, Goossens F, Scharpe S, Meltzer HY, Hondt P, Cosyns P. Lower serum prolyl endopeptidase enzyme activity in major depression: further evidence that peptidases play a role in the pathophysiology of depression. Biol Psychiatry 35:8 545–552, 1994.
26. Williams RS, Eames M, Ryves WJ, Viggars J, Harwood AJ. Loss of a prolyl oligopeptidase confers resistance to lithium by elevation of inositol (1,4,5) trisphosphate. EMBO J 8:10 2734–2745, 1999.
27. Kofman O, Belmaker RH Intracerebroventricular myoinositol antagonizes lithium-induced suppression of

28. Dixon JF, Lee CH, Los GV, Hokin LE Lithium enhances accumulation of [^{3}H]inositol radioactivity and mass of second messenger inositol 1,4,5-trisphosphate in monkey cerebral cortex. J Neurochem 59:2332–2335, 1992.
29. Belmaker RH, Agam G, Van Calker D, Richards MH, Kofman O. Behavioral reversal of lithium effects by four inositol isomers correlates perfectly with biochemical effects on the PI cycle: depletion by chronic lithium of brain inositol is specific to hypothalamus, and inositol levels may be abnormal in postmortem brain from bipolar patients. Neuropsychopharmacology 19(3):220–232, 1998.
30. Moore GJ, Bebchuk JM, Parrish JK, Faulk MW, Arfken CL, Strahl-Bevacqua J, Manji HK. Temporal dissociation between lithium-induced CNS myo-inositol changes and clinical response in manic-depressive illness. Am J Psychiatry 156:1902–1908, 1999.
31. Shamir A, Ebstein RP, Nemanov L, Zohar A, Belmaker RH, Agam G. Inositol monophosphatase in immortalized lymphoblastoid cell lines indicates susceptibility to bipolar disorder and response to lithium therapy. Mol Psychiatry 3(6):481–482, 1998.
32. Bersudsky Y, Einat H, Stahl Z, Belmaker RH. Epi-inositol and inositol depletion: two new treatment approaches in affective disorder. Curr Psychiatry 1:141–147, 1999.
33. De Montigny C, Cournoyer G. Lithium addition in treatment-resistant major depression. In: Treating Resistant Depression. J Zohar, RH Belmaker, eds. New York: PMA Publishing 1987:147–162.
34. Haddjeri N, Szabo ST, De Montigny C, Blier P. Increased tonic activation of rat forebrain 5-HT(1A) receptors by lithium addition to antidepressant treatments. Neuropsychopharmacology. 22: 346–356, 2000.
35. Redrobe JP, Bourin M. Evidence of the activity of lithium on 5-HT1B receptors in the mouse forced swimming test: comparison with carbamazepine and sodium valproate. Psychopharmacology (Berl) 141(4):370–377, 1999.
36. Massot O, Rousselle JC, Fillion MP, Januel D, Plantefl M, Fillion G. 5-HT1B receptors: A novel target for lithium. Possible involvement in mood disorders. Neuropsychopharmacology 21:530–541, 1999.
37. Dixon JF, Hokin LE. Lithium acutely inhibits and chronically up-regulates and stabilizes glutamate uptake by presynaptic nerve endings in mouse cerebral cortex. Proc Natl Acad Sci USA 95:8363–8368, 1998.
38. Kennedy ED, Challiss RAJ, Nahorsky SR. Lithium reduces the accumulation of inositol polyphosphate second messengers following cholinergic stimulation of cerebral cortex slices. J Neurochem 53:1652–1655, 1989.
39. Lee CH, Dixon JF, Reichman M, Moummi C, Los G, Hokin LE. Li$^+$ increases accumulation of inositol 1,4,5-trisphosphate and inositol 1,3,4,5-tetrakisphosphate in cholinergically stimulated brain cortex slices in guinea pig, mouse and rat. The increases require inositol supplementation in mouse and rat but not in guinea pig. Biochem J 1:28 (Pt 2):377–385, 1992.
40. Dixon JF, Lee CH, Los GV, Hokin LE. Lithium enhances accumulation of [^{3}H]inositol radioactivity and mass of second messenger inositol 1,4,5-trisphosphate in monkey cerebral cortex slices. J Neurochem. 59(6):2332–2335, 1992.
41. Dixon JF, Los GV, Hokin LE. Lithium stimulates glutamate "release" and inositol 1,4,5-trisphosphate accumulation via activation of the N-methyl-D-aspartate receptor in monkey and mouse cerebral cortex slices. Proc Natl Acad Sci USA 91:8358–8362, 1994.
42. Summers SA, Kao AW, Kohn AD, Backus GS, Roth RA, Pessin JE, Birnbaum MJ. The role of glycogen synthase kinase 3β in insulin-stimulated glucose metabolism. J Biol Chem 274:17934–17940, 1999.
43. Cui H, Meng Y, Bulleit RF. Inhibition of glycogen synthase kinase 3beta activity regulates proliferation of cultured cerebellar granule cells. Brain Res Dev Brain Res 111:177–188, 1998.
44. Salinas PC. Wnt factors in axonal remodelling and synaptogenesis. Biochem Soc Symp 65:101–109, 1999.
45. Agam G, Levine J. GSK-3 a new target for lithium's effects in bipolar patients? Hum Psychopharmacol Clin Exp 13:463–465, 1998.
46. Bijur GN, De Sarno P, Jope RS. Glycogen synthase kinase-3β facilitates staurosporine- and heat shock-induced apoptosis. Protection by lithium. J Biol Chem 275:7583–7590, 2000.
47. Stambolic V, Ruel L, Woodgett JR. Lithium inhibits glycogen synthase kinase-3 activity and mimics wingless signalling in intact. Curr Biol 6:1664–1668, 1996.
48. Chen G, Huang LD, Jiang YM, Manji HK. The mood stabilizing agent Valproate inhibits the activity of glycogen synthase kinase 3. J Neurochem 72: 1327–1330, 1999.
49. Klein PS, Melton DA. A molecular mechanism for the effect of lithium on development. Proc Natl Acad Sci USA 93:8455–8459, 1996.
50. Dierick H, Bejsovec A. Cellular mechanisms of wingless/Wnt signal transduction. Curr Top Dev Biol. 43:153–190, 1999.
51. Hedgepeth CM, Conrad LJ, Zhang J, Huang HC, Lee VM, Klein PS. Activation of the Wnt signaling pathway: a molecular mechanism for lithium action. Dev Biol 185:182–191, 1997.
52. Ryves WJ, Harwood AJ. Lithium inhibits glycogen synthase kinase-3 by competition for magnesium. Biochem Biophys Res Commun 280(3):720–275, 2001.
53. Yost, C, Farr GHI, Pierce SB, Ferkey DM, Chen M, Kimelman D. GBP, an inhibitor of GSK-3, is implicated in *Xenopus* development and oncogenesis. Cell. 93:1031–1041, 1998.
54. Hochman A, Liang H, Offen D, Melamed E, Sternin H. Developmental changes in antioxidant enzymes and oxidative damage in kidneys, liver and brain of bcl-2 knockout mice. Cell Mol Biol 46(1):41–52, 2000.

51

Mechanisms of Action of Anticonvulsants and New Mood Stabilizers

ROBERT M. POST
National Institute of Mental Health, Bethesda, Maryland, U.S.A.

ELZBIETA CHALECKA-FRANASZEK AND CHRISTOPHER J. HOUGH
Uniformed Services University of the Health Sciences, Bethesda, Maryland, U.S.A.

I. INTRODUCTION

With the recognition of the inadequacy of lithium carbonate treatment for a substantial proportion of patients with bipolar illness [1], the anticonvulsants have come to play an increasingly important alternative or adjunctive role in bipolar illness and related affective syndromes [2,3] (Table 1). The early demonstration of the efficacy of lithium in bipolar illness gave hope that these results would rapidly translate into better understanding of the drug's mechanisms of action and, secondarily, the neurobiological defects in the illness to which it was targeted. However, an expanding list of candidate mechanisms has been elucidated for lithium with no single mechanism being definitively linked to its mood-stabilizing effects [4]. These mechanisms can now be compared and contrasted with the putative mechanisms of the anticonvulsants involved in their psychotropic action. Electroconvulsive therapy (ECT) also exhibits potent anticonvulsant effects in many animal models as well as clinically [5,6]. As the seizures of ECT have stood the test of time for their excellent acute efficacy in both manic and depressive episodes, no single mechanism of action for their psychotropic effects in either phase of the illness has emerged among a long list of many candidates [7].

A. Anticonvulsant Versus Psychotropic Mechanisms

The use of anticonvulsants in bipolar illness has provided a surrogate marker for their mechanisms of action because one can readily investigate the mechanisms of their acute anticonvulsant effects [4,8] (Tables 2, 3). However, there are multiple caveats. The anticonvulsant mechanisms of action have not been clearly identified, and they may differ for the same drug as a function of seizure type. Moreover, there is considerable reason to believe that the anticonvulsant mechanisms (Fig. 1) may not be identical to the psychotropic ones as evidenced by dysjunctions in their time course of action and efficacy in different models. It is also clear from the effects of lithium, which is not a potent anticonvulsant in most models and tends to be pro-convulsant in many, that an anticonvulsant mechanism is not necessary for mood stabilization. The different temporal domains of carbamazepine's actions, for exam-

Table 1 Spectrum of Psychotropic Efficacy of the Anticonvulsants

	Mania	Depression	Prophylaxis	Other
VPA	+++	+	+++	Migraine, panic
GPN	—	(+)	?	Pain; restless leg OCD; anxiety; social phobia; alcohol withdrawal
TIA	—	?	?	
PRI	( )	( )	( )	Absence epilepsy
PHT	(+)	(+)	(+)	
CBZ	+++	+	+++	Paroxysmal pain syndromes; alcohol withdrawal; ?PTSD
OXC	+++	(+)	(+++)	Paraoxsymal pain syndromes
LTG	+?	+++	+++	Pain; ?PTSD
ZNS	(+)	?	?	
TPM	(±)	(+)	(++)	?PTSD
FBM	?	?	?	
LEV	?	?	?	

Abbreviations: VPA, valproate; GPN, gabapentin; TIA, tiagabine; PRI, primidone; PHT, phenytoin; CBZ, carbamazepine; OXC, oxcarbazepine; LTG, lamotrigine; ZNS, zonisamide; TPM, topiramate; FBM, felbamate; LEV, levetiracetam; OCD, obsessive-compulsive disorder; PTSD, posttraumatic stress disorder. Strength of evidence: +++, well recognized and documented; ++, substantial; +, weak to moderate evidence and efficacy; ±, equivocal; ?, unknown.

ple, illustrate a likely separation between its anticonvulsant and psychotropic effects [9].

The anticonvulsant effects of carbamazepine appear to be acute in most animal models, and clinical antiepileptic effects are readily achieved as adequate doses are administered (Fig. 2). The same appears to be the case for its antinociceptive effects in paroxysmal pain syndromes such as trigeminal neuralgia, in which the therapeutic effect occurs within 1 or 2 days. However, there is usually a delay of several days before carbamazepine exerts its initial efficacy in the treatment of acute mania, and often some weeks until maximum effect is achieved. Finally, as is typical in the time course of most antidepressants, although initial antidepressant effects of carbamazepine may be observed in the first several weeks, it is often 4–6 weeks before maximal effects are achieved [9]. Therefore, if one were examining mechanisms potentially related to antidepressant efficacy of carbamazepine, one would examine animal models and biochemical effects that required chronic administration and/or a considerable time period to develop [10]. Thus, the time required for a given biochemical action may be important in examining potentially relevant mechanisms of psychotropic action, in addition to critical pharmacokinetic variables necessary to a drug's pharmacodynamic effects, i.e., the achievement of clinically relevant blood levels sufficient to induce the mechanism postulated to be involved clinically.

B. Chronic Biochemical Effects as Candidates for Psychotropic Action

There is also a partial parallel between the acute to chronic temporal effects of the anticonvulsants and their presumed molecular targets. Mechanisms related to ion channel effects, neurotransmitter release, and receptor agonism/antagonism or modulation are likely to emerge acutely, whereas a variety of neuroadaptive effects may take place with an intermediate time course, and effects involving long-term changes in gene expression may evolve over longer time domains (in accordance with those changes more likely to be related to the antidepressant effects of these agents) (Fig. 3). An implied corollary of this postulate is that one might be able to find a more acutely active antidepressant if one were able to target the long-term adaptive changes more directly.

For example, it is thought that the cascade of antidepressant effects beginning at the blockade of neurotransmitter reuptake leads to receptor adaptations, changes in adenylate cyclase, the phosphorylation of cyclic AMP response element-binding protein (CREB), and the induction of neurotrophic factors such as brain-derived neurotrophic factor (BDNF) [11,12]. If BDNF were part of the final common pathway of antidepressant effects, one might suggest that direct application of BDNF to appropriate areas of brain could be clinically effective in a rapid fashion [11,13]. BDNF is

Table 2 Putative Mechanisms of Action of Anticonvulsants

Pre-synaptic Effects		Post-synaptic Effects	
Na$^+$ blockade	↓ Glutamate release	↓ Ca^{2+} influx NMDA$_R$	NMDA$_R$ block
(PHT) Phenytoin	(Li) Lithium	(Li) Lithium	(FBM) Felbamate
(CBZ) Carbamazepine	(PHT) Phenytoin	(CBZ) Carbamazepine	
(VPA) Valproate	(LTG) Lamotrigine	(VPA) Valproate	AMPA$_R$ block
			(TPM) Topiramate
(TPM) Topiramate	(CBZ) Carbamazepine	(LTG) Lamotrigine	
(LTG) Lamotrigine			
(ZNS) Zonisamide			
T-Type-Ca^{2+} *(absence seizures)*		GABA-benzodiazepine-Cl$^-$ *ionophore*	
(VPA) Valproate		(VPA) Valproate	(LOR) Lorazepam
(ETX) Ethosuximide		(GPN) Gabapentin	(KLN) Clonazepam
(ZON) Zonisamide		(TIA) Tiagabine	
		(LEV) Levetiracetam*	
Dihydropyridine L-type Ca^{2+} *(voltage sensitive)*			
(NIM) Nimodipine			
(AML) Amlodipine		Peripheral or Mitochondrial-type Benzodiazepine$_R$	
(ISR) Isradipine		(CBZ) Carbamazepine (antagonist)	
		(PK-11195) antagonist	
		(RO5-4864) agonist	
		* Modulatory via ↓ Zn^{2+} and beta-carboline inhibition	

Abbreviations: NMDA$_R$, N-methyl-D-aspartate receptors; AMPA, alpha-amino-3-hydroxy-5-methylisoxazole-4-propionate; GABA, gamma-amimobutryric acid; Na$^+$, sodium channel; Ca^{2+}, calcium channel; Cl$^-$, chloride channel.

positive in a variety of animal models of depression [14], and attempts are being made to find ways of administering BDNF or its analogs to patients for direct tests of this hypothesis.

Because there are not any well-established and convenient animal models of mania and depression [15], in contrast to the many available for the different types of epilepsies [16], one may have to wait until future developments in pharmacogenetics establish that a given mechanism is linked to a manifestation of affective illness, and this in turn is ameliorated by effective treatments and not by those that are ineffective.

One can also use anatomy/anatomical biochemistry to establish a mechanism of action, by confirming that a general defect in metabolism or specific alteration in neurotransmitter receptor function is ameliorated by a given agent in association with its therapeutic effects. As more specific anatomical and biochemical alterations are uncovered using functional brain imaging [17], this approach will likely become increasingly important.

C. Bimodal Effects from a Single Mechanism of Action

A final issue pertinent to considering mechanisms of action of mood stabilizers is their ability to stabilize both manic and depressive moods without exacerbating the other phase. This is in contrast to the unimodal antidepressants which, although effective in unipolar and bipolar depression, can precipitate a switch into mania or accelerate cycling [18,19]. Conversely, particularly with the older typical antipsychotics, although they have clear antimanic properties, some investigators have found that they could be associated with the induction of more severe, prolonged, or frequent depressions [20,21]. Thus, to the extent that one is seeking the mechanisms of mood stabilization as opposed to acute antimanic or acute antidepressant effects, it would appear that one should be looking for bidirectional or neuromodulatory effects on the one hand, or a single dampening mechanism of an overactive system in either an excitatory or an inhibitory part of the brain on the other.

Table 3 Mechanisms of Action of Anticonvulsants

	GABA levels	GABA$_A$-R (indirect)	↓ Na$^+$	Ca^{2+} T N P √	NMDA Ca^{2+}	Glutamate receptor block	Other
VPA[a]	↑		++	T √	↓		Multiple effects on GABA synthesis and catabolism, ↑ K efflux
GPN	↑	√		√			↓ Strychnine-insensitive glycine receptors
TIA	↑						
PRI			++				
PHT			++				
CBZ			++		↓		↑ AVP; ↑ Sub P; ↓ SRIF; ↓ Da T.O., ↑ K efflux
OXC			++	√			↑ K efflux
LTG[a]			++	N? √	↓		
ZNS[a]		√	++	T √			↑↓ DA, 5HT ++ (CA↓) free radical scavenger
TPM		√	++			+++$_{AMPA}$	Carbonic anhydrase ++ (CA ↓) inhibition
FBM[a]		√		√		+++$_{NMDA}$	
LEV[a]		(√)		N?	√		↓ Zn^{2+} and beta-carboline-negative modulation of GABA$_A$-R

[a] Broad-spectrum anticonvulsants.

Abbreviations: VPA, valproate; GPN, gabapentin; TIA, tiagabine; PRI, primidone; PHT, phenytoin; CBZ, carbamazepine; OXC, oxcarbazepine; LTG, lamotrigine; ZNS, zonisamide; TPM, topiramate; FBM, felbamate; LEV, levetiracetam; GABA, gamma-amino butyric acid; NMDA, N-methyl-D-asparate; K, potassium; AVP, activator protein-1; Sub P, substance P; SRIF, somatostatin; Da T.O., dopamine turnover; Ca^{2+}, calcium channel; Na$^+$, sodium channel; 5HT, serotonin; √, voltage dependent.

The latter proposition is highly convergent with the idea that anticonvulsant mechanisms of these drugs are surrogate markers for psychotropic ones. Clearly, seizures represent increased excitability or hypersynchrony of a given brain area and its associated pathways that one would seek to dampen with the use of appropriate anticonvulsant interventions which either decrease excitation or enhance inhibition (Fig. 1) or both. One could readily envision the occurrence of increased neural excitability in systems either enhancing activity or arousal more closely associated with the occurrence of mania, whereas a similar overactive process in largely inhibitory structures or neurotransmitter systems (i.e., those mediating behavioral inhibition) could be associated with the occurrence of depression. Both of these overactive processes could be moderated by the same anticonvulsant effect that decreases paroxysmal neuronal firing.

D. Kindling as a Nonhomologous Model for Affective Disorders

It has been argued elsewhere that the kindling model is clearly a nonhomologous one for the affective disorders in that there is not behavioral homology between seizures and affective episodes and, in fact, there are marked dysjunctions in their duration, inciting circumstances, likely neuroanatomy and chemistry, and clearly in their pharmacology [22]. There is no isomorphism between the agents that are effective in the different stages of kindled seizure evolution and those that are effective in the different stages of bipolar illness evolution. Nonetheless, it is clear that the kindling model reveals the principle that the neurochemistry and neuroanatomy of this pathological neurophysiological process changes as a function of time and stage of kindling evolution, and that drugs effective in one stage are not necessarily effective in another [23,24]. This model allows one to address the question of whether similar temporal distinctions are important in the different stages of affective illness, even though specific drugs that show differential efficacy as a function of stage of illness evolution may not be precisely or predictably parallel from kindled seizures to affective episodes.

Given these clear distinctions between the kindling model and the pharmacology of affective disorders, one might then ask why there is partial overlap

Anticonvulsants and New Mood Stabilizers

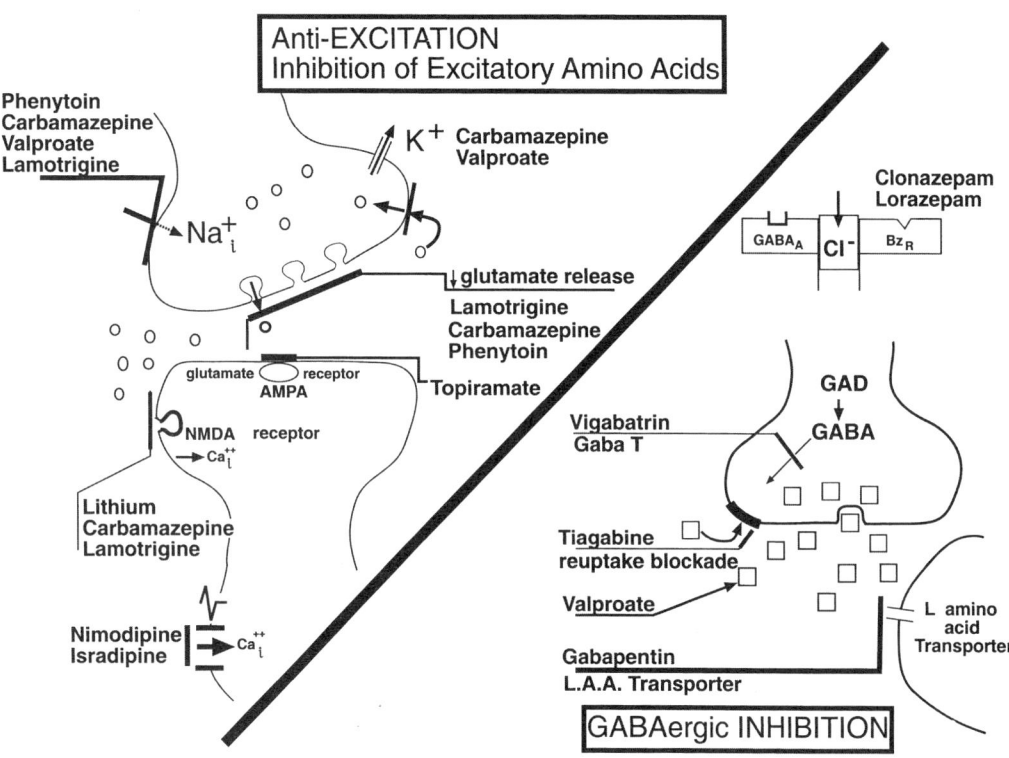

Figure 1 Dual targets of mood stabilizing drugs. NMDA = N-methyl-D-aspartate; GABA = gamma-aminobutyric acid; GAD = glutamate decarboxylase; Bz$_R$ = benzodiazepine receptor; AMPA = alpha-amino-3-hydroxy-5-methyl-4-isoxazolepropionate; L.A.A. = l-amino acid; KT, potassium channel; Na$^+$, sodium channel; Cl$^-$, chloride channel.

between many of the anticonvulsant medications and their ability to exert therapeutic actions in one or both phases of bipolar illness. In this regard, the authors would postulate that at one level of analysis, the principles of antiepileptogenesis and acute and prophylactic anticonvulsant effects that are relevant in the treatment of acute behavioral convulsions may nonetheless share some commonalities with those involved in longer phases of emotion dysregulation. Affective episodes do not involve a motor seizure as an end point, but more likely a more sustained process of regional increased or decreased excitability. It is perhaps this similar ability to dampen overactive circuits related to either the paroxysmal firing of a behavioral convulsion or a more sustained neuronal regional dysregulation pertinent to psychomotor and affective modulation that could relate to the large area of drug overlap with both inherent anticonvulsant and mood-stabilizing properties.

It will also be useful to consider the exceptions to this postulate, i.e., the drugs that are potent anticonvulsant agents which do not have clear antimanic or mood stabilizing properties. These exceptions may also give important hints in a negative sense to mechanisms not likely to be critically involved in psychotropic actions. For example, both tiagabine and gabapentin increase brain gamma-aminobutyric acid (GABA) [25] (Fig. 1; Table 3), but are ineffective in mania (Table 1) [26,27]. Thus, whereas valproate also increases brain GABA, it is likely that some of its other mechanisms are critical to its antimanic efficacy based on the ineffectiveness of tiagabine and gabapentin in mania despite their potent GABA-ergic effects.

The major focus of this chapter will be on the potential anticonvulsant and mood-stabilizing mechanisms of the commonly used medications valproate and carbamazepine, as well as on the most promising of the newer anticonvulsants such as lamotrigine and topiramate. We will also note the putative mechanisms of the newest anticonvulsants such as levetiracetam and zonisamide, even though they have not yet been systematically studied in affective illness. Potential molecular

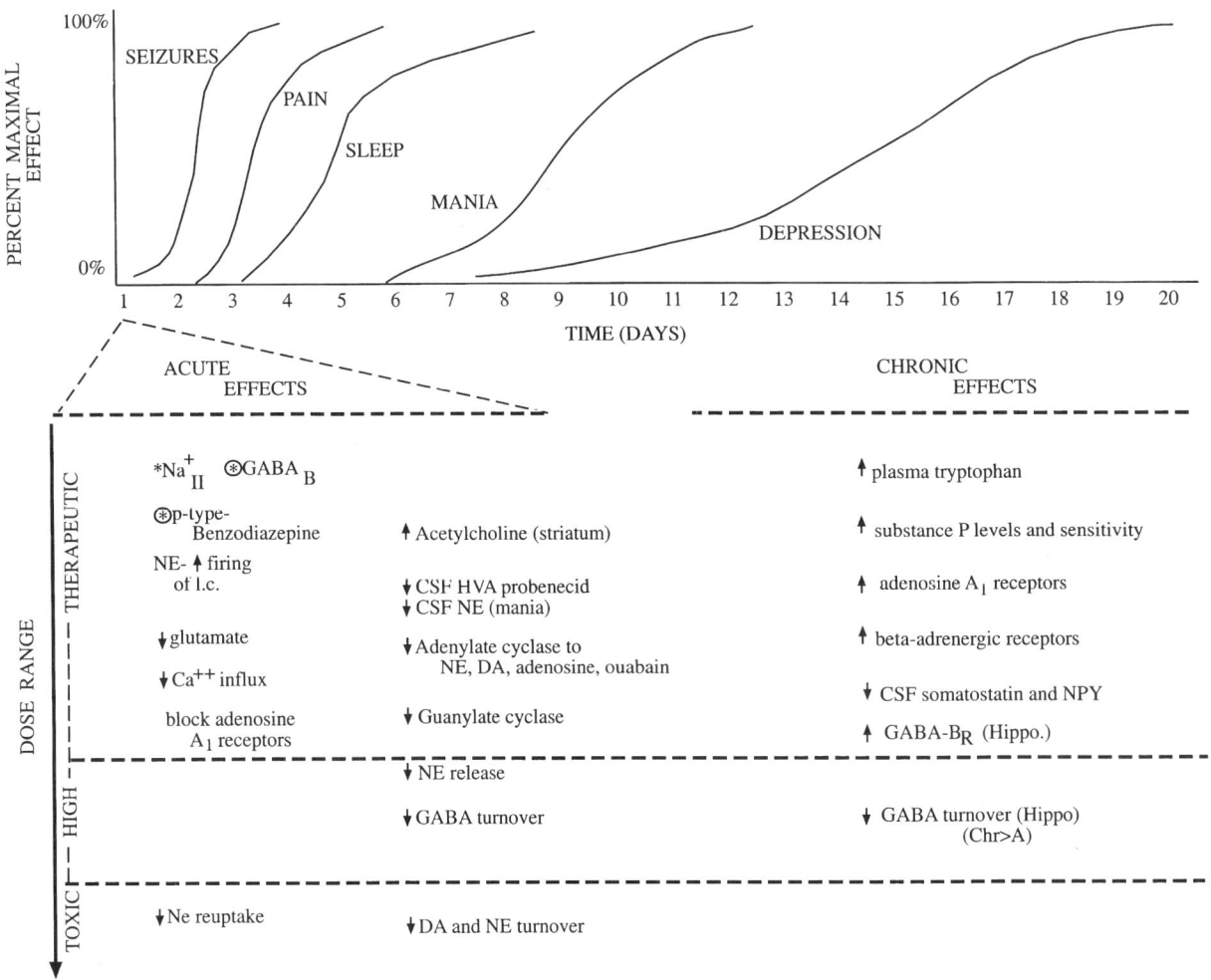

Figure 2 Time course of clinical and biochemical effects of carbamazepine. GABA = gamma-aminobutyric acid; NE = norepinephrine; l.c. = locus ceruleus; CSF = cerebrospinal fluid; HVA = homovanillic acid; DA = dopamine; NPY = neuropeptide Y; Hippo = hippocampus; Na$^+$, sodium channel; Hippo, hippocampus.

mechanisms involved in loss of anticonvulsant efficacy to these agents by tolerance mechanisms will also be reviewed, as these may be important in the possible development of clinical tolerance to the anticonvulsant, antinociceptive, or psychotropic effects of these agents. Relatively pure GABA-ergic drugs such as gabapentin and tiagabine appear less promising.

II. CARBAMAZEPINE AND OXCARBAZEPINE

There is a very substantial database supporting the psychotropic efficacy of carbamazepine [3,28] and a more preliminary database for oxcarbazepine [29–31]. However, the two drugs differ by only one oxygen molecule on the midring of the tricyclic structure and appear to have similar anticonvulsant, antinociceptive, and antimanic properties (on the basis of the few preliminary studies available for the latter findings) [29,30,32]. Thus, until evidence emerges otherwise, we will assume that oxcarbazepine is a similar congener or sister drug to carbamazepine and that many of the principles of their actions will be in parallel. However, it is clear that oxcarbazepine is a much less potent hepatic P450 enzyme inducer and therefore yields fewer pharmacokinetic interactions, and is clinically easier to use with other agents [33]. It may emerge

Anticonvulsants and New Mood Stabilizers

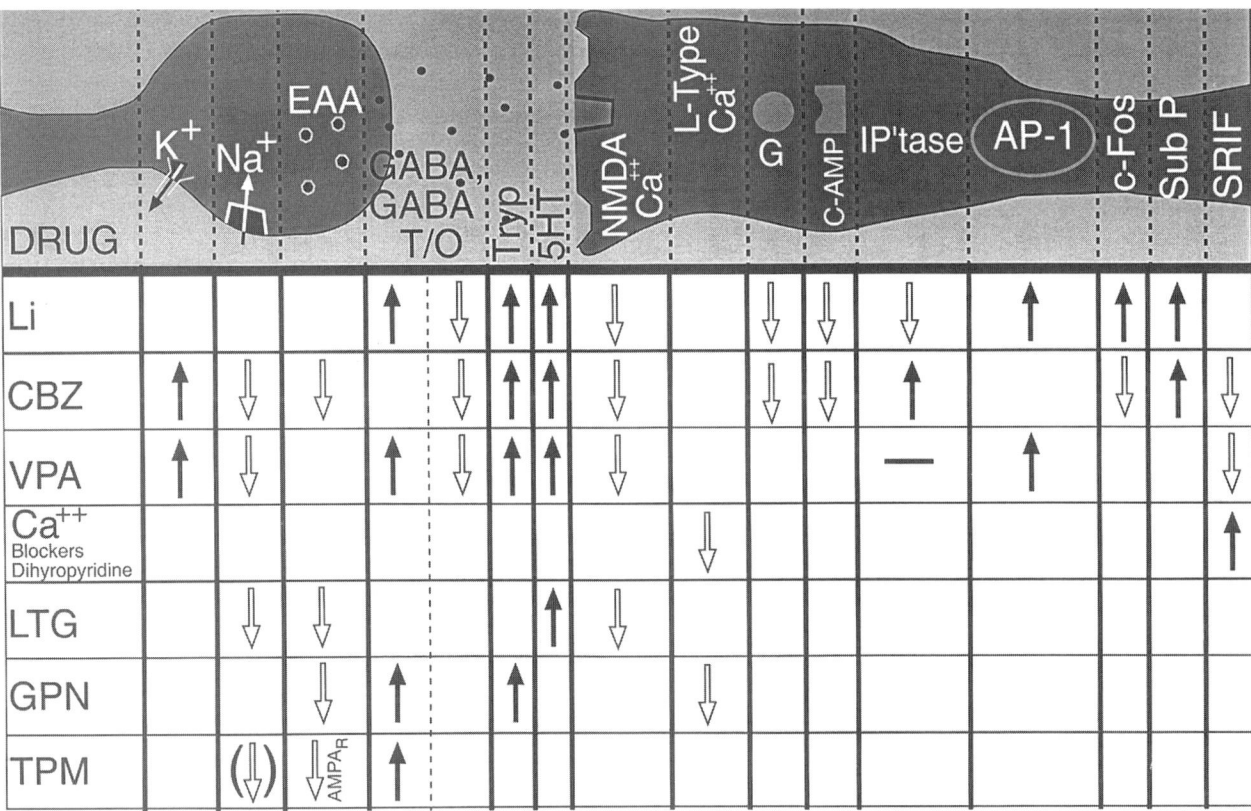

Figure 3 Mechanisms of mood stabilization. Depicted schematically at the top of the figure is a synapse with various types of channels, neurotransmitters, and proteins associated with the mechanisms of action of the mood stabilizers listed in the table below. Arrows indicate increases or decreases in substance/activity. *Row headings*: Li, lithium; CBZ, carbamazepine; VPA, valproate; Ca, calcium; LTG, lamotrigine; GPN, gabapentin; TPM, topiranmate. *Column headings*: K, potassium efflux; Na, sodium influx; EAA, excitatory amino acids; GABA, GABA t.o., gamma-aminobutyric acid, GABA turnover; Tryp, tryptophan; 5HT, serotonin; NMDA Ca, N-methyl-D-aspartate calcium channel; L-type Ca, L-type calcium channel; G, G protein; c-AMP, cyclic adenosine monophosphatase; IPtase, inositol monophosphatase; AP-1, activator protein-1; Sub P, substance P; SRIF, somatostatin.

that there are also substantial differences in pharmacodynamic effects as well as these major differences in catabolism.

Although carbamazepine, phenytoin, and lamotrigine show the ability to potently block batrachotoxin type-2 sodium channels [34,35] (Fig. 1) and therefore decrease release of excitatory amino acids and inhibit sustained rapid firing, there appear to be substantial differences in their clinical profiles. Carbamazepine is much more potent than phenytoin in inhibiting amygdala kindling compared with cortical kindling [36], a potential marker of clinical utility in complex partial seizures and other dysrhythmias of the limbic system.

In addition, whereas both phenytoin and carbamazepine can exacerbate *petit mal* or *absence* epilepsy, lamotrigine does not and may even be clinically useful in the syndrome as well [37]. Thus, some other mechanisms of action of these agents must account for these pharmacological and clinical differences.

Carbamazepine and lamotrigine both likely modulate calcium influx through the NMDA receptor [38,39] and lamotrigine may also affect N- or P-type calcium channels [40,41]. Carbamazepine also blocks peripheral-type benzodiazepine receptors (also called the mitochondrial-type benzodiazepine receptor) [42–44]. This receptor is thought to affect calcium influx not only at neural and glial membranes, but also at the mitochondrial permeability transition pore, modulating cholesterol transport [45–47] (Fig. 4).

Although noradrenergic effects are important to carbamazepine's anticonvulsant effects in some models, they do not appear to be directly related to its psychotropic effects. Carbamazepine's blockade of norepinephrine reuptake is weak [48], although it does block stimulation-induced release of norepinephrine at clinically relevant concentrations (a sodium channel-mediated event) [49] and may decrease norepinephrine turnover [50], as do many other antidepressant compounds.

However, many of carbamazepine's effects are not only uncharacteristic of, but even opposite to, those of traditional antidepressants. Instead of decreasing forebrain beta-adrenergic receptor expression, carbamazepine appears to increase it [51]. Most antidepressants decrease cortisol, presumably in part by downregulating corticotropin-releasing factor (CRF) receptors or upregulating glucocorticoid receptors, but carbamazepine appears to increase cortisol excretion as measured

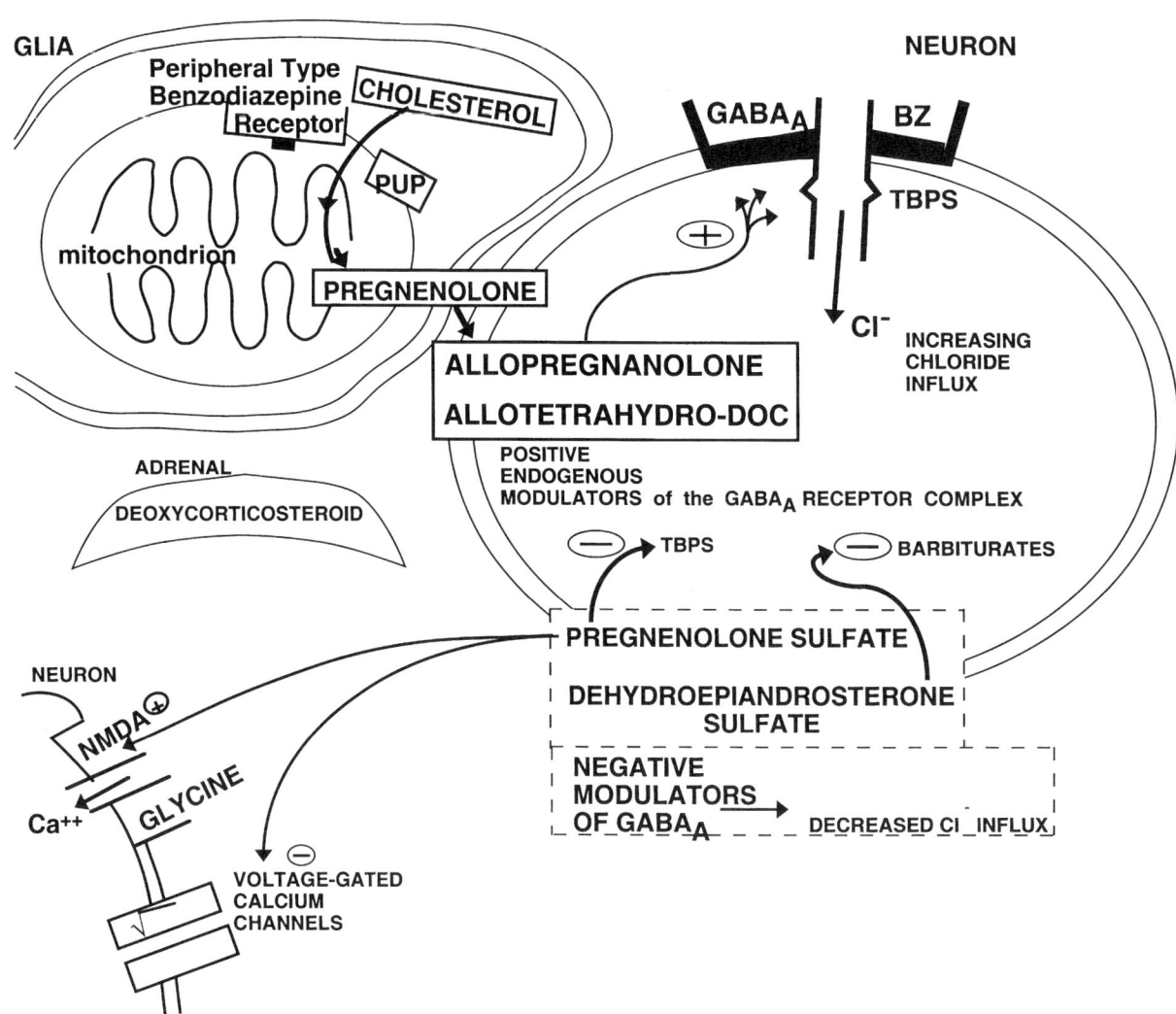

Figure 4 Peripheral-type benzodiazepine ligands modulate multiple receptors and ion channels via neurosteroids. GABA, gamma-aminobutyric acid; BZ, benzodiazepine; TBPS, [35S]-tert-butylbicyclophosphorothionate; NMDA, N-methyl-D-aspartate; Cl$^-$, chloride channel; Ca^{++}, calcium channel.

by urinary free cortisol [52]. At the same time, carbamazepine appears to decrease release of CRF in some *in vitro* hypothalamic preparations [53,54]. These or other differences from traditional antidepressants may account for the fact that carbamazepine can exert acute and prophylactic antidepressant effects in some unipolar and bipolar depressed patients who have not responded to more traditional antidepressant modalities [55,56].

In addition to these acute effects, carbamazepine has a variety of effects on neuropeptide systems that are likely to be pertinent to its profile of either therapeutic efficacy or side effects in the affective disorders (Fig. 3). Chronic administration of carbamazepine in patients with both seizure and affective disorders is associated with a decrease in somatostatin in cerebrospinal fluid (CSF) [57]. Presumably, this reflects a decrease in brain somatostatin, although the regional neurochemistry of this effect has not yet been delineated. This decrement in CSF somatostatin contrasts with the increases in CSF somatostatin observed following chronic administration of the dihydropyridine L-type calcium channel blocker nimodipine [58].

Carbamazepine and nimodipine also block calcium influx through different mechanisms [59] (Fig. 5), and appear to have different predictors and correlates of clinical response observed in clinical neuroimaging with deoxyglucose [60]. Affectively ill patients with evi-

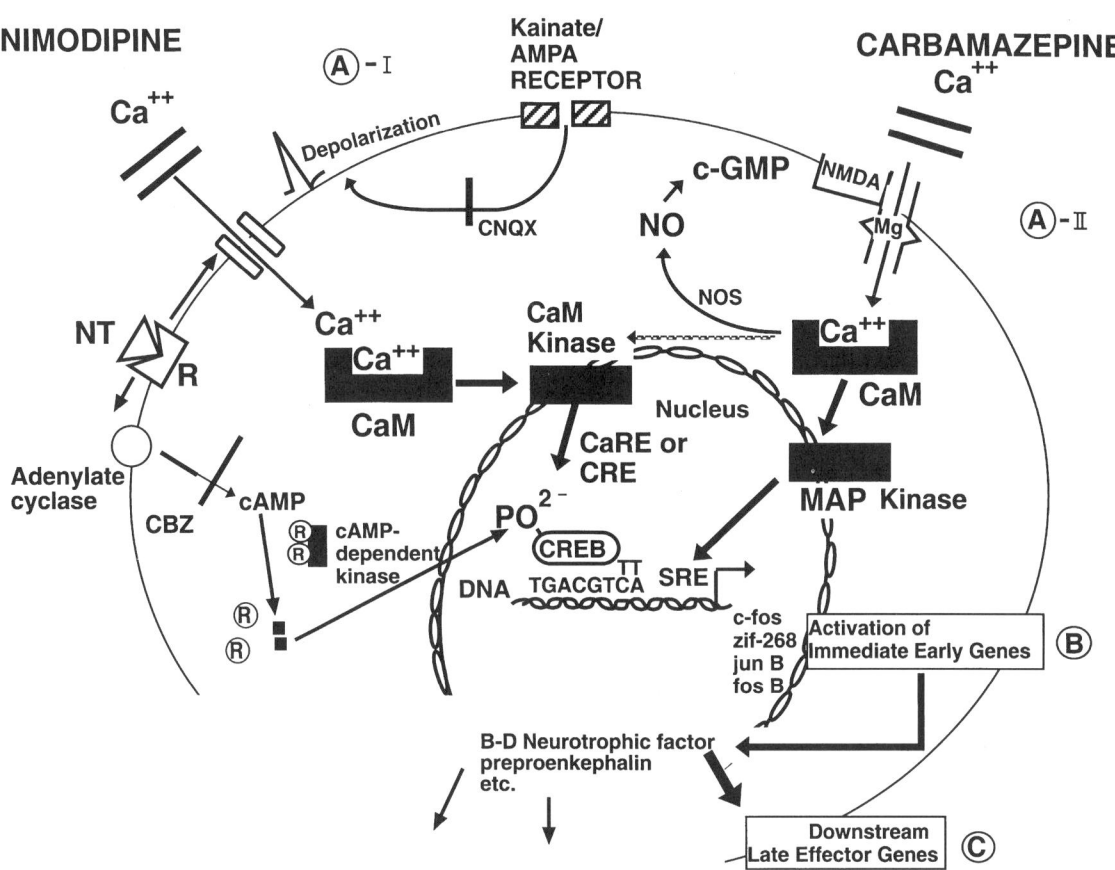

Figure 5 Differential targets of carbamazepine and nimodipine on intracellular calcium. AMPA, alpha-amino-3-hydroxy-5-methyl-4-isoxazolepropionate; B-D, brain derived; CaM, calmodulin; CaRE, calcium-response element; cGMP, cyclic guanosine monophosphate; CNQX, 6-cyano-7-nitroquinoxaline-2,3-dione; CRE, cyclic adenosine monophosphate (cAMP)-response element; CREB, cAMP response element-binding protein; MAP, mitogen-activated protein; NMDA, N-methyl-D-aspartate; NO, nitric oxide; NOS, nitric oxide synthase; NT, neurotrophin; R, receptor; SRE, serum response element; PO^2, phosphorylated CREB; CBZ, carbamazepine; Ca^{++}, calcium channel; Mg, magnesium.

dence of hypermetabolism, particularly in the left insula at baseline, appear to respond better to carbamazepine in association with normalization of this hyperactivity. Nimodipine shows the opposite pattern with better responses in those with baseline hypoactivity, which tends to normalize in association with treatment response. Whether these differential effects are directly or indirectly related to the alterations in somatostatin remains to be clarified. There is a direct positive correlation with the degree of metabolism in the subgenual anterior cingulate gyrus and the concentration of somatostatin in CSF [61]. The subgenual area of the cingulate has been one of the brain regions most closely associated with alterations not only in metabolism, but also in neuroanatomy, with substantial deficits reported in the number of glial cells in this area of brain in those with familial unipolar and bipolar affective disorders [62–64].

Carbamazepine increases striatal substance P levels and substance P sensitivity upon chronic (but not acute) administration, which is interesting in relation to observations that chronic, but not acute, treatment with lithium also increases substance P levels in the striatum [65–67] (Table 4). These observations, and a variety of antidepressants increase substance P sensitivity [68], and that a substance P antagonist [69] exhibited antidepressant effects equal to that of the conventional SSRI paroxetine (both were more effective than placebo), all suggest a potential role for substance P alterations in antidepressant effectiveness [70].

Carbamazepine's effects on vasopressinergic systems are more likely related to its side-effects profile than its therapeutic efficacy. Carbamazepine appears to indirectly enhance vasopressinergic function at or near the receptor, which may account for the fact that lithium's inhibition of vasopressin actions (by inhibiting transduction mechanisms at the level of adenylate cyclase inhibition, i.e., downstream of the receptor) is not able to be surmounted by carbamazepine [71]. Thus, carbamazepine will not reverse lithium-induced diabetes insipidus. In some animal models, carbamazepine is able to enhance some measures of learning and memory [72], and whether its vasopressinergic profile or some other effect accounts for these observations also needs to be further delineated. However, carbamazepine's ability to enhance antidiuretic effects at the vasopressin receptor is likely associated with its liability to induce hyponatremia [73–75]. Lithium is able to counter the effects of carbamazepine on hyponatremia, as is demeclocycline [76–78]. It remains to be directly assessed whether either of these agents would also be effective in ameliorating the hyponatremia of oxcarbazepine, which may occur in 1–3% of patients.

III. VALPROATE: SIMILARITIES AND DIFFERENCES FROM LITHIUM

Although valproate increases brain GABA through a variety of effects on GABA synthesis and degradation [32,79], there is considerable controversy as to whether this is directly related to its anticonvulsant or psychotropic efficacy [80]. Valproate also blocks sodium channel influx, and T-type calcium channels, and enhances potassium channel efflux [81–83]. It also shares a number of mechanisms of action with carbamazepine (Table 5), and with lithium carbonate, making these mechanisms candidate systems for its psychotropic efficacy, including the ability to inhibit protein kinase C (PKC) (Table 6) [84] and other downstream effects in this signal transduction cascade

Table 4 Effects of Lithium and Carbamazepine on Substance P

	Lithium	Carbamazepine
Acute Treatment		
↑ Substance P levels	None	None
↑ Substance P sensitivity	None	None
Chronic Treatment		
Substance P levels	↑ Striatum	↑ Striatum
	↑ Substantia nigra	↑ Substantia nigra
	↑ Nucleus accumbens	
	↑ Frontal cortex	
↑ Substance P is haloperidol-reversible	Yes	Yes
↑ Substance P sensitivity	?	Yes

Table 5 Comparative Effects of Two Anticonvulsant Mood Stabilizers in Bipolar Illness

	Carbamazepine	Valproate
GABA turnover[a]	↓	↓
GABA_B receptors[a] (hippocampus)	↑	↑
GABA levels	(↑)	↑
prepulse inhibition	0	↑
[^{3}H]-picrotoxinin binding	↓	↓
Dopamine turnover[a]	↓	↓
Na$^+$ influx	↓	↓
K$^+$ efflux	↑	↑
NMDA-mediated currents	(↓)	↓
NMDA-mediated Ca^{2+} influx	↓	
Release of aspartate	↓	↓
Somatostatin levels	↓	↓
Substantia nigra lesions block CBZ's anticonvulsant effects on kindling	++	0
Decrease AD in:		
Hippocampus	—	↓
Cortex	↓	—

[a] Effects shared by lithium.
Abbreviations: GABA, gamma-aminobutyric acid; NMDA, N-methyl-D-aspartate; CBZ, carbamazepine; AD, afterdischarge; Na$^+$, sodium channel; K$^+$, potassium channel; Ca^{2+}, calcium channel
Symbols: ↑, increase; ↓, decrease; ( ), equivocal; 0, none; —, not relevant, no evidence.

[85], inhibit glycogen synthase kinase-3 (GSK-3) [86,87], increase activator protein-1 (AP-1) binding [88,89], activate Akt (also known as protein kinase B) [90], and induce the neuroprotective factor Bcl-2 [91].

Recent studies have shown that lithium exerts neurotrophic or neuroprotective effects [92–94]. Moreover, it has been demonstrated in cultured neurons that lithium increases activity of the serine/theronine protein kinase Akt (Fig. 6) [90]. Akt is known as a key regulator of cellular survival [95]. The identification of Akt as a target for lithium may have significant implications for an understanding of its neuroprotective mechanism. Several targets of Akt have been recently identified that may underlie the ability of this regulatory kinase to promote survival. These substrates include two components of the intrinsic cell death machinery, BAD [96] and caspase-9 [97], transcription factors of the forkhead family [98], CREB [99], endothelial NOS [100], and a kinase, IKK, that regulates the NF-kB transcription factor [101]. Moreover, activated Akt is involved in the potentiation of L-type calcium channels [102], inhibition of the cytochrome C release from the mitochondria [103], and inactivation of a critical regulator of cellular metabolism GSK-3 [104]. It has been recently determined that not only lithium but also valproate induces activation of Akt in cultured neurons (Chalecka-Franaszek, unpublished information). Lithium also

Table 6 Drug Effects on Protein Kinase C (PKC) Isozymes and Substrates

	Lithium	VPA
PKC activity	↓	↓
PKC α	↓	↓
PKC ε	↓	↓
MARCKS levels	↓	↓
AP-1 binding activity	↑	↑
Inositol responsive	+	—

MARCKS, myristoylated alanine-rich C kinase substrate; AP-1, activator protein 1; VPA, valproate; ↑ increase; ↓ decrease; +, yes; —, unknown, no effect

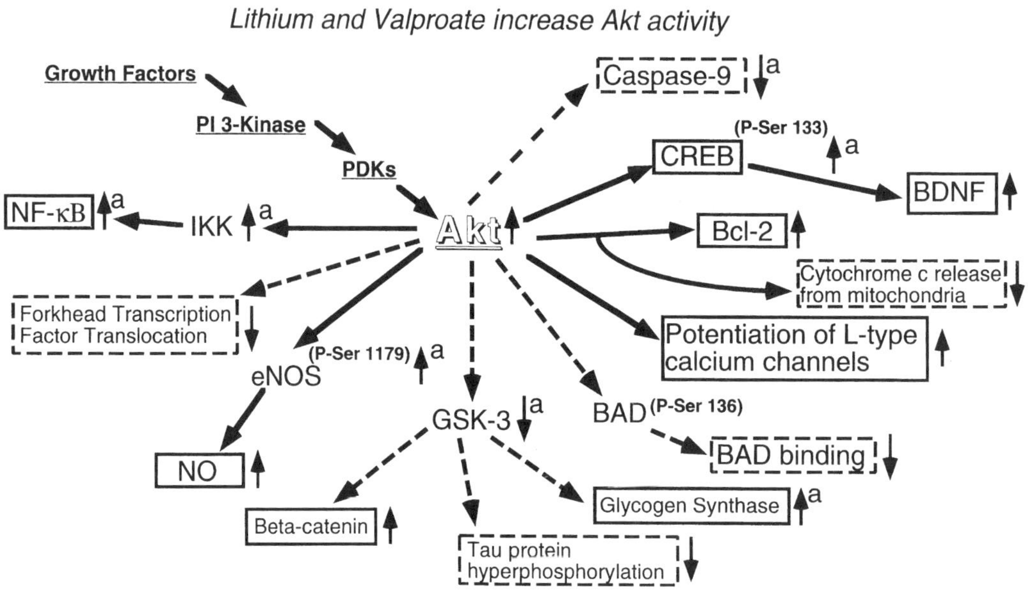

Lithium and Valproate increase Akt activity

Figure 6 Drug effects on Akt: possible downstream consequences. PI 3-kinase. phosphatidylinositol 3-kinase; PDKs, phosphoinositide-dependent kinases; NF-êB, nuclear factor-kappaB; IKK, IkappaB kinase; eNOS, endothelial nitric oxide synthase; NO, nitric oxide; GSK-3, glycogen synthase kinase-3; BDNF, brain-derived neurotrophic factor; CREB, cAMP response element-binding protein.

enhances neuroprotective factors such as brain-derived neurotrophic factor (BDNF) while inhibiting cell death factors such as Bax and p53 [92,105]. These and other neural intracellular mechanisms may account for lithium's apparent neuroprotective effects in a variety of animal models including stroke [93], Huntington's chorea [106], and in vitro protection for an AIDS-related neurodegenerative process [107]. Whether valproate and other putative mood-stabilizing anticonvulsants share lithium's apparent neuroprotective effects via mechanisms listed above, remains to be further delineated (Fig. 7). In addition, lithium has recently been shown to increase neurogenesis [108], an effect shared by some antidepressants [109] and opposite that of some stressors [110]. Together, these data may explain why lithium has recently been observed to increase human brain gray matter volume in subjects treated for 4 weeks [111] and to increase brain N-acetyl-aspartate (NAA) [112], a putative marker of neuronal viability and function.

Recently, lithium, carbamazepine, and valproate have all been shown to increase inositol transport, also raising the possibility that this could be a common mechanism involved in their mood-stabilizing properties [113].

IV. LAMOTRIGINE

Lamotrigine has particular promise as an effective treatment for the depressive phase of bipolar illness with evidence of mood stabilization in rapid-cycling patients [27,114,115]. Aside from the occurrence of serious rash in approximately one of every 500 patients [116], its side-effects profile is benign and well targeted toward many of the symptoms more prominently evident in bipolar depression. In contrast to lithium and valproate, lamotrigine does not increase weight and appears to be somewhat activating and able to decrease the hypersomnia of bipolar depression, rather than sedating and setting a psychomotor baseline slightly below normal.

As noted previously in Figure 1, lamotrigine is thought to block type 2 sodium channels [117], decrease release of glutamate [118], and inhibit calcium influx through the NMDA receptor (Hough et al., 1998, unpublished observations). However, it is likely to have other important mechanisms that could account for its additional effects in blocking absence seizures and a broader spectrum of both anticonvulsant and psychotropic actions than carbamazepine. Data suggest that lamotrigine may also be active at N- or P-type calcium channels [40,41], but

Anticonvulsants and New Mood Stabilizers

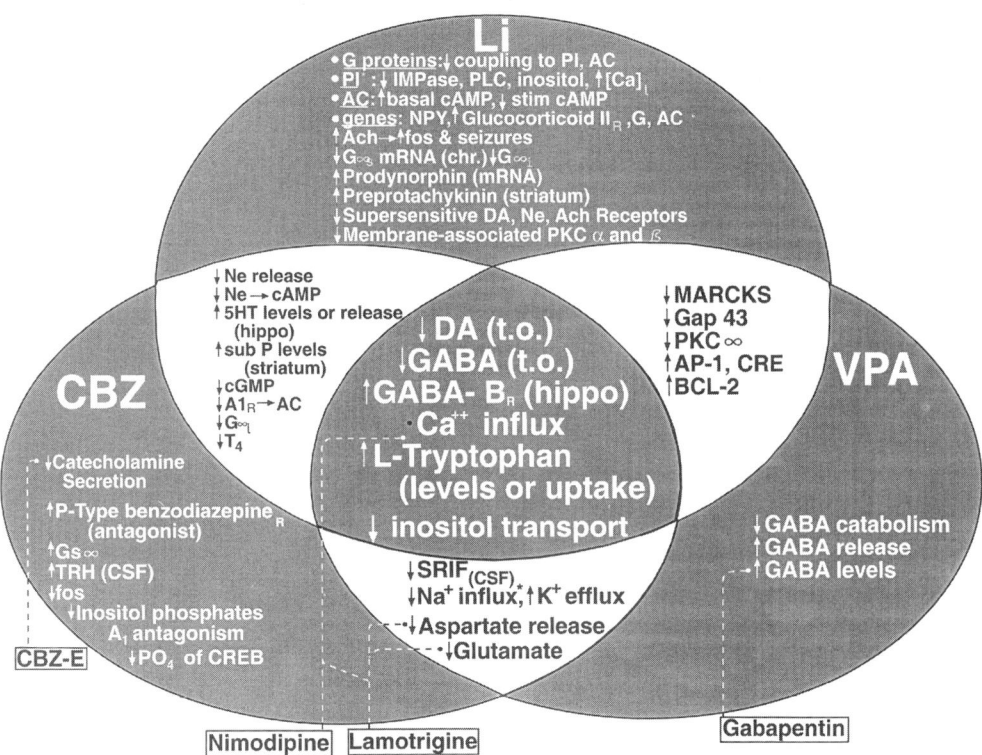

Figure 7 Common and differential mechanisms of mood stabilizers. PI, phosphoinositol; AC, adenylate cyclase; IMPase, inositol monophosphatase; PLC, phospholipase C; cAMP, cyclic adenosine monophosphate; NPY, neuropeptide Y; Ach, acetylcholine; $G\alpha_s$, G protein alpha (s) subunit; DA, dopamine; Ne, norepinephrine; PKC, protein kinase C; $A1_R$, adenosine A1 receptors; T_4, thyroxine; Gap 43, growth-associated protein 43; CRE, cyclic response element; CBZ, carbamazepine; TRH, thyrotropin-releasing hormone; CREB, cyclic response element-binding protein; VPA, valproate; SRIF, somatostatin; t.o., turnover; GABA, gamma-aminobutyric acid; CSF, cerebrospinal fluid; MARCKS, myristoylated alanine-rich C kinase substrate; cGMP, cyclic guanosine 3′,5′-monophosphate; CBZ-E, carbamazepine epoxide; PO_4, phosphorylation; 5HT, serotonin; sub P, substance P; cGMP, cyclic guanosine monophosphate; Na^+, sodium channel; K^+, potassium channel.

other differential mechanisms remain to be elucidated (Fig. 8).

V. TOPIRAMATE

Consistent with its broad spectrum of anticonvulsant action, topiramate has multiple putative mechanisms of action. In addition to its ability to block sodium channels and thus presumptively decrease glutamate and other excitatory amino acid release [119], topiramate indirectly enhances GABA-ergic mechanisms through an unclear molecular effect [120,121]. It also directly inhibits binding at the AMPA/kainate subtype of glutamate receptors [120], which may account for some of its broader spectrum of anticonvulsant action because AMPA receptor activity is necessary for the expression (as opposed to development) of long-term potentiation (LTP) [122]. This mechanism could account for topiramate's proclivity to impair some aspects of cognition, particularly upon rapid dose escalation [123,124]. This latter effect tends to involve speech and word-finding difficulties in a small percentage of patients. It is also possible that topiramate's ability to block AMPA receptors could account for other aspects of its psychotropic profile, including the preliminary report of its potential promise in the treatment of posttraumatic stress disorder (PTSD) [125]. To the extent that AMPA receptors are crucial to the maintenance of LTP, and PTSD involves an overactive replay of memory circuits, blockade of AMPA receptors could be of clinical importance.

As a carbonic anhydrase inhibitor, topiramate possesses an approximately 1% risk of causing renal calculi [126]. These are reportedly less frequent in women than in men, and are likely to respond rapidly to litho-

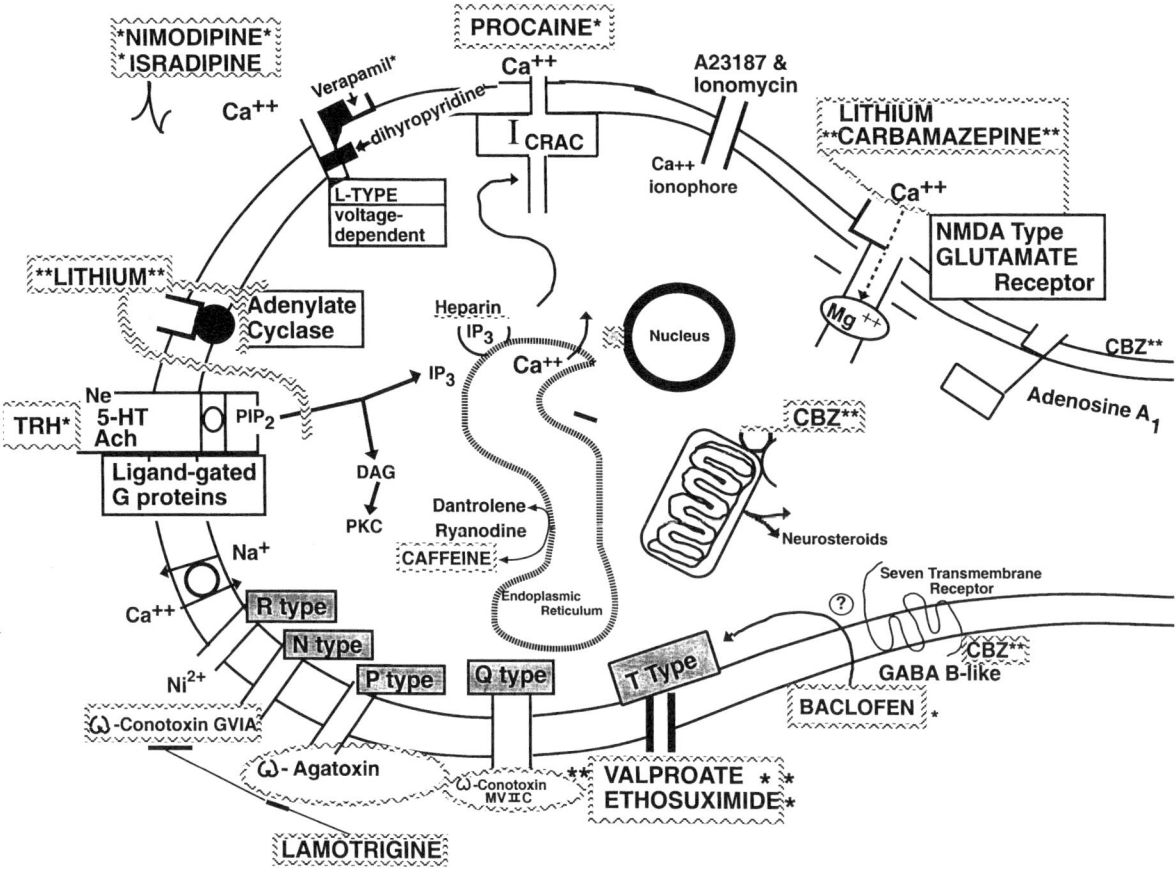

Figure 8 Calcium channel diversity and drug targets. CBZ, carbamazepine; 5-HT, serotonin; TRH, thyrotrophin-releasing hormone; Ach, acetylcholine; PKC, protein kinase C; DAG, diacylglycerol; IP$_3$, inositol 1,4,5-trisphosphate; MBR, mitochondrial (or peripheral-type) benzodiazepine receptor; NMDA, N-methyl-D-aspartate receptor; PIP$_2$, phosphatidylinositol-4,5-biphosphate; Ca^{++}, calcium channel; Na$^+$, sodium channel; Mg^{++}, magnesium channel.

tripsy treatment in an emergency room setting because the calculi are usually calcium based. It is noteworthy that in uncontrolled but long-term follow-up trials in clinical practice settings, more patients remained on topiramate than on gabapentin or lamotrigine [127], suggesting that for the sake of therapeutic efficacy, patients are willing to tolerate a modicum of side effects with this agent.

VI. GABAPENTIN AND TIAGABINE: ENHANCERS OF BRAIN GABA

Both gabapentin and tiagabine increase brain GABA [128] (Table 3). Tiagabine is a highly selective inhibitor of GABA reuptake. The mechanism of increasing GABA is somewhat obscure for gabapentin, although actions on the GABA transporter are thought to contribute. Gabapentin has other actions on calcium channels and on strychnine-insensitive glycine receptors [129]. Although it was originally synthesized as a GABA agonist, it possesses no direct effects at the GABA$_A$ receptor [129]. Whereas a series of open studies have suggested the efficacy of adjunctive gabapentin in bipolar disorders, two controlled studies do not support this conclusion for mania [27,130]. In the controlled trial of 6 weeks of monotherapy in patients with refractory mood disorders, the 28% response rate to gabapentin was not significantly (statistically) different from the 23% response rate achieved with placebo, and both were inferior to lamotrigine [27]. Moreover, in some patients, gabapentin appeared to exacerbate manic components of the illness, including cycle acceleration or increasing the severity of manic presentations. These data parallel those of Pande et al. [130], who reported that in a randomized double-blind study in acute mania, gabapentin augmentation did not exceed that of placebo.

Two studies suggest that tiagabine is not an effective antimanic or mood-stabilizing agent. Grunze and colleagues [26] treated 10 patients with tiagabine and none responded, and one patient who had not had a previous seizure disorder experienced a major motor seizure. Little evidence of efficacy was observed in an open add-on case series of 17 patients with bipolar illness (Suppes et al., 2000, unpublished observation). Again, there was one definitive occurrence of a seizure and another in which there was likely a seizure.

The findings that these two agents, which enhance brain GABA levels via two different mechanisms and are not likely to possess antimanic properties, suggest that the ability of valproate to increase brain GABA is not sufficient to account for its antimanic efficacy, and other candidate mechanisms should be sought. These data are, to some extent, convergent with the findings of lower CSF GABA in depressed patients, and increasing or normalizing CSF GABA with a switch into mania [131,132]. Perhaps these agents should be further explored in controlled trials of the depressive phase of the illness, given this putative deficit in brain GABA in this phase of the illness.

What might account for gabapentin's widespread use in the affective disorders, given its unlikely utility as an antimanic or mood-stabilizing agent? It is possible that effects of gabapentin on other symptoms and syndromes that are often comorbid in patients with bipolar illness may account for this phenomenon. For example, gabapentin is reported to be effective in controlled trials in the treatment of social phobia [133] and holds promise in other anxiety disorders [134,135]. Forty percent of the patients in the Stanley Foundation Bipolar Network have a comorbid anxiety disorder diagnosis [136,137]. Similarly, gabapentin has been suggested to have a role in the treatment of obsessive-compulsive disorder [138]; a variety of pain syndromes, tremor, and restless leg syndromes [139–141]; and perhaps parkinsonism [142].

In the NIMH clinical trial [27], although gabapentin response was not statistically significantly different from placebo, a positive clinical response was correlated with younger age, shorter duration of illness, and a lower weight at baseline entry into the study [143]. It is possible that the high doses that were used (averaging 3000–4000 mg/day) were too high for older patients, and more systematic controlled trials of both lower doses and younger populations would appear indicated.

VII. LEVETIRACETAM

Although, to our knowledge, there have been no case reports or systematic studies of the potential psychotropic effects of levetiracetam, it nonetheless remains a drug of considerable interest for further investigation. It appears to have a unique mechanism of action unshared by most of the other anticonvulsants, because it has not been shown to act at any neurotransmitter, receptor reuptake site, or ion channel among the many traditional candidates that have been tested based on the action of other psychotropic agents and anticonvulsants [144–146]. Recent data suggest that levetiracetam may decrease intracellular Ca^{2+}, but the precise site of action for this effect remains uncertain. Levetiracetam inhibits the ability of zinc ions and beta-carboline to negatively modulate $GABA_A$ receptors, thus enhancing chloride influx. It also decreases both neuronal hyperexcitability and hypersynchronization [147,148]. Additional support for its potential unique actions are the findings that it is not active in the traditional models for major motor and *absence* seizures, i.e., maximal electroshock (MES) and pentylenetetrazol, respectively [149]. Moreover, in contrast to many other agents, such as carbamazepine, phenytoin, and lamotrigine, which are not active in preventing the development of amygdala kindling (epileptogenesis), levetiracetam is an effective agent in preventing both the development and the expression of amygdala-kindled seizures [150]. These findings, taken with its apparently benign side-effects profile, make it an ideal candidate for further exploration in the affective disorders with the hope that its anti-epileptogenic properties in the initial phases of kindling may parallel other preventive effects in the affective disorders.

VIII. ZONISAMIDE

This recently approved adjunctive agent for partial onset seizures has multiple putative mechanisms of action. These include blockade of voltage dependent sodium channels; blockade of T-type, but possible enhancement of N-type channels; biphasic modulation of serotonin function; and free radical scavaging [151–155]. Kanba et al. [156] reported that open-label addition of zonisamide (100–600 mg/day) to other mood-stabilizing agents was associated with improvement in 80% of 15 acutely manic patients, but no controlled studies have been reported.

IX. LOSS OF ANTICONVULSANT EFFICACY: THE CONTINGENT TOLERANCE MODEL

A loss of efficacy to the prophylactic effects of a wide range of psychotropic agents is becoming increasingly evident in a small subgroup of affectively ill patients in the course of long-term treatment and followup. This has been noted for antidepressants and monoamine oxidase inhibitors [157,158] and the SSRIs [159].

Some of the molecular mechanisms of tolerance to the anticonvulsant effects of carbamazepine on amygdala-kindled seizures have been elucidated [160]. This type of tolerance is associative or "contingent" upon the drug's being present at the time of the seizure and is not based solely on repeated or chronic drug administration per se, i.e., pharmacodynamic tolerance (Fig. 9). Kindled seizures normally elicit a host of changes in gene expression leading to both pathological and adaptive (anticonvulsant) mechanisms, which lower and raise seizure threshold, respectively. During tolerance to the anticonvulsant effects of carbamazepine, some of the putative anticonvulsant mechanisms fail to be induced despite the occurrence of a full-blown seizure, because the presence of carbamazepine (Fig. 10). These include the failure of normal seizure-induced increases in the mRNA for TRH [161], the alpha-4 subunit of $GABA_A$ receptors (but not benzodiazepine receptors) [162], mineralocorticoid (but not glucocorticoid) receptors, and CRH and its binding protein CRH-BP [160]. Whereas CRH is usually thought to be proconvulsant, in the hippocampus, it is colocalized in GABA interneurons and thus could be part of an inhibitory pathway.

In tolerant animals, if seizures are induced in the absence of drug (either if it is discontinued or if it is administered immediately after the kindled stimulation rather than before), anticonvulsant efficacy (and the associated increase in seizure threshold produced by carbamazepine in the medication-free situation) is

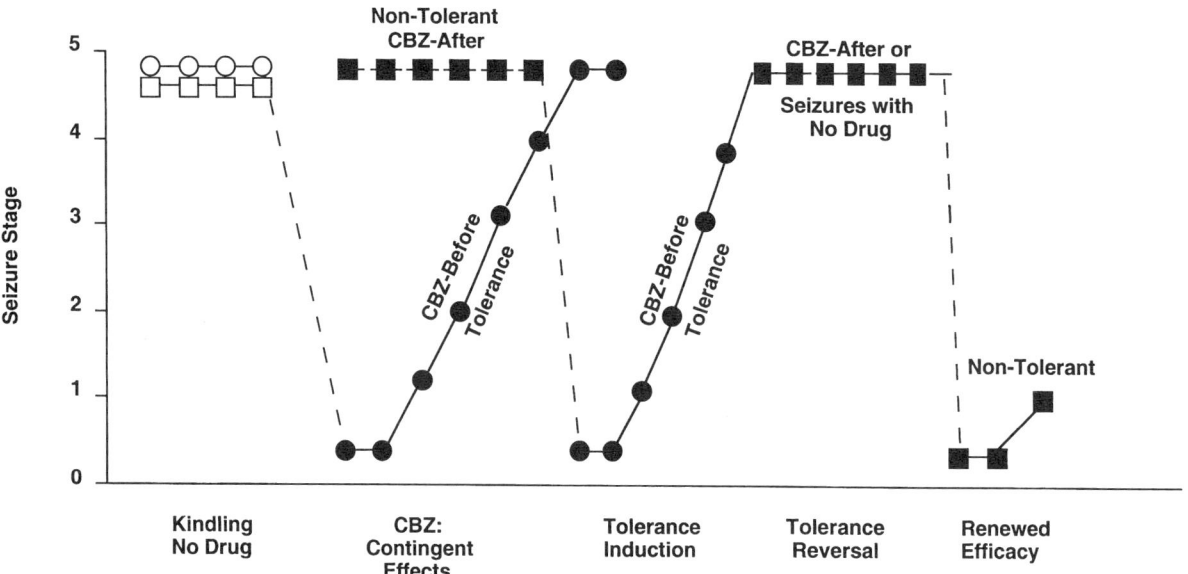

Figure 9 Schematic illustration of contingent tolerance to carbamazepine: development and reversal. In fully kindled animals (open circles), carbamazepine treatment (filled circles) inhibits kindled seizures. Repeated drug administration *before* (filled circles) but not after (filled squares), stimulation results in tolerance development. Tolerance induced in this manner can be reversed by a period of kindled seizures without drugs or with drug administration *after* each seizure (filled squares).

Anticonvulsants and New Mood Stabilizers

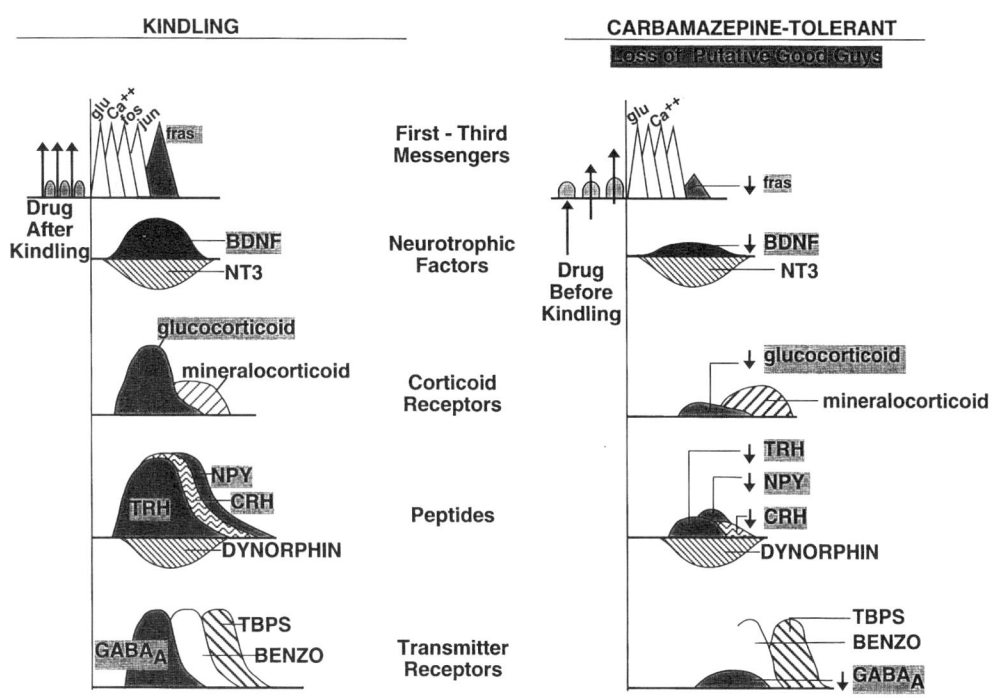

Figure 10 Competing pathological and adaptive endogenous responses to kindled seizures. Tolerance is associated with loss of selective kindling-induced effects on gene expression. Schematic illustration of potential transcription factor, neurotransmitter, and peptidergic alterations that follow repeated kindled seizures. Putative mechanisms related to the lasting primary pathological drive (i.e., kindled seizure evolution) are illustrated on top, and those thought to be related to the more transient secondary compensatory responses (i.e., anticonvulsant effects) are shown on the bottom. The horizontal line represents time. Sequential transient increases (above line) or decreases (below the line) in second messengers, immediate early genes, and neurotrophic factors are followed by longer-lasting alterations in peptides, neurotransmitters, and receptors or their mRNAs. Given the unfolding of these competing mechanisms in the evolution of seizures and their remission, the question arises as to whether parallel opposing processes also occur in the course of affective illness or other psychiatric disorders. Such endogenous adaptive changes may be exploited in the design of the new treatment strategies. fras, fos-related antigens; NT3, neurotrophin-3; BDNF, brain-derived neurotrophic factor; NPY, neuropeptide Y; CRH, corticotropin-releasing hormone; TRH, thyrotrophin-releasing hormone; TBPS, [35S]-tert-butylbicyclophosphorothionate; GABA, gamma-aminobutyric acid; BENZO, benzodiazepine receptors; glu, glutamate; Ca^{++}, calcium channel.

restored. This is presumably because some of the compensatory endogenous, seizure-induced anticonvulsant mechanisms have now been able to reemerge in the absence of carbamazepine and thus enable carbamazepine to again be more effective.

It is apparent that carbamazepine requires these increases in compensatory adaptive mechanisms in order to be an effective anticonvulsant. The seizure-induced increases in TRH mRNA and protein last ~ 4–5 days after a given seizure. If carbamazepine is administered after an interval of > 4 days from the last seizure, it is no longer effective [160]. These observations of the "time-off effect," taken in conjunction with those indicating that TRH administered directly into the hippocampus exerts anticonvulsant properties [163], suggest that this neuropeptide represents one of the factors that are transiently induced following a seizure that either are endogenously anticonvulsant in their own right or facilitate the actions of exogenous anticonvulsant drugs such as carbamazepine, diazepam, or lamotrigine achieving anticonvulsant efficacy.

In the anticonvulsant model of carbamazepine tolerance, the development of tolerance can be slowed by a variety of manipulations, as summarized in Table 7. Whether these are pertinent to the development of tolerance to the psychotropic effects of carbamazepine in

Table 7 Clinical Predictions (Left) to Be Explored Based on Observations from a Preclinical Model of Amygdala-Kindled Seizures (Right)

Preclinical studies	Future studies; is there predictive validity for clinical tolerance in affective illness?
Tolerance to anticonvulsant effects slowed by:	Would tolerance be slowed by:
Higher doses (except w/LTG)	Maximum tolerated doses
Not escalating doses	Stable dosing
More efficacious drugs (VPA > CBZ)	Different rate of treatment resistance (CBZ > VPA)?
Treatments initiated early in illness	Early institution of lithium treatment is more effective than late
Combination treatment (CBZ + VPA)	Combination > monotherapy?
Reducing illness drive	Treatment comorbidities
Treatment response restored by:	Treatment response restored by:
Period of drug discontinuation then re-exposure	Randomized study of continuation treatment vs. discontinuation and reexposure needed
Agents with different mechanisms of action, i.e., no cross-tolerance (cross tolerance from lamotrigine to CBZ, not VPA)	VPA should be more effective in those tolerant to LTG than would be CBZ

VPA, valproic acid; CBZ, carbamazepine; LTG, lamotrigine.

the recurrent affective disorders remains to be directly tested. Nonetheless, there are case observations suggesting that after a period of gradual loss of efficacy to carbamazepine via an apparent tolerance mechanism, therapeutic effects can again be achieved when the drug is reinstituted after a period of time off that medication [164]. A clinically more useful approach in the face of tolerance would be to use a drug with a different mechanism of action that does not display cross-tolerance. For example, carbamazepine shows cross-tolerance with PK-11195, lamotrigine, and (surprisingly) valproate, but not to diazepam, phenytoin, or clonazepam [160,165,166].

Although no systematic evidence has yet been offered that tolerance develops to the clinical anticonvulsant or psychotropic effects of lamotrigine, a number of preliminary case reports support this possibility. In this regard, it is noteworthy that lamotrigine, like carbamazepine, shows the rapid development of tolerance to its anticonvulsant effects on amygdala-kindled seizures [165]. There is essentially complete cross-tolerance between carbamazepine and lamotrigine, and vice versa. In contrast to a number of other agents in which higher doses appear to slow the development of tolerance, the converse appears to occur for lamotrigine [167]. Not only does lamotrigine in higher doses appear to propel a more rapid loss of efficacy, but the breakthrough seizures that are manifest become more severe, including stage VI type, with violent convulsions and running fits in rodents. Most interestingly, we have also observed that administration of either lamotrigine or carbamazepine in the initial stages of kindling development (when they are not effective in preventing the progression to full-blown seizures) rendered both of those drugs also ineffective on completed kindled seizures (when these drugs are ordinarily highly effective) [165].

We have begun to examine the possible dose and other drug administration parameters that would be most likely to slow tolerance development in this anticonvulsant model in the hope that they may provide paradigms that might also be effective in other clinical situations of tolerance development. Although both higher (20 mg/kg) and lower (5 mg/kg) doses of lamotrigine appear to be ineffective, alternating moderate and low doses on a daily basis (15 mg/kg on one day and 5 mg/kg on the next) appears to be the most effective in slowing tolerance to lamotrigine; however, the increased number of days until complete loss of efficacy was not very substantial.

Therefore, we examined other potential interventions, including use of anticonvulsants such as gabapentin, which have very different putative mechanisms of action and physiological effects. Lamotrigine (like carbamazepine) increases the threshold for seizure generation, whereas gabapentin affects its spread [168,169]. Gabapentin, at doses that in themselves were ineffective, appeared to slow tolerance development to the anticonvulsant effects of lamotrigine and to more notably inhibit the development of stage VI

Table 8 Differential Effects of Carbamazepine (CBZ) and Lamotrigine (LTG) on Anticonvulsant Tolerance Development

	CBZ (15 mg/kg)	LTG (16 mg/kg)
Rapid tolerance to anticonvulsant effects (amygdala kindling)	+++	+++
Cross-tolerance	+++	++
"Time-off" effect (seizures enhance efficacy)	+++ (4–5 days)	+++ (4–5 days)
Seizure threshold △ with tolerance	↓↓↓	↑↑ (possible residual drug effect)
High doses	Slow tolerance	Speed tolerance and are proconvulsant
Alternating high & low doses	?	Slows tolerance
Chronic noncontingent drug dosing	Slows tolerance	?
MK801 on tolerance development	No effect	Slows (NMDA implicated)
Cross tolerance to valproate	Yes	No
Valproate combination	Slows tolerance	?
Gabapentin augmentation (2 h pretreatment)	?	Slows tolerance
($\frac{1}{2}$ h pretreatment)	No effect	↓ VI seizures
Tolerance reversal	?	+++

NMDA, N-methyl-D-aspartate.

seizures manifest during lamotrigine treatment. A variety of other similarities and differences between carbamazepine and lamotrigine are summarized in Table 8. Whether any of these preclinical observations will generalize to the clinic remains to be directly studied and tested.

X. CONCLUSIONS

A variety of anticonvulsants have come to play a widely accepted and experimental role in the treatment of bipolar illness. Much further work is needed, not only to better understand their spectrum of therapeutic and mechanism of psychotropic action, but also most importantly, to develop better clinical and biological markers of therapeutic responsivity to these agents.

REFERENCES

1. Post RM, Frye MA, Denicoff KD, Leverich GS, Kimbrell TA, Dunn RT. Beyond lithium in the treatment of bipolar illness. Neuropsychopharmacology 19:206–219, 1998.
2. Post RM et al. A history of the use of anticonvulsants as mood stabilizers in the last two decades of the 20th century. Neuropsychobiology 38:152–166, 1998.
3. Post RM. Mood disorders: treatment of bipolar disorders. In: Sadock BJ, Sadock VA, eds. Comprehensive Textbook of Psychiatry, 7th ed. Baltimore: Lippincott Williams & Wilkins, 2000, pp 1385–1430,.
4. Post RM, Weiss SRB, Clark M, Chuang DM, Hough C, Li H. Lithium, carbamazepine, and valproate in affective illness: biochemical and neurobiological mechanisms. In: Manji H, Bowden CL, Belmaker RH, eds. Bipolar Medications: Mechanisms of Action. Washington: American Psychiatric Press, 2000, pp 219–248.
5. Fochtmann LJ. Animal studies of electroconvulsive therapy: foundations for future research. Psychopharmacol Bull 30:321–444, 1994.
6. Fink M. Convulsive therapy: a review of the first 55 years. J Affect Disord 63:1–15, 2001.
7. Sackeim HA. The anticonvulsant hypothesis of the mechanisms of action of ECT. Current status. J ECT 15:5–26, 1999.
8. Post RM, Chuang D-M. Mechanism of action of lithium: comparison and contrast with carbamazepine. In: Birch NJ, ed. Lithium and the Cell: Pharmacology and Biochemistry. London: Academic Press, 1991, pp 199–241.
9. Post RM. Time course of clinical effects of carbamazepine: implications for mechanisms of action. J Clin Psychiatry 49(suppl):35–48, 1988.
10. Post RM, Weiss SRB, Chuang D-M, Ketter TA. Mechanisms of action of carbamazepine in seizure and affective disorders. In: Joffe RT, Calabrese JR,

eds. Anticonvulsants in Mood Disorders. New York: Marcel Dekker. 1994, pp 43–92.
11. Duman RS. Novel therapeutic approaches beyond the serotonin receptor. Biol Psychiatry 44:324–335, 1998.
12. Thome J et al. cAMP response element-mediated gene transcription is upregulated by chronic antidepressant treatment. J Neurosci 20:4030–4036, 2000.
13. Fujimaki K, Morinobu S, Duman RS. Administration of a cAMP phosphodiesterase 4 inhibitor enhances antidepressant-induction of BDNF mRNA in rat hippocampus. Neuro-psychopharmacology 22:42–51, 2000.
14. Siuciak JA, Lewis DR, Wiegand SJ, Lindsay RM. Antidepressant-like effect of brain-derived neurotrophic factor (BDNF). Pharmacol Biochem Behav 56:131–137, 1997.
15. McKinney WT. Animal models of depression: an overview. Psychiatr Dev 2:77–96, 1984.
16. Loscher W. Animal models of intractable epilepsy. Prog Neurobiol 53:239–258, 1997.
17. Drevets WC. Functional neuroimaging studies of depression: the anatomy of melancholia. Annu Rev Med 49:341–361, 1998.
18. Altshuler LL, Post RM, Leverich GS, Mikalauskas K, Rosoff A, Ackerman L. Antidepressant-induced mania and cycle acceleration: a controversy revisited. Am J Psychiatry 152:1130–1138, 1995.
19. Post RM, Denicoff KD, Leverich GS, Frye MA. Drug-induced switching in bipolar disorder. Epidemiology and therapeutic implications. CNS Drugs 8:352–365, 1997.
20. Ahlfors UG et al. Flupenthixol decanoate in recurrent manic-depressive illness. A comparison with lithium. Acta Psychiatr Scand 64:226–237, 1981.
21. Kukopulos A, Reginaldi D, Laddomada P, Floris G, Serra G, Tondo L. Course of the manic-depressive cycle and changes caused by treatment. Pharmakopsychiatr Neuropsychopharmakol 13:156–167, 1980.
22. Weiss SR, Post RM. Caveats in the use of the kindling model of affective disorders. Toxicol Ind Health 10:421–447, 1994.
23. Post RM, Ketter TA, Speer AM, Leverich GS, Weiss SR. Predictive validity of the sensitization and kindling hypotheses. In: Soares JC, Gershon S, eds. Bipolar Disorders: Basic Mechanisms and Therapeutic Implications. New York: Marcel Dekker, 2000, pp 387–432.
24. Post RM, Weiss SRB. Kindling and stress sensitization. In: Joffe RT, Young LT, eds. Bipolar Disorder: Biological Models and Their Clinical Application. New York: Marcel Dekker, 1997, pp 93–126.
25. Ketter TA, Post RM, Theodore WH. Positive and negative psychiatric effects of antiepileptic drugs in patients with seizure disorders. Neurology 53:S53–S67, 1999.
26. Grunze H, Erfurth A, Marcuse A, Amann B, Normann C, Walden J. Tiagabine appears not to be efficacious in the treatment of acute mania. J Clin Psychiatry 60:759–762, 1999.
27. Frye MA et al. A placebo-controlled study of lamotrigine and gabapentin monotherapy in refractory mood disorders. J Clin Psychopharmacol 20:607–614, 2000.
28. Post RM, Denicoff KD, Frye MA, Leverich GS. Re-evaluating carbamazepine prophylaxis in bipolar disorder. Br J Psychiatry 170:202–204, 1997.
29. Emrich HM, Dose M, Von Zerssen D. The use of sodium valproate, carbamazepine and oxcarbazepine in patients with affective disorders. J Affect Disord 8:243–250, 1985.
30. Emrich HM, Altmann H, Dose M, Von Zerssen D. Therapeutic effects of GABA-ergic drugs in affective disorders. A preliminary report. Pharmacol Biochem Behav 19:369–372, 1983.
31. Post RM et al. The place of anticonvulsant therapy in bipolar illness. Psychopharmacology (Berl) 128:115–129, 1996.
32. Macdonald RL, Kelly KM. Antiepileptic drug mechanisms of action. Epilepsia 36(suppl 2):S2-S-12, 1995.
33. Ketter TA et al. The emerging role of cytochrome P450 3A in psychopharmacology. J Clin Psychopharmacol 15:387–398, 1995.
34. Willow M, Kuenzel EA, Catterall WA. Inhibition of voltage-sensitive sodium channels in neuroblastoma cells and synaptosomes by the anticonvulsant drugs diphenylhydantoin and carbamazepine. Mol Pharmacol 25:228–234, 1984.
35. Kuo CC. A common anticonvulsant binding site for phenytoin, carbamazepine, and lamotrigine in neuronal Na^+ channels. Mol Pharmacol 54:712–721, 1998.
36. Albright P, Burnham W. Effects of phenytoin, carbamazepine, and clonazepam on cortex- and amygdala-evoked potentials. Exp Neurol 81:308–319, 1983.
37. Fitton A, Goa KL. Lamotrigine. An update of its pharmacology and therapeutic use in epilepsy. Drugs 50:691–713, 1995.
38. Hough CJ, Irwin RP, Gao X-M, Rogawski MA, Chuang D-M. Carbamazepine inhibition of N-Methyl-D-aspartate-evoked calcium influx in rat cerebellar granule cells. J Pharmacol Exp Ther 276:143–149, 1996.
39. Grunze H, Von Wegerer J, Greene RW, Walden J. Modulation of calcium and potassium currents by lamotrigine. Neuropsychobiology 38:131–138, 1998.
40. Wang SJ, Huang CC, Hsu KS, Tsai JJ, Gean PW. Inhibition of N-type calcium currents by lamotrigine

in rat amygdalar neurones. Neuroreport 7:3037–3040, 1996.
41. Stefani A, Spadoni F, Siniscalchi A, Bernardi G. Lamotrigine inhibits Ca^{2+} currents in cortical neurons: functional implications. Eur J Pharmacol 307:113–116, 1996.
42. Marangos PJ, Daval JL, Weiss SRB, Post RM. Carbamazepine and brain adenosine receptors. In: Wasterlain CG, Vert P, eds. Neonatal Seizures. New York: Raven Press, 1990, pp 203–209.
43. Post RM, Weiss SRB, Clark M, Nakajima T, Ketter TA. Seizures as an evolving process: Implications for neuropsychiatric illness. In: Theodore WH, Devinsky O, eds. Epilepsy and Behavior. New York: Alan R. Liss, 1991, pp 361–387.
44. Weiss SRB, Post RM, Marangos PJ, Patel J. Peripheral-type benzodiazepines: behavioral effects and interactions with the anticonvulant effects of carbamazepine. In: Wada JA, ed. Kindling III. New York: Raven Press, 1986, pp 375–389.
45. Krueger KE. Molecular and functional properties of mitochondrial benzodiazepine receptors. Biochim Biophys Acta 1241:453–470, 1995.
46. Papadopoulos V et al. Peripheral benzodiazepine receptor in cholesterol transport and steroidogenesis. Steroids 62:21–28, 1997.
47. Syapin PJ, Skolnick P. Characterization of benzodiazepine binding sites in cultured cells of neural origin. J Neurochem 32:1047–1051, 1979.
48. Purdy RE, Julien RM, Fairhurst AS. Effect of carbamazepine on the in vitro uptake and release of norepinephrine in adrenergic nerves of rabbit aorta and in whole brain synaptosomes. Epilepsia 18:251–257, 1977.
49. Post RM et al. Effects of carbamazepine on noradrenergic mechanisms in affectively ill patients. Psychopharmacology (Berl) 87:59–63, 1985.
50. Maitre L, Baltzer V, Mondadori C. Psychopharmacological and behavioural effects of anti-epileptic drugs in animals. In: Emrich HM, Okuma T, Muller AA, eds. Anticonvulsants in Affective Disorders. Amsterdam: Excerpta Medica, 1984, pp 3–13.
51. Chen G, Hough C, Manji H, Chuang DM, Mefford IN, Potter WZ. Upregulation of beta-adrenergic receptors and beta2 mRNA by carbamazepine in vitro. Soc Neuroscie Abstr 1991, p 17.
52. Rubinow DR, Post RM, Gold PW, Uhde TW. Effect of carbamazepine on mean urinary free cortisol excretion in patients with major affective illness. Psychopharmacology (Berl) 88:115–118, 1986.
53. Kling MA et al. Effects of local anesthetics on experiential, physiologic and endocrine measures in healthy humans and on rat hypothalamic corticotropin-releasing hormone release in vitro: clinical and psychobiologic implications. J Pharmacol Exp Ther 268:1548–1564, 1994.
54. Calogero AE, Gallucci WT, Kling MA, Chrousos GP, Gold PW. Cocaine stimulates rat hypothalamic corticotropin-releasing hormone secretion in vitro. Brain Res 505:7–11, 1989.
55. Post RM, Uhde TW, Roy-Byrne PP, Joffe RT. Antidepressant effects of carbamazepine. Am J Psychiatry 143:29–34, 1986.
56. Post RM, Frye MA, Denicoff KD, Kimbrell TA, Cora-Locatelli G, Leverich GS. Anticonvulsants in the long-term prophylaxis of depression. In: Honig A, Van Praag HM, eds. Depression: Neurobiological, Psychopathological and Therapeutic Advances. Sussex, England: John Wiley & Sons, 1997, pp 483–498.
57. Rubinow DR, Post RM, Gold PW, Ballenger JC, Reichlin S. Effects of carbamazepine on cerebrospinal fluid somatostatin. Psychopharmacology (Berl) 85:210–213, 1985.
58. Pazzaglia PJ, George MS, Post RM, Rubinow DR, Davis CL. Nimodipine increases CSF somatostatin in affectively ill patients. Neuropsychopharmacology 13:75–83, 1995.
59. Post RM et al. Carbamazepine and nimodipine in refractory affective illness: Efficacy and mechanisms. In: Halbreich U, Montgomery S, eds. Pharmacotherapy for Mood, Anxiety, and Cognitive Disorders. Washington, DC: American Psychiatric Press, 2000 pp 77–110.
60. Ketter TA et al. Baseline cerebral hypermetabolism associated with carbamazepine response, and hypometabolism with nimodipine response in mood disorders. Biol Psychiatry 46:1364–1374, 1999.
61. Frye MA, Kimbrell TA, Willis MW, Ketter TA, George MS, Pazzaglia PJ, Dunn RT, Luckenbaugh D, Huggins T, Little JT, Vanderham L, Danielson A, Benson B, Davis C, Rubinow DR, Post RM. Low CSF somatostatin and cerebral hypometabolism in depression. Biol Psychiatry 41:32S–33S, 1997.
62. Ongur D, Drevets WC, Price JL. Glial reduction in the subgenual prefrontal cortex in mood disorders. Proc Natl Acad Sci USA 95:13290–13295, 1998.
63. Drevets WC, Ongur D, Price JL. Neuroimaging abnormalities in the subgenual prefrontal cortex: implications for the pathophysiology of familial mood disorders. Mol Psychiatry 3:220–221, 1998.
64. Drevets WC et al. Subgenual prefrontal cortex abnormalities in mood disorders. Nature 386:824–827, 1997.
65. Hong JS, Tilson HA, Yoshikawa K. Effects of lithium and haloperidol administration on the rat brain levels of substance P. J Pharmacol Exp Ther 224:590–593, 1983.
66. Le Douarin C, Oblin A, Fage D, Scatton B. Influence of lithium on biochemical manifestations

66. of striatal dopamine target cell supersensitivity induced by prolonged haloperidol treatment. Eur J Pharmacol 93:55–62, 1983.
67. Mitsushio H, Takashima M, Mataga N, Toru M. Effects of chronic treatment with trihexyphenidyl and carbamazepine alone or in combination with haloperidol on substance P content in rat brain: a possible implication of substance P in affective disorders. J Pharmacol Exp Ther 245:982–989, 1988.
68. Jones RS, Olpe HR. An increase in sensitivity of rat cingulate cortical neurones to substance P occurs following withdrawal of chronic administration of antidepressant drugs. Br J Pharmacol 81:659–664, 1984.
69. Kramer MS et al. Distinct mechanism for antidepressant activity by blockade of central substance P receptors. Science 281:1640–1645, 1998.
70. Nutt D. Substance-P antagonists: a new treatment for depression? Lancet 352:1644–1646, 1998.
71. Gold PW et al. Vasopressin in affective illness: direct measurement, clinical trials, and response to hypertonic saline. In: Post RM, Ballenger JC, eds. Neurobiology of Mood Disorders. Baltimore: Williams & Wilkins, 1984, pp 323–339.
72. Sudha S, Lakshmana MK, Pradhan N. Changes in learning and memory, acetylcholinesterase activity and monoamines in brain after chronic carbamazepine administration in rats. Epilepsia 36:416–422, 1995.
73. Joffe RT, Post RM, Uhde TW. Effects of carbamazepine on serum electrolytes in affectively ill patients. Psychol Med 16:331–335, 1986.
74. Uhde TW, Post RM. Effects of carbamazepine on serum electrolytes: clinical and theoretical implications. J Clin Psychopharmacol 3:103–106, 1983.
75. Yassa R, Iskandar H, Nastase C, Camille Y. Carbamazepine and hyponatremia in patients with affective disorder. Am J Psychiatry 145:339–342, 1988.
76. Brewerton TD, Jackson CW. Prophylaxis of carbamazepine-induced hyponatremia by demeclocycline in six patients. J Clin Psychiatry 55:249–251, 1994.
77. Ringel RA, Brick JF. Perspective on carbamazepine-induced water intoxication: reversal by demeclocycline. Neurol 36:1506–1507, 1986.
78. Vieweg WV, Yank GR, Rowe WT, Hovermale LS, Clayton AH. Increase in white blood cell count and serum sodium level following the addition of lithium to carbamazepine treatment among three chronically psychotic male patients with disturbed affective states. Psychiatr Q 58:213–217, 1986.
79. Motohashi N. GABA receptor alterations after chronic lithium administration. Comparison with carbamazepine and sodium valproate. Prog Neuropsychopharmacol Biol Psychiatry 16:571–579, 1992.
80. Bernasconi R. The GABA hypothesis of affective illness: influence of clinically effective antimanic drugs on GABA turnover. In: Emrich HM, Aldenhoff JB, Lux HD, eds. Basic Mechanisms in the Action of Lithium: Proceedings of a Symposium Held at Schloss Ringberg, Bavaria, F.R.G., October 4-6, 1981. Amsterdam: Excerpta Medica, 1982, pp 183–192.
81. McLean MH, Macdonald RL. Sodium valproate, but not ethosuximide, produces use- and voltage-dependent limitation of high frequency repetitive firing of action potentials of mouse central neurons in cell culture. J Pharmacol Exp Ther 237:1001–1010, 1986.
82. Slater GE, Johnston D. Sodium valproate increases potassium conductance in aplysia neurones. Epilepsia 19:379–384, 1978.
83. Walden J, Altrup U, Reith H, Speckmann E-J. Effects of valproate on early and late potassium currents of single neurons. Eur Neuropsychopharmacol 3:137–141, 1993.
84. Chen G, Manji HK, Hawver DB, Wright CB, Potter WZ. Chronic sodium valproate selectively decreases protein kinase C alpha and epsilon in vitro. J Neurochem 63:2361–2364, 1994.
85. Manji HK, Bebchuk JM, Moore GJ, Glitz D, Hasanat KA, Chen G. Modulation of CNS signal transduction pathways and gene expression by mood-stabilizing agents: therapeutic implications. J Clin Psychiatry 60(suppl 2):27–39, 1999.
86. Hong M, Chen DC, Klein PS, Lee VM. Lithium reduces tau phosphorylation by inhibition of glycogen synthase kinase-3. J Biol Chem 272:25326–25332, 1997.
87. Chen G, Huang LD, Jiang YM, Manji HK. The mood-stabilizing agent valproate inhibits the activity of glycogen synthase kinase-3. J Neurochem 72:1327–1330, 1999.
88. Ozaki N, Chuang DM. Lithium increases transcription factor binding to AP-1 and cyclic AMP–responsive element in cultured neurons and rat brain. J Neurochem 69:2336–2344, 1997.
89. Chen G, Yuan P, Hawver DB, Potter WZ, Manji HK. Increase in AP-1 transcription factor DNA binding activity by valproic acid. Neuro-psychopharmacology 16:238–245, 1997.
90. Chalecka-Franaszek E, Chuang DM. Lithium activates the serine/threonine kinase Akt-1 and suppresses glutamate-induced inhibition of Akt-1 activity in neurons. Proc Natl Acad Sci USA 96:8745–8750, 1999.
91. Chen G et al. The mood-stabilizing agents lithium and valproate robustly increase the levels of the neuroprotective protein bcl-2 in the CNS. J Neurochem 72:879–882, 1999.

92. Chen RW, Chuang DM. Long term lithium treatment suppresses p53 and Bax expression but increases Bcl-2 expression. A prominent role in neuroprotection against excitotoxicity. J Biol Chem 274:6039–6042, 1999.
93. Nonaka S, Chuang DM. Neuroprotective effects of chronic lithium on focal cerebral ischemia in rats. Neuroreport 9:2081–2084, 1998.
94. Manji HK, Moore GJ, Chen G. Clinical and preclinical evidence for the neurotrophic effects of mood stabilizers: implications for the pathophysiology and treatment of manic-depressive illness. Biol Psychiatry 48:740–754, 2000.
95. Datta SR, Brunet A, Greenberg ME. Cellular survival: a play in three Akts. Genes Dev 13:2905–2927, 1999.
96. Datta SR et al. Akt phosphorylation of BAD couples survival signals to the cell-intrinsic death machinery. Cell 91:231–241, 1997.
97. Cardone MH et al. Regulation of cell death protease caspase-9 by phosphorylation. Science 282:1318–1321, 1998.
98. Brunet A et al. Akt promotes cell survival by phosphorylating and inhibiting a Forkhead transcription factor. Cell 96:857–868, 1999.
99. Du K, Montminy M. CREB is a regulatory target for the protein kinase Akt/PKB. J Biol Chem 273:32377–32379, 1998.
100. Dimmeler S, Fleming I, Fisslthaler B, Hermann C, Busse R, Zeiher AM. Activation of nitric oxide synthase in endothelial cells by Akt-dependent phosphorylation. Nature 399:601–605, 1999.
101. Kane LP, Shapiro VS, Stokoe D, Weiss A. Induction of NF-kappaB by the Akt/PKB kinase. Curr Biol 9:601–604, 1999.
102. Blair LA, Bence-Hanulec KK, Mehta S, Franke T, Kaplan D, Marshall J. Akt-dependent potentiation of L channels by insulin-like growth factor-1 is required for neuronal survival. J Neurosci 19:1940–1951, 1999.
103. Kennedy SG, Kandel ES, Cross TK, Hay N. Akt/protein kinase B inhibits cell death by preventing the release of cytochrome c from mitochondria. Mol Cell Biol 19:5800–5810, 1999.
104. Cross DA, Alessi DR, Cohen P, Andjelkovich M, Hemmings BA. Inhibition of glycogen synthase kinase-3 by insulin mediated by protein kinase B. Nature 378:785–789, 1995.
105. Manji HK, Moore GJ, Rajkowska G, Chen G. Neuroplasticity and cellular resilience in mood disorders. Mol Psychiatry 5:578–593, 2000.
106. Wei H, Qin Z, Wei W, Wang Y, Qian Y, Chuang DM. Lithium suppresses excitotoxicity-induced striatal lesions in a rat model of Huntington's disease. Neuroscience 106:603–612, 2001.
107. Nonaka S, Katsube N, Chuang DM. Lithium protects rat cerebellar granule cells against apoptosis induced by anticonvulsants, phenytoin and carbamazepine. J Pharmacol Exp Ther 286:539–547, 1998.
108. Chen G, Rajkowska G, Du F, Seraji-Bozorgzad N, Manji HK. Enhancement of hippocampal neurogenesis by lithium. J Neurochem 75:1729–1734, 2000.
109. Malberg JE, Eisch AJ, Nestler EJ, Duman RS. Chronic antidepressant treatment increases neurogenesis in adult rat hippocampus. J Neurosci 20:9104–9110, 2000.
110. Gould E, Tanapat P. Stress and hippocampal neurogenesis. Biol Psychiatry 46:1472–1479, 1999.
111. Moore GJ, Bebchuk JM, Wilds IB, Chen G, Menji HK. Lithium-induced increase in human brain grey matter. Lancet 356:1241–1242, 2000.
112. Moore GJ et al. Lithium increases N-acetyl-aspartate in the human brain: in vivo evidence in support of bcl-2's neurotrophic effects? Biol Psychiatry 48:1–8, 2000.
113. Lubrich B, Van Calker D. Inhibition of the high affinity myo-inositol transport system: a common mechanism of action of antibipolar drugs? Neuropsychopharmacology 21:519–529, 1999.
114. Bowden CL et al. The efficacy of lamotrigine in rapid cycling and non-rapid cycling patients with bipolar disorder. Biol Psychiatry 45:953–958, 1999.
115. Calabrese JR et al. A double-blind, placebo-controlled, prophylaxis study of lamotrigine in rapid-cycling bipolar disorder. Lamictal 614 Study Group. J Clin Psychiatry 61:841–850, 2000.
116. Guberman AH et al. Lamotrigine-associated rash: risk/benefit considerations in adults and children. Epilepsia 40:985–991, 1999.
117. Zona C, Avoli M. Lamotrigine reduces voltage-gated sodium currents in rat central neurons in culture. Epilepsia 38:522–525, 1997.
118. Waldmeier PC, Baumann PA, Wicki P, Feldtrauer J-J, Stierlin C, Schmutz M. Similar potency of carbamazepine, oxcarbazepine, and lamotrigine in inhibiting the release of glutamate and other neurotransmitters. Neurology 45:1907–1913, 1995.
119. Perucca E. A pharmacological and clinical review on topiramate, a new antiepileptic drug. Pharmacol Res 35:241–256, 1997.
120. White HS, Brown SD, Woodhead JH, Skeen GA, Wolf HH. Topiramate enhances GABA-mediated chloride flux and GABA-evoked chloride currents in murine brain neurons and increases seizure threshold. Epilepsy Res 28:167–179, 1997.
121. White HS, Brown SD, Woodhead JH, Skeen GA, Wolf HH. Topiramate modulates GABA-evoked currents in murine cortical neurons by a nonbenzodiazepine mechanism. Epilepsia 41(suppl 1):S17–S20, 2000.

122. Muller D, Joly M, Lynch G. Contributions of quisqualate and NMDA receptors to the induction and expression of LTP. Science 242:1694–1697, 1988.
123. Aldenkamp AP et al. A multicenter, randomized clinical study to evaluate the effect on cognitive function of topiramate compared with valproate as add-on therapy to carbamazepine in patients with partial-onset seizures. Epilepsia 41:1167–1178, 2000.
124. Thompson PJ, Baxendale SA, Duncan JS, Sander JW. Effects of topiramate on cognitive function. J Neurol Neurosurg Psychiatry 69:636–641, 2000.
125. Berlant JL. Topiramate in post-traumatic stress disorder: preliminary clinical observations. J Clin Psychiatry 62 (Suppl 17); 60–63, 2001.
126. Shorvon SD. Safety of topiramate: adverse events and relationships to dosing. Epilepsia 37(suppl 2):S18–S22, 1996.
127. Lhatoo SD, Wong IC, Polizzi G, Sander JW. Long-term retention rates of lamotrigine, gabapentin, and topiramate in chronic epilepsy. Epilepsia 41:1592–1596, 2000.
128. Dalby NO, Nielsen EB. Comparison of the preclinical anticonvulsant profiles of tiagabine, lamotrigine, gabapentin and vigabatrin. Epilepsy Res 28:63–72, 1997.
129. Taylor CP et al. A summary of mechanistic hypotheses of gabapentin pharmacology. Epilepsy Res 29:233–249, 1998.
130. Pande AC, Crockatt JG, Janney CA, Werth JL, Tsaroucha G. Gabapentin in bipolar disorder: a placebo-controlled trial of adjunctive therapy. Gabapentin Bipolar Disorder Study Group. Bipolar Disord 2:249–255, 2000.
131. Gerner RH et al. CSF neurochemistry in depressed, manic, and schizophrenic patients compared with that of normal controls. Am J Psychiatry 141:1533–1540, 1984.
132. Post RM et al. Cerebrospinal fluid GABA in normals and patients with affective disorders. Brain Res Bull 5:755-759, 1980.
133. Pande AC et al. Treatment of social phobia with gabapentin: a placebo-controlled study. J Clin Psychopharmacol 19:341–348, 1999.
134. Pollack MH, Matthews J, Scott EL. Gabapentin as a potential treatment for anxiety disorders [letter]. Am J Psychiatry 155:992–993, 1998.
135. Chouinard G, Beauclair L, Belanger MC. Gabapentin: long-term antianxiety and hypnotic effects in psychiatric patients with comorbid anxiety-related disorders [letter]. Can J Psychiatry 43:305, 1998.
136. Suppes T, Leverich GS, Keck PE Jr, Nolen W, Denicoff KD, Altshuler LL, McElroy SL, Rush AJ, Kupka R, Bickel M, Post RM. The Stanley Foundation Bipolar Treatment Outcome Network: II. Demographics and illness characteristics of the first 261 patients. J Affect Disord, 67:45–59, 2001.
137. McElroy SL et al. Axis I psychiatric comorbidity and its relationship to historical illness variables in 288 patients with bipolar disorder. Am J Psychiatry 158:420–426, 2001.
138. Cora-Locatelli G, Greenberg BD, Martin J, Murphy DL. Gabapentin augmentation for fluoxetine-treated patients with obsessive-compulsive disorder. J Clin Psychiatry 59:480–481, 1998.
139. Merren MD. Gabapentin for treatment of pain and tremor: a large case series. South Med J 91:739–744, 1998.
140. Gironell A, Kulisevsky J, Barbanoj M, Lopez-Villegas D, Hernandez G, Pascual-Sedano B. A randomized placebo-controlled comparative trial of gabapentin and propranolol in essential tremor. Arch Neurol 56:475–480, 1999.
141. Adler CH. Treatment of restless legs syndrome with gabapentin. Clin Neuropharmacol 20:148–151, 1997.
142. Olson WL, Gruenthal M, Mueller ME, Olson WH. Gabapentin for parkinsonism: a double-blind, placebo-controlled, crossover trial. Am J Med 102:60–66, 1997.
143. Obrocea GV, Dunn RM, Frye MA, Ketter TA, Luckenbaugh DA, Leverich GS, Speer AM, Osuch EA, Jajodia K, Post RM. Clinical predictors of response to lamotrigine and gabapentin monotherapy in refractory affective disorders. Biol Psychiatry 51:253–260, 2002
144. Schachter SC. The next wave of anticonvulsants—focus on levetiracetam, oxcarbazepine and zonisamide. CNS Drugs 14:229–249, 2000.
145. Noyer M, Gillard M, Matagne A, Henichart JP, Wulfert E. The novel antiepileptic drug levetiracetam (ucb L059) appears to act via a specific binding site in CNS membranes. Eur J Pharmacol 286:137–146, 1995.
146. Klitgaard H, Matagne A, Gobert J, Wulfert E. Evidence for a unique profile of levetiracetam in rodent models of seizures and epilepsy. Eur J Pharmacol 353:191–206, 1998.
147. Georg MD, Klitgaard H. Inhibition of neuronal hypersynchrony in vitro differentiates levetiracetam from classical antiepileptic drugs. Pharmacol Res 42:281–285, 2000.
148. Margineanu DG, Wulfert E. ucb L059, a novel anticonvulsant, reduces bicuculline-induced hyperexcitability in rat hippocampal CA3 in vivo. Eur J Pharmacol 286:321–325, 1995.
149. Loscher W, Honack D. Profile of ucb L059, a novel anticonvulsant drug, in models of partial and generalized epilepsy in mice and rats. Eur J Pharmacol 232:147–158, 1993.
150. Loscher W, Honack D, Rundfeldt C. Antiepileptogenic effects of the novel anticonvulsant

151. Kawata Y et al. Effects of zonisamide on K$^+$ and Ca^{2+} evoked release of monoamine as well as K$^+$ evoked intracellular Ca^{2+} mobilization in rat hippocampus. Epilepsy Res 35:173–182, 1999.
152. Okada M et al. Biphasic effects of zonisamide on serotonergic system in rat hippocampus. Epilepsy Res 34:187–197, 1999.
153. Fromm GH, Shibuya T, Terrence CF. Effect of zonisamide (CI-912) on a synaptic system model. Epilepsia 28:673–679, 1987.
154. Okada M et al. Effects of zonisamide on dopaminergic system. Epilepsy Res 22:193–205, 1995.
155. Kito M, Maehara M, Watanabe K. Mechanisms of T-type calcium channel blockade by zonisamide. Seizure 5:115–119, 1996.
156. Kanba S et al. The first open study of zonisamide, a novel anticonvulsant, shows efficacy in mania. Prog Neuropsychopharmacol Biol Psychiatry 18:707–715, 1994.
157. Cohen BM, Baldessarini RJ. Tolerance to therapeutic effects of antidepressants. Am J Psychiatry 142:489–490, 1985.
158. Mann JJ. Loss of antidepressant effect with long-term monoamine oxidase inhibitor treatment without loss of monoamine oxidase inhibition. J Clin Psychopharmacol 3:363–366, 1983.
159. Fava M, Rappe SM, Pava JA, Nierenberg AA, Alpert JE, Rosenbaum JF. Relapse in patients on long-term fluoxetine treatment: response to increased fluoxetine dose. J Clin Psychiatry 56:52–55, 1995.
160. Weiss SR, Clark M, Rosen JB, Smith MA, Post RM. Contingent tolerance to the anticonvulsant effects of carbamazepine: relationship to loss of endogenous adaptive mechanisms. Brain Res Brain Res Rev 20:305–325, 1995.
161. Rosen JB, Weiss SR, Post RM. Contingent tolerance to carbamazepine: alterations in TRH mRNA and TRH receptor binding in limbic structures. Brain Res 651:252–260, 1994.
162. Clark M, Massenburg GS, Weiss SR, Post RM. Analysis of the hippocampal GABAA receptor system in kindled rats by autoradiographic and in situ hybridization techniques: contingent tolerance to carbamazepine. Brain Res Mol Brain Res 26:309–319, 1994.
163. Wan RQ, Noguera EC, Weiss SR. Anticonvulsant effects of intra-hippocampal injection of TRH in amygdala kindled rats. Neuroreport 9:677–682, 1998.
164. Pazzaglia PJ, Post RM. Contingent tolerance and reresponse to carbamazepine: a case study in a patient with trigeminal neuralgia and bipolar disorder. J Neuropsychiatry Clin Neurosci 4:76–81, 1992.
165. Krupp E, Heynen T, Li XL, Post RM, Weiss SR. Tolerance to the anticonvulsant effects of lamotrigine on amygdala kindled seizures: cross-tolerance to carbamazepine but not valproate or diazepam. Exp Neurol 162:278–289, 2000.
166. Weiss SR, Post RM, Sohn E, Berger A, Lewis R. Cross-tolerance between carbamazepine and valproate on amygdala-kindled seizures. Epilepsy Res 16:37–44, 1993.
167. Postma T, Krupp E, Li XL, Post RM, Weiss SR. Lamotrigine treatment during amygdala-kindled seizure development fails to inhibit seizures and diminishes subsequent anticonvulsant efficacy. Epilepsia 41:1514–1521, 2000.
168. Loscher W, Reissmuller E, Ebert U. Anticonvulsant efficacy of gabapentin and levetiracetam in phenytoin-resistant kindled rats. Epilepsy Res 40:63–77, 2000.
169. Ebert U, Reissmuller E, Loscher W. The new antiepileptic drugs lamotrigine and felbamate are effective in phenytoin-resistant kindled rats. Neuropharmacology 39:1893–1903, 2000.

52

Mechanisms of Action of New Mood-Stabilizing Drugs

JOSEPH LEVINE, YULY BERSUDSKY, CARMIT NADRI, YURI YAROSLAVSKY, ABED AZAB, ALEX MISHORI, GALILA AGAM, and ROBERT H. BELMAKER
Ben-Gurion University of the Negev, Beer-Sheva, Israel

I. INTRODUCTION

Several anticonvulsant (AC) compounds are useful in the treatment of bipolar disorder (BP). Carbamazepine and valproate were found to be effective treatments for BP [1,2]. Other ACs such as lamotrigine, topiramate, and more recently phenytoin also show promise [3–5]. However, much of the data regarding the clinical efficacy of the new AC depends on open, uncontrolled studies.

AC compounds have a multiplicity of pharmacological properties including GABA-agonistic effects, modulation of excitatory amino acids release, and blockade of sodium and calcium channels. A pharmacological dissection might be useful to identify the key mechanism for the mood-stabilizing effect of these drugs. In a pharmacological dissection, one first enumerates pharmacological properties at clinically relevant plasma concentrations. Second, one searches for common pharmacological properties. Third, one excludes properties not shared by all AC compounds or present in compounds showing no efficacy in BP.

In the following pages we will describe the pharmacological properties of AC reported to have antibipolar effects. Based on these data, we will propose that the shared common mechanism for antibipolar AC involves sodium channel–blocking activity. To illustrate this argument we will describe in detail the reported beneficial effects of phenytoin—a classical sodium channel blocker with relatively few other relevant pharmacological properties—in the manic phase of BP. We will attempt to demonstrate a relationship between clinical plasma therapeutic level of antibipolar AC and inhibition concentration 50% (IC_{50}) on sodium channels.

The preferential effect of phenytoin on the persistent sodium current allows for this AC to reduce late openings of sodium channels, while leaving early channel openings relatively intact. Speculatively, this could be the basis for an effect of phenytoin and other antibipolar ACs in diseases characterized by neuronal hyperexcitability (including manic states) while interfering minimally with normal function.

II. PHARMACOLOGICAL PROPERTIES OF MOOD-STABILIZING ANTICONVULSANT DRUGS

A. Carbamazepine

Carbamazepine has been demonstrated in open and double blind studies to have beneficial effects in bipolar illness [6,7] and is now routinely prescribed for this illness. Carbamazepine causes blockage of voltage-activated sodium channels, causing decreased electrical activity and, probably, a subsequent reduction in glutamate release [8]. This effect on sodium channels occurs at therapeutically relevant concentrations. This drug also inhibits benzodiazepine binding to peripheral type benzodiazepine receptors present on astrocytes [9]. Carbamazepine was also shown to bind to $GABA_A$ receptors, to potentiate chloride currents [10], and to prevent upregulation of cortical and hypothalamic $GABA_A$ receptors [11]. Another proposed mechanism of action of this drug involves an antagonistic activity at L-type cell membrane calcium channels; other findings suggest that it may also exert such an effect on N-type calcium channel [12]. Finally, there are reports that carbamazepine is an antagonist of A-type adenosine receptors [12].

B. Oxcarbazepine

Oxcarbazepine, 10-keto analog of carbamazepine, is indicated for the treatment of partial seizures with and without secondary generalization. There are data on the use of oxcarbazepine in patients with bipolar, schizoaffective, and schizophrenia-related disorders [13]. Macdonald and Kelly [14] suggested that its similarity in structure and clinical efficacy to carbamazepine suggests that its mechanism of action is similar to that of carbamazepine.

C. Valproate

Valproate is a branched-chain fatty acid. It is commercially available as the corresponding free acid, the sodium salt, and as divalproex sodium. Valproate causes blockage of voltage-operated sodium channels at therapeutic plasma levels [15]. Valproate is also reported to elevate brain GABA-ergic activity [16]. This mode of action may involve inhibition of GABA transaminase, an enzyme responsible for GABA metabolism, and it has also been suggested that valproate may inhibit succinic semialdehyde dehydrogenase [17], an enzyme that follows GABA transaminase in the process of GABA metabolism. The inhibition of the latter leads to product inhibition of GABA transaminase. Valproate has also been demonstrated to enhance the activity of glutamic acid decarboxylase, a key enzyme for GABA synthesis [18]. Thus, valproate increases synthesis of GABA and reduces its metabolism. It has also been reported that sodium valproate acts on T-type Ca^{2+} channels, and Franceschetti et al. [19] showed that this drug can suppress spontaneous epileptic activity in hippocampal slices by activating calcium and potassium conductance. An antagonistic action at the N-methyl-D-aspartate (NMDA) subtype of glutamate receptor has also been reported by several authors [20,21].

D. Topiramate

Topiramate is a sulfamate-substituted fructose derivative that is approved in several countries for the treatment of adult and pediatric epileptic disorders. Open studies suggest that topiramate may have mood-stabilizing properties for the treatment of bipolar disorder [22,23]. Topiramate, similarly to carbamazepine and valproate, blocks voltage-gated sodium channels [24]. Topiramate also potentiates GABA neuroinhibition [25], and increases cerebral GABA concentrations in healthy subjects [26]. In addition it has been reported to antagonize glutamate effects at NMDA receptors (AMPA/kainate type of glutamate receptor) [27], as well as to inhibit types II and IV isoenzymes of carbonic anhydrase [28]. Finally, topiramate has been reported to negatively modulate L- and N-type calcium channels, whereas its effects on T-type channels are still uncertain [28].

E. Lamotrigine

Lamotrigine is an antiepileptic drug of the phenyltriazine class. Recent studies suggest that lamotrigine may have beneficial effects in patients with BP [29,30]. Lamotrigine has been reported to stabilize type II sodium channels via selectively inhibiting sodium currents [31]. This drug interacts specifically with the slow inactivated state of the sodium channel. Davies [8] and Macdonald and Kelly [14] suggested that blockage of voltage-operated sodium channels by lamotrigine leads to decreased electrical activity and, probably, to a subsequent reduction in glutamate release. It has been also suggested that lamotrigine may modulate calcium and potassium channel currents [32]. Finally, this drug was reported to block the release of the excitatory amino acids glutamate and aspartate [33].

F. Gabapentin

Gabapentin was synthesized as an analog of GABA. It is approved as an adjunctive therapy for partial seizures with or without secondary generalization. Some preliminary data suggest that it may be effective for the acute or prophylactic treatment of bipolar illness [34,35]. However, a larger study did not demonstrate efficacy in bipolar disorder [36]. Gabapentin was reported to induce release of GABA from neurons and glia cells. Another mechanism offered was reversal of GABA transporter action, leading to increased extracellular GABA levels [37]. Yet another possibility is that this drug leads to increased synthesis of GABA [38]. Gabapentin also binds with high affinity to a brain binding site associated with an auxiliary subunit of voltage-sensitive Ca^{2+} channels, and it may thus modulate certain types of calcium current [39]. One could speculate that its lack of antibipolar activity in a double-blind controlled study [36] may be related to its clear lack of effect on sodium channels.

G. Tiagabine and Vigabatrin

Tiagabine is a nipecotic acid analog. There are anecdotal data regarding tiagabine's use for BP [40]. The drug enhances GABA-ergic activity by decreasing the uptake of GABA, leading to increased synaptic GABA content [41]. No affinity for a wide range of receptors was reported for this drug [42].

Vigabatrin increases synaptic concentration of GABA by inhibition of GABA aminotransferase [43]. Presumably, vigabatrin possesses only one mechanism of action, associated with this increased GABA-ergic activity [8]. There are still no reported studies of these drugs in BP at this time. We speculate that these two drugs, lacking an effect on sodium channels, will be devoid of beneficial activity in bipolar disorder.

H. Felbamate

Felbamate has been shown to block voltage-dependent sodium channels, to enhance GABA-mediated events, and to inhibit glutamatergic neurotransmission via action at the strychnine-insensitive glycine-binding site of the NMDA receptor [44,45]. There are as yet no reported studies of this drug in BP at this time. However, if sodium channel blockade is the primary mode of action of AC in BP, one would expect that this drug will show efficacy in BP.

I. Phenytoin

Phenytoin (5,5-diphenylhydantoin) mainly acts via blockade of voltage-dependent sodium channels, and it does not seem to modify GABA-ergic neural synaptic transmission [14]. Phenytoin at high concentrations, but not at therapeutically relevant concentrations, blocks depolarization-dependent calcium uptake in preparations of presynaptic nerve terminals [14], and it was suggested that it can at high concentrations inhibit calcium-calmodulin-dependent protein phosphorylation and regulate some neurotransmitter release [46]. Phenytoin was also reported to have little or no effect on T-type calcium channels in thalamic nuclei [14]. The blockade of sodium channels seems to be the main mode of action of this drug, and studies aiming at exploring the involvement of sodium channels blockade in the mode action of AC mood stabilizers may use phenytoin as a prototype drug for such exploration.

1. Phenytoin in Bipolar Illness

While numerous biochemical properties have been found for carbamazepine, valproate, lamotrigine, and topiramate, all seem to share with phenytoin, the classical anticonvulsant, powerful inhibition of voltage-activated sodium channels. It thus seemed of considerable theoretical importance to determine whether phenytoin is antibipolar. Early uncontrolled reports of improvement of mania with phenytoin exist [47], and its cognitive side effects have recently been reassessed favorably [48–50]. We therefore decided to conduct a trial of phenytoin in mania [5].

Based on our previous study of carbamazepine [51] and lithium [52] we used an add-on design to ongoing neuroleptic treatment. The study was approved by our Helsinki Committee, and all patients gave informed written consent. Patients could participate if they met DSM-IV criteria for mania or schizoaffective disorder, manic type, and had no serious physical illness. Only patients who had side effects or nonresponse to previous mood-stabilizing treatment were included.

Patients admitted to the study were treated with haloperidol at doses of physicians' discretion. Trihexyphenidyl was available as necessary for extrapyramidal symptoms and benzodiazepines for sleep. Phenytoin was begun at doses of 300 mg/day and increased to 400 mg after 4 days, with the first blood sample being drawn on the third day after that. Patients received phenytoin or identical capsules of placebo as assigned by the control psychiatrist according to random order; manic and schizoaffective manic patients were randomized separately. Weekly ratings by a psychiatrist blind to the study drug were conducted using the Brief Psychiatric Rating Scale (BPRS), the Young Mania Rating Scale (YMS), and the Clinical Global Impression (CGI). Blood was drawn weekly for phenytoin levels, and the results were reported to the control psychiatrist who created dummy levels for placebo patients and reported results to the treating physician, who adjusted dose of phenytoin accordingly.

Thirty-nine patients entered the study over 1 year and 30 completed at least 3 weeks. Patients completing at least 3 weeks were included in the data analysis on a last-value-carried-forward basis. Eighteen patients were schizoaffective manic and 12 were manic. Nine dropped out before 3 weeks: one with phenytoin toxicity (gait instability, blood level = 26 μg/mL); three refused to continue (one on phenytoin and two on placebo); three with exacerbation after 2 weeks on phenytoin; one on phenytoin after his brother's suicide; one on placebo violated the protocol with nonstudy medication.

Analyses were three-way MANCOVA, covariance for baseline (Greenhouse-Geisser corrected) for diagnosis, treatment, and time. For BPRS: Diagnosis, treatment and time showed a significant three-way interaction ($F = 5.09$, $df_{2.3, 60.6}$, $P = .006$), with a significant two-way interaction between treatment and time ($F = 3.83$, $df_{2.3, 60.6}$, $P = .02$) and significant two-way interaction between treatment and diagnosis ($F = 4.42$, $df_{1,25}$, $P = .046$). Tukey HSD posthoc comparisons show significant differences for manic patients only from week 3 to week 5 ($p_3 = .01$, $p_4 = .006$ and $p_5 = .001$) between phenytoin and placebo. The effect size of phenytoin improvement in manic patients and schizoaffective manic patients compares with similar figures for carbamazepine [51] in a similar acute add-on design.

Several patients illustrate the possible clinical utility of phenytoin in mania. A 44-year-old male with treatment resistance in previous episodes to lithium, valproate, carbamazapine, or Li-carbamazepine combination responded to haloperidol 15 mg/day plus phenytoin (blood level 19 μg/mL) by the end of week 2. He reached full remission but exacerbated rapidly when he stopped phenytoin at the end of the trial. A 26-year-old bipolar female with very long hospitalizations in the past improved on lithium within 2 weeks on haloperidol 25 mg/day plus phenytoin (blood level 17 μg/mL). She reached full remission within a month for the first time in her history. A 60-year-old male had never reached a stable remission, despite numerous hospitalizations on lithium, carbamazepine, or valproate with severe side effects. By the third week of haloperidol 10 mg plus phenytoin (blood level 15 μg/mL), he became completely euthymic and for the first time cooperative with treatment.

III. VOLTAGE-GATED SODIUM CHANNELS

We argued that voltage-gated sodium channels, playing a pivotal role in action potential generation in central neurons, may be the key target for AC mood stabilizers. In this section we will survey current knowledge on the nature of these channels.

A. Structure of Voltage-Sensitive Na$^+$ Channels

1. Protein Subunits

Sodium channels were the first ion channels whose structure has been characterized. Purified Na$^+$ channels were found to contain all the functional components necessary for electrical excitability: ion conductance and voltage-dependent gating. A variety of biochemical techniques such as: photoreactive derivatives of toxins that attach covalently to Na$^+$ channels in intact cell membrane, enabling identifying channel components without purification [53]; reversible binding of the toxins tetrodotoxin (TTX) and saxitoxin (STX) to their receptor to quantify the channel protein amount and functionality [56]; and solubilization of excitable membranes with nonionic detergents releasing the Na$^+$ channels in a form that retains their ability to bind TTX and STX with high affinity were used to identify the characteristics of the electrical exitability of the channels.

Toward understanding structure-function relationship of this channel, several groups identified a large glycoprotein (260 KDa) as the major subunit—the α-subunit. It is a transmembrane polypeptide composed of 1800–2000 amino acids and contains four repeated domains (designated I–IV) having ~ 50% amino acid sequence identity, resulting in similar secondary and tertiary structures [53]. Each domain contains six segments (designated 1–6) that form transmembrane α-helices and additional hydrophobic sequences that are thought to be membrane associated contributing to the formation of the outer pore. The four domains are connected by a relatively hydrophilic intracellular amino acid sequence. This structural motif of the voltage-gated sodium channel homologous domains is the building block of all the voltage-gated channels [54]. The α-subunit has sites for the attachment of carbohydrate chains and for the binding of neurotoxins on the external surface of the channel, as well as phosphorylation sites by cAMP-dependent protein kinase (PKA) on the intracellular surface [54]. In frog oocytes the α-subunit is sufficient to form an active channel by itself, emphasizing the importance of this subunit for the function of the channel [54]. In mammalian brain the α-subunit is associated with two additional polypeptides: the auxiliary β1-subunit (36 KDa) and β2-subunit (33 KDa). They are integral membrane proteins that interact with the phospholipid bilayer [53].

The β1-subunit consists of a large glycosylated, extracellular N-terminal segment, a single-transmembrane segment, and a short intracellular segment. The glycosylating groups are sialic acid, contributing to the strong net negative charge of the channel subunits. It consists of 218 amino acids and has a large extracellular domain with four potential sites of N-linked glycosylation, a single α-helical membrane spanning segment, and a very small intracellular domain [55]. The β1- and β2-subunits of Na$^+$ channels have similar overall structures but are not closely related in amino acid sequence. The β1-subunit is noncovalently attached to the α-subunit while the β2-subunit is covalently attached to the α-subunit via a disulfide bond. The β1- and β2-subunits reveal a probable structural relationship to the family of proteins that contain immunoglobulin-like folds [54]. This is a sandwich of two β-sheets held together by hydrophobic interactions, a unique structure among ion channels subunits.

A reentrant loop dipped in the transmembrane region of the sodium channel protein between the transmembrane segments S5 and S6 forms the outer pore of the channel. Relatively large extracellular loops were predicted in each homologous domain, connecting either the S5 or the S6 transmembrane segments to the membrane-reentrant loop. Even larger intracellular loops were predicted to connect the four homologous domains, and large N-terminal and C-terminal domains were also predicted to be intracellular.

2. Outer Pore and the Selectivity Filter

The movement of an ion across the membrane is a continual exchange of oxygen ligands as the ion passes through relatively free water molecules and polar groups that form the wall of the pore. This pore may interact with permeated ions as they approach and move through the channel. It is assumed that as the ion permeates polar and charged groups in the pore provide stabilization energy, compensating for water molecules that are left behind [54]. The pore is narrow enough to sense different ions and to distinguish among them. The channels also contain charged components that sense the electric field in the membrane and drive conformational changes that open and close "gates" controlling the permeability of the pore. A single channel handles up to 6×10^7 monovalent ions per second, implicating that the channel is indeed a pore [53].

Based on evidence from the blockade of the channels' permeability by lowering the pH of the external medium below 5.5, and from site-directed mutagenesis of aspartate and glutamate residues in cloned channels [54], these negatively charged residues were postulated to form outer and inner rings that serve as the receptor sites for TTX and STX and a selectivity filter in the outer pore of sodium channels. Mutational analysis identified glutamate 387 in the membrane reentrant loop in domain I, and another pair of important amino acid residues, mostly glutamate and aspartate, in analogous positions in all four domains near the C-terminal of the short hydrophobic segment between transmembrane α-helices S5 and S6, as crucial residues for the binding of the pore blockers TTX and STX [4]. Mutation of only two of the residues that are not negatively charged to glutamate (in domains III and IV) replaces the selectivity of the Na$^+$ channel into a Ca^{2+} selective channel [54].

3. The Voltage Sensor

A membrane protein responding to changes in membrane potential must have either charged or dipolar amino acid residues, or both, located within the membrane electric field, acting as a voltage sensor [53]. When the energy of the field-charge interactions is high, the protein may undergo a change to a new stable conformational state in which the net charge or the location of charge has been altered. Such movement of membrane-bound charges gives rise to a "gating" current [57].

The S4 segments of the homologous domains have been proposed as the voltage sensor of the Na$^+$ channel [58]. These segments are highly conserved in all voltage-gated channels, and consist of repeated triplets of two hydrophobic amino acids followed by positively charged residues. In the α-helical configuration they form a spiral of positive charge across the membrane, well suited for transmembrane movement of gating charges. Each positive charge is neutralized by a negative charge in one of the surrounding transmembrane segments.

It is suggested that the movement of the S4 helix in each domain initiates a more general conformational change in that domain. After taking place in all four domains, the transmembrane pore can open and conduct ions. Shortly after opening, the channel goes through inactivation.

Unlike activation, fast inactivation of the open state of Na$^+$ channels is not a strongly voltage-sensitive process. Apparently, regions of ion channels mediating inactivation are exposed to the intracellular surface of the membrane.

Treatment of the intracellular surface of the channel with proteolytic enzymes prevents inactivation [54]. The segment of the Na$^+$ channel between domains III and IV is proposed to serve as the inactivation gate by forming a hinged lid which folds over the intracellular pore after activation [54]. Antibodies against the intracellular segment connecting domains III and IV completely block inactivation [54]; expression of the Na$^+$ channel as two separate fragments cut between domains III and IV greatly attenuates inactivation [54]; phosphorylation of a single serin residue in this segment by protein kinase C slows inactivation [54]. Mutation of a cluster of three hydrophobic residues that is required for fast Na$^+$ channel inactivation, with three glutamine residues (hydrophilic amino acid), completely eliminates fast inactivation of Na$^+$ channels. Another essential residue is phenylalanine at position 1489. Its mutation to glutamine nearly blocks fast inactivation of the channel. The cluster of hydrophobic residues including Phe 1489 is thought to enter the pore and bind as a latch to keep the channel inactivated [53].

B. Gating Mechanism of the Na$^+$ Channel

Voltage-gated sodium channels, responsible for the rising phase of the action potential in the membranes of neurons and electrically excitable cells exhibit three key features: voltage-dependent activation, rapid inactivation, and selective ion conductance [54]. Together with K$^+$ channels they account for almost all the currents in axonal membranes.

Hodgkin and Huxley [57] suggested a kinetic model for the opening and closing steps of Na$^+$ channels: depolarization of the membrane is sensed by the voltage sensor and causes conformational reactions towards opening and activation of the channel. Repolarization or hyperpolarization causes closure and inactivation. An action potential due to a depolarizing stimulus begins with a transient, voltage-gated opening that allows Na$^+$ to enter the fiber and depolarize the membrane fully. This is followed by a transient voltage-gated opening of K$^+$ channels that allows K$^+$ to leave the cell and repolarize the membrane. In myelinated nerves, depolarization spreads from one excitable membrane patch to another by local circuit currents, but because of the insulating properties of the coating myelin, the excitable patches of axonal membrane (nodes of Ranvier) may be > 1 mm apart, and thus the rate of progression of the impulse is faster. Nodes of Ranvier have Na$^+$ channels similar to those of other axonal membranes, but nodal membranes have at least 10 times as many channels per area unit to depolarize the long, passive, intranodal myelin. The intranodal axonal membrane has K$^+$ channels but far fewer than Na$^+$ channels. Although hidden underneath the myelin, these K$^+$ channels may contribute to maintain resting potentials.

C. Pharmacological Agents Acting on the Na$^+$ Channels

The pharmacology of potent poisons targeted at the Na$^+$ channels aids in the definition of functional regions of the channel. At the outer end of the channel there is a site where the puffer fish poison, tetrodotoxin (TTX), and its analog saxitoxin (STX), a small lipid-insoluble charged molecule bind ($K_i = 1$–10 nM) and block Na$^+$ permeability [54].

Another class of Na$^+$ channel blockers is local anesthetics such as lidocaine and procaine and related antiarrhythmic agents. They are lipid-soluble amines with a hydrophobic end and a polar end; they bind to a hydrophobic site on the channel protein interacting with the inactivation gating machinery [54]. The relevant clinical actions of local anesthetics are fully explained by their mode of Na$^+$ channel blocking.

Two other classes of toxins that either open Na$^+$ channels spontaneously or prevent them from closing normally once they have opened are lipid-soluble steroids, such as batrachotoxin (BTX), aconitine, and veratridine, all acting at a site within the membrane; and peptide toxins from scorpion and anemone venom, which act at two sites on the outer surface of the membrane, blocking specifically the inactivation gating step [54]. The affinity of the Na$^+$ channels toward these agents is dependent on the gating conformation state of the channel.

D. Brain Voltage-Gated Sodium Channels

The physiological role and properties of ion channels may be expected to be similar in all tissues. However, brain, heart (cardiac), and skeletal muscles sodium channels differ, particularly in their selectivity. Studies using tetrodotoxin revealed that the difference in selectivity of different sodium channels is determined by a single amino acid residue located in domain I (the selectivity filter) [54].

Phosphorylation of brain sodium channels by cAMP-dependent protein kinase (PKA) on four sites in the intracellular loop connecting domains I and II in the α-subunit [54,59] causes a reduction in the peak of sodium currents in brain neurons, but does not alter Na$^+$ channel voltage dependence [54].

Membrane potential is a crucial determinant of the neuromodulation of hippocampal neurons sodium channels via PKA signal cascade. PKA is one of the signal cascades by which dopamine manifests its functions. Depolarization of the membrane, or activation of protein kinase-C (PKC) results in the amplification of D$_1$-dopaminergic effects and PKA activation. The localization of PKA near the sodium channel is essential to achieve phosphorylation of the α-subunit and to manifest dopaminergic-induced reduction in sodium currents.

Dopamine is also involved in excitation and firing of neurons in the striatonigral pathway. In addition, sodium currents in the nucleus accumbens are reduced after treatment with cocaine, a drug that blocks dopamine reuptake, implicating potential behavioral consequences of neuromodulation of sodium channels [53].

Activation of muscarinic acetylcholine receptors in hippocampal pyramidal neuron reduces peak sodium currents and slows inactivation of the Na$^+$ channels via activation of the PKC signal cascade [60]. Phosphorylation of specific sites in the intracellular loop between domains I and II reduces peak sodium currents, and phosphorylation of a site in the inactivation gate (intracellular loop connecting domains III and IV) slows Na$^+$ channels inactivation [53,54].

Several neurotransmitters, including dopamine and acetylcholine, activate brain G-proteins. Activation of G-proteins activates neuronal Na$^+$ channels. Thus, modulation of brain Na$^+$ channels by neurotransmission is apparently mediated via G-protein activation.

In conclusion, neuromodulatory processes of brain Na$^+$ channels affect excitability, overall conductance of neurons, and hence, their synaptic activity.

IV. RELATIONSHIP BETWEEN ANTIBIPOLAR AC PLASMA LEVEL AND IC$_{50}$ FOR SODIUM CHANNELS

Peroutka and Snyder [61] correlated the clinical potency of antipsychotic drugs and their in vitro dopamine receptor blockade activity, and demonstrated a high correlation between these two properties. Such a high correlation strongly supported the involvement of dopamine receptor blockade in the mode of action of antipsychotic drugs. We explored whether a correlation between antibipolar therapeutic plasma levels and their 50% inhibition concentration (IC$_{50}$) of sodium channels could be found for antibipolar AC. The antibipolar potencies of the AC were taken as the median effective clinical dosage used in the treatment of BP and the recommended therapeutic plasma level (Table 1).

The sodium channel blocking capacity of each drug was calculated by its IC$_{50}$ of sodium channels. In case the sodium blocking capacity varied between different studies (i.e., PHT and CBZ), the median IC$_{50}$ was taken as the representative value. Sodium channel blockade induced by CBZ and PHT was analyzed by Willow et al. [62] in mouse neuroblastoma cells using a patch voltage clamp procedure in a whole cell configuration. The IC$_{50}$ observed in this study was ~30 mM for each of these drugs. Another study—investigating the effect of CBZ, PHT, and LTG on voltage-activated sodium channels present in N4TG1 mouse neuroblastoma clonal cells—reported a tonic inhibition of sodium channels with IC$_{50}$ values of 140, 58, and 91 μM, respectively [63]. Taken together, these data showed IC$_{50}$ in the range of 30–58 μM (median = 44 μM) for PHT, and 30–140 μM (median = 85 μM) for CBZ, whereas the value for LTG was 91μM.

A study exploring sodium channel blockade by VPA in cultured rat hippocampal neurons using a whole-cell voltage clamp under conditions appropriate for isolating sodium currents [64], found that sodium

Table 1 Therapeutic Blood Levels and Sodium Channel Blockade

Compound	IC$_{50}$ (μM) [ref.]	Clinical dosage mg/day (median)	Plasma Level (μg/mL)
Carbamazepine (CBZ)	85 [62,63]	400–1600 (1000)	12
Sodium Valproate (VPA)	2400 [65]	1500–3000 (2250)	100
Lamotrigine (LTG)	91 [63]	50–200 (125)	~14
Topiramate (TPM)	48.9 [66]	200–400 (300)	~5
Phenytoin (PHT)	44 [63,64]	300–500 (400)	20

currents were reduced in a voltage-dependent manner. Even a large concentration (1 mM) of VPA did not lead to 50% inhibition of sodium currents. This effect of VPA was also determined by voltage and current clamp experiments in nodal membrane of peripheral nerve fibers of *Xenopus laevis*. Valproate was found to reduce sodium currents with IC_{50} of ~ 2.4 mM [65].

The half-maximal inhibition of sodium channels by TPM was examined in rat cerebellar granule cells, as measured by whole-cell current clamp recording. Topiramate was found to reduce the voltage-gated sodium channels with IC_{50} of 48.9 μM [66].

The effect of GBP on limiting the repetitive firing of sodium-dependent action potentials was examined in monolayer dissociated cell culture of mouse spinal cord and neocortical neurons [71]. These authors reported that GBP limited high-frequency action potential firing, but that this effect was not likely to be due to a blockade of sodium channels [71]. More than that, another study [72] showed that even a high concentration (200 mM) of GPB did not block voltage-dependent sodium currents. The anticonvulsant phenobarbital given in therapeutic doses did not seem to have an antibipolar effect [73] and did not inhibit sodium channels [74].

V. FUTURE DIRECTIONS

A. Prophylactic Study of Phenytoin in BP

In order to support the role of sodium channel blocking as a primary mechanism underlying the AC action in BP, prophylactic efficacy for phenytoin should be shown. We are conducting a 1-year double-blind crossover prophylactic study of phenytoin in BP illness. The study was approved by our Helsinki Committee, and patients gave informed written consent. Patients can participate if they meet DSM-IV criteria for mania or schizoaffective disorder, manic type, and have no serious physical illness. Patients can enter the study if they have been out of hospital for at least 1 month and had inadequate prophylaxis in the past on lithium, carbamazepine, or valproate, and had at least one episode per year for the last 2 years. All patients are evaluated by the clinical treating physician at baseline, weekly during the first month, and monthly thereafter. Ongoing prophylactic treatment is not changed (lithium, carbamazepine, valproate, or neuroleptic). Phenytoin or placebo (as randomized) is added slowly (100 mg per week) to ongoing antibipolar treatment. Blood levels of all antibipolar treatments are monitored weekly for the first month and adjusted as necessary. Ratings (BPRS, YMS, HDS, GAS) are done by the clinical treating psychiatrist at baseline and once monthly thereafter. After 6 months patients are crossed over during a month of weekly visits with one drug (phenytoin or placebo) being reduced by 100 mg weekly and the other increased by 100 mg weekly. This is done with individualized packets of capsules, such that the double-blind is maintained. Blood levels of all antibipolar drugs are monitored weekly during this adjustment phase, and doses adjusted as necessary. Blood levels are monitored monthly after the adjustment phase. The treating psychiatrist, who also performs the rating scales, is blind to whether the patient is on phenytoin or placebo. He receives from the control psychiatrist a bottle of tablets of phenytoin or placebo, according to prearranged random order. Blood levels of phenytoin are reported by the lab to the treating psychiatrist after "dummy" levels are assigned by the control psychiatrist to patients on placebo. The second phase also lasts for 6 months of monthly clinical ratings. Patients terminate from the study if hospitalization is necessary. Symptoms of sufficient severity to require addition of neuroleptic or antidepressant treatment are the major outcome variable, but will not terminate patients from the study.

Special attention is given to instruction of patients in dental hygiene, and patients showing signs of gingival hyperplasia will be dropped. Studies in epilepsy show that this side effect is surprisingly uncommon, despite wide publicity [75]. No cases were seen in our previous short-term study [5]. Nonlinear pharmacokinetics, drug interactions, and the consequent danger of toxicity will be handled by careful blood levels monitoring.

B. Intravenous Fosphenytoin in Acute Mania

There is a strong need in the clinical arena for fast-acting antimanic agents. Lithium loading has been reported [76]. Valproate loading has recently been reported to be promising [77]. Phenytoin is a drug with a long history of intravenous use in status epilepticus but has not yet been studied intravenously in mania.

Several authors explored the rapidity and magnitude of response of manic symptomatology in the hours following an intravenous administration of agents such as physostigmine or naloxone [77,78].

New Mood-Stabilizing Drugs

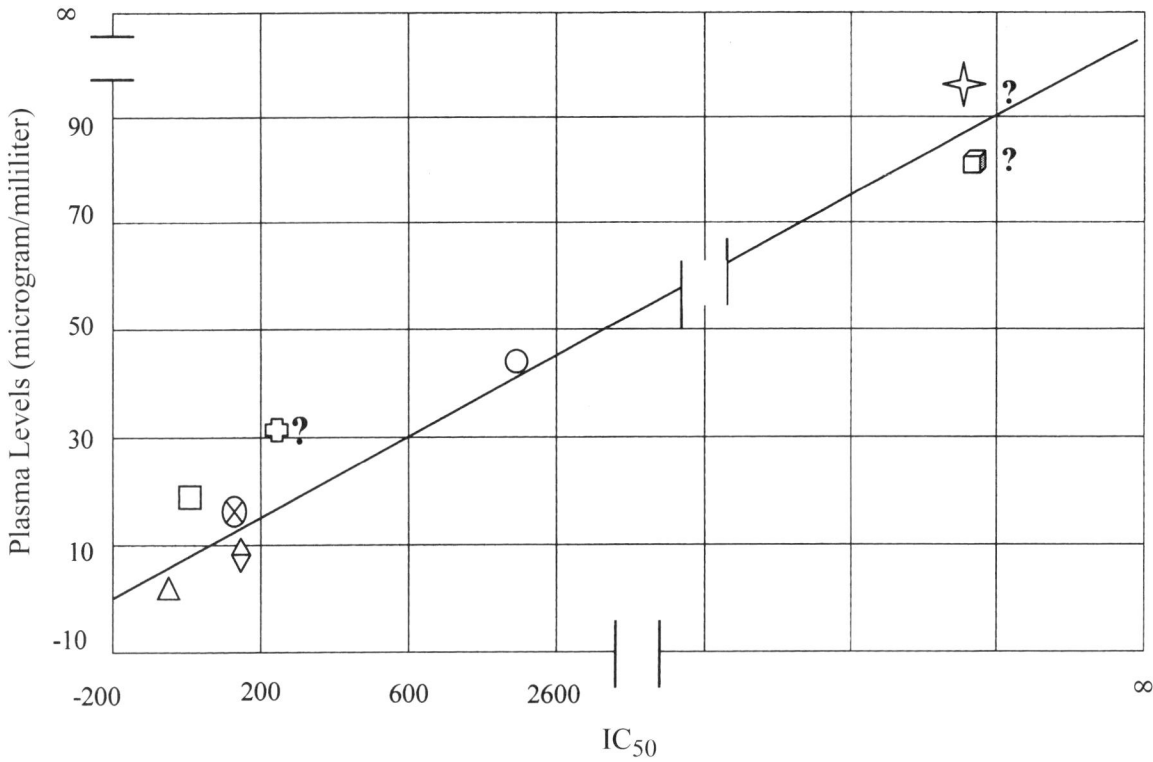

Figure 1 Relationship of IC$_{50}$ for sodium channels with therapeutic plasma levels. *Legend*: ○ = valproate; △ = carbamazepine; □ = phenytoin; ✧ = lorazepam; ⌐⌐ = gabapentin; ✢ = felbamate; ⊗ = lamotrigine; ◇ = topiramate.

Physostigmine given openly led to ~ 30% improvement in Pettersen Mania Rating Scale in the hour following its administration, which returned toward baseline 2–3 h later. Naloxone showed a more modest improvement up to 2 h following its administration. While physostigmine and naloxone IV have very limited clinical use today, they demonstrated that rapid improvement of manic symptoms is theoretically possible.

In the above pages we described beneficial effect of phenytoin in mania and have noted that sodium channel blockade is the primary mechanism of phenytoin. We are now performing a study of IV fosphenytoin in acute manic patients. We wish to explore whether such a strategy can induce rapid improvement in symptomatology of acute manic state without sedation. This may shed light on the possible role of sodium channel blockade as a primary therapeutic mechanism in mania.

Drugs used to treat status epilepticus must be tolerated when administered rapidly IV. Intravenous phenytoin is effective, and relatively free of sedation or respiratory suppression in the treatment of tonic-clonic status epilepticus [80]. However, intravenous phenytoin has a side-effect profile which compromises its tolerability. If administered IV too rapidly, it may lead to cardiac complications or skin necrosis at the injection site. Fosphenytoin sodium, a phosphate ester prodrug of phenytoin, was specifically developed for the replacement of parenteral phenytoin sodium. It has the same pharmacological properties as phenytoin, but has lower potential for local tissue irritation (e.g., burning and itching at the injection site) and cardiac toxicity than phenytoin. CNS effects are similar for the two drugs, but transient paresthesias are more common with fosphenytoin [81]. Unlike phenytoin, fosphenytoin is freely soluble in aqueous solutions. Fosphenytoin is metabolized to phenytoin by endogenous phosphatases (conversion half-life is ~ 15 min). Therapeutic unbound free and total plasma phenytoin concentrations are consistently demonstrated after IV administration of fosphenytoin loading doses. Fosphenytoin dosage is expressed as phenytoin sodium equivalents (PE). The standard loading dose for adults with status epilepticus is 15–20 mg PE/kg IV infused at 100–150 mg/min [82,83]. For nonemergency situations, a 10–20 mg PE/kg loading dose can be given IV [84], such as for anticonvulsant loading before a neurosurgical operation.

For our double-blind placebo-controlled study of IV fosphenytoin in acute manic patients, consenting manic patients with a score of > 20 points in Young Rating Mania Scale, with no psychiatric comorbidity and physically healthy, are administered fosphenytoin 5 mg/kg (half to quarter of the dose recommended for status epilepticus at a rate of 100 mg/min (similar to that given in status epilepticus). EKG, heart rate, and respiration are monitored during the drug administration and for 60 min after. Pettersen Mania Scale and Minimental Rating Scale will be rated at baseline and at 30 and 60 min after the IV fosphenytoin injection. Rapid relief of manic symptoms through use of this nonsedative sodium channel blocker would have theoretical as well as practical clinical significance.

C. Sodium Channel Abnormalities in Bipolar Patients

Several mutations have been reported in subunits of the sodium channel which may serve as candidate mutations in the search for the genetic etiology of BP illness. The rare autosomal-dominant disorder "generalized epilepsy with febrile seizures plus" was found to be associated with mutation in beta-1-subunit of the voltage-sensitive sodium channel [85]. This mutation changes a conserved cysteine residue, leading to disruption of a putative disulfide bridge which normally maintains an extracellular immunoglobulin-like fold. Based on their studies in *Xenopus laevis* oocytes these authors argue that this mutation interferes with the ability of the beta-1-subunit to modulate the channel-gating kinetics. Another rare autosomal-dominant disorder, "benign familial infantile convulsions," was not found to be associated with mutations encoded in intron 5 of the human sodium channel beta-1-subunit gene [86]. Makita et al. [87] reported the existence of an intragenic polymorphic (TTA)n repeat in the beta-1-subunit positioned between two tandem Alu repetitive sequences exhibiting five distinct alleles. Finally, Haug et al. [88] reported genetic variations in the human sodium channel beta-2-subunit gene which included for example a missense mutation in codon 209 (Asp 209 Pro) found in one of 92 patients with idiopathic generalized epilepsy but not found in an affected sibling of the index patient. These mutations, irrespective of their association with epileptic syndromes, may serve as candidate mutations for association studies of BP illness.

D. Relationship Between Antibipolar Potency and IC$_{50}$ Values for Sodium Channel Blocking

Figure 1 illustrates the relationship between sodium channel blockade and antibipolar potency of AC. Clearly, there is a group of highly potent sodium channel blockers such as phenytoin, carbamazepine, and lamotrigine. However, their spread of clinical dosages and therapeutic plasma levels does not allow a dissection of whether the therapeutic dosages and sodium channel blockade are truly related. Valproate requires higher clinical dosages and is also a less potent blocker of sodium channels, supporting our hypothesis. Further points on the graph between phenytoin and valproate are necessary, however, to truly support this hypothesis. We predict that drugs like gabapentin, phenobarbital, and lorazepam, which are unlikely to be effective sodium channel blockers, will also turn out to be poor antibipolar drugs. Phenobarbital is clearly an anticonvulsant in epilepsy, but its sedative nature sets it apart from nonsedative anticonvulsants like carbamazepine and phenytoin. It is clearly not antimanic. Benzodiazepines like lorazepam are clearly useful in mania and in agitated depression, but most clinicians would argue that this effect is essentially different from the true mood-stabilizing effect of lithium and the antibipolar AC. Clonazepam is felt by many neurologists to be a uniquely anticonvulsant benzodiazepine, so its effects in BP would be critical information. Unfortunately, convincing clinical data are lacking. Clinical use skyrocketed a few years back but has more recently greatly declined. We predict that it will turn out to be merely adjunctive as will other benzodiazepines that do not block sodium channels. Felbamate, as well as lamotrigine and topiramate, are high-potency sodium channel blockers, and our theory predicts true antibipolar efficacy for them.

It is important to note that not only clinical data are lacking in this field. Sodium channel blockade can vary across species, tissues, and experimental designs. The sodium channel, as discussed above, is a highly complex structure. Inhibition could occur at different steps in its opening and closing, which have different physiological meanings. Recent data in vivo on clozapine binding suggest that even the relatively simple dopamine receptor can be bound with differing degrees of reversibility in a way that could account for the unexpected excess efficacy of clozapine.

The sodium channel blockade hypothesis is heuristic and unifying, but clearly only a hypothesis. Manufacturers of new anticonvulsants have a clear interest in emphasizing the unique pharmacological properties of their new drugs, to encourage use in the many patients nonresponsive to existing drugs. This can be scientifically misleading, however, for an AC drug like topiramate with unique effects on carbonic anhydrase, for example, is also a very effective sodium channel blocker. We know that even AC, with very similar modes of action, such as phenytoin and carbamazepine, can synergize in a highly positive way in seizure disorders.

Preconceptions can also have negative effects on science. For example, phenytoin was almost universally dismissed as ineffective in BP for half a century and was simply not studied until recently. Clearly one controlled study of phenytoin is not enough, but its powerful sodium channel blockade surely justifies considerable further effort.

REFERENCES

1. Small JG, Klapper MH, Milstein V, Kellams JJ, Miller MJ, Marhenke JD, Small IF. Carbamazepine compared with lithium in the treatment of mania. Arch Gen Psychiatry 1991; 48(10):915–921.
2. Freeman TW, Clothier JL, Pazzaglia P, Lesem MD, Swann AC. A double-blind comparison of valproate and lithium in the treatment of acute mania. Am J Psychiatry 1992; 149(1):108–111.
3. Calabrese JR, Bowden CL, Sachs GS, Ascher JA, Monaghan E, Rudd GD. A double-blind placebo-controlled study of lamotrigine monotherapy in outpatients with bipolar I depression. Lamictal 602 Study Group. J Clin Psychiatry 1999; 60(2):79–88.
4. Marcotte D. Use of topiramate, a new anti-epileptic as a mood stabilizer. J Affect Disord 1998; 50(2-3):245–251.
5. Mishory A, Yaroslavsky Y, Bersudsky Y, Belmaker RH. Phenytoin as an antimanic anticonvulsant: a controlled study. Am J Psychiatry 2000; 157(3):463–465.
6. Post RM, Denicoff KD, Frye MA, Dunn RT, Leverich GS, Osuch E, Speer A. A history of the use of anticonvulsants as mood stabilizers in the last two decades of the 20th century. Neuropsychobiology 1998; 38(3):152–166.
7. Sachs GS, Printz DJ, Kahn DA, Carpenter D, Docherty JP. The Expert Consensus Guideline Series. Medication Treatment of Bipolar Disorder 2000. Postgrad Med 2000; Spec No:1–104.
8. Davies JA. Mechanisms of action of antiepileptic drugs. Seizure 1995; 4(4):276–271.
9. Bender AS, Hertz L. Evidence for involvement of the astrocytic benzodiazepine receptor in the mechanism of action of convulsant and anticonvulsant drugs. Life Sci 1988; 43(6):477–484
10. Granger P, Biton B, Faure C, Vige X, Depoortere H, Graham D, Langer SZ, Scatton B, Avenet P. Modulation of the gammaminobutyric acid type A receptor by the antiepileptic drugs carbamazepine and phenytoin. Mol Pharmacol 1995;47:1189–1196.
11. Galpern WR, Miller LG, Greenblatt DJ, Szabo GK, Browne TR, Shader RJ. Chronic benzodiazepine administration. IX. Attenuation of alprazolam discontinuation effects by carbamazepine. Biochem Pharmacol 1991; 42(suppl):S99–S104.
12. Schirrmacher K, Mayer A, Walden J, Dusing R, Bingmann D. Effects of carbamazepine on action potentials and calcium currents in rat spinal ganglion cells in vitro. Neuropsychobiology 1993; 27(3):176–179.
13. Emrich HM, Dose M, Von Zerssen D. The use of sodium valproate, carbamazepine and oxcarbazepine in patients with affective disorders. J Affect Disord 1985; 8(3):243–250.
14. Macdonald RL, Kelly KM. Antiepileptic drug mechanisms of action. Epilepsia 1995; 36(suppl 2):S2–S12.
15. McLean MJ, Macdonald RL. Sodium valproate, but not ethosuximide, produces use- and voltage-dependent limitation of high frequency repetitive firing of action potentials of mouse central neurons in cell culture. J Pharmacol Exp Ther 1986; 237(3):1001–1011.
16. Loscher W, Vetter M. Drug-induced changes in GABA content of nerve endings in 11 rat brain regions. Correlation to pharmacological effects. Neurosci Lett 1984; 47(3):325–331.
17. Fariello RG, Varasi M, Smith MC. Valproic acid. mechanisms of action. In: Levy RG, Mattson RG, Meldrum BS, eds. Antiepileptic Drugs, 4th ed. New York: Raven Press, 1995.
18. Wikinski SI, Acosta GB, Rubio MC. Valproic acid differs in its in vitro effect on glutamic acid decarboxylase activity in neonatal and adult rat brain. Gen Pharmacol 1996; 27(4): 635–638.
19. Franceschetti S, Hamon B, Heinemann U. The action of valproate on spontaneous epileptiform activity in the absence of synaptic transmission and on evoked changes in $[Ca^{2+}]o$ and $[K^{+}]o$ in the hippocampal slice. Brain Res 1986; 386(1-2):1–11.

20. Ko GY, Brown-Croyts LM, Teyler TJ. The effects of anticonvulsant drugs on NMDA-EPSP, AMPA-DPSP, and GABA-IPSP in the rat hippocampus. Brain Res Bull 1997(42):297–302.
21. Gean PW, Huang CC, Hung CR, Tsai JJ. Valproic acid suppresses the synaptic response mediated by the NMDA receptors in rat amygdalar slices. Brain Res Bull 1994; 33(3):333–336.
22. Chengappa KN, Rathore D, Levine J, Atzert R, Solai L, Parepally H, Levin H, Moffa N, Delaney J, Brar JS. Topiramate as add-on treatment for patients with bipolar mania. Bipolar Disord 1999; 1(1):42–53.
23. McElroy SL, Suppes T, Keck PE, Frye MA, Denicoff KD, Altshuler LL, Brown ES, Nolen WA, Kupka RW, Rochussen J, Leverich GS, Post RM. Open-label adjunctive topiramate in the treatment of bipolar disorders. Biol Psychiatry 2000; 47(12): 1025–1033.
24. Coulter DA, Sombati S, SeLorenzo RF. Selective effects of topiramate on sustained repetitive firing and spontaneous bursting in cultured hippocampal neurones. Epilepsia 1993; 34:123.
25. Petroff OA, Hyder F, Mattson RH, Rothman DL. Topiramate increases brain GABA, homocarnosine, and pyrrolidinone in patients with epilepsy. Neurology 1999; 52(3):473–478.
26. Kuzniecky R, Hetherington H, Ho S, Pan J, Martin R, Gilliam F, Hugg J, Faught E. Topiramate increases cerebral GABA in healthy humans. Neurology 1998; 51(2):627–629.
27. Coulter DA, Sombati S, DeLorenzo RF. Topirmate effects on excitatory amino acid mediated respoin cultured hippocampal neurones: selective blockade of kianate currents. Epilepsia 1995; 36:S40.
28. Shank RP, Gardocki JF, Vaught JL, et al. Topiramate: preclinical evaluation of structurally novel anticonvulsant. Epilepsia 1994; 35(2):450–460.
29. Calabrese JR, Suppes T, Bowden CL, Sachs GS, Swann AC, McElroy SL, Kusumakar V, Ascher JA, Earl NL, Greene PL, Monaghan ET. A double-blind, placebo-controlled, prophylaxis study of lamotrigine in rapid-cycling bipolar disorder. Lamictal 614 Study Group. J Clin Psychiatry 2000; 61(11):841–850.
30. Bowden CL, Mitchell P, Suppes T. Lamotrigine in the treatment of bipolar depression. Eur Neuropsychopharmacol 1999; 9(suppl 4):S113–S117.
31. Xie X, Lancaster B, Peakman T, Garthwaite J. Interaction of the antiepileptic drug lamotrigine with recombinant rat brain type IIA Na$^+$ channels and with native Na$^+$ channels in rat hippocampal neurones. Pflugers Arch 1995; 430(3):437–446.
32. Walden J, Wegerer J, Berger M. The antiepileptic drug lamotrigine may limit pathological excitation by modulating calcium and potassium currents: update on antiepileptic drugs in bipolar disorder. Second International Conference on Bipolar Disorder, Pittsburgh, 1997.
33. Messenheimer JA. Lamotrigine. Epilepsia 1995; 36(suppl 2):S87–S94.
34. Bennett J, Goldman WT, Suppes T. Gabapentin for treatment of bipolar and schizoaffective disorders. J Clin Psychopharmacol 1997; 17(2):141–142.
35. Vieta E, Martinez-Aran A, Nieto E, Colom F, Reinares M, Benabarre A, Gasto C. Adjunctive gabapentin treatment of bipolar disorder. Eur Psychiatry 2000; 15(7):433–437.
36. Pande AC, Crockatt JG, Janney CA, Werth JL, Tsaroucha G. Gabapentin in bipolar disorder: a placebo-controlled trial of adjunctive therapy. Gabapentin Bipolar Disorder Study Group. Bipolar Disord 2000; 2(3 Pt 2):249–255.
37. Gotz E, Feurerstein TJ. Effects of gabapentin on the release of gamma-aminobutyric acid from slices of rat neostriatum. Arzneimittelforchung 1993; 43:636–638.
38. Loscher W, Honack D, Taylor CP. Gabapentin increases aminooxyacetic acid induced GABA accumulation in several regions of rat brain. Neurosci Lett 1991; 128(2): 150–154.
39. Gee NS, Brown JP, Dissanayake VU, Offord J, Thurlow R, Woodruff GN. The novel anticonvulsant drug, gabapentin (Neurontin), binds to the alpha2delta subunit of a calcium channel. J Biol Chem 1996; 271(10):5768–5776.
40. Grunze H, Erfurth A, Marcuse A, Amann B, Normann C, Walden J. Tiagabine appears not to be efficacious in the treatment of acute mania. J Clin Psychiatry 1999; 60(11):759–762.
41. Braestrup C, Nielsen EB, Sonnewald U, et al. (R)-N-[4,4-bis(3-methyl-2-thienyl)but-3-en-1-yl]nipecotic acid binds with high affinity to the brain gamma-aminobutyric acid uptake carrier. J Neurochem 1990; 54(2):639–647.
42. Brodie MJ. Tiagabine pharmacology in profile. Epilepsia 1995; 36:S7–S9.
43. Lippert B, Metcalf BW, Jung MJ, Casara P. 4-Aminohex-5-enoic acid, a selective catalytic inhibitor of 4-aminobutyric-acid aminotransferase in mammalian brain. Eur J Biochem 1977; 74(3):441–445.
44. Ticku MK, Kamatchi GL, Sofia RD. Effect of anticonvulsant felbamate on GABA$_A$ receptor system. Epilepsia 1991; 32(3):389–391.
45. White HS, Harmsworth WL, Sofia RD, Wolf HH. Felbamate modulates the strychnine-insensitive glycine receptor. Epilepsy Res 1995; 20(1):41–48.
46. Delorenze RJ. Phenytoin: mechanism of action. In: Antiepileptic Drugs, eds Mattson R, Meldrum B. New York: Raven Press, 1995, pp 271–282.
47. Kalinowsky LB, Putnam TJ. Attempts at treatment of schizophrenia and other non-epileptic psychoses with Dilantin. Arch Neurol Psychiatry 1943; 49:414–420.

48. Devinsky O. Cognitive and behavioral effects of antiepileptic drugs. Epilepsia 1995; 35(suppl 2):S46–S65.
49. Dodrill CB, Troupin AS. Psychotropic effects of carbamazepine in epilepsy: a double-blind comparison with phenytoin. Neurology 1977; 27(11):1023–1028.
50. Dodrill CB, Troupin AS. Neuropsychological effects of carbamazepine and phenytoin: a reanalysis. Neurology 1991; 41(1):141–143.
51. Klein E, Bental E, Lerer B, Belmaker RH. Carbamazepine and haloperidol vs placebo and haloperidol in excited psychoses. A controlled study. Arch Gen Psychiatry 1984; 41(2):165–170.
52. Biederman J, Lerner Y, Belmaker RH. Combination of lithium carbonate and haloperidol in schizo-affective disorder: a controlled study. Arch Gen Psychiatry 1979; 36(3):327–333.
53. Catterall WA: From ionic currents to molecular mechanisms: the structure and function of voltage-gated sodium channels. Neuron 2000; 26(1):13–25.
54. Hille B, Catterall WA. Electrical excitability and ion channels. In: Basic Neurochemistry: Molecular, Cellular, and Medical Aspects. New York: Raven Press, 1994, pp 75–95.
55. Catterall WA. Modulation of sodium and calcium channels by protein phosphorylation and G proteins. Adv Second Messenger Phosphoprotein Res 997; 31:159–181.
56. Terlau H, Heinemann SH, Stuhmer W, Pusch M, Conti F, Imoto K, Numa S. Mapping the site of block by tetrodotoxin and saxitoxin of sodium channel II. FEBS Lett 1991; 293(1-2):93–96.
57. Hodgkin AL, Huxley AF. A quantitative description of membrane current and its application to conduction and excitation in nerve. J Physiol 1952; 117:500–544.
58. Stuhmer W, Conti F, Suzuki H, Wang XD, Noda M, Yahagi N, Kubo H, Numa S. Structural parts involved in activation and inactivation of the sodium channel. Nature 1989; 339(6226):597–603.
59. Costa MR, Catterall WA. Cyclic AMP-dependent phosphorylation of the alpha subunit of the sodium channel in synaptic nerve ending particles. J Biol Chem 1984; 259(13):8210–8218.
60. Cantrell AR, Ma JY, Scheuer T, Catterall WA. Muscarinic modulation of sodium current by activation of protein kinase C in rat hippocampal neurons. Neuron 1996; 16(5):1019–1026.
61. Peroutka SJ, Synder SH. Relationship of neuroleptic drug effects at brain dopamine, serotonin, alpha-adrenergic, and histamine receptors to clinical potency. Am J Psychiatry 1980; 137(12):1518–1522.
62. Willow M, Gonoi T, Catterall WA. Voltage clamp analysis of the inhibitory actions of diphenylhydantoin and carbamazepine on voltage-sensitive sodium channels in neuroblastoma cells. Mol Pharmacol 1985; 27(5):549–558.
63. Lang DG, Wang CM, Cooper BR. Lamotrigine, phenytoin and carbamazepine interactions on the sodium current present in N4TG1 mouse neuroblastoma cells. J Pharmacol Exp Ther 1993; 266(2):829–835.
64. Van den Berg RJ, Kok P, Voskuyl RA: Valproate and sodium currents in cultured hippocampal neurons. Exp Brain Res 1993; 93(2):279–287.
65. VanDongen AM, VanErp MG, Voskuyl RA. Valproate reduces excitability by blockage of sodium and potassium conductance. Epilepsia 1986; 27(3):177–182.
66. Shank RP, Gardocki JF, Streeter AJ, Maryanoff BE. An overview of the preclinical aspects of topiramate: pharmacology, pharmacokinetics, and mechanism of action. Epilepsia 2000; 41(suppl 1):S3–S9.
67. Catterall WA. Structure and regulation of voltage-gated Ca^{2+} channels. Annu Rev Cell Dev Biol 2000; 16:521–555.
68. Cabras PL, Hardoy MJ, Hardoy MC, Carta MG. Clinical experience with gabapentin in patients with bipolar or schizoaffective disorder: results of an open-label study. J Clin Psychiatry 1999; 60(4):245–248.
69. McElroy SL, Soutullo CA, Keck PE Jr, Kmetz GF. A pilot trial of adjunctive gabapentin in the treatment of bipolar disorder. Ann Clin Psychiatry 1997; 9:99–103.
70. Belmaker RH. Personal communication, 2002.
71. Wamil AW, McLean MJ. Limitation by gabapentin of high frequency action potential firing by mouse central neurons in cell culture. Epilepsy Res 1994; 17(1):1–11.
72. Taylor CP: The anticonvulsant lamotrigine blocks sodium currents from cloned alpha-subunits of rat brain Na^+ channels in a voltage dependent manner but gabapentin does not. Soc Neurosci Abstr 1993:19.
73. Brent DA, Crumrine PK, Varma R, Brown RV, Allan MJ. Phenobarbital treatment and major depressive disorder in children with epilepsy: a naturalistic follow-up. Pediatrics 1990; 85(6):1086–1091.
74. Willow M, Catterall WA: Inhibition of binding of [^{3}H]batrachotoxinin A 20-alpha-benzoate to sodium channels by the anticonvulsant drugs diphenylhydantoin and carbamazepine. Mol Pharmacol 1982; 22(3):627–635.
75. Zeitler DL, Zach GA. Diphenylhydantoin gingival hyperplasia: incidence and etiology. J Hosp Dent Pract 1980; 14(1):41–44.
76. Moscovich DG, Shapira B, Lerer B, Belmaker RH. Rapid lithiumization in acute manic patients. Hum Psychopharmacol 1992; 7:343–345.
77. Grunze H, Erfurth A, Amann B, Giupponi G, Kammerer C, Walden J. Intravenous valproate loading in acutely manic and depressed bipolar I patients. J Clin Psychopharmacol 1999; 19(4):303–309.

78. Davis KL, Berger PA, Hollister LE, Defraites E. Physostigmine in mania. Arch Gen Psychiatry 1978; 35(1):119–122.
79. Judd LL, Janowsky DS, Segal DS, Huey LY. Naloxone-induced behavioral and physiological effects in normal and manic subjects. Arch Gen Psychiatry 1980; 37:583–586.
80. DeToledo JC, Ramsay RE. Fosphenytoin and phenytoin in patients with status epilepticus: improved tolerability versus increased costs. Drug Saf 2000; 22(6): 459–466.
81. Devinsky O. Cognitive and behavioral effects of antiepileptic drugs. Epilepsia 1995; 36(suppl 2): S46–S65.
82. Fierro LS, Savulich DH, Benezra DA. Safety of fosphenytoin sodium. Am J Health Syst Pharm 1996; 53(22): 2707–2712.
83. Browne TR, Kugler AR, Eldon MA. Pharmacology and pharmacokinetics of fosphenytoin. Neurology 1996; 46(6 suppl 1):S3–S7.
84. Meek PD, Davis SN, Collins DM, et al. Guidelines for nonemergency use of parenteral phenytoin products: proceedings of an expert panel consensus process. Panel on Nonemergency Use of Parenteral Phenytoin Products. Arch Intern Med 1999; 159(22):2639–2644.
85. Wallace RH, Wang DW, Singh R, et al. Febrile seizures and generalized epilepsy associated with a mutation in the Na^+-channel beta1 subunit gene SCN1B. Nat Genet 1998; 19(4):366–370.
86. Moulard B, Buresi C, Malafosse A. Study of the voltage-gated sodium channel beta 1 subunit gene (SCN1B) in the benign familial infantile convulsions syndrome (BFIC). Hum Mutat 2000; 16(2):139–142.
87. Makita N, Sloan-Brown K, Weghuis DO, Ropers HH, George AL Jr. Genomic organization and chromosomal assignment of the human voltage-gated Na^+ channel beta 1 subunit gene (SCN1B). Genomics 1994; 23(3):628–634.
88. Haug K, Sander T, Hallmann K, Rau B, Dullinger JS, Elger CE, Propping P, Heils A. The voltage-gated channel beta2-subunit gene and idiopathic generalized epilepsy. Neuroreport 2000; 21(11):2687–2689.

53

Advances in Treatment and Perspectives for New Interventions in Mood and Anxiety Disorders

SANDEEP PATIL, SAEEDUDDIN AHMED, and WILLIAM ZEIGLER POTTER
Eli Lilly and Company, Indianapolis, Indiana, U.S.A.

I. BACKGROUND

During the past four decades, pharmacological treatment of mood and anxiety disorders has progressed dramatically, and clinicians have a bewildering number of choices among agents. We will focus first on mood disorders. To help clinicians in making decision judgments, algorithms for unipolar [1–4] and bipolar [5–7] disorders have been developed. The availability of safe and efficacious agents has reduced the disease burden of patients with mood disorders, and the gap between suffering and its treatment is narrower. However, this gap has not been closed, and the work of drug development continues.

During the upcoming decade, a variety of factors should influence the availability of newer pharmacological treatments for mood disorders. These include increases in knowledge of the pathophysiology of mood disorders and mechanisms of drug action, improvements in drug discovery and development technology, changes in the regulatory environment, and changes in reimbursement methods. New candidates for treatment of mood disorders face stiff market competition from many existing drugs, new chemical entities, and alternative therapies.

II. HOW DRUGS COME TO MARKET

"Drug development" is frequently a misnomer when applied to psychotropic drugs, because almost all available agents are products of accidental discoveries [8,9]. Most currently available psychotropic drugs were found to work, or work better than their predecessors, strictly by chance. Only then was their mechanism of action determined. This pattern of discovery has been repeated over and over again. However, this pattern appears to be changing for two main reasons. Firstly, our greater general understanding of molecular mechanisms has allowed "reasonable guesses" for cellular targets of drug action. Secondly, technological advancements have facilitated the fast production and assessment of greater numbers of potential drug candidates than ever before.

The progression of new chemical entities to marketed drugs is usually divided into two processes: drug discovery and drug development. Discovery yields "leads," or molecules that have promise as drug candidates. In the past, the most common method of producing leads was to make subtle changes to the structure of existing drugs and look for subsequent changes in activity that would be expected to improve efficacy or safety compared to the parent. Drug discovery has been greatly enhanced by computer aided drug design [10] and combinatorial chemistry [11–13]. The key to combinatorial chemistry is the formation of large libraries containing information on the constituent and reactive properties of many molecules. Miniaturization, efficiencies in cost, and availability of powerful computing resources have allowed such libraries to be effectively produced, which in turn have allowed systematic mass production of candidate molecules [14–16]. The candidate molecules then undergo "high-throughput" screening with in vitro and in vivo assays that can serve as predictors of drug disposition and chemical activity [17–19]. A well-designed combinatorial chemistry and high-throughput screening system can generate and test compounds cheaper, and about a thousandfold faster, than was possible 10 years ago [20].

In concert with developments in chemistry and information technology, the rapidly advancing fields of genomics and proteomics are providing vast numbers of lead molecules for the "engine" of high-throughput screening. Genomics has evolved from genetics and may be defined as the cellular and molecular biology of gene action [21]. Proteomics is a newer science than genomics, and refers to the ascertainment and application of protein expression and subcellular organization [22,23]. Genomics and proteomics complement each other, and have wide-ranging possibilities. One application is "pharmacogenomics," the study of variations in drug responses attributed to defined genomic changes [24]. Pharmacogenomics, which combines genomics techniques and molecular pharmacology, may be considered a progression of pharmacogenetics, which explored drug response differences at a macro level [25]. This new technology may eventually provide the ability to customize drug therapies to specific populations of patients.

A second application of genomics and proteomics is the identification of specific drug targets. The process is straightforward in principle, and is enabled by microarray and bioinformatic technology [26]. One approach is to characterize and analyze native biological samples (either from patient populations or animal models) to identify disease specific proteins and therapeutic targets. This amalgamation of technological advancements in discovery research has made it feasible to identify novel targets of drug action in a way not possible even a few years ago.

Another fruitful area has been the molecular cloning of receptor families [27], particularly G-protein-coupled receptors [28], and testing the action of various compounds of interest on these cloned receptors using both in vitro and in vivo systems.

After candidate molecules are generated, they enter the drug development process. There are two phases of development—nonclinical (animal studies) and clinical (human studies). Nonclinical development includes determination of the compounds toxicological properties in two or more animal species, basic pharmacokinetic parameters from in vitro and in vivo models, pharmacodynamic effects in animal models, and chemical synthesis considerations. Current animal models for assaying mood disorders continue to evolve, but their predictive value remains modest [29]. Based on data generated during nonclinical development, many potential drug candidates are removed from further consideration. By the time candidate drugs are first tested in humans, a substantial investment of research effort and money has been made over a period of several years.

Clinical development generally consists of three phases before a drug is "launched" (made available to the public in routine clinical settings), and a fourth postlaunch phase [30]. Phase I consists of clinical trials that are designed to test the safety of the compound within a specific dose range. The initial efficacy trials to determine the therapeutic effect of the drug are conducted in Phase II. Phase III trials are conducted after there is a high degree of certainty about dose and efficacy, and are designed to achieve regulatory approval and registration. A typical Phase III trial for major depression may involve up to 50 investigational sites in three to five countries, and cost many millions of dollars [29]. Many trials "fail", despite adequate sample size, owing to large placebo responses. In recent years, five or more Phase III trials have been required for successful drug launches [31]. Phase IV trials, conducted after registration, assess additional safety and efficacy issues, and are sometimes mandated by regulatory authorities. During Phase IV, other indications for the drug are often explored. Pharmaceutical companies differ somewhat in their definitions of Phases I–IV, and sometimes these are subdivided or combined depending on priorities, timelines, and knowledge about particular compounds and therapeutic areas.

The processes and techniques of drug development have not progressed as quickly as those of drug discovery, but some positive trends are becoming more and more noticeable. Pharmaceutical companies are making a concerted effort to reduce the overall time and cost of drug development. Established paradigms, such as fairly rigid separation of the four phases of development, are now being challenged. New "bridging strategies" are being adopted that emphasize testing drugs in patients as early as possible. Electronic data-capture methods are being used to speed the availability of information to help drive faster decisions. Methodological and statistical techniques are being refined, and biomarkers are being incorporated into clinical development plans to detect valid clinical "signals" in relatively small clinical trials.

One example of a biomarker approach is the use of radiolabeled ligands for determining receptor occupancy as a means of establishing dose ranges for clinical efficacy studies [32]. In general, the starting dose ranges for initial Phase I clinical trials in humans are based on animal behavioral pharmacology and toxicology studies. Subsequently, dose ceilings for initial efficacy studies are determined by the observed tolerability of the drug in humans derived from phase I studies. This is not a mechanistic approach, and can lead to major errors in dosing [33]. The availability of radiolabeled ligands for various receptors of interest has allowed for more rational dosing, by providing the ability to determine percentage of receptor binding as a function of drug plasma level. However, the widespread use of this methodology has been seriously hampered by the limited number of appropriate ligands, and by the number of investigational centers that are able to carry out this kind of research.

Serendipity continues to play a major role in drug development. However, greater knowledge and faster production and evaluation of new candidates have made it technically and economically feasible to evaluate chemical entities acting on novel targets. It could be argued that despite the risk of failure in linking these to efficacy, only compounds with novel mechanisms of action will provide "breakthrough" treatments with commensurate impact. Therefore, it is likely that the pharmaceutical industry will continue to shift its investments to such compounds. By attempting to treat disorders by targeting novel sites of drug action, it is hoped that better efficacy and safety profiles will be achieved.

III. WHY THE HUNT FOR NEW DRUGS FOR MOOD DISORDERS CONTINUES

Despite advances in drug discovery and development, no proven "breakthrough" treatments have yet emerged. Novel drugs are needed, as solo or adjunctive agents, to address some of the limitations of current treatments.

A. Speed of Onset

The time required to achieve clinical response is an enduring problem, particularly with antidepressant therapy. It has been frequently demonstrated that available antidepressants cause biochemical changes within minutes, yet clinical responses are not seen for $\sim$ 2–4 weeks. Claims for faster response have been made [34–39], but no antidepressant medication has been convincingly shown in prospective well-controlled studies to have a faster onset of action than other available agents. It is theoretically possible, however, to have a faster onset of action. Some somatic therapies do seem to work more quickly. These include electroconvulsive therapy [40,41], sleep deprivation [42,43], and perhaps transcranial magnetic stimulation [44] and light therapy in some patients [45]. One possible explanation is that all available antidepressants work through a very similar mechanism—alteration of synaptic monoamine concentrations—but this mechanism is not the immediate proximal cause of clinical response. Something else must occur. Current hypotheses about what this process could be focus on postreceptor signaling pathways, alterations in gene expression, and involvement of neuronal plasticity [46–49], as discussed later in this chapter. It is possible that ideal modulators of monoamine synaptic activity have not yet been discovered, and efforts continue to find them.

The more likely possibility is that other molecular targets must be engaged to achieve a faster clinical response. There is no guarantee, however, that drugs that cause a faster onset of action will also be better than (or as good as) current agents in maintaining clinical response. Quitkin and colleagues have highlighted the importance of differentiating "early onset" and "persistence" of clinical response [50]. Showing that an antidepressant has a fast onset of action is a complicated problem [51], and a successful demonstration of this phenomenon is likely to require a clinically significant and evident response in addition to a prospective statistically significant result. To make an impact, the drug should show convincing effects in hours and days, rather than in weeks.

B. Response

Of even greater importance than the speed of onset is the well-documented fact that a substantial percentage of patients with unipolar and bipolar mood disorders do not respond adequately to available pharmacologic agents. Estimates for major depressive disorders vary, but ∼ 30–45% of patients show partial or no response to available agents [52,53]. For bipolar disorders, historical response rates for an episode have been somewhat higher. There are indications, however, that these rates are declining, or are not sustained over repeated episodes, and more refractory patients are emerging [54].

Three important parameters relating to treatment effect are "response" (the fractional reduction in severity of symptoms), "remission" (sufficient reduction in symptoms to cross a predefined threshold for a period of time), and "recovery" (sustained remission). In clinical trials, response generally means a 50% or greater reduction in symptoms, as determined by standard rating scales. Remission and recovery have been given operational definitions as compiled by Frank and coworkers [55], who also proposed definitions for relapse (return during remission of symptoms sufficient to meet diagnostic criteria of disorder) and recurrence (return of symptoms during recovery sufficient to meet diagnostic criteria of disorder). Although response is the most often used endpoint in industry-sponsored clinical trials, the clinical goal of therapy is to achieve recovery, and the ultimate goal is to "cure" mood disorders.

C. Safety and Tolerability

A desired corollary of achieving better efficacy is to do so without side effects. All available treatments for mood disorders have limitations in safety and tolerability as well as some potential for drug-drug interactions. For unipolar depressive disorders, the leading agents for the last several years have been the selective serotonin reuptake inhibitors (SSRIs). These agents are widely used because, in the types of patients typically enrolled in large trials, they have comparable efficacy to tricyclic antidepressants (TCAs), but are much safer and are generally better tolerated. Although an improvement on TCAs and monoamine oxidase inhibitors, SSRIs are not free of troublesome side effects. These include sexual dysfunction, gastrointestinal disturbances, discontinuation syndromes, and neurological reactions [11,56–58]. Newer agents like bupropion, venlafaxine, and mirtazapine have not superceded the SSRIs because they don't offer obvious advantages for most patients; their safety profiles are no better than SSRIs [59]. Certain side-effect and efficacy advantages, however, may be seen, as in the case of fewer sexual side effects with bupropion [60] or greater overall antidepressant effects with higher doses of venlafaxine [61,62].

For patients who are first diagnosed with depression, there is another safety issue. Antidepressants can induce mania [63,64] or rapid cycling [65] in susceptible patients, as there is no way to be certain that an apparent unipolar depression is not the initial manifestation of bipolar disorder. An antidepressant medication that did not have this liability would be quite valuable. One could argue that such an antidepressant could be used for almost all cases of newly diagnosed depression. Ironically, such a drug may be available. Lithium has been shown to be effective in unipolar and bipolar depressions, although its equivalency to other agents is not established [66], and it carries no known risk of inducing mania. However, lithium's narrow therapeutic window, requirement for perpetual laboratory monitoring, and poor tolerability have precluded its use as a primary antidepressant. It may be that a drug that worked through the mechanisms of action of lithium relevant to antidepressant and mood-stabilizing effects, but without its liabilities, could be used in higher relative doses to achieve greater efficacy with wide benefit for the treatment of mood disorders. [67].

For the treatment of mania, there are no ideal choices. Clinicians generally choose between lithium and anticonvulsants, sometimes supplemented by benzodiazepines and antipsychotics, these treatment regimens are hampered by many troublesome side effects and safety concerns such as gastrointestinal disturbances, hepatotoxicity, hematotoxicity, neurological reactions, and many others [68,69]. Some of the novel molecular targets discussed later in this chapter could be explored in mania as well as depression.

D. Other Factors

Future drug candidates for mood disorders may be viable if they provide coverage for a wider spectrum of psychiatric and somatic conditions, show extraordinary efficacy for particular subsets of mood disorder patients, demonstrate improvements in quality of life, or have pharmacoeconomic benefits. Historically, expansion of drug indications has been beneficial for producers and consumers of pharmaceuticals. One major reason SSRIs were successful was their safety profile compared to previous agents. However, another reason is that they can treat conditions other than depression. Initially many conditions such as obsessive-compulsive disorder, posttraumatic stress disorder, late-luteal phase disorder, social phobia, and panic disorder were treated by SSRIs "off-label." In the past few years pharmaceutical companies that market individual SSRIs have conducted a sufficient number of studies in these indications to obtain regulatory approval for many of them. An emphasis on the discovery and development of compounds with novel mechanisms of action is likely to lead to drugs that may have many possible therapeutic indications in clinical syndromes that may not seem obviously related.

Drugs that have differential and/or greater efficacy in particular subsets of mood disorder syndromes may also have a role in the future. For drugs that are currently available, these differences have not been demonstrated compellingly. Regulatory authorities have been skeptical about superiority claims over competitor products. Nevertheless, in a market that has many similarly efficacious products, companies are likely to continue to invest in clinical studies that help promote superior efficacy claims.

The effects of drugs on the quality of life (QOL) of patients, and their pharmacoeconomic impact are two additional factors that have become better appreciated as important in the last decade. QOL implies overall sense of well being and, in assessing it, the subjective experiences of patients are important. Many clinical rating scale instruments have now been developed to assess effects of treatments on QOL [70]. These instruments encompass aspects of physical, psychological, social, and economic status.

Pharmacoeconomic analyses depend on two basic inputs—cost (direct and indirect) and outcome (defined by either traditional rating scales, by QOL instruments, or both). Two or more treatments may be compared using different types of pharmacoeconomic analyses [71]. These may include cost-benefit (converts of cost and outcome data to monetary values), cost-minimization (emphasizes cost determination and comparison, often outcome equivalence is assumed), cost-effectiveness (outcomes and costs are defined in their own units, then compared across treatments), and cost-utility measures (outcomes are defined by quality of life adjusted years, and outcomes and costs of different treatments are compared). These analytic methods have their individual strengths and weaknesses, and share difficulties in placing appropriate values on outcomes and costs. Patients, health care providers, payers, and even regulatory authorities [72] are becoming increasingly interested in obtaining and evaluating QOL and pharmacoeconomic data. Pharmaceutical companies are beginning to include suitable prospective studies into their clinical plans [73]. Such studies, however, are usually planned only after efficacy has been established using more traditional measures.

IV. MECHANISTIC APPROACHES TO BETTER ANTIDEPRESSANTS

The general application of molecular biology, cell biology, and combinatorial chemistry in new drug development has already been noted. These disciplines, coupled with improved brain imaging technologies, have increased our insight into the working of the human brain. The evolving knowledge of neurobiology and neurochemistry has now uncovered 50–100 neurotransmitters, compared to just acetylcholine and norepinephrine 50 years ago [74]. The neuroscience field has moved beyond just the serotonin and norepinephrine monoamine hypotheses to focus on more fundamental molecular and cellular processes that may reveal how current antidepressants work. The number of molecular sites identified as potential novel targets for antidepressant action already exceed our ability to evaluate them in a timely manner. The challenge is to select those candidates that are most likely to address the clinical needs, described above, for greater efficacy and tolerability. This will ultimately involve pharmacogenomics whereby individualized treatments are based on the genetic makeup of the patient.

A brief overview of targets being explored to advance the treatment of depression follows. A search of the clinical literature on new treatments in depression was performed using a number of databases: Medline-preMedline, the compound-specific Investigational Drug database (ID*db*), International Pharmaceutical abstracts, and Current Contents. This search was narrowed to specifically focus on the biochemical targets most likely to be clinically evaluated over the next few years. We chose to include serotonin receptor subtype agonists and antagonists, neurokinin-1 (substance P) antagonists, corticotrophin-releasing factor antagonists, N-methyl-D-aspartate antagonists, and nicotine agonists. Although a large number of alternative compounds targeted to other sites have been identified, no clinical data either are, or are likely to be, available in sufficient depth in the near future to draw firm conclusions.

A. Serotonin Augmentation by Targeting 5HT Receptor Subtypes

The neuropharmacological basis for the delay in the onset of antidepressant response remains to be determined. It is well known, for instance, that SSRIs rapidly increase serotonin concentration by blocking the serotonin transporter on the presynaptic membrane and on the cell bodies in the raphe nuclei [75–77]. Increased serotonin in the synaptic cleft stimulates the presynaptic serotonin autoreceptors ($5HT_{1B/D}$) and in the raphe stimulate the somatodendritic autoreceptor ($5HT_{1A}$). This inhibits serotonin release directly at the nerve ending and reduces firing of the cell bodies. This negative feedback mechanism prevents the optimal increase in serotonin concentration believed by many investigators to be necessary for "early" antidepressant effect. The time required to counter this effect, involving desensitization of the $5HT_{1A}$ somatodendritic autoreceptor, is proposed to be the cause of the so-called lag period, which can last several weeks [78–81]. Inhibition of the $5HT_{1A}$ serotonin autoreceptor is one approach proposed to eliminate the lag period.

Pindolol, a widely studied beta-adrenoceptor antagonist and a partial $5HT_{1A}$ antagonist, has been at the center of a heated debate as to the utility of this approach thanks to a number of positive and negative studies [78–88]. In studies that showed a negative effect, the potential cause for the pindolol failure has been proposed as follows: (1) Pindolol did not achieve sufficient concentration at the autoreceptor level to exert its effect (standard dose in most clinical trials was 2.5 mg TID); (2) partial agonism of pindolol at the autoreceptor level outweighed any antagonistic effect; (3) $5HT_{1A}$ postsynaptic receptor blockade counteracted benefits of increased intersynaptic serotonin; and (4) serotonin augmentation may not be relevant to enhancing antidepressant effects. Consistent with the first possibility, a study that utilized positron emission tomography (PET) in a small number of healthy subjects and patients demonstrated that higher doses of pindolol than previously employed are needed to achieve a substantial occupancy of the $5HT_{1A}$ autoreceptor [89]. A more recent study showed that estimates of $5HT_{1A}$ receptor occupancy, although low in other brain regions, averaged ~40% in the dorsal raphe nucleus after 1 week on 7.5 mg/day sustained-release pindolol [90]. A 30-mg dose increased mean occupancy to 64%. This may indicate a suboptimal dosing in the prior clinical trials. At higher dosages of pindolol, however, hypotension and dizziness may emerge.

Unpublished data from an Eli Lilly trial utilizing doses of pindolol from 4 to 32 mg/day in combination with fluoxetine does not provide evidence of quicker onset and greater efficacy, nor of significant side effects at the higher doses of pindolol. More recently, however, pindolol was reported to augment responses to electroconvulsive therapy (ECT). In a randomized, double-blind, placebo-controlled pilot study, the administration of pindolol (2.5 mg TID) was associated with antidepressant response to ECT within six treatments in four out of eight patients, while no response was seen in the placebo group in the same amount of time [91]. Pindolol did not enhance the ultimate efficacy of ECT treatment (as determined by the number of responders at the end of the study).

A clear answer to the role of the $5HT_{1A}$ autoreceptor in the onset of antidepressant effects is still elusive, and may have to wait until a more potent and selective antagonist is tested in properly powered clinical trials.

B. Substance P/Neurokinin (NK) Receptor Antagonist

Substance P (SP) belongs to a family of structurally related peptides, called tachykinins, which are involved in the regulation of many biologic processes. Tachykinins share a conserved carboxyl terminal sequence of Phe-X-gly-Leu-Met-NH2, but the amino terminal sequences are distinctive for each peptide. Although the existence of neuropeptide SP has been known since the 1970s [92], the exploration of many of its putative diverse therapeutic roles really began in earnest when selective, potent, nonpeptide analoges became available [93–95]. Actions of SP antagonists that would predictably lead to antidepressant effects remains to be established. However, there is some evidence that SP antagonists may modulate serotonergic or adrenergic systems in the brain and thereby link into monoaminergic mechanisms [96,97]. The SP neuropeptide colocalizes with the classical neurotransmitters (serotonin and norepinephrine) and other neuropeptides in the brain. In a recent preclinical report it was observed that neurokinin-1 (NK-1) antagonism and genetic deletion of the NK-1 receptors both lead to an enhanced serotonergic neurotransmission in the forebrain, a region believed to be involved in major depression [98,99]. NK-1 antagonists have also been shown to inactivate alpha-2 autoreceptors on the cell body of norepinephrine (NE) neurons in the locus coeruleus [98]. Several antidepressants, given chronically, decrease SP content in the striatum, substantia nigra, and amygdala [99]. Thus, NK-1 receptor antagonists may modulate NE and/or 5HT systems in the human brain. SP antagonists have also been hypothesized to be useful in anxiety disorders, irritable-bowel syndrome, migraine, chronic pain, and asthma [100,101].

The preclinical/clinical studies conducted with the SP receptor antagonist MK-869 have contributed to postulating a role for SP in the treatment of major depression [102]. In preclinical studies MK-869 was found to reduce or inhibit the vocalization of guinea pig pups observed following maternal separation [103]. In a double-blind placebo controlled Phase II study, MK-869 was found to be as effective as paroxetine in treating depressed patients [102]. The MK-869 compound was associated with an incidence of nausea and sexual dysfunction no different from placebo. The report that MK-869 is an effective antidepressant with a novel mechanism of action has generated considerable excitement. For the first time, it appeared that a new antidepressant had been discovered, the mechanism of which did not involve direct modulation of monoamines in the brain. Unfortunately, a much larger follow-up dose-finding study failed to show separation between active control, test drug, and placebo [102].

At issue with the new NK-1 antagonists is whether they can achieve a therapeutic concentration in the brain. Current on-going studies by at least two companies include NK-1 antagonist compounds, which are claimed to be more potent and/or achieve greater penetration into brain.

C. NMDA Receptor Antagonists

The N-methyl-D-aspartate (NMDA) receptors has long served as a tempting but challenging target for new antidepressant drug development. This ion channel receptor is stimulated by glutamate, the most widely distributed excitatory neurotransmitter in the brain. Activation of NMDA receptors requires glycine as a mandatory cofactor. In addition, NMDA receptors show a voltage-sensitive block by Mg^{2+} under resting conditions [104,105]. NMDA receptor antagonists have been proposed to be clinically useful in depression, epilepsy, motor neuron disease, traumatic brain injury, hyperalgesia, and anxiety. One of the main difficulties in targeting these receptors has been a constant threat of severe psychotomimetic effects as evidenced by the well-known actions of phencyclidine, an uncompetitive NMDA antagonist.

NMDA receptor antagonists show efficacy in various animal models used to evaluate potential antidepressant drugs. In addition, NMDA receptor antagonists have also been shown to be neuroprotective and anxiolytic in various animal studies [96,106,107]. An exploratory study with the uncompetitive NMDA antagonist ketamine supports a role for NMDA receptor-modulating drugs in the treatment of depression [108]. This small study, which is the only one of its kind, demonstrated that ketamine, but not placebo, infusion reduced Hamilton Depression Rating Scale scores by ~14 points. Although questions remain about the role of psychotomimetic effects in the antidepressant effect mediated by ketamine, future studies will clearly help in clarifying the role of glutamate in the neuropathology of depression.

There is also some preliminary evidence suggesting NMDA receptor modulation is a key factor in the delayed response to antidepressants. The ability of glycine to inhibit the binding of [^{3}H]5,7-dichlorokynurenic acid to strychnine-insensitive glycine receptors decreases after chronic antidepressant treatment [109–113]. This fact is suggestive of a "dampening" of NMDA receptors with chronic antidepressant treatment, and it has been proposed as a final common pathway utilized by all different antidepressants.

D. Nicotine Receptor Agonist in Depression

Nicotinic agonists have potential therapeutic uses in conditions such as depression, attention deficit hyperactivity disorder, eating disorder, Alzheimer's disease, a variety of cognitive disorders, pain, Tourette's, Parkinson's disease, and schizophrenia. Nicotinergic receptors belong to a large family of ligand-gated cation channels which, when stimulated by agonists, augment the release of numerous neurotransmitters such as dopamine, serotonin, norepinephrine, acetylcholine, gamma-aminobutyric acid, and glutamate. A strong link between smoking and depression has been reported in various epidemiological studies [103,104, 114–116]. In one study, the lifetime prevalence of depression in smokers was found to be twice that of nonsmokers [115]. Furthermore, depressed smokers had a harder time trying to stop smoking than nondepressed smokers.

There is preclinical and neurochemical evidence to support the role of nicotine agonists in depression. SIB-1508Y, a novel subtype-selective ligand for nicotinic acetylcholine receptors, was able to attenuate the learned helplessness deficit in rats which serves as a preclinical model for depression [117]. This was comparable to the effect produced by established antidepressants such as fluoxetine and imipramine. The rewarding effects of smoking and the beneficial effects of nicotine replacement therapy for depressed smokers may partially depend on genetic factors involved in dopamine transmission [118]. Interplay between the cholinergic and various monoaminergic systems might be relevant to any role of nicotinic agonists in the treatment of depression.

Data on nicotinic agonists from clinical trials for psychiatric or nonpsychiatric use is scarce. In one Phase II study, altinicline (a nicotinic receptor subtype ligand, SIBIA) was not superior to placebo in the treatment of Parkinson's disease [119]. It is still not clear whether it has been evaluated in depression. In a small pilot study, a nicotine patch applied to depressed nonsmokers decreased their Hamilton Depression Rating Scale scores an average of 44% [120]. Further studies are clearly indicated to explore nicotinic agonists in depression.

E. Corticotrophin-Releasing Factor (CRF) Antagonist and Depression

Elevated plasma corticosteroid concentrations, increased 24-h urinary free cortisol concentrations, and elevated cortisol metabolite levels in depressed patients have been noted for more than three decades [121–123]. Dexamethasone nonsuppression in a substantial proportion of depressed individuals is now well established [124–126]. Adrenocortical hyperactivity with associated elevated CRF concentrations in depressed patients has led to extensive research into the role of CRF in depression. CRF plays a major role in the regulation of cortisol secretion by being a primary physiological mediator of adrenocorticotrophic hormone (ACTH) secretion from the anterior pituitary [127]. CRF concentrations are elevated in the cerebrospinal fluid of depressed individuals [123,128–131]. The elevation seen in CRF concentration in major depression may be transient, as its level returns to normal after successful treatment [132–134]. In fact, symptomatic improvement in major depression not accompanied by a decrease in the elevated CRF concentration may indicate a poor prognosis [135].

CRF receptors are present in the pituitary and other neural tissue, and CRF peptide is considered to be a neurotransmitter playing a critical role in stress regulation. Clinical trial evidence supporting the role of a nonpeptide CRF receptor antagonist in the treatment of major depression is minimal. An open-label clinical trial conducted at the Max Planck Institute in Psychiatry in Munich, Germany, of a novel CRF antagonist, NBI 30775, was interpreted as supporting its efficacy in major depression [88]. It showed a dose-dependent decrease in HAM-D with 50% of patients responding in the low-dose group while 80% of patients responded in the high-dose group. Subsequent trials with this compound were discontinued because of a transient increase in hepatic enzymes observed in some patients studied in the United Kingdom. Studies are under way with other CRF-1 antagonists.

V. CELLULAR AND MOLECULAR MECHANISM OF ANTIDEPRESSANT ACTION

Could a final common pathway exist for the action of different antidepressants? The search for a possible common pathway for the action of disparate antidepressants continues. A multistep signal transduction pathway leading ultimately to modification in genetic expression and protein synthesis has been hypothesized as a possible underlying mechanism [47,48,111]. Most conventional antidepressants are known to stimulate adenyl cyclase via a G-protein dependent mechanism. The resulting elevation in cyclic-adenosine monophosphate (cAMP) leads to a corresponding activation of cAMP-dependent protein kinase A. A potentially relevant target for this enzyme is the cyclic AMP response element binding protein (CREB). The phosphorylated CREB is then thought to increase the expression of a brain-derived neurotrophic factor (BDNF) by modulating specific gene expression. Increased neuronal BDNF has been observed in the brain after chronic antidepressant treatment [74,136,137]. BDNF is considered to be a key factor in the protection of vulnerable neurons during chronic stress. Furthermore, in vitro long-term ($> 6\,h$) exposure of cerebellar granule cell neurons to BDNF reduced the mRNA for subunits of NMDA receptors [138]. A similar effect is seen with chronic imipramine treatment in mouse brain [139]. This temporal connection among BDNF, NMDA receptor function, and depression forms the basis of a cellular and molecular theory of major depression [47,48]. The most obvious potential therapeutic target in the above intracellular pathway is the prevailing CNS form of phosphodiesterase (PDE, type IV). Inhibition of PDE type IV increases cAMP levels [48,140]. There was some preliminary evidence that a type IV PDE inhibitor, rolipram, showed efficacy in depression [141], but gastrointestinal side effects apparently prevented further exploration of this compound. The recent preclinical findings that chronic ECS and imipramine increase PDE-IV mRNA [48,142] further implicate the cAMP pathway in the mechanism of action of antidepressant treatments. Currently, however, PDE-IV inhibitors under development are targeted only to the treatment of asthma because of difficulties in identifying compounds with sufficient brain activity and acceptable side effects.

Other possible intracellular sites of drug action that may be more feasible than previously imagined, emerge from studies on the mechanism of action of lithium. It has recently been proposed that lithium may actually have neuroprotective effects, achieved through lasting changes in cell-signaling pathways and gene expression. Chronic lithium administration produces a reduction in the expression of protein kinase C (PKC), as well as its major substrate, myristoylated alanine-rich c-kinase substrate (MARCKS). The MARCKS protein has been implicated in neuronal migration and development [67]. Other molecules affected by lithium include glycogen synthase kinase 3-beta (GSK-3β) and cytoprotective protein, bcl-2. Both of these proteins may play a major role in the long-term neuroprotective/neurotrophic effects of lithium [143–152].

Recently, with the aid of quantitative proton magnetic resonance spectroscopy, a significant increase in total brain N-acetyl-aspartate (NAA) concentration was noted ($P < .0217$) following 4 weeks of lithium treatment in bipolar patients [151]. NAA is believed to be a potential marker for neuronal viability, and has been followed to chart the course of neurodegenerative disorders. These findings have provided added support to the contention that chronic lithium increases neuronal viability/function in the human brain. Given its antidepressant, antimanic, and mood-stabilizing properties, finding how to duplicate the critical biochemical effects of lithium, while hopefully avoiding those that produce side effects, could have broad therapeutic benefits in the treatment of mood disorders. Compounds targeted to specific PKC enzymes and to GSK-3β should allow for this possibility to be tested. Such compounds that reach the CNS are not yet available for clinical studies, but should emerge in the next few years.

VI. BASIS OF NEW TREATMENTS FOR ANXIETY DISORDERS

There is substantial overlap of treatments for depression with treatments for anxiety since, as already noted, most "antidepressants" also show efficacy in anxiety disorders. However, anxiety disorders may be distinct from depression. "Anxiety" constitutes a range of psychiatric conditions characterized by irrational fears and behaviors that are expressed to avoid the associated distressing feelings. Normally, fear and anxiety function as warning signals to alert an individual to potential dangers. Pathological anxiety occurs when normal daily functioning is disrupted by apprehension of unknown threats (i.e., generalized anxiety disorder), or when an inappropriate fear response occurs out of context of the current environment (panic, posttraumatic stress disorder) [153]. The ideal anxiolytic drug would be pharmacologically selective for the causative mechanisms of anxiety, thus allowing the patient to lead a normal life with no drug-related CNS impairment.

Benzodiazepines are one of the most widely used drugs for the treatment of anxiety disorders. While highly efficacious in some anxiety disorders, their utility is greatly hampered by side effects that include CNS depression, drug interactions, cognitive impairment, dependence, and withdrawal liabilities [154]. In fact, this may be the primary reason why the SSRI drugs have replaced benzodiazepine as a first line of therapy for this indication. Specific SSRIs have recently been approved for the treatment of panic disorder (paroxetine), generalized anxiety disorder (paroxetine), obsessive-compulsive disorder (fluoxetine and fluvoxamine), PTSD (sertraline), and social anxiety disorder (paroxetine). Clomipramine, a tricyclic antidepressant with potent serotonin reuptake inhibition, has been effectively used for nearly three decades for the treatment of obsessive-compulsive disorder. The FDA approved buspirone, a partial $5HT_{1A}$ agonist for the treatment of generalized anxiety disorder (GAD) in 1986. Venlafaxine, a mixed 5HT and NE reuptake inhibitor, has also been recently approved for GAD.

For reasons specific to each class of compounds and diagnostic category, such as limited efficacy, side effects, and/or abuse potential, available medications are far from ideal, and the search for more selective and more effective treatments continues. Given the lack of understanding of the psychopathological mechanisms underlying anxiety disorders and the lack of validated objective measures or biomarkers to assess the efficacy of novel interventions, progress has been slow. Nevertheless, the success of early stage preclinical research has bought forward several new platforms for testing in the anxiety disorders. What follows is a brief overview of classes of new compounds targeted to molecular sites with potential application to anxiety disorders. Wherever possible, relevant preclinical and early clinical information is included.

A. Gamma-Aminobutyric Acid (GABA) Modulators

GABA, a ligand for $GABA_A$ receptors, is a major inhibitory neurotransmitter. Conversely, abnormal GABA receptor-mediated responses have been reported in anxiety patients who show reduced sensitivity to benzodiazepines (BZD). Benzodiazepine inverse agonists, such as beta-carbolines, can induce severe anxiety reactions in normal human subjects [155]. Benzodiazepine receptor density has also been reported to be low in the peripheral lymphocytes of anxious patients. Interestingly, this abnormality reverses after chronic diazepam treatment [156]. The synthesis rate of these receptors may also be decreased in anxious patients as evidenced by reduced levels of mRNA-encoding peripheral benzodiazepine receptors [157].

Interestingly, BZD receptor function has been shown to be affected by modulation of the serotonin and cholecystokinin (CCK) systems. $5HT_{1A}$ knockout mice exhibit BZD-resistant anxiety [158]. This was accompanied by abnormal BZD receptor α-subunit expression in the amygdala and hippocampus. One pathophysiological hypothesis is therefore that a $5_{HT_{1A}}$ receptor deficit may be linked to abnormal composition and levels of $GABA_A$ receptor subunits, resulting in BZD resistance and anxiety. In a different series of experiments, CCK antagonists have been shown to possess anxiolytic properties in the various animal models [159], as discussed later in greater detail. One can speculate that multiple pathways impacted by different molecular targets can modulate GABA levels and/or receptor function.

$GABA_A$ receptors display extensive structural heterogeneity since their assembly is based on a selection of at least 18 subunits (alpha1-6, beta1-3, gamma1-3, delta, varepsilon, and theta, rho1-3). Benzodiazepines are the allosteric modulators of $GABA_A$ receptors, and their effect can be attributed to specific $GABA_A$ receptor subtypes. Using in vivo gene dissection, it has been shown in preclinical models that anxiolytic action is mediated by the $alpha_2$ subtype, while the sedative and in part the anticonvulsant action are mediated by the $alpha_1$ subtype $GABA_A$ receptors [160,161]. It is thus hoped that a specific allosteric modulator of the relevant GABA receptor subtype for anxiety may be synthesized that does not produce the undesirable side effects of sedation, motor impairment, or abuse potential.

Currently there is only one compound fairly advanced in development that may have such properties. Pagoclone (IP 456, RP 62955), although classified as a nonspecific GABA partial agonist, is in Phase III development for panic disorder, and has reportedly shown efficacy with a superior tolerability profile to classical benzodiazepines (Interneuron Pharmaceutical Inc.). Pagoclone significantly reduced panic attack in a Phase II/III clinical trial (media release Aug. 17, 1998, 2 pp). Earlier, in a 277-patient double-blind, placebo-controlled, randomized study, pagoclone effectively reduced the frequency of panic attacks by 73% at a dose of 0.3 mg ($P = .021$).

B. Serotonin Receptor Agonists

A role for serotonin in various anxiety disorders is now well accepted. Treatment with SSRIs, SNRIs, TCAs, and MAOIs has been shown to be effective. A role for norepinephrine in the anxiety disorders is not as clear. With the advent of selective norepinephrine reuptake inhibitors, such as reboxetine and tomoxetine, it should now be possible to assess the potential of NE as a target.

Despite more than a decade of knowing that treatments which enhance intrasynaptic 5HT are efficacious, the role of specific 5HT receptor subtypes in anxiety has yet to be established. 5HT receptor subtypes such as $5-HT_{1A}$, $5-HT_{2A}$, and $5-HT_3$ have been associated with fear behavior in animal studies [162]. Decreased exploratory activity and increased fear of aversive environments is seen in mice bred without $5-HT_{1A}$ receptors, suggesting heightened anxiety [163]. Buspirone, marketed for the treatment of GAD, is believed to work as a partial $5HT_{1A}$ agonist. Interestingly, no new partial or full agonists of the $5_{HT_{1A}}$ receptor have been approved during almost a decade and a half since the approval of buspirone, despite intense efforts. From a drug development perspective, pursuit of a "just right" agonist for $5HT_{1A}$ has proved difficult. As many as 15 new chemical entities, in various stages of development, have failed to deliver [150]. Gepirone, a buspirone analog and a weak partial agonist at $5HT_{1A}$ receptors, may still be in development despite negative clinical results. A large trial showed that any anxiolytic effects of gepirone were delayed and accompanied by a poorer adverse-effects profile than diazepam [164]. Bristol Myers Squibb, which makes buspirone, has recently submitted a patent that relates to 6-hydroxy buspirone. This buspirone metabolite is believed to be largely responsible for the onset of therapeutic relief. If the patent is approved, then further delay in the development of azaspirone anxiolytics (precursors of 6-hydroxybuspirone), such as gepirone, is likely. New drugs based on 6-hydroxybuspirone could emerge with potentially increased efficacy, but could be limited by problems related to a favorable therapeutic index. In other words, as reviewed elsewhere, any real efficacy with $5HT_{1A}$ may come at the cost of unacceptable side effects [149]. Nevertheless, there is at least one other $5HT_{1A}$ agonist, lesopitron, reported to be in Phase II trials for GAD and panic disorder [48,142,165]. According to the manufacturers, a double-blind study in patients with GAD and long-standing GAD showed anxiolytic effects similar to those observed with lorazepam and a potentially superior adverse effect profile (company communication, Esteve, March 1998).

Therapeutic index may be less of a problem for repinotan hydrochloride (Bayer), a $5HT_{1A}$ agonist, currently in Phase III development for the IV treatment of stroke and traumatic brain injury. It may also have potential in depression and anxiety (21st CINP, Glasgow, 1998, PM01007). It is expected to be launched in 2002 (company communication, May 1996). This drug has shown a good tolerability profile, with headache being the most common adverse effect. Sarizotan hydrochloride (EMD-128130), a dual $5HT_{1A}$ agonist and dopamine D2 antagonist, is undergoing Phase II trial for treatment of dyskinesia in Parkinson's disease (Analysts' Conf, Merck KgaA, 2000). This compound is expected to be launched in 2005. Preclinical research suggests that this compound may have antianxiety effects and a low incidence of extrapyramidal effects (company communications, Feb 1995, Feb 1996).

C. Substance P Receptor Antagonists

The nonpeptide, substance P antagonists represent a potential new class of antidepressants and antianxiety agents with side-effects profiles superior to the current class of SSRIs and benzodiazepines. Two compounds from this class have come as far as Phase II for anxiety and/or depression—NKP 608 (Novartis) and MK 869 (Merck). The efficacy of MK 869 was evaluated in 213 patients with major depressive disorder and anxiety in a randomized, double-blind, placebo-controlled clinical trial. Patients received 6-week therapy with placebo, paroxetine (20 mg/day), or MK 869 (300 mg/day). Subjects receiving MK 869, as opposed to those on paroxetine, showed a side-effects profile almost indistinguishable from placebo. For instance, 25% of paroxetine recipients complained of sexual dysfunction in comparison with 3% of MK 869 recipients and 4% of placebo recipients. Recipients of MK 869 and paroxetine also had significant improvements, compared with placebo recipients, according to the Hamilton Anxiety Rating Scale on weeks 4 and 6 [102,103,143]. Unfortunately, Phase III development on MK 869 was stopped, as this compound failed to separate from placebo at lower doses, which presumably were the only ones judged to be economically feasible. Results from NKP 608 trials in anxiety or depression are not yet available.

V. METABOTROPIC GLUTAMATE RECEPTOR AGONISTS

Glutamate, the most abundant amino acid in the diet, is also a major excitatory neurotransmitter in the brain. Even though this has been known for about five decades, the putative role of glutamate in the neuropathology of various psychiatric illnesses is just beginning to be explored. The receptors for glutamate can be classified into a heterogeneous family of ionotropic and metabotropic receptors, the latter being localized to both pre- and postsynaptic sites. Metabotropic glutamate receptors (mGluR1, mGluR2, and mGluR3) belong to G-protein-coupled family of receptors and have been linked to presynaptic inhibition of excitatory and inhibitory amino acids, monoamines, and neuropeptides release [166]. Metabotropic glutamate (mGlu) may play important roles in the regulation of many physiological and pathological processes in the CNS. These include synaptic plasticity, learning and memory, motor coordination, pain transmission, and neurodegeneration [167]. Considerable excitement has been generated in the role of mGluR2 receptors in anxiety, schizophrenia, seizure disorder, and nicotine craving.

LY-354740 is a conformationally constrained analog of glutamate that is a potent systemically active agonist of group II mGlu receptors. It prevented lactate-induced paniclike response in panic-prone rats similar to alprazolam, suggesting an antipanic effect [168]. In the fear-potentiated startle and elevated plus maze models of anxiety LY-354740 was as effective as diazepam without the adverse effect of motor impairment. Antianxiety effects of LY-354740 are specific, as it was ineffective in behavioral models of depression including despair a-test and a-tail suspension test [169]. Immunohistochemical studies have demonstrated significant presence of mGluR2 receptors in basal ganglia, hippocampus, thalamus, and cerebellar cortex in the human brain [170]. Hippocampus has been considered to be a possible neuroanatomical site for anxiolytic effects of mGluR2 agonists [170]. LY-354740 is undergoing Phase II trials for anxiety disorder.

VI. OTHER POTENTIAL ANXIOLYTIC AGENTS

A. Cholecystokinin Receptor Antagonists

Until now the neurobiology and pharmacological treatment of anxiety disorders, like depression, have been heavily focused on the noradrenergic and serotonergic systems in the brain. More recently, with the development of nonpeptide ligands for CCK and SP receptors (both are present in significant quantities inside and out of the brain), novel approaches for the treatment of this condition have become a possibility. Systemic injection of CCK-8S, an octapeptide, has been shown to produce dose-dependent regional specific changes on GABA levels in brain. Furthermore, a selective CCK(B) receptor antagonist, PD 135,158, prevented the action induced by CCK-8S [97]. There is also some evidence that CCK receptors in the brain may be involved in panic disorders. This hypothesis is supported by the results of animal electrophysiological studies, animal models of anxiety, and challenge test using CCK fragments in humans [159]. Interestingly, the octapeptide CCK-8 concentrations were found to be significantly lower in the peripherral lymphocytes of the patients with panic disorder than in healthy controls [171]. This level did not correlate with the severity of panic attacks and was unchanged by chronic treatment with alprazolam. Benzodiazepines have been shown to antagonize the satiety and hypothermic effect of CCK8 in mice by an hitherto unknown mechanism [148,172,173].

Findings from the preclinical models have not definitively translated into the clinic. In preclinical studies, CI-988 (Parke-Davis) was shown to be an extremely potent and selective cholecystokinin B antagonist, with potent anxiolytic effects and a favorable tolerability profile. But clinical trials conducted in patients with anxiety disorder or panic disorder have been disappointing [174,175]. Sixteen patients with a principal DSM-III-R diagnosis of generalized anxiety disorder were enrolled in a study that involved two challenge tests. In this double-blind, placebo-controlled study, patients received a single oral dose of CI-988 followed 30 min later by an IV infusion of 0.1 mg/kg mCPP (meta-chlorophenyl-peperazine). CI-988 (100 mg) did not block the anxiety response to mCPP. Issues with brain penetration and poor pharmacokinetics make any interpretation from the data difficult. CI 1015 [*PD 145942*] is a second-generation molecule, developed by researchers at Parke-Davis (formerly a division of Warner-Lambert, now Pfizer) to improve on the low PO bioavailability. With an improved CI-1015 pharmacokinetic profile, it will be a better test compound for any proof of concept trial [176,177]

GW-150013 (GlaxoSmithKline) is another cholecystokinin-B receptor antagonist in Phase II development for the treatment of anxiety disorders. Similarly, LY-288513, a novel selective cholecystokinin B (CCK$_B$) antagonist, may have potential as an anxiolytic. In the animal model of benzodiazepine withdrawal, acute pretreatment with both diazepam and LY-288513 dose-dependently blocked withdrawal-induced increases in the auditory startle response [178].

B. Corticotrophin-Releasing Factor (CRF)

CRF has been implicated in both depression and anxiety disorder [135]. It is found in most of the regions of brain, with highest concentration in the hypothalamus where it is secreted by neurons in the hypothalamic paraventricular nucleus. One of the principal functions of CRF is to regulate the basal and stress-induced release of adrenocorticotrophic, beta-endorphin, and other pro-opiomelanocortin-derived peptides. CRF is found in moderate to low levels in the extrahypothalamic tissue, which includes cortical and limbic structures. At this time, two types of G-protein-linked CRF receptors have been found. The CRF-1 receptor is mainly found in the neocortical, cerebellar, and limbic structures, where CRF-2 receptor is typically localized in subcortical structures and some hypothalamic areas. Animal data have implicated the role of CRF in anxiety disorder [127,179–181], and CRF antagonists are currently under investigation as anxiolytics. NBI-30775 (Janssen) is the most researched and the first CRF antagonist to reach the clinic. This early study was argued to support its potential as an antidepressant and anxiolytic, but development was discontinued because of hepatic toxicity seen in two volunteers in an expanded safety study in the U.K.

CONCLUSION

The multiple efforts to develop new antidepressants and anxiolytics testify to the perceived medical need. In the absence of known pathophysiology for anxiety and depression, it is impossible to predict whether any of the novel mechanisms discussed above will result in improved therapeutic agents. Any relationships between improvement in efficacy and alternate mechanisms of action remain hypothetical. Would it be considered a significant improvement if a novel drug were successful in treating only 60% of a depressed population? Would it be worth investing hundreds of millions in developing such a drug? To what extent could a different mechanism of action ultimately be little more than a basis for marketing rather than a breakthrough in the treatment of depression?

These questions are even more relevant today since generic forms of the major antidepressants will be widely available in the near future. Nevertheless, there remain many reasons to invest in novel compounds. The promise and potential for improvements in the treatment of psychiatric disorders has never been higher as a consequence of the exponentially expanding number of probes and targets. The "me-too" era of the drugs in psychiatry is all but over. There is clearly no major medical need or good scientific basis for a new SSRI or a tricyclic antidepressant.

REFERENCES

1. Cornwall PL, Scott J. Which clinical practice guidelines for depression? An overview for busy practitioners. Br J Gen Pract 2000; 50(460):908–911.
2. Crismon ML, Trivedi M, Pigott TA, Rush AJ, Hirschfeld RM, Kahn DA, DeBattista C, Nelson JC, Nierenberg AA, Sackeim HA, Thase ME. The Texas Medication Algorithm Project: report of the Texas Consensus Conference Panel on Medication Treatment of Major Depressive Disorder. J Clin Psychiatry 1999; 60(3):142–156.
3. Rush AJ, Crismon ML, Toprac MG, Trivedi MH, Rago WV, Shon S, Altshuler KZ. Consensus guidelines in the treatment of major depressive disorder. J Clin Psychiatry 1998; 59:suppl 84.
4. Practice guideline for the treatment of patients with major depressive disorder (revision). Am J Psychiatry 2000; 157:1–45.
5. Goldberg JF. Treatment guidelines: current and future management of bipolar disorder. J Clin Psychiatry 2000; 61:suppl 8.
6. Motohashi N. Algorithms for the pharmacotherapy of bipolar disorder. Psychiatry Clin Neurosci 1999; 53:suppl 4.
7. Bauer MS, Callahan AM, Jampala C, Petty F, Sajatovic M, Schaefer V, Wittlin B, Powell BJ. Clinical practice guidelines for bipolar disorder from the Department of Veterans Affairs [see comments]. [Erratum appears in J Clin Psychiatry 1999; 60(5):341]. J Clin Psychiatry 1999; 60(1):9–21.
8. Peridis ACR. Mental disorder drug discovery. Nat Biotechnol 1999; 17:307–309.
9. Kaul PN. Drug discovery: past, present and future. Prog Drug Res 1998; 50:9–105.
10. Trophsa A. Recent trends in computer-aided drug discovery. Curr Opin Drug Discovery Dev 2000; 3:310–313.
11. Edwards JG, Anderson I. Systematic review and guide to selection of selective serotonin reuptake inhibitors [see comments]. [Erratum appears in Drugs 1999; 58(6):1207–1209]. Drugs 1999; 57(4):507–533.
12. Bohm HJ SM. Structure-based library design: molecular modelling merges with combinatorial chemistry. Curr Opin Chem Biol 2000; 4:283-286.
13. Terrett NK. Combinatorial synthesis—the design of compound libraries and their application to drug discovery. Tetrahedron Lett 1995; 51(8135):8173.
14. Hoplinger AJ DJ. Extraction of pharmacophore information from high-throughput screens. Curr Opin Biotechnol 2000; 11:97.
15. Willett P. Chemoinformatics—similarity and diversity in chemical libraries. Curr Opin Biotechnol 2000; 11:85–88.
16. Antel J. Integration of combinatorial chemistry and structure-based design. Curr Opin Drug Discovery Dev 1999; 2:224–233.
17. Panchagnula R, Thomas NS. Biopharmaceutics and pharmacokinetics in drug research. Int J Pharm 2000; 201:131–150.
18. Bajpal MAK. High-throughput screening for lead optimization: a rational approach. Curr Opin Drug Discovery Dev 2000; 3:63–71.
19. Hertzberg RP. High-throughput screening: new technology for the 21st century. Curr Opin Chem Biol 2000; 4:445–451.
20. Combinatorial chemistry. Nat Biotechnol 2000; 18(suppl):51–52.
21. Rosenthal A. Editorial review: genomics and proteomics. Curr Opin Mol Ther 1999; 1:669–670.
22. Parekh R. Proteomics and molecular medicine. Nat Biotechnol 1999; 17(suppl):19–20.
23. Proteomic analysis. Curr Opin Biotechnol 2000; 11:176–179.
24. Pharmacogenomics. Nat Biotechnol 2000; 18(suppl):40–42.
25. Vesell ES. Pharmacogenetics and pharmacogenomics. Pharmacol 2000; 61:118.
26. Stratowa C. Gene expression profiling in drug discovery and development. Curr Opin Mol Ther 1999; 1:671–679.
27. Herz JM, Thomsen WJ, Yarbrough GG. Molecular approaches to receptors as targets for drug discovery. J Receptor Signal Transduction Res 1997; 17(5):671–776.

28. Sautel M, Milligan G. Molecular manipulation of G-protein-coupled receptors: a new avenue into drug discovery. Curr Med Chem 2000; 7(9):889–896.
29. Keller MB. Antidepressants. In: Skolnick P. ed. Psychiatry. Totowa: Humana Press, 1997.
30. Spilker BPD. Guide to Clinical Trials, 1991.
31. Hooper MB Amsterdam JD. Do clinical trials reflect drug potential? A review of 5 FDA evaluations of new antidepressants. Depression Research Unit, University of Pennsylvania, Poster 2.
32. Hietala J. Ligand-receptor interactions as studied by PET: implications for drug development [see comments]. Ann Med 1999; 31(6):438–443.
33. Potter WZ. European cooperation in the field of scientific and technical research. Eur Commission 1998; 307–322.
34. Silverstone T. Relative speed of onset of the antidepressant effect of maprotiline. Clin Ther 1981; 3(5):374–381.
35. Quitkin FM. Mirtazapine onset of action appears more rapid than SSRIs. In 38th Annual Meeting of the American College of Neuropharmacology, Acapulco, Mexico, 1999.
36. Ban TA. Systematic studies with amoxapine, a new antidepressant. Int Pharmacopsychiatry 1982; 17:18–27.
37. Tollefson GD Holman SL. How long to onset of antidepressant action: a meta-analysis of patients treated with fluoxetine or placebo. Int Clin Psychopharmacol 1994; 9:245-250.
38. Montgomery SA. New developments in the treatment of depression. J Clin Psychiatry 1999; 60:suppl 5.
39. Montgomery SA. Rapid onset of action of venlafaxine. Int Clin Psychopharmacol 1995; 10: suppl 7.
40. Rodger CR, Scott AI, Whalley LJ. Is there a delay in the onset of the antidepressant effect of electroconvulsive therapy? [See comments.] Br J of Psychiatry 1994; 164(1):106–109.
41. Segman RH, Shapira B, Gorfine M, Lerer B. Onset and time course of antidepressant action: psychopharmacological implications of a controlled trial of electroconvulsive therapy. Psychopharmacology 1995; 119(4):440–448.
42. Post RM, Uhde TW, Rubinow DR, Huggins T. Differential time course of antidepressant effects after sleep deprivation, ECT, and carbamazepine: clinical and theoretical implications. Psychiatry Res 1987; 22(1):11–19.
43. Benedetti F, Barbini B, Lucca A, Campori E, Colombo C, Smeraldi E. Sleep deprivation hastens the antidepressant action of fluoxetine. Eur Arch Psychiatry Clin Neurosci 1997; 247(2):100–103.
44. Berman RM, Narasimhan M, Sanacora G, Miano AP, Hoffman RE, Hu XS, Charney DS, Boutros NN. A randomized clinical trial of repetitive transcranial magnetic stimulation in the treatment of major depression. Biol Psychiatry 2000; 47(4):332–337.
45. Kripke DF. Light treatment for nonseasonal depression: speed, efficacy, and combined treatment. J Affect Disord 1998; 49(2):109–117.
46. Duman RS, Malberg J, Thome J. Neural plasticity to stress and antidepressant treatment. Biol Psychiatry 1999; 46(9):1181–1191.
47. Duman RSP. A molecular and cellular theory of depression. Arch Gen Psychiatry 1997; 54(7):597–606.
48. Skolnick P. Antidepressants for the new millennium. Eur J Pharmacol 1999; 375(1-3):31–40.
49. Hyman SE, Nestler EJ. Initiation and adaptation: a paradigm for understanding psychotropic drug action. Am J Psychiatry 1996; 153(2):151–162.
50. Quitkin FM. Identification of true drug response to antidepressants. Arch Gen Psychiatry 1984; 41(782): 786.
51. Gershon S. Antidepressants: can we determine how quickly they work? Psychopharmacol Bull 1995; 31(21):22.
52. Fawcett J, Barkin RL. Efficacy issues with antidepressants. J Clin Psychiatry 1997; 58:suppl 9.
53. Fava M. New approaches to the treatment of refractory depression. J Clin Psychiatry 2000; 61:suppl 32.
54. Potter WZ, Ozcan ME. Methodological considerations for the development of new treatments for bipolar disorder. Aust NZ J Psychiatry 1999; 33:suppl 98.
55. Frank E, Prien RF, Jarrett RB, Keller MB, Kupfer DJ, Lavori PW, Rush AJ, Weissman MM. Conceptualization and rationale for consensus definitions of terms in major depressive disorder. Remission, recovery, relapse, and recurrence [see comments]. Arch Gen Psychiatry 1991; 48(9):851–855.
56. Spigset O. Adverse reactions of selective serotonin reuptake inhibitors: reports from a spontaneous reporting system. Drug Saf 1999; 20(3):277–287.
57. Coleman E, Gratzer T, Nesvacil L, Raymond NC. Nefazodone and the treatment of nonparaphilic compulsive sexual behavior: a retrospective study. J Clin Psychiatry 2000; 61(4):282–284.
58. Sternbach H. The serotonin syndrome. Am J Psychiatry 1991; 148(705):713.
59. Fava M. Management of nonresponse and intolerance: switching strategies. J Clin Psychiatry 2000; 61:suppl 2.
60. Ferguson JM. The effects of antidepressants on sexual functioning in depressed patients: a review. J Clin Psychiatry 2001; 62:suppl 34.
61. Einarson TR, Arikian SR, Casciano J, Doyle JJ. Comparison of extended-release venlafaxine, selective serotonin reuptake inhibitors, and tricyclic antidepressants in the treatment of depression: a meta-analysis of randomized controlled trials. Clin Ther 1999; 21(2):296–308.
62. Feiger RL. A double-blind, randomized, placebo-controlled trial of once-venlafaxine extended release (XR) and fluoxetine for the treatment of depression. Affect Disord 1999; 56:171–181.

63. Peet M. Induction of mania with selective serotonin reuptake inhibitors and tricyclic antidepressants [see comments]. Br J Psychiatry 1994; 164(4):549-550.
64. Howland RH. Induction of mania with serotonin reuptake inhibitors. J Clin Psychopharmacol 1996; 16(6):425–427.
65. Simpson HB, Hurowitz GI, Liebowitz MR. General principles in the pharmacotherapy of antidepressant-induced rapid cycling: a case series. J Clin Psychopharmacol 1997; 17(6):460–466.
66. Soares JC, Gershon S. The lithium ion: a foundation for psychopharmacological specificity. Neuropsychopharmacology 1998; 19(3):167–182.
67. Manji HK, McNamara R, Chen G, Lenox RH. Signalling pathways in the brain: cellular transduction of mood stabilisation in the treatment of manic-depressive illness. Aust NZ J Psychiatry 1999; 33(suppl):S65–S83.
68. Calabrese JR, Woyshville MJ. Lithium therapy: limitations and alternatives in the treatment of bipolar disorders. Ann Clin Psychiatry 1995; 7(2):103–112.
69. Vasudev K, Goswami U, Kohli K. Carbamazepine and valproate monotherapy: feasibility, relative safety and efficacy, and therapeutic drug monitoring in manic disorder. Psychopharmacology 2000; 150(1):15–23.
70. Spilker B. Introduction. In: Quality of Life and Pharmacoeconomics in Clinical Trials, 2nd ed. Philadelphia: Lippincott-Raven, 1996:1–10.
71. Reeder CE. Overview of pharmacoeconomics and pharmaceutical outcomes evaluations. Am J Health-System Pharm 1995; 52(19 suppl 4):8.
72. Glasziou PP. Use of pharmacoeconomic data by regulatory authorities. In: Quality of Life and Pharmacoeconomics in Clinical Trials, 2nd ed. Philadelphia: Lippincott-Raven, 1996:1141–1147.
73. Grabowski H. The effect of pharmacoeconomics on company research and development decisions. Pharmacoeconomics 1997; 11(5):389–397.
74. Snyder SH. Novel neurotransmitters and their neuropsychiatric relevance. Am J Psychiatry 2000; 157(11):1738–1751.
75. Fuller RW. Uptake inhibitors increase extracellular serotonin concentration measured by brain microdialysis. Life Sci 1994; 5(3):163–167.
76. Stahl SM. Mechanism of action of serotonin selective reuptake inhibitors. Serotonin receptors and pathways mediate therapeutic effects and side effects. J Affect Disord 1998; 51(3):215–235.
77. Broocks A, Briggs NC, Pigott TA, Hill JL, Canter SK, Tolliver TJ, Baldemore D, Murphy DL. Behavioral, physiological and neuroendocrine responses in healthy volunteers to m-chlorophenylpiperazine (m-CPP) with and without ondansetron pretreatment. Psychopharmacology (Berl)1997; 130:91–103.
78. Berman RM, Cappiello A, Anand A, Oren DA, Heninger GR, Charney DS, Krystal JH. Antidepressant effects of ketamine in depressed patients. Biol Psychiatry 2000; 47(4):351–354.
79. Blier PMP. Effectiveness of pindolol with selected antidepressant drugs in the treatment of major depression. J Clin Psychopharmacol 1995; 15(3):217–222.
80. Perez V. Randomised, double-blind, placebo-controlled trial of pindolol in combination with fluoxetine antidepressant treatment. Lancet 1997; 3349:1594–1597.
81. Romero L. Preferential potentiation of the effects of serotonin uptake inhibitors by 5-HT1 receptor antagonists in the dorsal raphe pathway: role of somatodendritic autoreceptors. J Neurochem 1997; 68(6):2593–2603.
82. Bordet R. Selective serotonin reuptake inhibitors plus pindolol [letter]. Lancet 1997; 350:289.
83. Zanardi RM. How long should pindolol be associated with paroxetine to improve the antidepressant response? J Clin Psychopharmacol 1997; 17(6):446–450.
84. Valenca A, Nascimento I, Nardi AE, Zin W, Guitmann G, Figueira I, Marques C, Andrade Y, Versiani M. Smoking, anxiety and depression. J Brasil Psiquiatria 1998; 47(5):243–250.
85. Vazquez FL, Becona E. Depression and smoking in a smoking cessation programme. J Affect Disord 1999; 55(2-3):125-132.
86. Wilhelm K. The relevance of smoking and nicotine to clinical psychiatry. Australasian Psychiatry 1998; 6(3):130–132.
87. Williams M. Nicotinic receptors: new targets for therapeutic agents. CNS Drug Rev 1999; 5(suppl).
88. Zobel AW, Nickel T, Kunzel HE, Ackl N, Sonntag A, Ising M, Holsboer F. Effects of the high-affinity corticotropin-releasing hormone receptor 1 antagonist R121919 in major depression: the first 20 patients treated. J Psychiat Res 2000; 34(3):171–181.
89. Rabiner EA, Gunn RN, Castro ME, Sargent PA, Cowen PJ, Koepp MJ, Meyer JH, Bench CJ, Harrison PJ, Pazos A, Sharp T, Grasby PM. Beta-blocker binding to human 5-HT(1A) receptors in vivo and in vitro: implications for antidepressant therapy. Neuropsychopharmacology 2000; 23(3):285–293.
90. Martinez D. Differential occupancy of somatodendritic and postsynaptic 5HT (1A) receptors by pindolol: a dose-occupancy study with [^{11}C]WAY 100635 and positron emission tomography in humans. Neuropsychopharmacology 2001; 20(373):378.
91. Shiah IS, Yatham LN, Srisurapanont M, Lam RW, Tam EM, Zis AP. Does the addition of pindolol accelerate the response to electroconvulsive therapy in patients with major depression? A double-blind, placebo-controlled pilot study. J Clin Psychopharmacol 2000; 20(3):373–378.
92. Chang MM, Leeman SE. Isolation of a sialogogic peptide from bovine hypothalamic tissue and its charac-

terization as substance P. J Biol Chem 1970; 245:4784–4790.
93. Hale JJ, Mills SG, MacCoss M, Finke PE, Cascieri MA, Sadowski S, Ber E, Chicchi GG, Kurtz M, Metzger J, Eiermann G, Tsou NN, Tattersall FD, Rupniak NM, Williams AR, Rycroft W, Hargreaves R, MacIntyre DE. Structural optimization affording 2-(R)-(1-(R)-3,5-bis(trifluoromethyl)phenylethoxy)-3-(S)-(4-fluoro)phenyl-4-(3-oxo-1,2,4-triazol-5-yl)methylmorpholine, a potent, orally active, long-acting morpholine acetal human NK-1 receptor antagonist. J Med Chem 1998; 41(23):4607–4614.
94. Snider RM, Constantine JW, Lowe JA III, Longo KP, Lebel WS, Woody HA, Drozda SE, Desai MC, Vinick FJ, Spencer RW. A potent nonpeptide antagonist of the substance P (NK1) receptor. Science 1991; 251:435–437.
95. Chen G, Hasanat KA, Bebchuk JM, Moore GJ, Glitz D, Manji HK. Regulation of signal transduction pathways and gene expression by mood stabilizers and antidepressants. Psychosom Med 1999; 61(5):599–617.
96. Bokesch PMMD. Neuroprotective, anesthetic, and cardiovascular effects of the NMDA antagonist, CNS 5161A, in isoflurane-anesthetized lambs. Anesthesiology 2000; 93(1):202–208.
97. Acosta GB. A possible interaction between CCKergic and GABAergic systems in the rat brain. Comp Biochem Physiol Toxicol Pharmacol 2001; 128(1):11–17.
98. Haddjeri N, Gobbi G, Santarelli L, Hen R, Blier P. Pharmacologic and genetic interference with the neurokinin 1 receptor enhances 5-HT transmission. American College of Neuropsychopharmacology, Scientific Abstract, 39th Annual Meeting, San Juan, Puerto Rico, Dec 10–14, 2000, p 307.
99. Shirayama Y, Mitsushio H, Takashima M, Ichikawa H, Takahashi K. Reduction of substance P after chronic antidepressants treatment in the striatum, substantia nigra and amygdala of the rat. Brain Res 1996; 739(1-2):70–78.
100. Kucharczyk N. Tachykinin antagonists in development. Expert Opin Invest Drugs 1995; 4(4):299–311.
101. Seward EM, Swain CJ. Neurokinin receptor antagonists. Expert Opin Ther Patents 1999; 9(5):571–582.
102. Kramer MS, Cutler N, Feighner J, Shrivastava R, Carman J, Sramek JJ, Reines SA, Liu G, Snavely D, Wyatt-Knowles E, Hale JJ, Mills SG, MacCoss M, Swain CJ, Harrison T, Hill RG, Hefti F, Scolnick EM, Cascieri MA, Chicchi GG, Sadowski S, Williams AR, Hewson L, Smith D, Rupniak NM. Distinct mechanism for antidepressant activity by blockade of central substance P receptors [see comments]. Science 1998; 281(5383):1640–1645.
103. Kramer MS. Update on Substance P (NK-1 receptor) antagonists in clinical trials for depression. Neuropeptides 2000; 34(5):255.

104. Kreimeyer A, Laube B, Sturgess M, Goeldner M, Foucaud B. Evaluation and biological properties of reactive ligands for the mapping of the glycine site on the N-methyl-D-aspartate (NMDA) receptor. J Med Chem 1999; 42(21):4394–4404.
105. Meldrum BS. Glutamate as a neurotransmitter in the brain: review of physiology and pathology. J Nutr 2000; 130(4S suppl):1007S–1015S.
106. Padovan CM, Del Bel EA, Guimaraes FS. Behavioral effects in the elevated plus maze of an NMDA antagonist injected into the dorsal hippocampus: influence of restraint stress. Pharmacol Biochem Behav 2000; 67:325–330.
107. Le Houezec J. Nicotine: abused substance and therapeutic agent. J Psychiatry Neurosci 1998; 23(2):95–108.
108. Berman RMM. Effect of pindolol in hastening response to fluoxetine in the treatment of major depression: a double-blind, placebo-controlled trial. Am J Psychiatry 1997; 154(1):37-43.
109. Nowak G, Legutko B, Skolnick P, Popik P. Adaptation of cortical NMDA receptors by chronic treatment with specific serotonin reuptake inhibitors. Eur J Pharmacol 1998; 342(2-3):367–370.
110. Nowak G, Trullas R, Layer RT, Skolnick P, Paul IA. Adaptive changes in the N-methyl-D-aspartate receptor complex after chronic treatment with imipramine and 1-aminocyclopropanecarboxylic acid. J Pharmacol Exp Ther 1993; 265(3):1380–1386.
111. Paul IA, Nowak G, Layer RT, Popik P, Skolnick P. Adaptation of the N-methyl-D-aspartate receptor complex following chronic antidepressant treatments. J Pharm Exp Ther 1994; 269:95–102.
112. Popoli M. Second messenger–regulated protein kinases in the brain: their functional role and the action of antidepressant drugs. J Neurochem 2000; 74(1):21.
113. Popik P, Wrobel M, Nowak G. Chronic treatment with antidepressants affects glycine/NMDA receptor function: behavioral evidence. Neuropharmacology 2000; 39(12):2278–2287.
114. Covey LS, Glassman AH, Stetner F. Cigarette smoking and major depression. J Addict Dis 1998; 17(1):35–46.
115. Glassman AH, Helzer JE, Covey LS, Cottler LB, Stetner F, Tipp JE, Johnson J. Smoking, smoking cessation, and major depression [see comments]. JAMA 1990; 264(12):1546–1549.
116. Quattrocki E, Baird A, Yurgelun-Todd D. Biological aspects of the link between smoking and depression. Harvard Rev Psychiatry 2000; 8(3):99–110.
117. Ferguson SM, Brodkin JD, Lloyd GK, Menzaghi F. Antidepressant-like effects of the subtype-selective nicotinic acetylcholine receptor agonist, SIB-1508Y, in the learned helplessness rat model of depression. Psychopharmacology 2000; 152(3):295–303.
118. Lerman C, Caporaso N, Main D, Audrain J, Boyd NR, Bowman ED, Shields PG. Depression and self-

medication with nicotine: the modifying influence of the dopamine D4 receptor gene. Health Psychology 1998; 17(1):56–62.
119. Cosford ND, Bleicher L, Vernier JM, Chavez-Noriega L, Rao TS, Siegel RS, Suto C, Washburn M, Lloyd GK, McDonald IA. Recombinant human receptors and functional assays in the discovery of altinicline (SIB-1508Y), a novel acetylcholine-gated ion channel (nAChR) agonist. Pharm Acta Helv 2000; 74:125–130.
120. Salin-Pascual RJ, Drucker-Colin R. A novel effect of nicotine on mood and sleep in major depression. Neuroreport 1998; 9(1):57–60.
121. Carpenter WT Jr, Bunney WE Jr. Adrenal cortical activity in depressive illness. Am J Psychiatry 1971; 128:31–40.
122. Sachar EJ, Hellman L, Fukushima DK, Gallagher TF. Cortisol production in depressive illness. A clinical and biochemical clarification. Arch Gen Psychiatry 1970; 23(4):289–298.
123. Banki CM, Bissette G, Arato M, Nemeroff CB. Elevation of immunoreactive CSF TRH in depressed patients. Am J Psychiatry 1988; 145:1526–1531.
124. Evans DL, Nemeroff CB. Use of the dexamethasone suppression test using DSM-III criteria on an inpatient psychiatric unit. Biol Psychiatry 1983; 18(4):505–511.
125. Schatzberg AF, Rothschild AJ, Bond TC, Cole JO. The DST in psychotic depression: diagnostic and pathophysiologic implications. Psychopharmacol Bull 1984; 20(3):362–364.
126. Artigas FP. Pindolol, 5-hydroxytryptamine, and antidepressant augmentation [letter]. Arch Gen Psychiatry 1995; 52:969–971.
127. Menzaghi F, Howard RL, Heinrichs SC, Vale W, Rivier J, Koob GF. Characterization of a novel and potent corticotropin-releasing factor antagonist in rats. J Pharmacol Exp Ther 1994; 269(2):564–572.
128. Arato M, Banki CM, Bissette G, Nemeroff CB. Elevated CSF CRF in suicide victims. Biol Psychiatry 1989; 25(3):355–359.
129. Nemeroff CB, Widerlov E, Bissette G, Walleus H, Karlsson I, Eklund K, Kilts CD, Loosen PT, Vale W. Elevated concentrations of CSF corticotropin-releasing factor–like immunoreactivity in depressed patients. Science 1984; 226(4680):1342–1344.
130. Aldenhoff J, Kell S, Koch J. Changes of CREB during recovery from major depression. American College of Neuropsychopharmacology, Scientific Abstract, 39th Annual Meeting, San Juan, Puerto Rico, Dec 10-14, 2000.
131. Anand AM. Attenuation of the neuropsychiatric effects of ketamine with lamotrigine: support for hyperglutamatergic effects of N-methyl-D-aspartate receptor antagonists. Arch Gen Psychiatry 2000; 57:270–276.
132. Barden N, Reul JM, Holsboer F. Do antidepressants stabilize mood through actions on the hypothalamic-pituitary-adrenocortical system? Trends Neurosci 1995; 18:6–11.
133. Pepin MC, Pothier F, Barden N. Antidepressant drug action in a transgenic mouse model of the endocrine changes seen in depression. Mol Pharmacol 1992; 42:991–995.
134. Bauer MPD. Double-blind, placebo-controlled trial of the use of lithium to augment antidepressant medication in continuation treatment of unipolar major depression. Am J Psychiatry 2000; 157:1429–1435.
135. Banki CM, Karmacsi L, Bissette G, Nemeroff CB. CSF corticotropin-releasing hormone and somatostatin in major depression: response to antidepressant treatment and relapse. Eur Neuropsychopharmacol 1992; 2:107–113.
136. Nibuya M, Morinobu S, Duman RS. Regulation of BDNF and trkB mRNA in rat brain by chronic electroconvulsive seizure and antidepressant drug treatments. J Neurosci 1995; 15(11):7539–7547.
137. Nibuya M, Nestler EJ, Duman RS. Chronic antidepressant administration increases the expression of cAMP response element binding protein (CREB) in rat hippocampus. J Neurosci 1996; 16(7):2365–2372.
138. Brandoli C, Sanna A, De Bernardi MA, Follesa P, Brooker G, Mocchetti I. Brain-derived neurotrophic factor and basic fibroblast growth factor downregulate NMDA receptor function in cerebellar granule cells. J Neurosci 1998; 18:7953–7961.
139. Boyer PA, Skolnick P, Fossom LH. Chronic administration of imipramine and citalopram alters the expression of NMDA receptor subunit mRNAs in mouse brain. A quantitative in situ hybridization study. J Mol Neurosci 1998; 10:219–233.
140. Engels P. Brain distribution of four rat homologues of the *Drosophila* dunce cAMP phosphodiesterase. J Neurosci Res 1995; 41:169–178.
141. Wachtel H. Potential antidepressant activity of rolipram and other selective cyclic adenosine $3',5'$-monophosphate phosphodiesterase inhibitors. Neuropharmacology 1988; 22(267):272.
142. Suda S, Nibuya M, Ishiguro T, Suda H. Transcriptional and translational regulation of phosphodiesterase type IV isozymes in rat brain by electroconvulsive seizure and antidepressant drug treatment. J Neurochem 1998; 71(4):1554–1563.
143. Chen G, Huang L, Jiang Y, Manji HK. The mood-stabilizing agent valproate inhibits the activity of glycogen synthase kinase-3. J Neurochem 1999; 72(3):1327–1330.
144. Chen G, Huang LD, Zeng WZ, Manji HK. Mood stabilizers regulate cytoprotective and mRNA-binding proteins in the brain: long-term effects on cell survival and transcript stability. Int J Neuropsychopharmacol 2001; 4(1):47–64.
145. Manji HK, Moore GJ, Chen G. Lithium at 50: have the neuroprotective effects of this unique cation

been overlooked? Biol Psychiatry 1999; 46(7):929–940.
146. Jetty PV, Charney DS, Goddard AW. Neurobiology of generalized anxiety disorder. Psychiatr Clin North Am 2001; 24(1):75–97.
147. Klodzinska A, Chojnacka-Wojcik E, Palucha A, Branski P, Popik P, Pilc A. Potential anti-anxiety, anti-addictive effects of LY 354740, a selective group II glutamate metabotropic receptors agonist in animal models. Neuropharmacology 1999; 38(12):1831–1839.
148. Kubota K, Matsuda I, Sugaya K, Uruno T. Cholecystokinin antagonism by benzodiazepines in the food intake in mice. Physiol Behav 1986; 36(1):175–178.
149. Levine LR, Potter WZ. The 5-HT1A receptor: an unkept promise? In: Briley M, Nutt D, eds. Anxioloytics. Secacus: Birkhauserverlag AG, 2000; 95–104.
150. Levine LR, Potter WZ. 5-HT1A agonists, partial agonists and antagonists in anxiety and depression: a lost cause? Curr Opin CPNS Invest Drugs 1999; 1(4):448–452.
151. Moore GJ, Bebchuk JM, Hasanat K, Chen G, Seraji-Bozorgzad N, Wilds IB, Faulk MW, Koch S, Glitz DA, Jolkovsky L, Manji HK. Lithium increases N-acetyl-aspartate in the human brain: In vivo evidence in support of bcl-2's neurotrophic effects? Biol Psychiatry 2000; 1:1–8.
152. Moore G, Chen G, Glitz DA, Bebchuk JM, Seraji-Bozorgzad N, Wilds IB, Zajac-Benitez C, Manji HK. Neurotrophic effects of mood stabilizers in the human brain. American College of Neuropsychopharmacology, Scientific Abstract, 39th Annual Meeting, San Juan, Puerto Rico, 2000:287.
153. Craig KJ, Brown KJ, Baum A. Environmental factors in the etiology of anxiety. In: Bloom FE, Kupfer DJ, eds. Psychopharmacology: the fourth generation of progress. New York: Raven Press, 1995; 1325–1339.
154. Woods JH, Katz JL, Winger G. Benzodiazepines: use, abuse, and consequences. Pharmacol Rev 1992; 44(2):155–338.
155. Dorow R, Duka T, Holler L, Sauerbrey N. Clinical perspectives of beta-carbolines from first studies in humans. Brain Res Bull 1987; 19:319–326.
156. Ferrarese C, Appollonio I, Frigo M, Perego M, Pierpaoli C, Trabucchi M, Frattola L. Characterization of peripheral benzodiazepine receptors in human blood mononuclear cells. Neuropharmacology 1990; 29(4):375–378.
157. Rocca P, Beoni AM, Eva C, Ferrero P, Zanalda E, Ravizza L. Peripheral benzodiazepine receptor messenger RNA is decreased in lymphocytes of generalized anxiety disorder patients. Biol Psychiatry 1998; 43(10):767–773.
158. Sibille E, Pavlides C, Benke D, Toth M. Genetic inactivation of the serotonin(1A) receptor in mice results in downregulation of major GABA(A) receptor alpha subunits, reduction of GABA(A) receptor binding, and benzodiazepine-resistant anxiety. J Neurosci 2000; 20(8):2758–2765.
159. Van Megen HJ, Den Boer JA, Westenberg HG. On the significance of cholecystokinin receptors in panic disorder. Prog Neuropsychopharmacol Biol Psychiatry 1994; 18(8):1235–1246.
160. Crestani F, Low K, Keist R, Mandelli M, Mohler H, Rudolph U. Molecular targets for the myorelaxant action of diazepam. Mol Pharmacol 2001; 59:442–445.
161. Rudolph U, Crestani F, Benke D, Brunig I, Benson JA, Fritschy JM, Martin JR, Bluethmann H, Mohler H. Benzodiazepine actions mediated by specific gamma-aminobutyric acid(A) receptor subtypes. [Erratum appears in Nature 2000; 404(6778):629.] Nature 1999; 401(6755):796–800.
162. Handley SL. 5-Hydroxytryptamine pathways in anxiety and its treatment. Pharmacol Ther 1995; 66(1):103–148.
163. Ramboz S, Oosting R, Amara DA, Kung HF, Blier P, Mendelsohn M, Mann JJ, Brunner D, Hen R. Serotonin receptor 1A knockout: an animal model of anxiety-related disorder [see comments]. Proc Nat Acad Sci USA 1995; 24:14476–14481.
164. Rickels K, Schweizer E, DeMartinis N, Mandos L, Mercer C. Gepirone and diazepam in generalized anxiety disorder: a placebo-controlled trial. J Clin Psychopharmacol 1997; (4):272–277.
165. Pagoclone, reduced the frequency of panic attacks in a Phase II/III US trial. SCRIP 1998; 2369:23.
166. Cartmell J, Schoepp DD. Regulation of neurotransmitter release by metabotropic glutamate receptors. J Neurochem 2000; 75:889–907.
167. De Blasi A, Conn PJ, Pin J, Nicoletti F. Molecular determinants of metabotropic glutamate receptor signaling. Trends Pharmacol Sci 2001; 22:114–120.
168. Shekhar A, Keim SR. LY354740, a potent group II metabotropic glutamate receptor agonist prevents lactate-induced panic-like response in panic-prone rats. Neuropharmacology 2000; 39(7):1139–1146.
169. Klodzinska A. Potential anti-anxiety, anti-addictive effects of LY 354740, a selective group II glutamate metabotropic receptors agonist in animal models. Neuropharmacology 1999; 38:1139–1156.
170. Phillips T, Rees S, Augood S, Waldvogel H, Faull R, Svendsen C, Emson P. Localization of metabotropic glutamate receptor type 2 in the human brain. Neuroscience 2000; 95(4):1139–1156.
171. Brambilla F, Bellodi L, Perna G, Garberi A, Panerai A, Sacerdote P. Lymphocyte cholecystokinin concentrations in panic disorder. Am J Psychiatry 1993; 150:1111–1113.
172. Sugaya K, Matsuda I, Kubota K. Inhibition of hypothermic effect of cholecystokinin by benzodiaze-

pines and a benzodiazepine antagonist, Ro 15-1788, in mice. Jpn J Pharmacol 1985; 39(2):277–280.

173. Pande AC, Greiner M, Adams JB, Lydiard RB, Pierce MW. Placebo-controlled trial of the CCK-B antagonist, CI-988, in panic disorder. Biol Psychiatry 1999; 46(6):860–862.

174. Goddard AW, Woods SW, Money R, Pande AC, Charney DS, Goodman WK, Heninger GR, Price LH. Effects of the CCK(B) antagonist CI-988 on responses to mCPP in generalized anxiety disorder. Psychiatry Res 1999; 3:225–240.

175. Pande AC, Greiner M, Adams JB, Lydiard RB, Pierce MW. Placebo-controlled trial of the CCK-B antagonist, CI-988, in panic disorder. Biol Psychiatry 1999; 46:860–862.

176. Trivedi BK, Padia JK, Holmes A, Rose S, Wright DS, Hinton JP, Pritchard MC, Eden JM, Kneen C, Webdale L, Suman-Chauhan N, Boden P, Singh L, Field MJ, Hill D. Second generation "peptoid" CCK-B receptor antagonists: identification and development of N-(adamantyloxycarbonyl)-alpha-methyl-(R)-tryptophan derivative (CI-1015) with an improved pharmacokinetic profile. J Med Chem 1998; 1:38–45.

177. Trivedi BK, Hinton JP. CI-1015. An orally active CCK-B receptor antagonist with an improved pharmacokinetic profile. Pharm Biotechnol 1998; 11:481–505.

178. Rasmussen K, Czachura JF, Kallman MJ, Helton DR. The CCK-B antagonist LY288513 blocks the effects of nicotine withdrawal on auditory startle. Neuroreport 1996 1996; 7(5):1050–1052.

179. Emoto H, Koga C, Ishii H, Yokoo H, Yoshida M, Tanaka M. A CRF antagonist attenuates stress-induced increases in NA turnover in extended brain regions in rats. Brain Res 1993; 627(1):171–176.

180. Heinrichs SC, Menzaghi F, Pich EM, Baldwin HA, Rassnick S, Britton KT, Koob GF. Anti-stress action of a corticotropin-releasing factor antagonist on behavioral reactivity to stressors of varying type and intensity. Neuropsychopharmacology 1994; 11(3):179–186.

181. Hennessy MB, O'Neil DR, Becker LA, Jenkins R, Williams MT, Davis HN. Effects of centrally administered corticotropin-releasing factor (CRF) and alpha-helical CRF on the vocalizations of isolated guinea pig pups. Pharmacol Biochem Behav 1992; 43(1):37–43.

54

Perspectives for Pharmacological Interventions in Eating Disorders

GUIDO K. FRANK
Western Psychiatric Institute and Clinic, University of Pittsburgh School of Medicine, Pittsburgh, Pennsylvania, U.S.A.

I. INTRODUCTION

Since their recognition as psychiatric disorders, eating disorders (EDs) have received a substantial amount of attention. Anorexia nervosa (AN) was found to have the highest mortality among all psychiatric disorders [1], and both AN and bulimia nervosa (BN) often have long and protracted courses [2]. Binge eating disorder (BED) has been identified more recently, and may be the most prevalent ED [3]. All three conditions are associated with high psychiatric or medical comorbidity, and cause significant impairment and distress for the affected individuals, as well as high treatment costs for the society [4].

The etiology of EDs is unknown. Sociocultural factors have been implicated in their development [5]; however, research over the past 20 years has shown that AN and BN are highly heritable disorders [6,7], and that neurotransmitters such as serotonin or dopamine are disturbed during the ill state and after recovery [8,9]. These findings suggest that a biological trait disturbance may predispose individuals to develop such illnesses. No specific medication for the treatment of EDs has been found. Most pharmacologic compounds used in the treatment of AN, BN, or BED were originally developed for other conditions, such as mood or anxiety disorders.

This chapter reviews past pharmacologic treatment approaches, reports on current treatment recommendations using drug treatment, and provides research perspectives for future drug trials based on current pilot studies and new neurobiological research findings.

II. ANOREXIA NERVOSA

The core symptoms of AN are (1) a refusal to maintain a minimally normal body weight; (2) an intense fear of gaining weight or becoming fat; (3) a body image disturbance, i.e., patients *feel* fat, even when being underweight; and (4) in postmenarcheal women, amenorrhea. A restricting type (AN-R), with food restriction and sometimes excessive exercising, has been distinguished from a binge-eating/purging type (AN-B/P), where episodes of binge eating and/or purging behavior such as self-induced vomiting or the use of laxatives, diuretics, or enemas, accompany fasting and overexercising [4]. AN patients typically have obsessive-compulsive features that are directly related to food and weight. However, obsessive-compulsive disorder (OCD) independent from AN-related content is also common. During the ill state and after recovery, individuals with AN frequently present with increased symptoms of depression and anxiety, and it has recently been recognized that anxiety disorders may be an antecedent in many patients with AN [10].

A. Appetite Stimulants

Early pharmacologic interventions targeted the core symptom of food refusal and low weight, trying to induce appetite and thus weight gain. In an open-label study [11], the antihistamine cyproheptadine (up to 32 mg/day) or placebo was given to 81 subjects with AN. In that study, cyproheptadine could induce weight gain only in a subgroup of more severe cases of AN. In a later double-blind, placebo-controlled study [12] in 72 subjects, where cyproheptadine (up to 32 mg/day, n = 24), or amitryptiline (up to 160 mg/day, n = 23) or placebo (n = 25) was administered to patients with AN, it was found that cyproheptadine slightly reduced the number of days needed to reach normal weight. Two findings stood out in that study. First, cyproheptadine appeared to be beneficial for the AN-R subtype only, whereas for the AN-B/P subtype it seemed to hinder positive treatment effects. Second, higher doses of cyproheptadine (12–32 mg/dL) reduced depressive symptoms but without the significant side effects that were seen in the amitryptiline group.

B. Classic Antidopaminergic Neuroleptic Agents

Food consumption is regulated by a complex interplay of monoamine neurotransmitters such as serotonin (5HT), dopamine (DA), and norepinephrine (NA), but also endogenous opioids, as well as a multitude of central-acting neuropeptides [13]. In this feedback circuit of food craving and hunger on one side and food reward and satiety on the other, DA plays an important role in the food reward circuit [14]. Patients with AN do not appear to get pleasure out of food, and a disturbance, e.g., a hyperactivity or a disturbed feedback mechanism of brain dopamine activity in AN, was hypothesized [15]. Studies using the neuroleptic and dopamine-blocking agents *pimozide* (4–6 mg/day, n = 18) and *sulpiride* (300 mg/day, n = 13; 400 mg/day, n = 5) in double-blind crossover designs, however, did not show a significant effect on eating behavior or weight gain in AN [16,17]. Recently, a study found reduced cerebrospinal fluid (CSF) levels of the DA metabolite homovanillin mandelic acid (HVA) in AN-R but not in AN-B/P [9], which suggests a DA disturbance in the restricting subtype of AN. Future studies are needed to investigate the involvement of the DA system in AN.

C. Opiates and Cannabinoids

Endogenous opiates are involved in the modulation of feeding, and Marrazzi et al. [18] suggested an "auto-addiction" model, where increased endogenous opioids were hypothesized to reduce the desire to eat in AN. A few studies investigated opiate antagonists in AN with the rationale that a removal of a suggested self-reward through endogenous opioids would stimulate food reward and thus eating. Moore et al. [19] found that a continuous infusion of naloxone (3.2–6.4 mg/day) over 1–11 weeks improved weight gain compared to before or after the infusion. A more recent study using naltrexone 100 mg/day in a double-blind crossover design over 6 weeks showed reduced binge/purge episodes compared to placebo [20] in AN-B/P patients. However, no effect of the drug on body weight was observed. The use of opioid antagonists in AN is quite questionable since such substances reduce food intake in most studies [21].

Endogenous cannabinoids enhance appetite, and most interestingly, a link has been established to the appetite-regulating peptide leptin, which is derived from body fat stores [22]. An early trial [23] studied 9-tetrahydrocannabinol (active study drug, up to 30 mg/day) or diazepam (as an active placebo, up to 15 mg/day) in 11 AN in a 4-week double-blind crossover design. All subjects participated in a behavior modification program. However, no beneficial effect was observed from 9-tetrahydrocannabinol compared to placebo. In fact, AN on the active study drug reported side effects such as severe dysphoria and sleep disturbances. We are not aware of other studies in AN using cannabinoids. However, the recent report of a down-regulation of endogenous cannabinoids by leptin [22,24] suggests that endogenous cannbinoids might be an interesting area of research for future pharmacologic interventions in AN, despite the disappointing results from Gross's [23] study.

D. Antidepressant Medication

Several antidepressant medications have been studied in AN. One rationale for this intervention is the observation that AN is very frequently associated with depressive symptoms. Depressive disorders are frequently associated with disturbed eating behavior. It has even been proposed that AN may be a variant of mood disorders [25].

The effect of the tricyclic antidepressant clomipramine (50 mg/day) on time to reach target weight was studied double-blindly in 16 inpatients with AN during an intensive behavioral treatment program [26,27]. Clomipramine increased hunger, appetite, and energy intake; however, it reduced the rate of weight gain. At 1 year follow-up there was no significant difference between groups. In a double-blind placebo-controlled design, Biederman [28] studied 11 patients on up to 175 mg/day amitryptiline (mean dose 2.9 mg/kg/day) and 14 patients on placebo, all in addition to behavioral psychotherapeutic inpatient treatment, and compared them to 18 patients treated with psychotherapy alone. Overall, amitryptiline-treated patients did not do better than unmedicated subjects. In fact, subjects on amitryptiline complained of side effects from the medication. In addition, the treated group did not report a reduction of depressive symptoms compared to the placebo group.

The monoamine serotonin most consistently has been shown to be disturbed in AN during the ill/underweight state as well as after refeeding and recovery [8]. Thus, with the advent of selective serotonin reuptake inhibitors (SSRIs), a promising new group of psychotropic medications for the treatment of AN seemed to be available. A pilot study in six subjects, using 20–60 mg/day fluoxetine, suggested reduced depressive symptoms and weight gain in the studied AN patients [29]. However, subsequent studies in underweight anorexic subjects could not replicate those initial findings. Attia et al. [30] conducted a double-blind, placebo-controlled study in 31 underweight inpatients over 7 weeks with a daily dose of 60 mg fluoxetine. They did not find statistically significant benefits regarding body weight, or general eating behavior from the medication over placebo. Similarly, Strober et al. [31] could not find a significant beneficial effect from fluoxetine administered over 6 weeks during inpatient treatment in underweight AN subjects compared to data from a matched historical control group.

A recent open-label study using citalopram in AN [32] reported beneficial effects regarding binge eating and a reduction of ED-related psychological symptoms. However, no weight increase was demonstrated. Moreover, a case report on eight patients treated with 20 mg/day of citalopram in addition to a course of psychotherapy showed a mean weight loss of 5.4 kg (range −0.7 to −11 kg) compared to a control group that lost on average 0.2 kg (range −4.7 to +2.4 kg) in the same treatment program but not on medication [33]. These findings suggest that citalopram should not be used during the underweight state in AN.

Studies in underweight AN showed a reduction of the serotonin (5HT) metabolite 5-hydroxyindole acetic acid (5HIAA) in CSF [34], suggesting a reduction of 5HT activity during the ill state. Brain 5HT is dependent on the brain uptake of the essential amino acid L-tryptophan (TRP), which is regulated by blood insulin levels as well as plasma concentrations of other large essential neutral amino acids (LNAAs) [35,36]. Anorexics severely restrict their food intake and supposedly reduce 5HT in the brain [37]. Since SSRIs act by increasing intrasynaptic 5HT via inhibiting 5HT presynaptic reuptake, this effect may not be functional in AN because of a low baseline brain 5HT availability. After recovery from AN however, *increased* levels of CSF 5HIAA were found [38].

AN patients show a substantial relapse rate, and medication trials *after refeeding* seemed to be a reasonable approach. An open trial of fluoxetine [39] in 31 AN patients after weight restoration and in outpatient treatment suggested a reduction of the usual relapse rate. By the time of follow-up (11 ± 6 months) 29 out of the 31 subjects were still at or above 85% of average body weight (ABW). Strober et al. [40] performed a study in 33 patients on variable doses of fluoxetine (mean 34 mg/day), and followed this group over 24 months. Patients on the active drug did not do significantly better than a group of matched historical controls. However, it should be noted that the median survival time for staying on target weight was 15 weeks for the fluoxetine group vs. 7 weeks for the non-medicated group, although this was not statistically significant. A recent double-blind study using flouxetine after weight restoration found an improved survival time with regard to healthy body weight in AN [41]. After inpatient weight restoration, 35 subjects were randomly assigned to fluoxetine (n = 16) or placebo (n = 19), and followed up over 1 year as outpatients. Ten subjects in the fluoxetine group (38 ± 21 mg/day fluoxetine at study end at 352 ± 5 total study days), whereas only three in the placebo group (368 ± 2 total study days) were considered treatment responders. The nonresponders, six subjects in the fluoxetine group (43 ± 15 mg/day fluoxetine at study end at 116 ±69 total study days), and 16 subjects in the placebo group (79 ± 32 total study days), relapsed and dropped out of the study. In addition to a reduced relapse rate, fluoxetine administration was associated with a significant reduction in obsessions and compulsions and a trend toward a reduction of depressive feelings. The relatively small sample size in this study limits the power of the results. In addition, since subjects were in outpatient treatment, those conditions could not be entirely standardized. However, this is the first double-blind controlled study that reports relapse prevention in AN. The approach of starting medication after weight restoration is appealing, and further studies seem to be warranted.

A recent case report series from our group in binge-eating/purging type AN [42] suggested that *sertraline* may be useful in this subgroup of AN. Two of the five subjects reported had failed on previous partial hospital and outpatient psychotherapy treatment with or without different additional antidepressants. Sertraline (between 100 and 150 mg/day) was added to psychotherapy treatment. All five subjects gained weight to between 92% and 100% of age-adjusted ABW. Sertraline administration was also associated with a reduction in ED-related behaviors, as well as depression and obsessional thoughts. As noted above, underweight subjects often do not respond to SSRIs. Moreover, it is difficult to get underweight people with an ED to gain weight outside of a hospital setting [43]. These case reports raise the question of whether sertraline shows some advantage over other SSRI medications in terms of helping ED subjects gain weight. Although SSRI medications have similarities in terms of blocking serotonin reuptake, these compounds have different molecular structures and may have different central nervous system effects. For example, sertraline has effects on noradrenergic transmission [44–46].

E. Mood Stabilizers

Lithium was among the first compounds studied [47]. In this 4-week double-blind study, Gross administered lithium carbonate (> 300 mg/day uptitrated to plasma levels of 0.9–1.4 mEq/L) to eight AN women and placebo to a matched AN group (all subjects were on an inpatient behavior modification program at the time of the study). The medicated group showed a limited weight gain. Considering the possibly severe side effects from this drug, the frequent repeated need for plasma level checkups, and the relatively small improvement found, lithium cannot be recommended for use in AN.

F. Atypical Neuroleptic Agents

With the discovery of the so-called atypical neuroleptic agents, a new and relatively safe group of medications was put on the market. An important side effect of several of those drugs is weight gain [48]. This effect may be related to alterations of central monoamine or histamine activity [49]. A few case reports have been published recently on olanzapine in AN. Hansen [50] first reported in 1999 on a patient with chronic AN who gained more than 20 kg over several months and who improved on mood and cognitive performance after initiation of treatment with 10 mg/day and later 5 mg/day (reduced due to side effects such as tiredness and dizziness) of olanzapine. La Via et al. [51] found in two severe cases of AN with a 5- and 6-year history of AN that administration of olanzapine in doses between 10 and 15 mg/day was associated with weight gain, and both patients were still at normal weight 4 and 6 months respectively after discharge from the hospital. Another case report, in three women with long-standing histories of AN treated with 5 mg olanzapine, indicated significant weight gain over several months and a normalization of ED-related thoughts [52]. A critical comment on that report is the authors' emphasis on psychotic experiences.

AN is not recognized as a psychotic disorder. Also, there was no mention of other treatments those subjects may have received in addition to the olanzapine administration. We recently assessed a group of 18 subjects retrospectively on their experience with olanzapine [53]. Subjects reported reduced anxiety and less difficulty eating; however, there was no effect on weight gain attributable to the drug. Our clinical experience is that AN patients feel more relaxed and less anxious on olanzapine, but no clear reduction of days needed to regain to their target weight has been observed, nor were anxiety or depressive feelings reduced on standardized instruments compared to placebo. However, further investigation is warranted, in particular for assessing the specific behavioral effects olanzapine has in ED subjects.

G. Other Agents

In addition to psychoactive drugs, a few controlled trials investigated drugs that supposedly had peripheral effects. Women with AN very frequently complain about gastric fullness and abdominal discomfort after meals during the refeeding process. A double-blind study [54] using the gastrointestinal motility drug cisapride (30 mg/day, n = 6) or placebo (n = 6) over 6 weeks reported increased gastric emptying for both groups, but a tendency to more improvement in the medicated group. More recently, a study [55] using a total of 30 mg/day of oral cisapride over 8 weeks studied 29 inpatients in a double-blind, placebo-controlled design. In that study, gastric emptying normalized similarly in both groups, although subjectively, AN subjects rated themselves as hungrier and overall improved. In addition, weight gain was similar in the two groups. Thus, the addition of this gastrointestinal motility drug for the treatment of AN does not seem to be justified.

Patients with AN show reduced zinc levels. This phenomenon is most likely a state related symptom that remits with normalization of food intake [56]. However, two double-blind and randomized studies found zinc supplementation beneficial for the treatment of AN. Katz et al. [57] found that zinc supplementation (50 mg/day) reduced symptoms of depression and anxiety AN patients, and Birmingham et al. [58] found in a double-blind, placebo-controlled study that 100 mg/day zinc supplementation doubled the rate of 10% BMI increase compared to the placebo group. However, in underweight women a 10% BMI increase is of very limited significance, and no further information exists about a beneficial effect beyond this early weight gain.

Since AN patients often show increased central and peripheral cortisol levels, a dysregulation of the hypothalamus–pituitary axis during the ill state has been suggested. A recent pilot study [59] attempted to counteract endogenous glucocorticoid hyperactivity in AN by administration of dexamethasone to five AN women and 10 healthy control women. The AN subjects showed some reduced depressive feelings but increased feelings of anxiety while on dexamethasone.

An important complication of AN is osteoporosis. Due to the reduced nutritional intake and impaired hormonal activity in AN, bone formation is significantly reduced but bone resorption is increased [60], leading to increased fracture risk [61]. Reduced bone density does not fully return to normal even after long-term recovery from AN [62]. In contrast to postmenopausal osteoporosis, hormone replacement therapy does not seem to be beneficial in AN [63]. The most accepted treatment for osteoporosis in AN beside weight restoration (resulting in a natural resumption of menses and improvement of bone density) is calcium supplementation [63]. The osteotrophic compound insulinlike growth factor I [64] administered in a controlled design at a dose of 100 μg/kg, increased markers of bone formation and resorption compared to placebo or a lower dose of 30 μg/kg. Future studies have to assess if long-term administration of such substances can improve bone mass in AN.

H. Recommendations

All medication trials performed were limited by relatively small sample sizes. No medication yet studied in controlled double-blind designs seemed to be able to specifically target core AN symptoms such as food refusal, body image distortion, or food- and weight-related obsessions. Similarly, depression- or OCD-related symptoms can often not effectively be treated during the underweight state. Studies with newer atypical neuroleptics appear to be encouraging despite the small groups and open-label application. Double-blind designs and control groups are needed for those agents in order to determine effects that are attributable to the medication. The supplementation of zinc and calcium during the underweight state might be an approach to complement other forms of treatment in an attempt, for example, to prevent associated conditions such as osteoporosis. Most promising at this point, appears to be the administration of fluoxetine—after weight restoration and at relatively normal food intake—for the reduction of relapse. Lastly, it might be necessary to study AN patients in pharmacological trials separated by their subtype and maybe even in relation to their comorbid conditions, since that may significantly determine the results.

III. BULIMIA NERVOSA

BN is characterized by recurrent episodes of binge eating followed by behaviors to counteract weight gain—so-called purging behaviors—such as self-induced vomiting, or the use of diuretics or laxatives (purging-type BN). Excessive exercising and fasting occur frequently in BN and can be the only measures for prevention of weight gain (nonpurging-type BN). Patients with BN, usually at normal weight or slightly overweight, present with a fear of gaining weight, body image distortions, and food- and body weight–related preoccupations similar to AN. During the ill state and after recovery, BN is usually associated with increased depressive and anxious feelings [8]. Impulsive behaviors as well as cluster B personality disorders are frequent [4]. During the ill state several neurotransmitters are altered and binge-purge frequency has been shown to directly reduce 5HIAA as well as HVA in CSF [65]. After long-term recovery, and to a higher degree than in AN, CSF 5HIAA has been found to be *increased* in BN.

No specific pharmacologic treatment has been established for BN. However, several compounds have been studied, targeting core behaviors such as bingeing and purging, and also depressive and anxious feelings. A major question was whether BN-specific pathology is related to mood alterations and major depressive disorder (MDD).

A. Antidepressant Agents

As with AN, the compounds most investigated are antidepressant agents. This choice may have been driven by the frequency of depressive symptoms in BN. Among the first drugs studied were the monoamine oxidase inhibitors (MAOs). Walsh et al. reported on groups of 20 [66], 30 [67], and 50 [68] BN women in placebo-controlled double blind-study designs using the irreversible MAO phenelzine. The medication was administered at 60 mg/day, or alternatively at 90 mg/day to patients who had previously not responded to the lower dose. Phenelzine was significantly more effective than placebo in reducing binge episodes. Those effects were not limited to subjects with comorbid depressive disorders. However, significant side effects occurred in 50% of study subjects, including sedation or severe blood pressure disturbances such as hypotension. Another MAO, isocarboxazid, was studied by Kennedy et al. [69] in a double-blind placebo-controlled crossover design in 18 BN women, at a dose that was gradually uptitrated from 10 mg/day to 60 mg/day. Similar to Walsh's studies, this MAO significantly reduced binge and purge frequency, independent of depressive symptoms.

In another double-blind, placebo-controlled study Kennedy et al. [70] investigated brofaromine, a selective reversible, and thus safer-to-use, MAO. Brofaromine administered over a period of 8 weeks at a dose of up 200 mg/day (n = 19) compared to placebo (n = 17) led to a body weight reduction in the active drug group. However, no differences in binge or purge frequency, or depression or anxiety ratings could be observed between groups. The reversible MAO moclobemide, studied in 52 BN women [71] in a double-blind placebo-controlled design at a dose of 600 mg/day, did not show to be superior to placebo in the reduction of BN pathology.

Among the first placebo-controlled double-blind studies in BN was the tetracyclic antidepressant mianserin [72] studied in an inpatient setting. Twenty-eight subjects dropped out of the study; 14 subjects on active drug (titrated to 60 mg/day) and 30 subjects on placebo completed the full study over a period of 8 weeks. Both groups improved significantly on core BN symptoms as well as anxiety and depression. Mianserin was not superior to placebo. Although the authors do not report on psychological treatments, it can only be speculated about the treatment effect of the hospitalization alone.

The TCA imipramine has been studied in a few placebo-controlled, double-blind studies. In a study with 22 BN women Pope et al. [74] reported that imipramine up to 200 mg/day was associated with a reduction of binge eating. Agras et al. [74] found imipramine over 16 weeks and with a maximum of 300 mg/day in 10 patients to be superior compared to placebo in 12 controls in reducing binge eating and purging behavior. A larger study by Mitchell et al. [75] studied 172 patients with or without intensive group psychotherapy, with imipramine (titrated to 200 mg/day) vs. placebo over a period of 12 weeks. All treatment groups were superior to placebo alone with respect to core ED behavior. Psychotherapy alone was superior to imipramine alone, but the combination of group therapy and imipramine resulted in greater improvement in symptoms of depression and anxiety.

Several research studies used desipramine in BN. In a double-blind, placebo-controlled study with desipramine treatment in a dose of 200 mg/day Hughes et al. [76] reported a 87% reduction of binge frequency; 68% of patients were totally abstinent from binge eating and purging at the end of the study, and there was a greater reduction of depressive symptoms in the desipramine group. Another study in 47 BN patients using a double-blind crossover design for 6 weeks [77] showed a significant reduction of binge/purge episodes in response to 150 mg/day desipramine. Scores on the Eating Disorders Inventory (EDI) or Symptom Checklist (SCL-90), however, did not change, nor was the improvement of bingeing or purging related to a reduction of depressive symptoms.

Blouin and colleagues [78] compared the effect of 150 mg/day desipramine or 60 mg/day fenfluramine (a central 5HT-releasing drug) with placebo in a double-blind design, and found both drugs beneficial in reducing binge eating and purging frequency. Interestingly, both drugs reduced the urge to binge as well as depressive feelings. Another study by Blouin et al. [79] in 24 BN women assessing the effect of 150 mg/day desipramine in relation to depressive symptoms in a double-blind, controlled, crossover design, found that desipramine was significantly superior to placebo, and more importantly the antibulimic effect was independent of its antidepressive action. Furthermore, a placebo-controlled double-blind study in 33 non-purging-type, in part obese, BN women (BMI 23–41) found a reduction of binge frequency [80] using 100–300 mg/day of desipramine (mean 188 mg/day) over a period of 12 weeks. A reduction in hunger ratings and increased dietary restraint in the active treatment group in that study led to the hypothesis that desipramine acts by suppressing appetite. No effect on depression was noted.

Walsh et al. [81] studied desipramine (200 mg/day) in 80 patients in a double-blind and placebo-controlled design. After an 8-week initiation phase, patients who had responded well to the active drug were then again randomly assigned to placebo or desipramine in order to assess longer-term effects of the medication. Desipramine was superior to placebo in reducing binge frequency. However, prolonged medication treatment was also associated with frequent relapse, suggesting that longer-term treatment with desipramine had significant limitations.

A comparison study of desipramine with cognitive behavioral therapy (CBT) [82] consisted of 71 BN patients randomly assigned to one of five groups, receiving either 15 sessions of CBT, desipramine alone over 16 or 24 weeks, or desipramine in addition to 15 sessions of CBT over 16 or 24 weeks. Desipramine was administered at doses of up to 350 mg/day, and the mean doses were 168 mg/day and 167 mg/day after 6 weeks and at the endpoint of the study respectively. After 16 weeks, both the CBT treatment group and the combined group (CBT plus 16 weeks of medication) were superior to medication alone. However, at week 32, only the combined treatment with desipramine over 24 weeks was superior to 16 week medication alone, and also reduced more effectively dietary preoccupation and hunger. A 1-year follow-up of that study [83] showed that the 16-week desipramine group did relatively poorly (18% in remission), and that the combined 24-week treatment regimen was the most beneficial, with 78% of that group being free of binge-purge episodes, and reduced emotional eating and dietary restraint.

Leitenberg et al. [84] conducted a small study in groups of seven subjects per condition (CBT, desipramine, and CBT plus desipramine) over a study period of 20 weeks and reassessed on follow-up after 6 months. Desipramine alone reduced binge and purge frequency but was inferior to CBT alone, and no benefit from the addition of desipramine to CBT over CBT alone was noted. However, the results were confounded by high dropout rates (60% in the desipramine and 30% in the CBT plus desipramine group) and very variable plasma levels of desipramine (170–447 ng/mL).

One study investigated amitryptiline in BN [85]. Thirty-two female outpatients were randomized in a double-blind design with 150 mg/day in the active treatment group. All subjects received a limited course of behavior therapy. Amitryptiline had a significant antidepressant effect, but was of no benefit over placebo regarding eating behavior.

Another TCA, trazodone, showed in an open-label design [86] a reduction in binge-purge frequency, as well as in scores on the Hamilton Depression Inventory (HAM-D) and EDI. Pope et al. [87] studied 42 women with BN in a double-blind placebo-controlled design over a 6-week treatment course with trazodone 400 mg/day, and reassessed [88] subjects 9–19 months after the initial 6-week period. Trazodone was superior to placebo in reducing the frequency of binge episodes and self-induced vomiting. On follow-up, 36% of subjects were in remission, 72% were considered improved, and most subjects were on trazodone or another antidepressant.

One double-blind and placebo-controlled study investigated the antidepressant bupropion in BN [89]. This medication has in general a low incidence of side effects and was shown to reduce hyperphagic episodes in depression in the past. Eighty-one subjects were enrolled, 55 of them on the active drug. Bupropion was superior to placebo in reducing binge-eating and purging episodes. However, four subjects (7%) in the bupropion group experienced grand mal seizures during the drug trial. The incidence of this side effect is much higher than in nonbulimic subjects, and might be attributable to electrolyte disturbances in BN due to bingeing and purging. Thus, the use of bupropion is contraindicated in both AN and BN.

The best-studied drug in the treatment of BN is the selective serotonin reuptake inhibitor (SSRI) fluoxetine. Early open-label data had suggested that fluoxetine could reduce binge and purge frequencies in BN [90]. The first double-blind placebo-controlled study [91] assessed 40 inpatients, randomized to 60 mg/day fluoxetine or placebo over 35 days. All subjects participated in an intensive CBT inpatient program. The addition of fluoxetine significantly reduced body weight; however, it was not superior to the psychotherapeutic inpatient program alone in reducing BN-related pathology. A large multicenter placebo-controlled study [92] in 387 BN women using fluoxetine either 20 or 60 mg/day over 8 weeks found that the drug significantly reduced episodes of binge eating and self-induced vomiting, as well as depressive symptoms and pathologic eating attitudes. Most interestingly, higher dosage was associated with more improvement. Side effects included mostly insomnia, nausea, asthenia, and tremor. A reassessment of those data [93] found that more of the subjects on the active drug showed an attitudinal change toward their eating behaviors, and this was independent of depression or anxiety.

A second large multicenter double-blind placebo-controlled study [94] using fluoxetine 60 mg/day over

16 weeks in 398 subjects found results similar to the previous study. Fluoxetine administration is save in BN and is associated with a significant reduction of binge-eating and vomiting episodes. A drawback, as in other studies, was the high attrition rate of > 40%. Those two multicenter studies were assessed post hoc on the dependence of symptom improvement on depressive symptoms at the time of the study [95]. This reassessment showed that the improvement of ED-related symptoms was independent of either depressive ratings at baseline or a history of a diagnosis of depression.

A recent study investigated medication benefits in BN in subjects that who had previously failed in psychotherapeutic treatment [96]. Twenty-two BN subjects, posttreatment failure or relapsed after psychotherapy, had been randomly and double-blindly assigned to fluoxetine or placebo. Most interestingly, binge eating and purging declined by > 80% in the active treatment group, whereas bingeing increased by 20% and purging by 150% in the placebo group. This suggests that fluoxetine may be a useful intervention in poor psychotherapy responders. However, the study was conducted over 8 weeks, and no long-term results exist. Another study [97] in 30 BN women using fluoxetine in a double-blind placebo-controlled design over 16 weeks also found a significantly reduced bingeing and purging frequency, together with a reduction of the cariogenic and thus tooth-eroding bacterium *Streptococcus sobrinus*. An additional aspect of disturbance in BN and its response to fluoxetine treatment was studied by Rissanen et al. [98], who found that BN women have increased cardiac vagal tone. Their study, a double-blind placebo-controlled design in 25 BN patients using fluoxetine 60 mg/day over 8 weeks, showed that drug treatment resulted in a normalization of cardiac vagal tone to the levels of healthy volunteer women. It was suggested that 5HT3 receptors may be involved in such disturbances in BN.

Another SSRI studied in BN is fluvoxamine. A few studies have reported reduced BN-related pathology in open-label study designs after fluvoxamine [Gardiner, 1993 #771; Ayuso-Gutierrez, 1994 #770]. The first double-blind, placebo-controlled study published assessed this drug for relapse prevention in 72 patients after intensive psychotherapeutic inpatient treatment [99]. Fluvoxamine was given over 15 weeks in a dose of 100–300 mg/day. In that study fluvoxamine was superior to placebo in its ability to reduce urges to binge, the actual number of binges, and scores on psychological rating scales such as the Structured Interview for Anorexia and Bulimia Nervosa (SIAB) or EDI. However, the study was limited by a high overall dropout rate (33%), that was particularly high in the fluvoxamine group (51%). Interestingly, fluvoxamine did not show a relapse-preventing effect in terms of depression or anxiety symptoms [100].

A recent study using the SSRI citalopram found, in an open label design in 12 BN patients, that the drug reduced bingeing in the treated group [32]. Another case report in 7 BN subjects [101] found that the noradrenegic antidepressant reboxetine (8 mg/day) administered over 12 weeks was beneficial in reducing bingeing by 73%, self-induced vomiting by 67%, and depressive symptoms by 50% in this group. However, three subjects (40%) dropped out prematurely, one after spontanoeus remission, and two after significant constipation and subsequent laxative use.

B. Mood Stabilizers

Mood instability and the frequent occurrence of impulsive behaviors warranted the trial of mood-stabilizing agents. An early report [102] on six BN women in a double-blind crossover design using carbamazepine (adjusted to plasma levels of 6–10 µg/mL) found a cessation of symptoms in one subject with a possible history of bipolar disorder. In another trial, in 91 BN patients [103], lithium administered in a double-blind randomized design over 8 weeks did not show the drug to be more effective than placebo for BN symptomatology.

C. Stimulants

Stimulants reduce appetite. Therefore it seemed reasonable to study such drugs for their effect on binge eating in BN. A small study using methylamphetamine supported this hypothesis [104]. This small double-blind controlled study found that the administration of methylamphetamine in eight patients with BN reduced hunger ratings as well as the amount of food eaten. BN is frequently associated with cluster B personality traits and disorder. Another case report [105], using methylphenidate in doses of 20 mg/day and 15 mg/day, in two subjects with BN and cluster B personality disorder, respectively, who had previously failed on SSRIs, found that methylphenidate treatment was effective in reducing bingeing and purging episodes.

D. Opioids

As mentioned earlier, endogenous opioids play an important role in appetitive behavior and food ingestion in humans [106]. Since endogenous opioids stimulate feeding behaviors, opiate blockade was hypothesized to reduce episodes of binge eating and associated purging behaviors. In an open-label study, Jonas and Gold [107] showed that naltrexone reduced bulimic episodes and that 200–300 mg/day was more effective than 50–100 mg/day. In a double-blind placebo-controlled crossover trial by Mitchell et al. [108] in 16 BN women, the opioid antagonist naltrexone 50 mg/day did not show a beneficial effect over placebo; however, this could have been due to the relatively low dose administered. In another study [109], naltrexone 100–150 mg/day reduced the duration of binge episodes in BN compared to placebo, but not the number of bulimic episodes. And naltrexone at 200 mg/day in a double-blind crossover design done by Marrazzi et al. [20] in 19 subjects showed a significant reduction of binge-and-purge episodes by the active drug over a 6-week period.

An investigational, more basic research-oriented study using intravenous naloxone, another opiate antagonist, found that this drug reduced consumption of both sweet and high-fat foods in binge-eating subjects [110], suggesting that the endogenous opioid system might be involved in the etiology of BN or, alternatively, that targeting the opioid system using medication might be beneficial in the reduction of BN symptoms. However, the higher risk-benefit ratio of those compounds compared to other effective medications makes those drugs not a first-line treatment of choice for BN at this point.

E. Other Agents

Increased central 5HT reduces food intake, and so fenfluramine, a 5HT-releasing agent, was investigated in several studies with the rationale that it would decrease binge-eating episodes. Robinson et al. [111] found in a double-blind, placebo-controlled study that fenfluramine 60 mg/day significantly reduced food intake, and that the amount of food eaten was inversely correlated with plasma fenfluramine levels. Another controlled trial studied fenfluramine in 42 subjects over a 12-week period [112]. In that study, fenfluramine did not prove to be beneficial. Fahy et al. [113] studying fenfluramine (45 mg/day) or placebo in addition to psychotherapy, found that the added drug treatment was not superior to psychotherapy alone. Fenfluramine was found to lead to pulmonary hypertension, cardiac abnormalities, and central nervous system damage and therefore was taken off the market [114].

Ondansetron is a 5HT3 receptor antagonist that is mainly used in the treatment of chemotherapy induced hyperemesis. Since in the past it was hypothesized that a vagal hyperactivity, possibly due to altered 5HT3 receptor activity, might contribute to the etiology of BN, ondansetron was studied in a double-blind placebo-controlled trial in 26 subjects after an initial placebo phase over 4 weeks [115]. A daily dose of 24 mg ondansetron was associated with a significantly reduced number of bingeing and purging episodes, and an increased number of normal meals.

Ipsapirone, a partial 5HT1A receptor agonist, was studied in an open label design over 4 weeks in 17 subjects [116]. The authors reported that after only 1 week of treatment with flexible doses between 7.5 and 12.5 mg/day ipsapirone, five subjects were free from bingeing and purging, and after 4 weeks 14 subjects showed 50% reduced bingeing and purging. The average binge frequency after 4 weeks was still 2.6 times per week; however, EDI scores decreased significantly, and subjects were on no other treatment regimen.

Myoinositol is involved in the second-messenger complex of brain 5HT receptors. It is possible that a modulation of this system could affect BN-related behaviors. Very recently, a report on inositol treatment in BN was published [117]. In this double-blind crossover study, 18 g/day inositol or placebo was administered over 6 weeks per condition to 24 nondepressed BN patients. Subjects on inositol scored significantly better on the EDI and on a visual analog scale of severity of binge eating. However, no information about the change of numbers of binge and purge episodes before and after inositol administration was presented.

F. Recommendations

Several antidepressant medications have been shown to be effective in the treatment of BN. Since SSRIs are of relatively low risk for side effects or intoxication toxicity compared to other medications such as tricyclic antidepressants, SSRIs are first-line drugs. Fluoxetine is the best-studied drug in BN. It has been shown that higher doses of fluoxetine (60 mg/day) are more effective and well tolerated. Fluoxetine is to date the only drug FDA approved for BN. It should be noted that not all BN patients respond to an antidepressant, so it is desirable to switch to another substance or drug class if one medication has not proved to be effective [118–120]. In addition, there is evidence that the combination of psychotherapy and antidepressant medication is superior to psychotherapy alone. It has to be noted that medication may cause significant side effects, resulting in cessation of drug treatment.

However, similar to studies in depression, tricyclics frequently lead to sedation, constipation, or dry mouth and may be lethal if consumed in overdose. SSRIs more frequently than placebo cause insomnia, nausea, and asthenia [121], but also sexual dysfunction [122]. At the beginning of pharmacologic interventions, patients should be carefully prepared for the possibility of occurrence and subsequent management of side effects. This may improve compliance. Long-term administration of medication is associated with significant dropout rates [123], and a reduction of efficacy over time may occur. Recently, Bacaltchuk and colleagues [124–126] reported on meta-analyses comparing drug treatment in BN with placebo or psychotherapeutic interventions. Consistent with single studies, antidepressant drug treatment was reported to be superior to placebo, with several drugs being effective. Psychotherapy is superior to drug treatment alone, but the difference between treatments may be small. Also, the efficacy of psychotherapy and medication combination treatment appears to be superior to single approaches. It has to be noted that the lengths of trials was between 5 and 24 weeks, and data on long-term results are very limited.

IV. BINGE-EATING DISORDER

BED has officially been recognized as a proposed diagnostic category for further research [4]. However, research criteria have been tentatively established, and several pharmacological studies have been conducted using those criteria. BED is characterized by (1) recurrent episodes of binge eating at least 2 days per week without compensatory behaviors; (2) a sense of lack of control over eating during eating binges; (3) at least three of the following symptoms during the binge episodes: eating much more rapidly than normal, eating until feeling uncomfortably full, eating large amounts of food when not feeling physically hungry, eating alone because of being embarrassed at how much one is eating, or feeling disgusted with oneself, depressed, or very guilty after overeating; (4) the condition is associated with marked distress; (5) it lasts at least 6 months; and (6) it does not occur exclusively during the course of AN or BN. A relatively small number of drug trials have been performed in BED, and these studies are thus described together.

With the notion that BED might respond to 5HT-specific drugs because food intake is related to brain serotonin activity [127], SSRIs were studied for reducing binge eating episodes and reducing weight gain in BED. Fluoxetine was among the first studied [128]. In that double-blind, placebo-controlled study, fluoxetine at 60 mg/day was associated with weight loss compared to placebo in both obese binge-eaters and non-binge-eaters. No effect of fluoxetine on EDI or depression scores could be observed. Greeno et al. [129] studied fluoxetine in a double-blind, placebo-controlled short-term design over 6 days and found that the drug treatment reduced eating in obese BED subjects as well as in non-BED subjects.

The 5HT-releasing and appetite suppressant drug fenfluramine (15–30 mg/day) administered over an 8-week period (Stunkard et al. 1996) in a double-blind placebo-controlled design in 28 BED patients reduced binge-eating episodes, but at 4 months follow-up post-fenfluramine, the medicated group was similar to the placebo group and thus similar to pretreatment severity, suggesting a very high relapse rate after discontinuation of the drug.

An open trial [130] studied fluoxetine (up to 60 mg/day) in combination with the appetite suppressant *phentermine* (up to 30 mg/day) over 20 weeks in addition to CBT treatment in 16 obese BED patients. Those subjects received monthly therapy sessions after this more intense treatment phase, and were followed up over 3 years. The dual-medication treatment was associated with reduction of binge eating. Between 3 and 23 months after medication discontinuation, patients' weight had returned to baseline, and a few subjects were binge-free whereas a few had more binge-eating episodes compared to pretreatment status.

The SSRI fluvoxamine (50–300 mg/day) was studied in a multicenter double-blind placebo-controlled investigation in 85 patients [131]. Fluvoxamine reduced binge-eating episodes, clinical global impression scores, and BMI. Interestingly, HAM-D scores were not affected by the active drug compared to placebo. However, significantly more subjects dropped out of the fluvoxamine group because of side effects. Another SSRI, sertraline, administered up to 200 mg/day in 34 patients in a double-blind placebo-controlled design over 6 weeks [132], reduced binge-eating frequency as well as BMI and global severity scores.

Marrazzi et al. [133] reported on the opioid antagonist naltrexone in one BED patient in a similar design as previously reported in BN [20]. He suggested that the addition of the drug to psychotherapy might improve the outcome over psychotherapy alone. Neumeister et al. [1999] recently reported on a case where, after failure of fluoxetine and psychotherapy alone, naltrexone 100 mg/day was added to this treatment regimen. The patient improved from at least one binge per day to two binges per month within 2 weeks, lost weight, and was stable until a reduction of naltrexone to 50 mg/day after 1 year of treatment. The patient then showed increased binge frequency, but was free of binges after returning to a naltrexone dose of 100 mg/day. No significant side effects were described in this report.

Another class of medication was tested with the antiepileptic topiramate that had been shown to be associated with reduced appetite and weight loss in the past. A case series in 13 subjects reported reduced binge eating and a positive relationship of topiramate plasma levels with the amount of weight lost in the studied subjects [134].

Sibutramine has been shown to be useful for weight loss and weight maintenance in the treatment of obesity [135]. A multicenter trial in BED subjects has been carried out recently, and data are currently under review.

Only very limited data exist on drug treatment in BED. The use of SSRIs seems to be a valid approach; however, relapse after medication discontinuation may have to be expected. The use of opiate receptor blockers appears to be a promising treatment possibility, but larger and controlled double-blind studies are needed to assess risks and benefits of such medications in BED. Sibutramine has been recognized in the treatment for obesity. However, results from the recent multicenter trial has to be reviewed before recommendation for the use in BED can be given.

V. CLOSING REMARKS

The etiology of EDs is unknown, and no medication studied in AN, BN, or BED seems to specifically target the etiologic factor that leads to their development. Central neurotransmitter systems show a close interaction with each other [136], and it is possible that the nonspecific administration of antidepressant medication in BN may lead to a normalization of the disrupted equilibrium between neurotransmitter systems, and reduce symptoms. This may be supported by the fact that several medications used in BN are effective at the beginning of therapy, but lose efficacy over time when the primary disturbance possibly regains its disturbing influence.

Substances such as opiate antagonists may reduce symptomatology, but it is not yet clear if this effect is simply a symptomatic treatment, or if a disturbance of those systems are involved in the etiology of EDs. Thus, future research studies, such as the use of brain-imaging techniques, need to target specific factors involved in the ill state, but even more important factors that could contribute to the etiology of EDs. In fact, 5HT1A and 5HT2A receptor alterations have been found after long-term recovery from AN and BN [137,138]. Such findings might open targets for future drug treatments. In addition, studies of other systems such a neuropeptides [139] or neuroactive steroids offer [140] promising areas for future research and possibly pharmacologic interventions. However, the absolute number of ED patients is relatively small, and to make trials comparable, uniform guidelines for pharmacologic trials in EDs should be developed [141]. This will also mean that since ED subtypes may have pathophysiologic traits that are distinct from each other, pharmacologic trials may have to be carried out in pure subgroups to be able to draw more meaningful conclusions.

REFERENCES

1. PF Sullivan. Mortality in anorexia nervosa. Am J Psychiatry 152(7):1073–1074, 1995.
2. DB Herzog, KM Nussbaum, AK Marmor. Comorbidity and outcome in eating disorders. Psychiat Clin North Am 19(4):843–859, 1996.
3. JF Kinzl, C Traweger, E Trefalt, B Mangweth, W Biebl. Binge eating disorder in females: a population-based investigation. International J Eating Disord 25(3):287–292, 1999.
4. American Psychiatric Association. Diagnostic and Statistical Manual of Mental Disorders IV. Washington: Author, 1994.
5. DM Garner. Pathogenesis of anorexia nervosa. Lancet 341(8861):1631–1635, 1993.
6. LR Lilenfeld, WH Kaye, CG Greeno, KR Merikangas, K Plotnicov, C Pollice, R Rao, M Strober, CM Bulik, L Nagy. A controlled family study of anorexia nervosa and bulimia nervosa: psychiatric disorders in first-degree relatives and effects of proband comorbidity. Arch Gen Psychiatry 55(7):603–610, 1998.
7. M Strober, R Freeman, C Lampert, J Diamond, W Kaye. Controlled family study of anorexia nervosa and bulimia nervosa: evidence of shared liability and

transmission of partial syndromes. Am J Psychiatry 157(3):393–401, 2000.
8. W Kaye, K Gendall, M Strober. Serotonin neuronal function and selective serotonin reuptake inhibitor treatment in anorexia and bulimia nervosa. Biol Psychiatry 44(9):825–838, 1998.
9. WH Kaye, GK Frank, C McConaha. Altered dopamine activity after recovery from restricting-type anorexia nervosa. Neuropsychopharmacology 21(4): 503–506, 1999.
10. NT Godart, MF Flament, Y Lecrubier, P Jeammet. Anxiety disorders in anorexia nervosa and bulimia nervosa: co-morbidity and chronology of appearance. Eur Psychiatry J Assoc Eur Psychiatrists 15(1):38–45, 2000.
11. SC Goldberg, KA Halmi, ED Eckert, RC Casper, JM Davis. Cyproheptadine in anorexia nervosa. Br J Psychiatry 134:67–70, 1979.
12. KA Halmi, E Eckert, TJ LaDu, J Cohen. Anorexia nervosa. Treatment efficacy of cyproheptadine and amitriptyline. Arch Gen Psychiatry 43(2):177–181, 1986.
13. SP Kalra, MG Dube, S Pu, B Xu, TL Horvath, PS Kalra. Interacting appetite-regulating pathways in the hypothalamic regulation of body weight. Endocrinol Rev 20(1):68–100, 1999.
14. W Schultz. Predictive reward signal of dopamine neurons. J Neurophysiol 80(1):1–27, 1998.
15. VC Barry, HL Klawans. On the role of dopamine in the pathophysiology of anorexia nervosa. J Neural Transm 38(2):107–122, 1976.
16. W Vandereycken, R Pierloot. Pimozide combined with behavior therapy in the short-term treatment of anorexia nervosa. A double-blind placebo-controlled crossover study. Acta Psychiatr Scand 66(6):445–450, 1982.
17. W Vandereycken. Neuroleptics in the short-term treatment of anorexia nervosa. A double-blind placebo-controlled study with sulpiride. Br J Psychiatry 144:288–292, 1984.
18. MA Marrazzi, J Mullings-Britton, L Stack, RJ Powers, J Lawhorn, V Graham, T Eccles, S Gunter. Atypical endogenous opioid systems in mice in relation to an auto-addiction opioid model of anorexia nervosa. Life Sci 47(16):1427–1435, 1990.
19. R Moore, IH Mills, A Forster. Naloxone in the treatment of anorexia nervosa: effect on weight gain and lipolysis. J R Soc Med 74(2):129–131, 1981.
20. MA Marrazzi, JP Bacon, J Kinzie, ED Luby. Naltrexone use in the treatment of anorexia nervosa and bulimia nervosa. Int Clin Psychopharmacol 10(3):163–172, 1995.
21. M de Zwaan, JE Mitchell. Opiate antagonists and eating behavior in humans: a review. J Clin Pharmacol 32(12):1060–1072, 1992.
22. V Di Marzo, SK Goparaju, L Wang, J Liu, S Baktkai, Z Jarai, F Fezza, GI Miura, RD Palmiter, T Sugiura, G Kunos. Leptin-regulated endocannabinoids are involved in maintaining food intake. Nature 410(6830):822–825, 2001.
23. H Gross, MH Ebert, VB Faden, SC Goldberg, WH Kaye, ED Caine, R Hawks, N Zinberg. A double-blind trial of delta 9-tetrahydrocannabinol in primary anorexia nervosa. J Clin Psychopharmacol 3(3):165–171, 1983.
24. R Mechoulam, E Fride. A hunger for cannabinoids. Nature 410:763–765, 2001.
25. W Vandereycken. Are anorexia nervosa and bulimia variants of affective disorders? Acta Psychiatr Belg 87(3):267–280, 1987.
26. JH Lacey, AH Crisp. Hunger, food intake and weight: the impact of clomipramine on a refeeding anorexia nervosa population. Postgrad Med J 56(suppl 1):79–85, 1980.
27. AH Crisp, JH Lacey, M Crutchfield. Clomipramine and "drive" in people with anorexia nervosa: an inpatient study. Br J Psychiatry 150:355–358, 1987.
28. J Biederman, DB Herzog, TM Rivinus, GP Harper, RA Ferber, JF Rosenbaum, JS Harmatz, R Tondorf, PJ Orsulak, JJ Schildkraut. Amitriptyline in the treatment of anorexia nervosa: a double-blind, placebo-controlled study. J Clin Psychopharmacol 5(1):10–16, 1985.
29. HE Gwirtsman, BH Guze, J Yager, B Gainsley. Fluoxetine treatment of anorexia nervosa: an open clinical trial. J Clin Psychiatry 51(9):378–382, 1990.
30. E Attia, C Haiman, BT Walsh, SR Flater. Does fluoxetine augment the inpatient treatment of anorexia nervosa? Am J Psychiatry 155(4):548–551, 1998.
31. M Strober, C Pataki, R Freeman, M DeAntonio. No effect of adjunctive fluoxetine on eating behavior or weight phobia during the inpatient treatment of anorexia nervosa: an historical case-control study. J Child Adolesc Psychopharmacol 9(3):195–201, 1999.
32. C Calandra, V Gulino, L Inserra, A Giuffrida. The use of citalopram in an integrated approach to the treatment of eating disorders: an open study. Eat Weight Disord 4(4):207–210, 1999.
33. C Bergh, M Eriksson, G Lindberg, P Sodersten. Selective serotonin reuptake inhibitors in anorexia [letter; comment]. Lancet 348(9039):1459–1460, 1996.
34. WH Kaye, HE Gwirtsman, DT George, DC Jimerson, MH Ebert. CSF 5-HIAA concentrations in anorexia nervosa: reduced values in underweight subjects normalize after weight gain. Biol Psychiatry 23(1): 102–105, 1988.
35. JD Fernstrom, RJ Wurtman. Brain serotonin content: increase following ingestion of carbohydrate diet. Science 174(13):1023–1025, 1971.
36. JD Fernstrom, RJ Wurtman. Brain serotonin content: physiological regulation by plasma neutral amino acids. Science 178(59):414–416, 1972.
37. S Haider, DJ Haleem. Decreases of brain serotonin following a food restriction schedule of 4 weeks in

male and female rats. Med Sci Monit 6(6):1061–1067, 2000.
38. WH Kaye, HE Gwirtsman, DT George, MH Ebert. Altered serotonin activity in anorexia nervosa after long-term weight restoration. Does elevated cerebrospinal fluid 5-hydroxyindoleacetic acid level correlate with rigid and obsessive behavior? Arch Gen Psychiatry 48(6):556–562, 1991.
39. WH Kaye, TE Weltzin, LK Hsu, CM Bulik. An open trial of fluoxetine in patients with anorexia nervosa. J Clin Psychiatry 52(11):464–471, 1991.
40. M Strober, R Freeman, M DeAntonio, C Lampert, J Diamond. Does adjunctive fluoxetine influence the post-hospital course of restrictor-type anorexia nervosa? A 24-month prospective, longitudinal follow-up and comparison with historical controls. Psychopharmacol Bull 33(3):425–431, 1997.
41. WH Kaye, T Nagata, TE Weltzin, LK Hsu, MS Sokol, C McConaha, KH Plotnicov, J Weise, D Deep. Double-blind placebo-controlled administration of fluoxetine in restricting- and restricting-purging-type anorexia nervosa. Biol Psychiatry 49(7):644–652, 2001.
42. GK Frank, WH Kaye, MD Marcus. Sertraline in underweight binge eating/purging-type eating disorders: five case reports. Int J Eat Disord 29(4):495–498, 2001.
43. A Deep-Soboslay, LM Sebastiani, WH Kaye. Weight gain with anorexia nervosa. Am J Psychiatry 157(9):1526, 2000.
44. DN Thomas, DJ Nutt, RB Holman. Sertraline, a selective serotonin reuptake inhibitor modulates extracellular noradrenaline in the rat frontal cortex. J Psychopharmacol 12(4):366–370, 1998.
45. CB Eap, P Baumann. Analytical methods for the quantitative determination of selective serotonin reuptake inhibitors for therapeutic drug monitoring purposes in patients. J Chromatogr B Biomed Appl 686(1):51–63, 1996.
46. CL DeVane. Differential pharmacology of newer antidepressants. J Clin Psychiatry 59(suppl 20):85–93, 1998.
47. HA Gross, MH Ebert, VB Faden, SC Goldberg, LE Nee, WH Kaye. A double-blind controlled trial of lithium carbonate primary anorexia nervosa. J Clin Psychopharmacol 1(6):376–381, 1981.
48. T Wetterling, HE Mussigbrodt. Weight gain: side effect of atypical neuroleptics? J Clin Psychopharmacol 19(4):316–321, 1999.
49. T Baptista. Body weight gain induced by antipsychotic drugs: mechanisms and management. Acta Psychiatr Scand 100(1):3–16, 1999.
50. L Hansen. Olanzapine in the treatment of anorexia nervosa. Br J Psychiatry 175:592, 1999.
51. MC La Via, N Gray, WH Kaye. Case reports of olanzapine treatment of anorexia nervosa. Int J Eat Disord 27(3):363–366, 2000.
52. VS Jensen, A Mejlhede. Anorexia nervosa: treatment with olanzapine. Br J Psychiatry 177:87, 2000.
53. A Malina, J Gaskill, C McConaha, GK Frank, M LaVia, L Scholar, WH Kaye. Olanzapine and anorexia nervosa: retrospective analyses of response to treatment. Int J Eat Disord (submitted).
54. G Stacher, TA Abatzi-Wenzel, S Wiesnagrotzki, H Bergmann, C Schneider, G Gaupmann. Gastric emptying, body weight and symptoms in primary anorexia nervosa. Long-term effects of cisapride. Br J Psychiatry 162:398–402, 1993.
55. GI Szmukler, GP Young, G Miller, M Lichtenstein, DS Binns. A controlled trial of cisapride in anorexia nervosa. Int J Eat Disord 17(4):347–357, 1995.
56. B Lask, A Fosson, U Rolfe, S Thomas. Zinc deficiency and childhood-onset anorexia nervosa. J Clin Psychiatry 54(2):63–66, 1993.
57. RL Katz, CL Keen, IF Litt, LS Hurley, KM Kellams-Harrison, LJ Glader. Zinc deficiency in anorexia nervosa. J Adolesc Health Care 8(5):400–406, 1987.
58. CL Birmingham, EM Goldner, R Bakan. Controlled trial of zinc supplementation in anorexia nervosa. Int J Eat Disord 15(3):251–255, 1994.
59. CM Gordon, SJ Emans, RH D uRant, C Mantzoros, E Grace, GP Harper, JA Majzoub. Endocrinologic and psychological effects of short-term dexamethasone in anorexia nervosa. Eat Weight Disord 5(3):175–182, 2000.
60. PS Powers. Osteoporosis and eating disorders. J Pediat Adolesc Gynecol 12(2):51–57, 1999.
61. AR Lucas, LJ Melton, CS Crowson, WM O'Fallon. Long-term fracture risk among women with anorexia nervosa: a population-based cohort study. Mayo Clini Proc 74(10):972–977, 1999.
62. D Hartman, A Crisp, B Rooney, C Rackow, R Atkinson, S Patel. Bone density of women who have recovered from anorexia nervosa. Int J Eat Disord 28(1):107–112, 2000.
63. S Grinspoon, D Herzog, A Klibanski. Mechanisms and treatment options for bone loss in anorexia nervosa. Psychopharmacol Bull 33(3):399–404, 1997.
64. S Grinspoon, H Baum, K Lee, E Anderson, D Herzog, A Klibanski. Effects of short-term recombinant human insulin-like growth factor I administration on bone turnover in osteopenic women with anorexia nervosa. J Clin Endocrinol Metab 81(11):3864–3870, 1996.
65. DC Jimerson, MD Lesem, WH Kaye, TD Brewerton. Low serotonin and dopamine metabolite concentrations in cerebrospinal fluid from bulimic patients with frequent binge episodes. Arch Gen Psychiatry 49(2):132–138, 1992.
66. BT Walsh, JW Stewart, SP Roose, M Gladis, AH Glassman. Treatment of bulimia with phenelzine. A double-blind, placebo-controlled study. Arch Gen Psychiatry 41(11):1105–1109, 1984.

67. BT Walsh, JW Stewart, SP Roose, M Gladis, AH Glassman. A double-blind trial of phenelzine in bulimia. J Psychiat Res 19(2-3):485–489, 1985.
68. BT Walsh, M Gladis, SP Roose, JW Stewart, F Stetner, AH Glassman. Phenelzine vs placebo in 50 patients with bulimia. Arch Gen Psychiatry 45(5):471–475, 1988.
69. SH Kennedy, N Piran, JJ Warsh, P Prendergast, E Mainprize, C Whynot, PE Garfinkel. A trial of isocarboxazid in the treatment of bulimia nervosa. J Clin Psychopharmacol 8(6):391–396, 1988.
70. SH Kennedy, D S Goldbloom, E Ralevski, C Davis, JD D'Souza, J Lofchy. Is there a role for selective monoamine oxidase inhibitor therapy in bulimia nervosa? A placebo-controlled trial of brofaromine. J Clin Psychopharmacol 13(6):415–422, 1993.
71. MO Carruba, M Cuzzolaro, L Riva, O Bosello, S Liberti, R Castra, R Dalle Grave, P Santonastaso, V Garosi, E Nisoli. Efficacy and tolerability of moclobemide in bulimia nervosa: a placebo-controlled trial. Int Clin Psychopharmacol 16(1):27–32, 2001.
72. EJ Sabine, A Yonace, AJ Farrington, KH Barratt, A Wakeling. Bulimia nervosa: a placebo-controlled double-blind therapeutic trial of mianserin. Br J Clin Pharmacol 15(suppl 2):195S–202S, 1983.
73. HG Pope Jr, JI Hudson, JM Jonas, D Yurgelun-Todd. Bulimia treated with imipramine: a placebo-controlled, double-blind study. Am J Psychiatry 140(5):554–558, 1983.
74. WS Agras, B Dorian, K B.G. Imipramine in the treatment of bulimia: a double-blind controlled study. Int J Eat Disord 6:29–38, 1987.
75. JE Mitchell, RL Pyle, ED Eckert, D Hatsukami, C Pomeroy, R Zimmerman. A comparison study of antidepressants and structured intensive group psychotherapy in the treatment of bulimia nervosa. Arch Gen Psychiatry 47(2):149–157, 1990.
76. PL Hughes, LA Wells, CJ Cunningham, D M Ilstrup. Treating bulimia with desipramine. A double-blind, placebo-controlled study. Arch Gen Psychiatry 43(2):182–186, 1986.
77. J Barlow, J Blouin, A Blouin, E Perez. Treatment of bulimia with desipramine: a double-blind crossover study. Can J Psychiatry 33(2):129–133, 1988.
78. AG Blouin, JH Blouin, EL Perez, T Bushnik, C Zuro, E Mulder. Treatment of bulimia with fenfluramine and desipramine. J Clin Psychopharmacol 8(4):261–269, 1988.
79. J Blouin, A Blouin, E Perez, J Barlow. Bulimia: independence of antibulimic and antidepressant properties of desipramine. Can J Psychiatry 34(1):24–29, 1989.
80. UD McCann, WS Agras. Successful treatment of nonpurging bulimia nervosa with desipramine: a double-blind, placebo-controlled study. Am J Psychiatry 147(11):1509–1513, 1990.
81. BT Walsh, CM Hadigan, MJ Devlin, M Gladis, SP Roose. Long-term outcome of antidepressant treatment for bulimia nervosa. Am J Psychiatry 148(9):1206–1212, 1991.
82. WS Agras, EM Rossiter, B Arnow, JA Schneider, CF Telch, SD Raeburn, B Bruce, M Perl, LM Koran. Pharmacologic and cognitive-behavioral treatment for bulimia nervosa: a controlled comparison [see comments]. Am J Psychiatry 149(1):82–87, 1992.
83. WS Agras, EM Rossiter, B Arnow, CF Telch, SD Raeburn, B Bruce, LM Koran. One-year follow-up of psychosocial and pharmacologic treatments for bulimia nervosa. J Clin Psychiatry 55(5):179–183, 1994.
84. H Leitenberg, JC Rosen, J Wolf, LS Vara, MJ Detzer, D Srebnik. Comparison of cognitive-behavior therapy and desipramine in the treatment of bulimia nervosa. Behav Res Ther 32(1):37–45, 1994.
85. JE Mitchell, R Groat. A placebo-controlled, double-blind trial of amitriptyline in bulimia. J Clin Psychopharmacol 4(4):186–193, 1984.
86. L Solyom, C Solyom, B Ledwidge. Trazodone treatment of bulimia nervosa. J Clin Psychopharmacol 9(4):287–290, 1989.
87. HG Pope J, PE Keck Jr, SL McElroy, JI Hudson. A placebo-controlled study of trazodone in bulimia nervosa. J Clin Psychopharmacol 9(4):254–259, 1989.
88. JI Hudson, HG Pope Jr, PE Keck Jr, SL McElroy. Treatment of bulimia nervosa with trazodone: short-term response and long-term follow-up. Clin Neuropharmacol 12(suppl 1):S38–S46; Discussion S47–S49, 1989.
89. RL Horne, JM Ferguson, HG Pope Jr, JI Hudson, CG Lineberry, J Ascher, A Cato. Treatment of bulimia with bupropion: a multicenter controlled trial. J Clin Psychiatry 49(7):262–266, 1988.
90. CP Freeman, M Hampson. Fluoxetine as a treatment for bulimia nervosa. Int J Obes 11(suppl 3):171–177, 1987.
91. MM Fichter, K Leibl, W Rief, E Brunner, S Schmidt-Auberger, RR Engel. Fluoxetine versus placebo: a double-blind study with bulimic inpatients undergoing intensive psychotherapy. Pharmacopsychiatry 24(1):1–7, 1991.
92. Fluoxetine Bulimia Nervosa Collaborative Study Group. Fluoxetine in the treatment of bulimia nervosa. A multicenter, placebo-controlled, double-blind trial. Arch Gen Psychiatry 49(2):139–147, 1992.
93. DS Goldbloom, MP Olmsted. Pharmacotherapy of bulimia nervosa with fluoxetine: assessment of clinically significant attitudinal change. Am J Psychiatry 150(5):770–774, 1993.
94. DJ Goldstein, MG Wilson, VL Thompson, JH Potvin, AH Rampey Jr. Long-term fluoxetine treatment of bulimia nervosa. Fluoxetine Bulimia Nervosa

Research Group. Br J Psychiatry 166(5):660–666, 1995.
95. DJ Goldstein, MG Wilson, RC Ascroft, M al-Banna. Effectiveness of fluoxetine therapy in bulimia nervosa regardless of comorbid depression. Int J Eat Disord 25(1):19–27, 1999.
96. BT Walsh, WS Agras, MJ Devlin, CG Fairburn, GT Wilson, C Kahn, MK Chally. Fluoxetine for bulimia nervosa following poor response to psychotherapy. Am J Psychiatry 157(8):1332–1334, 2000.
97. WA Bretz, DD Krahn, M Drury, N Schork, WJ Loesche. Effects of fluoxetine on the oral environment of bulimics. Oral Microbiol Immunol 8(1):62–64, 1993.
98. A Rissanen, H Naukkarinen, M Virkkunen, RR Rawlings, M Linnoila. Fluoxetine normalizes increased cardiac vagal tone in bulimia nervosa. J Clin Psychopharmacol 18(1):26–32, 1998.
99. MM Fichter, R Kruger, W Rief, R Holland, J Dohne. Fluvoxamine in prevention of relapse in bulimia nervosa: effects on eating-specific psychopathology. J Clin Psychopharmacol 16(1):9–18, 1996.
100. MM Fichter, C Leibl, R Kruger, W Rief. Effects of fluvoxamine on depression, anxiety, and other areas of general psychopathology in bulimia nervosa. Pharmacopsychiatry 30(3):85–92, 1997.
101. N El-Giamal, M de Zwaan, U Bailer, C Lennkh, P Schussler, A Strnad, S Kasper. Reboxetine in the treatment of bulimia nervosa: a report of seven cases. Int Clin Psychopharmacol 15(6):351–356, 2000.
102. AS Kaplan, PE Garfinkel, PL Darby, D M Garner. Carbamazepine in the treatment of bulimia. Am J Psychiatry 140(9):1225–1226, 1983.
103. LK Hsu, L Clement, R Santhouse, ES Ju. Treatment of bulimia nervosa with lithium carbonate. A controlled study. J Nerv Ment Dis 179(6):351–355, 1991.
104. YL Ong, SA Checkley, GF Russell. Suppression of bulimic symptoms with methylamphetamine. Br J Psychiatry 143:288–293, 1983.
105. MS Sokol, NS Gray, A Goldstein, WH Kaye. Methylphenidate treatment for bulimia nervosa associated with a cluster B personality disorder. Int J Eat Disord 25(2):233–237, 1999.
106. M de Zwaan, JE Mitchell. Opiate antagonists and eating behavior in humans: a review. J Clin Pharmacol 32(12):1060–1072, 1992.
107. JM Jonas, MS Gold. The use of opiate antagonists in treating bulimia: a study of low-dose versus high-dose naltrexone. Psychiatry Res 24(2):195–199, 1988.
108. JE Mitchell, G Christenson, J Jennings, M Huber, B Thomas, C Pomeroy, J Morley. A placebo-controlled, double-blind crossover study of naltrexone hydrochloride in outpatients with normal weight bulimia. J Clin Psychopharmacol 9(2):94–97, 1989.
109. SA Alger, MD Schwalberg, JM Bigaouette, AV Michalek, LJ Howard. Effect of a tricyclic antidepressant and opiate antagonist on binge-eating behavior in normoweight bulimic and obese, binge-eating subjects. Am J Clin Nutr 53(4):865–871, 1991.
110. A Drewnowski, DD Krahn, MA Demitrack, K Nairn, BA Gosnell. Naloxone, an opiate blocker, reduces the consumption of sweet high-fat foods in obese and lean female binge eaters. Am J Clin Nutr 61(6):1206–1212, 1995.
111. PH Robinson, SA Checkley, GF Russell. Suppression of eating by fenfluramine in patients with bulimia nervosa. Br J Psychiatry 146:169–176, 1985.
112. GF Russell, SA Checkley, J Feldman, I Eisler. A controlled trial of d-fenfluramine in bulimia nervosa. Clin Neuropharmacol 11(suppl 1):S146–S159, 1988.
113. TA Fahy, I Eisler, GF Russell. A placebo-controlled trial of d-fenfluramine in bulimia nervosa. [see comments]. Br J Psychiatry 162:597–603, 1993.
114. WS Poston, JP Foreyt. Scientific and legal issues in fenfluramine/dexfenfluramine litigation. [see comments]. Tex Med 96(2):48–56, 2000.
115. PL Faris, SW Kim, WH Meller, RL Goodale, SA Oakman, RD Hofbauer, AM Marshall, RS Daughters, D Banerjee-Stevens, ED Eckert, BK Hartman. Effect of decreasing afferent vagal activity with ondansetron on symptoms of bulimia nervosa: a randomised, double-blind trial [see comments]. Lancet 355(9206):792–797, 2000.
116. C Geretsegger, KV Greimel, IS Roed, JM Hesselink. Ipsapirone in the treatment of bulimia nervosa: an open pilot study. Int J Eat Disord 17(4):359–363, 1995.
117. D Gelber, J Levine, RH Belmaker. Effect of inositol on bulimia nervosa and binge eating. Int J Eat Disord 29(3):345–348, 2001.
118. JE Mitchell, RL Pyle, ED Eckert, D Hatsukami, C Pomeroy, R Zimmerman. Response to alternative antidepressants in imipramine nonresponders with bulimia nervosa. J Clin Psychopharmacol 9(4):291–293, 1989.
119. BT Walsh, GT Wilson, KL Loeb, MJ D evlin, KM Pike, SP Roose, J Fleiss, C Waternaux. Medication and psychotherapy in the treatment of bulimia nervosa. Am J Psychiatry 154(4):523–531, 1997.
120. WS Agras. Pharmacotherapy of bulimia nervosa and binge eating disorder: longer-term outcomes. Psychopharmacol Bull 33(3):433–436, 1997.
121. A Wood. Pharmacotherapy of bulimia nervosa— experience with fluoxetine. Int Clin Psychopharmacol 8(4):295–299, 1993.
122. AJ Rothschild. Sexual side effects of antidepressants. J Clin Psychiatry 61(suppl 11):28–36, 2000.
123. DS Goldbloom, M Olmsted, R Davis, J Clewes, M Heinmaa, W Rockert, B Shaw. A randomized controlled trial of fluoxetine and cognitive behavioral therapy for bulimia nervosa: short-term outcome. Behav Res Ther 35(9):803–811, 1997.
124. J Bacaltchuk, RP Trefiglio, IR de Oliveira, MS Lima, JJ Mari. Antidepressants versus psychotherapy for

125. J Bacaltchuk, P Hay, JJ Mari. Antidepressants versus placebo for the treatment of bulimia nervosa: a systematic review. Aust NZ J Psychiatry 34(2):310–317, 2000.
126. J Bacaltchuk, RP Trefiglio, IR Oliveira, P Hay, MS Lima, JJ Mari. Combination of antidepressants and psychological treatments for bulimia nervosa: a systematic review. Acta Psychiatr Scand 101(4):256–264, 2000.
127. MS Wallin, AM Rissanen. Food and mood: relationship between food, serotonin and affective disorders. Acta Psychiatr Scand Suppl 377:36–40, 1994.
128. MD Marcus, RR Wing, L Ewing, E Kern, M McDermott, W Gooding. A double-blind, placebo-controlled trial of fluoxetine plus behavior modification in the treatment of obese binge-eaters and non-binge-eaters. Am J Psychiatry 147(7):876–881, 1990.
129. CG Greeno, RR Wing. A double-blind, placebo-controlled trial of the effect of fluoxetine on dietary intake in overweight women with and without binge-eating disorder. Am J Clin Nutr 64(3):267–273, 1996.
130. MJ Devlin, JA Goldfein, JS Carino, SL Wolk. Open treatment of overweight binge eaters with phentermine and fluoxetine as an adjunct to cognitive-behavioral therapy. Int J Eat Disord 28(3):325–332, 2000.
131. JI Hudson, SL McElroy, NC Raymond, S Crow, PE Keck Jr, WP Carter, JE Mitchell, SM Strakowski, HG Pope Jr, BS Coleman, JM Jonas. Fluvoxamine in the treatment of binge-eating disorder: a multicenter placebo-controlled, double-blind trial. Am J Psychiatry 155(12):1756–1762, 1998.
132. SL McElroy, LS Casuto, EB Nelson, KA Lake, CA Soutullo, PE Keck Jr, JI Hudson. Placebo-controlled trial of sertraline in the treatment of binge eating disorder. Am J Psychiatry 157(6):1004–1006, 2000.
133. MA Marrazzi, KM Markham, J Kinzie, ED Luby. Binge eating disorder: response to naltrexone. Int J Obes Relat Metab Disord 19(2):143–145, 1995.
134. NA Shapira, TD Goldsmith, SL McElroy. Treatment of binge-eating disorder with topiramate: a clinical case series. J Clin Psychiatry 61(5):368–372, 2000.
135. WP James, A Astrup, N Finer, J Hilsted, P Kopelman, S Rossner, WH Saris, LF Van Gaal. Effect of sibutramine on weight maintenance after weight loss: a randomised trial. Sibutramine Trial of Obesity Reduction and Maintenance. Lancet 356(9248):2119–2125, 2000.
136. HH Berendsen. Interactions between 5-hydroxytryptamine receptor subtypes: is a disturbed receptor balance contributing to the symptomatology of depression in humans? Pharmacol Ther 66(1):17–37, 1995.
137. WH Kaye, GK Frank, CC Meltzer, JC Price, CW McConaha, PJ Crossan, KL Klump. Altered serotonin 2A receptor activity after recovery from bulimia nervosa. Am J Psychiatry 158(7):1152–1155, 2001.
138. GK Frank, WH Kaye, CC Meltzer, JC Price, CW McConaha, K Skovira. Presynaptic serotonin 1A receptor alterations in the brain after recovery from anorexia nervosa. Annual Eating Disorders Research Society Meeting, November 2000, Prien, Germany.
139. G Frank, W Kaye, A Sahu, J Fernstrom, C McConaha. Does reduced CSF galanin contribute to restricted eating in anorexia nervosa? (Submitted.)
140. P Monteleone, M Luisi, B Colurcio, E Casarosa, R Ioime, AR Genazzani, M Maj. Plasma levels of neuroactive steroids are increased in untreated women with anorexia nervosa or bulimia nervosa. Psychosom Med 63(1):62–68, 2001.
141. JE Mitchell, B Tareen, W Sheehan, S Agras, TD Brewerton, S Crow, M Devlin, E Eckert, K Halmi, D Herzog, M Marcus, P Powers, A Stunkard, BT Walsh. Establishing guidelines for pharmacotherapy trials in bulimia nervosa and anorexia nervosa. Int J Eat Disord 28(1):1–7, 2000.

# 55

Perspectives for New Pharmacological Treatments of Alcoholism and Substance Dependence

IHSAN M. SALLOUM, ANTOINE DOUAIHY, and SUBHAJIT CHAKRAVORTY
Western Psychiatric Institute and Clinic, University of Pittsburgh School of Medicine, Pittsburgh, Pennsylvania, U.S.A.

I. INTRODUCTION

Alcoholism and other addictive disorders are chronic relapsing illnesses that are similar to other chronic medical conditions in terms of genetic transmission, treatment response, and presenting clinical challenges such as treatment compliance and treatment adherence [1].

The Diagnostic and Statistical Manual of Mental Disorders fourth Edition (DSM-IV-TR) presents 13 categories of substance-related disorders for each of the 11 classes of drugs of abuse. These categories are arranged into two broad groups: a Substance Use Disorders group, which compromises substance abuse and substance dependence, and a Substance-Induced Disorders group, which includes intoxication, withdrawal, cognitive dysfunction (e.g., delirium, persisting dementia, and persisting amnestic disorders); psychotic, mood, and anxiety disorders; sexual dysfunction; and substance-induced sleep disorders [2]. Substance dependence is defined by the DSM-IV-TR as a cluster of cognitive, behavioral, and physiological symptoms indicating maladaptive pattern of substance use leading to significant impairment or distress [2].

Although disulfiram is one of the oldest medications to treat a behavioral disorder, the number of approved medications to treat addictive disorders is still very limited, and only three (nicotine addiction, alcoholism, and opiate addiction) of the 13 substances of abuse classified in DSM-IV-TR have indicated pharmacotherapy.

Pharmacotherapy for addictive disorders has recently received renewed fervor. The purpose of this chapter is to review recent advances in the psychopharmacology of nicotine dependence, alcoholism, and opioid and cocaine dependence.

II. PHARMACOTHERAPY OF NICOTINE DEPENDENCE

Tobacco use/nicotine dependence is a major public health problem in the United States. According to the latest Surgeon General's report dedicated to the health hazards of smoking published in 2000, tobacco smoking is responsible for a staggering direct medical cost of $50 billion a year. Tobacco use causes > 400,000 deaths each year, which is more than alcohol, drug abuse, AIDS, car crashes, murders, suicides, and fire-related deaths combined. Tobacco use remains the leading preventable cause of deaths in the United States [3].

Nicotine dependence is characterized by a chronic course with remissions and frequent relapses. Most people who quit smoking eventually relapse. It is estimated that only a little more than 2% successfully quit each year. Treatment increases the cessation rate dramatically from a low of 10% a year reported for limited interventions such as physician advice to a 25% cessation rate per year for combined pharmacological and behavioral counseling.

A salient feature of nicotine dependence, as noted by the DSM-IV-TR, is the continued use of nicotine products despite knowledge of medical problems related to smoking [2]. Nicotine is a highly rewarding substance. The rewarding effect of nicotine is believed to result from its action on dopaminergic and noradrenergic systems in the brain, particularly its action on the mesolimbic dopamine system. This system is believed to mediate the pleasure and reward circuits in the brain [4,5].

The action of nicotine or nicotinic cholinergic receptors in the brain enhances the release of a number of neurotransmitters [6], including dopamine, noradrenaline, acetylcholine, serotonin, vasopressin, β-endorphin, glutamate, and gamma-aminobutyric acid (GABA) [7]. Furthermore, nicotine exerts its effect on the locus ceruleus, which produces behavioral arousal [7].

Prolonged exposure to nicotine, however, produces a desensitization of nicotinic cholinergic receptors. This desensitization state may require the presence of nicotine to maintain normal functioning. Thus, smoking cessation may leave the individual in a state of subnormal neurotransmitter release, which produces the symptoms of withdrawal including inability to concentrate, irritability, restlessness, lethargy, and depression.

A. Pharmacotherapy of Nicotine Dependence

Although the focus of this section is on the pharmacotherapy of nicotine dependence, counseling strategies have been found to be helpful in smoking cessation. Particularly useful counseling strategies include those that focus on skill training and social support [8]. In spite of the availability of guidelines to smoking cessation, health care providers usually give advice to fewer than half the smokers they see. For example, a brief counseling session, even over the phone, may significantly enhance self-help interventions [8].

Several pharmacological approaches have been studied for the treatment of nicotine dependence and smoking cessation. These include nicotine replacement therapies using different methods of nicotine delivery and non-nicotine-based medications with diverse mechanisms of action to enhance smoking cessation [9,10].

Medications with established efficacy and safety and which have the U.S. Food and Drug Administration (FDA) approval for smoking cessation are considered first-line therapies. These include the various nicotine replacement therapies and the antidepressant bupropion. Second-line treatments are not FDA approved because of concerns regarding side effects. These medications, however, may be used as an alternative to first-line treatments [8].

1. Nicotine Replacement Therapy

Nicotine replacement therapy (NRT) has been until recently the main pharmacological approach to smoking cessation. The goal of NRT is to aid in initiating abstinence from cigarette smoking so that effective relapse prevention strategies may be developed. NRT reduces nicotine withdrawal symptoms, decreases craving, and dampens the reinforcing effects of cigarettes. These compounds lack the toxic substances associated with smoking such as tar, and they also have low abuse potential [11]. Further benefit of nicotine replacement may include positive effects on mood and attention states [12]. NRT suppresses hunger and weight gain associated with smoking cessation [13,14]. Nicotine replacement is now available in four different forms of delivery system: nicotine gum products, transdermal nicotine patches, nicotine nasal spray, and nicotine inhaler [15].

Nicotine gum is available in 2- and 4-mg doses and is available over the counter as a replacement product. Heavier smokers may benefit more from the higher dose of the gum. Nicotine patches, on the other hand, provide a constant infusion of nicotine in the bloodstream, while the nicotine as a spray delivers 0.5 mg of nicotine with each spray. The nicotine inhaler is available as a prescription medication. Smokers puff on the inhaler as they would a cigarette [8].

Nicotine replacement therapy in its various forms has been shown to enhance smoking cessation about twice as much as placebo [16,17]. However, it is estimated that 70–90% of smokers using nicotine replacement therapy fail to quit. Factors contributing to poor response to NRT include depression, weight gain, the use of other substances such as alcohol, stressful life events, and cognitive impairment [7]. Women smokers appear to be less responsive to NRT than men [18].

2. Non-Nicotine-Based Medications

A variety of non-nicotine-based medications have been tested for smoking cessation. These medications are based on different mechanisms of action to produce smoking cessation. These include medications that act on the neurotransmitter system to simulate the effects of nicotine, medications that block nicotine receptors, medications that influence the conditioned response associated with smoking, and medications that produce an aversive response to smoking. For example, medications that increase the brain levels of dopamine, noradrenaline, and serotonin may counteract the deficiency state produced by nicotine withdrawal. These drugs may also simulate the action of nicotine on the brain reward circuits. On the other hand, mecamylamine, a noncompetitive inhibitor of nicotine receptor [19,20], may block the reinforcing effects of nicotine. More recently, the use of vaccines to counteract the effects of nicotine has been proposed [9].

The use of sensory substitutes to target the significant conditioning to the smell, taste, and feel associated with cigarette smoking has also been tested. One sensory substitute, citric acid, has been shown to reduce withdrawal symptoms and cravings [21–23]. Also, dextrose has been proposed to reduce urges to smoking based on the theory that there is a mislabeling of a physiological desire for carbohydrates [24,25]. In one study, dextrose tablets produced significantly greater rates of abstinence than placebo whether taken alone or in combination with NRT [25].

Aversive therapy, on the other hand, aims at extinguishing the urge to smoking by pairing the pleasurable stimulus of smoking a cigarette with some unpleasant effect [26,27]. Rapid smoking and the use of silver acetate are examples of aversive therapy. The silver combination with tobacco produces a bad-tasting salt. These approaches, although they do not produce long-term benefit, are helpful when used in combination with NRT. Many non-nicotine-replacement medications have been tested alone and in combination with NRTs.

Clonidine

Clonidine is a α_2-adrenergic receptor agonist used as an antihypertensive medication. Clonidine inhibits the release of noradrenaline and the firing of the locus ceruleus. These effects produce sedation and decrease in anxiety [7,28]. This medication has been found to be useful in reducing alcohol and opiate withdrawal syndromes.

Clonidine reduces cravings and nicotine withdrawal symptoms such as anxiety, irritability, restlessness, and hunger in heavy cigarette smokers [28,29]. In a double-blind placebo-controlled study, the clonidine-treated group had more than double the success rates in smoking cessation than those treated with placebo [30]. A review of the literature and a meta-analysis of nine trials of clonidine showed that the clonidine-treated patients were more likely to quit smoking than those treated with placebo [31]. The skin patch delivery system was found to be more effective than the oral administration; also, clonidine was more effective in combination with behavioral therapy [31]. Patients with more severe nicotine dependence and high blood concentration of clonidine showed the most favorable response [7]. Female smokers appear to have a better response than male smokers to clonidine therapy [32].

Studies have also reported higher frequency of adverse effects, especially with increased levels of drowsiness, dry mouth, and fatigue. Furthermore, the abrupt discontinuation of clonidine may cause agitation, headache, tremors, nervousness, and rapid increase in blood pressure. These disadvantages limit the usefulness of clonidine for smoking cessation.

Antidepressants

Several studies have observed a strong link between depression, past history of depression, and smoking. Depressed mood predicts smoking relapse in many patients. Smokers are more likely to be depressed, and depressed patients are more likely to be dependent on nicotine and also have lower success rate at quitting [33,34]. Antidepressant medications are the most common non-nicotine-based medications used to treat nicotine dependence.

BUPROPION (AMFEBUTAMONE). The sustained-release bupropion, an antidepressant medication, is the first non-nicotine-based agent approved by the FDA (in 1997) for the treatment of nicotine dependence. The sustained-release formulation provides a slower absorption and allows for less frequent dose administration. It is hypothesized to aid in smoking cessation by blocking the reuptake of dopamine and noradrenaline and by decreasing the firing of the locus ceruleus [35,36]. Bupropion functions as a noncompetitive inhibitor of the nicotine receptor site producing a functioning blockade of the nicotine receptors [37]. Bupropion reduces the reinforcing effects of nicotine by its effects on the reward pathways through the dopaminergic system. It lessens nicotine withdrawal symptoms by its effects on the noradrenergic system.

A series of placebo-controlled studies have shown that bupropion is effective in smoking cessation as compared to placebo both in smokers who have depression and those without depression [38]. Studies have also demonstrated a dose response relationship. The 300-mg and 100-mg doses of the sustained-release formulation were found significantly more efficacious than placebo [39,40]. Sustained-release bupropion was also found superior to placebo on abstinence rate when tested with and without combination of NRT [38,40]. The effectiveness of the nicotine patch alone in those studies was no different from placebo.

Additional benefit of bupropion includes decrease in weight gain and improvement in the lethargy associated with nicotine withdrawal and smoking cessation [31,39]. Bupropion is well tolerated. Dry mouth and insomnia were the most commonly reported side effects, and there were no bupropion-induced seizures reported during those studies.

NORTRIPTYLINE. Nortriptyline is a tricyclic antidepressant. It blocks the reuptake of noradrenaline and serotonin and decreases the firing of the locus ceruleus. In addition it has anticholinergic activities that are sedating. However, nortriptyline does not block dopamine reuptake.

Two placebo-controlled studies have reported superiority of nortriptyline over placebo in smoking cessation with abstinence rates double that of placebo (24% vs. 12%) [41,42]. Additionally, nortriptyline improved depressive symptoms, although women with history of major depression had lower cessation rate than women without depression history. There were numerous side effects reported including dry mouth, tremors, blurred vision, and lightheadedness. Another disadvantage to nortriptyline is the serious risk of toxicity on overdose.

MOCLOBEMIDE. Moclobemide is a monoamine oxidase A (MAOA) inhibitor antidepressant that enhances dopamine activity [43]. A double-blind placebo-controlled study reported significant difference of moclobemide over placebo on self-report of smoking cessation. This difference, however, was not significant when the more objective serum cotinine concentration was examined [44,45].

Studies of other antidepressant agents have been conducted with some promising but mostly inconclusive evidence. Doxepin was reported to be superior to placebo in a small double-blind study [46]. Fluoxetine has been found ineffective in nondepressed smokers, although there is some suggestion that it may be helpful in smokers with symptoms of depression [7]. Similarly, buspirone does not appear to be helpful as a smoking cessation aid; however, one study suggested that buspirone may be helpful in reducing smoking in the initial phases of treatment of anxious individuals [47].

Mecamylamine

Mecamylamine is an antihypertensive medication that blocks the peripheral and central nervous system effects of nicotine. The nicotine antagonist properties of mecamylamine have been used to help with smoking cessation [48,49]. Studies have shown that mecamylamine was helpful in smoking cessation and also in reducing the withdrawal symptoms. Severe side effects were observed, however, such as constipation and urinary retention, resulting in high dropout rate [31]. Low doses of mecamylamine combined with nicotine patch, on the other hand, appear to be well tolerated and provide a significant advantage when compared to nicotine patch alone [50]. Mecamylamine combined with NRT blocks the reinforcing effect of nicotine, provides relief from withdrawal symptoms, and limits the increase in appetite associated with smoking cessation [50–52].

Opioid Antagonists

Mostly negative findings for smoking cessation were reported for the opioid antagonists naltrexone and naloxone. One study reported some benefit for female smokers with a history of major depression. High dropout rates were reported on naltrexone due to side effects which included drowsiness, disorientation, spaciness, problems with concentration, nausea, and abdominal pain [31].

In conclusion, there is substantial evidence to support the efficacy of bupropion in smoking cessation. Other medications may be effective in a limited subgroup of smokers. Combining medication with NRT may improve the outcome. Rates of relapse are quite high after the acute phase of treatment. The majority resume smoking within 6 months to 1 year after cessation of treatment. Subgroups of smokers, such as those with psychiatric comorbidity of depression and anxiety, may require a more targeted treatment strategy.

III. PHARMACOTHERAPY OF ALCOHOLISM

Alcohol use is highly prevalent, affecting 11–15% of adults throughout their lifetime [53,54], and is related to criminal activity, violence, accidental injuries, and both psychiatric and medical comorbidities. Research has enhanced our knowledge of the specific areas of the brain and the neurotransmitters associated with alcohol consumption, reinforcement, craving, and relapse. For examples, stress-induced craving has been associated with the serotonin-related mechanisms, while positive reinforcement and craving have been associated with the dopaminergic system [55].

Dopaminergic pathways projecting from the ventral tegmental area to the nucleus accumbens are associated with the pleasurable and stimulant effects of alcohol [57–59]. This pathway may be sensitized by continued, excessive alcohol ingestion, leading to development of dependence [57,60,61]. Thus, drugs targeting this dopaminergic system may reduce alcohol consumption [57].

Alterations in several neurotransmitter systems may be seen as part of an adaptive process to prolonged alcohol use, including downregulation of inhibitory neuronal γ-aminobutyric acid (GABA) receptors [57,64], upregulation of the excitatory glutamate receptors [56–68], and increased central norepinephrine (NE) activity [57,65]. Although there is no cure for alcohol dependence, both our understanding of this disorder and the drugs in our armamentarium have improved substantially.

The treatment of alcohol dependence may be conceptualized into three phases [66]:

1. Acute stabilization phase focuses on engaging the patient in treatment, inpatient or outpatient detoxification as deemed necessary, and treatment of any associated comorbid disorders. During this phase the patient is also enrolled in psychotherapy, which may include individual and/or group counseling

2. Continuation phase, which begins after the patient has achieved stability and is targeted at maintaining sobriety through continued use of medication and psychotherapy.

3. Maintenance phase aims at preventing relapse to alcohol, and it may also involve the use of psychotherapy and possibly medications.

Self-help programs and building a social support network are important objectives of treatment throughout these phases.

A. Medications Used to Treat Alcoholism

Medications used in the treatment of alcoholism and associated conditions have been classified as follow [53]:

1. Medications to reduce alcohol intake which include dopaminergic, serotonergic, and opioid antagonist agents.
2. Agents to induce aversion to alcohol.
3. Agents to treat acute alcohol withdrawal such as benzodiazepines and anticonvulsants.
4. Agents to treat protracted alcohol withdrawal.
5. Agents to decrease drinking by treating associated psychiatric pathology such as anxiolytics, antidepressants, and antipsychotics.
6. Agents to induce sobriety such as adenosine receptor antagonists.

1. Dopaminergic Agents

The two drugs that have been studied in this category are bromocriptine and tiapride. Studies involving bromocriptine, a dopaminergic agonist, have demonstrated varied results. Some studies have reported decreased craving, depression, and abstinence for > 6 months [53,67], while other studies reported no improvement in the incidence of relapse compared to placebo [53,68].

Tiapride, a D2 dopamine antagonist available in Europe since the 1970s, is an atypical neuroleptic and an anxiolytic drug. Tiapride reduces the symptoms of alcohol withdrawal [57,69], reduces the amount of alcohol consumed, increases the occurrence of abstinence, and decreases the reports of anxiety and depression [53,70,71]. This drug is approved in some European countries for the treatment of alcoholism.

Apomorphine has been used as an aversive agent and also to treat withdrawal, but no controlled trials are yet available [68,72].

In a case report, haloperidol has been suggested to decrease the alcohol-induced cravings among alcohol-dependent subjects [72,73]. Routine use of antipsychotic medications in the treatment of alcohol dependence, however, is not warranted other than to treat hallucinations associated with alcohol withdrawal, as these medications increase the risk of seizures and can produce severe hypotension. Despite these risks, patients currently taking antipsychotic medications for other indications should continue their use [53,74].

2. Opioid Antagonists

Animal studies have shown alcohol consumption to be increased by μ-opioid agonists and reduced by μ-opioid antagonists [53,75,76]. These findings led to clinical trials of naltrexone, and subsequently nalmefene, in the treatment of alcohol dependence.

Naltrexone hydrochloride, a pure, reversible opioid antagonist, is the first medication to have been approved by the FDA for alcohol dependence since the introduction of disulfiram over 50 years ago. This drug, as well as the other μ-opioid antagonists, blocks the release of dopamine secondary to alcohol use from the nucleus accumbens [53,78,79]. Naltrexone appears to decrease drinking, improve abstinence rates, reduce craving, and therefore reduce the risk for relapse [53,79–82]. Naltrexone use in social drinkers has been associated with increased sedation and unpleasant effects and decreased reward effects of alcohol [57,83]. Patients with alcoholism who continued to drink during treatment reportedly experienced less alcohol "high" and had decreased likelihood of progression to heavy drinking [57,82]. Naltrexone has been shown to reduce the craving for alcohol in alcohol-dependent patients as well as in social drinkers [57,84,85]. A posttreatment survey concluded that naltrexone is more effective in patients with higher craving and lower cognitive functioning [53,86].

Naltrexone is a synthetic congener of oxymorphone and is structurally related to naloxone. A 50-mg dose of naltrexone can block the effect of 25 mg of IV-injected heroin for up to 24 h [87,88]. Naltrexone is well absorbed orally. The pharmacologic activity is due to the parent compound as well as the 6-β-naltrexol metabolite. The mean half-lives of naltrexone and 6-β-naltrexol are 4 and 13 h, respectively. Although extrahepatic sites are postulated to exist, the drug is primarily metabolized by the liver and is excreted in the urine.

The most common side effects reported include nausea and headache [87,89]. Nausea may diminish on decreasing the dose. Hepatotoxicity has been seen at doses significantly higher than 50 mg [87,90] and is due to direct toxic effects on the liver rather than an idiosyncratic reaction [57]. Liver function tests (LFTs) should be performed prior to the onset of naltrexone and at regular intervals thereafter. An elevation of the liver enzymes (AST, ALT) greater than three times the normal limit and an elevated bilirubin level preclude the use of naltrexone. Other contraindications to the use of naltrexone include current use of opioids or opioid dependence, a failed naloxone challenge test, a positive urine screen for opioids, a history of sensitivity to naltrexone or related compounds, acute hepatitis, and hepatic failure [121].

Nalmephene is a μ- and κ-opioid antagonist; while chemically similar to naltrexone, nalmephene is less hepatotoxic. Nalmephene is approved by the FDA for reversal of opioid intoxication and overdose [57].

In a 12-week randomized, placebo-controlled trial of nalmephene (10 and 40 mg/day), a lower relapse rate was achieved with the higher dose of nalmephene [55,57,91].

3. GABA Agonists

Acamprosate or calcium acetyl homotaurinate, has excitatory effects on the GABA receptors and inhibits the N-methyl-d-aspartate receptors [57,92]. The normalization of the glutamatergic excitation that occurs in withdrawal and early abstinence may lead to a reduction in the craving, distress, and need to consume alcohol [57,93–95]. Several European trials have shown that abstinence rate on acamprosate over 3 months to a year is two times that of placebo [57,97–101]. Acamprosate is primarily excreted by the kidney and it is not metabolized in the body. It should thus be used with caution in patients with renal failure. The main side effects are headache and diarrhea [57,87]. Acamprosate is not available in the United States.

4. Serotonergic Agents

Sustained use of alcohol has been hypothesized to disrupt the serotonin system or cause a reduction in the neurotransmission of serotonin [53]. Therefore serotonergic compounds are potential treatments for alcoholism [53,102,103]. In recent years they have been used off-label for patients with comorbid depressive and anxiety disorders. The main drugs studied are ondansetron, buspirone, and selective serotonin reuptake inhibitors (SSRIs).

In one study, ondansetron, a 5HT3 antagonist, decreased the pleasurable effects of alcohol as well as the desire for drinking alcohol in healthy adult volunteers [53,104]. Likewise, another trial reported decreased alcohol consumption [53,105].

Buspirone, a 5HT1A agonist, was shown in one clinical trial to be associated with the subjects staying in treatment longer and drinking less than subjects on placebo [57,106]. Other studies have shown buspirone to be associated with reduced craving and consumption [53,106–108]. A 12-week placebo-controlled trial of patients with comorbid anxiety and alcoholism treated with buspirone showed that subjects remained in treatment longer and drank less than subjects on placebo [57,106]. On the contrary, a double-blind study of alcoholism and anxiety showed buspirone to be no more effective than placebo [57,109]. A review of the buspirone studies showed the only positive change in drinking behavior to be an increased time to the first drink [55].

Fluoxetine, citalopram, and other 5HT agonists (SSRTs) have been tested. Although some short-term studies in heavy social drinkers reported a modest decrease in alcohol use [110–112], studies of alcohol-dependent patients without comorbid major depression did not report an advantage of the SSRI fluoxetine over placebo [113–115]. However, in a randomized double-blind placebo-controlled study of fluoxetine in patients with comorbid major depression and alcohol dependence, fluoxetine decreased the depression as well as the total number of drinks consumed compared to placebo [57,116].

5. *Aversive Agents*

Aversive agents are compounds that when given alone produce no sensations but rather produce nausea and other unpleasant reactions if alcohol is consumed. The two common drugs in this group are disulfiram and calcium carbimide.

Disulfiram

Disulfiram, an antioxidant used in the rubber industry, was initially discovered by two Danish physicians to be a useful deterrent to drinking alcohol. Chemically bis(diethylthiocarbamoyl)disulfide, disulfiram is an irreversible inhibitor of the enzyme aldehyde dehydrogenase, which is responsible for the metabolism of acetaldehyde. The aversive effects of disulfiram is due to the disulfiram-ethanol reaction (DER) which develops as a consequence of the accumulation of acetaldehyde [87,117,137]. Disulfiram may also produce hypotension as a result of decreased norepinephrine synthesis, secondary to inhibition of the enzyme dopamine beta-hydroxylase [87].

DER develops within a few minutes after the ingestion of alcohol while on disulfiram maintenance. A mild DER may consist of increased heart rate and blood pressure, chills, nausea, vomiting, hypertension, and shortness of breath and may be treated with antihistamines. A moderate to severe DER may be associated with intense tachycardia and EKG changes. There may be ensuing vomiting, convulsions, congestive heart failure, and cardiovascular collapse. Other complications may include myocardial infarction, cerebrovascular accident, and cardiac arrest. Severe, delayed DERs have also been reported [87,118]. Management consists of supportive measures, anticholinergics, ascorbic acid, and 4-methylbyrazol, which blocks the acetaldehyde production by blocking the metabolism of alcohol. Other sources of alcohol, the so-called latent alcohols (e.g., cough syrups, facial lotions, wine vinegar, sauces, and some candies) may induce a similar reaction. Medications that may potentiate DER include amitriptyline, vasodilators, beta-adrenergic antagonists, MAO inhibitors, and antipsychotics [87,119,120]. Disulfiram is both slowly absorbed and slowly eliminated from the body and may be present about 2 weeks after the last dose is administered [121]. In the initial phase of treatment, a maximum of up to 500 mg/day may be given in a single dose for 1–2 weeks. While preferably taken in the morning, the medication may be taken at night for patients who experience a sedative effect. The maintenance dose is on average 250 mg/day with a range of 125–500 mg/day. Adverse effects from disulfiram include a number of potentially serious side effects, especially at higher dosages, warranting caution and frequent monitoring [87,119]. Careful monitoring may include liver function tests, patient education, and warnings pertaining to the potential side effects.

Side effects include transient mild drowsiness, fatigability, headache, decreased sexual desire, erectile dysfunction, skin eruptions, nickel dermatitis [53,122], a metallic or garlic aftertaste, restlessness, cholestatic and fulminant hepatitis, hepatic failure, optic neuritis, peripheral neuritis, polyneuritis, and psychotic reactions or unmasking of underlying psychosis. Disulfiram inhibits the metabolism of several medications including anticoagulants, phenytoin, and isoniazid [57].

The drug is contraindicated in patients concurrently consuming alcohol or receiving alcohol-containing preparations, metronidazole, or paraldehyde. Disulfiram is also contraindicated in patients who experience a hypersensitivity reaction to disulfiram or other thiuram derivatives or in the presence of psychoses, suicidal and impulsive behaviors [87], coronary artery occlusion, severe myocardial disease, or pregnancy [57,121]. Disulfiram may be particularly beneficial for motivated, older, and more severely affected subjects [56,123], and when used in conjunction with effective compliance-enhancing techniques [124,125]. Disulfiram implant trials have not shown satisfactory results aside from a reduction in the number of days that subjects consume alcohol [55].

Calcium Carbimide

Calcium carbimide was previously available in Canada and Australia but has been withdrawn from the market by the manufacturer. Although it has not been studied as well as disulfiram, calcium carbimide has shown no greater efficacy than placebo in clinical trials.

6. Benzodiazepines

Benzodiazepines are still the agents of choice for acute alcohol withdrawal [53,126–129]. They are particularly well suited as they treat both the anxiety and the seizures often seen in alcohol withdrawal [130]. The long-acting compounds chlordiazepoxide and diazepam and the intermediate-acting compounds lorazepam, oxazepam, and temazepam are most frequently used [87,119]. The long-acting compounds are most favorable since their long-acting metabolites allow less frequent dosing and produce a natural tapering effect. Adverse effects to the benzodiazepines include sedation, drowsiness, ataxia, dizziness, poor coordination, diplopia, vertigo, and impairment in motor performance. The long-acting benzodiazepines tend to produce these side effects due to their accumulation. Intermediate- and short-acting benzodiazepines are more likely to produce side effects from high peak levels as well as fluctuating blood levels. Episodes of severe agitation, hostility, and memory impairment have been reported [87,117,123,131,132].

7. Adrenergic Agents

The majority of the symptoms of alcohol withdrawal are related to heightened activity of the sympathetic nervous system, manifesting as hypertension, tremors, nausea, and anxiety. Mild to moderate withdrawal symptoms may be effectively managed with alpha-agonists but are associated with the adverse effects of sedation and hypotension [53,133–137]. Propranolol and atenolol have been shown to cause abatement of signs and symptoms with an earlier return to baseline, a reduction in the amount of benzodiazepines used, and a reduction in the length of inpatient stay [53,138]. Other studies have shown that propranolol and atenolol decrease the desire for alcohol, give rise to longer compliance with treatment, and cause fewer side effects compared to the other agents in this class [53,139–141]. However, both propranolol and atenolol may mask the severity of withdrawal [53,125] and may increase the occurrence of confusion and hallucinations during withdrawal [53,142–143]. For these reasons and because of the rapid development of tolerance to the anxiolytic effects of beta-blockers, their use is limited [53,144].

8. Calcium Channel Blockers

Calcium channel blockers of the dihydropyridine family (e.g., nimodipine and darodipine) decrease the severity of alcohol withdrawal in rodents [53,145–148]. Further research involving this class of compounds is warranted given that calcium channel blockers have potential benefits in the treatment of alcohol withdrawal.

9. NMDA-Receptor Channel Blockers

Some experimental evidence suggests that NMDA-receptor channel blockers such as MK-801 (dizocilpine) or related compounds might hold some promise for alcohol withdrawal, as MK-801 has been shown to decrease the frequency and severity of alcohol withdrawal-induced seizures [53,149,150].

10. Anticonvulsants

Although benzodiazepines are the preferred drugs for the control of seizures during alcohol withdrawal, other drugs that may be used include carbamazepine and valproate. Although more testing is warranted, both carbamazepine and valproate may be useful in the treatment of alcohol withdrawal [53,151,152].

Gabapentin has been reportedly used with some success in the detoxification from alcohol, in the treatment of alcohol-related sleep disorders, and in the augmentation of chlormethiazole, thereby decreasing the amount of chlormethiazole required for detoxification [153–156].

One important avenue of future direction may be to identify the genes that contribute to the risk for alcoholism and associated therapeutic response using the process of human genome sequencing [157–161].

IV. PHARMACOLOGICAL TREATMENT OF OPIOID DEPENDENCE

Opioid dependence has remained a costly and personally destructive national health problem. Epidemiological studies show that opioid addiction affects 810,000 people each year, touching all segments of American society, with annual costs around $21 billion [162]. Of the U.S. adult population, 0.4–0.7% will develop heroin dependence at some point in their lives [162]. About one-quarter of people who have ever used heroin develop dependence [162]. Dependent heroin users typically use heroin daily, become tolerant to its effects, and experience withdrawal manifestations on abrupt cessation of use. Heroin-dependent patients are at increased risk of premature death from drug overdose, HIV and hepatitis spread by sharing contaminated injecting equipment, violence, criminal behavior, and alcohol-related causes [163,164].

With the exception of naltrexone hydrochloride, opioid maintenance therapy remains the primary pharmacological approach to the treatment of opioid dependence. Opioid agonists, opioid antagonists, and more recently partial agonists, are the three primary types of medications available for the treatment of opioid dependence, all acting directly on opioid receptors, particularly μ-receptors.

A. Naltrexone Hydrochloride

Naltrexone hydrochloride is an opioid antagonist that blocks the subjective effects of opioids, thereby eliminating opioid-induced euphoria, diminishing the reinforcing effects of heroin [165], and potentially extinguishing the association between conditioned stimuli and opioid use [166]. Relative to other maintenance therapies, naltrexone has no abuse potential, has a benign side-effects profile, and can be prescribed without concerns about diversion (rarely traded in the illicit market) [167]. Moreover, approved by the FDA in 1984, naltrexone, available in tablet form for use in detoxified patients, is not subject to the restrictive regulatory requirements with methadone and levomethadyl acetate, and therefore can be prescribed in a wide range of settings.

Naltrexone displaces bound agonist and blocks the effects of heroin administration [166]. Peak plasma concentrations are achieved within 1 h, and antagonist effects can last up to 72 h [166]. Because of its long duration of action, standard dosages of naltrexone are 50 mg/day or 100 mg on Monday and Wednesday and 150 mg on Friday [166]. Potential side effects of naltrexone are similar to those described in the treatment of alcohol dependence. However, in opioid dependence, reported side effects of naltrexone may have been related to precipitation of the opiate withdrawal syndrome [168]. The most common side effects are nausea and headaches. Others include epigatric pain, dizziness, nervousness, fatigue or insomnia. Large doses (up to 300 mg/day) might increase the risk of hepatotoxicity [169].

Naltrexone has, despite its appealing properties, remained underused compared to methadone maintenance [170]. Its clinical usefulness has been limited [165,171] owing to problems with attrition and noncompliance. Induction can be difficult and early dropout is common. In one treatment program, 40% of patients dropped out during the first month of treatment and 60% dropped out by 3 months [172]. Randomized trials have shown low retention rates (2%), and one study demonstrated no efficacy in reducing opioid use compared to placebo [173,174].

Research on naltrexone has mostly focused on evaluating its utility in the treatment of selected populations (health care professionals and individuals mandated to treatment) [175]. Naltrexone has shown some efficacy in combination with fluoxetine and weekly drug counseling [176]. Since naltrexone lacks the pharmacological reward activity, contingency management (CM) and significant other (SO) involvement could be used to reward and provide incentives for retention and thus enhance naltrexone compliance [177]. A recent study evaluating CM and SO as treatments for recently detoxified opioid addicts taking naltrexone as maintenance treatment showed promising results which emphasized the importance of behavioral therapies targeting specific techniques to enhance compliance with pharmacological interventions [178].

B. Opioid Maintenance Therapy

Repeated exposure to opioids leads to major changes in the neurons in the locus ceruleus and mesolimbic areas of the brain producing the clinical phenomena of tolerance, dependence, craving, and supranormal stimulation of the reward circuitry [179]. These neurobiological changes explain the rationale for opioid agonist maintenance to stabilize these complex systems. Opioid agonist maintenance therapies offer many advantages including their slower onset of action which minimizes their euphoric effects, their competitive antagonism with heroin, and their ability to prevent withdrawal by cross-tolerance. Opioid agonist maintenance eliminates the risk for infections associated with intravenous drug injection [180].

1. Methadone Hydrochloride

Methadone hydrochloride is a synthetic long-acting opioid μ-receptor agonist. It is available in tablets or as a solution for oral or parenteral use in detoxification, maintenance, and treatment of severe pain. Methadone is taken once a day because its long duration of action eliminates opiate withdrawal symptoms for 24–36 h. Given in high doses, it reduces craving for heroin and blocks many of the euphoric effects of exogenously administered opioids [181], thereby breaking the cycle of seeking out, buying, and abusing heroin.

However, when injected, methadone has potential for abuse in persons who are less opioid dependent.

Long-term administration of methadone does not result in any adverse biochemical or tissue changes [182] but leads to tolerance to its analgesic, sedative, and euphoric effects [183], with minimal toxicity. Side effects usually appearing during the stabilization phase include constipation, sweating, and a skin rash (which may be transient), weight gain, decreased libido, menstrual irregularities (resulting from hyperprolactinemia), ankle edema, sedation (specially at higher doses) [184], and rare cases of reversible thrombocytopenia in patients with chronic hepatitis.

Since methadone undergoes extensive hepatic metabolism, it interacts with medications metabolized by the cytochrome P450 pathway: Levels of methadone can be increased by concomitant administration of such medications as erythromycine, ketoconazole, cimetidine, and fluvoxamine [185]. Induction of the CYP 450 enzyme activity leads to decreased plasma levels of methadone and withdrawal due to interactions with alcohol, phenytoin, barbiturates, carbamazepine, isoniazid, rifampin, ritonavir, nevirapine, and possibly efavirenz [185–188]. Methadone interferes with the metabolism of desipramine and other tricyclic antidepressants leading to elevated plasma levels of those agents and their active metabolites. Reduction in the dosages of those agents is warranted if patients are symptomatic, show signs of toxicity, or have elevated plasma levels. Methadone administration is considered to be the treatment of choice for pregnant women who are addicted to opiates. It is reportedly safe with mild effects on the offspring. Offspring may, however, develop neonatal abstinence syndrome after delivery [189].

The model of methadone maintenance treatment (MMT) originally proposed by Dole and Nyswander (high doses of methadone, long duration of treatment, intensive rehabilitative services) was modified during its popularization in the 1970s in the United States and Australia [190,191]. The goal of the programs moved from maintenance toward abstinence from all opioid drugs, including methadone [190]. The original study by Dole and Nyswander that demonstrated the efficacy of methadone in decreasing heroin use was conducted with daily doses ranging from 50 to 150 mg [192]. Some clinics use relatively low doses (< 30 mg), while others use 60 mg or more per day. Most studies have demonstrated that higher doses of methadone (> 50 mg) are more effective than lower doses and are associated with better treatment retention and decreased illicit drug use [193,194]. A recent 40-week randomized double-blind trial comparing the relative clinical efficacy of moderate (30–50 mg) versus high-dose (80–100 mg) methadone maintenance in 192 outpatients noted a greater decrease in illicit opioid use in the high-dose group [194]. Because of some degree of negativity and misconceptions about the methadone dose (195), many programs are reluctant to prescribe the optimal doses. Adopting a flexible dosing policy results in patients' feeling more positive about their treatment' and produces better retention rates [196,197].

The efficacy of methadone has been clearly demonstrated empirically in several experimental and observational studies [198–201]. An overview of 1-year follow-up outcomes in the Drug Abuse Treatment Outcome Study (DATOS) showed that in the 727 patients who started methadone treatment, weekly heroin use dropped from 89% before treatment to 28% at 1 year [196]. One recent study showed the advantages of methadone maintenance over a long detoxification program combined with enriched psychosocial treatment [202]. In addition to decreasing heroin use, methadone maintenance has also been shown to reduce risk behavior for HIV infection and seroconversion in injection drug users [203–206]. However, a series of studies from the Netherlands has documented the failure of "low-threshold" methadone programs to reduce HIV risk behavior and HIV transmission, which explains the importance of not just simply providing a suboptimal dose of methadone but also how treatment is delivered [207]. Parallel to the reduction in heroin use and risk of contracting HIV is a reduction in acquisitive crime that can be substantial [200,208]. Other benefits include a reduced risk of death and an improvement of well-being, and normalization of disruptions in immune and neuroendocrine functions caused by heroin use [209–211]. As documented in the Treatment Outcome Prospective Study, the major benefits of treatment (reductions in drug use and crime) are noted while patients continue to receive methadone [212].

Methadone has been almost exclusively provided through treatment programs since 1972, when the FDA created regulations that specified the types and amount of treatment services to be provided [200]. "Quality" of treatment is crucial. The quality of the staff-patient interactions and attitude of staff [200], good management of clinics, and quality of record keeping [213] are factors related to outcome of treatment. Abstinence from illicit drug use is monitored by urine toxicology screens in addition to patient's self-report. Continued illicit drug use is met with various strategies, including loss of privileges for take-home medication, increased frequency of clinic visits, and changes in medication dosage to address withdrawal manifestations.

2. L-Alpha-Acetylmethadol

L-alpha-acetylmethadol (LAAM) is a long-acting derivative of methadone that was approved by the FDA for maintenance treatment in 1993. It prevents the opiate withdrawal symptoms for up to 72 h [214,215] and reduces craving. It also increases tolerance to the opiate and thus blocks the "high" effects of abused opiates. It is available in oral and parenteral forms and is metabolized to more potent metabolites that have a prolonged duration of action. The main advantage of LAAM is its long-acting property (up to 92 h) which allows patients to receive doses every 2–3 days, instead of daily with methadone. Adverse effects of LAAM are similar to those of other μ-receptor agonists. Therefore these may be adverse events related to the development of dependence, withdrawal, risks of overdose, and side effects related to the physiological effects of LAAM [216]. Precautions must be undertaken in prescribing LAAM because its full effect is not felt for several days. Overdose on LAAM usually results from its combined use with other drugs, although overdose has also resulted from LAAM alone because of too-frequent dosing [217].

Comparative studies demonstrated similar rates of retention in treatment and opioid positive results on urine tests in patients receiving methadone and LAAM [218,219]. A recent meta-analysis of 14 randomized controlled trials comparing LAAM with methadone maintenance noted slightly greater treatment retention for methadone but a trend toward a greater decrease in illicit drug use with LAAM [220]. Recent trials have demonstrated that patients who received higher doses, a dose-related decrease in heroin use occurred [221,222]. However, they had greater incidence of adverse effects and dropout [221,223]. A recommended starting dose is 30 mg LAAM thrice weekly, with a dose increase by 10 mg every other day until a target of ∼70 mg is reached [223].

Despite the multiple advantages of LAAM, including the convenient dosing, sustained agonist activity, and decreased likelihood for diversion due to lack of "take-home" dosing, only a small proportion of patients enrolled in the maintenance programs receive it. Local and state regulatory processes and the delay in insurance reimbursement seem to be responsible for its slow acceptance in treatment programs [224].

3. Buprenorphine Hydrochloride

Buprenorphine hydrochloride is still an experimental medication for the treatment of opioid dependence. It is already available in Europe and is being considered for approval by the FDA. If approved, buprenorphine, unlike methadone and LAAM, may be available outside of regulated narcotic treatment programs, and in less stigmatized locations, most important, in office-based practices [225]. Buprenorphine is a high-affinity partial μ-agonist and a weak antagonist at the κ-receptor with a long duration of action [226,227]; thus, it may cause fewer withdrawal symptoms and have less potential for abuse, respiratory depression, and overdose [228–230]. It also has some advantages over methadone. Most notably, buprenorphine has a ceiling level on agonist activity, limiting adverse reactions at doses as high as 100 times the analgesic dose [231,232].

Buprenorphine exists in tablet form for sublingual administration, in parenteral form, and a new, sublingual tablet that combines buprenorphine with naloxone. Since the risk of diversion is significantly reduced by the combined buprenorphine-naloxone preparation, it has a great potential for use in office practice. Buprenorphine's lengthy half-life may allow it to be dispensed every 3 or even every 4 days [233]. It produces limited physical dependence of the opioid type. Because of its binding to the μ-receptor, the onset of the withdrawal symptoms after maintenance treatment is generally delayed for 24 h or more, and low symptom intensity may not worsen for 5 or more days. The major disadvantage of buprenorphine is its poor oral bioavailability; however, sublingual administration results in plasma concentrations that are 60–70% those of parenteral doses [230]. Its abuse potential limits its dispensing to home [230]. Buprenorphine has a more favorable safety profile than methadone. Buprenorphine appears to have a ceiling on pharmacodynamic effects in the presence of dose-proportionate plasma levels and has a high safety margin when given IV in the absence of other drugs [234]. The most common side effects include sedation or drowsiness, nausea, dizziness, headache, hypotension, miosis, and diaphoresis [235]. Constipation was the only significant side effect noted in a recent dose-ranging study of buprenorphine [225]. Buprenorphine is metabolized by the cytochrome P450 system, and potential drug-drug interactions may emerge between buprenorphine and benzodiazepines, fluoxetine, fluvoxamine, and ritonavir [187,236,237].

Early work and subsequent research have established buprenorphine's ability to suppress self-administration of heroin [238] and its effectiveness in opioid detoxification [239]. Clinical trials have demonstrated the efficacy of buprenorphine over placebo in decreasing illicit opioid use [240], and have shown that dosages ranging from 6 to 16 mg/day are as safe and effective as 60 mg methadone in stemming the use of opiates [225,241,242]. In addition, it has been shown that daily and alternate-day dosing have equivalent effects on opioid withdrawal syndrome and illicit drug use [243,244]. A 12-week randomized trial comparing the effects of thrice-weekly buprenorphine in a primary care setting with those in a traditional treatment program noted higher retention and lower illicit opioid use in the primary care setting group [245]. Another study demonstrated that buprenorphine administered three times weekly was similar to LAAM in terms of study retention and was similar to high-dose (60–100 mg) methadone in terms of abstinence [246].

C. Matching Pharmacological Approaches to Patients with Opioid Dependence

Federal requirements have evolved from fairly restrictive criteria to more flexible criteria. Initially, candidates for methadone maintenance were required to be 21–40 years of age, to have been addicted to heroin for at least 4 years, to have evidence of relapse with previous attempts at detoxification, and to have no major medical or psychiatric problems or polysubstance dependence. Current criteria for maintenance with methadone or LAAM specify that patients must be at least 18 years of age and have at least a 1-year history of opioid addiction and evidence of physiological dependence [256]. Comorbid psychiatric, substance abuse, and medical problems are not excluded, and pregnant women are eligible under modified criteria [256].

The decision to implement opioid agonist maintenance involves careful evaluation of the clinical characteristics including the risks and the benefits for every patient, within the regulations guidelines. For example, patients with a long history of severe dependence, previous failed attempts at detoxification, and substantial risk for infectious complications due to injection drug use would more likely benefit from an opioid agonist or partial agonist maintenance to reduce the harm associated with heroin and promote abstinence. Further research focusing on the roles and efficacy of maintenance therapies is warranted to identify the most appropriate strategies matching patients to treatment.

V. PHARMACOLOGICAL TREATMENT OF COCAINE DEPENDENCE

A number of drugs have been tried to treat cocaine-related problems, in part because of the postulated role of antecedent disorders in the genesis of chronic abuse, as well as the neurobiologic consequences of abuse and dependence. For example, since dysphoric mood is reported during and after the cessation of cocaine use, antidepressants were assessed for effectiveness in the treatment of cocaine dependence. The efficacy of medications is difficult to evaluate due to concurrent abuse of other drugs, and diversity of patterns of abuse and routes of administration. Many studies have examined pharmacological treatments for cocaine dependence, but no medication has been demonstrated to be clearly effective [247–254]. There has been a consideration of opioid agonists and antagonists, dopamine agonists, antidepressants, anticonvulsants, and the newer antipsychotics as antagonist agents [247,255,256]. Even though some agents showed early promising results, these results have not been replicated in subsequent studies [250,255,257–259]. Other agents, including gabapentine and mecamylamine, were reported to be reducing cocaine craving [260–262].

Transdermal selegeline seems to be safe and may be useful in the treatment of cocaine dependence [263]. Available agonists for cocaine dependence include methylphenidate and amphetamine analogs. Studies with methylphenidate showed no impact on retention or decrease in cocaine use [253,255,264,265]. A recent double-blind randomized clinical trial using sustained-release dextroamphetamine reported positive results for improved retention and reduction in illicit drug use in cocaine-dependent patients [266]. The work of others suggested that dextroamphetamine may likewise be of some use in amphetamine-abusing patients [256].

Other strategies explored in animal models, such as vaccination and manipulation of dopamine receptor subsets, offer potential possibilities for treatment of cocaine dependence [267–269].

ACKNOWLEDGEMENTS

This work was supported by USPHS Grants AA-10523 and AA-11929 from the National Institute of Alcohol Abuse and Alcoholism, Rickville, MD.

REFERENCES

1. McLellan AT, Lewis DC, O'Brien CP, Kleber HD. Drug dependence, a chronic medical illness: implications for treatment, insurance, and outcomes evaluation. JAMA 2000; 284(13):1689–1695.
2. American Psychiatric Association. DSM-IV-TR: Diagnostic and Statistical Manual of Mental Disorders. Fourth Edition, Text Revision. Washington: American Psychiatric Association, 2000.
3. U.S. Department of Health and Human Services. Reducing Tobacco Use: A Report of the Surgeon General. Atlanta: Centers for Disease Control and Prevention, 2000.
4. Di Chiara G. The role of dopamine in drug abuse viewed from the perspective of its role in motivation [erratum appears in Drug Alcohol Depend 1995; 39(2):155]. Drug Alcohol Depend 1995; 38(2):95–137.
5. Corrigall WA, Coen KM, Adamson KL. Self-administered nicotine activates the mesolimbic dopamine system through the ventral tegmental area. Brain Res 1994; 653(1–2):278–284.
6. Benowitz NL. Pharmacology of nicotine: addiction and therapeutics. Annu Rev Pharmacol Toxicol 1996; 36:597–613.
7. Benowitz NL, Wilson Peng Margaret. Non-nicotine pharmacotherapy for smoking cessation: mechanisms and prospects. CNS Drugs 2000; 13(4):265–285.
8. U.S. Department of Health and Human Services. Public Health Service. Treating Tobacco Use and Dependence. Clinical Practice Guideline. Rockville, MD: U.S. Public Health Service, 2000.
9. Vocci FJ, Chiang CN. Vaccines against nicotine: how effective are they likely to be in preventing smoking? CNS Drugs 2001; 15(7):505–514.
10. Pentel PR, Malin DH, Ennifar S, et al. A nicotine conjugate vaccine reduces nicotine distribution to brain and attenuates its behavioral and cardiovascular effects in rats. Pharmacol Biochem Behav 2000 1; 65(1):191–198.
11. Henningfield JE, Keenan RM. Nicotine delivery kinetics and abuse liability. J Consult Clin Psychol 1993; 61(5):743–750.
12. Henningfield, JE, Schuh LM, Jarvik ME. Pathophysiology of tobacco dependence. In: FE Bloom, DJ Kupfer, eds. Psychopharmacology: The Fourth Generation of Progress. New York: Raven Press, 1995, 1715–1729.
13. Gross J, Stitzer ML. Nicotine replacement: ten-week effects on tobacco withdrawal symptoms. Psychopharmacologia 1989; 98(3):334–341.
14. Dale LC, Schroeder DR, Wolter TD, Croghan IT, Hurt RD, Offord KP. Weight change after smoking cessation using variable doses of transdermal nicotine replacement. J Gen Intern Med 1998; 13(1):9–15.
15. Anonymous. Smoking cessation: information for specialists. Agency for Health Care Policy and Research. Clinical Practice Guideline—Quick Reference Guide for Clinicians 1996; 18B:1–10.
16. Henningfield JE. Nicotine medications for smoking cessation. N Engl J Med 1995; 333(18):1196–1203.
17. Hughes JR, Goldstein MG, Hurt RD, Shiffman S. Recent advances in the pharmacotherapy of smoking. JAMA 1999; 281(1):72–76.
18. Perkins KA. Smoking cessation in women. Special considerations. CNS Drugs 2001; 15(5):391–411.
19. Martin BR, Onaivi ES, Martin TJ. What is the nature of mecamylamine's antagonism of the central effects of nicotine? Biochem Pharmacol 1989; 38(20):3391–1087.
20. Takayama H, Majewska MD, London ED. Interactions of noncompetitive inhibitors with nicotinic receptors in the rat brain. J Pharmacol Exp Ther 1989; 251(3):1083–1089.
21. Westman EC, Behm FM, Rose JE. Dissociating the nicotine and airway sensory effects of smoking. Pharmacol Biochem Behav 1996; 53(2):309–315.
22. Behm FM, Schur C, Levin ED, Tashkin DP, Rose JE. Clinical evaluation of a citric acid inhaler for smoking cessation. Drug Alcohol Depend 1993; 31(2):131–138.
23. Rose JE, Behm FM, Levin ED. Role of nicotine dose and sensory cues in the regulation of smoke intake. Pharmacol, Biochem Behav 1993; 44(4):891–900.
24. West R, Courts S, Beharry S, May S, Hajek P. Acute effect of glucose tablets on desire to smoke. Psychopharmacologia 1999; 147(3):319–321.
25. West R, Willis N. Double-blind placebo controlled trial of dextrose tablets and nicotine patch in smoking cessation. Psychopharmacologia 1998; 136(2):201–204.
26. Hajek P, Stead LF. Aversive smoking for smoking cessation. Cochrane Database Syst Rev 2000; 2:CD000546.
27. Morrow R, Nepps P, McIntosh M. Silver acetate mouth spray as an aid in smoking cessation: results of a double-blind trial. J Am Board Fam Pract 1993; 6(4):353–357.
28. Gourlay SG, Benowitz NL. Is clonidine an effective smoking cessation therapy? Drugs 1995; 50(2):197–207.
29. Glassman AH, Jackson WK, Walsh BT, Roose SP, Rosenfeld B. Cigarette craving, smoking withdrawal, and clonidine. Science 1984; 226(4676):864–866.
30. Glassman AH, Stetner F, Walsh BT, Raizman PS, Fleiss JL, Cooper TB, Covey LS. Heavy smokers, smoking cessation, and clonidine. Results of a double-blind, randomized trial. JAMA 1988; 259(19):2863–2866.
31. Covey LS, Sullivan MA, Johnston JA, Glassman AH, Robinson MD, Adams DP. Advances in non-nicotine pharmacotherapy for smoking cessation. Drugs 2000; 59(1):17–31.

32. Glassman AH, Covey LS, Dalack GW, Stetner F, Rivelli SK, Fleiss J, Cooper TB. Smoking cessation, clonidine, and vulnerability to nicotine among dependent smokers. Clin Pharmacol Ther 1993; 54(6):670–679.
33. Hall SM, Munoz RF, Reus VI, Sees KL. Nicotine, negative affect, and depression. J Consult Clin Psychol 1993; 61(5):761–767.
34. Glassman AH, Helzer JE, Covey LS, Cottler LB, Stetner F, Tipp JE, Johnson J. Smoking, smoking cessation, and major depression. JAMA 1990; 264(12):1546–1549.
35. Cooper BR, Wang CM, Cox RF, Norton R, Shea V, Ferris RM. Evidence that the acute behavioral and electrophysiological effects of bupropion (Wellbutrin) are mediated by a noradrenergic mechanism. Neuropsychopharmacology 1994; 11(2):133–141.
36. Ascher JA, Cole JO, Colin JN, Feighner JP, Ferris RM, Fibiger HC, Golden RN, Martin P, Potter WZ, Richelson E. Bupropion: a review of its mechanism of antidepressant activity. J Clin Psychiatry 1995; 56(9):395–401.
37. Fryer JD, Lukas RJ. Noncompetitive functional inhibition at diverse, human nicotinic acetylcholine receptor subtypes by bupropion, phencyclidine, and ibogaine. J Pharmacol Exp Ther 1999; 288(1):88–92.
38. Holm KJ, Spencer CM. Bupropion: a review of its use in the management of smoking cessation. Drugs 2000; 59(4):1007–1024.
39. Hurt RD, Sachs DP, Glover ED, et al. A comparison of sustained-release bupropion and placebo for smoking cessation. N Engl J Med 1997; 337(17): 1195–1202.
40. Jorenby DE, Leischow SJ, Nides MA, et al. A controlled trial of sustained-release bupropion, a nicotine patch, or both for smoking cessation. N Engl J Med 1999; 340(9):685–691.
41. Prochazka AV, Weaver MJ, Keller RT, Fryer GE, Licari PA, Lofaso D. A randomized trial of nortriptyline for smoking cessation. Arch Intern Med 1998; 158(18):2035–2039.
42. Hall SM, Reus VI, Munoz RF, Sees KL, Humfleet G, Hartz DT, Frederick S, Triffleman E. Nortriptyline and cognitive-behavioral therapy in the treatment of cigarette smoking. Arch Gen Psychiatry 1998; 55(8):683–690.
43. Berry MD, Juorio AV, Paterson IA. The functional role of monoamine oxidases A and B in the mammalian central nervous system. Prog Neurobiol 1994; 42(3):375–391.
44. Berlin I, Said S, Spreux-Varoquaux O, Launay JM, Olivares R, Millet V, Lecrubier Y, Puech AJ. A reversible monoamine oxidase A inhibitor (moclobemide) facilitates smoking cessation and abstinence in heavy, dependent smokers. Clin Pharm Ther 1995; 58(4):444–452.
45. Berlin I, Said S, Spreux-Varoquaux O, Olivares R, Launay JM, Puech AJ. Monoamine oxidase A and B activities in heavy smokers. Biol Psychiatry 1995; 38(11):756–761.
46. Edwards NB, Murphy JK, Downs AD, Ackerman BJ, Rosenthal TL. Doxepin as an adjunct to smoking cessation: a double-blind pilot study. Am J Psychiatry 1989; 146(3):373–376.
47. Cinciripini PM, Lapitsky L, Seay S, Wallfisch A, Meyer WJ 3rd, van Vunakis H. A placebo-controlled evaluation of the effects of buspirone on smoking cessation: differences between high- and low-anxiety smokers [erratum appears in J Clin Psychopharmacol 1995; 15(6):408]. J Clin Psychopharmacol 1995; 15(3):182–191.
48. Rose JE, Sampson A, Levin ED, Henningfield JE. Mecamylamine increases nicotine preference and attenuates nicotine discrimination. Pharmacol Biochem Behav 1989; 32(4):933–938.
49. Stolerman IP, Goldfarb T, Fink R, Jarvik ME. Influencing cigarette smoking with nicotine antagonists. Psychopharmacologia 1973; 28(3):247–259.
50. Rose JE, Behm FM, Westman EC, Levin ED, Stein RM, Ripka GV. Mecamylamine combined with nicotine skin patch facilitates smoking cessation beyond nicotine patch treatment alone. Clin Pharmacol Ther 1994; 56(1):86–99.
51. Pomerleau CS, Pomerleau OF, Majchrzak MJ. Mecamylamine pretreatment increases subsequent nicotine self-administration as indicated by changes in plasma nicotine level. Psychopharmacologia 1987; 91(3):391–393.
52. Nemeth-Coslett R, Henningfield JE, O'Keeffe MK, Griffiths RR. Effects of mecamylamine on human cigarette smoking and subjective ratings. Psychopharmacologia 1986; 88(4):420.
53. Gatch MB, Lal H. Pharmacological treatment of alcoholism. Prog Neuropsychopharmacol Biol Psychiatry 1998; 22:917–944.
54. National Drug and Alcohol Treatment Unit Survey. Rockville, MD: U.S. Department of Health and Human Services, 1987, NIDA/NIAAA.
55. Garbutt JC, West SL, Carey TS, Lohr KN, Crews FT. Pharmacological treatment of alcohol dependence: a review of the evidence. JAMA 1999; 281(14):1318–1325.
56. Anton RF. Pharmacological approaches to the management of alcoholism. J Clin Psychiatry 2001; 62(S 20):11–17.
57. Swift RM. Drug therapy: drug therapy for alcohol dependence. N Engl J Med 1999; 340(19):1482–1490.
58. Koob GF, Weiss F. Neuropharmacology of cocaine and ethanol dependence. Recent Dev Alcohol 1996; 20:391–402.

59. Samson HH, Hodge CW. The role of the mesoaccumbens dopamine system in ethanol reinforcement: studies using the techniques of microinjection and voltammetry. Alcohol Alcohol Suppl 1993; 2:469–474.
60. Wise RA, Bozarth MA. A psychomotor stimulant theory of addiction. Psychol Rev 1987; 94:469–492.
61. Robinson TE, KC Berridge KC. The neural basis of drug craving: an incentive-sensitization theory of addiction. Brain research. Brain Res Rev 1993; 18:247–291.
62. Rohsenow DJ, Monti PM, Abrams DB, Rubonis AV. Cue elicited urge to drink and salivation in alcoholics: relationship to individual differences. Adv Behav Res Ther 1992; 14(3):195–210.
63. Anton RF, Moak DH, Latham PK. The obsessive compulsive drinking scale: a new method of assessing outcome in alcoholism treatment studies. Arch Gen Psychiatry 1996; 53:225–231.
64. Suzdak PD, Schwartz RD, Skolnick P, Paul SM. Ethanol stimulates gamma-aminobutyric acid receptor-mediated chloride transport in rat brain synaptoneurosomes. Proc Nat Acad Sci USA 1986; 83:4071–4075.
65. Linnoila M. NIH conference: alcohol withdrawal and noradrenergic function. Ann Intern Med 1987; 107:875–879.
66. Thase ME, Salloum IM, Cornelius JD. Comorbid alcoholism and depression: treatment issues. J Clin Psychiatry 2001; 62(S20):32–41.
67. Borg V. Bromocriptine in the prevention of alcohol abuse. Acta Psychiat Scand 1983; 68:100–110.
68. Dongier M, Vachon L, Schwartz G. Bromocriptine in the treatment of alcohol dependence. Alcohol Clin Exp Res 1991; 15:970–977.
69. Peters DH, Faulds D. Tiapride: a review of its pharmacology and therapeutic potential in the management of the alcohol dependence syndrome. Drugs 1994; 47:1010–1032.
70. Shaw GK, Majumdar SK, Waller S, MacGarvie J, Dunn G. Tiapride in the long-term management of alcoholics of anxious or depressive temperament. Br J Psychiatry 1987; 150:164–168.
71. Shaw GK, Waller S, Majumdar SK, Alberts JL, Latham CJ, Dunn G. Tiapride in the prevention of relapse in recently detoxified alcoholics. Br J Psychiatry 1994; 165:515–523.
72. Schuckit MA. Recent developments in the pharmacotherapy of alcohol dependence. J Consult Clin Psychol 1996; 64(4):669–676.
73. Modell JG, Mountz JM, Glaser FB, Lee JY. Effect of haloperidol on measures of craving and impaired control in alcoholic subjects. Alcohol Clin Exp Res 1993; 17:234–240.
74. Center for Substance Abuse Treatment. Intensive Outpatient Treatment for Alcohol and Other Drug Abuse TIP No. 8. Rockville, MD: U.S. Department of Health and Human Services, 1994.
75. Hubbell CL, Czirr SA, Hunter GA, Beaman CM, Lecann NC, Reid LD. Consumption of ethanol solution is potentiated by morphine and attenuated by naloxone persistently across repeated daily administrations. Alcohol 1986; 3:39–54.
76. Froehlich JC, Harts J, Lumeng L, Li TK. Naloxone attenuates voluntary ethanol intake in rats selectively bred for high ethanol preference. Pharmacol Biochem Behav 1990; 35:385–390.
77. Gessa GL, Muntoni F, Collu M, Vargiu L, Mereu G. Low doses of ethanol activate dopaminergic neurons in the ventral tegmental area. Brain Res 1985; 348:201–203.
78. Benjamin D, Grant E, Pohorecky LA. Naltrexone reverses ethanol-induced dopamine release in the nucleus accumbens in awake, freely moving rats. Brain Res 1993; 621:137–140.
79. O'Malley SS, Jaffe AJ, Chang G, Schottenfeld R, Meyer RE, Rounsaville B. Naltrexone and coping skills therapy for alcohol dependence. A controlled study. Arch Gen Psychiatry 1992; 49:881–887.
80. O'Malley SS, Jaffe AJ, Chang G, Rode S, Schottenfeld R, Meyer RE, Rounsaville B. Six month follow up of naltrexone and psychotherapy for alcohol dependence. Arch Gen Psychiatry 1996; 53:217–224.
81. Volpicelli JR, Alterman AI, Hayashida M, O'Brien CP. Naltrexone in the treatment of alcohol dependence. Arch Gen Psychiatry 1992; 49:876–880.
82. Volpicelli JR, Watson NT, King AC, Sherman CE, O'Brien CP. Effect of naltrexone on alcohol "high" in alcoholics. Am J Psychiatry 1995; 152:613–615.
83. Swift RM, Whelihan W, Kuznetsov O, Buongiorno G, Hsuing H. Naltrexone-induced alterations in human ethanol intoxication. Am J Psychiatry 1994; 151:1463–1467.
84. Monti PM, Rohsenhow DJ, Kent E, Swift RM, Mueller TI, Colby SM, Brown RA, Gulliver SB, Gordon A, Abrams DB. Naltrexone's effect on cue-elicited craving among alcoholics in treatment. Alcohol Clin Exp Res 1999; 23(8):1386–1394.
85. Davidson D, Swift RM, Fitz E. Naltrexone increases the latency to drink alcohol in social drinkers. Alcohol Clin Exp Res 1996; 20:732–739.
86. Jaffe AJ, Rounsaville B, Chang G, Schottenfeld RS, Meyer RE, O'Malley SS. Naltrexone, relapse prevention, and supportive therapy with alcoholics: an analysis of patient treatment matching. J Consult Clin Psychol 1996; 64:1044–1053.
87. Salloum IM, Cornelius JR. Management of side effects of drugs used in the treatment of alcoholism and drug abuse. In: Practical Management of the Side Effects of Psychotropics Drugs. Balon, R, ed. New York: Marcel Dekker, 1999, 169–197.

88. Physicians Desk Reference, 51st ed. R Arky, ed. Oradell, NJ: Medical Economics Co., 1997, 957–959.
89. Croop RS, Faulkner EB, Labriola DF. The safety profile of naltrexone in the treatment of alcoholism: results of a multicenter usage study. Arch Gen Psychiatry 1997; 54:1130–1135.
90. Sternbach HA, Annitto W, Pottash ALC, Gold MS. Anorexic effects of naltrexone in men. Lancet 1982; 1:388.
91. Mason BJ, Ritvo EC, Morgan RO, Salvato FR, Goldberg G, Welch B, Mantero-Atienza E. A double-blind, placebo-controlled pilot study to evaluate the efficacy and safety of oral nalmephene HCl for alcohol dependence. Alcohol Clin Exp Res 1994; 18:1162–1167.
92. Daoust M, Legrand E, Gewiss M, Heidbreder C, DeWitte P, Tran G, Durbin P. Acamprosate modulates synaptosomal GABA transmission in chronically alcoholised rats. Pharmacol Biochem Behav 1992; 41:669–674.
93. Samson HH, Harris RA. Neurobiology of alcohol abuse. Trends Pharmacol Sci 1992; 13:206–211.
94. Tsai G, Gastfriend DR, Coyle JT. The glutamatergic basis of human alcoholism. Am J Psychiatry 1995; 152:332–340.
95. Littleton J. Acamprosate in alcohol dependence: how does it work? Addiction 1995; 90:1179–1188.
96. Whitworth AB, Fischer F, Lesch OM, Nimmerrichter A, Oberbauer H, Platz T, Potgieter A, H Walter, Fleischhacker WW. Comparison of acamprosate and placebo in long-term treatment of alcohol dependence. Lancet 1996; 347:1438–1442.
97. Lhuintre JP, Moore N, Tran G, Steru L, Langrenon S, Daoust M, Parot Ph, Ladure PH, Libert C, Boismare F, Hillemand B. Acamprosate appears to decrease the alcohol intake in weaned alcoholics. Alcohol Alcohol 1990; 25:613–622.
98. Soyka M, Sass H. Acamprosate: a new pharmacolotherapeutic approach to relapse prevention in alcoholism-preliminary data. Alcohol Alcohol Suppl 1994; 2:531–536.
99. Sass H, Soyka M, Mann K, Zieglgansberger W. Relapse prevention by acamprosate: results from a placebo controlled study on alcohol dependence. Arch Gen Psychiatry 1996; 53:673–680.
100. Geerings PJ, Ansoms C, Van der Brink W. Acamprosate and prevention of relapse in alcoholics: results of a randomized, placebo-controlled, double-blind study in outpatient alcoholics in the Netherlands, Belgium and Luxembourg. Eur Addict Res 1997; 3:129–137.
101. Poldrugo F. Acamprosate treatment in a long-term community based alcohol rehabilitation programme. Addiction 1997; 92:1537–1546.
102. LeMarquand D, Pihl RO, Benkelfat C. Serotonin and alcohol intake, abuse and dependence: Clinical evidence. Biol Psychiatry 1994; 36:326–337.
103. Halliday G, Baker K, Harper C. Serotonin and alcohol-related brain damage. Metab Brain Dis 1995; 10:25–30.
104. Johnson BA, Campling GM, Griffiths P, Cowan PJ. Attenuation of some alcohol-induced mood changes and the desire to drink by 5-HT3 receptor blockade: a preliminary study in healthy male volunteers. Psychopharmacology 1993; 112:142–144.
105. Toneatto A, Romach MK, Sobell LC, Sobel MB, Somer GR, Sellers E. Ondansetron, a 5-HT3 antagonist, reduces alcohol consumption in alcohol abusers. Alcohol Clin Exp Res 1991; 15:382.
106. Kranzler HR, Burleson JA, Del Boca FK, Babor TF, Korner P, Brown J, Bohn MJ. Buspirone treatment of anxious alcoholics: a placebo-controlled trial. Arch Gen Psychiatry 1994; 51:720–731.
107. Bruno F. Buspirone in the treatment of alcoholic patients. Psychopathology 1989; 22(S1):49–59.
108. Kranzler HR, Meyer RE. An open trial of buspirone in alcoholics. J Clin Psychopharmacol 1989; 9:379–380.
109. Malcolm R, Anton RF, Randall CL, Johnston A, Brady K, Thevos A. A placebo-controlled trial of buspirone in anxious inpatient alcoholics. Alcohol Clin Exp Res 1992; 16:1007–1013.
110. Naranjo CA, Sellers EM, Sullivan JT, Woodley DV, Kadlec K, Sykora K. The serotonin uptake inhibitor citalopram attenuates ethanol intake. Clin Pharmacol Ther 1987; 41:266–274.
111. Naranjo CA, Poulos CX, Bremner KE, Lanctot KL. Fluoxetine attenuates alcohol intake and desire to drink. Int Clin Psychopharmacol 1994; 9:163–172.
112. Naranjo CA, Bremner KE. Serotonin-altering medications and desire, consumption and effects of alcohol-treatment implications. EXS 1994; 71:209–219.
113. Gorelick D, Pardes A. Effect of fluoxetine on alcohol consumption in male alcoholics. Alcohol Clin Exp Res 1992; 16:261–265.
114. Kabel D, Petty F. A double-blind study of fluoxetine in severe alcohol dependence: adjunctive therapy during and after inpatient treatment. Alcohol Clin Exp Res 1996; 20:780–784.
115. Kranzler HR, Burleson JA, Korner P, Del Boca FK, Bohn MJ, Brown J, Liebowitz N. Placebo-controlled trial of fluoxetine as an adjunct to relapse prevention in alcoholics. Am J Psychiatry 1995; 152:391–397.
116. Cornelius JR, Salloum IM, Ehler JG, Jarrett PJ, Cornelius MD, Perel JM, Thase ME, Black A. Fluoxetine in depressed alcoholics: a double-blind, placebo-controlled trial. Arch Gen Psychiatry 1997; 54:700–705.
117. Raby K. Relation of blood acetaldehyde level to clinical symptoms in the disulfiram-alcohol reaction. J Stud Alcohol 1954; 15:21–32.
118. Jacobsen E. The pharmacology of Antabuse (tetraethylthiuram disulfide). Br J Addict 1950; 47:26–40.
119. Ciraulo DA, Renner JA Jr. Alcoholism. In: Clinical Manual of Chemical Dependence. DA Ciraulo, RI

Shader, eds. Washington: American Psychiatric Press, 1991, pp 1–93.
120. Wright C, Moore RD, Grodin DM, Spyker DA, Gill EV. Screening for disulfiram-induced liver test dysfunction in an inpatient alcoholism program. Alcohol Clin Exp Res 1993; 17:184–186.
121. Physicians Desk Reference, 56th ed. Swifton DW, ed. Oradell, NJ: Medical Economics Co., 2002, pp. 2444–2447.
122. Forns X, Callaberia J, Bruguera M, Salmeron JM, Vilella A, Mas A, Pares A, Rodes J. Disulfiram-induced hepatitis. Report of four cases and review of literature. J Hepatol 1994; 21:853–857.
123. Fuller RK, Branchey L, Brightwell DR, Derman RM, Emrick CD, Iber FL, James KE, Lacoursiere RB, Lee KK, Lowenstam I, Maany I, Niederhiser D, Nocks JJ, Shaw S. Disulfiram treatment of alcoholism: a Veterans Administration cooperative study. JAMA 1986; 256:1449–1455.
124. Allen JP, Litten RZ. Techniques to enhance the compliance with disulfiram. Alcohol Clin Exp Res 1992; 16:1035–1041.
125. Chick J, Gough K, Falkowski W, Kershaw P, Hore B, Mehta B, Ritson B, Ropner R, Torley D. Disulfiram treatment of alcoholism. Br J Psychiatry 1992; 161:84–89.
126. Litten RZ, Allen JP. Pharmacotherapies for alcoholism: promising agents and clinical issues. Alcohol Clin Exp Res 1991; 15:620–633.
127. Jaffe JH, Kranzler HR, Ciraulo DA. Drugs used in the treatment of alcoholism. In: Medical Treatment and Diagnosis of Alcoholism. JH Mendelson, NK Mello, eds. New York: McGraw-Hill, 1992, 421–461.
128. Bohn M. Alcoholism. Psychiatr Clin North Am 1993; 16:679–692.
129. Miller NS. Pharmacotherapy in alcoholism. J Addict Dis 1995; 14:23–46.
130. Emmett-Oglesby MW, Mathis DA, Moon RTY, Lal H. Animal models of drug withdrawal symptoms Psychopharmacology 1990; 101:292–309.
131. Salzman C, Korchansky GE, Shader RI, et al. Is oxazepam associated with hostility? Dis Nerv Syst 1975; 36:30–32.
132. Angus WR, Romeny DM. The effect of diazepam on patient's memory. J Clin Psychopharmacol 1984; 4:203–206.
133. Wilkins AJ, Jenkins WJ, Steiner JA. Efficacy of clonidine in treatment of alcohol withdrawal state. Psychopharmacology 1983; 81:78–80.
134. Baumgartner GR, Rowen RC. Clonidine vs. chlordiazepoxide in the management of acute alcohol withdrawal syndrome. Arch Intern Med 1987; 147:1223–1226.
135. Cushman P, Forbes R, Lerner W. Alcohol withdrawal syndrome: clinical management with lofexidine. Alcohol Clin Exp Res 1985; 9:103–108.
136. Cushman P. Clonidine in alcohol-withdrawal. Adv Alcohol Substance Abuse 1988; 7:17–28.
137. Robinson BJ, Robinson GM, Maling TJB, Johnson RH. Is clonidine useful in the treatment of alcohol withdrawal? Alcohol Clin Exp Res 1989; 13:95–98.
138. Sellers EM, Zilm DH, Degani NC. Comparative efficacy of propanolol and chlordiazepoxide in alcohol withdrawal. J Stud Alcohol 1977; 38:2096–2108.
139. Kraus ML, Gottlieb LD, Horwitz RI, Anscher M. Randomized clinical trial of atenolol in patients with alcohol withdrawal. N Engl J Med 1985; 313:905–909.
140. Horwitz RI, Kraus ML, Gottlieb LD. The efficacy of atenolol and the mediating effects of craving in the outpatient management of alcohol withdrawal. Clin Res 1987; 35:348A.
141. Horwitz RI, Gottlieb LD, Kraus ML. The efficacy of atenolol in the outpatient management of the alcohol withdrawal syndrome. Arch Intern Med 1989; 149:1089–1093.
142. Kissin B. The use of psychoactive drugs in the long-term treatment of chronic alcoholics. Ann NY Acad Sci 1975; 252:385–395.
143. Jacob MS, Zilm DH, Macleod SM, Sellers EM. Propanolol-associated confused states during alcohol withdrawal. J Clin Psychopharmacol 1983; 3:185–187.
144. Center for Substance Abuse Treatment. Assessment and treatment of patients with coexisting mental illness and alcohol and other drug abuse. Rockville, MD: U.S. Department of Health and Human Services, 1994; TIP No. 9.
145. Whittington MA, Little HJ. A calcium channel antagonist stereo selectively decreases ethanol withdrawal hyper excitability but not that due to bicuculline, in hippocampal slices. Br J Pharmacol 1991; 103:1313–1320.
146. Little HJ, Dolin SJ, Whittington MA. Calcium channel antagonists prevent adaptive responses to ethanol. Alcohol Alcohol Suppl 1993; 2:263–266.
147. Rezvani AH, Pucilowski O, Grady DR, Janowsky D, O'Brien RA. Reduction of spontaneous alcohol drinking and physical withdrawal by levemopamil, a novel Ca^{2+} channel antagonist, in rats. Pharmacol Biochem Behav 1993; 46:365–371.
148. Colombo G, Agabio R, Lobina C, Reali R, Melis F, Fadda F, Gessa GL. Effects of the calcium channel antagonist darodipine on ethanol withdrawal in rats. Alcohol Alcohol 1995; 30(1):125–131.
149. Bhave SV, Snell LD, Tabakoff B, Hoffman PL, Hoffman P. Mechanism of ethanol inhibition of NMDA receptor function in primary cultures of cerebral cortical cells. Alcohol Clin Exp Res 1996; 20(5):934–934.
150. Riaz A, Faingold CL. Seizures during ethanol withdrawal are blocked by focal microinjection of excitant amino acid antagonists into the inferior colliculus and pontine reticular formation. Alcohol Clin Exp Res 1994; 18:1456–1462.

151. Butler D, Messiha FS. Alcohol withdrawal and carbamazepine. Alcohol Int Biomed J 1986; 3:113–129.
152. Malcolm R, Ballenger JC, Sturgis ET, Anton R. Double-blind controlled trial comparing carbamazepine to oxazepam treatment of alcohol withdrawal. Am J Psychiatry 1989; 146:617–621.
153. Shreeram SS, Dennison SJ. The future of pharmacologic interventions for addictive disorders. Psychiatr Ann 2001; 31(12):723–728.
154. Myrick H, Malcolm R, Brady KT. Gabapentin treatment of alcohol withdrawal. Am J Psychiatry 1998; 155:1632.
155. Bonnet U, Banger M, Leweke FM, Maschke M, Kowalski T, Gastpar M. Treatment of alcohol withdrawal syndrome with gabapentin. Pharmacopsychiatry 1999; 32:107–109.
156. Karam-Hage M, Brower KJ. Gabapentin treatment for insomnia associated with alcohol dependence. Am J Psychiatry 2000; 157:151.
157. Kranzler HR. Medications for alcohol dependence-new vistas. JAMA 2000; 284(8):1016–1017.
158. Collins FS. Shattuck lecture: medical and societal consequences of the human genome project. N Engl J Med 1999; 341:28–37.
159. Reich T, Edenberg HJ, Goate A, Williams JT, Rice JP, Eerdewegh PV, Faroud T, Hesselbrock V, Schuckit MA, Bucholz K, Porjesz B, Li TK, Conneally M, Nurnberger JI, Tischfield JA, Crowe RR, Cloninger CR, Wu W, Shears S, Carr K, Crosse C, Willig C, Begleiter H. Genome-wide search for genes affecting the risk for alcohol dependence. Am J Med Genet 1998; 81:207–215.
160. Thomasson HR, Edenberg HJ, Crabb DW, Mai XL, Jerome RE, Li TK, Wang SP, Lin YT, Lu RB, Yin SJ. Alcohol and aldehyde dehydrogenase genotypes and alcoholism in Chinese men. Am J Hum Genet 1991; 8:677–681.
161. Shen YC, Fan JH, Edenberg HJ, et al. Polymorphism of ADH and ALDH genes among four ethnic groups in China and effects upon the risk for alcoholism. Alcohol Clin Exp Res 1997; 21:1272–1277.
162. Anthony JC, Helzer JE. E Epidemiology of drug dependence. In. Tsuang MT, Tohen M, Zahner GE, eds. Textbook in Psychiatric Epidemiology. New York: Wiley-Liss, 1995, 361–406.
163. Goldstein A, Herrera J. Heroin addicts and methadone treatment in Albuquerque: a 22-year follow-up. Drug Alcohol Depend 1995; 40:139–150.
164. Hser Y, Anglin MD, Powers K. A 24-year follow-up of California narcotics addicts. Arch Gen Psychiatry 1993; 50:577–584.
165. Rounsaville BJ. Can psychotherapy rescue naltrexone treatment of opioid addiction? NIDA Res Monogr 1995; 150:37–52.
166. Kleber HD. Naltrexone. J Subst Abuse Treat 1985; 2:117–122.
167. Greenstein RA, Fudala PJ, O'Brien CP. Alternative pharmacotherapies for opiate addiction. In: Lowinsohn JH, Ruiz P, Millman RB, Langrod JG, eds. Comprehensive Textbook of Substance Abuse, 3rd ed. New York: Williams & Wilkins, 1997, 415–425.
168. Greenstein RA, Fudala PJ, O'Brien CP. Alternative pharmacotherapies for opiate addiction. In: Substance Abuse: A Comprehensive Textbook. JH Lowinson, P Ruiz, RB Millman, JG Langrod, eds. Baltimore: Williams & Wilkins, 1992, 562–573.
169. Atkinson PL, Berke LK, Drake CR, et al. Effects of long-term therapy with naltrexone on body weight in obesity. Clin Pharmacol Ther 1985; 38:419.
170. Rounsaville BJ. Can psychotherapy rescue naltrexone treatment of opioid addiction? In: Onken LS, Blain JD, eds. Potentiating the Efficacy of Medications. Rockville, MD: National Institute on Drug Abuse, 1995:37-52. NIDA Res Monogr 105.
171. Warner EA, Kosten TR, O'Connor PG. Pharmacotherapy for opioid and cocaine abuse. Med Clin North Am 1997; 81:909–925.
172. Greenstein RA, Arndt IC, McLellan AT, O'Brien CP, Evans B. Naltrexone: a clinical perspective. J Clin Psychiatry 1984; 45(9 Pt 2):25–28.
173. Clinical evaluation of naltrexone treatment of opiate-dependent individuals. Report of the National Research Council Committee on Clinical Evaluation of Narcotic Antagonists. Arch Gen Psychiatry 1978; 35:335–340.
174. San L, Pomarol G, Peri JM, Olle JM, Cami J. Follow-up after a six-month maintenance period on naltrexone versus placebo in heroin addicts. Br J Addict 1991; 86:983–990.
175. Ling W, Wesson DR. Naltrexone treatment for addicted health-care professionals: a collaborative private practice experience. J Clin Psychiatry 1984; 45(9 Pt 2):46–48.
176. Landabaso MA, Iraurgi I, Jimenez-Lerma JM, Sanz, et al. A randomized trial of adding fluoxetine to a naltrexone treatment program for heroin addicts. Addiction 1998; 93:739–744.
177. Budney AJ, Higgins ST. A Community Reinforcement Plus Vouchers Approach: Treating Cocaine Addiction. Rockville, MD: National Institute on Drug Abuse, 1998.
178. Carroll KM, Ball S, Nich C, et al. Targeting behavioral therapies to enhance naltrexone treatment of opioid dependence: efficacy of contingency management and significant other involvement. Arch Gen Psychiatry 2001; 58:755–761.
179. Nestler EJ, Aghajanian GK. Molecular and cellular basis of addiction. Science 1997; 278:58–63.
180. O'Connor PG, Selywn PA, Schottenffeld RS. Medical care for injection drug users with human immunodeficiency virus infection. N Engl J Med 1994; 331:450–459.

181. Dole VP, Nyswander ME, Kreek MJ. Narcotic blockade. Arch Intern Med 1966; 118:304–309.
182. Kreek MJ. Medical safety and side effects of methadone in tolerant individuals. J Psychoact Drugs 1991; 23:232–238.
183. Zweben JE, Payte JT. Methadone maintenance in treatment of opioid dependence. A current perspective. West J Med 1990; 152:588–599.
184. O'Connor LM, Woody G, Yeh HS, et al. Methadone and edema, J Subst Abuse Treat 1991; 8:153–155.
185. Kreek MJ. Drug interactions with methadone in humans. NIDA Res Monogr 1986; 68:193–225.
186. Kreek MJ. Opiate-ethanol interactions: implications for the biological basis and treatment of combined addictive diseases. NIDA Res Monogr 1988; 81:428–439.
187. Iribarne C, Berthou F, Carlhant D, et al. Inhibition of methadone and buprenorphine N-dealkykations by three HIV-1 protease inhibitors. Drug Metab Dispos 1998; 26:257–260.
188. Altice FL, Friedland GH, Cooney EL. Nevirapine induced opiate withdrawal among injection users with HIV infection receiving methadone. AIDS 1999; 13:957–962.
189. Rosen TS, Johnson HL. Long-term effects of prenatal methadone maintenance. Natl Inst Drug Res Monogr Ser 1985; 59:73–83.
190. Gerstein DR, Harwood HJ, eds. Treating Drug Problems, Vol I: A Study of the Evolution, Effectiveness, and Financing of Public and Private Drug Treatment Systems. Washington: National Academy Press, 1990.
191. Hall W, Ward J, Mattick RP. Introduction. In: Ward J, Mattick RP, Hall W, eds. Methadone and Other Opioid Replacement Therapies. Amsterdam: Harwood Academic 1998, 1–14.
192. Dole VP, Nyswander M. A medical treatment for diacetylmorphine (heroin) addiction. A clinical trial with methadone hydrochloride. JAMA 1965; 193:646–650.
193. Strain EC, Stitzer ML. Moderate- vs high-dose methadone in the treatment of opioid dependence. Ann Intern Med 1993; 119:23–27.
194. Strain EC, Bigelow GE, Liebson IA, Stitzer ML. Moderate-vs-high dose methadone in the treatment of opioid dependence: a randomized trial. JAMA 1999; 281:1000–1005.
195. Cooper JR. Ineffective use of psychoactive drugs. Methadone treatment is no exception. JAMA 1992; 267:281–282.
196. Brown BS, Waters JK, Iglehart AS. Methadone maintenance dosage levels and program retention. Am J Drug Alcohol Abuse 1982; 83,8:129–139.
197. Maddux JF, Desmond DP, Vogtsberger KN. Patient-regulated methadone dose and optional counseling in methadone maintenance. Am J Addict 1995; 4:18–32.
198. Newman RG, Whitehill WB. Double-blind comparison of methadone and placebo maintenance treatments of narcotic addicts in Hong Kong. Lancet 1979; 2:485–488.
199. Gunne LM, Gronbladh L. The Swedish methadone maintenance program: a controlled study. Drug Alcohol Depend 1981; 7:249–256.
200. Ball JC, Ross A. The Effectiveness of Methadone Maintenance Treatment: Patients, Programs, Services, and Outcomes. New York: Springer-Verlag, 1991.
201. Newman RG. Methadone treatment. Defining and evaluating success. N Engl J Med 1987; 317:447–450.
202. Sees KL, Delucchi KL., et al. Methadone maintenance vs. 180-day psychosocially enriched detoxification for treatment of opioid dependence: a randomized controlled trial. JAMA 2000; 283(10):1303–1310.
203. Ball JC, Lange WR, Myers CP, Friedman SR. Reducing the risk of AIDS through methadone maintenance treatment. J Health Soc Behav 1988; 29:214–226.
204. Metzger DS, Woody GE, McLellan AT, et al. Human immunodeficiency virus seroconversion among intravenous drug users in-and-out-of-treatment: an 18 month prospective follow-up. J Acquir Immune Defic Syndr 1993; 6:1049–1056.
205. Metzger DS, Navaline H, Woody GE. Drug abuse treatment as AIDS prevention. Public Health Rep 1998; 113(suppl 1):97–106.
206. Novick DM, Joseph H, Croxson TS, et al. Absence of antibody to human immunodeficiency virus in long-term, socially rehabilitated methadone maintenance patients. Arch Intern Med 1990; 150:97–99.
207. Anglin D, McGlothin WH. Outcome of narcotic addiction treatment in California. In: Timms FM, Luford JP, eds. Drug Abuse Treatment Evaluation: Strategies, Progress and Prospect (NIDA Res Monogr 51). Rockville, MD: National Institute on Drug Abuse, 1984, 106–128.
208. Bell J. Mattick RP, Chan J, et al. Methadone maintenance and drug related crime. J Subst Abuse Treat 1997; 9:15–25.
209. Gronbladh L, Ohlund LS, Gunne LM. Mortality in heroin addiction: impact of methadone treatment. Acta Psychiatr Scand 1990; 82(3):223–227.
210. Davoli M, Perucci CA, Forastiere F, et al. Risk factors for overdose mortality: a case control within a cohort of intravenous drug users. Int J Epidemiol 1993; 22:273–277.
211. Kreek MJ. Using methadone effectively: achieving goals by application of laboratory, clinical and evaluation research and by development of innovative programs. In: Pickens RW, Leukefeld CG, Schuster CR, eds. Improving Drug Abuse Treatment. Washington: U.S. Government Printing Office, 1991:245–266. (NIDA Res Monogr 16.)

212. Hubbard RL, Marsden ME, Rachel JV, et al. Drug abuse treatment: a national study of effectiveness. Chapel Hill: University of North Carolina Press, 1989.
213. Bell J, Ward J, Mattick RP, et al. An evaluation of private methadone clinics. Canberra: Australian Government Publishing Service, 1995. (National Drug Strategy Research report No. 4.)
214. Ling W, Compton P. Opiate maintenance therapy with LAAM. In: Stine SM, Kosten TR, eds. New Treatments for Opiate Dependence. New York: Guilford Press 1997, 286.
215. Blaine JD. Early clinical studies of levo-alpha acetylmethadol (LAAM): an opiate for use in the medical treatment of chronic heroin dependence. NIDA Res Monogr 1978; 19:249–259.
216. Jaffe JH, Martin WR. Opioid analgesics and antagonists. In: Goodman and Gilman's The Pharmacological Basis of Therapeutics, 8th ed. AG Gilman, TW Rall, AS Nies, eds.) New York: Pergamon, 1990, 485–521.
217. Physicians' Desk Reference, 51st ed. R Arky, ed. Oradell, NJ: Medical Economics Co., 1997, 2361–2365.
218. Ling W, Charuvastra C, Kaim SC, Klett CJ. Methadyl acetate vs. methadone as maintenance treatments for heroin addicts. A Veteran's Administration cooperative study. Arch Gen Psychiatry 1976; 33:709–720.
219. Senay EC, Dorus W, Renault PF. Methadyl acetate and Methadone. An open comparison. JAMA 1977; 237:138–142.
220. Glanz M, Klawansky S, McAullife W, Chalmers T. Methadone vs. L-alpha-acetylmethadol (LAAM) in the treatment of opiate addiction. A meta-analysis of the randomized controlled trials. Am J Addict 1997; 6:339–349.
221. Eissenberg T, Bigelow GE, Strain EC, et al. Dose-related efficacy of levomethadyl acetate for treatment of opioid dependence. A randomized clinical trial. JAMA 1997; 277:1945–1951.
222. Oliveto AH, Farren C, Kosten TR. Effect of LAAM dose on opiate use in opioid-dependent patients. A pilot study. Am J Addict 1998; 7:272–282.
223. Moore P. LAAM may be a good treatment option for opioid dependency. Lancet 1998; 352:629.
224. Rawson RA, Hasson Al, Huber AM, McCann MJ, Ling W. A 3-year progress report on the implementation of LAAM in the United States. Addiction 1998; 93:533–540.
225. Ling W, Charuvastra C, Collins JF, et al. Buprenorphine maintenance treatment of opiate dependence: a multicenter, randomized clinical trial. Addiction 1998; 93:475–486.
226. Bickel WK, Amass L. Buprenorphine treatment of opioid dependence: a review. Exp Clin Psychopharmacol 1995; 3:477–489.
227. Rance MJ, Dickens JN. The influence of drug-receptor kinetics on the pharmacological profiles of buprenorphine: In: Van Ree JM, Pereniums L, eds. Characteristics and Function of Opioids. Amsterdam: Elsevier, 1978, 65–66.
228. Bickel WK, Stitzer ML, Bigelow GE, Liebson IA, Jasinski DR, Johnson RE. A clinical trial of buprenorphine: comparison with methadone in the detoxification of heroin addicts. Clin Pharmacol Ther 1988; 43:72–78.
229. Walsh SL, Preston KL, Stitzer ML, Cone EJ, Bigelow GE. Clinical pharmacology of buprenorphine: ceiling effects at high doses. Clin Pharmacol Ther 1994; 55:569–580.
230. Jasinski DR, Fudala PJ, Johnson RE. Sublingual versus subcutaneous buprenorphine in opiate abusers. Clin Pharmacol Ther 1989; 45:513–519.
231. Bickel WK, Stitzer ML, Bigelow GE, Liebson IA, Jasinski D, Johnson R. Buprenorphine: dose-related blockade of opioid challenge effects in opioid dependent humans. J Pharmacol Exp Ther 19; 247:47–53.
232. Jasinski DR, Pevnick J, Griffith J. Human pharmacology and abuse potential of the analgesic buprenorphine. Arch Gen Psychiatry 1978; 35:501–516.
233. Petry NM, Bickel WK, Badger GJ. A comparison of four buprenorphine dosing regimens in the treatment of opioid dependence: clinical trial of daily versus alternate-day dosing. Drug Alcohol Depend 1995; 40:27–35.
234. Preston KL, Umbricht A, Huestis MA, Cone EJ. PI-114 intravenous buprenorphine: effects of 2 to 16 mg doses in nondependent opioid abusers. Clin Pharmacol Ther 2001; 69(2):29.
235. Physicians'Desk Reference, 51st ed. R Arky, ed. Oradell, NJ: Medical Economics Co., 1997, 2170–2172.
236. Tracqui A, Kintz P, Ludes B. Buprenorphine-related deaths among drug addicts in France: a report on 20 fatalities. J Anal Toxicol 1998; 22:430–434.
237. Iribarne C, Picart D, Dreano Y, Berthou F. In vitro interactions between fluoxetine or fluvoxamine and methadone or buprenorphine. Fundam Clin Pharmacol Exp Ther 1982; 12:194–199.
238. Mello NK, Mendelson JH, Kuehnle JC. Buprenorphine effects on the human heroin self-administration: an operant analysis. J Pharmacol Exp Ther 1982; 223(1):30–39.
239. Amass L, Bickel WK, Higgins ST, Hughes JR. A preliminary investigation of outcome following gradual or rapid burp detoxification. J Addict Dis 1994; 13:33:33–45.
240. Johnson RE, Eissenberg T. Stitzer ML, Strain EC, Liebson IA, Bigelow GE. A placebo controlled clinical trial of buprenorphine as a treatment for opioid dependence. Drug Alcohol Depend 1995; 40:17–25.

241. Johnson RE, Jaffe JH, Fudala PJ. A controlled trial of buprenorphine treatment for opioid dependence: clinical trial of dailys a treatment for opioid dependence. JAMA 1992; 267:2750–2755.
242. Kosten TR, Schottenfeld R, Ziedonis D, Falcioni J. Buprenorphine versus methadone in the treatment of opioid dependence. J Nerv Ment Dis 1993; 181:358–364.
243. Fudala PJ, Jaffe JH, Dax EM, Johnson RE. Use of buprenorphine in the treatment of opioid addiction. II. Physiologic and behavioral effects of daily and alternate-day administration and abrupt withdrawal. Clin Pharmacol Ther 1990; 47:525–534.
244. Johnson RE, Eissenberg T, Stitzer ML, Strain EC, Liebson IA, Bigelow GE. Buprenorphine treatment of opioid dependence clinical trial of daily versus alternate-day dosing. Drug Alcohol Depend 1995; 40:27–35.
245. O'Connor PG, Oliveto AH, Shi JM, et al. A randomized trial of buprenorphine maintenance for heroin dependence in a primary care clinic for substance users versus a methadone clinic. Am J Med 1998; 105:100–105.
246. Johnson RE, Chutuape MA, Strain EC, et al. A comparison of levomethadyl acetate, buprenorphine, and methadone for opioid dependence. N Engl J Med 2000; 343(18):1290–1297.
247. Kosten T, McCance E. A review of pharmacotherapies for substance abuse. Am J Addict 1996; 5:58–65.
248. Kosten TR. The pharmacotherapy of relapse prevention using anticonvulsants. Am J Addict 1998; 7:205–209.
249. Sofulglu M, Rentel PR, Bliss RL, et al. Effects of phenytoin on cocaine self-administration in humans. Drug Alcohol Depend 1999; 53:273–275.
250. Halikas JA, Crosby RD, Graves N. Double-blind carbamazepine enhancement in the treatment of cocaine abuse. Presented at the Annual Meeting of the American College of Neuropsychopharmacology, San Juan, Puerto Rico, December 1992. (Abstract 231.)
251. Hastukami D, Keenan R, Halikas JA, et al. Effects of carbamazepine on acute responses to smoked cocaine-base in human cocaine users. Psychopharmacology (Berl) 1991; 104:120–124.
252. Klein M. Research issues related to development of medications for treatment of cocaine addiction. Ann NY Acad Sci 1998; 844:75–91.
253. Gawain FH, Riordan C, Kleber H. Methylphenidate treatment of cocaine abusers without attention deficit disorder: a negative report. Am J Drug Alcohol Abuse 1985; 11:193–197.
254. Gawin FH, Kleber HD. Cocaine abuse treatment-open pilot trial with desipramine and lithium carbonate. Arch Gen Psychiatry 1984; 41:903–909.
255. Roache JD, Grabowski J, Schmitz JM, et al. Laboratory measures of methylphenidate effects in cocaine-dependent patients receiving treatment. J Clin Psychopharmacol 2000; 20:61–68.
256. Charnaud B, Griffiths V. Levels of intravenous drug misuse among clients prescribed oral dexamphetamine or oral methadone: a comparison. Drug Alcohol Depend 1998; 52:79–84.
257. Kuhn KL, Halikas JA, Kemp KD. Carbamazepine treatment of cocaine dependence in methadone maintenance patients with dual opiate cocaine addiction. NIDA Res Monogr 95. Proceedings of the College on Problems of Drug Dependence, Washington: Department of Health and Human Services, 1990:316–317.
258. Batki SL, Washburn A, Manfredi LB, Murphy J, Herbst M, Jones TA, Nanda N, Jacob P, Jones RT. Fluoxetine in primary and secondary cocaine dependence: outcome measured by quantitative benzoylecgonine concentration. NIDA Res Monogr Ser 141; NIH Publication No. 94-3749. Washington: National Institutes of Health, 1994:140.
259. Grabowksi J, Roache JD, Schmitz JM, Rhoades H, Creson D, Korszun A. Replacement medication for cocaine dependence. J Clin Psychopharmacol 1997; 17:485–488.
260. Galsor M, Ungard JT, Witkin JM. Preclinical evaluation of newly approved and potential antiepileptic drugs against cocaine-induced seizures. J Pharmacol Exp Ther 1999; 290:1148–1156.
261. Markowitz JS, Finkenbine R, Myrick H, King L, Carson WH. Gabapentin abuse in a cocaine user: implications for treatment? J Clin Psychopharmacol 1997; 17:423–424.
262. Reid MS, Mickalian JD, Delucchi KL, Berger SP. A nicotine antagonist, mecamylamine, reduces cue-induced craving in cocaine-dependent subjects. Neuropsychopharmacology 1999; 20:297–307.
263. Mendelson J, Dearborn AS, Uemura N, et al. PIII-54 pharmacologic interactions between transdermal selegiline and cocaine. Clin Pharmacol Ther 2001; 69(2):77.
264. Levin F, Kleber H. Attention-deficit hyperactivity disorder and substance abuse: relationships and implications for treatment. Harv Rev Psychiatry 1995; 2:246–258.
265. Grabowski J, Rhoades H, Schmitz J, et al. Dextroamphetamine for cocaine-dependence treatment: a double-blind randomized clinical trial. J Clin Psychopharmacol 2001; 21(5):522–526.
266. Grabowski J, Rhoades H, Silverman P, et al. Risperidone for the treatment of cocaine dependence: randomized, double-blind trial. J Clin Psychopharmacol 2000; 20(3):305–310.
267. Carrera MRA, Ashley JA, Parsons LH, Wirsching P, Koob GF, Janda KD. Suppression of psychoactive effect of cocaine by active immunization. Nature 1995; 378:727–730.

268. Ettinger R, Ettinger W, Harless W. Active immunizations with cocaine-protein conjugate attenuates cocaine effects. Pharmacol Biochem Behav 1997; 58:215–220.

269. Kantak KM, Collins SL, Lipman EG, Bond J, Giovanoni K, Fox BS. Evaluation of anti cocaine antibodies and a cocaine vaccine in a rat self-administration model. Psychopharmacology 2000; 148:251–262.

56

Perspectives on the Pharmacological Treatment of Dementia

BRUNO P. IMBIMBO
Chiesi Farmaceutici, Parma, Italy

NUNZIO POMARA
New York University School of Medicine, New York, and Nathan S. Kline Institute for Psychiatric Research, Orangeburg, New York, U.S.A.

I. INTRODUCTION

Alzheimer's disease (AD) is the most frequent cause of dementia in the elderly. Due to its high prevalence, AD is the type of dementia for which the most intensive efforts for the development of pharmacological treatments have been produced. Cholinergic deficits in AD, first demonstrated in 1976 by Davies and Maloney and subsequently replicated, provided the basis for the cholinergic hypothesis of memory dysfunction in AD and led to the marketing of the first effective drug therapy for the treatment of AD. Subsequent progress in the understanding of the pathophysiology of the disease was made in the 1990s and resulted in the so-called amyloid hypothesis and consequently a number of new therapeutic approaches have been developed.

It is estimated that there are currently 4 million people suffering from AD in the United States with associated direct and indirect costs of $100 billion per year. In the next 25 years, the proportion of the elderly population in the United States is expected to increase by ∼ 50%. This will lead to a dramatic rise in the prevalence of AD. Without effective therapeutic interventions, 14 million people are expected to develop AD by the year 2050 [Johnson 2000]. Although the available cholinesterase inhibitors represent a significant therapeutic achievement, there is still an urgent medical need of effective treatments able to interfere with the natural history of the disease. This is theoretically achievable, since typical histopathologic changes of AD begin to appear in the brain of patients many decades before the onset of clinical symptoms [Ohm 1997]. Thus, the present pharmacological research is directed to the identification of drugs able to slow or halt the progression of the disease during earlier, asymptomatic or minimally symptomatic stages. Progress has been limited by our incomplete understanding of the disease and the relatively slow and costly nature of new drug development. Nevertheless, a number of hypothetical mechanisms that are thought to be contributory to disease progression are being tested in the clinic.

Clinical trials for AD have evolved from short-term trials (3–6 months) adequate to test drug effects on symptoms, to longer trials (≥ 1 year) designed to test the ability of treatments to slow the disease process. The hypothesis that early intervention might reduce the prevalence of the disease has recently motivated the launch of trials directed at preventing or delaying the onset of AD. Due to practicality and costs considerations, most current prevention trials are focused on individuals considered at high risk for development of AD over the next 2–6 years. Risk factors are considered missense mutations in amyloid precursor protein, presenilin-1 and presenilin-2 genes, the ε4 allele of apolipoprotein *E* gene, advanced age, positive family history, gender, head trauma, memory complaints, or diminished memory performance on psychometric measures. These trials attempt to intervene while individuals are still asymptomatic or only minimally symptomatic, and are directed at preventing or delaying disease progression to clinically apparent AD.

Treatment of dementia can be divided as symptomatic treatment of cognitive or noncognitive symptoms and the treatment of underlying pathology, including prophylaxis. It should be emphasized, however, that certain approaches may have several effects; they may affect cognitive as well as noncognitive symptoms and theoretically also the underlying disease process. Some of these approaches may be appropriate for more than one type of dementia. This chapter reviews the major treatment strategies that are being pursued in dementia, especially in AD, and include anti-β-amyloid treatments, antiinflammatory drugs, antioxidants, estrogens, and statins.

II. TREATMENT OF ALZHEIMER'S DISEASE

In the AD brain there is selective loss of cholinergic neurons projecting from basal forebrain to cerebral cortex and hippocampus, the critical areas involved in cognition. In 1976, autopsy studies revealed that the activity of choline acetyltransferase, the biosynthetic enzyme for acetylcholine, was reduced in brains from patients with AD. The reduction in choline acetyltransferase activity correlated with the degree of cognitive impairment and senile plaque formation [Perry 1978]. These observations led to the hypothesis that it might be possible to improve memory and cognitive performance in patients with AD by augmenting cholinergic activity in the brain. A number of pharmacological strategies have been attempted to boost the central cholinergic activity of AD patients, the most successful being the development of acetylcholinesterase inhibitors. These agents increase cholinergic transmission by inhibiting the hydrolysis of acetylcholine at the synaptic cleft.

In addition to the dramatic decrease in the cholinergic innervation of cerebral cortex, a number of other neurotransmitters and neuropeptides are also reduced in the brain of patients with AD. These include noradrenaline, serotonin, glutamate, somatostatin, and corticotropin-releasing factor, among others. Although several drugs targeted at a correction of these deficits have been evaluated, only the glutamatergic transmission modulator memantine has been shown to improve symptoms of AD patients, specifically those severely impaired.

A. Acetylcholinesterase Inhibitors

Cholinesterase inhibitors are the only pharmacological agents repeatedly proved to be effective for the treatment of AD in large, double-blind placebo-controlled trials.

1. Approved Cholinesterase Inhibitors

Four acetylcholinesterase inhibitors have been approved by the U.S. Food and Drug Administration (FDA) for treatment of mild to moderate AD: tacrine, in 1993; donepezil, in 1996; and rivastigmine and galantamine, in 2000 (Table 1).

Statistically significant effects compared to placebo in cognitive functions, behavioral symptoms, and activities of daily living have been repeatedly demonstrated for these drugs in studies of generally 6-months' duration. The effects of donepezil on cognitive and functional decline have been also evaluated in two placebo-controlled studies of 1-year duration [Mohs 2001; Winblad 2001].

Although cholinesterase inhibitors have demonstrated statistically significant effects versus placebo in different symptom domains, dramatic clinical response has been observed in only 3–5% of patients. There are no major differences in terms of efficacy among the different drugs. The mean difference between drug and placebo effects on standardized psychometric scales is about 2–4 points on the cognitive subscale of the Alzheimer's Disease Assessment Scale (ADAS-Cog; a 70-point cognitive scale) and 0.2–0.5 points on the Clinician's Interview-Based Impression of Change with Caregiver Input (CIBIC-Plus; a 7-point global scale), or 5–14% of the average value of the scales (Table 1).

The beneficial effects of donepezil have also been recently demonstrated for more severe stages of AD. In a 24-week, placebo-controlled study in 290 AD patients with Mini-Mental State Examination score ranging between 5 and 17 at baseline, significant dif-

Table 1 Cholinesterase Inhibitors Approved by FDA for Treatment of Mild to Moderate Alzheimer's Disease

Drug	Effective dose (mg/day)	Dose frequency	Cognitive effect (ADAS-Cog[a])	Clinical global effect (CIBIC-Plus[a])	Main adverse events	Dropout rate[b]
Tacrine (Cognex)	80–160	QID	1.4–2.2	0.10–0.20	Elevated liver transaminases, nausea, vomiting, diarrhea, anorexia	36–40%
Donepezil (Aricept)	5–10	QD	1.5–2.9	0.28–0.44	Nausea, vomiting, diarrhea, myalgia, anorexia, asthenia	2–12%
Rivastigmine (Exelon)	6–12	BID	1.6–3.7	0.29–0.47	Nausea, vomiting, diarrhea, anorexia, weight loss, dizziness, abdominal pain, asthenia	20%
Galantamine (Reminyl)	16–24	BID	3.1–3.9	0.20–0.34	Nausea, vomiting, anorexia, weight loss, dizziness	5–13%

[a] Treatment differences from placebo based on intention-to-treat analysis; for tacrine a global scale without the caregiver input was used.

[b] Dropout rate in excess to that seen with placebo.

ferences in favor of donepezil on cognitive, functional, and behavioral performance were found (Feldman 2001). Another 6-month, placebo-controlled study indicated that AD patients residing in nursing home facilities treated with donepezil showed cognitive and behavioral responses [Tariot 2001]. In addition, observational studies suggested that cholinesterase inhibitors decrease the risk of nursing home admission but not the risk of death [Lopez 2002].

Although the positive effects of donepezil on cognitive and behavioral symptoms are able to significantly decrease the caregiver burden [Fillit 2000], this does not translate to an improvement of the quality of life (QOL) of the patient [Birks 2000]. On the other hand, the validity of self-ratings of QOL has been questioned for AD patients. A number of preliminary studies have demonstrated that the use of cholinesterase inhibitors results in reductions in the overall costs of care [Foster 1999]. Most health economic studies have focused only on comparison of the costs associated with paying for administering a treatment and the savings produced by postponed institutionalization. However, there is a growing realization that some measures of the QOL or well-being of both patient and caregiver should also be incorporated [Winblad 1999].

The most common adverse effects observed after administration of cholinesterase inhibitors are nausea, vomiting, diarrhea, dizziness, asthenia, and anorexia, symptoms linked to cholinergic overstimulation. These effects are dose related and largely depend on the degree of cholinesterase inhibition. Also important is the rate of onset of cholinesterase inhibition, which depends on the kinetics of enzyme inhibition, the presence and rate of titration, and the pharmacodynamic peak-to-trough fluctuations [Imbimbo 2001]. While the efficacy of different cholinesterase inhibitors is similar, their tolerability profiles differ. For example, the incidence of nausea [in excess of that seen with placebo] at cognitively effective doses ranges from 13–17% with donepezil [10 mg/day] to 37–40% with rivastigmine (6–12 mg/day) [Imbimbo 2001]. Rivastigmine has been associated with weight loss, so monitoring of patient weight is important when using this agent. Unpublished head-to-head comparative trials seem to confirm similar efficacy but better tolerability of donepezil versus rivastigmine and galantamine.

Differences in tolerability profile may be due to the extent of peripheral acetylcholinesterase inhibition needed to reach clinical efficacy. Indeed, while central acetylcholine levels are reduced up to 70% in AD patients [Tohgi 1994], maximal cognitive improvement in AD patients is associated to peripheral acetylcholinesterase inhibition ranging between 40% and 80% [Imbimbo 2001]. Other contributing pharmacodynamic factors are the rates of onset of and fluctuations in acetylcholinesterase inhibition at steady state.

2. New Cholinesterase Inhibitors

A number of new cholinesterase inhibitors are in development. Phenserine, TAK-147, and ganstigmine have reached clinical testing in AD patients.

Phenserine has been shown to protect rats against cognitive deficit induced by cholinergic lesions of basal forebrain. Interestingly, these studies have also evidenced that phenserine is able to inhibit the amyloidogenic pathway of the amyloid precursor protein [APP] processing in both lesioned and naive animals [Shaw 2001]. In particular, it seems that the compound reduces the βAPP protein expression with a posttranscriptional mechanism not associated with the anticholinesterase activity. A recent 12-week, placebo-controlled study in 72 AD patients showed a significant effect of phenserine 10 mg BID on cognitive performance of the patients, as measured by the Cambridge Neuropsychological Test Automated Battery [Kirby 2002].

TAK-147, another reversible inhibitor of acetylcholinesterase, has been described to possess partial antagonistic activity at the muscarinic M1 and M2 receptors [Hirai 1997]. Animal studies have shown that TAK-147 ameliorates learning and memory impairment without producing peripheral side effects [Miyamoto 1996]. In vitro experiments have claimed a nerve growth factor-like neurotrophic activity for TAK-147 [Ishihara 2000]. Although TAK-147 is indicated in Phase III clinical development in Japan, no clinical studies have been published [Mucke 2001].

Ganstigmine [CHF2819] is a novel acetylcholinesterase inhibitor that produces central cholinergic stimulation after oral administration in young and aged animals. Ganstigmine significantly attenuates scopolamine-induced amnesia in a passive avoidance task. Interestingly, in addition to acetylcholine, ganstigmine induces a significant elevation of extracellular concentrations of 5-hydroxytryptamine [Trabace 2000]. The stimulatory effect on central serotonergic functions might have a therapeutic potential for AD patients in whom the cognitive impairment is accompanied by a depressive syndrome [Trabace 2000]. Phase II studies with ganstigmine have shown dose-dependent inhibition of red blood cell cholinesterase activity after oral administration in AD patients. The pharmacodynamic half-life is ~15 h, allowing a once-a-day dosing [Shiovitz 2002].

B. Selective M1 Receptor Agonists

Muscarinic M1 cholinergic receptors are localized in brain regions associated with learning and memory, whereas other types of muscarinic receptors found in the periphery are thought to be responsible for such side effects as salivation, sweating, nausea, and vomiting. Several postsynaptic muscarinic receptor agonists have been developed aiming to counteract the cholinergic deficit associated with AD. Selective M1 agonists might be expected to be therapeutic at doses lower than those producing peripheral cholinergic side effects. A number of selective M1 muscarinic agonists have recently undergone testing in clinical trials. These include xanomeline [Bodick 1997], sabcomeline (Memric), [Loudon 1997], LU 25-109 [Thal 2000], AF102B [Nitsch 2000] milameline [Schwarz 1999], and talsaclidine [Wienrich 2001]. Unfortunately, none of these compounds have yet demonstrated a sufficient efficacy/tolerability balance for regulatory approval. Xanomeline, for example, was evaluated in a randomized, double-blind placebo-controlled trial of mildly to moderately impaired subjects with AD. A significant treatment effect was reported in the highest dose of xanomeline on the ADAS-Cog and CIBIC-Plus. Unfortunately, treatment at the highest dose also was associated with syncope and gastrointestinal side effects, requiring discontinuation of treatment in 52% of patients. It is presently unclear whether drugs of this class will yet emerge as viable treatments for AD. Of the compounds first mentioned, only talsaclidine is still in clinical development.

C. Nicotinic Acetylcholine Receptor Agonists

Nicotinic acetylcholine receptors are decreased in the brains of AD patients. In vitro, nicotinic stimulation is associated with increased presynaptic acetylcholine release. Nicotine has been shown to reverse spatial memory decline in rats with lesion in the medial septal nucleus and to show recovery on memory in aged monkeys. Nicotine also has effects on other transmitters like serotonin, dopamine, or GABA. Although nicotine has been reported to improve cognition in patients with AD [Parks 1996], its serious adverse effects do not allow clinical use. ABT-418, an analog of nicotine with cognition-enhancing properties, was unsuccessful in the clinic and its development has been discontinued [Potter 1999]. Nicotinic agonists, such as GTS-21 [Kem 2000] and SIB-1553A [Terry 2002] and others, are in development. It remains to be seen how they will perform in clinical trials.

D. Other Cholinergic Strategies

There are a number of compounds in development based on the cholinergic enhancement approach. They include XR-543, an acetylcholine release-enhancing agent [Earl 1998]; MKC-231, a choline uptake enhancer [Murai 1994]; and T-588, which stimulates acetylcholine and noradrenaline release [Nakada

2001]. Although these compounds are in clinical development, it is unlikely that they will produce dramatic beneficial effects in AD patients.

E. Adrenergic Compounds

There is evidence suggesting a facilitating role of noradrenaline on acetylcholine effects in the brain. Animal studies have shown that, noradrenergic activation through presynaptic α2-adrenoceptor blockade potentiate the effects of cholinesterase inhibitors on passive avoidance learning in the rat [Camacho 1996]. On the contrary, the presynaptic α2 receptor stimulation with clonidine has been shown to impair choice reaction time performance in healthy volunteers [Jakala 1999b] and disrupts attention and memory in AD patients [Riekkinen 1999]. Besipirdine, a combined α-adrenergic and cholinergic agonist, demonstrated some cognitive efficacy in a 3-month, placebo-controlled trial in 275 AD patients, although it did not affect clinical global rating [Huff 1996]. These data indicate that indirect cholinergic potentiation through postsynaptic adrenergic stimulation produce minor benefits in AD patients.

F. Serotoninergic Compounds

The serotoninergic system plays a complex role in learning and memory by interacting with the cholinergic, glutamatergic, dopaminergic, or GABA-ergic system. Serotonin receptors are primarily located in the septohippocampal complex and the nucleus basalis magnocellularis–frontal cortex. A better understanding of the role played by different serotonin receptor subtypes in learning and memory has been achieved from the availability of highly specific ligands and gene knockout mice [Buhot 2000]. While antagonism of $5HT_3$ receptors with ondansetron revealed ineffective in AD patients [Dysken 1998], animal studies suggest that specific antagonism of $5HT_{1A}$ receptors with WAY-100,635 may have a cognitive potential [Harder 2000]. Most importantly, recent in vitro studies have shown that activation of the human $5HT_4$ receptors stimulates the secretion of the non-amyloidogenic soluble form of the amyloid precursor protein [sAPPα]. Given the neuroprotective and enhancing memory effects of sAPPα, this approach could have some potential for the treatment of AD [Robert 2001]. Indeed, SL65.0102, a selective $5HT_4$ receptor agonist, was shown to improve learning and memory in rodents and is in clinical development [Moser 1998].

G. Excitatory Amino Acid Agonists and Antagonists

Ampakines are substances that enhance the glutamate activity by stimulating AMPA type of glutamate receptors. An ampakine derivative, CX516 (Ampalex), has been shown to improve memory in different animal models. Initial human studies in young and elderly healthy volunteers demonstrated favorable effects on memory functions [Ingvar 1997; Lynch 1997]. CX516 is currently being tested in a 12-week, double-blind placebo-controlled study in AD patients.

The N-methyl-D-aspartate (NMDA) receptor complex is a subtype of glutamate receptor with a complex function in different neurodegenerative diseases. The clinical development of several NMDA receptor antagonists in different clinical indications has been terminated mainly due to the severe psychomimetic adverse effects. Memantine is a non-competitive NMDA-receptor antagonist. It exerts a rapid, voltage-dependent blockade of NMDA receptors and is suggested to allow glutamatergic transmission under physiological conditions and inhibit the excitotoxicity when there is excessive glutamate release [Wenk 1994; Zajaczkowski 1997]. Memantine was found to protect from Aβ-induced neurotoxicity in hippocampus and improve learning in rats [Miguel-Hidalgo 1998]. The initial trials with memantine were short-term and included patients with AD, vascular or mixed dementia. Thus, the apparent benefits described in these studies are difficult to interpret [Jain 2000]. In the past few years, larger placebo-controlled studies have been carried out in moderately severe to severe AD patients and led to the recent approval in Europe for this specific subgroup of AD patients.

D-Cycloserine, a partial agonist at the glycine site of NMDA receptor, was found to facilitate activation of NMDA receptor-ionophore complex in the AD brain [Chessell 1991]. Clinical trials with D-cycloserine in AD produced mixed results with earlier studies at lower doses showing no beneficial effects [Fakouhi 1995] and more recent studies with higher doses, suggesting improvement in memory [Schwartz 1996] and cognition [Tsai 1999]. However, these observations involved a small number of patients and should be confirmed in large, long-term, controlled studies.

H. Antiamyloid Treatments

Neuritic plaques, the characteristic lesions found in the brain of AD patients, are composed mainly of aggregates of a protein with 39–43 amino acid residues known as β-amyloid (Aβ). The Aβ protein is the metabolic product of the processing of a complex transmembrane glycoprotein known as amyloid precursor protein (APP). APP may be processed according two metabolic pathways. In the so-called nonamyloidogenic pathway, the α-secretase enzyme cleaves APP within the Aβ sequence and releases its transmembrane fragment, APPα, which appears to exert neuroprotective activity. In the amyloidogenic pathway, the β-secretase enzyme releases APPβ plus a 12-kDa protein fragment (C99), which in turn is cleaved by the γ-secretase enzyme, giving way to Aβ.

The correlation among Aβ histopathologic lesions, brain cell death and cognitive deficiency in AD represents the so-called Aβ hypothesis of the disease. A number of important observations support this hypothesis:

1. Autopsies performed on the brain of AD patients consistently reveal Aβ deposits [McKhann 1984].

2. All of the dominating autosomic mutations associated with the familial early onset forms of AD are characterized by an overproduction of Aβ42 [Citron 1992; Scheuner 1996; Suzuki 1994; Citron 1997; Borchelt 1996].

3. The formation of Aβ plaques precedes the symptoms of the disease [Lippa 1998] and correlates with the cognitive deficit of AD patients [Naslund 2000].

4. The clearance of Aβ42 in the brain of patients appears to be reduced compared to controls [Motter 1995].

Several therapeutic approaches are being developed based on the amyloid hypothesis of AD. One of these includes selective β-secretase or γ-secretase inhibitors that block the metabolic generation of the Aβ peptide and thus the formation of Aβ plaques. Another approach involves the inhibition of Aβ aggregates with products that modify the secondary structure of the protein or that bind to specific regions of the protein itself. However, the most revolutionary approach is based on Aβ immunization that leads to an increase in the Aβ clearance from brain.

1. β-Secretase Inhibitors

The β-secretase enzyme, termed BACE [β-site-APP-cleaving enzyme], is a transmembrane aspartic protease. The enzyme was firstly characterized at Amgen in 1999 [Vassar 1999]. Later, the enzyme was found to be identical to that under investigation at GlaxoSmithKline (Asp 2) and Oklahoma Medical Research Foundation (memapsin 2). β-Secretase is considered to be a good therapeutic target for the prevention and treatment of AD. The enzyme catalyzes the initial step in Aβ production. The inhibition of β-secretase would shunt APP into the α-secretase pathway increasing the amount of αAPP that is considered to be neuroprotective [Mattson 1993] and to enhance memory and prevent learning deficits [Meziane 1998]. In addition, studies with BACE knockout mice revealed the absence of Aβ production but normal phenotype, suggesting that blocking β-secretase pharmacologically should effectively lower Aβ with minimal side effects [Luo 2001; Roberds 2001].

On the other hand, some concerns are raised by the discovery of a close β-secretase homolog, BACE2, strongly expressed in heart, kidney, and placenta [Bennett 2000]. Mice deficient in BACE2 should clarify the physiological role of this enzyme. In the case of important function of this enzyme, it might be critical to develop agents that selectively block BACE1 over BACE2.

However, despite strong interest and efforts, few inhibitors of β-secretase activity have been described up to now [Wolfe 2001]. Elan reported substrate-based inhibitors that ultimately were used to affinity purify the enzyme [Sinha 1999]. Ghosh and colleagues [2001] have recently reported peptidomimetics (OM99-1 and OM99-2) based on the Swedish mutated sequence of human APP. However, the selectivity of these prototype inhibitors with respect of other human aspartyl protease was poor. Recently, smaller substrate-based β-secretase inhibitors have been described [Tung 2002]. However, peptidomimetic compounds are not orally absorbed and are not able to cross the blood-brain barrier. Still, significant hurdles remain before the development of useful therapies. The recently solved structure of the enzyme-inhibitor complex should facilitate the identification of β-secretase inhibitors in the near future by using rational drug design.

2. γ-Secretase Inhibitors

Despite intense efforts, the γ-secretase enzyme has not yet been purified and cloned. This is mainly because γ-secretase appears to be a multiprotein complex, making its identification through conventional strategies, such as expression cloning, unlikely to succeed. In addition, the enzyme has unusual properties, the most peculiar being its ability to cut in the middle of the transmembrane region of its substrate. How hydrolysis takes place in what is otherwise a water-excluded environment is unclear. However, it has been established that γ-secretase is an aspartyl protease and requires presenilin 1 and 2 for activity that might be the catalytic component of the enzyme complex [Esler 2001].

Whether γ-secretase is a good target for treating AD remains an open question. The enzyme is known to play a role in the activation of an important receptor protein known as Notch. The Notch receptor is involved in cell-fate determinations during embryonic development and in hematopoiesis in adult age. Knockout mice for presenilin-1 do not show γ-secretase activity but die shortly after birth due to interference with Notch signaling [Shen 1997]. Treatment of thymus with γ-secretase inhibitors represses the development of CD8 T cells [Hadland 2001]. On the other hand, current evidence indicates that Notch processing can be blocked down to a certain threshold without affecting Notch signaling [Berezovska 2000]. If so, then Aβ production may be reduced to a substantial degree without untoward effects on Notch. Another source of concern is the increase in the APP C-terminal metabolite C99 generated by γ-secretase inhibition that could impair learning, as shown in transgenic mice overexpressing C99 [Nalbantoglu 1997]. However, the learning deficits in C99 transgenic mice may be due to resultant amyloid deposition [Nalbantoglu 1997].

The first γ-secretase inhibitor described in the literature [MW167] was a substrate-based peptidomimetic [Wolfe 1998]. This compound served as a starting point to develop several other peptidomimetic γ-secretase inhibitors [Esler 2000; Seiffert 2000]. One of these, L-685,458 was identified by screening compounds originally designed against HIV aspartyl protease and displayed a very potent in vitro activity ($IC_{50} = 0.3$ nM) [Shearman 2000]. At the same time, a number of nonpeptidic γ-secretase inhibitors were identified using high throughput screening on whole-cell assay. One of these compounds, DAPT, has been found to reduce Aβ levels in the brains of transgenic mice [Dovey 2001]. Administration of 100 mg/kg DAPT subcutaneously to young transgenic mice expressing mutated human APP (PDAPP) led to 30–50% reduction in total Aβ in several brain regions examined. Importantly, this level of efficacy was maintained after subchronic administration of a similar dose twice daily for 7 days.

Another nonpeptidic γ-secretase inhibitor with a sulfonamide scaffold has been described [May 2001]. Oral administration of this compound markedly decreases levels of total Aβ and Aβ42 in brain, cerebrospinal fluid, and plasma of young transgenic mice expressing mutated human APP (Tg2576). Interestingly, the compound does not seem to affect significantly Notch processing, the in vitro activity on Notch cleavage being 17 times lower than on γ-secretase. Phase I studies in normal volunteers showed a pharmacokinetic profile compatible with a once-daily dosing. The safety and tolerability of the compound after multiple ascending doses for 4 weeks is being evaluated in AD patients [Felsenstein 2002].

3. α-Secretase Activators

The shifting of the APP metabolism to the nonamyloidogenic pathway represents an alternative way to decrease brain Aβ burden in AD patients. Animal studies indicate that the product resulting from the α-secretase cleavage of APP, sAPPα, has potent memory-enhancing effects and block learning deficits induced by scopolamine [Meziane 1998]. Thus, augmenting α-secretase processing of APP to release sAPPα might be beneficial in treating AD.

Although cells contain a certain level of basal α-secretase activity, proteolysis by this enzyme can be increased pharmacologically. M1 and M3 muscarinic agonists have been shown to decrease Aβ levels in neocortex and hippocampus and to increase sAPPα in cerebrospinal fluid of normal and cholinergic denervated rats. The effects on APP processing correlated with cognitive performance of the animals [Lin 1999].

Talsaclidine, a selective M1 agonist, was recently shown in placebo-controlled study in 24 AD patients to decrease by 27% in 4 weeks the levels of total Aβ in cerebrospinal fluid [Hock 2000]. Lowering effects on total Aβ levels in cerebrospinal fluid were also described another selective M1 agonist, AF102B, in 19 AD patients [Nitsch 2000]. Unfortunately, M1-selective agonists are associated with important side effects, the most serious being syncope, which limit their clinical use.

Stimulation of α-secretase can be obtained by direct stimulation of protein kinase C with phorbol esters [Jacobsen 1994]. Activation of receptors that work through protein kinase C can augment α-secretase cleavage of APP as well. Agonists of the metabotropic glutamate receptors can lower Aβ by shunting APP toward the α-secretase pathway [Lee 1995].

4. Inhibitors of β-Amyloid Aggregation

Another strategy to reduce brain amyloid deposition is the development of inhibitors of Aβ aggregation. Aβ aggregation is a complex phenomenon that implies a nucleation and a deposition phase. The block of the initial steps of the formation of Aβ fibrils is an attractive objective, because the neuronal toxicity of Aβ is more linked to the oligomeric and protofibrillar forms than to the amyloid plaques. Interestingly, the initial observation that monoclonal antibodies raised against Aβ peptide inhibit its aggregation has prompted the later development of Aβ immunization strategies [Solomon 1996].

Several small organic molecules, synthetic peptides, and natural proteins have been shown to inhibit Aβ aggregation and neurotoxicity in vitro [Soto 1999]. These compounds include sulfonated dyes [Lorenzo 1994], anthracycline derivatives [Merlini 1995], rifampicin [Tomiyama 1996], porphyrins [Howlett 1997], benzofuran derivatives [Howlett 1999], tetracyclic and carbazole-type compounds [Howlett 1999], melatonin [Pappolla 2000], and a large variety of Aβ-derived peptides [Findeis 2000]. However, the large majority of these compounds have been tested in vitro. Few compounds have been shown to interfere with Aβ fibril formation in vivo and to possess pharmacokinetic characteristics compatible with their use in humans.

The best-documented compound is a pentapeptide (iAβ5) that mimics the 17-21 region of the Aβ peptide. iAβ5 was shown to prevent amyloid neurotoxicity in cell cultures and to reduce the formation of amyloid fibrils in a rat model of cerebral Aβ deposition [Soto 1998]. An end-protected derivative of this pentapeptide (iAβ5p) is able to cross the blood brain barrier and to reach pharmacological levels in the brain. The in vivo pharmacological activity of iAβ5p has been evaluated in double transgenic mice (APP-V717F/PS1-A246E) developing amyloid plaques at 6 months of age. The chronic (8 weeks) intraperitoneal administration of iAβ5p caused a 47% reduction of brain amyloid load and a 24% increase in neuronal survival. The astrocytosis and microglial activation associated with amyloid plaques was also reduced by the peptide treatment [Soto 2001]. Although iAβ5p has shown a good toxicological profile in rodents, its short plasma half-life (37 min) has limited the clinical development of the compound. A metabolic stabilized derivative of iAβ5p is being developed for treatment of AD [Soto 2002].

Histological studies have shown that proteoglycans and their constituent glycosaminoglycans are associated with Aβ deposits. Glycosaminoglycans are not simply involved in the lateral aggregation of fibrils or in nonspecific adhesion to plaques but promote the earliest stage of fibril formation [McLaurin 1999]. A small sulfonated compound (NC-531, Alzhemed) that mimics the anionic properties of glycosaminoglycans has been reported to significantly inhibit Aβ fibril formation and deposition in vitro. In transgenic mice expressing the human APP Swedish mutation (TgCRND8), chronic administration of NC-531 (100 mg/kg for 8 weeks) induced a 61% reduction in Aβ plasma levels and a 30% reduction in number and size of brain Aβ plaques [Gervais 2002]. A decrease of Aβ-associated inflammatory response was also observed. Phase I studies in young and elderly healthy subjects have established that maximum tolerated dose of NC-531 after single oral administration is 200 mg, the main adverse events being nausea, vomiting, dizziness, and headache. Multiple dose Phase I studies are ongoing [Garceau 2002].

PPI-1019 (Apan) is a modified peptide mimicking a particular region of Aβ peptide. It is a potent and selective inhibitor of Aβ polymerization that blocks the formation of neurotoxic species of Aβ. Studies in rats have shown that after intravenous administration, PPI-1019 reaches brain concentrations believed to be sufficient to block Aβ aggregation [Derr 2001]. The in vivo effects of PPI-1019 were studied in a rat model of AD obtained after continuous infusion of Aβ into the lateral ventricles. Compared to vehicle-treated animals, PPI-1019 reduced total Aβ burden in the brain [Harris-White 2001]. Studies in transgenic mice have shown that PPI-1019 significantly increases Aβ levels in the cerebrospinal fluid, suggesting a stimulatory effect of the compound on brain Aβ clearance. The safety and tolerability of PPI-1019 are being tested in healthy volunteers.

It is well known that zinc and copper ions are enriched in Aβ deposits in AD brain and that these heavy-metal ions catalyze the formation of Aβ fibrils in vitro. Clioquinol is a metal ion chelator with high affinity for these metal ions. This compound has been extensively used in the past as an oral antibiotic, but later withdrawn due to its association with subacute myelooptic neuropathy. These toxic effects are apparently due to brain depletion of vitamin B_{12} and believed to be preventable with B_{12} supplementation [Yassin 2000]. In a transgenic mice model of AD (Tg2576), clioquinol, given orally for 9 weeks, significantly decreased (by 49%) brain Aβ deposition [Cherny 2001]. Doses up 80 mg/day for 3 weeks were well tolerated in 30 AD patients [Regland 2001]. Recently a double-blind, placebo-controlled study of 9 months' duration was carried out in 36 AD patients. Clioquinol was administered at increasing oral doses with the concomitant administration of vitamin B_{12}. The study was completed by 32 patients and results indicated that clioquinol consistently decreased serum Aβ levels over time. Compared to placebo, there was a trend at the end of treatment in favor of clioquinol on cognitive performance (ADAS-Cog) that became significant in the 10 patients with severe disease at baseline [Masters 2002]. Although preliminary, this is the first study in AD patients reporting a biologic effect of an anti-β-amyloid agent.

5. β-Amyloid Immunization Approaches

The most revolutionary of the anti-Aβ approaches was proposed in 1999 by scientists at Elan Pharmaceuticals, which immunized against transgenic mice expressing human mutated APP (PDAPP) and spontaneously developing Aβ pathology [Schenk 1999]. The immunization was obtained by subcutaneous injections of a preaggregated form of the synthetic human Aβ42 emulsified with Freund's adjuvant, an immune stimulant. The vaccination caused a near complete inhibition of Aβ plaque formation in younger animals and a marked reduction of the Aβ burden in older animals. The effects on Aβ plaques were accompanied by the reduction of Aβ associated astrogliosis and neuritic dystrophy. These results were later confirmed by other groups [Lemere 2000] with similar vaccination protocols, which also demonstrated that Aβ immunization of transgenic animals normalizes or reduces the cognitive impairment associated to Aβ pathology [Morgan 2000; Janus 2000]. Interestingly, effective removal of brain Aβ plaques was also obtained administering peripherally Aβ antibodies [Bard 2000].

The mechanism with which the vaccine increases Aβ clearance is not fully understood. Centrally, the vaccine appears to activate Aβ phagocytosis by microglial monocytes [Bacskai 2001]. Peripherally, serum Aβ antibodies bind and sequester Aβ, thus altering its equilibrium between CNS and plasma [DeMattos 2001].

A vaccine preparation for human use (AN-1792) composed of preaggregated human Aβ42 peptide and a highly purified saponin derivative (QS-21) was developed by Elan Pharmaceuticals and Wyeth and tested in AD patients. Unfortunately, a Phase IIa study aimed at evaluating the safety and immunological activity of AN-1792 in 360 AD patients was discontinued because 15 subjects receiving the vaccine developed serious signs of CNS inflammation, including fever, headache, vomiting, altered consciousness, muscle weakness, and seizures [Schenk 2002]. Both central activation of cytotoxic T cells and autoimmune reactions were proposed as potential mechanisms of toxicity [Imbimbo 2002].

Other Aβ immunization strategies are being pursued. These include new antigens constituted by conjugation of Aβ fractions (epitopes) with immune carriers [Frenkel 2000; Sigurdsson 2001]. This approach employing nonendogenous proteins should induce a robust immune response without activating autoimmune reactions. Another, alternative strategy includes passive immunization with monoclonal antibodies [Bard 2000] or antibody fragments [Frenkel 2001]. This approach is based on the hypothesis that binding of antibodies to Aβ in plasma creates a peripheral sink which favors efflux of Aβ from the brain. This results in decreased levels of free Aβ in the brain and thus alters the kinetics of deposition favoring the dissolution of preexisting fibrils. This peripheral sink hypothesis should avoid central inflammatory responses.

Whether active or passive Aβ immunization approaches will work in humans is unknown. AD patients could develop tolerance or insufficient or inappropriate antibodies to Aβ antigen injection [Monsonego 2001]. Either active or passive Aβ immunization could provoke an inflammatory response [Grubeck-Loebenstein 2000]. Importantly, Aβ immunization might work effectively at preventing aggregation of amyloid in preasymptomatic patients, but not so well once the amyloid plaques are formed in frank AD patients. Finally, it remains possible that Aβ is not central to neuronal dysfunction and death but is, rather, a byproduct of the disease process. Despite these limitations, the revolutionary development of the first anti-Alzheimer vaccine has raised unprecedented hopes for an affective treatment of this devastating disease. A better understanding of the mechanism whereby Aβ immunization promotes Aβ clearance is needed in order to optimize the initial approach and render it successful in AD patients.

I. Approaches Against τ Hyperphosphorylation

Neurofibrillary tangles, the intracellular hallmark of the AD brain, consist mainly of abnormally phosphorylated τ proteins organized in paired helical filaments. Hyperphosphorylation of τ protein causes impaired neurite outgrowth, disturbed synaptic function, and reduced response to neurotrophic factors [Nuydens 1995]. There is a close correlation between the burden of τ-rich neurofibrillary lesions in selected telencephalic regions of the brain and the dementia severity in AD patients [Lee 1996]. Theoretically, both the inhibition of the kinases responsible for τ hyperphosphorylation and the stimulation of phosphatases able of dephosphorylating aberrant τ may have therapeutic potential [Iqbal 1996]. However, because of the ubiquity and multiplicity of kinases, the inhibition of their activity may impair other cellular functions. Dephosphorylation of τ by stimulation of phosphatases 2A and 2B may represent a better therapeutic option because these enzymes are overexpressed in the AD brain. Both phosphatases 2A and 2B were demonstrated to dephosphorylate protein τ in AD brain [Wang 1996] and phosphatase 2B was also found to dephosphorylate τ in rat brain cortex [Fleming 1995]. The muscarinic M_1 agonist AF150(S) was shown to selectively dephosphorylate the hyperphosphorylated protein τ [Genis 1999]. This effect was associated to a reversal of the cognitive and cholinergic deficits in ApoE-deficient transgenic mice [Fisher 1998], suggesting that muscarinic agonists may offer some therapeutic potential in this regard. It has recently been shown that chronic (4–6 weeks) administration of testosterone is able to prevent the heat shock-induced hyperphosphorylation of τ in female rats [Papasozomenos 2002]. This observation opens perspectives for the use of androgens for prevention or delay of AD.

J. ApoE-Based Approaches

Apolipoprotein E (apoE), a plasma apolipoprotein that plays a central role in lipoprotein metabolism, is localized in the senile plaques, congophilic angiopathy, and neurofibrillary tangles of AD. ApoE ε4 genotype has been found to be associated with a higher risk of AD whereas ApoE ε2 allele may provide protection or delay the onset of the disease. It is not clear the mechanism by which the different ApoE alleles contribute toward accelerating or retarding the disease process. Recent findings suggest that ApoE ε2 and ε3 have greater avidity than ApoE ε4 for the τ protein. Thus, the presence of ApoE ε2 and ε3 proteins may help prevent abnormal phosphorylation of τ [Huang 1994]. In addition, it has been demonstrated that ApoE ε4 allele binds to amyloid plaques and may accelerate Aβ deposition [Strittmatter 1993]. Finally, ApoE ε4 protein does not neutralize efficiently free radicals or ApoE ε2 and ε3 proteins [Miyata 1996]. Taken together, this evidence implies that drugs that alter the production of ApoE ε4 or the clearance of ApoE/Aβ complexes may be useful. Alternatively, therapeutic administration of ApoE ε2 or ε3 alleles through gene therapy or development of ApoE ε2 analogues can be pursued [Strittmatter 1994; Kaplitt 1996].

K. Neurotrophic Agents

Neurotrophic agents represent another potential treatment modality for AD. Neurotrophic factors are proteins that promote the growth and differentiation of neurons in the developing nervous system and promote survival of neurons in the adult.

1. Nerve Growth Factor

Nerve growth factor (NGF) has been considered in the past a very promising neurotrophic treatment for AD. NGF protects the cholinergic neurons from axotomy-induced degeneration [Gage 1988]. Intraventricular NGF infusion reverses the disappearance of axotomized cholinergic neurons in medial septum of adult rats [Hagg 1989] and improves retention of a spatial memory task in aged [Fischer 1987; Markowska 1994] and in lesioned rats [Dekker 1994]. Unfortunately, being a protein, NGF is inactive after oral administration and does not cross the blood brain barrier after intravenous administration. Nasal administration of NGF is not well tolerated. Thus, NGF has been administrated intraventricularly in few AD patients. Although some improvement in verbal episodic memory has been observed, the NGF infusions were associated with reversible back pain and weight loss [Eriksdotter Jonhagen 1998]. The results of these studies suggest that the intraventricular route of administration of NGF is associated with negative side effects that outweigh any potential benefit.

An alternative approach is the use of autologous transplants of skin fibroblasts genetically modified to express NGF. Similar techniques were shown to reverse atrophy of cholinergic neurons in the basal forebrain of aged monkeys [Smith 1999]. A Phase I study of this procedure in eight AD patients is ongoing. Cells are administered by stereotactic injection into the nucleus basalis of Meynert. Patients will be closely monitored for a year and then evaluated annually for an indefinite period. In April 2001, it was announced that the implantation was well tolerated by the first patient, but no efficacy data have been released.

2. AIT-082

AIT-082 (Neotrofin) is a neurotrophic agent under development as a potential treatment for AD. It is a metabolically stable derivative of the purine hypoxanthine and is able to cross the blood brain barrier [Taylor 2000]. In cell cultures, AIT-082 enhances NGF-mediated neurite outgrowth [Middlemiss 1995] and increases levels of synaptophysin, a marker of synaptic numbers and density [Lahiri 2000]. In mice, AIT-082 counteracts age-induced deficits in working memory, although the effect is not significant in animals with severe memory impairment [Glasky 1995]. In rats, AIT-082 decreases mortality and loss of hippocampal neurons induced by kainate administration [Di Iorio 2001]. Animals treated with AIT-082 demonstrate increased neurotrophin messenger RNA for NGF, basic fibroblast growth factor, and neurotrophin-3 in their cortex and hippocampus. The capacity of AIT-082 to selectively stimulate the production of a number of neurotrophins may be the basis of its ability to restore working memory deficits in aged animals.

Phase I studies in healthy volunteers indicated that AIT-082 is well tolerated [Grundman 2000]. However, Phase II double-blind placebo-controlled studies in AD patients employing doses up to 150 mg/day failed to demonstrate significant effects on cognitive performance. Additional trials with higher doses (500–1000 mg/day) are under way.

L. Antioxidants

Abnormal oxidative metabolism appears to be a fundamental process contributing to the neuronal death in AD. Oxidative stress generates free-radical species that damage cell membrane lipids, proteins, and DNA within the brain. A number of specific factors may promote oxidative damage in AD including Aβ deposition, microglia inflammation, abnormal τ hyperphosphorylation, and altered iron metabolism [Butterfield 2001]. The use of antioxidant agents to treat AD is based on their hypothesized neuroprotective properties. Although this is an area with encouraging promises, more controlled clinical trials need to be performed. It is not clear which agents may be effective and in what doses, or whether they may be more effective in combination with other treatments. Importantly, it not known whether antioxidant agents are effective in preventing AD or how many years before disease onset they need to be started to exert a protective effect.

1. Vitamin E

Epidemiologic studies suggest that antioxidant vitamin intake is associated with a lower incidence of cognitive impairment [Perrig 1997] or AD [Morris 1998]. Vitamin E protects neurons against the oxidative cell death caused by Aβ, hydrogen peroxide, and the excitatory amino acid glutamate [Behl 2000]. Vitamin E may provide neuroprotection in vivo through suppression of signaling events necessary for microglial activation [Li 2001]. Long-term (12 months) administration of vitamin E to aged apolipoprotein E-deficient mice significantly improves behavioural performance in the Morris water maze (Veinbergs 2000). In AD patients, supplementation with vitamin E significantly increases the concentrations of this vitamin in plasma and CSF [Kontush 2001]. The potential of vitamin E in AD was evaluated in a double-blind, placebo-controlled clinical trial of 2 years' duration involving 341 patients. Patients received either vitamin E (2000 IU/day), selegiline (10 mg/day), a combination of vitamin E and selegiline, or placebo. An analysis adjusted for baseline cognitive performance of the patients indicated that both vitamin E and selegiline delay progression to a more advanced disease state and subsequent institutionalization [Sano 1997].

The benefit found for vitamin E remains to be confirmed in additional studies. A clinical trial in people with mild cognitive impairment is under way to determine if vitamin E can prevent or delay a diagnosis of AD [Grundman 2000b]. Finally, the role of vitamin E together with vitamins A and C in the prevention of dementia and cognitive decline is also being evaluated within a large double-blind randomized controlled trial (the Heart Protection Study) in 20,500 cognitive normal subjects [Collins 2002].

2. Ginkgo Biloba

Ginkgo biloba extract is approved in Germany for the treatment of dementia and is available in many countries, including the United States, as a dietary supplement. Flavonoids and terpenoids that are present in ginkgo extracts are believed to have antioxidant and free radical–scavenging properties. Ginkgo extracts also contain ginkgolide B, a platelet aggregation inhibitor. In preclinical studies, a plethora of pharmacological effects have been attributed to ginkgo biloba, including reversal of age-related loss of muscarinic receptors, protection against ischemic neuronal death, increase of hippocampal high-affinity choline uptake, inhibition of the downregulation of hippocampal glucocorticoid receptors, enhancement of neuronal plasticity, and counteraction of the cognitive deficits induced by stress or traumatic brain injury [DeFeudis 2000].

In a 52-week, placebo-controlled trial in 309 AD patients, a modest benefit was reported for a particular extract of ginkgo biloba [EGb 761] at the dose of 40 mg TID [Le Bars 1997]. Fewer than half of the patients completed the trial. The modest cognitive improvement produced by the ginkgo biloba extract (1.4 points on the ADAS-Cog) was detected by the caregiver but not by the clinician. The incidence of adverse events with ginkgo was similar to placebo. In a post hoc analysis, the beneficial effects of ginkgo biloba seemed to be greater in patients with very mild to mild cognitive impairment at baseline [Le Bars 2002].

In another, 26-week, placebo-controlled study in 214 patients with either AD or vascular dementia or age-associated memory impairment, neither standard (120 mg/day) or high (240 mg/day) doses of EGb 761 showed significant effect on all the outcome measure of efficacy [Van Dongen 2000].

A dementia prevention trial in ∼ 3000 elderly individuals is being performed. This double-blind, placebo-controlled trial will follow subjects every 6 months for 5 years and determine whether ginkgo, at a dose of 240 mg/day, can reduce the incidence of dementia compared to placebo-treated subjects.

3. Idebenone

Idebenone is a benzoquinone derivative, structurally similar to coenzyme Q, with antioxidant and free radical scavenging properties. In vitro, idebenone protects cell membranes from lipid peroxidation [Bruno 1994; Wieland 1995] and neuronal cells against glutamate- and Aβ-induced neurotoxicity [Hirai 1996]. In vivo, idebenone stimulates synthesis of nerve growth factor and improves behavior in aged and basal forebrain-damaged rats [Nitta 1994]. Clinical trials with idebenone in AD patients produced conflicting results. Studies carried out in Germany reported beneficial effects on cognitive, noncognitive, and overall measures [Weyer 1997; Gutzmann 1998, 2002]. On the other hand, 1-year studies in the United States were suspended because of lack of sufficient efficacy [Grundman 2000]. Indeed, a number of methodological flaws (inadequate control groups, high dropout rates, lack of effects on global measures) characterize the studies carried out in Europe.

M. Anti-Inflammatory Agents

The brain in AD shows a chronic inflammatory response characterized by activated glial cells and increased expression of cytokines, complement factors, and acute-phase proteins surrounding amyloid deposits [McGeer 2001]. Inflammatory cytokines appear to directly interfere with APP processing and deposition of Aβ fibrils [Blasko 2000]. Anti-inflammatory approaches to AD are based on the idea that suppression of these mechanisms will lessen the rate of disease progression [Aisen 1994].

1. Glucocorticoids

Glucocorticoids suppress the acute-phase response and complement activation. A 1-year, double-blind, placebo-controlled trial of low doses of prednisone (10 mg daily) in 138 AD patients did not show any significant difference in cognitive decline between the prednisone and placebo treatment groups [Aisen 2000]. Patients treated with prednisone displayed a greater behavioral decline than those in the placebo group. These negative effects may be due ascribed to the dose of prednisone insufficient to suppress brain inflammatory activity or to potential hippocampal toxicity, previously described for glucocorticoids. Whatever the reasons, safety issues do not permit to test the hypothesis that higher doses of glucocorticoids may be effective in AD patients.

2. Nonsteroidal Anti-Inflammatory Drugs

Epidemiological studies have documented a reduced prevalence of AD among users of nonsteroidal anti-inflammatory drugs (NSAIDs), although not all studies are consistent. A recent population-based cohort study of 6989 subjects found a relative risk of AD of 0.95 in subjects with short-term use of NSAIDs, 0.83 in those with intermediate use, and 0.20 in those with long-term use. The use of NSAIDs was not found to be associated with a reduction in the risk of vascular dementia [in t' Veld 2001]. Thus, it seems that the long-term use of NSAIDs may protect against AD.

Recent studies indicate that the protective effects of NSAIDs may be independent from their anti-inflammatory activity but are linked to their ability to interfere with APP metabolism [Weggen 2001]. Specifically, ibuprofen, indomethacin, and sulindac were shown to inhibit the secretion of Aβ42 peptide in a variety of cultured cells. This effect was not seen in other NSAIDs and seems to be mediated by inhibition of γ-secretase. These observation were confirmed in vivo, where short-term administration of ibuprofen to transgenic mice expressing mutant human APP (Tg2576) lowered their brain levels of Aβ42 [Weggen 2001]. Other studies in transgenic animal models of AD (Tg2576) confirmed that chronic oral ibuprofen administration decreases the number and total area of Aβ deposits [Lim 2000] and ameliorates associated behavioral deficits [Lim 2001]. Finally, a nitric oxide–releasing derivative of flurbiprofen (NCX-2216), dramatically reduces both Aβ loads in doubly transgenic APP plus presenilin-1 mice [Jantzen 2002].

In AD patients, indomethacin (100–150 mg/day) was reported to slow cognitive decline in a 6-month, double-blind, placebo-controlled study [Rogers 1983]. However, the study involved only 44 patients, and many patients dropped out due to adverse events. Nonsignificant trends in favor of diclofenac (50 mg/day), coadministered with the gastroprotective misoprostol, were reported in a 6-month, double-blind, placebo-controlled study in 41 AD patients [Scharf 1999]. Again, the withdrawal rate was high in the active treatment group (12 of 24 patients), indicating that AD patients poorly tolerate standard prescription doses of NSAIDs.

The ability of the hydroxychloroquine to delay progression of AD was recently evaluated in an 18-month, double-blind, placebo-controlled study [Van Gool 2001]. Hydroxychloroquine is a potent anti-inflammatory drug widely used in the treatment of rheumatoid arthritis and able to cross the blood brain barrier [O'Dell 1998]. The study involved 168 patients and was completed by 92% of participants. Unfortunately, at the end of the 18-month treatment period there were no significant differences in the outcome measures of efficacy (activities of daily living, cognitive function, and behavioral abnormalities).

These results suggest that different NSAIDs may have different efficacy in AD patients depending to their specific chemical structure and ability to interfere with APP metabolism. However, it may be possible that anti-inflammatory treatment does not prevent further deterioration after a diagnosis of AD has been established.

3. Cyclo-oxygenase-2 Inhibitors

In brain, cyclo-oxygenase-2 (COX-2), the inducible isoform of cyclo-oxygenase, is selectively expressed in neurons of the cerebral cortex, hippocampus, and amygdala [McGeer 2000]. COX-2 is upregulated in the AD brain, and its expression in the hippocampal formation increases as the disease progresses [Ho 2001]. Transgenic mice overexpressing COX-2 show memory dysfunction, neuronal apoptosis, and astrocytic activation in an age-dependent manner [Andreasson 2001]. These studies suggest that COX-2 may contribute to the neurodegeneration occurring in AD brains and that inhibition of COX-2 may be a useful therapeutic target. COX-2 inhibitors would appear to be preferred agents over classic NSAIDs, given their better tolerability at full anti-inflammatory doses. Unfortunately, a 1-year, double-blind placebo-controlled study with the COX-2 inhibitor celecoxib (Celebrex) failed to demonstrate efficacy in slowing cognitive decline of AD patients [Sainati 2000]. Another 1-year, double-blind placebo-controlled study is ongoing in ~300 AD patients to compare the ability of rofecoxib (Vioxx), another COX-2 inhibitor, and naproxen in slowing cognitive deterioration [Grundman 2000].

N. Estrogens

A number of epidemiological studies suggest a protective effect of estrogen on development of AD. A meta-analysis of most of these observational studies indicated a 29% decreased risk of developing dementia among estrogen users [Yaffe 1998]. Several mechanisms have been suggested to explain how estrogens may affect neuropsychologic function [Yaffe 2001]. One mechanism is the modulation of neurotransmitters, particularly acetylcholine. Another possible mechanism is by promoting neuronal growth. In addition, estrogens may protect neurons by inducing vasodilatation, reducing platelet aggregation, or limiting oxidative stress-related injury induced by excitotoxins and Aβ. Finally, estrogen could reduce the risk of AD in humans via apolipoprotein E alterations.

Several open-label clinical trials and one placebo-controlled study [Asthana 1999] reported cognitive improvement in women with dementia who were receiving estrogen replacement therapy. These studies were all of brief duration and with relatively few subjects. Three larger controlled trials produced negative results. A 12-month, double-blind placebo-controlled study with two doses (0.625 and 1.25 mg/day) of conjugated equine estrogens (Premarin) was conducted in 120 hysterectomized women with AD [Mulnard 2000]. No differences were observed between the treatment groups in clinical global measure of efficacy. Deep-vein thrombosis was observed in four of the women assigned to estrogen (~5% incidence). A smaller, 16-week, placebo-controlled study of conjugated equine estrogens (1.25 mg/day) involving 42 women with AD similarly failed to find a beneficial effect for estrogen therapy [Henderson 2000]. Another, 12-week, placebo-controlled study in 50 female AD patients of conjugated estrogen (1.25 mg/day) did not show meaningful differences on all the outcome measures of efficacy between treatment groups. However, a recent 8-week, placebo-controlled study employing high doses (0.10 mg/day) of 17 β-estradiol in 20 postmenopausal women with AD showed significant effects of estrogen treatment on attention and on verbal and visual memory scales. Although the results of this small study must be extended to larger trials, it may be possible that high doses of estrogens are needed to produce significant benefits in AD patients.

Two prevention trials are under way to determine whether estrogen can prevent the onset of dementia in cognitively normal postmenopausal women. The first is an ancillary study, the Women's Health Initiative Memory Study [WHIMS] of the Women's Health Initiative Randomized Trial [Shumaker 1998]. This ancillary study will determine the effect of hormone replacement therapy on cognitive function and risk of developing dementia in ~ 8000 postmenopausal women treated for 10 years. The other prevention trial, Preventing Postmenopausal Memory Loss and AD with Replacement Estrogen (PREPARE), is enrolling ~ 1000 older women with a family history of AD. This study will determine whether women who are randomized to receive estrogen for 3 years have less risk of developing AD than those receiving placebo [Yaffe 2001].

O. Cholesterol-Lowering Agents

Statins are inhibitors of 3-hydroxy 3-methylglutaryl coenzyme A (HMG Co-A) reductase and are used to lower elevated low-density lipoprotein (LDL) cholesterol levels. Three epidemiological studies have recently found an association between statin therapy and a reduction in the occurrence of AD by as much as 70% [Wolozin 2000; Jick 2000; Rockwood 2002]. In addition, an observational study of 1037 postmenopausal women with coronary heart disease has shown that high LDL and total cholesterol levels are associated with cognitive impairment and that statin users have a trend for a lower likelihood of cognitive impairment [Yaffe 2002]. Although the association between statins and AD is still controversial [Muldoon 2001; Lesser 2001], these observations suggest that lipids may play an important role in the development of AD. Indeed, a known risk factor for AD, the ε4 allele of apolipoprotein E, also plays a role in cholesterol processing. In addition, many preclinical and some preliminary clinical studies indicate that statins may lower levels of Aβ through a stimulation of the nonamyloidogenic α-secretase cleaved of APP [Kojro 2001].

1. Lovastatin

Lovastatin reduces Aβ secretion in cell cultures of hippocampal and cortical neurons [Simons 1998; Fassbender 2001] and in APP-transfected human embryonic kidney cells [Frears 1999]. Lovastatin decreases brain cholesterol in normal mice but not in ApoE-deficient animals [Eckert 2001], suggesting that the effects of lovastatin are mediated by interaction with apolipoprotein E. In a 3-month, placebo-controlled study, human subjects with elevated LDL cholesterol received 10, 20, 40, or 60 mg once-daily doses of a controlled-release formulation of lovastatin (ADX-159, Altocor). Lovastatin dose-dependently reduced serum concentrations of Aβ [Friedhoff 2001]. The study did not measure cognitive impact, but these results support the need for further studies in AD patients.

2. Simvastatin

Simvastatin has been shown to reduce intracellular and extracellular levels of Aβ42 and Aβ40 peptides in primary cultures of hippocampal neurons and mixed cortical neurons [Fassbender 2001]. Guinea pigs treated with high doses of simvastatin showed a strong and reversible reduction of cerebral Aβ42 and Aβ40 levels in the cerebrospinal fluid and brain homogenate [Fassbender 2001]. A recent study in hypercholesterolemic patients demonstrated that chronic administration of simvastatin (80 mg/day) is able to lower by 53% circulating levels of brain-derived 24S-hydroxycholesterol [Locatelli 2002]. This study suggests that the simvastatin may reduce cholesterol turnover in the brain.

The ability of simvastatin to prevent dementia and cognitive decline is being tested in a large study (the Heart Protection Study) in which 20,500 subjects will receive for > 5 years 40 mg/day of the statin [Collins 2002].

3. Atorvastatin

A placebo-controlled study is ongoing to evaluate the role of atorvastatin in AD. The trial will enroll 120 patients with mild to moderate AD who will receive either 80 mg/day atorvastatin or placebo for 1 year. Results are expected in 2003 [Sparks 2002].

4. Other Approaches

Other approaches interfering with cholesterol metabolism are being explored as potential treatments of AD. Inhibition of 7-dehydrocholesterol delta-7 reductase, the enzyme catalyzing the last step of cholesterol biosynthesis, with BM15.766 produced a strong reduction of brain Aβ peptides and Aβ load in APP transgenic mice [Refolo 2001]. Inhibitors of acyl-coenzyme A:cholesterol acyltransferase, the enzyme that catalyzes the formation of cholesteryl esters, have been shown to inhibit the generation of Aβ through the control of the equilibrium between free cholesterol and cholesteryl esters [Puglielli 2001].

III. TREATMENT OF BEHAVIORAL SYMPTOMS

In addition to cognitive and functional decline, behavioral disturbances such as agitation, apathy, anxiety, aggression, disinhibition, and psychoses are frequently evident in AD patients. Such neuropsychiatric symptoms are the source of considerable patient and caregiver distress, and represent a major factor in the decision to transfer the care of patients into nursing homes.

Effectiveness of psychotropic medications in treating psychosis and behavioral symptoms in patients with AD has not been properly evaluated so far, and is being examined in conjunction with a federally funded project [Schneider 2001]. The existing literature consists mainly of clinical series and case reports, making interpretations of the efficacy of individual medications difficult. The few placebo-controlled studies have a small number of patients, showing at best very modest efficacy for study medication. Only in the last few years have a number of well-designed studies with large sample size been carried out.

The principal treatable behavioral disturbances in AD are agitation, psychosis, depression, anxiety, and insomnia. A variety of psychotropic medications can be used to treat these disturbances (Table 2). However, some of these medications, such as the benzodiazepines, can worsen the cognitive symptoms and lead to postural instability and gait disturbances which can result in falls and other serious adverse events [Pomara 1989, 1998]. In the past few years it appears evident that cholinesterase inhibitors, in addition to treating the cognitive deficits, possess favorable effects on behavioral symptoms of AD patients. They reduce particularly apathy and visual hallucinations, and in some cases a variety of other neuropsychiatric symptoms. The beneficial response is most likely mediated through limbic cholinergic structures [Cummings 2000].

Table 2 Psychotropic Medications Commonly Used for the Treatment of Neuropsychiatric Symptoms in Alzheimer's Disease

Class of symptom	Medication	Usual daily dose (range)
Delusions	Risperidone	1 mg (0.5–1.5 mg)
	Olanzapine	5 mg (5–20 mg)
	Quetiapine	200 mg (100–300 mg)
	Ziprasidone	40 mg (20–80 mg)
	Haloperidol	1 mg (0.5–3 mg)
Agitation/aggression	Risperidone	1 mg (0.5–1.5 mg)
	Olanzapine	5 mg (5–10 mg)
	Quetiapine	200 mg (100–300 mg)
	Ziprasidone	40 mg (20–80 mg)
	Haloperidol	1 mg (0.5–3 mg)
	Carbamazepine	400 mg (200–1200 mg)
	Divalproex	500 mg (250–3000 mg)
	Trazodone	100 mg (100–400 mg)
	Propranolol	120 mg (80–240 mg)
	Buspirone	15 mg (15–30 mg)
Depression	Citalopram	20 mg (10–30 mg)
	Sertraline	50 mg (50–200 mg)
	Fluoxetine	40 mg (20–80 mg)
	Nortriptyline	50 mg (50–100 mg)
	Venlafaxine	100 mg (50–300 mg)
	Mirtazapine	15 mg (7.5–30 mg)
Anxiety	Oxazepam	30 mg (20–60 mg)
	Lorazepam	1 mg (0.5–6 mg)
	Buspirone	30 mg (15–45 mg)
	Propranolol	120 mg (80–240 mg)
Insomnia	Trazodone	100 mg (50–200 mg)
	Zolpidem	10 mg (5–10 mg)
	Temazepam	20 mg (15–30 mg)
	Zaleplon	10 mg (5–20 mg)

A. Antipsychotics

Agitation and psychosis are common in AD. Psychosis has a cumulative incidence of ~50% and is manifested by delusions and less frequently by hallucinations. Benzodiazepines were frequently used in the past. Now the use of these drugs has declined since it was recognized that these medications often exacerbate behavioral disturbances and can produce marked cognitive toxicity. Sedating medications are frequently used in institutional environments to ease patient management by hospital staff. However, these medications have negative effects on patient movements, increasing the risk of falls and subsequent medical complications. Conventional neuroleptics such as haloperidol reduce psychotic symptoms but have a greater risk of inducing extrapyramidal side effects including parkinsonism and tardive dyskinesia. Atypical antipsychotics such as risperidone and olanzapine have been specifically evaluated in AD patients with controlled studies. They are the treatment of choice for patients manifesting psychotic symptoms because they cause less severe adverse events, especially extrapyramidal symptoms.

1. Haloperidol

Haloperidol is the most commonly used antipsychotic in AD. Since 1986, several small trials of haloperidol in AD patients have been published. The first relatively large double-blind, placebo-controlled study that evaluated the antipsychotic effects of haloperidol was published in 1998 [Devanand 1998]. This was a 12-week, placebo-controlled, crossover study comparing haloperidol at standard (2–3 mg/day) and low (0.50–0.75 mg/day) doses in 71 outpatients with AD. Standard-dose haloperidol was efficacious and superior to both low-dose haloperidol and placebo for scores on the Brief Psychiatric Rating Scale psychosis factor and on psychomotor agitation. However, moderate to severe extrapyramidal signs were observed more frequently with the haloperidol standard dose than with other treatments.

Another 16-week, double-blind placebo-controlled study compared the effects of haloperidol, trazodone, and behavior management techniques on agitation in 149 AD outpatients [Teri 2000]. Although there was a trend in favor of haloperidol compared to placebo in improving agitation, no significant differences were detected in all outcome measures of efficacy between treatment groups. Significantly fewer adverse events of bradykinesia and parkinsonian gait were evident in the behavior management techniques arm.

These studies indicate the modest behavioral effects of haloperidol in AD patients and point out its narrow therapeutic window.

2. Risperidone

Risperidone is an atypical antipsychotic that has been specifically evaluated in AD patients. A 12-week, double-blind placebo-controlled study was conducted in 625 institutionalized AD patients to evaluate the effects of different doses of risperidone on psychotic and behavioral symptoms [Katz 1999]. The higher doses of risperidone (1 and 2 mg/day) were superior to placebo in reducing total scores of behavioral symptoms on the BEHAVE-AD scale. The dose of 0.5 mg/kg significantly reduced aggression score. Adverse events were dose related and included extrapyramidal symptoms, somnolence, and mild peripheral edema. The frequency of extrapyramidal symptoms in patients receiving 1 mg/day of risperidone was not significantly greater than in placebo patients.

The effects of flexible dose of risperidone (0.5–4 mg/day) on behavioral symptoms of dementia were compared with that of haloperidol in a 13-week double-blind placebo-controlled study involving 344 patients [De Deyn 1999]. Both risperidone and haloperidol significantly reduced (compared to placebo) behavioral symptoms, particularly aggression. Frequency of extrapyramidal symptoms with risperidone did not differ significantly from that of placebo and was less than that of haloperidol.

Thus, risperidone appears effective in controlling agitation in patients with dementia and has a relatively benign adverse-effect profile, but more clinical trials are needed to elucidate its role for this indication [Falsetti 2000].

3. Olanzapine

Olanzapine is another atypical antipsychotic. The effects of olanzapine on psychosis and behavioral symptoms of AD were assessed in a 6-week, double-blind placebo-controlled study in 206 nursing home patients [Street 2000]. Patients were randomly assigned to placebo or a fixed dose of 5, 10, or 15 mg/day of olanzapine. Low-dose olanzapine (5 and 10 mg/day) produced a significant improvement compared with placebo on agitation, aggression, hallucinations, and delusions as assessed by the Neuropsychiatric Inventory Nursing Home Scale. The low dose of olanzapine [5 mg/day] positively affected (compared with placebo) the behavioral disturbance–associated distress of caregivers. Somnolence and gait disturbance were the most frequent adverse events of olanzapine. No significant cognitive impairment, increase in extrapyramidal symptoms, or central anticholinergic effects were found at any olanzapine dose relative to placebo.

Another double-blind, placebo-controlled study evaluated the efficacy of rapid-acting intramuscular olanzapine in treating acute agitation associated with AD and/or vascular dementia [Meehan 2002]. Both olanzapine (5 mg) and lorazepam (1 mg) showed superiority to placebo on the Cohen-Mansfield Agitation Inventory, but the effect of olanzapine appeared long-lasting. Drug treatments were well tolerated.

These studies indicate that that olanzapine (5 and 10 mg/day) is effective and relatively well tolerated in AD patients with agitation/aggression and psychosis. However, controlled studies of longer duration such as the ongoing NIMH CATIE trial [Schneider 2001] will provide data on the long-term efficacy and safety of olanzapine and other atypicals in the treatment of psychosis and behavioral disturbances associated with AD.

B. Antidepressants

Several studies have demonstrated marked atrophy of serotonin-containing neurites and serotonin uptake sites in AD brain. Depressive symptoms are frequent in AD, occurring in as many as 50% of individuals. Major depression is more unusual, occurring in 6–10% of patients with AD. Depression exacerbates functional disability in patients with dementia. Treatment of depressive symptoms in AD commonly utilizes selective serotonin reuptake inhibitors such as sertraline, citalopram, or fluoxetine. Alternatively, tricyclic antidepressants with few anticholinergic side effects such as nortriptyline or combined noradrenergic and serotonergic reuptake inhibitors such as venlafaxine have been utilized. Few double-blind, placebo-controlled trials have established the efficacy of antidepressants in the treatment of mood symptoms in AD.

1. Paroxetine

Paroxetine is the most commonly prescribed selective serotonin reuptake inhibitor (SSRI) in AD patients. Paroxetine and nortriptyline were compared in a 12-week, double-blind study of 116 elderly psychiatric patients who presented with a major depressive episode or melancholic depression [Mulsant 2001]. There were no significant differences between the rates of response of the paroxetine and nortriptyline groups (55% vs. 57%), but the discontinuation rate due to side effects was significantly lower with paroxetine than with nortriptyline (16% vs. 33%). Thus, although paroxetine shows efficacy similar to that of tricyclic antidepressants, it appears to be better tolerated.

2. Trazodone

Trazodone is commonly used when sedation is needed to aid in sleep or manage agitation. A 9-week, double-blind study compared the trazodone and haloperidol in 28 patients with dementia and agitated or aggressive behaviors [Sultzer 2001]. Cohen-Mansfield Agitation Inventory scores improved in each treatment group. In the trazodone treatment group, improvement in agitation was higher in patients with higher depressive symptoms at baseline. Mild depressive symptoms in patients with dementia and agitated behavior were associated with greater behavioral improvement by trazodone-treated patients. However, the hypothesis that trazodone corrects behavioral and affective disturbance induced by serotonin depletion in AD requires confirmation in double-blind placebo-controlled trials.

3. Citalopram

There are many trials evaluating the antidepressant effects of citalopram in demented patients, but most of them are open label studies. Unfortunately, the controlled studies involved heterogeneous patient populations and employed short-term observation periods. In a 4-week, double-blind placebo-controlled study, the efficacy of citalopram was investigated in 98 patients with AD or vascular dementia [Nyth 1990]. AD patients treated with citalopram showed a significant improvement, compared to placebo, in emotional bluntness, confusion, irritability, anxiety, fear/panic, depressed mood, and restlessness.

There were no significant improvements in patients with vascular dementia. Citalopram was associated with few and mild side effects. Another double-blind, placebo-controlled study of 6-weeks' duration involved 149 depressed elderly patients with or without dementia [Nyth 1992]. Patients treated with citalopram improved more than those on placebo on both depression and clinical global scales. A 12-week, double-blind study compared citalopram (20–40 mg/day) and mianserin (30-60 mg/day) in 336 elderly depressed patients with or without dementia [Karlsson 2000]. Demented patients treated with the two drugs showed similar improvements on the Montgomery-Asberg Depression Rating Scale. Fatigue and somnolence were more frequent with mianserin, while insomnia was more frequent with citalopram. In a double-blind, placebo-controlled study involving 85 nondepressed patients undergoing short-term hospitalization, the acute effects of citalopram on psychotic symptoms and behavioral disturbances were compared to those of the neuroleptic perphenazine [Pollock 2002]. Patients treated with citalopram showed significantly greater improvement in the total Neurobehavioral Rating Scale score and in agitation/aggression scores.

4. Sertraline

Initial studies with sertraline in dementia involved patients with advanced stage of disease. An open study in 10 severely impaired AD patients found encouraging effects of sertraline on food refusal [Volicer 1994]. However, an 8-week, double-blind placebo-controlled study in 31 female nursing home patients with late-stage AD failed to show significant effects of sertraline on objective scales of depression, although differences on the "knit-brow" facial measure approached statistical significance [Magai 2000]. Another 12-week, double-blind placebo-controlled study in 22 AD patients evaluated the efficacy and safety of sertraline in the treatment of major depression [Lyketsos 2000]. Patients given sertraline had significantly greater mean declines from baseline in the Cornell Scale for Depression in Dementia scores.

5. Fluoxetine

Again, for fluoxetine there are few and small controlled studies in patients with dementia. A recent double-blind, placebo-controlled study in 41 AD patients with major or minor depression, failed to show a significant effect of fluoxetine (40 mg/day) on Hamilton Depression Scale scores [Petracca 2001]. Complete remission of depression was found in 47% of patients treated with fluoxetine and in 33% of subjects treated with placebo, the difference not being significant. Another, 6-week, double-blind study comparing the effects of fluoxetine and amitriptyline on major depression in 37 AD patients did not show significant differences between the two drugs [Taragano 1997]. However, more patients on amitriptyline than on fluoxetine failed to complete the study (58% vs. 22%). Finally, a small double-blind placebo-controlled study comparing fluoxetine and haloperidol on reduction of agitation in 15 AD patients did not show significant differences compared to placebo [Auchus 1997].

C. Anxiolytics

Anxiety is a common symptom in AD, present in 40–50% of individuals at some point in the course of the illness. Most patients do not require pharmacologic treatment of anxiety. For those requiring pharmacologic management, benzodiazepines are best avoided, given their potential adverse effects on cognition. Nonbenzodiazepine anxiolytics such as buspirone are preferred. Although the efficacy of buspirone has been well documented in generalized anxiety disorder, no placebo-controlled trials have been conducted with this agent in demented patients [Apter 1999].

D. Hypnotics

Insomnia occurs at some point in the course of the illness in many patients with AD. Patient insomnia may disturb the sleep of caregivers, thus increasing the family burden. Although few well-designed studies have been conducted, specific management strategies are recommended mainly based on clinical experience and case reports from the literature [Boeve 2002]. Anticholinergic hypnotics should be avoided in patients with AD, given the presence of an underlying cholinergic deficiency. Sedating antidepressants such as trazodone or low doses of atypical antipsychotics, such as Seroquel, may be useful in managing insomnia. Sleep hygiene measures, such as limiting daytime napping, morning exposure to sunlight, adequate treatment of pain, and limiting nighttime fluids, should be implemented.

IV. TREATMENT OF VASCULAR DEMENTIA

Vascular dementia (VaD) is the second most common cause of dementia after AD. In VaD cognitive decline is caused by a single localized stroke or a series of strokes. VaD is directly correlated with risk factors for stroke, including high blood pressure, diabetes, elevated cholesterol levels, and smoking. VaD differs from AD in that there is no specific neurotransmitter deficiency. In contrast to patients with AD who often experience a gradual, progressive decline, patients with VaD typically experience a stepwise decline in function. However, some of the treatment approaches developed for AD have also been evaluated for VaD including antioxidants and neurotrophic and neuroprotective agents. Several other compounds have been recently tested in clinical studies. However, specific drugs have not been approved. Although many trials have been published, few of them were carried out according to a randomized, double-blind, placebo-controlled design. Most of these studies had major limitations regarding the definition of the patient population, the limited sample size, the short treatment duration, the unclear definition of outcome measures of efficacy, the incomplete description of patient accountability, and the lack of intention-to-treat analysis. Finally, the positive results observed in some studies were not replicated in further trials.

Recently large, well-designed studies with cholinesterase inhibitors have been reported with positive results, supporting the existence of some degree of overlap between pathology AD and VaD [Kalaria 1999].

A. Calcium Channel Blockers

The role played by calcium in regulating brain functions is well known. The calcium ion links membrane excitation to subsequent intracellular response. Change in calcium homeostasis is one important effect of aging with consequences on higher cortical functions. The primary action of calcium channel blockers is to reduce the number of open channels, thus restricting influx of calcium ions into the cell.

Initial open studies with nimodipine, a calcium channel blocker able to cross the blood brain barrier, suggested beneficial effects of nimodipine in VaD [Parnetti 1993; Pantoni 1996]. A later, 26-week, double-blind placebo-controlled study of nimodipine in 259 patients with multiinfarct dementia (DSM-III-R criteria) failed to show a significant effect of nimodipine on cognitive or global assessments although some trend favored the calcium channel blocker [Pantoni 2000]. A recent review reported that there is no convincing evidence that nimodipine is a useful treatment for the symptoms of either VaD or AD [Lopez-Arrieta 2001].

Nicardipine, another calcium antagonist, was also evaluated in VaD. In a pilot study, nicardipine was compared with placebo over a 6-month period in 40 patients who had a previous transient ischemic attack. Although no significant differences were found, patients on nicardipine tended to perform better in certain tests [Molto 1995]. A larger double-blind, placebo-controlled study in 156 patients with VaD adopted as primary efficacy variable the loss of > 10 % of the basal score on the Mini-Mental State Examination after 1 year [Anonymous 1999]. At the end of the study, 35% of patients with placebo and 21% with nicardipine reached the endpoint, the difference not reaching statistical significance. These studies suggest a modest benefit, if any, of nicardipine in VaD.

B. Xanthine Derivatives

Methylxanthine derivatives are phosphodiesterase inhibitors with vasodilating properties. They also inhibit platelet aggregation and thromboxane A2 synthesis, decrease the release of free radicals, and may be neuroprotective. Methylxanthine derivatives have been evaluated mainly in peripheral vascular diseases, but a number of studies have been carried out in VaD and even in AD.

Positive results with pentoxifylline have been reported in a double-blind placebo-controlled study in 80 patients with symptoms of VaD [Blume 1992]. A well-designed placebo-controlled study in 64 patients meeting the DSM-III criteria for multi-infarct dementia showed borderline significance in favor of pentoxifylline on the rate of cognitive deterioration over a 36-week period [Black 1992]. There were no significant effects on global function of patients. Similarly, another 9-month, placebo-controlled study on pentoxifylline in 289 patients with multi-infarct dementia (DSM-III-R criteria) approached statistical significance on the primary outcome measure of efficacy [Gottfries-Brane-Steen scale] in the intent-to-treat analysis [Anonymous 1996].

Propentofylline, another xanthine derivative, was reported to increase regional cerebral glucose metabolism in the motor cortex of patients with VaD in a 3-month, placebo-controlled study [Mielke 1996]. These effects were coupled to positive trends on cognitive performance of the patients. Another placebo-controlled trial in 190 patients with unspecified mild dementia also showed beneficial effects of propentofylline on the Gottfries-Brane-Steen scale [Saletu 1990]. In a further, 12-month, placebo-controlled study in 260 patients with VaD and AD, treatment differences in favor of propentofylline for both clinical global measures and cognitive scales were also reported [Marcusson 1997]. A review of clinical trials of propentofylline in VaD concluded that, although propentofylline appear to affect positively cognitive and global function, no benefits could be demonstrated for activities of daily living [Kittner 1999].

C. Nootropics

So far, no generally accepted mechanism of action has emerged for piracetam-like nootropics [piracetam, oxiracetam, pramiracetam, and aniracetam]. Some indications seem to suggest cholinergic mechanisms [Gouliaev 1994]. A 12-week, placebo-controlled study of oxiracetam in 289 patients suffering from VaD or AD reported significant effects in favor of oxiracetam on Blessed Dementia Scale [Maina 1989]. Positive results were also described in a double-blind placebo-controlled study of oxiracetam in a mixed group of 65 demented patients treated for 12 weeks [Bottini 1992]. In another 3-month study in 60 patients with VaD and AD, significant improvements in patients treated with oxiracetam compared to placebo were observed on a number of cognitive tests [Villardita 1992]. However, a recent meta-analysis of all available studies of another nootropic, piracetam, concluded that there is no evidence supporting the use of piracetam in the treatment of people with dementia or cognitive impairment [Flicker 2001].

Nicergoline, an ergoloid derivative, is an α-adrenergic blocker claimed to possess activities on cell energy metabolism and platelet aggregation. In a 6-month, placebo-controlled study, nicergoline was found to improve cognitive and overall functions in 252 patients with VaD [Herrmann 1997]. A previous study of shorter duration (8 weeks) in 112 patients with VaD and AD also reported positive results [Saletu 1995]. A meta-analysis of controlled clinical trials of nicergoline in VaD and AD was recently published [Fioravanti 2001]. The analysis provides some evidence of positive effects of nicergoline on cognition and behavior in patients with VaD. In particular, the analysis found a difference in favor of nicergoline in reducing the behavioral symptoms as assessed by the Sandoz Clinical Assessment Geriatric Scale, but the effect size was minimal (4% of the scale range). Other outcome measures including functional scales failed to demonstrate statistically significant effects of nicergoline.

D. Cholinesterase Inhibitors

Studies in rats with tandem occlusion of left middle cerebral and common carotid arteries have shown that central cholinesterase inhibition improves cerebral blood flow in the ischemic brain [Scremin 1997]. The stimulating effects of cholinesterase inhibitors of regional cerebral blood flow and glucose metabolism have been confirmed in AD patients receiving long-term treatment with tacrine [Nordberg 1998] and donepezil [Nakano 2001]. These observations have opened the possibility to test cholinesterase inhibitors in VaD.

A post hoc analysis of studies with rivastigmine in AD, revealed a larger effect size on cognitive measures in patients with concurrent vascular risk factors at baseline (Modified Hachinski Ischemic Score > 0) [Kumar 2000]. Preliminary clinical experience with donepezil in VaD showed encouraging results [Mendez 2000]. Recently two large double-blind, placebo-controlled trials of donepezil in VaD found statistically significant effects of the drug on both cognitive and clinical global scales [Pratt 2002]. In both studies diagnosis of probable or possible VaD was made according to NINDS-AIREN criteria. The two studies involved 616 and 603 patients, respectively, randomized to receive placebo or donepezil 5 mg or 10 mg daily for 24 weeks. In both studies, both doses of donepezil produced significant effects on cognitive measures of efficacy (ADAS-Cog and MMSE). On the clinical global measure of efficacy significant effects were observed with the 5-mg dose in Study 308 (CIBIC-Plus) and with the 10-mg dose in Study 307 (CDR-SB), indicating different sensitivities of the two scales to drug dose. The donepezil safety profile did not differ from that of previous AD trials. These studies are probably the best-designed and best-conducted clinical trials in VaD published so far.

Positive effects in VaD were also recently shown with galantamine but in a less homogeneous population [Erkinjuntti 2002]. Five hundred ninety-two patients with a diagnosis of probable VaD or AD combined with cerebrovascular disease participated at this 6-month, double-blind placebo-controlled study. Galantamine (24 mg/day) showed greater efficacy than placebo on cognitive (ADAS-Cog), clinical global (CIBIC-Plus), activities of daily living (Disability Assessment in Dementia), and behavioral [Neuropsychiatric Inventory] measures of efficacy. Galantamine was well tolerated. This study confirms the therapeutic role of cholinesterase inhibitors in VaD.

V. TREATMENT OF DEMENTIA WITH LEWY BODIES

Dementia with Lewy bodies (DLB) is a common form of dementia in the elderly, characterized clinically by fluctuating cognitive impairment, attention deficits, visual hallucinations, parkinsonism, and other neuropsychiatric features. Many deficits in cholinergic neurotransmission are seen in the brains of patients with DLB. Thus, drugs enhancing central cholinergic function represent a rationally based therapeutic approach to this disorder.

The effects of the cholinesterase inhibitor rivastigmine in DLB were initially evaluated in a preliminary open-label study [McKeith 2000] and later in a double-blind, placebo-controlled study in 120 patients [McKeith 2000]. Subjects were given up to 12 mg rivastigmine or placebo daily for 20 weeks. Patients on rivastigmine had significant improvement with regard to apathy, anxiety, delusions, and hallucinations. About twice as many patients on rivastigmine (38%) as on placebo (18%), showed at least a 30% improvement from baseline. Cognitive effects of rivastigmine were detected with a computerized assessment system and with neuropsychological tests. Nausea, vomiting, and anorexia were seen more frequently with rivastigmine than with placebo.

Recently, a post hoc analysis was carried out in a subgroup of patients with DLB included in a placebo-controlled trial of olanzapine for the treatment of psychosis in AD patients [Cummings 2001]. Patients meeting the clinical criteria for DLB and exhibiting parkinsonism and visual hallucinations were selected from the initial study. Patients treated with 5 mg olanzapine showed significant reductions in delusions and hallucinations, while patients treated with 10 mg showed a significant improvement in the Neuropsychiatric Inventory/Nursing Home delusion subscale score. This post hoc analysis suggests that olanzapine reduces psychosis in patients with DLB without worsening parkinsonism.

VI. TREATMENT OF FRONTOTEMPORAL DEMENTIA

Patients with frontotemporal dementia [FTD] include those who suffer from Pick's disease or corticobasal degeneration, as well as the infrequent families with FTD and parkinsonism associated with chromosome 17. This type of dementia is clinically characterized by behavior and personality disorders, more than cognitive alterations. Behavioral symptoms (disinhibition, aggression, hyperorality, and speech disturbance) may trouble caregivers and present a safety risk to the individual suffering from the disease.

Treatment approaches to FTD are still in their infancy. Many of the therapies developed for AD may not work for FTD because the two disorders have different behavioral, cognitive, neurochemical, and molecular features. The recent discovery of mutations in the τ gene and the development of mouse models for FTD should eventually lead to more rational therapies. However, the treatment of frontotemporal dementia is currently directed toward the psychiatric alterations that characterize this disorder [Perry 2001]. Atypical antipsychotics have improved "positive symptoms" such as logorrhea, wandering, agitation, and aggression, without impairing cognitive function. There is some evidence from open trials that SSRIs improve depressive symptoms, compulsions, food craving, and disinhibition [Swartz 1997].

VII. TREATMENT OF MILD COGNITIVE IMPAIRMENT

Mild cognitive impairment (MCI) is the term used to describe a condition with isolated memory deficits in individuals who do not have significant impairment of other cognitive domains (beyond that expected for their age and level of education) and have normal basic activities of daily living. MCI represents the transitional zone between normal aging and AD. As many as 60–80% of patients with MCI may progress to AD over a 5-year period. Specific memory deficit, apolipoprotein E status, and hippocampus atrophy on magnetic resonance imaging are predictors of a more rapid progression [Petersen 2001].

It has been estimated that there are from 2.5 million to 4 million people in the United States with MCI, and probably an equivalent number in Western Europe. In March 2001, the U.S. Food and Drug Administration recognized MCI as an indication that could be defined and that was separate from AD.

At present, no treatments are recommended for MCI. The only published controlled clinical trial in MCI regards piribedil, a dopamine receptor agonist [Nagaraja 2001]. This study was based on the hypothesis that cognitive decline in healthy elderly individuals is associated with age-related decrease in dopamine receptors [Wang 1998]. The 3-month, double-blind placebo-controlled study was carried out in 60 patients with clinically diagnosed MCI and a MMSE score of 21–25 at baseline. At 3 months, 19 patients (63%) of those taking piribedil and 8 (27%) of those treated with placebo had increases in MMSE scores to 26 or more, the difference being significant.

Current major efforts are aimed to find drugs able to impede the progression of MCI to AD. A number of clinical trials on potential therapies are under way. These refer mainly to drugs developed for AD, specifically cholinesterase inhibitors and COX-2 inhibitors [Sramek 2001]. One of these studies is assessing the ability of donepezil, compared to vitamin E and placebo, in reducing the conversion of amnestic MCI to AD [Doody 2002]. In another study, rofecoxib is being studied in individuals with MCI to see if it can delay the onset of AD in this population [Grundman 2000].

Finally, in a large prevention study, the Alzheimer's Disease Anti-Inflammatory Prevention Trial (ADAPT), cognitively normal individuals at risk for AD (age > 70 years and first-degree relative with dementia) are being randomized to receive a traditional NSAID or a COX-2 inhibitor or placebo [Sparks 2002]. They will be assessed yearly for 7 years. The major endpoint is conversion to dementia. In the Ancillary Study on Cholesterol and Statin parameters, yearly cholesterol levels will be determined in subjects where statin use is known at entry. Conversion to dementia and changes in yearly cognitive indices will be correlated to changes in cholesterol levels and use of statins.

VIII. CONCLUSIONS

Because of its high prevalence, AD is the type of dementia for which the most intensive efforts for the development of pharmacological treatments have been directed. These efforts have resulted in the introduction of cholinesterase inhibitors which have been shown to produce a temporary amelioration of cognitive symptoms and delay of functional decline of the patients. The pharmacological treatments of the behavioral and psychotic disturbances of AD patients have been less systematically addressed. However, a number of clinical trials using atypical antipsychotics have recently been conducted or are in progress. The development of pharmacological treatments for other types of dementia is at earlier stages, with encouraging results in VaD and LBD, again with cholinesterase inhibitors. Neurotransmitter substitution therapy of AD will probably soon reach its limits and is not likely to provide additional efficacy with the novel compounds that are being developed. The major breakthrough in terms of therapeutic success is expected from approaches directed toward the interference with the so-called β-amyloid cascade. The testing of the β-amyloid hypothesis in clinical trials is likely to be achieved within the next 5 years. The most exciting products include β-amyloid immunization, although a putative β-amyloid vaccine has recently discontinued owing to central inflammation adverse events. Therapeutic efforts are also being concentrated on prevention of dementia. The large ongoing studies with estrogens (WHIMS) and NSAIDs (Alzheimer's Disease Anti-Inflammatory Prevention Trial) will probably determine their prophylactic potential in the next few years. Randomized, placebo-controlled prospective studies with certain statins are also expected to provide definitive results on their potential. Finally the 20,500-patient Heart Protection Study of simvastatin and vitamins A, C, and E will assess the role of lipid reduction and antioxidants in the prevention of dementia and cognitive decline. Other promising approaches for the treatment and prevention of Alzheimer's disease may involve the use of antiglucocorticoid agents such as Mifepristone [Pomara et al. 2002].

REFERENCES

Aisen PS, Davis KL. Inflammatory mechanisms in Alzheimer's disease. Implications for therapy. Am J Psychiatr 1994; 151:1105–1113.

Aisen PS, Davis KL, Berg JD, Schafer K, Campbell K, Thomas RG, Weiner MF, Farlow MR, Sano M, Grundman M, Thal LJ. A randomized controlled trial of prednisone in Alzheimer's disease. Alzheimer's Disease Cooperative Study. Neurology 2000; 54:588–593.

Andreasson KI, Savonenko A, Vidensky S, Goellner JJ, Zhang Y, Shaffer A, Kaufmann WE, Worley PF, Isakson P, Markowska AL. Age-dependent cognitive deficits and neuronal apoptosis in cyclooxygenase-2 transgenic mice. J Neurosci 2001; 21:8198–8209.

Anonymous. European Pentoxifylline Multi-Infarct Dementia Study. Eur Neurol 1996; 36:315–321.

Anonymous. An experimental, randomized, double-blind, placebo-controlled clinical trial to investigate the effect of nicardipine on cognitive function in patients with vascular dementia. Spanish group of nicardipine study in vascular dementia. Rev Neurol 1999; 28:835–845.

Apter JT, Allen LA. Buspirone: future directions. J Clin Psychopharmacol 1999; 19:86–93.

Asthana S, Craft S, Baker LD, Raskind MA, Birnbaum RS, Lofgreen CP, Veith RC, Plymate SR. Cognitive and neuroendocrine response to transdermal estrogen in postmenopausal women with Alzheimer's disease: results of a placebo-controlled, double-blind, pilot study. Psychoneuroendocrinology 1999; 24:657–677.

Auchus AP, Bissey-Black C. Pilot study of haloperidol, fluoxetine, and placebo for agitation in Alzheimer's disease. J Neuropsychiatry Clin Neurosci 1997; 9:591–593.

Bacskai BJ, Kajdasz ST, Christie RH, Carter C, Games D, Seubert P, Schenk D, Hyman BT. Imaging of amyloid-β deposits in brains of living mice permits direct observation of clearance of plaques with immunotherapy. Nat Med 2001; 7:369–372.

Bard F, Cannon C, Barbour R, Burke RL, Games D, Grajeda H, Guido T, Hu K, Huang J, Johnson-Wood K, Khan K, Kholodenko D, Lee M, Lieberburg I, Motter R, Nguyen M, Soriano F, Vasquez N, Weiss K, Welch B, Seubert P, Schenk D, Yednock T. Peripherally administered antibodies against amyloid β-peptide enter the central nervous system and reduce pathology in a mouse model of Alzheimer disease. Nat Med 2000; 6:916–919.

Behl C. Vitamin E protects neurons against oxidative cell death in vitro more effectively than 17-beta estradiol and induces the activity of the transcription factor NF-kappaB. J Neural Transm 2000; 107:393–407.

Bennett BD, Babu-Khan S, Loeloff R, Louis JC, Curran E, Citron M, Vassar R. Expression analysis of BACE2 in brain and peripheral tissues. J Biol Chem 2000; 275:20647–20651.

Berezovska O, Jack C, McLean P, Aster JC, Hicks C, Xia W, Wolfe MS, Kimberly WT, Weinmaster G, Selkoe DJ, Hyman BT. Aspartate mutations in presenilin and γ-secretase inhibitors both impair Notch1 proteolysis and nuclear translocation with relative preservation of Notch1 signaling. J Neurochem 2000; 75:583–593.

Birks JS, Melzer D. Donepezil for mild and moderate Alzheimer's disease. Cochrane Database Syst Rev 2000; 2:CD001190.

Black RS, Barclay LL, Nolan KA, Thaler HT, Hardiman ST, Blass JP. Pentoxifylline in cerebrovascular dementia. J Am Geriatr Soc 1992; 40:237–244.

Blasko I, Veerhuis R, Stampfer-Kountchev M, Saurwein-Teissl M, Eikelenboom P, Grubeck-Loebenstein B. Costimulatory effects of interferon-γ and interleukin-1β or tumor necrosis factor α on the synthesis of Aβ1-40 and Aβ1-42 by human astrocytes. Neurobiol Dis 2000; 7:682–689.

Blume J, Ruhlmann KU, De la Haye R, Rettig K. Treatment of chronic cerebrovascular disease in elderly patients with pentoxifylline. J Med 1992; 23:417–432.

Bodick NC, Offen WW, Levey AI, Cutler NR, Gauthier SG, Satlin A, Shannon HE, Tollefson GD, Rasmussen K, Bymaster FP, Hurley DJ, Potter WZ, Paul SM. Effects of xanomeline, a selective muscarinic receptor agonist, on cognitive function and behavioral symptoms in Alzheimer disease. Arch Neurol 1997; 54:465–473.

Boeve BF, Silber MH, Ferman TJ. Current management of sleep disturbances in dementia. Curr Neurol Neurosci Rep 2002; 2:169–177.

Borchelt DR, Thinakaran G, Eckman CB, Lee MK, Davenport F, Ratovitsky T, Prada CM, Kim G, Seekins S, Yager D, Slunt HH, Wang R, Seeger M, Levey AI, Gandy SE, Copeland NG, Jenkins NA, Price DL, Younkin SG, Sisodia SS. Familial Alzheimer's disease-linked presenilin 1 variants elevate Aβ1-42/1-40 ratio in vitro and in vivo. Neuron 1996; 17:1005–1013.

Bottini G, Vallar G, Cappa S, Monza GC, Scarpini E, Baron P, Cheldi A, Scarlato G. Oxiracetam in dementia: a double-blind, placebo-controlled study. Acta Neurol Scand 1992; 86:237–241.

Bruno V, Battaglia G, Copani A, Sortino MA, Canonico PL, Nicoletti F. Protective action of idebenone against excitotoxic degeneration in cultured cortical neurons. Neurosci Lett 1994; 178:193–196.

Buhot MC, Martin S, Segu L. Role of serotonin in memory impairment. Ann Med 2000; 32:210-221.

Butterfield DA, Drake J, Pocernich C, Castegna A. Evidence of oxidative damage in Alzheimer's disease brain: central role for amyloid β-peptide. Trends Mol Med 2001; 7:548–554.

Camacho F, Smith CP, Vargas HM, Winslow JT. Alpha 2-adrenoceptor antagonists potentiate acetylcholinesterase inhibitor effects on passive avoidance learning in the rat. Psychopharmacology 1996; 124:347–354.

Cherny RA, Atwood CS, Xilinas ME, Gray DN, Jones WD, McLean CA, Barnham KJ, Volitakis I, Fraser FW, Kim Y, Huang X, Goldstein LE, Moir RD, Lim JT, Beyreuther K, Zheng H, Tanzi RE, Masters CL, Bush AI. Treatment with a copper-zinc chelator markedly and rapidly inhibits beta-amyloid accumulation in Alzheimer's disease transgenic mice. Neuron 2001; 30:665–676.

Chessell IP, Procter AW, Francis PT, Bowen DM. D-cycloserine, a putative cognitive enhancer, facilitates activation of the N-methyl-D-aspartate receptor-ionophore complex in Alzheimer brain. Brain Res 1991; 565:345–348.

Citron M, Oltersdorf T, Haass C, McConlogue L, Hung AY, Seubert P, Vigo-Pelfrey C, Lieberburg I, Selkoe DJ. Mutation of the β-amyloid precursor protein in familial Alzheimer's disease increases β-protein production. Nature 1993; 360:672–674.

Citron M, Westaway D, Xia W, Carlson G, Diehl T, Levesque G, Johnson-Wood K, Lee M, Seubert P, Davis A, Kholodenko D, Motter R, Sherrington R, Perry B, Yao H, Strome R, Lieberburg I, Rommens J, Kim S, Schenk D, Fraser P, St George Hyslop P, Selkoe DJ. Mutant presenilins of Alzheimer's disease increase production of 42-residue amyloid β-protein in both transfected cells and transgenic mice. Nat Med 1997; 3:67–72.

Collins R, Peto R, Armitage J. The MRC/BHF Heart Protection Study: preliminary results. Int J Clin Pract 2002; 56:53–56.

Cummings JL. Cholinesterase inhibitors: a new class of psychotropic compounds. Am J Psychiatry 2000; 157:4–15.

Cummings JL, Street J, Masterman D, Clark WS. Efficacy of olanzapine in the treatment of psychosis in dementia with Lewy bodies. Dement Geriatr Cogn Disord 2002; 13:67–73.

Davies P, Maloney AJ. Selective loss of central cholinergic neurons in Alzheimer's disease. Lancet 1976; 2:1403.

De Deyn PP, Rabheru K, Rasmussen A, Bocksberger JP, Dautzenberg PL, Eriksson S, Lawlor BA. A randomized trial of risperidone, placebo, and haloperidol for behavioral symptoms of dementia. Neurology 1999; 53:946–955.

DeFeudis FV, Drieu K. Ginkgo biloba extract [EGb 761] and CNS functions: basic studies and clinical applications. Curr Drug Targets 2000; 1:25–58.

Dekker AJ, Winkler J, Ray J, Thal LJ, Gage FH. Grafting of nerve growth factor–producing fibroblasts reduces behavioral deficits in rats with lesions of the nucleus basalis magnocellularis. Neuroscience 1994; 60:299–309.

DeMattos RB, Bales KR, Cummins DJ, Dodart JC, Paul SM, Holtzman DM. Peripheral anti-Aβ antibody alters CNS and plasma Aβ clearance and decreases brain Aβ burden in a mouse model of Alzheimer's disease. Proc Natl Acad Sci USA 2001; 98:8850–8855.

Derr SM, Phillips K, Komar SA, Hill SE, Lazarus DD, Hayward NJ. Basic in vivo pharmacology of the amyloid polymerization inhibitor PPI-1019. Society of Neuroscience, 31st Annual Meeting, San Diego, Nov. 10–15, 2001.

Devanand DP, Marder K, Michaels KS, Sackeim HA, Bell K, Sullivan MA, Cooper TB, Pelton GH, Mayeux R. A randomized, placebo-controlled dose-comparison trial of haloperidol for psychosis and disruptive behaviors in Alzheimer's disease. Am J Psychiatry 1998; 155:1512–1520.

Di Iorio P, Virgilio A, Giuliani P, Ballerini P, Vianale G, Middlemiss PJ, Rathbone MP, Ciccarelli R. AIT-082 is neuroprotective against kainate-induced neuronal injury in rats. Exp Neurol 2001; 169:392–399.

Doody R. Donepezil across the spectrum of Alzheimer disease (AD). Seventh International Geneva/Springfield Symposium on Advances in Alzheimer Therapy, Geneva, April 3-6, 2002. Abstract p 50.

Dovey HF, John V, Anderson JP, Chen LZ, et al. Functional γ-secretase inhibitors reduce β-amyloid peptide levels in brain. J Neurochem 2001; 76:173–181.

Dysken MW, Kuskowski M. Ondansetron in the treatment of cognitive decline in Alzheimer's dementia. Neurobiol Aging 1998; 19(4S):178.

Earl RA, Zaczek R, Teleha CA, Fisher BN, Maciag CM, Marynowski ME, Logue AR, Tam SW, Tinker WJ, Huang SM, Chorvat RJ. 2-Fluoro-4-pyridinylmethyl analogues of linopirdine as orally active acetylcholine release-enhancing agents with good efficacy and duration of action. J Med Chem 1998; 41:4615–4622.

Eckert GP, Kirsch C, Mueller WE. Differential effects of lovastatin treatment on brain cholesterol levels in normal and apoE-deficient mice. Neuroreport 2001; 12:883–887.

Eriksdotter Jonhagen M, Nordberg A, Amberla K, Backman L, Ebendal T, Meyerson B, Olson L, Seiger, Shigeta M, Theodorsson E, Viitanen M, Winblad B, Wahlund LO. Intracerebroventricular infusion of nerve growth factor in three patients with Alzheimer's disease. Dement Geriatr Cogn Disord 1998; 9:246–257.

Erkinjuntti T, Kurz A, Gauthier S, Bullock R, Lilienfeld S, Damaraju CV. Efficacy of galantamine in probable vascular dementia and Alzheimer's disease combined with cerebrovascular disease: a randomised trial. Lancet 2002; 359:1283–1290

Esler WP, Kimberly WT, Ostaszewski BL, Diehl TS, Moore CL, Tsai JY, Rahmati T, Xia W, Selkoe DJ, Wolfe MS. Transition-state analogue inhibitors of γ-secretase bind directly to presenilin-1. Nat Cell Biol 2000; 2:428–434.

Esler PW, Wolfe MS. A portrait of Alzheimer secretases. New features and family faces. Science 2001; 293:1449–1454.

Fakouhi TD, Jhee SS, Sramek JJ, Benes C, Schwartz P, Hantsburger G, Herting R, Swabb EA, Cutler NR. Evaluation of cycloserine in the treatment of Alzheimer's disease. J Geriatr Psychiatry Neurol 1995; 8:226–230.

Falsetti AE. Risperidone for control of agitation in dementia patients. Am J Health Syst Pharm 2000; 57:862–870.

Fassbender K, Simons M, Bergmann C, Stroick M, Lutjohann D, Keller P, Runz H, Kuhl S, Bertsch T, von Bergmann K, Hennerici M, Beyreuther K, Hartmann T. Simvastatin strongly reduces level of Alzheimer's disease β-amyloid peptides Aβ 42 and Aβ 40 in vitro and in vivo. Proc Natl Acad Sci USA 2001; 98:5856–5861.

Feldman H, Gauthier S, Hecker J, Vellas B, Subbiah P, Whalen E, Donepezil MSAD Study Investigators Group. A 24-week, randomized, double-blind study of donepezil in moderate to severe Alzheimer's disease. Neurology 2001; 57:613–620.

Felsenstein K. Aβ modulation: what is the best target for therapeutic intervention, Geneva/Springfield Symposium on Advances in Alzheimer Therapy. Geneva, April 3–6, 2002. Abstract p 57.

Fillit HM, Gutterman EM, Brooks RL. Impact of donepezil on caregiving burden for patients with Alzheimer's disease. Int Psychogeriatr 2000; 12:389–401.

Findeis MA. Approaches to discovery and characterization of inhibitors of amyloid β-peptide polymerization. Biochim Biophys Acta 2000; 1502:76–84.

Fioravanti M, Flicker L. Efficacy of Nicergoline in dementia and other age associated forms of cognitive impairment [Cochrane Review]. Cochrane Database Syst Rev 2001; 4:CD003159.

Fischer W, Wictorin K, Bjorklund A, Williams LR, Varon S, Gage FH. Amelioration of cholinergic neuron atrophy and spatial memory impairment in aged rats by nerve growth factor. Nature 1987; 329:65–68.

Fisher A, Brandeis R, Chapman S, Pittel Z, Michaelson DM. M1 muscarinic agonist treatment reverses cognitive and cholinergic impairments of apolipoprotein E–deficient mice. J Neurochem 1998; 70:1991–1997.

Fleming LM, Johnson GV. Modulation of the phosphorylation state of τin situ: the roles of calcium and cyclic AMP. Biochem J 1995; 309:41–47.

Flicker L, Grimley Evans G. Piracetam for dementia or cognitive impairment. Cochrane Database Syst Rev 2001; [2]:CD001011.

Frears ER, Stephens DJ, Walters CE, Davies H, Austen BM. The role of cholesterol in the biosynthesis of β-amyloid. Neuroreport 1999; 10:1699–1705.

Foster RH, Plosker GL. Donepezil. Pharmacoeconomic implications of therapy. Pharmacoeconomics 1999; 16:99–114.

Frenkel D, Katz O, Solomon B. Immunization against Alzheimer's β-amyloid plaques via EFRH phage administration. Proc Natl Acad Sci USA 2000; 97:11455–11459.

Frenkel D, Kariv N, Solomon B. Generation of auto-antibodies towards Alzheimer's disease vaccination. Vaccine 2001; 19:2615–2619.

Friedhoff LT, Cullen EI, Geoghagen NS, Buxbaum JD. Treatment with controlled-release lovastatin decreases serum concentrations of human β-amyloid (Aβ) peptide. Internat J Neuropsychopharmacol 2001; 4:127–130.

Gage FH, Armstrong DM, Williams LR, Varon S. Morphological response of axotomized septal neurons to nerve growth factor. J Comp Neurol 1988; 269:147–155.

Garceau D, Gurbindo C, Lurin J. Safety, tolerability and pharmacokinetic profile of Alzhemed™, an anti-amyloid agent for Alzheimer disease, in healthy volunteers. Seventh International Geneva/Springfield Symposium on Advances in Alzheimer Therapy, Geneva, April 3–6, 2002. Abstract 27C, p 187.

Genis I, Fisher A, Michaelson DM. Site-specific dephosphorylation of tau of apolipoprotein E-deficient and control mice by M1 muscarinic agonist treatment. J Neurochem 1999; 72:206–213.

Gervais F, Paquette J, Morisette C, Kryskowski P, Yu M, Kong X, Tremblay P. A low molecular weight GAG mimetic compound reduces brain amyloid burden in hAPP transgenic mice. Seventh International Geneva/Springfield Symposium on Advances in Alzheimer Therapy, Geneva, April 3–6, 2002. Abstract 28C, p 188.

Ghosh AK, Bilcer G, Harwood C, Kawahama R, Shin D, Hussain KA, Hong L, Loy JA, Nguyen C, Koelsch G, Ermolieff J, Tang J. Structure-based design: potent inhibitors of human brain memapsin 2 (β-secretase). J Med Chem 2001; 44:2865–2868.

Glasky AJ, Melchior CL, Pirzadeh B, Heydari N, Ritzmann RF. Effect of AIT-082, a purine analog, on working memory in normal and aged mice. Pharmacol Biochem Behav 1994; 47:325–329.

Gouliaev AH, Senning A. Piracetam and other structurally related nootropics. Brain Res Rev 1994; 19:180–222.

Grubeck-Loebenstein B, Blasko I, Mark FK, Trieb I. Immunization with β-amyloid: could T-cell activation have a harmful effect? Trends Neurosci 2000; 23:114.

Grundman M, Thal LJ. Treatment of Alzheimer's disease: rationale and strategies. Neurol Clin 2000a; 18:807–828.

Grundman M. Vitamin E and Alzheimer's disease. The basis for additional clinical trials. Am J Clin Nutr 2000b; 71(suppl 2):630S–637S.

Gutzmann H, Hadler D. Sustained efficacy and safety of idebenone in the treatment of Alzheimer's disease: update on a 2-year double-blind multicentre study. J Neural Transm Suppl 1998; 54:301–310.

Gutzmann H, Kuhl KP, Hadler D, Rapp MA. Safety and efficacy of idebenone versus tacrine in patients with Alzheimer's disease: results of a randomized, double-blind, parallel-group multicenter study. Pharmacopsychiatry 2002; 35:12–18.

Hadland BK, Manley NR, Su D, Longmore GD, Moore CL, Wolfe MS, Schroeter EH, Kopan R. γ-Secretase inhibitors repress thymocyte development. Proc Natl Acad Sci USA 2001; 98:7487–7491.

Hagg T, Fass-Holmes B, Vahlsing HL, Manthorpe M, Conner JM, Varon S. Nerve growth factor (NGF) reverses axotomy-induced decreases in choline acetyltransferase, NGF receptor and size of medial septum cholinergic neurons. Brain Res 1989; 505:29–38.

Harder JA, Ridley RM. The 5-HT1A antagonist, WAY 100 635, alleviates cognitive impairments induced by dizocilpine (MK-801) in monkeys. Neuropharmacology 2000; 39:547–552.

Harris-White ME, Frautschy SA, Miller SA, Hu W, Talamantes V, Balverde Z, Centrella PA, Phillips K, Grace ML, Findeis MA, Hayward NJ. The amyloid polymerization inhibitor PPI-1019 reduces β-amyloid burden in a rat model of Alzheimer's disease. Society of Neuroscience, 31st Annual Meeting, San Diego, Nov. 10–15, 2001.

Henderson VW, Paganini-Hill A, Miller BL, Elble RJ, Reyes PF, Shoupe D, McCleary CA, Klein RA, Hake AM, Farlow MR. Estrogen for Alzheimer's disease in women: randomized, double-blind, placebo-controlled trial. Neurology 2000; 54:295–301.

Herrmann WM, Stephan K, Gaede K, Apececche M. A multicenter randomized double-blind study on the efficacy and safety of nicergoline in patients with multi-infarct dementia. Dement Geriatr Cogn Disord 1997; 8:9–17.

Hirai K, Hayako H, Kato K. Idebenone protects against oxidative stress mediated neuronal cell death by coupling with the mitochondrial electron transport system. Soc Neurosci 1996; 22:200.

Hirai K, Kato K, Nakayama T, Hayako H, Ishihara Y, Goto G, Miyamoto M. Neurochemical effects of 3-[1-(phenylmethyl)-4-piperidinyl]-1-(2,3,4,5-tetrahydro-1H-1-benzazepin-8-yl)-1-propanone fumarate (TAK-147), a novel acetylcholinesterase inhibitor, in rats. J Pharmacol Exp Ther 1997; 280:1261–1269.

Ho L, Purohit D, Haroutunian V, Luterman JD, Willis F, Naslund J, Buxbaum JD, Mohs RC, Aisen PS, Pasinetti GM. Neuronal cyclooxygenase 2 expression in the hippocampal formation as a function of the clinical progression of Alzheimer disease. Arch Neurol 2001; 58:487–492.

Hock C, Maddalena A, Heuser I, Naber D, Oertel W, von der Kammer H, Wienrich M, Raschig A, Deng M, Growdon JH, Nitsch RM. Treatment with the selective muscarinic agonist talsaclidine decreases cerebrospinal fluid levels of total amyloid beta-peptide in patients with Alzheimer's disease. Ann NY Acad Sci 2000; 920:285–291.

Howlett DR, Perry AE, Godfrey F, Swatton JE, Jennings KH, Spitzfaden C, Wadsworth H, Wood SJ, Markwell RE. Inhibition of fibril formation in beta-amyloid peptide by a novel series of benzofurans. Biochem J 1999; 340:283–289.

Howlett DR, George AR, Owen DE, Ward RV, Markwell RE. Common structural features determine the effectiveness of carvedilol, daunomycin and rolitetracycline as inhibitors of Alzheimer beta-amyloid fibril formation. Biochem J 1999; 343:419–423.

Howlett D, Cutler P, Heales S, Camilleri P. Hemin and related porphyrins inhibit β-amyloid aggregation. FEBS Lett 1997; 417:249–251.

Huang DY, Goedert M, Jakes R, Weisgraber KH, Garner CC, Saunders AM, Pericak-Vance MA, Schmechel DE, Roses AD, Strittmatter WJ. Isoform-specific interactions of apolipoprotein E with the microtubule-associated protein MAP2c: implications for Alzheimer's disease. Neurosci Lett 1994; 182:55–58.

Huff FJ. Preliminary evaluation of besipirdine for the treatment of Alzheimer's disease. Besipirdine Study Group. Preliminary evaluation of besipirdine for the treatment of Alzheimer's disease. Besipirdine Study Group. Ann NY Acad Sci 1996; 777:410–414.

Imbimbo BP. Pharmacodynamic-tolerability relationships of cholinesterase inhibitors for Alzhcimcr's disease. CNS Drugs 2001; 15:375–390.

Imbimbo BP. Toxicity of β-amyloid vaccination in Alzheimer's patients. Ann Neurol 2002 51:794.

Ingvar M, Ambros-Ingerson J, Davis M, Granger R, Kessler M, Rogers GA, Schehr RS, Lynch G. Enhancement by an ampakine of memory encoding in humans. Exp Neurol 1997; 146:553–559.

in t' Veld BA, Ruitenberg A, Hofman A, Launer LJ, Van Duijn CM, Stijnen T, Breteler MM, Stricker BH. Nonsteroidal antiinflammatory drugs and the risk of Alzheimer's disease. N Engl J Med 2001; 345:1515–1521.

Iqbal K, Grundke-Iqbal I. Molecular mechanism of Alzheimer's neurofibrillary degeneration and therapeutic intervention. Ann NY Acad Sci 1996; 777:132–138.

Ishihara Y, Goto G, Miyamoto M. Central selective acetylcholinesterase inhibitor with neurotrophic activity: structure-activity relationships of TAK-147 and related compounds. Curr Med Chem 2000; 7:341–354.

Jacobsen JS, Spruyt MA, Brown AM, Sahasrabudhe SR, Blume AJ, Vitek MP, Muenkel HA, Sonnenberg-Reines J. The release of Alzheimer's disease beta amyloid peptide is reduced by phorbol treatment. J Biol Chem 1994; 269:8376.

Jain KK. Evaluation of memantine for neuroprotection in dementia. Expert Opin Investig Drugs 2000; 9:1397–1406.

Jakala P, Sirvio J, Riekkinen M, Koivisto E, Kejonen K, Vanhanen M, Riekkinen P Jr. Guanfacine and clonidine, alpha 2-agonists, improve paired associates learning, but not delayed matching to sample, in humans. Neuropsychopharmacology 1999; 20:119–130.

Jantzen PT, Connor KE, DiCarlo G, Wenk GL, Wallace JL, Rojiani AM, Coppola D, Morgan D, Gordon MN. Microglial activation and beta-amyloid deposit reduction caused by a nitric oxide-releasing nonsteroidal anti-inflammatory drug in amyloid precursor protein plus presenilin-1 transgenic mice. J Neurosci 2002; 22:2246–2254.

Janus C, Pearson J, McLaurin J, Mathews PM, Jiang Y, Schmidt SD, Chishti MA, Horne P, Heslin D, French J, Mount HT, Nixon RA, Mercken M, Bergeron C, Fraser PE, St George-Hyslop P, Westaway D. Aβ peptide immunization reduces behavioural impairment and plaques in a model of Alzheimer's disease. Nature 2000; 408:979–982.

Jick H, Zornberg GL, Jick SS, Seshadri S, Drachman DA. Statins and the risk of dementia. Lancet 2000; 356:1627–1631.

Johnson N, Davis T, Bosanquet N. The epidemic of Alzheimer's disease. How can we manage the costs? Pharmacoeconomics 2000; 18:215–223.

Kalaria RN, Ballard C. Overlap between pathology of Alzheimer disease and vascular dementia. Alzheimer Dis Assoc Disord 1999; 13(suppl 3):S115–S123.

Kaplitt M, Gouras GK, Makimura H, Jovanovic J, Sweeney D, Greengard P, Relkin NR, Gandy S. Apolipoprotein E, A β-amyloid, and the molecular pathology of Alzheimer's disease. Therapeutic implications. Ann NY Acad Sci 1996; 802:42–49.

Karlsson I, Godderis J, Augusto De Mendonca Lima C, Nygaard H, Simanyi M, Taal M, Eglin M. A randomised, double-blind comparison of the efficacy and safety of citalopram compared to mianserin in elderly, depressed patients with or without mild to moderate dementia. Int J Geriatr Psychiatry 2000; 15:295–305.

Katz IR, Jeste DV, Mintzer JE, Clyde C, Napolitano J, Brecher M. Comparison of risperidone and placebo for psychosis and behavioral disturbances associated with dementia: a randomized, double-blind trial. Risperidone Study Group. J Clin Psychiatry 1999; 60:107–115.

Kem WR. The brain alpha7 nicotinic receptor may be an important therapeutic target for the treatment of Alzheimer's disease: studies with DMXBA [GTS-21]. Behav Brain Res 2000; 113:169–181.

Kirby LC, Baumel B, Eisner LS, Safirstien BE, Burford RG. The efficacy of phenserine tartrate following twelve [12] weeks of treatment in Alzheimer disease patients. Seventh International Geneva/Springfield Symposium on Advances in Alzheimer Therapy, Geneva, April 3–6, 2002. Abstract 43A, p 203.

Kittner B. Clinical trials of propentofylline in vascular dementia. European/Canadian Propentofylline Study Group. Alzheimer Dis Assoc Disord 1999; 13(suppl 3):S166–S171.

Kontush A, Mann U, Arlt S, Ujeyl A, Luhrs C, Muller-Thomsen T, Beisiegel U. Influence of vitamin E and C supplementation on lipoprotein oxidation in patients with Alzheimer's disease. Free Radic Biol Med 2001; 31:345–354.

Kojro E, Gimpl G, Lammich S, Marz W, Fahrenholz F. Low cholesterol stimulates the nonamyloidogenic pathway by its effect on the alpha-secretase ADAM 10. Proc Natl Acad Sci USA 2001; 98:5815–5820.

Kumar V, Anand R, Messina J, Hartman R, Veach J. An efficacy and safety analysis of Exelon in Alzheimer's disease patients with concurrent vascular risk factors. Eur J Neurol 2000; 7:159–169.

Lahiri DK, Ge YW, Farlow MR. Effect of a memory-enhancing drug, AIT-082, on the level of synaptophysin. Ann NY Acad Sci 2000; 903:387–393.

Le Bars PL, Katz MM, Berman N, Itil TM, Freedman AM, Schatzberg AF. A placebo-controlled, double-blind, randomized trial of an extract of ginkgo biloba for dementia: North American Egb Study Group. JAMA 1997; 278:1327–1332.

Le Bars PL, Velasco FM, Ferguson JM, Dessain EC, Kieser M, Hoerr R. Influence of the severity of cognitive impairment on the effect of the ginkgo biloba extract EGb 761 in Alzheimer's disease. Neuropsychobiology 2002; 45:19–26.

Lee RK, Wurtman RJ, Cox AJ, Nitsch RM. Amyloid precursor protein processing is stimulated by metabotropic glutamate receptors. Proc Natl Acad Sci USA 1995; 92:8083–8087.

Lee VM. Regulation of tau phosphorylation in Alzheimer's disease. Ann NY Acad Sci 1996; 777:107–113.

Lemere CA, Maron R, Spooner ET, Grenfell TJ, Mori C, Desai R, Hancock WW, Weiner HL, Selkoe DJ. Nasal Aβ treatment induces anti-Aβ antibody production and decreases cerebral amyloid burden in PD-APP mice. Ann NY Acad Sci 2000; 920, 328–331.

Lesser GT, Libow LS. Statin-Alzheimer disease association not yet proven. Arch Neurol 2001; 58:1022–1023.

Li Y, Liu L, Barger SW, Mrak RE, Griffin WS. J Neurosci Res 2001; 66:163–170.

Lim GP, Yang F, Chu T, Chen P, Beech W, Teter B, Tran T, Ubeda O, Ashe KH, Frautschy SA, Cole GM. Ibuprofen suppresses plaque pathology and inflammation in a mouse model for Alzheimer's disease. J Neurosci 2000; 20:5709–5714.

Lim GP, Yang F, Chu T, Gahtan E, Ubeda O, Beech W, Overmier JB, Hsiao-Ashec K, Frautschy SA, Cole GM. Ibuprofen effects on Alzheimer pathology and open field activity in APPsw transgenic mice. Neurobiol Aging 2001; 22:983–991.

Lin L, Georgievska B, Mattsson A, Isacson O. Cognitive changes and modified processing of amyloid precursor protein in the cortical and hippocampal system after cholinergic synapse loss and muscarinic receptor activation. Proc Natl Acad Sci USA 1999; 96:12108–12113.

Lippa CF, Nee LE, Mori H, St George-Hyslop P. Aβ-42 deposition precedes other changes in PS-1 Alzheimer's disease. Lancet 1998; 352:1117–1118.

Locatelli S, Lutjohann D, Schmidt HH, Otto C, Beisiegel U, Von Bergmann K. Reduction of plasma 24S-hydroxycholesterol [cerebrosterol] levels using high-dosage simvastatin in patients with hypercholesterolemia: evidence that simvastatin affects cholesterol metabolism in the human brain. Arch Neurol 2002; 59:213–216.

Lopez-Arrieta JM, Birks J. Nimodipine for primary degenerative, mixed and vascular dementia. Cochrane Database Syst Rev 2001; [1]:CD000147

Lopez OL, Becker JT, Wisniewski S, Saxton J, Kaufer DI, DeKosky ST. Cholinesterase inhibitor treatment alters the natural history of Alzheimer's disease. J Neurol Neurosurg Psychiatry 2002; 72:310–314.

Lorenzo A, Yankner BA. β-amyloid neurotoxicity requires fibril formation and is inhibited by Congo Red. Proc Natl Acad Sci USA 1994; 91:12243–12247.

Loudon JM, Bromidge SM, Brown F, Clark MS, Hatcher JP, Hawkins J, Riley GJ, Noy G, Orlek BS. SB 202026: a novel muscarinic partial agonist with functional selectivity for M1 receptors. J Pharmacol Exp Ther 1997; 283:1059–1068.

Luo Y, Bolon B, Kahn S, Bennett BD, Babu-Khan S, Denis P, Fan W, Kha H, Zhang J, Gong Y, Martin L, Louis JC, Yan Q, Richards WG, Citron M, Vassar R. Mice deficient in BACE1, the Alzheimer's beta-secretase, have normal phenotype and abolished beta-amyloid generation. Nat Neurosci 2001; 4:231–232.

Lyketsos CG, Sheppard JM, Steele CD, Kopunek S, Steinberg M, Baker AS, Brandt J, Rabins PV. Randomized, placebo-controlled, double-blind clinical trial of sertraline in the treatment of depression complicating Alzheimer's disease: initial results from the Depression in Alzheimer's Disease study. Am J Psychiatry 2000; 157:1686–1689.

Lynch G, Granger R, Ambros-Ingerson J, Davis CM, Kessler M, Schehr R. Evidence that a positive modulator of AMPA-type glutamate receptors improves delayed recall in aged humans. Exp Neurol 1997; 145:89–92.

Magai C, Kennedy G, Cohen CI, Gomberg D. A controlled clinical trial of sertraline in the treatment of depression in nursing home patients with late-stage Alzheimer's disease. Am J Geriatr Psychiatry 2000; 8:66–74.

Maina G, Fiori L, Torta R, Fagiani MB, Ravizza L, Bonavita E, Ghiazza B, Teruzzi F, Zagnoni PG, Ferrario E. Oxiracetam in the treatment of primary degenerative and multi-infarct dementia: a double-blind, placebo-controlled study. Neuropsychobiology 1989; 21:141–145.

Marcusson J, Rother M, Kittner B, Rossner M, Smith RJ, Babic T, Folnegovic-Smalc V, Moller HJ, Labs KH. A 12-month, randomized, placebo-controlled trial of propentofylline (HWA 285) in patients with dementia according to DSM-III-R. The European Propentofylline Study Group. Dement Geriatr Cogn Disord 1997; 8:320–328.

Markowska AL, Koliatsos VE, Breckler SJ, Price DL, Olton DS. Human nerve growth factor improves spatial memory in aged but not in young rats. J Neurosci 1994; 14:4815–4824.

Masters CL, Beyreuther K. Alzheimer disease: the next wave of Aβ amyloid therapeutic targets. Seventh International

Geneva/Springfield Symposium on Advances in Alzheimer Therapy, Geneva, April 3–6, 2002. Abstract p 86.

Mattson MP, Cheng B, Culwell AR, Esch FS, Lieberburg I, Rydel RE. Evidence for excitoprotective and intraneuronal calcium-regulating roles for secreted forms of the β-amyloid precursor protein. Neuron 1993; 10:243–254.

May PC. Current progress on new therapies for Alzheimer's disease. Drug Discov Today 2001; 6:459–462.

McGeer PL. Cyclo-oxygenase-2 inhibitors: rationale and therapeutic potential for Alzheimer's disease. Drugs Aging 2000; 17:1–11.

McGeer PL, McGeer EG. Inflammation, autotoxicity and Alzheimer disease. Neurobiol Aging 2001; 22:799–809.

McKeith IG, Grace JB, Walker Z, Byrne EJ, Wilkinson D, Stevens T, Perry EK. Rivastigmine in the treatment of dementia with Lewy bodies: preliminary findings from an open trial. Int J Geriatr Psychiatry 2000; 15:387–392.

McKeith I, Del Ser T, Spano P, Emre M, Wesnes K, Anand R, Cicin-Sain A, Ferrara R, Spiegel R. Efficacy of rivastigmine in dementia with Lewy bodies: a randomised, double-blind, placebo-controlled international study. Lancet 2000; 356:2031–2036.

McKhann G, Drachman D, Folstein M, Katzman R, Price D, Stadlan EM. Clinical diagnosis of Alzheimer's disease: report of the NINCDS-ADRDA Work Group under the auspices of Department of Health and Human Services Task Force on Alzheimer's Disease. Neurology 1984; 34:939–944.

McLaurin J, Franklin T, Zhang X, Deng J, Fraser PE. Interactions of Alzheimer amyloid-β peptides with glycosaminoglycans effects on fibril nucleation and growth. Eur J Biochem 1999; 266:1101–1110.

Meehan KM, Wang H, David SR, Nisivoccia JR, Jones B, Beasley CM, Feldman PD, Mintzer JE, Beckett LM, Breier A. Comparison of rapidly acting intramuscular olanzapine, lorazepam, and placebo. A double-blind, randomized study in acutely agitated patients with dementia. Neuropsychopharmacology 2002; 26:494–504.

Mendez MF, Younesi FL, Perryman KM. Use of donepezil for vascular dementia: preliminary clinical experience. J Neuropsychiatry Clin Neurosci 1999; 11:268–270.

Merlini G, Ascari E, Amboldi N, Bellotti V, Arbustini E, Perfetti V, Ferrari M, Zorzoli I, Marinone MG, Garini P, Diegoli M, Trizio D, Ballinari D. Interaction of the anthracycline 4'-iodo-4'-deoxydoxorubicin with amyloid fibrils: inhibition of amyloidogenesis. Proc Natl Acad Sci USA 1995; 92:2959–2963.

Meziane H, Dodart JC, Mathis C, Little S, Clemens J, Paul SM, Ungerer A. A memory-enhancing effect of secreted forms of the β-amyloid precursor protein in normal and amnestic mice. Proc Natl Acad Sci USA 1998; 95:12683–12688.

Middlemiss PJ, Glasky AJ, Rathbone MP, Werstuik E, Hindley S, Gysbers J. AIT-082, a unique purine derivative, enhances nerve growth factor mediated neurite outgrowth from PC12 cells. Neurosci Lett 1995; 199:131–134.

Mielke R, Kittner B, Ghaemi M, Kessler J, Szelies B, Herholz K, Heiss WD. Propentofylline improves regional cerebral glucose metabolism and neuropsychologic performance in vascular dementia. J Neurol Sci 1996; 141:59–64.

Miguel-Hidalgo JJ, Alvarez XA, Quack R, Cacabelos R. Protection by memantine against Aβ (1-40)-induced neurodegeneration in the CA1 subfield. Neurobiol Aging 1998; 19(4 suppl):129.

Miyamoto M, Takahashi H, Kato K, Hirai K, Ishihara Y, Goto G. Effects of 3-[1-(phenylmethyl)-4-piperidinyl]-1-(2,3,4,5-tetrahydro-1-H-1-benzazepin-8-yl)-1-propanone fumarate (TAK-147), a novel acetylcholinesterase inhibitor, on impaired learning and memory in animal models. J Pharmacol Exp Ther 1996; 277:1292–1304.

Miyata M, Smith JD. Apolipoprotein E allele-specific antioxidant activity and effects on cytotoxicity by oxidative insults and beta-amyloid peptides. Nat Genet 1996; 14:55–61.

Mohs RC, Doody RS, Morris JC, Ieni JR, Rogers SL, Perdomo CA, Pratt RD, "312" Study Group. A 1-year, placebo-controlled preservation of function survival study of donepezil in AD patients. Neurology 2001; 57:481–488.

Molto JM, Falip R, Martin R, Insa R, Pastor I, Matias-Guiu J. Comparative study of nicardipine versus placebo in the prevention of cognitive deterioration in patients with transient ischemic attack. Rev Neurol 1995; 23:54–58.

Monsonego A, Maron R, Zota V, Selkoe DJ, Weiner HL. Immune hyporesponsiveness to amyloid β-peptide in amyloid precursor protein transgenic mice: implications for the pathogenesis and treatment of Alzheimer's disease. Proc Natl Acad Sci USA 2001; 98:10273–10278.

Morgan D, Diamond DM, Gottschall PE, Ugen KE, Dickey C, Hardy J, Duff K, Jantzen P, DiCarlo G, Wilcock D, Connor K, Hatcher J, Hope C, Gordon M, Arendash GW. Aβ peptide vaccination prevents memory loss in an animal model of Alzheimer's disease. Nature 2000; 408:982–985.

Morris MC, Beckett LA, Scherr PA, Hebert LE, Bennett DA, Field TS, Evans DA. Vitamin E and vitamin C supplement use and risk of incident Alzheimer disease. Alzheimer Dis Assoc Disord 1998; 12:121–126.

Moser PC, Bergis OE, Santamaria R. SL65.0102, a novel and selective partial agonist at 5-HT4 receptors, improves learning and memory in rodents. Neurobiol Aging 1998; 19(4s):262.

Motter R, Vigo-Pelfrey C, Kholodenko D, Barbour R, Johnson-Wood K, Galasko D, Chang L, Miller B, Clark C, Green R. Reduction of β-amyloid peptide42 in the cerebrospinal fluid of patients with Alzheimer's disease. Ann Neurol 1995; 38:643–648.

Mucke H. TAK-147 [Takeda]. Curr Opin Invest Drugs 2001; 2:1595–1599.

Muldoon MF. Report on statins and dementia disputed. Arch Neurol 2001; 58:1166–1167.

Mulnard RA, Cotman CW, Kawas C, Van Dyck CH, Sano M, Doody R, Koss E, Pfeiffer E, Jin S, Gamst A, Grundman M, Thomas R, Thal LJ. Estrogen replacement therapy for treatment of mild to moderate Alzheimer disease: a randomized controlled trial. Alzheimer's Disease Cooperative Study. JAMA 2000; 283:1007–1015.

Mulsant BH, Pollock BG, Nebes R, Miller MD, Sweet RA, Stack J, Houck PR, Bensasi S, Mazumdar S, Reynolds CF 3rd. A twelve-week, double-blind, randomized comparison of nortriptyline and paroxetine in older depressed inpatients and outpatients. Am J Geriatr Psychiatry 2001; 9:406–414.

Murai S, Saito H, Abe E, Masuda Y, Odashima J, Itoh T. MKC-231, a choline uptake enhancer, ameliorates working memory deficits and decreased hippocampal acetylcholine induced by ethylcholine aziridinium ion in mice. J Neural Transm 1994; 98:1–13.

Nagaraja D, Jayashree S. Randomized study of the dopamine receptor agonist piribedil in the treatment of mild cognitive impairment. Am J Psychiatry 2001; 158:1517–1519.

Nakada Y, Tamura R, Kuriwaki J, Kimura T, Uwano T, Nishijo H, Ono T. Ameliorative effects of a cognitive enhancer, T-588, on place learning deficits induced by transient forebrain ischemia in rats. Physiol Behav 2001; 74:227–235.

Nakano S, Asada T, Matsuda H, Uno M, Takasaki M. Donepezil hydrochloride preserves regional cerebral blood flow in patients with Alzheimer's disease. J Nucl Med 2001; 42:1441–1445.

Nalbantoglu J, Tirado-Santiago G, Lahsaini A, Poirier J, Goncalves O, Verge G, Momoli F, Welner SA, Massicotte G, Julien JP, Shapiro ML. Impaired learning and LTP in mice expressing the carboxy terminus of the Alzheimer amyloid precursor protein. Nature 1997; 387:500–505.

Naslund J, Haroutunian V, Mohs R, Davis KL, Davies P, Greengard P, Buxbaum JD. Correlation between elevated levels of amyloid β-peptide in the brain and cognitive decline. JAMA 2000; 283:1571–1577.

Nitsch RM, Deng M, Tennis M, Schoenfeld D, Growdon JH. The selective muscarinic M1 agonist AF102B decreases levels of total Aβ in cerebrospinal fluid of patients with Alzheimer's disease. Ann Neurol 2000; 48:913–918.

Nitta A, Murakami Y, Furukawa Y, Kawatsura W, Hayashi K, Yamada K, Hasegawa T, Nabeshima T. Oral administration of idebenone induces nerve growth factor in the brain and improves learning and memory in basal forebrain-lesioned rats. Naunyn Schmiedebergs Arch Pharmacol 1994; 349:401–407.

Nordberg A, Amberla K, Shigeta M, Lundqvist H, Viitanen M, Hellstrom-Lindahl E, Johansson M, Andersson J, Hartvig P, Lilja A, Langstrom B, Winblad B. Long-term tacrine treatment in three mild Alzheimer patients: effects on nicotinic receptors, cerebral blood flow, glucose metabolism, EEG, and cognitive abilities. Alzheimer Dis Assoc Disord 1998; 12:228–237.

Nuydens R, De Jong M, Nuyens R, Cornelissen F, Geerts H. Neuronal kinase stimulation leads to aberrant tau phosphorylation and neurotoxicity. Neurobiol Aging 1995; 16:465–475.

Nyth AL, Gottfries CG. The clinical efficacy of citalopram in treatment of emotional disturbances in dementia disorders. A Nordic multicentre study. Br J Psychiatry 1990; 157:894–901.

Nyth AL, Gottfries CG, Lyby K, Smedegaard-Andersen L, Gylding-Sabroe J, Kristensen M, Refsum HE, Ofsti E, Eriksson S, Syversen S. A controlled multicenter clinical study of citalopram and placebo in elderly depressed patients with and without concomitant dementia. Acta Psychiatr Scand 1992; 86:138–145.

O'Dell JR. Triple therapy with methotrexate, sulfasalazine, and hydroxychloroquine in patients with rheumatoid arthritis. Rheum Dis Clin North Am 1998; 24:465–477.

Ohm TG. Does Alzheimer's disease start early in life? Mol Psychiatry 1997; 2:21–25.

Pantoni L, Carosi M, Amigoni S, Mascalchi M, Inzitari D. A preliminary open trial with nimodipine in patients with cognitive impairment and leukoaraiosis. Clin Neuropharmacol 1996; 19:497–506.

Pantoni L, Bianchi C, Beneke M, Inzitari D, Wallin A, Erkinjuntti T. The Scandinavian Multi-Infarct Dementia Trial: a double-blind, placebo-controlled trial on nimodipine in multi-infarct dementia. J Neurol Sci 2000; 175:116–123.

Papasozomenos SC, Shanavas A. Testosterone prevents the heat shock-induced overactivation of glycogen synthase kinase-3 β but not of cyclin-dependent kinase 5 and c-Jun NH2-terminal kinase and concomitantly abolishes hyperphosphorylation of τ: implications for Alzheimer's disease. Proc Natl Acad Sci 2002; 99:1140–1145.

Pappolla MA, Chyan YJ, Poeggeler B, Frangione B, Wilson G, Ghiso J, Reiter RJ. An assessment of the antioxidant and the antiamyloidogenic properties of melatonin: implications for Alzheimer's disease. J Neural Transm 2000; 107:203–231.

Parks RW, Becker RE, Rippey RF, Gilbert DG, Matthews JR, Kabatay E, Young CS, Vohs C, Danz V, Keim P, Collins GT, Zigler SS, Urycki PG. Increased regional cerebral glucose metabolism and semantic memory performance in Alzheimer's disease: a pilot double blind transdermal nicotine positron emission tomography study. Neuropsychol Rev 1996; 6:61–79.

Parnetti L, Senin U, Carosi M, Baasch H. Mental deterioration in old age: results of two multicenter, clinical trials with nimodipine. The Nimodipine Study Group. Clin Ther 1993; 15:394–406.

Perrig WJ, Perrig P, Stahelin HB. The relation between antioxidants and memory performance in the old and very old. J Am Geriatr Soc 1997; 45:718–724.

Perry EK, Tomlinson BE, Blessed G, Bergmann K, Gibson PH, Perry RH. Correlation of cholinergic abnormalities with senile plaques and mental test scores in senile dementia. Br Med J 1978; 2:1457–1459.

Perry RJ, Miller BL. Behavior and treatment in frontotemporal dementia. Neurology 2001; 56(suppl 4):S46–S51.

Petersen RC, Doody R, Kurz A, Mohs RC, Morris JC, Rabins PV, Ritchie K, Rossor M, Thal L, Winblad B. Current concepts in mild cognitive impairment. Arch Neurol 2001; 58:1985–1992.

Petracca GM, Chemerinski E, Starkstein SE. A double-blind, placebo-controlled study of fluoxetine in depressed patients with Alzheimer's disease. Int Psychogeriatr 2001; 13:233–240.

Pollock BG, Mulsant BH, Rosen J, Sweet RA, Mazumdar S, Bharucha A, Marin R, Jacob NJ, Huber KA, Kastango KB, Chew ML. Comparison of citalopram, perphenazine, and placebo for the acute treatment of psychosis and behavioral disturbances in hospitalized, demented patients. Am J Psychiatry 2002; 159:460–465.

Pomara N, Deptula D, Medel M, Block RI, Greenblatt DJ. Effects of diazepam on recall memory: relationship to aging, dose and duration of treatment. Psychopharmacol Bull 1989; 25:144–148.

Pomara N, Tun H, DaSilva D, Hernando R, Deptula D, Greenblatt DJ. The acute and chronic performance effects of alprazolam and lorazepam in the elderly: relationship to duration of treatment and self-rated sedation. Psychopharmacology 1998; 34(2):139–153.

Pomara N, Doraiswamy M, Tun H, Ferris, S. Mifepristone (RU 486) for Alzheimer's Disease. Neurology 2002; 58:1436.

Potter A, Corwin J, Lang J, Piasecki M, Lenox R, Newhouse PA. Acute effects of the selective cholinergic channel activator (nicotinic agonist) ABT-418 in Alzheimer's disease. Psychopharmacology 1999; 142:334–342.

Pratt RD, Perdomo CA, The Donepezil 308 VaD Study Group. Cognitive and global effects of donepezil in vascular dementia: results from study 308, a 24-week, randomized, double-blind, placebo-controlled trial. Seventh International Geneva/Springfield Symposium on Advances in Alzheimer Therapy, Geneva, April 3-6, 2002. Abstract 72A, pp 232–233.

Puglielli L, Konopka G, Pack-Chung E, Ingano LA, Berezovska O, Hyman BT, Chang TY, Tanzi RE, Kovacs DM. Acyl-coenzyme A: cholesterol acyltransferase modulates the generation of the amyloid β-peptide. Nat Cell Biol 2001; 3:905–912.

Refolo LM, Pappolla MA, LaFrancois J, Malester B, Schmidt SD, Thomas-Bryant T, Tint GS, Wang R, Mercken M, Petanceska SS, Duff KE. A cholesterol-lowering drug reduces β-amyloid pathology in a transgenic mouse model of Alzheimer's disease. Neurobiol Dis 2001; 8:890–899.

Regland B, Lehmann W, Abedini I, Blennow K, Jonsson M, Karlsson I, Sjogren M, Wallin A, Xilinas M, Gottfries CG. Treatment of Alzheimer's disease with clioquinol. Dementia 2001; 12:408–414.

Riekkinen P Jr, Laakso MP, Jakala P, Riekkinen P Jr. Clonidine impairs sustained attention and memory in Alzheimer's disease. Neuroscience 1999; 92:975–982.

Roberds SL, Anderson J, Basi G, et al. BACE knockout mice are healthy despite lacking the primary β-secretase activity in brain: implications for Alzheimer's disease therapeutics. Hum Mol Gen 2001; 10:1317–1324.

Robert SJ, Zugaza JL, Fischmeister R, Gardier AM, Lezoualc'h F. The human serotonin 5-HT4 receptor regulates secretion of non-amyloidogenic precursor protein. J Biol Chem 2001; 276:44881-44888.

Rogers J, Kirby LC, Hempelman SR, Berry DL, McGeer PL, Kaszniak AW, Zalinski J, Cofield M, Mansukhani L, Willson P. Clinical trial of indomethacin in Alzheimer's disease. Neurology 1993; 43:1609–1611.

Rockwood K, Kirkland S, Hogan DB, MacKnight C, Merry H, Verreault R, Wolfson C, McDowell I. Use of lipid-lowering agents, indication bias, and the risk of dementia in community-dwelling elderly people. Arch Neurol 2002; 59:223–227.

Sainati SM, Ingram DM, Talwalker S, Geis G. Results of a double-blind, randomized, placebo-controlled study of celecoxib in the treatment of progression of Alzheimer's disease. Sixth International Stockholm/Springfield Symposium on Advances in Alzheimer Therapy, Stockholm, Sweden, April 5–8, 2000. Abstract, p 180.

Saletu B, Moller HJ, Grunberger J, Deutsch H, Rossner M. Propentofylline in adult-onset cognitive disorders: double-blind, placebo-controlled, clinical, psychometric and brain mapping studies. Neuropsychobiology 1990; 24:173–184.

Saletu B, Paulus E, Linzmayer L, Anderer P, Semlitsch HV, Grunberger J, Wicke L, Neuhold A, Podreka I. Nicergoline in senile dementia of Alzheimer type and multi-infarct dementia: a double-blind, placebo-controlled, clinical and EEG/ERP mapping study. Psychopharmacology 1995; 117:385–395.

Sano M, Ernesto C, Thomas RG, Klauber MR, Schafer K, Grundman M, Woodbury P, Growdon J, Cotman CW, Pfeiffer E, Schneider LS, Thal LJ. A controlled trial of selegiline, alpha-tocopherol, or both as treatment for Alzheimer's disease. The Alzheimer's Disease Cooperative Study. N Engl J Med 1997; 336:1216–1222.

Scharf S, Mander A, Ugoni A, Vajda F, Christophidis N. A double-blind, placebo-controlled trial of diclofenac/misoprostol in Alzheimer's disease. Neurology 1999; 53:197–201.

Scremin OU, Li MG, Scremin AM, Jenden DJ. Cholinesterase inhibition improves blood flow in the ischemic cerebral cortex. Brain Res Bull 1997; 42:59–70.

Seiffert D, Bradley JD, Rominger CM, et al. Presenilin-1 and 2 are molecular targets for γ-secretase inhibitors. J Biol Chem 2000; 275:34086–34091.

Shaw KT, Utsuki T, Rogers J, Yu QS, Sambamurti K, Brossi A, Ge YW, Lahiri DK, Greig NH. Phenserine regulates translation of beta-amyloid precursor protein mRNA by a putative interleukin-1 responsive element, a target for drug development. Proc Natl Acad Sci USA 2001; 98:7605–7610.

Shearman MS, Beher D, Clarke EE, Lewis HD, Harrison T, Hunt P, Nadin A, Smith AL, Stevenson G, Castro JL. L-685-458, an aspartyl protease transition state mimic, is a potent inhibitor of amyloid β-protein precursor γ-secretase activity. Biochemistry 2000; 39:8698–8704.

Shen J, Bronson RT, Chen DF, Xia W, Selfoe DJ, Tonegawa S. Skeletal and CNS defects in presenilin-1-deficient mice. Cell 1997; 89:629–639.

Schenk D, Barbour R, Dunn W, et al. Immunization with amyloid-β attenuates Alzheimer-disease-like pathology in the PDAPP mouse. Nature 1999; 400:173–177.

Schenk D. Immunization in neurodegenerative disease: a new paradigm. IPSEN Foundation Conference. Immunization Against Alzheimer's Disease and Other Neurodegenerative Disorders, Paris, March 13, 2002.

Scheuner D, Eckman C, Jensen M, et al. Secreted amyloid β-protein similar to that in the senile plaques of Alzheimer's disease is increased in vivo by the presenilin 1 and 2 and APP mutations linked to familial Alzheimer's disease. Nat Med 1996; 2:864–870.

Schneider LS, Tariot PN, Lyketsos CG, et al. National Institute of Mental Health Clinical Antipsychotic Trials of Intervention Effectiveness (CATIE): Alzheimer's disease trial methodology. Am J Geriatr Psychiatry 2001; 4:346–360.

Schwartz BL, Hashtroudi S, Herting RL, Schwartz P, Deutsch SI. d-Cycloserine enhances implicit memory in Alzheimer patients. Neurology 1996; 46:420–424.

Schwarz RD, Callahan MJ, Coughenour LL, Dickerson MR, Kinsora JJ, Lipinski WJ, Raby CA, Spencer CJ, Tecle H. Milameline (CI-979/RU35926): a muscarinic receptor agonist with cognition-activating properties: biochemical and in vivo characterization. J Pharmacol Exp Ther 1999; 291:812–822.

Shiovitz T, Monici P, Pietra C, Fabbri L, Piccinno A, Jhee SS, Zarotsky V, Tan E. A double-blind, placebo-controlled evaluation of the safety and tolerability of increasing doses of CHF 2891.01 (ganstigmine) in patients with probable Alzheimer's disease (AD). Seventh International Geneva/Springfield Symposium on Advances in Alzheimer Therapy, Geneva, April 3–6, 2002. Abstract p 114.

Shumaker SA, Reboussin BA, Espeland MA, Rapp SR, McBee WL, Dailey M, Bowen D, Terrell T, Jones BN. The Women's Health Initiative Memory Study (WHIMS): a trial of the effect of estrogen therapy in preventing and slowing the progression of dementia. Control Clin Trials 1998; 19:604–621.

Sigurdsson EM, Scholtzova H, Mehta PD, Frangione B, Wisniewski T. Immunization with a nontoxic/nonfibrillar amyloid-β homologous peptide reduces Alzheimer's disease–associated pathology in transgenic mice. Am J Pathol 2001; 159:439–447.

Simons M, Keller P, De Strooper B, Beyreuther K, Dotti CG, Simons K. Cholesterol depletion inhibits the generation of beta-amyloid in hippocampal neurons. Proc Natl Acad Sci USA 1998; 95:6460–6464.

Sinha S, Anderson JP, Barbour R, et al. Purification and cloning of amyloid precursor protein β-secretase from human brain. Nature 1999; 402:537–540.

Smith DE, Roberts J, Gage FH, Tuszynski MH. Age-associated neuronal atrophy occurs in the primate brain and is reversible by growth factor gene therapy. Proc Natl Acad Sci USA 1999; 96:10893–10898.

Solomon B, Koppel R, Hanan E, Katzav T. Monoclonal antibodies inhibit in vitro fibrillar aggregation of the Alzheimer β-amyloid peptide. Proc Natl Acad Sci USA 1996; 93:452–455.

Soto C. Plaque busters: strategies to inhibit amyloid formation in Alzheimer's disease. Mol Med Today 1999; 5:343–350.

Soto C, Sigurdsson EM, Morelli L, Kumar RA, Castano EM, Frangione B. β-Sheet breaker peptides inhibit fibrillogenesis in a rat brain model of amyloidosis: implications for Alzheimer's therapy. Nat Med 1998; 4:822–826.

Soto C, Adessi C, Saborio GP, Fraga S, Frossard MJ, Dewatcher I, Van Dorpe J, Banks WP, Van Leuven F, Permanne B. β-sheet breaker peptide for treatment of amyloidosis in Alzheimer disease. Seventh International Geneva/Springfield Symposium on Advances in Alzheimer Therapy, Geneva, April 3–6, 2002. Abstract p 118.

Soto C, Adessi C, Saborio GP, Fraga S, Frossard MJ, Van Dorpe J, Banks WA, Van Leuven F, Bermanne B. Sheet breaker peptide reduces amyloid load and cerebral damage in an Alzheimer's transgenic animal model. Society of Neuroscience, 31st Annual Meeting, San Diego, November 10–15, 2001.

Sparks DL. Cholesterol in AD: the AD atorvastatin treatment trial and the ancillary ADAPT trial. Seventh International Geneva/Springfield Symposium on Advances in Alzheimer Therapy, Geneva, April 3–6, 2002. Abstract p 119.

Sramek JJ, Veroff AE, Cutler NR. The status of ongoing trials for mild cognitive impairment. Expert Opin Invest Drugs 2001; 10:741–752.

Street JS, Clark WS, Gannon KS, Cummings JL, Bymaster FP, Tamura RN, Mitan SJ, Kadam DL, Sanger TM, Feldman PD, Tollefson GD, Breier A. Olanzapine treatment of psychotic and behavioral symptoms in patients with Alzheimer disease in nursing care facilities: a double-blind, randomized, placebo-controlled trial. The HGEU Study Group. Arch Gen Psychiatry 2000; 57:968–976.

Strittmatter WJ, Weisgraber KH, Goedert M, Saunders AM, Huang D, Corder EH, Dong LM, Jakes R, Alberts MJ, Gilbert JR. Hypothesis: microtubule instability and paired helical filament formation in the Alzheimer disease brain are related to apolipoprotein E genotype. Exp Neurol 1994; 125:163–171.

Strittmatter WJ, Weisgraber KH, Huang DY, Dong LM, Salvesen GS, Pericak-Vance M, Schmechel D, Saunders AM, Goldgaber D, Roses AD. Binding of human apolipoprotein E to synthetic amyloid beta peptide: isoform-specific effects and implications for late-onset Alzheimer disease. Proc Natl Acad Sci USA 1993; 90:8098–8102.

Sultzer DL, Gray KF, Gunay I, Wheatley MV, Mahler ME. Does behavioral improvement with haloperidol or trazodone treatment depend on psychosis or mood symptoms in patients with dementia? J Am Geriatr Soc 2001; 49:1294–1300.

Suzuki N, Cheung TT, Cai XD, Odaka A, Otvos L Jr, Eckman C, Golde TE, Younkin SG. An increased percentage of long amyloid β protein secreted by familial amyloid beta protein precursor (βAPP717) mutants. Science 1994; 264:1336–1340.

Swartz JR, Miller BL, Lesser IM, Darby AL. Frontotemporal dementia: treatment response to serotonin selective reuptake inhibitors. J Clin Psychiatry 1997; 58:212–216.

Taragano FE, Lyketsos CG, Mangone CA, Allegri RF, Comesana-Diaz E. A double-blind, randomized, fixed-dose trial of fluoxetine vs. amitriptyline in the treatment of major depression complicating Alzheimer's disease. Psychosomatics 1997; 38:246–252.

Tariot PN, Cummings JL, Katz IR, Mintzer J, Perdomo CA, Schwam EM, Whalen E. A randomized, double-blind, placebo-controlled study of the efficacy and safety of donepezil in patients with Alzheimer's disease in the nursing home setting. J Am Geriatr Soc 2001; 49:1590–1599.

Taylor EM, Yan R, Hauptmann N, Maher TJ, Djahandideh D, Glasky AJ. AIT-082, a cognitive enhancer, is transported into brain by a nonsaturable influx mechanism and out of brain by a saturable efflux mechanism. J Pharmacol Exp Ther 2000; 293:813–821.

Teri L, Logsdon RG, Peskind E, Raskind M, Weiner MF, Tractenberg RE, Foster NL, Schneider LS, Sano M, Whitehouse P, Tariot P, Mellow AM, Auchus AP, Grundman M, Thomas RG, Schafer K, Thal LJ. Alzheimer's Disease Cooperative Study. Treatment of agitation in AD: a randomized, placebo-controlled clinical trial. Neurology 2000; 55:1271–1278.

Terry AV Jr, Risbrough VB, Buccafusco JJ, Menzaghi F. Effects of (+/−)-4-{[2-(1-methyl-2-pyrrolidinyl)ethyl]thio}phenol hydrochloride (SIB-1553A), a selective ligand for nicotinic acetylcholine receptors, in tests of visual attention and distractibility in rats and monkeys. J Pharmacol Exp Ther 2002; 301:284–292.

Thal LJ, Forrest M, Loft H, Mengel H. Lu 25-109, a muscarinic agonist, fails to improve cognition in Alzheimer's disease. Lu25-109 Study Group. Neurology 2000; 54:421–426.

Tohgi H, Abe T, Hashiguchi K, Saheki M, Takahashi S. Remarkable reduction in acetylcholine concentration in the cerebrospinal fluid from patients with Alzheimer type dementia. Neurosci Lett 1994; 177:139–142.

Tomiyama T, Shoji A, Kataoka K, Suwa Y, Asano S, Kaneko H, Endo N. Inhibition of amyloid β protein aggregation and neurotoxicity by rifampicin. Its possible function as a hydroxyl radical scavenger. J Biol Chem 1996; 271:6839–6844.

Trabace L, Cassano T, Steardo L, Pietra C, Villetti G, Kendrick KM, Cuomo V. Biochemical and neurobehavioral profile of CHF2819, a novel, orally active acetylcholinesterase inhibitor for Alzheimer's disease. J Pharmacol Exp Ther 2000; 294:187–194.

Tsai GE, Falk WE, Gunther J, Coyle JT. Improved cognition in Alzheimer's disease with short-term D-cycloserine treatment. Am J Psychiatry 1999; 156:467–469.

Tung JS, Davis DL, Anderson JP, Walker DE, Mamo S, Jewett N, Hom RK, Sinha S, Thorsett ED, John V. Design of substrate-based inhibitors of human β-secretase. J Med Chem 2002; 45:259–262.

Van Dongen MC, van Rossum E, Kessels AG, Sielhorst HJ, Knipschild PG. The efficacy of ginkgo for elderly people with dementia and age-associated memory impairment: new results of a randomized clinical trial. J Am Geriatr Soc 2000; 48:1183–1194.

Van Gool WA, Weinstein HC, Scheltens P, Walstra GJ, Scheltens PK. Effect of hydroxychloroquine on progression of dementia in early Alzheimer's disease: an 18-month randomised, double-blind, placebo-controlled study. Lancet 2001; 358:455–460.

Vassar R, Bennett BD, Babu-Khan S, Kahn S, Mendiaz EA, Denis P, Teplow DB, Ross S, Amarante P, Loeloff R, Luo Y, Fisher S, Fuller J, Edenson S, Lile J, Jarosinski MA, Biere AL, Curran E, Burgess T, Louis JC, Collins F, Treanor J, Rogers G, Citron M. β-Secretase cleavage of Alzheimer's amyloid precursor protein by the transmembrane aspartic protease BACE. Science 1999; 286:735–741.

Veinbergs I, Mallory M, Sagara Y, Masliah E. Vitamin E supplementation prevents spatial learning deficits and dendritic alterations in aged apolipoprotein E–deficient mice. Eur J Neurosci 2000; 12:4541–4546.

Villardita C, Grioli S, Lomeo C, Cattaneo C, Parini J. Clinical studies with oxiracetam in patients with dementia of Alzheimer type and multi-infarct dementia of mild to moderate degree. Neuropsychobiology 1992; 25:24–28.

Volicer L, Rheaume Y, Cyr D. Treatment of depression in advanced Alzheimer's disease using sertraline. J Geriatr Psychiatry Neurol 1994; 7:227–229.

Wang JZ, Grundke-Iqbal I, Iqbal K. Restoration of biological activity of Alzheimer abnormally phosphorylated τ by dephosphorylation with protein phosphatase-2A, -2B and -1. Brain Res Mol Brain Res 1996; 38:200–208.

Wang PN, Liao SQ, Liu RS, Liu CY, Chao HT, Lu SR, Yu HY, Wang SJ, Liu HC. Effects of estrogen on cognition, mood, and cerebral blood flow in AD: a controlled study. Neurology 2000; 54:2061–2066.

Wang Y, Chan GL, Holden JE, Dobko T, Mak E, Schulzer M, Huser JM, Snow BJ, Ruth TJ, Calne DB, Stoessl AJ. Age-dependent decline of dopamine D1 receptors in human brain: a PET study. Synapse 1998; 30:56–61.

Weggen S, Eriksen JL, Das P, Sagi SA, Wang R, Pietrzik CU, Findlay KA, Smith TE, Murphy MP, Bulter T, Kang DE, Marquez-Sterling N, Golde TE, Koo EH. A subset of NSAIDs lower amyloidogenic Aβ42 independently of cyclooxygenase activity. Nature 2001; 414:212–216.

Wenk GL, Danysz W, Mobley SL. Investigations of neurotoxicity and neuroprotection within the nucleus basalis of the rat. Brain Res 1994; 655:7–11.

Weyer G, Babej-Dolle RM, Hadler D, Hofmann S, Herrmann WM. A controlled study of 2 doses of idebenone in the treatment of Alzheimer's disease. Neuropsychobiology 1997; 36:73–82.

Wieland E, Schutz E, Armstrong VW, Kuthe F, Heller C, Oellerich M. Idebenone protects hepatic microsomes against oxygen radical-mediated damage in organ preservation solutions. Transplantation 1995; 60:444–451.

Wienrich M, Meier D, Ensinger HA, Gaida W, Raschig A, Walland A, Hammer R. Pharmacodynamic profile of the M1 agonist talsaclidine in animals and man. Life Sci 2001; 68:2593–2600.

Winblad B, Wimo A. Assessing the societal impact of acetylcholinesterase inhibitor therapies. Alzheimer Dis Assoc Disord 1999; 13(suppl 2):S9–S19.

Winblad B, Engedal K, Soininen H, Verhey F, Waldemar G, Wimo A, Wetterholm AL, Zhang R, Haglund A, Subbiah P, Donepezil Nordic Study Group. A 1-year, randomized, placebo-controlled study of donepezil in patients with mild to moderate AD. Neurology 2001; 57:489–495.

Wolfe MS, Citron M, Diehl TS, Xia W, Donkor IO, Selkoe DJ. A substrate-based difluoro ketone selectively inhibits Alzheimer's γ-secretase activity. J Med Chem 1998; 41:6–9.

Wolfe MS. γ-Secretase inhibitors as molecular probes of presenilin function. J Mol Neurosci 2001; 17:199–204.

Wolfe MS. Secretase targets for Alzheimer's disease: identification and therapeutic potential. J Med Chem 2001; 44:2039–2060.

Wolozin B, Kellman W, Ruosseau P, Celesia GG, Siegel G. Decreased prevalence of Alzheimer disease associated with 3-hydroxy-3-methyglutaryl coenzyme A reductase inhibitors. Arch Neurol 2000; 57:1439–1443.

Yaffe K, Sawaya G, Lieberburg I, Grady D. Estrogen therapy in postmenopausal women: effects on cognitive function and dementia. JAMA 1998; 279:688–695.

Yaffe K. Estrogens, selective estrogen receptor modulators, and dementia: what is the evidence? Ann NY Acad Sci 2001; 949:215–222.

Yaffe K, Barrett-Connor E, Lin F, Grady D. Serum lipoprotein levels, statin use, and cognitive function in older women. Arch Neurol 2002; 59:378–384.

Yassin MS, Ekblom J, Xilinas M, Gottfries CG, Oreland L. Changes in uptake of vitamin B(12) and trace metals in brains of mice treated with clioquinol. J Neurol Sci 2000; 173:40–44.

Zajaczkowski W, Frankiewicz T, Parsons CG, Danysz W. Uncompetitive NMDA receptor antagonists attenuate NMDA-induced impairment of passive avoidance learning and LTP. Neuropharmacology 1997; 36:961–971.

57

Pharmacological Interventions in Psychiatric Disorders Due to Medical Conditions

E. SHERWOOD BROWN and DANA C. PERANTIE
University of Texas Southwestern Medical Center, Dallas, Texas, U.S.A.

I. INTRODUCTION

Psychiatric illnesses, particularly mood and anxiety disorders, are clearly more common in patients with general medical conditions than in the general population [1]. However, the nature, course, and treatment of psychiatric disorders in general medical conditions have been the subject of relatively little research. In this chapter, the relationship between psychiatric disorders and general medical conditions is divided into three categories. The first category is psychiatric illnesses, primarily mood and anxiety disorders, associated with but not necessarily secondary to a general medical condition. In the Diagnostic and Statistical Manual of Mental Disorders, 4th ed. Text Revision (DSM-IV-TR) [2], these are classified as major depressive disorder, dysthymic disorder, and panic disorder, as are similar symptoms with persons without a general medical condition. The second category of psychiatric illnesses includes not only depression and anxiety disorders, but also mania and psychosis—those thought to be etiologically linked to the general medical condition. These are classified as mood disorders or psychotic disorders due to a general medical condition in the DSM-IV-TR [2].

The third category consists of psychiatric disturbances associated with medications used to treat general medical conditions. These are classified as substance-induced disorders in DSM-IV-TR [2]. The treatment of each of these categories of illnesses will be discussed.

Several general principles useful in the treatment of psychiatric disorders in general medical conditions are outlined in Table 1. The first is to consider possible drug interactions between the psychotropic agent and medications used to treat the general medical condition. The second is to consider possible side effects of the psychotropic agent which might exacerbate symptoms of the general medical condition. Third, titration or dosage of psychotropic medications may need to be adjusted in those patients with illnesses affecting drug metabolism, such as liver or kidney disease. Also, some medications used to treat medical conditions may induce or exacerbate psychiatric symptoms. An additional consideration is that an improvement in psychiatric symptoms may result in an improvement or perceived improvement in the medical condition. These principles will be discussed as individual disorders and agents are reviewed.

Table 1 General Principles in Treating Psychiatric Disorders in General Medical Conditions

Interactions may exist between psychotropic medications and those being used to treat the medical condition.
Psychiatric medications may affect the general medical condition (positively or negatively).
Certain medical conditions (e.g., hepatic and renal disease) affect the metabolism of psychotropic medications, so dosage and/or titration may need to be adjusted.
Some medications used to treat general medical conditions can induce or exacerbate psychiatric symptoms.
Improvement in psychiatric symptoms may positively influence the outcome of the medical illness.

II. PHARMACOTHERAPY OF PSYCHIATRIC DISORDERS ASSOCIATED WITH MEDICAL CONDITIONS

Most research related to the pharmacotherapy of psychiatric illnesses associated with general medical conditions involves the treatment of depression, although a few studies have examined the treatment of anxiety disorders. A summary of controlled antidepressant trials in general medical conditions is provided in Table 2. A summary of findings in individual medical illnesses is given below.

A. Cardiovascular Diseases

Several investigations have shown a strong though complex relationship between cardiovascular disease and depression. Depression following a myocardial infarction appears to be a risk factor for death, and depressive symptoms appear to also predict future development of cardiovascular disease [3–5]. Therefore, the use of antidepressants in patients with coronary artery disease or at risk for coronary artery disease is an area of great interest. However, thus far only two controlled trials of an antidepressant have been published in the peer-reviewed literature. Veith et al. [6] examined the use of imipramine versus doxepin versus placebo in a group of 24 depressed patients with heart disease. Antidepressant therapy was more effective than placebo for depressive symptoms; however, the use of antidepressants had no effect on ejection fraction although imipramine appeared to reduce premature contractions. More recently, Roose et al.

Table 2 Controlled Trials of Antidepressant Medications in Medical Conditions

Medical condition	Medication(s) investigated	Psychiatric benefits	Benefits to Medical condition [Ref]
Heart disease	TCAs	(+) (6,7)	(+) [6]
	SSRI	(+) (7)	(+/−) [7]
Arthritis	TCAs	(+) (12)	(+) [11–13]
		(−) (11,13)	(−) [14]
		n/a (14)	
Fibromyalgia	TCAs	(−) (17,18)	(+) [17–20,22–24]
		n/a (19–24)	(−) [21]
	SSRIs	(+) (25,26)	(+) [18,26]
		(−) (18,27)	(−) [25,27]
Diabetes	nortriptyline	(+) (28)	(−) [28]
	fluoxetine	(+) (29)	(+) [29]
HIV/AIDS	TCAs	(+) (34,37,41)	(−) [34,39–41]
		n/a (39,40)	n/a [37]
	SSRIs	(+) (35,36,41)	(−) [35,41]
			n/a [36]
Cancer	Mianserin (tetracyclic)	(+) (52,53)	n/a [52,53]
Renal disease	Fluoxetine	(+) (54)	n/a [54]
COPD	nortriptyline	(+) (55)	subjective measures: (+) [55]
			objective measures: (−) [55]
Asthma	tianeptine (atypical TCA)	n/a (57)	(+) [57]

n/a = Not assessed.
(+) = Benefit reported.
(−) = Absence of benefit, which is not meant to imply the treatment was harmful.

compared paroxetine to nortriptyline in 81 depressed patients with ischemic heart disease [7]. Both antidepressants appeared effective for treatment of depressive symptoms. However, nortriptyline was associated with an 11% increase in heart rate, a decrease in orthostatic blood pressure, and suppression of ventricular arrhythmia, while paroxetine had no clinically significant effects on these variables. The rate of cardiac events that required intervention by a cardiologist and discontinuation of the medication was 17% in nortriptyline-treated patients, but only 2% in the paroxetine-treated patients.

Although the data in this area are relatively limited, the lack of cardiovascular effects of the selective serotonin reuptake inhibitors (SSRIs) has led some experts in the field to recommend these as first-line treatment of depression in patients with heart disease [8,9]. However, there are significant drug interactions between several SSRIs and also nefazodone, with digoxin (10). In addition, citalopram appears to potentiate the effects of beta-blockers [10].

B. Collagen Vascular Diseases

1. Rheumatoid Arthritis

Four placebo-controlled trials have examined the use of a tricyclic antidepressant (TCA) in patients with rheumatoid arthritis. In one study, Ash et al. examined the use of dothiepin versus placebo in a group of 48 female outpatients with rheumatoid arthritis and depression [11]. The study found a significant reduction in disability scores, duration of early morning stiffness, and pain in the dothiepin group. The reductions in pain were significantly correlated with reduction in depression and anxiety scores, but no significant difference was found at 12 weeks in depression scores between dothiepin- and placebo-treated groups. However, in a 4-week study of dothiepin and ibuprofen versus placebo and ibuprofen in 60 rheumatoid arthritis patients, Sarzi Puttini et al. found that the patients receiving dothiepin who were classified as depressed at baseline had a significant reduction in depression scores, in addition to a reduction in daytime pain [12]. In another placebo-controlled study, Macfarlane et al. examined the use of low-dose trimipramine in 36 patients with arthritis who were depressed according to a self-rated depression scale [13]. Joint pain and tenderness were found to be significantly reduced, while depression scores did not change. These studies are among only a few that demonstrate an improvement in symptoms of the general medical condition with antidepressant treatment. Amitriptyline has also been examined by Grace et al. in a controlled study in 36 arthritis patients, but no differences were found between amitriptyline and placebo in joint pain or tenderness [14]. The above data suggest TCAs are useful in depressed patients with arthritis. However, Bird et al. recently reported in a placebo-controlled trial (n = 76) that both paroxetine and amitriptyline were effective for both depressive and arthritic symptoms, but side effects were much more common in the amitriptyline group [15]. Thus, as with cardiovascular disease patients, improved tolerability over TCAs suggest SSRIs may be appropriate first line treatment for arthritis patients.

2. Fibromyalgia

Numerous controlled trials of antidepressants have been conducted in patients with fibromyalgia as recently reviewed by Arnold et al. [16]. In fact, more controlled antidepressant trials may have been conducted in fibromyalgia patients than in all other general medical conditions combined. In general, the trials have shown some improvement in symptoms of fibromyalgia including pain, stiffness, tenderness, fatigue, and sleep quality with the use of antidepressants [17–24]. The use of second-generation antidepressants (e.g., SSRIs) has generally shown either negative results or very modest improvement in symptoms of the disease [18,25–27]. Therefore, despite their side effect burden, TCAs appear at present to remain first line agents in fibromyalgia patients.

C. Diabetes

Two controlled studies have examined the use of antidepressants in depressed patients with diabetes. Lustman et al. examined nortriptyline versus placebo in 68 depressed patients with diabetes, finding significantly greater reduction in depressive symptoms in the nortriptyline-treated group [28]. However, nortriptyline was not superior to placebo in reducing glycosylated hemoglobin levels (a measure of diabetic control). The lack of improvement in glycemic control with nortriptyline was attributed to a direct effect of nortriptyline to worsen glycemic control even though improvement in depression appeared to have a beneficial effect on glycosylated hemoglobins in the subjects studied. More recently, Lustman et al. examined fluoxetine versus placebo in depressed patients (n = 60) with diabetes [29]. The fluoxetine-treated group had a significant improvement in depression compared to placebo, and a trend toward a reduction in glycosylated hemoglobin levels ($p = .13$). Thus, in the limited diabetes literature available, both TCAs and SSRIs appear to be effective for depressive symptoms. However, only SSRIs appear to be associated with improvement in glycosylated hemoglobin levels.

D. HIV and AIDS

The psychiatric disorders associated with human immunodeficiency virus (HIV) infection are highly variable in presentation and include depressive or anxiety symptoms possibly related to the disability and life-threatening nature of the illness. Psychiatric symptoms may also be related to direct effects of the virus on the central nervous system or side effects of antiviral medications [30]. The medications used to treat HIV infections can be associated with psychiatric symptoms [31,32]. Thus, HIV infection includes all three categories of psychiatric illnesses in general medical conditions contained in the introduction to this chapter. The treatment of psychiatric disorders in patients with HIV has been the subject of several investigations. Recently the American Psychiatric Association released practice guidelines for the treatment of patients with HIV and acquired immunodeficiency syndrome (AIDS) [33]. These guidelines emphasize starting with low doses and slow upward titration of medications when possible, avoiding medications with unfavorable side-effects profiles, and an awareness of the many potential drug interactions of antiviral drug regimens used in HIV-affected persons.

Several placebo-controlled trials have examined the use of antidepressants in HIV-positive patients with depression. In general, these studies suggest that antidepressant therapy including TCAs and SSRIs is effective for depressive symptoms in HIV [34–41]. However, the SSRIs appear to be better tolerated than TCAs in this population [41]. The studies that examined variables of immune functioning such as CD4 cell count found that immunity was not affected by the psychotropic medications [34,35,41,42]. Although the studies suggest that antidepressants are useful for depressive symptoms, no controlled trials to date have shown improvement in measures of severity of HIV illness or disease progression. However, finding a significant improvement in somatic symptoms on an HIV Symptom Scale in an open-label trial of SSRIs in 33 depressed, HIV-positive patients, Ferrando et al. suggest that depression significantly affects the perception of symptom severity, even in late stage HIV illness [43].

Although no controlled studies are available for the treatment of other psychiatric disorders in HIV-positive patients, anecdotal reports and small open studies suggest that valproic acid, clonazapam, phenytoin, and carbamazepine may be useful in some patients with mania [44,45]. Buspirone and fluoxetine may be useful for anxiety disorders [46,47], and low doses of antipsychotics may be useful for psychotic symptoms [48–51].

E. Cancer

As with HIV-positive patients, appreciation of the numerous drug interactions and side effects of the many chemotherapeutic agents available is important in treating patients with cancer and depression. Surprisingly few data are available in the form of controlled studies on the treatment of depression in patients with cancer. Costa et al. examined mianserin versus placebo in 73 women with cancer and depression, finding that antidepressant therapy was superior to placebo [52]. Van Heeringen and Zivkov found that mianserin was superior to placebo for depressive symptoms in 57 women with breast cancer and depression [53]. No controlled trials using SSRIs were found in our literature search.

F. Renal Diseases

One small placebo-controlled trial of an antidepressant in depressed patients (n = 14) on dialysis has been reported. Blumenfield et al. found a significant reduction in depression with fluoxetine compared to placebo at 4 weeks but not at 8 weeks [54]. In treating patients with renal disease, caution is required particularly with medications metabolized by the kidneys (e.g., lithium, gabapentin). Slow dose titration and careful monitoring of blood levels may be necessary when prescribing medications metabolized by the renal system in this population.

G. Pulmonary Diseases

One double-blind, placebo-controlled study examined the use of antidepressants in depressed patients with lung disease. Borson et al. examined the use of 12 weeks of nortriptyline versus placebo in 30 patients with chronic obstructive pulmonary disease, finding an improvement in mood and subjective but not objective symptoms of airway obstruction [55]. Although numerous studies suggest that depressive symptoms are common and may be associated with medication noncompliance and even sudden death from asthma, no placebo-controlled trials of antidepressants in depressed asthma patients have been published [56]. However, one study using tianeptine, a serotonin reuptake enhancer, in children with asthma found a substantial improvement in asthma symptoms [57]. Given the at least partially reversible nature of the airway obstruction in asthma patients, controlled trials of antidepressants in depressed asthma patients are needed, examining both changes in mood and asthma symptoms.

III. PSYCHIATRIC DISORDERS ETIOLOGICALLY RELATED TO GENERAL MEDICAL CONDITIONS

Some medical conditions in which psychiatric disturbance appear to frequently occur include porphyria, thyroid abnormalities, and hypothalamic-pituitary-adrenal axis disorders. The treatment of psychiatric disturbances secondary to general medical conditions should begin with the appropriate treatment of the general medical condition. However, this is not always sufficient to ameliorate the psychiatric disturbance, necessitating the use of psychotropic medications. The literature on the use of psychotropic medications for psychiatric illnesses secondary to general medical conditions consists of case reports and small open studies.

Two of these medical conditions have had an influence on psychopharmacology of idiopathic mood disorders. For many years, physicians have noted that persons with hypothyroidism and Cushing's disease often have affective symptomatology which resolves with successful treatment of the endocrine abnormality [58–60]. In addition, a subset of patients with mood disorders have subtle abnormalities of the neuroendocrine system including a blunted thyrotropin (TSH) response to thyrotropin-releasing hormone (TRH) [61] and nonsuppression on the dexamethasone suppression test (DST) [62], leading to the use of thyroid supplementation and antiglucocorticoid medications (i.e., ketoconazole, metyrapone) in patients with mood disorders [63–66]. However, the treatment of psychiatric disturbance associated with these endocrine disorders has not been a topic of systematic investigation, although the symptoms appear to frequently resolve with successful treatment of the general medical condition [58–60].

IV. PSYCHIATRIC DISTURBANCES SECONDARY TO MEDICATIONS USED TO TREAT MEDICAL CONDITIONS

A wide variety of medications has been implicated in psychiatric disturbances including digoxin, antihypertensives, antibiotics, corticosteroids, interferon alpha, and thyroid supplements. The treatment of psychiatric disturbances secondary to a medication begins with dose reduction or discontinuation of the medication or a switch to a different medication when possible. Minimal data are available on the pharmacotherapy of medication-induced psychiatric disturbances. Almost all reports consist of anecdotal evidence or small open case series. Medication-induced psychiatric disturbances are of historical interest in that reports of depressive symptomatology with reserpine in the 1950s were consistent with norepinephrine theories of depression which were put forward at that time [67,68].

This section will focus on data on the treatment of two medications that appear to be frequently associated with psychiatric disturbances: interferon alpha and oral corticosteroids. In recent years, it has become clear that interferon alpha, used to treat hepatitis C and other disorders, is frequently associated with the development of depressive symptoms. A report by Miyaoka et al. found that 37% of patients free of mood disturbance developed a major depressive episode during interferon alpha therapy [69]. Case reports of the successful use of fluoxetine 20 mg/day or low-dose nortriptyline (25–50 mg/day) for interferon alpha–induced depression have been published [70,71]. Gleason and Yates presented five cases of interferon alpha–induced depression which were successfully treated with SSRIs or a TCA [72]. In perhaps the only placebo-controlled study on the treatment of a medication-induced psychiatric disorder to date, Miller et al. reported the successful use of paroxetine as a prophylactic agent to prevent depression during alpha interferon [73].

Corticosteroids are frequently prescribed medications given for a variety of diseases mediated by the immune system. Despite their use for > 50 years, no controlled trials have examined the treatment of psychiatric disorders associated with their use [74,75]. Anecdotal reports suggest that lithium [76–81], neuroleptics [82–84], atypical antipsychotics [85,86], valproic acid [87], and lamotrigine [88] may be useful for psychiatric symptoms associated with corticosteroids. Falk et al. pretreated 27 patients in an open design with lithium carbonate and found none of these patients developed severe psychiatric disturbances, but 6/44 patients (14%) not receiving lithium developed mania or depression with psychotic features [76]. Anecdotal data suggest that TCAs may in some cases lead to a worsening of mood symptoms in patients with steroid-induced depressions [83,89]. In contrast, a single case report found that fluoxetine may improve depressive symptoms in patients on steroids [90]. In general, the evidence seems to support treating corticosteroid-induced psychiatric symptoms with agents effective for bipolar disorder (i.e., mood stabilizers).

V. CONCLUSION

Some psychiatric symptoms and disorders appear to be more common in general medical settings than in the general population. However, the treatment of these disorders has been the topic of relatively little attention. The SSRIs appear to be the agents of first choice for depression in some, but not all, general medical conditions. Almost no data are available on the treatment of anxiety in medical settings. Future studies are needed to examine the efficacy, tolerability, and acceptability of standard psychotropic agents in these medical settings. Of particular interest is whether treatment of psychiatric symptoms leads to improvement in the general medical condition or, conversely, treatment of the medical symptoms improves the psychiatric disorder.

REFERENCES

1. W Katon, MD Sullivan. Depression and chronic medical illness. J Clin Psychiatry 51(suppl):3–11, 1990.
2. American Psychiatric Association. Diagnostic and Statistical Manual of Mental Disorders, 4th ed text revision. Washington: American Psychiatric Association, 2000.
3. N Frasure-Smith, F Lesperance, M Talajic. Depression following myocardial infarction. Impact on 6-month survival. JAMA 270:1819–1825, 1993.
4. J Hippisley-Cox, K Fielding, M Pringle. Depression as a risk factor for ischaemic heart disease in men: population based case-control study. BMJ 316:1714–1719, 1998.
5. DE Ford, LA Mead, PP Change, L Cooper-Patrick, NY Wang, MJ Klag. Depression is a risk factor for coronary artery disease in men: the precursors study. Arch Intern Med 158:1422–1426, 1998.
6. RC Veith, MA Raskind, JH Caldwell, RF Barnes, G Gumbrecht, JL Ritchie. Cardiovascular effects of tricyclic antidepressants in depressed patients with chronic heart disease. N Engl J Med 306:954–959, 1982.
7. SP Roose, F Laghrissi-Thode, JS Kennedy, JC Nelson, JT Bigger Jr, BG Pollock, A Gaffney, M Narayan, MS Finkel, J McCafferty, I Gergel. Comparison of paroxetine and nortriptyline in depressed patients with ischemic heart disease. JAMA 279:287–291, 1998.
8. SP Roose, E Spatz. Treatment of depression in patients with heart disease. J Clin Psychiatry 60(suppl 20):34–37, 1999.
9. AH Glassman. Cardiovascular effects of antidepressant drugs: updated. J Clin Psychiatry 59(suppl 15):13–18, 1998.
10. Physician's Desk Reference. 54th ed. Oradel, NJ: Medical Economics Co., 2000.
11. G Ash, CM Dickens, FH Creed, MIV Jayson, B Tomenson. The effects of dothiepin on subjects with rheumatoid arthritis and depression. Br Soc Rheumatol 38:959–967, 1999.
12. P Sarzi Puttini, M Cazzola, L Boccassini, G Ciniselli, S Santandrea, I Caruso, C Benvenuti. A comparison of dothiepin versus placebo in the treatment of pain in rheumatoid arthritis and the association of pain with depression. J Int Med Res 16:331–337, 1988.
13. JG Macfarlane, S Jalali, EM Grace. Trimipramine in rheumatoid arthritis: a randomized double-blind trial in relieving pain and joint tenderness. Curr Med Res Opin 10:89–93, 1986.
14. EM Grace, N Bellamy, Y Kassam, WW Buchanan. Controlled, double-blind, randomized trial of amitriptyline in relieving articular pain and tenderness in patients with rheumatoid arthritis. Curr Med Res Opin 9:426–429, 1985.
15. H Bird, M Broggini. Paroxetine versus amitriptyline for treatment of depression associated with rheumatoid arthritis: a randomized, double-blind parallel group study. J Rheumatol 27:2791–2979, 2000.
16. LM Arnold, PE Keck Jr, JA Welge. Antidepressant treatment of fibromyalgia. Psychosomatics 41:104–113, 2000.
17. WJ Reynolds, H Moldofsky, P Saskin, FA Lue. The effects of cyclobenzaprine on sleep physiology and symptoms in patients with fibromyalgia. J Rheumatol 18:452–454, 1991.
18. D Goldenberg, M Mayskiy, C Mossey, R Ruthazer, C Schmid. A randomized, double-blind crossover trial of fluoxetine and amitriptyline in the treatment of fibromyalgia. Arthritis Rheum 39:1852–1859, 1996.
19. S Carette, MJ Bell, WJ Reynolds, et al. Comparison of amitriptyline, cyclobenzaprine, and placebo in the treatment of fibromyalgia. A randomized, double-blind clinical trial. Arthritis Rheum 37:32–40, 1994.
20. S Carette, GA McCain, DA Bell, AG Fam. Evaluation of amitriptyline in primary fibrositis. A double-blind placebo-controlled study. Arthritis Rheum 29:655–659, 1986.

21. S Carette, G Oakson, C Guimont, M Steriade. Sleep electroencephalography and the clinical response to amitriptyline in patients with fibromyalgia. Arthritis Rheum 38:1211–1217, 1995.
22. LG Quimby, GM Gratwick, CD Whitney, SR Block. A randomized trial of cyclobenzaprine for the treatment of fibromyalgia. J Rheumatol 19(suppl):140–143, 1989.
23. L Caruso, PC Sarzi Puttini, L Boccassini, S Santandrea, M Locati, R Volpato, F Montrone, C Benvenuti, A Beretta. Double-blind study of dothiepin versus placebo in the treatment of primary fibromyalgia syndrome. J Int Med Res 15:154–159, 1987.
24. RM Bennett, RA Gatter, SM Campbell, RP Andrews, SR Clark, JA Scarola. A comparison of cyclobenzaprine and placebo in the management of fibrositis. A double-blind controlled study. Arthritis Rheum 31:1535–1542, 1988.
25. F Wolfe, MA Cathey, DJ Hawley. A double-blind placebo controlled trial of fluoxetine in fibromyalgia. Scand J Rheumatol 23:255–259, 1994.
26. UM Anderberg, I Marteinsdottir, L von Knorring. Citalopram in patients with fibromyalgia—a randomized, double-blind, placebo-controlled study. Eur J Pain 4:27–35, 2000.
27. J Norregaard, H Volkmann, B Danneskiold-Samsoe. A randomized controlled trial of citalopram in the treatment of fibromyalgia. Pain 61:445–449, 1995.
28. PJ Lustman, LS Griffith, RE Clouse, KE Freedland, SA Eisen, EH Rubin, RM Carney, JB McGill. Effects of nortriptyline on depression and glycemic control in diabetes: results of a double-blind, placebo-controlled trial. Psychosom Med 59:241–250, 1997.
29. PJ Lustman, KE Freedland, LS Griffith, RE Clouse. Fluoxetine for depression in diabetes: a randomized double-blind placebo-controlled trial. Diabetes Care 23:618–623, 2000.
30. RS el-Mallakh. Mania in AIDS: clinical significance and theoretical considerations. Int J Psychiatry Med 21:383–391, 1991.
31. MJ Brouilette, G Chouinard, R Lalonde. Didanosine-induced mania in HIV infection. Am J Psychiatry 151:1839–1340, 1994.
32. JM Wright, PS Sachdev, RJ Perkins, P Rodriguez. Zidovudine-related mania. Med J Aust 150:339–341, 1989.
33. American Psychiatric Association. Practice guideline for the treatment of patients with HIV/AIDS. Am J Psychiatry 157(suppl 11):1–62, 2000.
34. JG Rabkin, R Rabkin, W Harrison, G Wagner. Effect of imipramine on mood and enumerative measures of immune status in depressed patients with HIV illness. Am J Psychiatry 151:516–523, 1994.
35. JG Rabkin, GJ Wagner, R Rabkin. Fluoxetine treatment for depression in patients with HIV and AIDS: a randomized, placebo-controlled trial. Am J Psychiatry 156:101–107, 1999.
36. S Zisook, J Peterkin, KJ Goggin, P Sledge, JH Atkinson, I Grant. Treatment of major depression in HIV-seropositive men. HIV Neurobehavioral Research Center Group. J Clin Psychiatry 59:217–224, 1998.
37. JC Markowitz, JH Kocsis, B Fishman, LA Spielman, LB Jacobsberg, AJ Frances, GL Klerman, SW Perry. Treatment of depressive symptoms in human immunodeficiency virus-positive patients. Arch Gen Psychiatry 55:452–457, 1998.
38. EF Targ, DH Karasic, PN Diefenbach, DA Anderson, A Bystritsky, FI Fawzy. Structured group therapy and fluoxetine to treat depression in HIV-positive persons. Psychosomatics 35:132–137, 1994.
39. K Kieburtz, D Simpson, C Yiannoutsos, MB Max, CD Hall, RJ Ellis, CM Marra R McKendall, E Singer, GJ Dal Pan, DB Clifford, T Tucker, B Cohen. A randomized trial of amitrityline and mexiletine for painful neuropathy in HIV infection. Neurology 51:1682–1688, 1998.
40. JC Shlay, K Chaloner, MB Max, B Flaws, P Reichelderfer, D Wentworth, S Hillman, B Brizz, DL Cohn. Acupuncture and amitriptyline for pain due to HIV-related peripheral neuropathy: a randomized controlled trial. JAMA 280:1590–1595, 1998.
41. AJ Elliott, KK Uldall, K Bergam, J Russo, K Claypoole, PP Roy-Byrne. Randomized, placebo-controlled trial of paroxetine versus imipramine in depressed HIV-positive outpatients. Am J Psychiatry 155:367–372, 1998.
42. JG Rabkin, R Rabkin, Wagner G. Effects of fluoxetine on mood and immune status in depressed patients with HIV illness. J Clin Psychiatry 55:92–97, 1994.
43. SJ Ferrando, JD Goldman, WE Charness. Selective serotonin reuptake inhibitor treatment of depression in symptomatic HIV infection and AIDS. Improvements in affective and somatic symptoms. Gen Hosp Psychiatry 19:89–97, 1997.
44. MH Halman, JL Worth, DM Sanders, PR Renshaw, GB Murray. Anticonvulsant use in the treatment of manic syndromes in patients with HIV-1 infection. J Neuropsychiatry Clin Neurosci 5:430–434, 1993.
45. JA RachBeisel, E Weintraub. Valproic acid treatment of AIDS-related mania. J Clin Psychiatry 58:406–407, 1997.
46. SL Batki. Buspirone in drug users with AIDS or AIDS-related complex. J Clin Psychopharmacol 10 (suppl):111S–115S, 1990.
47. J McDaniel, K Johnson. Obsessive-compulsive disorder in HIV disease: response to lfuoxetine. Psychosomatics 36:417–418, 1995.
48. W Breitbart, RF Marotta, P Call. AIDS and neuroleptic malignant syndrome. Lancet 2:1488–1489, 1988.
49. M Maccario, DW Sharre. HIV and acute onset of psychosis. Lancet 2:342, 1987.

50. LR Belzie. Risperidone for AIDS-associated dementia—a case series. AIDS Patient Care and STDs 10:246–249, 1996.
51. F Fernandez, L Joel. The use of molidone in the treatment of psychotic and delirious patients infected with the human immunodeficiency virus: case reports. Gen Hosp Psychiatry 15:31–35, 1993.
52. D Costa, I Mogos, T Toma. Efficacy and safety of mianserin in the treatment of depression of women with cancer. Acta Psychiatr Scand 320(suppl):85–92, 1985.
53. K van Heeringen, M Zivkov. Pharmacological treatment of depression in cancer patients. A placebo-controlled study of mianserin. Br J Psychiatry 169:440–443, 1996.
54. M Blumenfield, NB Levy, B Spinowitz, C Charytan, CM Beasley, AK Dubey, RJ Solomon, R Todd, A Goodman, RF Bergstrom. Fluoxetine in depressed patients on dialysis. Int J Psychiatry Med 27:71–80, 1997.
55. S Borson, J Gwendolyn, RN McDonald, MD Terence-Gayle, M Deffebach, S Lakshminarayan, MD VanTuinen. Improvement in mood, physical symptoms and function with nortriptyline for depression in patients with chronic obstructive pulmonary disease. Psychosomatics 33:190–201, 1992.
56. TA Zielinski, ES Brown, VA Nejtek, DA Khan, JJ Moore, AJ Rush. Depression in asthma: prevalence and clinical implications. Primary Care Companion J Clin Psychiatry 2:153–158, 2000.
57. F Lechin, B van der Dijs, B Orozco, H Jara, I Rada, ME Lechin, AE Lechin. Neuropharmacologic treatment of bronchial asthma with the antidepressant tianeptine: a double-blind, crossover placebo-controlled study. Clin Pharmacol Ther 64:223–232, 1998.
58. VK Jain. A psychiatric study of hypothyroidism. Psychiatr Clin 5:121–130, 1972.
59. J McGaffee, MA Barnes, S Lippmann. Psychiatric presentations of hypothyroidism. Am Fam Physician 23:129–133, 1981.
60. MN Starkman, DE Schteingart, MA Schork. Cushing's syndrome after treatment: changes in cortisol and ACTH levels, and amelioration of the depressive syndrome. Psychiatry Res 19:177–188, 1986.
61. PT Loosen, AJ Prange. Serum thyrotropin response to thyrotropin-releasing hormone in psychiatric patients: a review. Am J Psychiatry 139:405–416, 1982.
62. GW Arana, D Mossman. The dexamethasone suppression test and depression. Endocrinol Metabol Clin North Amer 17:21–39, 1988.
63. ES Brown, L Bobadilla, AJ Rush. Ketoconazole in bipolar patients with depressive symptoms: a case series and literature review. Bipolar Disord (in press).
64. OM Wolkowitz, VI Reus. Treatment of depression with antiglucocorticoid drugs. Psychosom Med 61:698–711, 1999.
65. BEP Murphy. Antiglucocorticoid therapies in major depression: a review. Psychoneuroendocrinology 22(suppl):S125–S132, 1997.
66. OM Wolkowitz, VI Reus, T Chan, F Manfrdi, W Raum, R Johnson, J Canick. Antiglucocorticoid treatment of depression: double-blind ketoconazole. Biol Psychiatry 45:1070–1074, 1999.
67. JJ Schildkraut. The catecholamine hypothesis of affective disorders: a review of supporting evidence. Am J Psychiatry 122:509–522, 1965.
68. WE Bunney Jr, JM Davis. Norepinephrine in depressive reactions: review. Arch Gen Psychiatry 13:483–494, 1965.
69. H Miyaoka, T Otsubo, K Kamijima, M Ishii, M Onuki, K Mitamura. Depression from interferon therapy in patients with hepatitis C. Am J Psychiatry 156:1120, 1999.
70. JL Levenson, HJ Fallon. Fluoxetine treatment of depression caused by interferon-alpha. Am J Gastroenterol 88:760–761, 1993.
71. LS Goldman. Successful treatment of interferon alpha-induced mood disorder with nortriptyline. Psychosomatics 35:412–413, 1994.
72. OC Gleason, WR Yates. Five cases of interferon-alpha-induced depression treated with antidepressant therapy. Psychosomatics 40:510-512, 1999.
73. AH Miller, DL Musselman, BD Pearce, S Penna, CB Nemeroff. Pretreatment with the antidepressant, paroxetine, attenuates development of sickness behavior during high dose interferon alpha therapy (abstr). Presented at XXXth Congress of International Society of Psychoneuroendocrinology, Orlando, FL, 1999.
74. ES Brown, T Suppes. Mood symptoms during corticosteroid therapy: a review. Harv Rev Psychiatry 5:239–246, 1998.
75. ES Brown, DA Khan, VA Nejtek. The psychiatric side effects of corticosteroids. Ann Allergy Asthma Immunol 83:495–504, 1999.
76. WE Falk, MW Mahnke, DC Poskanzer. Lithium prophylaxis of corticotropin-induced psychosis. JAMA 241:1011–1012, 1979.
77. VI Reus, K Dark, HVS Puke, R Johnson, O Wolkowitz. Lithium prophylaxis of steroid-induced changes in behavior and biochemistry. Biol Psychiatry 29(suppl):162A, 1991
78. DG Blazer, WM Petrie, WP Wilson. Affective psychosis following renal transplant. Dis Nerv Syst 37:663–667, 1976.
79. K Kemp, JR Lion, G Magram. Lithium in the treatment of a manic patient with multiple sclerosis: a case report. Dis Nerv Syst 38:210–211, 1977.
80. T Terao, T Mizuki, T Ohji, K Abe. Antidepressant effect of lithium in patients with systemic lupus erythematosus and cerebral infarction, treated with corticosteroid. Br J Psychiatry 164:109–111, 1994.

81. SS Sharfstein, DS Sack, AS Fanci. Relationship between alternate-day corticosteroid therapy and behavioral abnormalities. JAMA 248:2987–2989, 1982.
82. DA Lewis, RE Smith. Steroid-induced psychiatric syndromes: a report of 14 cases and a review of the literature. J Affect Disord 5:319–332, 1983.
83. RCW Hall, MK Popkin, RN Stickney, E Gardner. Presentation of the steroid psychosis. J Nerv Mental Dis 167:229–236, 1979.
84. G Fricchione, M Ayyala, VF Holmes. Steroid withdrawal psychiatric syndromes. Ann Clin Psychiatry 1:99–108, 1989.
85. ES Brown, DA Khan, T Suppes. Treatment of corticosteroid-induced mood changes with olanzapine [letter]. Am J Psychiatry 156:968, 1999.
86. TM Kramer, EM Cottingham. Risperidone in the treatment of steroid-induced psychosis. J Child Adolesc Psychopharmacol 9:315–316, 1999.
87. A Abbas, R Styra. Valproate prophylaxis against steroid induced psychosis. Can J Psychiatry 39:188–189, 1994.
88. A Preda, A Fazeli, BG McKay, MB Bowers Jr, CM Mazure. Lamotrigine as prophylaxis against steroid-induced mania. J Clin Psychiatry 60:708–709, 1999.
89. RC Hall, MK Popkin, B Kirkpatrick. Tricyclic exacerbation of steroid psychosis. J Nerv Ment Dis 166:738–742, 1978.
90. AA Wyszynski, B Wyszynski. Treatment of depression with fluoxetine in cortico-steroid-dependent central nervous system Sjogren's syndrome. Psychosomatics 34:173–177, 1993.

58

Perspectives on Treatment Interventions in Paraphilias

FLORENCE THIBAUT

Rouen University Hospital, Rouen, France

I. INTRODUCTION

A variety of interventions have been attempted to reduce sexual violence. These include strengthening sanctions for punishment, establishing laws and a registry of offenders, and of course, treatment of offenders. Soothill and Gibbens [1], in a study on sex offenders with a 22-year follow-up, found that the recidivism rate rose by ∼ 3% per year and that at the end of the follow-up period, 48% of the sample had recidivated. The strongest predictor of sexual reoffence was sexual interest in children as measured by plethysmography. Indeed, homosexual pedophiles are more likely to recidivate (53.4%) as compared with a rate of 33% in heterosexual pedophiles [2]. Some sexually deviant acts are classified as paraphilias. Others arise in the context of neurological or psychiatric diseases, alcohol, or drug abuse.

The term paraphilia involves the sexual fixation on an unusual object (e.g., animals, underwear), a child or other nonconsenting person, or an act that leads to the suffering or humiliation of oneself or one's partner. The most common paraphilias are pedophilia, exhibitionism, voyeurism, sadomasochism, fetishism, or transvestism. Rape is not included in this classification. However, a small number of rapists may meet the criteria for having a paraphilia as well (often exhibitionism or pedophilia). The focus of a paraphilia is usually very specific and unchanging. Furthermore, there is considerable comorbidity among the paraphilias (one-third of pedophiles are also exhibitionists) [3].

The actual incidence and prevalence of the paraphilias remain unknown. Most sex offenders are male, but studies have estimated that up to 20% of abusers of boys and 5% of abusers of girls are women. In some of these cases, but not all, the abuse is carried out with, or under the influence of, a male partner [4]. The onset of paraphilic sexual interest usually occurs prior to age 18, and primary prevention in adolescence for paraphilias might be suggested.

In spite of years of research, not much is known about the etiology of paraphilias. Nevertheless, paraphilias seem to be of multifactorial origin. Paraphilic subjects rarely seek treatment unless an arrest or discovery by a family member traps them into it. Paraphilia treatment studies are difficult to conduct and much of the research has been done on male paraphilias. For ethical reasons, double-blind placebo-controlled studies are not conducted in violent or recidivist sex offenders. Usual treatment approaches have included traditional psychoanalysis and behavior therapy techniques, but often they have not been very successful. Pharmacological treatment had historically been based on studies that involved the surgical castration of sex offenders. Traditionally, the pharmacological treatment of sexually deviant behavior was based on the assumption that suppression of the sexual drive would decrease paraphilic sexual behavior. Ideally, successful treatment would mean that deviant sexual behaviors were suppressed, while conventional sexual fantasies and urges would be maintained or enhanced. Antiandrogen treatments, which either drastically lower testosterone levels or antagonize the action of testosterone at the receptor level, have been used alone or in conjunction with other treatment modalities. Psychotropic drugs and, more recently, serotoninergic antidepressants have also been used in the treatment of paraphilias.

In the first part of this review we will evoke the efficacy of psychotropic drugs in some types of paraphilias; in a second part, we will focus on hormonal therapies.

II. BACKGROUND

A. Testosterone

Approximately 95% of the testosterone is produced in the testes, the other 5% by the adrenal glands. The secretion of testosterone is regulated by a feedback mechanism in the hypothalamus-pituitary-testis axis. The hypothalamus produces gonadotrophin hormone-releasing hormone (GnRH), which stimulates the pituitary gland to produce luteinizing hormone (LH). LH stimulates the release of testosterone from the testes. Testosterone has an inhibiting effect on the hypothalamus and the pituitary.

The physiological effects of testosterone (and of its reduced metabolite 5α-dihydrotestosterone) are mediated through their actions on the intracellular androgen receptor. In humans, testosterone plays a major role not only in the development and maintenance of male sexual characteristics but also in sexuality and aggression [for review, see 5].

Testosterone has been shown to restore nocturnal penile tumescence responses in hypogonadal men with impaired nocturnal penile tumescence. A certain level of testosterone is necessary for sexual desire in males, above which testosterone levels does not seem to be correlated with levels of sexual drive. However, the threshold remains questionable. Although rigidity and detumescence seem to be androgen dependent to a certain degree, erections in response to visual erotic stimuli are not dependent on androgens, but erections in response to auditory stimuli possibly are [6]. Whether, or to what extent, erections as a result of fantasies and tactile stimulation are androgen dependent remains controversial.

The role of testosterone and its influence on general aggression remains unclear. In animals, testosterone plays a significant role in facilitating aggression among males [7]. In humans, more aggressive acts are often associated with high testosterone levels, but these levels remain in the normal range [5].

Although androgen-depleting agents are useful in controlling paraphilia, there is neither evidence that sex offenders have higher testosterone levels nor data indicating an increased androgen receptor activity. The expected benefit of decreasing testosterone activity (by lowering testosterone levels or by competing with testosterone at the receptor level) is probably derived from decreasing nonspecifically sexual arousal and behavior. However, Gaffney and Berlin [8] reported a marked hypersecretion of LH in response to GnRH in pedophiles, as compared to controls and other paraphilias, whereas baseline LH and testosterone values were in the normal range.

B. Estrogens and Progesterone

Most studies suggest that estrogens have little direct influence on sexual desire in either males or females. In men, relatively high levels of exogenous estrogens have been effective in inhibiting sexual desire among sex offenders [9]. Few studies have examined the effects of progesterone on male sexuality; some authors have used progesterone treatment to reduce excessive sexual desire in men [10].

C. Serotonin

In humans, selective serotonin reuptake inhibitors (SSRIs) are associated with sexual side effects such as decreased libido and impaired ejaculation. It is not known why SSRIs produce sexual side effects, but some authors suggest that activation of the $5HT_2$ receptors impairs sexual functioning and stimulation of the $5HT_{1A}$ receptors facilitates sexual functioning [for review see 11].

D. Brain Regions Involved in Sexual Behavior

Animal studies indicate that lesions to the medial preoptic area, which is connected to the limbic system and brainstem, significantly impairs male copulatory behavior by impairing the animal's ability to recognize a sexual partner. Electrical stimulation of the paraventricular nucleus elicits penile erections [11].

Recently, positron emission tomography (PET) was used to study the brain areas activated in eight healthy males during visually evoked sexual arousal [12]. They reported the following pattern of activation: (1) a bilateral activation of the inferior temporal cortex (a visual association area); (2) an activation of the right insula and right inferior frontal cortex (two paralimbic areas relating highly processed sensory information with motivational states); and (3) the activation of the left anterior cingulate cortex (another paralimbic area known to control autonomic and endocrine functions). Activation of some of these areas was positively correlated with plasma testosterone levels.

III. BEHAVIOR THERAPY

Sex offenders employ distorted patterns of thinking which allow them to rationalize their behavior. These attitudes include, for example, the belief that children can consent to sex with an adult and that victims are responsible for being sexually assaulted. Behavior therapy programs for sex offenders seek to tackle and change these distorted attitudes as well as other major factors which can contribute to sexual offending, including inability to control anger (anger serves as the primary motivation for many sex crimes, especially for rapists), inability to express feelings and communicate effectively, problems in managing stress, alcohol and drug abuse, or deviant sexual arousal.

The offenders who have the most distorted thoughts and attitudes toward children are fixated pedophiles. The aims of such programmes are to (1) counter the offender's distorted beliefs; (2) increase their awareness of the effects of their crimes on victims; (3) get offenders to accept responsibility for the results of their actions; and (4) assist offenders to develop ways of controlling their deviant behavior, preventing relapse and avoiding high-risk situations. Research studies in the United States into these treatment programs in prisons and in the community have identified substantial reductions in reoffending rates [for review see 13].

IV. PSYCHOTROPIC DRUGS

A. SSRIs

Several authors have conceptualized hypersexuality and some paraphilias as related to obsessive-compulsive disorders (OCD), or even impulsive control disorders [14]. In addition, there is a very high comorbidity of depression in the paraphilic patients. Since 1990, numerous uncontrolled single-case studies have reported the efficacy of SSRIs or clomipramine in the treatment of paraphilias, as well as hypersexuality without paraphilia [for review see 15–17]. One of the first reports on the efficacy of an antidepressant in a male exhibitionist was accidental. This man was suffering from dysphoria which was treated and the paraphilic behavior concomitantly decreased. The starting doses of SSRIs are low and may be progressively increased to the dosages usually prescribed in OCD. The maximal reduction of the symptoms occurs after 1–3 months. In most studies that have reported on the duration of treatment, the treatment period varied between 3 to 12 months.

Coleman et al. [18], Kafka [19], and Greenberg et al. [20] conducted several open clinical trials reporting the efficacy of SSRIs in paraphilia. In Kafka's study [19], paraphilic and hypersexual male nonresponders to sertraline for at least 4 weeks (100 mg/day) were offered fluoxetine (50 mg/day), and two-thirds (six of nine subjects) showed clinical improvement. No pedophiles were included in this study. Most subjects had comorbid mood disorders. Greenberg et al. [20] have found fluvoxamine, fluoxetine, and sertraline equally effective in a retrospective study of 58 paraphilic male subjects for 12 weeks. However, Stein et al. [14] reported that fluvoxamine (200–300 mg/day) or fluoxetine (60–80 mg/day) did not improve five paraphilic subjects after 2–10 months of treatment. However, comorbid nonsexual OCD symptoms improved in these patients. With the exception of Stein's study, SSRIs had improved paraphilic patients.

Kafka and Prentsky [21] reported that fluoxetine (40 mg/day for 12 weeks) reduced the frequency of paraphilic behaviors preferentially, and they hypothesized that SSRIs may even facilitate normal sexual arousal. In the same way, Bradford [3] reported that the physiologic measures of sexual arousal (penile plethysmography) showed a decrease in pedophilic arousal (by 53%) and an improved or maintained normophilic arousal after 12 weeks of sertraline treatment (130 mg/day).

Interestingly, Kruesi et al. [22], in a double-blind crossover study, have observed that clomipramine (25–250 mg/day) and desipramine (25–250 mg/day) reduced equally paraphilic behavior in 8 subjects (7 of 15 dropped out). These results indicate that there was no preferential response to the more specific serotoninergic antidepressant.

In many studies, heterogeneous groups of paraphilic subjects were included. Exhibitionism, compulsive masturbation, and pedophilia were the most frequent paraphilias in which SSRIs have shown improvement. In most cases, other psychiatric diagnoses were associated to paraphilias (mostly affective disorders or OCD). These studies draw attention to a new option for treating paraphilias that are accompanied by OCD, impulse control disorders, or depressive disorders. However, despite the increasing clinical use of SSRIs for paraphilia and hypersexuality, double-blind placebo-controlled trials with these agents are lacking and, in addition, the use of SSRI in adolescents deserves investigations.

B. Other Psychotropic Drugs

Various phenothiazines such as thioridazine, fluphenazine, or butyrophenones such as benperidol, have been used in sex offenders [23,24]. Their incomplete efficacy and the risk of tardive dyskinesia have limited their prescription in the treatment of paraphilia. However, antipsychotic agents may benefit sex offenders with comorbid psychotic disorders; indeed, in these patients hormonal therapy may even exacerbate psychosis. Anecdotal reports have reported the quick response observed with lithium in different types of paraphilia (within 1–10 days). Most of these subjects had paraphilia comorbid with mood disorders [18].

V. SURGICAL TREATMENTS

A. Surgical Castration

Castration has been practiced on human beings in all cultures for thousands of years. In ancient China and Oriental sagas, eunuchs served as chamberlains or guards of women's quarters. In Europe, castration was done on modern psychiatric indication for the first time in Switzerland in 1892, as an "imbecile" was cured from his neuralgic pains from the testes and his hypersexuality. Heim and Hursch [25], in their review of European literature, reported that populations of surgically castrated sex offenders (follow-up max 20 years) showed recidivism rates of 2.5–7.5% (1200 sex offenders), as opposed to recidivism rate of 60–84% before castration, and of 39% in 685 sex offenders who were not castrated. Reoffence rates were usually based on rearrest or conviction. The decline of the nonsexual crimes after castration was less obvious. In castrated subjects, there was no change in the object of the offender's sexual desire or sexual orientation. Unfortunately, these studies were not controlled.

Forty percent to 50% of subjects were content with the outcome of castration, whereas 30% of patients complained of undesirable side effects. Twenty percent to 40% of castrates felt calmer after castration, whereas 20–30% complained that they were often depressed since castration. A substantial percentage of surgical castrates retain sexual functioning (sex drive and potency) (35% of young subjects). Moreover, Eibl [26] reported that 19 of 38 castrated sex offenders whose penile erections were measured while viewing a sex movie, exhibited full erections.

In the United States (in several states) and in Europe (in Germany and Czechoslovakia), surgical castration is allowed in place of chemical castration. In some countries (e.g., Germany) the Law on Voluntary Castration provided that voluntary castration be available in men aged at least 25 years. This would be available in the case of seriously disturbed and dangerous sexual offenders. A board of experts is required to review the request in order to establish that castration is necessary for the prevention of further sexual offences. The incidence of surgical castration in Germany is small (five cases per year). California passed a law in 1996 that mandated chemical castration for repeat child molesters. Several other states have considered passing such laws (Colorado, Florida, Louisiana, Massachusetts, Michigan, Texas, and Washington). Castration has increasingly been seen as ethically problematic. However, Bailey and Greenberg [27] argued that offering castration as an option to sex offenders in exchange for sentence reduction is not unethical.

The results obtained using surgical castration have motivated further research in antiandrogenic treatment.

B. Neurosurgery

Stereotactic neurosurgery has previously been attempted in sex offenders. Because of the level of invasiveness of this technique, it has not been practical to any extent.

VI. HORMONAL THERAPIES

A. Estrogens

Historically, estrogens were the first hormonal agents used for the treatment of sex offenders. Despite their clinical efficacy, their adverse effects (gynecomastia, increased occurrence of thrombosis, testes atrophy, carcinoma of breast) rapidly limited their use [28].

B. Medroxyprogesterone Acetate (Depo-Provera) and Cyproterone Acetate (Androcur)

Medroxyprogesterone acetate (MPA) is a progesterone derivative. MPA is already used as a contraceptive, and as a treatment for endometriosis or breast cancer. The first report of its efficacy in reducing sexual drive was published in 1958 in healthy males [29]. MPA may be prescribed as a depot preparation (300–500 mg/week) or PO [50–100 mg/day) (oral administration may sometimes be used even if its absorption is less erratic) [30].

MPA reduces testosterone by inhibiting its production through reducing LH. MPA induces the testosterone reductase which accelerates testosterone metabolism, and reduces plasma testosterone by enhancing its clearance. In addition, MPA also has an effect in increasing testosterone binding to testosterone hormone-binding globulin (TeBG), which reduces the availability of free testosterone, and finally, MPA may also bind to androgen receptors [31]. The drug was first noted for its efficacy in the treatment of one case of paraphilia by Money in 1968 [32].

Cyproterone acetate (CPA) is already used as a treatment for precocious puberty and as a treatment for carcinoma of the prostate. CPA is a synthetic steroid, similar to progesterone, which acts directly on all androgen receptors (including brain receptors), where it blocks intracellular testosterone uptake and the intracellular metabolism of the androgen. Indeed, CPA is a competitive inhibitor of testosterone and dihydrotestosterone at androgen receptor sites. In addition, it has a strong progestational action which causes an inhibition of GnRH secretion. CPA may be given either by injection (depot form: 200–400 mg once weekly or every 2 weeks) or by tablets (100–200 mg/day).

The first clinical use of CPA in sex offenders (predominantly exhibitionists) occurred in Germany [33], which reported efficacy of CPA in 80% of the cases in an open study. Moreover, in 80% of the cases, 100 mg/day oral CPA was sufficient. Depending on dosage, the authors suggested that CPA could be used as a chemical castration agent or as a reductor of sexual drive, allowing erecting ability in nondeviant sexual behavior.

MPA is available in the United States; CPA is used predominantly in Canada, the Middle East, and Europe.

Numerous uncontrolled case studies involving several hundreds of patients and some controlled studies (alternating antiandrogens with placebo and using each subject as his own control) have repeatedly reported the efficacy of MPA and CPA in the treatment of paraphilias [10,34–36; for review see 15,16,37].

Both CPA and MPA, along with reduction of active testosterone levels, significantly decreased self-reported deviant sexual behavior or fantasies and frequency of masturbation within 2–4 weeks in 80% of patients. Morning erections, ejaculations, and spermatogenesis were decreased. The efficacy was maintained while on treatment for up to 8 years. Meyer and Cole [38] have examined the reoffence rates for 127 individuals taking CPA and have found a mean rate of 6% at the end of the follow-up period, as compared with 85% before treatment from seven studies; the duration of follow-up varied from 2 months to 4.5 years. Many of the reoffences were committed by individuals who did not comply with therapy. In addition, a significant number of patients reoffend after stopping therapy. The reoffence rate for 334 individuals taking depot MPA was greater than with CPA with a mean rate of 27% at the end of the follow-up period, as compared with 50% before treatment (follow-up 6 months to 13 years) [38]. Five studies reported increased recidivism after MPA was stopped.

Money et al. [39], using MPA, reported no reduction in nonsexual crimes in sex offenders with antisocial behavior. However, some studies have reported reduced anxiety and irritability with CPA or MPA in their patients [10,36].

The results of the evaluation of penile responses to a variety of erotic stimuli, using plethysmography, for CPA and MPA, have been less impressive than when subjective measures of improvement have been used. Using visual erotic stimuli, Bancroft et al. [9], Langevin et al. [40], and Cooper et al. [10] found that CPA or MPA had no significant or more variable effects on the erectile responses of sex offenders. These results are in accordance with the view that erections in response to visual stimuli are less androgen dependent. By contrast, Bradford and Pawlak [36], using CPA, have reported a consistent trend toward preferential suppression of deviant arousal during phallometric measures in a group of pedophiles with high levels of testosterone (within the normal range).

The adverse effects of CPA, in addition to those related to hypoandrogenism (such as bone mineral loss), include gynecomastia (20% of cases, reversible), depression, fatigue, weight gain, leg cramps, decreased glucose tolerance, increased level of prolactin, and hepatocellular damage (which may be rarely fatal). Adrenal suppression has been described primarily in adolescents with CPA [41]. The adverse effects of MPA include weight gain, hypertension, gynecomastia, lethargy, leg cramps, bone mineral loss, hot and cold flashes, diabetes mellitus, gallstones, adrenal suppression, and thromboembolic phenomena. Pulmonary embolism is the most severe side effect reported.

CPA and MPA treatment have to be carefully managed medically, via physical examination, especially for the effects of feminization. Biochemical monitoring of liver function is required when CPA is used. The treatment effects of CPA or MPA were completely reversible, 1 or 2 months after medication withdrawal.

CPA treatment has been compared with estrogens, MPA, and GnRHa treatments in sex offenders. Brancroft et al. [9] compared the effects of 100 mg/day CPA and of 0.01 mg ethinylestradiol twice a day. The two treatments equally decreased sexual interest, sexual activity, and objective measurement of sexual arousal with no major side effects.

Cooper et al. [10] reported the first double-blind comparison of MPA (100–200 mg/day) and CPA (100–200 mg/day) and concluded that MPA and CPA performed equally in seven sex offenders with no side effects except for those related to hypoandrogenism. Cooper and Cernovsky [42] described a significantly greater decrease in self-report and objective measure of sexual arousal with leuprolide (7.5 mg IM per month), as compared with previous CPA treatment (after a 10-week washout period), in one case of pedophilia. Although there is no consensus on the optimal duration of CPA or MPA treatment, many authors have written that 3–5 years of treatment are necessary [for review, see 15]. Unfortunately, MPA and CPA have rarely been used in women with paraphilia [43].

C. GnRH Analogs or GnRH Agonists (GnRHa) [Triptorelin (Decapeptyl-CR), Leuprolide (Lupron), and Gosereline (Zoladex)]

After an initial stimulation, these long-acting GnRH analogs cause rapid desensitization of GnRH receptors, resulting in reduction of LH (and to a lesser extent of FSH) and testosterone to castration levels. They do not interfere with the action of androgens of adrenal origin. Somehow, only 40% of normal controls reported reduction in normal sexual desire with GnRH treatment [44]. In addition, GnRH-containing neurons project into pituitary and extrapituitary sites, such as the olfactory bulb or the amygdala. At these latter sites, GnRH is believed to act as a neuromodulator and, through this action, may be involved in sexual behavior [45,46]. Moreover, the intracerebroventricular administration of GnRH suppresses aggression in male rats [47].

Leuprolide (Lupron) and gosereline (Zoladex) are already approved by the U.S. Food and Drug Administration for prostate cancer, central precocious puberty, and endometriosis. Rousseau et al. [48] reported the first case of a male severe exhibitionist who has been successfully treated for 26 weeks with the combination of a short-acting GnRHa and the antiandrogen flutamide. The assessment of the patient's sexual fantasies and activities was achieved through self-reports. Concurrently with the decrease of testosterone, a sharp decline in the patient's deviant sexual activities and fantasies was observed. The patient's deviant activities completely ended after 2–4 weeks. Two months after discontinuation of the treatment, the patient relapsed.

Dickey [49] reported the case of a male patient with multiple paraphilias, successfully treated for 6 months with a long-acting GnRH agonist (leuprolide acetate), and observed that suppression of androgen of testicular origin alone was sufficient for treatment.

Thibaut et al. [50] reported the first open study describing the efficacy of triptorelin (3.75 mg IM monthly) in five out of six cases of severe male paraphilia (four cases of pedophilia, one case of severe exhibitionism, one case of sexual sadism). In all patients, CPA treatment had been initiated 1 week before GnRHa and concurrently prescribed for at least 10 days with GnRHa in order to control the early and transient increase in plasma testosterone level, and possibly in sexual drive, due to an initial stimulation effect of GnRHa. In five cases, concurrent with the decrease of plasma testosterone, LH, and estradiol levels within the first month, we observed a parallel drop of deviant sexual interest and activities (using self-reports), and the deviant behavior ended. The TeBG remained unchanged, which leads to a decrease in free testosterone level. The beneficial effect of the treatment was maintained during follow-up periods varying from 7 months to 3 years. Apparently, the remaining secretion of androgens of adrenal origin did not interfere with the efficacy of GnRHa, and the addition of a pure antiandrogen did not seem useful. However, the remaining low levels of testosterone of adrenal origin might have played a role in the failure of GnRHa in one patient. In this case, the combination of CPA and GnRHa might have been effective.

Rösler and Witztum [51], using a similar methodology, reported the efficacy of GnRHa (triptorelin, 3.75 mg IM monthly) in 30 men (25 pedophiles) with severe, long-standing paraphilia, in an open study, with a duration of follow-up of 12–42 months. They did not use CPA to counter the possible initial increase in deviant sexual behavior during the first weeks of GnRHa treatment. In five cases of paraphilia, a diagnosis of paranoid schizophrenia was reported. The maximal reduction in sexual desire and activity occurred after 3–10 months according to patients. The authors reported a decrease of 50% of baseline testicular volume after 36 months of treatment.

The duration of antiandrogen treatment necessary to achieve a definite disappearance of deviant sexual behavior and the conditions of treatment interruption remain unanswered. In most studies, the duration of antiandrogenic treatment is < 1 year, except for the study by Davies [52], which reported no recidivism during 3 years of follow-up after cessation of 5 years' CPA treatment in different types of paraphilias. In Rousseau's study [48], they reported recidivism when successful GnRHa treatment was abruptly stopped at the 26th week. In Thibaut's study [53], the authors described recidivism of deviant sexual behavior within 8–10 weeks in two cases, when successful GnRHa treatment was abruptly interrupted after 12 and 34 months, respectively. In one case, GnRHa treatment was reintroduced and the deviant behavior disappeared. In Rösler's study [51], in eight cases, treatment was interrupted after 8–10 months (owing to unspecified intolerable side effects in three cases). In five cases, in whom follow-up was possible, paraphilia resumed. In men who interrupted treatment, serum testosterone returned to baseline level within 2 months.

In these three studies, the patients' recidivism might have been encouraged by the abrupt withdrawal of GnRHa and might have resulted from a release of testosterone interacting with hypersensitive androgen receptors. By contrast, in Thibaut's study [53], in a third case, after 4.5 years of effective GnRHa treatment, testosterone was gradually added to GnRHa in order to avoid the "rebound effect" in sexual behavior, which could be observed 4–6 weeks after abrupt antiandrogen treatment withdrawal, when a transient increase in testosterone levels to above baseline levels appeared [48,53,54]. In our case, the deviant sexual behavior did not return when GnRHa and testosterone were interrupted, after 10 months of concurrent prescription, as soon as testosterone level was back in the normal range. Maintenance of the beneficial effect of antiandrogen treatment after interruption could be the result of a conditioned behavioral response, or it could result from changes in androgen-receptor sensitivity.

In summary, concurrent with the decrease in testosterone levels, GnRHa treatment was effective in 37 out of 38 cases of severe paraphilia with a maximal follow-up duration of 6 years [55]. Twenty-one patients out of 38 were convicted for sexual offences prior to treatment. GnRHa treatment was more potent than CPA or MPA: 13 patients out of 38 were previously unsuccessfully treated with CPA (150–300 mg/day for up to 10 years) or MPA, and seven patients were previously unsuccessfully treated with SSRIs. The use of long-acting GnRHa excluded the uncontrolled breaks in the therapy often observed with oral CPA treatment (depot CPA is not available in France).

In addition, GnRHa treatment can lead to reversible castration without further side effects than those related to hypoandrogenism (i.e., hot flashes, asthenia, depression, decrease in normal sexual behavior, and decrease in bone mineral density, which needs to be closely monitored, especially after a duration of 2 years of antiandrogen treatment, and treated if necessary). These studies do not support the specificity of GnRHa treatment in reducing sex drive for deviant versus normal stimuli. However, while treated, 14 patients out of 37 maintained lower erectile capacity and were able to maintain some masturbation and coital activities; this was proportional to age. The direction of the sexual drive was not affected.

Some people may argue that sex offenders may try to revive their libidos by obtaining exogenous testosterone. We can answer that many paraphilic men feel their paraphilia as unwanted and experience the diminution of their deviant behavior as relief. In addition, these patients could be subject to random blood tests which could detect excess testosterone.

However, none of these studies utilized placebo, because of the potential for the men to continue to offend without active medication. Moreover, none of these studies used objective measurements of sexual activity. The need for controlled studies, using large samples of well-defined paraphilic patients, to confirm these promising results is urgent.

VII. CONCLUSION

Most people recognize that incarceration alone will not solve sexual violence. Treating the offenders is critical in an approach to preventing sexual violence and reducing victimization. A recent meta-analysis of factors predicting recidivism, based on 61 follow-up studies, including 23,400 sex offenders, found that failure to complete treatment was associated with higher risk of recidivism of sex offences [56]. However, it is not possible at this time to identify those individuals who will not have any recurrence compared with those who may. Sex offenders with intellectual disabilities or sequella of head injury are particularly susceptible to reoffend after stopping therapy. Alcohol and drug abuse have also been reported as risk factors of reoffences. By contrast, self-referred or highly motivated subjects are best responders to chemical treatment.

Paraphilic men may be ordered by the judge to undergo psychiatric treatment as part of the rehabilitative aspect of sentencing, but these situations should leave treatment options up to the professionals. In case of antiandrogen treatment, it may include freely given informed consent. Indeed, these treatments must remain a choice for the patient to make on the basis of medical advice. Somehow, in some cases, failure of the offender to participate in treatment could lead to sanctions by the court. Prior to treatment, each individual should be carefully examined by at least one mental health professional, in order to identify and evaluate sex offenders and, if necessary, protect offenders who are suffering from a major mental illness or mental retardation. However, little is known about which treatments are most effective, for which offenders, over what duration, or in what combination.

Because of ethical issues, the great majority of pharmacological studies are uncontrolled studies with methodological problems. One major difficulty is the identification of standardized and reliable measures of sexual behavior. Sex offenders' self-reports of their sexual activity and arrest records reports are usually used, but they do not constitute reliable indices of deviant or nondeviant sexual behavior. In addition, the definition of recidivism is often different from one study to another. In the same way, the validity and reliability of the evaluation of sexual response via penile plethysmography, which measures penile erectile responses to various visual erotic stimuli in a laboratory, are still a subject of debate. In any case, plethysmography should be used to predict further sex offences or to make a diagnosis.

Moreover, various types of sex offenders are included in the same studies and makes it difficult to draw definite conclusions owing to the great heterogeneity of the samples of patients. Duration of follow-up periods is another source of variability among studies. Large international controlled studies including big samples of well-defined paraphilic patients are clearly needed to confirm these preliminary data, reporting the efficacy of pharmacological treatments in paraphilias.

In accordance with Gijs and Gooren [15], we may propose the following guidelines:

1. Not every sex offender is a candidate for antiandrogen treatment, even if it has the benefit of being reversible once discontinued. For paraphilias characterized by intense and frequent deviant sexual desire and arousal, which highly predispose the patient to severe paraphilic behaviors (such as pedophilia or rape), a hormonal intervention may be needed. Antiandrogens have to be prescribed by a physician after appropriate medical assessment and after informed consent is given. These medications should be used after other alternatives are ruled out or when there is a high risk of sexual violence. However, hormonal agents cannot be easily used in the treatment of sexually deviant adolescents owing to possible interference with the development or course of puberty.

2. Antiandrogens significantly reduce the intensity and frequency of sexual arousal but do not change the content of paraphilias. However, MPA and CPA treatments are associated with high dropout rates [16]. In spite of their efficacy, there are associated with a high percentage of side effects which have considerably limited their use, especially for MPA, in Europe. In addition, uncontrolled breaks in the therapy are often observed with oral CPA treatment. Long-acting GnRHa is more potent than CPA or MPA. Moreover, it induces fewer side effects, except for those related to hypoandrogenism. Long-acting GnRHa may be administered parentally once every 1–3 months. GnRHa treatment probably constitutes the most promising treatment for sex offenders at high risk of sexual violence, such as pedophiles or rapists. In spite of these new treatments, which induce chemical reversible castration, in the United States (in several states) and in Europe (in Germany and Czechoslovakia), surgical castration is still allowed in place of chemical castration for repeat child molesters.

3. SSRIs are useful in paraphilias associated with obsessive-compulsive disorders, impulse control disorders, or depressive disorders. Some paraphilic subjects clearly suffer from an inability to resist their sexual urges, which has a strong compulsive element and

often causes considerable subjective distress. SSRIs can be effective in these cases, which are usually not associated with dangerous sex offending.

4. Pharmacological interventions should always be part of a more comprehensive treatment plan including psychotherapy and, in most cases, behavior therapy.

It would be informative for future research to include a focus on all sex offenders including women and adolescents.

REFERENCES

1. KL Soothill, TCN Gibbens. Recidivism of sexual offenders: reappraisal. Br J Criminol 18:267–275, 1978.
2. PH Gebhard, JH Gagnon, WB Pomeroy, CV Christeason. Sex Offenders: An Analysis of Types. New York: Harper and Row, 1965, pp 811–812.
3. JMW Bradford. The paraphilias, obsessive compulsive spectrum disorder, and the treatment of sexually deviant behaviour. Psychiatr Q 70(3):209–219, 1999.
4. M Elliott. Female sexual abusers: the ultimate taboo. In: M Elliott, ed. Female Sexual Abusers: The Ultimate Taboo. London: J. Wiley and Sons, 1993.
5. DR Rubinow, PJ Schmidt. Androgens, brain and behavior. Am J Psychiatry 153:974–984, 1996.
6. C Carani, J Bancroft, A Granata, G Del Rio, P Marrama. Testosterone and erectile function, nocturnal penile tumescence and rigidity, and erectile response to visual erotic stimuli in hypogonadal and eugonadal men. Psychoneuroendocrinology 17(6):647–654, 1992.
7. RM Rose, JW Holaday, IS Bernstein. Plasma testosterone, dominance rank and aggressive behaviour in male rhesus monkeys. Nature 231:366–368, 1972.
8. GR Gaffney, FS Berlin. Is there hypothalamic-pituitary-gonadal dysfunction in paedophilia? Br J Psychiatry 145:657–660, 1984.
9. J Bancroft, G Tennent, K Loucas, J Cass. The control of deviant sexual behavior by drugs. I. Behavioral changes following estrogens and antiandrogens. Br J Psychiatry 125:310–315, 1974.
10. AJ Cooper, S Sandhu, S Losztyn, ZZ Cernovsky. A double-blind placebo controlled trial of medroxyprogesterone acetate and cyproterone acetate with seven pedophiles. Can J Psychiatry 37:687–693, 1992.
11. CM Meston, PF Frohlich. The neurobiology of sexual function. Arch Gen Psychiatry 57:1012–1030, 2000.
12. S Stoléru, MC Grégoire, D Gérard, J Decety, E Lafarge, L Cinotti, F Lavenne, D Le Bars, E Vernet-Maury, H Rada, C Collet, B Mazoyer, MG Forest, F Magnin, A Spira, D Comar. Neuroanatomical correlates of visually evoked sexual arousal in human males. Arch Sex Behav 28(1):1–21, 1999.
13. LS Grossman, B Martis, CG Fichter. Are sex offenders treatable? A research overview. Psychiatr Serv 50:349–391, 1999.
14. DJ Stein, E Hollander, DT Anthony, FR Schneier, B Fallon, MR Liebowitz, DF Klein. Serotonergic medication of sexual obsessions, sexual addictions, and paraphilias. J Clin Psychiatry 53:267–271, 1992.
15. L Gijs, L Gooren. Hormonal and psychopharmacological interventions in the treatment of paraphilias: an update. J Sex Res 33(4):273–290, 1996.
16. JMW Bradford, DM Greenberg. Pharmacological treatment of deviant sexual behaviour. Annu Rev Sex Behav 7:283–306, 1996.
17. R Balon. Pharmacological treatment of paraphilias with a focus on antidepressants. J Sex Marital Ther 24:241–254, 1998.
18. E. Coleman, J Cesnik, AM Moore, SM Dwyer. An exploratory study of the role of psychotropic medications in treatment of sexual offenders. J Off Rehab 18:75–88, 1992.
19. MP Kafka. Sertraline pharmacotherapy for paraphilias and paraphilia-related disorders: an open trial. Ann Clin Psychiatry 6:189–195, 1994.
20. DM Greenberg, JMW Bradford, S Curry, A O'Rourke. A comparison of treatment of paraphilias with three serotonin reuptake inhibitors: a retrospective study. Bull Am Acad Psychiatry Law 24:525–532, 1996.
21. MP Kafka, R. Prentsky. A comparative study of non-paraphilic sexual addictions and paraphilias in men. J Clin Psychiatry 53: 345–350, 1992.
22. MP Kruesi, S Fine, L Valladares, RA Phillips, J Rapoport. Paraphilias : a double bind cross-over comparison of clomipramine versus desipramine. Arch Sex Behav 21:587–593, 1992.
23. P Sterkman, F Geerts. Is benperidol (RF 504) the specific drug for the treatment of excessive and disinhibited sexual behaviour? Acta Neurol Psychiatr 66:1030–1040, 1966.
24. AA Bartholomew. A long-acting phenothiazine as a possible agent to control deviant sexual behavior. Am J Psychiatr 124:917–923, 1968.
25. N Heim, CJ Hursch. Castration for sex offenders: treatment or punishment? A review and critique of recent European literature. Arch Sex Behav 8(3):281–304, 1979.
26. E Eibl. Treatment and after-care of 300 sex offenders, especially with regard to penile plethysmography. Justizministerium Baden-Württemberg. Proceedings of the German Conference on Treatment Possibilities for Sex Offenders in Eppingen, Stuttgart, 1978.
27. JM Bailey, AS Greenberg. The science and ethics of castration: lessons from the Morse case. Northwestern Law Rev 92: 266–277, 1998.
28. LH Whittaker. Estrogens and psychosexual disorders. Med J Aust 2:547–549, 1959.

29. CG Heller, M Laidlaw, HT Harvey, DL Nelson. The effects of the progestational compounds on the reproductive processes of the human male. Ann NY Acad Sci 71:649–655, 1958.
30. HG Gottesman, DS Schubert. Low-dose oral medroxyprogesterone acetate in the management of the paraphilias. J Clin Psychiatry 54(5):182–188, 1993.
31. AL Southren, GG Gordon, J Vittek, K Altman. Effect of progestagens on androgen metabolism. In: L Martini, M Motta, eds. Androgens and antiandrogens. New York: Raven Press, 1977, pp 263–279.
32. J Money. Discussion on hormonal inhibition of libido in male sex offenders. In: RP Michael, ed. Endocrinology and Human Behavior. London: Oxford University Press, 1968, p 169.
33. U Laschet, L Laschet. Psychopharmacotherapy of sex offenders with cyproterone acetate. Pharmacopsychiatr Neuropsychopharmacol Adv Clin Res 4:99–110, 1971.
34. AJ Cooper A placebo controlled trial of the antiandrogen cyproterone acetate in deviant hypersexuality. Compr Psychiatry 22:458–465, 1981.
35. TA Kiersch. Treatment of sex offenders with Depo-Provera. Bull Am Acad Psychiatry Law 18:179–187, 1990.
36. JMW Bradford, A Pawlak. Double-blind placebo cross-over study of cyproterone acetate in the treatment of paraphilias. Arch Sex Behav 22:383–402, 1993.
37. A Rösler, E Witztum. Pharmacotherapy of paraphilias in the next millennium. Behav Sci Law 18:43–56, 2000.
38. WJ Meyer, CM Cole. Physical and chemical castration of sex offenders: a review. J Off Rehab 25(3/4):1–18, 1997.
39. J Money, C Wiedeking, P Walker, C Migeon, W Meyer, D Borgaonkar. 47,XYY and 46,XY males with antisocial and/or sex-offending behavior: antiandrogen therapy plus counselling. Psychoneuroendocrinology 1:165–178, 1975.
40. R Langevin, D Paitich, S Hucker, S Newman, G Ramsey, S Pope, G Geller, C Anderson. The effect of assertiveness training, Provera, and sex of therapist in the treatment of genital exhibitionism. J Behav Ther Exp Psychiatry 10:275–282, 1979.
41. F Neumann. Pharmacology and potential use of cyproterone acetate. Horm Metab Res 9:1–13, 1977.
42. AJ Cooper, ZZ Cernovski. Comparison of cyproterone acetate and leuprolide acetate (LHRH agonist) in a chronic pedophile: a clinical case study. Biol Psychiatry 36(4):269–271, 1994.
43. AJ Cooper, S Swaminath, D Baxter, C Poulin. A female sex offender with multiple paraphilias: a psychological, physiologic (laboratory sexual arousal) and endocrine case study. Can J Psychiatry 35:334–337, 1990.
44. PT Loosen, SE Purdon, SN Pavlou. Effects on behavior of modulation of gonadal function in men with gonadotrophin releasing hormone antagonists. Am J Psychiatry 151:271–273, 1994.
45. KM Kendrick, AF Dixson. Luteinizing hormone releasing hormone enhances proceptivity in a primate. Neuroendocrinology 41:449–453, 1985.
46. RL Moss, CA Dudley. Luteinizing hormone–releasing hormone (LHRH): peptidergic signals in the neural integration of female reproductive behavior. In: JM Lakoski, JR Perez-Polo, DK Rassin, eds. Neural Control of Reproductive Function. New York: Liss, 1989, pp 485–499.
47. T Kadar G Telegdy, AV Schally. Behavioral effects of centrally administered LH-RH agonist in rats. Physiol Behav 50:601–605, 1992.
48. L Rousseau, M Couture, A Dupont, F Labrie, N Couture. Effect of combined androgen blockade with an LHRH agonist and flutamide in one severe case of male exhibitionism. Can J Psychiatry 35:338–341, 1990.
49. R Dickey. The management of a case of treatment-resistant paraphilia with a long-acting LHRH agonist. Can J Psychiatry 37:567–569, 1992.
50. F Thibaut, B Cordier, JM Kuhn. Effect of a long-lasting gonadotrophin hormone–releasing hormone agonist in six cases of severe male paraphilia. Acta Psychiatr Scand 87:445–450, 1993.
51. A Rösler, E Witztum. Treatment of men with paraphilia with a long-acting analogue of gonadotropin-releasing hormone. N Engl J Med 338:416–422, 1998.
52. TS Davies. Cyproterone acetate for male hypersexuality. J Int Med Res 2:159–163, 1974.
53. F Thibaut, B Cordier, JM Kuhn. Gonadotrophin hormone releasing hormone agonist in cases of severe paraphilia: a lifetime treatment? Psychoneuroendocrinology 21(4):411–419, 1996.
54. JM Bradford. Organic treatment for the male sexual offender. Ann NY Acad Sci 528:193–202, 1998.
55. F Thibaut, JM Kuhn, B Cordier, M Petit. Les traitements hormonaux de la délinquance sexuelle. Encéphale XXIV:132–137, 1998.
56. RK Hanson, MT Bussiere. Predicting relapse: a meta-analysis of sexual offender recidivism studies. J Consult Clin Psychol 66:348–362, 1998.

59

Potential of Repetitive Transcranial Magnetic Stimulation in the Treatment of Neuropsychiatric Conditions

THOMAS E. SCHLAEPFER
University of Bern, Bern, Switzerland, and Johns Hopkins University School of Medicine, Baltimore, Maryland, U.S.A.

MARKUS KOSEL
University of Bern, Bern, Switzerland

I. INTRODUCTION

Transcranial magnetic stimulation (TMS) is a noninvasive technique to stimulate the human brain in vivo using very strong, pulsed magnetic fields. Owing to recent technical advances, the needed equipment is comparatively affordable and no surgery and/or anesthesia is needed in contrast to other new methods of direct brain stimulation, like magnetic seizure therapy (MST), vagus nerve stimulation (VNS), and deep brain stimulation (DBS). These techniques have received considerable research and clinical interest in recent years because there are indications that they might have effects in neuropsychiatric disorders, especially affective disorders.

MST is a novel approach in which a focal magnetic stimulus applied to the cortex is used to elicit generalized convulsions in patients under general anesthesia and muscle relaxation, similar to electroconvulsive therapy (ECT). At the present moment, it is clearly an experimental procedure, since no results from trials assessing its clinical efficacy are available. However, the general feasibility in human patients has been established [1]. VNS is a method approved by the FDA in 1997 for the management of medically refractory partial-onset epileptic seizures. Stimulation electrodes are attached to the left vagus nerve at the cervical level and linked to an implanted nerve stimulator—in function and size similar to a cardiac pacemaker—which is inserted in a pouch in the left chest wall. Applications in psychiatry are currently being investigated, and first multicenter studies for the treatment of depression have been completed [2]. DBS is a method of treating motor symptoms, mainly in Parkinson's disease, where stimulatory electrodes are placed in appropriate structures of the brain and linked to a nerve stimulator similar to those used for VNS. Studies of its potential efficacy in patients suffering from depressive disorder and obsessive-compulsive disorder (OCD) are being conducted at the moment.

TMS refers to the delivery of a magnetic pulse to the cortex of a subject trough a handheld stimulating coil, which is directly applied to the head (Figs. 1, 2). The magnetic pulses pass unimpeded through scalp and skull and induce an electrical current in the underlying tissue, which in turn is able to depolarize neurons. The main advantages of this stimulation

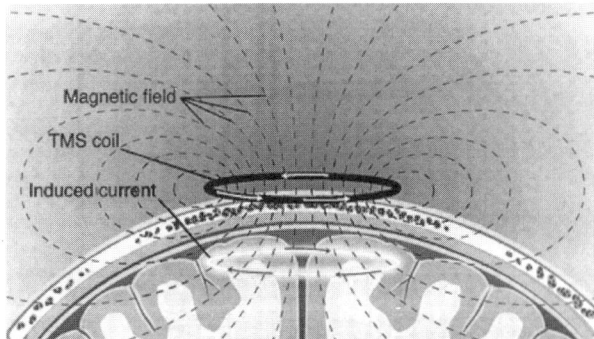

Figure 1 *Transcranial magnetic stimulation: principle of action.* A transient current in a magnetic stimulating coil over the scalp induces a small current in the brain, which is able to activate neural elements in the motor cortex.

method are its relative noninvasiveness and the possibility to stimulate very focused. With recent technology, single or paired pulse technique which are used to assess brain physiology and pathophysiology [3], as well as repetitive transcranial magnetic stimulation (rTMS) (high- frequency rTMS: stimulation faster than 1 Hz; low-frequency rTMS: stimulation at 1 or less Hz) up to 80 Hz can be delivered.

At the moment, clinical interest in the rTMS technique originates mainly from ∼ 15 placebo-controlled clinical studies involving up to 70 subjects [4] where rTMS was delivered to patients suffering from treatment refractory depression. However, results are not yet conclusive with respect to clinical efficacy. It has been demonstrated that rTMS has effects on the brain, but whether its properties are clinically useful and constitute meaningful alternatives to already available treatment modalities remains to be investigated. Today rTMS seems to be a very interesting and potentially promising technique in search of useful applications in neuropsychiatry.

We focus this review on practical details concerning the delivery of rTMS and on the current state of knowledge concerning its clinical applications in neuropsychiatric disorders. We will give an overview of TMS to the clinical psychiatrist. After a brief historical overview, results of application of rTMS in patients suffering mainly from mood disorders are discussed. Then we will discuss practical issues of rTMS application in volunteers and patients, its side effects and safety issues, and data on putative mechanisms of action. We will finish with a brief outlook on future developments.

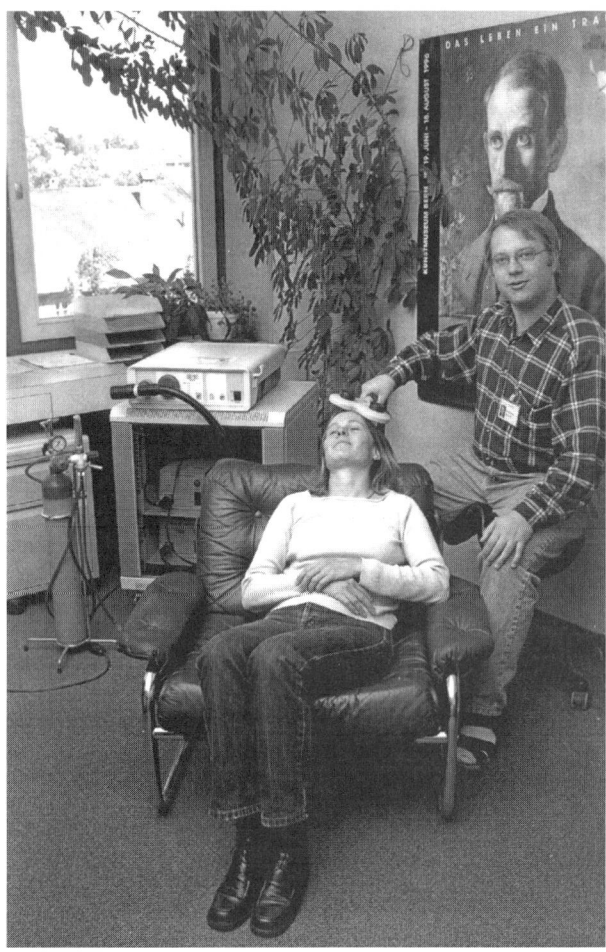

Figure 2 *Practical use of repetitive transcranial magnetic stimulation.* This is a usual setting for nonconvulsive rTMS studies. Patients are awake, sitting relaxed in a chair while stimulation (here to the left dorsolateral prefrontal cortex) is applied. A typical stimulator, here with four booster modules affording high-frequency stimulation, is used. Note the oxygen tank nearby, which would be used as most important therapy in the event of a seizure developing.

II. HISTORICAL OVERVIEW

With the observation of Faraday in 1831 that a time-varying magnetic field can induce a current in a nearby conductor, the theoretical basis of inducing depolarizing currents by electromagnetic coils was established. The French scientist d'Arsonval reported on the first human application of TMS in 1896. He was able to induce phosphenes (flickering-light sensation, not elicited by visual perception), vertigo, and syncope in subjects whose head was placed in a large electromagnetic coil [5]. In 1959, Kolin demonstrated for the first time that an alternating magnetic field is able to stimulate a sciatic frog nerve and could induce contractions of the gastrocnemic muscle [5]. In 1965, Bickford was able to induce muscle twitching in humans by applying a pulsed magnetic field with a maximum field strength of 20,000–30,000 Gauss to ulnar, peroneal, and sciatic nerves [5].

The induction of muscle potentials by magnetic stimulation of the central nervous system was first demonstrated by Barker in 1985 [6]. He induced muscle twitching with a coil of 10 cm diameter placed on the scalp over the motor cortex. A brief pulse of 110 μs with a peak current of 4000 amps was applied and pulses at a maximal rate of 0.33 Hz were delivered.

With the possibility of stimulating the motor cortex noninvasively (Fig. 2), TMS replaced high-voltage transcutaneous electrical stimulation used in clinical studies, mainly to measure central motor conduction time. This variable may be altered by a variety of neurological disorders such as multiple sclerosis, amyotrophic lateral sclerosis, cervical myelopathy, and degenerative ataxic disorders. It seems that TMS has great potential in the intraoperative monitoring of the integrity of motor tracts during surgery of the brain and spinal tract [7]. TMS has subsequently found diagnostic use in neurology for disorders such as demyelinating diseases involving the excitability and the connections of the motor cortex with other parts of the nervous system involved in motor pathways [8].

In 1987 Bickford made an observation that changed the whole field of neuropsychiatric TMS research: He described transient mood elevation in several normal volunteers receiving single-pulse stimulations to the motor cortex [9]. This was the starting point of the scientific investigation of effects of depolarizing magnetic fields on a variety of neuropsychiatric disorders. Subsequently, unblinded pilot studies of TMS with depressed patients were done using single pulse stimulations at frequencies < 0.3 Hz [10–12]. In these studies relatively large areas under the vertex were stimulated bilaterally, and all involved only few subjects. More recent work has suggested that rTMS at 1 Hz with a round coil may have some value in depression [4].

After studies on mood alteration in healthy volunteers and open studies involving only very few subjects, the first subject-blinded rTMS study involving 17 patients suffering from treatment-resistant major depression, psychotic subtype, was published by Pascual-Leone [13]. More recently, larger studies were conducted and researchers attempted to establish meaningful sham conditions. These include stimulations at different cortical sites (e.g., right prefrontal vs. left prefrontal cortex in depression), and holding of the stimulation coil not tangentially to the head but tilted at 45° or 90°.

With technical advances in the past 2 years, it has been possible to develop stimulators that were able to deliver strong pulses at high frequency. Therapeutic effects were investigated not only in mood disorders, but also in other psychiatric disorders, such as anxiety, schizophrenia, and tic disorders. Other studies investigated the basic neurobiology of TMS effects at different levels. TMS techniques also allowed investigations of neuronal connectivity and functionality of neural circuits [8,14]. An important recent development is the combination of TMS with functional imaging; this approach affords testing of important novel hypotheses on TMS effects.

III. PUTATIVE CLINICAL APPLICATIONS OF RTMS

Today, rTMS is not indicated as a clinical treatment approach to any of the neuropsychiatric conditions. The only disorder for which a substantial body of information about clinical efficacy is available is major depression. For other disorders, only preliminary results are available, or only small, nonconclusive studies have been conducted. rTMS has mainly been delivered to adult subjects, older than 20 and younger than 60 years old. For instance, in a study with adolescent depressive patients, a group that would particularly benefit from a treatment with a favorable side-effects profile, only very preliminary data on the application of rTMS to seven adolescents suffering from bipolar disorder (1 subject), major depression (3 subjects), or schizophrenia (3 subjects), between 16 and 18 years old, were found. All subjects showed improvement except for the patient suffering from bipolar disorder and one subject suffering from major depression [15].

A. Affective Disorders

rTMS as a putative treatment in neuropsychiatry has been researched thoroughly in affective disorders and especially in major depressive disorders. There are studies about the use of single-pulse TMS, slow rTMS, and fast rTMS. Different locations of TMS application have been studied as well. At the present time, there is still controversy about the effectiveness of TMS as a potential treatment. This is not astonishing, since only a small part of the full parameter space of possible stimulation conditions has been explored, and the total number of patients studied falls far short of the numbers in registration trials for new drug treatments. Many technical details as where to stimulate, at which frequency, the total number of stimuli, the duration of the treatment, etc., have yet to be resolved. Double-blind, thoroughly controlled multicenter studies involving large numbers of patients are lacking. This is the reason why rTMS cannot be considered as a treatment option in depressive disorder and even less as an alternative to already established treatments at the present time.

The dorsolateral prefrontal cortex (DLPFC) has been the most important target for stimulation in depression. Converging evidence from different areas of research supports the hypothesis that mood is regulated by a interconnected network of brain regions encompassing prefrontal, cingulate, parietal, and temporal cortical regions an well as parts of the striatum, thalamus, and hypothalamus. Lesions of this network from tumor, infarction, or transient disruption may result in mood changes. In addition, alterations of cerebral blood flow and metabolism in the dorsolateral, ventrolateral, orbitofrontal, and mediofrontal regions, as well as the subgenual prefrontal and anterior cingulate cortex, have been demonstrated in patients suffering from major depression [16,17]. Studies of rTMS in mood in healthy subjects [18] and treatment-refractory major depression selected the DLPFC as a region that is both a key part of the network discussed above and at the same time accessible to focally limited effects of TMS.

George reported the first open study of the antidepressant effects of rTMS in six treatment-resistant depressed patients treated with five daily rTMS sessions to the left DLPFC [19]. He demonstrated that two patients in this study experienced substantial improvement as assessed by a drop of 26% in Hamilton Rating Scale for Depression (HRSD) scores. Open and blinded studies of rTMS to the left DLPFC followed with varying results. Figiel showed in a comparatively large open study that 42% of 56 patients responded to five daily rTMS sessions with a considerably lower response rate in the elderly [20]. Triggs demonstrated in a study of 2 weeks' treatment a 41% drop in HRSD in another open trial [21]. It is important to note that there have been open studies that have failed to find any antidepressant activity of rTMS [22].

Effect sizes have varied considerably in controlled single blinded studies of rTMS in treatment resistant depression. George found only modest antidepressant efficacy of rTMS in a within-subject crossover sham-controlled study of 12 depressed patients whom he treated for 2 weeks with stimulation to the left DLPFC [23]. Berman found an antidepressant response in 20 subjects that was statistically different from sham stimulation using similar stimulation parameters in a parallel design, but still only of modest clinical impact [24]. Both George and Berman used a low stimulation intensity of 80% of motor threshold. Generally, it seems that higher intensity may be more effective; however, Loo found no differences between active and sham rTMS using 110% of motor threshold [25]. In a study looking at low-frequency rTMS Klein demonstrated in a sham-controlled trial of 71 patients that 1 Hz stimulation to the *right* DLPFC was significantly more effective than sham [4]. It is unclear whether stimulation of the *left* hemisphere at these parameters would have had the same effect.

More recent work on rTMS treatment of acute mania suggests that right-hemisphere treatment may be more effective in that condition [26]. In a study looking at the effect of frequency, Padberg randomized 18 patients to single-pulse TMS, 10 Hz rTMS, and sham rTMS delivered to the left DLPFC, and demonstrated a mild antidepressant effect with single-pulse TMS [27]. George recently reported a sham-controlled trial in which 20 patients were randomly assigned to receive an equivalent number of pulses at 5 Hz or 20 Hz over 2 weeks. Both active groups had a 45% response, and no patients responded to sham stimulation [28]. This suggests that lower frequencies may have therapeutic efficacy as well, which is important because slow rTMS is associated with a lower risk of seizure. An analysis of treatment response and cerebral metabolism suggests that patients with hypometabolism at baseline may respond better to high-frequency stimulation (20 Hz), whereas those with baseline hypermetabolism respond better to 1 Hz stimulation [29]; however, the effects of rTMS on mood examined in this study were not statistically significant.

Contrary to depression, in which disorder several studies about the efficacy of TMS have been performed, there is only one study on mania in which right prefrontal cortex stimulation was compared with left prefrontal cortex stimulation in manic patients [26]. The results suggest that rTMS of right prefrontal cortex might have some therapeutic effect in mania. In one case report a treatment-resistant patient was treated with right prefrontal rTMS, and she responded well to the treatment [30]. These results have to be considered as very preliminary.

There is some indication that TMS stimulation at higher amplitudes might be more efficacious. This observation, together with the established fact that therapeutic seizures have a strong and reliable effect in depression, leads to another which uses rTMS at convulsive levels as a more targeted form of ECT. Efficacy and side effects of ECT seem to depend on the path of the current passed through the brain [31,32]; this is why targeting seizures to focal cortical areas, such as regions of the prefrontal cortex, may reduce some side effects of convulsive treatment. Magnetic seizure therapy (MST) has now been tested in proof-of-concept studies both in nonhuman primates and patients [1,33], and preliminary results on cognitive side effects of the treatment compared to those of ECT have been obtained [34]. Much additional research is needed to evaluate the putative clinical efficacy of this approach and to determine if it has significant advantages over ECT.

In conclusion, the key findings in depression have not been systematically replicated, and effect sizes have often been small and variable. Sources of variability across studies include differences in stimulation parameter settings, concomitant medications, and patient sample characteristics. In addition, simple and economical methods for precise and reliable coil placement are needed, as this factor is likely important for effectiveness [35]. In much of this work, the magnitude of antidepressant effects, while often statistically significant, has been below the threshold of clinical usefulness [24] and has not lived up to expectations raised by encouraging results in animal studies. The disparity between the human and animal studies on depression may relate to the differences in amount and site of stimulation between humans and rodents (see section on animal studies above). Furthermore, the persistence of antidepressant effects beyond the 1- to 2-week treatment period has rarely been examined. Initial evidence suggests that the beneficial effects may be transitory, making the development of maintenance strategies important if rTMS is to move to the clinic

Establishing whether nonconvulsive rTMS has antidepressant properties aside from their clinical usefulness is of theoretical importance, since positive data support the notion that focally targeted manipulations of cortical function can result in mood improvement. Nonetheless, as a clinical antidepressant intervention, the future of rTMS is far from certain. More work and larger studies are needed to establish its efficacy, the optimal treatment paradigm, and the appropriate patient population. The main problems that need to be dealt with in order to gain more conclusive data are:

1. The establishment of true double blind conditions of delivering TMS, implying that no one getting in contact with the subjects knows whether real or sham TMS is applied. In addition, subject's sensations during the application of TMS may not significantly differ between real and sham conditions.

2. Large multicenter studies assessing the therapeutic efficacy of TMS for instance in major depression disorder are in urgent need. To date, effects on mood improvement of TMS have not been compared in blinded studies against established treatments, such as pharmacotherapy and ECT.

B. Anxiety Disorders

Preliminary results of the application of rTMS in anxiety disorders are available for obsessive-compulsive disorder (OCD) and posttraumatic stress disorder (PTSD) only. The results from two case reports and an open study in patients suffering from PTSD are somewhat encouraging. Concerning OCD, an open study showed improving when rapid rTMS was applied to the right prefrontal cortex; however, in a double-blinded, placebo-controlled study no differences could be found between the sham and the real condition.

1. Obsessive Compulsive Disorder

In a study involving 12 patients suffering from OCD effects of rTMS at the right and left prefrontal cortex were compared. rTMS at 80% motor threshold was applied at 20 Hz. Compulsive urges decreased significantly for 8 h after right lateral prefrontal repetitive transcranial magnetic stimulation [36]. In a double-blind, sham-controlled study, slow rTMS was applied at 110% of motor threshold for 6 weeks to 10 subjects. Sham rTMS (circular coil held perpendicular to the head) was given to eight subjects at 20% of motor threshold. Assessments were carried out at baseline, every week during the treatment, and 4 weeks after the treatment as assessed with the Yale-Brown obsessive-compulsive scale. No difference in the outcome was found between the two groups [37].

2. Posttraumatic Stress Disorder

In an open study, slow rTMS was applied first to one side of the vertex (motor cortex) and after 5 min to the other side. Compared to baseline assessment (prior to the treatment), avoidance, anxiety and somatization symptoms improved transiently and were at baseline level after 7 days of treatment [38]. Application of slow rTMS to the right frontal cortex of to two patients was also encouraging: symptoms improved during 1 month but returned to the level at baseline 1 month after end of treatment [39].

C. Schizophrenia

Compared to depression, only a few studies are available for schizophrenia. A very important finding which was established in a double-blinded cross-over design study of rTMS to the dorsolateral cortex in 12 schizophrenic patients was a decrease in the brief psychiatric rating scale score [40]. In another study six right-handed patients suffering from chronic schizophrenia negative symptoms showed a general decrease for all patients that could be documented in the Positive and Negative Symptom Scale negative-symptoms subscale [41]. Ten schizophrenic patients were given 15 stimuli over the frontal area on each side at 100% stimulus intensity, at 1 Hz. Measured with the Brief Psychiatric Rating Scale scale, an improvement of symptoms could be documented 1, 7, and 28 days after rTMS [42].

However, these encouraging findings could not be confirmed in another randomized placebo controlled study in which 15 patients received sham and 16 real treatment. Stimulation occurred at the right prefrontal cortex, at 10% above motor threshold, at 1 Hz. No statistical significant differences in Clinical Global Impression Scale, Positive and Negative Symptom Scale, or Brief Psychiatric Rating Scale could be found by comparing the placebo group with the real treatment group at the end of the treatment and after 1 week [43]. In this study positive findings reported earlier by the same group could not be replicated [44].

Probably more relevant than the up-to-date controversial and still very preliminary findings about therapeutic efficacy are the strong results on influencing the key symptom in schizophrenia of hallucinations: 12 right-handed schizophrenic patients, all receiving antipsychotic medication, with hallucinations were treated in a double-blind crossover study with 1 Hz stimulation at 80% motor threshold over the left temporoparietal area. There was a significant decrease in hallucination score 12 and 16 min after active stimulation, and not after sham stimulation. In the follow-up assessment, the effect of rTMS on hallucinations lasted maximally for 2 months in one patient. Other positive and negative symptoms did not vary much [45]. This study confirmed preliminary findings reported earlier in three patients [46].

In summary, these studies show that TMS at the chosen parameters clearly has an effect on the brain and consecutively psychotic symptoms, but a general therapeutic effect has not been established. This is encouraging and should provide impetus for further studies in this area.

IV. PRACTICAL APPROACH, SIDE EFFECTS, AND SAFETY CONSIDERATIONS

A. Delivery of TMS

The equipment necessary for delivering TMS consists basically of two parts: (1) a stimulator, which generates brief pulses of strong electrical currents (frequency and intensity of the current pulses, train duration, and intertrain interval can be varied); and (2) stimulation coil connected to the stimulator.

The TMS stimulus interfering with the brain consists of very strong pulsating magnetic fields changing amplitude from 0 to 1.5 Tesla in a few milliseconds. The shape of the magnetic field depends on the design of the coil. There are circular coils with a cylinder-shaped field, figure-8 coils with a more focal field (maximum strength at the intersection of the two circles), and iron core coils that also generate focal fields with a maximum strength in the center of the coil. The magnetic field generated by the coil is perpendicular to its surface and passes unimpeded through the skin and the skull. Since the strength of magnetic fields declines exponentially with distance from the inducing conductor, depolarization of neurons occurs only to a distance of 2–3 cm from the surface of the coil. This is why only superficial structures of the brain can be directly interfered with. However, distant effects of the application of TMS, for example, on regional cerebral blood flow, can be measured and might be important for biologic effects. Older coil models that use water or air-cooling have to be connected to water circulation or a ventilating system. The costs of a device capable of delivering fast rTMS amount to $10,000–40,000.

Subjects and patients undergoing rTMS treatment should first be carefully evaluated and informed about side effects as outlined below (Sec. IV.2; safety considerations). During stimulation, which should always be done in the presence of a person trained to manage eventual emergency situations (mainly epileptic seizure), subjects should be seated comfortably so as to eliminate the risk of accidental falling or hurting oneself even by ample movements. To endure a stimulation session, which may last for up to 30 min, a head holder should support the head, which should not be moved during the application. The rTMS coil is directly held to the head of the subject and placed over the brain region, which is intended to be stimulated (Fig. 2). This can be done by an administrator or by a specially designed coil holder.

The exact site of stimulation can be determined using either anatomical or functional landmarks. In clinical studies on mood disorder, the preferred site of stimulation is the prefrontal cortex. In practice, this place is found by first identifying the spot of inducing movements of contralateral finger muscles, the abductor pollicis brevis, or extensor digiti minimi. The stimulation occurs 5 cm anterior to the spot of maximum response in a line parallel to the midsagittal line. The intensity of stimulation is expressed as percentage of the motor threshold, which can be defined in different ways, for example, as the intensity to elicit evoked motor potentials in the above-mentioned contralateral finger muscles of 50 μV in 50% of the applied pulses, e.g., in 5 out of 10. The practical value of determining the motor threshold is to establish safe stimulation amplitudes, which are much below the seizure threshold.

B. Side Effects and Safety Considerations

Compared to ECT, MST, DBS, and VNS, rTMS can be considered as relatively safe since (1) it is noninvasive, and (2) the induction of convulsions is not required for a treatment. Therefore, side effects linked to anesthesia and convulsion do not occur. However, there are side effects directly linked to the application of rTMS or occurring a few hours later. Of major concern are involuntarily induced epileptic seizure, local pain during application, changes in the auditory performance due to the noise generated in the coil by the passing electrical current, and headache as well as the concern of alterations of cognitive functions. Until now, in research applications, mainly short-term problems (application of TMS, follow-up of a few weeks) were addressed. Long-term concerns have also to be addressed. These might include long-lasting cognitive impairment which includes the most frequent unwanted long-term side effect of ECT, sleep problems, or, potentially, problems linked to effects of the influence of the strong magnetic fields on the brain.

1. Immediate and Short-Term Risks

Seizures

The risk of causing a seizure is the primary safety concern with TMS. Even if this risk is primarily associated with rTMS, single-pulse stimulation also has been reported to produce seizures in patients with large cerebral infarcts, contusions, or other structural brain lesions. According to Wassermann [47], in patients with completely subcortical lesions, no seizures are reported. According to the same author, there are a few articles reporting the induction of seizures in epilepsy patients without gross lesions.

In at least six normal volunteers, and at least two patients with depression, inadvertent seizure occurred during rTMS stimulation [47]. None of the subjects who experienced rTMS-induced seizures suffered lasting sequelae. EEG recordings became normal after at least 2 days. Recorded effects were mild recall deficits, which returned to normal after 24 h in two individuals, and significant anxiety in one subject concerning the possibility of a recurrent seizure.

Until today, several thousand individuals have been subjected to rTMS treatments. It seems reasonable to assume that under observation of the safety guidelines as discussed below, a development of seizure activity is extremely unlikely.

Cognitive Impairment

Mainly short-term observations concerning cognitive function after TMS administration are available. rTMS can produce transient disruption of various cerebral functions, depending on the site of stimulation. Observations reported include a significant decrease in a memory subtest within an hour after stimulation with 150 trains of rTMS at 15 Hz and 120% motor threshold delivered at four different positions [48]. Commenting on these results, Lorberbaum concludes that these cognitive effects were due to subconvulsive epileptic activity or that the threshold for adverse effects on memory might be near that of seizure [49]. Loo reported results from a study in wich 12 subjects suffering from major depression received rTMS during 4 weeks. No significant changes in neuropsychologic functioning after 4 weeks were observed [50].

Cardiovascular Effects

No significant changes in blood pressure or heart rate have been reported during and after the administration of rTMS [51].

Hearing

No significant changes in auditory threshold were observed in a study involving 12 depressed subjects undergoing rTMS over 4 weeks when assessed for 4 weeks after the end of the study [50].

Headache

The application of TMS may cause local pain resulting from direct stimulation of muscles underlying the coil and from stimulation of facial and scalp nerves. It is generally more painful at higher intensities and frequencies. About 5–20% of subjects subsequently experience tension headache [52].

Special Conditions

"Special conditions" refers to subjects who have risk factors which are investigated by the proposed questionnaire (pregnancy, medical implants in the head, implanted medical devices such as pacemakers, or drug delivery pumps). We would advise care in administering rTMS to such subjects, since until now, rTMS cannot be considered as treatment of choice in a medical condition. There are no systematic studies about the application of rTMS to subjects presenting with special conditions. However, there are some isolated reports which might indicate that TMS might be administered to pregnant subjects [53], or to subjects with some implanted medical devices [54,55].

2. *Potential Long-Term Effects*

There is, of course, legitimate concern that the application of rTMS might cause brain damage in the widest sense. Mechanisms discussed are heating of neuronal tissue, excitotoxicity, and any influences of magnetic fields. As with other side effects, besides the occurrence of seizure, there are very few data and no thorough investigations available which address these questions. There are, however, after the administration of TMS and rTMS to many thousand subjects, no indications that their application might cause brain damage.

The kind of low-frequency, high-strength magnetic fields delivered to the human brain during rTMS are not known from other applications. Considerable evidence has accumulated about constant, strong static magnetic fields with the introduction of MRI techniques in medicine. These fields have about the same strength as those produced by rTMS. Since the introduction of MRI, more than 150,000,000 examinations have been performed and only seven deaths occurred due to these procedures [56]. One involved a ferromagnetic cerebral aneurysm clip, and five examinations involved patients with cardiac pacemakers.

High-frequency (~ 1000 MHz) electromagnetic fields as generated by cellphones raised concern in the public about adverse health effects. They are known to induce changes in sleep EEG patterns 20–50 min after electromagnetic fields were applied to awake subjects [57]. In rTMS, very different energies and frequencies of electromagnetic fields are applied to the human brain. In a safety study, rTMS at therapeutic parameters has been demonstrated to have no significant effects on sleep EEG [58].

3. *Safety Guidelines and Assessment of Subjects Undergoing rTMS*

The widely accepted safety guidelines on rTMS application are based on the report of the International Workshop on the Safety of Repetitive Transcranial Magnetic Stimulation,1996 [59]. Absolute contraindications retained are metal in cranium, intracardial lines, and increased intracranial pressure.

Relative contraindications are pregnancy, heart disease, cardiac pacemaker, medication pump, ongoing medication with tricyclic antidepressants or neuroleptics, and family history of epilepsy. Since inadvertent seizures may develop during rTMS and even TMS, one has to prepare for their management on site. Seizures in nonepileptic patients are always self-limiting. The risk of permanent damage to the brain is minimal and can be reduced considerably by prompt administration of oxygen. Diazepam 10 mg might be administered to end a seizure lasting > 2 min.

Keel [60] proposed a transcranial magnetic stimulation adult safety screen (TASS) which consists of the following 14 yes-or-no questions:

Have you ever:

1. Had an adverse reaction to TMS?
2. Had a seizure?
3. Had an EEG?
4. Had a stroke?
5. Had a head injury (including neurosurgery)?
6. Do you have any metal in your head (outside of the mouth), such as shrapnel, surgical clips, or fragments from welding or metalwork?
7. Do you have any implanted devices, such as cardiac pacemakers, medical pumps, or intracardiac lines?
8. Do you suffer from frequent or severe headaches?

9. Have you ever had any other brain-related condition?
10. Have you ever had any illness that caused brain injury?
11. Are you taking any medications?
12. If you are a woman of childbearing age, are you sexually active, and if so, are you not using a reliable mode of birth control?
13. Does anyone in your family have epilepsy?
14. Do you need further explanation of TMS and its associated risks?

A positive screen is any "yes" answer, indicating further investigation by the clinician (but not indicating exclusion from TMS). Subjects assessed with this questionnaire and subjected to rTMS within the proposed safe limits of the stimulation parameters are very unlikely to experience a seizure. Maximum recommended train durations are displayed in Table 1. According to Chen et al. [61], the following intertrain intervals are proposed as reasonably safe: in rTMS below 20 Hz, 5 sec intertrain interval seems to be safe below a stimulation intensity of 110% of motor threshold. Above, no data were available. Intertrain intervals of 0.25 and 1 sec were not considered to be safe. They advised intertrain intervals of 1 min at an intensity of < 120% of motor threshold.

V. BASIC EFFECTS INDUCED BY TMS

The generated magnetic fields are interacting with an extremely complex biological system where essential interactions between brain and mind take place [62,63]. It seems obvious that the impact of these magnetic fields on the underlying brain structures is difficult to evaluate, since monitoring the functions of the living human brain is only possible by assessing summation responses which are determined by the action of many thousand or more cells. The actual psychopathological models of psychiatric disorders are integrating so-called functional systems at molecular, cellular, neurotransmitter, organ, systemic, or individual and social levels that are not known in detail. Presenting the mechanisms of action of TMS as a research or treatment tool challenges old hypotheses of aspects of the function of the brain and, hopefully, allows the construction of new ones. Several acute and chronic alterations at different levels, ranging from changes in gene expression of cells in the central nervous system to alterations in mood and behavior, have been documented during and after the application of TMS. Among the many interesting approaches, where valuable studies are available, only a few examples are cited.

Ji recently reported that one single train of rTMS applied to rats in vivo induced c-fos and c-jun expression in different brain regions and among them in key regions controlling circadian biological rhythms [64]. Similar stimulation parameters have earlier been shown to have efficacy in an animal model of depression [65]. These findings might point to a possible antidepressant mode of action of TMS effects via circadian rhythms. The finding that immediate to early gene expression is modified by TMS has been replicated and further examined recently by other authors, in vivo as well as in vitro [66,67].

Keck measured modulatory effects of frontal rTMS in rat brain in vivo using intracerebral microdialysis [68]. There was a continuous reduction in arginine vasopressin release of up to 50% within the hypothalamic paraventricular nucleus in response to rTMS. In contrast, the release of taurine, aspartate, and serine was selectively stimulated within this nucleus by rTMS. Furthermore, in the dorsal hippocampus the extracel-

Table 1 Maximum Safe Duration (sec) for Single Trains of rTMS

Frequency (Hz)	Intensity (% of stimulator output at motor threshold												
	100	110	120	130	140	150	160	170	180	190	200	210	220
1	>1800	>1800	360	>50	>50	>50	>50	27	11	11	8	7	6
5	>10	>10	>10	>10	7.6	5.2	3.6	2.6	2.4	1.6	1.4	1.6	1.2
10	>5	>5	4.2	2.9	1.3	0.8	0.9	0.8	0.5	0.6	0.4	0.3	0.3
20	2.05	1.6	1.0	0.55	0.35	0.25	0.25	0.15	0.2	0.25	0.2	0.1	0.1
25	1.28	0.84	0.4	0.24	0.2	0.24	0.2	0.12	0.08	0.12	0.12	0.08	0.08

Indicated are durations of single rTMS trains, after which no after discharge or spread of excitation has been encountered at the specified conditions (frequency, intensity). Numbers preceded by > are the longest durations tested.
Source: Ref. 59.

lular concentration of dopamine was elevated in response to rTMS.

By using PET scanning, a diminished ^{11}C raclopride binding to dopamine receptors in the left dorsal caudate nucleus could be measured in eight volunteers after left dorsolateral prefrontal cortex rTMS. This implies that rTMS can trigger dopamine release in these brain structures [69].

Several studies documented the effect of rTMS on human blood hormone levels. They include effects on cortisol, prolactin, and TSH. Actual results cannot be considered as conclusive. They indicate, however, that TMS might significantly influence endocrine functions of the brain [70–72].

TMS can transiently disrupt or induce activity in focal brain regions, depending on the region stimulated. Applied to the visual cortex, for example, strong TMS can produce phosphenes, and a stimulus of lower intensity can induce transient scotomas [73]. Other functions, such as linguistic processing, can also be investigated with rTMS [48]. Peinemann reported a neuromodulatory effect of subthreshold high frequency rTMS in 10 subjects. After 1250 stimulations at 90% motor threshold, an intracortical inhibition could be measured which lasted at least 10 min after the rTMS stimulation [74].

The combination of noninvasive stimulation of the brain coupled with functional neuroimaging techniques offers new opportunities to investigate functions of the human brain. It also allows visualization of effects of TMS which are documented to occur at distant sites from the stimulation [75]. In another study, 10 medication-free subjects suffering form major depression (eight unipolar, two bipolar) received rTMS in a crossover, randomized study at the left prefrontal cortex, at 100% motor threshold at 20 Hz or 1 Hz. With 20 Hz, an increase in rCBF in the prefrontal cortex left > right, cingulated gyrus left ≫ right, left amygdala, bilaterally insula, basal ganglia, uncus hippocampus, parahippocampus, thalamus, cerebellum was observed, with a 1 Hz only decreases in rCBF: right prefrontal cortex, left medial cortex, left basal ganglia, left amygdala. Individuals who improved in one frequency concerning their depressive symptoms worsened in the other [76].

All these approaches from different areas of neuroscience convergingly show that TMS has prominent and reproducible effects on the brain, which is certainly encouraging and puts TMS apart from some other putative approaches to treat neuropsychiatric disorders [73]. The problem is that the connection from cellular levels to complex behavioral changes—such as those observed in depression—is difficult to do. The field has suffered somewhat from a "top-down" approach in which early promising results in depression have led to enthusiasm for clinical studies without sufficient neuroscientific foundations. Approaches integrating findings from all levels of biologic systems are extremely important and should be undertaken in order to support the ongoing clinical research.

VI. DISCUSSION AND OUTLOOK

rTMS is a relatively affordable and—if the safety precautions are followed—safe method to apply magnetic fields noninvasively to the human brain. As has been discussed in this chapter, research into different clinical applications for rTMS in neuropsychiatric disorders remains active and has the potential to provide useful data, but as of yet there is no consensus among the blinded controlled trials that rTMS has beneficial effects that replace or even match the effectiveness of conventional treatments in any disorder. From the viewpoint of the *clinician*, the following comments can be made:

1. Today data on clinical efficacy of rTMS in mood disorders are not unequivocal, and results on other psychiatric disorders, such as schizophrenia and anxiety disorders, have to be considered as very preliminary but nevertheless interesting and encouraging.

2. For the therapeutic application in mood disorders rigorously controlled and double-blinded multicenter trials are needed to address the question of the clinical efficacy of TMS. Even before that, technical problems in the application of TMS have to be solved; e.g., more satisfactory sham conditions have to be developed. Today, using analogies to pharmacological drug development, valid Phase II trials have still to be conducted. Crucial open questions remain regarding medium- and long-term efficacy of TMS, prevention of relapse, and medium- and long-term side effects. There are virtually no data on these issues since most trials assessed only treatment response after 2 weeks. rTMS has not been demonstrated to be clinically superior or even equal to pharmacological treatment or to ECT. Double-blinded Phase III trials, comparing established drug treatments and ECT with TMS, have still to be conducted.

3. There is no consensus at all about possible mechanisms of action of antidepressant effects of TMS. However, this is also the case for many other treatments in psychiatry. rTMS research is basically

empirical. Many variables play a role in rTMS, and a large parameter space has therefore to be carefully explored in order to find the most efficacious treatment. This complicated process will likely be very slow, since there is not a large amount of funding for such studies. Nevertheless, rTMS has clearly effects on the brain—which is certainly remarkable—and it might be that rTMS is a treatment modality in search of a suitable application in psychiatry. Therefore it is of utmost importance to continue on the long and difficult path of research on clinical rTMS applications.

4. Today, different TMS methodologies have a place as diagnostic tools in neurological disorders, where neural conductivity is assessed in different, mainly demyelinating disorders.

From the viewpoint of the neuroscientist, TMS is a methodology with great potential as a research tool [14,73]. This technique, by itself and combined with other methods such as EEG and neuroimaging, may be useful to test functional connectivity, neuroplasticity, information processing (for example in the visual system), indirect and direct motor control, and aspects of mood control. It affords testing of both general hypotheses of the function of the brain at different levels and hypotheses of the underlying pathology of neuropsychiatric disorders. Even if the early enthusiasm, which prevailed after early studies of clinical effects in the treatment of mood disorders settled down somewhat, rTMS will be even more useful as an investigational tool of basic and clinical research.

REFERENCES

1. SH Lisanby, TE Schlaepfer, HU Fisch, HA Sackeim. Magnetic seizure therapy of major depression. Arch Gen Psychiatry 58:303–304, 2001.
2. MS George, HA Sackeim, JA Rush, LB Marangell, Z Nahas, MM Husain, SH Lisanby, T Burt, J Goldman, JC Ballenger. Vagus nerve stimulation: a new tool for brain research and therapy? Biol Psychiatry 47:287–295, 2000.
3. LS Boylan, HA Sackeim. Magnetoelectric brain stimulation in the assessment of brain physiology and pathophysiology. Clin Neurophysiol 111:504–512, 2000.
4. E Klein, I Kreinin, A Chistyakov, D Koren, L Mecz, S Marmur, D Ben Sachar, M Feinsod. Therapeutic efficacy of right prefrontal slow repetitive transcranial magnetic stimulation in major depression. Arch Gen Psychiatry 56:315–320, 1999.
5. LA Geddes. History of magnetic stimulation of the nervous system. J Clin Neurophysiol 8:3–9, 1991.
6. AT Barker, R Jalinous, IL Freeston. Noninvasive magnetic stimulation of human motor cortex. Lancet 2:1106–1107, 1985.
7. NMF Murray. Magnetic stimulation of cortex: clinical applications. J Clin Neurophysiol 8:66–76, 1991.
8. U Ziemann, M Hallett. Basic neurophysiological studies with TMS. In: Transcranial Magnetic Stimulation in neuropsychiatry, eds. George MS, Belmaker RH. Washington: American Psychiatric Press, 2000.
9. RG Bickford, M Guidi, P Fortesque, M Swenson. Magnetic stimulation of human peripheral nerve and brain: response enhancement by combined magnetoelectrical technique. Neurosurgery 20:110–116, 1987.
10. N Grisaru, Y Yaroslavsky, JM Abarbanel, T Lamberg, R Belmaker. Transcranial magnetic stimulation in depression and schizophrenia. Eur Neuropsychopharmacol 4:287–288, 1994.
11. G Höflich, S Kasper, A Hufnagel, S Ruhrmann, HJ Möller. Application of transcranial magnetic stimulation in the treatment of drug-resistant major depression: a report of two cases. Hum Psychopharmacol 8:361–365, 1993.
12. HM Kolbinger, G Höflich, A Hufnagel, HJ Möller, S Kasper. Transcranial magnetic stimulation (TMS) in the treatment of major depression. Hum Psychopharmacol 10:305–310, 1995.
13. A Pascual-Leone, B Rubio, F Pallardo, MD Catala. Rapid-rate transcranial magnetic stimulation of left dorsolateral prefrontal cortex in drug-resistant depression. Lancet 348:233–237, 1996.
14. SH Lisanby, B Luber, HA Sackeim. Transcranial magnetic stimulation: application in basic neuroscience and neuropsychopharmacology. Int J Neuropsychopharmacol 3:259–273, 2000.
15. G Walter, JM Tormos, JA Israel, A Pascual-Leone. Transcranial magnetic stimulation in young persons: a review of known cases. J Child Adolesc Psychophrmacol 11:69–75, 2001.
16. JC Soares, JJ Mann. The functional neuroanatomy of mood disorders. J Psychiatr Res 31:393–432, 1997.
17. HS Mayberg, SK Brannan, RK Mahurin, PA Jerabek, JS Brickman, JL Tekell, JA Silva, S McGinnis, TG Glass, CC Martin, PT Fox. Cingulate function in depression: a potential predictor of treatment response. Neuroreport: 8:1057–1061, 1997.
18. UP Mosimann, T Rihs, J Engeler, HU Fisch, TE Schlaepfer. Mood effects of repetitive transcranial magnetic stimulation of left prefrontal cortex in healthy volunteers. Psychiatry Res 94:251–256, 2000.
19. MS George, EM Wasserman, WA Williams, A Callahan, TA Ketter, P Basser, M Hallett, RM Post. Daily repetitive transcranial magnetic stimulation (rTMS) improves mood in depression. Neuroreport 6:1853–1856, 1995.
20. GS Figiel, C Epstein, WM McDonald, J Amazon-Leece, L Figiel, A Saldivia, S Glover. The use of

rapid-rate transcranial magnetic stimulation (rTMS) in refractory depressed patients. J Neuropsychiatry Clin Neurosci 10:20–25, 1998.
21. WJ Triggs, KJM McCoy, R Greer, F Rossi, D Bowers, S Kortenkamp, SE Nadeau, KM Heilmann, WK Goodman. Effects of left frontal transcranial magnetic simulation on depressed mood, cognition, and corticomotor threshold. Biol Psychiatry 45:1440–1445, 1999.
22. EA Schouten, AA D'Alfonso, WA Nolen, EH De Haan, J Wijkstra, RS Kahn. Mood improvement from transcranial magnetic stimulation. Am J Psychiatry 156:669–670, 1999.
23. MS George, EM Wassermann, TA Kimbrell, JT Little, WE Williams, AL Danielson, BD Greenberg, M Hallet, RM Post. Mood improvement following daily left prefrontal repetitive transcranial magnetic stimulation in patients with depression: a placebo-controlled crossover trial. Am J Psychiatry 154:1752–1756, 1997.
24. RM Berman, N Narashiman, G Sanacora, AP Miano, RE Hoffman, XS Hu, DS Charney, NN Boutros. A randomized clinical trial of repetitive transcranial magnetic stimulation in the treatment of major depression. Biol Psychiatry 47:332–337, 2000.
25. C Loo, P Mitchell, P Sachdev, B McDarmont, G Parker, S Gandevia. Double-blind controlled investigation of transcranial magnetic stimulation for the treatment of resistant major depression. Am J Psychiatry 156:946–948, 1999.
26. N Grisaru, B Chudakov, Y Yaroslavsky, R Belmaker. Transcranial magnetic stimulation in mania: a controlled study. Am J Psychiatry 155:1608–1610, 1998.
27. F Padberg, P Zwanzger, H Thoma, N Kathmann, C Haag, BD Greenberg, H Hampel, HJ Möller. Repetitive transcranial magnetic stimulation (rTMS) in pharmacotherapy-refractory major depression: comparative study of fast, slow and sham rTMS. Psychiatry Res 88:163–171, 1999.
28. MS George, Z Nahas, M Molloy, AM Speer, NC Oliver, XB Li, GW Arana, SC Risch, JC Ballenger. A controlled trial of daily left prefrontal cortex TMS for treating depression. Biol Psychiatry 48:962–970, 2000.
29. TA Kimbrell, JT Little, RT Dunn, MA Frye, BD Greenberg, EM Wassermann, JD Repella, AL Danielson, MW Willis, BE Benson, AM Speer, E Osuch, MS George, RM Post. Frequency dependence of antidepressant reponse to left prefrontal repetitive transcranial magnetic stimulation (rTMS) as a function of baseline cerebral glucose metabolism. Biol Psychiatry 46:1603–1613, 1999.
30. A Erfurth, N Michael, C Mostert, V Arolt. Euphoric mania and rapid transcranial magnetic stimulation. Am J Psychiatry 157:835–836, 2000.
31. HA Sackeim, J Prudic, DP Devanand, MS Nobler, SH Lisanby, S Peyser, L Fitzsimons, BJ Moody, J Clark. A prospective, randomized, double-blind comparison of bilateral and right unilateral electroconvulsive therapy at different stimulus intensities. Arch Gen Psychiatry 57:425–434, 2000.
32. HA Sackeim, J Prudic, DP Devanand, JE Kiersky, L Fitzsimons, BJ Moody, MC McElhiney, EA Coleman, JM Settembrino. Effects of stimulus intensity and electrode placement on the efficacy and cognitive effects of electroconvulsive therapy. N Engl J Med 328:839–846, 1993.
33. SH Lisanby, B Luber, HA Sackeim, AD Finck, C Schroeder. Deliberate seizure induction with repetitive transcranial magnetic stimulation in nonhuman primates. Arch Gen Psychiatry 58:199–200, 2001.
34. SH Lisanby, B Luber, L Barriolhet, E Neufeld, TE Schlaepfer, HA Sackeim. Magnetic seizure therapy (MST)—acute cognitive effects of MST compared with ECT. J ECT (in press).
35. FA Kozel, Z Nahas, C deBrux, M Molloy, JP Lorberbaum, D Bohning, SC Risch, MS George. How coil-cortex distance relates to age, motor threshold, and antidepressant response to repetitive transcranial magnetic stimulation. J Neuropsychiatry Clin Neurosci 12:376–384, 2000.
36. BD Greenberg, MS George, JD Martin, J Benjamin, TE Schlaepfer, M Altemus, EM Wassermann, RM Post, DL Murphy. Effect of prefrontal repetitive transcranial magnetic stimulation in obsessive-compulsive disorder: a preliminary study. Am J Psychiatry 154:867–869, 1997.
37. P Alonso, J Pujol, N Cardoner, L Benlloch, J Deus, JM Menchon, A Capdevila, J Vallejo. Right prefrontal repetitive transcranial magnetic stimulation in obsessive compulsive disorder: a double-blind, placebo-controlled study. Am J Psychiatry 158:1143–1145, 2001.
38. N Grisaru, M Amir, H Cohen, Z Kaplan. Effect of transctranial magnetic stimulation in posttraumatic stress disorder: a preliminary study. Biol Psychiatry 44:52–55, 1998.
39. UD McCann, TA Kimbrell, CM Morgan, T Anderson, M Geraci, BE Benson, EM Wassermann, MW Willis, RM Post. Repetitive transcranial magnetic stimulation for posttraumatic stress disorder. Arch Gen Psychiatr 55:276–279, 1998.
40. JD Rollnik, TJ Huber, H Mogk, S Siggelkow, S Kropp, R Dengler, HM Emrich, U Schneider. High frequency transcranial magnetic stimulation (rTMS) of the dorsolateral prefrontal cortex in schizophrenic patients. Neuroreport 11:4013–4015, 2000.
41. E Cohen, M Bernardo, J Masana, FJ Arrufat, V Navarro, J Vallas-Sole, T Boget, N Barrantes, S Catarineu, M Font, FJ Lomena. Repetitive transcranial magnetic stimulation in treatment of chronic negative schizophrenia: a pilot study. J Neurol Neurosurg Psychiatry 67:129–130, 1999.
42. V Geller, N Grisaru, JM Abarbanel, B Lemberg, R Belmaker. Slow magnetic stimulation of prefrontal

cortex in depression and schizophrenia. Prog Neuro-Psychopharmacol Biol Psychiatry 21:105–110, 1997.
43. E Klein, Y Kolsky, M Puyerovsky, D Koren, A Chistyakov, M Feinsod. Right prefrontal slow repetitive transcranial magnetic stimulation in schizophrenia: a double-blind sham-controlled pilot study. Biol Psychiatry 46:1451–1454, 1999.
44. M Feinsod, B Kreinin, A Chistyakov, E Klein. Preliminary evidence for beneficial effect of low-frequency, repetitive transcranial stimulation in patients with major depression and schizophrenia. Depress Anxiety 7:65–68, 1998.
45. RE Hoffman, NN Boutros, S Hu, RM Berman, JH Krystal, DS Charney. Transcranial magnetic stimulation and auditory hallucinations in schizophrenia. Lancet 355:1073–1075, 2000.
46. RE Hoffman, NN Boutros, RM Berman, E Roessler, A Belger, JH Krystal, DS Charney. Transcranial magnetic stimulation of left temporoparietal cortex in three patients reporting hallucinated "voices". Biol Psychiatry 46:130–132, 1999.
47. EM Wasserman. Side effects of repetitive transcranial magnetic stimulation. Depress Anxiet: 12:124–129, 2000.
48. SS Flitman, J Grafman, E Wassermann, BA Cooper, J O'Grady, A Pascual-Leone, M Hallett. Linguistic processing during repetitive transcranial magnetic stimulation. Neurology 50:175–181, 1998.
49. JP Lorberbaum, EM Wasserman. Safety concerns of TMS. In: Transcranial Magnetic Stimulation in Neuropsychiatry. eds. George MS, Belmaker R. Washington: American Psychiatric Press, 2000, pp 141–161
50. C Loo, P Sachdev, H Elsayed, B McDarmont, P Mitchell, M Wilkinson, G Parker, S Gandevia. Effects of a 2- to 4-week course of repetitive transcranial magnetic stimulation (rTMS) on neuropsychologic functioning, electroencephalogram, and auditory threshold in depressed patients. Biol Psychiatry 49:615–623, 2001.
51. A Foerster, JM Schmitz, S Nouri, D Claus. Safety of rapid-rate transcranial magnetic stimulation: heart rate and blood presuure changes. Electroencephalogr Clin Neurophysiol 104:207–212, 1997.
52. MS George, SH Lisanby, HA Sackeim. Transcranial magnetic stimulation: applications in neuropsychiatry. Arch Gen Psychiatry 56:300–311, 1999.
53. Z Nahas, DE Bohning, M Molloy. Safety and feasibility of repetitive transcranial magnetic stimulation in the treatment of anxious depression in pregnancy: a case report. J Clin Psychiatry 60:50–52, 1999.
54. M Kofler, AA Leis, AM Sherwood, JS Delapasse, JA Halter. Safety of transcranial magnetic stimulation in patients with abdominally implanted devices. Lancet 338:1275–1276, 1991.
55. M Kofler, AA Leis. Safety of transcranial magnetic stimulation in patients with implanted equipment. Electroencephalogr Clin Neurophysiol 107:223–224, 1998.
56. JF Schenck. Safety of strong, static magnetic fields. J Magn Reson Imag 12:2–19, 2000.
57. R Huber, T Graf, KA Cote, L Wittmann, E Gallmann, D Matter, J Schuderer, N Kuster, AA Borbely, P Achermann. Exposure to pulsed high-frequency electromagnetic field during waking affects human sleep EEG. Neuroreport 11:3321–3325, 2000.
58. T Graf, J Engeler, P Achermann, UP Mosimann, R Noss, H Fisch, TE Schlaepfer. High frequency repetitive transcranial magnetic stimulation (rTMS) of the left dorsolateral cortex: EEG topography during waking and subsequent sleep. Psychiatry Res Neuroimag 107:1–9, 2001.
59. EM Wassermann. Risk and safety of repetitive transcranial magnetic stimulation: report and suggested guidelines from the International Workshop on the Safety of Repetitive Transcranial Magnetic Stimulation, June 5–7, 1996. Electroencephalogr Clin Neurophysiol 108:1–16, 1998.
60. JC Keel, MJ Smith, EM Wasserman. A safety screening questionnaire for transcranial magnetic stimulation. Clin Neurophysiol 112:2000.
61. R Chen, C Gerloff, J Classen, EM Wasserman, M Hallett, LG Cohen. Safety of inter-train intervals for repetitive transcranial magnetic stimulation and recommendations for safe ranges of stimulation parameters. Electroencephalogr Clin Neurophysiol 105:415–421, 1997.
62. ER Kandel. A new intellectual framework for psychiatry. Am J Psychiatry 155:457–469, 1998.
63. ER Kandel. Biology and the future of psychoanalysis: a new intellectual framework for psychiatry revisited. Am J Psychiatry 156:505–524, 1999.
64. RR Ji, TE Schlaepfer, CD Aizenman, CM Epstein, D Qiu, JC Huang, F Rupp. Repetitive transcranial magnetic stimulation activates specific regions in rat brain. Proc Natl Acad Sci USA 95:15635–15640, 1998.
65. A Fleischmann, K Prolov, J Abarbanel, RH Belmaker. The effect of transcranial magnetic stimulation of rat brain on behavioral models of depression. Brain Res 699:130–132, 1995.
66. W Doi, D Sato, H Fukuzako, M Takigawa. c-Fos expression in rat brain after repetitive transcranial magnetic stimulation. Neuroreport 12:1307–1310, 2001.
67. A Hausmann, J Marksteiner, H Hinterhuber, C Humpel. Magnetic stimulation induces neuronal c-fos via tetrodotoxin-sensitive sodium channels in organotypic cortex brain slices in rat. Neurosci Lett 310:105–108, 2001.
68. ME Keck, I Sillaber, K Ebner, T Welt, N Toschi, ST Kaehler, N Singewald, A Philippu, GK Elbel, CT Wotjak, F Holsboer, R Landgraf, M Engelmann. Acute transcranial magnetic stimulation of frontal brain regions selectively modulates the release of vaso-

pressin, biogenic amines and amino acids in the rat brain. Eur J Neurosci 12:3713–3720, 2000.
69. AP Strafellea, T Paus, J Barrett, A Dagher. Repetitive transcranial magnetic stimulation of the human prefrontal cortex induces dopamine release in the caudate nucleaus. J Neurosci 21:151–154, 2001.
70. S Cohrs, F Tergau, J Korn, W Becker, G Hajak. Suprathreshold repetitive transcranial magnetic stimulation elevates thyroid-stimulationg hormone in healthy male subjects. J Nerv Ment Dis 189:393–397, 2001.
71. MP Szuba, JP O'Reordon, AS Rai, J Snyder-Kastenberg, JD Amsterdam, DR Gettes, E Wassermann, DL Evans. Acute mood and thyroid stimulating hormone effects of transcranial magnetic stimulation in major depression. Biol Psychiatry 50:22–27, 2001.
72. MS George, EM Wasserman, WA Williams, J Steppel, A Pascual-Leone, P Basser, M Hallet, RM Post. Changes in mood and hormone levels after rapid-rate transcranial magnetic stimulation (rTMS) of the prefrontal cortex. 8:172–180, 1996.
73. M Hallett. Transcranial magnetic stimulation and the brain. Nature 406:147–150, 2000.
74. A Peinemann, C Lehner, C Mentschel, A Münchau, B Conrad, HR Siebner. Subthreshold 5-Hz repetitive transcranial magnetic stimulation of the human primary motor cortex reduces intracortical paired-pulse inhibition. Neurosci Lett 296:21–24, 2000.
75. T Paus, R Jech, CJ Thompson, R Comeau, T Peters, AC Evans. Transcranial magnetic stimulation during positron emission tomography: a new method for studying connectivity of the human cerebral cortex. J Neurosci 17:3178–3184, 1997.
76. AM Speer, TA Kimbrell, EM Wasserman, JD Repella, MW Willis, P Herscovitch, RM Post. Opposite effects of high and low frequency rTMS on regional brain activity in depressed patients. Biol Psychiatry 48:1133–1141, 2000.

60

Pharmacokinetic Principles and Drug Interactions

AHSAN Y. KHAN and SHELDON H. PRESKORN
University of Kansas School of Medicine, Wichita, Kansas, U.S.A.

I. INTRODUCTION

This chapter is dedicated to explaining the basic concepts of clinical pharmacokinetics to aid the prescriber in avoiding adverse drug-drug interactions (DDIs) and practice rationale therapeutics (i.e., prescribing drugs to maximize the chances of efficacy and to minimize drug-induced illness). These concepts are important for patients in general and in particular in those on antidepressants because of their high likelihood of being on other medications. That is true regardless of the type of medical setting in which they are being seen (Table 1).

In this era of medicine, polypharmacy is common. This frequency is a natural consequence of the increase in drug discovery. The Food and Drug Administration currently approves an average of 25 new chemical entities per year. Physicians typically learn about new drugs from pharmaceutical company–sponsored lunches and/or dinners, colleagues, and other sources. These may all lack scientific details. The general focus is on the pharmacology alone. However, most patients on an antidepressant are also on other medications.

This issue is important because the more drugs a patient is taking, the greater the risk that they will experience a DDI. Such interactions can be intended or unintended, beneficial, or adverse. In fact, augmentation and combination drug strategies are planned DDIs with the goal of increasing efficacy and/or tolerability. Conversely, adverse DDIs can result in patient morbidity, patient mortality, and reduced efficacy. All of the above in turn increases health care costs.

II. WHAT IS A DRUG-DRUG INTERACTION?

A DDI is a measurable change in magnitude, nature, or duration of the action of one drug as a result of prior or concomitant administration of another drug. DDIs are not limited to any specific therapeutic class, and drugs from different therapeutic classes can nevertheless interact.

Knowledge about pharmacokinetic drug interactions (i.e., the effects of one drug on the absorption, distribution, metabolism, or elimination of another, coadministered drug) is critical for the safe and effective use of drug combinations. A point central to this chapter is understanding that a patient's response to any drug treatment is determined by the relationship of three variables: the drug's pharmacodynamics (Pd), the drug's pharmacokinetics (Pk), and the biological variance between patients as shown in Eq. (1).

Table 1 Percentage of Patients on Antidepressants Having the Potential to Experience a Drug-Drug Interaction as a Function of Treatment Setting

Clinical	Number of patients	Prescribed only an antidepressant	Prescribed at least one other medication	Prescribed three or more other medications
Primary-care setting	2045	28%	72%	34%
Psychiatry clinic	224	29%	71%	30%
VA medical clinics	1076	7%	93%	68%
HIV clinic	66	2%	98%	77%

Other medications include a systemically taken, prescription drug from any therapeutic class. Does not include over-the-counter medications, topicals, or herbs.
Source: Ref. 46.

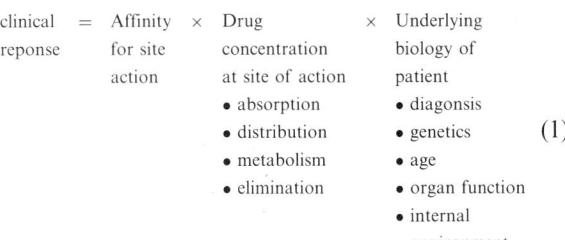

Pd is what the drug does to the body, i.e., the drug's affinity for its sites of action, whereas Pk is what the body does to the drug, i.e., the factors that determine the drug concentration at the site of action. The third variable in Eq. (1) is critical to understanding why different patients respond differently to the same dose of the same medicine. The prescriber usually cannot change the diagnosis, genetics, or age or organ function of a patient; however, the prescriber can change the internal environment of the patient by the drugs they prescribe. These drugs become part of the biology of the patient and can alter their response, either quantitatively or qualitatively, to another drug.

That is the essence of what is meant by a drug-drug interaction. DDIs can be grouped into two major classes: pharmacodynamics or pharmacokinetics. Both types are important, but this chapter will focus only on pharmacokinetically mediated DDIs and will explain how one drug can affect the absorption, distribution, metabolism, and elimination of another drug and how that in turn can change the effect observed in the patient [Eq. (1)]. This chapter will first review general pharmacokinetic principles to set the stage and will then discuss the relevance of the specific principles to specific types of DDIs.

III. RELATIONSHIP BETWEEN DOSE AND CONCENTRATION

Following systemic administration, a drug achieves a certain concentration in plasma. That concentration ultimately determines and is in equilibrium with the concentration of drug at its site of action. The latter in combination with the binding affinity of the drug for different targets, determines which sites of action of the drug (variable 1) in Eq. (1) are engaged and to what degree. That in turn determines the nature and the magnitude of the drug's effect (i.e., whether beneficial or adverse).

Drug concentration is directly proportional to the dosing rate and inversely related to the clearance, as expressed in Eq. (2):

$$\text{Drug concentration} = \frac{\text{Dosing rate}}{\text{Clearance}} \quad (2)$$

The relationship between dose of the drug and its concentration in plasma is the second variable in Eq. (1), and is determined by the pharmacokinetics of drug in that specific patients in relationship to the dose of the drug ingested by the patient as a function of time (e.g., usually the daily dosing rate). As mentioned before, pharmacokinetics of a drug is what the body does to the drug. Pharmacokinetics can be divided into four phases: absorption, distribution, metabolism, and elimination. Each of these phases will be described beginning with a case vignette that illustrate the relevance of that phase in understanding and thus avoiding the risk of an intended and unintended DDI.

A. Absorption

Case Example. A 47-year old schizoaffective patient was treated with thioridazine (100 mg orally QID), phenytoin (100 mg orally QID), and amitriptyline (50 mg orally q.i.d.). The patient had been stabilized on this regimen for several weeks, but then complained of daytime sedation. The treating physician therefore combined all three into a single bedtime regimen. The patient expired the first night of the new schedule from acute cardiac arrest.

In this case, each of the drugs the patient was taking was individually capable of slowing the intracardiac conduction in a concentration-dependent manner. The patient died as a result of their additive effects. Those individual effects were in turn amplified by the decision to give each drug as a single nighttime dose, and all at the same time. As a result of that decision, the peak concentration of each drug was substantially increased. That in turn resulted in a fatal arrhythmia.

Absorption of the drugs depends upon route of administration, the state of the patient, and factors related to drug itself. Common routes of administration include oral, intramuscular, and intravenous. While many drugs can be administered using any one of these routes, different routes can result in somewhat different concentrations of the drug.

Most drugs, including psychiatric medications, are taken orally, with absorption generally occurring in the small bowel. Drugs then pass into the portal circulation and enter the liver. Most psychiatric medications are highly lipophilic, and hence readily cross the blood brain barrier to enter the central nervous system.

When a drug is given by intravenous (IV) route it completely and immediately enters the systemic circulation (i.e., 100% bioavailability). Thus, bioavailability usually refers to the percentage of total orally administered dose which reaches systemic circulation. Factors that can influence bioavailability include:

1. Formulation of the product.
2. Physiochemical characteristics of the drug.
3. Disease states that affect gastrointestinal function (e.g., slower transit time in small intestine delays drug absorption and peak levels; lowers peak blood concentration).
4. Lower acidic environment (which can increase absorption of weak bases (e.g., TCAs, BZDs, some antipsychotics).
5. Precipitation of a drug at the injection site.
6. Ingestion of drugs with food which generally increases their bioavailability through transient increase in hepatic blood flow and transient inhibition of drug metabolism associated with eating (e.g., food-drug interaction while using monoamine oxidase inhibitors).
7. Coadministration with a drug capable of enhancing or retarding the entrance of the drug from the gastrointestinal tract into the central compartment.

When drugs are given by any route other than IV, the extent of absorption and bioavailability may be incomplete and must be understood to prescribe the drug rationally and to make adequate adjustments if the route of administration is changed. For example, a patient whose pain is under control on demerol 75 mg IV every 4 h might need an oral dose of 300 mg because of the change in route of administration which affects bioavailability.

The state of the patient is also important in determining absorption of the drug. Patients in shock have decreased blood flow to subcutaneous tissues and variable rate of flow through skeletal muscles. Therefore, intramuscular and subcutaneous routes should not be used in case of emergencies.

For orally administered drugs, rate of absorption can be manipulated by altering the physicochemical properties of the tablets or capsules. With rapid-release formulations there is a higher peak concentration (C_{max}) and a shorter time (T_{max}) i.e., as a general rule, C_{max} is inversely related to T_{max}. Sustained-release formulations typically produce a lower peak (C_{max}) that is reached later (T_{max}). This information about the drug can help the physician to avoid DDIs related to the peak concentration, especially when the drug has narrow therapeutic index, or if the patient is on two rapid-release formulations.

Fast absorption may not always be desirable, because adverse effects may be a function of C_{max}. In the case example at the beginning of this section on absorption, failure to appreciate the effect of rate of absorption on the magnitude of the effect resulted in the death of the patient. Cardiotoxicity, due to stabilization of excitable membranes, is as much a function of the peak plasma concentration as it is of steady-state tissue concentration.

Case Example. A 22-year-old woman was admitted to the emergency room with palpitations and dizziness. Her past medical and psychiatric history was negative. She had been taking terfenadine (Seldane) 120 mg/day for 5 days and ketoconazole (Nizoral) 200 mg/day also for 5 days, for allergic rhinitis and a fungal infection of the skin. She claimed to have taken no other medications. The 12-lead resting electrocardiogram recorded on admission showed sinus rhythm with prolonged QT (0.58 sec) and QTc (0.52 sec) intervals. Multiple premature ventricular complexes with a long coupling interval (> 500 msec) were observed. Slight exercise during the physical examination provoked palpitation with syncope, and torsades de pointes were identified on the electrocardiogram. The patient was transferred to ICU and all medications were withdrawn. During the next 5 days QT and QTc intervals slowly returned to normal values (0.44 sec for QT and 0.42 sec for QTc) [1].

"First-pass" refers to the metabolism of a drug before it reaches the systemic circulation. During the absorption stage of an orally administered drug, first-pass metabolism may occur either in the bowel wall or in the liver. Gut wall metabolism of many drugs is extensively accomplished by cytochrome P450 (CYP) enzymes in the luminal epithelium of the small intestine, particularly CYP3A3/4. Drugs that pass to the liver may be taken up by hepatocytes and then biotransformed by CYP enzymes. The parent drug and any metabolites (which may have similar or substantially different Pk or Pd in relation to the parent drug) that survive these two processes, then enter the systemic circulation [2,3].

A large number of commonly prescribed drugs are subject to significant first-pass metabolism either via the gut wall or the liver and thus have low oral bioavailability (e.g., propranolol, amitriptyline, imipramine, morphine) [4,5]. These drugs have a high extraction ratio and high intrinsic gut wall and/or hepatic clearance [5]. For such drugs oral bioavailability can be altered by:

1. Decrease liver blood flow as seen in cirrhosis, persistent hepatitis, and portacaval shunting [6,7].
2. Congestive heart failure.
3. Drugs inhibiting or inducing cytochrome P-450 (CYP) enzymes (e.g., alcohol, ketoconazole) [1,4,8,9]. Antacids like magnesium hydroxide or aluminium hydroxide can also decrease the bioavailability of some drugs such as gabapentin (an anticonvulsant) by 20% [10].
4. Ingestion of drugs with food.
5. Even the dose (i.e., the concentration) of the drug itself can alter the extent of its first-pass metabolism (e.g., nefazodone in a dose-dependent fashion inhibits its own first-pass metabolism) [4,11].

Once first-pass metabolism has occurred, metabolites may be excreted back into the small bowel. Metabolites that are sufficiently lipid soluble can then be reabsorbed into the portal circulation, eventually entering the systemic circulation. First-pass metabolism is extensive with the TCAs [4,5,12]. Acute ingestion of alcohol can impair hepatic extraction of TCAs, increasing the amount reaching the target tissue, and thus cause concentration- (or dose-) dependent toxicity [8,13]. This information about drug-alcohol interactions can help physicians avoid adverse events from concomitant use of alcohol or other drugs. In fact, it is part of the basis for commonly advising patients to not combine their drugs with alcohol.

As mentioned previously, CYP3A is an enzyme responsible for a substantial amount of first pass metabolism of a number of drugs [4,6]. Substantial inhibition of this enzyme by drugs such as the antifungal ketoconazole or the antidepressant nefazodone can substantially elevate the amount of a coprescribed drug reaching the systemic circulation [4,11,14]. That in turn can substantially increase the effect of that coprescribed drug. It can also alter the ratio of the parent drug to its metabolite.

In the case example which began this section, that was the problem. Terfenadine (Seldane), the parent drug, was relatively inactive as an antihistamine but more active at slowing intracardiac conduction [1,15,16]. The reverse was true of its active metabolite, fexofenadine (Allegra). When terfenadine was given alone, it was essentially completely biotransformed by CYP3A in the bowel wall and liver during its absorption (i.e., first-pass metabolism) to the active and safe fexofenadine [1,15]. When given concomitantly with ketoconazole or comparable CYP3A inhibitor, terfenadine was not biotransformed during absorption and thus directly enter the systemic circulation from where it could reach the heart and could slow intracardiac conduction sufficiently to cause sudden death [1,15].

B. Distribution

Case Example. A 44-year-old healthy, physically active, white man developed major depressive disorder. He was started on an oral dose of 20 mg/day fluoxetine. On 23rd day of treatment, the patient developed hives believed to be due to fluoxetine, which was discontinued. The patient was given an oral dose of 25 mg of diphenhydramine as needed. The hives persisted for 11 days after fluoxetine discontinuation [17].

The treatment plan was to wait for at least 48 h after the disappearance of all hives and then to start a structurally dissimilar serotonin selective reuptake inhibitor (SSRI) such as sertraline. However, 36 h into the hive-free period, the patient took an oral dose of two tablets of (650 mg) of acetylsalicylic acid for an unrelated painful joint condition, and the hives reappeared. Despite the recurrence of hives, he continued to take two tablets of ASA every 6 h. The hives eventually resolved. At that point, sertraline was started after a 48-hour hives-free period without subsequent problems [17].

In this case, the authors attributed the initial occurrence of hives to an allergic reaction to fluoxetine. The persistence of the hives for 11 days after the fluoxetine discontinuation is consistent with the long half-life of fluoxetine (3–5 days) and its active metabolite, norfluoxetine (7–15 days). The authors invoked displacement of the highly bound fluoxetine and norfluoxetine by ASA and its metabolite, salicylic acid, as the mechanism explaining the recurrence of hives when the patient took ASA 36 h after resolution of the hives. Their hypothesis was that this displacement produced sufficiently elevated free levels of fluoxetine and/or norfluoxetine to cause the recurrence of the allergic reaction [17].

This case thus illustrates the issue of DDIs mediated by changes in drug distribution. The authors proposed that there was an increase in the free level of drug (i.e., the concentration "seen" by the site of action) rather than the total concentration (i.e., free + bound).

Drug distribution begins as soon as the drug reaches the systemic circulation. Many factors affect how a drug distributes within the body. Factors that favor a high ratio of drug in plasma versus tissue include low lipid solubility, low tissue protein binding, and increased plasma protein binding. Factors that encourage greater tissue accumulation include high lipid solubility, high tissue protein binding, and decreased plasma protein binding either due to decreased circulating plasma proteins (e.g., malnutrition) or due to displacement as a result of DDIs.

Most psychotropic drugs are tightly bound to plasma proteins [18,19]. Such bound drugs often account for > 90% of the total plasma concentration. Although the free fraction is small, that concentration determines the concentration of the drug at the site of action and hence is important [18,19]. For this reason, a small change in the percent bound, from 95% to 90%, doubles the effective concentration at the site of action from 5% to 10% [19,20]. Drugs that are highly bound in plasma therefore have the potential for a displacement DDI from this carrier protein by another drug with higher affinity for the same protein, resulting in an increase in the free concentration of the displaced drug.

There are also populations at increased risk for such a phenomenon. For example, protein binding is lower in women than in men [20–22]. Also, exogenous hormone and pregnancy can alter protein binding and are reduced in the elderly and in patients with chronic hepatic and renal diseases, as well as due to displacement DDIs [14,19].

An example of the latter is the fact that valproate free concentration can be increased upto fourfold in the presence of aspirin compared to valproate alone [23]. In addition to increasing the free concentration of drug, changes in plasma protein binding can cause large apparent changes in volume of distribution (Vd), and clearance (Cl) based on total drug concentration [18–20].

Vd refers to the apparent volume into which the drug must have been distributed to reach a specific concentration. Many psychotropic drugs have much larger apparent volumes of distribution than would be expected based on physical size of the body, because the drugs dissolve disproportionately more in lipid and protein compartments (i.e. tissue) than in the body's water compartment. The Vd can be calculated as shown in Eq. (3).

$$\text{Volume of distribution (Vd)} = \text{Dose/Plasma concentration} \quad (3)$$

C. Metabolism

Case Example. A 52-year-old male was being seen by four different prescribers and was on eight medications: acetaminophen, cimetidine, codeine, erythromycin, ibuprofen, metoprolol, paroxetine, and thiothixene. As a result of the interaction among these medications, this patient could present with a worsening of his depressive syndrome [29].

For simplicity, the discussion of this case will focus only on the following four drugs codeine, erythromycin, metoprolol, and paroxetine (Table 2). The DDIs among these drugs can be seen in Figure 1. Codeine is an inactive prodrug that must be converted by CYP2D6 to morphine to produce analgesia [24–26]. On the other hand, metoprolol is a beta blocker

Table 2 Medication Regimen of a Patient Seeing Four Physicians[a]

Drug	Indication	Prescriber
Codeine	Pain	Primary care physician
Erythromycin	Infection	Infectious disease specialist
Metoprolol	Hypertension	Cardiologist
Paroxetine	Depression	Psychiatrist

[a] These medications could have been prescribed by a single physician in any one of these specialities, but in this case, the patient happened to be seeing four different prescribers
Source: Ref. 29.

whose clearance is dependent on CYP2D6-mediated biotransformation [26,27]. Paroxetine produces substantial inhibition of CYP2D6 under usual dosing conditions [3,4,6]. While paroxetine is metabolized by CYP2D6 at low concentrations, but at higher concentrations is most likely dependent on CYP3A-mediated biotransformation for its elimination [4,6,28], CYP3A is substantially inhibited by erythromycin under usual dosing conditions [4,28]. The inhibition of CYP3A by erythromycin should produce an increase accumulation of paroxetine, which in turn would lead to less conversion of codeine to morphine and more accumulation of metoprolol [27,29].

Due to inhibition of the conversion of codeine to morphine, the patient should have less than optimal pain control. A sufficient accumulation of metoprolol can lead to profound hypotension as a result of reduced cardiac output [27,29]. More modest increases in metoprolol levels might simply present as fatigue. Elevated levels of paroxetine can cause sexual dysfunction including decreased libido, and can interfere with sleep, causing insomnia and daytime tiredness. As a result of all these effects, the patient might clinically appear ironically to be more depressed. This case makes the point that DDIs can be complex, can cross therapeutic classes, can occur across prescribers, and can present in masked ways.

As a result of the patient's looking more depressed, the prescriber might conclude that the patient was in need of more paroxetine or a switch to a different antidepressant or the addition of an augmentation or combination treatment. Thus, DDIs ironically can result in more rather than less polypharmacy as prescribers add drugs to treat the symptoms caused by the DDI.

The metabolism of most drugs occurs principally in the liver and involves the conversion of an active, lipophilic drug into inactive polar metabolites through the process of oxidative biotransformation [2–4]. The resultant polar metabolites are then cleared by the kidneys. The necessary biotransformation steps may involve one or several of the following steps: hydroxylation, demethylation, oxidation, and/or sulfoxide formation [3,4,6].

Many drugs undergo extensive biotransformation (phase 1 reaction), and are susceptible to factors that can alter the rate of drug metabolism, as phase 1 oxidation reactions occur through a large group of cytochrome P450 enzymes [3,30]. For example, in the case that began this section, an important fact was that codeine itself is not a potent analgesic. To be effective,

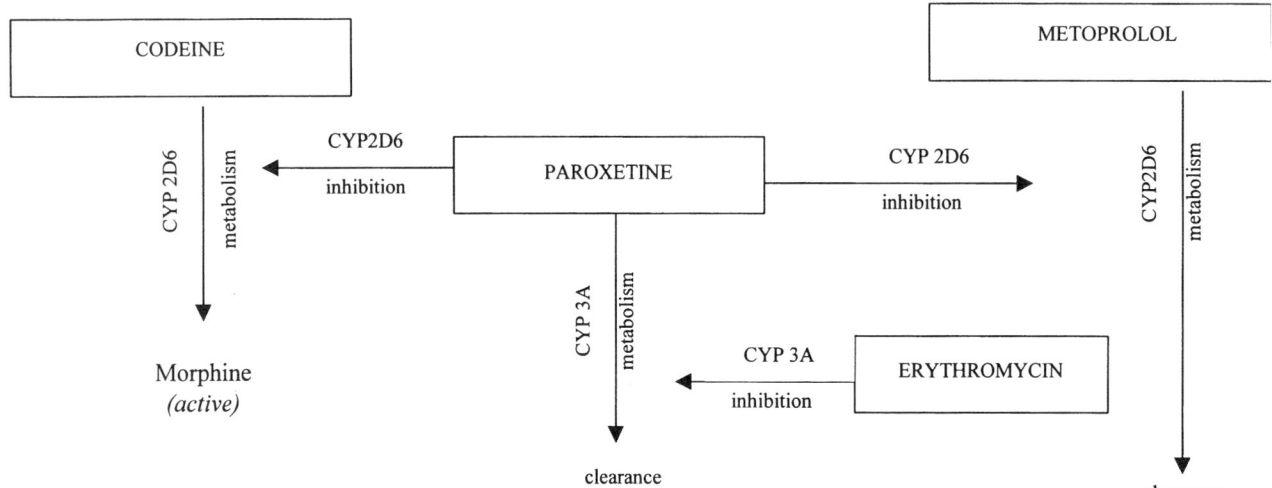

Figure 1 Cytochrome P450 (CYP)-mediated drug-drug interactions among codeine, erythromycin, metoprolol, and paroxetine. Source: Ref. 29.

codeine needs to be converted to morphine [24,31]. This transformation requires the action of CYP2D6 [24,29]. The addition of paroxetine, a substantial inhibitor of CYP2D6 [3,4,6,28] could cause codeine to become ineffective as an analgesic, and the patient could be interpreted to be drug seeking.

Another example is the coadministration of lorazepam with probenecid resulting in increased plasma concentration of lorazepam by impairing the glucuronidation and in turn clearance of lorazepam [23].

Oxidative biotransformation results in the formation of metabolites whose pharmacologic profile may be same as or different from the parent compound and may themselves be toxic [3,4]. For example, trazodone is converted to its active metabolite, metacholorophenylpiperazine (mCPP), through CYP3A4 [3,4,14]. mCPP has a different pharmacologic profile from the parent compound [11,28]. It is highly anxiogenic through its 5HT2C agonism [6,11,32]. Elimination of mCPP is dependent on CYP2D6 [11,14]. Coadministration of trazodone with fluoxetine can result in a DDI where fluoxetine-induced CYP2D6 inhibition can increase levels of mCPP by blocking its excretion from the body. As norfluoxetine has essentially the same activity as fluoxetine in terms of both serotonin uptake blockade and inhibition of CYP enzymes [4,28,33,34], this inhibition will continue as long as norfluoxetine is in the body because fluoxetine-induced inhibition of CYP enzymes is competitive and concentration dependent. This DDI between trazodone and fluoxetine can result in increased concentration of mCPP which in turn produces more 5HT2C stimulation and worsening of anxiety. The long half-life of fluoxetine and norfluoxetine in combination with their inhibition of multiple CYP enzymes makes this antidepressant particularly prone to causing DDIs. For that reason, fluoxetine has fallen out of favor as a first-line antidepressant and should generally be avoided, particularly in patients on other medications.

Knowledge of phase 1 metabolism has expanded substantially over the past decade as a result of improved understanding of cytochrome P450 (CYP) enzymes (Table 2). These advances came as a result of molecular biology, which permitted identification and cloning of the genes that encode specific CYP enzymes. Studies are now directed at identifying which CYP enzymes are involved in the biotransformation of specific drugs and also determining whether specific drugs can induce or inhibit specific CYP enzymes (Table 3). In addition to such in vitro studies, the metabolism of the drug can be assessed in individuals who are genetically deficient in a specific enzyme, but this approach is limited to those CYP enzymes that have a genetic polymorphism, such as CYP2D6 and CYP2C19 [2,4,6,28].

1. CYP Enzyme Induction

This phenomenon refers to an increase in the clearance as a result of increase in the drug-metabolizing capacity of the individual generally by increasing the production of the enzyme mediating the metabolism of the drug. As a result, the plasma concentration of the affected drug will fall unless there is a compensatory increase in the dosing rate. Induction refers to inducing the expression of the gene that makes the enzyme. This

Table 3 Inhibitory Effect of Newer Antidepressants at Their Usually Effective Minimum Dose on Specific CYP Enzymes

	No or minimal effect (< 20%)	Mild (20–50%)	Moderate (50–150%)	Substantial (> 150%)
Citalopram	1A2, 2C9/10, 2C19, 3A3/4	2D6	—	—
Fluoxetine	1A2	3A3/4	2C19	2D6, 2C9/10
Fluvoxamine	2D6	—	3A3/4	1A2. 2C19
Nefazodone	1A2, 2C9/10, 2C19, 2D6	—	—	3A3/4
Paraxetine	1A2, 2C9/10, 2C19, 3A3/4	—	—	2D6
Sertraline	1A2, 2C9/10, 2C19, 3A3/4	2D6	—	—
Venlafaxine	1A2, 2C9/10, 2C19, 3A3/4	2D6	—	—

Mirtazapine based on in vitro modeling is unlikely to produce clinically detectable inhibition of these five cytochrome P450 (CYP) enzymes. However, no in vivo studies have been done to confirm that prediction
Source: Ref. 4.

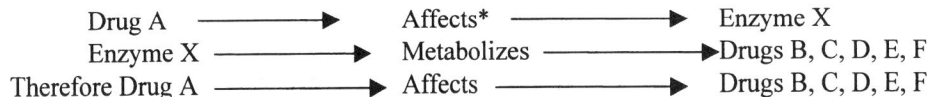

Figure 2 How knowledge of drug-metabolizing enzymes will simplify understanding of pharmacokinetic interactions. (From Ref. 4.)

process takes time as the enzyme concentration reaches a new steady-state level as a result of the increased production. As the concentration of the enzyme increases, the clearance of drugs metabolized by that enzyme increases and the levels of those drugs decrease. The achievement of the new steady-state level of the enzyme and the new clearance takes ~ 2 weeks. When the inducer is stopped, the levels of the enzyme fall back to baseline as does the clearance of drugs metabolized by that enzyme. That process also takes ~ 2 weeks as the basal (or noninduced) steady-state level of the enzyme is achieved. Thus, there is a delay in onset and offset of the induction phenomenon [6,35]. This delay must be taken into account by the prescriber when starting or stopping an inducer.

The starting of an inducer is like stopping an inhibitor in terms of change in the clearance of the affected drug, and stopping an inducer is like starting an inhibitor in terms of change of clearance. The prescriber must keep those facts in mind as well.

The time course of induction is considerably longer than inhibition, which occurs immediately. However, the magnitude of the inhibition is a function of reaching the steady state of the inhibitor. In the case of fluoxetine and its active metabolite, norfluoxetine, that can take weeks to months during which time the magnitude of the effect on the clearance of the drugs and hence their levels is increasing.

Induction is often the equivalent of dropping the dose which can lead to a loss of efficacy. For example, certain anticonvulsants (e.g., CBZ, phenobarbital) potently induce psychotropics resulting in a fall in their levels because of an acceleration in their metabolism [14,30]. Thus, the addition of carbamazepine to control mood swings in a psychotic patient previously stabilized on an antipsychotic may precipitate a psychotic exacerbation or relapse unless the dose is adjusted to compensate. For example, quetiapine (Seroquel) is principally metabolized by CYP3A [35–37]. The addition of an inducer like carbamazepine could decrease the levels of quetiapine below its minimum threshold for efficacy [30,35]. Another example of enzyme induction is concomitant use of carbamazepine with sertraline which resulted in a lack of efficacy of sertraline as an antidepressant at doses two to four times higher than its usually effective minimum dose (i.e., 50 mg/day). This lack of sertraline efficacy was the result of a DDI with carbamazepine but might simply have been interpreted as the patient being "resistant" to the antidepressant effects of sertraline [38,39]. DDIs are not restricted to prescription drugs but can involve drugs such as alcohol, illicit drugs, herbs, and dietary substances. Acute alcohol ingestion has complex effects on the metabolism of drugs. Acute alcohol ingestion can reduce first-pass metabolism and thus increase the plasma concentration of some drugs with usually high first-pass metabolism [8,40]. Subchronic alcohol use on a regular basis for several weeks to months can induce CYP enzymes, resulting in lower plasma levels of drugs that undergo oxidative biotransformation as a necessary step in their elimination [3,6]. Chronic alcohol use can result in cirrhosis, reducing hepatic CYP enzyme concentration and liver mass and cause portacaval shunting [3,6,28]. Cirrohosis can also decrease circulating protein binding, resulting in an increase in the free drug fraction particularly for psychiatric drugs which as a group are usually highly protein bound (venlafaxine being an exception to this general rule). The amount and activity of biotransformation are dependent on the rate of delivery of the drugs to the liver which in turn are dependent on hepatic arterial flow. Drugs like cimetidine and propranolol decrease arterial flow, slowing the clearance of various drugs that undergo extensive oxidative biotransformation [3,39,40]. The effect of these drugs is comparable to the effect of a metabolic inhibition even though the mechanism is different.

2. CYP Enzyme Inhibition

As mentioned previously, inhibition is usually a competitive process, so the magnitude of the inhibitors is a direct and immediate function of the concentration of the drug and its potency for inhibiting the enzyme. As mentioned earlier, the terfenadine story is the tragic example of CYP enzyme inhibition and had by 1996 resulted in the death of > 125 otherwise healthy individuals and eventually resulted in the removal of the drug from the market [41]. Terfenadine is a pro-drug whose conversion to an active antihistamine required metabolism by CYP3A4 [15]. The principal effect of potent 3A4 inhibitors (e.g., ketoconazole, nefazodone) was to massively increase the levels of the parent drug, terfenadine, reaching the systemic circulation by blocking its first-pass metabolism [1,11,28,32]. However, these inhibitors also slowed the clearance of terfenadine following absorption and thus prolonged the period that the patient was at risk for a potentially fatal arrhythmia. Recall, as mentioned earlier, that the half life of the inhibitor drug is important because it determines that how long the inhibitor must be administered before its full effect on the clearance of other drugs is achieved and how long after its effects on their clearance will persist after its discontinuation.

Individuals receiving antipsychotic medications often receive concurrent drug therapy because of coexisting depression, anxiety, or other syndromes that necessitate the administration of antidepressants, anxiolytics, or hypnotics. Thus, the potential for a pharmacokinetically mediated DDI is considerable. An example is an increase in plasma levels of clozapine and norclozapine after addition of nefazodone [42]. In this case, the patient's psychosis was under control with clozapine, and nefazodone was started to treat persistent negative symptoms of schizophrenia. A week later, on this combination, the patient reported increased anxiety and dizziness with mild hypotension. Therapeutic drug monitoring showed increased levels of clozapine and norclozapine consistent with a DDI between clozapine and nefazodone. The clearance of clozapine and norclozapine was reduced by nefazodone through its substantial inhibition for CYP3A4, one of the several enzymes involved in the metabolism of clozapine [42–44].

Drugs such as bupropion, fluoxetine, quinidine, nefazodone, paroxetine, and antipsychotics can under usual dosing conditions produce substantial inhibition of CYP2D6-, CYP2C9/10-, CYP3A3/4-, and CYP2C19-specific CYP enzymes and can produce an average of a 500% increase in the levels of coprescribed drugs which are principally dependent on those inhibited CYP enzymes for their clearance (Table 3). An increase of this magnitude in the levels of coprescribed drugs can lead to serious and even fatal DDIs particularly if the drug has a narrow therapeutic index and its dose is not adjusted for the change in clearance.

D. Elimination

Case Example. A 48-year-old bipolar woman, stabilized on lithium 1200 mg/day for the past 6 months, had a plasma level that varied between 0.8 and 1.0 mEq/L. She developed a recurrence of her rheumatoid arthritis, for which her internist prescribed ibuprofen (800 mg TID). A week later she was brought to the emergency room in a confused, disoriented, and lethargic state. She was also ataxic and had periodic generalized myoclonic jerks. TDM revealed a lithium level of 4.0 mEq/L, and despite a rapid fall to under 0.5 mEq/L with plasma dialysis, her neurological status continued to deteriorate. After 5 days, she died.

Failure to account for a critical drug interaction, affecting the renal clearance of lithium, resulted in an otherwise avoidable fatality. Caution should be used when lithium and diuretics or angiotensin-converting enzyme (ACE) inhibitors are used concomitantly because sodium loss may reduce the renal clearance of lithium and increase serum lithium levels with risk of lithium toxicity [45]. When such combinations are used, the clinician may need to decrease the dose of lithium and do more frequent monitoring of lithium plasma levels.

The simplest definition for elimination is the body's ability to rid itself of a drug. For the sake of simplicity, one can think of the human body as a central compartment connected to at least two important pump and filter systems—the liver and the kidneys. The final clearance of most psychotropics occurs via kidney. At this stage, most psychotropic drugs, which are almost invariably highly lipophilic, have been converted into more hydrophobic metabolites, which facilitates their final clearance via kidneys. The process of clearance by the kidneys involves a combination of glomerular filtration, tubular secretion, and sometimes tubular reabsorption as well. Concomitant drugs can affect the ability of the renal tubules to excrete a drug and results in the accumulation of higher concentration of polar metabolites. These polar metabolites can be less efficacious, more toxic, or both relative to the parent compound depending on the pharmacological profile of these metabolites. Two examples are the effect of loop diuretics and nonsteroidal antiinflammatory agents on renal clearance of lithium.

Dehydration can result in the same outcome by diminishing glomerular filtration rate.

This chapter has sought to explain why it is important for the clinicians to understand the third variable of Eq. (1) (i.e., interindividual biological variance which is in part determined by concomitant drugs, and dietary substance as well as genetics; concomitant cardiac, renal, and liver diseases; and age). All these factors, by altering the biology of a given patient, shift the dose-response curve for a specific drug in that specific patient to a clinically meaningful degree can result in DDIs by simply increasing or decreasing the rate of clearance of the drug from the body.

Half-life and steady state are two pharmacokinetic terms which summarize the major concepts presented in this chapter.

1. Half-Life

The half-life of a drug is determined by characteristics of the drug and the patient. It is the time necessary to eliminate half of the drug from the body or decrease the concentration of drug in the plasma by 50%. Half-life determines how much time will be needed to achieve steady-state concentration of drug in plasma. The general rule is that the time to reach steady-state concentration of a drug is five times the drug's half-life, not five times the dosing interval. The half-life of a drug is proportional to the volume of distribution (Vd) of the drug and inversely proportional to the clearance, as shown in Eq. (4).

$$\text{Half life } (t_{1/2}) = \frac{\text{Volume of distribution (Vd)}}{\text{Clearance (Cl)}} \quad (4)$$

2. Steady State

When successive doses of a drug are administered, the concentration of the drug in the body accumulates until equilibrium is achieved: The amount of drug administered during a dosing interval equals the amount of drug eliminated during the dosing interval. That condition is steady state. The time to reach steady state depends on the half-life of the drug. Once steady state is reached, the drug concentration in various body compartments (e.g., adipose tissue, the brain) is at equilibrium.

For most clinical purposes, measurement of drug levels under steady state is preferred because the drug level with subsequent doses will remain the same as long as the sample is drawn at the same time in the dosing interval. In addition, if peak and trough levels are measured at steady state, patient's pharmacokinetic variables such as half-life and Vd can be calculated from just two serum levels [4,6]. In contrast, if peak and trough levels are determined before steady state is achieved, one would get only a "snap shot in time" of the serum levels with that particular dose because the levels will change with the next dose.

The length of the drug's half-life determines the time needed to reach steady state, and that can be important in determining the magnitude and nature of the response to the drug (i.e., efficacy versus toxicity). Half-life also determines the time needed to clear the drug.

These concepts are important to the issue of DDIs. Drugs interact not so long as they are prescribed but as long as they persist in the body. A lady who had a seizure 10 weeks after the addition of fluoxetine to imipramine is an example of how the time to steady state affects when an adverse event due to a DDI will occur [6,28,34]. In this case, the long half-life of fluoxetine and its active metabolite, norfluoxetine, meant that it took weeks for these substances to reach their eventual steady-state levels [4,6,12,28]. Over this time, the activity of CYP2D6 progressively fell as a result of the competitive inhibition caused by fluoxetine and norfluoxetine [6]. As that enzyme became progressively less functional, the clearance of imipramine progressively diminished and its levels progressively increased [5,12]. In essence, the half-life of imipramine became a function of the half-life of fluoxetine and norfluoxetine. The levels of imipramine increased to the point that it produced its classic concentration-dependent adverse effects which in this case was a grand mal seizure. [12,35].

Returning to Eq. (1), the patient biology (variable 3) was affected by the addition of fluoxetine and norfluoxetine (i.e., progressive CYP2D6 inhibition). That reduced the clearance of imipramine (variable 2), so that the levels of this drug increased to the point that it began affecting ion channels (variable 1) to the point that a clinically meaningful change in clinical effects was observed (i.e., a grand mal seizure) [12].

IV. CONCLUSION

This chapter reviewed important pharmacokinetic principles and their relationship to DDIs. Understanding the pharmacokinetics of a drug is not only essential to the safe and effective prescribing of medications when used alone but can also helps clinicians to avoid adverse DDIs. Rational clinical therapeutics depends on identification and understanding of clinically important DDIs. The topic of DDIs, once a medical curiosity, is now one of great clinical importance and growing public interest. The legal profession is also becoming more attentive to the role played by the DDIs in issues of medical liability. For these and other reasons, the clinicians must be attentive to the possibility of adverse DDIs, not only between the drug he or she prescribes, but also between these medications and those prescribed by other physicians, those available over the counter, and those provided by well-intentioned friends and relatives.

REFERENCES

1. Zimmerman M, Duruz H, Guinand O, et al. Torsades de pointes after treatment with terfenadine and ketoconzaole. Eur Heart J 1992; 13:1002–1003.
2. Coutts RT, Urichuk LJ. Polymorphic cytochromes P450 and drugs used in psychiatry. Cell Mol Neurobiol 1999; 19:325–354.
3. Preskorn SH. Clinically relevant pharmacology of selective serotonin reuptake inhibitors. An overview with emphasis on pharmacokinetics and effects on oxidative drug metabolism. Clin Pharmacokinet 1997; 32:1–21.
4. Preskorn SH. Outpatient Management of Depression: A Guide for the Primary-Care Practitioner. Caddo, OK: Professional Communications Inc., 1999, p 256.
5. Rudorfer MV, Potter WZ. Metabolism of tricyclic antidepressants. Cell Mol Neurobiol 1999; 19:373–409.
6. Preskorn SH. Clinical Pharmacology of Selective Serotonin Reuptake Inhibitors. Caddo, OK: Professional Communications, 1996, pp. 1–255.
7. Tegeder I. Pharmacokinetics of opiods in liver disease. Clin Pharmacokinet 1999; 37:17–40.
8. Weller R, Preskorn SH. Psychotropic drugs and alcohol: pharmacokinetic and pharmacodynamic interactions. Psychosomatics 1984; 25:301–309.
9. Albengres E, Le LH, Tillement JP. Systemic antifungal agents. Drug interactions of clinical significance. Drug Saf 1998; 18:83–97.
10. Anonymous. Gabapentin package insert. In: Physician Desk Reference. Montvale, NJ: Medical Economics Company, 2001, pp 2458–2459.
11. Rotzinger SE. Cytochrome P450 enzymes and the metabolism of trazodone and nefazodone. Dissertation Abstracts International 1999; Section B, Sciences & Engineering 60:0143–0143.(Abstract).
12. Preskorn SH, Fast GA. Tricyclic antidepressant induced seizures and plasma drug concentration. J Clin Psychiatry 1992; 53:160–162.
13. Rubino FA. Neurologic complications of alcoholism. Psychiatr Clin North Am 2001; 15:359–359.
14. Loiseau P. Treatment of concomitant illnesses in patients receiving anticonvulsants: drug interactions of clinical significance. Drug Saf 1998; 19:495–510.
15. Monahan BP, Ferguson CL, Killeavy ES, Lloyd BK, Troy J, Cantilena LR Jr. Torsades de pointes occurring in association with terfenadine use. JAMA 1990; 264:2788–2790.
16. Honig PK, Woosley RL, Zamani K, Conner DP, Cantilena LR. Changes in the pharmacokinetics and electrocardiographic pharmacodynamics of terfenadine with concomitant administration of erythromycin. Clin Pharmacol Ther 1992; 52: 231–238.
17. Shad MU, Harvey AT. A possible pharmacokinetic interaction between fluoxetine and acetylsalicylic acid. J Clin Psychiatry 1997; 58:549–550.
18. Wallace SM, Verbeek RK. Plasma protein binding of drugs in the elderly. Clin Pharmacokinet 1987; 12:41–72.
19. Routledge PA. The plasma protein binding of basic drugs. Br J Clin Pharmacol 1986; 22:499–506.
20. Goulden KJ, Dooley JM, Camfield PR, Fraser AD. Clinical valproate toxicity induced by acetylsalicylic acid. Neurology 1987; 37:1392–1394.
21. Thurmann PA, Hompesch BC. Influence of gender on the pharmacokinetics and pharmacodynamics of drugs. Int J Clin Pharmacol Ther 1998; 36:586–590.
22. Woodhouse KW, Mutch E, Williams FM, Rawlins MD, James OFW. The effect of age on pathways of drug metabolism in human liver. Age Ageing 1984; 13:328–334.
23. Anonymous. Lorazepam package insert. In: Physician Desk Reference. Montvale, NJ: Medical Economics Company, 2001, pp 3346–3347.
24. Chen ZR, Irvine RJ, Bochner F, Somogyi AA. Morphine formation from codeine in rat brain: a possible mechanism of codeine analgesia. Life Sci 1990; 46:1067–1074.
25. Cantwell DP. Attention deficit disorder: A review of the past 10 years. J Am Acad Child Adolesc Psychiatry 1996; 35:978–987.
26. Carlson A, Morris L. Coprescription of terfenadine and erythromycin or ketaconazole: an assessment of potential harm: pharmacists can be key in changing prescribing behavior to avoid drug-drug interactions. Sci Prac 1996; NS36:263–269.
27. Belpaire FM, Wignant P, Temmerman A, Rasmussen BB, Brosen K. The oxidative metabolism of metoprolol in human liver microsomes: inhibition by the selective serotonin reuptake inhibitors. Eur J Clin Pharmacol 1998; 54:261–264.
28. Greenblatt DJ, von Moltke LL, Harmatz JS. Drug interactions with newer antidepressants: role of human cytochromes P450. J Clin Psychiatry 2001; 59:19–27.
29. Preskorn S, Silkey B. Multiple medications, multiple considerations. J Psychiatr Pract 2001; 7:48–52.

30. Spina E, Pisani F, Perucca E. Clinically significant pharmacokinetic drug interactions with carbamazepine. An update. Clin Pharmacokinet 1996; 31:198–214.
31. Sindrup SH, Brosen K, Bjerring P, et al. Codeine increases pain thresholds to copper vapor laser stimuli in extensive but not poor metabolizers of sparteine. Clin Pharmacol Ther 1990; 48:686–693.
32. Barbhaiya RH, Shukla UA, Kroboth PD, Greene DS. Coadministration of nefazodone and benzodiazepines. II. A pharmacokinetic interaction study with triazolam. J Clin Psychopharmacol 1995; 15:320–326.
33. Walley T, Pirmohamed M, Proudlove C, Maxwell D. Interaction of metoprolol and fluoxetine. Lancet 1993; 341:967–968.
34. Bhatara VS, Magnus RD, Paul KL, Preskorn SH. Serotonin syndrome induced by venlafaxine and fluoxetine: a case study in polypharmacy and potential pharmacodynamic and pharmacokinetic mechanisms. Ann Pharmacother 1998; 32:432–436.
35. Tanaka E, Hisawa S. Clinically significant pharmacokinetic drug interactions with psychoactive drugs: antidepressants and antipsychotics and the cytochrome P450 system. J Clin Pharm.Ther 1999; 24:7–16.
36. Weiden PJ. Queitiapine (seroquel) a new atypical antipsychotic. J Prac Psych Behav Health 1997; 368–374.
37. Anonymous. Queitapine package insert. In: Physician Desk Reference. Montvale, NJ: Medical Economics Company, 2001, pp 639–642.
38. Khan A, Shad MU, Preskorn SH. Lack of sertraline efficacy probably due to an interaction with carbamazepine [letter]. J Clin Psychiatry 2000; 61:526–527.
39. Harvey A, Preskorn SH. Cytochrome P450 enzymes: interpretation of their interactions with selective serotonin reuptake inhibitors. Part II. J Clin Psychopharmacol 1996; 16:345–355.
40. Harvey A, Preskorn SH. Cytochrome P450 enzymes: interpretation of their interactions with selective serotonin reuptake inhibitors Part I. J Clin Psychopharmacol 1996; 16:273–285.
41. Anonymous. Drug interactions, cardiac toxicity, and terfenadine: from bench to clinic. J Clin Psychopharmacol 1996; 16:101.
42. Khan AY, Preskorn SH. Increase in plasma levels of clozapine and norclozapine after administration of nefazodone. J Clin Psychiatry 2001; 62:375–376.
43. Cohan LG, Chesley S, Eugenio L, et al. Erythromycin induced clozapine toxic reaction. Arch Intern Med 1996; 156:675–677.
44. Eirmann B, Engel G, Johansson I, et al. The involvement of CYP1A2 and CYP3A4 in the metabolism of clozapine. Br J Clin Pharmacol 1997; 444:439–446.
45. Stein GS, Robertson M, Nadarajah J.: Toxic interactions between lithium and non-steroidal anti-inflammatory drugs. Psychol Med 1998; 18:535–543.
46. Preskorn SH. Do you feel lucky? J Prac Psych Behav 1998; 4:37–40.

Index

AAMR, 57
Academic deficits
  mental retardation, 58
ACC, 228, 283
Acetylcholine (ACh), 26
  affective disorders, 347–357
  Alzheimer's disease, 543–544
  catecholamine, 353–355
  neuromodulator interactions, 352–353
  neurotransmitter interactions, 352–353
  personality disorder, 646
  second-messenger, 356–357
  serotonin, 355–356
Acetylcholinesterase inhibitors
  Alzheimer's disease, 866–867
Acetylmethadol
  opioid dependence, 853
ACh. *see* Acetylcholine (ACh)
Acquired immunodeficiency syndrome (AIDS), 902
ACTH, 177, 455
Activation positron emission tomography
  aging, 487
  Alzheimer's disease, 487
Acute/brief psychotic disorder
  DSM and ICD definition, 74
  refining, 76–77
Acute mania
  fosphenytoin, 800–801
Acute stress disorder (ASD), 61
  classification, 93
AD. *see* Alzheimer's disease (AD)

ADAPT, 885
ADC, 102–103
Addicted brain
  PET, 597–604
Addiction Severity Index (ASI), 590
Addictive disorders
  animal models, 624
  genetics, 615–624
  treatment optimization, 591
Addictive drugs
  mechanisms of action, 586–587
  neurotransmitters, 583
  pharmacokinetics, 584
  rewarding effects, 584
ADHD. *see* Attention deficit hyperactivity disorder (ADHD)
Adolescent anxiety disorders. *see* Childhood anxiety disorders
Adolescent mania
  outcome, 154
Adolescent mood disorders. *see* Childhood mood disorders
Adolescent psychotic disorders. *see* Childhood psychotic disorders
Adoption studies, 15
  alcoholism, 616–618
  suicidal behavior, 702
Adrenergic agents
  alcoholism, 850
  Alzheimer's disease, 869
Adrenocorticotropic hormone (ACTH), 177, 455

Adrenomedullary axes
  cholinergic mechanisms, 351–352
Adventurous temperament type
  pharmacological treatment, 142–143
Affective disorders
  ACh, 347–357
  imaging studies, 335–342
  kindling, 770–771
  putative clinical applications, 921–923
  serotonin markers, 400–401
African-Americans
  comorbid depression, 554
Aggression, 744–745
  genetics, 676–677
  neuroanatomical correlates, 675–676
  neurobiology, 671–677
  serotonin, 672–675
Aging
  activation PET, 487
  brain
    characterization, 478
    metabolism, 482–484
  healthy
    definition, 477–478
  immaturity, 129
  PET
    image processing, 481–482
  structural imaging studies, 336
Agitation
  childhood depressive disorders, 150
Agoraphobia, 91
  clinical genetics, 467–469
  comorbidity, 467–468
  epidemiology, 467–468
  panic disorder, 472
AIDS, 902
AIDS Dementia Complex (ADC), 102–103
AIT-082 (Neotrofin)
  Alzheimer's disease, 874–875
Alarm system, 89
Alcohol
  craving, 565
  emotional attachment, 565
  mechanisms of action, 586
  neurotransmitters, 583
  obsession, 564–565
  reward centers, 566–569
Alcohol abuse
  PET, 604
Alcohol/cocaine abuse
  simultaneous
    PET, 600–601
Alcohol dependence, 554
  GABA, 570
  plasma GABA, 365
  TCA, 554

Alcoholic dementia, 103
Alcohol intoxication
  characterization, 564
Alcoholism, 128–129
  amygdala, 568
  biological features, 565–566
  brain pathways, 567
  clinical features, 564–565
  dementia, 103
  denial, 565
  disorders genetically related to, 618–619
  dopamine, 573–574
  drug abuse
    familial relationships, 619–620
  etiologic marker studies, 623–624
  GABA, 569–571
  gene identification, 620–622
  genetics, 565, 615–619
  glutamate, 571–572
  neurobiology, 563–576
  pharmacotherapy, 846–850
  progression, 565
  racial groups, 565
  serotonin, 572–573
Alcohol-non-craving animals, 575
Alcohol reward
  GABA, 570
Alcohol tolerance, 564
Alcohol use disorder (AUD), 553–558
  future directions, 557
Alcohol withdrawal, 564
  GABA, 570
  signs and symptoms, 564
Allele sharing methods, 19–20, 20
Allopregnanolone, 570
Allostatic dysregulation model
  compulsive drug use, 584–585
Allostatis, 451
Alpha-acetylmethadol
  opioid dependence, 853
Alpha-secretase inhibitors
  Alzheimer's disease, 871
Alpha-synucleinopathies, 107–108
Alprazolam
  sexual dysfunction, 659
Alzheimer's disease (AD), 100–101, 865
  activation PET, 487
  apoptosis, 543
  behavioral symptoms
    treatment, 879–882
  biomarkers, 543
  brain
    pathology, function and structure, 484–486
  brain imaging, 499–503
    functional, 501–503
    genotyping, 503

Index

[Alzheimer's disease]
    structural, 499–501
  brain metabolism, 484–486
  characterization, 478
  chromosome 9 gene, 529–530
  chromosome 10 gene, 529
  chromosome 12 gene, 527–529
  cost, 521
  vs. frontosubcortical dementia, 108
  vs. frontotemporal dementia, 501
  genetics, 104, 521–530
  incidence, 521, 537
  mild cognitive impairment
    pathological correlates, 545–546
  neurobiology, 537–546
  neuronal death, 543
  neurotransmitter abnormalities, 543–545
  pathological diagnosis, 542
  pathology, 521–522
  pathophysiology, 107
  PET, 480, 484–485
  prevalence, 537
  sleep, 718
  structural abnormalities, 538–542
  treatment, 866–879
  vs. vascular dementia, 505
  in vivo imaging techniques, 478–479
Amantadine
  cocaine dependence, 589
  sexual dysfunction, 662
Amenorrhea
  antipsychotics, 659
American Association of Mental Retardation (AAMR), 57
American Psychiatric Association (APA)
  bipolar disorder practice guidelines, 160
Amfebutamone. *see* Bupropion (Amfebutamone)
Amitriptyline
  bulimia nervosa, 833
  childhood mood disorders, 159
Amphetamine
  model, 324
  neurotransmitters, 583
  psychoses, 318, 320–321
Amygdala, 179
  aggression, 675–676
  alcoholism, 568
  hyperresponsivity, 453
  measurement, 337
  PTSD, 451–453, 453
  viscerosensory information, 441
Amyloid
  aggregation inhibitors, 871–873
  immunization, 873
  protein, 544
Amyloid-beta protein, 108

Amyloid deposition
  inflammatory reaction
    Alzheimer's disease, 540
Amyloid metabolism
  Alzheimer's disease, 538–540
Amyloid precursor protein (APP)
  early-onset Alzheimer's disease, 522
  metabolism, 541
Androgens
  sexual dysfunction, 660
Angular gyrus syndrome, 102
Animal models, 1–10
  changing role, 7–8
  cholinergic-behavioral effects, 347–348
  definitional/conceptual issues, 4–5
  ethological context, 3–4
  genetics, 8–9
  historical context, 3
  new therapies, 9
  psychoses, 317–329
    developmental viral infection, 326
    early limbic lesion models, 325
    evoked immune response, 326
    perinatal distress models, 326
    pharmacological, 323
  schizophrenia, 319
    future directions, 328
  significance, 6
  types, 4–5
  validation criteria, 5–6
Animal rights, 9
Anorexia nervosa, 633
  behavioral traits, 635
  course, 634–635
  genetics, 635–636
  neurotransmitters, 636–639
  osteoporosis, 831
  pharmacological intervention, 827–831
  phenomenology, 634
ANP, 436
Anterior cingulate cortex (ACC), 228, 283
Antiamyloid treatments
  Alzheimer's disease, 869–873
Antibiotics, 903
Anticholinergic agents
  antidepressants, 350–351
Anticipation
  trinucleotide repeat sequences, 401–402
Anticonvulsants
  alcoholism, 850
  bimodal effects, 769–770
  biochemical effects, 768–769
  contingent tolerance model, 782–785
  mechanisms of action, 767–785
  vs. psychotropic mechanisms, 767–768
  sexual dysfunction, 661

Antidepressants, 95
  Alzheimer's disease, 881–882
  anorexia nervosa, 828–829
  bulimia nervosa, 832–834
  cellular and molecular mechanism, 814–815
  mechanistic approaches, 811–814
  nicotine dependence, 845–846
  response studies, 340
  sexual dysfunction, 657–659
Antidopaminergic neuroleptic agents
  anorexia nervosa, 828
Antiepileptics
  childhood bipolar disorders, 162
Antihypertensives, 903
Anti-inflammatory agents
  Alzheimer's disease, 876–877
Anti-Inflammatory Prevention Trial (ADAPT), 885
Antioxidants
  Alzheimer's disease, 875–876
Antipsychotics
  Alzheimer's disease, 879–881
  childhood psychotic disorders, 201–202
  receptor effects, 734
  receptor occupancy, 245–246
  receptor pharmacology, 733
  sexual dysfunction, 659–660
  side effects, 201–202, 734
  weight gain, 747–748
Antisocial personality, 142–143
Antisocial personality disorders (ASPD), 647
Anxiety disorder proneness, 471
  alcoholism, 618
Anxiety disorders, 61–62, 128–129, 923–924
  benzodiazepine, 815
  childhood, 175–188
  vs. childhood mood disorders, 153
  with childhood mood disorders, 152
  classification, 89–97
    current, 90–91
  comorbid SUDs, 555–556
  new treatments, 815–816
Anxiolytics
  Alzheimer's disease, 882
  sexual dysfunction, 659
APA
  bipolar disorder practice guidelines, 160
Apolipoprotein E (ApoE)
  Alzheimer's disease, 874
  late-onset Alzheimer's disease, 524–527
  racial groups, 526
  structure, 525
Apoptosis
  Alzheimer's disease, 543
  prevention, 757–758
APP
  early-onset Alzheimer's disease, 522

[APP]
  metabolism, 541
Appetite
  childhood depressive disorders, 151
Appetite stimulants
  anorexia nervosa, 828
Aretaeus of Cappadocia, 69
Arginine vasopressin (AVP)
  personality disorder, 646
Aripiprazole
  schizophrenia, 737
Arizona Sexual Experiences Scale (ASEX), 663
ASD, 61
  classification, 93
ASEX, 663
ASI, 590
Asians
  alcoholism, 565
ASPD, 647
Asperger's disorder, 59
  neurobiology, 211–212
Association studies, 17–18, 298–299, 397–398
Atorvastatin
  Alzheimer's disease, 878
Atrial natriuretic peptide (ANP), 436
Attention deficit hyperactivity disorder (ADHD), 18, 55–56, 61
  with childhood bipolar disorders, 152
  vs. childhood mood disorders, 153
  comorbidity, 56
  prevalence, 56
Attention deficits
  schizophrenia, 225–226
Atypical antipsychotics
  pathological gambling, 693
  schizophrenia
    dopamine hypothesis, 261
Atypical neuroleptic agents
  anorexia nervosa, 830
AUD, 553–558
Autism, 59
  biochemical factors, 206–207
  electroencephalography, 207–208
  eye movement, 208
  functional MRI, 210
  genetic factors, 206
  immunological factors, 208
  magnetic resonance spectroscopy, 209
  morphometric neuroimaging, 209
  neurobiology, 205–211
  neuroimaging, 208–210
  neurophysiology, 207–208
  pathology, 206
  positron emission tomography, 209–210
  quantitative MRI, 208–209
  single-photon emission computed tomography, 209–210

Index

[Autism]
  therapeutic intervention, 210–211
Aversive therapy
  alcoholism, 849–850
  nicotine dependence, 845
Avoidant personality, 141
AVP
  personality disorder, 646

Baddeley's model of working memory, 226
Basal ganglia, 735
BDNF, 778
Behavioral inhibition, 180
Behavioral similarity models, 4
Behavioral therapy, 911
  Rett's disorder, 213
Benperidol, 912
Benzodiazepines, 95
  alcoholism, 570, 850
  anxiety disorders, 815
  childhood social phobia, 181
  comorbid SUDs
    and anxiety disorders, 556
  obsessive personality, 140
  panic disorder, 438–439
  psychotic disorders, 735
  PTSD, 458
  sexual dysfunction, 659, 660–661
Beta-amyloid
  aggregation inhibitors, 871–873
  immunization, 873
  protein, 544
Beta blockers
  performance anxiety, 181
Beta-endorphin
  alcoholism, 565
Beta-secretase inhibitors
  Alzheimer's disease, 870
Binswanger's disease, 102
Biobehavioral animal models, 2
Biochemical signaling, 308
Biofeedback
  sleep, 720
Biogenic amine
  reuptake, 27–33
  transport, 28
  transporters, 32, 741
    mechanisms, 31
Biological markers
  Alzheimer's disease, 543
  family studies, 468
  panic disorder, 442
Biological preparedness theory, 92
Biopsychosocial view, 1
Bipolar disorders, 60–61
  adolescents

[Bipolar disorders]
  prevalence, 150
  childhood, 151–152, 160–164
    outcome, 154
    trauma, 650
  comorbid SUDs, 555
  cyclic AMP-generating pathway, 372
  cyclic AMP-signaling pathway, 380–381
  ERK/MAP kinase signaling pathway, 376
  functional imaging, 341–342
  GABA system, 279–281, 367–368
  gene expression regulation, 385
  GH, 409
  G-proteins, 378–380
  hyperintensities, 341
  imaging studies, 340–342
  intracellular calcium signaling, 373–375, 383–385
  intracellular responses
    integration, 376
  phenytoin, 795–796
    prophylactic study, 800
  phosphoinositide pathway, 372–373, 381–383
  prevalence
    adolescents, 150
  signal transduction abnormalities, 371–386, 378–385
  sodium channel abnormalities, 802
  structural imaging studies, 340–341
    clinical significance, 341
  vs. unipolar disorder, 407–415
  volumetric studies, 340–341
Bleuler, Eugen, 70
Blockers. *see also* Calcium channel blockers
  performance anxiety, 181
Blood oxygen level dependent (BOLD), 687
BOLD, 687
Borderline personality, 140–141
Brain
  aging
    characterization, 478
  function
    exploration, 479–481
  5HT, 676
  hypometabolism
    Alzheimer pattern, 485–486
  metabolism, 479
    aging, 482–484
    Alzheimer's disease, 484–486
    atrophy corrected, 486–487
  pathology, function and structure
    Alzheimer's disease, 484–486
  phospholipid metabolism
    spectroscopy studies, 312
  tumors
    dementia, 103
Brain-derived neurotrophic factor (BDNF), 778
Brain voltage-gated sodium channels, 798–799

Brief psychotic disorder
  DSM and ICD definition, 74
  refining, 76–77
Brofaromine
  bulimia nervosa, 832
Bromocriptine
  alcoholism, 847
  cocaine dependence, 589
Bulimia nervosa, 633, 831–836
  behavioral traits, 635
  course, 634–635
  genetics, 635–636
  neurotransmitters, 636–639
  phenomenology, 634
Buprenorphine (Subutex)
  opioid dependence, 588, 853–854
Bupropion (Amfebutamone)
  bulimia nervosa, 833
  childhood bipolar disorders, 164
  cocaine dependence, 589
  cyclothymic-dependent personality, 144
  histrionic personality, 143
  nicotine dependence, 845–846
  sexual dysfunction, 658, 661, 663
  sustained-release
    nicotine dependence, 589
Buspirone
  alcoholism, 848
  autism, 211
  childhood social phobia, 181
  comorbid SUDs
    and anxiety disorders, 555–556
  generalized anxiety disorder, 815
  nicotine dependence, 589
  sexual dysfunction, 659, 661

CADASIL, 105
Calcium
  differential target, 775
Calcium-binding peptides
  cerebral cortex, 282
  GABA system
    schizophrenia, 281–282
  hippocampus, 282
Calcium carbimide
  alcoholism, 849–850
Calcium channel blockers
  alcoholism, 850
  childhood bipolar disorders, 163
  vascular dementia, 883
Calcium signaling pathway abnormalities, 384
Cancer, 902
Candidate chromosomal regions, 398–400
Candidate genes, 398–400
  alcoholism, 620–621
  panic disorder, 470

[Candidate genes]
  panic syndrome, 442
Cannabinoids
  anorexia nervosa, 828
  mechanisms of action, 587
Carbamazepine
  alcoholism, 850
  anticonvulsant effects, 768
  anticonvulsant tolerance, 785
  bipolar disorders
    comorbid SUDs, 555
  bulimia nervosa, 834
  childhood bipolar disorders, 162
  contingent tolerance model, 782–783
  differential target, 775
  drug interactions, 742
  mechanism of action, 772–776
  pharmacological properties, 793–794
  Rett's disorder, 213
  sexual dysfunction, 661
  substance P, 776
Carbon dioxide hypersensitivity, 434
Cardiovascular disease
  pharmacological interventions, 900–901
Castration
  surgical, 912
Catatonic type schizophrenia, 200
Catecholamines
  ACh interactions, 353–355
  stress-induced increases, 177
Cautious temperaments, 137, 141
CBD, 105
  brain imaging, 509
  pathophysiology, 107
CBF. *see* Cerebral blood flow (CBF)
CBT. *see* Cognitive behavior therapy (CBT)
CCK-4, 470–471
CDD, 59
  neurobiology, 213–214
Cell death. *see* Apoptosis
Central choline
  imaging studies, 350
Central nervous system
  immune system, 410
Central pathways
  panic disorder, 435
Central sleep apnea syndrome, 719
CERAD, 542
Cerebral autosomal-dominant angiopathy subcortical
    infarcts and leucoencephalopathy (CADASIL), 105
Cerebral blood flow (CBF), 439–440, 479, 480
  model, 480
Cerebral cortex
  calcium-binding peptides, 282
Cerebral hyperintensity
  depression, 337

Index

Character, 644
  psychobiology, 117–148
  psychotherapy, 136, 137
  scores, 118
  vs. temperament, 119
  treatment guidelines, 134–148
Character immaturity
  mental disorder, 126–129
Character traits
  psychobiological summary, 129
Chemical neuroimaging
  development, 46–49
Childhood anxiety disorders, 175–188
Childhood bipolar disorders, 151–152, 160–164
  outcome, 154
Childhood depressive disorders
  symptoms, 150–151
Childhood disintegrative disorder (CDD), 59
  neurobiology, 213–214
Childhood generalized anxiety disorder, 178–180
Childhood mania, 61
Childhood mood disorders, 149–164
  biology, 154–159
  clinical characteristics, 149–150
  comorbidity, 152–153
  differential diagnosis, 153
  epidemiology, 149–150
  future directions, 164
  future research, 188
  natural course, 153–154
  pharmacotherapy, 159–160
  prevalence, 150
  psychotherapy, 160
  signs and symptoms, 150–151
  treatment, 159–164
    guidelines, 160
Childhood obsessive-compulsive disorder, 182–185
  brain chemistry/glutamate, 184–185
  volumetric studies, 182–184
Childhood panic disorder, 181
Childhood posttraumatic stress disorder, 185–187
  with separation anxiety, 186
Childhood psychiatric disorders
  classification, 55–59
Childhood psychotic disorders, 63, 197–202
  clinical picture, 198–200
  etiology, 200–202
  historical background, 198
  neuroimaging, 200–201
  pathophysiology, 200–202
  treatment, 201–202
    guidelines, 202
Childhood schizophrenia, 198
  delusions, 63
Childhood social anxiety disorder, 180–181
Childhood social phobia, 180–181

Childhood specific phobias, 187–188
Childhood trauma
  bipolar disorders, 650
Children's Medication Algorithm Project, 161
Chlordiazepoxide
  alcoholism, 850
  sexual dysfunction, 659
Chlorpromazine
  cocaine dependence, 589
Cholecystokinin receptor antagonists, 818
Cholecystokinin tetrapeptide (CCK-4), 470–471
Cholesterol
  aggression, 675
  personality disorder, 646–647
Cholesterol-lowering agents
  Alzheimer's disease, 878–879
Choline, 349
Cholinergic innervation
  Alzheimer's disease, 544
Cholinergic neurons
  Alzheimer's disease, 544
Cholinergic pathways, 47
Cholinergic receptors
  Alzheimer's disease, 544
Cholinesterase inhibitors
  Alzheimer's disease, 867–868
  vascular dementia, 884
Cholinomimetics
  mood-depressing effects, 348–349
Chromosome 4, 400–401
Chromosome 5, 399
Chromosome 11, 399–400
Chromosome 12, 401
  linkage studies, 527
Chromosome 18, 398–399
Chromosome 19
  late-onset Alzheimer's disease, 524–527
Chromosome 21, 401
Chromosome 9 gene
  Alzheimer's disease, 529–530
Chromosome 10 gene
  Alzheimer's disease, 529
Chromosome 12 gene
  Alzheimer's disease, 527–529
Chromosome X, 398
Chronic alcoholism
  dementia, 103
Cigarette smoking
  comorbidity, 557
  genetics, 619
Cisapride
  anorexia nervosa, 830–831
Citalopram
  alcoholism, 849
  Alzheimer's disease, 881
  anorexia nervosa, 829

[Citalopram]
  bipolar disorders, 413
  bulimia nervosa, 834
  childhood obsessive-compulsive disorder, 184
  obsessive personality, 139
Citric acid
  nicotine replacement, 845
CJD, 103
  brain imaging, 510
Classification systems
  future research, 76–77
  validity, 75
Clinical diagnoses, 74–76
Clinical disorders
  animal models, 7–8
Clioquinol
  Alzheimer's disease, 872–873
Clomipramine, 911–912
  anorexia nervosa, 828–829
  autism, 211
  OCD, 815
  pathological gambling, 686
  schizophrenia, 740–741
  serotonin, 738
Clonazepam
  childhood obsessive-compulsive disorder, 184
  sexual dysfunction, 659
Clonidine, 455
  childhood panic disorder, 181
  nicotine dependence, 589, 845
  panic disorder, 437
Clozapine
  childhood bipolar disorders, 163
  pharmacological profile, 732
  schizophrenia, 259–260, 731–732, 735, 736
    dopamine hypothesis, 261
  serotonin receptors, 271
  sexual dysfunction, 659
Cluster A personality disorders, 647
Cocaine, 27
  administration
    pharmacokinetics, 584
  mechanisms of action, 586
  neurotransmitters, 583
  time activity curves, 596
Cocaine abuse
  comorbidity, 556–557
Cocaine addiction
  PET, 598–600
Cocaine/alcohol abuse
  simultaneous
    PET, 600–601
Cocaine dependence
  pharmacological treatment, 854
  pharmacotherapy, 589–590

Cogeners
  mechanisms of action, 586
Cognition
  repetitive transcranial magnetic stimulation, 925
Cognitive behavior therapy (CBT)
  for childhood generalized anxiety disorder, 179
  childhood mood disorders, 160
  childhood social phobia, 181
  pathological gambling, 690
Cognitive catastrophe, 435
Cognitive deficit model
  compulsive drug use, 585
Cognitive deficits
  schizophrenia, 223–231
    amphetamine-induced DA release, 242–244
    baseline DA release, 244
    clinical significance, 229–230
    DA transporters, 244
    DOPA decarboxylase, 242
    functional imaging, 239–240
    imaging DA transmission, 240
    MRS, 246–249
    neurochemical imaging, 240–249
    neuropharmacological imaging, 240–249
    nondopaminergic receptors, 244–245
    PET, 240–246
    phosphorus spectroscopy, 246–247
    prefrontal DA transmission, 244
    proton spectroscopy, 247–248
    resting-state studies, 239–240
    SPECT, 240–246
    striatal DA transmission, 240–242
    task-related activation studies, 239–240
Cognitive disability
  schizophrenia
    treatment, 230–231
Cognitive disorders
  protein aggregation, 106
Cognitive therapy
  sleep, 720
Collagen vascular disease, 901
Collimator, 46
Combat-related posttraumatic stress disorder (PTSD), 455
Combat-related PTSD, 455
Communication disorders, 58–59
Comorbid AUDs
  and bipolar disorders, 555
Comorbid depression
  African-Americans, 554
Comorbid SUDs
  and anxiety disorders, 555–556
  and bipolar disorders, 555
  psychiatric disorders, 554
  psychotic disorders, 556
Complex genetics, 296

Index

Complex phenotype, 296–297
Compulsions, 92
Compulsive drug use
   biological theory, 584–585
Computed tomography (CT)
   advent of, 44
   childhood mood disorders, 157
   personality disorder, 649
Conduct disorder, 56
   with childhood bipolar disorders, 152
   vs. childhood mood disorders, 153
Confusional arousals, 722
Congenital hypoventilation syndrome, 177
Consortium to Establish a Registry for Alzheimer's Disease (CERAD), 542
Construct validity, 5
Continuous-performance task (CPT), 225
Convergence, 4
Cortex
   GABAergic interneurons, 277–279
Cortical dementia, 109
Corticobasal degeneration (CBD), 105
   brain imaging, 509
   pathophysiology, 107
Corticosteroids, 903
   immune response, 411
Corticostriatothalamocortical circuits
   OCD, 424
Corticotrophin-releasing factor (CRF), 177, 436, 455, 818
   antagonist
     depression, 814
Cortisol, 455, 457
   aggression, 675
Cost
   Alzheimer's disease, 521
CPA, 913
CPT, 225
Craving
   alcohol, 565
Creutzfeldt-Jakob disease (CJD), 103
   brain imaging, 510
CRF. see Corticotrophin-releasing factor (CRF)
CT. see Computed tomography (CT)
Cushing's syndrome, 457
Cyanocobalamin
   dementia, 103
Cyclic AMP-generating pathway
   bipolar disorders, 372
Cyclic AMP-signaling pathway
   bipolar disorders, 380–381
Cyclo-oxygenase-2 inhibitors
   Alzheimer's disease, 877
Cyclothymic-dependent personality, 144
Cyclothymic type, 137
CYP
   drug-drug interactions, 938–939

[CYP]
   enzyme induction, 939–940
   enzyme inhibition, 940–941
Cyproheptadine
   sexual dysfunction, 662, 663
Cyproterone acetate (CPA), 913
Cytochrome P450 (CYP)
   drug-drug interactions, 938–939
   enzyme induction, 939–940
   enzyme inhibition, 940–941
Cytogenetic abnormalities, 300–301
Cytokines
   mood disorders, 412

DA. see Dopamine (DA)
d-amphetamine
   psychoses, 318, 320–321
DAT, 27
DBS, 919
DBT, 651
Declarative memory, 227
Deep brain stimulation (DBS), 919
Degenerative dementia, 100–102
Delusional disorder
   DSM and ICD definition, 74
Delusions, 199
   childhood schizophrenia, 63
Dementia
   brain imaging, 497–511
     functional, 498–499
     structural, 497–498
   classification, 99–110
     clinical profile, 109
     etiology, 100
   clinical classification, 108–110
   definition, 99
   etiology, 99–104
   genetics, 104–105, 106
   pathophysiology, 105–108, 107
   pharmacological treatment, 865–886
   protein aggregation, 106
Dementia infantilis. see Childhood disintegrative disorder
Dementia praecox, 70
Dementia syndromes
   brain imaging
     abnormalities, 512
     contributions, 513
Dementia with Lewy bodies (DLB), 101, 884–885
   brain imaging, 506
Demyelinating disorders, 103–104
Denial
   alcoholism, 565
Deoxyglucose model, 480–481
Dependence, 845–846
Dependent personalities, 137
Depo-Provera, 913

Depot neuroleptics, 748–749
Depression, 60
　alcoholism, 618
　animal models, 366–367
　cerebral hyperintensity, 337
　comorbid
　　African-Americans, 554
　CRF antagonist, 814
　functional imaging studies, 339–340
　GABA, 364
　GH, 409
　imaging studies, 335
　muscarinic interactions, 352
　neuroimaging
　　clinical significance, 338–339
　nicotine receptor agonist, 813–814
　nicotinic interactions, 352
　regional brain measurements, 336–338
　sleep, 714–716
　structural imaging studies, 336
　valproate, 366
Depressive disorders
　childhood
　　symptoms, 150–151
Desipramine
　bulimia nervosa, 832, 833
　cocaine dependence, 589
　comorbid major depressive disorder
　　and alcohol use disorder, 554
DESNOS, 450
Developmental coordination disorder, 58
Developmental models
　implications, 327–328
Deviant personalities
　vs. normal personalities, 120–122
Dexamethasone, 457
Dexamethasone suppression test (DST), 408
Dextroamphetamine
　sexual dysfunction, 663
DFP, 8, 348
Diabetes, 901–902
　antipsychotics, 748
Diagnosis
　threshold
　　international differences, 74
Diagnostic and Statistical Manual of Mental Disorders
　　(DSM), 71–73
　challenges, 93–95
　comorbidity, 94–95
　treatment discrimination, 95
Diagnostic and Statistical Manual of Mental Disorders-1
　　(DSM-1), 71
Diagnostic and Statistical Manual of Mental Disorders-II
　　(DSM-II), 72
Diagnostic and Statistical Manual of Mental Disorders-III
　　(DSM-III), 73

Diagnostic and Statistical Manual of Mental Disorders-IIIR
　　(DSM-IIIR), 73
Diagnostic and Statistical Manual of Mental Disorders-IV
　　(DSM-IV), 73–74
Diagnostic and Statistical Manual of Mental Disorders-IV-
　　TR (DSM-IV-TR), 73–74
Diagnostic criteria
　DSM, 71–73
　ICD, 73–74
　international differences, 74–75
Diagnostic hierarchies
　international differences, 74
Dialectical Behavior Therapy (DBT), 651
Diazepam
　sexual dysfunction, 659
Diffusion tensor imaging (DTI), 46
DiGeorge syndrome, 301
Digoxin, 903
Dihydroxyphenylacetic acid (DOPAC)
　pathological gambling, 687
Di-isopropylfluorophosphate (DFP), 8, 348
Discriminant analysis, 487
Disintegrative disorder
　childhood, 59, 213–214
Disintegrative psychosis. see Childhood disintegrative
　　disorder
Disorders of Extreme Stress (DESNOS), 450
Disorganized type schizophrenia, 200
Disruptive behavior disorders, 55
Dissocial alcoholics, 648
Distractibility
　childhood bipolar disorders, 152
Disulfiram
　alcoholism, 849
　cocaine dependence, 589–590
　schizophrenia
　　comorbid SUDs, 556
Divalproex
　autism, 211
　childhood bipolar disorders, 162
　side effects, 162
DLB, 101, 884–885
　brain imaging, 506
DLPFC, 228
DMD
　gene, 16
DNA
　epigenetic manipulations, 327
Donepezil, 354
　Alzheimer's disease, 867
　autism, 211
DOPAC
　pathological gambling, 687
Dopamine (DA), 25, 26, 27
　aggression, 674
　alcohol, 565

Index

[Dopamine]
    alcoholism, 573–574
    Alzheimer's disease, 545
    anorexia nervosa, 828
    autism, 207
    bipolar disorders, 413–414
    D3 receptor genes, 299–300
    eating disorders, 639
    histrionic personality, 143
    neuroimaging studies
        pathological gambling, 687–688
    pathological gambling, 687–688
        genetics studies, 688
    personality disorder, 646
Dopamine model
    compulsive drug use, 585
Dopaminergic agonists
    cocaine dependence, 589
Dopaminergic neuroleptic agents
    anorexia nervosa, 828
Dopaminergic pathways, 47
Dopaminergic reward system
    regulation, 597
Dopaminergic system, 735–738
    PTSD, 454
Dopamine transporter (DAT), 27
Dorsolateral prefrontal cortex (DLPFC), 228
Dothiepin, 901
Douchene muscular dystrophy (DMD)
    gene, 16
Doxapram
    panic disorder, 437
Drug abuse
    alcoholism
        familial relationships, 619–620
    definition, 581–582
    genetics, 619
Drug-addicted individuals
    clinical assessment of, 588–591
Drug addiction
    biological basis, 581–591
    definition, 581–582
    neural substrates, 582–584
Drug dependence
    definition, 581–582
    gene identification, 622–623
    understanding, 596–597
Drug-drug interactions, 933–934
    cytochrome P450, 938–939
Drug holiday, 661
Drugs
    absorption, 934–936
    addictive, 583–587
    development, 807–811
        rationale, 809–811

[Drugs]
    discovery, 9
    distribution, 936–937
    dosage *vs.* concentration, 934–942
    elimination, 941–942
    mechanism
        PET, 597–604
    metabolism, 937–941
Drug user
    with psychiatric comorbidity, 590–591
DSM. *see* Diagnostic and Statistical Manual of Mental Disorders (DSM)
DST, 408
DTI, 46
Dysthymia, 60

Early-onset Alzheimer's disease, 522–524
    APP gene, 522
    presenilin genes, 522–523
Eating disorders. *see also* Anorexia nervosa; Bulimia nervosa
    biological basis, 633–639
    etiology, 633
    pharmacological intervention, 827–837
ECA study, 553
Ecstasy. *see* Methylenedioxymethamphetamine
ECT, 919
EEG, 50
    autism, 207–208
Ejaculation
    dysfunction, 658
Electroconvulsive therapy (ECT), 919
Electroencephalography (EEG), 50
    autism, 207–208
Electrogenic process, 29
Elevated mood
    childhood bipolar disorders, 151
Emotional core, 119
Empirical validity models, 5
Endogenous opiate
    PTSD, 458
Endogenous opioid peptide (EOP)
    alcohol, 566
    pathways
        drug addiction, 582
Endorphin
    alcoholism, 565
    self-injurious behavior, 646
Enkephalin-containing neurons
    alcoholism, 574
Environment
    immaturity prevention, 134–135
EOP
    alcohol, 566
    pathways
        drug addiction, 582

Epidemiologic Catchment Area (ECA) study, 553
Erectile dysfunction
  haloperidol, 663
ERK/MAP kinase signaling pathway
  bipolar disorders, 376
ERPs, 50
Esquirol, Jean Etienne, 69
Estrogen, 910, 913
  Alzheimer's disease, 877–878
Event-related potentials (ERPs), 50
Evoked immune response
  animal models
    psychoses, 326
Excessive worry, 90
Excitatory amino acids, 761–762
  agonists
    Alzheimer's disease, 869
Expansive mood
  childhood bipolar disorders, 151
Explosive temperament type, 140–141
Extreme harm avoidance
  pharmacological treatment, 139–142
Extreme temperament variants
  causal pharmacotherapy, 138–139
  pharmacological guidelines, 138–139
  pharmacotherapy guidelines, 137
  symptomatic pharmacotherapy, 137–138
Eye movement
  autism, 208

Face validity, 5
Facilitation, 226
FAD, 522
False alarm, 91
False suffocation alarm hypothesis, 434–435
Familial Alzheimer's disease (FAD), 522
Familiality
  genetic risk, 295–296
Family-based linkage studies
  alcoholism, 621–622
  drug dependence, 622–623
Family studies, 14
  affective disorders, 702
  alcoholism, 615–616
  biological markers, 468
  depression, 702
  eating disorders, 635–636
  panic disorder, 468
  suicidal behavior, 702–703
Fatal familial insomnia, 103
Fatigue
  childhood depressive disorders, 151
Fatty acids
  childhood bipolar disorders, 163
Fear
  structures, 188

Fear processing
  structures involving, 180
Feedback, 277
Feedforward, 277
Felbamate
  pharmacological properties, 795
Fenfluramine
  aggression, 672
  autism, 211
  bulimia nervosa, 832, 835
Fibromyalgia, 901
Field trials
  clinical diagnoses, 75
5-hydroxytryptamine (5HT), 25, 26, 27
  transporter, 27
Flickering-light sensation, 920–921
Flinders Resistant Line (FRL), 348
Flinders-sensitive line (FSL) rats, 8
Fluoxetine, 911–912
  alcoholism, 849
  Alzheimer's disease, 882
  bipolar disorders, 413
  bulimia nervosa, 833
  childhood mood disorders, 159
  childhood obsessive-compulsive disorder, 184
  cocaine abuse
    comorbidity, 556–557
  comorbid major depressive disorder
    and alcohol use disorder, 554
  drug holiday, 661
  obsessive personality, 139
  OCD, 815
  pathological gambling, 690–692
  pindolol, 812
Fluphenazine, 912
Fluvoxamine
  autism, 211
  bipolar disorders, 413
  bulimia nervosa, 834
  for childhood generalized anxiety disorder, 179
  childhood social phobia, 181
  drug interactions, 742
  obsessive personality, 139
  OCD, 815
  pathological gambling, 692
fMRI. see Functional magnetic resonance imaging (fMRI)
Food restriction, 638
Fosphenytoin, 802
  acute mania, 800–801
Freud's project, 650–652
FRL, 348
Frontal cortex, 735
Frontal lobe
  measurement, 336
Frontosubcortical dementia (FSCD), 108
  vs. Alzheimer's disease, 108

Index

Frontotemporal dementia (FTD), 101
  vs. AD, 501
  brain imaging, 506–507
  genetics, 104–105
  treatment, 885
FSCD, 108
FSL rats, 8
FTD. *see* Frontotemporal dementia (FTD)
Functional magnetic resonance imaging (fMRI)
  autism, 210
  childhood mood disorders, 157
  dopamine
    pathological gambling, 687
  personality disorder, 649
Functional neuroimaging, 49–51
  childhood mood disorders, 158

GABA. *see* Gamma-aminobutyric acid (GABA)
GABAergic interneurons
  cortex, 277–279
  discriminative processing, 279–280
  hippocampus, 277–279
  network oscillations, 279
  phenotypical differentiation, 279
GABAergic pathways, 47
  PET, 48
GABAergic terminals
  markers, 282–284
Gabapentin, 780–781, 784
  alcoholism, 850
  borderline personality, 141
  childhood bipolar disorders, 163
  pharmacological properties, 794–795
GABHS infections, 182
GAD. *see* Generalized anxiety disorder (GAD)
Galanin (GAL), 35
Galantamine
  Alzheimer's disease, 867
Gamblers Anonymous (GA), 689–690
Gambling
  defined, 683–684
Gambling Symptom Assessment Scale (G-SAS), 692
Gamma-aminobutyric acid (GABA), 95, 364–365, 816
  alcohol, 565
  alcohol dependence, 365
  alcoholism, 569–571
  Alzheimer's disease, 545
  bipolar disorders, 414
  depression, 364
  nicotine dependence, 844
  panic disorder, 438–439
  pathological gambling, 689
  personality disorder, 646
  pharmacology, 365–366
  plasma, 364–365
  receptor-binding, 284–285
  system

[Gamma-aminobutyric acid]
  altered inputs, 285–286
  bipolar disorders, 279–281, 367–368
  cell migration, 286
  cortical lamination, 286
  extrinsic afferents postnatal ingrowth, 286–287
  hippocampus
    activity driven changes, 287
  neurodevelopmental hypothesis, 286–287
  reelin, 286
  schizophrenia, 279–281
    postmortem evidence, 281–286
  stress, 287
Gamma-secretase inhibitors
  Alzheimer's disease, 870–871
Gene expression
  gene expression regulation, 376–378
  regulation
    bipolar disorders, 376–378
Generalized anxiety disorder (GAD), 61–62
  buspirone, 815
  childhood, 178–180
  classification, 90
  paroxetine, 815
  SAD, 177
  venlafaxine, 815
Genes
  identification, 14
Genetic knockout, 32
Genetic models, 5
Genetic panic syndrome
  comorbid medical conditions, 441–442
Genetic risk
  familiality, 295–296
Genetics, 2. *see also* Adoption studies; Family studies; Twin studies
  addictive disorders, 615–624
  alcoholism, 565, 615–619
  Alzheimer's disease, 521–530
  animal models, 8–9
    psychoses, 326–327
  anorexia nervosa, 635–636
  autism, 206
  bipolar disorder, 648
  childhood mood disorders, 155
  childhood psychotic disorders, 201
  epidemiology, 295–296, 395–396
  panic disorder, 440–442
  personality disorder, 647–648
  phospholipid metabolism, 312–313
  psychotic disorders, 295–302
  schizophrenia
    serotonergic dysfunction, 267–268
  smoking, 619
Genetic studies
  classification, 96
  dopamine

[Genetic studies]
    pathological gambling, 688
    pathological gambling, 686, 689
    suicidal behavior, 702–705
Genome scan studies
    panic disorder, 470–471
Genotyping
    brain imaging
        Alzheimer's disease, 503
Gerstmann-Straussler-Scheinker disease, 103
Gerstmann syndrome, 102
Ginkgo biloba
    Alzheimer's disease, 875–876
    sexual dysfunction, 664
Ginseng
    sexual dysfunction, 664
Glucocorticoids
    Alzheimer's disease, 876
    stress-induced increases, 177
Glucose dysregulation
    antipsychotics, 748
Glutamate, 200
    alcoholism, 571–572
    Alzheimer's disease, 545
    panic disorder, 439
Glutamate excitatory amino acid system
    schizophrenia, 739–740
Glutamatergic function
    schizophrenia
        cognitive disability, 231
Glutamate systems
    panic disorder, 438–439
Glutamine
    bipolar disorders, 414
Glycine cycloserine
    schizophrenia
        cognitive disability, 231
Glycogen synthase kinase-3, 762–763
GnRH analogs, 914
Gosereline (Zoladex), 914
G-proteins, 372
    bipolar disorders, 378–380
Grandiosity
    childhood bipolar disorders, 151
Granulovacuolar degeneration
    Alzheimer's disease, 542
Group A beta-hemolytic streptococcal (GABHS) infections, 182
Growth hormone
    bipolar disorders, 409
    depression, 409
    mood disorders, 350
G-SAS, 692
Guam-Parkinson-dementia complex, 541
Guanine-nucleotide binding proteins. *see* G-proteins

Guided imagery
    sleep, 720
Guilt
    childhood depressive disorders, 150

Haloperidol
    Alzheimer's disease, 880
    childhood obsessive-compulsive disorder, 184
    cocaine dependence, 589
    erectile dysfunction, 663
    schizophrenia, 741–742
Haloperidol-clozapine
    childhood psychotic disorders, 201
Haplotype Relative Risk (HRR), 18–19, 397–398, 469
Hard-wired transmission, 25–27
Harm avoidance
    psychobiological correlates, 130
    psychobiology, 129–130
HD
    brain imaging, 508
    gene, 21
    genetics, 105
Headache
    repetitive transcranial magnetic stimulation, 926
Healthy aging
    definition, 477–478
Hearing
    repetitive transcranial magnetic stimulation, 926
Heart period variability (HPV), 436
Heinroth, Johann Christian, 70
Heller, Theodor, 213
Hereditary dysphasic dementia
    pathophysiology, 106–107
High blood pressure
    panic attacks, 436
High harm avoidance, 137
High novelty seeking
    pharmacological treatment, 142–144
High reward dependence
    high harm avoidance, 137
    pharmacological treatment, 144
Hippocampus
    calcium-binding peptides, 282
    GABAergic interneurons, 277–279
    GABA system
        activity driven changes, 287
        schizophrenia, 281–282
    measurement, 337
    neuritic plaques, 539
    normal afferent connections, 539
    PTSD, 457
Hirano bodies
    Alzheimer's disease, 541
Histrionic personality, 143–144

Index

HIV-related dementia (HRD), 102–103, 902
  brain imaging, 511
Homology, 4
Homovanilic acid (HVA)
  pathological gambling, 687
Hormonal therapy, 913–915
HPV, 436
HRD, 102–103, 511, 902
HRR, 18–19, 397–398, 469
Human Genome Project, 18
Huntington's chorea, 282
Huntington's disease (HD)
  brain imaging, 508
  gene, 21
  genetics, 105
HVA
  pathological gambling, 687
5-Hydroxytryptamine (5HT), 25, 26, 27
  transporter, 27
Hyperactivity
  alcoholism, 618
Hyperglycemia
  antipsychotics, 748
Hyperintensity
  location, 338
Hyperphosphorylation
  Alzheimer's disease, 873–874
Hyperresponsivity
  amygdala, 453
Hypersomnia
  childhood depressive disorders, 150–151
Hypertension
  panic attacks, 436
Hypnotics
  Alzheimer's disease, 882
  mechanisms of action, 586
Hypothalamic-growth hormone axis, 409
Hypothalamic-pituitary-adrenal axis, 407–408, 408–409, 451
  cholinergic mechanisms, 351–352
  drug addiction, 582
  hyperactivity, 408
  panic disorder, 436–437
Hypothalamic-pituitary-gonadal axis, 410
Hypothyroidism
  dementia, 103

Iatrogenic sexual dysfunction, 657–665
Ibuprofen, 901
ICD. *see* International Classification of Diseases (ICD)
Idebenone
  Alzheimer's disease, 876
Iloperidone
  schizophrenia, 740
Imagery, 92

Imipramine
  bulimia nervosa, 832
  childhood mood disorders, 159
  sexual dysfunction, 659
Immature character
  relative risk, 123
Immature fantasy, 199
Immaturity
  age, 129
  prevention, 134–135
Immune response
  mood disorders, 411
  PTSD, 459
  stress, 410–411
Immune system
  central nervous system, 410
  mood disorders, 410–411
  PTSD, 458–459
Impaired cognition
  schizophrenia, 228–230
Impaired executive functions
  schizophrenia, 228–229
Impulses, 92
Impulsive aggression
  serotonin, 645–647
  tryptophan hydroxylase, 648
Incentive-sensitization model
  compulsive drug use, 585
Independent temperament type
  pharmacological treatment, 144–145
Infectious agents
  genes, 13
Inflammatory reaction
  amyloid deposition
    Alzheimer's disease, 540
Inflated self-esteem
  childhood bipolar disorders, 151
Inhalant abuse
  PET, 603
Inositol, 778
Inositol depletion hypothesis, 759–761
Insomnia
  childhood depressive disorders, 150–151
Interference, 226
International Classification of Diseases (ICD), 73
International Classification of Diseases-9 (ICD-9)
  vs. International Classification of Diseases-10 (ICD-10), 73–74
International Classification of Diseases-10 (ICD-10)
  vs., 73–74
  vs. International Classification of Diseases-9 (ICD-9), 73–74
Interpersonal therapy (IPT)
  childhood mood disorders, 160
Intracellular calcium signaling
  bipolar disorders, 373–375, 383–385

Intracellular responses
　integration
　　bipolar disorders, 376
Intravenous immunoglobulin
　autism, 211
Ipsapirone, 645
　bulimia nervosa, 835
IPT
　childhood mood disorders, 160
Irritability
　childhood bipolar disorders, 151
　childhood depressive disorders, 150

Kernberg's Transference Focused Therapy, 650–651
Ketamine, 322
　mimicking schizophrenia, 739
　schizophrenia, 318
Ketamine abuse
　PET, 602
Ketoconazole, 903
　cardiovascular safety, 747
Ketogenic diet
　Rett's disorder, 213
Kindling, 770–771
Kraeplin, Emil, 70
Kraeplin's systematic classification of psychoses, 70
Kuru, 103

Laboratory
　advances, 21
Lacunar state, 102
L-alpha-acetylmethadol
　opioid dependence, 853
Lamotrigine, 778–779, 784, 903
　anticonvulsant tolerance, 785
　autism, 211
　childhood polar disorders, 162
　pharmacological properties, 794
　side effects, 162
Late-onset Alzheimer's disease, 522, 524–530
　apolipoprotein E gene, 524–527
　chromosome 19, 524–527
　susceptibility genes, 524
LC, 35, 454–455
LDP, 279
Learning disorders, 58–59
Leuprolide (Lupron), 914
Levetiracetam, 781
Lewy bodies
　Alzheimer's disease, 542
　dementia, 884–885
LHPA, 451, 456
Life events, 135
Light
　absorption, 51
　scattering, 51

Limbic-hypothalamic-pituitary-adrenal (LHPA), 451, 456
Linehan's Dialectical Behavior Therapy, 651
Linkage disequilibrium, 297–298
　isolated populations, 20–21
Linkage method, 396–397
Lipska-Weinberger model, 325
Lithium, 757–764, 903
　Bcl-2 upregulation, 758
　bipolar disorders
　　comorbid SUDs, 555
　childhood bipolar disorders, 160–162, 163–164
　loading, 800
　neurotrophic effects, 777
　pathological gambling, 693
　serotonin, 761
　sexual dysfunction, 660–661
　side effects, 162
　substance P, 776
　vs. valproate, 776–778
Locus coeruleus (LC), 35
　PTSD, 454–455
　stress, 454–455
Long-term depression (LDP), 279
Long-term memory
　models, 226
Long-term potentiation (LTP), 279
Lorazepam, 802
　psychotic disorders, 735
Lovastatin
　Alzheimer's disease, 878
Low character variants
　psychotherapy guidelines, 134
Low harm avoidance
　high reward dependence, 137
Low reward dependence
　pharmacological treatment, 144–145
Loxapine
　schizophrenia, 742
LSD
　schizophrenia, 318
LTP, 279
Lupron, 914
Lysergic acid diethylamide (LSD)
　schizophrenia, 318

Magnetic resonance imaging (MRI), 45
　advent, 44
　autism, 208–209
　brain
　　Alzheimer's disease, 500
　childhood mood disorders, 157
　clinical application, 46
　personality disorder, 649
　quantitative
　　autism, 208–209
　quantitative volumetric

Index

[Magnetic resonance imaging (MRI)]
    brain
        Alzheimer's disease, 500
Magnetic resonance spectroscopy (MRS), 48, 312
    autism, 209
    childhood mood disorders, 157, 158
    childhood psychotic disorders, 201
    cognitive deficits
        schizophrenia, 246–249
Magnetic seizure therapy (MST), 919
Magnetization transfer imaging (MTI), 49
Magnetoencephalography (MEG), 51
Major depression, 554
    comorbidity, 554–555
    vs. panic disorder, 436–437
    TCA, 554
Major depressive disorder (MDD), 60, 128–129
    comorbidity, 60
Maladaptation, 122
Mania
    childhood, 61
    fosphenytoin, 800–801
MAO
    pathological gambling, 686–687
MAOIs
    comorbid SUDs
        and anxiety disorders, 556
    cyclothymic-dependent personality, 144
    sexual dysfunction, 658
Marchiafava-Bignami, 103
Marijuana
    neurotransmitters, 583
Marijuana abuse
    PET, 603
Mature character
    protecting against personality disorder, 122
Maturity
    higher level, 129
Mazindol
    cocaine dependence, 589
McCrae and Costa's model of personality, 645
m-CPP
    pathological gambling, 686
MDD, 60, 128–129
MDMA, 27
    mechanisms of action, 587
    neurotransmitters, 583
Mecamylamine
    nicotine dependence, 589, 846
Mechanistic models, 5
Medial prefrontal cortex
    PTSD, 453–454
Medication. *see* Drugs
Meditation
    sleep, 720
Medroxyprogesterone acetate (MPA), 913

MEG, 51
Melancholy
    definition, 69
Melatonin
    childhood bipolar disorders, 163
Membranes
    biology, 307–308
    phospholipid metabolism
        phospholipase A2, 308–310
    remodeling, 308
Memory
    neurobiology, 226–228
Mendelian inheritance, 16–17
Menstrual irregularities
    antipsychotics, 659
Mental disorder
    character immaturity, 126–129
Mental retardation, 57–58
    comorbidity, 57
Mental rituals, 92
Mescaline
    schizophrenia, 318
Mesolimbic dopamine
    drug addiction, 582
    pathways, 584
Metabolic dementia, 103
Metabotropic glutamate, 437
    receptor agonists, 817–818
Metachlorophenylpiperazine (m-CPP)
    pathological gambling, 686
Methadone
    opioid dependence, 588, 851–853, 854
Methamphetamine
    mechanisms of action, 586
Methamphetamine abuse
    PET, 601
Methodical temperament type, 139–140
Methylenedioxymethamphetamine (MDMA), 27
    mechanisms of action, 587
    neurotransmitters, 583
Methylphenidate
    cocaine dependence, 854
    histrionic personality, 143
    mechanisms of action, 586
    sexual dysfunction, 663
Metyrapone, 903
Mianserin
    bulimia nervosa, 832
    sexual dysfunction, 662
MID, 102
Milameline
    Alzheimer's disease, 868
Mild cognitive impairment
    Alzheimer's disease
        pathological correlates, 545–546
    treatment, 885

Mild personality disorder, 128–129
Mirtazapine
    autism, 211
    sexual dysfunction, 658, 662
Mitral valve prolapse (MVP), 441
Mixed expressive-receptive disorder, 58
Moclobemide
    nicotine dependence, 589, 846
    sexual dysfunction, 658
Molecular genetics, 297–300
    aggression, 677
Monoamine
    neuropeptides, 34
    transporter structures, 27
Monoamine oxidase inhibitors (MAOIs)
    comorbid SUDs
        and anxiety disorders, 556
    cyclothymic-dependent personality, 144
    sexual dysfunction, 658
Monoamine oxidase (MAO)
    pathological gambling, 686–687
Monoaminergic
    regulation, 25–36
Monoaminergic neurotransmission
    neuropeptide modulation, 33–36
Monodrug user, 590
Mood disorders, 60–61
    childhood. see Childhood mood disorders
    cytokines, 412
    GAMA, 363–369
    growth hormone, 350
    hypothalamic-pituitary-gonadal axis, 410
    immune response, 411
    immune system, 410–411
    molecular genetics, 395–402
Mood disturbance, 199
Mood stabilizers
    anorexia nervosa, 830
    bulimia nervosa, 834
    mechanisms, 773, 779
    pathological gambling, 692–693
    sexual dysfunction, 660–661
Morel, Benedict Augustin, 70
Motive circuit
    alcoholism, 569
Motor disorders, 58–59
Motor stereotypy, 320
MPA, 913
MRI. see Magnetic resonance imaging (MRI)
MRS. see Magnetic resonance spectroscopy (MRS)
MS, 103–104
MSA, 107
    brain imaging, 510
MST, 919
MTI, 49
Multifinality, 126

Multi-infarct dementia (MID), 102
Multiple sclerosis (MS), 103–104
Multiple system atrophy (MSA), 107
    brain imaging, 510
MVP, 441
Myocardial infarction
    panic attacks, 436
Myoinositol
    bulimia nervosa, 835

Nalmephene
    alcoholism, 848
Naloxone
    personality disorder, 646
    PTSD, 458
Naltrexone (Trexan)
    alcoholism, 848
    autism, 211
    bulimia nervosa, 835
    opioid dependence, 588, 851
    pathological gambling, 692
    personality disorder, 646
Narcolepsy, 720–721
NARP, 76–77
National Comorbidity Survey (NCS), 553, 554
NCS, 553, 554
NE. see Norepinephrine (NE)
Nefazodone
    sexual dysfunction, 658
Neoplastic dementia, 103
Neostigmine, 354
Neotrofin
    Alzheimer's disease, 874–875
Nerve growth factor
    Alzheimer's disease, 874
NET, 27
Neumann, Heinrich, 70
Neural circuitry
    selective vulnerability, 537–538
Neurobiological insights
    classification, 96–97
Neurobiological status, 2
Neuroendocrine hypothesis, 407
Neuroendocrine studies
    childhood mood disorders, 156–157
Neurofibrillary tangles (NFRTs), 100
    Alzheimer's disease, 538, 540
Neuroimaging
    childhood mood disorders, 157–158
    classification, 95–96
Neuroleptics
    psychotic disorders, 735
Neuromodulator
    ACh interactions, 352–353
Neuronal death
    Alzheimer's disease, 543

Neuropeptides, 33–34
  autism, 207
  bipolar disorders, 415
  monoamines, 34
  OCD, 427–428
  schizophrenia, 740–741
Neuropeptide Y (NPY), 35
  galanin
    norepinephrine, 35–36
Neuropil threads
  Alzheimer's disease, 541
Neuropsychiatric disorders
  repetitive transcranial magnetic stimulation, 919
  sleep, 714–718
Neurosciences
  animal models, 7
Neurosurgery, 912
Neurotensin
  schizophrenia, 740–741
Neurotransmitter
  ACh interactions, 352–353
  bipolar disorders, 415
Neurotransmitter studies
  childhood mood disorders, 155–156
Neurotrophic agents
  Alzheimer's disease, 874–875
Neurotrophins
  autism, 207
New-variant CJD (vCJD), 103
NFRTs, 100
  Alzheimer's disease, 538, 540
Nicardipine
  vascular dementia, 883
Nicergoline
  vascular dementia, 884
Nicotine
  mechanisms of action, 586–587
  neurotransmitters, 583
Nicotine abuse
  PET, 601
Nicotine dependence
  pharmacotherapy, 588–589, 843–846
Nicotine gum, 844
Nicotine receptor agonist
  depression, 813–814
Nicotine replacement therapy, 588–589, 844
Nicotine use
  genetic studies, 623
Nicotinic acetylcholine receptor agonists
  Alzheimer's disease, 868
Nightmares, 722–723
Nimodipine
  childhood bipolar disorders, 163
  differential target, 775
  vascular dementia, 883
NMDA. see N-methyl-D-aspartate (NMDA)

N-methyl-D-aspartate (NMDA), 457
  glutamate receptor antagonists
    psychoses, 318, 321–323
  receptor antagonists, 813
  receptor channel blockers
    alcoholism, 850
NMR
  advent of, 44
Nonaffective acute remitting psychosis (NARP), 76–77
Nonalcohol SUDs
  comorbidity, 556–557
Nondegenerative dementia, 102–104
Nonparametric methods, 17–19
Nonsteroidal anti-inflammatory drugs (NSAIDs)
  Alzheimer's disease, 876–877
Nootropics
  vascular dementia, 883–884
Noradrenaline
  Alzheimer's disease, 545
Norepinephrine (NE), 25, 27
  aggression, 674
  anorexia nervosa, 828
  bipolar disorders, 415–416
  histrionic personality, 143
  personality disorder, 646
Norepinephrine transporter (NET), 27
Normal personalities
  vs. deviant personalities, 120–122
Normal pressure hydrocephalus (NPH), 102
Normal sleep, 713–714
Nortriptyline
  childhood mood disorders, 159
  nicotine dependence, 589, 846
  vs. paroxetine, 901
Novelty seeking
  psychobiological correlates, 131
  psychobiology, 130–131
NPGi, 437
NPH, 102
NPY, 35
  galanin
    norepinephrine, 35–36
NREM parasomnias, 721–722
NSAIDs
  Alzheimer's disease, 876–877
Nuclear magnetic resonance (NMR)
  advent of, 44
Nucleus accumbens, 596
Nucleus paragigantocellularis (NPGi), 437
Nutrition
  genes, 13

Obsession
  alcohol, 564–565
Obsessive-compulsive disorder (OCD), 61–62, 911–912, 923–924

[Obsessive-compulsive disorder (OCD)]
  autoimmune pathology, 425–426
  childhood, 182–185
  classification, 92–93
  clomipramine, 815
  dopaminergic systems, 427
  fluoxetine, 815
  functional studies, 424–425
  neuroanatomical models, 423–425
  neurobiology, 423–428
  neurochemistry, 426–428
  neuropeptides, 427–428
  neuropharmacology, 426–428
  serotonin, 426–427
  structural studies, 424
Obsessive personality, 139–140
Obstructive sleep apnea syndrome, 719
OCD. see Obsessive-compulsive disorder (OCD)
ODD. see Oppositional defiant disorder (ODD)
Olanzapine
  Alzheimer's disease, 880–881
  childhood bipolar disorders, 163
  dementia with Lewy bodies, 885
  pathological gambling, 693
  psychotic disorders, 735
  schizophrenia, 737, 742, 746
  serotonin, 738
  sexual dysfunction, 660
Olivopontocerebellar atrophy, 107
Omega-3 fatty acids
  childhood bipolar disorders, 163
Ondansetron
  alcoholism, 573, 848
  bulimia nervosa, 835
Opiate abuse
  PET, 602
Opiates
  anorexia nervosa, 828
Opioid
  alcoholism, 574–576
  bulimia nervosa, 834–835
  mechanisms of action, 587
  neurotransmitters, 583
  pathological gambling, 689
  self-injurious behavior, 646
Opioid antagonists
  alcoholism, 847–848
  nicotine dependence, 846
  pathological gambling, 692
Opioid dependence
  pharmacological treatment, 850–854
  pharmacotherapy, 588
Opioid maintenance therapy, 851–854
Opioid pathways, 47
Oppositional defiant disorder (ODD), 56–57
  vs. childhood mood disorders, 153

[Oppositional defiant disorder (ODD)]
  comorbidity, 57
  prevalence, 56
Orgasm
  dysfunction, 658
Osteoporosis
  anorexia nervosa, 831
Overanxious disorder. see Generalized anxiety disorder
Oxcabamazepine
  childhood bipolar disorders, 163
Oxcarbazepine
  mechanism of action, 772–776
  pharmacological properties, 794

Pallidal-thalamocortical pathway
  alcoholism, 569
Panic attacks, 62, 436
  situationally bound, 433
  symptoms, 91
Panic disorder (PD), 61–62, 91
  agoraphobia, 472
  biological markers, 442
  biological systems, 434–439
  candidate gene studies, 470
  central pathways, 435
  childhood, 181
  classification, 90–91
  clinical genetics, 467–469
  comorbidity, 440–442, 467–468
  epidemiology, 467–468
  future directions, 442
  GABA/glutamate systems, 438–439
  genetics, 440–442
  genome scan studies, 470–471
  heritability, 468
  molecular studies, 470–471
  neurobiology, 433–443
  neuroimaging studies, 439–440
  noradrenergic system, 437–438, 438
  paroxetine, 815
  respiratory physiology, 434–436
  risk loci, 469–470
  SAD, 177
  sighing, 435
  SSRI, 439
  syndrome, 471
  trait markers
    neurodevelopmental studies, 434
Panic syndrome
  candidate gene, 442
PAP phosphatase, 758–759
Paracrine transmission, 25–27
Paralimbic system
  OCD, 423–424
Parametric methods, 15–17

Parametric stress tests, 487
Paranoid type schizophrenia, 200
Paraphilias, 909
Parkinson's disease, 101–102
    sleep, 718
Parkinson's disease with dementia
    brain imaging, 509–510
Paroxetine
    Alzheimer's disease, 881
    bipolar disorders, 413
    childhood mood disorders, 159
    childhood social phobia, 181
    drug holiday, 661
    vs. nortriptyline, 901
    obsessive personality, 139
    panic disorder, 815
    pathological gambling, 690–692
    social anxiety disorder, 815
Partial volume effect (PVE)
    correction, 482–484
Passionate temperament type, 143–144
Passionate type, 137
Passive-aggressive personality, 142
Passive-aggressive temperaments, 137
Pathological gambling, 683–693
    behavioral treatment, 690
    classification, 685–686
    comorbidity, 684–685
    conceptualization, 685–686
    defined, 684–685
    definition, 683–685
    diagnostic criteria, 684
    genetic studies, 686, 689
    high-risk groups, 685
    neurobiology, 686–689
    neurochemical studies, 686
    norepinephrine systems, 688–689
    opioid antagonists, 692
    opioid systems, 689
    pharmacological challenge studies, 686
    pharmacotherapy, 690–693
    prevalence, 684
    self-help, 689–690
    treatment, 689–693
PCOS, 661
    divalproex, 162
PCP. see Phencyclidine (PCP)
PD. see Panic disorder (PD)
Pedigree
    linkage analysis, 16
Pentoxifylline
    vascular dementia, 883
Peptides neurotransmitters
    Alzheimer's disease, 545
Performance anxiety
    beta blockers, 181

Persistence
    psychobiological correlates, 133
    psychobiological data, 132–133
Personality
    production, 120
Personality development
    fifteen-step, 127
    hierarchical model, 128
Personality disorder
    biological basis, 643–652
    categorical and dimensional assessment, 124
    genetics, 647–648
    life events, 649–650
    neuroimaging studies, 649
    neurotransmitters, 645–647
    psychobiological integration of treatment, 145–148, 146–147
    social vs. clinical diagnosis, 124–125
    symptoms
        predictors, 121
Pervasive developmental disorder not otherwise specified, 59
    vs. childhood mood disorders, 153
    neurobiology, 214
Pervasive developmental disorders, 59
PET, 46
Pettersen Mania Rating Scale, 801, 802
PFC
    aggression, 675
    alcohol, 566
    OCD, 423
Pharmacoeconomics
    drug development, 811
Phasic/tonic dopamine model
    compulsive drug use, 585
Phencyclidine (PCP), 322, 324
    abuse
        PET, 602
    mechanisms of action, 587
    mimicking schizophrenia, 739
    neurotransmitters, 583
    schizophrenia, 318
Phenelzine
    bulimia nervosa, 832
Phenobarbital, 802
Phenotypes
    definition, 14, 644
Phenytoin
    bipolar disorders, 795–796
        prophylactic study, 800
    drug interactions, 742
    pharmacological properties, 795–796
Phonological disorder, 58
Phosphoadenosine phosphate (PAP) phosphatase, 758–759
Phosphoinositide pathway
    bipolar disorders, 372–373, 381–383

Phospholipase A2
  membrane phospholipid metabolism, 308–310
Phospholipids
  metabolism
    genetic studies, 312–313
    molecular structure, 308
    schizophrenia, 310–313
Phosphomonoesters (PME), 312
Physostigmine, 801
  bipolar disorders, 349
Pick's disease, 101
  pathophysiology, 106
Pilocarpine
  supersensitive pupillary responses, 351
Pimozide
  autism, 210–211
  childhood obsessive-compulsive disorder, 184
Pindolol
  fluoxetine, 812
  obsessive personality, 139
Pinel, Philippe, 69
Piribedil
  mild cognitive impairment, 885
PKC
  alcoholism, 570
  drug effects, 777
Plasma GABA, 364–365
  alcohol dependence, 365
PM, 396
31P magnetic resonance spectroscopy, 312
PME, 312
Polycystic ovarian syndrome (PCOS), 661
  divalproex, 162
Polydrug user, 590
Polygenic Model (PM), 396
Polymorphism, 18, 32
Population stratification, 469
Positron emission tomography (PET), 46
  activation, 487
  AD, 480, 484–485
  aging, 487
  Alzheimer's disease, 487
  autism, 209–210
  childhood mood disorders, 157, 158
  childhood psychotic disorders, 201
  cognitive deficits
    schizophrenia, 240–246
  dopamine
    pathological gambling, 687
  image processing
    aging, 481–482
  personality disorder, 649
  PTSD, 453
  scanner, 47
Posttraumatic stress disorder (PTSD), 61–62, 185–187, 455, 923–924

[Posttraumatic stress disorder (PTSD)]
  amygdala, 451–453
  benzodiazepine, 458
  childhood, 185–187
  vs. childhood mood disorders, 153
  classification, 93
  clinical factors, 450–451
  combat-related, 455
  dopamine system, 454
  endogenous opiate, 458
  epidemiology, 449–450
  hippocampus, 457
  HPT, 459–460
  immune system, 458–459
  LHPA axis, 455–457
  locus ceruleus, 454–455
  medial prefrontal cortex, 453–454
  neurobiology, 449–460
  vs. panic disorder, 436–437
  with separation anxiety, 186
  serotonin system, 457–458
  sertraline, 815
  trauma, 459–460
PPA, 109
PPI, 225, 320
Precession, 45
Predictive validity, 5
Prefrontal cortex, 283
Prefrontal cortex (PFC)
  aggression, 675
  alcohol, 566
  OCD, 423
Preparatory attention, 225
Prepulse inhibition (PPI), 225, 320
Primary insomnia, 719–720
Primary progressive aphasia syndrome (PPA), 109
Prion diseases, 102–103
Problem gambling
  defined, 684–685
  prevalence, 684
Progesterone, 910
Programmed cell death. see Apoptosis
Progressive muscle relaxation
  sleep, 720
Progressive supranuclear palsy (PSP), 108–109
  brain imaging, 508–509
  vs. frontotemporal dementia, 501
  genetics, 105
  tau lesions, 107
Prolactin
  schizophrenia, 260
Prolyloligopeptidase, 760
Propanolol
  autism, 211
Propentofylline
  vascular dementia, 883

Index

Propositional memory, 119
Protein kinase C (PKC)
  alcoholism, 570
  drug effects, 777
Proton MRS
  childhood mood disorders, 158
PSP. *see* Progressive supranuclear palsy (PSP)
Psychiatric comorbidity, 553–558
Psychiatric disorders
  childhood
    classification, 55–59
    comorbid SUDs, 554
    genes predisposing to, 15–21
    genetic etiology, 14–15
    medical conditions, 903
      pharmacological interventions, 899–904
    most common, 554
Psychiatric genetics
  methodological advances, 13–22
Psychiatric neuroimaging
  developments, 43–52
Psychobiological model, 644
Psychoses, 127–128
  animal models, 317–329
    early limbic lesion models, 325
    pharmacological, 323
  drug-induced models, 318–323
Psychosocial stresses
  genes, 13
Psychostimulants
  mechanisms of action, 586
Psychotherapy
  advanced stages, 137
Psychotic disorders, 62–63
  childhood. *see* Childhood psychotic disorders
  comorbid SUDs, 556
  genetic findings, 295–302
  membrane abnormalities, 307–313
Psychotropic drugs, 911–912
Psychotropic-induced sexual dysfunction
  treatment, 661–662
PTSD. *see* Posttraumatic stress disorder (PTSD)
Pulmonary disease, 902–903
PVE
  correction, 482–484

Quality of life
  drug development, 811
Quantitative MRI
  autism, 208–209
Quantitative trait loci (QTL), 21
Quantitative volumetric MRI
  brain
    Alzheimer's disease, 500
Quetiapine
  childhood bipolar disorders, 163

[Quetiapine]
  schizophrenia, 259, 736, 740
  serotonin, 738
  sexual dysfunction, 659

Rabi, Isaac, 44
Racial groups
  alcoholism, 565
  apolipoprotein E gene, 526
Racing thoughts
  childhood bipolar disorders, 152
Raclopride
  schizophrenia
    dopamine hypothesis, 261
rCBF, 49
Reactive psychosis, 76
  psychobiological correlates, 132
Reelin protein, 326
Regional cerebral blood flow (rCBF), 49
Region of interest (ROI), 45
Relaxation techniques
  sleep, 720
Reliability
  clinical diagnoses, 75
Reliable temperament type
  pharmacological treatment, 144
REM sleep behavior disorder, 723–724
Renal disease, 902
Repetitive transcranial magnetic stimulation (rTMS)
  effects induced by, 927–928
  neuropsychiatric disorders, 919–929
  safety guidelines, 926–927
  side effects, 925–926
Residual type schizophrenia, 200
Resting studies, 339–340
Restless legs syndrome/periodic limb movement disorder, 721
Rett's disorder, 59
  neurobiology, 212–213
Reversible monoamine oxidase A inhibitor (RIMA)
  sexual dysfunction, 658
Reward
  addictive drugs, 584
Reward dependence
  psychobiological data, 132
  psychobiology, 131
Rheumatoid arthritis, 901
Rifampin
  drug interactions, 742
RIMA
  sexual dysfunction, 658
Risperidone
  Alzheimer's disease, 880
  childhood bipolar disorders, 163
  childhood obsessive-compulsive disorder, 184
  serotonin, 738
  sexual dysfunction, 659, 660

Ritanserin
    schizophrenia
        dopamine hypothesis, 261
        serotonin receptors, 271
Rivastigmine
    Alzheimer's disease, 867
RLA, 348
ROI, 45
Roman Low Avoidance rats (RLA), 348
rTMS. *see* Repetitive transcranial magnetic stimulation (rTMS)

Sabcomeline
    Alzheimer's disease, 868
Sabril, 605
    pharmacological properties, 795
SAD, 62, 177–178
Safety
    drug development, 810
Salivary cortisol, 436
SANS, 200, 238
Scale for the Assessment of Negative Symptoms (SANS), 200, 238
Scanditronix PC 1024-7B, 484
Schizoaffective disorder, 63
    DSM and ICD definition, 74
    erectile dysfunction, 663
Schizoid personality
    pharmacological treatment, 144–145
Schizophrenia, 62–63, 924
    affective symptoms, 746–748
    animal models, 319
        future directions, 328
    attention deficits, 225–226
    catatonic type, 200
    childhood, 198
        delusions, 63
    classification systems, 69–77, 199–200
        diagnostic criteria, 71–73
        evolution, 69–70
        symptoms, 71
        twentieth century, 70–71
    clozapine, 259–260
    cognitive deficits, 223–231
        amphetamine-induced DA release, 242–244
        antipsychotic drugs, 245–246
        baseline DA release, 244
        clinical significance, 229–230
        DA transporters, 244
        DOPA decarboxylase, 242
        functional imaging, 239–240
        imaging DA transmission, 240
        MRS, 246–249
        neural basis, 228–229
        neurochemical imaging, 240–249
        neuropharmacological imaging, 240–249

[Schizophrenia]
    nondopaminergic receptors, 244–245
    PET, 240–246
    phosphorus spectroscopy, 246–247
    prefrontal DA transmission, 244
    proton spectroscopy, 247–248
    resting-state studies, 239–240
    SPECT, 240–246
    striatal DA transmission, 240–242
    task-related activation studies, 239–240
cognitive disability
    treatment, 230–231
cognitive symptoms, 746
comorbid SUDs, 556
D2 block, 262
developmental manipulations, 323–328
disorganized behavior, 746
dopamine depletion, 260
dopamine hypothesis, 259–263
    atypical antipsychotics, 261
    effect lag, 260–261
    isomers, 260
    molecular genetics, 263
dopamine receptors, 262–263
D1 receptor, 263
drug-induced, 318
ejaculatory dysfunction, 659
GABA system, 279–281
genetic model, 328
glutamate excitatory amino acid system, 739–740
impaired cognition, 228–230
impaired executive functions, 228
international pilot study, 75–76
negative symptoms, 745–746
neuroimaging findings, 237–240
perceptual disturbances, 224–225
pharmacological treatment, 731–750
    genotyping, 748
    older, 732–738
    switching patients, 742–744
phospholipids, 310–313
positive symptoms, 744–745
prolactin elevation, 260
psychopathology, 319
quetiapine, 259
serotonergic dysfunction, 267–272
    atypical antipsychotics, 271–272
    challenge studies, 268
    genetics, 267–268
    serotonin receptors, 268–271
    serotonin transporters, 271
serotonin, 738–739
sleep, 717–718
SPD, 647
structural imaging, 237–239
symptoms, 732

Index

[Schizophrenia]
    categories, 318
    cross-cultural groups, 75–76
School performance
    childhood depressive disorders, 151
Secretase inhibitors
    Alzheimer's disease, 870, 871
Sedatives
    mechanisms of action, 586
    neurotransmitters, 583
Segregation analysis, 15
    panic disorder, 469
Seizures
    repetitive transcranial magnetic stimulation, 925
Selective attention, 226
Selective breeding, 8
Selective M1 receptor agonists
    Alzheimer's disease, 868
Selective serotonin uptake inhibitors (SSRIs), 138, 901, 911–912
    aggression, 673
    alcoholism, 573
    borderline personality, 140–141
    cautious temperaments, 141
    childhood mood disorders, 159
    childhood obsessive-compulsive disorder, 185
    cocaine dependence, 589
    comorbid SUDs
        and anxiety disorders, 556
    cyclothymic-dependent personality, 144
    obsessive personality, 139
    panic disorder, 439
Selegeline
    cocaine dependence, 854
Self-deprecation
    childhood depressive disorders, 150
Self-injurious behavior
    endorphin system, 646
    opioids, 646
Selye, Hans, 451
Semantic priming tasks, 227
Senile plaques (SPs), 100
    Alzheimer's disease, 538
Sensitive temperament type, 142
Separation anxiety disorder (SAD), 62, 177–178
Serotonin, 25, 910
    ACh, 355–356
    aggression, 672–675
    agonists, 324
        psychoses, 321
    alcoholism, 572–573, 848–849
    Alzheimer's disease, 545, 869
    anorexia nervosa, 828, 829
    augmentation, 811–812
    autism, 206–207
    bipolar disorders, 413

[Serotonin]
    eating disorders, 636–639
    lithium, 761
    markers
        affective disorders, 400–401
    OCD, 426–427
    pathological gambling, 686–689
    pathways, 47
    personality disorder, 645–647
    PTSD, 457–458
    receptor agonists, 816–817
        psychoses, 318
    receptors, 299
        schizophrenia
            serotonergic dysfunction, 268–271
    schizophrenia, 738–739
    transporter gene
        suicidal behavior, 704
    transporters
        schizophrenia, 271
Serotonin reuptake inhibitors (SRIs), 95
    autism, 211
    pathological gambling, 690–692
Sertraline, 911–912
    Alzheimer's disease, 881–882
    anorexia nervosa, 830
    bipolar disorders, 413
    childhood mood disorders, 159
    comorbid major depressive disorder
        and alcohol use disorder, 554–555
    drug holiday, 661
    obsessive personality, 139
    PTSD, 815
    sexual dysfunction, 658
Severely disorganized behaviors, 127–128
Severe personality disorders, 128
Sex hormone binding globulin (SHBG)
    sexual dysfunction, 661
Sexual behavior
    brain regions, 910–911
Sexual dysfunction
    antidepressants, 657–659
    anxiolytics, 659
    iatrogenic, 657–665
    pharmacotherapy, 661–664
    treatment, 661–662, 665
SHBG
    sexual dysfunction, 661
Shprintzen syndrome, 301
Shy-Drager syndrome, 107
Shyness, 92
Sibpair analysis, 20, 397
Sighing
    panic disorder, 435
    social phobia, 435

Signal transduction abnormalities
    bipolar disorders, 371–386
Signal transduction systems, 371–372
Sildenafil
    sexual dysfunction, 663–664
Simultaneous cocaine/alcohol abuse
    PET, 600–601
Simvastatin
    Alzheimer's disease, 878
Single Major Locus (SML) model, 396
Single-photon emission computed tomography (SPECT), 46
    autism, 209–210
    childhood mood disorders, 157, 158
        cognitive deficits
            schizophrenia, 240–246
        personality disorder, 649
        scanner, 47
Situationally bound panic attacks, 433
Sleep
    cholinomimetic effects, 349–350
    neuropsychiatric disorders, 714–718
Sleep apnea syndrome, 718–719
Sleep disorders, 713–724
Sleep disturbance
    childhood bipolar disorders, 151
    childhood depressive disorders, 150–151
Sleep restriction therapy, 720
Sleep studies
    childhood mood disorders, 157
Sleep terrors, 722
Sleepwalking, 722
SML model, 396
Smoking
    comorbidity, 557
    genetics, 619
SNS, 451
Social anxiety disorder
    childhood, 180–181
    paroxetine, 815
Social functioning, 2
Socialization
    childhood depressive disorders, 151
Social phobia, 61–62
    childhood, 180–181
    classification, 91–92
    clinical genetics, 467–469
    comorbidity, 467–468
    epidemiology, 467–468
    sighing, 435
Sodium channel
    abnormalities
        bipolar disorders, 802
    antibipolar AC plasma level, 799–800
    antibipolar potency, 802–803
    gating mechanism, 798
    pharmacological agent, 798

Somatic complaints
    childhood depressive disorders, 151
Somatostatin
    bipolar disorders, 415
Specific phobias
    categories, 92
SPECT. *see* Single-photon emission computed tomography (SPECT)
Spinning, 45
Spin-spin relaxation, 45
Spontaneous panic attacks, 91
Spontaneous panic disorder, 433
Sporadic Alzheimer's disease, 522
SPs, 100
    Alzheimer's disease, 538
SRIs, 95
    autism, 211
    pathological gambling, 690–692
SSRIs. *see* Selective serotonin uptake inhibitors (SSRIs)
Stage fright
    beta blockers, 181
Statistical parametric mapping, 481–482
Stepwise character development, 135–136
Stevens-Johnson syndrome, 162
STG, 200
Stimulants
    bulimia nervosa, 834
    sexual dysfunction, 663
Stimulus control therapy
    sleep, 720
Stress
    immune response, 410–411
    locus ceruleus, 454–455
    plasma cortisol, 459
Stress vulnerability
    animal models, 7
Striatonigral degeneration, 107
Striatum
    OCD, 424
Stroke
    panic attacks, 436
Stroop task, 226, 453
Structural MRI, 45
Structural neuroimaging
    childhood mood disorders, 157–158
    development, 44–46
Subcortical dementia, 108–109
Subcortical gray matter
    measurement, 337
Substance abuse disorders (SUDs), 553–558
    and anxiety disorders, 555–556
    comorbidity, 554–555
    future directions, 557
    pathological gambling, 684–685
    psychiatric disorders, 554
    psychotic disorders, 556

[Substance abuse disorders (SUDs)]
  treatment strategy
   PET, 604–606
Substance P
  antagonists
   antidepressant/anxiolytic drugs, 34–35
  bipolar disorders, 415
  carbamazepine, 776
  lithium, 776
  neurokinin receptor antagonist, 812–813
  receptor antagonists, 817
  schizophrenia, 740–741
Substance use
  with childhood mood disorders, 152
Subutex
  opioid dependence, 588, 853–854
SUDs. *see* Substance abuse disorders (SUDs)
Suicidal behavior
  cholesterol, 706
  future directions, 707
  genetic studies, 702–705
  molecular genetic research, 702–705
  postmortem studies, 705–706
  psychotropic medications, 706–707
  stress-diathesis model, 701–702
  in vivo biochemical studies, 705
Suicidal comorbid populations, 557
Suicidal ideation
  childhood depressive disorders, 151
Suicide
  genetics, 648
  neurobiology, 701–707
Superior temporal gyrus (STG), 200
Surgical castration, 912
Susceptibility genes
  late-onset Alzheimer's disease, 524
Sustained-release bupropion
  nicotine dependence, 589
Sympathetic nervous system (SNS), 451
Symptom domain, 138
Synapse loss
  Alzheimer's disease, 540–541
Synuclein family, 107
Synucleinopathies, 107–108

Tachycardia, 436
Tacrine
  Alzheimer's disease, 867
Talairach space, 481
Talkative
  childhood bipolar disorders, 151–152
Talsaclidine
  Alzheimer's disease, 868, 871
Tauopathies
  pathophysiology, 105–107
TBI, 103

TCAs. *see* Tricyclic antidepressants (TCAs)
TCI, 118
  scales, 120
TDT, 19, 469
Technetium-99m hexamethylpropylene amine oxime
  childhood mood disorders, 158
Teenagers. *see* Adolescent
Temperament
  vs. character, 119
  character outcome, 125–126
  protecting against personality disorder, 122–124
  psychobiology, 117–148, 129–133
  scores, 118
  stimulus-response patterns, 125
  treatment guidelines, 134–148
Temperament and Character Inventory (TCI), 118
  scales, 120
Temporal lobe
  aggression, 676
  atrophy
   Alzheimer's disease, 500
  epilepsy, 453
  measurement, 336–337
Testosterone, 910
  aggression, 674
Thalamus, 183
Theory-driven models, 4–5
Thiamine deficiency
  dementia, 103
Thioridazine, 912
  cardiovascular safety, 747
  childhood psychotic disorders, 201
  sexual dysfunction, 659
Thiothixene
  childhood psychotic disorders, 201
31P magnetic resonance spectroscopy, 312
Thyroid hormone
  metabolism, 459–460
Tiagabine, 780–781
  childhood bipolar disorders, 163
  pharmacological properties, 795
Tiapride
  alcoholism, 847
Tics, 177
TMS, 919–929
Tobacco
  mechanisms of action, 586–587
  neurotransmitters, 583
Tolerability
  drug development, 810
Tonic dopamine model
  compulsive drug use, 585
Topiramate, 779–780
  childhood bipolar disorders, 163
  pharmacological properties, 794
Tourette syndrome, 17

Tower of London, 229
Toxic dementia, 103
Toxic epidermal necrolysis, 162
Toxins
  genes, 13
Transcranial magnetic stimulation (TMS), 919–929
Transmission disequilibrium test (TDT), 19, 469
Transporters, 27–33
  anatomical localization, 29–30
  models, 27–29
  regulation, 30–33
Trauma, 451
  childhood
    bipolar disorders, 650
  neurobiology, 451
  PTSD, 459–460
Traumatic brain injury (TBI), 103
Traumatic stress response
  neurobiology, 452
Trazodone
  Alzheimer's disease, 881
  bulimia nervosa, 833
  sexual dysfunction, 658
Trexan. see Naltrexone (Trexan)
Tricyclic antidepressants (TCAs)
  autism, 211
  childhood mood disorders, 159
  cocaine dependence, 589
  comorbid major depressive disorder
    and alcohol use disorder, 554
  comorbid SUDs
    and anxiety disorders, 556
  cyclothymic-dependent personality, 144
  sexual dysfunction, 658
Trinucleotide repeats
  anticipation, 300
  sequences
    anticipation, 401–402
Triptorelin, 914
Tryptophan hydroxylase, 637, 638
  impulsive aggression, 648
  suicidal behavior, 704
Tuberoinfundibular projections, 735–736
Tuberous sclerosis, 471
Twin studies, 15
  aggression, 676
  alcoholism, 616
  eating disorders, 636
  panic disorder, 468
  suicidal behavior, 702

Undifferentiated type schizophrenia, 200
Unexpected panic disorder, 433
Unipolar disorder
  vs. bipolar disorder, 407–415
Universal addiction site, 566–567

Upper-airway resistance syndrome (UARS), 719
Urinary free cortisol (UFC), 455

Vagus nerve stimulation (VNS), 919
Valproate, 364
  alcoholism, 850
  bipolar disorders
    comorbid SUDs, 555
  depression, 366
  vs. lithium, 776–778
  loading, 800
  pharmacological properties, 794
  sexual dysfunction, 661
Vancomycin
  autism, 211
Vascular dementia, 102
  vs. Alzheimer's disease, 505
  brain imaging, 503–506
    functional, 504
    structural, 504
    white matter changes, 504–505
  treatment, 882–884
Vascular depression, 339
Vasopressin
  aggression, 674
  bipolar disorders, 414–415
vCJD, 103
Velocardiofacial syndrome (VCFS), 301, 471
Venlafaxine
  for childhood generalized anxiety disorder, 179
  generalized anxiety disorder, 815
Ventral tegmentum (VTA), 596
  alcohol, 566
VietNam Era Twin Registery, 689
Vietnam veterans
  PTSD, 459
Vigabatrin (Sabril), 605
  pharmacological properties, 795
Vineland Adaptive Behavior Scales, 58
Violence
  neurobiology, 671–677
Vitamin B12 deficiency
  dementia, 103
Vitamin E
  Alzheimer's disease, 875
VNS, 919
Voltage-gated sodium channels, 796–799
Voltage-sensitive sodium channels
  structure, 796–798
Volume transmission (VT), 25–27
VTA, 596
  alcohol, 566

Weight
  antipsychotics, 747–748
  childhood depressive disorders, 151

Index

Wernicke-Korsakoff syndrome, 103
Wilson's disease
  genetics, 105
Wistar Kyoto (WKY) rats, 8
Wolfram syndrome, 471
Women's Health Initiative Memory Study (WHIMS), 878
Women's Health Initiative Randomized Trial, 878
Working memory, 226
Worthlessness
  childhood depressive disorders, 150

Xanomeline
  Alzheimer's disease, 868
Xanthine derivatives
  vascular dementia, 883

Yohimbine
  childhood panic disorder, 181
  panic disorder, 437
  sexual dysfunction, 662–663
Young Rating Mania Scale, 802

Zinc
  anorexia nervosa, 831
Ziprasidone
  cardiovascular safety, 746
  psychotic disorders, 735
  schizophrenia, 737
Zoladex, 914
Zonisamide, 781–782
  childhood bipolar disorders, 163

About the Editors

JAIR C. SOARES is Associate Professor of Psychiatry and Chief, Division of Mood and Anxiety Disorders, University of Texas Health Science Center, San Antonio. The author or coauthor of many journal articles, book chapters, and books, including *Bipolar Disorders* and *Brain Imaging in Affective Disorders* (both titles, Marcel Dekker, Inc.), Dr. Soares is a member of the American Psychiatric Association, the International Society for Neuroimaging in Psychiatry, the Society for Neurosciences, the Society of Biological Psychiatry, the International Society for Bipolar Disorders, and the Society for Nuclear Medicine. He received the M.D. degree (1990) from the University of São Paulo School of Medicine, Brazil.

SAMUEL GERSHON is Professor of Psychiatry, Western Psychiatric Institute and Clinic, University of Pittsburgh School of Medicine, Pittsburgh, Pennsylvania. The author or coauthor of numerous journal articles, book chapters, and books, including *Bipolar Disorders* and *Pharmacotherapy for Child and Adolescent Psychiatric Disorders, Second Edition* (both titles, Marcel Dekker, Inc.), Dr. Gershon is a Fellow of the American College of Neuropsychopharmacology, the Royal College of Psychiatrists, U.K. He received the M.B.B.S. degree (1950) from the Faculty of Medicine, University of Sydney, Australia.

ISBN 0-8247-0835-0

90000

WITHDRAWN